CHPt 27 153, 54

Clinical Certified Medical Assistant

AAH

D0138444

KINN'S

THE MEDICAL ASSISTANT

An Applied Learning Approach

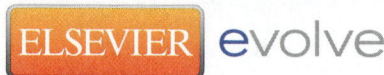
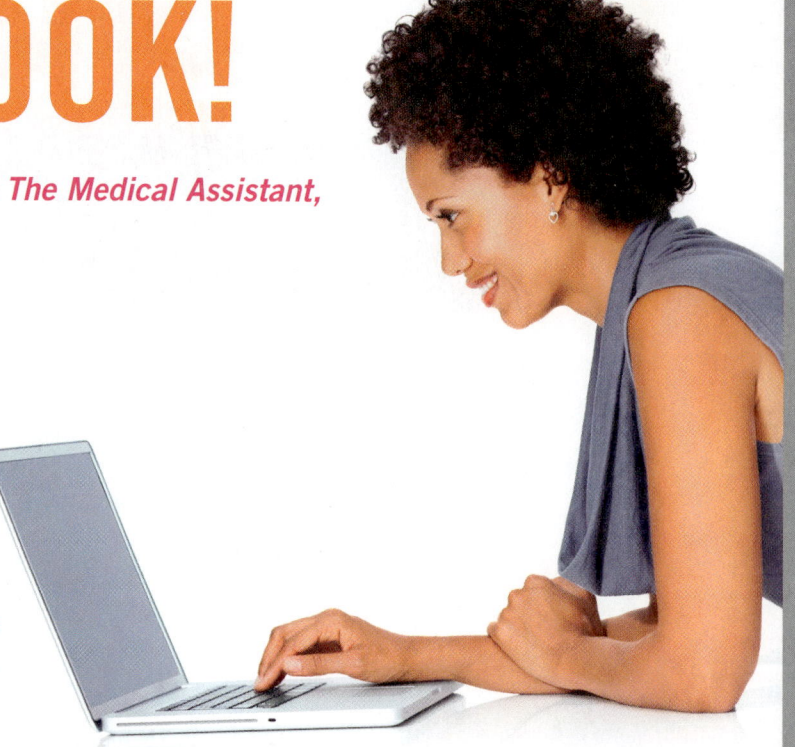

KINN'S

THE MEDICAL ASSISTANT

An Applied Learning Approach

Deborah B. Proctor, EdD, RN
Adjunct Faculty Member
Butler County Community College
Butler, Pennsylvania

Alexandra Patricia Adams, MA, BA, RMA, CMA (AAMA)
Former Health Information Specialist Program Director & Administrative
    Medical Assisting Instructor
Ultrasound Diagnostic School (now Sanford-Brown College)
Professional Writer
Grand Prairie, Texas

TWELFTH EDITION

12

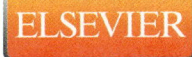

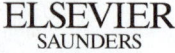

ELSEVIER
SAUNDERS

3251 Riverport Lane
St. Louis, Missouri 63043

KINN'S THE MEDICAL ASSISTANT: AN APPLIED LEARNING APPROACH   ISBN: 978-1-4557-2678-3

Notices

Knowledge and best practice in this field are constantly changing. As new research and experience broaden our understanding, changes in research methods, professional practices, or medical treatment may become necessary.

Practitioners and researchers must always rely on their own experience and knowledge in evaluating and using any information, methods, compounds, or experiments described herein. In using such information or methods they should be mindful of their own safety and the safety of others, including parties for whom they have a professional responsibility.

With respect to any drug or pharmaceutical products identified, readers are advised to check the most current information provided (i) on procedures featured or (ii) by the manufacturer of each product to be administered, to verify the recommended dose or formula, the method and duration of administration, and contraindications. It is the responsibility of practitioners, relying on their own experience and knowledge of their patients, to make diagnoses, to determine dosages and the best treatment for each individual patient, and to take all appropriate safety precautions.

To the fullest extent of the law, neither the Publisher nor the authors, contributors, or editors, assume any liability for any injury and/or damage to persons or property as a matter of products liability, negligence or otherwise, or from any use or operation of any methods, products, instructions, or ideas contained in the material herein.

Previous editions copyrighted 2011, 2007, 2003, 1999, 1993, 1988, 1981, 1974, 1967, 1960, 1956

ISBN: 978-1-4557-2678-3

Vice President and Publisher: Andrew Allen
Executive Content Strategist: Jennifer Janson
Content Developmental Specialist: Laurie Vordtriede
Publishing Services Manager: Julie Eddy
Senior Project Manager: Richard Barber
Design Direction: Paula Catalano

Printed in Canada

Last digit is the print number: 9 8 7 6 5 4 3 2 1

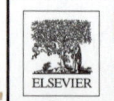

Working together
to grow libraries in
developing countries

www.elsevier.com • www.bookaid.org

To Susan Cole, Executive Editor, whom we lost far too soon.
Susan was greatly respected by her peers and was a dedicated professional at
Elsevier. We dedicate this edition to her memory.

To the students who will use this textbook as they begin their careers
in the medical profession. It is our hope that they will use this text as a reference
manual during their studies, their externship, and throughout their careers.

To my children, Jimmie, Stacey, Jonathan, and Jessica.
Thank you for your patience as your mom spent hours at the computer
working on "the book."

To my loving husband, Bentley Adams. Your hugs are the best part of my day!
I love you for your support, your guidance, your care, and your patience.
I'm looking forward to our rocking chair days!

Alexandra Patricia Adams, MA, BBA, RMA, CMA (AAMA)

To the medical assistant students who will use this text to help learn the crucial
clinical skills needed to be successful in the healthcare environment.
I hope Kinn helps you reach your goals and that providing high-quality care
for your patients will always be your primary professional focus.

To my children and grandchildren…you are the light of my life.

To my husband, whose unfailing love, patience, and support
provide me the freedom to reach for the stars.

To my baby sister, Jeannette, who continues her battle for health…your strength
is a model for us all.

To Susan Cole, our dedicated editor, who passed from this world much too early.
Wishing her family peace and happiness.

Deborah B. Proctor, EdD, RN

PREFACE

Medical assisting as a profession has changed dramatically since *The Office Assistant in Medical and Dental Practice,* by Portia Frederick and Carol Towner, was first published in 1956. Each subsequent edition of this textbook has reflected the age in which it was published. Now, *Kinn's The Medical Assistant: An Applied Learning Approach,* twelfth edition, continues to represent a long-standing commitment to high-quality medical assisting education with its engaging, straightforward writing style and demonstrated positive outcomes. Hundreds of instructors in classrooms across the country have used this text to teach thousands of students over the years. Many of these students have gone on to teach students of their own with this very same trusted resource. To continue the use and growth of this text and its features, the twelfth edition continues to offer the most comprehensive, up-to-date, and innovative approach to teaching this subject today. We appreciate the opportunity to explore the exciting field of medical assisting with you!

DISTINCTIVE FEATURES OF OUR APPROACH

This textbook has endured throughout the years because it has been able to keep pace with an ever-changing profession while producing students who are well trained and qualified to enter medical practices across the country. This dependability is the reason the market continues to rely on this text, edition after edition. Underlying this dependability is a foundation of pedagogic features that has stood the test of time and that has been expanded and improved upon yet again in this latest edition. Such features include the following:

- An easy-to-read, highly interactive writing style that engages students through practical applications of medical assistant competencies.
- An emphasis on skill development, with procedural steps outlining each skill, supported by rationales that provide meaning to each step.
- An organizational approach that addresses each body system with its own chapter, with additional chapters dedicated to specialty medical assistant skills.
- Each clinical chapter begins with a review of that system's anatomy and physiology, then moves to the common disorders found in that system, and concludes with patient education and legal and ethical issues.
- A pedagogic framework based on the use of learning objectives, vocabulary terms, and supportive student supplements.
- A package of supportive materials to accommodate a wide variety of student learning types and instructor teaching styles.

KEY FEATURES IN THIS EDITION

This edition of *Kinn's The Medical Assistant* incorporates a unique approach that is reflected in the subtitle: *An Applied Learning Approach.* Learning is believed to take place only when students are engaged, and when the learning requires something from them in response to the information being imparted to them.

This "applied" theme is set upfront in the first chapter, which introduces students to the concepts of critical thinking and the effect of individual learning styles on student success. This, in turn, transitions into time management and problem-solving skills, as well as effective study skills and test-taking strategies. The text develops from there, true to the original Kinn textbook, with its distinctive administrative and clinical sections, and is rounded out by the last chapter, which helps the student focus on preparing for and nurturing a career as a medical assistant.

This pedagogic theme and other new enhancements can be found throughout the book and its supplements in the following new features of the twelfth edition:

- The artwork throughout has been updated and modernized, providing a more attractive textbook for student use. Many new photographs throughout better support the revised content and are more relevant to the actual medical office. Many photographs were replaced with new images that show up-to-date equipment, provide more disease examples, and better illustrate key procedural steps.
- Separate chapters covering paper medical records and electronic medical records teach students about the intricacies of each system.
- Customer service is heavily stressed throughout the chapters. As patients become more involved in their healthcare, medical assistants must realize that the healthcare field is a service industry and that patients should be treated as customers.
- New compliance regulations in medical billing and coding have put a far greater emphasis on reimbursement practices than ever before. The billing and coding unit has been updated to include the basics of diagnostic coding, basics of procedural coding, basics of health insurance, and the health insurance claim form, as well as a brief introduction to ICD-10 coding.
- The sections on emergency preparedness have expanded so that medical assistants will know what to do in emergency situations. This critical information benefits not only the medical assistant but also aids patients, other staff members, and physicians in the medical facility.
- The Connections heading at the end of each chapter integrates text content with the accompanying Evolve Resources website and Student Study Guide.

EVOLVE

The Evolve site features a variety of student resources, including Chapter Quizzes and Review Activities, Clinical Skills Videos, Medical Terminology, Audio Glossary, practice CMA and RMA exams, and much more! The instructors' Evolve Resources site consists of TEACH Instructor Resources, including Lesson Plans, PowerPoint Presentations, Answer Keys for Chapter Quizzes and

Review Activities, and an extensive Test Bank with more than 5000 questions.

To access this comprehensive online resource, the student can simply go to the EVOLVE home page at *http://evolve.elsevier.com* and enter the user name and password provided by the instructor. If your instructor has not set up a Course Management System, you can still access all the learning resources available free with this textbook by going to http://evolve.elsevier.com/Kinn/.

STUDY GUIDE AND PROCEDURE CHECKLISTS

The Study Guide provides students with the opportunity to review and build on information they have learned in the text through vocabulary reviews, case studies, workplace applications, and more. The updated Procedure Checklists include CAAHEP and ABHES competencies that can be traced to the online correlation grid, and work products in the study guide ensure that students grasp all the medical assisting competencies.

KINN'S MEDICAL ASSISTING ONLINE

The Medical Assisting Online course closely maps content from the text to CAAHEP and ABHES competencies. Each module is competency focused and outcome oriented, providing the proof and documentation needed to demonstrate the student's knowledge to accrediting organizations.

SPECIAL FEATURES

A Scenario is presented at the beginning of each chapter so that the student can think about a real-world situation when reading the chapter content.

Each chapter contains a Vocabulary with definitions.

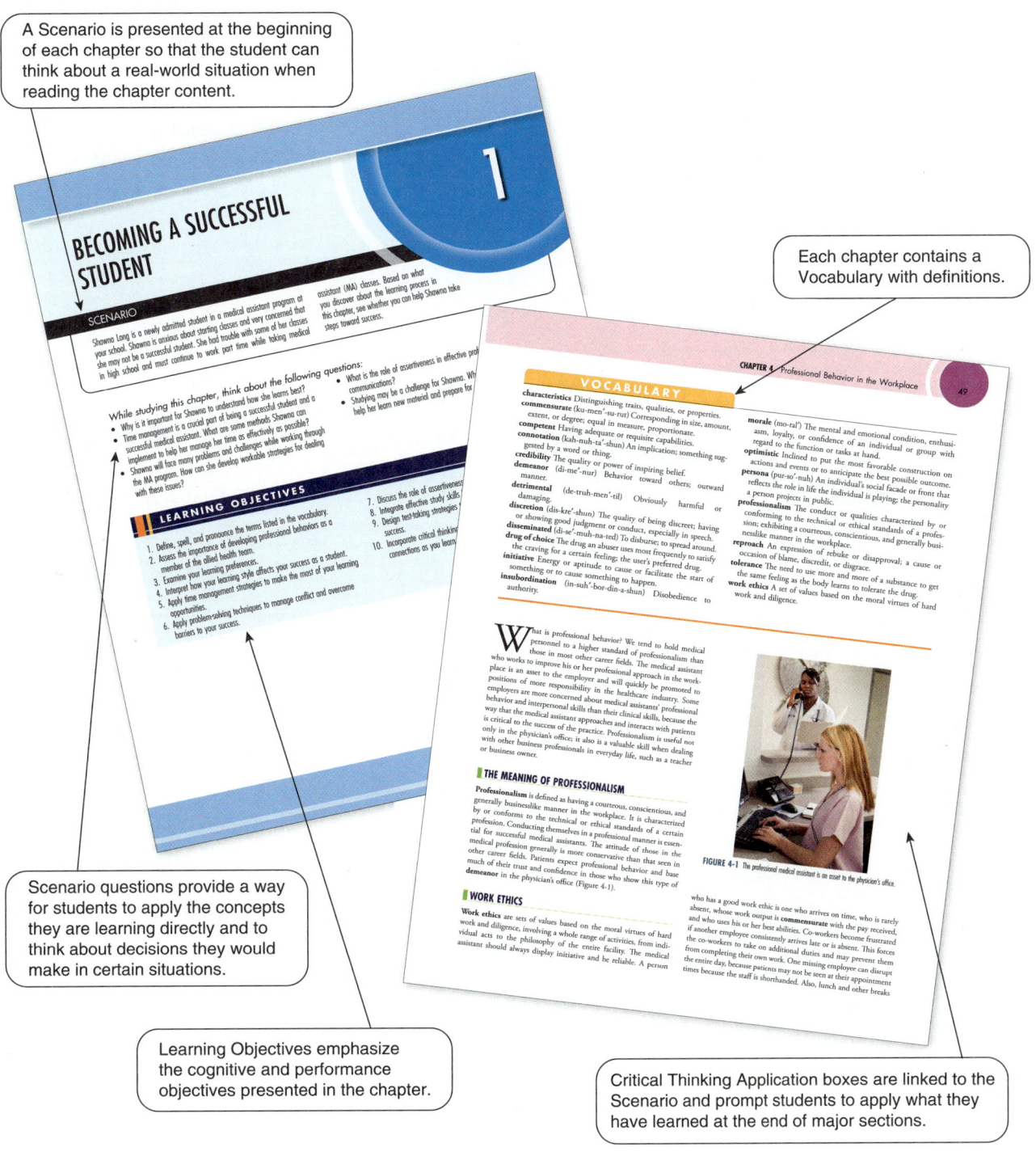

Scenario questions provide a way for students to apply the concepts they are learning directly and to think about decisions they would make in certain situations.

Learning Objectives emphasize the cognitive and performance objectives presented in the chapter.

Critical Thinking Application boxes are linked to the Scenario and prompt students to apply what they have learned at the end of major sections.

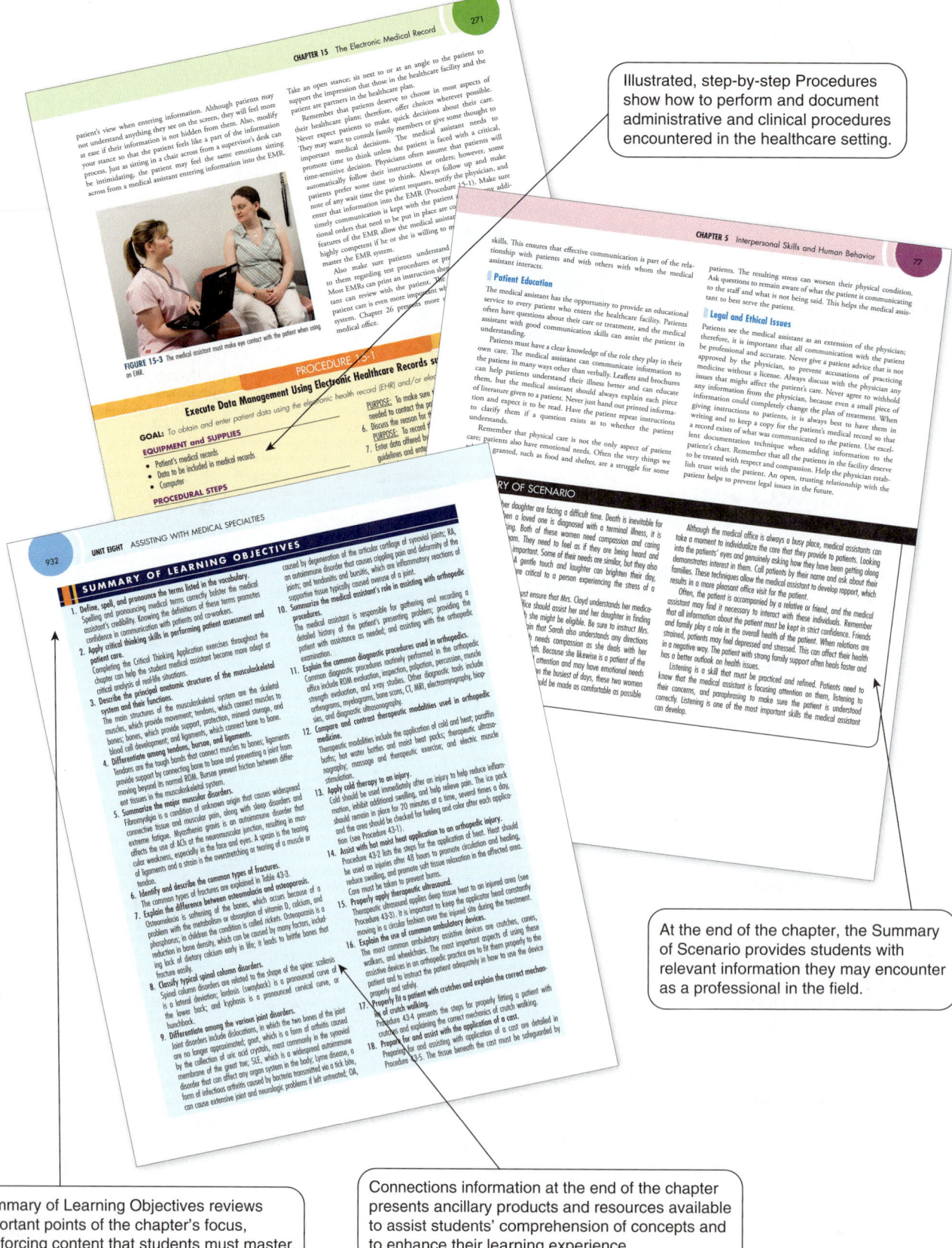

Illustrated, step-by-step Procedures show how to perform and document administrative and clinical procedures encountered in the healthcare setting.

At the end of the chapter, the Summary of Scenario provides students with relevant information they may encounter as a professional in the field.

Summary of Learning Objectives reviews important points of the chapter's focus, reinforcing content that students must master.

Connections information at the end of the chapter presents ancillary products and resources available to assist students' comprehension of concepts and to enhance their learning experience.

REVIEWERS

Kathy Cline, RN, ASN MA
Instructor
Blue Cliff College
Alexandria, Louisiana

Nelda Davis, RN, RMA
Program Director, Medical Assisting
Northeast Texas Community College
Mount Pleasant, Texas

Ruth E. Dearborn, CCS, CCS-P
Instructor
University of Alaska Southeast
Sitka, Alaska

Brian Dickens, MBA, RMA, CHI
Regional Program Director, Medical Assisting
Keiser Career College
Greenacres, Florida

Debra Downs, LPN, AAS, RMA (AMT)
Instructor and Program Director, Medical Assisting
Okefenokee Technical College
Waycross, Georgia

Deborah S. Gilbert, RHIA, CMA
Program Director, Medical Assisting
Dalton State College
Dalton, Georgia

Jen Gouge, XRT
Coordinator, Medical Assistant Program
Peninsula College
Port Angeles, Washington

Susanna M. Hancock, AAS-MOM, RMA, CMA, RPT, COLT
Retired Medical Assistant Director and Instructor
American Institute of Health Technology
Boise, Idaho

Carolyn Rowe Helms, BS, RMA
Extern Coordinator/Instructor
Atlanta Technical College
Atlanta, Georgia

Judith Kimelman-Kline, CMA, RMA
Instructor
Miami Lakes Educational Center (MDPS)
Miami Lakes, Florida

Colleen A. Lace, BLS, AA, LPN
Instructor and Allied Health Program Director
Moraine Park Technical College
Fond du Lac, Wisconsin

Loreen W. MacNichol, CMRS, RMC, CCS-P
Faculty, Health Science Department
Kaplan University
Portland, Maine

Laura Melendez, BS, RMA, RT BMO
Instructor
Keiser Career College
Greenacres, Florida

Maureen E. Russell Messier, CMA, RMA, AS, BA
Instructor
Branford Hall Career Institute, a division of Premier Education Group
Southington, Connecticut

Joyce A. Minton, Ed.S, CMA (AAMA), RMA
Director, Medical Assisting Health Sciences
Wilkes Community College
Wilkesboro, North Carolina

Kim Smith Norris, BSM, CPC
Instructor
Everest University
Orange Park, Florida

Julie Pepper, CMA (AAMA), BS
Instructor
Chippewa Valley Technical College
Eau Claire, Wisconsin

Andrea Potteiger, CCS, CCS-P, CPC, CHI, CMAA, CBCS
Lead Healthcare Instructor
New Horizons Harrisburg
Mechanicsburg, Pennsylvania

Macie Rubida, CPC, AA, LPN, BA
Instructor
Kaplan University
Council Bluffs, Iowa

Lynn G. Slack, BS, CMA (AAMA)
Director, Business Programs and Medical Programs
Kaplan Career Institute
Pittsburgh, Pennsylvania

Judith D. Symons, MA, Voc Ed Cert
Medical Assistant
Geisinger Medical Center
Danville, Pennsylvania
Former Instructor
McCann School of Business and Technology
Pottsville, Pennsylvania

Amy D. Tabak, MBA/HR, CPC, CMAA, CBCS
Full-Time Online Instructor
Ultimate Medical Academy Online
Tampa, Florida

Gail Van Grieken, CCMA-C
Teacher, Medical Assistant Program
San Joaquin County Office of Education
Stockton, California

Shannon Ydoyaga, MS, BBA
Associate Dean of Health Professions, School of Mathematics
   Science and Health Professions Richland College
Dallas, Texas

La Tanya Young, PA-C, MMSc, MPH, CHES
Assistant Professor, College of Professional Studies
Coordinator, Medical Assisting Program
Clayton State University
Morrow, Georgia

ACKNOWLEDGMENTS

Years before I became the author of this book, I used it to teach my own students. All medical assistants owe a great debt to the original author, Mary E. Kinn. Her contributions to this discipline changed the playing field for our medical assisting students, and my gratitude to her is heartfelt and sincere.

I would like to express appreciation to the Elsevier Team, including Susan Cole, Laurie Vordtriede, Richard Barber, all the sales professionals who introduce us to instructors and program managers all over the country, as well as the other employees who worked on the text. We appreciate your insight and assistance as Deb and I do our best to make the Kinn text the finest medical assisting text available.

Deb Proctor has now been my partner for almost 12 years as we revise, rewrite, and rethink the ideas that have made this an outstanding textbook. I appreciate that Deb is so well informed and so willing to share of herself so that medical assisting students gain the knowledge they need to become successful in the medical field. It's been a great 12 years getting to know you and your family and sharing bits and pieces of life with you. I look forward to many more years of working together.

Without our families, writers could not do the work we are called to do. I would like to thank my brothers and sisters, LaNell Crumley, Alisha Crumley, Karry Chapman, Dr. Terry Watson, and Shawn Crumley, and their families for their support. Many thanks to my mom, Patricia Crumley, and my dad, Jim Crumley, for all the things they taught me. Without my mom using flashcards to help me with medical terminology, I might never have become a medical assistant! My dad, who was an attorney and a veteran of the Korean War, instilled a love for law and ethics in me, as well as a strong work ethic. I so appreciate the patience and support that my kids give to me. Jimmie, Stacey, Jonathan, and Jessica consistently stick with me when I have to be at the computer instead of being out and about with them. There are no words to describe my appreciation for my husband, Bentley. You truly take great care of me and are so supportive of my work. Those "rocking chair days" are soon to come! Thank you all for your belief in me and my abilities as a writer. Thank you for making our home a haven where love exists and grows every day.

To all medical assistants using this text: never doubt that you can accomplish your goals. You are the only person who can make a difference in your life, and your life will influence generations to come. Refuse to allow anything to keep you from realizing your dreams. Never stop setting new goals and striving to reach them.

Alexandra Patricia Adams, MA, BBA, RMA, CMA (AAMA)

A complex project like this text cannot be completed by only one person. The editorial team for the twelfth edition gave extensive feedback and support throughout the development process, and I thank each of them for his or her significant contributions. This is especially true for Laurie Vordtriede, who provided the consistency needed in the editorial team throughout Susan Cole's illness and eventual replacement. My co-author, Tricia Adams, offered a sounding board for issues throughout the project and repeatedly came up with creative ideas and resolutions to burgeoning problems—thank you, Tricia, for your support and consistent professional approach to this project.

My students continue to be my inspiration. They are the reason I fell in love with teaching. My dedication to teaching led me to earn a Doctorate in Education, and my Doctorate led to my working on the Kinn text. So thank you to my past, current, and future students, who have opened so many doors for me.

Finally, I give my heartfelt thanks to my family. We have experienced many significant events since the last edition—weddings, new homes, graduate degrees, and grandbabies—and through it all, you have understood that Mom had to keep working on the "book." Thank you for your support and for being proud of my work. Last of all, to my husband: at the risk of sounding corny—you complete me.

Deborah B. Proctor, EdD, RN

CONTENTS

PROCEDURES

BECOMING A SUCCESSFUL STUDENT

SCENARIO

Shawna Long is a newly admitted student in a medical assistant program at your school. Shawna is anxious about starting classes and very concerned that she may not be a successful student. She had trouble with some of her classes in high school and must continue to work part time while taking medical assistant (MA) classes. Based on what you discover about the learning process in this chapter, see whether you can help Shawna take steps toward success.

While studying this chapter, think about the following questions:

- Why is it important for Shawna to understand how she learns best?
- Time management is a crucial part of being a successful student and a successful medical assistant. What are some methods Shawna can implement to help her manage her time as effectively as possible?
- Shawna will face many problems and challenges while working through the MA program. How can she develop workable strategies for dealing with these issues?
- What is the role of assertiveness in effective professional communications?
- Studying may be a challenge for Shawna. What skills can she use to help her learn new material and prepare for examinations?

LEARNING OBJECTIVES

1. Define, spell, and pronounce the terms listed in the vocabulary.
2. Assess the importance of developing professional behaviors as a member of the allied health team.
3. Examine your learning preferences.
4. Interpret how your learning style affects your success as a student.
5. Apply time management strategies to make the most of your learning opportunities.
6. Apply problem-solving techniques to manage conflict and overcome barriers to your success.
7. Discuss the role of assertiveness in effective communication.
8. Integrate effective study skills into your daily activities.
9. Design test-taking strategies that help you take charge of your success.
10. Incorporate critical thinking and reflection to help you make mental connections as you learn material.

VOCABULARY

critical thinking The constant practice of considering all aspects of a situation when deciding what to believe or what to do.

empathy (em'-puh-the) Sensitivity to the individual needs and reactions of patients.

learning style The way an individual perceives and processes information to learn new material.

perceiving (pur-sev'-ing) How an individual looks at information and sees it as real.

processing (pro'-ses-ing) How an individual internalizes new information and makes it his or her own.

professional behaviors Actions that identify the medical assistant as a member of a healthcare profession, including being dependable, providing respectful patient care, exercising initiative, demonstrating a positive attitude, and working as an effective team member.

reflection (re-flek'-shun) The process of considering new information and internalizing it to create new ways of examining information.

You have taken the first step toward becoming a successful student by choosing your profession and field of study. The medical assistant profession is both challenging and rewarding. Becoming a medical assistant opens the doors to a wide variety of opportunities in both administrative and clinical practice at ambulatory or institutional healthcare facilities. Medical assistants are important members of the healthcare team, and as a healthcare professional, you will be expected to practice certain **professional behaviors** (Figure 1-1). These professional behaviors include demonstrating dependability, respectful patient care, **empathy,** initiative, a positive attitude, and teamwork. To become a successful medical assistant, you first must become a successful student. This chapter helps you discover the way you learn best and provides multiple strategies to assist you in your journey toward success.

CRITICAL THINKING APPLICATION   1-1

Consider your history as a student. What do you think helped you to succeed? What do you think needs improvement? Create a plan for improvement that includes two or three ways you can become a more successful student. Be prepared to share this plan with your classmates.

WHO YOU ARE AS A LEARNER: HOW DO YOU LEARN BEST?

Think about what you do when you are faced with something new to learn. How do you go about understanding and learning the new material? Over time you have developed a method for **perceiving** and **processing** information. This pattern of behavior is called your **learning style.** Learning styles can be examined in many different ways, but most professionals agree that a student's success depends more on whether the person can "make sense" of the information than on whether the individual is "smart." Determining your individual learning style and understanding how it applies to your ability to learn new material are the first steps toward becoming a successful student (Figure 1-2).

Learning Style Inventory

For you to learn new material, two things must happen. First, you must *perceive* the information. This is the method you have developed over time that helps you examine new information and recognize it as real. Once you have developed a method for learning about the new material, you must *process* the information. Processing the information is how you internalize it and make it your own.

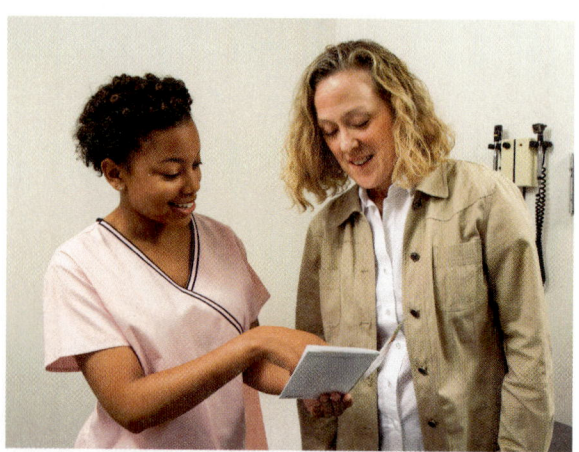

FIGURE 1-1 Professional interaction with patient.

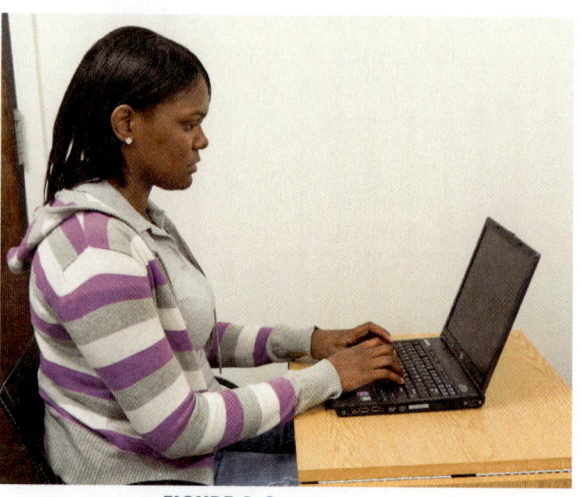

FIGURE 1-2 Student learning.

Researchers believe that each of us has a preferred method for learning new material. By investigating your learning style, you can figure out how to combine different approaches to perceiving and processing information that will lead to greater success as a student.

The first step in learning new material is determining how you perceive the information. When faced with a new learning experience, students decide how they will go about learning the new material; that is, either by watching and observing the new activity or by doing something active to learn about it. Individuals who learn by analysis, observation, and **reflection** are considered *abstract perceivers*. Abstract learners analyze new material as ideas that require thought to process. They study the information and build theories to help them understand it. Abstract perceivers prefer structured learning situations and use a step-by-step approach to problem solving.

Individuals who learn by "doing" are *concrete perceivers,* who learn information through direct experiences of acting, sensing, or feeling the new material. Concrete learners prefer to learn things that have a personal meaning or that they believe are relevant, and they rely on detailed information to learn new material.

The second step in learning new material is information processing, which is the way learners internalize the new information and make it their own. New material can be processed by two methods. *Active processors* prefer to jump in and start doing things immediately. They make sense of the new material by using it immediately. They look for practical ways to apply the new material and typically do not mind taking risks to get the desired results. They learn best with practice and hands-on activities. *Reflective processors* have to think about the information before they can internalize it. They prefer to observe and consider what is going on. The only way they can make sense of new material is to spend time thinking and learning a great deal about it before acting. Complete the activity in the Student Study Guide to help you determine your learning style preference.

CRITICAL THINKING APPLICATION   1-2

- Consider the two ways to perceive new material. Are you a concrete perceiver, who ties the information to a personal experience, or are you an abstract perceiver, who likes to analyze or reflect on the meaning of the material? Choose the type you think most accurately describes your method of investigating new information.
- Now, think about the way you process learning. Are you an active processor, who always looks for the practical applications of what you learn, or are you a reflective processor, who has to think about new material before internalizing it?
- After completing this activity, write down the combination of your perceiving and processing learning styles and share it with your instructor.

Using Your Learning Profile to Be a Successful Student: Where Do I Go from Here?

No one falls completely into one or the other of the categories just discussed. However, by being aware of how we generally prefer first to perceive information and then to process it, we can be more

sensitive to our learning style and can approach new learning situations with a plan for learning the material in a way that best suits our learning preferences.

Your preferred perceiving and processing learning profile will fall into one of the following four stages of the Learning Style Inventory, which was created by David Kolb of Case Western Reserve University.

- *Stage 1* learners have a *concrete reflective* style. These students want to know the purpose of the information and have a personal connection to the content. They like to consider a situation from many points of view, observe others, and plan before taking action. They feel most comfortable watching rather than doing, and their strengths include sensitivity toward others, brainstorming, and recognizing and creatively solving problems. If you fall into this stage, you enjoy small-group activities and learn well in study groups.
- *Stage 2* learners have an *abstract reflective* style. These students are eager to learn just for the sheer pleasure of learning, rather than because the material relates to their personal lives. They like to learn lots of facts and arrange new material in a clear, logical manner. Stage 2 learners plan studying and like to create ways of thinking about the material, but they do not always make the connection with its practical application. If you are a stage 2 learner, you prefer organized, logical presentations of material and therefore enjoy lectures and readings and generally dislike group work. You also need time to process and think about new material before applying it.
- *Stage 3* learners have an *abstract active* style. Learners with this combination learning style want to experiment and test the information they are learning. If you are a stage 3 learner, you want to know how techniques or ideas work, and you also want to practice what you are learning. Your strengths are in problem solving and decision making, but you may lack focus and may be hasty in making decisions. You learn best with hands-on practice by doing experiments, projects, and laboratory activities. You enjoy working alone or in small groups (Figure 1-3).
- *Stage 4* learners are *concrete active* learners. These students are concerned about how they can use what they learn to make a difference in their lives. If you fall into this stage, you like to relate new material to other areas of your life. You have leadership capabilities, can create on your feet, and usually are vocal in a group, but you may have difficulty completing your work on time. Stage 4 learners enjoy teaching others and working in groups and learn best when they can apply new information to real-world problems.

To get the most out of knowing your learning profile, you need to apply this knowledge to how you approach learning. Each of the learning stages has pluses and minuses. When faced with a learning situation that does not match your learning preference, see how you can adapt your individual learning profile to make the best of the information. For example, if you are bored by lectures, look for an opportunity to apply the information being presented to a real problem you are facing in the classroom or at home. If you are an abstract perceiver, take time outside of class to think about new information so that you are ready to process it into your learning system. If you benefit from learning in a group, make the effort to organize review sessions and study groups. If you learn best by

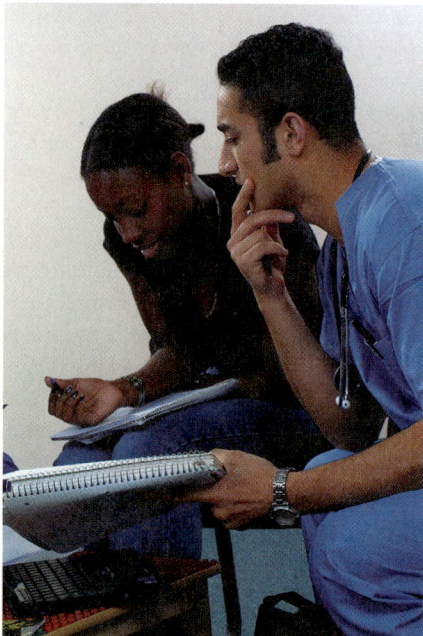

FIGURE 1-3 Learning in a small group.

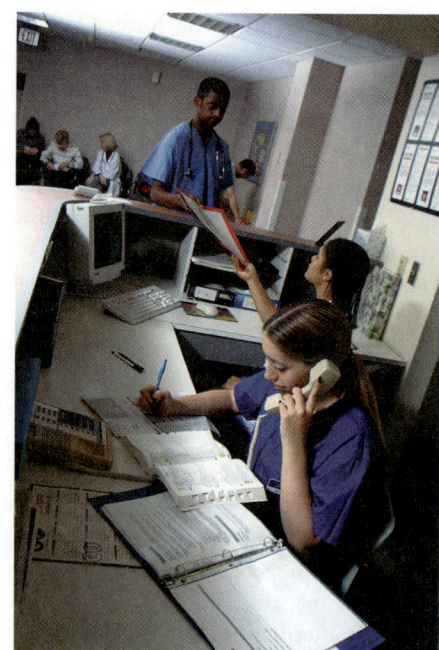

FIGURE 1-4 Time management in a busy medical practice.

teaching others, offer to assist your peers with their learning. By taking the time now to investigate your preferred method of learning, you will perceive and process information more effectively throughout your school career.

CRITICAL THINKING APPLICATION   **1-3**

Take a few minutes to reflect on a time when you really enjoyed learning about something new. How was the material presented, and what did you do to "make it your own"? What do you need to do to become a more effective learner?

▌TIME MANAGEMENT: PUTTING TIME ON YOUR SIDE

One of the most complicated tasks for a professional medical assistant is to manage time effectively. No other workplace can compete with the distractions and demands of a busy healthcare practice. Do you think you practice effective time management skills? Do you believe that you are in control of your time, or do you think that other people or situations control it? How frequently do you say that you just do not have enough time to do what you are supposed to do, let alone those things you would like to do? Time management gives you the opportunity to spend time in the way you choose. Effective time management is also crucial to your success as a student and as a future healthcare professional (Figure 1-4).

▌How to Put Time on Your Side

The following time management skills are designed to help you deal effectively with the demands on your time. Highlight the ones that you think will be most useful in helping you deal with your situation.

1. **Determine your purpose.** What do you want to accomplish this semester, in this course, or in this unit of study? What do you

want to achieve as a student? What is one thing you can do to help achieve your goals?

2. **Identify your main concern.** Besides school, what other demands do you have on your time? Based on the learning goals you have established, what do you need to do to accomplish your goals?
   - *Plan time:* Schedule projects in advance, and make notes to yourself on deadlines.
   - *Use down time:* Take your work with you everywhere you go. Do small bits at every opportunity.
   - *Guard time:* Avoid distractions (e.g., television, music) that interfere with your concentration. Notice how others abuse your time. Learn to say no to outside demands on your time.
   - *Discover time:* Steal time from other activities in your schedule.
   - *Assign time:* Ask for help when you need it from friends and family.

3. **Be organized.** What materials (e.g., books, research, supplies) do you need to have an effective study session? What preparation is needed to make the most of your time?
   - *Record time:* Use a day planner or calendar, either paper or electronic, to note the due dates for assignments and tests. If a paper or project is due on a specific date, put a reminder in your day planner to start the project on a specific date so that you are sure to have it done when it is due.
   - *Optimal time:* Take advantage of the time of day when you study and learn the best. Schedule study time during your peak performance time. If you are an early riser, make time for homework first thing in the day; if you are a night owl, do your homework at night. Plan on dedicating at least some of your optimal time to your school work.

4. **Stop procrastinating.** If you avoid working on your goals, you may not achieve them. Examine the following suggestions as ways to break the procrastination cycle.

- *Make the work meaningful:* What is important about the work you are putting off and what are the benefits of getting it done? Reflect on your long-range goals. Is it important to do a good job on the work so you can earn an acceptable grade, do well in the course, complete the medical assisting program, and ultimately find employment?
- *Plan work deadlines:* Break assignments into achievable sections that can be completed in the time slots available. Schedule those work sections in your day planner so that you do not forget deadlines for assignments.
- *Ask for help:* Let your support system know you have work to get done. Ask them for encouragement to stay on track. If you have school-age children, you can set an excellent example by planning "family" homework sessions. You can get some of your work done while acting as a role model for learning behaviors for your children. Let your partner know when due dates are looming or tests are scheduled. Ask for help in meeting day-to-day demands so that you can study or prepare for school.
- *Prioritize:* If you keep avoiding a certain task, re-evaluate its priority. If it is really worth worrying about, get started now, not later. Don't waste time worrying about how you are going to get things done. Spend that time actually working on the projects that worry you the most.
- *Reward yourself:* Create a reward that is meaningful and something for which you will work. If you want to spend time with your family or friends on the weekend, develop a plan and stick to it so that you can share that special time as a reward.

5. **Remember you.** It is very easy to become overwhelmed with responsibilities both in school and at home. Part of successful time management includes setting aside time to do things you enjoy. You have chosen a profession that can be very demanding. Now is the time to remember that you have to take care of yourself in addition to meeting your professional and personal responsibilities.

CRITICAL THINKING APPLICATION   1-4

How do you spend your time? For 3 days this week, write down the amount of time you spend on each activity. How much television do you watch? How much time do you spend talking on the phone? How about driving time, visiting time, work time for family and friends, and so on? At the end of the 3-day period, add up the amount of time you spend on your daily activities. Do you recognize any time you might be wasting? Can you implement any of the suggested time management strategies to make more time available?

PROBLEM SOLVING AND CONFLICT MANAGEMENT

As a future member of the healthcare team, you frequently will face problems and conflict. Although we usually look at these situations as negative factors in our lives, problem solving and conflict management actually give us the opportunity to affect a potentially negative situation in a positive way. Learning how to manage problems can be very useful for your practice as a medical assistant, as well as for your success as a student.

The first step in reaching an equitable solution to a problem or conflict is to identify the central issue. How many times have you known that you were upset about something but were not really sure why you felt that way? You cannot solve a problem or resolve a negative situation unless you are sure of what is at the root of your feelings. You need to understand the problem and gather as much information about the situation as possible before you decide to act. One way of doing this is to ask yourself these questions:

- When does the situation occur and under what circumstances?
- How does it make me feel?
- Is someone else involved?
- What interferes with making a decision or resolving the conflict?

Once you understand the situation and how you feel about it, you need to decide whether it is worth the effort to resolve it. Prioritize your involvement. Sometimes situations and problems may arise that you are unable to resolve or that you may decide are not important enough to act on. For example, if one of your co-workers refuses to take out the garbage when it is his or her turn, does that really bother you? If it does, you need to deal with the issue. However, if the individual helps out in other ways, then perhaps the garbage isn't worth the effort to resolve the conflict.

After you have gathered the details about the problem or conflict and you have decided it is important enough to act on, it is time to determine possible solutions. One way to do this is to ask for advice or brainstorm ideas with individuals you respect. Sometimes another person can give you special insight into the problem that you were unable to see on your own. After brainstorming for possible solutions, you should then get feedback regarding the workability of the suggested solutions. An alternative to brainstorming possible solutions to the problem is to list on a piece of paper the pros and cons of possible solutions. Simply looking at a list of the positive and negative aspects of the solution may clarify how you could solve the problem. Before deciding on a particular solution, make sure you critically analyze the consequences of each proposed solution: Which one best meets your needs and has the potential for providing an outcome you can live with?

Finally, you are ready to implement the chosen solution. However, your work is not over yet. You need to evaluate the outcome of your decision and see whether it truly did meet your needs. If not, it may be time to review other possible solutions and try another approach.

Conflict management requires some additional consideration. If you are in conflict with a peer, an instructor, or a co-worker, it is important to follow certain guidelines. You should attempt to solve the conflict in a private place at a prescheduled time. This ensures that the person will meet with you and that neither one has to worry about others overhearing the conversation. At the meeting, clearly state your feelings about the conflict and how you would like it resolved. Then try to come to an agreeable solution. The best way to deal with conflict situations is through open, honest, assertive communication. However, just as with problem solving, it is important to follow up on the decided course of action to see whether it effectively dealt with the source of the conflict (Figure 1-5).

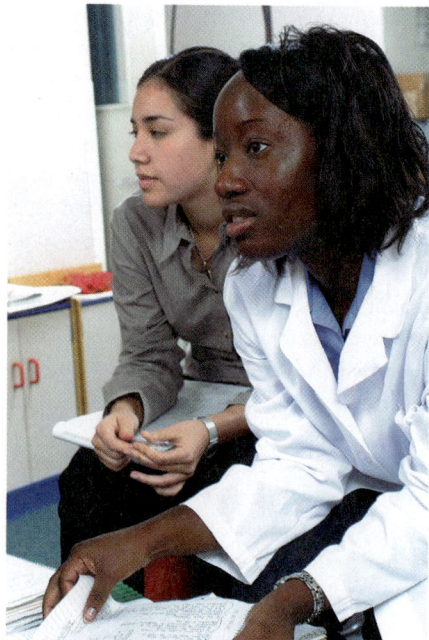

FIGURE 1-5 Dealing with conflict.

Assertive Communication

One of the challenges faced by workers in a healthcare environment is acting assertively when necessary. Assertive communication allows you to express your thoughts and feelings honestly and enables you to stand up for yourself in a reasonable, rational manner without an emotional scene. However, most of us are not born assertive; it is a behavior that must be learned, and many of us must practice it over and over again before it becomes a natural response.

Passive, or nonassertive, individuals often feel hurt when they are taken advantage of or are anxious about dealing with conflict. Just because they comply with what they are told to do or do not argue when they are treated unfairly does not mean that they are not upset about the situation. Often these individuals internalize their hurt and anxiety and eventually have an angry outburst because of built-up stress. Aggressive individuals, on the other hand, take advantage of others, appear self-righteous, and act in a superior way to get what they want. People who act aggressively may humiliate or hurt others to achieve their goals or to have their own needs satisfied.

NONASSERTIVE AND AGGRESSIVE BEHAVIORS AND LANGUAGE

An individual with nonassertive body language displays the following behaviors when attempting to deal with conflict and may use some of the following words:

- Keeps eyes downcast
- Shifts weight when talking
- Has a slumped posture or wrings the hands
- Whines or uses a hesitant tone of voice
- May use the following phrases:
  - "Maybe" or "I guess"
  - "I wonder if you could…"
  - "Would you mind very much if…"
  - "It's not really important."

An aggressive person displays the following behaviors:

- Leans forward and points a finger when talking
- Raises the voice or sounds arrogant
- May use the following phrases:
  - "You'd better…"
  - "If you don't watch out…"
  - "Do it or else!"
  - "You should do it this way!"

Learning how to respond assertively in a potentially challenging situation enables us to be honest and direct with others while at the same time being emotionally honest with ourselves. The goal of assertive behavior is to treat others with respect while acknowledging our own feelings about the problem.

The first step in becoming assertive is to describe the situation and how it makes you feel. Perhaps you have a co-worker who is taking advantage of you; coming to work late, taking long breaks, not answering the phones, and so on. How does that make you feel? Are you angry, hurt, or disappointed? Decide which word best describes your feelings and, using an "I" sentence, clearly state how you feel about the situation. Be specific about the problem. If your statement is too general (e.g., "I am very hurt when you act like that"), the person you are confronting can either misunderstand or ignore you, because the individual does not know specifically what is wrong. A statement such as, "I am very hurt that you take advantage of me by consistently being late for work, taking long breaks, and not helping with answering the phones," makes the problem very clear and how you feel about it.

Acting assertively takes practice, practice, practice. In addition, just because you deliver a clear, concise, assertive message does not mean that the problem will be solved that quickly. Your assertive words must be combined with assertive body language to deliver a clear message about how serious you consider the situation. Remember, 80% to 90% of a message is nonverbal. Therefore, your "I" message must be accompanied by assertive behavior, including establishing eye contact and slightly raising your voice to get the individual's attention. And just because you deliver the perfect message does not mean you will always get what you want. The message may have to be repeated; do you really think someone who is habitually late for work is going to start showing up on time because of one assertive message? However, regardless of the outcome, you will feel better because you have honestly communicated how you feel about the situation, and you are working on a resolution of the problem.

STUDY SKILLS: TRICKS FOR BECOMING A SUCCESSFUL STUDENT

So far in this chapter, we have looked at the influence of individual learning styles and time management on learning success. Now we will investigate some ideas that are useful for learning new material. These study skills include memory techniques, active learning, brain tricks, reading methods, and note-taking strategies.

Several techniques can help you store and remember information. The first of these involves organizing information into recognizable groups so that the brain can find it easily. You can organize information by getting the big picture first before trying to learn the details. One way to implement this strategy is to skim a reading assignment before actually reading and taking notes on the material, thus getting a general impression of what you need to learn before tackling the details. Depending on your learning style, it may also help to find a way of making the new information meaningful. Think about your educational goals and how the new material will help you achieve those goals. Another way of remembering material is to create an association with something you already know. If new material is grouped with already stored material, the brain remembers it much more easily.

A useful study skill for some learners is to be physically active while learning. Some students learn best if they walk or talk out loud while studying. Besides encouraging learning, moving and talking while studying relieves boredom and keeps you awake. Another way to be actively involved in learning is to use pictures or diagrams to represent the material you are studying. Some people are visual learners, and creating pictures of the material is the easiest method for them to retain the information. Other students find that rewriting notes or making lists of information helps them retain the material. Writing also helps students who need to "do" something to learn.

Studying goes much more smoothly if you work *with* your brain rather than *against* it. If you tend to get anxious and worried while studying, you may be acting as your own worst enemy. One way of dealing with a topic you are anxious about is to overlearn it. If material is overlearned, you are much less likely to experience test anxiety. Another method for remembering material is to review it quickly after class. This minireview helps the new information become part of your long-term memory system. Many students find creating songs, dances, or word associations an effective way to learn and remember new material. Putting details into a familiar song and moving to it can help trick the brain into remembering the information. This is especially helpful when trying to learn anatomy and physiology. Another excellent way of learning information is to actually teach it to someone else. Teaching requires you to have a good understanding of the material and the ability to describe it for others. It can be an effective reinforcement of complicated material.

A great deal of the learning process is expected to take place from assigned readings. You can use several methods to make reading assignments more meaningful. If you find a reading assignment challenging or difficult to understand, the first step is to take the time to read it again. Sometimes the first time through the material is not enough to gain understanding. As you read, highlight important words or thoughts and stop periodically to summarize the material. If you get bored while reading, use your body; walk or talk your way through the assignment. Take the time to look up words

or terms you do not understand or ask your instructor or tutor for help. Outlining the material can help you create a brief overview of what you need to learn. The best way to determine whether you have learned anything from your reading is to try to explain the material to someone else. If you can do that effectively, you know you have acquired the knowledge needed from the reading assignment.

Many students find effective note taking a challenge. The big question is, "How much of what the instructor says do I actually need to write down?" The first step in effective note taking is to come to class prepared. The more familiar you are with the material, the easier it will be to determine the important parts of the instructor's lecture. Pay attention to the instructor and look for clues to what he or she thinks is important. Ask questions about the material if you do not understand it, rather than writing down information that makes no sense to you. Think critically about what you hear before you write it down so you can start to build relationships among the things you want or need to know.

When it comes to actual note taking, some strategies can make the process of recording notes an active learning tool. Organize the information as much as possible while you are writing or typing, either in an outline or a paragraph format. If you take notes directly into a laptop or tablet, make sure your keyboarding skills are good enough for you to keep up with the flow of information and that you review your notes shortly after class to fill in any missing details. If you take notes on paper, use only one side of the page (for easier reading) and leave blank spaces where needed to fill in details later. Use key words to help you remember the material, and create pictures or diagrams to help visualize it. If permitted, use tape recorders when appropriate and make sure you have any handouts or notes that cover material written on the board or provided in a PowerPoint presentation. If your instructor refers the class to a YouTube video, make sure you have transcribed the site address correctly to refer to it at a later time. Another helpful tool is to develop your own system of abbreviations to help simplify the note-taking process.

The most effective way to use your notes is to review them shortly after class. This is the time to add details, clarify information, or make notes about asking the instructor for explanations during the next class. You could even exchange notes with students you trust to compare information (Figure 1-6). Some students find it beneficial to type their notes (if they took them on paper) or to rewrite them. This can give you an opportunity to learn the material as you

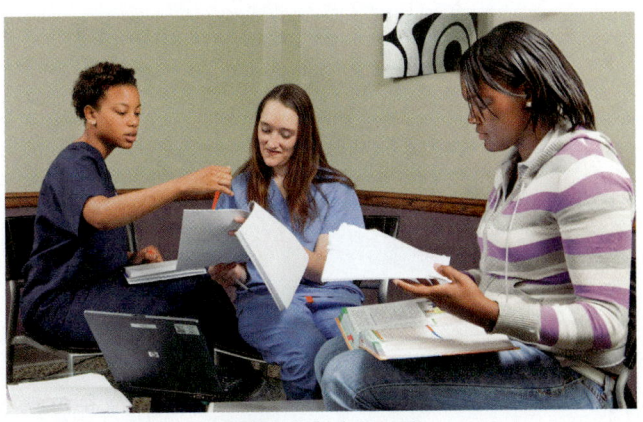

FIGURE 1-6 Sharing notes.

transcribe it. As you are reviewing your notes, you also can draw mind maps of the information or diagram outlines to help you better understand and remember the material.

Creating mind maps is a way of representing the main idea of a topic and supporting important details with a figure or picture. Healthcare textbooks present complicated concepts with multiple main ideas, each with its own important details. Mind maps are a way of consolidating complex details and organizing them into a format that is easier to remember. The spider map (Figure 1-7) presents a method for including several main ideas with details in one study guide. The fishbone map (Figure 1-8) can be used to learn complicated causes of disease. The chain-of-events map (Figure 1-9) displays the cause and effect of events, such as infection control or the history of medicine. The cycle map (Figure 1-10) shows the connection between factors, such as in the chain of infection.

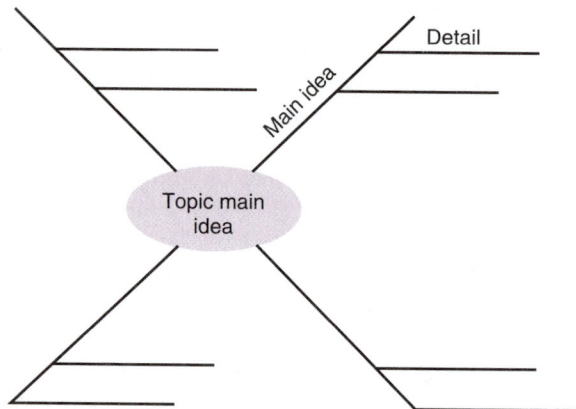

FIGURE 1-7 Spider map showing multiple main ideas with supporting details.

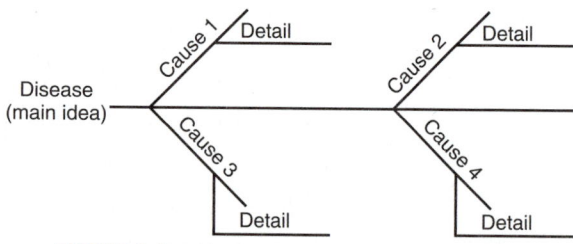

FIGURE 1-8 Fishbone map used to describe causes of disease.

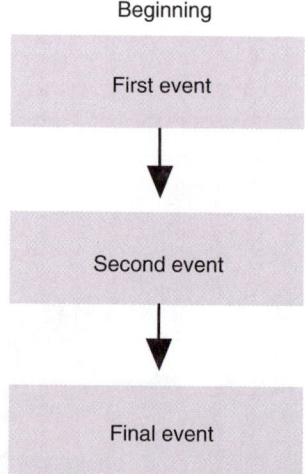

FIGURE 1-9 Chain-of-events map showing the cause and effect of events.

Creating your own mind maps is a way of making the information more meaningful and easier for you to understand.

Although many techniques can help you study, perhaps the most important one is your attitude toward learning. Some students fall into the "I can't possibly learn this material" trap. That type of attitude only leads to self-defeat. The way to overcome barriers is first to recognize that they exist. Once you know your weak spots, use the suggested study skills to improve in those areas. Do not be afraid to ask questions or to ask for help if you do not understand the material. Use as many different strategies as necessary to become a successful student.

TEST-TAKING STRATEGIES: TAKING CHARGE OF YOUR SUCCESS

What happens when you do not know the answer to the first question on a test? What if you do not know the next one? Are you able to go on without panicking? Many people find taking tests the most challenging part of being a successful student. Multiple approaches are available that you can use to take charge of your success and improve your ability to take tests. These include such strategies as adequate preparation, controlling negative thoughts during test time, and understanding ways to manage various types of questions.

The first step is to go into a test adequately prepared. Use the time management skills already outlined in this chapter to prepare for the big day. Recognize and use your preferred learning style to overlearn the material and increase your confidence. Use memory tools (e.g., flash cards, checklists, and mind maps) to help you visualize the material. Form a study group if you are the type of learner who benefits from studying in groups. Schedule and plan study time, and reward yourself for your hard work. It also is important to go

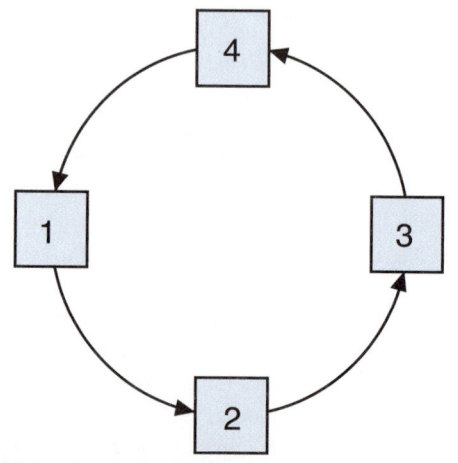

FIGURE 1-10 Cycle map illustrating the way one action leads to another.

into the test rested and relaxed; therefore, you should eat, exercise to relieve stress, and sleep before the test so that you are as alert as possible.

Before you start the test, make sure you read the directions carefully. If possible, begin with the easiest or shortest questions to build your confidence. Be aware of the amount of time allotted for the examination, and pace yourself accordingly. As you go through the test, look for clues to answers in other questions. During test time, remember to use positive self-talk at the first indication of panic. Repeatedly remind yourself that you are well prepared; relax and think about the material before you get worried. You need to stop negative thoughts as soon as they arise and instead visualize yourself being successful. Use slow, deep breathing to relax and, if helpful, close your eyes for a minute and visualize a relaxing place before you go on with the test. You may find it helpful to wear a thick rubber band on your wrist and snap it as soon as you start to think negatively. The sting of the rubber band provides a physical reaction that interferes with the power of your negative thoughts and serves as a reminder to focus on the exam and not on your anxiety.

Certain strategies are useful for answering different types of questions. With multiple choice questions, try to identify key words or clues in each question. Read the question carefully and answer it in your head before you review the provided answers. If you are not absolutely sure of the answer, make an educated guess or follow your instincts in choosing an answer. "True or false" questions give you a 50/50 chance of being correct. Remember that if any part of the question is not true, then the statement is false. Again, check the statements for key words that help indicate the direction of the answer. Look for qualifying terms (e.g., *always, never, sometimes*) that are the key to understanding the meaning of the true or false statement.

CRITICAL THINKING APPLICATION   1-8

Think about a time you experienced test anxiety. Write down the details of the situation and how you felt. Choose four test-taking strategies you think would be beneficial in handling similar situations in the future.

BECOMING A CRITICAL THINKER: MAKING MENTAL CONNECTIONS

The ability to process information and arrive at reasonable conclusions is crucial to all healthcare workers. The process of **critical thinking** involves (1) sorting out conflicting information, (2) weighing your knowledge about that information, (3) ignoring or letting go of personal biases, and (4) deciding on a reasonable belief or action. Critical thinking is actually an active search for the truth.

Critical thinking could be described as thorough thinking, because it requires learners to keep an open mind to all possibilities. Successful students are thorough thinkers, because they must determine the facts about the topic being learned and come to logical conclusions about the material. Critical thinkers also are inquisitive learners, who constantly analyze and sort out conflicting information to reach conclusions.

A crucial step in critical thinking is evaluating the results of your learning. Reflection is the key to critical thinking. "How did I learn what I learned?" and "What does it mean in my life?" are questions that must be asked consistently to continue to learn. Becoming a successful student, and ultimately a successful member of the allied health team, requires critical thinking skills.

SUMMARY OF SCENARIO

One of the things Shawna can do to improve her learning is to determine her individual learning style. By understanding how she typically perceives and processes new information, she can plan the best methods for learning the material. In addition to understanding who she is as a learner, Shawna needs to practice successful time management skills to keep up with school and work responsibilities. Effective problem solving and developing study skills that work for her are also keys to her success as a student.

SUMMARY OF LEARNING OBJECTIVES

1. **Define, spell, and pronounce the terms listed in the vocabulary.**
   Spelling and pronouncing medical terms correctly bolster the medical assistant's credibility. Knowing the definitions of these terms promotes confidence in communication with patients and co-workers.

2. **Assess the importance of developing professional behaviors as a member of the allied health team.**
   Medical assistants play a vital role on the healthcare team and are expected to show such professional behaviors as being dependable, practicing respectful patient care, displaying empathy, showing initiative, demonstrating a positive attitude, and functioning as an effective member of the healthcare team.

3. **Examine your learning preferences.**
   Learning preferences are the ways you like to learn and that have proven successful in the past.

4. **Interpret how your learning style affects your success as a student.**
   Your learning style is determined by your individual method of perceiving or examining new material and the way you process it or make it your own. People are either concrete or abstract perceivers and either active or reflective processors.

5. **Apply time management strategies to make the most of your learning opportunities.**
   Effective time management strategies, such as setting goals, prioritizing, getting organized, and avoiding procrastination, will make you a more successful student and an effective medical assistant.

6. **Apply problem-solving techniques to manage conflict and overcome barriers to your success.**
   Problem-solving and conflict management techniques are crucial to your success. First, identify the central issue and how you feel about it; then, consider possible solutions and their potential results, implement the chosen solution, and analyze the results.

7. **Discuss the role of assertiveness in effective communication.**
   Assertive communication allows you to express your thoughts and feelings honestly and enables you to stand up for yourself in a reasonable, rational manner without an emotional scene. Learning how to respond assertively in a potentially challenging situation enables us to be honest and direct with others while at the same time being emotionally honest with ourselves. The goal of assertive behavior is to treat others with respect while acknowledging our own feelings about the problem.

8. **Integrate effective study skills into your daily activities.**
   Study skills, such as memory techniques, active learning, brain tricks, effective reading methods, note-taking strategies, and mind maps, all help students to be more successful.

9. **Design test-taking strategies that help you take charge of your success.**
   Test-taking strategies include preparing adequately for the examination, controlling negative thoughts during the examination, and understanding how to deal with different types of questions.

10. **Incorporate critical thinking and reflection to make mental connections as you learn material.**
    Critical thinking can be defined as thorough thinking, because it considers all sides of the information without bias. Reflection is the process of thinking about or reviewing information before acting.

CONNECTIONS

Study Guide Connection: Go to the Chapter 1 Study Guide. Read and complete the activities.

Evolve Connection: Go to the Chapter 1 link at *evolve.elsevier.com/ kinn* to complete the Chapter Review and Chapter Quiz. Check out the other resources listed for this chapter to make the most of what you have learned from Becoming a Successful Student.

THE HEALTHCARE INDUSTRY

2

SCENARIO

Carlos Santos, CMA, is a medical assisting instructor with 10 years' experience in the clinical area. He worked for a group of family practitioners and for an allergist during his career as a medical assistant before becoming an instructor. Mr. Santos believes that it is very important to give his students an overview of the history of medicine early in their training. He knows that it is exciting to show them the progress of medicine and to introduce students to the pioneers who contributed to the field. This helps the student to understand where he or she fits into the whole picture as a medical assistant. Often Mr. Santos assigns the students a short report on one person who played a role in the progress of medicine. He finds that this is a good way to encourage students to use the Internet and to conduct research right from the start of their training; also, the students get a chance to grow more comfortable speaking in front of a group when they give their reports in class. Mr. Santos knows that his students will develop an appreciation for those who contributed to the medical profession, which will influence their own dedication to both peers and patients.

Mr. Santos knows that his students must recognize the different members of the healthcare team and their responsibilities. Once the students begin their externship or practicum, they will be able to work effectively with each person in the facility and understand each one's role in the treatment of patients. Mr. Santos also introduces them to the current types of facilities available for patient care on both a national and a local level. The knowledge the students gain about the different areas of patient care will be useful once they graduate and begin working in a healthcare facility. All of these skills will make Mr. Santos' students more versatile and valuable to their eventual employers.

While studying this chapter, think about the following questions:

- What recent events could be included as groundbreaking discoveries in medicine?
- Why are continuing medical education and research so important to the healthcare industry and specifically to the medical assistant?
- How can the individual medical assistant contribute to the progress of medicine in today's world?
- What is the value of gaining an overview of the history of medicine as one begins a career in medical assisting?

LEARNING OBJECTIVES

1. Define, spell, and pronounce the terms listed in the vocabulary.
2. Identify the ancient cultures that contributed a major portion of our medical terminology.
3. Distinguish between and describe the staff of Aesculapius and the caduceus.
4. Explain the philosophy behind the phrase "physicians must learn to despise money."
5. Explain why a medical education at Johns Hopkins University School of Medicine was considered superior, even in its early years.
6. List several medical pioneers and discuss the importance of their contributions to the medical profession.
7. Explain the roles of the national health organizations.
8. Identify the role of the Centers for Disease Control and Prevention (CDC) regulations in healthcare settings
9. Discuss the various types of ambulatory care.
10. Name the three main provider portals of entry into the healthcare system and distinguish among the different types of physicians and medical practices.
11. Become familiar with the medical specialties recognized by the American Board of Medical Specialties.
12. Understand both the allied health professions and how they relate to medical assisting.

VOCABULARY

accreditation (u-kre-duh-ta′-shun) The process through which an organization is recognized for adherence to a group of standards that meet or exceed the expectations of the accrediting agency.

advent Coming into being or use.

allopathic (al-o-path′-ik) A term used to contrast homeopathic medicine with mainstream medicine; allopathic medicine is characterized by an effort to counteract the symptoms of a disease by administration of treatments that produce effects opposite to the symptoms.

ambulatory (am′-bu-la-to-re) Able to walk about and not be bedridden.

amenities Things that contribute to comfort, enjoyment, or convenience.

case management The process of assessing and planning patient care, including referral and follow-up, to ensure continuity of care and quality management.

chiropractic (ki′-ruh-prak-tik) A medical discipline that focuses on the nervous system and involves manual adjustment of the vertebral column to affect the nervous system, and thereby treat various disorders, as well as to promote patient wellness.

cited Quoted by way of example, authority, or proof or mentioned formally in commendation or praise.

complementary and alternative medicine (CAM) A group of diverse medical and healthcare systems, practices, and products that are not generally considered part of conventional medicine. Complementary medicine is used in combination with conventional medicine (allopathic or osteopathic); alternative medicine is used instead of conventional medicine.

contamination (kun-ta-mu-na′-shun) The process by which something is made impure, unclean, or unfit for use by the introduction of unwholesome or undesirable elements.

conventional medicine Medicine as practiced by holders of the Doctor of Medicine (MD) and Doctor of Osteopathy (OD) degrees and by their allied health professionals, such as physical therapists, psychologists, and registered nurses.

credentialing (kri-den′-shuh-ling) The process of extending professional or medical privileges to an individual; the process of verifying and evaluating that person's credentials.

dissection (di-sek′-shun) The separation into pieces and exposure of parts for scientific examination.

encounter Any contact between a healthcare provider and a patient that results in treatment or evaluation of the patient's condition; it is not limited to in-person contact.

fermentation (fur-men-ta′-shun) An enzymatically controlled transformation of an organic compound.

holistic (ho-lis′-tik) A health viewpoint that considers all the systems of the body and their interdependence, rather than breaking down the body into discrete parts.

homeopathy (ho-me-uh′-puh-the) A type of alternative medicine that attempts to stimulate the body to recover by itself; a system of therapy based on the concept that disease can be treated with minute doses of drugs thought capable of producing the same symptoms in healthy people as the disease itself.

hospice (hos′-pus) A concept of care that involves health professionals and volunteers who provide medical, psychological, and spiritual support to terminally ill patients and their loved ones.

indicators An important point or group of statistical values that, when evaluated, indicates the quality of care provided in a healthcare facility.

indicted (in-di′-ted) Charged with a crime by the finding of a jury according to due process of law.

indigent (in′-di-junt) A needy or poor person who is unable to provide the basic necessities of life; totally lacking in something of need.

innate Existing in, belonging to, or determined by factors present in an individual since birth.

innocuous (i′-nuh-kyu-wus) Having no effect, adverse or otherwise; harmless.

integrated Formed, coordinated, or blended into a functioning or unified whole; to incorporate into a larger unit.

integrated delivery system (IDS) A network of healthcare providers and organizations that provides or arranges to provide a coordinated continuum of services to a defined population and is willing to be held clinically and fiscally accountable for the clinical outcomes and health status of the population served.

mysticism The experience of seeming to have direct communication with God or ultimate reality.

naturopathy (na-chu-ra′-puh-the) An alternative to conventional medicine in which holistic methods are used, in addition to herbs and natural supplements, with the belief that the body will heal itself. Naturopathic physicians currently can be licensed in 15 states, Puerto Rico, and the Virgin Islands.

osteopathic (us-te-uh-path′-ik) A term describing the type of medicine that is based on the theory that disturbances in the musculoskeletal system affect other bodily parts, causing many disorders that can be corrected by various manipulative techniques in conjunction with conventional medical, surgical, pharmacologic, and other therapeutic procedures.

pandemic (pan-de′-mik) A condition in which most people in a country, a number of countries, or a geographic area are affected.

peer review organizations (PROs) Groups of medical reviewers contracted by the Centers for Medicare and Medicaid Services (CMS) to ensure quality control and the medical necessity of services provided by a facility.

philanthropist (fu-lan′-thruh-pist) An individual who makes an active effort to promote human welfare.

putrefaction (pyu-truh-fak′-shun) Decomposition of animal matter, which results in a foul smell.

robotics Technology dealing with the design, construction, and operation of robots in automation.

staff privileges The permission granted by a facility to a healthcare professional to practice in that facility.

standards Items or indicators used as a measure of quality or compliance with a statutory or accrediting body's policies and regulations.

subluxations (suh-bluk-sa′-shuns) Slight misalignments of the vertebrae or a partial dislocation.

telemedicine The use of telecommunications in the practice of medicine to compensate for the great distances that can separate healthcare professionals, colleagues, patients, and students.

teleradiology The use of telecommunication devices to enhance and improve the results of radiologic procedures.

treatises (tree′-te-ses) Systematic expositions or arguments in writing, including a methodic discussion of the facts and principles involved and the conclusions reached.

triage (tree′-azh) Identification of the severity of patients' conditions and the allocation of treatment according to a system of priorities, which is designed to maximize the number of survivors and provide treatment for the sickest patients first.

The growth of today's healthcare industry seems unstoppable. Thanks to modern technologic advances, medicine speeds forward faster than ever in its quest to improve the health of humankind. Modern advances, such as **telemedicine**, are experiencing significant growth, and the images produced with **teleradiology** have vastly improved in their resolution. **Robotics** is assisting healthcare professionals in surgery and even delivers drugs to hospital floors using laser sensors. Education in medicine has grown exponentially: computers, the Internet, and video have enabled an instructor in New York to communicate with a student in Los Angeles. The key to this technology lies in the development and widespread use of elaborate information systems that have revolutionized the way medicine is practiced today. Technology is advancing at an astounding rate; the healthcare environment of the future is barely imaginable. This chapter looks back at the history of medicine, gazes at its present, and glances toward its future.

THE HISTORY OF MEDICINE

Medical Language and Mythology

Today's medical professional uses words with origins stemming from the romance and fantasy of classical and ancient languages. The study of anatomy reaches back to the dawn of recorded history. Today's modern terms often are similar to their original versions. Some terms are inaccurate when translated literally, because the ancients did not fully understand bodily functions. The word *artery*, for example, which comes from the Greek word *arteria*, literally means "a windpipe." The early Greeks believed that the arteries carried air, not blood. Greek and Roman mythologies have contributed a major portion of our medical terminology, but we have also borrowed liberally from Arabic, Anglo-Saxon, and Germanic sources. Several terms originate from the Bible.

The human head rests on the first cervical vertebra, which is called the *atlas*. Atlas was the famous Greek Titan who was condemned by Zeus to bear the heavens on his shoulders. Achilles' mother held him by the heel as she dipped him into the river Styx so that he would become invulnerable. However, his heel was not immersed, and he later died from a wound in that area. *Achilles heel* is a common expression used today to indicate a point of weakness. Aphrodite, the Greek goddess of love and beauty, is the source of the name for drugs used to enhance sexual arousal, called *aphrodisiacs*. The equivalent Roman goddess of love, Venus, is associated with lustful desires. A portion of the female anatomy, the mons *veneris* (mons pubis), and *venereal* diseases were named after her.

Aesculapius, the son of Apollo, was revered as the god of medicine. The early Greeks worshiped the healing powers of Aesculapius and built temples in his honor where patients were treated by trained priests. His daughters were Hygeia, goddess of health, and Panacea, goddess of all healing and restorer of health. Our modern word *hygiene* has its origin in Hygeia, and the modern meaning for *panacea* is "a remedy for all ills and difficulties." The staff of Aesculapius is a common medical icon. It depicts a serpent encircling a staff and signifies the art of healing. The staff of Aesculapius has been adopted by the American Medical Association as the symbol of medicine. The mythological staff belonging to Hermes, the messenger of the gods, is the caduceus, which was thought to have magical powers. The caduceus is a winged staff encircled by two serpents. This icon is the medical insignia of the U.S. Army Medical Corps, although it often is misused as a symbol of the medical profession (Figure 2-1).

Medicine in Ancient Times

Although religious and mythological beliefs were the basis for care for the sick in ancient times, evidence suggests that drugs, surgery, and other treatments based on theories about the body were used as early as 5000 BC. In the well-developed societies of the Egyptians, Babylonians, and Assyrians, certain men acted as physicians and used the little knowledge they had to try to treat illness and injury.

Moses presented rules of health to the Hebrews in approximately 1205 BC. He was the first advocate of preventive medicine and is considered the first public health officer. Moses knew that some animal diseases could be passed to humans and that **contamination** existed; therefore a religious law was developed forbidding humans to eat or drink from dirty dishes. The people of that era believed that doing so would defile their bodies and they would lose their souls.

Hippocrates, known as the Father of Medicine, is the most famous of the ancient Greek physicians (Figure 2-2). He was born in 450 BC on the island of Cos in Greece. He is best remembered for the Hippocratic Oath, which has been administered to physicians

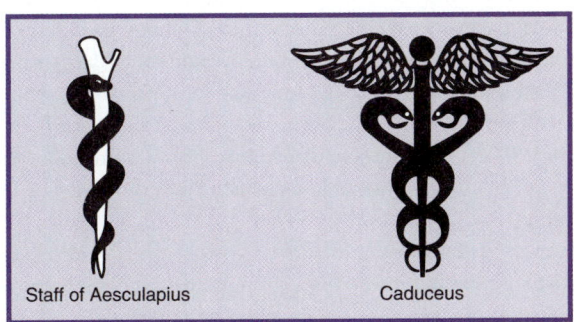

Staff of Aesculapius   Caduceus

FIGURE 2-1 Staff of Aesculapius and the caduceus.

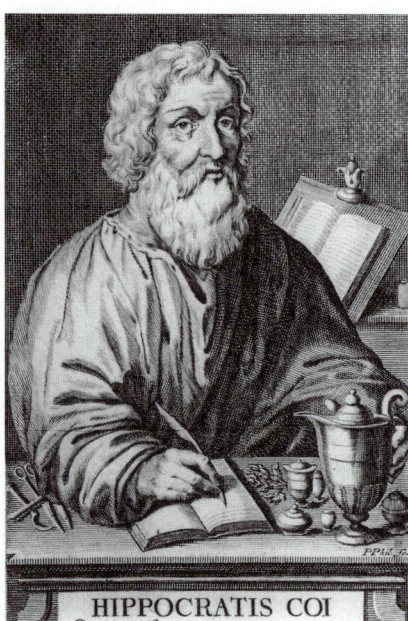

FIGURE 2-2 Hippocrates is known as the Father of Medicine. (Courtesy National Library of Medicine, Bethesda, Md.)

for more than 2,000 years. Hippocrates is credited with taking **mysticism** out of medicine and giving it a scientific basis. During this period of history, most believed that illness was caused by demonic possession; for the illness to be cured, the demon had to be removed from the body. Hippocrates' clinical descriptions of diseases and his volumes on epidemics, fevers, epilepsy, fractures, and instruments were studied for centuries. He believed that the body had the capacity to heal itself and that the physician's role was to help nature. He described four "humors"—blood, phlegm, yellow bile, and black bile—that he believed must be in balance for the body to maintain a healthy state.

Galen was a Greek physician who migrated to Rome in AD 162 and became known as the Prince of Physicians. He is said to have written more than 500 **treatises** on medicine. He wrote an excellent summary on anatomy as it was known at the time, but his work was faulty and inaccurate, because it was largely based on the **dissection** of apes and swine. He is considered the Father of Experimental Physiology and the first experimental neurologist. He was the first to describe the cranial nerves and the sympathetic nervous system, and he performed the first experimental section of the spinal cord, producing hemiplegia. Galen was a champion of medical ethics; he thought that physicians "must learn to despise money," and that if a physician was interested in profit, he was not serious in his devotion to the art of medicine. Galen's beliefs about monetary profit from medicine parallel the views of many modern healthcare professionals, who understand the nature of the healthcare crisis the world faces today. Although much of what he believed about the body was incorrect, Galen's teachings remained intact until human dissections began and physicians were able to visualize exactly what was inside the human body.

Because both Hippocrates and Galen were highly respected, the authority of their observations went unquestioned. This had a negative effect on the progress of science throughout the Dark Ages and well into the sixteenth century. Their theories and descriptions were considered immutable principles; therefore, few physicians were innovative and curious enough to challenge them. Those who did experiment in medicine were scorned by their colleagues, and physicians continued to use methods that were at best ineffectual or **innocuous** and at worst harmful to the patient. However, the establishment of universities led to a study of theories of disease rather than observation of the sick.

Early Development of Medical Education

Medical knowledge developed slowly, and distribution of such knowledge was poor. Before the printing press was invented in the middle of the fifteenth century, very little exchange of scientific knowledge and ideas occurred; scientists were not well informed about the investigations of other scientists. The printing press allowed books to be distributed faster and over a widespread area.

In the seventeenth century, European academies or societies were established, consisting of small groups of men who met to discuss subjects of mutual interest. The academies provided freedom of expression that, with the stimulus of exchanging ideas, contributed significantly to the development of scientific thought. One of the earliest of the academies was the Royal Society of London, formed in 1662. The development of communication during this era was important, and these societies contributed to the exchange of information.

In the United States, medical education was greatly influenced by the Johns Hopkins University School of Medicine in Baltimore, Maryland, established in the early 1890s. The school admitted only college graduates with at least one year's training in the natural sciences. The clinical education at Johns Hopkins was superior, because the school partnered with Johns Hopkins Hospital, which had been created expressly for teaching and research by members of the medical faculty.

The earliest medical school **accreditation** resulted from a report published by Abraham Flexner. He received a grant from the Carnegie Foundation Commission to study the quality of medical colleges in the United States and Canada. His report, called the Flexner Report, resulted in the closure of many low-ranking schools and the upgrading of others. These events legitimized medical education and opened new doors for many individuals to the world of medicine.

CRITICAL THINKING APPLICATION   2-1

- Mr. Santos asks his class to identify which of the individuals involved in early medicine have had the greatest impact on modern healthcare. Whom would you choose and why?
- The students point out that early research often was viewed in a negative manner. How does research affect us now, and how is it viewed by the public?

Early Medical Pioneers

Andreas Vesalius (1514-1564) was a Belgian anatomist known as the Father of Modern Anatomy (Figure 2-3). At the age of 29, he published his great *De Corporis Humani Fabrica,* in which he described the structure of the human body. This work marked a turning point by breaking with the traditional belief in Galen's theories. Vesalius introduced many new anatomic terms, but because of his radical

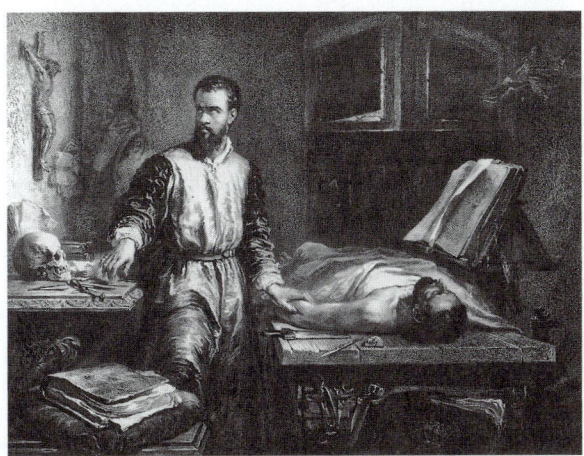

FIGURE 2-3 Andreas Vesalius is known as the Father of Modern Anatomy. (Courtesy National Library of Medicine, Bethesda, Md.)

approach, he was subjected to persecution by his colleagues, teachers, and pupils.

Other important advances and discoveries took place throughout the world. Gabriele Fallopius (1523-1562), an Italian student of Vesalius, also was an accurate dissector. He described and named many parts of the human anatomy. He named the fallopian tubes after himself and also named the vagina and placenta. In 1628 English physician William Harvey (1578-1657) announced his discovery that the heart acts as a muscular pump, forcing and propelling the blood throughout the body. He revealed that the blood's motion is a continuous cycle. He based his conclusion on his experimental vivisection, ligation, and perfusion, as well as brilliant reasoning. Harvey's writings were recognized in Germany before the English permitted their publication at home. Modern England considers Harvey its medical Shakespeare.

The unseen world of microorganisms was first revealed by Anton van Leeuwenhoek (1632-1723), a Dutch linen draper and haberdasher. He ground more than 400 lenses during his lifetime, some of which were no larger than a pinhead. In the grinding process, Leeuwenhoek learned how to use a simple biconvex lens to magnify the minute world of organisms and structures never before seen. Leeuwenhoek was the first ever to observe bacteria and protozoa through a lens, and his accurate interpretations of what he saw led to the sciences of bacteriology and protozoology.

Marcello Malpighi (1628-1694) was born near Bologna, Italy, and attended the University of Bologna, where he earned a doctorate in both medicine and philosophy. He pioneered the use of the microscope in the study of plants and animals. Microscopic anatomy became a prerequisite for advances in physiology, embryology, and practical medicine. In 1661 he described the pulmonary and capillary network connecting the smallest arteries with the smallest veins. This was one of the most important discoveries in the history of science, and it validated Harvey's work. Malpighi is commonly regarded as the first histologist.

Medical Advances in the Eighteenth and Nineteenth Centuries

English scientist John Hunter (1728-1793) is known as the Founder of Scientific Surgery. An army surgeon, he became an expert on gunshot wounds and experimented with tissue transfer. His surgical procedures were soundly based on pathologic evidence. He was the first to classify teeth in a scientific manner, and he introduced artificial feeding by means of a flexible tube passed into the stomach. He provided a classic description of the syphilitic chancre, which sometimes is called a *hunterian chancre.* During his studies of venereal diseases, he inoculated himself with what he thought was gonorrhea, but instead he acquired syphilis. His results in this study actually caused confusion in the medical community, because he mistakenly thought that gonorrhea was a symptom of syphilis. This misconception was not corrected until the beginning of the twentieth century. His collection of anatomic and animal specimens formed the basis for the museum of the Royal College of Surgeons. Hunter is considered the Founder of Scientific Surgery, and today, the John Hunter Hospital in Australia serves more than 600 inpatients and 1,000 outpatients a day.

Edward Jenner (1749-1823) was a student of John Hunter and a country physician from Dorsetshire, England. He is considered one of the immortals of preventive medicine for his development of the smallpox vaccine. While Jenner was serving as an apprentice, he assisted in treating a dairymaid. Smallpox was mentioned, and she commented, "I cannot take that disease, for I have had cowpox." Smallpox at that time was a deadly **pandemic**. Jenner observed that those who had contracted cowpox never contracted smallpox. Later, as a practicing physician, Jenner continued investigating the relationship between cowpox and smallpox almost obsessively, but the medical society members grew bored with his obsession and threatened to expel him from their ranks. On May 14, 1796, Dr. Jenner took purulent matter from a pustule on the hand of Sarah Nelmes, a dairymaid, and inserted it through two small superficial incisions into the arm of James Phipps, a healthy 8-year-old boy. This was the first vaccination. Phipps' vaccination kept him safe from the dreaded disease, and Jenner's method of vaccination spread throughout the world. Today smallpox has been eradicated worldwide as a result of a planned program of global vaccination.

Austrian physician Leopold Auenbrugger (1722-1809) developed the use of percussion in diagnosis. Although scorned and ignored by his contemporaries, his techniques later made him famous and are still used today during physical examinations. René Laënnec (1781-1826) was a French physician who developed the stethoscope in 1819. At first he used only a cylinder of rolled paper in his hands; later he used a wooden device because of its sound-conducting properties. With today's sophisticated stethoscopes, physicians are able to hear sounds in the body, including a fetus inside the mother. Laënnec's book, *Treatise on Mediate Auscultation and Diseases of the Chest,* was readily accepted and translated into many languages. The book is said to be the most important treatise on diseases of the thoracic organs ever written.

Several men of the early 1800s are remembered for their fight against puerperal fever and their concern for women's health. Puerperal fever, an infectious disease that can be contracted during childbirth, was also called *puerperal sepsis* or *childbed fever.* The term *puerperal,* denoting a woman in childbed, originates from the Latin *puer,* "a child," and *pario,* "to bring forth."

The best known of these men was the Hungarian physician Ignaz Philipp Semmelweis (1818-1865); history has called him the Savior of Mothers. His fight against puerperal fever is a sad story

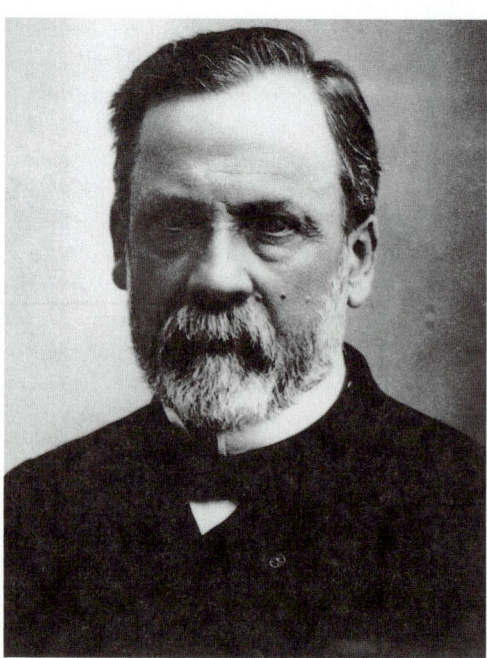

FIGURE 2-4 Louis Pasteur was a brilliant chemist who made numerous contributions to medicine. (Courtesy National Library of Medicine, Bethesda, Md.)

of hardships. His theories were resisted by many professionals, including his instructors. Semmelweis noted that the fever often attacked women who were delivered by medical students coming straight from the autopsy or dissecting rooms. Semmelweis directed that in his wards the students were to wash and disinfect their hands before going to examine the women and deliver the children. As his theories were proved correct, Semmelweis felt an incredible guilt that doctors themselves had caused so many deaths. He died at the age of 47, ironically, from the very disease he had fought. He was infected with puerperal fever from a cut on his finger during an autopsy. His grave had hardly been closed when scientists began to understand the causes of this disease, largely as a result of the investigations of two great scientists, Louis Pasteur and Joseph Lister.

Louis Pasteur (1822-1895) was a Frenchman who did brilliant work as a chemist, but it was his studies in bacteriology that made him one of the most famous men in medical history (Figure 2-4). The title of Father of Bacteriology was bestowed on him, and he also has been honored as the Father of Preventive Medicine. Pasteur's adventures included studying the difficulties involved in the **fermentation** of wine. He averted disaster in France's critical winemaking industry by a process he developed, now called *pasteurization*. This achievement alone would have made him an immortal among the French. Through a process of supplying enough heat to destroy microorganisms, wine was prevented from turning to vinegar. Pasteur's research efforts were impeded when he was stricken with hemiplegia, but after a long, difficult recovery, he was able to continue with a stiff hand and a limp.

Convinced that the infinite world of bacteria held the key to the secrets of contagious diseases, Pasteur left chemistry again to continue studying his theory. Many renowned scientists denied the germ theory of disease and devoted themselves to degrading Pasteur's theories and experiments. In the midst of this controversy, he became involved in the prevention of anthrax, which threatened the health of cattle and sheep. Pasteur eventually was honored for his work with many other diseases, such as rabies, chicken cholera, and swine erysipelas. He devoted the last 7 years of his life to the Pasteur Institute, which was founded as a clinic for rabies treatment, a research center for infectious disease, and a teaching center. The Pasteur Institute still exists. Pasteur died in 1895, with his family at his bedside. It is said that his last words were, "There is still a great deal to do."

Joseph Lister (1827-1912) revolutionized surgery through the application of Pasteur's discoveries. He understood the similarity between infections in postsurgical wounds and the processes of **putrefaction**. Pasteur proved that these processes were caused by microorganisms. Before this time, surgeons accepted that infections in surgical wounds were inevitable. Lister reasoned that microorganisms must be the cause of infection and should be kept out of wounds. His colleagues were indifferent to his theories, because most believed infections were God-given and natural. Lister disagreed, and he developed antiseptic methods by using carbolic acid for sterilization. By spraying the rooms with a fine mist of the acid, soaking instruments in carbolic solutions, and washing his hands in a similar solution, he was able to prove his theories. He is honored as the Father of Sterile Surgery. Pasteur and Lister met after years of great mutual admiration. The meeting was filled with emotion, and it was written in *Pathfinders in Medicine* that "a new star should have appeared in the heavens to commemorate the event." Medicine truly owes a deep gratitude to these two pioneers for the knowledge they imparted to the art.

Robert Koch (1843-1910) was a German physician, famous for his Koch's Postulates; that is, his theory of rules that must be followed before an organism can be accepted as the causative agent in a given disease. He introduced many of the tools used in the laboratory, such as the culture plate method of isolating bacteria. He discovered the cause of cholera and demonstrated its transmission by food and water. This discovery completely transformed health departments and proved the importance of bacteriology in everyday life. Koch's greatest disappointment was his failure to find a cure for tuberculosis, but in his attempt, he isolated tuberculin, the substance produced by tubercle bacteria. Its use as a diagnostic aid was of immense value to medicine. He became a Nobel Laureate in 1905.

One of Koch's students was a German physician named Paul Ehrlich (1854-1915). He pioneered the fields of bacteriology, immunology, and especially chemotherapy. Ehrlich was only 28 when he wrote his first paper on typhoid, but his greatest gift to humanity was called his "magic bullet," or formula 606, which was designed to fight syphilis. With the organism identified by scientists Bordet and Wasserman, Ehrlich set out to find a chemical that would destroy the organism but not harm the host, specifically, the human body. The six hundred sixth drug Ehrlich tried finally brought about healing. He called it *salvarsan,* because he believed that it offered humankind salvation from the disease. This endeavor also marked the beginning of the practice of injecting chemicals into the body to destroy a specific organism. In 1908 Ehrlich shared the Nobel Prize with Eli Metchnikoff, who is remembered for his theory of phagocytosis and immunology.

Crawford Williamson Long (1815-1878) was the first to use ether as an anesthetic agent. Early in 1842, a group of students would have a social gathering after chemistry lectures and inhale ether, a chemical commonly found in chemistry laboratories, as a form of amusement. Ether, an intoxicant similar to nitrous oxide, functions as a *soporific,* or sleep-inducing agent. However, at one of these "ether frolics," as they were called, Dr. Long also observed that people under the influence of ether did not seem to feel pain. After considerable thought, he decided to use ether for a surgical procedure. In March, 1842, he removed a tumor from the neck of James M. Venable after placing him under the influence of ether. Dr. Horace Wells was a dentist who reported using nitrous oxide as an anesthetic in 1844. Another dentist, Dr. William T. G. Morton, reported using ether in 1846 when he extracted a tooth from a patient, and he also used the gas at Massachusetts General Hospital for a surgical procedure.

Surgeons are grateful to Wilhelm Konrad Roentgen (1845-1923), a professor of physics at the University of Wurzburg, Germany. Roentgen discovered the x-ray in 1895 while experimenting with electrical currents passed through sealed glass tubes. He was awarded the Nobel Prize in Physics in 1901. Although he called it an *x-ray,* history has honored him by calling it the *roentgen ray.* Marie and Pierre Curie discovered radium in 1898, and they were awarded the 1902 Nobel Prize in Physics for their work on radioactivity. Unfortunately, Pierre was killed 3 years later while crossing a street in a rainstorm. Marie was awarded his teaching position at the Sorbonne, a medical university in France; no woman had taught at the school in its 650-year history. In 1911 she was awarded the Nobel Prize for her discoveries of radium and polonium, the first person to receive the award twice. She died in 1934 from pernicious anemia, which was believed to have been caused by her overexposure to radiation and years of overwork.

Nineteenth Century Women in Medicine

Many women made great contributions to medicine in the early nineteenth century, at a time when women were not considered to be as capable as men outside the home environment. Florence Nightingale (1820-1910) is known as the founder of nursing and is fondly called the Lady with the Lamp (Figure 2-5). She was of noble birth, and somewhat late in life she sought nursing training in both England and Europe. By the dawn of the Crimean War in 1854, she

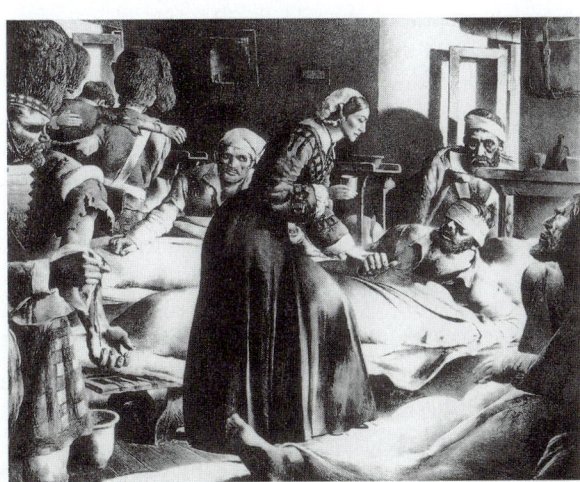

FIGURE 2-5 Considered the founder of nursing, Florence Nightingale is also known as the Lady with the Lamp. (Courtesy National Library of Medicine, Bethesda, Md.)

had established a fine reputation for her work in hospital organization. She was invited by the British Secretary of War to visit the Crimea to help correct the terrible conditions that existed in caring for the wounded. She created the Women's Nursing Service in Scutari and Balaklava. The physicians treated her and the other 38 nurses poorly until a crisis brought thousands of wounded and sick soldiers to the army hospitals. The bravery and competence of the nurses helped the doctors realize their value to the medical profession. In 1860 she founded the Nightingale School and Home for Nurses in London, which marked the beginning of professional nursing education.

Clara Barton (1821-1912), an American, began her nursing career early in life. When she was 11 years of age, her brother fell from the roof of their barn, and Clara nursed him back to health over a 2-year period. She later was a battlefield nurse and **philanthropist**, whose work during the Civil War led her to recognize that very poor records were kept in Washington to aid in the search for missing men who were wounded or killed in combat. Her efforts to remedy this led to the formation of the Bureau of Records. Her organization and recruitment of supplies for the wounded led to her eventual involvement with the Red Cross in the Franco-Prussian War. In 1881 she organized a Red Cross Committee in Washington, the original formation of the American Red Cross. She served as its first president, from 1881 to 1904. She retired at the age of 82, just after personally leading dangerous expeditions to help victims of fires, hurricanes, and floods. The American Red Cross remains a vital organization to this day.

Elizabeth Blackwell (1821-1910) was the first woman in the United States to receive the Doctor of Medicine degree from a medical school. She began her medical education by reading medical books and later obtained private instruction. Medical schools in New York and Pennsylvania initially refused her applications for formal study, but finally, in 1847, she was accepted at the Geneva Medical College in New York.

Lillian Wald (1867-1940), a social worker and nurse, made great contributions to medical care when she founded the Henry Street Settlement in New York City. Wald operated a visiting nurse service from this establishment. When one of her nurses was assigned to the city's public schools in 1902, the New York City Municipal Board of Health established the world's first public school nursing system.

Margaret Sanger (1883-1966) was born in Corning, New York, and trained as a nurse at the White Plains Hospital. She became the American leader of the birth control movement. While working among the poor in New York City, she came to understand the public's need for information about contraception. In 1873 the federal Comstock Law declared it illegal to import or distribute any device, medicine, or information designed to prevent conception or induce abortion or to mention in print the names of sexually transmitted diseases. Nurses and physicians were legally prohibited from providing this information to their patients. In 1914 Sanger was **indicted** for circulating the magazine *The Woman Rebel,* in which she attacked the legislative restrictions of the Comstock Law. The case was dismissed 2 years later. In the same year, she established the first American birth control clinic; this led to her arrest, conviction, and incarceration in the county jail. She continued her work, and after World War II, she successfully advocated research into hormonal contraception because of the newfound concern about population growth. This research ultimately led to development of the birth control pill. When the Planned Parenthood Federation of America was formed in 1941, she was named honorary chairperson.

CRITICAL THINKING APPLICATION   **2-2**

Mr. Santos asks his students to tell him which of these early pioneers they would most like to have worked with. Whom would you choose and why?
- What difficulties would these early medical workers have faced as they explored medicine?
- What difficulties do researchers face today?

MODERN MILESTONES IN MEDICINE

In recognition of the achievements of scientists of the past, Sir Isaac Newton spoke of our innovative ability in the medical field. He humbly said, "If I have seen a little further than others, it is because I have stood on the shoulders of giants." Great strides in medicine occurred in the twentieth century, and technology began to advance rapidly. Medical leaders continued their contributions, and knowledge, treatment, and research grew by leaps and bounds.

Walter Reed, a U.S. Army pathologist and bacteriologist, proved that yellow fever was transmitted by the bite of a mosquito. Individuals with diabetes should be grateful to Sir Frederick Grant Banting, a Canadian physician who isolated insulin for treatment, along with Charles Herbert Best, a Canadian physiologist. In 1928 Sir Alexander Fleming discovered penicillin accidentally while researching influenza and working with staphylococcal bacteria. He found a substance in mold that prevented the growth of bacteria even when the substance was diluted 800 times.

Cardiologist Helen Taussig and surgeon Alfred Blalock explored the health issues of children born with cyanosis resulting from a malformed heart. Dr. Taussig collaborated with Dr. Blalock to develop a lifesaving operation for these children, called "blue babies." History often omits the contributions of Vivien Thomas, an African-American man who was Dr. Blalock's surgical research technician at Johns Hopkins Hospital. Thomas was a former carpenter who constructed several of the medical instruments used in the Blalock-Taussig procedure. Thomas actually created the blue baby condition in dogs, on which he regularly practiced the surgical procedure. When Dr. Blalock and Dr. Taussig performed the first blue baby operation at Johns Hopkins University, Thomas stood over Blalock's shoulder and advised him during the procedure, because Thomas had done the surgery several more times than Blalock. This happened at a time when African-Americans were not allowed on the main floors of the hospital, much less in the surgical suite. This surgery became known as the Blalock-Taussig procedure, and although the first blue baby operation prolonged the patient's life by only 2 months, subsequent operations were successful, and children were able to leave the hospital with the hope of a healthy life.

Jonas Edward Salk and Albert Sabin almost eradicated poliomyelitis, once the killer and crippler of thousands in the United States. Salk's injectable vaccine was developed in 1952, and after wide-scale testing in 1954, it was distributed nationally, greatly reducing the incidence of the disease. Sabin's live-virus vaccine, in a form that could be swallowed, became available less than a decade later.

Werner Forssmann, a German surgeon, originated a cardiac technique called *catheterization* that is used in the diagnosis and treatment of heart disease. Christiaan Barnard, a South African surgeon, performed the first human heart transplantation in 1967. Dr. Elisabeth Kübler-Ross, a Swiss-born psychiatrist who died in 2004, was shocked at the treatment of terminally ill patients at her hospital in New York. She wrote the best-selling book *On Death and Dying,* which helped professionals and laypersons alike understand the stages of grief.

Edwin Carlyle "Carl" Wood is best known for his pioneering work developing and commercializing the technique of in vitro fertilization (IVF). Although some of Dr. Wood's work was controversial, his medical career spanned over 50 years. He wrote 23 books, 59 chapters, and over 400 papers in refereed medical and scientific journals.

Some diseases, conditions, and anatomical structures are named for the person who first discovered them or pioneered the disease. Dr. Virginia Apgar (1909-1974) founded neonatology. She developed the Apgar score, which is a method of assessing the health of newborns at the time of birth. The assessment has greatly reduced infant mortality by quickly determining whether a newborn needs immediate medical treatments. Henry Jay Heimlich, MD, is credited for the Heimlich maneuver, which uses abdominal thrusts to relieve choking. Aloysius Alzheimer (1864-1915) was a German physician who was credited with identifying the first published case of presenile dementia, later known as Alzheimer's disease. Parkinson's disease is named for Dr. James Parkinson, an English surgeon, geologist, and paleontologist. Down's syndrome, which is a chromosomal condition caused by an extra twenty-first chromosome, was first described by British doctor John Langdon Haydon Down. Asperger syndrome was named for Hans Asperger of Austria, who wrote hundreds of publications about autism. Asperger's is characterized by significant difficulties in social interaction along with restricted and repetitive patterns of behavior and interests. Thomas Hodgkin (1798-1866) was considered one of the most prominent pathologists of his time and pioneered preventative medicine. Dr. Hodgkin provided the first description of Hodgkin's disease or Hodgkin's lymphoma, characterized by the orderly spread of disease from one lymph node to another and by the development of systemic symptoms with advanced disease. Those familiar with the common diseases related to human immunodeficiency virus infection (HIV) and acquired immunodeficiency syndrome (AIDS) will recognize Kaposi's sarcoma, a skin tumor discovered by Hungarian physician Moritz Kaposi. In the 1980s, Kaposi's sarcoma, or KS, was determined to be caused by a viral infection and became widely known as one of the AIDS-defining illnesses.

CRITICAL THINKING APPLICATION   **2-3**
- During a class discussion, Mr. Santos points out that the leaders in the healthcare industry had specific goals for their careers and achieved worldwide recognition for their contributions. What individuals have made contributions to medicine in recent years?
- How can the individual medical assistant make a contribution to medicine?

Many modern physicians are making important discoveries in and contributions to the field of medicine. Dr. David Ho is considered by many to be one of the most brilliant minds in medicine today, helping to piece together the puzzle of HIV. A professor at Rockefeller University, Ho is the scientific director and chief executive officer (CEO) of the Aaron Diamond AIDS Research Center in New York City, which is the largest private HIV/AIDS research organization in the world. He was born in Taiwan and his family immigrated to the United States when he was 12 years old. He eventually entered college to study physics—medicine was actually his second choice—but once he discovered molecular biology and the concept of gene splicing, he decided to become a researcher. In 2011, he won the Avant-Garde Award, presented by the National Institute on Drug Abuse, which contributes $500,000 per year for 5-years. The award is given to stimulate high-impact research that may lead to groundbreaking opportunities for the prevention and treatment of HIV/AIDS in drug abusers.

Dr. C. Everett Koop graduated from Cornell University as a medical doctor in 1941 and spent most of his career as a pediatric surgeon. During his terms as the U.S. Surgeon General, he became a proponent of tobacco awareness, insisting that tobacco advertisements must be less attractive to the youth of today. Dr. Koop is a professor at Dartmouth Medical School. He founded the Koop Institute, an organization that has a mission to "promote the health and well-being of all people." Dr. Koop has been honored with many awards, including 41 honorary doctorates.

Dr. Marcia Angell is the former editor in chief of the *New England Journal of Medicine* (NEJM), one of the most prestigious medical publications in the United States. Her career with NEJM began in 1979, and her excellent articles spanned a variety of subjects, from the pharmaceutical companies' profit margins to the effects of socioeconomic status on Americans seeking healthcare services. Dr. Angell was named one of the 25 most influential Americans in 1997 by *Time* magazine. She has written and contributed to several books, including *Science on Trial: The Clash of Medical Evidence and the Law in the Breast Implant Case*. Dr. Angell is a board-certified pathologist and currently serves as senior lecturer in the Department of Global Health and Social Medicine at Harvard Medical School.

As the director of the National Institute of Allergy and Infectious Diseases at the National Institutes of Health (NIH), Dr. Anthony Fauci leads research efforts on immune-mediated disorders. Many of his studies now relate to HIV and the body's response to AIDS, in addition to ways to improve HIV treatment and prevention, including the development of an HIV vaccine. In 2003, an Institute for Scientific Information study indicated that in the 20-year period from 1983 to 2002, Dr. Fauci was the 13th-most-cited scientist among the 2.5 to 3 million authors in all disciplines throughout the world who published articles in scientific journals during that time frame. Dr. Fauci was the world's 10th-most-cited HIV/AIDS researcher in the period between 1996 to 2006. He received his MD degree from Cornell University Medical College, and his career with the NIH has spanned more than 40 years. In 2009, *Forbes* magazine named Dr. Fauci one of the seven most powerful people in medicine.

Vice Admiral Regina M. Benjamin, MD, the current Surgeon General of the United States, took office in 2006 (Figure 2-6). She

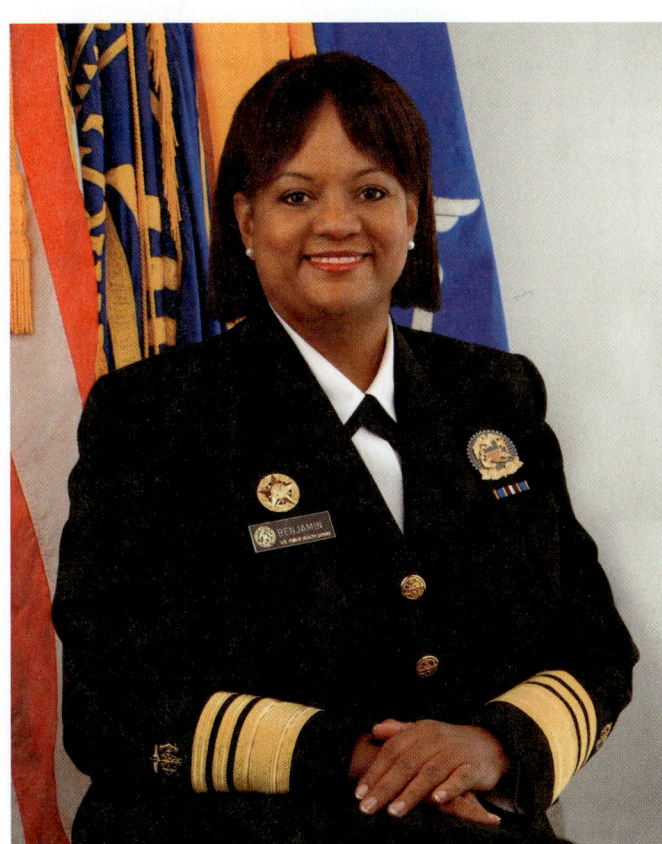

FIGURE 2-6 Vice Admiral Regina Benjamin was the first female and first African-American to be elected to the American Medical Association board of directors. Dr. Benjamin is the current Surgeon General of the United States.

earned her bachelor's degree in chemistry at Xavier University in New Orleans, her MD from the University of Alabama at Birmingham, and her MBA from Tulane University in New Orleans; she also holds 18 honorary degrees. In 1995, she was the first female and first African-American woman to be elected to the American Medical Association's board of directors. After establishing a clinic in a small fishing village in Alabama, Dr. Benjamin persevered through Hurricanes Georges and Katrina, in addition to a devastating fire, often contributing her own money to keep the clinic open. She became nationally prominent for her business acumen and her humane approach to preventative medicine.

Armando E. Giuliano, MD, is the executive vice-chair of surgery and surgical oncology at Cedars-Sinai Medical Center in Los Angeles, California. The co-director of the Saul and Joyce Brandman Breast Center, Dr. Giuliano has been honored extensively for his treatment and research on breast cancer. His most recent research on breast cancer was published in the *Journal of the American Medical Association*.

Ching-Hon Pui, MD, is the chair of the Department of Oncology at St. Jude's Children's Research Hospital in Memphis, Tennessee. Dr. Pui received his medical education in Taiwan and uses his experience as a pediatrician, educator, and humanitarian to advance the cure rate and understanding of acute lymphoblastic leukemia in children. Many of his research findings have stimulated changes in clinical practice that are now widely accepted in the global pediatric oncology community. He has authored more than 700 original articles and chapters, edited seven books and monographs, and serves as section editor or editorial board member for several prestigious journals. He is also one of the most highly cited authors in clinical medical research. A series of Dr. Pui's innovative treatment protocols boosted cure rates at St. Jude from about 70% in the early 1980s to an unprecedented 90% in the past decade.

The director of the Center to Advance Palliative Care, a national organization devoted to increasing the number and quality of palliative care programs in the United States, Dr. Diane E. Meier has served as professor of medical ethics at Mount Sinai School of Medicine in New York City, where she has served on the faculty since 1983. Dr. Meier has published extensively in all major peer-reviewed medical journals, including the *New England Journal of Medicine* and the *Journal of the American Medical Association*. She edited the first textbook on geriatric palliative care and four editions of *Geriatric Medicine*. Dr. Meier has appeared on television and in print, including ABC World News Tonight, *The New York Times*, the *Los Angeles Times*, and *Newsweek*.

Keith Black, MD, is the chairman of the Department of Neurosurgery at Cedars-Sinai Medical Center in Los Angeles. Throughout his medical career, Dr. Black has been fascinated with the human brain. He hopes to change cancer treatment by reducing and possibly eliminating the need for chemotherapy, surgery, and radiation treatments, believing that the body's immune system was critical in fighting tumors. His aggressive treatments and leadership have made Cedars-Sinai one of the top neurosurgical centers in the country.

One of the nation's top obstetricians, Dr. Linda Bradley, is considered an innovative leader in the field of obstetrics and gynecology. She has researched hysterectomy alternatives and abnormal uterine bleeding extensively and pioneered the use of hysteroscopy and new procedures such as endometrial ablation and myomectomy. Dr. Bradley is the vice chairman of obstetrics, gynecology, and the Women's Health Institute at the Cleveland Clinic.

THE NATIONAL VIEW OF HEALTHCARE

World Health Organization

The World Health Organization (WHO), founded in 1948, is a specialized agency of the United Nations. The organization promotes cooperation among nations in their efforts to control and eliminate diseases worldwide. The purposes of WHO are:

- To provide worldwide guidance in the field of health
- To set global standards for health
- To cooperate with governments in strengthening national health programs
- To develop and transfer appropriate health technology, information, and standards

One of the greatest accomplishments of this agency was the eradication of smallpox. Other diseases, such as polio and leprosy, are on the verge of eradication. The agency also created and maintains the International Classification of Diseases (ICD) coding system. ICD-9 is used today to identify diseases and conditions with a specific code number (ICD-10 goes into effect in fall 2013). The original purpose of this system was to track worldwide morbidity and mortality statistics. WHO is committed to research and delivery of needed drugs and medical supplies to various areas of the world.

In addition, WHO promotes the sharing of health information, and WHO officials meet with the leaders of the worldwide health industry to discuss various ethical and moral implications that face today's healthcare professionals.

U.S. Department of Health and Human Services

The Department of Health and Human Services (DHHS) is the principal U.S. agency for providing essential human services and protecting the health of all Americans, especially those unable to help themselves. The DHHS is made up of more than 300 programs involved in:

- Medical and social science research
- Immunization services
- Financial assistance for low-income families
- Child support enforcement services
- Improvement of infant and maternal health
- Child and elder abuse prevention services
- Assistance programs for elderly Americans

The DHHS also oversees the Medicare and Medicaid programs. Medicare is the nation's largest health insurer, and the DHHS processes more than 1 billion claims every year.

U.S. Army Medical Research Institute of Infectious Diseases

The primary focus of the U.S. Army Medical Research Institute of Infectious Diseases (USAMRIID) is to protect members of the military, but the institute conducts key research programs in national defense and infectious diseases that benefit everyone (Figure 2-7). USAMRIID, located at Fort Detrick in Maryland, works extensively with the Centers for Disease Control and Prevention (CDC) and WHO. USAMRIID also controls an internationally known reference laboratory with state-of-the-art facilities. This laboratory is instrumental in identifying biologic threats and the diseases those threats produce. USAMRIID is the only laboratory facility operated by the Department of Defense that is equipped to study biosafety level IV viruses and pathogens, the most deadly organisms.

Four biosafety levels are commonly accepted among laboratory professionals. Biosafety level I includes well-known agents that pose a minimal or low biohazard potential to laboratory personnel and

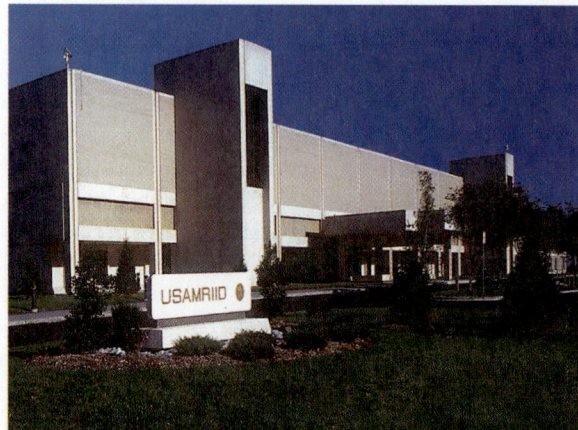

FIGURE 2-7 U.S. Army Medical Research Institute of Infectious Diseases in Fort Detrick, Maryland. (Courtesy USAMRIID, Fort Detrick, Md.)

to the environment as a whole. At this level, the laboratory is not necessarily separated from the regular areas of the facility. Examples of level I pathogens include *Pneumococcus* and *Salmonella* organisms. In the biosafety level II section of the laboratory, substances with a moderate biohazard potential are studied. For biosafety level I and level II areas, laboratory personnel receive specific training in handling pathogens, and specialized equipment is used to prevent splashes and splatters. Pathogens classified as biosafety level II include the hepatitis, Lyme disease, and influenza viruses.

Personnel working in the biosafety level III section receive very specific training in working with the potentially deadly pathogens found at this level. All procedures performed on level III pathogens have a high biohazard risk and are done inside protective safety cabinets. Laboratory personnel are required to wear heavy personal protective equipment. Special regulations concerning exhaust air and ventilation are strictly followed, and access to the laboratory is limited when work is in progress. HIV; *Bacillus anthracis,* which causes anthrax; and *Rickettsia typhi* and *Rickettsia prowazekii,* which cause typhus, are some of the pathogens classified as biosafety level III.

Biosafety level IV includes the most deadly pathogens, which often produce incurable diseases. The biohazard risk of transmission of these agents is extreme and includes the risk of airborne transmission. Laboratory personnel are highly trained in the manipulation and handling of these dangerous pathogens. Laboratory access is strictly controlled in this section. Some of the pathogens studied at biosafety level IV include the Ebola virus, Lassa virus, and hantavirus.

Centers for Disease Control and Prevention

The headquarters of the CDC is in Atlanta, Georgia (Figure 2-8). The CDC is the principal U.S. federal agency concerned with the health and safety of people throughout the world and is part of the DHHS. It is a clearinghouse for information and statistics associated with healthcare. Several divisions in the CDC focus on specific health-related issues, such as the National Center for HIV, STD, and TB Prevention; the Public Health Practice Program Office; the National Center on Birth Defects and Developmental Disabilities; and the National Center for Health Statistics. Branch offices

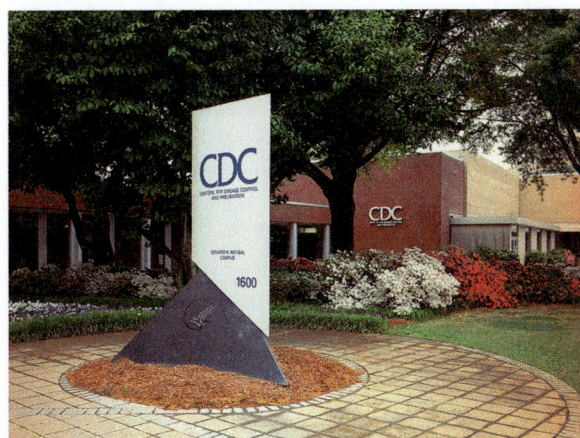

FIGURE 2-8 Headquarters of the Centers for Disease Control and Prevention (CDC) in Atlanta, Georgia. (Courtesy Centers for Disease Control and Prevention, Atlanta, Ga.)

are located throughout the United States and in several foreign countries. The CDC provides regulations that affect all healthcare facilities. When the virus now known as HIV was discovered, the CDC was one of the first organizations to research and attempt to isolate the virus. When a pandemic begins, the CDC information services offer guidelines that help facilities ensure the health of their employees, patients, and the public at large. The agency also conducts research into the origin and occurrence of diseases and develops methods to control and prevent them. In addition, it develops immunization services and aids in the training of healthcare workers.

National Institutes of Health

The NIH began as a one-room laboratory in the Marine hospital on New York's Staten Island in 1887. Its first major contribution to medicine was the isolation of the bacterium that causes cholera. In 1930 the laboratory became the NIH, an agency of the DHHS. The mission of the NIH is to develop knowledge that will lead to better health for everyone. As a part of the public health service, it seeks to improve the health of the American people, supports and conducts biomedical research into the causes and prevention of diseases, and uses a modern communications system to furnish biomedical information to the healthcare professions.

The NIH moved from Washington, D.C., to Bethesda, Maryland, in 1938 and today occupies more than 60 buildings covering 30 acres. It consists of 27 different institutes and centers, in addition to the National Library of Medicine. Thousands of research projects are underway in NIH laboratories and clinics at any given time. The NIH also provides support to other research projects conducted at universities, medical schools, and hospitals.

TYPES OF HEALTHCARE FACILITIES

Hospitals

Hospitals are classified according to the type of care and services they provide to patients, as well as by the type of ownership. *Acute care* hospitals offer intensive care units and emergency or trauma departments and are equipped to handle the most severely ill or injured patients. *Subacute care* hospitals offer patient care for those who do not require extensive services but still need hospital supervision and treatment. *Specialty* hospitals, such as a psychiatric hospital, offer specific services. *Teaching* hospitals provide a learning environment and often also have research departments. These hospitals usually are affiliated with medical schools, and interns or residents provide care supervised by licensed physician instructors. *Community* hospitals provide care in rural areas or in specific areas within a metropolis. *Regional* hospitals usually are acute care facilities and serve a large area in which intensive care may not be offered in local communities.

Private hospitals are run by a corporation or other organization and usually are designed to produce a profit for the owners or stockholders. *Nonprofit* hospitals exist to serve the community in which they are located and are normally run by a board of directors. The term *nonprofit* sometimes is misleading, because "profit" is different from "making money." A nonprofit hospital or organization may make money in a campaign or fund raiser, but all of the money is returned to the organization. Nonprofit hospitals and organizations must follow strict guidelines in the area of finance and must account to the government for the money brought in and the purposes for which it is used.

A *hospital system* is a group of facilities that are affiliated and work toward a common goal. Hospital systems may include a hospital and a cancer center in a small community or may consist of a group of separate hospitals in a specific geographic region. Many hospital systems are designed as integrated health delivery systems. An integrated delivery system (IDS) is a network of healthcare providers and organizations that provides or arranges to provide a coordinated continuum of services to a defined population and is willing to be held clinically and fiscally accountable for the clinical outcomes and health status of the population served. An IDS may own or could be closely aligned with an insurance product, such as a type of insurance policy. Services provided by an IDS can include a fully equipped community and/or tertiary hospital, home healthcare and hospice services, primary and specialty outpatient care and surgery, social services, rehabilitation, preventive care, health education and financing, usually using a form of managed care. An IDS can also be a training location for health professional students, including physicians, nurses, and allied health professionals.

Sometimes the term *county hospital* is used to designate the hospital to which **indigent** patients are taken. These hospitals provide emergency care to those who cannot pay for medical expenses. Today, however, many people without insurance go to the emergency department (ED or ER) for routine illnesses. This is one reason EDs are busy and full. If patients have no other options, the ED physicians become primary care providers. This is a major cause of the long waiting times in hospital EDs. Managed care has eased this problem somewhat by refusing to cover visits to the ED that are not true emergencies. **Triage**, performed by physicians, nurses, and some other licensed medical professionals, determines which patients have the most severe conditions and should be seen first.

Hospitals have various departments that are organized to provide efficient patient care. The admissions department gathers information and enters it into a computer for use by the rest of the hospital staff. Nursing service supervises all of the nursing care given to the patients and is involved in **case management**. The laboratory provides diagnostic testing on blood, body fluids, and tissues, and the radiology or nuclear medicine department offers diagnostic imaging and radiographic services. The respiratory services department offers a broad spectrum of diagnostic tests and various treatments. Most hospitals also have a physical medicine and rehabilitation department, which offers both physical and occupational therapy. The dietary department employs professionals who carefully plan menus to meet the needs of each patient served. Most modern hospitals have a surgery department, and many offer day surgery services that allow patients to undergo a procedure and return home the same day, if they recover as expected. The medical records department is responsible for the patient records related to every **encounter** that takes place in the facility. Social services works with patients to ensure continuity of care, patient education, and social intervention, all of which assist patients with emotional, economic, and social concerns.

Hospital administrators manage the hospital on a day-to-day basis, and human resource responsibilities usually are a part of the administration department. Almost every hospital has a board of directors to assist the administrators in governing the hospital; in addition, a medical staff committee, led by the hospital's chief of staff, usually assists in the management of the facility and the credentialing process for the physicians who have **staff privileges**. **Credentialing** involves determining whether a practitioner should be allowed to practice medicine in a facility, based on his or her education, license, past performance, and other qualifications.

The National Practitioner Data Bank (NPDB) also gathers information that helps healthcare facilities ensure that physicians who might be brought on staff are competent. The intent of the NPDB is to improve the quality of healthcare by encouraging state licensing boards, hospitals, healthcare entities, and professional societies to identify and discipline those who engage in unprofessional behavior and to restrict the ability of incompetent physicians to move from state to state without disclosure or discovery of previous medical malpractice payment or adverse action history. NPDB provides information about physicians who have had licensure problems, made malpractice settlements, had clinical privileges revoked or restricted, or had action taken against them by a professional society to registered entities, but not to the general public.

Peer review organizations (PROs) are also critical to good healthcare facility management. A medical peer review is defined by the American Medical Association as a process conducted by physicians to ensure that other physicians consistently maintain optimum standards of fitness to practice medicine. Peer review also can be applied to other medical professionals. Credentialing, as mentioned, is the verification process that takes place before assignment or reappointment of staff privileges; peer reviews help ensure that physicians or other medical professionals maintain the high standards necessary to practice medicine in an accurate and effective way.

Accreditation is considered the highest form of recognition for the quality of care a facility or organization provides. Not only does it indicate to the public that the facility is concerned with providing high-quality care, it also provides professional liability insurance benefits and plays a role in regulatory agency relicensure and certification efforts. Hospitals and other healthcare facilities are often accredited by the Joint Commission, an organization concerned with the quality of care in healthcare facilities. **Standards** or **indicators** have been developed that help determine when patients are receiving high-quality care. The term *quality* refers to much more than whether the patient liked the food served or had to wait to have a procedure or test performed. Categories of compliance include:

- Assessment and care of patients
- Use of medication
- Plant, technology, and safety management
- Orientation, education, and training of staff
- Medical staff qualifications
- Patients' rights

Ratings from 1 to 5 are given to the facility on its performance in specific areas. A 1 rating means that the facility is in full compliance with that standard, and the other ratings indicate levels of noncompliance. The DHHS also regulates healthcare facilities, as does the federal Occupational Safety and Health Administration (OSHA), a division of the U.S. Department of Labor that enforces many laws related to workplace safety.

CRITICAL THINKING APPLICATION   2-4

- Mr. Santos has assigned his students to groups and asked them to investigate local hospitals. What types of hospitals are found in your local area, and what services do they provide? How might a hospital board decide what services to offer to the community?
- How might Mr. Santos' students find out whether a physician has staff privileges at a certain hospital?
- What areas or populations are underserved, and why might this be the case?

Ambulatory Care

Many other types of healthcare facilities operate in the industry today. **Ambulatory** care centers include a wide range of facilities that offer healthcare services to patients who are able to walk around (are not bedridden). Physicians' offices, group practices, and multispecialty group practices are common types of ambulatory care facilities. Group practices may involve a single specialty, such as pediatrics, or may be multispecialty. A multispecialty practice might consist of an internal medicine specialist, an oncologist, a family practitioner, and an endocrinologist. Usually the physicians in the practice refer patients to each other when indicated. This is not only more convenient for the patients, but also more profitable for the physicians in the practice. A patient seeing a physician for the first time is considered a *new* patient, whereas a patient who has seen the physician on previous occasions is called an *established* patient. Most physicians charge new patients more than established patients, because the levels of decision making, the extent of the physical examination, and the complexity of the medical history require that more time be directed toward the new patient. This information is critical to the coding process (see Chapters 18 and 19).

Occupational health centers are concerned with helping patients return to work and productive activity. Often, physical therapy is used in conjunction with rehabilitation services that assist the patient in regaining as much of his or her previous level of ability as possible. Also, freestanding rehabilitation centers can assist patients with a wide range of services. Pain management centers help patients deal with discomfort associated with their condition. Sleep centers diagnose and treat people with sleep problems. As is pain, difficulty sleeping is a symptom, and the cause of the disturbance must be found so that proper treatment can be provided. Freestanding urgent or emergency care centers provide patients with an alternative to hospital EDs. They are less expensive, have a shorter waiting time, and are conveniently located in many areas. Most have flexible hours, many are open well into the evening, and walk-in appointments usually are accepted.

Surgery has become more convenient because of the number of ambulatory surgical centers that exist today. Day surgery performed in hospitals continues to provide patients with alternatives to overnight hospital care after surgery. Many insurance companies now prefer day surgery, because it is more cost-effective. Not many years ago, the only alternative to inpatient surgery was the same hospital's day surgery department. Today, more and more freestanding surgical centers are becoming available. Patients can be treated with laser surgery, radial keratotomy, and cataract removal during the day and

recover at home the same evening. Plastic surgeons are becoming very innovative in the physical structure of their offices and the types of surgery they offer on an outpatient basis. Many plastic surgeons offer breast augmentation and reduction and even abdominoplasty ("tummy tuck") and liposuction in the office. Not long ago, an abdominoplasty meant staying in the hospital for several days. The new trend is becoming more accepted, partly as a result of the "office-based surgery" accreditation offered by the Ambulatory Care Accreditation Program of The Joint Commission.

A number of rehabilitation services are available to patients, based on their need and the type of illness or injury. Rehabilitation services may be obtained from acute care hospitals, rehabilitation hospitals, or various ambulatory rehabilitation facilities. Patients may use these services for a few weeks after an illness or injury or may continue them for several years. Rehabilitation usually involves several members of the healthcare team working together to ensure that the patient recovers to the greatest extent possible.

Dialysis centers offer services to patients with severe kidney disorders, and many of the larger cities across the country have cancer centers for patients who need treatment by oncologists. Many other types of ambulatory care facilities exist, including centers that provide magnetic resonance imaging (MRI), student health clinics, dental clinics, endoscopy centers, community health centers, mobile health services, podiatric care centers, and women's health centers.

Geriatric and long-term patients have more options today for ambulatory care than ever before. In the past, nursing homes were the only alternative to keeping elderly patients in their own homes. These nursing homes provided care for residents who needed more than just assistance with day-to-day activities. Now, many attractive options to traditional nursing homes or skilled nursing facilities are available. One of the most popular is assisted living. Most assisted-living facilities provide 24-hour supervision of their residents, most meals, and a broad range of services, from the very basic, such as transportation to physician office visits and errand running, to the extravagant, such as shopping trips and daylong outings. Most also provide exercise programs, social services, laundry and linen services, and housekeeping. The cost ranges from approximately $1,000 to $3,000 per month, depending on the location and the **amenities** desired by the resident. Many new assisted-living facilities are designed specifically for patients with Alzheimer's disease or other impaired memory conditions. Independent retirement communities offer residents the opportunity to come and go as they please. Many have a resortlike design, catering to the desire of retirees to enjoy their golden years. Usually the communities consist of apartments or duplex units, and some even offer small cottages.

Other Healthcare Facilities

Several other types of healthcare facilities deserve attention in the broad overview of the healthcare industry. Diagnostic laboratories offer testing services for patients referred by their physicians. Since the enactment of the Clinical Laboratory Improvement Act (CLIA) in 1967 and its amendment i in 1988, many physicians have stopped providing laboratory tests in their offices. These types of laboratories are called *physician office laboratories* (POLs). CLIA was enacted to ensure high-quality laboratory testing. The regulations set forth by both OSHA and CLIA rules often made it more cost-effective to have the patient go to an outside laboratory to have the tests done. The medical assistant should note that, as mentioned previously, OSHA is an organization and division of the U.S. Department of Labor that enforces many laws related to workplace safety. CLIA is a law, not an agency. However, both influence safety and quality testing. (CLIA is discussed in more detail in Chapter 7).

Home health agencies were tremendously successful in the late 1980s to the mid-1990s, but cuts in Medicare funding have caused them to suffer severe losses in recent years. This concept of care is very popular. Unfortunately, the influx of too many home health agencies and the subsequent drop in payments made to them have resulted in fewer home healthcare providers over the past several years. In addition, many hospitals began offering home healthcare, which added to the already heavy competition that smaller firms faced. Home healthcare offers its patients home care, therapy services, administration of and assistance with medications, and other services so that the patient can remain at home yet still obtain the care needed.

Medical suppliers are retail operations that offer all types of medical devices and products. Patients with diabetes can purchase glucose monitoring machines. Special hospital beds can be ordered for those who need them. All types of durable medical equipment (DME), such as bedpans, crutches, bathing assistance devices, wheelchairs, and walkers, are available, often without a physician's prescription. Most medical suppliers serve both the public and the profession.

Hospice centers play an important role in the acceptance of terminal illnesses. These facilities are designed to care for the patient with a terminal disease and provide support to family members. The goal of hospice is to provide peace, comfort, and dignity while controlling pain and promoting the best possible quality of life for the patient. Most patients involved in hospice care have a life expectancy of less than 6 months.

TYPES OF MEDICAL PRACTICE

Medical practices today generally are organized according to one of three types of business structures: the sole proprietorship, the partnership, or the corporation. Sole proprietorships dominated medical practice until the last quarter of the twentieth century. These practices are on the decline as a result of the **advent** of managed care, which favors the multispecialty group practice.

Sole Proprietorship

A sole proprietor is an individual who holds exclusive right and title to all aspects of the medical practice. The sole proprietor may employ other physicians to participate in the practice. The employed physician is entitled to employee benefits; the owner, however, is not considered an employee and is not so entitled. In addition, the owner is potentially liable for all the acts of his or her professional employees and staff members. Although practicing alone has many advantages, including flexibility and independence, it also has significant disadvantages. For example, the owner has total responsibility for covering the practice 24 hours a day, 7 days a week. In an unincorporated solo practice, the business dies when the owner leaves it unless it is sold to someone else. Many modern

physicians do not see sole proprietorship as an avenue for a decent income as a doctor, because managed care companies often offer participation to group practices over the single-practice physician, enabling them to provide more options to the patients. Some doctors organize associate practices. In this case, physicians share office space and often equipment and employees, but they operate their practices as sole proprietorships. Agreements such as these should always be put in writing to prevent misunderstandings and legal problems.

Partnership

When two or more physicians elect to associate in the practice of medicine, they may enter into a partnership agreement. This agreement specifies all the rights, obligations, and responsibilities of each partner. The participants have a greater potential for profit as a partnership than they would in practice as sole proprietors, because various expenses are shared and resources are pooled. Each physician has more freedom, because the doctors rotate an "on call" schedule so that each has some time away from the office and patients. One disadvantage of the partnership is the liability of each for the actions and conduct of all the others. In a partnership arrangement, the partners often pool employees, equipment, insurance, facilities, and even profits, and these resources are divided according to the specifications of the partnership agreement or contract.

A *group practice* is a body of at least three licensed physicians who engage in full-time practice in a formally organized and legally recognized entity. A group practice may take the form of a partnership, or it may be formed as a corporation. The group may share income and expenses, equipment, records, and personnel and may combine patient care and business management. The group practice may be an association of the same specialty or may be a multispecialty organization. Usually a group practice takes the form of a partnership or corporation.

Corporation

A *corporation* may be defined as an artificial entity having a legal and business status that is independent of its shareholders or employees. Corporations are regulated by the statutes of the state in which the incorporation takes place. In most cases the physician shareholders are employees of the corporation. Even a physician in a solo practice can incorporate the practice. All employees of the corporation receive income and tax advantages. Corporations are usually able to offer better benefits packages, which may include pension and profit-sharing plans, medical expense reimbursement, life insurance, disability income insurance, and many other benefits.

HEALTHCARE PROFESSIONALS

Physicians and providers are portals of entry (first contacts) into the healthcare system. Patients who have a medical problem go to a physician or provider to obtain help. Some patients must be referred to a medical specialist for further examinations and treatments. Many insurance policies will not pay for a patient to see a specialist without first consulting with their primary provider. Medical doctors, osteopathic doctors, and chiropractors are three of the portals of entry into the healthcare system.

Title of "Doctor"

Doctors of Medicine

Medical doctors (Doctor of Medicine [MD]) are considered **allopathic** physicians and are the most widely recognized type of physician. They diagnose illness and disease and prescribe treatment for their patients. MDs are allowed to write prescriptions and perform surgery. They offer advice on nutrition and preventive medicine. Becoming an MD usually requires 4 years of undergraduate training (premed) and 4 years of medical school. Some extraordinary students are allowed entry after 3 years of undergraduate studies; however, because competition for entry into medical school is intense, grades and other experience in healthcare are strongly considered. Premed students study biology, physics, organic and inorganic chemistry, mathematics, English, humanities, and social sciences. There are approximately 125 allopathic medical schools in the United States. After medical school, the student faces 3 to 8 years of internship and residency programs. An *intern* is a medical student still in training at medical school who treats patients under the supervision of licensed physicians. A *residency* is a graduate medical education program, often in a specialty, and usually is a paid, on-the-job training hospital position.

Often MDs specialize in a certain field, such as cardiology or pediatrics. These doctors usually invest 3 to 6 years of training in the specialty after medical school and can obtain board certification in one or more of 24 different specialty areas recognized by the American Board of Medical Specialties (ABMS) (Table 2-1). An MD must have a state license to practice, and continuing education is required to maintain the license. Graduates of foreign medical schools usually can obtain a license in the United States after passing an examination and completing a residency program in this country.

Doctors of Osteopathy

Osteopathic physicians (Doctor of Osteopathy [DO]) complete requirements similar to those of MDs to graduate and practice medicine. Osteopaths use medicine and surgery, in addition to osteopathic manipulative therapy (OMT), in treating their patients. Andrew Taylor Still is considered the Father of Osteopathic Medicine, which he began in 1874. He believed in a more **holistic** approach to medicine, and although he was an MD, he founded the American School of Osteopathy in Kirksville, Missouri. The school originally was chartered to offer an MD degree but later focused more on the osteopathic approach. DOs stress preventive medicine and holistic patient care, in addition to a special focus on the musculoskeletal system and OMT. Osteopathic medicine also promotes the **innate** ability of the body to heal itself, and many osteopaths tend to take a more conservative approach to using medications and surgical procedures than allopathic physicians. Many DOs practice **homeopathy**, believing in the body's ability to heal itself. Premed students moving toward osteopathic medicine study biology, physics, organic and inorganic chemistry, mathematics, English, humanities, and social sciences. They also usually complete 4 years of undergraduate studies and then begin 4 years of medical studies at a school for osteopathic medicine. Most DOs participate in a 12-month rotating internship in the various specialty areas before entering a residency program that lasts 2 to 6 years, and they are eligible for board certification through either the American Board of Medical Specialists or the American Osteopathic Association. Approximately one in 20 physicians in the United States is a DO. DOs participate in continuing education programs to renew their licenses annually.

Doctors of Chiropractic

Chiropractors (Doctor of Chiropractic [DC]) typically are thought of as "bone doctors," but they actually focus on the nervous system to help patients live healthier lives. The nervous system is the master system of the body, controlling and coordinating all the other systems. Information from the environment, both internal and external, moves through the spinal cord to get to the brain, and in the same manner, information from the brain moves through the spinal cord to reach the body in a two-way flow of communication. The intention of the **chiropractic** adjustment is to remove any disruptions or distortions of this energy flow that may be caused by slight misalignments, which chiropractors call **subluxations**. Chiropractic colleges require undergraduate studies in biology, organic and inorganic chemistry, physics, English, and the humanities and then 3 to 4 years studying chiropractic. Each state offers licensing. Some chiropractors devote their practices to a specialty, but more often they practice general chiropractic. Continuing education is required for relicensure. Chiropractic is one of the most common fields of **complementary and alternative medicine (CAM)**. Chiropractic can be used along with both allopathic and osteopathic medicine to enhance the results of treatment.

Hospitalists

Hospitalists are physicians whose primary professional focus is the general medical care of hospitalized patients. Most hospitalists are employed by the healthcare facility instead of having individual free-standing offices in which patients are seen and treated. Perhaps the most attractive benefit of becoming a hospitalist is the quality of life for the physician and his or her family. Hospitalists work a specific, set number of hours each week and do not directly experience the economic pressures of managed care, because they usually are placed on a salary. Although the hospitalist is in charge of the patient while the person is in the hospital, if the patient has a primary care provider (PCP), he or she may still visit the patient. Of course, the patient is not required to use the services of a hospitalist and may be cared for by the PCP. However, patients admitted from the emergency department or those in a location away from the PCP may find the hospitalist to be an excellent alternative to their regular physician.

CRITICAL THINKING APPLICATION **2-5**

- Mr. Santos challenges his new medical assisting students to interview several types of doctors at some point during their studies. The class discusses the different philosophies of medicine among allopathic, osteopathic, and chiropractic physicians. Discuss with your class the similarities and differences of these three aspects of medicine.
- Most of Mr. Santos' students have visited one or more of these types of doctors. What experiences have you had with medical doctors (MDs), osteopaths (DOs), or chiropractors (DCs)?

TABLE 2-1 Examples of Medical Specialties Recognized by the American Board of Medical Specialties

SPECIALTY	PRACTITIONER'S TITLE	DESCRIPTION
Allergy and Immunology	Allergist/ Immunologist	Allergists/immunologists are trained to evaluate disorders and diseases of the immune system. This includes conditions such as adverse reactions to drugs and food, anaphylaxis, and problems related to autoimmune diseases, asthma, and insect stings.
Anesthesiology	Anesthesiologist	Anesthesiologists provide pain relief and pain management during surgical procedures and also for patients with long-standing conditions accompanied by pain such as cancer patients. Anesthesiologists also provide critical care and resuscitation for patients during cardiac or respiratory emergencies.
Colon and Rectal Surgery	Colon and rectal surgeon	Colorectal surgeons diagnose and treat conditions affecting the intestines, rectum, and anal area, in addition to organs affected by intestinal disease. They often treat cancers that appear in these areas. They also treat disorders such as hemorrhoids and fissures.
Dermatology	Dermatologist	Dermatologists work with adult and pediatric patients in treating disorders and diseases of the skin, hair, nails, and related tissues. Dermatologists are specially trained to manage conditions such as skin cancers, cosmetic disorders of the skin, scars, allergies, and other disorders, both malignant and benign.
Emergency Medicine	Emergency physician	Emergency physicians are experts in triage and treating a patient to prevent the patient's death or serious disability. This physician gives immediate care to stabilize the patient, and then refers to the appropriate professional for further care. These physicians are usually found in hospital emergency rooms or freestanding emergency centers.
Family Medicine	Family practitioner	Family practitioners offer care to the whole family, from newborns to elderly adults. They are familiar with a wide range of disorders and diseases. However, preventive care is their primary concern. This is one of the specialties most often chosen by physicians.
General Surgery	Surgeon	General surgeons correct deformities and defects and treat diseases or injured parts of the body by means of operative treatment. A general surgeon must be familiar with the various specialties to treat patients effectively. General surgery includes all aspects of surgery other than those classified into a subgroup specialty.
Genetics	Medical geneticist	Geneticists are physicians trained to diagnose and treat patients with conditions related to genetically linked diseases. They also may provide genetic counseling when indicated. Often associated with research projects, geneticists may participate in screening programs for defects and abnormalities, sometimes before the birth of an infant.
Internal Medicine	Internist	Internists are concerned with comprehensive care, often diagnosing and treating those with chronic, long-term conditions. They also offer treatment for common illnesses and preventive care. Internists must have a broad understanding of the body and its ailments to be able to diagnose conditions and provide treatment.
Neurological Surgery	Neurosurgeon	Neurosurgeons provide surgical and nonsurgical care for patients with conditions of the central, autonomic, and peripheral nervous systems, including the supporting structures and vascular supplies of related organs.
Neurology/Psychiatry	Neurologist/ psychiatrist	Neurologists diagnose and treat disorders of the brain, spinal cord, and nerves and the blood vessels that support those organs. Generally, neurologists manage infectious, metabolic, degenerative, and systemic involvement of the nervous system. Psychiatrists are physicians who specialize in the diagnosis and treatment of people with mental, emotional, or behavioral disorders. A psychiatrist is qualified to conduct psychotherapy and to prescribe medications when necessary.
Nuclear Medicine	Nuclear medicine specialist	Specialists in nuclear medicine use radioactive substances to diagnose and treat disease. Radiation and imaging instruments are used to detect diseases often before the organ is assessed as abnormal by other methods. Nuclear medicine specialists are aware of the effects of radiation on various structures and are educated in the fundamental principles of radiation and physics.

TABLE 2-1 Examples of Medical Specialties Recognized by the American Board of Medical Specialties—cont'd

SPECIALTY	PRACTITIONER'S TITLE	DESCRIPTION
Obstetrics and Gynecology	Obstetrician/ gynecologist	Obstetricians provide care to women of childbearing age and monitor the progress of the developing child. They deliver the baby and care for the mother for approximately 6 weeks after birth. Gynecologists are concerned with the diagnosis and treatment of the female reproductive system.
Ophthalmology	Ophthalmologist	Ophthalmologists diagnose, treat, and provide comprehensive care for the eye and its supporting structures. These physicians also offer vision services, including corrective lenses. Screening tests are promoted as preventive care.
Otolaryngology	Otolaryngologist	Otolaryngologists treat diseases and conditions that affect the ear, nose, and throat and structures related to the head and neck. Problems that affect the voice and hearing are also referred to this specialist.
Pathology	Pathologist	Pathologists study the causes of diseases that affect the body and determine what may have caused a patient's death. These physicians study tissues and cells, body fluids, and the organs themselves to aid in the diagnosis of a patient's ailments. Pathologists often perform autopsies.
Pediatrics	Pediatrician	Pediatricians promote preventive medicine and treat diseases that affect children and adolescents. They monitor the child's growth and development and provide a wide range of health services to keep their patients healthy.
Physical Medicine and Rehabilitation	Physiatrist	Physiatrists assist patients who have physical disabilities, which may include rehabilitation; patients with musculoskeletal disorders; and patients suffering from pain as a result of injury or trauma. Their primary goal is to restore the patient to the state of health he or she had before the injury or trauma, as nearly as possible, through rehabilitation.
Plastic Surgery	Plastic surgeon	Plastic surgeons work with patients who have a physical defect as a result of some type of injury or condition. These surgeons perform reconstructive procedures using grafts, flaps, and tissue transfer and replanting. They also provide cosmetic enhancements and elective procedures.
Preventive Medicine	Preventive medicine specialist	Preventive medicine specialists are concerned with preventing mental and physical illness and disability. They also analyze current health services and plan for future medical needs. Preventive medicine consists of several components, including biostatistics, environmental studies, occupational studies, and clinical preventive medicine activities.
Radiology	Radiologist	Radiology is a specialty in which x-rays are used to diagnose and treat disease. A diagnostic radiologist specializes in using x-rays, ultrasound, nuclear medicine, computed tomography, and magnetic resonance imaging to detect abnormalities throughout the body.
Thoracic Surgery	Thoracic surgeon	Thoracic surgeons are concerned with the operative treatment of the chest and chest wall, lungs, and respiratory passages. They also are involved with heart surgery, including both valvular and coronary heart surgery.
Urology	Urologist	Urologists are concerned with the treatment of diseases and disorders of the urinary tract. They diagnose and manage problems with the genitourinary system and practice endoscopic and percutaneous procedures related to these structures.

Data from http://www.abms.org/who_we_help/physicians/specialties.aspx.

Dentists

The two basic types of dentists in the United States are Doctors of Dental Medicine (DMDs) and Doctors of Dental Surgery (DDSs). Dentists treat and prevent problems of the teeth and gums and the tissue surrounding them. They can perform oral surgery and write prescriptions for antibiotics and analgesics. Some specialist dentists perform straightening, called *orthodontics,* and some perform root canal therapy, called *endodontics.* Dental school usually lasts 4 years after completion of undergraduate studies, and state licensing is required.

Optometrists

The optometrist (OD) is trained and licensed to examine the eyes to test visual acuity and to treat vision defects by prescribing correctional lenses and other optical aids. A program of exercise may be planned for the patient's eyes. Optometrists study at accredited schools of optometry for 4 years after completing undergraduate studies in the sciences, mathematics, and English. They must be licensed in the state in which they practice. Optometrists should not be confused with ophthalmologists, who are licensed MDs.

Podiatrists

Podiatrists (Doctors of Podiatric Medicine [DPMs]) are educated in the care of the feet, including surgical treatment. Most people spend an extraordinary amount of time on their feet, resulting in wear and tear and chronic pain. Podiatrists are trained to find pressure points and weight-distribution problems. These doctors train for 4 years at accredited colleges after undergraduate studies in the sciences.

Other Doctorates

Other individuals may be called "doctor" based on the degree they have earned in their field. For instance, a person with a PhD has a doctor of philosophy degree in his or her field of expertise and may be addressed as "doctor." This individual might work as a professor at a university or in a field related to his or her discipline. An individual with a PsyD degree is a doctor of psychology, and someone with an EdD degree is a doctor of educational psychology. Doctors who practice **naturopathy**, called *naturopathic physicians,* use only natural means to help the body to heal. These medical professionals are licensed in 15 states.

Nurses

Registered Nurses

The RN has many career options. Many nurses work in an administrative capacity as managers in hospitals or other types of healthcare facilities. They also provide direct patient care, a role in which they are vital for assessing the patient and providing a care plan. Nurses usually find a specialty area that they enjoy and practice within that area, although they may also "float" to different departments in the hospital. Some function as home health nurses, visiting patients and providing home care. Others work in nursing homes, in public health, or in physicians' offices.

Licensed Practical and Vocational Nurses

Licensed practical nurses (LPNs) and licensed vocational nurses (LVNs) offer bedside care, assisting with the day-to-day personal care required by inpatients. They assess patients, chart their progress, and administer medications and intravenous fluids where allowed by law. They often work in hospitals or skilled nursing facilities and also are found in physicians' offices. They sometimes supervise nursing assistants and may also provide patient education services.

Nurse Practitioners

Nurse practitioners (NPs) provide basic patient care services, including diagnosing and prescribing medications for common illnesses. These professionals must have advanced academic training beyond the registered nurse (RN) degree and also have vast clinical experience. Nurse practitioners usually focus on preventive care and disease prevention. An NP is allowed to practice independently or as a part of a team of healthcare professionals.

Nurse Anesthetists

Nurse anesthetists are registered nurses (RNs) who administer anesthetics to patients during care by surgeons, physicians, dentists, or other qualified health professionals. They practice in many different settings, including offices, traditional hospitals, labor and delivery units, ophthalmology offices, plastic surgery offices, and many others. This practice is quite advanced, and they are compensated well for their skills. Nurse anesthetists can be found in both metropolitan and rural communities.

Other Healthcare Professionals

Many different healthcare professionals contribute to the patient's care and recovery. Some work in a hospital setting, and others perform their duties in other types of medical facilities or in the patient's home. The *Healthcare Careers Directory,* published by the American Medical Association, lists many of the various allied healthcare professionals who provide care to patients (Table 2-2). Additionally, more information about licensed healthcare professionals is available in Table 2-3.

CLOSING COMMENTS

The healthcare industry is certainly one of the most exciting career fields in today's world. The constant change in and development of new technology and theories make medicine an attractive option for career choices. The needs of medicine extend far beyond the boundaries of the United States, and collaborative efforts among countries promote a faster move forward, with new discoveries and hope for those affected by disease. Headlines daily grace newspapers and computer screens, detailing stories of human cloning, "designer" babies, genetic discoveries, and computer capabilities that amaze us all. Medications are being developed that will bring us to the brink of eliminating certain diseases. The mapping of the human genome may lead to incredible breakthroughs in the study of colon, breast, and ovarian cancers, cystic fibrosis, neurologic degeneration, sickle cell anemia, and countless other conditions. There has never been a more thrilling time to become part of the world of medicine and to make a contribution as a healthcare professional.

Patient Education

Some patients have very little knowledge about the healthcare industry and may need instruction and explanations about details important to their healthcare. For instance, many patients do not understand that they may receive several bills after a hospital stay. They often call the physician's office with questions; therefore medical assistants must understand hospital systems to be able to help the patients. Become familiar with community resources to make referrals for patients that need help from various sources. If a patient seems to have a need, speak with him or her privately and determine whether any agency or organization could help with the issues at hand. Patients will appreciate the medical assistant's willingness to look for ways to help when confronted with problems. Always have an attitude of enthusiasm at every opportunity to assist a patient.

Legal and Ethical Issues

The medical assistant should have a good understanding of the history of medicine and develop an appreciation of those who paved the way to the achievement of today's level of medical technology. These pioneers of medicine should be respected for their efforts to expand and improve healthcare, because many of them sacrificed their reputations and even their lives to prove their theories. Often,

TABLE 2-2 Allied Health Occupations Recognized by the American Medical Association

TITLE	CREDENTIAL	JOB DESCRIPTION
Anesthesiologist Assistant	AA	Functions as a specialty physician assistant under the direction of a licensed and qualified anesthesiologist; assists in developing and implementing the anesthesia care plan.
Art Therapist	ATR	Uses drawings and other art and media forms to assess, treat, and rehabilitate patients with mental, emotional, physical, and/or developmental disorders.
Athletic Trainer	ATC	Provides a variety of services, including injury prevention, assessment, immediate care, treatment, and rehabilitation after physical injury or trauma.
Audiologist	CCC-A	Identifies individuals with symptoms of hearing loss and other auditory, balance, and related neural problems; assesses the nature of those problems and helps individuals manage them.
Blindness and Visual Impairment professionals	LVT, O&M, VRT	Help people learn to use their vision more efficiently, both with and without optical devices; provide training and offer recommendations to help patients function more successfully in their environments.
Blood Bank Technology Specialist	SBB	Performs routine and specialized tests in blood center and transfusion services, using methods that conform to the accepted standards in the blood bank industry.
Diagnostic Cardiovascular Sonographer/Technologist	RDCS, RVT	Using invasive or noninvasive techniques (or both), performs diagnostic examinations and therapeutic interventions for the heart and blood vessels at the request of a physician.
Clinical Laboratory Science/ Medical Technologist	MT, MLT	In conjunction with pathologists, performs tests to diagnose the causes and nature of disease; also develops data on blood, tissues, and fluids of the human body using a variety of methodologies.
Counseling-related professional	LPC, LMHC	Deals with human development through support, therapeutic approaches, consultation, evaluation, teaching, and research; practices the art of helping people to grow.
Cytotechnologist	CT	Works with pathologists to evaluate cellular material from all body sites, primarily through use of the microscope; examines specimens for normal and abnormal cytologic changes, including malignancies.
Dance Therapist	DTR, ADTR	Uses the psychotherapeutic properties of movement as a process that furthers the emotional, cognitive, social, and physical integration of the patient as a tool for healing.
Dental Assistant, Dental Hygienist, Dental Laboratory Technician	CDA, RDH, CDT	Performs a wide range of tasks, from assisting the dentist to teaching patients how to prevent oral disease and maintain oral health.
Diagnostic Medical Sonographer	RDMS	Uses medical ultrasound to gather sonographic data, which can aid the diagnosis of a variety of conditions and diseases; also monitors fetal development.
Dietician, Dietetic Technician	DTR	Integrates and applies the principles of food science, nutrition, biochemistry, physiology, food management, and behavior to achieve and maintain health status.
Electroneurodiagnostic Technologist	REEG-T	Records and studies the electrical activity of the brain and nervous system; obtains interpretable recordings of patients' nervous system function.
Emergency Medical Technician, Paramedic	EMT, Paramedic	Provides medical care to people who have suffered an injury or illness outside the hospital setting, most often in an emergency; provides basic or advanced life support (or both).
Genetics Counselor	IGC	Provides genetic services to individuals and families seeking information about the occurrence or risk of a genetic condition or birth defect.
Health Information Management professional	RHIA, RHIT	Provides expert assistance in the systems and processes for health information management, including planning, engineering, administration, application, and policy making.
Kinesiotherapist	RKT	Provides rehabilitation exercise and education designed to reverse or minimize debilitation and enhance the functional capacity of medically stable patients.

Continued

TABLE 2-2 Allied Health Occupations Recognized by the American Medical Association—cont'd

TITLE	CREDENTIAL	JOB DESCRIPTION
Massage Therapist	MT	Applies manual techniques, and may apply adjunctive techniques, with the intention of positively affecting the health and well-being of a patient or client.
Medical Assistant	CMA, RMA	Functions as a member of the healthcare delivery team and performs both administrative and clinical procedures and duties; a multiskilled health professional.
Medical Illustrator	MI	Specializes in the visual display and communication of scientific information; creates visuals and designs communication tools for teaching both medical professionals and the public.
Music Therapist	MT-BC	Uses music in a therapeutic relationship to address the physical, emotional, cognitive, and social needs of individuals of all ages; assesses the strengths and needs of clients and patients.
Nuclear Medicine Technologist	RT	Uses the nuclear properties of radioactive and stable nuclides to make diagnostic evaluations of anatomic or physiologic conditions of the body; also provides therapy with unsealed radioactive sources.
Occupational Therapist	OTR	Uses purposeful activity and interventions to achieve functional outcomes, thereby maximizing the independence and maintaining the health of those limited by physical injury or illness.
Ophthalmic Laboratory Technician, Medical Technician/Technologist	COT, COMT	Collects data and performs clinical evaluations; performs tests and protocols required by ophthalmologists; assists in the treatment of patients.
Orthoptist	CO	Performs a series of diagnostic tests and measurements on patients with visual disorders; helps design a treatment plan to correct disorders of vision, eye movements, and alignment.
Orthotist/Prosthetist	RTO, RTP, RTPO	Designs and fits devices (orthoses) to patients who have disabling conditions of the limbs and spine and/or partial or total absence of a limb.
Perfusionist	CCP	Operates extracorporeal circulation and autotransfusion equipment during any medical situation where the patient's respiratory or circulatory function must be supported or temporarily replaced.
Pharmacy Technician	CPhT	Assists pharmacists with duties that do not require the expertise or judgment of a licensed pharmacist.
Physical Therapist	PT	Helps to improve a patient's strength and mobility, relieve pain, and prevent or limit permanent physical disabilities; takes a personal, direct approach to meeting individual health goals.
Physician Assistant	PA	Practices medicine under the direction and supervision of a licensed doctor of medicine or osteopathy; makes clinical decisions and provides a range of services.
Radiation Therapist, Radiographer	RRTD	Delivers prescribed dosages of radiation to patients for therapeutic purposes; provides appropriate patient care and maintains accurate records of the treatment provided.
Rehabilitation Counselor	CRC	Determines and coordinates services to assist people with disabilities in moving from psychological and economic dependence to independence.
Respiratory Therapist, Respiratory Therapy Technician	RRT, CRT, RPFT, CPFT	Evaluates, treats, and manages patients of all ages with respiratory illnesses and other cardiopulmonary disorders; advanced respiratory therapists exercise considerable independent judgment.
Surgical Assistant	CSA	Assists in exposure, hemostasis, closure, and other intraoperative technical functions that help the surgeon carry out a safe operation with optimal results for the patient.
Surgical Technologist	ST, CST	Helps prepare patients for surgery and maintains the sterile field in the surgical suite, making sure all members of the surgical team follow sterile technique.
Therapeutic Recreation Specialist	CTRS	Uses treatment, education, and recreation services to help people with illnesses, disabilities, and other conditions develop and use their leisure in ways that enhance their health.

TABLE 2-3 Licensed Healthcare Professions

TITLE	CREDENTIAL	JOB DESCRIPTION
Physician Assistant	PA	Physician assistants provide direct patient care services under the supervision of licensed physicians. They are trained to diagnose and treat patients as directed by the physician, and in 46 states and the District of Columbia, they are allowed to write prescriptions. These professionals take patient histories, order and interpret tests, perform physical examinations, and even make diagnostic decisions. They work in physicians' offices and hospitals, on military bases, and in other healthcare facilities.
Nurse Practitioner	NP	Nurse practitioners provide basic patient care services, including diagnosing and prescribing medications for common illnesses. These professionals must have advanced academic training, beyond the registered nurse (RN) degree, and also must have extensive clinical experience. Nurse practitioners usually focus on preventive care. A nurse practitioner is allowed to practice independently as part of a team of healthcare professionals.
Nurse Anesthetist	NA	Nurse anesthetists are registered nurses who administer anesthetics to patients during care provided by surgeons, physicians, dentists, or other qualified health professionals. They practice in many different settings, including offices, traditional hospitals, labor and deliver units, ophthalmology offices, and plastic surgery offices. This practice is quite advanced, and nurse anesthetists are compensated well for their skills. They can be found in both metropolitan and rural communities.
Registered Nurse	RN	A registered nurse has many career options. Many nurses work in administration as managers in hospitals or other types of healthcare facilities. They also provide direct patient care, a role in which they are vital for assessing the patient and providing a care plan. Nurses usually find a specialty area that they enjoy and practice in that area, although they may also "float" to different departments in the hospital. Some function as home health nurses, visiting patients at home and providing home care. Others work in nursing homes, in public health, or in physicians' offices.
Licensed Practical or Vocational Nurse	LPN or LVN	Licensed practical nurses (LPNs) and licensed vocational nurses (LVNs) offer bedside care, assisting with the day-to-day personal care required by inpatients. They assess patients, chart their progress, and administer medications and intravenous fluids where allowed by law. They often work in hospitals or skilled nursing facilities and also are found in physicians' offices. They sometimes supervise nursing assistants and may also provide patient education services.
Medical Technologist	MT	Medical technologists perform diagnostic testing on blood, body fluids, and other types of specimens to assist the physician in arriving at a diagnosis. These professionals work with bacteria and viruses and use their technical skills, combined with their knowledge of disease, to perform their duties. They can make quality control decisions and can act independently in their profession. Hospitals, teaching universities, research organizations, and laboratories employ most of the medical technologists. These professionals usually have a Bachelor of Science (BS) degree in addition to certification or licensure.
Medical Laboratory Technician	MLT	Medical laboratory technicians perform most of the same test procedures that the medical technologist performs; the difference between the two is that the MLT does not work independently. MLTs usually are supervised by an MT and have at least an associate's degree and certification or a licensure. MLTs work in the same types of facilities as MTs.
Physical Therapist	PT	Physical therapists assist patients in regaining their mobility and improving their strength and range of motion, which may have been impaired by an accident or injury or as a result of disease. After assessing the patient, the physical therapist devises a treatment plan in conjunction with the patient's physician. The goal of the physical therapist is to improve how the patient functions at work and at home.
Respiratory Therapist	RT	Most respiratory therapists work in hospitals. All types of patients receive respiratory care, including newborns and geriatric patients. Respiratory therapists commonly use oxygen therapy to assist with breathing, and they also perform diagnostic tests that measure lung capacity.
Occupational Therapist	OT	Occupational therapists work with patients who have developed conditions that disable them developmentally, emotionally, mentally, or physically. Occupational therapists assist in helping the individual to compensate for loss of function; their goal is to bring patients to a functional level where they can live healthy, productive lives.

Continued

TABLE 2-3 Licensed Healthcare Professions—cont'd

TITLE	CREDENTIAL	JOB DESCRIPTION
Diagnostic Cardiac Sonographer or Vascular Technologist	DCS or DVT	Diagnostic cardiac sonographers (DCSs) or vascular technologists (DVTs) assist in the diagnosis and treatment of cardiac and vascular diseases and disorders. They perform noninvasive tests, including echocardiographs and electrocardiographs. Often the cardiovascular technician uses ultrasonography to assist the physician in identifying malfunctions of the heart and its structures.
Radiology Technician	RT	Radiology technicians use various machines to help the physician diagnose and treat certain diseases. These machines may include x-ray equipment, ultrasonographic machines, and magnetic resonance imaging (MRI) scanners. Radiology technicians explain procedures to patients. They also are knowledgeable about the correct positioning techniques used for each examination; these techniques ensure that the images recorded are accurate and helpful for the diagnosing physician.
Paramedic	Paramedic	Paramedics are specially trained to provide emergency care to patients in life-threatening situations. Paramedics are highly efficient and well versed in the functions of the body. They perform advanced skills and, with more experience, are able to supervise or direct the operations of an emergency care ambulance facility.
Emergency Medical Technician	EMT	Emergency medical technicians progress through several levels of training, each providing more advanced skills. Their medical education encompasses managing respiratory, cardiac, and trauma cases and often emergency childbirth. Some states also recognize specialties in the EMT field, such as EMT-Cardiac, which includes training in cardiac arrhythmias, and EMT–Shock Trauma, which includes starting intravenous fluids and administering specific medications.
Registered Dietician	RD	Registered dieticians are thoroughly trained in nutrition and the different types of diets patients require to improve or maintain their condition. They use the advice of the physician and information about the patient to design healthy diets during hospital stays and even help plan menus for home use. In addition, they teach patients about their recommended diet and also about alternatives that can help the patient choose attractive foods.

Modified from the American Medical Association: *Healthcare careers directory (2012-2013)*. Accessed [02-19-2013] at http://www.ama-assn.org/ama/pub/education-careers/careers-health-care/directory.page

they broke the laws of the time to advance medical science. Their historical legacy represents enormous endeavors by these discoverers of new principles, theories, treatments, and cures.

Ethical medical assistants must always strive to serve the patient above the call of duty and continuously work within their scope of practice. Patients expect everyone in the medical field to have ethics above reproach; remember that all actions are under an ethical microscope and must be professional, accurate, and performed in a competent manner. Put the patient first every day at work and always treat the individual with respect and compassion.

SUMMARY OF SCENARIO

Mr. Santos is an effective instructor, and one who is concerned about providing interesting material for his students. He wishes to instill a strong respect in the students for the people who played a role in early medical advances. His classroom discussions will help the students to think about what it was like to present new ideas to the public and often be ridiculed.

In addition to teaching his students about the history of medicine and the state of healthcare today, he provides opportunities for the students to work together in discussion groups and present information to the class. He encourages Internet research, a valuable skill that will help the medical assisting student in many areas of training. By allowing the students to speak in front of the class to give reports on the medical pioneers, Mr. Santos teaches them to be more at ease when speaking in public and when articulating instructions and details to patients and co-workers. All of these skills make a well-rounded medical assistant who will become a great asset to the facility in which he or she is employed.

Mr. Santos explains that continuing medical research is critical to the healthcare industry, because new and more effective drugs and treatments are necessary, and because many diseases and conditions do not as yet have a cure. Medical research constantly looks for better ways to make patients well and continually strives to find cures for diseases that medicine has not yet conquered. Medical assistants may work for physicians who are involved in research projects, and this may afford them the opportunity to contribute to medical research.

By providing his students with an overview of the healthcare industry, Mr. Santos helps them to become more familiar with the professionals whom they will encounter in various medical facilities and to have a better awareness of their duties and responsibilities.

SUMMARY OF LEARNING OBJECTIVES

1. **Define, spell, and pronounce the terms listed in the vocabulary.**
   Spelling and pronouncing medical terms correctly bolster the medical assistant's credibility. Knowing the definition of these terms promotes confidence in communication with patients and co-workers.

2. **Identify the ancient cultures that contributed a major portion of our medical terminology.**
   Greek and Roman mythology contributed the major portion of the medical terms we use today. Terms have also been borrowed from Anglo-Saxon, German, Arabic, and other sources, including the Bible.

3. **Distinguish between and describe the staff of Aesculapius and the caduceus.**
   The American Medical Association adopted the staff of Aesculapius as the symbol of medicine. The symbol is a staff encircled by a serpent. The caduceus often is mistakenly used to represent medicine but is actually the medical insignia of the U.S. Army Medical Corps. This icon is a winged staff encircled by two serpents.

4. **Explain the philosophy behind the phrase "physicians must learn to despise money."**
   Galen was a champion of medical ethics and believed that physicians could not truly be devoted to the practice of medicine if they were concerned about profit. Many modern medical professionals agree with Galen's theory and argue that physicians must base their decisions on what is best for the patient as opposed to focusing on monetary profit.

5. **Explain why a medical education at Johns Hopkins University School of Medicine was considered superior, even in its early years.**
   Johns Hopkins University School of Medicine has been recognized as a leader in healthcare education for more than a century. The university was one of the first institutions to partner with a hospital for training purposes, resulting in its superior medical education. The School of Medicine also had a research department, where faculty members investigated new methods and treatments for patients. The combination of a medical education with readily available patients brought the discovery of illness and disease into a new light for those early medical students. Today, the Johns Hopkins medical system is a multibillion-dollar organization, incorporating three acute care hospitals and other facilities into an integrated healthcare system.

6. **List several medical pioneers and discuss the importance of their contributions to the medical profession.**
   Numerous early pioneers made tremendous contributions to the medical field. Constant growth and research have pressed the medical profession forward, and with the assistance of technology, the growth speeds along today faster than ever.

7. **Explain the roles of the national healthcare organizations.**
   National healthcare organizations provide information, medication, and personnel to attempt to eradicate diseases and treat the diseases for which no cure exists. Many of these organizations operate with restricted funding and rely often on donations and volunteer workers to operate. These agencies often work together in an effort to solve problems of epidemics effectively and learn more about diseases. All of the national healthcare organizations are a vital part of the medical industry today.

8. **Identify the role of the Centers for Disease Control and Prevention (CDC) regulations in healthcare settings.**
   The CDC is a clearinghouse for information and statistics associated with healthcare. Several divisions within the CDC focus on specific health-related issues, such as the National Center for HIV, STD, and TB Prevention; the Public Health Practice Program Office; the National Center on Birth Defects and Developmental Disabilities; and the National Center for Health Statistics. Branch offices are located throughout the United States and in several foreign countries. The CDC provides regulations that affect all healthcare facilities. When the virus now known as HIV was discovered, the CDC was one of the first organizations to research and attempt to isolate the virus. When a pandemic begins, the CDC information services offer guidelines that help facilities ensure the health of their employees, patients, and the public at large.

9. **Discuss the various types of ambulatory care.**
   Physicians' offices, group practices, and multispecialty group practices are a few types of ambulatory care. This division of medicine also includes occupational health centers, dialysis centers, rehabilitation clinics, and sleep centers. Patients who are ambulatory are able to move from place to place, usually on their own or with the assistance of a wheelchair or walker.

10. **Name the three main provider portals of entry into the healthcare system and distinguish among the different types of physicians and medical practices.**
    The three main provider portals of entry into the healthcare system are medical doctors, osteopathic physicians, and chiropractic physicians. These different disciplines have some similar training, but osteopathic physicians usually use a holistic approach, and chiropractors concentrate many of their efforts on the alignment of the spine in an effort to promote healing of the body. Most physicians work in a sole proprietorship, a group practice, or a healthcare corporation.

11. **Become familiar with the medical specialties recognized by the American Board of Medical Specialties.**
    Numerous specialties focus on particular areas of the practice of medicine. The American Board of Medical Specialties recognizes 24 specialty groups, which support various organizations designed to promote that particular branch of medicine. Although other specialties and subspecialties of medicine exist, the most common and most generally recognized are those associated with the American Board of Medical Specialties.

12. **Understand both the allied health professions and how they relate to medical assisting.**
    The American Medical Association recognizes more than 60 allied health-care occupations. These allied health professionals contribute to the field of medicine, each playing a specific role in the healthcare industry. The medical assistant works as a part of the healthcare team with all of these professionals.

CONNECTIONS

Study Guide Connection: Go to the Chapter 2 Study Guide. Read and complete the activities.

Evolve Connection: Go to the Chapter 2 link at evolve.elsevier.com/kinn to complete the Chapter Review and Chapter Quiz. Check out the other resources listed for this chapter to make the most of what you have learned from The Healthcare Industry.

THE MEDICAL ASSISTING PROFESSION

3

SCENARIO

Sandra Ramirez is a single mother who has decided on medical assisting as a career. She has always been interested in the medical field and wants a job that will allow her to spend evenings and weekends with her 3-year-old son, Roberto. The idea of working in a physician's office appeals to her, and she has applied to a school that is close to her apartment and day care provider. She plans to attend day classes and work part-time after school until it is time to pick up her son.

Sandra is very excited about her new career and has set several goals for her training. First, she hopes to attain perfect attendance, and second, she would like to graduate with honors. She has budgeted her study time and plans to ask her instructors during the first 2 weeks of school for suggestions on how she can better prepare for classes and examinations. Sandra will find medical assisting to be a rewarding career and respected profession.

While studying this chapter, think about the following questions:

- What obstacles might prevent Sandra from attending all her classes, and how can she prepare in advance to overcome them?
- How can Sandra begin to explore the type of physician's office in which she would enjoy being employed after graduation?
- What goals might Sandra have at the commencement of her training? At the end of training?
- How can Sandra make the most of her time attending school to become a medical assistant?

LEARNING OBJECTIVES

1. Define, spell, and pronounce the terms listed in the vocabulary.
2. Briefly discuss the history of medical assisting as a profession.
3. Discuss the versatility of a career in medical assisting.
4. Differentiate between administrative and clinical medical assisting duties and recognize the importance of becoming knowledgeable about the general responsibilities of the medical assistant.
5. Comprehend the current employment outlook for the medical assistant.
6. Give the reasons that hiring an individual with no formal training often is more expensive than hiring a professional medical assistant.
7. Identify several considerations to keep in mind, other than financial compensation, when choosing a position as a medical assistant.
8. Discuss the aspects of the medical assistant's performance on a successful externship.
9. List three unacceptable behaviors on the externship site.
10. Explain why continuing education is so important to the medical assistant.
11. Understand medical assistant credentialing requirements, the importance of credentialing, and the process of obtaining credentials.
12. Discuss the difference between a CMA and a RMA.

VOCABULARY

allied health fields Occupational disciplines in which professionals involved with the delivery of healthcare or related services assist physicians with the diagnosis, treatment, and care of patients in many different specialty areas.

benefits Services or payments provided under a health plan, employee plan, or some other agreement, including programs such as health insurance, pensions, retirement planning, and many other options that may be offered to employees of a company or organization.

certification (ser-tuh-fuh-ka´-shun) The attesting of something as being true as represented or as meeting a standard; the result of having been tested, usually by a third party, and awarded a certificate based on proven knowledge.

continuing education units (CEUs) Credits for courses, classes, or seminars related to an individual's profession that are designed to promote education and to keep the professional up to date on current procedures and trends in the field; CEUs often are required for licensing.

cross-training Training in more than one area so that a multitude of duties may be performed by one person or so that substitutions of personnel may be made in an emergency or at other necessary times.

externship (or **internship**) A training program that is part of the medical assisting course of study in an educational institution. This part of training is taken in the actual business setting of that field of study; the terms are interchanged in some areas of the country.

intangibles (in-tan´-juh-buls) Qualities that cannot be perceived, especially by touch, or cannot be precisely identified or realized by the mind.

invasive Involving entry into the living body, as by incision or insertion of an instrument.

perks Extra advantages or benefits of working in a specific job that may or may not be commonplace in that particular profession; a shortened form of perquisites.

phlebotomy (fli-bah´-tuh-me) An invasive procedure used to obtain a blood specimen for testing, experimentation, or diagnosis of disease.

practicum Another word for the externship; a training program that is a part of the medical assisting course of study in the actual business setting of a medical office or facility. (This term is used by the Commission on Accreditation of Allied Health Education Programs [CAAHEP] to designate the externship.)

profit sharing Offer of a part of a company's profits to employees or other designated individuals or groups.

stock options Offers of stocks for purchase to a certain group of individuals or certain groups, such as employees of a for-profit hospital.

versatile (vur´-suh-til) Embracing a variety of subjects, fields, or skills; having a wide range of abilities.

According to the U.S. Department of Labor's *Occupational Outlook Handbook,* medical assisting employment will grow 31% in the decade between 2010 and 2020, making this career field one of the fastest growing occupations in the United States. Much of this growth will be the result of an increase in the number of group practices, clinics, and other facilities that need a high number of support personnel. This makes the medical assistant who can handle both clinical and administrative duties particularly valuable to the physician.

A career as a medical assistant is challenging and offers job satisfaction, opportunities for service, financial reward, and possibilities for advancement. Men and women can be equally successful as medical assistants. Individuals considering the medical assisting discipline must be dedicated and committed and must have a strong desire to become caregivers. Caregivers are people who have the ability to put the needs of the patient first, and they have a sincere concern for those who are not at their best. A caregiver must feel an obligation to assist the patient in whatever way possible and must have patience with those who, at times, are more difficult. This strong inner desire is one of the most important qualities of the successful professional medical assistant. Through the development of this "care giving" mentality, many personal rewards will follow, as will a long and beneficial career.

THE HISTORY OF MEDICAL ASSISTING

The first medical assistant was probably a neighbor of a physician who was called on to help when an extra pair of hands was needed. As time passed and the practice of medicine became more organized and more complicated, some physicians hired nurses to help in their office practices. Gradually, record keeping, data reporting, and an increasing number of business details became important to physicians, and they realized a need for an assistant with both administrative and clinical training. Nurses were likely to have training only in clinical skills; therefore, many physicians began training them or other individuals to assist with all of the office duties. Community and junior colleges began offering training programs that focused on both administrative and clinical skills in the late 1940s. Medical assistant organizations at the local and state levels began developing around 1950, and soon after, certifying examinations became available. Today medical assisting is one of the most respected **allied health fields** in the industry, and training is readily available through community colleges, junior colleges, and private educational institutions throughout the United States.

The American Association of Medical Assistants (AAMA) was co-founded by Mary E. Kinn, who served as the organization's president in 1958. She helped to establish a certifying program for members of the AAMA and chaired the certifying branch in 1959. Kinn authored this textbook from 1967 through 1999 and then retired. She is greatly respected for her contributions to the field of medical assisting.

THE SCOPE OF PRACTICE OF A MEDICAL ASSISTANT

Today's medical assistant is a **versatile** professional. The duties that medical assistants perform vary not only from office to office, but even within the same office. Medical assistants perform routine duties within the offices of many types of health professionals, including physicians, chiropractors, podiatrists, and others. According to the *Occupational Outlook Handbook,* more than half of the total number of medical assistants work in a physician's office. Individuals with medical assisting training can accomplish various jobs in the hospital environment, and some are employed by freestanding emergency centers or surgery centers. Opportunities for medical assistants are growing because of the constant change within the medical profession and the surge of **cross-training**, which means that one individual is trained to do a variety of duties. Medical assistants work under the direct supervision of a physician in the office and perform tasks delegated by the doctor or supervisor.

The AAMA once defined the scope of practice as the "performance of delegated clinical and administrative duties within the supervising physician's scope of practice consistent with the medical assistant's education, training, and experience." This definition remains accurate today. The duties performed by the medical assistant do not constitute the practice of medicine. Students should review the definition and requirements of the scope of practice for medical assistants in their individual states.

The two major categories of duties that medical assistants perform are administrative tasks and clinical tasks (Figure 3-1). On the administrative end of the spectrum, medical assistants greet patients who arrive in the office or clinic and obtain basic registration information. They may enter information into a computer and assemble the patient's paper or electronic medical record. They are trained to do office bookkeeping, which may be done electronically or manually. The medical assistant is trained in filing procedures and in proper techniques for adding information to the medical record. A

basic knowledge of procedure and diagnosis coding is important today, and some medical assistants concentrate strictly on the billing and coding career option. They are able to complete insurance claim forms and determine insurance coverage and limitations for the patient. Medical assistants answer telephones, schedule appointments, update medical records, and handle all types of correspondence. Often the medical assistant schedules outpatient procedures and hospital admissions and may coordinate consultations with physicians. Those who enjoy the administrative side of the profession often enter office management positions.

The clinical duties that medical assistants perform are just as broad as the administrative duties. These professionals prepare patients and the equipment needed before examinations and assist the physician during patients' office visits. They assist with or perform basic testing procedures and are usually proficient in **phlebotomy**. Medical assistants are trained in first aid skills and cardiopulmonary resuscitation. They collect and prepare laboratory specimens, and they know how to follow the regulations established by the U.S. Occupational Safety and Health Administration (OSHA) and the Clinical Laboratory Improvement Amendments (CLIA). Often medical assistants working in the clinical area are responsible for inventorying and ordering supplies. When directed by a physician and allowed by the state, they may administer various types of medications and perform x-ray examinations, if trained to do so. Medical assistants also perform electrocardiograms and prepare patients for x-ray evaluations. They assist in minor surgical procedures, prepare sterile trays, and perform autoclave sterilization procedures for instruments. Other clinical duties involve taking medical histories from patients, patient teaching, and obtaining and recording vital signs. Medical assistants who enjoy the clinical side of the profession may become office managers or may supervise other medical assistants.

Duties and restrictions related to medical assisting vary from state to state, but in most of the United States, the medical assistant performs as an agent of the physician and is under the physician's supervision. This means that the medical assistant performs actions that he or she is told to perform by the physician and that the physician is responsible for those actions. The command may be relayed to the medical assistant from the physician verbally, through a

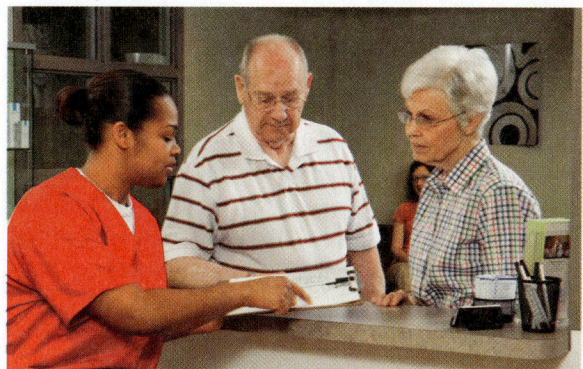
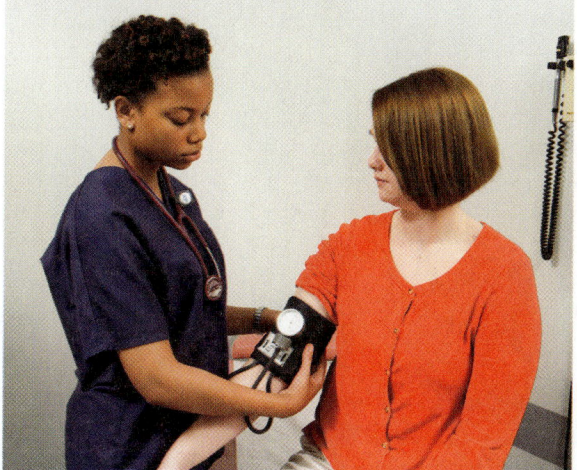

FIGURE 3-1 The responsibilities of a medical assistant include both administrative and clinical duties.

supervisor, or by way of the office policy and procedure manual. *Respondeat superior* is a Latin term meaning "let the master answer." Physicians are responsible not only for their own actions, but for the actions of employees performing within the scope of their employment.

CRITICAL THINKING APPLICATION 3-1

■ Sandra is not sure whether she would enjoy administrative or clinical assisting more. How can she begin to explore both avenues during her classroom training? During her externship or practicum?

■ How could Sandra explore the medical specialties and determine what areas might be of interest to her as a career?

A CAREER IN MEDICAL ASSISTING

Trained medical assistants are equipped with a flexible, adaptable career in which they experience the rewards of helping other people (Figure 3-2). The skills acquired by the medical assistant are valuable, and employment is readily available anywhere in the world where medicine is practiced. Many medical assistants pursue their careers far beyond the usual retirement age, because physicians realize the value of the experienced, mature employee. This career attracts the nontraditional student who may be older than the average postsecondary student by a decade or more. Although many older students feel intimidated by the classroom, they often have excellent experiences in school and reach the top of the class. Medical assisting is more than suitable for the student just exiting high school. Many individuals plan to work as medical assistants to earn a viable income while pursuing further academic studies.

The practice of medicine has changed dramatically in the past several decades. Increasing costs have created a trend away from hospital-based treatment and toward the delivery of care in physicians' offices and in outpatient ambulatory clinics. Although physicians have employed medical assistants in their practices for many years, computerization and technologic advances have created more

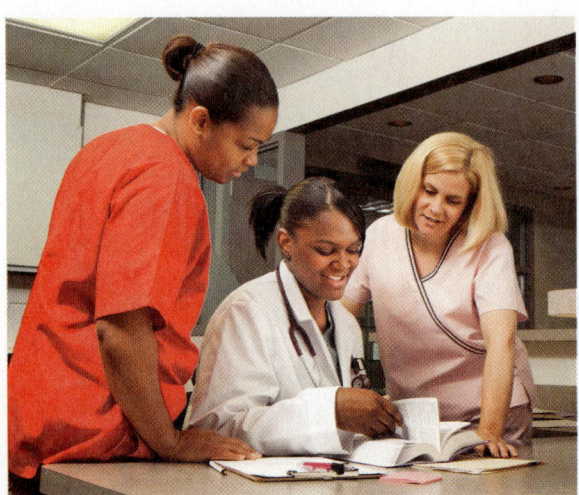

FIGURE 3-2 Medical assisting is a career with many benefits and perks, not to mention the innate rewards of assisting patients in need.

opportunities for formally trained medical assistants, and their responsibilities have similarly increased. Clearly defined educational requirements have been established, and this has resulted in improvement of the quality and accessibility of medical assistant training. These requirements have also helped create a healthy respect for medical assistants, who are considered an integral part of today's allied health field.

Employment for medical assistants is abundant. As mentioned previously, the Labor Department projects that the medical assisting field will grow much faster than the average for all occupations; a growth of 31% is expected in the medical assisting field between 2010 and 2020. In 2010, medical assistants held approximately 527,600 jobs in the United States, and about one half of those were in physicians' offices. The projected employment for 2020 is 690,400 medical assistants. According to the Department of Labor, job growth will be so great because of the increasing number of group practices, clinics, and other healthcare facilities that need a high proportion of support personnel, particularly medical assistants who can handle both administrative and clinical duties. Additionally, the movement toward electronic medical records has resulted in a strong demand for medical assistants who can manage health information. Jobs may also be available with federal agencies, such as the Department of Veterans Affairs, the Public Health Service, and armed forces clinics or hospitals.

Most medical assistants derive a high degree of satisfaction from their work. Job turnover among medical assistants is surprisingly low; some begin working with a physician when the practice is opened and stay until the physician's retirement. In the past, physicians often would hire any individual to perform office and clinical duties, but these people frequently were untrained and unprofessional; they therefore could be paid a minimum amount for their work. Most physicians have learned that hiring an untrained person to work in the medical office usually is more expensive in the long run. Untrained assistants often make errors that are costly to the practice, and these assistants require much more supervision; this means that the supervisor's time is not used for the duties that he or she would normally perform because the medical assistant is not completely able to work alone. Formal training and **certification** are valuable not only to the medical assistant, but also to the physician-employer.

Medical assistants are compensated in various ways, some by hourly wages and some by salary. The earnings vary from place to place. Overall, medical assistants can expect a healthy return on their investment in training, experience, and skills. Most physicians realize that a good medical assistant is worth a higher than average wage, and a medical assistant with formal training is almost always compensated on a higher scale than one with no training. The *Occupational Outlook Handbook* reports statistics on the average salaries for many different career fields, including medical assisting. (This information can be accessed at www.bls.gov/oco. Annual salary updates are also available on the Web site.) More information on salaries may be obtained by monitoring the local classified advertisements and by checking online job information on sites such as Yahoo! Careers. Medical assistants must determine a realistic entry-level salary for their geographic area. Often graduates expect to make a much higher salary than is reasonable right after graduation with little or no experience.

The medical field offers great **benefits** to employees. Usually, the larger the organization, the better the benefits and **perks**. Most employers offer a health insurance plan or managed care plan to their employees. Often a life insurance program is included, and dental insurance is always a valuable benefit. Some companies have **profit-sharing** plans and **stock options**, as well as a retirement plan. Some organizations give their employees access to credit unions, and many have discount options at local businesses, such as uniform shops. Other benefits may include uniform stipends or reimbursement, tuition reimbursement, and continuing education allowances.

Remember that you should consider benefits and perks when contemplating a job opportunity. Many medical assistants may choose to work for less money if the benefits and the opportunities for advancement are good. Consider driving time, holidays, paid parking, sick days, vacation days, and facilities when choosing a job. Do the co-workers seem to enjoy one another's company and get along? Is the physician friendly or more aloof? All of these should be weighed carefully before the final decision is made as to which position to accept. Some facilities pay more and offer fewer benefits, whereas others pay less and offer more benefits. It is a truism that "money is a byproduct of services rendered." Nowhere is this more accurate than in the medical field. When the patients are served well, the medical assistant becomes more and more valuable to the employer and is compensated accordingly.

CRITICAL THINKING APPLICATION   3-2

- Sandra knows that she needs certain benefits as a single mother. What might she need to look for in a job after she graduates?
- What are some ways Sandra can compare positions and opportunities?
- What types of Web sites might help Sandra learn about opportunities in her geographic location?

PROFESSIONAL APPEARANCE

A well-groomed medical assistant in appropriate attire has a positive psychological effect on patients. The essentials of a professional appearance are good health, good grooming, and suitable dress.

Good health requires adequate sleep, balanced meals, and enough exercise to keep fit. Medical assistants can set a good example by living a sensible, healthy lifestyle that includes regular checkups for their own physical condition, both medical and dental. A radiantly healthy office staff presents the best possible public relations image for the physician.

Good grooming is little more than attention to the details of personal appearance. Personal cleanliness, which includes taking a daily bath or shower, using deodorant, and practicing good oral hygiene, is vital. Perfume and aftershave cologne should not be used or should be applied lightly, because patients and co-workers may be allergic to some scents. Makeup should be conservative and applied moderately. Heavy or exaggerated makeup is out of place in the professional office; subtle eye and lip makeup is best. Clear or muted shades of nail polish are best, and long nails are not only inappropriate but can be dangerous to the patient and the medical assistant. Nails must be kept clean and at a very conservative length.

The medical assistant's hair should be shiny, clean, neatly styled, and off the collar.

Medical assistants usually wear a uniform or laboratory coat; this not only presents a professional appearance, but also identifies the assistant as a member of the healthcare team (Figure 3-3). Medical professionals rarely wear traditional white in today's medical facilities, although it is appropriate if allowed in the office policy manual. Fashionable styling makes it possible for the medical assistant's uniform to be both practical and attractive. Women may choose to wear pantsuits, which are available in white or a variety of colors; a two-piece dress uniform in white or a color; an attractively styled traditional white uniform; or a scrub set. Scrubs have become increasingly popular and much more attractive over the past decade. They now are often made of pretty fabrics in rich colors and patterns and are much better suited for the professional office than the old green or blue scrubs worn in the surgical suites of hospitals.

Men may also wear the newer scrubs or may choose white slacks with a white or colored shirt, jacket, or pullover top. If it is acceptable in the facility, a lab coat may be worn over street clothes, but it is important that the lab coat be buttoned when **invasive** procedures are performed. Uniforms should be laundered daily and neatly pressed, because medical assistants are exposed to ill patients throughout the workday. Shoes should be appropriate for a uniform, spotless, and comfortable. Many attractive styles that resemble running or tennis shoes are available at uniform shops, specially conditioned for the medical professional who is on his or her feet most of the day. White shoes must be kept white by daily cleaning and touchups. Remember that if laced shoes are worn, the laces also need cleaning.

In some facilities, the physician prefers that the staff not wear uniforms. Some psychiatrists and some pediatricians, for example, believe that the clinical appearance of a uniform may affect patients adversely. However, today's uniforms reflect so many styles and patterns that the right one for the particular office should be readily available. Some of the fabrics depict cartoon characters or drawings that will appeal to children yet still function as a durable uniform. A medical assistant who does not wear a uniform should follow the dictates of good taste and should be conservative in choosing a

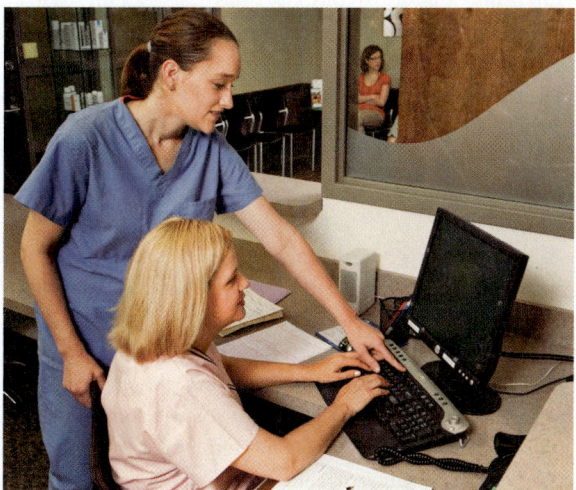

FIGURE 3-3 Medical assistants must have a professional appearance and demeanor in the medical office.

professional wardrobe. Jeans are rarely acceptable in the medical facility, unless the office is extremely casual or it is a special day.

The garments worn while on duty must be comfortable, allow for easy movement, and still look fresh at the end of a busy day. Whatever uniform style the assistant chooses, it should be personally becoming and worn over appropriate undergarments. The lines, colors, and ornamentation of the undergarments should not be seen through the uniform; therefore, it is best to wear undergarments that have a neutral color and not a pattern. Thongs and high-cut underwear should be avoided. When a uniform is worn, jewelry should be limited to an engagement ring, wedding band, and professional pin. No more than two earrings per ear lobe should be worn, and the clothing or hairstyle should always cover tattoos.

Facial and tongue piercings are unacceptable in the medical setting and must be removed during working hours. A name badge will help patients identify each staff person by name.

Make sure the dress code required in the office setting is clearly understood. Adherence to that code is a demonstration of responsibility and willingness to cooperate with office rules. Compliance with office regulations is a factor in decisions on office promotions.

EDUCATION AND TRAINING

Ideally, a medical assistant should have both administrative and clinical skills, although he or she may have a personal preference for one over the other. The physician's staff must be able to handle all responsibilities of the office except those requiring the services of the physician or another licensed professional. In an office with several assistants, each should be able and willing to substitute in an emergency for any of the others, and all should be cross-trained to perform each others' duties. Teamwork is a very important part of any occupation and even more so in the medical environment.

Certain knowledge and skills are expected of a trained medical assistant. The skills mentioned in this chapter are not all-inclusive; rather, they suggest what may be expected on entry into employment as a professional medical assistant.

Classroom Training

Formal training is essential for today's medical assistant. Many community colleges, junior colleges, and private career institutions offer courses in medical assisting. After satisfactory completion of the program, the student usually receives a certificate or diploma. Private career institutions offer training that usually takes 7 to 10 months to complete, and they offer enrollment as often as monthly. Students who attend community colleges, junior colleges, and some private career institutions to study medical assisting may complete the educational requirements to obtain an associate's degree in medical assisting. Courses at the community college level usually take 1 to 2 years to complete and offer enrollment from every few weeks to two or three times a year.

Currently the trend is toward offering the medical assisting program in modules, so that the student receives some clinical training, some administrative training, and some theory in each module. Some classes are taught in traditional classrooms, and the clinical aspect usually is taught in a laboratory at the school. Much of the equipment the medical assistant will use in practice is found in the

laboratory, such as an autoclave, medical instruments and trays, and specimen collection equipment. Medical assistant training usually involves the study of medical terminology, anatomy and physiology, aseptic technique, clinical procedures, medical law and ethics, principles of pharmacology, insurance billing and coding, receptionist and telephone technique, patient communication, human relations, management duties, and receptionist duties, among other subjects.

Instructors are important allies of medical assisting students, and the relationship between instructor and student should be one of mutual respect. Students must realize that instructors have a strong desire to share their knowledge and that they want each student to succeed. Individual schools have certain rules and regulations that must be enforced, many of them a result of state or federal regulation or legislation. The guidelines that students must follow are not designed to hinder their education, but rather to ensure that graduates are competent medical assistants. Students should complete assignments accurately, turn them in on time, and take pride in all the work they do for class. They should never miss school days unless absolutely necessary, and they should develop good habits in school so that they become valuable assets to future employers.

> ### CRITICAL THINKING APPLICATION   3-3
> - How can Sandra develop a positive, nurturing relationship with her instructors?
> - What should she do if she has difficulty in the classroom or if her grades begin to fall?
> - How can Sandra study effectively and prepare for examinations?

Externship (Practicum)

Medical assistant training programs require an **externship** or a **practicum** before the student graduates. Some schools call this the **internship**. This on-the-job training allows students to put the skills they have learned in the classroom to use with real patients and staff members. In most cases, externships are unpaid positions that are part of the medical assistant training program, not a separate entity. Most accreditation organizations do not allow student externs to be paid.

The physician, probably more than any other employer, expects employees to carry out their duties independently, with little or no direct supervision. Someone at the externship site is designated as the student's supervisor. Medical assisting students should consult frequently with their externship supervisors to determine what is expected of them and the progress they are making (Figure 3-4).

The student must be open to constructive criticism and must be a willing learner. Techniques may be learned on the externship that were not included in the classroom training, or optional methods may be taught for various procedures. The medical assisting student should never argue with the staff at the clinical site that a method taught by the school is the only correct way. Often several methods can be used to obtain the same result. The medical assisting student should treat the externship experience as if it were a probationary period on an actual job. Remember, the externship often is the first medical reference the student will be able to list on the resume.

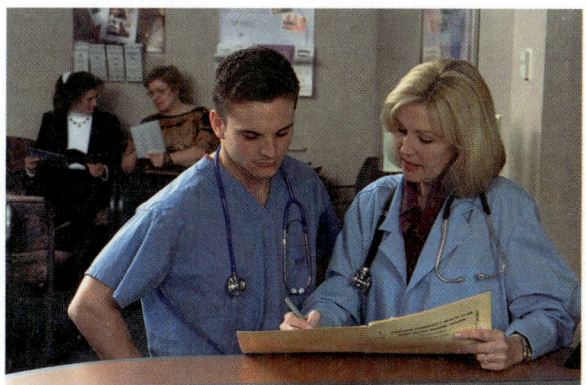

FIGURE 3-4 The externship or internship provides practical experience in the skills learned in the classroom. It is usually listed first on the medical assistant graduate's resumé; therefore, it is vital to perform well and make a good impression.

Several general rules must be remembered on the externship site. First, the medical assisting student must gain the trust of the employees there. The student should perform the assigned duties eagerly, in a timely manner, and to the best of his or her ability. If questions arise at any time, the student should ask the externship supervisor for clarification instead of assuming or performing the duties incorrectly.

It often is helpful to read the job description of the medical assistant in the facility so that the student will understand what is expected. The student medical assistant must show responsibility and dependability. The student must remain busy while at the externship site. If all assigned duties have been completed, the extern should offer to assist others in their duties or ask for additional responsibilities. Counters always need cleaning, and filing always needs to be done. The student who performs these duties without being told shows initiative and a strong work ethic. In addition, all the rules for professional appearance apply to the site and should be followed meticulously, because the student medical assistant will be working with actual patients.

The medical assistant may find it necessary to educate the patient about what a medical assistant is and does. Patients often assume that those assisting in the office are nurses, but medical assistants should never represent themselves as such. When making introductions or assisting with patients, the student medical assistant should state, "I am Sandra Ramirez, Dr. Patrick's medical assistant extern," or "I am Sandra, a medical assistant intern here in Dr. Patrick's office." These words accurately portray the duties performed and let patients know who is caring for them in the physician's office.

Externs need to know a few other rules. A medical assisting student must never attempt to form a romantic relationship with patients or co-workers on the externship site. Patient confidentiality must be respected at all times; therefore, anything the student discovers about a patient must not be revealed or discussed under any circumstances. The student can never use any of the drug samples at the office unless specifically given permission by the physician. The student should not go to the drug storage area alone without permission or unless directed to do so by the supervisor or physician. Externs should be extremely careful if asked to handle petty cash in the office. No student wants to be accused of any impropriety while performing externship duties. Students must never ask the physician to treat them or any members of their family or friends. If the

physician offers this as a benefit, it is acceptable, but it must not be assumed that the physician is available for and willing to give free treatment. An extern must not ask the physician to provide prescriptions; for liability reasons, most physicians will not prescribe medications for people who are not their patients.

The extern should bring to the physician's office **intangibles** that are not found in any job description. Courtesy toward others, a capacity for teamwork, a positive attitude, enthusiasm, initiative, and dedication are important personal attributes for the professional medical assistant. After becoming comfortable with the expectations of the externship, the student should concentrate on developing his or her skills and learning as much as possible during this short period. An extern becomes a valuable team player by assisting others and by being reliable. By performing at peak level, the student gains the respect and trust of those on the externship site, and these people can serve as excellent references when the search begins for that first paid position. Remember, the professional services of a medical assistant are extremely personal. Therefore, the manner in which these services are performed can affect the health and welfare of a patient in either a positive or a negative way. When medical assisting students do their best to make sure all contact with patients is positive, they win the praise of patients, supervisors, and co-workers alike.

BENEFITS OF AN EXTERNSHIP

- The school has a line of communication to the community and is better able to assess the needs and expectations of the public for which it is training prospective employees.
- The externship agency benefits from the new ideas and methods that the trainee may introduce. If the facility is looking for additional help, this is an ideal way to evaluate the performance of a trainee without involvement in the hiring process.
- The trainee benefits most of all by exposure to practical experience in a variety of settings. This experience in the real world removes a great deal of the anxiety that might otherwise be present in a first employment situation.

CRITICAL THINKING APPLICATION   3-4

- If Sandra has any difficulty on her externship, whom should she contact?
- What should Sandra do when she has completed her normal duties for the day at the externship site but it is not yet time to leave the clinic?
- How can Sandra gain more knowledge from her co-workers during her externship?

Continuing Education

Education does not end with the completion of formal training. The amount of medical knowledge gained in a given year is astounding. The practicing medical assistant must keep current with the rapid changes in the profession. Most physicians appreciate medical assistants who ask questions about unfamiliar conditions and procedures, and they are willing to teach students about the functioning of the body and treatments that benefit the patient. Much can be learned by reading or reviewing the medical literature that arrives in the daily mail or articles that appear in newspapers, magazines, and medically related newsletters.

Continuing education classes are available to enhance the knowledge of the professional medical assistant. **Continuing education units (CEUs)** may be required to maintain the medical assistant's certification. These credits can be obtained through many sources, including the AAMA, the American Medical Technologists (AMT), and various other agencies and educational institutions. Professional seminars and workshops often offer CEUs. Notices of continuing education classes are sent in bulk to medical facilities and physicians' offices, and staff members should watch for courses that pertain to their particular job duties and take advantage of them.

PROFESSIONAL ORGANIZATIONS

By joining a professional organization and taking part in the activities it offers, a medical assistant can grow personally and professionally, keeping abreast of current trends. Participation in a recognized professional organization shows that the employee takes his or her career seriously and wants to be an asset to the employer. Often, a medical assistant is qualified to sit for more than one type of exam; for instance, a medical assistant with 1,020 hours of clinical experience, including venipuncture, skin puncture, and specimen processing, may be able to take the phlebotomy exam. A medical assistant with 2 years' experience working as an administrative medical assistant may be eligible to take the Certified Medical Administrative Specialist (CMAS) exam. Several billing and coding certifications are available (these are discussed in more detail in Chapter 16). National organizations, state chapters of these organizations, and local groups meet to promote the profession of medical assisting. The organizations offer many benefits to members. Some offer health, disability, and malpractice insurance programs. Some offer credit card options and discount programs that are exclusive to their membership. All extend an opportunity for continuing education and learning beyond the classroom. Some schools that offer medical assistant training form local or school-based chapters of professional organizations. Both the AAMA and AMT offer discounted student memberships.

CRITICAL THINKING APPLICATION   3-5

- When should Sandra get involved with professional organizations for medical assistants?
- How can she contribute to professional organizations in her area once she has graduated and secured a position as a medical assistant?
- Why is it important that Sandra participate in volunteer organizations?

American Association of Medical Assistants and Certified Medical Assistants

The AAMA was organized formally in 1955 as a federation of several state associations that had been functioning independently. Today, the AAMA has 45 state societies and 250 local chapters. The organization, which has its national headquarters in Chicago, was the driving force behind the establishment of a national certification program for medical assistants. The AAMA also has been instrumental in the accreditation of medical assistant training programs in community colleges and private career institutes and in setting the minimum standards for entry-level medical assistants. At meetings held on national, state, and local levels, medical assistants can participate in workshops, learn about all types of advancement in the field, listen to prominent speakers, and network with other medical assistants from other parts of the country. The AAMA publishes a bimonthly journal, *CMA Today*, which includes articles with tests that may be submitted for CEU credit.

Since 1963, the AAMA has administered the Certified Medical Assistant (AAMA) examination. Those who pass the examination are awarded the CMA (AAMA) credential (Figure 3-5). Examinations are computerized and are offered continuously, year-round, at Prometric Testing and Assessment Centers throughout the United States. Certification is available to graduates of medical assisting programs accredited by the Commission on Accreditation of Allied Health Education Programs (CAAHEP) or by the Accrediting Bureau of Health Education Schools (ABHES). Recertification is required every 5 years and can be accomplished through CEUs or re-examination. Exam applications and additional information are available on the AAMA's Web site at www.aama-ntl.org.

American Medical Technologists and Registered Medical Assistants

In the early 1970s, the AMT, a national certifying body for laboratory professionals, began offering a certifying examination for medical assistants. This led to the formation of the Registered Medical Assistant (RMA) program within the AMT in 1976. The AMT offers this credential to medical assistants who meet established standards and pass the certifying examination (Figure 3-6).

Several other certification examinations are offered by the AMT that may be of interest to medical assistants. The Certified Office Laboratory Technician (COLT) examination is available to those who have completed certain educational and work experience requirements. Most medical assistants who work in the clinical area and have at least 6 months of experience are qualified to take the examination. Medical assistants also may qualify to take the examination for certification as a Registered Phlebotomy Technician (RPT), which is offered by the AMT, after meeting

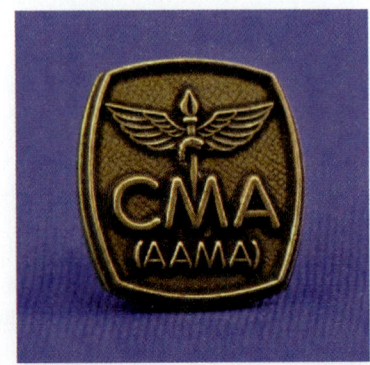

FIGURE 3-5 This pin is worn by the Certified Medical Assistant (AAMA). (Courtesy American Association of Medical Assistants, Chicago, Ill.)

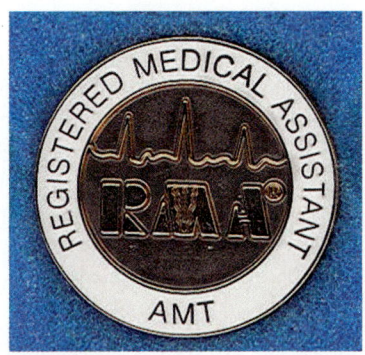

FIGURE 3-6 This pin is worn by the Registered Medical Assistant. (Courtesy RMA/American Medical Technologists, Park Ridge, Ill.)

specific work-related requirements. The examination for Certified Medical Administrative Specialist (CMAS) is offered to those who have graduated from an accredited administrative program or who have 5 years of experience in the field. RMAs with 2 years of administrative experience may also take the examination. All of these exams are computerized and can be taken at Pearson VUE centers throughout the United States. More information about the RMA examination is available on the American Medical Technologists' Web site at www.americanmedtech.org.

The AMT provides societal benefits, including publications such as *AMT Events,* a quarterly magazine with useful information and articles relating to the professions served by the organization. The AMT also offers national, state, and local meetings to enhance the knowledge and networking opportunities of its members. CEU credits are available to help increase a medical assistant's level of competence and are a requirement for those who first became certified (or will recertify) after January 1, 2006. (For more information on the AMT, visit the Evolve Web site at *evolve.elsevier.com/kinn*).

National Healthcareer Association

Some schools also offer certification through the National Health-career Association (NHA). Examinations and credentials available from the NHA include those for Certified Medical Administrative Assistant (CMAA), Certified Clinical Medical Assistant (CCMA), Certified Billing and Coding Specialist (CBCS), and Certified Medical Transcriptionist (CMT). The cost for these certification examinations ranges from about $100 to $150. More information is available on the NHA Web site at www.nhanow.com.

American Registry of Medical Assisting

The purpose of the American Registry of Medical Assistants (ARMA) is to certify and advance the position of the qualified medical assistant, to provide updated medical and social information of interest to the medical assistant through publications, and to be of service to its members. This registry is accomplished through a recommendation system, and medical assistants are not required to test to receive the registration designation; however, the organization does require CEUs. More information can be obtained on the ARMA Web site at www.arma-cert.org.

National Center for Competency Testing

The National Center for Competency Testing (NCCT) is an independent certification agency that has tested more than 240,000 individuals since 1989. The organization offers certification as a medical assistant, billing and coding specialist, medical office assistant, phlebotomy technician, patient care technician, and electrocardiography (ECG) technician. To earn an NCCT credential, candidates must meet all eligibility requirements and pass an examination based on the knowledge, skills, and abilities required at job entry. The NCCT's Web site is www.ncctinc.com.

Taking Certification Examinations

Both the CMA and RMA certifications are national credentials. As mentioned, the CMA credential is offered by the AAMA, and the RMA credential is offered by the AMT. Because medical assistants are not required to be licensed, both of these examinations are voluntary. A medical assistant may practice in the United States without either certification, but most employers today require at least one certification. Both organizations have committees that develop their certifying examinations, which are based on the roles that medical assistants fulfill in the workplace.

Students should take the examination soon after graduation; the intricate knowledge gained in school is easier to recall the sooner the exam is taken. In addition, the fee for the CMA examination goes up 1 year after the graduation date. Although the graduate is not guaranteed higher wages with certification or registration, most employers are willing to pay more for a graduate who has been through formal training and the certification or registration procedure. By registering for certification examinations soon after beginning the medical assistant training, the student can prepare throughout the classroom experience.

The CMA examination covers three general categories, including administrative, clinical, and transdisciplinary competencies. The examination is scored by tallying correct responses; therefore, making a guess does not count against the student. The minimum score to obtain the CMA credential currently is 425, and students are allowed 3 hours to complete the examination. Once the student has been approved to take the exam, the AAMA sends a testing center scheduling permit to the candidate, who then schedules the exam. The test can be scheduled at the candidate's convenience within a 90-day assigned period of the student's choice. The AAMA offers two practice tests on its Web site; these tests cover anatomy and physiology and include a medical terminology review. The AAMA requires either continuing education credits or re-examination to maintain the CMA credential.

The RMA examination can be scheduled nearly every day of the year other than Sundays and holidays at more than 200 testing centers throughout the United States, its territories, and Canada. Applicants for the RMA examination must be graduates of a medical assisting course accredited by ABHES or CAAHEP, or they must meet requirements related to their experience. The RMA examination covers administrative skills, clinical skills, and general skills and comprises more than 200 questions. Examinees are allowed 3 hours to take the test. Scoring is based on a scale, and the minimum passing score is 70. Practice examinations are available on the AMT Web site.

The AMT recently mandated a point system to prove compliance with continuing education requirements. RMAs, CMASs, and COLTs are required to earn 30 points, and RPTs are required to earn 20 points. Points can be earned through continuing education, employer evaluations, professional and formal education, and various other methods.

THE MEDICAL ASSISTANT CREED

I believe in the principles and purposes of the profession of medical assisting.
I endeavor to be more effective.
I aspire to render greater service.
I protect the confidence entrusted to me.
I am dedicated to the care and well-being of all patients.
I am loyal to my physician-employer.
I am true to the ethics of my profession.
I am strengthened by compassion, courage, and faith.

The Difference Between CMAs and RMAs

The two major differences between the CMA and RMA credentials are the examination consultant organizations and the cost. The current CMA examination fee is $125 for recent CAAHEP or ABHES graduates. The fee is $250 for nonrecent graduates and individuals who are not members of the AAMA, which administers this exam. The annual membership fees for the AAMA vary from state to state and are substantially lower if a person joins while still a student. The cost of student membership ranges from $20 to approximately $35, but the student must apply for membership before graduating. Annual dues thereafter are $67 to $107, depending on the state association. The RMA examination fee is $95, which includes the first year's dues. Annual dues thereafter currently are $50. Table 3-1 presents a detailed comparison of the CMA and RMA.

CRITICAL THINKING APPLICATION   3-6

- Why is it important for Sandra to obtain one of the medical assisting certifications after graduation?
- How important are continuing education units to the new graduate?
- How might certification help her career as a medical assistant?
- When and where can the tests be taken in your area?

CLOSING COMMENTS

This chapter has presented the advantages of becoming a trained medical assistant and some of the many career opportunities available. The skills that must be developed and the general knowledge that must be acquired to perform the duties of a medical assistant effectively have been presented. However, skills and knowledge alone do not ensure success. Personality traits and professional appearance are also critical. Professional societies and continuing education are vital to the medical assistant's career. The individual who chooses this career must be willing to accept the responsibilities inherent in its standards. The importance of obtaining national certification cannot be stressed enough.

Patient Education

Medical assistants may find it necessary to educate the patient about their scope of practice. Patients often assume that those assisting in the office are nurses, but medical assistants should never present themselves in this manner. When making introductions, the medical assistant should state, "I am Sandra Ramirez, Dr. Patrick's medical assistant." These words accurately portray the medical assistant's role and help the patient identify who is who in the physician's office.

Medical assisting has grown into one of the most respected professions in the allied health field. When asked, medical assistants should share information about their roles in the office and the training that has prepared them for their duties. Some of those who ask may be interested in a career change or have the desire to enter the medical field. Medical assistants should always be good ambassadors for their profession.

Legal and Ethical Issues

In the course of medical assistants' daily work, they must deal with a vast amount of personal and intimate information about the patients who have entrusted their care to the physician and those employed by the practice. Such information must be held in strict confidence and must never be discussed with or relayed to others, including professional associates, unless the lack of knowledge would hinder the patient's care.

On an externship or practicum, a medical assisting student should expect to observe all the office protocols of regular attendance, punctuality, and dress code. The extern should hold the rules and regulations of the office in high regard and not expect special treatment. Never expect or ask for payment for serving as an extern, because this is a part of the school curriculum.

During the externship, medical assisting students should restrict their practice to areas in which they have been trained. Know the boundaries within which medical assistants are expected to perform and do not exceed them. Some medical assistants carry their own malpractice or medical liability insurance policies; externs may be covered by a blanket policy held by their school. Remember, if ever in doubt about what is acceptable during the externship, or even in actual practice as a medical assistant, ask the physician or supervisor.

TABLE 3-1   Differences Between the Certified Medical Assistant and the Registered Medical Assistant

	CERTIFIED MEDICAL ASSISTANT (CMA)	REGISTERED MEDICAL ASSISTANT (RMA)
Credentialing organization	American Association of Medical Assistants (AAMA)	American Medical Technologists (AMT)
Address of certification or registration organization	American Association of Medical Assistants 20 N. Wacker Drive, Suite 1575 Chicago, IL 60606-2903 Telephone: 800-228-2262 or 1-312-899-1500	American Medical Technologists 10700 W. Higgins Road, Suite 150 Rosemont, IL 60018 800-275-1268 1-847-823-5169
Organization Web site	www.aama-ntl.org	www.americanmedtech.org
Mailing address for certification applications	AAMA Certification 7999 Eagle Way Chicago, IL 60678-1079	RMA Certification/AMT 10700 W. Higgins Road, Suite 150 Rosemont, IL 60018
Requirement for certification or registration	Federal licensing is not required; certification or registration is optional in most states.	Federal licensing is not required; certification or registration is optional in most states.
Qualifications for taking the examination	Applicants must fall into one of three categories to qualify to take the CMA examination: • Category one: Graduating student or recent graduate of a medical assisting program accredited by the Commission on Accreditation of Allied Health Education Programs (CAAHEP) or the Accrediting Bureau of Health Education Schools (ABHES) • Category two: Non-recent graduate of a medical assisting program accredited by CAAHEP or ABHES • Category three: Recertificant	• Good moral character and at least 18 years old • High school graduate or acceptable equivalent • Graduate of or scheduled to graduate from one of the following: Must meet one of five eligibility routes, including: ○ Route 1—Education: a recent graduate of, or scheduled to graduate from, an accredited medical assistant program; ○ Route 2—Military: a recent graduate of, or scheduled to graduate from, a formal medical services training program of the United States Armed Forces; ○ Route 3—Work Experience: employed as a medical assistant for five of the last seven years, no more than two years as a medical assisting instructor; ○ Route 4—Instructor: must be currently instructing and must have completed a course of instruction in a healthcare discipline related to medical assisting; ○ Route 5—Passed another certifying organization's certification exam approved by the AMT Board of Directors • Must have 5 years of work experience unless graduated from the medical assisting program within the last 3 years
Examination approval organization	National Board of Medical Examiners (NBME) www.nbme.org	National Commission for Certifying Agencies (NCCA) www.noca.org/ncca/ncca.htm
Cost of examination	AAMA members and recent graduates: $125 Non-recent graduates and nonmembers: $250	$95 (membership in the AMT is not required)
Duration of examination	3 hours	3 hours
Content of examination	200 computerized questions covering general or transdisciplinary skills, clinical skills, and administrative skills	More than 200 computerized questions covering general subject areas, clinical areas, and administrative areas
Testing sites	More than 200 centers throughout the United States; applicants are assigned to a center after they have been approved to take the examination. A list of testing sites is available at www.prometric.com.	More than 200 centers throughout the United States A list of testing sites is available at www.pearsonvue.com/amt.
Web sites for obtaining a practice test	www.aama-ntl.org/becomeCMA/exam_outline.aspx	AMT Web site: www.amt1.com
Testing dates	Apply for a 90-day window, then schedule the exam within that window at a convenient date and time. Testing dates are ongoing and are arranged at Prometric Testing and Assessment Centers throughout the United States.	Testing dates are ongoing and are arranged at Pearson VUE Centers throughout the United States.

SUMMARY OF SCENARIO

Sandra has chosen to embark on an exciting career and will find her work rewarding. She knows that she will be proud of her efforts and looks forward to becoming a respected member of the healthcare team in a physician's office. She has set goals for her class work and attendance and is determined to meet them. Obstacles usually arise whenever a person embarks on a new project, and Sandra must plan for the days that she or her child may be ill or her transportation fails. She should have a backup plan in place to help her overcome minor setbacks.

Many opportunities exist for the medical assistant in both administrative and clinical positions, and as Sandra progresses through her training, she will find areas that appeal to her more than others. However, all her courses will be vital to her development as a versatile medical assistant, able to perform front-office and back-office duties. She will be exposed to various duties during her externship, and these experiences will help her determine where she might enjoy working once she graduates. It is important that Sandra gain as much experience and knowledge as possible while in school, so that she will have more options after her training.

Sandra should develop a good relationship with her instructors and go to them when she has questions or concerns. These professionals are anxious to share their knowledge and experience with students to best prepare them for the work environment. If Sandra's grades ever drop or if she is struggling, she should seek the advice of the instructor to determine how to improve her performance. The externship also is crucial, because it usually is the first medical reference a new graduate will have. Sandra should bring any difficulties at the externship site to the attention of the externship supervisor or an instructor at her school. Learning to set goals will help her achieve more throughout her education, and this is a habit she should carry into her career.

With so many benefits available at different facilities in the medical field, Sandra must carefully weigh what she needs for herself and her son before taking any position. Many physicians' offices now offer evening and weekend hours; Sandra may have to adjust her schedule to fit those working hours, or she may stick to her original desire to find a job without evening or weekend shifts. She should look at all of her options and choose the best one after careful evaluation.

For now, Sandra should spend her time in school getting to know her instructors and understanding their expectations. In addition, she should study hard, learn to budget time and money, and discover as much as possible about the field of medical assisting. These efforts will pay off in satisfaction with her chosen career and in the job she ultimately accepts.

SUMMARY OF LEARNING OBJECTIVES

1. **Define, spell, and pronounce the terms listed in the vocabulary.**
   Spelling and pronouncing medical terms correctly bolster the medical assistant's credibility. Knowing the definition of these terms promotes confidence in communication with patients and co-workers.

2. **Briefly discuss the history of medical assisting as a profession.**
   The first medical assistants probably were neighbors and friends of the physician. The field has grown into one of the most respected and versatile professions in allied health.

3. **Discuss the versatility of a career in medical assisting.**
   Medical assistants are versatile enough to work in many different settings. Most are employed in physicians' offices, but they also work in hospitals, insurance companies, clinics, laboratories, and many other facilities. The combination of administrative and clinical training makes the medical assistant quite valuable to the employer.

4. **Differentiate between administrative and clinical medical assisting duties and recognize the importance of becoming knowledgeable about the general responsibilities of the medical assistant.**
   Administrative duties involve running the office, such as scheduling appointments and filing insurance claims. Administrative medical assistants usually spend most of the day in the front office of the facility. Clinical duties include more patient contact and assisting the physician in the back office. New graduates often move toward one or the other division, but they should always be ready and willing to adapt to new duties or to substitute in other areas when necessary.

5. **Comprehend the current employment outlook for the medical assistant.**
   According to the Department of Labor, the medical assisting field is projected to grow much faster than the average for all occupations, with a 35% expected growth from 2006 to 2016. The projected employment for 2016 is 565,000 medical assistants.

6. **Give the reasons that hiring an individual with no formal training often is more expensive than hiring a professional medical assistant.**
   Untrained assistants often make errors that are costly to the practice, and these assistants require much more supervision; this means that the supervisor's time is not used for the duties that he or she would normally perform, because the medical assistant is not completely able to work alone. Formal training and certification are valuable not only to the medical assistant, but also to the physician-employer.

7. **Identify several considerations to keep in mind, other than financial compensation, when choosing a position as a medical assistant.**
   The medical assistant should consider many factors other than the salary when choosing a position. Location, perks, benefits, and the atmosphere of the office all are important. Many assistants are interested in growth within the organization and welcome those opportunities. Working for a friendly, caring physician and/or supervisor is invaluable. Sometimes, taking a lesser position in a well-known and reputable facility is

temporarily worth a lower wage because of future opportunities. Consider all aspects of a position before accepting a job offer.

8. **Discuss the aspects of the medical assistant's performance on a successful externship.**

   The medical assisting externship offers the student an opportunity to put the skills learned in the classroom to good use. If completed successfully, the externship is an excellent reference for the resumé. Students should perform at the optimal level and never hesitate to complete duties assigned. Offer to go above and beyond to secure the support of the externship site as the job search begins.

9. **List three unacceptable behaviors on the externship site.**

   A student medical assistant extern should never attempt to form relationships with patients outside the office or read patients' charts for personal information. Do not ask the physician to treat family members, and do not take medications without explicit permission from the physician or supervisor. Be very careful when handling cash and drugs in the office. The student should make every effort never to be late to the externship site unless a true emergency occurs.

10. **Explain why continuing education is so important to the medical assistant.**

    Continuing education is important to medical assistants because it enables them to learn the latest trends and information and understand how to use them. Take advantage of local seminars and continuing education classes. Often the employer will agree to pay for classes or seminars that the medical assistant takes if they relate to his or her employment at the facility. Some employers will provide tuition reimbursement for college expenses, often even if the college courses are not related to the position the employee holds at the facility.

11. **Understand the medical assistant credentialing requirements, the importance of credentialing, and the process of obtaining credentials.**

    Most physicians prefer a credentialed medical assistant when making hiring decisions. Information about the credentialing process is available from the AAMA and AMT Web sites and from other certifying organizations.

12. **Discuss the difference between a CMA and a RMA.**

    The main difference between the CMA and RMA credentials is the agency that provides the certification. The CMA credential is awarded by the AAMA, and the RMA credential is awarded by the AMT. Both are nationally recognized certifications.

CONNECTIONS

Study Guide Connection: Go to the Chapter 3 Study Guide. Read and complete the activities.

Evolve Connection: Go to the Chapter 3 link at *evolve.elsevier.com/kinn* to complete the Chapter Review and Chapter Quiz. Check out the other resources listed for this chapter to make the most of what you have learned from The Medical Assisting Profession.

4

PROFESSIONAL BEHAVIOR IN THE WORKPLACE

Karen Yon has wanted to work in the medical field for most of her adult life. She studied very hard in high school and graduated with honors. She volunteered in a local hospital and then, after working as a server in restaurants for 3 years, she enrolled in medical assisting classes. After her externship, she was asked to continue as a regular employee at a family practice in her area.

Karen strives to perform all her duties professionally and compassionately. She maintains a professional image for patients and co-workers. She had found it difficult to learn to be professional at all times and show compassion to patients through just the classroom experience. However, she knew that these were important aspects of her job, and she was able to gain valuable experience in these areas during her externship. Because this is her first job in the medical field, she wants to make a good impression on her employer and to be a team player.

Throughout most of Karen's training as a medical assistant, her grandmother was confined to a rehabilitation center after a stroke. Although she has progressed well with treatment, Karen is the only relative who lives close to the rehabilitation center, and her family depends on her to check on her grandmother from time to time. Karen enjoys spending time at the center reading to her grandmother, because they are close. Still, Karen realizes that the stroke has caused permanent damage, and her grandmother's health seems to be declining.

While studying this chapter, think about the following questions:

- How do professional medical assistants put aside personal issues and devote themselves to the patients in the office?
- How can Karen meet her family and work obligations equally well?
- What steps should Karen take to ensure that both her family and her supervisors understand her obligations to the other?
- How can Karen exhibit professional behavior and compassion for patients on a daily basis at the physician's office?

LEARNING OBJECTIVES

1. Define, spell, and pronounce the terms listed in the vocabulary.
2. Explain the reasons professionalism is important in the medical field.
3. Discuss several of the characteristics of professionalism.
4. Explain why confidentiality is so important in the medical profession.
5. Discuss the importance of the medical assistant's attitude in caring for patients.
6. List some examples of office politics.
7. Identify specific ways teamwork can be promoted in the physician's office.
8. Discuss the meaning of *insubordination* and why it is grounds for dismissal.
9. Identify and implement time management principles to maintain efficient office function.
10. Talk about goal setting and how it helps a person achieve career success.
11. Discuss how substance abuse can impact the medical assistant's employment.

VOCABULARY

characteristics Distinguishing traits, qualities, or properties.

commensurate (ku-men′-su-rut) Corresponding in size, amount, extent, or degree; equal in measure, proportionate.

competent Having adequate or requisite capabilities.

connotation (kah-nuh-ta′-shun) An implication; something suggested by a word or thing.

credibility The quality or power of inspiring belief.

demeanor (di-me′-nur) Behavior toward others; outward manner.

detrimental (de-truh-men′-til) Obviously harmful or damaging.

discretion (dis-kre′-shun) The quality of being discreet; having or showing good judgment or conduct, especially in speech.

disseminated (di-se′-muh-na-ted) To disburse; to spread around.

drug of choice The drug an abuser uses most frequently to satisfy the craving for a certain feeling; the user's preferred drug.

initiative Energy or aptitude to cause or facilitate the start of something or to cause something to happen.

insubordination (in-suh′-bor-din-a-shun) Disobedience to authority.

morale (mo-ral′) The mental and emotional condition, enthusiasm, loyalty, or confidence of an individual or group with regard to the function or tasks at hand.

optimistic Inclined to put the most favorable construction on actions and events or to anticipate the best possible outcome.

persona (pur-so′-nuh) An individual's social facade or front that reflects the role in life the individual is playing; the personality a person projects in public.

professionalism The conduct or qualities characterized by or conforming to the technical or ethical standards of a profession; exhibiting a courteous, conscientious, and generally businesslike manner in the workplace.

reproach An expression of rebuke or disapproval; a cause or occasion of blame, discredit, or disgrace.

tolerance The need to use more and more of a substance to get the same feeling as the body learns to tolerate the drug.

work ethics A set of values based on the moral virtues of hard work and diligence.

What is professional behavior? We tend to hold medical personnel to a higher standard of professionalism than those in most other career fields. The medical assistant who works to improve his or her professional approach in the workplace is an asset to the employer and will quickly be promoted to positions of more responsibility in the healthcare industry. Some employers are more concerned about medical assistants' professional behavior and interpersonal skills than their clinical skills, because the way that the medical assistant approaches and interacts with patients is critical to the success of the practice. Professionalism is useful not only in the physician's office; it also is a valuable skill when dealing with other business professionals in everyday life, such as a teacher or business owner.

THE MEANING OF PROFESSIONALISM

Professionalism is defined as having a courteous, conscientious, and generally businesslike manner in the workplace. It is characterized by or conforms to the technical or ethical standards of a certain profession. Conducting themselves in a professional manner is essential for successful medical assistants. The attitude of those in the medical profession generally is more conservative than that seen in other career fields. Patients expect professional behavior and base much of their trust and confidence in those who show this type of **demeanor** in the physician's office (Figure 4-1).

WORK ETHICS

Work ethics are sets of values based on the moral virtues of hard work and diligence, involving a whole range of activities, from individual acts to the philosophy of the entire facility. The medical assistant should always display initiative and be reliable. A person

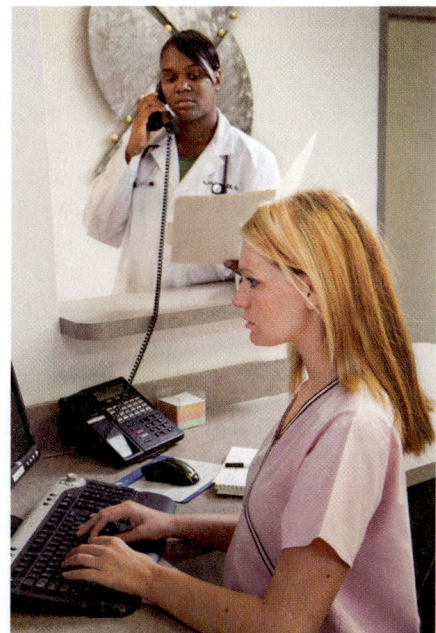

FIGURE 4-1 The professional medical assistant is an asset to the physician's office.

who has a good work ethic is one who arrives on time, who is rarely absent, whose work output is **commensurate** with the pay received, and who uses his or her best abilities. Co-workers become frustrated if another employee consistently arrives late or is absent. This forces the co-workers to take on additional duties and may prevent them from completing their own work. One missing employee can disrupt the entire day, because patients may not be seen at their appointment times because the staff is shorthanded. Also, lunch and other breaks may be shortened because the staff cannot process cases as quickly when an employee does not show up. All employees should know the attendance policies in their facility as outlined in the policy and procedure manual.

Most new hires have a probationary period that may last 30 to 90 days. Any absences or tardiness during the probationary period can be grounds to terminate the employee once the probationary period is up or even before that if multiple attendance issues arise. If the medical assistant has an emergency and must be absent or tardy, he or she should make sure to notify the supervisor according to office policy. All employees must be on time and in attendance every day in the medical office. Physicians and patients alike expect this reliability.

Work ethics also apply to other situations. If another employee is seen taking drugs from the supply cabinet or money from the cash box, the act should certainly be reported. However, if the guilty employee is also a close friend of the person who witnesses the act, an ethical dilemma arises. A medical assistant must always act in such a way that his or her actions are above **reproach**.

CHARACTERISTICS OF PROFESSIONALISM

Many **characteristics** make up the professionalism required of medical assistants. Student medical assistants should begin developing these characteristics while in school; these qualities do not appear magically when the student begins working with actual patients. Although we might think that we would always behave appropriately during an externship or in a job setting, the habits developed in school will carry over into these experiences. If the behavior is unacceptable, it will be **detrimental** to the medical assistant's professional career. If the medical assistant wishes to advance and receive wage increases, promotions, and the trust of the employer, the characteristics discussed in the following sections must be a part of his or her **persona**.

> ### CRITICAL THINKING APPLICATION   4-1
> - How can students practice professional behavior while still in the classroom situation?
> - When students are practicing clinical skills, how can they demonstrate proficiency in professional behavior?

Loyalty

Loyalty is faithfulness or allegiance to a cause, ideal, custom, institution, or product. Loyalty to an employer means that the employee is appreciative of the opportunity provided by the job and supports the company by giving the best effort possible. Many individuals today are interested only in what the employer can provide for them. However, this is an immature approach to take toward a job. When a person is employed by a company, use of skills is exchanged for different types of compensation. Each benefits the other. Often we forget that experience alone is a great benefit from working. Loyalty to the employer is important, and in return the employee should feel a sense of loyalty from the company.

> ### CRITICAL THINKING APPLICATION   4-2
> - How can Karen demonstrate loyalty to her employer?
> - What are some ways her employer can reciprocate Karen's loyalty?

Dependability

One of the most valuable traits of a successful medical assistant is dependability. The physician and supervisors must know that they can depend on the medical assistant to perform all of the assigned duties each day. A medical assistant must follow through when the physician or supervisor gives an order. Be responsible enough to know the job description and what is expected on a daily, weekly, and monthly basis. Supervisors should be confident that once given a task to do, the medical assistant will carry it out accurately and in a timely manner.

Courtesy

Show courtesy to the patients and your co-workers in the physician's office. Kind words and compassion go far in building trust between the medical assistant and patients (Figure 4-2). All visitors and staff members in the office should be shown kindness and consideration. The fact that a medical assistant is having a bad day is no excuse for inflicting anger or irritation onto patients. Always demonstrate a good attitude and offer patients and visitors a sincere smile.

Initiative

Lack of **initiative** is one of the more common complaints from supervisors about employees. Taking initiative means that the medical assistant looks for opportunities to be of help, assisting others as the workload demands. Instead of waiting to be told to perform a task, the **competent** medical assistant looks for jobs that need to be completed. Never remain idle. Employees can always find tasks to complete in the medical office. For example, filing is a continual need. Supplies can be inventoried, ordered, or restocked when extra time is available. Cleaning countertops and straightening areas as work is done helps keep the facility tidy. The medical assistant should also keep an eye on the reception area, which may need attention several times during the day.

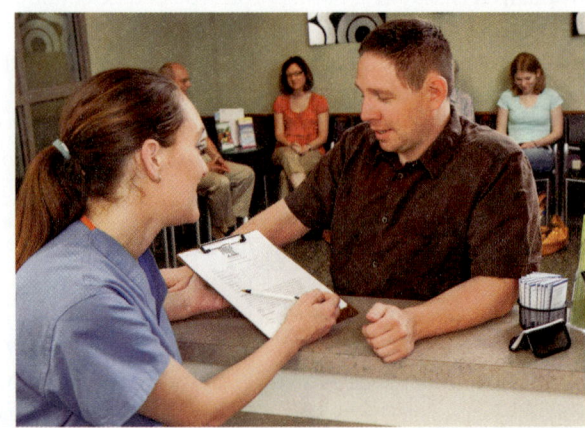

FIGURE 4-2 Taking a few moments to explain forms and bills to a patient is a courteous way to prevent misunderstandings and to promote goodwill.

CRITICAL THINKING APPLICATION   4-3
- How can Karen show her initiative on the job?
- What types of duties can she perform if she has finished her work for the day and some time is left before she is scheduled to leave?

Flexibility

A medical assistant must be able to adapt to a wide variety of situations. An emergency could occur in the office, and the staff must be flexible enough to adjust the schedule and care for all patients. Being flexible also means that staff members are willing to assist one another in the performance of their duties. No one in the physician's office should ever say, "That's not my job." The patients must come first, and every staff member must be willing to lend a hand where needed. Some medical assistants trade or rotate their duties. If one assistant does not particularly enjoy doing a certain task, perhaps another assistant would be willing to trade tasks. This way, both are more satisfied with their jobs. If the medical assistant is able to adapt to various situations quickly and cheerfully, he or she becomes a valuable asset to the office.

Credibility

Credibility is the perceived competence or character of a person, leading to the belief that the individual can be trusted. Because trust is a vital component of the physician-patient relationship, the credibility of the physician and those who assist in the office should be strong. The information provided to patients must be accurate. Patients expect that the physician and medical assistant instruct them in a manner that enhances their health and provides positive results. A medical assistant must take care in giving any advice to patients, because they view the medical assistant as an agent of the physician. Patients may not distinguish between the medical assistant's comments and the physician's orders. Remember that giving anything that could be construed as medical advice is outside the scope of the duties of the medical assistant. To avoid facing charges of practicing medicine without a license, a medical assistant must be sure to suggest only what the physician has authorized.

Confidentiality

The importance of confidentiality in the medical environment cannot be stressed enough. Patients are entitled to privacy where their health is concerned, and they should be confident that medical professionals use information only to care for them. Never reveal any information about any patient to anyone without specific permission to do so. Always verify that the person seeking information has the right to see it and that the patient has signed a consent form allowing a third party to view the record. Casual conversations in hallways, elevators, and break rooms between staff members can be overheard by a family member or friend of the patient. Confidentiality is often breached in these areas of the medical office.

The rules regarding confidentiality extend beyond the medical office. At home, medical assistants should not discuss details about patients with their families and friends. Those outside the medical profession do not understand how vital it is to keep information confidential and may pass along private or damaging facts to others. Medical assistants must make it a rule never to discuss a patient with

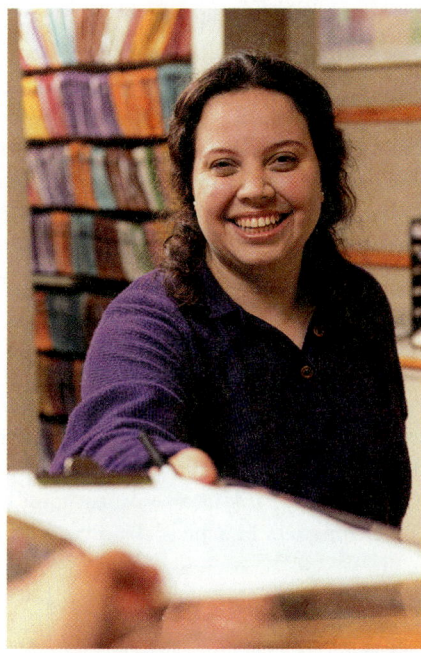

FIGURE 4-3 A good attitude goes a long way in supporting good patient and staff relationships.

anyone unless information must be shared for the patient's care and treatment. The Health Insurance Portability and Accountability Act (HIPAA) was passed in part to ensure patient confidentiality. (HIPAA is discussed in more detail in later chapters.)

Attitude

Possibly the most important asset a medical assistant brings to the office is a good attitude. A good attitude is characterized by courtesy and kindness to others, refraining from jumping to conclusions, giving the other person the benefit of the doubt, and being **optimistic**. This trait alone can influence promotions, terminations, and the entire atmosphere of the office (Figure 4-3). Individuals are able to control their attitudes with practice. It takes skill to react calmly to people who are very upset rather than to respond in kind, especially if you are being harassed or accused. Speaking in an even tone and perhaps a little softer than normal forces the listener to lower his or her voice to hear. Offer to help resolve the problem and attempt to move to a private room to talk, out of the hearing of other patients. Always have a good attitude with co-workers and be willing to assist them with their duties, especially on hectic days.

OBSTRUCTIONS TO PROFESSIONALISM

At times it is not easy to be a professional. Sometimes patients, co-workers, and supervisors try our patience, and it can be difficult to maintain a professional attitude in these cases. Some of the obstructions to professional behavior are discussed in this section.

Personal Problems and "Baggage"

Everyone has a life outside the workplace, and sometimes we face challenges and difficult times that are hard to put aside. During working hours, our thoughts should be on the job at hand, especially when we are dealing with patients. However, some situations in our lives may be so critical or distracting that we find ourselves thinking of them constantly. This personal baggage can interfere with our ability to perform job duties properly.

When a situation intrudes on our thoughts at work, it often is best to take the time to talk with a supervisor. It is not always necessary to share the intimate details, but a quick explanation that some difficulties are occurring outside of work helps the supervisor to understand any changes in habit or attitude. Some supervisors are uncaring and are concerned only with satisfactory job performance. The medical assistant must use some **discretion** in discussing private affairs with the supervisor.

The professional medical assistant never transfers personal problems or baggage to anyone at the medical facility, especially patients. The workday should be centered around patient care; therefore, do not allow personal business to impinge on time that should be spent assisting patients and the physician. The patient must be the prime concern of all the employees in a medical facility.

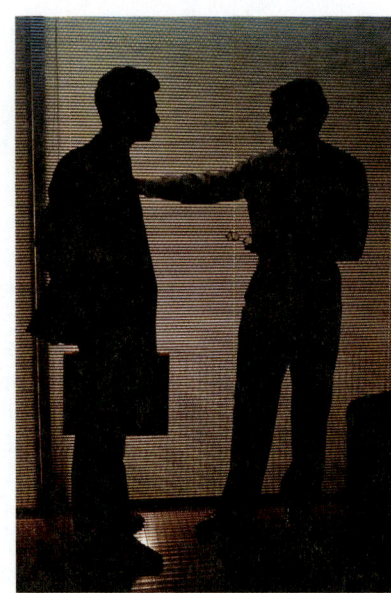

FIGURE 4-4 Gossip and rumors have no place in the medical profession. Avoid employees who participate in this type of activity.

> ### CRITICAL THINKING APPLICATION   4-4
> It often is difficult to keep from thinking about a problem while you are working. How can Karen do this if she is concerned about a grandmother who is critically ill?

Rumors and the "Grapevine"

A rumor is talk or widely **disseminated** opinion with no discernible source, or a statement that is not known to be true. The definition alone suggests that spreading rumors should be avoided. Most people enjoy working in an environment in which employees cooperate and get along with each other, but rumors can cause problems with employee **morale** and often are great exaggerations or manipulations of the truth. By promoting the grapevine, rumors are passed along and become more and more outrageous with each retelling. A medical assistant should refuse to participate in the office rumor mill and should attempt to be cordial and friendly to everyone at work (Figure 4-4). Supervisors regard those who spread or discuss rumors as unprofessional and untrustworthy. Avoid passing along work-related rumors to patients, family, and friends.

Personal Phone Calls and Business

The medical assistant should not take unnecessary phone calls from friends and family at the office. The office phone is a business line and must be used as such, except in emergencies. Using personal cell phones during working hours is not acceptable. Use breaks and lunch hours to take care of business on the phone. Never take a personal call or respond to text messages on a cell phone while working with a patient. If a phone must be carried, place it on the vibrate setting and always step into a hall or break area if a call absolutely must be taken. This should happen only in rare cases. Visitors should not frequent the office, especially the area where the medical assistant is working. If someone must come to the office, always offer the reception area as a waiting room. Visitors should never be allowed to enter patient areas.

Checking personal e-mail also should be avoided in the work-place. Any type of personal business, such as studying, looking up information on the Internet for personal use, Internet shopping,

or balancing a personal checkbook should be done at home and not in the office. All of these actions distract the medical assistant from the job at hand; the focus should be on serving the patients in the office at all times. Many employees are fired each year for surfing or shopping on the Internet for personal reasons or for checking personal e-mail. Make sure all personal business is handled outside of business hours.

> ### CRITICAL THINKING APPLICATION   4-5
> - Karen has a friend who works in a video store a few doors down from her office. Her friend has started stopping in daily on her lunch hour to chat with Karen. How can Karen politely discourage this?
> - Karen feels the need to check on her grandmother's condition as often as possible during the days she is ill. How might she accomplish this in a professional way?

Office Politics

Most people associate office politics with some underhanded scheme or plans to move upward in the company in whatever way possible, whether the methods used are ethical or not. The tendency is to give the word *politics* a negative **connotation**, and that is usually correct. Politics can be defined as the art or science of influencing and guiding government or some other organization. The same can be applied to medical office politics. When an individual wishes to move upward in an organization, he or she may use a positive or negative strategy. Many people develop a specific plan regarding how they will advance and in what time period they will accomplish their goals. Medical assistants who want to advance should be productive workers, accept responsibility, be dependable, and always conduct themselves in a professional manner. Using underhanded techniques and instigating trouble is not an effective method of career advancement. Those who use negative office politics often find that their methods turn into disasters and they lose the support of co-workers

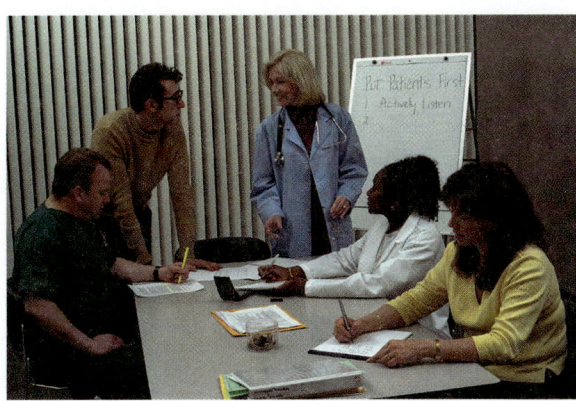

FIGURE 4-5 Teamwork is a vital part of the medical profession. All staff members must work together to care for the patient and perform required duties in the physician's office.

and supervisors, making the work environment tense and anxious. Often, they seek other employment, but if they continue negative office politics in their new office, they will likely face the same results and find themselves without a job.

PROFESSIONAL ATTRIBUTES

Teamwork

If managers were asked to name the most important attributes for medical professionals, teamwork would be high on the list (Figure 4-5). Staff members must work together for the good of the patients. They must be willing to perform duties outside the formal job description if they are needed in other areas of the office. Many supervisors frown on employees who state, "That's not in my job description." Any order that is given by a supervisor becomes mandatory, and an individual who refuses to perform an assigned task can have his or her employment terminated for **insubordination**. A medical assistant should perform the duty and later discuss with the supervisor any valid reasons that the task should have been assigned to someone else. However, if the task is illegal, unethical, or places the patient or anyone else in danger, it should not be done. Discuss the situation with the supervisor above the one who ordered the task; in many cases, this would be the physician.

Although we all would enjoy working in an office where everyone gets along and likes every other employee, this does not always happen. Personal feelings must be set aside at work, and all employees must cooperate with others to get the job done efficiently. If a medical assistant has an issue with another employee, the first move would be to discuss it privately with the other person. If the situation does not improve, perhaps a supervisor should be involved for further discussions.

Time Management

We have often heard the expression "work smart." This means that we are to use our time efficiently and concentrate on the most important duties first. To do this, we must first prioritize our duties and arrange our schedules to ensure that these duties can be performed. The first way to improve time management is to plan the tasks that need to be done that day. Taking 10 minutes to write down the tasks for the day helps ensure that they are done. Then, stay on

schedule throughout the day, unless you are interrupted by emergencies. Even then, when office days are well planned, allowances can be made for emergencies and most tasks can still be completed. The key to managing time is prioritizing.

Prioritizing

Prioritizing is simply deciding which tasks are most important. Many people make a "to do" list for the day's activities, but the secret to success is prioritizing those activities into categories that give order to the tasks.

Most tasks can be prioritized into three general categories: those that *must* be done that day, those that *should* be done that day, and those that *could* be done if time permits. Once a general list of tasks has been established, review the list and further prioritize it, using a code such as *M* for must, *S* for should, and *C* for could (or this might be further simplified by using the letters *A*, *B*, and *C*). Once the tasks have been divided into these categories, they can be further classified in each section. For instance, if category *A* (must be done that day) has six tasks, they can be numbered in the order they should be performed. The same process is completed with the tasks in categories *B* and *C*. As the tasks are completed, they are checked off for that day. Other categories can be added to customize the list. For example, an *H* category can be used for duties to perform at home, *P* could represent phone calls that need to be made, *E* could represent errands to run, and *EM* might represent e-mails to be sent. Customizing the categories makes the list more user-friendly and helps the user to meet his or her individual needs.

Setting Goals

Individuals who succeed in life are planners and goal setters. The first step in becoming a proficient goal setter is to take the time to really think about what is to be accomplished throughout one's lifetime. These goals must be written down and reviewed often. Goals should be set for all areas in a person's life, including personal growth, career, home life, family, spiritual needs, and any others that apply to the individual. The goals should not be unreasonable. They should be measurable and specific, with written steps detailing how they will be reached. Determination and persistence in reaching the goals helps make them happen, along with hard work. The goals should be reviewed often and progress evaluated. Reset goals whenever necessary and celebrate accomplishments.

> **CRITICAL THINKING APPLICATION   4-6**
> - What are some goals Karen might set regarding her behavior on the job?
> - List several goals for the new medical assistant to work toward during his or her first year on the job.

KNOWING THE FACILITY AND ITS EMPLOYEES

A much-circulated story tells of a college professor who used to end a critical test with the question, "What is the name of the woman who cleans our wing of the building?" This would perplex most students, but the question makes a good point. A professional medical assistant should attempt to get to know the people who work in the facility and should have a good idea of

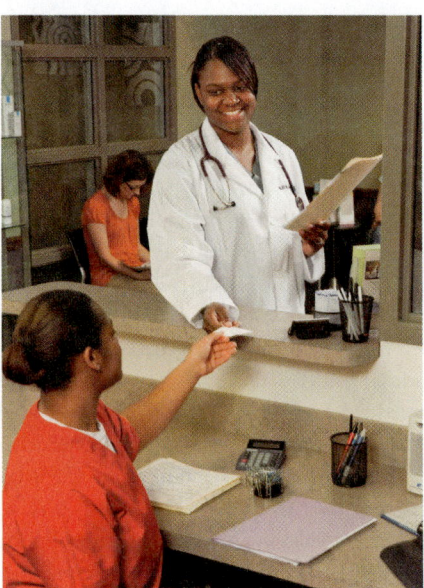

FIGURE 4-6 Knowing which employee to call when help is needed promotes goodwill among employees and often gets a task done more efficiently.

who handles which duties (Figure 4-6). When patients have specific problems with which they need help, they can be referred to the person who knows the most about that particular issue. It is wise to express appreciation to others whenever possible. Say "thank you" or "I appreciate your help" often when working with others. This makes co-workers more likely to assist at other times when their help is needed.

DOCUMENTATION

From the standpoint of professional behavior, documentation skills are vital to medical assistants. Charting accurately with legible, neat handwriting can make a difference in the perception of professionalism in the medical office. Complete, accurate EMR entries are critical as well, and a thorough knowledge of the computer program used in the office will enhance the providers' ability to provide competent patient care. Be complete in any narrative regarding patients. Be sure to state facts, not opinions, and never use sarcastic remarks when charting. Phone messages must be documented carefully as well and handled in a professional manner. Never use sarcasm when reporting messages to the physician or anyone else in the office. Use conservative speech, proper wording, and good grammar in all situations in the medical facility.

Note Taking

Whenever office meetings or seminars are held, be prepared by having a pad and pencil ready for note taking. A medical assistant should never be without paper and pen so that accurate information from the meeting can be jotted down for future reference. It is wise to keep a notebook or file on office meetings for reference in case clarification of an order or a point is needed. Keep a small spiral notebook in a pocket with a pen so that if an order is given in passing by the physician, you have a place to jot it down until you have access to the patient's chart. This can help you avoid administering incorrect dosages of medication or forgetting to order a laboratory test, in addition to many other errors that could be made by relying on memory. If notebook, pad, or personal desk assistants (PDAs) are used, notes can be easily uploaded and organized in whatever manner the medical assistant finds helpful. However, do not hold up meetings or disrupt them as information is typed into the machines (long nails are especially disruptive and should be kept trimmed and neat).

INTERPERSONAL SKILLS

Interpersonal skills are paramount in working with patients and other health professionals. A medical assistant should work to perfect his or her communication techniques. Often the success of a business is directly related to the ability of its employees to communicate effectively.

When speaking to patients and providing them with information, remember that most do not have any medical background and do not understand many of the phrases used by the medical community. A medical assistant must be patient and explain in a courteous manner any aspect of the instructions or details that the patient does not understand. When educating the patient, the medical assistant should have a professional attitude of concern and helpfulness. Assure the patient that medical assistants and the rest of the staff in the facility are bound by rules of patient confidentiality if the patient seems concerned about revealing information.

SUBSTANCE ABUSE

All employees of medical facilities must avoid drug and alcohol abuse (also called *substance abuse*), which is defined as the repeated and excessive use of a substance, despite its destructive effects, to produce pleasure and escape reality. Substance abuse includes the use of illegal and legal drugs. Many facilities require screening before employment, and some perform screenings randomly during employment. Because drugs and alcohol remain in the body for various lengths of time, an individual who uses on a Sunday afternoon may still have residual effects on Monday. This can prevent a medical assistant from performing at maximum capacity and can cause mistakes that may even be life-threatening to the patient. Also, the drive to and from work can result in an accident. Fatal or not, anytime substance abuse results in harm to another person, the user is at risk of lawsuits and legal problems. By abusing drugs even once, the medical assistant can damage his or her career irreparably.

A person is considered to have a substance abuse problem if at least one of the following four criteria is met:
- Continued use despite social or interpersonal problems
- Repeated use that results in failure to fulfill obligations at work, school, and/or home
- Repeated use that results in physically hazardous situations
- Use that results in legal problems

Before a person is labeled an abuser, however, the medical assistant should understand the differences between use, dependence, abuse, and addiction. Most people use some type of drug or supplement, many on a daily basis. If a patient takes a blood pressure medication, he or she uses that drug for a specific purpose that provides a health benefit. Physical dependence is not always part of the definition of addiction. Some drugs cause a physical dependence but not an addiction, such as a medication for diabetes. The patient depends on the drug to relieve the symptoms of the disease, but the drug usually is not abused or used in a way that would be considered an addiction. *Abuse* is the use of illegal drugs or the misuse of prescription and over-the-counter drugs.

Anyone who experiences at least three of the following seven criteria in the same 12-month period could be considered an abuser and should seek drug and alcohol counseling:

- Tolerance for the drug
- Withdrawal symptoms
- Difficulty controlling drug use
- Negative consequences from drug use
- Significant time or emotional energy spent seeking drugs
- Neglect of regular activities
- A desire to cut down on the use of a certain drug

Addiction is the compulsive use of a substance despite its negative and sometimes dangerous effects. The abuse of prescription drugs is a growing concern in the United States. Many of these drugs alter brain activity and are highly addictive, and as a result, the user's behavior changes. Opioids, central nervous system depressants, anti-anxiety drugs, and stimulants are the most common categories of prescription drug abuse. Once users are addicted, their ability to make voluntary decisions changes and a craving leads to a state of constantly seeking the **drug of choice**. Most physicians are opposed to hiring a person with a history of or convictions for substance abuse. Often, personal relationships and careers are destroyed, and this can lead to theft to buy drugs or alcohol. (For more information on the most commonly abused drugs and symptoms of substance abuse, visit the Evolve site at *evolve.elsevier.com/kinn.*)

According to the National Institute on Alcohol Abuse and Alcoholism (NIAAA), alcohol abuse is a disease that has the following four symptoms:

- *Craving*—a strong urge or need to drink
- *Loss of control*—the inability to stop drinking once it has begun
- *Physical dependence*—the occurrence of withdrawal symptoms after drinking (e.g., shakiness, nausea, sweating, and anxiety)
- **Tolerance**—the need to increase the amount of alcohol taken in to get the same effect

The potential to abuse alcohol is partly inherited, and the individual lifestyle may also influence whether a person becomes an alcoholic. This does not mean that a person who is a child of an alcoholic will definitely become an alcoholic, but the risk is greater when alcoholism is prevalent in the family. Treatment for alcoholism works for many people. Some never drink again, but others may go for months or years without drinking and still suffer a relapse; still others are simply unable to stop drinking for any length of time.

In the physician's office, one question opens the door to talk about alcoholism and helps to diagnose patients, including employees, with alcohol problems. That question is, "On any single occasion in the past 3 months, have you had more than five drinks containing alcohol?" A positive answer should lead to more questions about the individual's drinking habits. Detecting abuse issues early leads to the initiation of treatment, and this can help a person avoid becoming an alcoholic. The earlier in life abuse issues are identified, the

more likely it is that treatment will be effective and further abuse will be prevented.

Substance abuse has the potential to end a medical assistant's career and can lead to incarceration. A medical assistant who is under the influence of controlled substances or alcohol can easily make medication errors and fail to document correctly and, in addition, cannot care for the patient to his or her optimal ability. Almost all physicians report missing medications to the police, and in subsequent investigations, the medical assistant may be arrested and jailed. Convictions for substance abuse can make finding a job in a healthcare facility almost impossible. Many facilities conduct pre-employment and random drug testing, and the chances of not being caught are extremely slim, especially if a substance is still in the system several days after use. Avoid any behavior that can threaten loss of a career in the medical field and legal action.

CLOSING COMMENTS

Patients expect and deserve professional behavior from those who work in medical facilities. Always show compassion, caring, and consideration for a person who comes to the office, whether a patient, visitor, or co-worker. By displaying these traits, the medical assistant earns the respect of co-workers and becomes indispensable to the physician-employer. Behaving in a professional manner in the medical office helps gain the patient's trust. Trust is one of the most important factors in preventing cases of medical professional liability. The medical assistant must never be judgmental when dealing with patients who have substance abuse problems; these patients have a disease just as difficult as cancer or any chronic illness. They deserve empathy and concern. Treating patients with care and not subjecting them to poor attitudes keeps the patient-physician relationship strong and conducive to the health and recovery of the patient.

Patient Education

Remember that most patients do not have any medical background and do not understand many of the phrases used by the medical community. Always be patient and courteously explain any aspect of the instructions or details the patient does not understand. Project a professional attitude of concern and helpfulness. If the patient seems concerned about revealing pertinent information, assure the person that medical assistants and the rest of the staff in the facility are bound by rules of patient confidentiality. Before the patient leaves the exam room, make sure to ask, "Do you have any questions?" This gives patients the opportunity to get all their questions answered before they leave the office.

A professional medical assistant does not share personal information with anyone at the medical facility. Refrain from passing along rumors of any type to patients or their families.

Legal and Ethical Issues

Confidentiality is perhaps the most important aspect of professionalism. Release of any information about patients without their permission is not only unethical, it is against the law. The American Medical Association (AMA) suggests that the purpose of a physician's ethical duty to maintain patient confidentiality is to allow the patient to feel free to make a full and frank disclosure of information to the physician, knowing that the physician will protect the confidential nature of the information. Patients must feel that their confidences will be protected by each member of the physician's staff, including the medical assistant. The workday should be centered around

patient care, so never allow personal business to intrude on time that should be spent assisting patients and the physician. Otherwise, the patient may be left with the impression that the medical assistant, or the entire staff, is unprofessional and this often leads to trust issues between physician and patient.

SUMMARY OF SCENARIO

Karen is happy to be employed in a family practice in which providing quality patient care is paramount. She is learning to be careful of what she says and to remain focused on the patient instead of any difficulties she may be having. Karen knows it is her responsibility to be a team player and to assist the other staff members as much as possible. She maintains a good attitude, even when personal issues could distract her from her duties. Karen gets a strong sense of pride from being a member of the medical profession. She is meticulous about presenting a neat appearance and arrives on time for each workday. She always asks others whether they need help when she has any extra time throughout the day. Karen looks forward to a long relationship with her employer. The rewards she feels as a member of the health team are second to none.

Although Karen is concerned about her grandmother's health, those concerns must be minimally intrusive on her work duties and her attitude toward her

patients and co-workers. By taking time to speak with her supervisor and explaining the situation with her grandmother, Karen takes a proactive role in ensuring that the supervisor understands the pressures Karen is facing. Most supervisors are sympathetic and understanding when issues outside the practice affect employees; however, this should not happen on a regular basis. By encouraging Karen to call and check on her grandmother periodically, the supervisor helps Karen to feel more confident and less distracted during the day. Because she has found her supervisor to be a supportive ally, Karen can relax and carry out her duties professionally and competently throughout the workday. Karen puts the patients first, and this is a fine example of both professionalism and patient compassion.

SUMMARY OF LEARNING OBJECTIVES

1. **Define, spell, and pronounce the terms listed in the vocabulary.**
   Spelling and pronouncing medical terms correctly bolster the medical assistant's credibility. Knowing the definition of these terms promotes confidence in communication with patients and co-workers.

2. **Explain the reasons that professionalism is important in the medical field.**
   Professionalism is the characteristic of conforming to the technical or ethical standards of a profession. It involves showing courtesy, being conscientious, and conducting oneself in a businesslike manner at the workplace. Professionalism is vital in the medical profession, because patients expect and deserve to be treated in a professional way. When the medical assistant acts in a professional way, he or she creates trust with the patient. Patients notice professional behavior, even when it is not directed at them specifically. They notice how others are treated in the reception room and in other areas of the office. Always act in a professional manner while at work.

3. **Discuss several of the characteristics of professionalism.**
   Some of the characteristics of professionalism are loyalty, dependability, courtesy, initiative, flexibility, credibility, confidentiality, and a good attitude.

4. **Explain why confidentiality is so important in the medical profession.**
   Confidentiality is crucial in the medical profession, because patients depend on medical personnel to keep their health information private. Breach of patient confidentiality is one reason an employee could be

terminated immediately and can result in litigation between the patient and the physician-employer.

5. **Discuss the importance of the medical assistant's attitude in caring for patients.**
   Because most patients are not at their best when visiting the physician's office, the attitude of the staff plays an important role in patients' attitudes while in the office. Medical assistants need patience when working with those who are ill. A smile or a reassuring pat on the back goes a long way and can be encouraging.

6. **List some examples of office politics.**
   Office politics can be negative or positive. A person who uses others to gain promotion in the company or who takes credit for a team effort may be using office politics in a negative way; a person who strategically plans advancement through outstanding performance, dependability, and teamwork uses office politics in a positive manner. Knowing when to speak and when to listen helps the medical assistant play the game of politics well in the medical facility.

7. **Identify specific ways teamwork can be promoted in the physician's office.**
   Teamwork makes any job easier to complete. By helping those who may be overwhelmed with duties, the medical assistant may find willing co-workers who will help when the situation is reversed in the future. If two assistants both have duties they dislike, they might trade the duties, to the satisfaction of both. All must work together for the good of the facility and the patients it serves.

8. **Discuss the meaning of insubordination and why it is grounds for dismissal.**

   Insubordination is disobedience to any type of authority figure, usually the supervisor, and it can be grounds for immediate dismissal. When given a task to complete, the medical assistant should carry out the order unless it is unlawful or unethical. If the medical assistant does not carry out an order, the patient's life may be at risk. If the medical assistant feels that the duty should be performed by someone else or should not be performed for some reason, he or she should consult the supervisor. Discuss the issue and attempt to reach an agreement about the appropriateness of performing the task in the future.

9. **Identify and implement time management principles to maintain efficient office function.**

   Prioritizing tasks can help the medical assistant accomplish more tasks. Prioritizing can be used for work, home, and extracurricular activities. Tasks can be identified as those that must, should, or could be done that day. Then, within each of these categories, the tasks can be numbered in the order in which they should be completed. Prioritizing tasks is the most important time management principle.

10. **Talk about goal setting and how it helps a person achieve career success.**

    Goals should be written down and reviewed often to check progress. Taking small steps toward goals helps ensure that they eventually are reached. Individuals should set goals in each area of their lives, breaking the tasks down into manageable parts. Goals should not be unreasonable or unattainable, but rather should provide the opportunity for small successes along the way to reaching the ultimate goal.

11. **Discuss how substance abuse can impact the medical assistant's employment.**

    Substance abuse can lead to arrest and conviction. The medical assistant may face legal action if he or she is abusing drugs or alcohol. This can lead to the end of a career in the healthcare industry. Additionally, the medical assistant could injure a patient by giving incorrect doses of medication or failing to document information properly in the medical record. In extreme cases, patients could die from the medical assistant's actions while under the influence of controlled substances. Any medical assistant struggling with a substance abuse problem should seek professional help immediately.

CONNECTIONS

Study Guide Connection: Go to the Chapter 4 Study Guide. Read and complete the activities.

Evolve Connection: Go to the Chapter 4 link at *evolve.elsevier.com/ kinn* to complete the Chapter Review and Chapter Quiz. Check out the other resources listed for this chapter to make the most of what you have learned from Professional Behavior in the Workplace.

5

INTERPERSONAL SKILLS AND HUMAN BEHAVIOR

Many types of patients seek medical attention and care in the physician's office. Each has different needs and different concerns, even if the diagnoses are similar. Communication and interpersonal skills are vital in meeting these needs and providing optimum care to the patient. However, the patient is not the only individual to consider. Family members often are crucial to the health and well-being of the patient.

Lucille Cloyd is an 83-year-old patient who has been diagnosed with pancreatic cancer and is seeing Dr. Neill for treatment. Her daughter, Sarah Smithson, helps to care for her; she is close to her mother emotionally. Sarah also is Dr. Neill's patient. Although Sarah does not want to see her mother in pain,

she suffers with the knowledge that life will be very different without her. Mrs. Cloyd is widowed and visits the physician once a month in addition to receiving hospice services. She is a good-humored woman who feels that she has led a fruitful life, yet she has moments of depression. She has been living with Sarah and her family for 2 months and enjoys interacting with her two grandchildren and the family's pets.

The medical assistant must consider not only Mrs. Cloyd, but also her extended family. Compassion and sensitivity are necessary to care for this patient, in addition to excellent listening skills. A good knowledge of human relations helps the medical assistant make Mrs. Cloyd's medical care as pleasant as possible under the circumstances.

While studying this chapter, think about the following questions:

- How can the medical assistant treat patients as individuals during a busy workday?
- How does the medical assistant effectively communicate with a patient's family members?
- How will developing good listening skills make the medical assistant more effective?
- How do friends and family members play a role in the health of the patient?

LEARNING OBJECTIVES

1. Define, spell, and pronounce the terms listed in the vocabulary.
2. Explain why first impressions are crucial.
3. Differentiate between verbal and nonverbal communication.
4. Identify styles and types of verbal communication.
5. Explain the different levels of spatial separation.
6. Analyze the effect of hereditary, cultural, and environmental influences on communication.
7. Discuss the value of touch in the communication process.
8. Recognize the elements of oral communication using a sender-receiver process.
9. Explain the value of active listening.
10. Define and understand abnormal behavior patterns.
11. Recognize commonly used defense mechanisms.
12. Discuss the role of assertiveness in effective professional communication.
13. Identify the roles of self-boundaries in the healthcare environment.
14. List several ways to deal with conflict.
15. Recognize communication barriers.
16. Identify techniques for overcoming communication barriers.
17. Differentiate between adaptive and nonadaptive coping mechanisms.
18. Identify common stages that terminally ill patients go through and discuss the support that can assist them and their families during their struggle.
19. Discuss using empathy when treating terminally ill patients.
20. Identify resources and adaptations that are required based on individual needs.
21. List and explain the levels of Maslow's hierarchy of needs.
22. Discuss why physical and emotional needs affect our daily performance at work.

VOCABULARY

adage (a'-dij) A saying, often in metaphoric form, that embodies a common observation.

aggressive Forceful or intended to dominate; hostile, injurious, or destructive, especially when referring to a behavior caused by frustration.

ambiguous (am-bi'-gu-wus) Capable of being understood in two or more possible senses or ways; unclear.

animate To fill with life; to give spirit and support to expressions.

battery An offensive touching or use of force on a person without his or her consent.

caustic (kos'-tik) Marked by sarcasm.

channels Means of communication or expression; courses or directions of thought.

comfort zone A place in the mind where an individual feels safe and confident.

congruent (kun-gru'-unt) Being in agreement, harmony, or correspondence; conforming to the circumstances or requirements of a situation.

decodes Converts, as in a message, into intelligible form; recognizes and interprets.

defense mechanisms Psychological methods of dealing with stressful situations that are encountered in day-to-day living.

encodes Converts from one system of communication to another; converts a message into code.

encroachments Actions that advance beyond the usual or proper limits.

enunciate (e-nun'-se-at) To utter articulate sounds; the act of being very distinct in speech.

external noise Sounds or factors outside the brain that interfere with the communication process.

externalization The attribution of an event or occurrence to causes outside the self.

feedback The transmission of evaluative or corrective information to the original or controlling source about an action, event, or process.

grief Reaction to an unfortunate outcome; a deep distress caused by bereavement, a loss, or a perceived loss.

internal noise Factors inside the brain that interfere with the communication process.

language barrier Any type of interference that inhibits the communication process and is related to languages spoken by the people attempting to communicate.

litigious (luh-ti'-jus) Prone to engage in lawsuits.

malediction (ma-luh-dik'-shun) Speaking evil or the calling of a curse.

media A term applied to agencies of mass communication, such as newspapers, magazines, and telecommunications.

paraphrasing To express an idea in different wording in an effort to enhance communication and clarify meaning.

perception Capacity for comprehension; an awareness of the elements of the environment.

physiologic noise Internal interferences comprised of biological factors within a speaker or listener that hinder effective and accurate communication.

pitch Highness or lowness of a sound; the relative level, intensity, or extent of some quality or state.

proxemics (prok-se'-miks) The study of the nature, degree, and effect of the spatial separation individuals naturally maintain.

sarcasm A sharp and often satirical response or ironic utterance designed to cut or inflict pain.

stereotype Something conforming to a fixed or general pattern; a standardized mental picture that is held in common by many and represents an oversimplified opinion, prejudiced attitude, or uncritical judgment.

stressors Stimuli that cause stress.

subtle Difficult to understand or perceive; having or marked by keen insight and ability to penetrate deeply and thoroughly.

thanatology (tha-nuh-tah'-luh-je) The study of the phenomena of death and of psychological methods of coping with death.

vehemently (ve'-uh-ment-le) In a manner marked by forceful energy; intensely, emotionally.

volatile (vah'-luh-til) Easily aroused; tending to erupt in violence.

The interpersonal skills developed by the medical assistant help to set the tone of a medical office. Interpersonal skills include the communications process and how we relate to one another during that process. Human relations can be defined as the study of the problems that arise from organizational and interpersonal contact. The two entities intersect, and the successful medical assistant continually works to enhance these attributes. Patients who visit the healthcare facility may not be at their best, and the way in which the medical assistant reacts to and interacts with them can make an incredible difference in their **perception** of the office, the physician, and the medical staff. These interactions may also affect the patient's treatment and recovery.

FIRST IMPRESSIONS

Our elders have stressed all our lives that first impressions are lasting ones, and this old **adage** is still true! The opinions formed in the early moments of meeting someone remain in our thoughts long after the first words have been spoken. The first impression involves much more than just physical appearance or dress; it includes attitude and compassion, and the all-important smile (Figure 5-1).

One of the primary objectives of the professional medical assistant is to care for and about the people being served. Patients are the reason the facility exists, and they should be offered the best customer service possible. They must be welcomed warmly, and it is

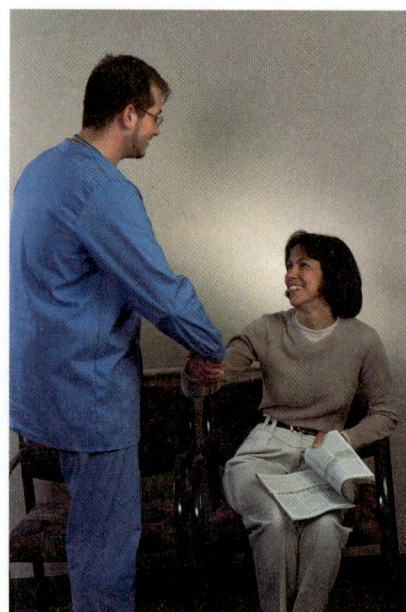

FIGURE 5-1 First impressions are critical in gaining the patient's trust.

important to call patients by their names. People enjoy hearing their names, and it gives a patient confidence that the medical staff members know for whom they are caring.

Think for a moment about how it feels to be a new patient entering the unknown territory of the physician's office. Staff members of the facility are in familiar surroundings and already have some information about the new patient. However, the patient knows nothing about the staff members. One way to break that barrier is to have all staff members wear name badges, with letters large enough to be read at a distance of 3 feet. Include the staff position if several divisions of responsibility exist (e.g., "medical assistant," "insurance biller," and "office manager"). When the patient approaches, if you are wearing a name badge, make introductions and smile. Smiles should show in the voice and the eyes. Genuinely welcome the patient to the office. This small effort helps put the patient at ease in the office environment.

Some physicians make brief notes in the medical record about the personal life of the patient. When the patient arrives for an appointment, the physician can ask about a recent trip abroad or a new grandchild. This tells the patient that the doctor and the office staff see him or her as more than just an illness or a medical record number. It gives the impression that they truly care, and that impression should be an accurate one. Once an impression is formed in the patient's mind, it is very difficult to change; therefore, make the first impressions of your office positive ones. The events in a patient's life can drastically influence the person's health, and any information that would be beneficial to the physician in treating the patient belongs in the medical record.

PATIENT-CENTERED CARE

Healthcare professionals have embraced patient-centered care, an innovative approach to plan, deliver, and evaluate healthcare that is grounded in mutually beneficial partnerships among healthcare providers, patients, and families. Patient- and family-centered care applies to patients of all ages and may be practiced in any healthcare

setting. Each patient that seeks care from the physician has a unique set of needs, including clinical symptoms that require medical attention and issues specific to the individual that can affect his or her care. As patients navigate the healthcare delivery system, physicians and their employees must be prepared to identify and address not just the clinical aspects of care, but also the spectrum of each patient's demographic and personal characteristics. Good communication skills are vital to meeting the needs of the patient and his or her support system.

COMMUNICATION PATHS

Verbal Communication

Peter Urs Bender suggests several types of verbal communication in his book "Guide to Strengths and Weaknesses of Personality Types," including:

1. Expressive – talkative, excited, enthusiastic.
2. Decisive – domineering, controlling, authoritarian.
3. Amiable – nurturing, positive, helpful.
4. Analytical – supportive, questioning, perfectionist.

The medical assistant can develop enough perception to determine the type of verbal communication that a patient uses most often. Then, by studying these four types, it will be easier to communicate verbally with each of the personality types. Think about family members and close friends – what personality type might they be?

The **pitch** of the voice is a part of verbal communication. The voice lifts at the end of a question. It drops at the end of a statement. Usually when a speaker intends to continue a statement, the voice holds the same pitch, the head remains straight, and the eyes and hands are unchanged. This is not an appropriate time to interrupt. If the message is interrupted, the train of thought may not be completed. The tone of voice and choice of words also affect messages.

The medical assistant should speak clearly and **enunciate** words properly. Speak loudly enough that the patients are able to hear clearly, and pay particular attention to those who wear some type of hearing assistance device. It is wise to note this information on the patient's medical record to jog the memory when a patient with a hearing problem visits the office. Never assume that just because a patient is elderly, he or she has a hearing problem. When talking with patients, be sure to use the volume of speech to an advantage. Always speak at a clearly audible level, but at times it will be necessary to increase or decrease the volume of speech. When a patient is upset, for instance, it often helps to lower the volume of speech, because the patient tends to get quieter to hear the person speaking.

Eye contact is critical, especially in the age of electronic medical records. Look at the person to whom you are speaking and do not forget a genuine smile. Look at the person more than at the computer. Many people feel that a person who speaks and cannot look another in the eyes is being deceptive. It also can mean that the speaker is very shy and has little self-confidence. Use gestures where appropriate to liven speech and **animate** the conversation.

Medical assistants must become aware of how they express themselves and how they affect the feelings of others. The tone of voice is vital. **Sarcasm** and **caustic** remarks have no place in the medical office. For example, telling a patient, "I hope you can manage to be on time for your next appointment" is needless and rude. The

PROCEDURE 5-1

Recognize and Respond to Verbal Communications

GOAL: *To be able to recognize verbal communication and respond to it in a professional manner.*

EQUIPMENT and SUPPLIES

• Cards with various patient scenarios (available on Evolve)

PROCEDURAL STEPS

1. Select a classmate as a partner who will play the role of a patient for this procedure. Use patients of varying cultural backgrounds and ability to communicate in English while practicing the procedure. Make sure your partner understands the patient's role on the card.
   PURPOSE: To practice communication with a patient whose responses will not be predictable.

2. Taking turns, draw a card and role-play the scenario described on it.

3. State the message to your patient. Demonstrate sensitivity appropriate to the message being delivered.
   PURPOSE: To send a clearly communicated message.

4. Demonstrate empathy and be impartial when communicating with patients, family, and staff.
   PURPOSE: To treat each person fairly and with professionalism.

5. Demonstrate awareness of the territorial boundaries of the person with whom you are communicating.
   PURPOSE: To recognize and protect personal boundaries in communicating with others.

6. Allow your patient to respond to the sent message. Apply active listening skills.

PURPOSE: To make sure your patient understood your message and to allow him or her to communicate a response.

7. Restate your patient's response.
   PURPOSE: To make sure you understand the patient's message.

8. Clarify any issues that are unclear.
   PURPOSE: To make sure the meaning of each message sent is understood.

9. Demonstrate awareness of diversity in providing patient care.
   PURPOSE: To respect the diversity of the patient population.

10. Refrain from using slang or other unprofessional terms.
    PURPOSE: To maintain professional communication.

11. Demonstrate recognition of the patient's level of understanding in communications.
    PURPOSE: To ensure that the message sent is worded or expressed in a way the patient can understand and to communicate on the recipient's level of comprehension.

12. Continue to communicate back and forth, making sure that your message to each patient is understood correctly.

13. Analyze communications in providing appropriate responses and feedback.
    PURPOSE: To continually improve the communications process between healthcare professionals, other staff members, and patients.

medical assistant must be conservative when speaking and must not be too familiar. The patient expects professionalism and has the right to demand this in the healthcare setting. Never make an inappropriate remark and follow with "I was just kidding." This is never used in a medical facility or in any type of interpersonal communication. Take special care not to hurt anyone's feelings with words and phrases. Be very careful about what is said, especially to patients (Procedure 5-1).

Remember that patients are in the facility to be treated by the physician and staff. They usually are concerned about their illness and may have great apprehension and fear about the future. It is completely out of place for the medical assistant to talk about his or her personal life and challenges with the patients. Allow the patient to speak, and listen instead of offering personal information. Often patients casually mention details to the medical assistant that might influence their care. The saying that we are given "one mouth and two ears" stresses which should get more use!

Nonverbal Communication

Both verbal and nonverbal communications are important in the art of expression, and both are needed to succeed in the communication exchange. Nonverbal communication involves messages conveyed without the use of words. They are transmitted by body language, gestures, and mannerisms that may or may not be in agreement with the words the person speaks. Body language is partly instinctive, partly taught, and partly imitative. It involves eye contact, facial expression, hand gestures, grooming, dress, space, tone of voice, posture, touch, and much more. We are often unaware of our own nonverbal signals and consciously recognize only a small number of the signals sent by others. Our ability to help others increases as we hone our own skills in interpreting nonverbal communication; it is almost always more accurate than verbal communication and tends to convey our true feelings and beliefs (Procedure 5-2).

Appearance is an integral part of nonverbal communication. Our appearance influences the way others view us and can present a conflicting message, or even a totally incorrect message. When we see someone who dresses or grooms in a way that is very different from our own style, we tend to assume that the personalities are also very different. This is not always true. Although we should not judge people by the way they dress, it is difficult not to form opinions based on what we see. Visible piercings and tattoos often are regarded unfavorably in the medical profession, as are long, brightly painted nails. Although these do not signify that the wearer is not professional, many patients, especially older patients, are uncomfortable with these trends. For this reason alone, the medical assistant who is less conservative may diminish his or her chances for certain jobs and advancements. Expressing oneself is healthy, yet in the medical profession, a conservative appearance is mandatory so as not to raise obstacles to communication.

PROCEDURE 5-2

Recognize and Respond to Nonverbal Communications

GOAL: *To be able to recognize nonverbal communication and respond to it in a professional way.*

EQUIPMENT and SUPPLIES

- Cards with various statements that can be communicated in a nonverbal way (available on Evolve)

PROCEDURAL STEPS

1. Select a classmate as a partner who will play the role of a patient for this procedure. Use patients of varying cultural backgrounds and ability to communicate in English while practicing the procedure.
   <u>PURPOSE:</u> To practice nonverbal communications with a patient whose responses will not be predictable.

2. Taking turns, draw a card and communicate the thought on the card to your patient.

3. Use appropriate body language and other nonverbal skills in communicating with patients, family, and staff.
   <u>PURPOSE:</u> To make certain that the nonverbal communication sends the same message as the verbal communication.

4. Demonstrate respect for individual diversity, incorporating awareness of one's own biases in areas including gender, race, religion, age, and economic status. Refrain from influencing the patient toward personal ethics and beliefs.
   <u>PURPOSE:</u> To demonstrate awareness of diversity when providing patient care and to avoid offending patients of any culture.

5. Determine whether the receiver understood the message correctly.
   <u>PURPOSE:</u> To send a nonverbal message that is understood by the receiver.

6. Continue to communicate back and forth, making sure each message sent is conveyed to the receiver accurately. Remain impartial and show empathy when dealing with patients.

7. Analyze communications in providing appropriate responses and feedback.
   <u>PURPOSE:</u> To continually improve the communications process between healthcare professionals, other staff members, and patients.

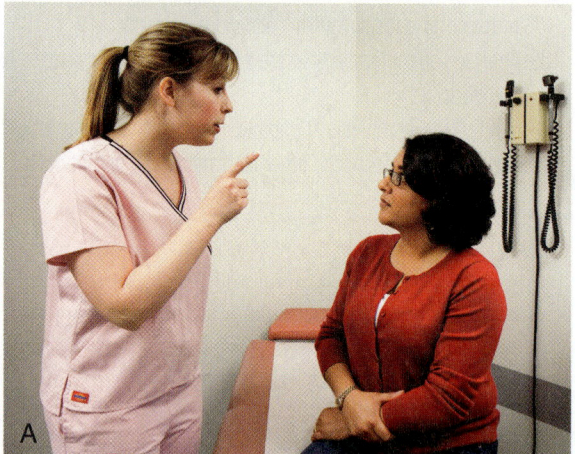 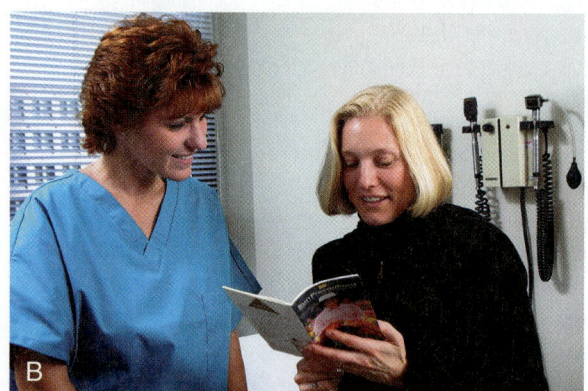

FIGURE 5-2 A, Pointing often is an accusatory gesture and causes discomfort. **B,** A bright smile helps to put the patient at ease and to relax.

The successful medical assistant expresses self-esteem and confidence by stance, vocabulary, facial expression, and a caring attitude. The experience of speaking to someone who does not make eye contact helps one realize the importance of greeting the patient with the eyes as well as the voice and body language. Facial expressions often convey our true feelings and are not masked by the words we use. Our eyes often tell the truth when our words are misleading or false. Use an open body stance when dealing with patients. Crossed arms and legs hint that you are "closed" to the person to whom you are speaking, and this may be construed as disinterest or disbelief. Nonverbal and verbal communication are interdependent (Figure 5-2); they must be in harmony to convey an accurate message that the receiver can easily interpret. If the two are not **congruent**, the nonverbal presentation usually is dominant and expresses the true message.

The need for boundaries, or personal space, is demonstrated by how patients in the reception area choose a seat. **Proxemics** is the study of the nature, degree, and effect of the spatial separation individuals naturally maintain and how this separation relates to heredity, cultural, and environmental factors. Seldom does a person sit in a space next to a stranger if another option is available. Although the need for space varies with the individual culture, some might even remain standing to satisfy the need for personal space. Public space usually is accepted as a distance of 12 to 25 feet, and social space usually is considered to be 4 to 12 feet. Personal space ranges from 1½ to 4 feet, and intimate contact includes physical touching to approximately 1½ feet. The medical assistant often can tell when he or she has invaded someone's personal space, because the person tends to back up a step or two. If this happens, take a small step back and respect the boundaries being set. The more familiar and

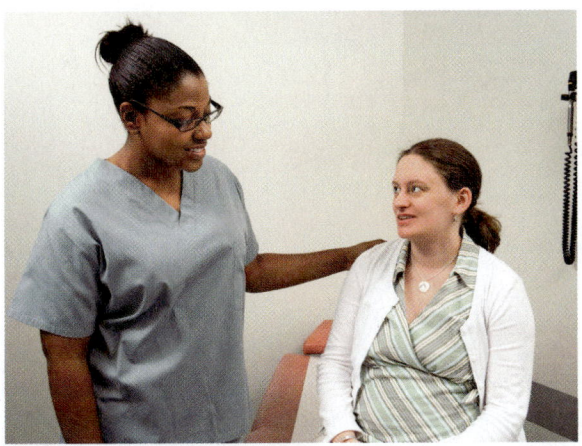

FIGURE 5-3 Touching the patient communicates care and compassion. Careful listening and asking questions helps the patient express thoughts and feelings.

CRITICAL THINKING APPLICATION   **5-1**
- How might touch be an important communication tool with Mrs. Cloyd?
- How can using touch affect Sarah?
- Could laughter affect either of these women as they deal with death?

THE PROCESS OF COMMUNICATION

Anyone who works in the realm of public service should develop good communication skills. It is important to be able to interact with others and to put them at ease so that their comfort level increases and they develop trust. To communicate well, we first must have a general understanding of the process of communication. Once a message has been sent, it cannot be retrieved and restated or expressed in a different way. Especially in the medical profession, communication must be clear and concise, and the message we intend to send must match what the receiver understands.

Although many different scientific models of communication exist, the one that best fits most types of communication is the transactional communication model. Before students can understand how this model works, they must understand the elements we use to communicate.

When two people interact, both people usually act as senders and as receivers (or communicators). The sender is the person who sends a message through a variety of different channels. **Channels** can be spoken words, written messages, and body language. The sender **encodes** the message, which simply means that he or she chooses a specific means of expression using words and other channels. The receiver **decodes** the message according to his or her understanding of what is being communicated. However, sometimes the receiver misunderstands the message. This often is a result of *noise,* which is anything that interferes with the message being sent. It can be literal noise, such as a radio or a jackhammer on the street outside; this is called **external noise.** Or it can be **internal noise,** which includes the receiver's own thoughts or prejudices and opinions. **Physiologic noise** also interferes with communication. This includes any biologic factor that would prevent the communicator from sending or receiving accurate messages, such as not feeling well or being overly tired. **Feedback** can be given through verbal expressions or body language, such as a simple nod of understanding. The perception of the receiver is very important and is discussed later in this chapter.

The transactional communication model (Figure 5-4) depicts "communicators" instead of one sender and one receiver. If two people are communicating, both are sending and receiving messages and both are encoding and decoding messages. Even when two people are speaking one at a time, messages are continually sent with words, body language, facial expressions, and gestures. Various channels of communication are used, and both communicators offer feedback, including subconscious feedback. Noise may or may not be present, but even the best communicators experience some type of noise, even if that is only thinking of what to say next.

Listening

Listening is just as important to good communication as the spoken word. *Hearing* is the process, function, or power of perceiving sound,

comfortable patients are with the medical assistant, the closer the space they allow. Other types of boundaries are discussed later in the chapter.

Touch is a powerful communicator. The soft acceptance of shaking someone's hand, to the good-natured pat on the back, to the harsh slap on the face all relay different messages that need no words to express accurately. In the medical profession, as in any business, touch can be comforting or can lead to a sexual harassment suit. Individuals who have experienced sexual abuse or other traumatic experiences may not want to be touched at all. Unfortunately, one must be extremely careful when using this effective communication tool. In today's **litigious** society, any nonconsensual touching may be considered **battery,** and touch should be used with great discretion and caution.

The medical assistant should not be afraid to touch patients appropriately, such as giving a pat on the back or a squeeze of the hand (Figure 5-3). Some patients are receptive to a brief sideways hug, whereas others would take this as an intrusion into their personal space. Certainly patients with serious illnesses appreciate touch as an expression of empathy. Never be afraid to touch sick patients, especially those with diseases such as acquired immunodeficiency syndrome (AIDS), as long as proper precautions are followed where indicated. If unsure, ask a patient whether he or she minds being hugged. These patients need to feel acceptance, and the attitude of the medical staff members they encounter directly influences their adherence to keeping their appointments with the physician. If they do not feel accepted and cared for, they will not return to the physician's office. A gentle touch and a smile do wonders for showing care and concern.

Posture can signal depression, excitement, anger, or even an appeal for help. When the physician sits at the front of the chair and leans forward, he or she is sending a message of care and interest. Positioning also is important. Sitting behind a desk promotes an air of authority. Standing or sitting across a room may convey a negative message of denying involvement or reluctance to talk. Sitting side by side with a patient helps initiate trust and promote open conversation. The medical assistant should practice good postural techniques as a part of projecting a positive image and for personal health reasons.

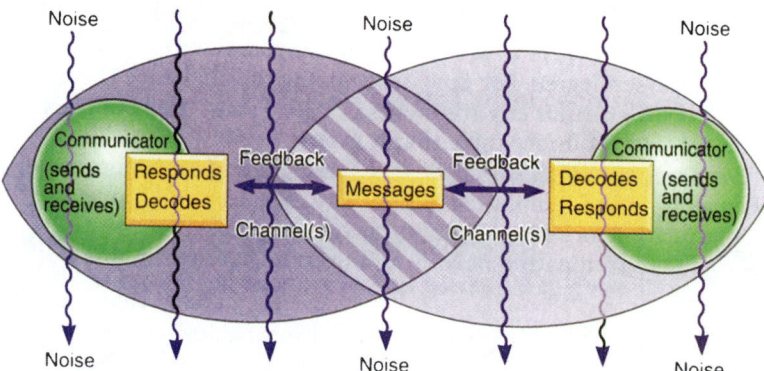

FIGURE 5-4 The transactional communication model. (From Adler RB, Towne N: *Looking out, looking in: interpersonal communication,* San Antonio, 1996, Harcourt Brace.)

whereas *listening* is defined as paying attention to sound or hearing something with thoughtful attention. Patients need to know that the medical assistant is listening. This is actually true in all interpersonal relationships, including husband-wife, parent-child, supervisor-employee, and doctor-patient interactions. When listening to someone who is attempting to communicate, the first rule is to look at the speaker and pay attention. Sometimes it is important not to respond immediately but to remain silent and offer an understanding and reassuring nod.

Sometimes it is hard to listen. We may not be able to listen effectively, because we are distracted by our own thoughts. Perhaps the situations occurring in our own lives make the conversation we are hearing seem meaningless and unimportant. Or so many messages may be attacking at once that we are unable to focus on any specific one to listen to what is being communicated. At other times, such as in anger, we are so rapidly preparing our response that we cannot listen to what is being said. We may simply be too tired to listen, or we may have prejudged the speaker and decided that we do not need to listen. However, while working with patients, the medical assistant must be diligent not only in *hearing* the words being spoken, but also in *listening* to them and to what the patient is attempting to communicate.

Active listening is a skill that enables a person to paraphrase and clarify what the speaker has said. **Paraphrasing** is listening to what the sender is communicating, analyzing the words, and restating them to confirm that the receiver has understood the message as the sender intended. This process clarifies the speaker's thoughts and helps indicate that a common understanding of the message exists between the speaker and the receiver. When communicating in this way, the receiver should reword what the sender has said and then ask a clarifying question. Consider the following example:

| Patient: | *"I haven't been feeling well lately."* |
| Medical assistant: | *"You say you have not been feeling well. What exactly is the trouble?"* |

This type of communication may seem awkward at first, because most of us believe that listening involves lack of speech. *Active listening* means that the speaker's words are heard, and a restatement is used to verify that the message was understood correctly. This statement gives the speaker the opportunity to correct any misconceptions or misunderstandings. Consider the following example:

Patient:	*"My back hurts."*
Medical assistant:	*"Where does it hurt?"*
Patient:	*"In the middle."*
Medical assistant:	*"Can you point to exactly where it hurts?"*
Patient:	*"Yes, right here (points)."*
Medical assistant:	*"Is it a sharp or dull pain?"*
Patient:	*"Very sharp."*
Medical assistant:	*"How often does it occur?"*
Patient:	*"Several times a day."*
Medical assistant:	*"Can you tell me on an average day how many times it bothers you?"*
Patient:	*"About six times."*
Medical assistant:	*"How long does it last?"*
Patient:	*"About 10 or 15 minutes."*
Medical assistant:	*"How long have you felt this pain?"*
Patient:	*"For about 2 weeks."*
Medical assistant:	*"So you have had a sharp pain in this part of your back about six times a day lasting for up to 15 minutes for 2 weeks? Is that correct?"*
Patient:	*"Yes."*

It would have been easier if the patient had said, "I have had a sharp pain in my back that lasts up to 15 minutes, and it happens about six times a day." This example shows how the medical assistant can continue clarifying until the answer is specific enough, which is critical when obtaining information from the patient.

It also is best to ask "open" rather than "closed" questions. An open question requires more than a "yes" or "no" answer. It forces the patient to provide more detail and expand on his or her thoughts. A closed question can be answered with "yes" or "no" and compels the medical assistant to spend more time obtaining the answers needed to document the patient's needs thoroughly.

CRITICAL THINKING APPLICATION   5-2

■ How can the medical assistant be sure that Mrs. Cloyd understands how she is to take her medication?

■ Often older patients do not appreciate instructions being given to their caregiver instead of directly to them. How can the medical assistant place the primary focus on communicating with Mrs. Cloyd, yet at the same time make sure Sarah understands the instructions and care?

Often when a person or patient is talking with the medical assistant, the person is looking for a specific type of response. Some patients want advice, some want sympathy, and others are looking for reassurance. Many patients open up more quickly and more completely to the medical assistant than to the physician. This can be a very positive aspect of the relationship the medical assistant has with patients, because it is important to build good rapport with them. However, the medical assistant should never agree to withhold information from the physician under any circumstances. If the patient asks that the assistant not reveal something to the physician, the medical assistant should politely explain that he or she has an ethical obligation to report any and all pertinent information to the physician, especially if it affects medical care. For example, if the patient asks the medical assistant not to tell the physician that the patient has been smoking against medical advice, the assistant could be jeopardizing the patient's care if the information is not reported.

This does not mean that specific details must always be aired. If the patient reveals that her stress levels have been high because she has filed a sexual harassment suit against her boss, but she does not want to share each detail with the physician, the medical assistant could report to the physician that the patient is having some legal problems that have resulted in additional stress at work. The physician will understand that the patient's stress level is elevated and can effectively treat the patient without knowing the specific, intimate details of the acts between the patient and her employer. However, the medical assistant must *never* agree to lie to the physician. The patient must understand that if the physician questions any information given by the patient, it must be revealed so that the physician is assured that the care provided is appropriate. Remember that the physician may have worked with the patient for a long time and has a better understanding of the patient's needs than the medical assistant. One patient may be able to handle a high stress level, and another may crumble at the first sign of stress. Good physicians know their patients and keep accurate, complete records that aid decision making in these situations.

If the medical assistant is ever in doubt about telling the physician something a patient has said, the best solution is to tell. Medical professionals are legally bound to confidentiality, and the patient may need to be reminded of this. Encourage the patient to talk to the physician and communicate all concerns, no matter how insignificant they may seem. Never display a judgmental attitude or express negativity about the patient's activities, thoughts, or behavior. Offer to be with the patient, if he or she desires, during difficult discussions with the physician or to make arrangements for a special counseling session with the physician if this is indicated. Some patients are hesitant to initiate a conversation with the physician because they feel they are taking too much time. The medical assistant can help ensure that critical issues receive the doctor's attention.

WARNINGS AGAINST ADVISING A PATIENT

The medical assistant must be extremely careful when making suggestions or comments to a patient to prevent legal accusations of practicing medicine without a license. Often a patient asks for an opinion as to which course of action to take. Medical assistants are not qualified to give any type of advice to a patient. Strict laws in most states prohibit anyone other than a licensed physician from offering medical advice. Even if the patient asks what the medical assistant would do if presented with the same options, the assistant cannot encourage the patient to choose one option over another. The assistant can offer a listening ear, though, and help the patient process his or her own thoughts. This can be done in much the same way as using active listening techniques. When a patient expresses a concern, the medical assistant should restate the concern and then ask a clarifying question. For example:

Patient: *"I don't know whether I should take the chemotherapy treatments the doctor wants me to have."*

Medical assistant: *"You seem worried about the treatments. What are you concerned about specifically?"*

Patients must make their own decisions about treatment options when faced with a medical decision. The medical assistant often is looked upon not only as an authority figure, but also as an extension of the physician. Patients may mistakenly think that the medical assistant has the same opinion as the physician. All communication with the patient must be professional and accurate. Always attempt to get the patient to discuss all concerns and fears openly with the physician.

The medical assistant should never agree to withhold any information from the physician, because even a small detail could completely change the plan of treatment. When giving instructions to patients, offer them in writing and keep a copy for the patient's medical record so that a written record of what was communicated to the patient is available. Use excellent documentation technique when adding information to the patient's medical record. Remember that all the patients in the facility deserve to be treated with respect and compassion. Help the physician establish trust with the patient. An open, trusting relationship helps to prevent legal issues in the future.

CRITICAL THINKING APPLICATION   5-3
- How should the medical assistant handle Sarah's questions about the various aspects of her mother's treatments?
- How does her mother's decision not to have chemotherapy affect Sarah? What barriers to communication might exist between them?

OBSERVING CAREFULLY

In the fast-paced world of medicine, medical professionals sometimes miss the nonverbal signals sent by patients; however, these signals play a critical role in patients' care. If the patient hesitates when speaking, it may be an indication that he or she has more to say. As mentioned previously, the inability to look a person directly in the eyes sometimes, but not always, indicates deception. The medical assistant must pay close attention both to what is seen and what is heard when communicating with the patient. Look into the patient's eyes and watch intently for signs of trouble.

When a patient cries, the medical assistant should always question what is causing the tears. Some patients may refuse to discuss the issue or insist that nothing is wrong, but tears are always a sign of some emotion, whether anger, frustration, fear, pain, or some other concern. Do not allow patients who are obviously emotionally upset to leave the office without reasonable assurance that they are going to be safe. The medical assistant might wish to suggest that a friend come to the office and escort the patient home. On rare occasions, it is better to be firm with the patient and insist on help getting home if the person is in a **volatile** state. This action may save patients from hurting themselves or someone else. Careful observation of the patient as a whole is worth the time investment and may even save the patient's life. By using observational skills, the medical assistant can begin to identify abnormal behaviors and use these observations to provide better patient-centered care. Remember that any observations that the medical assistant makes and documents in the medical record cannot be misconstrued as diagnoses. Communicate with the physician if there is any question or concern about proper documentation methods.

PSYCHOLOGICAL DISORDERS

A *psychological disorder* is defined as a psychological or behavior pattern that occurs in an individual and is thought to cause distress or disability that is not expected as a part of normal development and culture. The roots of psychology extend to beliefs in witchcraft and demon possession, but today, the science of psychology is a vast field involving the study of the brain and how it works.

Numerous abnormal behavior patterns affect humans. Some are better understood than others, and many can be controlled with medications. In his introductory psychology textbook, Rod Plotnik argues that treating abnormal behavior is accomplished by using one or more of three basic methods: the psychoanalytic, the cognitive-behavioral, and the medical-model approaches. When using a psychoanalytic approach, a psychiatrist or psychologist engages in therapy with the patient, usually face-to-face. The patient identifies and discusses the issues or conflicts that cause his or her abnormal behavior in an effort to understand it; then the psychiatrist or psychologist and the patient explore alternative actions that may allow the patient to live normally with the abnormal behavior or to eliminate it completely. The cognitive-behavioral approach is based upon the belief that mental disorders result from a deficit in a thought process and that the patient suffers from maladaptive thinking processes, so treatment focuses on changing the patient's maladaptive thoughts and behaviors. The medical-model approach involves using psychoactive drugs to treat mental disorders.

The *Diagnostic and Statistical Manual of Mental Disorders* contains standard classifications of mental disorders as used by mental health professionals in the United States. Some of the abnormal behaviors include:

- *Phobia:* An exaggerated, usually inexplicable and illogical fear of a particular object or situation
- *Obsessive-compulsive disorder:* An anxiety disorder characterized by recurrent, unwanted thoughts and/or repetitive behaviors
- *Antisocial behavior:* An inability to distinguish right from wrong or to feel remorse, characterized by dysfunctional thinking and perception of situations
- *Panic disorder:* Sudden, sometimes chronic, episodes of intense fear that develops for no apparent reason

- *General anxiety disorder:* An ongoing anxiety that interferes with day-to-day activities and relationships
- *Major depressive disorder:* A condition affecting both mind and body that can cause a variety of emotional and physical problems

DEFENSE MECHANISMS

Anxiety or stress causes the human body to react in many different ways. Some people handle **stressors** more easily than others. Most people use **defense mechanisms** when they feel pressured or attacked in some way. These often are subconscious reactions designed for emotional protection; they help us deal with whatever difficult event has triggered such a response. Often people may not even realize that they are using these mechanisms and may **vehemently** deny that they are doing so. Many types of defense mechanisms exist; the medical assistant should be familiar with them to better communicate with patients and others with whom they come in contact in the course of their duties.

Verbal Aggression

When a person verbally attacks another without addressing the original complaint, or disregards it, he or she is being verbally **aggressive** (Figure 5-5). Such people may attack, or they may change the subject. Some individuals get very angry at any suggestion of wrongdoing. They lash out, usually quite loudly, and attack quickly in hopes of diminishing their role in any wrongdoing. For example:

"When are you going to clean the drug sample closet?"

"Who are you to ask me that? You haven't finished your duties today, either!"

Handling Verbal Aggression

When a person is verbally aggressive, diffuse the situation by using communication techniques. Some people wildly exaggerate with accusations such as, "You always act that way…" You can partially agree by responding with, "I sometimes say things like that, but…" Giving the aggressor an unsatisfying agreement, such as, "You may be right" or "You have a point," will not add to the argument but will not indicate agreement, either.

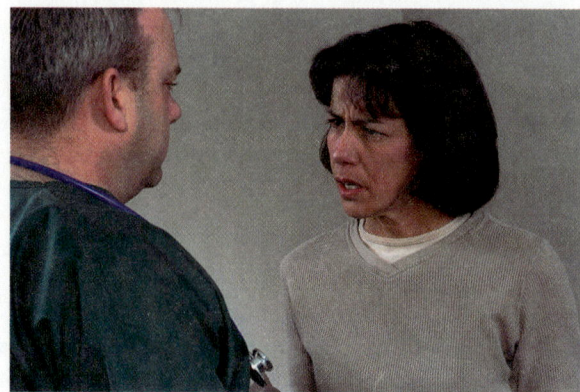

FIGURE 5-5 Remain calm even if a patient becomes verbally aggressive. Attempt to calm the person by listening and expressing empathy whenever possible.

Sarcasm

The word *sarcasm* comes from the Greek word *sarkasmos,* which means "to tear flesh" or "to bite the lips in rage." This is quite an accurate definition of the nature of sarcasm. It is a biting edge added to words that a person states with the intent to cause pain or anger. Sarcasm is hostile and cruel in most cases, and some individuals use it constantly, thinking it is quite witty. On the contrary, it often makes bitter enemies of its victims. For example, "Of course it's a nice dress, if you like tents."

Handling Sarcasm

Although ignoring the sarcasm is often suggested, it is not always effective. Sarcasm is a type of bullying, and the best way to deal with any kind of bullying is to stand up to it. For instance, if a co-worker makes a sarcastic remark, even if it is done in front of others, the medical assistant might say, "That was an awfully sarcastic remark…" Just the open confrontation itself may cause the person to rethink making such statements in public.

Rationalization

Rationalizing is attributing actions to rational and credible motives without analyzing underlying methods. When people rationalize their behavior, they are offering excuses for what has been done or said and trying to convince others that the behavior was completely justified. For example, "He only hits me because he is stressed at work."

Handling Rationalization

Often, when a person is rationalizing, the medical assistant can simply ask a more probing question, such as, "Now, is that the real reason that you were late for work, or did you wake up late?" Often the person will immediately admit the real reason for his or her actions.

Compensation

A person who compensates makes up for one behavior by stressing another. Compensation is a psychological mechanism through which feelings of inferiority, frustration, or failure in one area are counterbalanced by achievement in another. Compensation is not always a negative response, but it often is used as an excuse for not accomplishing what should be accomplished. For example, "I know I gained 5 pounds, Dr. George, but I exercised three times last week."

Handling Compensation

Using the method of further questioning, described previously, also is effective in dealing with a person who is compensating for his or her behavior. Say, "How long did you exercise?" or "What was your diet like last week?" Often, by asking questions and not making judgmental statements, the person will realize that he or she was compensating and will eventually admit inappropriate behavior.

Regression

Regression is the reversion to an earlier mental or behavioral level. Some people regress to a childlike state or period or exhibit qualities inherent to an earlier time in life. This can include making excuses for not doing a certain thing, saying that it cannot be done, instead of telling the truth, which is that the person does not want to do it. Replacing the word "can't" with "won't" is a good gauge of the use of regression. For example, "I'd like to get better grades, but I can't find time to study."

Handling Regression

Preceding your response with a positive statement may make the person exhibiting regression feel more comfortable admitting inappropriate behavior. For instance, reply to the statement about grades, in the preceding section, by saying, "I know you are really smart, and I'll bet you can make more time to study if you look for opportunities to do your reading and other work."

Repression

The process whereby unwanted desires or impulses are excluded from the consciousness and left to operate in the unconscious is called *repression.* Blocking a problem from the mind and changing the subject when it is mentioned are both types of repression. The repressed urges or desires may seethe beneath the surface, absorbing energy, and force continual repression of the desires, which takes more and more concentration to do successfully. For example, "I had a fight with my brother and I should phone him, but I just can't deal with that now."

Handling Repression

A person who is repressing his or her feelings may truly be unable to handle stressful situations temporarily. The best approach may be to simply be supportive and lend an ear if the person is willing to talk. Say, "I understand that you're in a difficult situation. If you want to talk about it, I will be there to listen." Severe cases may prompt a referral to a professional counselor.

Apathy

Apathy is a lack of feeling, emotion, interest, or concern. It is an indifference to what is happening or a pretense of not caring about a situation. Usually, apathy is not a true reflection of the inner feeling. It is a defense mechanism similar to repression but with a more flippant attitude. For example, "I don't care what grade I got on the test, because I am not going to pass the class anyway."

Handling Apathy

Attempt to get past the pretense that the person is expressing by saying, "Now, I know you really do care about your grades and of course you can pass the class. How can I help you study and prepare?" When you express confidence, the person may open up about the true concerns or may eventually develop more confidence in his or her abilities.

Displacement

Displacement is the redirection of an emotion or impulse from its original object, such as an idea or person, to another object. When challenged or attacked by one person or event, the person uses displacement to channel negative feelings to some other area, which gives a false sense of control over issues that may not be controllable. The venting of hostile feelings is directed somewhere other than where it should be directed; however, this usually is a result of a lack of confidence in addressing the true issues at hand. For example, "I have enough problems at work; I don't need to come home to a nagging wife!"

Handling Displacement

Sometimes, simply stating, "Are you really mad at me or are you upset about issues at work?" will diffuse a person using displacement. However, if displacement is used often, professional counseling may be indicated.

Denial

Denial is a psychological defense mechanism in which a person avoids confronting a personal problem or reality by denying the existence of the problem or reality. The common expression, "He's in denial," originates from this situation. For whatever reason, the person is unable to cope with the stress of a situation and completely pushes it away, and any person or thing representing it. For example, "I can't possibly have cancer; I just had a checkup, and I'm completely healthy."

Handling Denial

Listening is an important technique to use when a person is in denial. Express empathy, using phrases such as, "I know it is devastating to receive a cancer diagnosis, especially in an otherwise healthy patient. What concerns do you have about the diagnosis and what lies ahead for you?" This technique gently brings the person back to dealing with the situation and moving his or her thought process forward to deal with the issues at hand. Avoid suggesting that you "know how he feels," because no patient wants to hear about another person's problems or experiences when trying to deal with a major life event.

Physical Avoidance

Some events are so painful that a person may completely avoid any representation of the event. This could be a person, a place, an object, or just about anything that serves as a reminder of the event that induces the negative feelings. If the problem is a person, that person may be avoided forever. If it is a place, such as a home that a couple lived in before one of them died, the other person may move. In some cases, such as physical abuse, the avoidance may be necessary, but it also can be quite unhealthy and may need to be explored further through therapy. For example, "I will never go to that restaurant again, because that's where my ex-husband told me he wanted a divorce."

Handling Physical Avoidance

Being unwilling to revisit painful experiences is not always unhealthy. A person who doesn't want to be in a physical place that brings painful memories really should not have to confront those feelings unless physical avoidance becomes a pattern of behavior. Say, "Let's go to that new Mexican restaurant and just start new memories." This may be a more positive move forward than insisting on confronting old hurt.

Projection

Projection, as a defense mechanism, is the attribution of one's own ideas, feelings, or attitudes to other people or to objects. This especially includes the **externalization** of blame, guilt, or responsibility

as a defense against anxiety. Some people project their feelings about a certain issue onto others, who may not be affected by the negative connotations the first person feels. Projection is a way to avoid dealing with the root issues of a problem. For example, "Everyone else is always late, so why am I getting reprimanded for it?"

Handling Projection

Bring the person back to dealing with his or her behavior. Say, "We are dealing with your behavior right now. I realize that situations will make us late periodically, but this has become a pattern that we need to deal with." Insist that the conversation remain about only this person's behavior.

CONFLICT

Conflict is defined as the struggle resulting from incompatible or opposing needs, drives, or wishes or external or internal demands. We deal with conflict in our lives in some capacity almost daily. Knowing how to recognize the signs of conflict and the patterns people use to deal with conflict can be of great benefit to the medical assistant. This enables the professional to be understanding and empathetic to patients, co-workers, supervisors, and others in the day-to-day work environment.

Conflict is not always negative; sometimes it is beneficial to relationships. It can be constructive and allow people to learn more about each other. This may promote a stronger understanding and deeper levels of intimacy. Unless both parties are aware that a problem exists between them, no conflict exists. The conflict begins when both realize that a problem needs to be resolved. People handle conflict in different ways. Some avoid it at all costs; on the other end of the spectrum, some seem to thrive on conflict.

The knowledge of some of the many types of conflict can help the medical assistant understand the thought processes of others and how best to respond to them and also to discern how others respond. Of itself, assertion is not conflict; assertion is stating or declaring positively. Often being forcefully assertive or aggressive can be very productive. Assertive people often receive job promotions and reach the goals they set for their lives. However, too much aggression can make a person seem pushy; therefore, it should be controlled and used at the appropriate times. Remember, there is a difference between assertion and aggression, which are discussed in the following paragraphs.

Nonassertion is the inability to express needs and thoughts or the refusal to express them. Some avoid conflict and some accommodate by putting others' desires before their own. Sometimes nonassertion is justifiable. Anyone who has been involved in a long-term relationship realizes that sometimes the other person's needs must come first. Many have learned the truth of the old saying, "Choose your battles wisely."

> ## CRITICAL THINKING APPLICATION   5-4
> - Why might Mrs. Cloyd and Sarah experience conflict at this stage in their lives?
> - How might each deal better with disagreements, especially regarding Mrs. Cloyd's decisions about her medical care?

Aggression is defined in several ways. It can be a hostile, injurious, or destructive behavior or outlook, especially when caused by frustration. It is also the practice of making attacks or **encroachments**, especially if the acts are unprovoked. In the realm of psychological studies, there are different types of aggression. Direct aggression occurs when a person directly attacks another, whether by criticism, **malediction**, ridiculing, or other methods. This behavior causes the victim to feel embarrassment, shame, anger, or a range of other emotions. *Passive aggression* is a familiar term, but many may not know its definition. A passive-aggressive person expresses himself or herself in an obscure, **ambiguous** way. People who experience passive aggression may have feelings of rage, inadequacy, or resentment that they cannot articulate in a direct manner. Unfortunately, this behavior does not usually provide the results needed or expected.

Resolving Conflict

Conflict exists in all relationships, whether they are at work, home, or in social situations. In most cases, the person or persons involved in conflict do not intend to cause problems, and the conflict should not be considered personal. The first impulse in response to conflict is often the fight-or-flight response, either to attack or retreat. Professionalism dictates that the first response be put aside so that the medical assistant can apply logical thought to the situation. Personal beliefs are developed based on each individual's unique experiences and perspectives.

Resolving conflict can range from being simple to excruciatingly difficult. Also, the medical assistant must remember that conflict presents an opportunity for growth and increased maturity at the workplace. The following tips can help resolve conflicts.

- Expect conflict, because people do not agree on every viewpoint or situation all the time. Do not dread or fear conflict.
- Realize that conflict can be a healthy process that allows input from various points of view. That input can lead to better decisions.
- Accept that others have legitimate, viable opinions that they should be allowed to express.
- Listen to other opinions and then consider them in an honest, fair manner. People are rarely wrong 100% of the time.
- Never attack a person with a different opinion. Instead, keep the focus on the situation at hand and how it can be resolved.
- Do not insist on being right all the time. Welcome input from those with alternative, original ideas.
- Avoid judgment or assigning blame; do not immediately assume that the other person is wrong.
- Deal with conflict as it happens. Never let several situations build up to an explosion. Do not say that nothing is wrong when hurt feelings are quietly accumulating.

BOUNDARIES

Remember that a patient has physical boundaries or personal space, as discussed earlier in this chapter. The patient's personal space ranges from 1½ to 4 feet, so be aware of any nonverbal communication from the patient that you may be infringing on his or her space.

Keep in mind, too, that spacial boundaries are not the only ones that affect patients.

Boundaries indicate a limit or fixed extent. Setting boundaries at work helps prevent awkward situations and misunderstandings. The first step in setting boundaries is to perform a self-inventory. Determine what is important in the work environment and the type of environment most conducive to strong performance on the job.

Life Coach David B. Bohl suggests five steps in setting self-boundaries at work:

1. Know how you expect to be treated and be clear about it with others. If you prefer to be called "Ms. Roberts" instead of "Linda," correct anyone who uses your first name directly and politely.
2. Do not feel that you have to offer explanations for your boundaries. Adults should respect the preferences of other adults in the workplace. Do not feel that you have to explain boundary choices.
3. Be respectful, thoughtful, and responsible when setting boundaries. Do not make unreasonable demands, and consider your motives in each situation. For instance, do not insist that the staff call you by your last name simply to remind them that you are the boss, but do use last names when promoting a more professional environment for workers and patients alike.
4. Respect other people's boundaries if you want yours to be respected, even if you do not agree with their boundaries. If boundaries are incompatible, work toward an acceptable, fair compromise. If the person with whom you share office space enjoys listening to country music during the day and you prefer classical music, compromise by listening to country in the morning and classical in the afternoon or determine another fair arrangement. Or, both could agree to wear earphones if that is allowed in the office policies manual.
5. Be proactive when dealing with other people's boundaries. If unsure, ask. Do not make assumptions when unsure. Ask co-workers questions, such as how they prefer to receive communications and how they prefer to be addressed.

Self-Boundaries

Individuals also may want to set self-boundaries in the workplace, forming a sort of "rule book" for personal actions when on the job or standards of behavior that the individual will or will not accept. For instance, a medical assistant may decide to pair up with another employee whenever each one takes a medication from the supply closet or takes money from the petty cash drawer, serving as each other's witness. This may take some cooperation and time management skills, but it makes each accountable to the other and provides a witness in case of some impropriety in those areas. Of course, always team with a co-worker who has a track record of being trustworthy. A medical assistant may decide to avoid checking personal e-mail at work or to refrain from Internet use unless completing a job duty. Additionally, some medical assistants may prefer to be addressed by just their first name, whereas others prefer their last name. Self-boundaries allow medical assistants to keep their focus on work duties and concentrate on performing at an optimum level every day.

The Crazy-Makers: Passive-Aggressive Communication

In their book, *Looking Out, Looking In: Interpersonal Communication,* Ronald B. Adler and Neil Towne discuss the concept of "crazy-makers," which is credited to psychologist George Bach. Bach developed the theory of creative aggression; he nicknamed this passive-aggressive behavior "crazy-making." According to Bach, two types of aggression exist: clean fighting and dirty fighting. Crazy-making was his name for dirty fighting, which is a detrimental behavior for all involved. The term *partner* is used loosely to indicate the opposite side or victim of the crazy-maker. Bach described the characteristic types of passive-aggressive individuals:

The Avoider

Avoiders refuse to fight. When a conflict arises, they leave, fall asleep, pretend to be busy at work, or keep from facing the problem in some other way. This behavior makes it difficult for the partner to express feelings of anger and hurt, because avoiders will not fight back.

The Pseudoaccommodator

Pseudoaccommodators refuse to face up to a conflict either by giving in or by pretending nothing is wrong. This drives the partner crazy, because the partner definitely feels a problem exists; the partner also feels guilty and resentful toward the pesudoaccommodator for having brought up the situation for discussion in the first place.

The Guilt-Maker

Instead of saying straight out that they do not want or do not approve of something, guilt-makers try to make their partners feel responsible for causing pain. A guilt-maker's favorite line is, "It's okay, don't worry about me…," followed by a long sigh.

The Subject Changer

The subject changer is an avoider who escapes facing up to aggression by shifting the conversation whenever it approaches an area of conflict. Because of their tactics, subject changers and their partners never have the chance to explore their problems and do something about them.

The Distracter

Rather than come out and express their feelings about an object of dissatisfaction, distracters attack other parts of their partners' lives. Thus they never have to share what is really on their minds and can avoid dealing with painful parts of their relationships.

The Mind Reader

Instead of allowing their partners to express feelings honestly, mind readers go into character analysis, explaining what the other person really means or what is wrong with the other person. By behaving this way, mind readers refuse to handle their own feelings and leave no room for their partners to express themselves.

The Trapper

Trappers play an especially dirty trick by setting up a desired behavior for their partners; then, when the behavior is manifested, they attack the very thing they requested. For example, the trapper may say, "Let's be totally honest with each other," then attack the partner's words of honesty.

The Crisis Tickler

Crisis ticklers bring what is bothering them almost to the surface but never quite express their true feelings. For instance, instead of admitting concern about the finances, they innocently ask, "Gee, how much did that cost?" dropping a rather obvious hint but never really dealing with the crisis.

The Gunnysacker

Gunnysackers do not respond immediately when angry. Instead, they put their resentment into a gunnysack, which after a while begins to bulge with both large and small gripes. Then, when the sack is about to burst, the gunnysacker pours out all the pent-up aggression on the overwhelmed and unsuspecting partner.

The Trivial Tyrannizer

Instead of honestly sharing their resentments, trivial tyrannizers do things they know will bother their partners, such as leaving dirty dishes in the sink, clipping fingernails in bed, belching out loud, turning up the television too loud, and so on.

The Beltliner

Everyone has a psychological "beltline," and below it are subjects too sensitive to be approached without damaging the relationship. Belt-lines may have to do with physical characteristics, intelligence, past behavior, or deeply ingrained personality traits a person is trying to overcome. In an attempt to "get even" or hurt their partners, beltliners use intimate knowledge to hit below the belt, where they know it will hurt.

The Joker

Because they are afraid to face conflicts squarely, jokers kid around when their partners want to be serious, thus blocking the expression of important feelings.

The Blamer

Blamers are more interested in finding fault than in resolving a conflict. Needless to say, they usually do not blame themselves. Blaming behavior almost never resolves a conflict and is an almost surefire way to make partners defensive.

The Contract Tyrannizer

Contract tyrannizers do not allow their relationships to change from the way they once were. Whatever the agreements the partners had for roles and responsibilities at one time, they will remain unchanged.

The Kitchen Sink Fighter

Kitchen sink fighters are so named because in an argument, they bring up things that are totally off the subject, as in everything, including the kitchen sink. Perhaps it is the way the other person behaved last New Year's Eve, or bad breath, or the unbalanced checkbook; any past imperfection is fair game for picking a fight.

The Withholder

Instead of expressing their anger honestly and directly, withholders punish their partners by holding something back, such as courtesy, affection, good cooking, humor, or sex. Such withholding is likely to build up even greater resentments in the relationship.

The Benedict Arnold

Benedict Arnolds get back at their partners by sabotage, by failing to defend them from attackers, and even by encouraging ridicule or disregard from outside the relationship.

BARRIERS TO COMMUNICATION

Physical Impairment

Patients may have physical conditions that impair their ability to communicate effectively. This could be a vision or hearing problem or one of many other conditions that make communicating a bit more difficult than usual. The medical assistant should use more descriptive language when speaking with the patient who has a visual disturbance. This helps the patient "see" what is being discussed. The person with diminished hearing may be very sensitive and in denial of the condition. Make sure you have his or her attention and that you are face-to-face with the person while speaking. People who are hearing impaired often are very dependent on lip reading for comprehension.

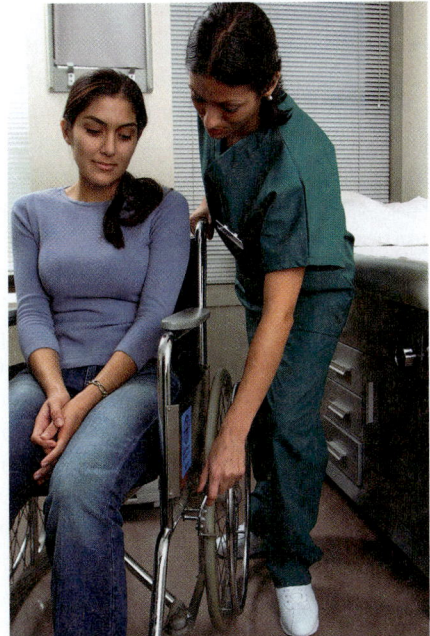

FIGURE 5-6 Bilingual staff members are valuable in ensuring accurate communication with patients who speak a different language.

> **CRITICAL THINKING APPLICATION   5-5**
> ■ What must be considered when communicating verbally with Mrs. Cloyd? With Sarah?
> ■ How can the medical assistant show compassion to a terminally ill patient during her appointment when the office is extremely busy?

Language

With non-English-speaking patients, the medical assistant may need to use gestures and more body language to convey messages. In such cases, be alert to the possibility of misunderstanding. Confirm that the message sent is the message the listener received by asking for feedback. Ask the listener to repeat the message, and if family members are present, make sure they, also, have a good understanding of what was communicated.

The clinic may employ a bilingual staff member to reduce the chance of miscommunication with those who speak a different language (Figure 5-6).

Prejudice

Personal and social bias, or prejudice, brings about discrimination. Discrimination is unfair treatment of a person because of race, gender, religious affiliation, or handicap or for any other reason. Discrimination is unethical, morally and socially wrong, and in many situations illegal; it also prevents us from communicating effectively.

Some discrimination is very **subtle** and is not expressed openly or in a blatant manner. Subtle discrimination is based on a person's appearance, values, lifestyle, or some other personal factor. Examples include discrimination against those who are obese, divorced individuals, homosexuals, welfare recipients, or those with sexually transmitted diseases. Sometimes we are not aware that our words or actions reflect subtle discrimination against others.

Personal prejudices must be recognized before one can change them. Medical professionals are exposed to a wide variety of people who need excellent medical care. The professional cannot allow personal prejudice to affect the care of any individual. Everyone has the right to be honored as a human being and treated respectfully. This enforces the Golden Rule: treat others as you would wish to be treated. Realize the worth of each individual and allow that attitude to be reflected in all actions taken with a patient.

Stereotyping

Stereotyping is defined as the application of a standardized mental picture that is held in common by members of a group; it represents an oversimplified opinion, prejudiced attitude, or uncritical judgment. It is unfair to **stereotype** anyone or categorize the person based on preconceived and often incorrect assumptions. Although sometimes an assumption based on stereotypic categories may have a degree of truth, people should not be judged before you have gotten to know them as individuals. The medical assistant should push preconceived notions aside and look at the individual when forming and building a relationship. In the medical profession, stereotypic categories should not be considered when caring for patients and developing good rapport with them.

Perception

Perhaps one of the most important issues to consider when discussing barriers to communication is the concept of perception. Perception is the capacity for comprehension or the discernment of what is being communicated according to the message receiver's point of reference. When we discussed the transactional communication model earlier in the chapter, it was obvious that because of different types of noise and channels, the message sent sometimes would be distorted; the receiver would not always get the message the sender meant to send. The receiver's perceptions could completely alter the message, no matter how clearly it was sent. If the receiver believes that all attorneys are corrupt, he or she will probably be unable to get past this perception when speaking with one and therefore may not be able to trust any attorney.

Often our perceptions stem from some experience that happened in the past with a certain group of people. This perception goes unresolved or has affected us so strongly that we group all people from that walk of life into a negative category. This is an unfair way to deal with people; everyone should be viewed as an individual, not as a part of a stereotypic group. Remember, perception is an individual's point of view, right or wrong. The issue of interpretation also plays a role: the determination of what is meant by a certain message. An attempt must be made to understand both points of view, and the participants must be willing to discuss them calmly, even when discussing subjects that evoke anger. Most people do not truly enjoy conflict. Have a healthy respect for others' opinions. The differences among individuals are part of what makes each of us unique.

OVERCOMING BARRIERS TO COMMUNICATION

We know that communication barriers exist – but how do we overcome them? Most people who enter the medical field have a natural sense of caring and empathy, but the medical assistant can nurture their skills in using patience, perception, and listening skills. If a patient has a physical impairment, being observant will help with communication issues. Often, these patients want to be self-sufficient, so they may not appreciate help with simple tasks while at the physician's office. Be patient with them, as well as those who have a language barrier. Encourage these patients to bring an interpreter so that accurate, quality information can be placed into the medical records. Prejudice can be overcome with facts about the source of the social bias, and the same is true for stereotyping and perception issues. Even highly abrasive patients can be tolerated when the medical assistant wants to be an effective communicator with all patients. If nothing seems to work, talk to the office manager or physician. In severe cases, the physician may have to speak to the patient, or even suggest that he or she seek a different provider.

COMMUNICATION DURING DIFFICULT TIMES

Communication is not an art that comes easily to everyone. It often is difficult to express feelings in an honest, open way. When a crisis occurs, it is much harder to communicate effectively, and we sometimes say things we do not mean. Medical assistants must develop communication skills that can be used in times of trouble. They must be able to understand the reason or reasons a patient or co-worker is unable to communicate.

Patience is important, too, because people are not always at their best when they are concerned about their condition or that of a loved one. Always remain calm when dealing with a person who is experiencing a traumatic event or has any depressive condition. Remember that he or she may be reacting to many emotions, such as fear, anger, doubt, inadequacy, or many others. The key is to listen, to determine the best way to help the patient out of any

immediate danger and to help him or her establish some type of support system.

Anger

One of the most difficult times to communicate is when we are angry. Anger is a normal emotion that all of us feel at one time or another. Usually the expression of anger is a healthy thing. Some people bottle up their emotions and do not express what they truly feel inside. If this is done repeatedly, at some point the anger erupts, possibly over a tiny event or at an inappropriate time. Others explode over every little situation; people who do this need anger management skills and training.

Anger, like most emotions, can cause physiologic changes. When a person feels anger, the blood pressure rises and the heart rate increases. Many things can trigger anger, from a simple traffic backup to a real or perceived betrayal, the diagnosis of a disease, or the death of a close relative. "Road rage" is one example of anger out of control and is a serious problem on our public highways today. Unexpressed anger can cause or contribute to all types of health problems, including depression and hypertension.

The medical assistant can help pacify an angry patient by speaking calmly and refusing to return the emotion. If the volume is gradually lowered with every sentence spoken, the angry person also must lower the volume to hear what the assistant is saying. Suggest that the person breathe deeply and stop talking for a few minutes. Remember that the anger being expressed usually is not directed intentionally at the medical assistant. Be a good listener and allow the person to speak, as long as it is not abusive speech. Using logic with the angry individual may also help. Some use words such as *never* and *always;* for example, "My wife never balances the checkbook!" or "You always make me wait for my appointment!" These statements are broad generalizations and usually untrue. Using a logical approach and maintaining a calm attitude help the angry individual.

Address the root of the problem and be willing to admit it if the physician's office has made a mistake or contributed to a problem. Do not be afraid to say, "I'm sorry, I/we made an error." If you made the mistake, own it and apologize. Arguing never resolves the situation and only increases the intensity of the patient's feelings. Four words that often can disarm an angry person are, "Let me help you." Sometimes in a medical professional's career, a patient, a co-worker, or even the physician will lash out, even though the medical assistant is not the cause of the anger. Realize that this is a part of being human, and be as caring and kind as possible. If the anger becomes abusive, either refer the situation to a supervisor or, if that is not possible, tell the patient that you can no longer discuss the situation and offer to schedule an appointment so that the matter can be discussed at a later time. By then, the patient probably will have calmed down and will be able to discuss the situation rationally.

Shock

When an event or a circumstance arises that is especially painful, an individual may experience emotional shock. This may happen when a person has just been told that a family member has been killed in an automobile accident or some other catastrophe has taken place. Many different types of shock occur, but in this chapter, the emotional aspect is discussed. Often the person cannot think or move, and other coping reactions may take place. One person may scream in agony, whereas another may sit down and begin to talk about a completely unrelated subject. The person who appears calm is probably more at risk, because in addition to shock, he or she may be experiencing denial. We never really know in advance how we will react to events that are traumatic. Also, our reactions may differ from time to time. A person is able to cope with a traumatic event based on the other stressors in his or her life at the time.

David Straker, in his book, *Changing Minds*, describes adaptive and nonadaptive coping mechanisms. An adaptive coping mechanism is one that offers some type of positive help. Logically, a nonadaptive coping mechanism would be negative in nature. Consider the sleep requirement. A person who is in some type of shock may have some insomnia and needs to sleep. Getting several nights of recuperative sleep is an adaptive coping mechanism. If, however, he or she begins to sleep consistently during the day and at night, sleep may be considered a nonadaptive coping mechanism, because the individual is using sleep to avoid stressful issues.

Never leave a person in emotional shock alone. If the healthcare professional cannot stay close by, arrangements should be made for someone to stay near, especially during the early stages, if at all possible. Because the thought processes the person is experiencing may not be under control, he or she could be a danger to himself or herself or others.

The medical assistant should watch for several signs of emotional shock, including hyperactivity, disruptions in breathing patterns, blank staring, sudden hysterics, and shaking. Humans have an innate sense of threat or danger, and this sense may initiate the fight-or-flight syndrome. When a person feels a threat of some kind, the hormone adrenaline is released in the body quickly, producing an increased heart rate and blood pressure. The oxygen level in the body increases, which prepares the muscles to help the body flee. Awareness is increased, as are energy and performance. The individual either runs, avoiding the danger, which is the "flight" aspect, or stays to "fight," facing the stressors or threat. With either choice, the body must have this increased energy level and awareness to deal with the situation. When the immediate period of shock abates, the individual may feel a debilitating, drained sensation as the hormonal levels return to normal.

CRITICAL THINKING APPLICATION   5-6

- Is it possible that Sarah might experience shock months after her mother's death?
- How can the medical assistant help Sarah deal with these emotions?

Death and Dying

Years ago patients who were considered terminally ill were placed in hospital wards and left to their demise. The medical community did not focus on understanding the fears and concerns of the dying, and very few measures were offered to them that preserved their dignity. However, in 1969, Dr. Elisabeth Kübler-Ross, a Swiss psychiatrist, wrote a ground-breaking book, *On Death and Dying*. Kübler-Ross, who studied **thanatology**, realized that terminally ill patients were somewhat ignored, even by medical professionals, and she spent many hours interviewing these patients and discovering their fears and concerns. Kübler-Ross listened to them and realized that patients passed through certain stages as they dealt with their impending death. She held seminars, during which she interviewed dying patients as medical students listened. When the book was published, she was recognized internationally as an authority on the subject of death. She wrote more than 20 books about the process of dying. In *Life Lessons,* she shares many of the truths she had learned from the dying to encourage us to live. Kübler-Ross died in August, 2004.

Kübler-Ross believed that the process of dealing with death or loss has five specific stages: denial, bargaining, anger, depression, and acceptance. She believed that all people go through each stage in the grieving process, but they may not go through the stages in the same order. A stage could take days to work through or several months. Although she related these stages to dying patients, they are not exclusively limited to those who are dying. Anyone experiencing **grief** may progress through these five stages, and having a good understanding of them can help the medical assistant to better care for the patient.

On Death and Dying identifies denial as the first stage, during which the patient or grieving person denies the issue that is causing the grief and thinks, "No, not me." The person is shocked and rejects the facts. The denial is a defense mechanism that helps the individual deal with the news. The second stage is anger, when the dying patient begins to ask, "Why me?" The anger often is directed at others, who may include the people in the family taking care of the patient or healthcare workers who cannot produce a cure. In the third stage, the patient begins to bargain in an attempt to postpone death or eliminate it altogether. This bargaining usually is with God, and the patient may pray to see a child marry or to witness some other upcoming event. The event is not the true hope of the patient, but life itself is. These patients say, "Yes, me, but…" in the attempt to postpone death. The fourth stage is depression. During this stage, patients realize that they are going to die and may feel regret for the goals they did not accomplish or for not taking better care of themselves. These patients say, "Yes, it's me…" and they must be allowed this period of grieving. However, family and friends should watch the patient carefully for signs of deep depression. The final stage of grief is acceptance, during which the patient is able to say, "Yes, me, and I'm ready." The reality of the impending death or distressing situation is accepted, and although the patient may continue to experience some depression, he or she is better equipped to deal with the arrangements that have to be made and may even demonstrate good humor during this time.

Patients who are dying must be treated with empathy, dignity, and respect. This does not mean that they are unable to laugh and enjoy the life they are still living. Gentle touch and kind words reassure patients that the medical assistant cares for them. It is important to be careful with words and phrases around dying patients, but be natural in your conversations with them and do not be afraid to laugh. Never suggest to such patients that you "know how they feel." This phrase belittles their situation, and we never truly know how another person feels. Asking questions is a good method of communication when you are unsure about what to say. Use questions such as, "How do you feel about that?" or "What does your family think about your plans to discontinue treatment?" Then listen to the patient and make eye contact with him or her as you listen. You may also ask, "How can I help you?" as opposed to "Is there anything I can do?" There will be a natural tendency for the patient to say "No" to the second question. However, if you ask specifically how to help, they may open up and allow you or the office staff to be of help. They may simply need suggestions about who could cut their grass or how to contact Meals on Wheels. Hospice services provide terminally ill patients and their families with care and support, often from the point of diagnosis to bereavement. Many have found hospice services invaluable in the process of coping with a loved one close to death. The medical office should have listings of community resources to assist in these types of situations. Always use empathy when talking with the patient by being aware of, and sensitive to, the feelings that the patient may be experiencing.

CRITICAL THINKING APPLICATION   5-7

- People often put off writing a will. Could this be procrastination or a fear of death?
- When is it important to have a will?
- How can the medical assistant help Sarah to deal with her mother's impending death?
- What stage of grief might Mrs. Cloyd currently be experiencing? What stage might Sarah be experiencing?

MULTICULTURAL ISSUES

Cultural differences influence the way we deal with people from various parts of the world. We often become isolated in our thinking and incorrectly assume that people all over the world think and do things the same way we do. However, vast differences in cultures exist from country to country, and even in areas within the same country.

We sometimes stereotype people of other cultures and think we understand what they are like and how they live. Often, the **media** have influenced our thinking. Much can be learned from other cultures, and sharing is a way to gain an understanding of experiences in other places.

EXAMPLES OF CULTURAL TRADITIONS

- A husband speaks for his wife. The wife does not speak to the physician.
- The palm of the hand, facing down, is used to beckon someone. The hand motion signaling one to come or follow, performed with the back of the hand toward the patient, is used only when calling an animal. An open hand is used to point, rather than one finger.
- A female's clothing is not removed without the presence of another female family member.
- Emotional crying and sobbing denote femininity.
- Going to the doctor is a sign of weakness.
- The female medical assistant never touches the male patient.
- Acquaintances are not permitted to stand within 3 feet of the patient; only immediate family members are permitted to stand within this space.
- The Chinese do not like to be touched by people they do not know.
- The Laotian's "yes" response may not mean "yes," because it is considered rude to say "no" to others or to cause conflict.

- A native of Cambodia, as well as a Laotian, will not look into the eyes of the person being addressed because long eye contact means disrespect and is impolite.
- Cambodians do not like to have their blood drawn, because they believe it will weaken them.
- Afghans and Mexicans have a concept of time that is less precise than in the United States.
- Vietnamese consider the head to be a sacred part of the body and are offended by being touched on the head or shoulders. Only the elderly may touch the head of a child without giving offense.

Communicating with People of Other Cultures

People from other cultures want to be treated just as you would like to be treated if you were visiting another country; they want to be respected and treated fairly. Much can be learned about the background of others, and much can be shared about the culture we know, too. Cultural differences are responsible for many misunderstandings. We must make an attempt to understand people from other walks of life.

When we speak with those from a foreign country, a **language barrier** may exist. Even if the person knows some English, some words and phrases may not make sense in the way we use them in the United States.

It is important to be sensitive to and aware of the beliefs of the many cultures represented in the patient population. If you work in a practice that predominantly serves a distinct ethnic group, discuss possible cultural differences with the physician and with influential people in the cultural group. Learning to understand cultural differences helps you gain the confidence and respect of patients. Always use language and verbal skills that enable patients to understand the details of their medical care. Even if the traditions and cultures are vastly different and difficult to understand, the medical assistant must demonstrate respect for diversity in approaching patients and their families.

Communicating with patients who speak another language is difficult without an interpreter. If the physician serves a large population of non-English speakers, he or she should make certain that at least one staff member is bilingual and available to assist with interpreting when necessary. If none of the employees are bilingual, the appointment scheduler should tell patients to bring a friend or relative to their office visits to assist with paperwork and interpreting. The office policy should state that an interpreter must be present for the physician to treat the patient, so that the entire staff is able to communicate properly with the patient. Appropriate communication is vital to ensure that the patient understands the physician and the instructions to be followed, especially medication dosages.

COMMUNICATING DURING THE PATIENT ENCOUNTER

Remember that patients often are apprehensive during their appointments with the physician. Some questions can elicit information the patient has not voiced aloud. Many hospitals have added the phrase "Are you safe at home?" to their basic intake to ensure that the patient is not being abused or is the victim of violence. Even the simplest tasks, such as collecting a urine specimen, can cause nervousness and

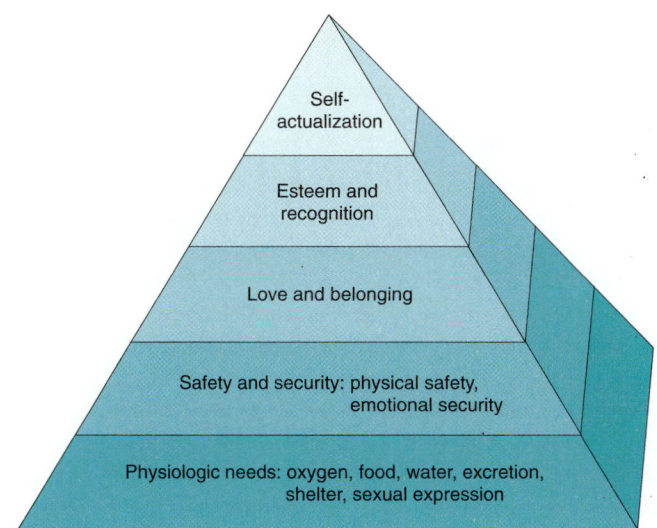

FIGURE 5-7 Maslow's hierarchy of needs. (From Adler RB, Towne N: *Looking out, looking in: interpersonal communication*, San Antonio, 1996, Harcourt Brace.)

anxiety. Always explain the purpose of tests the physician orders, and when performing treatments, explain each step to put the patient more at ease. Patients may not understand that a "blood glucose" simply means a blood sugar test in lay terms. Be sensitive to the patient rights and feelings when collecting specimens.

Maslow's Hierarchy of Needs

Psychologist Abraham Maslow created what he called the "hierarchy of needs" (Figure 5-7). A *hierarchy* is defined as things arranged in order, rank, or a graded series. Maslow believed that our human needs can be categorized into five levels and that the needs on each level must be satisfied before we can move to the next level. These levels often are depicted as a triangle, with the most basic needs at the bottom and the highest potential for growth as a human being at the top.

The needs we have as humans, at the most basic level, are those that involve our physical well-being: food, rest, sleep, water, air, and sex. The second level includes issues related to our safety. We need to feel safe and secure in our homes and our environments, as well as the places where we work. The third level involves our social needs for love, a sense of belonging, and interaction with others. The fourth level relates to our self-esteem. We have an inner need to feel good about ourselves and to know that others view us in a positive manner. The last level is the self-actualization stage, in which we maximize our potential. In this level, we attempt to be at our best and to live our lives to the fullest extent possible.

People adapt to life based on their individual needs, and many entities influence that adaptation, such as cultural and other elements of the environment, language abilities, and even physical threats, such as situations in which a woman refuses to leave her abusive husband for fear of harm. The medical assistant should actively investigate the resources that will allow patients to adapt to situations that affect their health status, and almost any life event can influence the patient's well-being.

Approval, Acceptance, and Achievement

Three specific needs that we have, apart from Maslow's hierarchy of needs, are critical to our happiness. These three are approval,

acceptance, and achievement. Although most would agree that we do not need everyone's approval at all times, we do seek the approval of specific people. Children usually want to please their parents, even when the child is an adult. We seek to please our supervisors, and even our own children. However, the need to please can be taken too far. Various books address personalities called *pleasers,* who often place their own needs second to the needs of those they feel they must please to feel of worth.

We have a healthier self-esteem if we feel accepted by others. This resembles the sense of belonging discussed earlier but is a bit more extensive. A feeling of acceptance includes the belief that our actions, words, dress, mannerisms, and other personality traits are acceptable to others we wish to impress.

Last, we have an inner need for achievement. Most humans want to do something great and contribute to their world in some way. A great thing to one person may be winning an Olympic race, but to another it may be reading to an elderly grandmother at a nursing home. We all enjoy praise for a job well done, or for losing weight, or for passing a difficult examination. Everyone benefits when legitimate praise is shared freely and appreciated. This is especially true in our close relationships but is just as important in the workplace. It is much easier to work for a supervisor who praises for work well done than for one who never offers a pat on the back.

A Good Night's Sleep

Many of us do not realize the value of our sleep time. Sleep is one of the most important physical needs we have, and it is the one most often sacrificed during busy, stressful periods. This is called *sleep deprivation.* Human beings need approximately 8 hours of sleep each night, although many can function for a period of time with less sleep. Eventually this lack of sleep takes a physical and emotional toll on the body.

Healthy Nutrition

We have been taught since we were children that good nutrition is vital to a healthy body. Our bodies are machines, and their performance depends on good health. We care for the body with a balance of good nutrition, activity, and healthcare. A balanced diet is essential to ensure that the organs and systems within us function at optimal levels. When the body is not receiving the nutrients and vitamins it needs, various parts may malfunction, and this can lead to conditions or diseases or to worsening of problems already present.

> ### CRITICAL THINKING APPLICATION   5-8
> - Could Sarah's sleep and nutrition habits affect her ability to care for her mother?
> - How might these affect Sarah's personal stress levels, and how can she ensure that she is caring for herself, when her thoughts are primarily on her mother?

Positive Relationships

As mentioned earlier in this chapter, all of us need to feel approval, acceptance, and achievement. These also are vital components of our relationships. When we are involved in a relationship that is not going well, it naturally is reflected in our attitude, our opinions, and our sense of self-esteem. This can greatly influence our performance at work. Often, because of infatuation, we find ourselves in a situation that might not be a positive one. Once the relationship is in progress, it sometimes is difficult to end it and find a connection with a supportive, caring individual.

Many individuals really have not determined what they need from a relationship. It is helpful to make a list of what you are looking for in a partner and to commit to refusing to compromise on the critical points. The sparks and fireworks that appear in the beginning of a relationship may lose their intensity as time goes on, and a firm foundation must be present after the newness wears off. Choose carefully and wisely, and the chances of becoming involved in healthy relationships greatly increase. In addition, more and more individuals are choosing to remain single and are enjoying life to the fullest. Certainly this choice is better than being a part of a destructive partnership.

Harmful relationships are not always just between partners. Often we experience stress and strain with relatives, friends, and co-workers. Sometimes contact with the person causing the discontent cannot be avoided, at least for a period of time. In these cases, we must learn coping techniques for dealing with the difficult relationship. Open, honest communication is paramount. By making wise relationship choices, medical assistants may prevent additional stress and worry during working hours, which can help keep their focus on the patients and duties to be performed and not on stressful situations outside of work.

CRITICAL THINKING APPLICATION   5-9

- Often survivors feel a sense of "unfinished business" with a person who has died, and they have a more difficult time bringing closure to the relationship. How might Sarah spend high-quality time with her mother and come to terms with her death in a positive way?
- Is there anything that should not be discussed with a terminally ill patient?

Healthy Self-Esteem

Self-esteem is confidence and satisfaction in oneself. To have high self-esteem, an individual must also be self-aware, and that takes some honesty. It means taking a look at your strengths and your weaknesses and knowing what you have to offer as a person. To feel well and accomplish goals in life, you must develop positive attitudes and positive responses to the pressures in life. It sometimes can be difficult to keep a positive attitude when others are being negative. Some people believe that if they inflict their bad feelings on others, they will feel better about themselves. It is important to remember, though, that no one can make you feel a certain way; it is a choice you make. Blaming others for one's situation in life or negative emotions is self-defeating.

We are able to control two things in life: our attitude and our actions. Even when faced with a potentially volatile situation, our attitude and reactions are decisions we make. These decisions should be made with careful thought, even if the reaction must be a swift one. Think before speaking. Pause a moment, if needed, before

reacting. Take a timeout. Choose your battles wisely. All of these suggestions can help you react in a more positive, constructive way when faced with a difficult situation.

Improving Yourself

No matter how great a person's training or how many opportunities are placed in front of the individual, fear and doubt can sabotage efforts to improve one's self-image, confidence, and potential. Almost every failure or mistake can be traced to fear or doubt; either we are afraid to take a specific action, or we doubt our own abilities. Blaming the circumstances around us is no excuse for a poor performance. It also is important to remember that small, daily decisions make a huge impact on our lives, sometimes even more than what we consider critical life decisions. For example, a student decides not to study for 30 minutes daily for an upcoming major examination, then fails it. This small decision to do something other than study results in failing an examination, which may force course repetition and delay the graduation date.

Self-esteem improves if a person is able to adapt to situations well. To be human is to be a changing, growing, imperfect but amazing living creation. Adapting means being flexible and open to the actions of others. Although we should have empathy for others, we cannot allow others to ruin our day or lower our confidence level. Inventor-philanthropist Charles Kettering once said, "The only time you can't afford to fail is the last time you try." Our failures often teach us much more than our successes. The important thing is to get up, evaluate why the failure occurred, then move forward armed with the new knowledge gained from mistakes.

Procrastination is often a symptom of the fear of failure and the fear of success. Many people procrastinate because they feel it gives them an excuse for their failure. They say, "There is no way I could pass that test; I only had 2 days to study!" Others are perfectionists and put off doing a job or delegating because they feel no one can do it as well as they can. The best way to stop procrastinating is to do something! Divide projects into small steps and complete one at a time. This makes tasks much less overwhelming.

Comfort Zones

We all have comfort zones. When faced with new ideas or changes, many of us tend to be a bit unsure of ourselves. Think back to the first day of school, the first day on a new job, the first time at a fancy restaurant, a first date; these events often made us feel a bit uncomfortable. New experiences may be outside our comfort zone. Psychologists often speak about a **comfort zone**, which is a place in the mind where we feel safe and comfortable, where we can perform comfortably and confidently. For most goals, however, we have to move outside our comfort zone to reach them.

CLOSING COMMENTS

Interpersonal skills are critical to success as a medical assistant. Communication is a part of all interactions throughout the day, and the better developed these skills are, the better the medical assistant can serve the patients in the facility. Every attempt should be made to enhance the interpersonal and human relations skills the medical assistant currently has and to strive continually to better these skills. This ensures that effective communication is part of the relationship with patients and with others with whom the medical assistant interacts.

Patient Education

The medical assistant has the opportunity to provide an educational service to every patient who enters the healthcare facility. Patients often have questions about their care or treatment, and the medical assistant with good communication skills can assist the patient in understanding.

Patients must have a clear knowledge of the role they play in their own care. The medical assistant can communicate information to the patient in many ways other than verbally. Leaflets and brochures can help patients understand their illness better and can educate them, but the medical assistant should always explain each piece of literature given to a patient. Never just hand out printed information and expect it to be read. Have the patient repeat instructions to clarify them if a question exists as to whether the patient understands.

Remember that physical care is not the only aspect of patient care; patients also have emotional needs. Often the very things we take for granted, such as food and shelter, are a struggle for some patients. The resulting stress can worsen their physical condition. Ask questions to remain aware of what the patient is communicating to the staff and what is not being said. This helps the medical assistant to best serve the patient.

Legal and Ethical Issues

Patients see the medical assistant as an extension of the physician; therefore, it is important that all communication with the patient be professional and accurate. Never give a patient advice that is not approved by the physician, to prevent accusations of practicing medicine without a license. Always discuss with the physician any issues that might affect the patient's care. Never agree to withhold any information from the physician, because even a small piece of information could completely change the plan of treatment. When giving instructions to patients, it is always best to have them in writing and to keep a copy for the patient's medical record so that a record exists of what was communicated to the patient. Use excellent documentation technique when adding information to the patient's chart. Remember that all the patients in the facility deserve to be treated with respect and compassion. Help the physician establish trust with the patient. An open, trusting relationship with the patient helps to prevent legal issues in the future.

SUMMARY OF SCENARIO

Mrs. Cloyd and her daughter are facing a difficult time. Death is inevitable for everyone, but when a loved one is diagnosed with a terminal illness, it is particularly distressing. Both of these women need compassion and caring from the medical team. They need to feel as if they are being heard and that their opinions are important. Some of their needs are similar, but they also have differing needs. A gentle touch and laughter can brighten their day, and these expressions are critical to a person experiencing the stress of a devastating illness.

The medical assistant must ensure that Mrs. Cloyd understands her medications and treatments. The office should assist her and her daughter in finding community resources for which she might be eligible. Be sure to instruct Mrs. Cloyd primarily, and make certain that Sarah also understands any directions her mother should follow. Sarah needs compassion as she deals with her mother's illness and impending death. Because she likewise is a patient of the clinic, she should be given care and attention and may have emotional needs or periods of great stress also. Even on the busiest of days, these two women deserve warmth from the staff and should be made as comfortable as possible as they seek medical care.

Although the medical office is always a busy place, medical assistants can take a moment to individualize the care that they provide to patients. Looking into the patients' eyes and genuinely asking how they have been getting along demonstrates interest in them. Call patients by their name and ask about their families. These techniques allow the medical assistant to develop rapport, which results in a more pleasant office visit for the patient.

Often, the patient is accompanied by a relative or friend, and the medical assistant may find it necessary to interact with these individuals. Remember that all information about the patient must be kept in strict confidence. Friends and family play a role in the overall health of the patient. When relations are strained, patients may feel depressed and stressed. This can affect their health in a negative way. The patient with strong family support often heals faster and has a better outlook on health issues.

Listening is a skill that must be practiced and refined. Patients need to know that the medical assistant is focusing attention on them, listening to their concerns, and paraphrasing to make sure the patient is understood correctly. Listening is one of the most important skills the medical assistant can develop.

SUMMARY OF LEARNING OBJECTIVES

1. **Define, spell, and pronounce the terms listed in the vocabulary.**
   Spelling and pronouncing medical terms correctly bolster the medical assistant's credibility. Knowing the definition of these terms promotes confidence in communication with patients and co-workers.

2. **Explain why first impressions are crucial.**
   First impressions are crucial in the medical profession because dress, attitude, and appearance all influence the credibility of the medical assistant. The medical assistant should always treat patients and visitors to the office as individuals who deserve the best in customer service.

3. **Differentiate between verbal and nonverbal communication.**
   Verbal communication depends on words and sound, whereas nonverbal communication consists of messages conveyed to another without the use of words. Body language, eye contact, facial expressions, and hand gestures are some of the many ways we use body language. Sometimes our body language conflicts with verbal communication, and a mixed signal is sent to the receiver. Often we are unaware of nonverbal signals and notice only a small number of the signals that other people send.

4. **Identify styles and types of verbal communication.**
   Medical assistants communicate casually in day-to-day life but use a professional style when communicating in the medical facility. Tone and diction are important. All information must be clear and accurate when communicating with patients. Although a personal or casual type of verbal communication is used in normal discussion, professional verbiage and attitude are required in medical facilities.

5. **Explain the different levels of spatial separation.**
   Spatial separation can be defined as the space of comfort between individuals. Public space usually is considered to be 12 to 25 feet, whereas social space is approximately 4 to 12 feet. Personal space is a range of 1½ to 4 feet, and intimate space includes touching up to approximately 1½ feet.

6. **Analyze the effect of hereditary, cultural, and environmental influences on communications.**
   Communication is affected by heredity when an individual inherits a gene that plays a part in the communication process; for example, a person with delayed speech and language skills may find it more difficult to communicate with others. Many conditions, such as autism, affect communication and social interaction. A patient's cultural heritage may prevent or hinder communication, depending on the beliefs related to culture that are held by the patient. Additionally, our environment may hinder communication. A person who is physically or emotionally abused may refuse to share information about the abuser.

7. **Discuss the value of touch in the communication process.**
   Touch is important in the process of communication because it projects an air of care and compassion to the receiver. The medical assistant should never be afraid to touch patients, as long as precautions are taken with those who are contagious. Touching the patient shows empathy and often can be more eloquent than the spoken word.

8. **Recognize the elements of oral communication using a sender-receiver process.**
   The transactional communication model includes a sender and a receiver, who offer messages to each other using various channels. The sender encodes a message, then the receiver decodes it to the best of his or her ability. Often some type of noise interferes, such as internal, external, and physiologic noise. Perception is important when communicating, because messages sometimes can be easily misinterpreted.

9. **Explain the value of active listening.**
   Listening is one of the most important skills the medical assistant can develop. Listening involves not only silence, but also active feedback. Open-ended questions help the medical assistant restate what the patient is saying to make sure the patient is understood clearly.

10. **Define and understand abnormal behavior patterns.**
    Patients may exhibit various abnormal behavior patterns that affect their physical and emotional health, such as phobias, obsessive-compulsive disorder, antisocial behavior, panic disorder, general anxiety disorder, and major depressive disorder. Some degree of knowledge about each of these disorders can help the medical assistant understand individual patients and allows the medical assistant to approach patients with empathy and professionalism.

11. **Recognize commonly used defense mechanisms.**
    Defense mechanisms are psychological methods of dealing with stressful situations. They include sarcasm, denial, repression, compensation, and several others. Often these mechanisms are our only way of dealing with circumstances with which it is difficult to cope.

12. **Discuss the role of assertiveness in effective professional communication.**
    There is a difference between assertion and aggression. Being assertive can mean that a person is forcefully stating his or her beliefs or point of view, often with no support or attempt at proof. An aggressive individual is acting in a forceful, dominant, hostile, injurious, or destructive manner. However, being either assertive or aggressive can be positive and productive. Assertive people often receive job promotions and reach the goals they set for their lives. However, too much aggression can make a person seem pushy; therefore, it should be controlled and used at the appropriate times.

13. **Identify the roles of self-boundaries in the healthcare environment.**
    Self-boundaries can include the physical space between people, but they also can apply to communications in a way that affects interaction with others. Each medical assistant must determine the workplace boundaries that are personally important to him or her; such as the use of first or last names, off-the-clock interactions with co-workers and supervisors, and e-mail forwarding of inappropriate materials.

14. **List several ways to deal with conflict.**
    Everyone experiences conflict in daily living; therefore, it is necessary to develop skills in dealing with conflict in as positive a way as possible. Conflict is not always negative and can be quite beneficial to relationships. Knowing the different types of conflict and the ways people

attempt to process conflict help the medical assistant to recognize patterns and respond appropriately. Some individuals deal with conflict by being aggressive, assertive, or nonassertive. In addition, many passive-aggressive methods of dealing with conflict can be used, such as avoidance, changing the subject, distraction, blaming, and several others.

15. **Recognize communication barriers.**

Some of the barriers to communication include physical impairment, language differences, prejudice, stereotyping, and perception. Barriers may also be present during difficult times, such as when a crisis occurs, when a person is angry or in shock, or when a patient or family member is experiencing an impending death or illness or has experienced a serious accident.

16. **Identify techniques for overcoming communication barriers.**

The medical assistant who approaches the patient with understanding and respect often wins the trust of the patient, who in turn will offer the information needed to help the person. Sincerity, empathy, and kindness make a difference, and a caring attitude also helps to overcome communication barriers.

17. **Differentiate between adaptive and nonadaptive coping mechanisms.**

An adaptive coping mechanism is one that offers some type of positive help. Logically, a nonadaptive coping mechanism would be negative in nature. Consider the sleep requirement. A person who is in some type of shock may have some insomnia and needs to sleep. Getting several nights of recuperative sleep is an adaptive coping mechanism. If, however, he or she begins to sleep consistently during the day and at night, sleep may be considered a nonadaptive coping mechanism, because the individual is using sleep to avoid stressful issues.

18. **Identify common stages that terminally ill patients pass through and discuss the support that can assist them and their families during their struggle.**

Dr. Elisabeth Kübler-Ross suggested that the process of grief has five stages: denial, bargaining, anger, depression, and acceptance. She believed that all stages are experienced while grieving, but not necessarily in the same order. A medical assistant with a good understanding of the grieving process can better care for the patient and the patient's loved ones.

19. **Discuss the use of empathy when treating terminally ill patients.**

Empathy is the ability to understand another person's feelings, situation, or motives. The medical assistant should look at situations from the patient's point of view and be considerate of his or her wishes at all times, even if the patient's needs and desires differ from the medical assistant's opinions. Terminally ill patients should never be pushed toward unwanted treatments or procedures by the healthcare professional.

20. **Identify resources and adaptations that are required based on individual needs.**

Each medical office should keep accurate, up-to-date information about available resources on hand so that it can be accessed quickly when needed. Be sure to check the physician's notes to determine whether he or she made a referral for a patient, and follow up to make sure the patient sought assistance from the person or organization named in the referral.

21. **List and explain the levels of Maslow's hierarchy of needs.**

Maslow's hierarchy of needs includes five levels, beginning with our most basic needs, such as food, rest, sleep, water, and anything that involves our physical well-being. The second level is related to safety issues; and the third, to our social needs, such as love and interaction with others. The fourth level deals with our self-esteem, and the fifth is self-actualization, where our potential is maximized.

22. **Discuss why physical and emotional needs affect our daily performance at work.**

Everyone needs physical and emotional rest to function throughout the day. A good night's sleep, consisting of at least 8 hours; regular exercise; and healthy nutrition help keep the medical assistant fit for duty. When these needs are not met, work performance may suffer, and the medical assistant may not be able to give proper attention and care to patients. Exhaustion affects the ability to perform, as do pressing concerns that linger in the mind. Make every effort to clear all negative thoughts and completely focus on the patients.

CONNECTIONS

Study Guide Connection: Go to the Chapter 5 Study Guide. Read and complete the activities.

Evolve Connection: Go to the Chapter 5 link at *evolve.elsevier.com/kinn* to complete the Chapter Review and Chapter Quiz. Check out the other resources listed for this chapter to make the most of what you have learned from Interpersonal Skills and Human Behavior.

6

MEDICINE AND ETHICS

Monica Johnson has been employed for 6 months as a medical assistant in a family practice. She works as the clinical medical assistant for Dr. Richard Wray. One of Dr. Wray's patients, Anna Walsh, recently adopted a baby after 8 years of trying to conceive a child. The baby, Delaney Gracelia, was born to a single mother, Susan, who participated in an open adoption in which she and the Walshes met and got to know each other during her pregnancy. Susan dated the baby's father for about 6 months before discovering that she was pregnant, and they are no longer dating. Susan wanted to make a good decision for the baby and decided to place her for adoption. Dr. Wray performed some genetic testing on Delaney, and the adoptive parents were involved throughout the pregnancy, even meeting Delaney's birth mother for physician appointments from time to time. Monica observed both Susan and the Walshes and saw many benefits from the arrangement, noticing that everyone was primarily concerned with Delaney and her happiness and well-being. However, some periods were difficult for both sides. This prompted Monica to give some thought to her own feelings and ideas about many different ethical situations and issues and how she would react in the face of having to make ethical decisions.

While studying this chapter, think about the following questions:

- What difficulties do patients placing their babies for adoption face?
- What difficulties do adoptive parents face when participating in an open adoption?
- How can the medical assistant be supportive of both the adoptive parents and the birth mother?
- Should the medical assistant discuss personal beliefs about ethical situations with patients?

LEARNING OBJECTIVES

1. Define, spell, and pronounce the terms listed in the vocabulary.
2. Differentiate between legal, ethical, and moral issues affecting healthcare.
3. Compare personal, professional, and organizational ethics.
4. Identify the effect personal ethics may have on professional performance.
5. Recognize the role of patient advocacy in the practice of medical assisting.
6. Explain rights and duties as related to ethics.
7. List and define the four types of ethical problems.
8. Discuss the process used to make an ethical decision.
9. Detail the impact of the American Medical Association's Council on Ethical and Judicial Affairs (CEJA) on the ethical decisions made by healthcare professionals.
10. Discuss several of the CEJA's opinions and how they might differ from the views of the class as a whole.
11. Explore the role of confidentiality as it applies to the medical assistant.
12. Discuss the role of cultural, social, and ethnic diversity in ethical performance of medical assisting practice.
13. Describe the way unique identifiers can help patients infected with the human immunodeficiency virus (HIV) avoid discrimination.
14. Note some of the concerns about ethics that apply to genetic information.

VOCABULARY

advocate (ad′-vuh-kat) One who pleads the cause of another; one who defends or maintains a cause or proposal.

allocating (a′-luh-ka-ting) Apportioning for a specific purpose or to particular persons or things.

annotations (a-nuh-ta′-shuns) Notes added by way of comment or explanation.

beneficence (buh-ne′-fuh-sens) The act of doing or producing good, especially performing acts of charity or kindness.

clinical trials Research studies that test how well new medical treatments or other interventions work in the subjects, usually human beings.

disparities (di-spar′-uh-tes) Marked differences or distinctions.

disposition (dis-puh-zi′-shun) The tendency of something or someone to act in a certain manner under given circumstances.

duty Obligatory tasks, conduct, service, or functions that arise from one's position, as in life or in a group.

euthanasia (yu-thuh-na′-zhe-uh) The act or practice of killing or permitting the death of hopelessly sick or injured individuals in a relatively painless way for reasons of mercy.

fidelity (fuh-de′-luh-te) Faithfulness to something to which one is bound by pledge or duty.

gametes (ga′-mets) Mature male or female germ cells, usually possessing a haploid chromosome set and capable of initiating formation of a new diploid individual; a sex cell, whether sperm or ovum.

genome (jeh′-nom) The genetic material of an organism.

idealism The practice of forming ideas or living under the influence of ideas.

impaired Being in a less than perfect or less than whole condition; it includes having handicaps or functional defects and being under the influence of drugs, alcohol, and/or controlled substances.

infertile Not fertile or productive; not capable of reproducing.

introspection (in-truh-spek′-shun) An inward, reflective examination of one's own thoughts and feelings.

justice With regard to medical ethics, the fair distribution of benefits and burdens among individuals or groups in society with legitimate claims on those benefits.

nonmaleficence (non-mal-fe′-zens) Refraining from the act of harming or committing evil.

opinions Formal expressions of judgment or advice by an expert; formal expressions of the legal reasons and principles on which a legal decision is based.

philosopher A person who seeks wisdom or enlightenment; an expounder of a theory in a certain area of experience.

postmortem Done, collected, or occurring after death.

procurement (pro-kuhr′-ment) To get possession of, to obtain by particular care and effort.

public domain The realm embracing property rights that belong to the community at large, are unprotected by copyright or patent, and are subject to use or appropriation by anyone.

ramifications (ra-muh-fuh-ka′-shuns) Consequences produced by a cause or following from a set of conditions.

reparations (re-puh-ra′-shuns) Amends, acts of atonement, or satisfaction given as a result of a wrong or injury.

sociologic Oriented or directed toward social needs and problems.

surrogate (suhr′-uh-gat) A substitute; to put in place of another.

unique identifiers Codes used instead of names to protect the confidentiality of the patient in a method of anonymous HIV testing.

veracity (vuh-ra′-suh-te) A devotion to or conformity with the truth.

Ethics can be defined as the thoughts, judgments, and actions on issues that have implications of moral right and wrong. Various beliefs exist about what is and is not ethical in everyday life and in the medical profession. The decisions that people make based on ethical beliefs can quite possibly alter the course of human existence. Ethics are different from legal issues mainly because something that is legal is not necessarily ethical. Ethics is considered a higher authority than legality. The American Medical Association's Council on Ethical and Judicial Affairs (CEJA) clarifies the relationship between law and ethics as follows: Ethical values and legal principles are usually closely related, but ethical obligations typically exceed legal duties. In some cases, the law mandates unethical conduct. In general, when physicians believe a law is unjust, they should work to change the law. In exceptional circumstances of unjust laws, ethical responsibilities should supersede legal obligations. Ethics and morals are more closely related, although ethics often are attributed to professional interactions, whereas morals are usually personal in nature. Medical assistants not only must have a strong knowledge base about ethical issues they might face throughout their careers, they also must come to terms with some of the deeply rooted value systems that have been a part of their lives since youth. The trials and tribulations we have experienced, as well as the joys, all influence our thought patterns when we are faced with an opportunity to make a good ethical decision.

Personal, professional, and organizational ethics all contribute to the way the medical assistant approaches the patient. For instance, if a medical assistant personally believes that a patient should be taken off life support when there are no signs of brain activity, he or she must understand that professionally, this decision must be left to the patient's family members. The medical assistant must not force his or her personal ethical beliefs on the patient or family members. Organizations will offer ethical guidelines as well in the form of policies and procedures; for example, each medical assistant is required to maintain patient confidentiality. This practice reflects the organizational ethic that all patients have the right to confidentiality of their information and records (Procedure 6-1). Personal and professional ethics must be kept separate so that patients can make their own decisions regarding their healthcare (Procedure 6-2).

PROCEDURE 6-1

Respond to Issues of Confidentiality

GOAL: *To ensure that medical assistants treat all information regarding patient care as completely confidential.*

Unless otherwise noted, all equipment and supplies are to be provided by the instructor.

EQUIPMENT and SUPPLIES

- Copy of the Code of Ethics of the American Association of Medical Assistants (AAMA)
- Copy of the Medical Assistant Creed
- Copy of the Oath of Hippocrates
- Copy of the guidelines from the Health Insurance Portability and Accountability Act (HIPAA)
- Notepad and pen
- Patient medical record
- Patient role-play cards (provided by instructor)

PROCEDURAL STEPS

1. Read through each document, paying particular attention to the references to confidentiality.
   PURPOSE: To gain insight into documents that stress confidentiality as a critical aspect of the healthcare process, to reinforce the importance of patient confidentiality, and to understand the roots of ethical behavior.
2. Select a student with whom to role-play as a patient. The patient should present with a situation or an illness that he or she wants to keep confidential.
   PURPOSE: Apply ethical behaviors, including honesty and integrity, in performance of medical assisting practice.
3. Greet each patient by name.
4. Take the patient to a private exam room or other area suitable for a private conversation and attend to his or her needs and questions.
   PURPOSE: To restrict the conversation to medical personnel and the patient.

5. Listen carefully to what the patient says, taking notes if necessary, asking clarifying questions, and using restatement to clear up any misunderstandings.
   PURPOSE: To demonstrate to patients an interest in what they say and to make sure all their concerns are addressed and answered.
6. Assure the patient that his or her concerns and health issues are confidential.
   PURPOSE: To put the patient at ease, so that he or she feels comfortable in sharing each detail of the condition or of the concerns that need to be discussed.
7. Explain to the patient that information cannot be kept from the physician.
   PURPOSE: To make sure the medical assistant will not be asked to withhold information from the physician.
8. Discuss the information with the physician or ask the physician to speak personally with the patient, depending on which is appropriate to the circumstances.
   PURPOSE: To act only with authorization from the physician.
9. Instruct the patient according to the physician's orders, if necessary.
10. Document the patient's concerns, information given by the patient, and the physician's orders in the medical record.
    PURPOSE: To provide a record of the conversation and the circumstances of the patient's concerns and the physician's plan for resolution.
11. Do not share information about the patient with anyone not directly related to the patient's care.
    PURPOSE: To ensure complete patient confidentiality.

PROCEDURE 6-2

Develop a Plan for Separating Personal and Professional Ethics

GOAL: *To determine one's ethical views before having to confront an ethical decision.*

Unless otherwise noted, all equipment and supplies are to be provided by the instructor.

EQUIPMENT and SUPPLIES

- Pen and paper
- Copy of the Council on Ethical and Judicial Affairs Opinions
- Patient Role-Play Cards (provided by instructor)

PROCEDURAL STEPS

1. Set aside time to study and consider the ethical issues outlined in this chapter (e.g., abuse, abortion, organ donation, stem cell research, and so on).

PURPOSE: To make any ethical decision, research the subject and give thought to each issue so that the decision is credible.
2. For each issue, make notes regarding personal thoughts, paying particular attention to whether you agree with the current opinion of the Council on Ethical and Judicial Affairs.
   PURPOSE: To examine the impact that personal ethics and morals may have on the medical assistant's practice.

PROCEDURE 6-2—cont'd

3. Look at each issue as a separate ethical problem and apply the ethical decision-making process to each.
   PURPOSE: To consider each issue in an organized way.
4. Gather relevant information by researching each problem.
   PURPOSE: To make certain that all facts are considered when determining personal views about each issue.
5. Identify the type of ethical problem that each issue represents.
   PURPOSE: By accumulating information about the issue and matching it with an ethical problem, the medical assistant will be able to apply knowledge and determine personal views more easily.
6. Determine the ethical approach to use.
   PURPOSE: Knowing the type of problem that each ethical issue represents helps the medical assistant to determine the best approach to each decision.
7. Explore practical alternatives.
   PURPOSE: Considering all practical alternatives helps the medical assistant make the best ethical decisions.
8. Decide your personal stand on each issue.
   PURPOSE: By gathering information, identifying the problem and the best ethical approach to use, then considering all practical alternatives, the medical assistant can arrive at a sound ethical decision about his or her personal stand on each issue.
9. Determine the Council on Ethical and Judicial Affairs stance on each issue.

PURPOSE: By determining the personal stance and knowing the professional stance for each ethical issue, the medical assistant will not be faced with having to make a decision on the spot.

10. Continue the process until each ethical issue has been addressed.
11. Conduct further research about other ethical issues using the American Medical Association Web site.
    PURPOSE: To discover additional ethical issues that medical assistants may face throughout their career.
12. Refrain from inflicting personal ethical views on any patient.
    PURPOSE: To ensure that patients determine their own ethical views and make medical decisions based on their own views as opposed to those of the medical staff.
13. Interact with patients in a professional way, regardless of their or your own ethical views.
    PURPOSE: All patients must be treated in a professional way, regardless of their ethical views or healthcare choices.
14. Re-evaluate personal ethical views periodically and apply new knowledge and experience to determine whether ethical views have changed.
    PURPOSE: To be open to change based on experience in the medical field and new discoveries or technology. Healthcare is an ever-changing profession; therefore a medical assistant must develop an attitude of being a lifelong learner. New trends may change the medical assistant's position on ethical issues.

HISTORY OF ETHICS IN MEDICINE

From earliest recorded history, humans have pondered ethics, or the judgment of right and wrong. Ethics should not be confused with etiquette. *Etiquette* refers to courtesy, customs, and manners, whereas *ethics* explores the moral right or wrong of an issue. It is not surprising that for centuries, the field of medicine has set for itself a rigid standard of ethical conduct toward patients and professional colleagues.

The earliest written code of ethical conduct for medical practice was conceived in approximately 2250 BC by the Babylonians. It was called the Code of Hammurabi. It elaborated on the conduct expected of a physician and even set the fees a physician could charge. The code was quite lengthy and detailed, which is probably the reason it did not survive the ages. In approximately 400 BC Hippocrates developed a brief statement of principles that remains an inspiration to the physicians of today. The Oath of Hippocrates has been administered to many medical graduates. The most significant contribution to medical ethics after Hippocrates was made by Thomas Percival, an English physician, **philosopher**, and writer. In 1803 he published his Code of Medical Ethics. Percival was very concerned about **sociologic** matters and took great interest in the study of ethical concepts as they related to the medical profession.

In 1846, as the American Medical Association (AMA) was being organized in New York City, medical education and medical ethics already were considered important aspects of the profession. At the first annual AMA meeting in 1847, a Code of Ethics was formulated and adopted. It specifically acknowledged Percival's code as its foundation, and this document became a part of the fundamental standards of the AMA and its components. Even today, sections of the AMA Code of Ethics stem from Percival's writings.

WHO DECIDES WHAT IS ETHICAL?

When we weigh the question of who decides what is ethical, the answer is evident: you do. Every day medical professionals face the task of making ethical decisions. As with any important choice, the short- and long-term effects and consequences must be considered. Although depending on groups and committees to guide ethical decisions is a completely acceptable practice, the responsibility for making these decisions ultimately rests with the individual (Figure 6-1).

Organizations that study ethical dilemmas may decide that a concept such as abortion is an ethical medical practice. But if an individual does not find abortion to be an acceptable practice for religious or other reasons, abortion is not ethical for that individual. A great freedom that Americans often take for granted is that we can exercise free will in decisions related to individual conscience in this country and that we can choose from a variety of options; however, we must exercise this responsibility carefully.

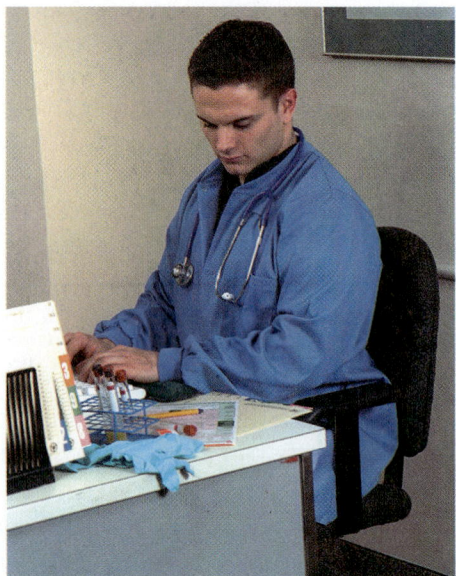

FIGURE 6-1 Medical assistants may find themselves making ethical decisions on a daily basis.

THE ROLE OF THE AMERICAN MEDICAL ASSOCIATION AND ITS COUNCIL ON ETHICAL AND JUDICIAL AFFAIRS IN ISSUES OF ETHICS

The AMA serves physicians as a national organization that provides various types of information and support. One of the most important facets of the AMA is its Council on Ethical and Judicial Affairs. The CEJA consists of nine active members of the AMA, including one resident physician member and one medical student member. It is responsible for interpreting the *AMA Principles of Medical Ethics* as adopted by the House of Delegates of the AMA. The AMA's Code of Ethics has four components:

- Principles of medical ethics
- The fundamental elements of the patient-physician relationship
- Current opinions of the CEJA with **annotations**
- Reports of the CEJA

The *Code of Medical Ethics: Current Opinions with Annotations* contains the first three components, with discussion of more than 135 ethical issues encountered in medicine. A separate publication, *Reports of the Council on Ethical and Judicial Affairs,* discusses the rationale of the council's **opinions**. The *AMA Principles of Medical Ethics* has been revised several times to take into account

developments in medicine, but the moral intent and overall **idealism** of these principles have not changed.

MAKING ETHICAL DECISIONS

An understanding of a few of the elements of ethics, the different types of ethical problems, and how a good ethical decision is made is important before we discuss the opinions of the CEJA. Then, as some of the opinions are presented in this text, students can begin to evaluate their own positions on each issue. This section enables the medical assistant to recognize the types of ethical problems that might arise in the physician's office and provides a pattern to follow in making an ethical decision.

Elements of Ethics

Dr. Ruth Purtilo, an authority on ethics in medicine, has written a book on the subject, *Ethical Dimensions in the Health Professions.* She presents three general elements of ethics: duties, rights, and character traits. A **duty** is an obligation a person has or perceives himself or herself to have. A daughter may feel the obligation to care for her elderly parents, or a husband who has hurt his spouse may feel an obligation to somehow make up for his act.

Purtilo mentions several types of duties related to the medical profession. **Nonmaleficence** means refraining from harming oneself or another person. **Beneficence** means bringing about good. **Fidelity** is the concept of keeping promises, and **veracity** is the duty of telling the truth. **Justice**, in relation to medical ethics, deals with the fair distribution of benefits and burdens among individuals or groups in society having legitimate claims on those benefits. When a person has wronged another, he or she has a duty to make **reparations**, or right the wrong. Last, a person should feel grateful if he or she is a beneficiary of someone else's goodness. This also is a type of duty.

Rights are defined as claims a person or group makes on society, a group, or an individual. The Bill of Rights appended to the U.S. Constitution guarantees certain liberties that we enjoy as American citizens. However, some individuals think that they have rights, but those rights are actually privileges. For instance, Americans do not have the "right" to healthcare services. Individuals may expect to be cared for when sick, but this is not a right guaranteed to anyone in America. Some countries provide medical care to all their citizens, but the United States is not one of those countries. A right applies to all people within a group, without prejudice.

Purtilo defines *character traits* as a **disposition** to act a certain way. A person who believes that honesty is an important character trait usually can be trusted to speak the truth. One who feels comfortable with taking small items from work for use at home may not be able to resist an opportunity to take something more valuable. Character traits certainly do not always indicate how a person will react in all situations. No human being is perfect, and we sometimes are unpredictable. Stress also can interfere with our normal reactions, and other factors, such as depression or anger, influence how we act. The phrase that someone is acting "out of character" usually means that the person is deviating from his or her normal behavior patterns.

With an understanding of these basic elements of ethics, we have a good foundation to help us look more objectively at ethical problems and solve them to the best of our ability.

Types of Ethical Problems

Purtilo presents four basic types of ethical problems (Figure 6-2):

- Ethical distress
- Ethical dilemmas
- Dilemma of justice
- Locus of authority issues

Ethical distress is a problem in which a certain course of action is indicated, but some type of hindrance or barrier prevents that action. A professional knows the right thing to do but for some reason cannot do it.

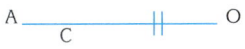

WHAT SHOULD BE DONE?

---

1. **Ethical Distress**

   I know which course of action I (the "agent") should take for the patient's benefit, but there is a structural barrier to my being able to do it.

   $$A \underset{C}{\rule{3cm}{0.4pt}} \| \rule{1cm}{0.4pt} O$$

   A = Agent
   C = Course of Action
   O = Outcome

2. **Ethical Dilemma**

   There are two (or more) courses of action, each of which is right (or wrong). No matter which one I (the "agent") choose, something of value will be compromised.

   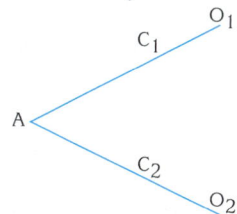

3. **Distributive Justice**

   There are benefits to be distributed among several potential beneficiaries. Not everyone can receive a full measure of the benefit. On what basis should the distribution be made?

   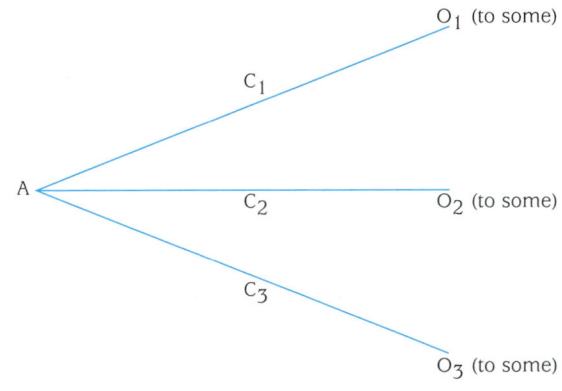

WHO SHOULD DO IT?

---

4. **Locus of Authority**

   There are 2 (or more) agents or "authorities" in this situation. Each believes he or she knows what outcome will benefit the patient the most, but only one authority will prevail.

   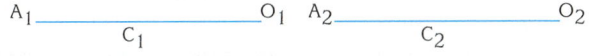

FIGURE 6-2 Summary of the types of ethical problems. (From Purtilo R: *Ethical dimensions in the health professions,* ed 4, Philadelphia, 2005, WB Saunders.)

An *ethical dilemma* is a situation in which an individual is faced with two or more acceptable or correct choices, but doing one precludes another. A choice must be made, and something of value may be lost if a second choice is eliminated. This could be viewed as the proverbial "being caught between a rock and a hard place," when the effect of a choice made may be greater than is immediately obvious.

The third type of ethical problem is the *dilemma of justice.* This problem focuses on the fair distribution of benefits to those who are entitled to them. Choices must be made regarding who receives these benefits and in what proportion. Examples include organ donation and distribution of scarce or costly medications.

In *locus of authority issues,* two or more authority figures have their own ideas about how a situation should be handled, but only one of those authorities can prevail. If one physician feels that a patient should have surgery and another does not, how does the patient decide?

Recognizing the type of ethical problem is not always easy. Sometimes an issue is a mixture of one or more types of ethical problems. When possible, it is wise to take time to weigh the courses of action before making an important decision. Unfortunately, with the fast pace of the medical profession, this is not always possible. Some decisions must be made in a split second; therefore, having a thorough grasp of ethical decision making before the need arises is important.

The Ethical Decision-Making Process

Purtilo proposes a five-step process for ethical decision making:

1. Gathering relevant information
2. Identifying the type of ethical problem
3. Determining the ethical approach to use
4. Exploring the practical alternatives
5. Completing the action

To gather information, a medical professional should ask questions, review charts, talk to the patient and other professionals, and search for other data so that the entire situation is available for scrutiny. Once the information has been gathered, the medical professional must decide which ethical problem or problems are presented. In determining the ethical approach to use, we must consider the duties, rights, and character traits of all the individuals involved, paying close attention to the **ramifications** of all possible decisions. All of the alternatives must be considered and evaluated, after which an action should be taken.

Although taking time to give these areas some thought is best, it may not be possible. Therefore, those entering the medical profession should take stock of their core beliefs. Scan the newspapers and search professional journals for ethical situations, think about the facts, then decide how you would react to each one. This is excellent preparation for the day you are faced with making a quick ethical decision.

CRITICAL THINKING APPLICATION   6-2

- What are the ramifications of an open adoption such as Delaney's? What problems might occur during the first year of her life?
- How might these problems be prevented?
- What are the positive aspects of the adoption?

CURRENT OPINIONS OF THE COUNCIL ON ETHICAL AND JUDICIAL AFFAIRS AND MEDICINE'S ETHICAL ISSUES

Now, armed with a basic knowledge of the types of ethical problems and the process for solving them, we take a look at some of the CEJA's opinions. Remember, physicians and other medical professionals are not bound to abide by these opinions. They are free to make their own decisions, but many of the medical professionals in our country tend to agree with the decisions made by the council. In the study guide, students will find cases to discuss relating to many of these ethical situations.

Abortion

In 1973 the U.S. Supreme Court heard the case of *Roe v. Wade.* Norma McCorvey (using the name Jane Roe) petitioned the court for permission to have an elective abortion when, at age 21, she found herself pregnant with her third child. The class action suit she filed against Henry Wade, then the district attorney in Dallas, Texas, eventually was appealed to the Supreme Court. Although she won her case, it was too late for her to have an abortion, and her child was born and placed for adoption. McCorvey went public with her true identity in the early 1980s and later became a staunch opponent of abortion and has spent many years promoting the overturn of *Roe v. Wade.*

Since the ruling was handed down in 1973, abortion has been one of the most volatile issues in medical ethics. According to the *AMA Principles of Medical Ethics,* the AMA does not prohibit a physician from performing an abortion in accordance with good medical practice and under circumstances that do not violate the law. In recent years laws have been passed in some states requiring mandatory parental notification of a minor's intent to have an abortion. In some cases this means that the minor must have parental consent, and in others, parents only must be notified of their daughter's intent to have an abortion. Some states also require a 24-hour or longer waiting period after the notification. However, the CEJA states that the patient, even if an adolescent, should ultimately be in control of the decision on whether parents should be involved in the abortion decision.

The AMA strongly encourages physicians to attempt to persuade the minor to seek counseling from someone she trusts, such as a school counselor, teacher, or relative, if the minor's parent will not be involved in the abortion decision. However, the AMA agrees that the physician should not feel compelled to require minors to involve the parent in the decision. Medical professionals must be aware of the laws in their respective states that deal with the mandatory notification requirements and should contact the medical societies in their region to determine what constitutes proper notification.

Abuse

The AMA requires that a physician be familiar with the signs of physical, psychological, and sexual abuse of spouses, children, mentally incompetent persons, and the elderly. Discovery of abuse creates a difficult situation for a medical professional. The patient may be the object of abuse but may deny its existence because of fear of further attacks. The law requires that abuse be reported, and if the physician does not report abuse, ethical standards have been breached. In addition, the abuse may continue. Any medical assistant who suspects abuse must report this information to the physician immediately. Then, the physician must determine whether the incident is reportable by law and take action. If the physician does not take action, but the medical assistant is confident that abuse has happened, he or she is responsible for making a report to the proper authority in the city or state.

Allocation of Health Resources

Sometimes society must decide who receives care when serving all who need care is not possible. Decisions must be made fairly and should be weighed carefully. The criteria to consider when **allocating** health resources include urgency of need, likelihood of benefit, duration of benefit, amount of resources required for successful treatment, and potential for change in the quality of life. Nonmedical criteria should not be considered; these include ability to pay, the social worth of the individual, age, obstacles to treatment, and the patient's contribution to the illness. The physician must remain the patient's **advocate** and should not be involved in making allocation decisions for that patient. Procedures for such allocations are determined in an objective manner by the institutions involved in the patient's care.

Artificial Insemination/In Vitro Fertilization

Any individual or couple considering artificial insemination or in vitro fertilization must be thoroughly counseled and must endure lengthy screening procedures for communicable and genetic diseases that the donor and/or recipient may have. Artificial insemination is performed when donated sperm is used to impregnate a woman. Egg cells are fertilized outside the womb and then, if fertilization takes place, the embryo is placed inside the woman's uterus. Before in vitro fertilization can happen, the physician must determine the woman's most fertile time in the month and harvest the eggs at that time. The technique of in vitro fertilization and embryo transplantation enables certain couples previously incapable of conception to bear a child. The CEJA holds that because of serious ethical and moral concerns, any fertilized egg that has the potential for human life and that will be implanted in the uterus of a woman should not be subjected to laboratory research. All fertilized ova not used for implantation that are maintained for research purposes must be handled with the strictest adherence to the *AMA Principles of Medical Ethics,* to the guidelines for research and medical practice expressed in the CEJA's opinion on fetal research, and to the highest standards of medical practice.

Informed consent must be provided, and further regulations are based on the marital status of the people involved. If the recipient is married to the donor, the resultant child has all the rights of a child naturally conceived. If the donor is anonymous, the husband must sign a consent if he is to become the legal father of the resultant child. If the donor and recipient are not married, the recipient is considered the sole parent, unless both parties agree to recognize a right to paternity. Providing artificial insemination or in vitro fertilization to a single woman or a woman who is part of a homosexual couple is not considered unethical. It usually is considered unethical to offer compensation to donors other than reimbursement of actual expenses and/or compensation for the donor's time.

Much discussion is ongoing about the use of extra embryos harvested for reproductive purposes. The control and use of these **gametes** logically should be left to the man and woman who produced them, but the AMA agrees that both must give their consent to how they are used. Artificial insemination/in vitro fertilization is considered an ethical procedure.

Stem Cell Research

Many organizations believe that using human embryos for stem cell research destroys the most vulnerable of beings, and laws have been passed to protect these embryos. Others want to explore the possibility of developing cures from this research for conditions such as Alzheimer's disease, diabetes, Parkinson's disease, and heart disease. Stem cell research continues to be an area of disagreement because of the controversy regarding the point at which life begins. Those who believe that life begins at conception usually oppose stem cell research, because it involves experimentation and testing on a "viable human being." Many physicians believe that their commitment is first to "living persons," as opposed to embryos, and therefore support stem cell research.

Surrogate Motherhood

Surrogate motherhood introduces many different ethical, legal, and social problems for the individuals involved. However, it may be the only opportunity for an **infertile** couple to have a child. The benefits of surrogacy must be heavily weighed against the possible risks and psychological problems that might arise. The AMA believes that the birth mother must be given a period during which she can reverse her decision to give up the child she has delivered and void the contract. However, in cases of gestational surrogacy, the legality and ethical implications are more complicated. In gestational surrogacy, the child is not genetically linked to the birth mother. Usually the couple engaging the surrogate mother are the genetic parents of the resultant child. One must also consider what will happen if the child is born with a deformity or handicap. This is a contract that should never be enacted without strong forethought and counseling.

Genetic Counseling

Genetic counseling is another area in which the AMA recommends caution. Through genetic counseling, parents of tomorrow may be able to choose eye color, talents, and intellect levels for their children. Human beings already have been conceived as "designer babies." In 1980 the Repository for Germinal Choice (more commonly known as the "Genius Sperm Bank") was founded. Although it was not established to create a perfect "master race," it did attempt to produce leaders and creators. As with cloning, the AMA recommends that much more research be done before genetic counseling is instituted on a global scale.

CRITICAL THINKING APPLICATION   6-3
- How might the genetic testing done in Delaney's case have caused an ethical dilemma?
- Discuss whether genetic testing can be counted on to predict disease.
- How many in your class would have genetic testing done on their own child before birth?

Family and Intimate Partner Violence

The CEJA believes that all forms of family and intimate partner violence are major public health issues and urges the profession, both individually and collectively, to work with other interested parties to prevent such violence and to address the needs of victims. Physicians have a major role in lessening the prevalence, scope, and severity of child maltreatment, intimate partner violence, and elder abuse, all of which fall under the rubric of family violence. To support physicians in practice, the AMA will continue to campaign against family violence and remains open to working with all interested parties to address violence in American society. The AMA's efforts are guided, in part, by its Advisory Council on Family Violence.

Ethical Responsibility to Study and Prevent Error and Harm

In the context of healthcare, an error is an unintended act or omission or a flawed system or plan that harms or has the potential to harm a patient. Patient safety can be enhanced by studying the circumstances surrounding healthcare errors. According to the CEJA, physicians should participate in the development of reporting mechanisms that emphasize education and systems change, providing a substantive opportunity for all members of the healthcare team to learn. Physicians also must show professional and compassionate concern for patients who have been harmed, regardless of whether the harm was caused by a healthcare error.

Physician-Assisted Suicide

The AMA believes that physician-assisted suicide interferes with the fundamental purpose of being a physician—to be a healer. The CEJA advocates that physicians aggressively provide care and treatment alternatives for those near the end of life but that they avoid promoting or providing the means by which patients could end their own lives. Such means include not only assisting the patient to inject chemicals that induce death, but also prescribing drugs and providing information about lethal doses or administering a lethal dose of a drug to a patient to promote death. This is sometimes called **euthanasia**, or mercy killing.

Surrogate Decision Making

According to the CEJA, physicians should encourage patients to document their preferences about advance directives through a living will or durable power of attorney. However, many patients do not have any type of documentation of their wishes available when tragedy strikes. In these cases, a surrogate may be asked to make decisions for the patient about medical treatment. Even when such provisions have been made, the documents sometimes are unavailable in an emergency; therefore, patients should discuss treatment options in advance with those who may be called on to act as a surrogate decision maker. If patients cannot make medical decisions for themselves and documented advance directives are unavailable or nonexistent, absent any state regulation to the contrary, the physician should approach the patient's family, domestic partner, or a close friend to act as the surrogate decision maker. In some cases family members may disagree about decisions necessary for the patient's health and well-being. In these instances the physician should work to resolve the conflict through mediation or should consult the facility's ethics committee. The physician's ultimate goal is to act in the best interests of the patient, and in the absence of any other basis for interpreting how a patient would wish to proceed with treatment, the physician should make the decision that, in the physician's professional opinion, would most benefit the patient.

Withholding or Withdrawing Life-Prolonging Treatment

A physician is committed to saving life and relieving suffering. Sometimes these two goals are incompatible, and a choice between them must be made. If possible, the patient should decide what treatment is given. Often the patient makes his or her wishes known to a responsible relative or other representative in case the patient becomes incapacitated. Some patients want a "do not resuscitate" (DNR) or "no code" order added to their charts. Usually such an order is established so that no heroic measures are taken in a situation in which a patient would be unable or incompetent to make a decision. In any case, the decision to withdraw life support should be made before any mention of organ donation is made by the medical professionals tending the patient. In the best situation, the patient has formally completed advance directives. Two types of advance directives usually are used in the United States: a living will and a durable power of attorney. These documents are written instructions for healthcare and are strongly recommended by the AMA.

A durable power of attorney is a legal document that allows the patient to appoint someone who is trusted to make medical decisions for the patient in the event the patient cannot. This person is sometimes called a *patient advocate* or *healthcare proxy*. Federal law requires that patients be given information about advance directives by all facilities that participate in the Medicare and Medicaid programs.

Quality of Life

Physicians sometimes must participate in or advise others on decisions affecting the fate of a person whose prognosis is poor, such as a deformed newborn or a person of advanced age with many physical problems. The first thought may be the burden that the patient's care places on the family or society. However, the AMA insists that the physician's primary consideration must be what is best for the patient.

Fees for Medical Services

Concern for the quality of patient care should be the physician's first consideration. However, the physician should be conscious of costs and should not provide or prescribe unnecessary services. Access to an adequate level of healthcare for all members of our society is now a moral expectation but certainly not a right. Cost must be considered when these services are provided, in addition to the degree of benefit to the patient, the duration of the benefit, and the number of people who will benefit.

Organ Donation

Organ donation is not only considered ethical by the AMA, it is encouraged. However, it is considered unethical to participate in proceedings in which the donor receives payment, except reimbursement of expenses directly incurred in the removal of the donated organ. The rights of the patient and the donor must be protected equally. If the donor is deceased, the death must be certified by a physician other than the recipient's physician.

Because the need for donated organs is so extreme, protocols have been established by healthcare facilities to determine when it is proper to harvest organs. Organ **procurement** may be performed immediately after a person has died, or it may be done after a patient has been kept alive artificially for a time. Hospitals also have specific guidelines for the donation of organs from living donors, such as a kidney donation. When donations are made from one living person to another, both patients must have an advocate team that includes a physician, so that the interests and well-being of each patient are addressed. Payment to a living donor other than legitimate expenses incurred in connection with removal of the organ is considered unethical. Blood donations probably are the most common form of organ donation.

The CEJA has recommended consideration of two proposals with regard to organ donation: the mandated choice model and the presumed consent model. These proposals are aimed at increasing organ donations and would change the approach to consent for deceased donations. The mandated choice model would require individuals to express their preferences about organ donation when they perform some state-regulated task, such as renewing a driver's license. This method would be ethically appropriate only if the individual's choice was made in accordance with the principles of informed consent. Under the presumed consent model, deceased individuals would be presumed to be organ donors unless they had indicated a refusal to donate.

> ## CRITICAL THINKING APPLICATION   6-4
> - Monica has often thought about being an organ donor. She is very much in favor of organ donation because of her interest in the medical field. Her parents are very opposed to this because of their religious beliefs. How can Monica deal with this conflict within her family?
> - If Monica dies before her parents do, how can she ensure that her wishes are carried out?

Capital Punishment

The CEJA does not consider participation by a physician in the act of capital punishment to be ethical. The physician may certify the person's death but should not administer a lethal injection or induce death in any way. This will conflict with the physician's role as a healer, much in the same manner as does physician-assisted suicide.

Potential Patients

According to the CEJA, physicians must keep their professional obligations to provide care to patients in accord with their prerogative to choose whether to enter into a patient-physician relationship and must respond to the best of their ability in cases of medical emergency. The Emergency Medical Treatment and Active Labor Act (EMTALA) is a statute that ensures public access to emergency services regardless of ability to pay. Physicians also cannot refuse to care for patients based on race, gender, sexual orientation, gender identity, presence of infectious diseases, or any other criteria that would constitute discrimination. However, if a physician does not feel he or she is qualified to treat a certain condition or disease, the patient can ethically be referred to a more qualified physician.

Withholding Information from Patients

The practice of withholding pertinent medical information from patients in the belief that disclosure is medically contraindicated is known as "therapeutic privilege." It creates a conflict between the physician's obligations to promote patients' welfare and respect for their autonomy by communicating truthfully. Withholding medical information from patients without their knowledge or consent is ethically unacceptable. Physicians should encourage patients to specify their preferences regarding communication of their medical information, preferably before the information becomes available. Moreover, physicians should honor patients' requests not to be informed of certain medical information or to convey the information to a designated proxy, provided these requests appear to genuinely represent the patient's own wishes.

Healthcare Fraud and Abuse

The following guidelines encourage physicians to play a key role in identifying and preventing fraud: (1) Physicians must renew their commitment to the Principles of Medical Ethics, which state that "a physician shall deal honestly with patients and colleagues, and strive to expose those physicians deficient in character, competence, or who engage in fraud or deception"; and (2) physicians should make no intentional misrepresentations to increase the amount of payment they receive or to secure noncovered health benefits for their patients.

National Health Information Technology

The AMA supports the development, adoption, and implementation of national health information technology standards through collaboration with public and private interests and consistent with current efforts to establish health information technology standards for use by the federal government.

Genetic Information and the Criminal Justice System

The release of genetic information from a physician's records without the consent of the patient constitutes a breach of confidentiality. However, according to the CEJA, the confidentiality laws acknowledge that law and overriding social considerations may permit physicians to disclose confidential information in limited circumstances. Physicians should follow the AMA's guidelines when releasing information to criminal justice authorities.

Gifts to Physicians from Industry

Many gifts given to physicians by companies in the pharmaceutical, device, and medical equipment industries serve an important and socially beneficial function. However, there is a growing concern about certain gifts from industry to physicians. To avoid the acceptance of inappropriate gifts, physicians should observe the following guidelines: (1) Any gifts accepted by the physicians individually should primarily be of benefit to patients and not be of substantial value; (2) individual gifts of minimal value are permissible as long as the gifts are related to the physician's work (e.g., pens and notepads); (3) gifts for conferences or meetings must meet the CEJA's definitions; and (4) subsidies from industry must contribute to patient care. If a question ever arises as to the ethics regarding acceptance of any gift from industry, the physician or office manager should consult the AMA.

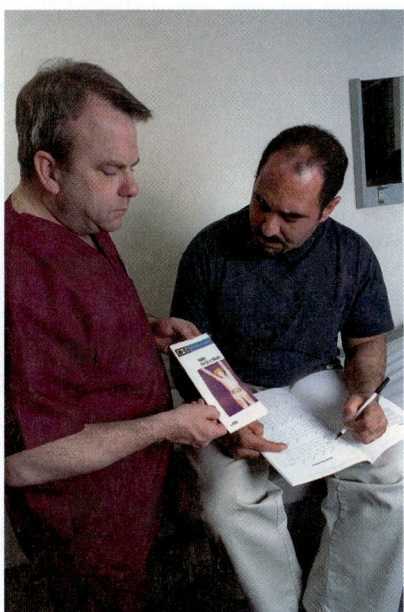

FIGURE 6-3 One of the duties of a medical assistant is to ensure that the patient understands the instructions given. Only when the patient fully understands the choices available can he or she make sound decisions.

Informed Consent

The patient's right of self-decision can be effectively exercised only if the patient possesses enough information to enable an informed choice (Figure 6-3). The CEJA holds that the patient should make his or her own determination about treatment. The physician's obligation is to present the medical facts accurately to the patient or to the individual responsible for the patient's care and to make recommendations for management in accordance with good medical practice. The physician has an ethical obligation to help the patient make choices from among the therapeutic alternatives consistent with good medical practice. Physicians should also sensitively and respectfully disclose all relevant information to patients.

Interprofessional Relationships

If a medical assistant recognizes or suspects an error in a physician's orders, he or she has an ethical obligation to report this to the physician. A possible error must be questioned, even if it means risking the physician's or supervisor's displeasure. This could save a life or prevent a lawsuit.

Physicians often refer a patient to another physician for diagnosis and treatment. Physicians should make these referrals only when they are confident that the patient will receive competent treatment. Offering a financial incentive or other valuable consideration to patients in exchange for recruitment of other patients is unethical.

Unless the state imposes legal restrictions, a physician in private practice is free to choose whom he or she will treat. Although private practitioners may refuse certain patients, they must treat those who have already been accepted in the practice or face possible charges of neglect. This does not include referring a patient to another physician for a condition that is not within the scope of practice of the original physician.

A sports medicine physician must keep in mind that the professional responsibility at a sporting event is to protect the health and

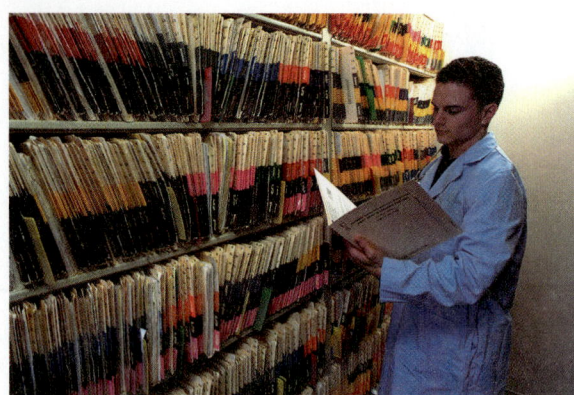

FIGURE 6-4 Confidentiality applies to all information about the patient, including what is charted and what is said between the patient and the medical assistant.

safety of the participants, and personal judgments are governed only by medical considerations. Players should not be allowed to play and risk injury to ensure that a game is won.

In years past, it was considered unethical for a physician to have any type of romantic relationship with nurses or assistants in the office or hospital. Although this is not as stringent a rule today, fraternizing with co-workers, especially subordinates, is unwise.

Confidentiality and Patient Privacy

Confidentiality is one of the cardinal rules of the medical profession. It is completely unethical and unacceptable to divulge any information about a patient to any other person not directly related to the patient's care. The places where confidentiality often is breached are elevators, hallways, waiting or reception areas, break rooms, and lunch rooms. A relative may be standing behind the medical assistant, listening to conversations that are inappropriate for those not personally involved in the patient's care to hear. Breach of patient confidentiality is grounds for immediate termination from a healthcare facility or physician's office.

Confidentiality restrictions apply to information in a patient's records and charts and also to what the medical assistant is told by the patient or the patient's family (Figure 6-4). Never investigate a patient's record strictly for curiosity. All information in the record must be kept in confidence. If records are computer based, accessing records of patients who do not fall directly under the medical assistant's realm of duty also is considered unethical. Never share information about patients with anyone outside the medical facility or office, including your own immediate family.

The prime objective of the medical profession is to render service to humanity, and this also must be a medical assistant's first concern. The importance of respecting the confidentiality of information learned from or about patients in the course of employment cannot be overemphasized. It is unethical to reveal patient confidences to anyone, including family members, a spouse, best friends, and other medical assistants. A medical assistant must never mention the names of patients outside the place of employment, because sometimes the doctor's specialty reveals the patient's reason for consultation. Confidential papers, case histories, and even the appointment book should be kept out of sight of curious eyes.

Outside observers should be present during the patient's encounters with the physician only with the patient's explicit permission.

Outside observers may include a friend who drove the patient to the physician's office or a medical student or intern observing in the clinic. This permission should be documented in the patient's chart.

Never discuss one patient's case with another patient. If curious patients ask questions about others, simply explain that medical assistants are obligated to keep all patient information confidential. This can be done in a tactful, kind manner. Patients who ask questions of a medical nature about their own case should be referred to the physician for information and instructions unless the physician has authorized the medical assistant to provide this information. When minors request confidential services, physicians should encourage them to include their parents. However, if the minor does not want to involve them and the law does not require otherwise, physicians should allow competent minors to consent to medical care and should not notify the parents without the minor's consent.

Remember that the Health Insurance Portability and Accountability Act (HIPAA) has established strict regulations for patient confidentiality and disclosure of private health information. Make sure the physician's office is abiding by its own privacy policy and that all patients have been given a chance to review that policy. A document stating that the patient has read and understands the privacy policy or that he or she has refused to sign should be part of the patient's medical record.

Patients may not always understand the ethical standards to which physicians and medical assistants adhere. They may ask questions about their own health or the health of a fellow patient. Medical assistants must educate patients about the issues of confidentiality in such a way that patients are not offended; they should explain that all patients deserve to have their medical and personal information kept private. Now more than ever, the medical assistant's obligation to keep information private is not only an ethical but also a legal responsibility. All patients should understand that they are entitled to confidential treatment of their records and that the facility is dedicated to that principle.

CRITICAL THINKING APPLICATION   6-5

- Susan, Delaney's birth mother, comes to the office for a checkup 6 weeks after the baby was born. She looks a little sad, and when Monica questions her, she asks how Delaney is doing. What should Monica tell her?
- How can the office protect itself from issues involving confidentiality in this unusual adoption scenario?

Advertising

The only restrictions on advertising by physicians are those that specifically protect the public from deceptive practices. Standards on advertising and publicity have been liberalized over the years, but any advertisement or publicity must be true and not misleading. Testimonials of patients, for instance, should not be used in advertising, because they are difficult to verify or measure by objective standards. Statements regarding the quality of media services are highly subjective and difficult to verify.

Communication with the Media

Although information about some patients, such as celebrities and politicians, may be considered news, the physician cannot discuss any patient's condition with the press without authorization from the patient or the patient's legal representative. The physician may release only authorized information or that which is public knowledge. Certain kinds of news are part of public records; such news in the **public domain** includes births, deaths, accident reports, and police cases.

A medical assistant must be aware that only the physician is authorized to release information, and under no circumstances should the medical assistant violate the confidential nature of the physician-patient relationship. It is unethical even to certify or verify that a patient is under the physician's care without the patient's permission. A policy must be in place for every medical office regarding how media inquiries should be handled and to whom they should be referred. Never voluntarily speak to the press without authorization from the physician. Communication with the media falls under the HIPAA guidelines. Do not release a patient's health information without written permission.

Physician Obligations in Emergency Preparedness and Response

Physicians are ethically obligated to provide urgent medical care during disasters. Because extensive physician involvement is required during national, state, regional, and local disasters, physicians are expected to contribute both their time and their skills in such emergencies. Examples of instances when physicians would be obligated to act include natural disasters, epidemics, terrorist attacks, and emergencies on a local and national scale.

Malevolent Use of Biomedical Research

Because biomedical research may produce information that has potential for both harmful and beneficial applications, the physician must assess the possible ramifications of participation in such research before engaging in projects. One of the most harmful uses of biomedical research involves biologic weapons. Physicians are expected to hold public trust as sacred and consider the welfare of society as a whole, in addition to the welfare of individual patients.

Racial and Ethnic Healthcare Disparities

No **disparities** in medical care based on race or ethnic background are acceptable. Patients are entitled to the same quality of care regardless of their race or ethnic background. The CEJA demands that physicians strive to eliminate biased behavior toward patients. Discrimination toward any patient or patient group cannot be tolerated. In addition, physicians must take into account any language barriers that might hinder effective treatment of the patient. Every effort must be made to ensure that the patient understands the physician and vice versa. The medical assistant must recognize that patients will have cultural, social, and ethnic diversities and that these diversities should be respected.

Diagnostic Imaging on Request

Patients may request diagnostic imaging services for reasons such as determination of a baby's gender. Physicians should perform diagnostic imaging only when they believe the benefits of the imaging service outweigh the risks involved.

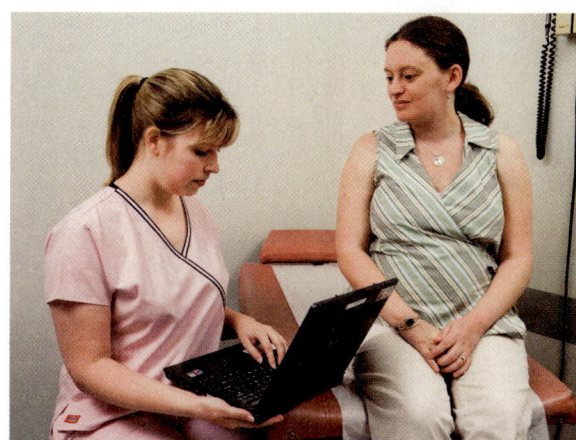

FIGURE 6-5 With the advent of advanced computer technology, a medical assistant must be particularly careful about using information about patients on the computer.

Computers

The expanding uses of computer technology permit the accumulation of an unlimited amount of medical information. With the use of computers in the physician's office and the employment of computer service organizations, confidentiality becomes even more difficult to maintain. In general, all information must be entered and accessed only by authorized personnel, and a tracking system should be used to identify which employees access information. Breaches in computer policies should be considered a breach of patient confidentiality, and the consequences should be stringent enough to deter employees from accessing information to which they are not entitled (Figure 6-5). Computerized information should be disseminated only to those with a legitimate need for it.

Fees and Charges

Charging or collecting an illegal or excessive fee is unethical. The medical assistant is responsible for keeping informed about current billing regulations and to see that they are followed conscientiously.

Requesting that payment be made at the time of treatment is entirely appropriate and very common in today's medical offices. Often, managed care patients are asked to remit their co-payment before seeing the physician on the day of the visit. If the patient is notified in advance, adding interest or other reasonable charges to delinquent accounts also is considered ethical. Most offices use a patient information booklet, which provides a written reference for all policies, that is given to new patients on the first visit. A reasonable fee may be charged for duplicating patients' records.

Physicians should never base their decision whether to order a diagnostic test on the patient's insurance coverage. If an expensive diagnostic test is needed, such as a magnetic resonance imaging (MRI) scan, the physician should order it instead of withholding the order for financial reasons. However, if the physician is aware of a way that the patient could get financial assistance with the test, he or she should relay that information to the patient.

Fee Splitting and Contingent Fees

If a physician accepts payment from another physician solely for referral of a patient, both are guilty of an unethical practice called *fee splitting.* This practice is unethical whether it involves another physician, a clinic, a laboratory, or a drug company.

Although attorneys often accept a case on a contingency fee basis, it is unethical for a physician to engage in this practice. The fee in this case is contingent on a successful outcome, but a physician should never set his or her fee on the successful outcome of medical treatment. A physician's fee must always be based on the value of service provided to the patient.

Insurance Forms

Although in times past physicians' offices willingly filed insurance claims for their patients, some have changed to a payment up front system and give patients the information needed to file the claim themselves. Many offices still file at least one insurance claim for established patients, but they may charge for multiple or complex insurance filing. This practice is entirely ethical if it conforms to local custom.

Waiver of Insurance Co-Payments

Physicians may opt to write off or waive co-payments to facilitate a patient's access to medical care. If access to care is directly threatened because the patient cannot make the co-payment, the physician may forgive the payment. However, routine waiver of co-payments may violate the policies of some insurers, both public and private. Physicians should ensure that their policies on co-payments are consistent with applicable law and within the legal boundaries of their contracts with insurers.

Professional Courtesy

Professional courtesy is defined as the provision of medical care to physician colleagues or their families and staff free of charge or at a reduced fee. This is a long-standing tradition but certainly not an ethical requirement. Physicians make the decision as to who receives professional courtesy in their offices, and this should be written into the office policy manual. In some cases, extending professional courtesy is contrary to insurance and/or managed care contracts. In addition, some physicians have stopped offering professional courtesy because of the rising costs of healthcare and shrinking reimbursements.

Appointment Charges

It is ethical for a physician to charge for a missed appointment or one that was not cancelled within a stated time if the patient was fully advised in advance that such a charge may be made. Discretion should be used in applying such charges, however, because the patient may have encountered an emergency. Often, adding a missed appointment charge to the bill of a patient who never cancels in advance prompts a call in the future when the appointment cannot be kept.

Prescribing Drugs and Devices

The physician should not be influenced in the prescription of drugs, devices, or appliances by a direct or indirect financial interest in the supplier. A physician may own or operate a pharmacy but generally may not ethically refer his or her patients to that pharmacy. Patients should enjoy the same freedom of choice in deciding who fills their prescriptions as they do in choosing a physician.

Professional and Contractual Relationships

Physicians often enter into contractual relationships, which may be as simple as monthly pest control services for the office. However, contracts can be quite complicated and contain numerous provisions, requiring an attorney's assistance. Physicians should negotiate the wording of contracts so that no question exists of financial incentives for the physician that would in any way compromise professional judgment or integrity.

Physician Ownership of a Health Facility

A physician ethically may own or have a financial interest in a for-profit or other healthcare facility, such as a freestanding clinic or health club. However, before admitting or referring a patient to that facility, the physician has an ethical obligation to reveal such ownership to the patient. In general, physicians should not refer patients to a health facility outside their office practice and at which they do not directly provide care or services.

Ghost Surgery

Substitution of another surgeon without the patient's consent is called *ghost surgery.* Patients have the right to choose their own physician or surgeon. Ghost surgery may happen when the patient has already received anesthesia and has no idea that a substitution has been made. To make a substitution without consulting the patient is deceitful and unethical.

Discipline Within Medicine

A physician should expose incompetent, corrupt, dishonest, or unethical conduct on the part of members of the profession without fear of loss of favor. A physician may be subject to civil or criminal liability, including loss of license to practice medicine, for violating government laws. Expulsion from membership is the maximum penalty that may be imposed by a medical society for violation of ethical standards.

Physician Health and Wellness

Physicians are responsible for maintaining their own good health and for being well enough to treat their patients. When physicians are not well, both physically and mentally, their health can interfere with the ability to provide good care to patients and engage in the safe execution of professional medical activities and decision making. Physicians not in such good health are said to be **impaired**.

The CEJA recommends that all physicians have their own personal doctor, who will use uncompromised objectivity in caring for the physician's health. Healthcare providers are expected to intervene promptly when the health or wellness of a colleague appears to have become compromised. The CEJA suggests types of intervention, such as offers of encouragement and referrals to physician health programs or other programs that restore and maintain the physician's health and wellness.

Substance Abuse

It is unethical for a physician to practice medicine while under the influence of a controlled substance, alcohol, or other chemical agents that could impair the ability to care for the patient properly or perform procedures. The physician's staff also must avoid all types of substance abuse. Healthcare providers who are aware of other providers or staff members with substance abuse problems must take action to ensure patients' safety, which may include reporting the user to the appropriate authority in the city or state in which the person practices medicine or works in the medical industry.

Unethical Conduct by Members of the Health Professions

In rare instances, a medical assistant is faced with a situation in which the physician-employer's conduct appears to violate established ethical standards Before making any judgments, the medical assistant must be absolutely sure of all the information and circumstances. If unethical conduct occurs, the medical assistant must then make his or her own decision about continued employment in the facility and whether the unethical behavior should be reported to a law enforcement agency, the local medical society, or the hospital where the physician has been granted privileges. Would it be wise to remain in the office under the circumstances? Would it be better to seek other employment? Would remaining adversely affect future opportunities for employment with another physician?

These decisions are difficult, especially if the relationship and employment conditions have been favorable and congenial. An ethical medical assistant does not want to participate in known substandard or unlawful practices, especially those that might be harmful to patients. In addition, the medical assistant must never make inaccurate reports regarding unethical behavior and should realize that some states can prosecute individuals who file a false report. Be absolutely certain of the facts before making such accusations against any health professional. When the physician's ethical standards conflict with those of the medical assistant, the medical assistant must decide whether staying with the physician is the best option. That decision may require a degree of soul searching and perhaps listing the pros and cons of each decision. Never compromise ethical standards for monetary gain. Remember that we must live with the decisions we make today, tomorrow.

ETHICAL ISSUES REGARDING HIV

Infection with the human immunodeficiency virus (HIV) creates a whole new world of ethical concerns for patients and those who support and care for them. When the HIV crisis first came to public attention, much about the virus was unknown, and a wealth of misinformation resulted. Those infected with the virus often were forced to leave their homes and lost their jobs; they were shunned by society, and they faced rejection seemingly everywhere they turned, all because of fear of the illness.

Clinical trials currently are underway for vaccinations against HIV, but clinical trials need volunteers for testing. Because vaccinations often are made of an *attenuated,* or weakened, strain of a virus, serious concerns exist about who receives the vaccination. Researchers have considered testing the vaccines in several Third World countries with a high number of prostitutes and a thriving sex industry. These people, who have no intention of changing their lifestyle regardless of the risks, may see vaccination trials as a chance to avoid contracting HIV. However, this raises the ethical question of whether testing should be done on people from disadvantaged countries rather than our own citizens.

Even today, people infected with HIV face discrimination. Consequently, problems arise with testing in some states in which the names of patients who test positive for HIV are reported to various health departments and agencies. Although the stated intention is to ensure that these patients receive care, the accompanying effect is the risk of discriminatory practices. Some states use code systems, called **unique identifiers**, to help maintain the confidentiality of those tested. However, other states insist by statute that the names be reported. Some states require mandatory HIV testing for prisoners and those who have committed sex crimes. Insurance is a difficult issue when a person is infected with HIV, and some policies can be cancelled if HIV infection is discovered. This may prompt providers who want to treat patients infected with HIV to delay reporting the infection as long as possible, using other diagnoses regarding symptoms as opposed to the underlying cause of the patient's problems. Many details are involved when HIV is a factor, even the reporting of HIV-positive status on the **postmortem** report. All of these ethical issues are difficult to resolve, and great care must be taken in making decisions that affect a patient who tests positive for HIV.

ETHICS AND THE HUMAN GENOME

The mapping of the human **genome** has been in the news for several years. The genome project formally began in 1990 with the goals of identifying all 20,000 to 25,000 genes present in the human body; determining the sequences of the 3 billion chemical base pairs that make up human deoxyribonucleic acid (DNA); and finding ways to catalog this information in databases to make it readily available to those who need it. The project was completed in 2003, but the data discovered during the 13 years of the project will be studied for years.

The mapping of the human genome and the information provided have raised concerns about privacy and confidentiality issues. Who actually owns genetic information, and who will be allowed to control it? Logically, the patient would seem to own his or her own genetic information; however, if that is so, the patient should be able to control access to it. Also, decisions must be made regarding fair use of genetic information. Employers, schools, courts, insurance companies, adoption agencies, and the military are just a few examples of organizations that might misuse genetic information and discriminate against those whom they may wish to target for inclusion or exclusion. Reproductive issues also arise, along with questions about the reliability of genetic testing.

CLOSING COMMENTS

Medical assistants have an ethical obligation to keep abreast of current developments that affect the practice of medicine and the care of patients. Membership in a professional organization provides access to continuing education for maintaining knowledge and skills pertaining to the performance of medical assisting.

The study of ethics requires much thought and honest appraisal of what the medical assistant believes. Sometimes **introspection** of this type is difficult. Often our beliefs are a result of our environment, upbringing, and other factors that have influenced our thinking and actions from the time we were small children to our current age. It is important that our belief system be one that we have created personally, not just a set of beliefs accepted from another source.

Medical assistants should take a serious look at the thoughts and concepts that make up their own concepts of ethics. It is important to approach ethical decisions calmly, logically, and without haste.

Patient Education

Patients may not always understand the ethical standards to which physicians and medical assistants adhere. They may ask medical assistants questions about their own health or the health of a fellow patient. Medical assistants must educate patients about confidentiality in such a way that the patient does not take offense, explaining that all patients deserve to have their medical and personal information kept private. Now more than ever, ethical obligations for privacy, in addition to legal ones, are imperative. A medical assistant must be certain that all patients understand that they are entitled to confidential treatment of their records and that the facility is dedicated to that principle.

Legal and Ethical Issues

The prime objective of the medical profession is to render service to humanity, and this also must be a medical assistant's first concern.

The importance of respecting the confidentiality of information learned from or about patients in the course of employment cannot be overemphasized. It is unethical to reveal patient confidences to anyone, including family members, a spouse, best friends, and other medical assistants. Never mention patient names outside the place of employment; sometimes, the physician's specialty reveals the patient's reason for consultation.

Do not discuss one patient's case with another patient. If curious patients ask questions about others, simply explain that the staff is obligated to keep all patient information confidential. This can be done in a tactful and kind manner. Patients who ask questions of a medical nature about their case should be referred to the physician for information and instructions unless the physician has authorized the medical assistant to provide such information. A medical assistant should never give advice of a personal or professional nature to the patient, because patients tend to identify remarks made by any of the assistants as reflecting the advice of the physician. By avoiding these situations, medical assistants protect themselves, the physician, and the patient. Confidential papers, case histories, and even the appointment book should be kept out of sight from curious eyes.

SUMMARY OF SCENARIO

Pregnancy usually is a joyous time, but Monica has learned that even such an anticipated event can bring ethical issues to light. She has realized that every situation has two or more sides and that she must be open and willing to look at all sides when making an ethical decision.

Medical assisting is a rewarding career, but sometimes the decisions medical professionals face are quite difficult. Monica must learn to be nonjudgmental and not to inflict her opinions on her patients. They must make their own decisions about their health and emotional well-being, and the medical assistant should not influence their thinking unfairly.

Monica must continue to evaluate her own ideas and beliefs throughout her career as a medical assistant. Periodic self-evaluation is good for everyone, and she will grow emotionally from the experiences that patients bring about where ethical issues are concerned.

Patients who place their babies for adoption often feel the same type of grief experienced on the death of a loved one. Sometimes this loss does not register with the patient for many years after the event. Adoptive parents also face many fears, such as the concern that the adoptive mother will change her mind about the proceedings and want the child back. Some families find the adjustment to having an adopted child in the family a difficult one. Siblings may be less than accepting of the new child, and later in life other children may tease the adopted child. However, adoption is most often a positive event in the life of a family.

The medical assistant should be supportive of both the adoptive parents and the birth mother. Personal beliefs should be set aside, so that the patient and others involved are able to make the best decisions they can for their own lives.

SUMMARY OF LEARNING OBJECTIVES

1. **Define, spell, and pronounce the terms listed in the vocabulary.**
   Spelling and pronouncing medical terms correctly bolster the medical assistant's credibility. Knowing the definition of these terms promotes confidence in communication with patients and co-workers.

2. **Differentiate between legal, ethical, and moral issues affecting healthcare.**
   Legal issues are related to an actual law or a regulation that affects medical practice. Ethical issues are not as strict as laws and vary from person to person, but most physicians follow the ethical guidelines set forth by the AMA. Moral issues are related to a person's concept of right and wrong.

3. **Compare personal, professional, and organizational ethics.**
   Personal ethics are those beliefs held by an individual. Professional ethics are those generally held by most people in a profession. Organizational ethics are closely related to professional ethics and are outlined by organizations as policy.

4. **Identify the effect personal ethics may have on professional performance.**
   The medical assistant may hold personal ethical beliefs that contradict professional ethics. However, the medical assistant must agree to the ethical policies and procedures set forth by the employer and follow them in every situation. If the ethical policies and procedures differ greatly

from personal ethical beliefs, the medical assistant should look for employment opportunities that are more in line with those personal beliefs.

5. **Recognize the role of patient advocacy in the practice of medical assisting.**

All medical professionals should be patient advocates, providing support as the patient makes decisions related to his or her health. Personal ethical opinions and beliefs cannot be forced upon patients or used to coerce the patient's decisions.

6. **Explain rights and duties as related to ethics.**

Ethics are judgments of right and wrong or actions on issues that have implications of a moral right and wrong. *Etiquette* deals with courtesy, customs, and manners. A *duty* is an obligation that a person has or perceives himself or herself to have. *Rights* are claims made by a person or a group on society, a group, or an individual. Although these terms have different definitions, the concepts are interrelated, and often all are involved in ethical questions.

7. **List and define the four types of ethical problems.**

Ethical distress is caused when a problem has an obvious solution but some type of barrier hinders the action that needs to be taken. An *ethical dilemma* is a situation that has two or more solutions, but if one is chosen, something of value is lost in not choosing the other. A *dilemma of justice* involves allocation of benefits and how they are to be distributed fairly. Two or more authority figures, each with his or her idea of how to handle a certain situation, are the center of the *locus of authority* ethical problem. Only one of the authority figures can prevail. Often an ethical problem has several aspects, and more than one type of problem is presented.

8. **Discuss the process used to make an ethical decision.**

Making an ethical decision is easier when the situation is approached logically and considered using a five-step process. First, relevant information is gathered; then the type of problem is identified. After the ethical approach to use has been determined, alternatives are explored. Finally, all that is left is to complete the action and make the decision.

9. **Detail the impact of the American Medical Association's Council on Ethical and Judicial Affairs on the ethical decisions made by health-care professionals.**

Although healthcare professionals do not have to abide by the opinions of the CEJA, the council's opinions are highly regarded, and many professionals practice in accordance with these opinions. Often providers abide by the opinions to prevent controversy, but many still openly oppose the decisions of the CEJA.

10. **Discuss several of the CEJA's opinions and how they might differ from the views of the class as a whole.**

The opinions put forth by the CEJA are just one group of opinions. Class members may share very differing views based on culture, experience, or serious consideration of the issues. Each individual is entitled to an opinion, and these opinions should be discussed and shared calmly and respectfully.

11. **Explore the role of confidentiality as it applies to the medical assistant.**

Confidentiality is of major importance in the medical profession. The patient's privacy should be a prime concern of the medical assistant. It is a serious enough issue that a breach of patient confidentiality is sufficient reason for immediate termination of an employee. Because confidentiality is such a critical aspect of patient care, it is considered highly unethical to reveal any information about a patient to anyone else. All medical assistants are required and expected to uphold the confidentiality of the information with which they come in contact.

12. **Discuss the role of cultural, social, and ethnic diversity in ethical performance of medical assisting practice.**

Our cultural, social, and ethical beliefs are all related to our personal views. When practicing their profession, medical assistants must set aside personal beliefs if they conflict with the patient's care, and the patient's cultural, social, and ethical beliefs must be honored.

13. **Describe the way unique identifiers can help patients infected with HIV avoid discrimination.**

Unique identifiers maintain the confidentiality of patients who are tested for HIV. Some individuals might hesitate to be tested if they are concerned that their names would be reported to various agencies. If unique identifiers are used, patients may have much more confidence that the chances of discrimination because of HIV status are reduced.

14. **Note some of the concerns about ethics that apply to genetic information.**

Many ethical concerns apply to genetic testing. Many patients are concerned about how the information gained will be used and who will have access to it. Questions arise about the ownership of the information. When negative information is found, other ethical problems arise that must be addressed. Knowledge of a person's genetic blueprint could lead to discrimination. Countless issues must be examined before the use of genetic information becomes widespread.

CONNECTIONS

📖 **Study Guide Connection:** Go to the Chapter 6 Study Guide. Read and complete the activities.

ℯ **Evolve Connection:** Go to the Chapter 6 link at *evolve.elsevier.com/kinn* to complete the Chapter Review and Chapter Quiz. Check out the other resources listed for this chapter to make the most of what you have learned from Medicine and Ethics.

7

MEDICINE AND LAW

SCENARIO

Barbara Johnson is the new office manager for two neurologists in an urban area. Recently she was subpoenaed to appear in court with medical records to testify about a patient. This particular patient was referred to one of the physicians in the clinic, Dr. Rebecca Patrick. Dr. Patrick saw the patient several years ago, and the patient has brought a medical professional liability case against a surgeon in another city. Barbara is considered the custodian of medical records and will take them to court and answer questions about the information in them.

One of Barbara's first priorities at her new job is to make sure the office is operating in compliance with the legal regulations that affect the facility. She is knowledgeable about the requirements of the Occupational Safety and Health Administration (OSHA), as well as other legal issues. She is familiar with legal issues and has testified as a custodian of records several times during her tenure as an office manager.

Two of the employees Barbara supervises, Samantha and Lynda, are newly graduated from medical assisting school and are anxious to learn more about the statutes and laws that affect the physicians' office. Barbara is more than happy to share what she has learned with them. She is excited about her new job and eager to be a great success.

While studying this chapter, think about the following questions:

- How can the medical assistant help the staff comply with legal regulations in the medical office?
- How can new graduates learn about the laws that affect them in their state?
- What are some ways medical professional liability suits can be prevented?
- What should the medical assistant do if the employer is not in compliance with legal regulations?

LEARNING OBJECTIVES

1. Define, spell, and pronounce the terms listed in the vocabulary.
2. Discuss all levels of government legislation and regulation as they apply to medical assisting practice, including regulations established by the U.S. Food and Drug Administration (FDA) and the federal Drug Enforcement Administration (DEA).
3. Discuss the legal scope of practice for medical assistants.
4. Distinguish among an act, a statute, and an ordinance.
5. Compare criminal and civil law as they apply to the practicing medical assistant.
6. Explain the three basic categories of criminal law.
7. Distinguish which type of civil law deals with medical professional liability.
8. Provide an example of tort law as it would apply to a medical assistant.
9. Describe liability, professional and personal injury, and third-party insurance.
10. Explain the four essential elements of a valid contract.
11. Distinguish between interrogatories and depositions.
12. List three things to remember when testifying in court.
13. Discuss the advantages of arbitration.
14. Differentiate among malfeasance, misfeasance, and nonfeasance.
15. Explain the "four Ds" of negligence.
16. Define the types of damages.
17. Compare and contrast physician and medical assistant roles in terms of standard of care.
18. Explain the importance of informed consent.
19. List several legal disclosures the physician must make.
20. Identify where to report illegal and/or unsafe activities and behaviors that affect the health, safety, and welfare of others.
21. Explain how the medical assistant's practice is affected by negligence, malpractice, statutes of limitation, Good Samaritan laws, the Uniform Anatomical Gift Act, Living Wills/Advanced Directives, and the Medical Durable Power of Attorney.
22. Summarize the Patient's Bill of Rights.
23. Describe the implications of the Health Insurance Portability and Accountability Act (HIPAA) for the medical assistant in various medical settings.
24. Describe personal protective equipment.
25. Discuss requirements for responding to hazardous materials disposal.
26. Describe the importance of Material Safety Data Sheets (MSDS) in a healthcare setting.
27. Distinguish between the OSHA and CLIA; indicate which one is an actual agency.
28. Identify how the Americans with Disabilities Act (ADA) applies to the medical assisting profession.

VOCABULARY

abandonment To withdraw protection or support; in medicine, to discontinue medical care without proper notice after accepting a patient.

act The formal action of a legislative body; a decision or determination of a sovereign state, a legislative council, or a court of justice.

allegation (a-li-ga'-shun) A statement by a party to a legal action of what the party undertakes to prove; an assertion made without proof.

appeal A legal proceeding by which a case is brought before a higher court for review of the decision of a lower court.

appellate (uh-pe'-lut) Having the power to review the judgment of another tribunal or body of jurisdiction, such as an appellate court.

arbitration (ar-buh-tra'-shun) The hearing and determination of a cause in controversy by a person or persons either chosen by the parties involved or appointed under statutory authority.

arbitrator (ar-buh-tra'-ter) A neutral person chosen to settle differences between two parties in a controversy.

assault An intentional, unlawful attempt of bodily injury to another by force.

assent To agree to something, especially after thoughtful consideration.

bailiff An officer of some U.S. courts who usually serves as a messenger or usher and who keeps order at the request of the judge.

battery A willful and unlawful use of force or violence on the person of another.

Code of Federal Regulations (CFR) A coded delineation of the rules and regulations published in the Federal Register by the various departments and agencies of the federal government. The CFR is divided into 50 titles that represent broad subject areas and chapters that provide specific detail.

concurrently Occurring at the same time.

contributory negligence Statutes in some states that may prevent a party from recovering some damages if he or she contributed in any way to the injury or condition.

damages Loss or harm resulting from injury to person, property, or reputation; compensation in money imposed by law for losses or injuries.

decedent (di-se'-dent) A legal term for a deceased person.

defendant A person required to answer in a legal action or suit; in criminal cases, the person accused of a crime.

docket A formal record of judicial proceedings; a list of legal cases to be tried.

due process A fundamental constitutional guarantee that all legal proceedings will be fair; that one will be given notice of the proceedings and an opportunity to be heard before the government acts to take away life, liberty, or property; a constitutional guarantee that a law will not be unreasonable or arbitrary.

emancipated minor A person under legal age who is self-supporting and living apart from parents or a guardian; a mature minor considered by the courts to possess a sufficient understanding of self-care and responsibility.

expert witnesses People who provide testimony to a court as experts in certain fields or subjects to verify facts presented by one or both sides in a lawsuit, often compensated and used to refute or disprove the claims of one party.

felony A major crime, such as murder, rape, or burglary; punishable by a more stringent sentence than that given for a misdemeanor.

fine A sum imposed as punishment for an offense; a forfeiture or penalty paid to an injured party or the government in a civil or criminal action.

guardian ad litem Legal representative for a minor.

implied consent Presumed consent, such as when a patient offers an arm for a phlebotomy procedure.

implied contract A legally enforceable agreement that arises from conduct, from assumed intentions, from some relationship among the immediate parties, or from the application of the legal principle of equity.

informed consent A consent, usually written, which states understanding of what treatment is to be undertaken and of the risks involved, why it should be done, and alternative methods of treatment available (including no treatment) and their attendant risks.

infractions (in-frak'-shuns) Breaking the law; minor offenses against the rules, usually punishable by fines.

judicial (ju-di'-shuhl) Of or relating to a judgment, the function of judging, the administration of justice, or the judiciary.

jurisdiction (jur-uhs-dik'-shun) A power constitutionally conferred on a judge or magistrate to decide cases according to law and to carry sentence into execution; jurisdiction is original when it is conferred on the court in the first instance, called original jurisdiction; or it is appellate when an appeal is given from the judgment of another court.

jurisprudence (jur-uhs-proo'-dens) The science or philosophy of law; a system or body of law or the course of court decisions.

law A binding custom or practice of a community; a rule of conduct or action prescribed or formally recognized as binding or enforceable by a controlling authority.

liable (li'-uh-buhl) Obligated according to law or equity; responsible for an act or circumstance.

libel A written defamatory statement or representation that conveys an unjustly unfavorable impression.

litigious (luh-ti'-juhs) Prone to engage in lawsuits.

manifestation (ma-nuh-fuh-sta'-shun) Something that is easily understood or recognized by the mind.

misdemeanor (mis-duh-me'-nuhr) A minor crime, as opposed to a felony, punishable by fine or imprisonment in a city or county jail rather than in a penitentiary.

municipal (myu-ni'-suh-puhl) **courts** Courts that sit in some cities and larger towns and that usually have civil and criminal jurisdiction over cases arising within the municipality.

negligence (ne'-gli-jents) Failure to exercise the care a prudent person usually exercises; implies inattention to one's duty or business; implies want of due or necessary diligence or care.

ordinance (or'-di-nens) Authoritative decree or direction; law set forth by a governmental authority, specifically, municipal regulation.

other potentially infectious materials (OPIM) Substances or materials other than blood that have the potential to carry infectious pathogens, such as body fluid, urine, semen, and others.

perjured testimony The voluntary violation of an oath or vow either by swearing to what is untrue or by omission to do what has been promised under oath; false testimony.

physician office laboratories (POLs) Laboratories owned by a private physician or corporation, such as the laboratory inside a physician's office or a freestanding laboratory.

plaintiff The person or group bringing a case or legal action to court.

precedence (pre-sed'-ens) To surpass in rank, dignity, or importance; to be, go, or come ahead or in front of.

precedents (pre'-suh-dens) A person or thing that serves as a model; something done or said that may serve as an example or rule to authorize or justify a subsequent act of the same kind.

preponderance of the evidence Evidence of greater weight or more convincing than the evidence offered in opposition to it; evidence that as a whole shows that the fact sought to be proven is more probable than not.

prudent Marked by wisdom or judiciousness; shrewd in the management of practical affairs.

reasonable doubt Doubt based on reason and arising from evidence or lack of evidence; it is not doubt that is imagined or conjured up, but doubt that would cause reasonable persons to hesitate before acting.

reciprocity The mutual exchange of privileges; a recognition of one state or institution of the licenses or privileges granted by the other.

recourse A turning to something or someone for help or protection.

relevant Having significant and demonstrable bearing on the matter at hand.

respondent (ri-spahn'-dunt) The person required to make answer in a civil legal action or suit; similar to a defendant in a criminal trial.

slander Oral defamation; a harmful, false statement made about another person.

statutes (sta-choots) Laws enacted by the legislative branch of a government.

stipulate To specify as a condition or requirement of an agreement or offer; to make an agreement or covenant to do or forbear from doing something.

subpoena (suh-pe'-nuh) A writ or document commanding a person to appear in court under a penalty for failure to appear.

subpoena duces tecum A legally binding request to appear in court and provide records or documents that pertain to a particular case.

testimony A solemn declaration usually made orally by a witness under oath in response to interrogation by a lawyer or authorized public official.

Uniform Commercial Code (UCC) A unified set of rules covering many business transactions; it has been adopted in all 50 states, the District of Columbia, and most U.S. territories. It regulates the fields of sales of goods; commercial paper, such as checks; secured transactions in personal property; and particular aspects of banking, letters of credit, warehouse receipts, bills of lading, and investment securities.

verdict The finding or decision of a jury on a matter submitted to it in trial.

The **law** is a fascinating subject. When law is applied to medicine, it can provoke interesting case studies and complex decisions. In today's **litigious** society, medical assistants, in addition to physicians and other staff members, must take steps to protect themselves from lawsuits. Legal issues underlie many aspects of the provision of healthcare in a physician's office. Although the wording of **statutes** and regulations often is long and complicated, medical assistants must stay abreast of the rules governing medical facilities and do everything possible to remain in compliance with the standards and regulations for all organizations that oversee the medical industry.

Generally, the law holds that every person is **liable** for the consequences of his or her own **negligence** when another person is injured as a result. In some situations, this liability also extends to the employer. Physicians may be held responsible for the mistakes of those who work in their healthcare facility, and sometimes they must pay **damages** for the negligent acts of their employees.

Under the doctrine of *respondeat superior,* physicians are legally responsible for the acts of their employees when the employees are acting within the scope of their duties or employment. Physicians are also responsible for the acts of assistants who are not their own employees if the assistant commits acts of negligence in the presence of the physician while under the physician's immediate supervision. *Respondeat superior* is a Latin term meaning "let the master answer." When physicians practice as partners, they are liable not only for their own acts and those of their partners, but also for the negligent acts of any agent or employee of the partnership. A medical assistant acting within the scope of the employment contract is considered an agent of the employer.

Medical assistants guilty of negligence are liable for their own actions, but the injured party generally sues the physician, because the chance of collecting damages is greater. However, even an assistant who has no money can be liable for any negligent action. This fact illustrates the continuing importance of exercising extreme care in performing all duties in the professional office and maintaining liability coverage once employed in the healthcare industry.

JURISPRUDENCE AND THE CLASSIFICATIONS OF LAW

Jurisprudence, the science and philosophy of law, comes from the Latin words *juris,* which means "law, right, equity, or justice," and *prudentia,* which means "skill or good judgment."

Law is a custom or practice of a community. It is a rule of conduct or action prescribed or formally recognized as binding or enforceable by a controlling authority. Law is the system by which society gives order to our lives. The U.S. Constitution is the supreme law of the United States; it takes **precedence** over federal statutes, court opinions, and state constitutions. The state constitution is the supreme law within the boundaries of each state unless it conflicts with the U.S. Constitution. States cannot pass laws that conflict with the U.S. Constitution, nor can local governments pass laws that conflict with the state constitution.

A law enacted at the federal level, which must be passed by Congress, is called an **act**. *Statutes* are laws that have been enacted by state legislatures. Local governments create and enact **ordinances**. Much of our law is based on previous **judicial** and jury decisions, which are called **precedents**. Often judges and juries follow precedents when making a decision on a case. The two basic categories of jurisprudence are criminal law and civil law.

Criminal Law

Criminal law governs violations of the law punishable as offenses against the state or the federal government. Such offenses involve the welfare and safety of the public as a whole rather than of one individual. Criminal offenses are classified into three basic categories: misdemeanors, felonies, and treason. To ensure fair treatment under the law, all physicians are entitled to **due process**, which guarantees that the accused will have an opportunity to defend himself or herself against any charges brought in opposition. Several crimes can be committed **concurrently**, such as a criminal who robs and assaults a convenience store clerk or a man who commits rape and murder.

Misdemeanors

A minor crime is called a **misdemeanor**. Such a crime is punishable by **fine** or imprisonment in a city or county jail rather than in a penitentiary. Misdemeanors vary from state to state and often are divided into subgroups or classes, such as class A, class B, or class C misdemeanors. In most states the subgroups are divided from most serious offenses to lesser offenses. Some states have created a subcategory of misdemeanors for **infractions**, which often are called *violations*. Infractions are minor offenses, such as traffic tickets, which are punishable only by a fine.

Felonies

A **felony** is a major crime, such as murder, rape, or burglary. It is punishable by a more stringent sentence than for misdemeanors. Federal law and most state statutes classify felonies as crimes punishable by imprisonment for more than 1 year, whereas misdemeanors are punishable by imprisonment for 1 year or less. Usually a convicted felon cannot vote, hold public office, or own a firearm. Felonies often are divided into subgroups or degrees, such as first degree, second degree, and third degree. A first-degree offense is normally the most serious.

Treason

Treason, the most serious crime, is the offense of attempting to overthrow the government. High treason constitutes a serious threat to the stability or continuity of the government, such as an attempt to kill the president. The president of the United States has the right to declare an action against the United States an act of war rather than an act of treason, which is considered a crime. For instance, although the terrorist attacks of September 11, 2001, were certainly a threat against the United States, they were declared acts of war.

Civil Law

Civil law is concerned with acts that are not criminal in nature but involve relationships of individuals with other individuals, organizations, or government agencies. Many types of civil law address numerous issues. The three that most directly affect the medical profession include tort law, contract law, and administrative law.

Tort Law

Tort law provides a remedy for a person or group that has been harmed by the wrongful acts of others. Four elements must be established in every tort action: (1) the **plaintiff** must establish that the **respondent** or **defendant** was under a legal duty to act in a particular fashion; (2) the plaintiff must demonstrate that the defendant breached this duty by failing to conform his or her behavior accordingly; (3) the plaintiff must prove that the breach of the legal duty proximately caused some injury or damage; and (4) the plaintiff must prove *damages,* the injury or loss suffered. Medical professional liability, or medical malpractice, falls into the category of tort law. **Libel** and **slander** are common complaints that fall into the category of tort law. When a person is liable for an act, he or she is obligated or responsible according to the law. Professional and personal injuries are types of torts, meaning that a person or group has injured someone or something else. Physicians carry professional liability insurance, a type of third-party insurance, to help guard them from liability costs. Medical assistants can also invest in liability insurance. Remember, "libel" and "liable" are defined differently although they sound the same. Refer to the vocabulary list for clarification.

Contract Law

A contract is an agreement that creates an obligation. Contract law touches our lives in many ways practically every day, but we usually do not give much thought to its influences. If a person parks a car in a parking garage for a monthly fee and signs a contract for a year, then begins parking elsewhere and refuses to pay the fee, the person may be liable for the fees for the duration of the entire contract. If the person's vehicle is damaged while parked in the garage, the garage may be responsible for reimbursement, if the contract does not **stipulate** otherwise. A contract does not have to be formalized in writing to be binding on the parties involved. Oral contracts also are valid in many states in most situations. The **Uniform Commercial Code (UCC)** is a long, elaborate act that attempts to harmonize the law of sales and other commercial transactions in all 50 states. This code directly affects contract law.

Administrative Law

Administrative law involves regulations set forth by governmental agencies. For example, the Internal Revenue Service (IRS) has thousands of regulations and codes, and the typical American does not understand all of them, which may result in errors when filing taxes. The laws that allow the IRS to collect taxes and pursue restitution are administrative laws. Other agencies that are involved with administrative law are the Social Security Administration (SSA),

Citizenship and Immigration Services (USCIS), and the Centers for Medicare and Medicaid Services (CMS).

ANATOMY OF A MEDICAL PROFESSIONAL LIABILITY LAWSUIT

A medical liability case often stems from a breach of trust or miscommunication between the physician and the patient. These cases fall into the category of tort law. Even when the physician has made an error, often the level of trust between the physician and patient determines whether a lawsuit is pursued. First, the physician-patient relationship must be formed. Before this relationship can be discussed, the requirements for a valid, enforceable contract must be understood.

What Constitutes a Valid Contract?

A valid legal contract has four essential elements. First, a **manifestation** of **assent** or "meeting of the minds" must exist. This element is proven by an "offer" and the "acceptance" of that offer. The parties to the contract must understand and agree on the intent of the contract. Second, the contract must involve legal subject matter. An obligation that requires an illegal action, such as a gambling contract, is not an enforceable contract. Third, both parties must have the legal capacity to enter into a contract. This means that each party must be an adult of sound mind or an emancipated minor. Fourth, some type of consideration must be involved. Consideration is an exchange of something of value (e.g., money) for the physician's time.

> **CRITICAL THINKING APPLICATION   7-1**
>
> Barbara works for Dr. Rebecca Patrick, who saw the patient bringing the lawsuit against the surgeon as a referral patient. Does Dr. Patrick have a contract with the patient, based on a physician-patient relationship? Why or why not?

The physician-patient relationship is generally held by courts to be a contractual relationship that is the result of three steps:

- The physician invites an offer by establishing his availability (e.g., posting office hours or making himself available during office hours).
- The patient accepts the appointment and makes an offer by arriving for or requesting treatment.
- The physician accepts the patient's offer by examining the patient and beginning treatment. Physicians also accept the offer by exercising independent medical judgment on behalf of the patient.

Before accepting a patient, the physician is under no obligation, and no contract exists. However, once the physician has accepted the patient, an **implied contract** exists (Figure 7-1). An implied contract in this case assumes that the physician will treat the patient using reasonable care and that the physician has a degree of knowledge, skill, and judgment that might be expected of any other physician in the same locality and under similar circumstances. It is extremely important that no express promise of a cure be made by anyone in the office, including the physician, because this would become a part of the contract.

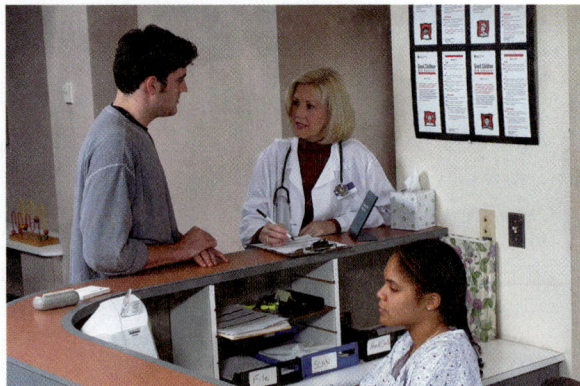

FIGURE 7-1 The physician-patient relationship is built on a strong foundation of trust, but it also is a contractual relationship.

The patient's responsibility in this agreement includes the liability of payment for services and a willingness to follow the advice of the physician. Most physician-patient contracts are implied contracts. Although many forms may be completed by the patient before he or she is accepted by the physician, they do not in most cases constitute a formal contract for each specific visit to the physician.

> **CRITICAL THINKING APPLICATION   7-2**
>
> - If the patient does not pay for the services rendered by the physician, does this negate the physician-patient contract?
> - How might Barbara, Samantha, and Lynda ensure that patients understand that they are expected to follow the advice of the physician?

After the physician-patient relationship has been established, the physician is obligated to attend the patient as long as attention is required, unless the physician or patient terminates the contract. When a physician terminates the contract, the patient must be given notice of the physician's intentions so that the patient has sufficient time to secure another physician. The physician may write a letter of withdrawal from medical care of the patient, and it should be delivered by certified mail, return receipt requested. A copy of the letter and the return receipt should be attached to the patient's chart and permanently retained. Reasonable time should be allowed for the patient to secure other medical care.

To protect the physician against a lawsuit for **abandonment**, the details of the circumstances under which the physician is withdrawing from the case should be included in the patient's medical chart. The letter of withdrawal does not have to specify a reason for withdrawal unless the physician so chooses. However, some physicians include a brief reason in the letter, such as missing appointments or failing to comply with treatment orders. In either case, the letter should state the following:

- That professional care is being discontinued
- That the physician will provide copies of the patient's records to another physician on request
- That the patient should seek the attention of another physician as soon as possible

A patient who wants to terminate the physician-patient relationship simply no longer seeks the physician for treatment. The patient does not have to inform the office; however, if this is done, the office manager or physician should follow up with a confirmation letter, stating that the patient has ended the relationship.

Breach of Contract

An unjustifiable failure to perform all or some part of a contractual duty is a breach of contract. For example, if a surgeon prepares a surgery estimate and says that the fee will be no more than $6,500, but then charges the patient $7,200, a breach of contract exists. Although most physicians state that the document is just an estimate, this particular physician stated a clear amount that the surgery costs would not exceed.

The Statute of Frauds

In 1677 a statute was adopted in England to reduce the occurrence of **perjured testimony**. It provided that certain contracts could not be enforced if they depended on the **testimony** of witnesses alone and were not evidenced in writing. The provisions of this English statute have been closely followed by statutes adopted in all 50 states in the United States.

A promise to pay the debts of another person is an example of a contract that usually must be made in writing. If a third party who is not otherwise legally responsible for a patient's medical bills agrees to pay them, the agreement cannot be enforced unless it is in writing. If a physician were to enter into an agreement to perform a series of treatments for a given sum and this series covered a time span of more than 1 year, the contract would have to be in writing to be enforceable.

CRITICAL THINKING APPLICATION   7-3
- For what reasons might a physician not want to accept a patient?
- Must the physician treat every patient who attempts to make an appointment?
- How might Barbara tactfully explain that the physician will not accept the patient into treatment?

Preliminaries of Litigation

Lawsuits are filed in a variety of different courts, and different states have different types of courts at various levels. The state judiciary has several branches. At the local level are usually **municipal courts**. These are courts in a city or town that usually deal with ordinance violations. Municipal judges may issue search and arrest warrants. Some states also have justice of the peace courts, which have **jurisdiction** over many misdemeanors and some civil matters, in addition to concurrent jurisdiction over some matters along with the municipal courts. The judges that preside over justice of the peace courts may also issue search and arrest warrants. They often function as small claims courts, with which the medical assistant may have contact in cases of patients who do not pay their bills. Both municipal and justice of the peace courts are local trial courts with limited jurisdiction.

County courts are higher than municipal and justice of the peace courts. These courts handle misdemeanors and civil matters up to a certain monetary limit. District courts have unlimited jurisdiction in criminal and civil matters. They are the highest state courts, other than **appellate** courts. If one party to a lawsuit is dissatisfied with a lower court's decision, it has the right to **appeal** to a higher court

for review and possible reversal of the decision. Most states have an appellate court for both criminal and civil matters. The U.S. District Court handles federal matters of a criminal or a civil nature. States also have Supreme Courts that handle a limited number of appellate cases.

Under Article III, Section One of the U.S. Constitution, the U.S. Supreme Court has the authority to ensure equal justice under the law (Figure 7-2). The Supreme Court interprets and guards the Constitution. The court's one chief justice and eight associate justices are appointed by the president and confirmed by Congress. Approximately 8,000 cases are on the **docket** per term, which runs from the first Monday in October to the first Monday in October of the next year. Only 80 to 90 cases are chosen each year for full oral argument in front of the justices.

CRITICAL THINKING APPLICATION   7-4
Samantha and Lynda are curious as to how Supreme Court's decisions affect the individual physician's office. What Supreme Court decisions have affected the medical profession?

Preparing for Court

Medical professional liability suits are far from rare, and every physician faces the probability of being sued at least once during his or her career. When a suit is filed, preparation for court should start expeditiously. A medical assistant may be involved in preparing materials for court and scheduling or participating in depositions. The best advice for a medical assistant in this position is to remember to tell the truth. Attorneys help prepare the defense of the physician and the staff, but everyone should be truthful in answering in court to prevent the loss of his or her credibility in the trial and charges of perjury. Be especially careful to present a true, complete statement to the representing attorney. Unless he or she knows the whole truth, an appropriate defense cannot be prepared.

Interrogatories

Before the trial, the physician may be asked to complete an interrogatory, which is a list of questions from each party to the other in the lawsuit. Answers to the interrogatory must be provided within

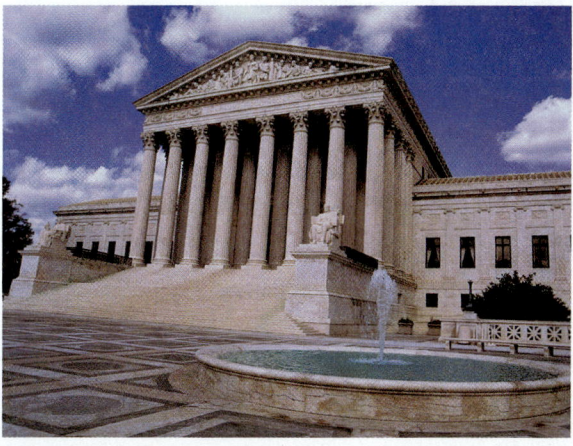

FIGURE 7-2 The U.S. Supreme Court. The Supreme Court decides cases that involve interpretation of the Constitution of the United States.

a specified time, and the answers are considered to be given under oath. Only the parties named in the lawsuit may be questioned through interrogatories.

Depositions

A deposition is testimony taken from a party or witness to the litigation and is not limited to the parties named in the lawsuit. A witness who is not a party to the lawsuit may be summoned by **subpoena** for the deposition. The deposition usually is taken in an attorney's office in the presence of a court reporter and is taken under oath. The person giving the deposition is called the *deponent*. The transcribed deposition, once finished, is sent to the deponent for review, and the deponent is at liberty to request any necessary changes or corrections in the document.

CRITICAL THINKING APPLICATION   7-5
- Samantha and Lynda are anxious to hear about Barbara's previous experiences in testifying in court. She mentions that attorneys often advise witnesses to "answer the question, then be quiet." What might be meant by this advice?
- Discuss the phrase, "the truth, the whole truth, and nothing but the truth."

Subpoenas

A subpoena is a document issued by a court that requires a person to be in court at a specific time and place to testify as a witness in a lawsuit, either in a court proceeding or in a deposition. A **subpoena duces tecum** is a legally binding request to provide records or documents to appear in court and usually is issued to the person considered the custodian of the records. This may be the medical assistant or office manager. A fee may be demanded for the time spent in compiling the records and for photocopying charges, but this fee must be requested at the time the subpoena duces tecum is served, or it is considered to be waived. Physician approval must be obtained to release or to copy any patient records. Original records should never be released under any circumstances. If an original record is demanded in the subpoena, it usually is taken to court or to mediation by the physician or an employee of the physician's office. Copies can be released in advance of the court date. Release only the information requested in the subpoena and provide only information that originated in the physician's office. Do not provide records sent from previous or consulting physicians. Those records must be subpoenaed separately from the originating office.

Before responding to a subpoena, make sure it is valid. Although variances may occur from state to state, some general rules can be used to judge the validity of a subpoena:

- A subpoena issued in one state court generally is not valid in another state. Always verify the state in which the subpoena was issued.
- A subpoena issued by a federal court in one state generally is not valid in another state unless a federal statute authorizes nationwide service of process.
- Any duly authorized law officer may execute a valid subpoena anywhere in the same state. The officer notifies the issuing court once the subpoena has been served.

- Generally, the person or entity subpoenaed has 21 days to respond, but this period can differ from place to place.
- A subpoena duces tecum should be filed no less than 15 days before a trial. One served less than 15 days before a trial should not be honored.

Read the subpoena carefully to determine exactly what records are requested. The physician should always be notified of subpoenas served to the medical facility. Never copy records required in a subpoena without bringing the matter to the attention of the physician or office manager, or both. It also is advisable to keep a log of subpoenas served to the office, what records were involved, and the disposition of the request, including when the records were presented to the court. Always inform the physician about the subpoena, because he or she may want to present the document to an attorney for review before any information is released.

Discovery

Discovery is the pretrial disclosure of pertinent facts or documents by one or both parties to a legal action or proceeding. Many states have extensive discovery statutes that require each side to reveal to the other the facts that they "discover" while investigating the case. Discovery is also considered the process of uncovering facts in a lawsuit before the court proceedings.

Presentation of evidence may be done by testimony. A witness is called who has some information about an aspect of the case and is asked questions by one or both attorneys. The witness does not know about every part of the case, but something the person knows is **relevant**.

Another type of evidence may be documentary evidence. This is any type of evidence brought before the court by document or display. It could be a patient's chart, a letter, a laboratory result, or a photograph. All of these are usually entered into evidence and numbered for easy reference.

CRITICAL THINKING APPLICATION   7-6
Samantha wonders what she should do if she ever finds information during a medical professional malpractice case that might harm her employer's defense. What advice would you offer? Would it be considered an obligation or a choice to report the employer for wrongdoing?

Preparing Witnesses and Testifying

Attorneys prepare witnesses who may be called to testify during the court proceedings. They review the questions that will be asked and potential questions the opposite side may present. The attorney helps the witness to clarify the answers he or she gives so that they are sharp and succinct. One of the first rules law students learn is never to ask a question to which they do not already know the answer.

Witnesses should always be on time for a court appearance, because the judge and jury may frown on those who appear late; and that frown may include a fine or confinement in jail for contempt of court! It is critical that witnesses dress conservatively and in a manner that shows respect for the court. If any documents are to be referenced while testifying, the witness should review the documents before the court appearance if possible, so that the needed information is easy to locate and discuss. The witness should speak clearly and at a volume audible to the attorneys and parties to the suit, the judge, the jury, and the court reporter. The witness should always answer each question aloud, because the court reporter must record those answers and cannot specify that the witness "nodded yes" as a response to a question.

If a question is confusing, the witness should ask the attorney to restate or repeat it. If the witness does not know the answer to a question or does not recall, that should be stated clearly and confidently. Above all, the parties involved are expected to tell the truth and must be seen as credible witnesses (Figure 7-3). Lying under oath constitutes perjury, which carries stiff penalties. Listening is as important as speaking; therefore the witness should be sure to listen to the question and answer it, elaborating only if the attorney asks for more details.

If an attorney lodges an objection to a question, the witness should be silent until the judge rules on the objection. The objection may be sustained or overruled. Sustaining the objection means that the judge agrees with the objection and will not allow the question stated in that manner. If the judge allows the question, he or she will overrule the objection. Then the witness will be allowed to answer. The witness should never display a combative or hostile attitude and should not make sarcastic remarks while testifying in court. The witness should be professional at all times and restrain inappropriate comments and belligerent behavior. Using "yes, sir" and "no, ma'am" is appropriate in the courtroom. Always address the judge as "Your Honor."

Inside the Courtroom

Today's courtrooms are a far cry from the ones depicted on television shows representing the Old West. Modern courtrooms are equipped with computer and video equipment, and elaborate security systems often monitor those entering the building. The advent of truTV has changed the way Americans see the justice system. By simply turning on our televisions, we can watch justice at work.

Knowing the role of each person in a court of law can be helpful. The person or body bringing the lawsuit to court is referred to by different terms, depending on the type of case. In a criminal court, the government brings the case and is represented by a prosecutor. For example, in criminal cases, legal documents read, *The State of Texas v. Robert Smith*. In this case, the fictitious Robert Smith is the defendant. In civil court, the person or group bringing the case to court is called the *plaintiff* (or *complainant* in some court systems), and the opposite party is called the *defendant* or *respondent*. A judge presides over the case, giving instructions concerning the law to the jury, if a jury is present. If no jury is present, the judge decides the case; this is called a *bench trial*. A witness is a person who knows some pertinent information about the case and gives testimony. Often a court reporter takes notes of the proceedings, and a **bailiff** may be present, who assists in keeping order. All of these individuals should be treated with respect and courtesy.

Burden of Proof

In a criminal case the burden of proof is on the prosecution, which must prove guilt beyond any **reasonable doubt**. Reasonable doubt is defined as the level of certainty a juror must have to find a defendant guilty of a crime. It is real doubt, based on reason and common sense after careful and impartial consideration of all the evidence, or lack of evidence, in a case.

Civil cases must be proven by a **preponderance of the evidence**. This means that the greater weight of evidence must point to the defendant or respondent as being responsible for the act involved in the case.

To understand the difference between reasonable doubt and preponderance of the evidence, think of the scales of justice (Figure 7-4). For a case to be proven beyond a reasonable doubt, the scales should tip heavily toward either guilt or innocence. However, for a case to be proven by preponderance of the evidence, the scales need tip only slightly one way or the other.

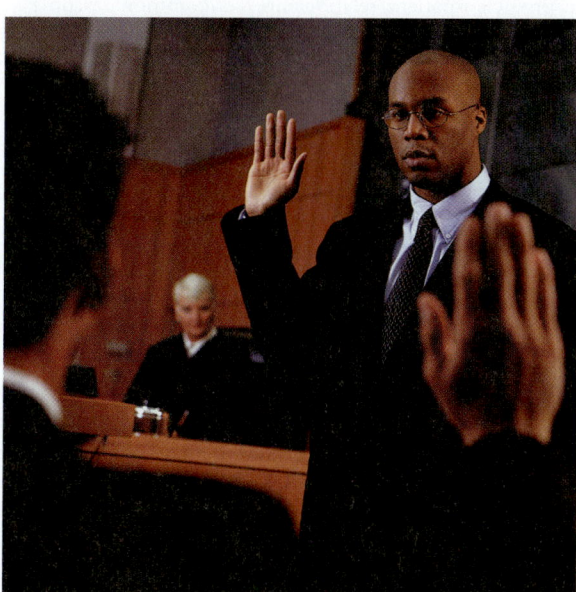

FIGURE 7-3 Witnesses must be credible and must tell the truth on the stand in court to avoid charges of perjury.

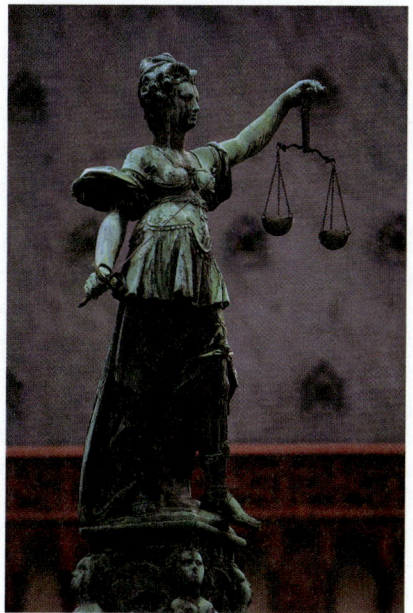

FIGURE 7-4 Lady Justice. Justitia was the Roman goddess of justice and is the figure depicted in statues across the world, often holding both scales and a sword. Her scales imply the weighing of justice, and the blindfold represents the impartiality of justice.

To illustrate the difference in the burden of proof in criminal and civil cases, consider *The People of the State of California v. Orenthal James Simpson*. In O.J. Simpson's criminal trial, much circumstantial evidence was presented; however, enough doubt also existed that the scales could not tip heavily toward a **verdict** of guilty, and Mr. Simpson was acquitted. In the civil trial brought by family members of Nicole Brown Simpson and Ron Goldman after the criminal trial had ended, just enough evidence existed to tip the scales in favor of the families' claim that Mr. Simpson was somehow responsible for the deaths of the two victims. This is the equivalent of a preponderance of the evidence.

CRITICAL THINKING APPLICATION   7-7

A discussion of the burden of proof prompts Barbara, Samantha, and Lynda to discuss the case of O.J. Simpson. Discuss whether reasonable doubt existed in his criminal trial.

▎Outcome of the Case

Once both sides have presented their case to the judge or jury, they usually are given the opportunity to present a final summation of their case. The jury then retires to consider the verdict. This can take minutes, hours, days, or weeks. After the jury reaches a decision, the judge may enter it as a final verdict or may disregard it if the evidence does not support the jury's decision. The judge may also revise the verdict to comply with statutes, such as statutory limits on the amount of punitive damages. The final decision of the trial court is reflected in the judgment, signed by the judge.

Either side normally has the right to appeal the decision to a higher court. However, not all appellate courts are required to hear all cases. For instance, the U.S. Supreme Court chooses the cases it hears each year, and it is restricted to cases that involve interpretation of the Constitution and how that interpretation affects the people it governs.

In criminal cases, if the defendant is found guilty of the crime, a sentencing date is set, usually a few weeks to a few months after the verdict is announced. At this time the punishment is announced.

▎ARBITRATION

Arbitration is an alternative to trial in which a third party is chosen to hear evidence and make a decision because of the individual's familiarity with or knowledge of the law or the issues involved. Arbitration is common in modern business life. It is recognized by statute in most states and usually is available to the medical profession, offering an alternative for resolving legal disputes between physician and patient. Many physicians and attorneys see arbitration as one way to solve the crisis of litigation in this country. Court battles can take years and can be extremely expensive, and much of the money reverts to the attorneys rather than the victors in the lawsuit.

In arbitration, the patient and the physician agree to submit the dispute to an **arbitrator** in an informal hearing. The arbitrator renders a legally binding decision based on very specific rules of arbitration. Arbitration applies essentially the same rights and the

same measure of damages as a court. It is fair, less expensive, faster, and more confidential than court litigation.

The staff of each medical office should know whether arbitration statutes exist in the state where the office conducts business. The state medical board or local medical society should be able to provide this information. An arbitration agreement is a contract and is subject to the judgment of the courts only as to the fairness of the agreement. The agreement is precisely worded by an attorney and should not be paraphrased when explained to a patient. Signing the agreement is a voluntary act by the patient, who has a grace period in which to revoke the agreement if he or she later decides against it. Likewise, a physician always has the option to decide not to care for a patient but must formally notify a patient if the decision is made to no longer render care.

If a physician elects to implement an arbitration agreement procedure with patients, every member of the physician's staff should know the details of the agreement, how and when the patient should sign up, and how to answer the patient's questions. The way the program is presented to the patient and the office staff's willingness to answer the patient's questions play a large part in whether courts uphold the arbitration agreement as fair and legal.

The patient and the physician both have the opportunity to agree on who will arbitrate the case, so that one side is not favored over the other. By prior agreement, the arbitrator (or arbitrators) may be appointed by or from the American Arbitration Association, which is a neutral, private, nonprofit association dedicated to the advancement of out of court remedies. Its panels of arbitrators are made up of people from business, the professions, and public interest groups.

▎MEDICAL PROFESSIONAL LIABILITY AND NEGLIGENCE

When a patient is injured as a result of a physician's negligence, the patient may initiate a malpractice lawsuit to recover financial damages. However, experience has shown that the incidence of malpractice claims is directly related to the personal relationship and trust that exist between the physician and the patient. Deterioration of the physician-patient relationship is a common reason patients sue physicians for malpractice, even when the patient has sustained no real injury.

Medical professional liability, commonly called *medical malpractice,* is governed by the law of torts. The term *medical professional liability* encompasses all possible civil liability that can be incurred during the delivery of medical care. Medical professional liability is much more easily prevented than defended.

To understand medical malpractice, the term *negligence* first must be understood. Negligence, in general, implies inattention to one's duty or business, or the implication of a lack of necessary diligence or care. In medicine, negligence is defined as the performance of an act that a reasonable and **prudent** physician would not do or the failure to do an act that a reasonable and prudent physician would do. This, of course, also applies to any other healthcare professional. The standard of prudent care and conduct is not defined by law but is left to the determination of a judge or jury, usually with the help of **expert witnesses**. Expert witnesses are members of the profession involved—in this case, medicine. To be considered an expert witness, a person usually belongs to a certifying or qualifying organization, against which the defendant's qualities may be compared.

Professional negligence in medicine falls into one of three general classifications:

- *Malfeasance,* or performance of an act that is wholly wrongful and unlawful
- *Misfeasance,* or improper performance of a lawful act
- *Nonfeasance,* or failure to perform an act that should have been performed

A physician who performs an operation carelessly or fails to render care that should have been given may be found to have been negligent. Although a medical assistant acts as an agent of the physician in carrying out most of his or her duties, the medical assistant may perform an act that can result in litigation. For instance, if the medical assistant gives a patient the wrong medication or the wrong dose of medication, both the physician and the medical assistant can be held liable for the error. Some states limit the scope of practice of medical assistants where medications are involved; however, if medical assistants are performing within the realm of duties for which they have received training and the physician is accepting responsibility for the actions of those in the medical office, they usually are allowed to dispense and administer medications unless prohibited by state law. The medical assistant should always practice within the legal boundaries of the state (Procedure 7-1).

CRITICAL THINKING APPLICATION   **7-8**

Lynda is curious as to whether a physician is guilty of medical professional liability if he or she makes a mistake in diagnosing a patient. When might this be considered malpractice and when might it not be considered malpractice?

What if the patient makes his or her condition worse? Is the physician then fully responsible? **Contributory negligence** exists when the patient contributes to his or her own condition, and it can lessen the damages that can be collected or even prevent them from being collected altogether.

The Four Ds of Negligence

Negligence is not presumed; it must be proven. The Committee on Medicolegal Problems of the American Medical Association (AMA) has determined that patients must present evidence of four elements before negligence has been proven. These elements have become known as the four Ds of negligence:

1. *Duty:* Duty exists when the physician-patient relationship has been established. The patient has sought the assistance of the

---

PROCEDURE 7-1

Perform Within the Scope of Practice

GOAL: *To perform duties within legal boundaries and within the scope of practice in the state where employed as a medical assistant.*

EQUIPMENT and SUPPLIES

- Computer with Internet access
- Access to text of laws and regulations affecting the practice and scope of practice for medical assistants

PROCEDURAL STEPS

1. Read the laws and regulations that apply to medical practices thoroughly.
   PURPOSE: To understand the content and intent of the laws and regulations.
2. Become familiar with the laws that affect medical practices in your state.
   PURPOSE: To understand which laws apply to the employer's facility.
3. Obtain additional training on compliance with the laws and regulations, if necessary.
   PURPOSE: To make sure all actions and procedures in the office are in compliance with the current applicable laws.
4. Read journals and other information, either in print or on the Internet, about the laws and regulations.
   PURPOSE: To remain current in compliance activities.
5. Stay aware of licensure issues that affect the physician, including:
   - Licensure
   - Registration
   - Certification
   - Suspension
   - Revocation
   PURPOSE: To ensure that the physician is practicing medicine legally according to all laws and regulations.
6. Know the scope of practice for a medical assistant.
   PURPOSE: To ensure that the medical assistant is practicing legally according to the scope of practice.
7. Make certain information is available on current laws and regulations at all times.
8. Perform all activities in accordance with applicable laws and regulations.
   PURPOSE: To ensure compliance with applicable laws and regulations.
9. Demonstrate an awareness of the consequences of not working within the legal scope of practice.
   PURPOSE: Follow the laws and regulations to ensure compliance in the medical facility.
10. Prepare a brief report for your instructor summarizing the laws in your state that apply to medical offices or choose one specific law to summarize. Turn in the report to your instructor.

physician, and the physician has knowingly undertaken to provide the needed medical service.

2. *Dereliction:* Dereliction is failure to perform a duty. Proof must exist that the physician somehow neglected the duty to the patient.

3. *Direct cause:* Proof must exist that the patient was harmed directly because of the physician's actions or failure to act and that the harm would not otherwise have occurred.

4. *Damages:* The patient must prove that a loss or harm has resulted from the physician's actions.

If all four of these elements exist, the patient may obtain a judgment against the physician in a medical professional liability case.

Types of Damages

Five types of damages are common in tort cases: nominal, punitive, compensatory, general, and special damages.

Nominal damages are small awards that are token compensations for the invasion of a legal right in which no actual injury was suffered. For instance, if an unauthorized medical facility employee accesses a patient's medical record and is discovered but has not revealed any of the information in the record, the patient has not actually been harmed but may be awarded nominal damages in a lawsuit for the invasion of the patient's privacy.

Punitive damages are designed to punish the party who committed the wrong in such a way so as to deter repetition of the act; these are sometimes called *exemplary damages*. These damages were historically set so that the amounts would discourage intentional wrongdoing, misconduct, and outrageous behavior. The amount of damages awarded coincides in some percentage with the wealth of the defendant. Tort reform, currently a much-discussed subject, would cap the amount of money that could be collected during personal injury litigation, including medical malpractice cases. A specific monetary figure (e.g., $500,000) has been suggested as a limit on punitive damages; some believe that plaintiffs should be allowed to collect only up to three times the amount of compensatory damages. Some states have passed legislation that caps one or more of the categories of damages.

CRITICAL THINKING APPLICATION   7-9

Samantha and Lynda disagree as to whether punitive damages should be awarded in medical professional liability cases. Samantha believes that nothing compensates for certain losses, but Lynda believes that monetary compensation is reasonable when a loss has been suffered. Discuss both sides of the issue, and whether providers should be punished AND compensated if the liability proves to be true.

Compensatory damages are designed to compensate for any actual damages caused by the negligent person. They are intended to make the injured person "whole." Of course, nothing can substitute for the loss of an arm or a leg, for example, but compensatory damages help the patient or the family recover from the loss.

General damages include compensation for pain and suffering, for loss of a bodily member or faculty, for disfigurement, or for other similar direct losses or injuries. The fact of the losses has to be proven, but the monetary value does not.

Special damages are awarded for injuries or losses that are not a necessary consequence of the physician's negligent act or omission. These may include the loss of earnings or costs of travel. Both the fact of these losses and the monetary value must be proven.

Standard of Care

The standard of care as it pertains to a medical assistant must be distinguished from the medical assistant's scope of practice. From a legal perspective, each medical assistant is required to perform all duties in a manner that meets or exceeds that of a reasonably competent and knowledgeable medical assistant. Also, medical assistants cannot perform any duties for which they have not been trained. A medical assistant should treat every chart touched as if it will end up in a court of law. Remember, if it is not in the chart, there is no way to prove an event happened. The courts hold that a physician must do the following:

- Use reasonable care, attention, and diligence in the performance of professional services
- Follow his or her best judgment in treating patients
- Have and exercise reasonable skill and care that are commonly had and exercised by other reputable physicians in the same type of practice in the same or a similar locality

In the worst case, a physician or medical facility may be faced with wrongful death litigation. A wrongful death **allegation** is one in which the physician or medical facility is blamed for the death of a patient because of error or inappropriate treatment. A wrongful death suit usually is brought by the family of the **decedent** against the physician or others involved with the patient.

Consent

A physician must have consent to treat a patient, even though this consent usually is implied by the patient's appearance at the office for treatment. This **implied consent** is sufficient for common or simple procedures generally understood to involve little risk, such as phlebotomy and taking vital signs. When more complex procedures are anticipated, the physician must obtain the patient's **informed consent**. A physician who fails to secure some formal expression of consent could be charged with the crime of **battery**. Make sure the patient's identity has been verified before asking him or her to sign the consent form.

Informed consent involves a deeper understanding of the patient's condition and a full explanation of the plan for treatment. Informed consent is not satisfied merely by having the patient sign a form. A discussion must occur during which the physician provides the patient or the patient's legal representative with enough information to decide whether the patient will undergo the treatment or seek an alternative. The medical assistant cannot hold this conversation about consent with the patient; the discussion must be initiated by the physician. However, the medical assistant can witness the document and ask the patient to sign the consent form. After such discussion, the patient either consents to the proposed therapy and signs a consent form or refuses to consent. According to the AMA's standards for informed consent, the discussion should include at least the following elements:

- Patient's diagnosis, if known
- Nature and purpose of the proposed treatment or procedure
- Risks and benefits of the proposed treatment or procedure

- Alternative treatments or procedures, regardless of the cost or the extent to which the treatment options are covered by health insurance
- Risks and benefits of the alternative treatment(s) or procedure(s)
- Risks and benefits of not receiving or undergoing a treatment or procedure

The discussion should be fully documented in the patient's medical record, and a copy of the signed form should be placed in the record. Treatment may not exceed the scope of the consent that the patient has given. Often the consent forms are lengthy and mention excessive possibilities and complications. Some language may attempt to be all inclusive (e.g., "included, but not limited to") when risks are listed. It is wise to have an attorney review the forms used for informed consent, because those that are too broad or too specific can be detrimental to the physician in a medical professional liability case.

Patients cannot be forced to undergo any type of medical treatment or care. The ultimate decision about care must be left to the patient, and although medical professionals should disclose information to help the patient make a good, informed decision, the patient should never be persuaded to act in any manner or accept any treatment with which he or she does not agree. Should the patient decide not to undergo treatment the physician feels is necessary, an informed refusal of treatment or care should be signed. This should be a statement similar to the informed consent, but it indicates that the patient has elected not to undergo treatment. Some physicians discontinue all treatment if a patient does not participate in the care the physician recommends. This document, once signed, should be added to the patient's medical record.

Each state has its own consent laws. Some states and insurance programs require a certain period to pass between the signing of the consent and the actual medical procedure; for instance, Medicaid sometimes requires a 30-day waiting period between the signing of a consent for a tubal ligation and performance of the procedure. Medical assistants should be familiar with the laws in their own state that apply to their particular facility. Most of the laws can be found easily by searching on the Internet. More information about consent can be found in Chapter 17, along with a sample consent form.

CRITICAL THINKING APPLICATION   7-10

Barbara stresses to Samantha and Lynda that at some time in their professional career, a patient will ask for their advice regarding whether the patient should undergo a certain procedure or treatment. Barbara explains that patients often consider advice from the medical assistants in the office to be an extension of the physician's opinions. How might they handle such questions from patients? Should a medical assistant offer any type of advice?

Giving Consent to Medical Procedures

Mentally competent adults certainly are able to consent to medical procedures. However, if an act is unlawful, the consent is invalid.

For instance, if an abortion is performed in a state where abortion is illegal, the consent to that procedure is null. Consent is also invalid if it is given by a person who is unauthorized to do so or if it is obtained by misrepresentation or fraud.

In an emergency, one may render aid or care to prevent loss of life or serious illness or injury. However, implied consent in this circumstance lasts only as long as the emergency exists, and formal consent must be obtained for further treatment as soon as the emergency has passed.

Physicians sometimes are reluctant to render aid in an emergency to someone who is not their patient for fear they will later be charged with negligence or abandonment. In 1959 California passed the first Good Samaritan law. Under this law, volunteers at the scene of an accident are given immunity to liability for any civil damages resulting from the rendering of emergency care. Most states now have either Good Samaritan or Volunteer Protection statutes. As long as the emergency care is given in good faith and without gross negligence, and the healthcare worker provides only emergency care that he or she has been trained to provide, the likelihood of a successful lawsuit against that individual is very slim.

Adults who have been found by a court to be insane or incompetent usually cannot consent to medical treatment. Consent must be obtained from the guardian, except in emergency situations.

Generally, when the patient is a minor, consent for surgery or treatment must be obtained from a parent, guardian, or **guardian ad litem**, except in an emergency requiring immediate treatment. If the parents are legally divorced or separated, consent should be obtained from the custodial parent, but if the child is visiting the second parent, consent may be obtained from that parent, because in such a situation that parent has temporary custody.

Consent is not required for minors in the following circumstances:

- When consent may be assumed, such as in a life-threatening situation
- When a certain treatment is required by law, such as a vaccination or x-ray evaluation for school entry or safety
- When a court order has been issued, as in a situation in which parents withhold consent for a necessary treatment because of religious reasons

In many states, treatment of sexually transmitted diseases, drug abuse, alcohol dependency, pregnancy, or providing birth control measures does not require parental consent. Even if there are age of consent laws, physicians can still treat minors with these issues; the fact that the patient disregarded age statutes does not mean that he or she cannot receive medical treatment.

Emancipation is defined by statute and varies from state to state. An **emancipated minor** is a person younger than the age of majority (usually 18 to 21 years) who meets one or more of the following conditions:

- Married
- In the armed forces
- Living separately and apart from parents or a legal guardian
- Self-supporting

Some states include a minimum age for emancipation. Unless a statute declares otherwise, a minor who has the right to consent to treatment is entitled to the protection of his or her confidences, even from parents.

Statute of Limitations

A statute of limitations is a period after which a lawsuit cannot be filed. The statute of limitations varies from state to state and differs for various types of litigation. Many states have a 2-year statute of limitations for medical malpractice issues. However, in some instances, the statute of limitations may be extended because of a delay in the discovery of an injury. For example, a patient has surgery to replace a valve in the heart, and the surgery seems successful. Two years later, the patient undergoes a routine echocardiogram and the physician discovers that the surgeon mistakenly replaced the aortic valve when the surgery was intended for the pulmonary valve. Although 2 years have already passed, the statute of limitations begins at the point of discovery of the injury; therefore the patient could now bring suit against the surgeon for the error.

Confidentiality

Confidentiality is one of the most sacred trusts the patient places in the hands of the physician and staff (Figure 7-5). Breach of patient confidentiality is grounds for immediate dismissal of a healthcare professional. The strictest care must be taken when handling patient records and discussing information about patients.

In many special cases, patient confidentiality plays a vital role. A patient who tests positive for the human immunodeficiency virus (HIV) may face discrimination if the information surfaces. Physicians who treat such patients may want to take extra care when leaving phone messages or sending mail. Instead of leaving a message for a patient from "Dr. Watson's office," the medical assistant could say that the message is from "Terry Watson's office." This could indicate an attorney, accountant, or real estate broker. Curious co-workers or relatives may not grow as suspicious as they might if they were to encounter a message from a physician's office.

Patients receiving treatment for substance abuse are protected by federal statutes. Confidentiality also is of utmost importance to patients receiving treatment for mental health issues, sexually transmitted diseases, sexual **assault**, and any type of abuse.

■ LAW AND MEDICAL PRACTICE

Law affects the physician's day-to-day practice. Some of the ways the medical assistant encounters legal issues in the physician's office are discussed in this section. Medical assistants must comply with both state and federal laws and regulations while performing the duties associated with their job (Procedure 7-2).

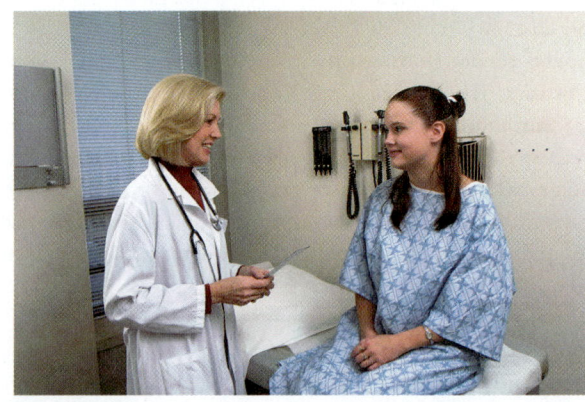

FIGURE 7-5 Patient confidentiality is the most important trust that exists between the physician and the patient.

PROCEDURE 7-2

Practice Within the Standard of Care for a Medical Assistant

GOAL: *To perform duties within the standard of care in the state where employed as a medical assistant.*

EQUIPMENT and SUPPLIES

- Computer with Internet access
- Access to text of laws and regulations affecting the standard of care for medical assistants

PROCEDURAL STEPS

1. Become familiar with the standard of care expected of a medical assistant in your state.
   PURPOSE: To make certain that the laws and regulations that apply to the specific practice are applied with each patient.
2. Approach every patient, every day, in a professional manner.
3. During your introduction, identify yourself as a medical assistant.
   PURPOSE: To ensure that the patient understands the medical assistant's position.
4. Use reasonable care, attention, and diligence during each encounter with patients.
   PURPOSE: To make certain that each patient is treated carefully and with the utmost professionalism during each encounter.

5. Follow your best judgment while working with each patient.
   PURPOSE: To ensure that patients are given optimum care.
6. Exercise reasonable skill and care, as would be expected from other area physicians' medical assistants in the same practice area.
   PURPOSE: Each patient must be treated with equal quality care.
7. Stay abreast of medical developments and techniques.
   PURPOSE: To consistently provide patients with the best care available.
8. Refrain from performing a procedure or treatment if it is beyond the scope of technical skill and/or training.
   PURPOSE: To ensure that the patient's care is provided by those who are confident and competent in their work.
9. Document treatments and care as required in the patient's medical record.
   PURPOSE: To provide a legal, permanent record of the patient's care.
10. Follow this standard of care while performing the remainder of the procedures in this chapter.

Legal Disclosure

The physician is charged with safeguarding patient confidences within the constraints of the law, but according to state laws, which vary somewhat across the nation, certain disclosures must be made. Frequently the medical assistant is involved with the responsibility for reporting these events.

Births and deaths must be reported. In some states, detailed information about stillbirths is required. Physicians also must report cases that may have been a result of violence, such as gunshot wounds, knife injuries, or poisonings. Any death from accidental, suspicious, or unexplained causes must also be reported. In some states, occupational diseases and injuries must be reported within specific time limits.

Sexually transmitted diseases are reportable in every state. All 50 states require that patients with confirmed cases of acquired immunodeficiency syndrome (AIDS) be reported by name to the local health department. Furthermore, more than half of the 50 states require that patients who test positive for HIV be reported. Individuals are reported either by name or by unique identifiers. A continuing controversy exists as to whether the reporting prompts patients to receive care or deters individuals in high-risk groups from seeking care.

Child abuse is a leading cause of death among children younger than 5 years of age, and healthcare professionals are required by law to report any suspected cases of child abuse. The report should be made as soon as evidence is discovered that gives the physician "cause to believe" that abuse or neglect has occurred. Even if the evidence is uncertain, the physician should report it and allow the government to investigate and determine what action to take to protect the child. However, it is essential to make every attempt to ensure that the report is legitimate, because it could lead to the child's being removed from the home and placed in foster care. Cases of spousal and elder abuse are difficult, because the person being abused often is reluctant to report the situation for fear of further mistreatment. The law requires that suspected cases of abuse of children, the elderly, or any others at risk be reported to the authorities.

Local health departments publish lists of reportable diseases and the method to use in reporting them. Often this can be done by telephone or mail. Appropriate forms must be used for mail reporting and are supplied by the health departments or available on their Web sites. County and state health departments periodically issue bulletins that are sent to healthcare providers with information about disease outbreaks and various statistics. Local health departments should be consulted for specific procedures and reporting protocols.

Patient Self-Determination Act

The Patient Self-Determination Act of 1990 brought the term *advance directives* to the forefront of medical care. This act requires healthcare facilities to develop and maintain written procedures that ensure that all adult patients receive information about living wills, durable powers of attorney for healthcare, and advance directives. These documents place the decision-making power in the hands of the patient and the family, providing them with written notification of their right to consent to or refuse medical treatment.

Patient's Bill of Rights

In March of 1998, President Bill Clinton received the final report from the President's Advisory Commission on Consumer Protection and Quality in the Healthcare Industry. The commission was created to advise the president on current issues in the healthcare industry and to make recommendations to ensure that patients would receive high-quality healthcare services. The report, "Quality First: Better Healthcare for All Americans," led to the development of a Consumer Bill of Rights and Responsibilities for the healthcare industry. This usually is called the Patient's Bill of Rights. The document, which has eight sections, lists three specific goals:

1. To strengthen consumer confidence by ensuring that the healthcare system is fair and responsive to consumers' needs, provides consumers with credible and effective mechanisms to address their concerns, and encourages consumers to take an active role in improving and ensuring their health
2. To reaffirm the importance of a strong relationship between patients and their healthcare professionals
3. To reaffirm the critical role consumers play in safeguarding their health by establishing rights and responsibilities for all participants in improving their health

Most healthcare facilities have adopted a Patient's Bill of Rights that provides a condensed version of the entire report. Often this information is presented to patients when they are admitted to healthcare facilities, or it may be posted in a prominent place in the facility. The medical assistant must consider the rights of the patient in each encounter. Explain procedures to patients and make sure they consent to treatment. The Patient's Bill of Rights is honored when written consent is obtained from patients, but the medical staff must always consider the patient and his or her individual desires and preferences in all phases of medical treatment. Office information booklets or bulletin board postings often contain information on where a patient may make a complaint about the care received at a facility. Policies and procedures should honor the provisions of the Patient's Bill of Rights that apply in that particular medical facility (Procedure 7-3).

PATIENT'S BILL OF RIGHTS

I. Information Disclosure
You have a right to receive accurate and easily understood information about your health plan, healthcare professionals, and healthcare facilities. If you speak another language, have a physical or mental disability, or just don't understand something, assistance will be provided so you can make informed healthcare decisions.

II. Choice of Providers and Plans
You have the right to a choice of healthcare providers that is sufficient to provide you with access to appropriate high-quality healthcare.

III. Access to Emergency Services
If you have severe pain, an injury, or a sudden illness that convinces you your health is in serious jeopardy, you have the right to receive screening and stabilization emergency services whenever and wherever needed, without prior authorization or financial penalty.

IV. Participation in Treatment Decisions

You have the right to know all your treatment options and to participate in decisions about your care. Parents, guardians, family members, or other individuals whom you designate can represent you if you cannot make your own decisions.

V. Respect and Nondiscrimination

You have a right to considerate, respectful, and nondiscriminatory care from your doctors, health plan representatives, and other healthcare providers.

VI. Confidentiality of Health Information

You have the right to talk in confidence with healthcare providers and to have your healthcare information protected. You also have the right to review and copy your own medical record and request that your physician amend your record if it is not accurate, relevant, or complete.

VII. Complaints and Appeals

You have the right to a fair, fast, and objective review of any complaint you have against your health plan, doctors, hospitals, or other healthcare personnel. This includes complaints about waiting times, operating hours, the conduct of healthcare personnel, and the adequacy of healthcare facilities.

VIII. Consumer Responsibilities

In a healthcare system that protects consumer rights, it is reasonable to expect and encourage consumers to assume reasonable responsibilities. Greater individual involvement by consumers in their care increases the likelihood of achieving the best outcomes and helps support a quality-improvement, cost-conscious environment.

AFFORDABLE CARE ACT OF 2010

The Affordable Care Act, signed into law in March of 2010, was designed to provide better health security by enacting comprehensive health insurance reforms that hold insurance companies accountable, lower healthcare costs, guarantee more choice, and enhance the quality of care for all Americans. The law restricts the use of annual limits and bans lifetime limits on healthcare benefits; for example, if a patient has cancer, the insurance company cannot put a limit on the amount of coverage provided to that patient, even if it is a catastrophic amount. Additionally, the act prohibits discrimination against children with pre-existing conditions.

Additional benefits went into effect on September 23, 2011, including:

- Preventive services, such as mammograms, colonoscopies, immunizations, prenatal and new baby care, will be covered and insurance companies will be prohibited from charging co-payments or co-insurance for these services.
- Patients will have the right to appeal coverage decisions to a third party.
- Patients are guaranteed their choice of primary care physicians and do not have to get a referral for an obstetrician/gynecologist or pediatrician.

Health insurers and employers are also now required to provide clear and consistent information about health plans, including an easy-to-understand Summary of Benefits and Coverage and a uniform Glossary of terms commonly used in health insurance coverage. More benefits will take effect through 2014.

Controlled Substances Act

On May 1, 1971, the Controlled Substances Act of 1970 became effective. In October, 1973, the Drug Enforcement Administration became a part of the U.S. Department of Justice. The DEA works with local, state, federal, and international agencies and organizations to address and regulate the serious issues of drug use and abuse in the United States.

Before administering, prescribing, or dispensing any drugs, a physician is required to register with the regional office of the DEA. This registration is renewable every 3 years. If a physician works from more than one office, he or she must register each individual office. Regulations on the writing, telephoning, and refilling of prescriptions vary, depending on which drug schedule is involved.

Under the Controlled Substances Act, drugs are categorized into schedules I to V. Drugs in schedule I have the highest potential for abuse and addiction, and those in schedule V have the lowest abuse potential.

Schedule I substances have no accepted medical use in the United States (e.g., heroin and lysergic acid diethylamide [LSD]). Only a physician involved in research with such drugs is concerned with schedule I substances.

Schedule II drugs have a high abuse potential, with severe risk of mental and physical dependence. These include certain narcotic, stimulant, and depressant drugs (e.g., opium, morphine, codeine, and methylphenidate [Ritalin]). Controlled substances in schedule II can be obtained only with a federal triplicate order form obtained from the DEA. A special inventory must be maintained on controlled substances and retained for 2 to 3 years, depending on state requirements. When a controlled substance is removed from inventory, it must be recorded. The record must show the date, the name of the drug, the dosage, and the name of the patient, physician, and employee involved. Substances in schedules III, IV, and V do not require triplicate forms.

Schedule III substances have an abuse potential that is lower than that of drugs in the first two schedules. They include compounds that have limited amounts of certain narcotic drugs combined with nonnarcotic substances (e.g., acetaminophen [Tylenol] with codeine, hydrocodone (Lortab, Norco, Vicodin), butalbital with aspirin and caffeine (Fiorinal) and several steroids.

Schedule IV substances have still lower potential for abuse; for example, phenobarbital, diazepam (Valium), propoxyphene (Darvon and Darvocet), alprazolam (Xanax), chlordiazepoxide (Librium), and pentazocine lactate (Talwin).

Schedule V substances have lower abuse potential than those in schedule IV but still warrant control. They include preparations that contain moderate amounts of certain narcotics, as may be found in cough medicines and antidiarrheal products.

The physician may call in a prescription to the pharmacist, but the pharmacist must transcribe it in writing before filling it. With permission from the physician, the medical assistant may orally transmit a prescription for controlled substances only in schedules

PROCEDURE 7-3

Incorporate the Patients' Bill of Rights into Personal Practice and Medical Office Policies

GOAL: *To ensure that the patient's rights are honored in the daily procedures performed and policies enacted in the physician's office.*

Unless otherwise noted, all equipment and supplies are to be provided by the instructor.

EQUIPMENT and SUPPLIES

- Copy of the Patient's Bill of Rights
- Office policy and procedure manuals
- Patient Role-Play Cards (provided by instructor)

PROCEDURAL STEPS

1. Review the eight points in the Patient's Bill of Rights.
   PURPOSE: To become familiar with the points and content of the document.
2. Review the office policy regarding information disclosure to make sure patients have the right to receive information about their health plan, professionals, facilities, and personal care.
   PURPOSE: To comply with the first article in the Patient's Bill of Rights.
3. Review the office policy regarding choice of providers, realizing that some patients may have restrictions on those choices according to their insurance plan.
   PURPOSE: To comply with the second article in the Patient's Bill of Rights.
4. Review the office policy regarding emergency treatment, paying close attention to the procedures for referral to emergency facilities and for emergency treatment in the office.
   PURPOSE: To comply with the third article in the Patient's Bill of Rights.
5. Review the office policy regarding consent for treatment and discussion of healthcare options to ensure that patients are given the ultimate choice in making decisions about their medical care.
   PURPOSE: To comply with the fourth article in the Patient's Bill of Rights.

6. Review the office policy regarding discrimination to make sure the policy is nondiscriminatory and that all employees are expected to be courteous and considerate to every patient and visitor to the office.
   PURPOSE: To comply with the fifth article in the Patient's Bill of Rights.
7. Review the office policy's sections on confidentiality to make certain that they comply with the patients' right to see their records and to expect confidential treatment of their healthcare information.
   PURPOSE: To comply with the sixth article in the Patient's Bill of Rights.
8. Review the office policy regarding patients' complaints and appeals (if applicable) to ascertain whether patients are given information about filing such grievances.
   PURPOSE: To comply with the seventh article in the Patient's Bill of Rights.
9. Review the office policy regarding quality improvement and cost-consciousness to make certain the office maintains the utmost level of quality while remaining cost-conscious.
   PURPOSE: To comply with the eighth article in the Patient's Bill of Rights.
10. Consider each of the eight articles while completing daily duties and performing patient care and treatment in the medical facility.
    PURPOSE: To incorporate the Patient's Bill of Rights into everyday practice.
11. Demonstrate sensitivity to patients' rights.
    PURPOSE: To reassure patients so that they know healthcare professionals are sensitive to their needs and desires.
12. Explain the Patient's Bill of Rights while role-playing with another student.

III, IV, or V, and the dispensing pharmacist must put the prescription into writing before filling it. The medical assistant cannot under any circumstances orally transmit a prescription for a schedule II drug. These prescriptions must be presented in writing to the pharmacist on the appropriate form.

Stored controlled substances must be kept in a locked cabinet or safe. Any loss of controlled drugs by theft must be reported to the regional office of the DEA when the theft is discovered. If a physician discovers that his or her DEA number is being used in the unauthorized prescription of controlled substances, he or she should report the incident to the DEA, to the state regulatory agency, and to the local police. This is especially important in the case of employees whose employment has been terminated and who are suspected of drug theft in the office. In numerous cases fired employees have

retaliated by reporting to the DEA exactly what they themselves took, but they accuse the physician or other staff members of taking the controlled substances. This results in messy investigations and months of follow-up; therefore any suspected employee drug use or abuse should be documented and reported to the local authorities. Periodic drug testing of employees is one way to help prevent office drug abuse. Many states now have laws to prevent the filing of false reports; therefore, if the physician is wrongly accused by a disgruntled employee, the physician often has some **recourse**.

A physician who discontinues medical practice must return the registration certificate and any unused order forms and triplicate prescription pads to the nearest office of the DEA. The regional DEA office advises the physician on the disposition of any controlled drugs still on hand.

CRITICAL THINKING APPLICATION   7-11
Barbara explains the importance of reporting any employee who is suspected of using drugs or taking drugs from the office. This may be difficult, because co-workers often are friendly with one another and may hesitate to report such acts. Discuss ways to handle this situation.

The Uniform Anatomical Gift Act

The Uniform Anatomical Gift Act was approved by the National Conference of Commissioners on Uniform State Laws in 1968. Although many states already had passed laws that permitted living persons to make a gift of their body or portions of it after death, the laws were so different from state to state that arrangements for a donation in one state might not be recognized in another. All states have adopted the Uniform Anatomical Gift Act or similar legislation.

Essentially, the model law for donation states the following:

- Any person of sound mind and 18 years of age or older may give all or any part of his or her body after death for research, transplantation, or placement in a tissue bank.
- A donor's valid statement of gift is paramount to the rights of others except when a state autopsy law may prevail.
- If a donor has not indicated an intent to donate during his or her lifetime, his or her survivors, in a specified order of priority, may do so.
- Physicians who accept organs or tissues, relying in good faith on the documents, are protected from lawsuits. The physician attending at the time of death, if acquainted with the donor's wishes, may dispose of the body under the Uniform Anatomical Gift Act.
- The time of death must be determined by a physician who is not involved in the transplantation, and the attending physician cannot be a member of the transplant team.
- The donor may revoke the gift, or the gift may be rejected by the proposed recipient.

The most important clause of the act permits the donation to be made by a will (without waiting for probate) or by other written or witnessed documents, such as a card designed to be carried by the person or a Uniform Donor Card (Figure 7-6). The Uniform Donor Card is considered a legal document in all 50 states. Many states now list donor preference on the driver's license as well.

The provisions of the Uniform Anatomical Gift Act are so designed that the offer is exercised only after death. Therefore, donors should reveal their intentions to as many of their relatives and friends as possible and to their physician. Because the human body and its parts are not commodities in commerce, no money can be exchanged in making an anatomic donation itself. Fees are charged for performing the transplant and various procedures, but organs cannot be bought and sold. It also is important to note that family members should be prepared to receive the body of the person who has donated his or her entire body to research once the research facility has completed its study. This can often be a traumatic experience that rekindles the grief process, so the procedures and final disposition of the body should be decided at the time of the donation to avoid this difficult situation.

The Health Insurance Portability and Accountability Act

HIPAA was signed into law on August 21, 1996, and all healthcare providers were required to comply with HIPAA's privacy standards by April 2003. Its history began in the Clinton healthcare reform proposals. HIPAA was designed for several purposes, with many goals in mind. Limiting the administrative costs of healthcare and privacy issues and preventing fraud and abuse are of primary importance in the HIPAA regulations. The law has two provisions: Title I (Insurance Reform) and Title II (Administration Simplification). The use of electronic transmissions ideally lowers the administrative costs of providing healthcare, but it has led to problems with privacy regarding health information. The law also had to provide security and confidentiality guarantees for the individual patient. Extensive privacy rules, including the use of unique identifiers, have shaped the law.

The final regulations regarding the privacy legislation sections of HIPAA were published in December, 2000, after the Centers for Medicare and Medicaid Services (CMS) reviewed more than 50,000 comments on and concerns about this important subject. All healthcare organizations that transmit any health information electronically must comply with HIPAA; fines as well as prison terms can be imposed on those who do not comply with the regulations.

HIPAA has had a tremendous effect on the healthcare industry. All healthcare providers, clearinghouses, and health plans that use electronic information must comply with HIPAA regulations. The benefits of HIPAA compliance include:

- Lower administrative costs
- Increased accuracy of data
- Increased patient and consumer satisfaction
- Reduced revenue cycle time
- Improved financial management

Title I, which deals with insurance reform, includes several provisions that protect individuals and their insured dependents if they change jobs or lose a job.

Title II details the process of administrative simplification. Standardization of the exchange of healthcare data is one way HIPAA promotes computer-to-computer transactions. This standardization process helps reduce the number of forms and methods used in the claims processing cycle, including electronic transactions and standard code sets (e.g., diagnosis, procedure, and supply codes). It also provides for unique identifiers for providers, employers, health plans, and patients. Medical professionals who access medical information must use log-in and password systems that prevent unauthorized individuals from accessing protected health information.

DONOR   DONOR CARD

I _____, have spoken to my family about organ and tissue donation. I wish to donate:
__ any needed organs and tissue
__ only the following organs and tissue: _____
The following people have witnessed my commitment to be a donor.
donor signature _____ date _____
witness_____
witness_____
next of kin _____ ph _____

FIGURE 7-6 Organ donation card.

The Occupational Safety and Health Act and the Bloodborne Pathogens Standard

In 1970 President Richard Nixon signed the Occupational Safety and Health Act, which created what has become the Occupational Safety and Health Administration. OSHA is a division of the U.S. Department of Labor, and since its creation, workplace injuries, illnesses, and fatalities have been reduced significantly. OSHA's mission is to ensure workplace safety and a healthy environment in the workplace.

OSHA commonly is considered the regulatory agency that requires steel-toe boots and hard hats; however, the medical industry moved into the OSHA spotlight in the late 1980s, when the threat of HIV infection extended to healthcare workers. Hepatitis and other pathogens already were a concern for healthcare workers, but when HIV, the virus that causes AIDS, was identified, action was needed to better protect the individuals who cared for patients with these infectious diseases. OSHA's Final Ruling on Bloodborne Pathogens became fully effective in July, 1992, and since then various additions have been made to update the regulations in light of new information about blood-borne pathogens.

The law requires medical facilities to comply with the Bloodborne Pathogens standard and to be able to prove their compliance to OSHA inspectors if necessary. The actual standard can be found in 29 **Code of Federal Regulations (CFR)** 1910.1030. The following information details the legal requirements of the OSHA standard as it pertains to the physician's office.

General Duty Clause

No law can cover every single situation that may arise in the course of daily living. Because of this, OSHA's general duty clause is a catchall regulation that fits almost any situation not specified in any other section of the law. The general duty clause simply states that a workplace must be free of any hazard that might cause serious harm or death. For example, one breach of the general duty clause is failure of a facility to provide reasonable security procedures at a retail store. Although not a specific breach of any regulation, this fits nicely into the general duty clause.

Emergency Preparedness

OSHA requires that all facilities with more than 10 employees have a written emergency action plan in place. The plan must include procedures that cover:

- Reporting a fire or other emergency
- Performing an emergency evacuation, including the type of evacuation and exit route assignments
- Establishing rules for employees who remain to run critical equipment before they evacuate
- Accounting for all employees after evacuation
- Establishing procedures to be followed by employees performing rescue or medical duties
- Providing the name or title of the person (or persons) to be contacted for information about the plan or an explanation of the individual's duties under the plan
- A list of the Personal Protective Equipment (PPE) to be used by each employee who will be exposed to bloodborne pathogens, such as lab coats, protective glasses, or gloves, as well as an indication of which tasks require what PPE

The plan also must have an alarm system to notify employees in case of an emergency, and the system must use a separate, distinct signal for each type of emergency. The employees must be trained in safe evacuation procedures. Also, the employer must review the plan with each employee at four specific times: (1) when the plan is developed, (2) when the employee is initially assigned to a job, (3) when the employee's responsibilities change, and (4) and when the plan is changed.

Facilities with more than 10 employees also must have a written fire prevention plan. The fire prevention plan must include:

- A list of all major fire hazards and the proper handling and storage of each
- The type of fire prevention equipment necessary to control each major hazard
- Procedures to control accumulations of flammable and combustible waste materials
- Procedures for regular maintenance of safeguards installed on heat-producing equipment to prevent the accidental ignition of combustible materials
- The name or job title of the person responsible for maintaining equipment, preventing or controlling sources of ignition or fires, and controlling fuel source hazards.

Employers must tell employees about the fire hazards associated with their job, in addition to ways the employee can protect himself or herself. The office policy manual should include information about procedures to follow during natural disasters, such as hurricanes, tornadoes, and other weather-related events, and during crime incidents at the facility (e.g., robbery and vandalism). Large-scale events, such as terrorist attacks or bioterrorism, also should be addressed, because medical professionals will be called upon to help in these situations. Obtain a copy of the local hospital's emergency preparedness plan and use it as a guideline if the office needs a written plan. (More information about emergency preparedness can be found in Chapters 27 and 58.)

OSHA inspectors can recommend fines when a facility is found to be out of compliance with an OSHA standard. One of the most common infractions involves a facility that has an Exposure Control Plan but is not using it or following its procedures and policies. This could cause an inspector to declare the facility willfully negligent. Willful negligence exists when "an employer representative was aware of the requirements of the [OSHA] Act, or the existence of an applicable standard or regulation, and was also aware that the condition or practice was in violation of those requirements, and did not abate the hazard." Fines for noncompliance can quadruple for willful negligence.

COMMON OSHA VIOLATIONS

- No eyewash facilities available
- No labeling or improper labeling of hazardous chemicals
- No MSDS for each hazardous chemical
- Storage of contaminated laboratory coats with clean ones
- Not communicating hazards to employees
- No documentation of initial employee training
- No documentation of annual employee training

- No annual hazard assessment
- Having an Exposure Control Plan but not following it
- No proof of destruction of hazardous waste
- No Emergency Action Plan in the facility
- No written Exposure Control Plan
- OSHA Form 300 not posted during required period
- No records of hepatitis B vaccinations or declination forms

MSDS, Material Safety Data Sheet; *OSHA*, Occupational Safety and Health Administration.

Exposure Control Plan

The Exposure Control Plan can be a part of the regular safety plan written for the medical facility or a stand-alone document, but it must cover all the elements required by OSHA. The plan must be put in writing, must be reviewed annually, and written documentation must exist that the plan was reviewed and updated or revised, if needed. A hard copy must be provided to employees on their request within 15 working days, and the plan must be available at all times in the workplace.

The plan must delineate the tasks employees perform in which the risk of blood exposure is present. It also must classify jobs in the facility according to the likelihood of exposure. For instance, some job duties always expose the employee to blood or **other potentially infectious materials (OPIM)**, often on a daily basis. Some duties only occasionally expose the employee, and other duties never expose the employee to blood or OPIM. Employees must be told to which category they belong and what duties they will perform that could lead to exposure. In addition, a clear follow-up procedure must be in place that details how the medical facility will track employee exposures. The employee cannot be abandoned after an exposure incident. Periodic counseling must take place in which the facility determines and documents the progress of the employee who has had an exposure, including laboratory tests and medical treatment received.

The Exposure Control Plan must contain a Waste Management section that details how waste is removed from the facility and destroyed. Most medical offices contract with companies that specialize in removing and destroying hazardous medical waste. The office must keep the receipts given by the company that prove that the waste was taken away from the facility and then incinerated or otherwise destroyed.

The plan must also contain a section on Hazardous Materials Communication, which explains what substances in the facility are hazardous and how to handle a spill or exposure to those products. Only the manufacturer of a chemical can determine whether it is hazardous, and Material Safety Data Sheets must be kept on almost all chemicals and reagents in the facility. Recent rulings have exempted some chemicals, but without the MSDS information, a medical assistant could not determine what type of health, reactivity, flammability, or other risks the chemical could have.

If the facility has equipment for x-ray studies, a Radiation Safety Plan must also be written and followed. All facilities should have an Emergency Action Plan in place, which provides procedures in case of tornadoes, fires, floods, or any other type of emergency that might occur in the office. This plan should contain floor plans of the facility, diagrams depicting the most efficient exits from the building, and the chain of command in an emergency. Diagrams with exit routes should be posted in every room of the medical office. At least annually, a hazard assessment must be performed on the entire facility. The hazard assessment is an inspection for problem areas in which the facility might be out of compliance. The facility must have documentation that the hazard assessment was done.

OSHA Record-Keeping Regulations

An injury or illness is considered to be work related when an event or exposure in the work environment contributed to or caused the condition or significantly aggravated a pre-existing condition. OSHA made several changes in the regulations covering record keeping on work-related injury to simplify forms, protect employee privacy, encourage employee involvement, and enable computer use for meeting OSHA requirements. The revised rules took effect January 1, 2002. Three basic forms now are used to keep records on injuries, accidents, and illnesses related to the workplace.

- OSHA Form 300—Log of Work-Related Injuries and Illnesses: Information is posted on form 300 regarding work-related deaths and every work-related injury or illness that involves loss of consciousness, restricted work activity or job transfer, days away from work, or medical treatment beyond first aid. An OSHA Form 301 (Injury and Illness Incident Report) should be completed for each entry on the log.
- OSHA Form 300A—Summary of Work-Related Injuries and Illnesses: Form 300A must be completed even if no injuries or illnesses that were work related occurred during the year. It must be posted in a common area for viewing by all employees, and provides the total number of accidents, illnesses, and injuries in the facility for the previous year. The length of time that this information must be posted has increased from 1 month to 3 months, specifically from February 1 to April 30 each year. An additional change is the certification of the form. A company executive must examine the document and certify that it is accurate.
- OSHA Form 301—Injury and Illness Incident Report: Form 301 is used to report what actually happened when an employee suffers a work-related injury or illness. This form, or an acceptable substitute, such as a state worker's compensation form, must be completed within 7 calendar days after notification of the illness or injury. The form should be completed as quickly as possible so that an exact recollection of events can be documented (Procedure 7-4). Now that the new record-keeping regulations have become effective, employees are guaranteed access to their OSHA 301 forms for the first time.

The log and summary forms must be kept on file for a minimum of 5 years. Only the Summary should be posted during the specified period from February 1 to April 30 each year, reflecting information from the previous calendar year. The forms are not sent to OSHA unless specifically requested. (To view these forms, visit the Evolve site at *evolve.elsevier.com/kinn*)

CRITICAL THINKING APPLICATION 7-12

Barbara quickly realizes that the office is using older versions of OSHA forms 300 and 301. Where might she look for or go to find updated information and forms?

PROCEDURE 7-4

Complete an Incident Report

GOAL: *To fill out an accurate, complete incident report that provides all legally required information.*

Unless otherwise noted, all equipment and supplies are to be provided by the instructor.

EQUIPMENT and SUPPLIES

- OSHA Form 301 (or other incident report form)
- Pen
- Notes taken regarding incident (Patient Role-Play Cards on Evolve)

PROCEDURAL STEPS

1. Interview the employee(s) involved in the incident using Patient Role-Play cards (choose cards that detail an employee or patient incident).
2. Review the notes taken by those who witnessed the incident.
   PURPOSE: To gain an understanding of what happened during the incident.
3. Interview those who may have additional information or those who provided the original notes, if clarification on the issues is needed.
   PURPOSE: To be clear about the exact sequence of events during the incident.
4. Read through OSHA Form 301 before filling out any sections.
   PURPOSE: To avoid making mistakes while putting the information in the spaces on the form.
5. Complete information about the employee(s) and the healthcare professional who treated the employee(s).
   PURPOSE: To document the incident and the principles involved.
6. Detail the information requested about the incident, including the actual injury or illness, a narrative of what happened, and what object(s) was involved in the injury.
   PURPOSE: To document the incident and the sequence of events.
7. Sign the report and, if possible, review it with the employee(s).
   PURPOSE: To prove that the report was submitted and reviewed by a supervisor.
8. If the injured employee(s) completes the incident report, make sure it is reviewed and signed by a supervisor.
   PURPOSE: Some facilities have incident reports the employee completes that detail the events surrounding the incident. These must be reviewed by a supervisor.
9. Make sure the incident was reported in a timely manner and within any state regulatory times.
10. Refer the employee(s) to the proper persons for medical care.
    PURPOSE: To make sure the employee(s) obtains timely and proper medical care.
11. Submit the completed report to your instructor.

It is wise to keep a communication log of calls to OSHA in which questions were asked or information verified. Note the day and time called, the first and last name of the person spoken to, the person's title, and the question asked and response given. Take detailed notes while discussing the issue on the phone. This log could be invaluable if a question ever arises about a subject discussed with a local OSHA official. It may make the difference when an OSHA inspector suggests a hefty fine. If the medical facility can show documentation that a certain procedure was discussed with an OSHA official and decisions were made based on that discussion, the facility may have sufficient evidence that the law was considered and the facility did its best to comply.

Needlestick Safety and Prevention Act

An estimated 600,000 to 800,000 injuries occur annually among healthcare workers. One third of these injuries happen during the disposal process. In an effort to reduce these injuries, which can lead to exposure to HIV, hepatitis B virus (HBV), or other blood-borne pathogens, OSHA revised its Bloodborne Pathogens standard to comply with the Needlestick Safety and Prevention Act, which became law on November 6, 2000. The regulations became effective on April 18, 2001.

Employers are now required to involve employees in the selection of needle safety devices. The facility must be able to prove that consideration was given to various types of devices that promote needle safety, what led to the decision to choose the device currently in use, and which employees were involved in these decisions. A list should be kept of which employees contributed to the selection decisions. Minutes from meetings, copies of employee response forms, and the forms used to solicit input are good methods of proving that employees were involved in the selection process.

> ### CRITICAL THINKING APPLICATION 7-13
> Barbara needs input about the needle safety devices used in the facility. Should she call a meeting of the entire office or should just specific employees present? If so, discuss who should have input in these decisions.

A needlestick and sharps injury log must also be kept in the medical facility. At a minimum, the log must include the following information:

- Description of the incident
- Type and brand of device used when the incident took place
- Location of the incident

The regulations that took effect in 2001 require all needlestick and sharps injuries to be reported and documented, not just the ones that result in injury or illness.

OSHA Training Requirements

All employees, including full-time, part-time, and temporary employees with a risk of occupational exposure, must receive training in the facility in which they are employed at two very specific times. Initial training must be conducted before a new employee starts any work-related duties. In addition, training must be conducted annually to update and inform employees about new regulations and procedures related to OSHA compliance. The initial training requirement is one of the most frequently breached regulations, yet it is critical to the employee's safety. Training must include the following:

- Making accessible a copy of the regulatory text of the OSHA standard and an explanation of its content.
- General discussion of blood-borne diseases and their transmission
- Universal precautions and body substance isolation
- The Exposure Control Plan
- Engineering and work practice controls, including handling of needles and sharps
- Personal protective equipment
- Hepatitis B vaccine
- Response to emergencies involving blood
- Potential sources of infection and tasks that might pre-empt exposure
- Written schedules for cleaning
- Handling of contaminated laundry
- Handling of exposure incidents and spills
- Post-exposure evaluation and follow-up program
- Reading of MSDS, signs, labels, and color coding (Figure 7-7) and the locations of these items

The employee must be given an opportunity to ask questions and receive answers, and the trainer must be knowledgeable about the subject matter. Documentation of the training sessions should be kept in each employee's personnel file or a special file for OSHA-related information.

CRITICAL THINKING APPLICATION   7-14

Barbara reviews the employee files and finds that neither Samantha nor Lynda received OSHA training when they were initially hired. How might Barbara rectify this, and what documentation would be helpful?

Hepatitis B Vaccination

The hepatitis B vaccination series must be offered to employees at risk of occupational exposure at no cost to the employee. The employee cannot be asked to pay in advance for the vaccination and be reimbursed, nor can the employee be asked to put the vaccination series on his or her personal health insurance policy. It must be made available to the employee within 10 working days of initial hire or assignment. The vaccination series can be declined by the employee, who must sign a declination form. If at any time the employee decides to receive the vaccination series, this must still be offered at no cost. The employee does not have to offer a reason for the declination. Prescreening and postvaccination serologic tests cannot be required.

The vaccination series is completed within a 6-month period. The second vaccination is given 1 month after the first, and the third 5 months after the second. Documentation should be provided to the employee for each vaccination received. Currently a booster dose of the hepatitis B vaccine is not required. However, if a routine booster is recommended by the U.S. Public Health Service in the future, it must be made available at no cost to employees.

CRITICAL THINKING APPLICATION   7-15

Lynda has not disclosed to anyone at the facility that she has had a case of hepatitis. Should she discuss this matter with Barbara? Is Lynda required to discuss this matter with Barbara? Is Lynda placing her patients at risk? If Lynda declines the hepatitis vaccination, must she explain why on the declination form?

Clinical Laboratory Improvement Amendments

The Clinical Laboratory Improvement Amendments (CLIA) were the result of a congressional investigation of **physician office laboratories (POLs)** and the deficiencies in the quality of the services and results provided by these laboratories. A set of minimum standards for laboratories was established, which improved the quality of test procedures. Quality control and assurance, as well as personnel and proficiency testing, are of utmost importance to the facility complying with CLIA.

CLIA regulations set the minimum standard for laboratory practice and quality. Remember that CLIA is not a governmental agency, but a law. CLIA is enforced by the Department of Health and Human Services (DHHS). OSHA is both a law (Occupational Safety and Health Act) and an agency (Occupational Safety and Health Administration). This is an important difference between CLIA and OSHA.

Some tests conducted in the laboratory are exempt from CLIA standards:

- Nonautomated dipstick or tablet urinalysis
- Fecal occult blood
- Ovulation using visual color comparison
- Urine pregnancy using visual color comparison
- Erythrocyte sedimentation rate
- Hemoglobin by copper sulfate method
- Spun microhematocrit
- Blood glucose testing using certain devices cleared by the U.S. Food and Drug Administration (FDA) for home use
- Specialized self-contained hemoglobin tests

Offices that perform only these tests may obtain a certificate of waiver and are not routinely inspected for CLIA compliance. Tests of moderate or high complexity must be performed by trained personnel with education and experience in the test areas in which they are working. A list of the moderate- and high-complexity procedures can be found in the July 26, 1993, issue of the *Federal Register*, and updates are published periodically that detail any changes in the list or regulations for testing procedures. Laboratories apply for a CLIA certificate through their local health departments and are periodically inspected for compliance.

Material Safety Data Sheets communicate hazards to employees about the products and chemicals used in the medical office. They also inform the employee as to what to do in case of an exposure. OSHA requires that MSDS are kept on all hazardous chemicals, unless exempted. Only the manufacturer can determine if a product is hazardous. MSDS can be obtained from either the manufacturer or the medical supply company from which the product was ordered. They must be provided after requested from the manufacturer within 30 days. Keep copies of requests to prove that an attempt has been made to obtain the MSDS information.

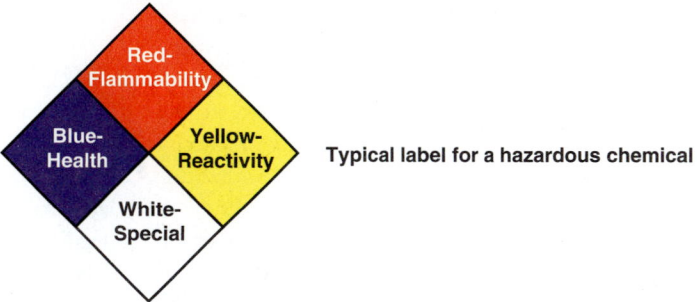

Typical label for a hazardous chemical

The appropriate number should be placed inside each box that applies in the figure above. Most offices use the National Fire Protection Association Rating System. Many MSDS provide the labeling information on the sheet. Others must be read thoroughly to determine how the labels should be completed. If the MSDS says that a chemical has a "moderate to high" hazard, label it high. If it says "low to moderate," label it moderate. Never guess at the numbers used for the label—always consult the MSDS. If individual containers are labeled, the facility is said to always be out of compliance, because it is easy to miss a container that may have just arrived in a shipment. Many medical facilities place labels on a permanent fixture next to where the product is stored, but it must be permanently stored in that area.

Simple Rating Guide

0—no hazard
1—slight hazard
2—moderate hazard
3—high hazard
4—extreme hazard

NFPA Rating Summary						
Health (Blue)			**Reactivity (Yellow)**			
4	Danger	May be fatal on short exposure. Specialized protective equipment required.	4	Danger	Explosive material at room temperature.	
3	Warning	Corrosive or toxic. Avoid skin contact or inhalation.	3	Danger	May be explosive if shocked, heated under confinement, or mixed with water.	
2	Warning	May be harmful if inhaled or absorbed.	2	Warning	Unstable or may react violently if mixed with water.	
1	Caution	May be irritating.	1	Caution	May react if heated or mixed with water but not violently.	
0		No unusual hazard.	0	Stable	Not reactive when mixed with water.	
Flammability (Red)			**Special Notice Key (White)**			
4	Danger	Flammable gas or extremely flammable liquid.	W		Water reactive.	
3	Warning	Flammable liquid flash point below 100° F.	Oxy		Oxidizing agent.	
2	Caution	Combustible liquid flash point of 100° to 200° F.				
1		Combustible if heated.				
0		Not combustible.				

FIGURE 7-7 Labeling and the National Fire Protection Association (NFPA) Rating System. (Courtesy National Fire Protection Association, Quincy, Mass.)

Americans with Disabilities Act

In 1990 the Americans with Disabilities Act (ADA) was signed into law with the intent of eliminating discrimination against individuals with disabilities. The act is comprehensive legislation that addresses many areas in which a person might experience discrimination, including telecommunications, housing, public transportation, air carrier access, voting accessibility, education, and rehabilitation. The physician's office falls in the category of public accommodations, which are defined as private entities that own, lease, lease to, or operate public facilities.

Public accommodations must comply with basic nondiscrimination requirements that prohibit exclusion, segregation, and unequal treatment. They also must comply with specific requirements related to architectural standards for new and altered buildings; reasonable modifications to policies, practices, and procedures; effective communication with people with hearing, vision, or speech disabilities;

and other access requirements. Public accommodations also must remove barriers in existing buildings, where it can be done without much difficulty or expense given the public accommodation's resources.

These regulations affect the physician's office because individuals with disabilities must be able to enter and exit the facility without difficulty. This means that individuals in wheelchairs need a ramp to enter and exit the building. They also must be able to navigate throughout the office without major barriers. Any facility with 15 or more employees must comply with the ADA. To be protected by the act, a person must have a disability or a relationship or association with an individual with a disability. An individual with a disability is defined by the ADA as a person who has a physical or mental impairment that substantially limits one or more major life activities; a person who has a history or record of an impairment; or a person who is perceived by others as having an impairment. The ADA does not specifically name all the impairments covered. Every medical facility must comply with the ADA. The law requires that public medical facilities must allow persons with disabilities to easily and safely:

- Reach door handles for opening and closing
- Enter and exit buildings
- Move through doors and hallways
- Use drinking fountains, phones, and restrooms
- Move from floor to floor (elevators are required for multilevel buildings)
- Do everything the general public can do in a public place

HITECH Act of 2009

The Health Information Technology for Economic and Clinical Health was signed into law in February, 2009, to promote the adoption and meaningful use of health information technology. The law encourages physicians and healthcare entities to comply with HIPAA regulations by enacting stiff penalties for noncompliance. Physicians who do not adopt electronic medical records will eventually be penalized in Medicare payments. The HITECH Act also imposes data breach notification requirements for unauthorized uses and disclosures of "unsecured PHI"; in other words, patients must be notified if there is a breach that exposes the patient's protected health information (PHI) (Procedures 7-5, 7-6).

PROCEDURE 7-5

Apply Local, State, and Federal Healthcare Laws and Regulations for Medical Assisting

GOAL: To be aware of local, state, and federal, laws and regulations that apply to the employer's facility and recognize the importance of compliance with such laws and regulations.

EQUIPMENT and SUPPLIES

- Computer
- Access to organizational Web sites that have established legislation and regulations that pertain to medical facilities
- Information about changes to and new federal and state legislation and regulations

PROCEDURAL STEPS

1. Consistently review applicable legislation and regulations that apply to the facility.
   PURPOSE: To ensure compliance with the law.
2. Discover the federal and state ramifications of issues related to healthcare workers, such as:
   - Regulatory bodies
   - Education and credentials
   - Scope of practice
   - Job qualifications
   - Continuing education unit (CEU) requirements
   - Loss of credentials
   PURPOSE: To ensure full compliance in the medical facility.
3. Review and understand federal and state legislation and regulations related to:
   - Americans with Disabilities Act
   - Controlled substance schedules
   - Occupational Safety and Health Administration (OSHA)
   - Centers for Disease Control and Prevention (CDC)

- Local Public Health Departments
- Material Safety Data Sheets (MSDS)
   PURPOSE: To ensure full compliance in the medical facility.
4. Review and understand accrediting agency requirements that affect the facility.
   PURPOSE: To recognize the importance of local, state, and federal legislation and regulations in the practice setting.
5. Stay aware of new state and federal legislation and regulations and the consequences of noncompliance.
6. Always follow office policy when performing any action at the facility.
   PURPOSE: To ensure full compliance in the medical facility.
7. Apply all local, state, and federal regulations to the daily duties of the medical facility.
   PURPOSE: To ensure full compliance with laws and regulations that affect the medical facility.
8. Report new or changed regulations to the appropriate supervisor in the medical facility.
   PURPOSE: To incorporate new regulations or changes into the office policy manual.
9. Facilitate or attend training sessions that explain new or changed regulations.
   PURPOSE: To ensure full compliance with laws and regulations that affect the medical facility.
10. Research one federal or state law that has recently been updated or changed. Prepare a report summarizing the change and submit it to your instructor.

Report Illegal and/or Unsafe Behaviors That Affect Health, Safety, and Welfare of Others to Proper Authorities

GOAL: *To provide a proper procedure for the medical assistant to follow when legal or ethical regulations have been breached.*

EQUIPMENT and SUPPLIES

- Contact information for regulatory and law enforcement agencies.
- Written reports or documentation of breaches of regulations, if available.

PROCEDURAL STEPS

1. Compile a list of all regulatory and law enforcement agencies that have jurisdiction over the medical facility.
2. Construct an office directory of contact information for each agency.
   PURPOSE: To have contact information close at hand when needed.
3. Document any illegal and/or unsafe act that occurs in the medical office.
   PURPOSE: To have a record of questionable incidents so that the medical assistant will not have to rely on memory.
4. Consider each aspect of the incident and make sure that it was truly a breach of law or ethics before acting. If unsure, discuss the situation with a trusted peer.
   PURPOSE: To prevent false accusations and the filing of a false report.
5. Report the incident to the direct supervisor and give him or her an opportunity to act.
   PURPOSE: To follow the chain of command.
6. If the situation is not resolved, report the incident to the next person in the chain of command unless the situation is critical and could cause harm to the patient.
   PURPOSE: To follow the chain of command.
7. If the situation still is not resolved, report the incident to the proper authorities, depending on the nature of the incident.
   PURPOSE: To comply with the law and ethical standards for medical practice.
8. Turn in your directory to your instructor.

CLOSING COMMENTS

Most patients never entertain the thought of taking legal action against their physicians, and a medical assistant should not develop an attitude of skepticism. However, a medical assistant can play an important role in preventing medical claims.

- Give scrupulous attention to the needs of each patient and do not leave patients alone for long periods. This especially applies to young children and elderly patients. Do not criticize other physicians or healthcare facilities. Never give out any information about the patient without written consent, and verify the identity of anyone asking for information about a patient.
- Use discretion in phone and office conversations. One never knows who may be standing nearby. Be aware of tone of voice and attitude during spoken conversations. Communicate office policies and procedures to patients clearly before treatment whenever possible.
- Keep accurate records that show exactly what was done to the patient and when it was done. The medical assistant must never make any promises as to the outcome of treatment. Record cancelled and no-show appointments and record the facts if a patient discontinues treatment.
- Check office equipment often to ensure that it is working properly. Keep drug samples and prescription pads out of sight. Never diagnose, prescribe, or offer a prognosis. Perform only the tasks for which you are trained and keep abreast of new findings and procedures in healthcare. Correctly follow all federal and state regulations.

- Play a positive part in the prevention of medical liability claims. Take care of the patient in a compassionate and competent way, and malpractice will not be a frequent issue in the medical facility.

Patient Education

Perhaps the most important detail to remember with regard to patient education and law is patience. Many medical forms are complicated, and regulations change often. Patients usually are not as well educated as the medical assistant on matters concerning legal policies and procedures. Often patients become frustrated with the number of changes with which they are expected to contend, and they unintentionally may project this frustration onto the medical assistant. Remain calm and answer questions, offering as much assistance to the patient as possible.

Legal and Ethical Issues

Generally, the law holds that every person is liable for the consequences of his or her own negligence when another person is injured as a result. In some situations, this liability extends to the employer. Physicians may be held responsible for the mistakes of those who work in their healthcare facility, and sometimes they must pay damages for the negligent acts of their employees.

Under the doctrine of *respondeat superior,* physicians are legally responsible for the acts of their employees when they are acting within the scope of their duties or employment. Physicians also are responsible for the acts of assistants who are not their own employees if they commit acts of negligence in the presence of the physician while under the physician's immediate supervision. When physicians practice as partners, they are liable not only for their own acts and those of their partners, but also for the negligent acts of any agent or employee of the partnership.

Medical assistants guilty of negligence are liable for their own actions, but the injured party generally sues the physician, because the chances of collecting damages are better. However, even assistants with no money can be held liable for any negligent action, and liens can be placed on their property in anticipation of its sale and potential profit. This fact illustrates the continuing importance of exercising extreme care in performing all duties accurately and professionally in the healthcare facility.

SUMMARY OF SCENARIO

Barbara is enthusiastic about her new job and duties. She is confident about appearing in court to represent Dr. Patrick and discuss the contents of the medical record of the patient suing his surgeon. Dr. Patrick is not a party to the lawsuit but has a physician-patient relationship with the patient just the same. An offer existed, as did the acceptance of that offer. The relationship was based on legal subject matter, and the physician and the patient had the legal capacity to enter into a contract. Consideration also existed, because the patient paid for services and the physician treated the patient. Both received something of value. Samantha and Lynda would like to accompany Barbara to the court proceedings to watch and learn.

Even if a patient does not pay for treatment, a contract still exists. The physician may elect to terminate the physician-patient relationship if the patient does not pay, but the trust that the patient places in the physician can be considered a thing of value.

Patients should understand their role in their treatment and their responsibilities to the physician. Often this information is communicated in the patient policy brochure, or it may be discussed orally with the patient. Physicians are not required to accept all patients; for instance, not all physicians deliver babies. Some physicians do not treat patients with workers' compensation claims. Physicians do have the right to see the types of patients they want to and are competent to treat, but they should never discriminate on the basis of race, gender, or any other protected status.

A physician may not always be correct in his or her diagnoses, but this does not mean that the physician has committed malpractice. However, if expert witnesses feel that the physician should have made a different diagnosis based on the case, then the physician might be held liable for negligence. If an employee has information about a case that is damaging to the physician, he or she is ethically obligated to report the information, but rarely legally liable to speak up unless a law has been broken.

Samantha and Lynda have learned many new concepts about law from Barbara and are anxious to follow the court proceedings. They will learn more by watching the actual process of law at work. Barbara looks forward to sharing more knowledge with the employees as they continue to work together.

Medical assistants can help the physician comply with legal regulations in the office by making sure that they understand the policies and procedures required by the facility. Rules are made to ensure compliance so that both patients and employees are kept safe and risks in the office are kept to a minimum. Patient confidentiality is one of the most important rules to remember. New graduates can learn about the laws that affect medical facilities in their area by discussing them with their supervisors and by attending seminars and training. Much information is available on the Internet regarding legal issues.

Trust is a critical factor in avoiding medical professional liability lawsuits. When the patient trusts the physician, he or she is much more likely to work through issues that otherwise might lead to legal action against the physician. Keeping accurate patient records and documenting all information required in the patient chart helps prove that the physician adequately cared for the patient. Clearly, legible handwriting is vital in this process.

The medical assistant may find that the physician is not in compliance with certain rules and regulations. Never jump to conclusions and assume that the physician has no intention of complying. There are various reasons for noncompliance, and any issues should be brought to the attention of the office manager or the physician for clarification. It is the medical assistant's responsibility to question noncompliance and make every effort to bring the facility into compliance with the cooperation of supervisors, co-workers, and the physician. As a team, medical professionals can remain in compliance and deliver excellent care to all patients.

SUMMARY OF LEARNING OBJECTIVES

1. **Define, spell, and pronounce the terms listed in the vocabulary.**
   Spelling and pronouncing medical terms correctly bolster the medical assistant's credibility. Knowing the definition of these terms promotes confidence in communication with patients and co-workers.

2. **Discuss all levels of government legislation and regulation as they apply to medical assisting practice, including regulations established by the FDA and the DEA.**
   An exhaustive listing of government legislation and regulation is available to the medical assistant through Internet research, useful for those situations when asked to keep the facility in compliance with the law. The person charged with this duty must be able to interpret lengthy legalese and determine the exact tasks and precautions required of the facility. Some offices form a compliance committee to help ensure that all pertinent laws that govern the medical practice are followed meticulously.

3. **Discuss the legal scope of practice for medical assistants.**
   From a legal perspective, each medical assistant is required to perform all duties in a manner that meets or exceeds that of a reasonably competent and knowledgeable medical assistant. Also, medical assistants cannot perform any duties for which they have not been trained.

4. **Distinguish among an act, a statute, and an ordinance.**
   Different types of laws and regulations affect us, depending on the origination of the law. *Acts* are introduced at the federal level and must be passed by Congress. State legislative bodies develop *statutes*, and local governments create *ordinances*.

5. **Compare criminal and civil law as they apply to the practicing medical assistant.**
   Criminal law governs violations punishable as offenses against the state or government. *Civil law* is concerned with acts that are not criminal but involve relationships between individuals and other individuals, groups, or government agencies. The medical assistant needs to understand the differences between the types of law and how they affect the physician's medical practice. Medical assistants must personally review those laws that influence medical assistant practice and make sure that they are followed on a constant basis, with documentation to prove so if necessary in a courtroom.

6. **Explain the three basic categories of criminal law.**
   Infractions are the lowest on the criminal law scale, usually resulting in a fine. *Misdemeanors* are minor crimes punishable by a fine or imprisonment in a city or county jail. *Felonies* are major crimes, such as rape, murder, or burglary. Most felonies carry punishment of imprisonment for at least 1 year, and they are divided into subgroups, usually first-, second-, and third-degree felonies. *Treason* is a higher crime, usually an attempt to overthrow the government. High treason constitutes a serious threat to the stability of the government, such as an attempt on the life of the president.

7. **Distinguish which type of civil law deals with medical professional liability.**
   Tort law is the division of civil law that deals with medical professional liability. Tort law provides relief for those who have suffered harm from the actions of others. The plaintiff must establish duty, breach of duty, and damages as a result of the breach of duty, and the extent of the damages suffered.

8. **Provide an example of tort law as it would apply to a medical assistant.**
   If a medical assistant committed a breach of patient confidentiality, his or her error would fall under the category of tort law, and the medical assistant could be held liable for the error, resulting in damages being paid to the patient by the physician and/or his liability insurer.

9. **Describe liability, professional and personal injury, and third-party insurance.**
   When a person is liable for an act, he or she is obligated or responsible according to the law. Professional and personal injuries are types of torts, meaning that a person or group has injured someone or something else. Physicians carry professional liability insurance, a type of third-party insurance, to help guard them from liability costs. Medical assistants can also invest in liability insurance.

10. **Explain the four essential elements of a valid contract.**
    Four elements are essential to a valid legal contract: (1) there must be a "meeting of the minds," or manifestation of assent; (2) the contract must involve legal subject matter; (3) the parties to the contract must have the legal capacity to enter into a contract; and (4) some type of consideration must be offered.

11. **Distinguish between interrogatories and depositions.**
    Interrogatories are lists of questions directed from each party of a lawsuit to the other. Interrogatories are answered under oath and directed only to the parties actually named in the lawsuit. *Depositions* can be taken from any witness or party to the lawsuit. They also are taken under oath, and often witnesses are subpoenaed to offer a deposition.

12. **List three things to remember when testifying in court.**
    Testifying in court can be an intimidating experience, but good preparation can alleviate many anxieties. Discussing potential questions with the attorney helps prepare the witness for giving testimony. Always tell the truth to prevent charges of perjury. Speak clearly and distinctly, and do not hesitate to ask the attorney to repeat a question. A brief pause to think about an answer causes no harm. Dress conservatively, know the location and room of the court in advance, and always arrive on time. Credibility is critical in a medical professional liability trial.

13. **Discuss the advantages of arbitration.**
    Arbitration is a popular alternative to court trials. It involves the use of a third party familiar with law or the issues at hand. It is recognized by statute in most states and provides a faster, confidential, fair, and less expensive resolution to a dispute.

14. **Differentiate among malfeasance, misfeasance, and nonfeasance.**
    Malfeasance, misfeasance, and nonfeasance are types of negligence often involved in medical professional liability cases. *Malfeasance* is performing an act that is completely wrong or unlawful. *Misfeasance*, comparable to a mistake, is the improper performance of a lawful act. *Nonfeasance* is the failure to perform some act that should have been performed.

15. **Explain the "four Ds" of negligence.**

The four Ds of negligence are (1) the *duty* to care for the patient; (2) *dereliction,* or failure to perform that duty; (3) proof that this failure was the *direct* cause of a patient's injury; and (4) proof that the patient suffered *damages* from the injury.

16. **Define the types of damages.**

Nominal damages are token compensations for invasion of a legal right. *Punitive damages* are designed to punish an offender and discourage repetition of an act. *Compensatory damages* are designed to compensate for the actual damages suffered, whereas *general damages* include compensation for pain and suffering, loss of a body member, disfigurement, and other similar losses. *Special damages* can include such losses as earnings or travel costs.

17. **Compare and contrast physician and medical assistant roles in terms of standard of care.**

Physicians are highly trained and skilled professionals who are licensed to diagnose and treat patients. Medical assistants cannot diagnose, treat, or advise patients toward any course of action and must be careful to remain within the medical assistant scope of practice when carrying out their duties at work.

18. **Explain the importance of informed consent.**

Informed consent gives the patient a full understanding of the condition that has been diagnosed, including what could happen if the patient undergoes treatment, refuses treatment, or delays treatment. It provides the patient with information on the advantages and risks of a medical procedure and alternative treatments the patient may want to consider. Informed consent places control in the hands of the patient, who is given the opportunity to make the decisions about his or her healthcare. Patients can never be forced to undergo any type of procedure or treatment.

19. **List several legal disclosures the physician must make.**

The physician must make several types of legal disclosures with regard to a patient's health that do not require the patient's consent. Information about births and deaths, injuries or illnesses as a result of violence, accidental or suspicious deaths, sexually transmitted diseases, and any type of abuse are examples of legal disclosures that must be made by healthcare professionals.

20. **Identify where to report illegal and/or unsafe activities and behaviors that affect the health, safety, and welfare of others.**

In any emergency situation, the medical assistant should call 911. Keep a list of contact information for agencies that provide community assistance. Hospitals often keep an exhaustive list of agencies that can help patients receive various types of assistance. Government agencies are usually listed in the blue pages of a telephone directory and can be easily found using Internet search engines.

21. **Explain how the medical assistant's practice is affected by negligence, malpractice, statutes of limitations, Good Samaritan acts, the Uniform Anatomical Gift Act, Living Wills/Advanced Directives, and the Medical Durable Power of Attorney.**

Because medical assistants are required to perform all duties in a manner that meets or exceeds that of a reasonably competent and knowledgeable medical assistant, they must be aware of state and federal laws and regulations that affect their practice. Many physicians keep copies of the laws that affect the practice in the policy and procedure manual. All employees are responsible for knowing the law and following procedures that are outlined in the policy manual.

22. **Summarize the Patient's Bill of Rights.**

The Patient's Bill of Rights was designed to (1) strengthen consumer confidence by ensuring that the healthcare system is fair and responsive to consumers' needs; (2) provide consumers with credible and effective mechanisms to address their concerns; (3) encourage consumers to take an active role in improving and ensuring their health; (4) affirm the importance of a strong relationship between patients and their healthcare professionals; and (5) affirm the critical role consumers play in safeguarding their health by establishing rights and responsibilities for all participants in improving patients' health.

23. **Describe the implications of the Health Insurance Portability and Accountability Act (HIPAA) for the medical assistant in various medical settings.**

Passage of the Health Insurance Portability and Accountability Act (HIPAA) in 1996 established extensive privacy rules and regulations for the healthcare profession concerning the electronic transfer of information. The act also limited administrative costs by supporting the use of electronic transfer of information and presented guidelines for preventing fraud and abuse. However, the privacy issues raised by HIPAA have been the most discussed and debated topics related to this law.

24. **Describe personal protective equipment.**

Personal protective equipment is designed to protect the wearer from blood-borne pathogens and/or other potentially infectious materials. OSHA requires that employers provide personal protective equipment (PPE) if the employee is at risk of exposure to blood-borne pathogens.

25. **Discuss requirements for responding to hazardous materials disposal.**

Hazardous materials must be disposed of according to the information provided on the MSDS. Spill kits, used to dispose of waste safely, are required in medical facilities. Most biologically hazardous waste is disposed of by waste removal companies and is usually incinerated. The medical facility is provided with receipts both when the waste is picked up and when it is finally incinerated. OSHA requires that these receipts be kept for a specific time.

26. **Describe the importance of the Material Safety Data Sheet (MSDS) in a healthcare setting.**

The Material Safety Data Sheet (MSDS) provides vital information about a product or chemical used in the medical facility. The MSDS explains the proper use of the product and the appropriate action when a spill occurs.

27. **Distinguish between OSHA and CLIA; indicate which one is an actual agency.**

The Occupational Safety and Health Administration (OSHA) is an agency, a division of the U.S. Department of Labor. More than 2,300 employees work for OSHA, and the agency runs on an annual budget of approximately $443 million as of 2002. Twenty-six states have their own OSHA programs, which adds 3,100 employees. The Occupational Safety and

Health Act of 1970 created this agency to ensure safety in the workplace. The Clinical Laboratory Improvement Amendments (CLIA) is a law that regulates the quality of services provided by laboratories. CLIA is enforced by the Department of Health and Human Services.

28. **Identify how the Americans with Disabilities Act (ADA) applies to the medical assisting profession.**

Medical assistants must comply with the ADA as it applies to the medical facility employer. Know the provisions of the act and assist in making certain that the facility is in full compliance. Assist patients with disabilities as they make their way into, through, and out of the facility. Offer to help with disrobing and dressing before assuming that the patient needs assistance.

CONNECTIONS

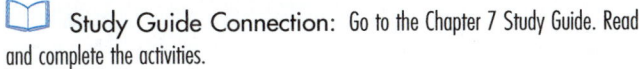 **Study Guide Connection:** Go to the Chapter 7 Study Guide. Read and complete the activities.

Evolve Connection: Go to the Chapter 7 link at *evolve.elsevier.com/ kinn* to complete the Chapter Review and Chapter Quiz. Check out the other resources listed for this chapter to make the most of what you have learned from Medicine and Law.

8

COMPUTER CONCEPTS

Dr. Michael Bouchard is aware of the advantages of networking his office computers and having Internet access to meet the needs of his facility. Every day he and his staff send and receive many important e-mail messages to and from patients and other individuals. His staff members use the computer for communications and to access sources of online information. Patient tracking, accounting functions, and health information retrieval are immensely faster on a computer than with a paper-based system. The scheduling features of the software are a distinct advantage, because the schedule is shared; everyone in the office knows the doctor's schedule, which prevents double-booking and miscommunication. Dr. Bouchard sends his staff members for regular computer training so that all of them can use the computers in the most efficient ways.

The requirements of the Health Information Portability and Accessibility Act (HIPAA) have altered the methods by which information may be used in medical facilities. No employee is allowed to access information in the clinic that is not necessary for that employee to provide patient care and assistance. Dr. Bouchard takes the HIPAA guidelines seriously and makes sure that his entire staff understands the importance of keeping health information secure.

While studying this chapter, think about the following questions:

- How do computers help the physician's office to run more efficiently?
- Can an employee in the physician's office invade a patient's right to privacy by accessing medical records?
- How can information on the computer be kept secure from curious employees who do not need to access the information for the purpose of patient care?
- How does logging in and logging out of the office network help ensure proper access to medical records?
- How could the computer be considered a co-worker in the medical office?

LEARNING OBJECTIVES

1. Define, spell, and pronounce the terms listed in the vocabulary.
2. List several ways the computer can be effective in a medical office.
3. Explain the basic functions a computer performs.
4. Explain the basic parts of a computer.
5. List the three elements that differentiate microprocessors.
6. Discuss the differences among various types of printers.
7. Explain the importance of a motherboard.
8. Explain and give examples of peripheral devices.
9. List and discuss several types of file formats.
10. Explain the concept of computer networking.
11. Define the function of browsers.
12. Discuss the importance of computer security.
13. Locate the keys on a keyboard.

VOCABULARY

application software Computer programs designed to perform specific tasks.

artificial intelligence The aspect of computer science that deals with computers taking on the attributes of humans, such as mimicking human thought. For example, expert systems can make decisions, such as software designed to help a physician diagnose a patient, given a set of symptoms.

backup Any type of storage that prevents the loss of files with hard disk failure.

bits The smallest units of information inside the computer, each represented either by the digit "0" or "1"; 8 bits equal 1 byte.

bookmark A command in a browser that marks the Internet protocol (IP) address of a Web site so that it can be saved and recalled quickly without typing the entire Web address.

browsers Software programs that allow users to view Web pages on the Internet (e.g., Internet Explorer, Firefox).

byte A unit of data that contains 8 binary digits, or bits.

cache (kash) Special, high-speed storage that either can be part of the computer's main memory or a separate storage device. One function of a cache is to store Web sites visited in the computer memory for faster recall the next time the Web site is requested.

CD burner A device that can "write" data on a blank compact disk (CD) or copy data from one CD to a blank CD.

cookies Messages sent to a Web browser from a Web server that identify users and can prepare custom Web pages for them, possibly displaying their name on return to the site.

cursor A symbol on the monitor screen that shows the location of the next character to be typed.

cyberspace The nonphysical space of the online world of computer networks in which communication takes place.

database A collection of related files that serves as a foundation for retrieving information.

device driver The program or commands given to a device connected to a computer that enable the device to function. For instance, a printer may come equipped with software that must be loaded onto the computer first so that the printer will work.

digital subscriber line (DSL) A high-speed, sophisticated modulation scheme that operates over existing copper telephone wiring systems; often referred to as "last-mile technologies," because DSL is used for connections from a telephone switching station to a home or office and not between switching stations.

digital video disk (DVD) An optical disk that holds approximately 28 times more information than a CD; a DVD is most commonly used to hold full-length movies. Compared with a CD, which holds approximately 600 megabytes, a DVD can hold approximately 4.7 gigabytes. Also called a *digital versatile disk.*

disk drives Devices that load a program or data stored on a disk into the computer.

domain name The initial part of a URL listing; the domain and name of the host or server, indicating the publisher of a Web page or site.

e-commerce Short for *electronic commerce;* used to describe the sale and purchase of goods and services over the Internet; doing business over the Internet.

e-mail Short for *electronic mail;* communications transmitted via computer or computer network.

environment The state of a computer, usually determined by the programs running and hardware and software characteristics.

flash drive A small, portable device that can carry 2 to 8 gigabytes or more of information and that plugs into a USB port; also called a *thumb drive, jump drive,* or *portable drive.*

gigabyte (GB) Approximately 1 billion bytes.

hard copy The readable paper copy or printout of information.

hardware The physical components of the computer system, such as the central processing unit (CPU), monitor, and printer.

HTML The acronym for *hypertext markup language,* the language used to create documents for the Internet.

HTTP The acronym for *hypertext transfer protocol,* which defines how messages are formatted and transmitted over the Internet. When a URL is entered into the computer, an HTTP command tells the Web server to retrieve the requested Web page.

hub A common connection point for devices in a network with multiple ports, often used to connect segments of a local area network (LAN).

icons Pictures, often on the monitor screen "desktop," that represent programs or objects. Clicking on an icon directs the user to the program.

input Information entered into and used by the computer.

kilobyte (KB) Approximately 1,024 bytes.

megabyte (MB) Approximately 1 million bytes.

megahertz (MHz) The measuring device for microprocessors. A megahertz is 1 million cycles of electromagnetic currency alternation per second and is used as a unit of measure for the clock speed of computer microprocessors.

modem Short for *modulator-demodulator;* a device that allows information to be transmitted over telephone lines at speeds measured in bits per second (bps). The modem speed generally is listed somewhere on the unit.

multimedia The presentation of graphics, animation, video, sound, and text on a computer in an integrated way or all at once. CD-ROMs are efficient multimedia devices.

notebook Although often used interchangeably with "laptop," this term was created to identify a smaller, thinner, and lighter device, partially designed to fit on tray tables on airplanes.

output Information processed by the computer and transmitted to a monitor, printer, or other device.

personal digital assistant (PDA) A handheld computer capable of functions such as mobile telephony, Web browsing, and media playing. PDAs typically include an appointment calendar, to-do list, address book, note programs, and e-mail and/or Web capabilities.

queries Requests for information from a database.

router (rau'-ter) A device used to connect any number of LANs, which communicate with other routers and determine the best route between any two hosts.

scanner A device that reads text or illustrations on a printed page and can translate the information on that page into a form the computer can understand.

search engines Programs that search documents for keywords and return a list of documents containing those words.

server A computer or device on a network that manages shared network resources.

switch In networks, a device that filters information between LAN segments and reduces overall network traffic and increases speed and bandwidth use efficiency.

system software The operating system and all utility programs that allow the computer to function and perform operations.

tablet A wireless, portable personal computer with a touch screen interface, usually smaller than a notebook but larger than a smart phone (e.g., Apple iPad, Samsung Galaxy, Dell Streak).

TCP/IP The acronym for *transmission control protocol/Internet protocol;* a suite of communications protocols used to connect users or hosts to the Internet.

telecommunications The science and technology of communication by transmission of information from one location to another via telephone, television, telegraph, or satellite.

terabyte (TB) Approximately 1 trillion bytes.

URL The acronym for *uniform resource locator;* specifies the global address of documents or information on the Internet. The URL provides the IP address and the domain name for the Web page, such as microsoft.com.

virtual reality An artificial environment presented to a computer user that feels as if it were a real environment, often involving use of special gloves, earphones, and goggles to enhance the experience.

Today's business world is almost unimaginable without computers, although the computer industry is less than a century old. Within this short time, a computer upsurge has taken place, and today our lives are affected by computers daily. Personal computers (PCs), laptops or notebook computers, and cell phones that send and receive **e-mail** are commonplace. Our world is now one of enhanced **telecommunications**, where faster processing of information is both needed and expected. Advances in technology happen daily; as soon as one "new and improved" device is on the market, its "better and faster" competitor is released. Most people venture into **cyberspace** on a daily basis, where a world of information is waiting with the simple click of a mouse!

Computers are critical in the physician's office and in other types of healthcare facilities. The development of medically specific software, the decrease in the cost of computer **hardware**, and the time savings the computer brings to the office make it well worth the investment. A medical assistant must have more than computer literacy; a good understanding of the way computers work and their capabilities is essential in a medical office.

Since the emergence of the electronic medical record (EMR), patients are likely to see physicians using laptops, tablets, smart phones, and/or personal digital assistants (PDAs) in the exam room, an indication that the entire medical industry is steadily moving toward a paperless environment. The EMR makes the physician's office more efficient and patient information more accessible. The EMR is covered extensively in Chapter 15; before the medical assistant can grasp the concepts of the EMR, he or she needs a strong foundation in basic computer operation. In the current economy, many displaced workers who have found themselves without employment have had to improve their computer skills to be marketable. Some have worked in fields that required little or no computer use, and certainly in any medical facility, computer skills will be mandatory.

COMPUTER BASICS

Getting Started

Even with a basic knowledge of a computer's components and capabilities, without hands-on knowledge the beginner may have some

initial fear of the unknown. The most basic setup of a computer system includes a microprocessor, monitor, keyboard, and mouse (Figure 8-1). The computer is only a machine that takes direction from the operator, performing the tasks it is told to do. A computer can simulate the thought process and make decisions, but most computers found in medical facilities wait for commands that prompt it to act. Dialog boxes appear that ask for **input** from the user; this is how the computer communicates with the user. Computers assist workers in medical offices in several ways, such as:

- Performing repetitive tasks
- Reducing errors
- Speeding up production
- Recalling information on command
- Saving time
- Reducing paperwork and storage space
- Allowing for more creative and productive use of workers' time

The more familiar medical assistants become with the computer, the better skilled they become in its use. Occasionally errors are made, and the computer may respond with an error message. However, the monitor's screen normally indicates what to do next.

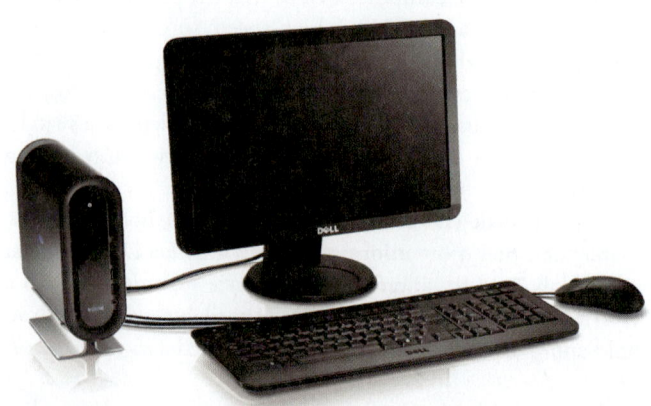

FIGURE 8-1 Computers are an invaluable tool for today's medical office. This photograph shows *(left to right)* a CPU, monitor, keyboard, and mouse. The keyboard and mouse are types of input devices that allow data to be entered into the computer, where they are processed. (Courtesy Dell Corp., Round Rock, Texas.)

The computer usually allows the operator the opportunity to figure out the correct information and input it. A help menu can always be accessed, or the instruction manual can be consulted; help lines and technical support also are available when problems occur. The problem may be with the software or with the computer itself. Usually, determining which has caused the problem is fairly easy.

Rarely does a computer "break," although this is a common fear among new users. Records are unlikely to be destroyed by accident; usually, very specific commands are needed to delete stored information. However, a medical assistant must take care not to shut off the computer without saving the information that has been entered. By using a computer in the classroom and practicing at home or at a library, if possible, the medical assistant can become familiar with computer operation and gain confidence that it can be mastered. However, mastery is accomplished only through practice.

With a knowledge of computer terms, the ability to follow step-by-step instructions, and reasonable expertise with a keyboard, a medical assistant can rapidly learn and use almost any computer system. Although computers and software may vary from facility to facility, basic computer operation is similar, and if the instructions given by the computer are carried out, the user should be successful in the tasks attempted.

Although it seems elementary, the first step in computer use is to turn on the system. If nothing happens when the power button is pressed, the primary troubleshooting protocol is to make sure the system is plugged into the power outlet. If a surge protector or an uninterruptible power supply (UPS) is used, be sure this device has power. Then, check all the cords that attach the hardware to determine whether they are fastened securely. Once the power is on, the computer goes through a process called *booting*. The boot sequence is a set of operations the computer performs to load the operating system and prepare it for use.

Once the computer is on, the desktop appears, along with several **icons**. To open a certain program, double-click on its icon. Once a program has been opened, many functions can be performed, such as creating a document, a spreadsheet, or a presentation or maintaining a **database**. Some basic computer functions include:

- *Opening a document.* A document stored on the computer can be opened by clicking on its icon, if the icon appears on the desktop. If the document is stored in a folder, open the folder and click on the document icon.
- *Saving a document.* Most toolbars have a button that allows a document to be saved to a folder or to the desktop. Click the button, then name the file so that it can be easily found when it is needed. Word processing programs also usually have a "Save As" option so that a document can be saved and edited without changing the original file. Be sure to check the compatibility of the versions of the software being used. Most programs are backward compatible; for instance, MS Office 2010 can open MS Office 2007, but older software versions cannot open newer versions.
- *Creating a folder.* Folders in which documents can be stored are easily created. For instance, in a Windows **environment**, a folder can be created on the desktop. To do this, right-click on the desktop away from other files, folders, and icons, then select the command "New." When the second dialog box appears, select "Folder." Click "Folder" and a folder titled "New Folder" will appear on the desktop. To rename it, click twice on the words "New Folder" and type in the words "Study Guides" or whatever title is to be used. The folder is ready for use. To move documents into the folder, click on the document icon and hold the left mouse button down while dragging the document on top of the folder. This is called "drag and drop" or sometimes "click and drag." To place documents not on the desktop in the folder, use the "Save As" feature and save the document to the desired folder. Or the document can be saved to the desktop, after which the "drag-and-drop" feature can be used to place it in the desired folder.
- *Copying, moving, deleting, and renaming files.* Most word processing programs allow the user to copy, move, delete, and rename files. In Windows, a file may be copied easily by right-clicking on the document icon and then clicking "Copy." Then, open the folder to which the file is to be copied, right-click inside the folder, and click "Paste." A copy of the file will appear in the folder. Files can be moved from one place to another by using the drag-and-drop method. To delete a file, right-click on the document icon and click "Delete." A dialog box will open that confirms the user's choice to delete the file. The file remains in the Recycle bin on the desktop for a brief period once deleted; therefore, if a mistake was made and the file is needed, the user should look to see whether it is still available. Renaming files is as simple as clicking twice on the file name and typing in the new one. The user also can right-click on the document icon and select "Rename," which will allow the user to change the name of the document.
- *Cutting, copying, and pasting text.* Text can be moved from one place to another by cutting and pasting. First, highlight the text to be moved, then press the "Cut" button. This function can also be accomplished by right-clicking the mouse and selecting "Cut." Next, place the **cursor** at the point where the text should be inserted, then click the "Paste" or right-click the mouse and select "Paste." Text is copied in the same manner. Instead of clicking the "Cut" button, press the "Copy" button. These functions allow the user to be more efficient when creating documents.
- *Finding files.* Computers have a search mechanism that allows the user to search for a file with certain keywords or extensions. In the Windows environment, click the "Start" button, then click on "Search." The dialog box that appears asks the user for what to search (e.g., picture, audio file, document, or other file type). An option to search all files and folders also is available. Enter keywords that pertain to the desired file, and click "Search."
- *Copying an entire disk.* An entire diskette or compact disk (CD) can be copied. First, click on "Start" and then click on "My Computer." Find the drive that has the diskette or CD and right-click on that icon. Then, click on "Copy." Open the folder to which the contents should be copied, and click "Paste." The actual diskette or CD could also be opened, then under the "Edit" drop-down menu, the user can choose "Select All." This allows all the files on the diskette or CD to be copied or permanently moved to another location.
- *Exiting a program.* Click on the "X" button in the upper right corner of the document to exit a program. If the work has not

yet been saved, the user is prompted either to save the document or cancel the action. The user also can exit the program by clicking on "File" then "Close."

When the user has finished with the computer for the day, it always should be shut down properly. To do this, click the "Start" icon, then click "Shut down Computer." The dialog box that appears allows the user to turn off the computer, restart it, stand by, or cancel the action. The restart function is helpful when the computer "freezes" or fails to function as it should. This takes the computer back through the booting sequence and often corrects problems and allows the user to continue working. Never attempt to fix problems on the computer that are beyond the medical assistant's scope of knowledge. Often a technical assistance desk can guide the user through various steps to correct basic issues. Always report computer malfunctions to the proper person or department.

Computer systems have user manuals which can usually be easily accessed and referenced online, and can usually be saved to the local computer system or the computer desktop. These manuals can be consulted when functions do not perform as they should or when a user is working with an unfamiliar system. Tutorials may be available to help the new user learn the system or to refresh the skills of the experienced user. Software programs have a *help* function, usually accessed on the tool bar. The help function allows the user to type in keywords to search for instructions on using certain features or to reference an index of help topics. The help function is written into the program, and users do not pay a fee for its use. However, most of the major software programs, such as Microsoft Office and Adobe Creative Suite, have entire books devoted to details about the use and capabilities of the software, and classes often are available.

▌ PROCESSING INFORMATION

A computer is a machine designed to accept, store, process, and provide information (Figure 8-2). Computers serve the following basic functions:

- *Input:* Input includes any information that enters the computer. It can take a variety of forms, from commands entered from the keyboard to data from another computer or device, such as a **scanner**. The device that feeds data into a computer, such as a mouse, scanner, keyboard, or voice recognition system, is called an *input device.*
- *Processing:* Processing is the act of manipulating the data that are currently inside the computer to carry out a certain task.
- *Output:* **Output** is anything that exits the computer. Output can appear in many forms, such as binary numbers, characters, pictures, printed pages, or a simple image on the computer screen. Output devices include monitors, speakers, printers, scanners, and modems.
- *Storage:* The act of retaining data or applications is called *storage.* Data can be stored on the hard drive, on CDs, or on separate drives, such as an external hard drive or a **flash drive** (two different types of storage devices). The type of storage device used depends on the amount of information that needs to be saved and where it needs to be used. CDs and flash drives are common portable storage devices used in the business world.

> **CRITICAL THINKING APPLICATION   8-1**
>
> - Dr. Bouchard plans to send two of his employees to a training class on using a new software program designed to perform all computer functions needed for his practice. Although he can send only two employees, how can the others learn the system?
> - Would it be beneficial or detrimental to close the office for a day to educate the other employees about the system? What should the physician consider before losing a day of patient visits?

▌ TYPES OF COMPUTERS

Various types of computers meet the needs of staff in today's medical office. The most common type is the desktop computer, which usually consists of a central processing unit (CPU), monitor, mouse, and keyboard. The laptop, **notebook**, **tablet**, and **personal digital assistant (PDA)** have grown in popularity because they are compact and portable (Figures 8-3 and 8-4). Some physicians and office employees carry the computer from room to room while treating patients. Information can be entered directly into the computer, which saves time and is much more efficient than handwritten or transcribed notes. The PDA and some tablets are small enough to carry in a pocket or purse. Physicians may use this device when treating patients or making hospital rounds, because it is lighter and even more convenient than a laptop. The PDA also organizes personal information, such as addresses and phone numbers, and most models allow the user to access the Internet and read e-mail. The PDA also can be used as a day planner to keep track of appointments, meetings, and other important events.

Embedded computers are computers inside another device, such as an ultrasound unit or electrocardiograph (ECG). These computers allow data input and output and usually analyze information.

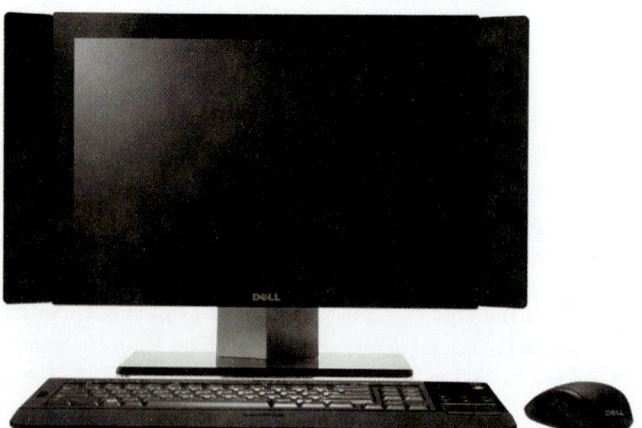

FIGURE 8-2 The keyboard and mouse are types of input devices that allow data to be entered into the computer, where they are processed. These are the main two types of input devices used with computer systems, although the evolution of technology continually provides faster, easier methods of getting data from outside the computer system to its internal processing system. (Courtesy Dell Corp., Round Rock, Texas.)

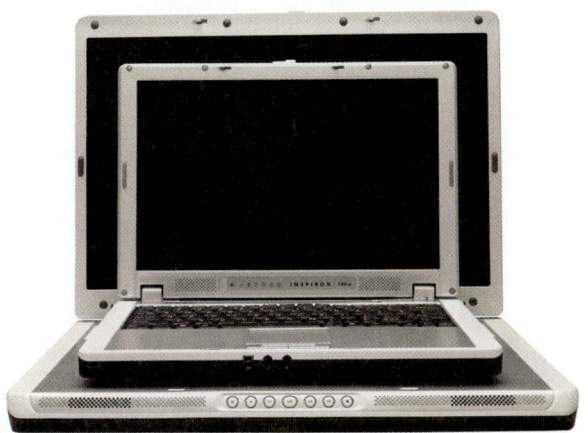

FIGURE 8-3 Laptop computers vary in size and weight and are easily portable. (Courtesy Dell Corp., Round Rock, Texas.)

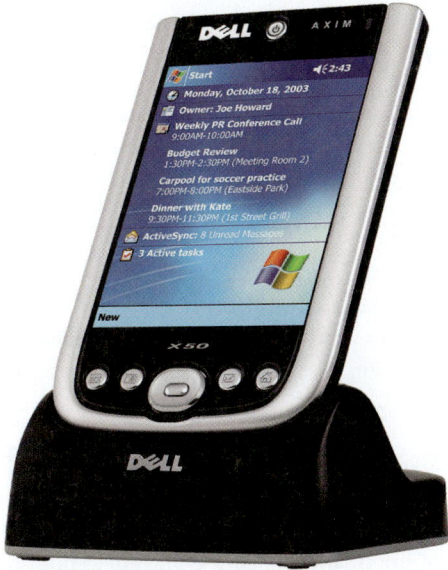

FIGURE 8-4 The personal digital assistant (PDA) is a handheld device that usually contains an address, a phone book, and a personal organizer and allows the user to access the Internet. (Courtesy Dell Corp., Round Rock, Texas.)

PARTS OF THE COMPUTER

A medical assistant must understand the function of the different parts of a computer. The physical pieces that can be touched and seen are called *hardware.* Computers using Windows software have an option in the control panel for adding hardware. This shortcut makes adding new equipment easy and provides instruction all along the way. Many types of software have an automatic setup that allows for installation and an uninstall feature; for example, Microsoft also has installation Wizard to assist in installation of programs. Hardware provides the medium on which software can be used. Most PCs have a microprocessor, monitor, keyboard, and mouse, and many are connected to a printer.

Microprocessor

The microprocessor is housed inside the casing of the main computer hardware. The microprocessor is the central unit of the computer; it contains the logic circuitry, which carries out the instructions of a computer's programs. It is considered the most important piece of hardware in a computer system. Microprocessors act as the brain of the computer and interpret instructions from a program. Microprocessors, sometimes called *CPUs,* are differentiated by three basic elements:

- *Bandwidth:* Bandwidth is the amount of information that can be sent over a connection at one time or how many **bits** can be processed in a single instruction. *Bits* (short for binary digits) are the smallest pieces of information on the computer. Eight bits make up 1 **byte.** A **kilobyte (KB)** is approximately 1,024 bytes, and a **megabyte (MB)** is approximately 1 million bytes. A **gigabyte (GB)** consists of approximately 1 billion bytes. A **terabyte (TB)** provides a huge amount of storage, consisting of approximately 1 trillion bytes.
- *Clock speed:* Clock speed determines how many instructions per second the processor can handle. Clock speed is measured in **megahertz (MHz)**. One megahertz equals 1 million cycles per second; therefore, a processor that operates at 300 MHz executes 300 million cycles per second.
- *Instruction set:* The instruction set is the set of instructions the microprocessor can execute.

The higher the bandwidth and clock speed, the faster and more powerful the microprocessor. For instance, a 32-bit microprocessor that runs at 50 MHz is more powerful than a 16-bit microprocessor that runs at 25 MHz.

A microprocessor contains memory consisting of electronic and magnetic cells, each of which contains information. The two kinds of memory are read-only memory (ROM) and random-access memory (RAM). ROM is internal memory, which contains a portion of the operating system and computer language; this is sometimes known as *main memory.* Data that have been "burned" onto a ROM chip cannot be removed and can only be read, similar to a CD-ROM, unless the CD is a "rewriteable" type. With this permanent memory, much less information has to be transferred from a disk to start the computing process. ROM cannot be overwritten and is not erased when the power is shut off. RAM can be thought of as an internal scratch pad for the computer. It contains the program instructions and the data currently processing. RAM normally is erased when the power is shut off.

> **CRITICAL THINKING** APPLICATION **8-2**
>
> A colleague of Dr. Bouchard has mentioned that he knows of a Web site with several computer programs that can be downloaded for free. Dr. Bouchard investigates the site and realizes that the software has been pirated. What concerns could this cause if he uses the software in his office? What would happen if any of this software were to malfunction?

Monitor

A monitor, which looks very much like a television screen, is a device used to display computer-generated information. Monitors can be adjusted for brightness, sharpness, and other settings of the user's choice. Many are high-definition monitors that rival the best plasma TV screens. Color monitors allow for a high-quality display, and the more advanced models have resolutions capable of reproducing high-quality pictures good enough for viewing a **digital video disk (DVD)**. The monitor provides the user with instant feedback on entries into the computer. Monitors sometimes are referred to as *displays*.

Keyboard

For most computers, the keyboard is the primary text input device. Keyboards have special function keys, such as the escape key, tab key, cursor movement keys, numeric keys, shift keys, and control keys. Additional function keys, numbered F1 to F12, are used to perform specific word processing or other computer-related operations. Used alone, a function key may create bold print, underline, indent, or call up a help screen. Used in conjunction with the Ctrl, Alt, or Shift key, the function keys can produce other effects, such as activating the printer, inserting the current date into a document, retrieving a file, or moving a designated block of text. Wireless keyboards are a popular alternative that allow the user to move around more freely while operating the computer. Wave keyboards, and others designed with ergonomics in mind, also are popular.

Mouse

A wireless mouse allows the user to manipulate the cursor without a cord attached. The mouse is a pointing device with a ball on the bottom that is moved by rolling it on a flat tabletop or mouse pad. An optical mouse has a photosensor instead of the rolling ball device. Some computers, especially laptops, have a built-in device, called a *trackball,* that is moved with the finger or thumb and serves the same function as a mouse. Other computers have a touchpad or trackpoint that is manipulated to control the cursor. The cursor is a pointer or flat bar that appears on the monitor to show where the next character will appear (i.e., the insertion point). The mouse allows the user to navigate around the screen quickly and to click on links to access Web sites.

Printer

Printers are output devices. Documents on the monitor may be directed to a printer to produce a printout, or **hard copy**, of a document. Many printers are bidirectional, which means they print from both left to right and right to left. The type of printer used should depend on the job being performed.

Impact printers are inexpensive and produce a fair to moderate quality hard copy. They form letters or shapes that they are directed to print by arranging patterns of dots on the paper. They often operate faster than letter-quality or color machines, but the print lacks the clarity generally desired for a truly professional look. These printers are often used in laboratories and larger departments in healthcare facilities that run lengthy reports or produce output that does not need a pristine appearance.

Inkjet printers use an ink cartridge that feeds an array of nearly microscopic tubes, each of which has a heating element that is energized during the printing process. The ink cartridge may be black or color. Inkjet printers cost less than laser printers, but the ink cartridges they use are fairly expensive and increase the operating cost.

Laser printers use xerographic technology similar to that in photocopiers; therefore, a laser printer can produce an almost limitless variety of forms and sizes as well as complex graphics. One disadvantage of inkjet and laser printers is that they cannot produce multiple copies with carbon sets or multicopy forms, which often are used by insurance companies for their filing forms.

Some printers today are multifunctional, serving as printers, fax machines, scanners, and copiers. Although these are excellent for home offices, they may not be the best investment for offices that use these machines often during the day. Many larger offices have networked printers that allow users to send jobs to a specific printer from any point within the network.

INSIDE THE COMPUTER

A basic knowledge of the parts of a computer and their function can help a medical assistant deal with minor technical issues and more easily communicate with technical support personnel.

Motherboard

A motherboard is the main circuit board for the computer, to which other devices can be attached. Usually it contains the processor, the memory, and other controllers and devices that allow the system to operate and function.

Disk Drives

Today's computers have various **disk drives** on which information can be stored or accessed. The hard disk or hard drive is a magnetic disk inside the computer that holds approximately 10 MB to 400 to 500 GB of information (Figure 8-5). Application software normally is saved to the hard disk and stored there on the computer for use when needed. This is commonly called the *C drive.*

CDs normally are used in the computer's A drive, although the drives can have different names or labels, depending on the brand of computer. Flash drives make transporting information from one computer to another quick and easy.

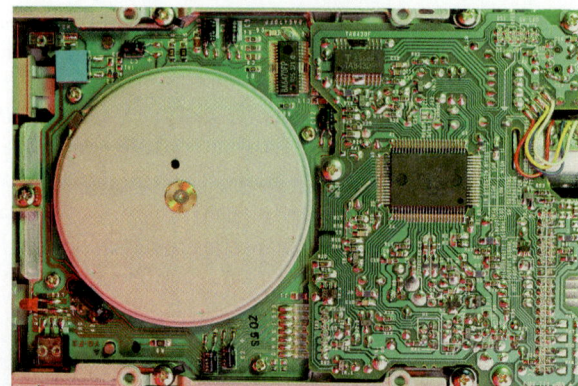

FIGURE 8-5 Hard drives store data and applications for fast, effective access and retrieval. Although a program installed on a hard drive can be removed, most are intended for permanent use, such as Microsoft Office or Peachtree Accounting.

CRITICAL THINKING APPLICATION 8-4

Dr. Bouchard mentions that he noticed CD-R disks on sale over the weekend. The price was $30 for 100 CD-Rs. One of the medical assistants noticed a 30-pack of CD-Rs for $7.99. Which is the better buy?

CD-ROM

Most of today's PCs are equipped with CD-ROM drives, which allow the storage of data on a CD. CDs hold much more information than their predecessors, floppy disks. A single CD can store the equivalent of about 300,000 text pages. A CD-RW is one on which data can be written, erased, and rewritten. Computers with a **CD burner**, or CD-R drive, can take information from one CD or another source and write it to a second CD. The computer must also have software that enables the burner to work. Software installed on a computer to allow a hardware device to function is called a **device driver**. Unlike most other storage media, CDs can easily be mailed in a flat envelope.

Software

Software comprises the programs and utilities loaded onto or inside a computer that carry out the work performed by the machine. The two types of software are system software and application software.

System software serves as the operating system of the computer and allows it to run and carry out the functions the computer performs. For instance, Windows XP is a type of operating system software. **Application software** refers to the programs loaded onto the computer that carry out the work for the actual users of the computer. Examples of application software are Microsoft Office, MediSoft, and Medical Manager. Applications (programs) are designed to perform specific tasks, such as word processing, billing, accounting, appointment setting, insurance form preparation, payroll, and database management. Many software applications are available for complete medical practice management (Procedure 8-1).

Modems

A **modem**, short for *modulator-demodulator,* is a device over which data can be transmitted via telephone lines and other media, such as a coaxial cable. Modems can be internal or external. An internal modem is built into or added to the inside of the computer casing. A cable modem operates over cable TV lines and uses the coaxial cable to provide faster Internet access. **Digital subscriber line (DSL)** modems operate over phone lines, as do normal modems, but they use a different frequency; as a result, the telephone can be used while the computer is accessing the Internet. Often a filter is attached to the phone that removes other frequencies in which the DSL is working; this prevents interference with the telephone line operation.

PROCEDURE 8-1

Use Office Hardware and Software to Maintain Office Systems

GOAL: *To use the office computer system to maintain the hardware and software systems used in the physician's office.*

EQUIPMENT and SUPPLIES

- Computer system
- Computer software applications
- Software manuals
- Description of office systems
- Hardware user manuals
- Patient data
- Business data

PROCEDURAL STEPS

1. Determine the types of data the physician's office needs to computerize.
   PURPOSE: To effectively plan the needs of the physician's office.
2. List these data in a Word document.
3. Research each type of data and determine how often it should be backed up to maintain accuracy and follow regulations.
   PURPOSE: To make certain that the office is in compliance with all rules and regulations regarding the data produced in the medical office.
4. Research computer systems and software that can handle the tasks that need to be completed daily in the physician's office.

5. Determine a schedule for maintaining the hardware of the computer system.
   PURPOSE: To comply with manufacturers' recommendations for hardware maintenance.
6. Determine a reasonable backup schedule for the data contained on the office computer system.
   PURPOSE: To plan a workable time period in which data should be backed up.
7. Develop a spreadsheet that includes a timeline for hardware and software maintenance in the physician's office.
8. Discuss the spreadsheet and the choices with the instructor, including any changes that might be indicated.
   PURPOSE: To receive input on the spreadsheet and suggestions for changes, if indicated.
9. Revise the spreadsheet if necessary.
10. Submit the spreadsheet to the instructor.

Speakers and Microphones

Some computers have external speakers to provide a higher quality sound from the computer. Many computers also have built-in speakers that provide a fair quality of sound. Microphones can be built in or attached so that the user can speak directly into the computer, even to someone on the other side of the world!

PERIPHERAL DEVICES

Peripheral devices are those that are not essential to the operation of the computer. For instance, the computer can operate without a modem, although a modem is necessary to access the Internet. Even a mouse is considered a peripheral device, because everything the mouse can access also can be reached by pressing certain buttons on the keyboard, although often multiple keys must be pressed at once. This section discusses some of the peripheral devices in use today.

Scanners

Scanners read text, illustrations, or photographs printed on paper and put them into a format the computer can understand. Photographs can be placed in the scanner, saved on the computer, and then used in a document. Some advanced scanners are used like highlighters and can collect notes from printed text.

Digital Cameras

Many digital cameras can be attached directly to a computer or printer, and photographs can be downloaded directly from the camera. Other cameras use a disk to load the pictures onto the computer.

> **CRITICAL THINKING APPLICATION   8-5**
>
> How might a digital camera be of use to a physician in the medical practice? What care should be taken when the camera is used with a patient?

Flash Drives

Individuals who use numerous computers in different places find the flash drive to be a convenient way to transfer files. The flash drive (also known as a *thumb drive* or *jump drive*) allows the user to save files from the originating computer to the drive so that only the drive is transported to the second computer (Figure 8-6). To use the device, after a document is completed, use the "Save As" function and find the flash drive in the "My Computer" location. After the file has been saved to the flash drive, it can be removed from the computer. Flash drives can be carried in a pocket or purse and have a cap that should be left on to protect the USB mechanism. Flash drives commonly have a storage capacity of 2 to 4 GB and can be purchased with a capacity of 64 GB or more.

External Hard Drives

An external hard drive is a disk drive with a very high storage capacity that is attached externally to a computer. These drives are used as a **backup** device for important data. The first external hard drives

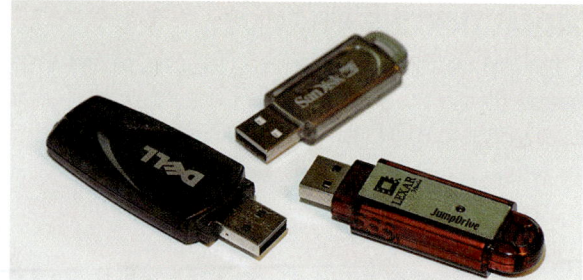

FIGURE 8-6 A flash drive (also called a *thumb* or *jump drive*) allows the user to store documents for use on a different computer.

were called Zip drives, which held 100 to 250 MB of data. Today's internal hard drives can hold 400 to 500 GB, whereas high-end external hard drives commonly hold 500 GB. Some are sold with two drives in one unit, which have a capacity of a terabyte or more. These drives can even be stored somewhere other than the facility so that they are safe in case of fire or some other destructive event. Some external hard drives can be set up to back up the main hard drives at a specific date and time.

ADDING A PROGRAM TO A COMPUTER

Adding or loading a program onto a computer is relatively easy. Most programs today come on a CD-ROM. The program usually includes instructions for loading it onto the computer. Watch the monitor for steps to complete and information about the user's preferences, then follow all the directions.

In a Windows environment, the Control Panel provides an option to "Add/Remove Programs." Once clicked, this allows the program in the CD disk drive to be loaded onto the computer. At several points the computer may ask the user questions about his or her preferences for the program. Often the computer needs to be restarted after installation.

To remove a program from the computer, access the "Add/Remove Programs" icon and follow the directions for removing the program. This may be the only way to remove the program completely from the computer system.

FILE FORMATS

A file is a collection of data. Computers use many types of files. A text file, for example, contains some type of text, which is the main body of printed words or written matter on a page. Often an extension is used at the end of the filename to designate the type of file. A few of the common file extensions include the following:

- *jpg:* JPG (or JPEG) stands for "joint photographic experts group"; this format often is used for photographs.
- *gif:* GIF stands for "graphics interchange format," which supports color and often is used for scanned images and illustrations rather than photographs.
- *doc:* The extension .doc usually indicates a file created by a word processor or word processing software; *doc* stands for document.
- *txt:* A text file usually has the extension .txt.
- *rtf:* RTF stands for "rich text format."

- *bmp:* Bit-mapped graphics are indicated by the extension .bmp. These are compiled by a graphics image set in rows or columns of dots.

A medical assistant familiar with these types of files can save and open them correctly and use the computer to the fullest advantage in the medical office.

COMPUTER NETWORKING

A network is a group of two or more computer systems that are linked together. Several types of networks exist:

- *LAN:* A *local area network,* or a computer network spanning a relatively small area. Most LANs are contained in a single building or group of buildings and are connected by a **router**, but LANs can be connected to other LANs even at a distance. A **hub** is a device that connects several computers or networks, and a **switch** is designed to help the LAN run more efficiently by controlling local network traffic.
- *MAN:* A *metropolitan area network.* A MAN spans an area that does not exceed a metropolitan area or city and connects several LANs.
- *WAN:* A *wide area network,* which spans a relatively large geographic area. Typically, a WAN consists of two or more LANs or MANs. These networks can be connected through public networks, such as a telephone system, or through leased lines or satellites. The largest WAN is the Internet.
- *HAN:* A *home area network,* which connects computers inside a user's home.
- *CAN:* A *campus area network,* often used on college campuses and sometimes on military bases.

A computer network enables resource and information sharing. A group of computers may be liked to one printer, and print jobs are completed as they are requested by users, one at a time. Computers may also be linked by a network to an insurance company database, so that insurance claims can be transmitted electronically. A group of businesses operating in different locations may also share a network. All networks are designed to make computer systems more efficient.

SERVERS

A **server** is important to the network, because it is the computer that manages the shared network resources. Several types of servers exist. When many computers are connected to one printer, often a print server manages these printers. File servers are used for file storage, and database servers are used to process database **queries**.

THE INTERNET

The Internet is a global network that connects millions of computers. This fascinating structure has made the world a smaller place. Through chat programs one can talk with individuals literally on the other side of the world and be introduced to cultures that 20 years ago would never have been understood. Through Web pages, we can visit different parts of the world and learn and see many things that previously were impossible for the average person to experience. **E-commerce** allows us to shop on the Internet, from the most

exclusive stores in Beverly Hills to the corner grocer. The Internet has changed the way we learn, do business, communicate, and entertain ourselves.

Each computer connected to the Internet is called a *host* and is independent of all the others. The users of each computer determine which services to make available to other users on the Internet. Often a company or organization also has an Intranet, which is a local network that uses Internet technology within a company or single location but does not have access to the Internet directly.

Internet service providers (ISPs) are companies that provide access to the Internet (e.g., AT&T, America Online, Verizon, Earthlink, Yahoo, and scores of others). ISPs issue each user an IP address, which is a unique identifier for that user's particular computer on a transmission control protocol/Internet protocol (**TCP/IP**) network. An IP address is a 32-bit number written as four numbers separated by a period. Each number can be zero to 255; therefore a valid IP address could be 10.145.32.254. Messages are defined and transmitted over the Internet when a uniform resource locator (**URL**) is entered into the browser and a hypertext transfer protocol (**HTTP**) command tells the Web server to retrieve the requested Web page (Box 8-1).

A **domain name** identifies an IP address, such as microsoft.com or ama-assn.org. A limited number of top-level domains are available

---

BOX 8-1 READING A WEB SITE URL ADDRESS

URL is an acronym for *uniform resource locator.* A URL specifies the global address of documents or information on the Internet. An example of a URL is: http://www.hhs.gov/policies/index.html

Using this example, the information in the Web site address can be broken down as follows:

http://www.hhs.gov/

http:

Hypertext Transfer Protocol: This allows the user to access a server that stores Web pages.

ftp:

File Transfer Protocol: This allows the user to access a section of a Web site onto which files and documents can be uploaded.

mailto:

Mailto: This initiates an outgoing message to the e-mail address that follows

http://www.hhs.gov/policies/index.html

This section of the URL defines the Web address and is the part that is usually typed into the address bar to reach the Web site.

http://www.hhs.gov/**policies/**index.html

This section of the URL is the pathname, containing directory/subdirectory names, indicating where information can be found on a server's hard drive.

http://www.hhs.gov/policies/**index.html**

This section represents the filename (index) and the format, or extension (.html); it indicates what the Web browser is to do with the downloaded file. Other examples of filename extensions include .htm, .exe, .jpg, and .gif.

to which a domain name can be attached. Some of these top-level domains are *.com* (familiarly called *dot-com*) for commercial businesses; *.org* for organizations, usually nonprofit; *.edu* for educational institutions; *.gov* for government agencies; and *.net* for network organizations. Others include *.biz, .info, .tv, .name,* and *.pro.* The IP address can also be used to locate information on a computer; for instance, if the IP address reads as follows: *www.smithclinic.com/documents/mailings/patient_address_list/* then the list used for sending mailings to patients can be found in the Documents section in a file named Mailings, and the document is named patient_address_list.

Most Internet sites use a language called *hypertext markup language* (**HTML**), which was one of the first and is still one of the most popular languages used to create Web pages.

Hotspots are locations that offer an access point, providing public wireless broadband network services. They are found in places such as airports, libraries, convention centers, and hotels. Users may be able to connect to the network for no charge or may be required to place a credit card number on file or make a deposit. This service is convenient for the medical professional who is traveling or attending events away from the office.

Many physicians and health organizations offer a Web site with information about their services. In today's data-driven society, this is an excellent way to educate the public about the services the organization offers and to provide all types of information to the audience the organization wants to reach. To obtain a domain name, the desired name must be available, and one must pay a small fee to have the name registered and added to a central database. Companies such as register.com or verisign.com offer domain name registration services.

A word of caution: Because most medical offices have some type of connection to the Internet, the medical assistant may be tempted to check personal e-mail, "surf" the Web, or participate in instant messaging during working hours. Remember, personal business should not be conducted while at work. Supervisors appreciate the medical assistant who is honest with his or her time and spends it in productive, work-related activities.

BROWSERS

Web **browsers** are software applications that allow the user to locate and display Web pages. Two commonly used browsers are Microsoft Internet Explorer and Mozilla Firefox. These browsers can display graphics and text and can also present **multimedia** information, the quality of which depends on the computer system in use and the Internet connection speed. Browsers also have a **bookmark** capability that allows the user to mark a certain Web page and then easily return to it by clicking on its link in a drop-down box in the browser's menu. The **cache** allows quick retrieval of previously viewed sites, because the computer remembers and saves the information on the hard drive. **Cookies** are stored information about individual users, such as screen names and passwords.

Browsers and other Web sites also have **search engines**. These are programs in which a topic, word, or group of words can be entered, and the program searches the Internet for matches. A listing of those matches appears, and the user can click on each match to reference information and perform research. Information on just about any subject can be found by using search engines.

CRITICAL THINKING APPLICATION   8-6

Dr. Bouchard wants all employees to have Internet access at his office, but he is concerned about occasional misuse. He does not want the staff to use the computer for personal business, but he does not mind if they check their personal e-mail on a break or at lunch.

- What are some reasonable policies for office Internet use?
- How would an office manager develop a fair policy on personal computer use at the office? Does the employee have a right to be able to access the Internet at work?
- Because much of today's business involves the Internet, how does an employee balance Internet use at work?

USING A PHONE TO PERFORM COMPUTER FUNCTIONS

Most of today's cell phones have Web browsing capabilities. The costs depend on what services are ordered. Smart phones offer advanced capabilities, often with PC-like functionality. Some mobile phones and most smart phones allow the user to read and edit business documents in a variety of formats, such as .doc and .pdf. PDAs are handheld computers and can have the same capabilities as a mobile phone or smart phone. Even the telephony industry has difficulty defining the differences among these three items, but in general, they differ in how they are built and what they can do. A physician can see magnetic resonance imaging (MRI) reports on some devices, which eliminates the need to sit at a computer to make medical decisions, allowing the physician more mobility. The medical assistant can expect to see these devices become almost standard in the future.

THE COMPUTER AS A CO-WORKER

The computer is a valuable tool in the medical office. It can assist in filing insurance claims by sending information from the computer in the office to the computers at the insurance company via a modem. Electronic processing of insurance claims not only saves time but also provides immediate information as to whether a claim will be accepted. Errors in coding or procedure are immediately evident, and many rejections can be avoided even before the claim is transmitted. Most insurance companies require that providers file claims electronically.

A patient's demographics can appear on computerized patient ledgers, listing the name, address, telephone number, and insurance information. As services are rendered, charges are entered into the computer, and payments also are displayed. This helps the medical facility maintain an accurate balance of all patient accounts.

At the appropriate time each month, the computer can print a patient's billing statement, which shows a detail of charges, payments, adjustments, and the current balance. In addition, the computer can be programmed to age the accounts according to any criteria selected and to include this information on the billing statement. A series of collection letters can be developed and personalized for individual patients as they are needed.

Database software makes it possible to organize a large volume of information, which can be used in a number of ways. One of the most practical uses is the organization of identifying information on each patient. The computer also can store clinical information about patients using much less space and with greater security than papers in a patient's chart. Access to records can be limited with passwords.

The computer has virtually replaced the appointment book in many medical offices today. Software for setting appointments ranges from relatively simple programs to very sophisticated systems. An advantage of computer scheduling is that more than one person can access the system at one time, and the same information is available to all users.

Computers are even being used as marketing tools and virtual secretaries in some modern medical offices (Figure 8-7). Computers can be used for functions such as automatic routing to call all patients with appointments for the next day and remind them to visit the doctor, or perhaps to call all patients due for a 6-month eye or dental examination. The program often gives the patient the opportunity to cancel and reschedule before the 24-hour cutoff time. As a marketing tool, computers can be programmed to call all phone numbers in a certain area code with a prerecorded message about a new procedure available at the office or a new physician in the area. Although many individuals are annoyed by the telemarketing concept and being called by a computer, the success rate is good. Computers can call thousands upon thousands of phone numbers, relay a message, and track replies within a matter of hours. Even if only a handful of new patients are obtained, over the life of the patients, the doctor may see a strong profit. Remember, the physician's office is a business, and businesses need to make a profit to survive. This number of calls could never be accomplished in the same time period by humans. These methods of using the computer open all kinds of doors for the medical practice of the future.

The medical office should routinely perform a file backup to make sure valuable data can be retrieved in the event of a system failure. Many medical office computer programs have an automatic backup function, but some must be backed up manually. It is wise to keep backup copies of the database and other critical documents off the premises in case of fire or other tragedy.

COMPUTER SECURITY

Patients are entitled to the utmost confidentiality with respect to their medical records and the release of any information of a personal nature. Computer technology allows the accumulation and storage of a vast amount of data that may be accessible to a variety of individuals, making it imperative that guidelines be set up for the protection of such data.

Encryption is the translation of data into a code that is not readily understood by most users. It is one effective way to achieve data security. To access or read an encrypted file, the user must have a password that enables the code to be decrypted. Once the code has been decrypted, the file can be used by the application. Encrypted data are called *cipher text.*

Some individuals attempt to access information in a computer without the owner's consent. These people may intend to use the information just for fun or may have a malicious intent, such as to steal or corrupt the data. Although these people are commonly called *hackers,* computer enthusiasts insist that the correct term for individuals who break into computers with dishonorable intent is *crackers.* The term *hacker* originally simply described a person who enjoyed learning about using computers and becoming proficient in their use.

Various methods may be used to protect networks, computers, and data from unauthorized access. Firewalls are systems designed for just such a purpose and can be integrated into both the hardware and the software of the computer. Firewalls often are used to prevent individuals from accessing private networks. Each message sent and received is examined, and the firewall blocks those that do not meet specific security criteria. Passwords, frequent password changes, and user logs also help protect data and the integrity of the database.

Viruses are programs or pieces of code that are loaded onto a computer, usually without the owner's knowledge, and can act like a physical virus in that they can make the computer "sick." Viruses can replicate themselves, copying themselves over and over again, and can be passed to other computers through e-mails, usually without the sender's knowing that a virus was passed along. Even simple viruses can quickly use all available memory and bring the system to a standstill; some can completely corrupt the computer's hard drive. More dangerous types of viruses can transmit over networks, bypassing security systems and destroying valuable data. This is why antivirus software is an important part of any computer system. Check for updates to the antivirus program at least weekly.

HIPAA REGULATIONS AND COMPUTERS

The Health Insurance Portability and Accountability Act (HIPAA) was passed in part to ensure that patient health information would be kept private and confidential. The wide use of computers in healthcare facilities sometimes makes this a difficult goal. The law limits who can look at and/or receive a patient's health information. Health information may be used and shared as follows:

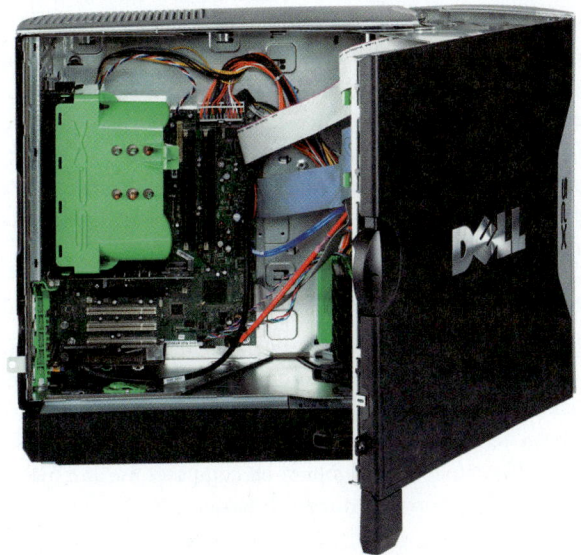

FIGURE 8-7 Inside a computer. Today's microprocessors are designed so that memory, additional drives, and other hardware can easily be added to the system. (Courtesy Dell Corp., Round Rock, Texas.)

- For patient care and treatment coordination
- To pay physicians and facilities for healthcare
- With family, friends, and relatives whom the patient has identified as being involved in the patient's healthcare
- To make sure good care is provided in clean facilities
- To protect public health
- To make required reports to law enforcement officials

Health information cannot be shared or used without the patient's permission in most cases. Specifically, the provider cannot:

- Give health information to a patient's employer
- Use or share health information for marketing purposes
- Share mental health information obtained in counseling sessions

The healthcare facility must train those who use computer systems in what information can and cannot be shared. Individual computer users should have their own log-in names and passwords that are not provided to anyone else. All users should be required to use the log-in name and password every time they use the computer system. Patient information must not be accessed unless the user needs to know the contents of the patient's file to provide care. Be careful when releasing any type of medical information to anyone. Questions should be directed to the office manager or physician. Additional information about HIPAA can be found in Chapter 17.

ELECTRONIC SIGNATURES

Electronic signature programs are offered both as stand-alone products and as part of computerized medical record systems. After a report has been reviewed for accuracy, a physician can use a password and personal identification number (PIN) to electronically "sign" the document by clicking on an icon. Once the document has been signed, it cannot be altered; only additions are allowed.

COMPUTERS AND ERGONOMICS

The increased use of computers in the workplace has underscored the need to choose comfortable, safe furniture and equipment. Repetitive strain injury (RSI) accounts for most work-related injury claims. This includes a number of conditions caused by repeatedly straining certain nerves, muscles, or tendons. Carpal tunnel syndrome is an example of an RSI.

To prevent such injuries, office staff should use posture chairs that support the lumbar section of the back, with a correct angle of the knee and the feet resting on the floor. Of the many designs for keyboards available, one should be chosen that allows the correct angle at the elbow and the wrist to be held in a neutral position. Learn where all of the keys are located, because the last computer in use may have had a different key placement. Practicing keyboard skills and typing speed are the best way to learn key location. If work stations are shared, know how to adjust the components so that they are in the best position each day.

Eyestrain is another danger arising from continuous use of a computer. The monitor should be just below eye level and an arm's length away. At least once an hour, the user should take a break from looking at the monitor. (Ergonomics is discussed in more detail in Chapter 12 and on the Evolve Web site.)

CLOSING COMMENTS

Computers should be considered additional workers in the office. A medical assistant who learns how best to use the computer and discovers as many of its capabilities as possible is a valuable employee.

Read the manuals that accompany equipment and programs and try new applications for old procedures. Computers are designed to save time, so look for ways to make the day's workload lighter by taking full advantage of the computer.

The future promises more rapid technologic advances; computer equipment can become archaic in as short a time as 6 months after purchase. **Artificial intelligence**, voice recognition, **virtual reality**, and retinal scanning, seen mostly in the movies, will become commonplace in our homes and businesses. These tools will make the work environment even faster and more efficient as the world becomes a smaller place.

The evolution of computers will continue to bring about changes in medical facilities of the future. Medical staffs will find themselves educating their patients about computer use, because numerous programs in development will allow patients to "check in" once they arrive at the office and verify their identity. A medical assistant will need patience to teach these procedures and assure the patients that these new methods will increase their security and the protection of their medical records.

Patient Education

Patients commonly enter the physician's office having researched their symptoms and illnesses on the Internet. This practice is an indication that the patient is interested in health matters and in being part of the process of maintaining their health. No patient should substitute their regular physician for information obtained on the Internet. The medical assistant can encourage patients who are interested in learning about their condition but should remind them to discuss any concerns and questions with the physician.

With the growing number of medical databases online, physicians now can use information on the Internet to help educate their patients about the illnesses they face right from the exam room. While consulting with the patient, with a few clicks of the mouse the physician can print excellent information, which often can assist the patient with referrals to help agencies and suggestions for better healthcare.

Legal and Ethical Issues

The medical assistant should use the computer at work for business purposes only. Never allow it to become a distraction from doing the job at hand. Many medical assistants and other office personnel have been terminated for using the office computer for personal reasons. Always follow office policy on computer use and make sure patients are the priority during office hours.

SUMMARY OF SCENARIO

Dr. Bouchard is a progressive physician who believes that the use of technology will assist him in the care of his patients and help his office run more efficiently. The computer helps the staff complete tasks in a timely manner and provides records of business transactions. Staff members are able to function much faster than when records were kept by hand. Dr. Bouchard understands the need to train his staff and to keep them up-to-date on the latest versions of their computer software. His willingness to close his office for staff-wide training demonstrates his commitment. He is cost conscious and looks for the best available equipment for the investment he is willing to make.

Dr. Bouchard often uses digital camera equipment to take "before" and "after" pictures of his patients, but only with their special written consent. He also uses the computer to send his patients a monthly e-mail newsletter with health information and special news about the practice.

He monitors his staff's Internet use but is reasonable about allowing them a small degree of personal access on breaks and at lunch. The doctor cautions his staff about accessing medical records that they are not actively involved with in patient care to avoid invading the patient's privacy. The computer system prints a daily log of all employees and what information they accessed throughout the day, and he stresses the importance of logging on and off the computer using their individual passwords and log-on IDs. Dr. Bouchard's employees realize the importance of keeping medical information private. Unless a staff member needs to know the information in the chart to care for the patient, he or she may be accused of invading the patient's privacy when accessing medical information.

Dr. Bouchard is very interested in new developments for healthcare facilities, such as those that will allow his patients to check themselves in and gain access to limited information about their own medical record. He has a vision that one day his patients will be able to download their statements or perhaps their child's immunization records from their home computers, reducing the staff's workload and providing instant access to some information for his patients. Insightful physicians such as Dr. Bouchard see the computer as a co-worker in the medical facility.

SUMMARY OF LEARNING OBJECTIVES

1. **Define, spell, and pronounce the terms listed in the vocabulary.**
   Spelling and pronouncing medical terms correctly bolster the medical assistant's credibility. Knowing the definition of these terms promotes confidence in communication with patients and co-workers.

2. **List several ways the computer can be effective in a medical office.**
   The computer performs repetitive tasks, reduces errors, speeds up production, recalls information on command, saves time, reduces paperwork, and allows for more creative and productive use of staff members' time.

3. **Explain the basic functions a computer performs.**
   The computer performs four basic functions: input, processing, output, and storage. *Input* includes information that is put into the computer, and *output* is information that comes out of the computer. *Processing* is the manipulation of data that occurs between input and output. *Storage* is the retention of data in the computer or on storage media.

4. **Explain the basic parts of a computer.**
   The *microprocessor* is the brains of the system that interprets the instructions given to it by an application program. The *monitor* allows the user to see immediate output on a screen, and *printers* allow the output to be produced as a hard copy. The *keyboard* and *mouse* are input devices.

5. **List the three elements that differentiate microprocessors.**
   (1) The *bandwidth* describes the amount of information that can be sent over a connection at one time; (2) the *clock speed* determines the number of instructions per second the processor can handle; (3) the *instruction set* is the instructions the microprocessor can execute.

6. **Discuss the differences among various types of printers.**
   Three main types of printers are used in medical offices. *Impact* printers produce output of moderate quality and are inexpensive. *Inkjet* printers use a cartridge and a heating element to produce an image on a page. *Laser* printers use technology similar to a photocopier.

7. **Explain the importance of a motherboard.**
   The motherboard is the main board to which all other devices are connected inside the computer. It holds all the essential wiring and expansion devices needed to operate the computer and the battery that keeps the clock and calendar running when the computer is turned off.

8. **Explain and give examples of peripheral devices.**
   Peripheral devices (e.g., scanners, Zip drives) perform special functions but are not necessary to the computer's functioning.

9. **List and discuss several types of file formats.**
   The *file format* is the extension just after the file name that describes the method used to save the file. It also helps identify the type of file. For example, a *.jpeg* file often is used for photographs, a *.gif* file is used for scanned illustrations or images, and a *.txt* file is usually specifically for text for a printed page.

10. **Explain the concept of computer networking.**
    Computer networks are groups of two or more computers linked together. These networks can be local or can cover a city or wide geographic area. Some are limited to a few buildings. Networks often share resources, such as printers.

11. **Define the function of browsers.**

Browsers are software applications that allow a user to find information on the Internet. They can show graphics and often multimedia (e.g., videos). Internet Explorer and Netscape Navigator are commonly used browsers.

12. **Discuss the importance of computer security.**

Computer security is critical, especially because confidential patient information is stored on computers in medical facilities. Several methods may be used to enhance computer security, such as firewalls and antivirus programs. Restrictions on who may log in and the use of passwords also help the facility ensure that only authorized individuals have access to confidential information.

13. **Locate the keys on a keyboard.**

Examine the keyboard used in the educational or medical facility and determine the location of the keys. The medical assistant may need to adjust to different keyboard types at various work stations.

CONNECTIONS

📖 **Study Guide Connection:** Go to the Chapter 8 Study Guide. Read and complete the activities.

℮ **Evolve Connection:** Go to the Chapter 8 link at *evolve.elsevier.com/kinn* to complete the Chapter Review and Chapter Quiz. Check out the other resources listed for this chapter to make the most of what you have learned from Computer Concepts.

TELEPHONE TECHNIQUES

9

SCENARIO

Ashlynn McDowell, a recent graduate of a medical assisting program, has begun her first position as a receptionist in an obstetrician's office. Ashlynn's lifelong goal has been to work in obstetrics, and she is determined to perform to the best of her abilities. However, she has never held a job in a professional office. She knows that she needs to practice all the skills she learned in school to be an effective receptionist.

Ashlynn works for Dr. Stella Frank, who is customer-service oriented and wants her patients to feel cared for and special. She insists that all their concerns be taken seriously. Ashlynn is anxious to build trust with the patients and offer them help with the problems they encounter that fall into her realm of responsibility.

Dr. Frank recently purchased computer software that allows Ashlynn to record phone messages on the computer, and these messages are automatically routed both to an inbox for the physician and as an entry in the patient's medical record.

Although the system is new to everyone in the office, Ashlynn is determined to become proficient at its use as quickly as possible.

She knows that she must speak clearly and distinctly and must be adept at follow-up skills. She plans to dress professionally each day so that she projects the right image to the patients with whom she comes in contact. Ashlynn will strive to be the type of employee who has a willingness to learn, an ability to adapt, and a heart full of compassion for the patient. She is a team player who sincerely wants to cooperate with other staff members who might need her help.

Dr. Frank is pleased that she has found such an eager person to add to her staff and will assist and guide Ashlynn as she learns how to make the patients feel like a part of the clinic family. Ashlynn's self-esteem has increased because she feels she is making a great contribution to healthcare.

While studying this chapter, think about the following questions:

- How can Ashlynn's telephone demeanor convince patients she wants to help them?
- Why does the tone of voice play an important role in patient perception?
- How does the medical assistant speaking to patients on the telephone strike a balance between too much and too little time?
- How can the medical assistant reduce patients' frustration with telephone issues?

LEARNING OBJECTIVES

1. Define, spell, and pronounce the terms listed in the vocabulary.
2. Determine and discuss the source of incoming and outgoing calls to a physician's office.
3. Describe how to develop a pleasing telephone voice.
4. Demonstrate the correct way to hold a telephone handset.
5. Explain why courtesy is so important when speaking on the telephone.
6. Demonstrate the correct way to answer the telephone in the office.
7. Discuss different ways to handle callers who want to speak to the physician.
8. List the seven elements of a correctly handled telephone message.
9. Demonstrate the correct way to record a message accurately and take a request for action.
10. Demonstrate the most efficient way to call in a prescription or a prescription refill to a pharmacy.
11. Discuss how the medical assistant should handle callers who have a complaint.
12. Explain how angry callers might be handled.
13. List several questions to ask when handling an emergency call.
14. Discuss several useful sections of the introductory pages of the phone directory.

VOCABULARY

clarity The quality or state of being clear.

competent Having adequate abilities or qualities; having the capacity to function or perform in a certain way.

cultivate To foster the growth of; to improve by labor, care, or study.

diction The choice of words, especially with regard to clearness, correctness, or effectiveness.

enunciation (e-nun-se-a′-shun) The utterance of articulate, clear sounds.

inflection (in-flek′-shun) A change in the pitch or loudness of the voice.

invariably (in-var′-e-uh-buh-le) Consistently; not changing or capable of change.

jargon The technical terminology or characteristic idiom of a particular group or special activity, as opposed to lay terms.

monotone A succession of syllables, words, or sentences in an unvaried key or pitch.

multitasking Performing multiple tasks at the same time.

pitch The property of a sound, especially a musical tone, that is determined by the frequency of the waves producing it; the highness or lowness of sound.

provider An individual or company that provides medical care and services to a patient or the public.

salutation (sal-yu-ta′-shun) An expression of greeting, goodwill, or courtesy by words or gestures.

screen Something that shields, protects, or hides; to select or eliminate through a screening process.

STAT Medical abbreviation for immediately; at this moment.

tactful Having a keen sense of what to do or say to maintain good relations with others or to prevent offense.

tedious (te′-de-yus) Tiresome because of length or dullness.

The telephone is the lifeline of a medical practice and a powerful public relations tool. Most patients seen in a medical facility make the initial appointment by telephone. When used appropriately, the telephone can help build a medical practice from its beginning and throughout its life (Figure 9-1). If used inappropriately, it can destroy a flourishing practice. Always remember that the voice on the other end of the line is that of the patient, and telephone calls can never be considered an interruption of the workday. The patients are the reason the practice exists.

Most incoming calls are from the following sources:

- Established patients calling for appointments or to ask questions
- New patients making a first contact with the physician's office
- Patients and medical workers reporting treatment results or emergencies
- Other physicians making referrals or discussing a patient
- Laboratories reporting vital patient information
- Pharmacies and patients calling in to refill prescriptions

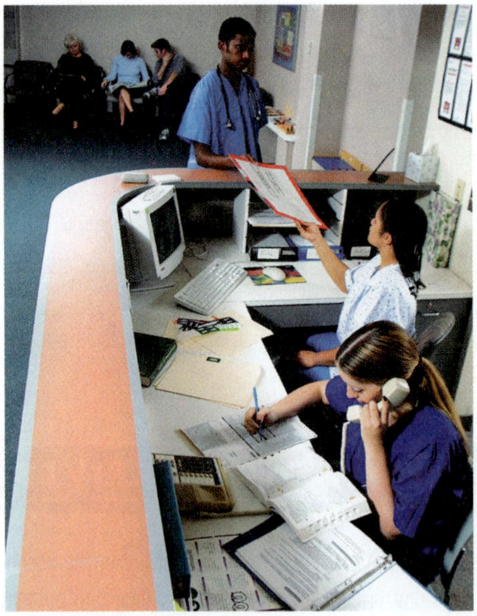

EFFECTIVE USE OF THE TELEPHONE

Active Listening

Although great emphasis is placed on rules for speaking, the importance of active listening often is overlooked. The same attention should be given to a telephone conversation that would be given to a face-to-face conversation (Box 9-1). Concentration is not always easy for a medical assistant who is juggling several duties at once in the medical office; therefore, he or she must practice focusing on the call at hand. Effective active listening also provides vital information about the nature of the call—whether the caller is distressed, agitated, or has a concern that must be addressed immediately. Review listening skills in Chapter 5.

FIGURE 9-1 The telephone plays a vital role in the success of a medical practice.

Developing a Pleasing Telephone Voice

Individuals who call a physician's office should be greeted by a pleasant, friendly voice. A common sales technique is to make sure the caller "hears a smile." Customer service is critical in today's medical offices, and this technique is quite useful for medical assistants, because they are likely to be the caller's first point of contact with the practice. Be sure to enunciate clearly, pronouncing each word separately and distinctly. **Diction**, **pitch**, and **clarity** also are important. Avoid speaking in a **monotone**; instead, use **inflection**, or a change in the pitch and loudness of the voice. This helps the speaker emphasize certain points during the conversation.

When a telephone call is received from a stranger, one usually tries to visualize that person's appearance and perhaps forms an opinion of the individual's personality. The caller may sound mature, somewhat

BOX 9-1   HOW TO LISTEN

- Quiet the mind to absorb what the speaker is saying.
- Focus on the conversation.
- Look at the speaker's eyes.
- Don't interrupt.
- Allow the speaker to express the complete thought.
- Repeat your interpretation of what has been said, using the speaker's words when possible.
- Ask whether the interpretation is correct.
- Respond to the speaker.
- Don't look at a watch or clock or answer a cell phone when listening.
- Remain on the speaker's subject.
- Respect differing opinions.
- Be empathetic.

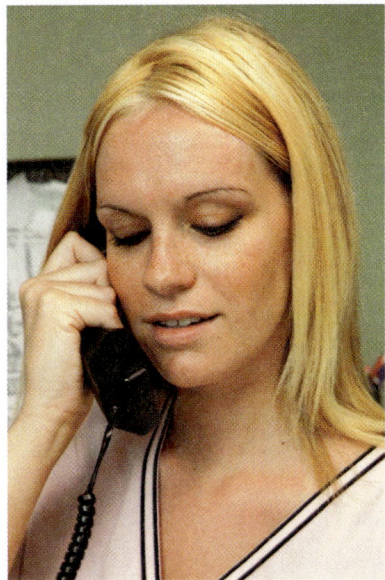

FIGURE 9-2 The handset should be held in the center, with the mouthpiece approximately 1 inch in front of the lips.

worried, well educated, or frantic. Because communication is a two-way street, the caller also forms an impression of the person answering the phone. Sometimes these impressions are incorrect, but much can be inferred from what is heard on the telephone.

The tone of voice used by the medical assistant and other medical staff members plays a role in the patient's attitude. A study by Harvard University claims that the tone of voice used by surgeons is directly linked to medical professional liability claims. How something is said to a patient is just as important as what is said. Always use a friendly, warm tone of voice and project confidence when speaking with patients. Be courteous and **tactful** and choose your words carefully. Every caller should be made to feel that the medical assistant has time to attend to his or her needs. If the medical assistant is rushed to pick up the telephone, he or she should wait a few seconds until able to answer graciously without seeming breathless or impatient.

Be alert and interested in the person calling. Always give your full attention to the caller, and do not allow distractions to interfere with the conversation. Build a pleasant, friendly image for the office. Talk naturally and avoid repetition of mechanical words or phrases, such as "uh-huh" and "you know." Do not use professional **jargon**, such as referring to *otalgia* when the patient reports an earache. Using correct grammar adds to a favorable impression. Speak distinctly; clear pronunciation and **enunciation** are vital. Move the lips, tongue, and jaw freely. Talk directly into the mouthpiece. Never answer the telephone while eating, drinking, or chewing gum. A well-modulated voice carries best. Use a normal tone of voice, neither too loud nor too soft. Talk at a moderate rate, neither too quickly nor too slowly. Be expressive, and vary the tone of voice.

CRITICAL THINKING APPLICATION   9-1

Ashlynn has a tendency to speak a little fast in her normal conversations. How will she need to adjust as she is answering phones in the medical office? She also is a friendly person and enjoys talking on the phone. What precautions should she take so that this does not become an issue on the job?

This brings out the meaning of sentences and adds color and vitality to what is said.

Holding the Telephone Handset Correctly

A medical assistant must develop professional telephone habits and correct the more casual ones that are used at home. The handset should be placed so that the medical assistant's voice is relayed distinctly and accurately. Practice holding the handset around the middle, with the mouthpiece approximately 1 inch from the lips and directly in front of the teeth (Figure 9-2). Never hold it under the chin. Check the proper distance by taking the first two fingers and passing them sideways through the space between the lips and the mouthpiece. If the fingers just squeeze through, the lips are the correct distance from the telephone and the voice will go over the line in as close to its natural tone as possible. When using a headset, speak directly into its mouthpiece, positioning it the same distance from the mouth as a telephone handset.

Speak directly into the telephone immediately after removing it from its cradle. When turning to face another part of the room, make sure the handset moves, too; otherwise, the voice will be lost. A medical assistant who speaks too quickly, enunciates poorly, or fails to speak directly into the transmitter may not be easily understood by the person on the other end of the line.

Maintaining Confidentiality

Keep in mind that all communications in a healthcare facility are confidential. If others are nearby, use discretion when mentioning the name of the caller. Be careful about being overheard when repeating any symptoms or other information received by telephone. Never use a speaker phone to listen to voice mail or hold a phone conversation within the hearing range of others. Do not place patients on speaker phone at any time. Another individual may hear private medical information, which is a violation of regulations established by the Health Insurance Portability and Accountability Act (HIPAA).

CRITICAL THINKING APPLICATION   9-2

Ashlynn hears an employee speaking on the intercom to a patient. How should she handle this situation? To whom, if anyone, should Ashlynn report this activity and why? What problems might be caused if this type of conversation is overheard?

Each employee must be courteous on the phone since it is the lifeline of the office. The medical assistant's phone manner sets the tone for the caller's perception of the entire practice. Patients expect good customer service, and because they can decide who their providers are, courtesy must be a part of every patient encounter. Additionally, if patients are happy with the experience they had, they may refer others to the physician's office.

Thinking Ahead

Always think ahead when an important call must be made. Have the patient's chart or the bill in question at hand before dialing the phone and a pen and pad nearby ready to take notes. Write down a list of questions to ask or goals for the conversation. Keep the call short and simple, then free the line for other calls.

Most offices keep a list of frequently called phone numbers both for staff use and to offer to patients. A list of local pharmacies, hospitals, and their departments is helpful. All of these are time-savers that help the medical assistant better serve patients.

MANAGING TELEPHONE CALLS

A medical office receives many calls during the course of a single day. Each deserves the medical assistant's complete and **competent** attention, no matter how busy the office. The following section can assist the medical assistant with managing and following up on common incoming calls.

Answering Promptly

Whenever possible, answer the telephone on the first ring and always by the third ring. If the facility has several incoming lines or more than one telephone, a conversation sometimes must be interrupted to answer another call. It is courteous to say, "Excuse me just a moment; the other line is ringing." Answer the second call and determine who is calling. If it is not an emergency, ask that person to hold while the first call is completed. If possible, get the phone number of the second caller, but do not allow that request to turn into a lengthy conversation. Do not make the mistake of continuing with the second call while the first caller waits. Return to the first call as soon as possible and apologize briefly for the interruption. Think of what would happen during a face-to-face conversation. A second person who approaches people involved in a conversation should not expect to interrupt and be heard at length. However, if the second call is an emergency, take a moment to return to the first line and alert the caller that he or she will have to be kept waiting or be called back.

Never answer a call by saying, "Please hold" without first finding out who is calling. The call could be an emergency, and this type of greeting is extremely discourteous. It takes only a moment to be polite. If the call is an emergency, prompt attention to it could save

a life. The medical assistant must know how to activate emergency medical services (EMS) in his or her area. Usually this is as easy as calling 911; however, each medical assistant should be able to communicate quickly and efficiently with the EMS staff.

Keep the focus on the call. Do not attempt to multitask while answering the telephone, because this practice takes attention away from the patient. Callers can hear keyboard strokes and other office activity; a caller therefore might assume that the medical assistant is not giving full attention to the person on the phone. Treat the phone call just as if the patient were standing in the office (Procedure 9-1).

Identifying the Facility

The medical assistant should identify the facility first, then state his or her name. Numerous telephone greetings can be used. Discuss which are best with the physician or office manager. Some physicians prefer a very formal statement when answering the phone, whereas others allow a more casual script. Always follow the procedure outlined in the policy manual. Examples of telephone greetings include:

"This is Dr. Frank's office, Miss McDowell speaking. How may I help you?"

"Frank Maternal Health Clinic, this is Ashlynn McDowell. How may I help you?"

"Stella Frank's office, this is Miss McDowell. How may I help you?"

"Dr. Frank's office, this is Ashlynn. How may I help you?"

Some physicians avoid using the title "Doctor" to protect their patient's confidentiality. For instance, if a physician needs to call a work number and leave a message for a patient, curious co-workers might attempt to investigate what type of physician is being seen. Dropping the "Doctor" when leaving messages and when answering the telephone can be an effective means of protecting a patient's privacy. However, merely saying "Hello" is unsatisfactory; the name of the facility should always be mentioned to callers. Otherwise, the caller **invariably** asks if he or she has reached the physician's office, which wastes time, and the opportunity to create a favorable impression of the facility has been lost.

The use of a **salutation** in telephone identification is optional. Sometimes adding "Good morning" or "Good afternoon" to the identification is awkward. A rising inflection or a questioning tone of voice indicates interest and a willingness to assist and eliminates the need for an additional greeting. When the type of greeting has been chosen, practice until it can be said easily and smoothly. Never rush, so that all callers can clearly understand exactly what is said.

CRITICAL THINKING APPLICATION   9-3

Most offices dictate how the phone is to be answered. What should Ashlynn do if she is very uncomfortable with the way she is asked to answer the phone? Who ultimately should decide how the phone is answered?

Identifying the Caller

If the caller does not identify himself or herself, ask who is calling. Write the name down immediately on a pad of paper or phone message form. Repeat the caller's name by using it in the

PROCEDURE 9-1

Demonstrate Telephone Techniques

GOAL: *To answer the telephone in a physician's office in a professional manner and respond to a request for action.*

EQUIPMENT and SUPPLIES

- Telephone
- Message pad
- Pen or pencil
- Appointment book
- Computer
- Notepad

PROCEDURAL STEPS

1. Demonstrate telephone techniques by answering the telephone by the third ring, speaking directly into the mouthpiece, which should be positioned 1 inch from the mouth.
   PURPOSE: To convey interest in the caller by answering promptly. Proper positioning of the handset allows for an audible tone and carries the voice well.

2. Speak distinctly with a pleasant tone and expression, at a moderate rate, and with sufficient volume for the person to understand every word.

3. Identify the office and/or physician and yourself.
   PURPOSE: To assure the caller that the correct number has been reached and to identify the staff member.

4. Verify the identity of the caller, and if using a computerized messaging system, bring the patient's medical record to the active screen of the computer.
   PURPOSE: To confirm the origin of the call.

5. Screen the call if necessary.
   PURPOSE: To determine whether the caller has an emergency and needs immediate attention or referral to a hospital emergency department.

6. Apply active listening skills to assess whether the caller is distressed or agitated and to determine the concern to be addressed.
   PURPOSE: To make sure the medical assistant hears and understands the message being sent by the patient and to show that the patient has the medical assistant's full attention.

7. Determine the needs of the caller and provide the requested information or service if possible. Provide the caller with excellent customer service. Be as helpful as possible.
   PURPOSE: To allow the medical assistant to handle many calls and conserve the physician's and staff members' time and energy.

8. If unable to assist the caller, transfer the call to the appropriate person. However, first provide the person to whom the call is being transferred with as much information as possible about the caller and his or her needs.
   PURPOSE: To provide good customer service and be as helpful to the caller as possible.

9. Take a proper message for further action, if required, and suggest a time the patient will likely get an answer from the physician's office.
   PURPOSE: Not all calls can be resolved immediately.

10. Terminate the call in a pleasant manner and replace the receiver gently. Always allow the caller to hang up first.
    PURPOSE: To promote good public relations, provide excellent customer service, and ensure that the caller has no further questions.

---

conversation as soon as possible. Individuals like to hear their own names, and name repetition assures the patient that he or she has been identified correctly. Try to use the person's name at least three times during the call, and remember other courteous expressions, such as "thank you," "please," and "you're welcome," as often as possible. However, if other patients are within the range of your voice, remember that the caller's privacy must be respected.

Occasionally a caller refuses to identify himself or herself to the medical assistant and may be quite insistent on speaking with the physician. The individual could be a patient; therefore, every attempt to identify the patient and assist him or her should be made. Such callers may also be salespersons who are fully aware that if their identity is revealed, they will never get the opportunity to speak to the physician. These people may be firmly told, "Dr. Frank is busy with a patient and has asked that we take messages for her. If you

will not leave a message, you may wish to write a letter to her and mark it 'personal.'" This phrase usually prompts the caller to provide his or her name, and the call then can be handled according to office policy. Rarely does the caller choose to write a letter to the physician and deal with the wait time that course of action requires. If the patient agrees, the situation may be best handled with a regular appointment, during which the patient can speak privately with the physician.

Screening Incoming Calls

Most physicians expect the medical assistant to **screen** all telephone calls. The physician and office manager provide guidance on the type of calls to be routed to the physician and those that he or she will return at a later time. The medical assistant should become familiar with their preferences and also use good judgment, much of which comes with experience, in deciding whether to put through a call to the physician.

If it is office policy, put calls from other physicians through at once. If the physician is busy and cannot possibly come to the telephone, explain this briefly and politely, then say that the physician will return the call as soon as possible.

Many callers ask, "Is the doctor in?" or "May I speak to the doctor?" Avoid answering with a simple "Yes" or "No" or by responding with the question, "Who is calling, please?" If the physician is not in, say so before asking the identity of the caller. Otherwise, the impression may be created that the physician is just not willing to talk with this person.

If the physician is away from the office, the rule of offering assistance still holds. The medical assistant may say, "No, I am sorry, Dr. Frank is not in. May I take a message?" or "No, I am sorry, but Dr. Frank will be at the hospital most of the morning. May I ask her to return your call after 1 o'clock?"

If the physician is in and is available for telephone calls, a typical response would be, "Yes, Dr. Frank is in; may I say who is calling, please?"

When physicians prefer to keep telephone calls to a minimum, say, "Yes, Dr. Frank is in the office, but she is not free to come to the phone. May I take a message, please?" By responding in this way, the physician is not committed to taking the call.

During the time a physician is examining a patient, he or she will not wish to be interrupted with a routine call. In such cases you might say, "Yes, Dr. Frank is in, but she is with a patient right now. May I help you?" or "Yes, Dr. Frank is in, but she is with a patient right now. Is there anything you would like me to ask her?"

Try to guard against being overprotective. A patient should be able to talk with the physician when absolutely necessary, but unless it is an emergency, the patient probably is willing to do so at the physician's convenience. The medical assistant who answers the telephone acts as a screen, not a roadblock.

Although no one wants to sit next to a telephone waiting on a physician to call, this is the reality in most cases. In fact, physicians almost always rely on their staff to give them messages from patients and then follow up on the instructions the physician gives for each patient. Staff members should provide an approximate time frame within which the patient's call will be returned, but they must always stress that the time is an estimate. Emergencies cannot be predicted, and it may be impossible to abide by that time frame. Always ask for the patient's cell phone number, if available, then ask him or her to keep the phone handy for the rest of the day. Make every effort to return calls by noon for morning messages and by the time the office closes for afternoon messages. By cross-training all employees to take accurate messages and document calls, any employee can return calls, even if he or she did not take the original message.

Find out exactly how calls are to be handled when the physician is out of the office and under what circumstances he or she can be interrupted when on the premises. **Cultivate** a reputation for being helpful and reliable. A medical assistant can save the physician many interruptions if patients develop confidence in the medical assistant's ability to help them and have faith in his or her promises to take messages and deliver them properly. (For more tips on handling telephone calls, visit the Evolve site at *evolve.elsevier.com/kinn.*)

CRITICAL THINKING APPLICATION   9-4

Ashlynn answers the phone; the caller is a male pharmaceutical representative who has been visiting the clinic for several months. She cheerfully greets him and asks if he is calling to make an appointment. He states that he wants to make an appointment with Ashlynn—for a date. How should she handle this call? What problems could arise if this were a patient and Ashlynn were to accept the date?

Minimizing Wait Time

When a call cannot be put through immediately, ask, "Would you prefer to wait, or should I call you back when Dr. Frank is free?" If the caller elects to wait, remember that waiting with a silent telephone can be irritating and **tedious**. The waiting time always seems long, no matter how brief it really is. Many of today's phones are equipped with timers that tell the caller exactly how long they have been waiting on hold. The longer they wait, the more irritated they may become. Let no more than 1 minute pass without breaking in with some reassuring comment. For instance: "I'm sorry, Dr. Frank is still busy. Would you like to continue to hold?" or "I'm sorry to keep you waiting so long, Ms. Hughes. Would you prefer to have me return your call when Dr. Frank is free?" If the wait is longer than expected, the caller may wish to reconsider and call back at another time or have the call returned. By going back on the line at frequent intervals, the medical assistant allows the caller an opportunity to express such concerns. In any event, be considerate and remember that irritation can be lessened each time the medical assistant returns to the call by saying, "Thank you for waiting, Ms. Hughes."

When it is necessary to leave the telephone and obtain information, ask the caller, "Will you please wait while I get the information?" Listen for a reply. If getting the information will take longer than a few seconds, give some estimate of the time required and offer to call back. When returning to the telephone, always thank the caller for waiting. Requests that might require pulling the patient's chart from the files are best handled with a call back to the patient.

Remember that leaving a person on hold ties up one of the physician's telephone lines, and an emergency call could be coming through or new patients might be attempting to call. Most phone calls to a physician's office during the day are important, therefore the lines should be kept clear as much as possible.

Transferring a Call

Always ask the patient's permission to place him or her on hold and to transfer the call. Identify the person on the phone when a call is transferred to the physician or another person in the facility. Transferring the call to a co-worker's voice mail without warning the caller that the person is not available is considered poor customer service. Any person who refuses to give a name should not be put through unless the medical assistant has been specifically instructed to do so. If the person is not immediately available, ask the caller whether he or she would prefer to be put through to voice mail. Some callers simply believe their call will receive more attention if a human takes the message. If the caller insists, take a written message and deliver it to the proper person as soon as possible.

All medical assistants should learn "who does what" in the medical facility. Knowing about the functions of the office and which person is responsible for which areas makes a significant difference in the customer service provided to the patient. For example, suppose that the medical office employs one insurance receptionist, named Sarah, and three insurance billers. Opel handles names that begin with A through G, David handles names that begin with H through P, and Andrea handles names that begin with Q through Z. If a call comes to the office and the patient has an insurance question, the medical assistant could put the call through to Sarah. However, better customer service dictates that the medical assistant ask the name of the patient and put the call through to the person who handles that patient's particular claims. If the patient's name is Rebecca Whitehead, the medical assistant should call Andrea and ask if she may transfer Ms. Whitehead's call to her. The fewer times the caller is transferred, the happier the caller.

When the caller is a patient, the physician or clinical medical assistant probably will need his or her medical record at hand during the conversation. Remember, protecting the patient's right to privacy is vital. If others are in hearing range, take the chart to the person responsible for the call and say, "This patient is waiting on the telephone." Because the physician's office often is a hectic place, most require that a message be taken so that the medical record can be reviewed, the patient's request considered, and the patient called back with questions or instructions from the doctor.

Taking a Telephone Message

If the office uses a manual message-taking system, always have a pen or pencil in hand and a message pad nearby when answering the telephone. Several calls may be answered before an opportunity arises to relay a message or carry out a promise of action. The telephone message, whether taken through a computer system or by hand, is a vital part of competent patient care (Procedure 9-2).

Many types of message pads are available today (Figure 9-3). Ordinary spiral-bound notebooks are inexpensive, sturdy, and well proportioned. These usually lie flat on a desk and can be filed for future reference. Never use small scraps of paper for messages; they are too easily lost. Message books should be kept indefinitely in the medical office, because they could be used as evidence in a court of law. Once the caller's request has been acted upon, a copy of a phone message could be added to the patient's chart, or at a minimum the information could be noted in the chart if it concerns the patient's medical care.

A minimum of seven items are needed to take a telephone message correctly:

1. Name of the person to whom the call is directed
2. Name of the person calling

PROCEDURE 9-2

Take a Telephone Message

GOAL: To take an accurate telephone message and follow up on the requests made by the caller.

EQUIPMENT and SUPPLIES

- Telephone
- Computer
- Message pad
- Pen or pencil
- Notepad

PROCEDURAL STEPS

1. Demonstrate telephone techniques by answering the telephone using the guidelines in Procedure 9-1.
   PURPOSE: To answer promptly and courteously, which conveys interest in the caller and promotes good customer service.
2. Using a message pad or the computer, take the phone message (either on paper or by data entry into the computer) and obtain the following information:
   - Name of the person to whom the call is directed
   - Name of the person calling
   - Caller's telephone number
   - Reason for the call
   - Action to be taken
   - Date and time of the call
   - Initials of the person taking the call
   PURPOSE: To have accurate information, which allows the staff member to address the caller's issues quickly and efficiently.

3. Apply active listening skills and repeat the information back to the caller after recording the message.
   PURPOSE: To verify that all the information was recorded accurately.
4. Provide the caller with an approximate date and time the call will be returned, if possible.
   PURPOSE: To show consideration for the patient's time and to prevent the person from sitting by the phone, awaiting a call.
5. End the call and wait for the caller to hang up first.
6. Deliver the phone message to the appropriate person. Separate trays or slots for each staff member are helpful.
7. Follow up on important messages.
   PURPOSE: To make sure important issues are addressed in a timely manner.
8. Keep old message books for future reference. Carbonless copies allow the facility to keep a permanent record of phone messages.
   PURPOSE: To have a permanent source of messages in case a number is needed after the paper message has been discarded.
9. File pertinent phone messages in the patient's medical record. Make sure the computer record is closed after the documentation has been done.
   PURPOSE: To keep a permanent record of important information in the patient's chart.

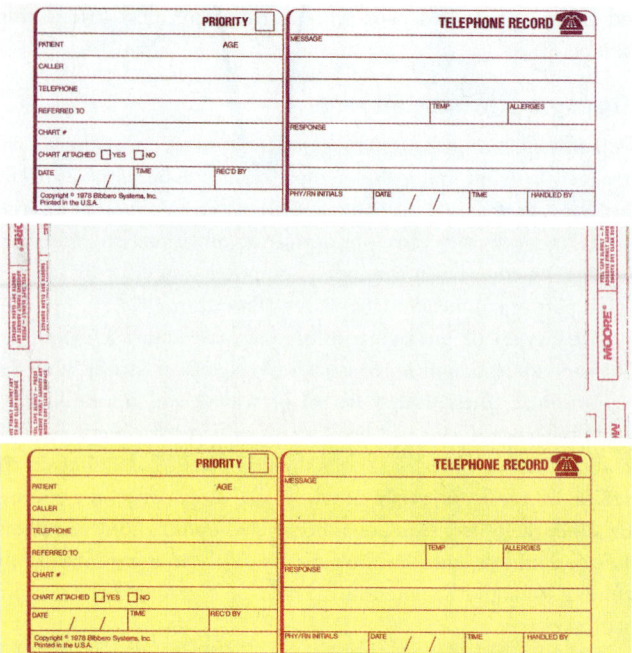

FIGURE 9-3 Phone message forms with self-adhesive backing make charting calls easier and more time efficient. (Courtesy Bibbero Systems, Petaluma, Calif.)

3. Caller's daytime, evening, and/or cell phone number
4. Reason for the call
5. Action to be taken
6. Date and time of the call
7. Initials of the person taking the call

Impression-sensitive message pads, which provide a copy of each page, ensure that no message is forgotten and are the best way to keep track of handwritten messages. These pads also provide a copy of the message in case one is lost, and they help ensure that all messages are delivered and receive follow-up action. Make certain that the handwriting on all phone messages is legible.

Electronic software systems usually populate the name, address, phone number, date, and time of a message; therefore, the medical assistant needs only to type in the reason for the call and what the patient would like the physician to do. The software may also offer ways to flag the messages for various actions once it has been taken, such as a flag for a call back or for a prescription refill. Electronic flags also can indicate the message's level of urgency.

The nature of the message determines whether it should be reported immediately. The person who completes the call must sign and date the message. If the call is from a patient and relates in any way to the medical history or if any instructions were given or queries answered, this information must be placed in the patient's medical record. Message forms are available that have a self-adhesive backing and can be placed permanently in the patient's case history.

Taking Action on Telephone Messages

The message procedure is not complete until the necessary action has been taken. Place notations on the memo pad or in the computerized day planner to carry over to the following day if they have not been completed, but this should be a rare occurrence. Do not trust to memory messages that were not attended to from previous days; always carry them forward either electronically or in writing.

Make brief notations of patients' attitudes while talking to them on the telephone, if they are significant. The physician does not require a character study, but it is helpful to know when a patient appears fearful, apprehensive, or nervous. If a patient shows such symptoms, it may be wise to consult with or transfer the call to the physician or clinical medical assistant.

Ending a Call

When a caller's requests have been satisfied, do not encourage inappropriate chatting or permit the call to monopolize your time unnecessarily. The telephone lines should be cleared for other calls. Thank the person for calling, close the conversation with some form of "good-bye," and replace the telephone on its cradle gently. Allow the caller to hang up first.

Retaining Records of Telephone Messages

Each office must develop a policy on the retention of telephone message records. Electronic medical record systems will likely be capable of sending message information directly to the computerized medical record. Many offices elect to keep handwritten message pads for the same period that the statute of limitations runs for medical professional liability cases. Remember that phone records include telephone bills, especially those that detail long-distance charges. Keeping message records can be of assistance in proving any number of claims, including the number of times patients called the office and the fact that calls to the patient were attempted or returned. Make sure accurate telephone records are kept to ensure good patient care and customer service.

TYPICAL INCOMING CALLS

Medical assistants answer incoming calls to spare the physician unnecessary interruptions during visits with patients. Outgoing calls may be made to follow up with patients or to conduct the general business of the office, such as ordering supplies and obtaining laboratory results. Many calls relate to the administrative aspects of the office and actually can be better handled by the medical assistant. The policy on handling calls should be clearly set forth in the office procedures manual.

New Patients and Return Appointments

Procedures for handling appointments for new patients and scheduling return appointments are discussed in Chapter 10. Always provide excellent customer service to the caller. Remember that the routine questions that may be asked should be answered in a polite, cheerful manner. Health matters are important to the individual patients whom the practice serves. Follow the designated office procedure as to what information should be gathered and recorded when appointments are made.

Directions

Each office should have a clear set of directions written out that can be read to the caller who requests directions. Prepare them from various points in the area; for instance, one set would guide a patient who is coming from the north, and another set would be for a patient coming from the south. Place these directions close to the telephone so that all employees can access them easily. Not all employees live close to the clinic or are familiar with the area; therefore, the written set of directions will be helpful to all staff members and those who call the facility. Place a map on the office Web site and direct patients there for printable instructions. Never simply suggest that the caller refer to an Internet map when he or she asks for directions.

Inquiries about Bills

A patient may ask to speak with the physician about a recent bill. Ask the caller to hold for a moment while the ledger is obtained from the computer or files. If nothing irregular is found on the ledger, return to the telephone and say, "I have your account in front of me now. Perhaps I can answer your question." Most likely the caller will have some simple inquiry, such as whether the insurance has paid, or he or she may want to delay making a payment until the next month. Not all patients realize that the medical assistant usually makes such decisions and is the best person with whom to discuss these matters. When necessary, create a note in the electronic medical record (EMR) or the physical ledger card about the patient's call, such as a promise to pay on a certain date.

A patient may have a question about a statement that came in the mail. If billing matters are handled by another employee, tell the patient that the call will be transferred to the billing office. If you are responsible for billing, politely ask the patient to hold the line while you obtain the patient ledger. On returning to the line, thank the patient for waiting and explain the charges carefully. If an error has occurred, apologize and say that a corrected statement will be sent out at once. Always remember to thank the patient for calling. If patients are properly advised about charges at the time services are rendered, the number of these calls can be reduced considerably.

Inquiries about Fees

Fees vary widely in each medical office, and quoting an exact fee before the physician sees the patient is difficult. However, a good estimate should be given to the patient as to what they should expect to pay, especially on the first visit. Asking a patient to just appear at the office without having any idea of the cost is unreasonable. Discuss with the physician or office manager what range should be quoted to the patient, then follow your quotes with the statement that the fees vary, depending on the patient's condition and tests the physician orders. If fees are regularly discussed on the telephone, write a suggested script in the policy manual. Do not be evasive. Have a schedule of fees available.

Participating Provider

Patients may call the office to inquire whether the physician is a participating **provider** with their particular insurance plan or managed care organization. The physician should keep a carefully updated list of which plans are valid. This is important, because insurance benefits vary for participating and nonparticipating providers, and a claim will be denied or reimbursement lessened if the physician is not a provider for the patient's insurance company.

Requests for Assistance with Insurance

In today's environment of managed care, co-pays, Medicaid, and Medicare, insurance claims will more than likely be completed and filed by the healthcare facility. Nevertheless, patients may call to inquire about their coverage or ask whether any response to claims has been made. A medical assistant or member of the staff responsible for insurance filing must have the knowledge to answer these inquiries. Be patient with these inquiries; insurance is a difficult subject to understand, even for trained individuals familiar with the various forms and procedures. Some patients, especially elderly ones, can become quite confused when dealing with insurance companies. Help them as much as possible so that they can collect the benefits to which they are entitled.

Radiology and Laboratory Reports

When results are urgently needed, laboratory and radiologic findings may be telephoned, faxed, or e-mailed to the physician's office on the day the procedures are performed. The medical assistant should take these reports and relay them to the physician. If the test has been marked **STAT**, which means that the physician wants the results immediately, reports may be faxed to the physician's office. Original reports usually are delivered by mail for the medical record. Some facilities are equipped to receive laboratory results directly from the laboratory by computer.

Satisfactory Progress Reports from Patients

Physicians sometimes ask patients to phone the office to report on their condition a few days after the office visit. The medical assistant can take such calls and relay the information to the physician if the report is satisfactory. Assure the patient that you will inform the physician about the call. The physician should always be immediately informed about unsatisfactory progress reports. The doctor should provide instructions for the patient to follow in such situations.

Routine Reports from Hospitals and Other Sources

Routine calls may be received from hospitals and other sources reporting a patient's progress. Take the message carefully and make sure that the physician sees it. The message should then be placed in the patient's medical record.

Office Administration Matters

Not all calls concern patients. Calls may come from the accountant or the auditor or about banking procedures, office supplies, or office maintenance, most of which the medical assistant can handle or refer to the appropriate person. For some of these calls, the medical assistant may need to gather additional information and return the call.

Requests for Referrals

Physicians who are liked and respected by their patients frequently are called for referrals to other specialists. If the physician has furnished the medical assistant with a list of practitioners for this purpose, these inquiries may be handled without consulting the physician, unless the patient's insurance plan requires a written referral. However, the physician should always be informed of such requests. Document referrals in the patient's medical record.

Some managed care organizations require a physician referral before a patient may see a specialist. This referral should come from the physician, unless he or she has authorized automatic referrals. Most physicians require the patient to come in for an office visit to discuss the referral. Afterward, a staff member calls the referral physician and notifies the office staff of the referral. Handle these calls as

Call the Pharmacy with New or Refill Prescriptions

GOAL: *To call in an accurate prescription to the pharmacy in the most efficient manner.*

EQUIPMENT and SUPPLIES

- Prescription information
- Notepad
- Patient medical record
- Telephone
- Computer and/or fax machine

PROCEDURAL STEPS

1. Receive the call from the patient or a fax from a pharmacy requesting a prescription; use appropriate telephone technique.
   PURPOSE: To provide consistently good customer service when speaking with callers.
2. Obtain the following information from the patient:
   - Patient's name
   - Telephone number where he or she can be reached
   - Patient's symptoms and current condition
   - History of this condition
   - Treatments the patient has tried
   - Pharmacy name, telephone number, and/or fax number
   PURPOSE: To have the information the physician will need to determine whether a prescription will be called in for the patient or whether the person needs to come to the office to be seen by the doctor.
3. Write in the patient's chart the prescription the physician wants the patient to have. Be very careful to transcribe the information correctly. Analyze communications in providing appropriate responses and feedback by reading it back to the physician.
   PURPOSE: To have a permanent record of the prescription in the chart and to make sure the prescription is exactly what the physician wants the patient to take, eliminating errors in medication name and dosage.
4. If the prescription is a refill, give the physician the patient's chart with the message requesting a refill attached, along with the information in step 2.

PURPOSE: To have the patient's chart as a reference and to provide the physician with the information needed to determine whether the medication requested should be refilled.
5. Note the comments the physician writes in the chart. If the prescription is written or a refill is approved, call the patient's pharmacy and ask to speak to a member of the pharmacy staff. (If the prescription was requested by fax, complete the requested information and send the fax back to the pharmacy.)
6. Ask the pharmacy staff member to repeat the prescription back to you.
   PURPOSE: To verify that the pharmacy staff member took down the prescription accurately.
7. Note in the chart the date and time the prescription was called to the pharmacy.
   PURPOSE: To create a permanent record of the medication being called to the pharmacy, along with the correct dose and frequency of doses.
8. Call the patient to notify him or her that the prescription has been called in. Provide any information about the prescription doses, frequency, and so on requested by the physician. Tell the patient when to return to the office, if necessary. Ask the patient to write this information down.
   PURPOSE: To inform the patient of the dosage and frequency, so that if an error is made by the pharmacy, the patient will note the discrepancy and the error can be corrected before the patient takes any of the medication.
   NOTE: Many physicians use an electronic medical record system that allows them to use e-prescribing functions. E-prescribing works in a similar way to electronic faxing. The physician usually enters the desired prescription information into the patient's electronic record while in the exam room. The patient's pharmacy is listed in the record, so once the prescription is completed, the physician clicks "send" and it is on its way to the pharmacy. This method is becoming more common and helps to eliminate prescribing errors and forged prescriptions.

---

quickly as possible so that the patient may make an appointment to see the referral physician.

Prescription Refills

Pharmacies periodically call the physician's office to obtain approval for a patient to refill a prescription. Prescriptions have a specific notation as to the number of times the prescription can be refilled. However, the physician may have noted in the chart that a certain medication is to be taken for 6 months, but the prescription was written only for 1 to 2 months. Any prescription refills should be authorized only with the physician's approval. Tell the pharmacist that you will have to check with the physician and call back. Many pharmacies today handle prescription refills by fax so that they

have a written record that the refill was authorized. Make sure state regulations and procedures are followed any time you deal with prescription refills or calls (Procedure 9-3). Some medications require a written prescription.

SPECIAL INCOMING CALLS

Patients Refusing to Discuss Symptoms

Occasionally patients call and want to talk with the physician about symptoms they are reluctant to discuss with a medical assistant. Patients have a right to privacy, but the physician cannot be expected to take numerous calls from patients who do not want to speak to the medical assistant. If the patient refuses to discuss any symptoms, suggest that he or she make an appointment with the physician to discuss the problem in person.

Unsatisfactory Progress Reports

If a patient under treatment reports that he or she is still not feeling well or that the prescription the doctor provided is not helping, do not practice medicine illegally by giving the patient medical advice. Make detailed notes about the patient's comments, then present them to the physician. He or she may make a medication change or may decide that the patient should return to the office. Follow up with the patient and convey the physician's instructions.

Requests for Test Results

When the physician orders special tests for the patient, the patient may be told to call the office in a couple of days for the results. It is ultimately the responsibility of the physician to notify the patient of test results, especially if they are abnormal. Make sure the physician has seen the results and has given permission before sharing the results with the patient. If specified in the office policy, the medical assistant can give test results to the patient. Patients do not always understand that the medical assistant does not have the privilege of giving out information without the permission of the physician. If the result is unfavorable, the physician should be the one to inform the patient and give further instructions. This call must be handled tactfully; otherwise, the patient may feel as if the staff is concealing information.

Most physicians prefer that medical assistants provide only normal test results to the patients. However, the medical assistant may provide abnormal test results if authorized by the physician. For example, when a patient has a questionable Pap smear, the medical assistant usually is the person who calls the patient with the results and further instructions from the physician. If the patient then has any questions about the test results, he or she must be referred to the physician. The medical assistant needs good communication skills to relay information such as this without crossing the line of practicing medicine without a license.

The best policy for dealing with more serious abnormal test results is to schedule an appointment for the patient to see the physician. These results are best related in person instead of on the telephone. Human immunodeficiency virus (HIV) test results should never be given on the telephone; the physician should always insist that the patient return to the office to obtain these results.

Patients who call the office for test results must be appropriately identified before the results are given. Some offices use a special code that is written in the chart, and knowledge of this code or password gives the person access to the information. Make sure the right individual is on the line before offering test results. Especially be careful in situations in which the family includes a "Senior" and "Junior." If the medical assistant calls and asks for Robert Smith, the elder Mr. Smith may answer, whereas the younger Mr. Smith is the one who came to the office for tests. Staff members may breach HIPAA regulations if they do not identify the patient accurately.

Requests for Information from Third Parties

The patient must give written permission before any member of the physician's staff can give information to third-party callers. This includes insurance companies, attorneys, relatives, neighbors, employers, and any other third party.

Complaints about Care or Fees

A medical assistant may be able to offer a satisfactory explanation to a patient who complains about the care he or she received or the fee charged. Often, the patient simply does not understand a charge, and the medical assistant can provide assistance by reviewing the bill. If a patient seems angry, offer to pull the chart, research the problem, and if needed, discuss it with the physician. Four magic words often calm the angry patient: "Let me help you." This reassures the patient that someone is willing to talk about the problem. However, if you are unable to appease the patient easily, the physician or office manager may prefer to talk directly to the patient.

Calls from the Physician's Family and Friends

Personal calls to the physician from family members or friends are handled in accordance with instructions from the physician. If the physician does not want to take the calls, the medical assistant must tactfully tell the caller that the physician cannot be disturbed at that time.

Calls from Staff Members' Family and Friends

The telephone lines should never be burdened with an excess of personal calls to the staff. A call is necessary in emergencies, but staff members should never monopolize the telephone for personal business and conversations. Emergency calls could be coming through, and the lines must be clear. Keep personal calls to an absolute minimum.

HANDLING DIFFICULT CALLS

Angry Callers

No matter how efficient the medical assistant is on the telephone or how well liked the employer may be, sooner or later an angry caller will be on the line. The anger may have a legitimate cause, or the caller's irritation may have resulted from a misunderstanding. Handling such calls is a real challenge. First, take the required action, even if it is to say that the matter will be discussed with the physician as soon as possible and the patient will be called back later. If answers are not readily available, a friendly assurance that the situation is important and that every attempt will be made to find the answer quickly usually calms the angry feelings.

The medical assistant may find that lowering the tone of voice and volume of speech may force the angry caller to do the same to hear. This method does not always work, but it usually is true that when dealing with an angry person, calm promotes calm. Some patients may misread this method and become even angrier, thinking that their complaint is not being taken seriously. Interpersonal skills are critical when dealing with other individuals, because the more skilled the medical assistant becomes, the better able he or she is to deal with multiple types of personalities.

Always avoid getting angry in response and try to get to the root of the real problem. Express interest and understanding, take careful notes, and follow through with the problem to the most appropriate resolution. Never "pass the buck" by saying, "That isn't my job," or "I am not the person who filed that insurance claim." No matter whose fault the problem is, it is best to deal with it and find a solution instead of placing blame.

CRITICAL THINKING APPLICATION   9-5

An angry caller raises his voice at Ashlynn over an issue that happened before she began to work at the facility. She suggests that he speak with the office manager, but he refuses and continues to berate Ashlynn.

- What choices does Ashlynn have in this situation?
- Should she simply hang up on the patient?
- How can the call be handled diplomatically?

Aggressive Callers

Aggressive callers insist that they receive whatever action they feel is necessary, and they usually insist on action immediately. Treat these callers with a calm, poised attitude, but do not allow the caller's aggression to initiate inappropriate action. Reassure the caller that the concern being shared is valid and will receive the full attention of the right person. Explain when the caller can expect a response from the office, and be sure to follow up that the appropriate action was taken.

Unauthorized Inquiry Calls

Some individuals call the physician's office requesting information to which they are not entitled. These callers must be told politely but firmly that such information cannot be provided to them because of privacy laws. Insistent callers should be referred to the office manager or physician.

Sales Calls

Sales calls often are thought of as an interruption to the physician's busy day, but some salespersons may have important information on products, equipment, or services the office uses regularly. Do not completely disregard salespersons, but do not allow them to monopolize time or telephone lines, either. Keep these calls quick and to the point. Most professional salespersons realize that the physician's and staff's time is extremely valuable and respect this. Developing a good rapport with representatives ("reps") from the companies whose products are frequently used in the practice may result in discounted prices and first news of sales and promotions. In turn, these people rarely waste the time of office personnel.

Physician Shopping

Some calls are from prospective patients seeking information about the office and the types of illnesses or conditions the physician treats. Because managed care plans require the patient to choose a primary care provider, patients may call to obtain an idea of the physician's background before selecting him or her to be their physician. Often patients must choose from a list of physicians they do not know. Consider these callers future patients or as people who may refer patients to the office. Always be polite and answer questions respectfully. Remember, even if the caller does not become a patient, he or she may share his or her impressions of the practice with another prospective patient.

Not to be confused with physician shopping, "doctor shopping" has become a serious issue in the medical community. Patients who see multiple physicians requesting prescriptions for narcotics without the provider's knowledge of the other prescriptions, are said to be doctor shopping, which is now illegal in many states. The Center for Disease Control defines this act as obtaining drugs through fraud, deceit, misrepresentation, or concealment. Over a period of time, the medical assistant who answers the phone will learn to spot many drug seekers when they call for an initial appointment. Always share any concerns or suspicious activity with the physician or the office manager.

If reference needed for above information: http://www.cdc.gov/homeandrecreationalsafety/Poisoning/laws/dr_shopping.html Accessed on 5-15-2013

Complaints

When callers complain, use an approach similar to the one used with angry callers. Do not attempt to blame someone else and never argue with the patient. Find the source of the problem, then present the options to the caller as to how the situation can be resolved. Remember to treat callers in the same manner that you would wish to be treated. A complaint may seem small and insignificant to the office staff, but to the patient it could be paramount. Provide good customer service to patients, and complaints will be few and far between.

Callers with Difficulty Communicating

Occasionally, calls will come to the office from patients or family members who have difficulty with the English language. In some cases, English is not the caller's primary language, so the medical assistant must use listening skills to ensure understanding. If a certain language is predominant in the area, the physician should consider hiring a medical assistant who is bilingual. Some patients speak English, but have a heavy accent, so listen carefully and ask questions to be sure that he or she is properly understood. Some physicians may have a population of deaf patients and will need to either employ an individual who uses sign language or have access to some other type of device designed to communicate with the hearing impaired.

EMERGENCY CALLS

Many emergency calls require judgment on the part of the person answering the phone in the medical practice. Good judgment comes from experience and proper training by the physician with regard to what constitutes a real emergency in each type of practice and how such calls should be handled. The person answering the telephone first should determine whether the call is truly urgent. If so, never hang up the phone until an ambulance reaches the patient or other help arrives. When necessary, ask another staff member to call 911 while remaining on the line with the patient. Emergency calls could include such conditions and/or symptoms as chest pain, profuse bleeding, severe allergic reactions, cessation of breathing, injuries resulting in loss of consciousness, and broken bones. An urgent call could be an adult patient with a fever over 102° F, an animal bite, or an increasingly painful ear infection. Emergency calls are life-threatening, whereas an urgent call requires prompt attention but is not life-threatening. Often the physician instructs the patient to go straight to the closest hospital emergency department instead of the office. Policy and procedure manuals should dictate the action to take in emergency situations.

If the physician is in, the call may need to be transferred to him or her immediately. All offices should have a written plan of action for the times the physician is not physically present in the office to handle the call. The physician and medical assistant may also jointly develop typical questions to ask the caller to determine the validity and disposition of an emergency. Some examples of questions to ask include:

- At what telephone number can you be reached?
- Where are you located?
- What are the chief symptoms?
- When did they start?
- Has this happened before?
- Are you alone?
- Do you have transportation?

Screening Guidelines

In a facility with multiple employees, the physician may designate one individual as the screening nurse or assistant. In the managed care environment, every physician would be wise to have a written telephone protocol for handling urgent situations and emergencies. The protocol should state that the employees are bound by the written guidelines and that any giving of advice by unauthorized personnel may be grounds for dismissal.

A special sheet of instructions listing specific medical emergencies, such as chest pain, heavy bleeding, fainting, seizure, and poisoning, should be posted by each telephone. The phone numbers for the nearest poison control center, hospital, and ambulance should be listed. Such calls should be routed to a physician immediately. Additional instructions should include what action to take if no physician is available, such as sending the patient to an emergency department or calling an ambulance. Most offices have some means of constant contact with the physician, whether by pager, cell phone, or another method.

Getting the Information the Physician Needs

As the medical assistant gains experience and knows the physician better, he or she begins to have a sense of the questions the physician will have for patients who call the facility. For instance, the physician is interested in how long the patient has had symptoms, what makes the symptoms better or worse, what remedies have been tried, what has worked and not worked, and other specifics about the condition. If the patient complains of painful urination, the medical assistant learns to ask about pain in the back, blood in the urine and/or stool, and cramping. One way to learn about questions to ask is to listen to the physician carefully as he or she questions patients about their symptoms. This can help the medical assistant learn more about signs and symptoms and enable him or her to be a better assistant to the physician.

Remember to always be "patient with your patients." Those who call the medical office for help are almost never at their best. When feeling ill, people often are short-tempered and even display poor manners. Some can be verbally abusive. Care for patients as if they were family members, and they will feel care and compassion in the medical facility.

TYPICAL OUTGOING CALLS

Most outgoing calls in a physician's office are responses to the incoming calls. The same rules for courtesy and diction apply to calls made from the office to patients, other individuals, and businesses.

It is helpful to plan outgoing calls in advance. For instance, if the medical assistant is placing an order for office supplies, a list should be made that includes the product, the price, the quantity needed, and a catalog page number, if applicable. Questions about the various products ordered should be noted so that they can be asked while the sales representative is on the phone.

Some medical assistants find it helpful to make all outgoing calls at once, when possible. This way the calls can be made one after another, and if a call back is necessary, the medical assistant is likely to still be by the phone. Organizing calls helps increase office efficiency.

Never be rude to an individual on the phone. Remember to treat those on the other end of the phone as you would wish to be treated. Do not forget that the medical assistant is a representative of the physician and should behave in a professional manner at all times.

TELEPHONE SERVICES

Voice Mail

Voice mail is widely used in today's business offices because it affords an around-the-clock method for receiving patient messages. Unfortunately, it can prove frustrating to those who find themselves speaking to an electronic device more often than a human being. Voice mail allows the caller to hear a recorded message that may also provide information about what to do in case of an emergency. Similar to an answering machine, voice mail records a caller's message, which can later be retrieved, and allows special temporary greetings when the user is away from the office. Keep patients happy by answering voice mail messages promptly.

Answering Services

Because a physician's telephone is an all-important tool of the practice, someone must be able to answer it at all times, day and night, weekends and holidays. This presents no problem during weekdays, but nights and weekends require special attention. Most physicians subscribe to telephone answering services that provide round-the-clock coverage. Answering services normally provide an operator (rather than a recording device) to answer the phones, which often is preferred over standard voice mail. Two types of operator-answered services are available. With the first type, physician-subscribers leave messages with or obtain patients' messages from a service for which a number appears in the local telephone directory after the physician's number, with a notation to call the second number after hours. This form of service is somewhat inconvenient for the patient but is far better than no coverage at all. With the second type, the answering service has a direct connection with the office telephone. When the telephone rings in the physician's office or at home, it also signals on the switchboard of the answering service. As long as the telephone rings, it continues to signal at the answering service. If no one answers within a certain agreed-on number of rings (or immediately in some cases), the answering service operator takes the call. This method provides continuous live telephone coverage.

Even during the day, such an answering service can function effectively. Sometimes the staff members may be assisting the physician and unable to answer the telephone. Not answering the telephone is extremely poor policy; therefore, if the office has an agreement with the answering service, its operators accept calls in such situations. With this direct-wire answering method, the operator answers the telephone in the same manner as the regular staff.

The answering service greatly appreciates receiving a call every day from a member of the physician's staff before leaving the office with information on where the physician will be during the evening or other special messages. The next morning, a staff member should call the service and ask for any messages that may have been taken or collect the messages through e-mail. Usually there will be messages from patients who called after office hours but whose calls were not urgent enough to merit an emergency call to the physician. An answering service can act as a buffer for the physician and help eliminate too frequent, unnecessary calls during the late evening or night hours. Some physicians in smaller practices or in rural areas have a recorded message that plays after hours. The message directs patients with an emergency either to go to the nearest emergency department or to call a secondary number to reach the physician on call. In rare cases, a physician's message simply states to call back during regular office hours.

Automatic Call Routing

In automatic call routing, a call is answered by an automated operator's message that presents a list of options, such as "If you are calling about your account, press 1; to make an appointment, press 2 …" and so forth. The impersonal nature of automation does not lend itself well to answering the telephone in a small to medium-sized physician's office, but the medical assistant encounters it frequently when placing outgoing calls. Some larger clinics and hospitals may use automatic call routing on a daily basis.

> **CRITICAL THINKING APPLICATION   9-6**
> Ashlynn has had many complaints from patients about the new call routing system, because it takes so long to "get to a human being." How can she get her patients to be more accepting of modern call routing systems? What methods might help elderly patients to deal with automated call routing more easily?

Call Forwarding

Call forwarding allows the user to forward calls to another designated number, such as a cell phone. Usually a code is entered, then the phone number to which the calls should be forwarded. This prevents the user from missing important calls when away from the main telephone.

Caller ID

Caller ID allows the user to see who is calling before picking up the handset to answer the phone. The caller's phone number and name appear on a screen, and the user can decide whether to take the call.

If the user subscribes to call-waiting services, another benefit called call-waiting caller ID is often available. Call-waiting caller ID allows the user to see who is calling even when the user is already on the phone.

Caller ID Blocking

Patients may have a feature on their phones that prevents anonymous or private calls from connecting and ringing. The feature, which works with caller ID, shows the words "anonymous," "private," "out of area," or "unavailable." The user has several options when using this feature. He or she can accept the call, reject the call, or send it directly to voice mail. Some physicians often use a blocker (e.g., *67) before calling patients, so that the patient will not have access to the physician's personal phone numbers. The caller hears a message stating that the person being called does not accept unidentified calls and then must choose from several menu options. This system is most commonly used when a patient calls a physician after hours and the physician subsequently returns the patient's call. Patients may need to be educated about this procedure so that the physician can reach them easily when calling after established office hours.

Cellular Phones

Considered a luxury item only 10 years ago, cellular (or cell) phones have become commonplace. Many people no longer have a home phone because of the expense of having two phones, and the cell phone usually is the better buy for the money. Several of the more popular cell phone companies offer free long distance calls in the United States and may provide users free night and weekend minutes as a bonus. Most of today's advanced cell phones even allow the user to access the Internet and check e-mail through the telephone. Cell phone companies usually offer a text messaging service, which allows the user to type a message with the cell phone keys, which then is sent directly to a cell phone number. Encourage staff members who use mobile telephones to take advantage of Bluetooth technology for hands-free talking.

Fax Machines

A fax machine can be a great time and labor saver in conveying patient information from physician to physician or from physician to hospital. It allows its user to send and receive copies of printed documents over telephone lines to other facilities that have fax machines (Figure 9-4). Most offices find this machine indispensable. Unless precautions are taken to ensure the security of information arriving by fax, the danger of loss of confidentiality is present. When sensitive material is sent, it is wise to telephone ahead to alert the receiver that this information will be arriving so that the appropriate person is on hand to receive it. A fax cover sheet should be used that instructs individuals who receive faxes in error to destroy them and states that the information contained in the fax is strictly confidential. Many offices use a printer that also functions as a fax, scanner, and copier. Fax services are also available online, such as Ring Central, through which documents are uploaded from the computer but sent to a fax machine. These services also usually offer a fax number, so that a fax sent from a machine to that fax number will be received in the e-mail inbox. The cost of these services varies and is usually quite affordable; however, the user must still have access

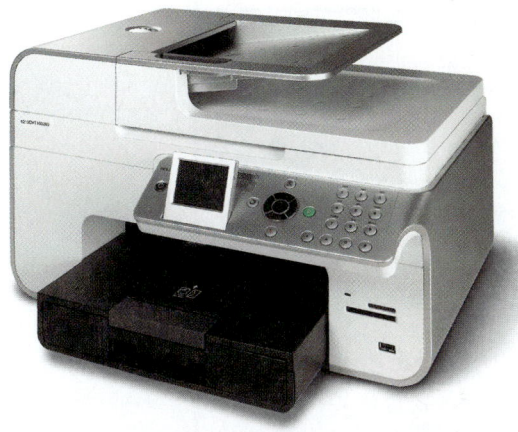

FIGURE 9-4 Fax machines allow written data to be transferred from one place to another simply by dialing a telephone. (Courtesy Dell Corp., Round Rock, Texas.)

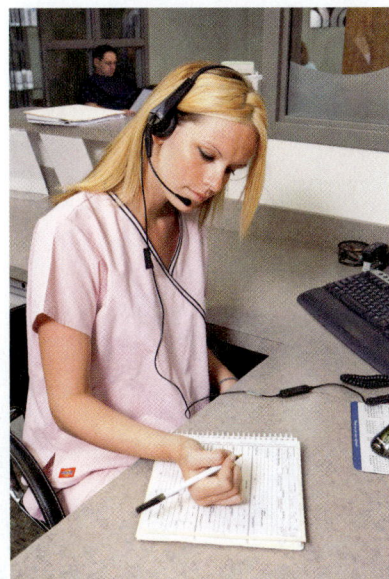

FIGURE 9-5 Using a headset helps the medical assistant keep the hands free while using the telephone and is better ergonomically.

to a scanner to fax documents that are not loaded onto the computer, such as a request for records that the patient has signed.

Headsets

In today's world of **multitasking**, the headset helps a medical assistant keep hands free while speaking on the phone. A popular headset is a very lightweight plastic earphone and microphone combination that allows the wearer to move about the room with the hands free (Figure 9-5). Some units weigh less than 1 ounce and are worn behind the ear or clipped to the wearer's glasses. Some headsets can be equipped with a cord that allows for easy mobility. Some also have a quick-disconnect feature that allows the user to separate the headset even during a call without breaking the connection.

USING LONG DISTANCE AND SPECIAL SERVICES

Long distance calls are simple to place, usually inexpensive, and efficient. When information is needed in a hurry, telephoning is much more expedient. Before placing a long distance call, have the

correct number ready. If you do not have the number, you may obtain directory assistance by dialing 1, then the area code of the party you are calling, followed by 555-1212. In some areas, numbers are available by calling 1-411. Directory assistance is now an automated service in many regions, and you will be asked for the name of the city and the person you are calling. Often a fee is charged for using directory assistance, so look for the phone number using free sources whenever possible.

The Internet makes searching for phone numbers much easier. Try to find phone numbers through the Internet (try *www.yellowpages.com* or *www.whitepages.com*) or use a printed phone book to avoid directory assistance charges on the monthly phone bill. A search for the business or physician needed may yield the information. If the company has a Web site, there is usually a "Contact Us" page that directs the user to the individual departments and even personnel who can assist in finding the correct phone numbers. Some Internet services allow the user to call long distance, and sometimes even internationally, through the computer with no long distance charges.

Time Zones

The continental United States is divided into four standard time zones: Pacific, Mountain, Central, and Eastern (Figure 9-6). When it is noon Pacific time, it is 3 PM Eastern time. When calling from San Francisco to New York, plan to make the call no later than 2 PM if the call is to a business or professional office. When it is 2 PM on the West Coast, it is 5 PM on the East Coast.

International Service

International Direct Distance Dialing (IDDD) is available in many areas. International dialing codes are the same for all companies offering IDDD. Depending on the long distance company, additional numbers or codes may preface the international access, country, and city codes. IDDD is still not available in all areas. If it is available, you may place international station-to-station calls by dialing the following in sequence:

1. International code 011
2. Country code
3. City code
4. Local telephone number
5. The pound sign (#) button if the telephone is touchtone

After dialing any international code, allow at least 45 seconds for the ringing to start. Consult the Internet for updates on international calling procedures and country or city codes.

Wrong Numbers

One slip in direct distance dialing can mean a call to Los Angeles or New York instead of Dallas. If you reach a wrong long distance number, be sure to obtain the name of the city and state that was called. Report this information promptly to the local operator so that the facility will not be charged for the call. If you are cut off before terminating a call, also report this. The operator will either reconnect the call or adjust the charge.

Conference Calls

Conference telephone service is of great value to the medical profession in notifying and explaining to a family how a patient is

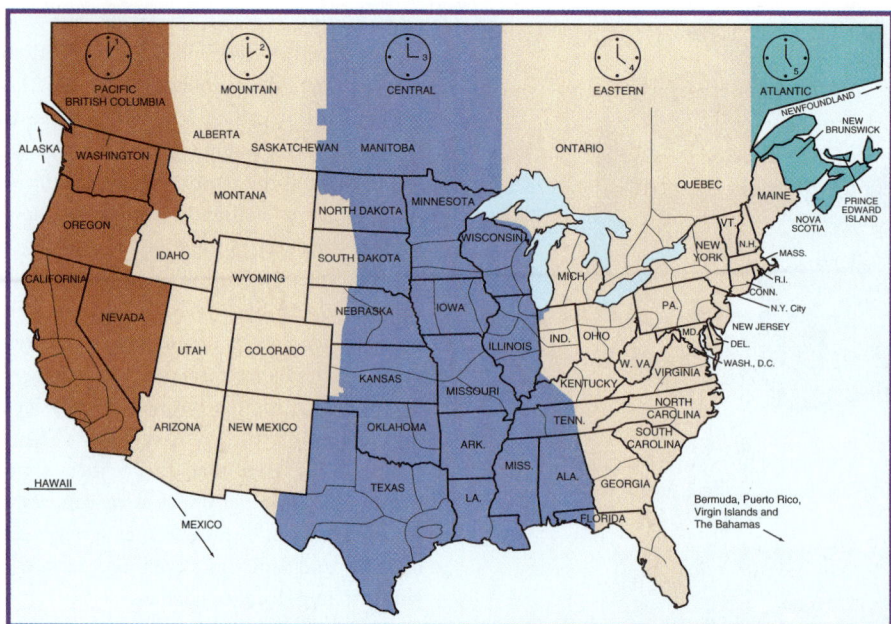

FIGURE 9-6 Time zones across the United States.

progressing. It has exceptional value in family conferences, at which a quick decision by the entire family regarding a patient's condition is required.

This service can connect numerous points for a conference in which each person can hear or talk to all others participating. Conference calls may be local or long distance. Charges are added for the number of places connected, the distance between parties, and the length of the conversation.

Conference calls can be set up by a normal long distance operator or through conference call services, many of which can be found online. To schedule a call, contact either an operator or the calling service and relay the pertinent information about time, date, and the individuals who are to be included in the call. Many businesses have conference call capabilities on their phone or computer systems. Notify everyone participating in the call of the time, date, number to call, and subjects to discuss. If prior arrangements are made with all parties, there is a better chance of reaching everyone and having a successful conference.

Operator-Assisted Calls and Services

Operator-assisted calls include the following:

- Person to person
- Billing to a third party
- Collect calls
- Requests for time and charges
- Certain calls placed from hotels
- Credit for wrong numbers
- Conference calls
- Some international calls

Operator-assisted calls through most phone service providers have an initial charge and a service charge. Fewer and fewer calls are operator assisted in today's business world, because the cost for these calls often is high. Try other alternatives before making an operator-assisted call.

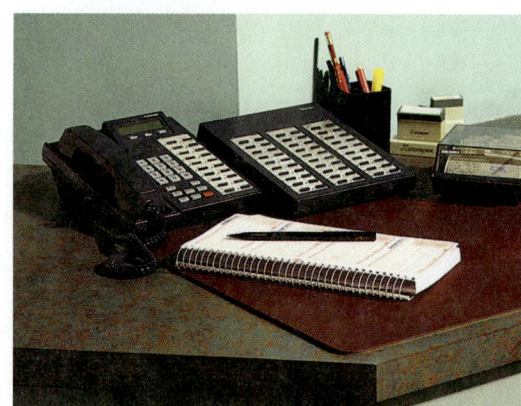

FIGURE 9-7 Multiline telephones allow numerous calls to come into the office at once. Each call deserves the same kind of attention and care from the medical assistant.

OFFICE TELEPHONE EQUIPMENT NEEDS

Number and Placement of Telephones

Familiarity with a multiple-line telephone system is a must for medical assistants. Few healthcare facilities can get along with just one telephone line. Two incoming lines, along with a private outgoing line with a separate number for the physician's exclusive use, is the minimum recommended number of lines.

One medical assistant can handle no more than two incoming lines; therefore, the addition of more lines may involve additional staffing (Figure 9-7). If a staff member is assigned solely to dealing with insurance and billing, a separate line and listing in the telephone directory for this service may considerably lessen the load on the main incoming lines.

Telephones should be placed where they are accessible but private. Some facilities also place a telephone in the reception room for the convenience of patients and to prevent their asking to use the facility's phones. However, recent trends suggest that a separate telephone line with a limited calling area for the convenience of patients who need to call out may be preferable. This telephone should not be in the reception room but in an area available to patients on request. It should be placed low enough for use by patients in wheelchairs. Wherever possible, other telephones should be placed on the wall to conserve desk space.

USING A TELEPHONE DIRECTORY

As previously mentioned, online telephone directories are convenient and provide the user with a fast response after a query. Some television programming systems provide service right on the television screen, which is helpful to patients. To use the television-based service, the remote control guides the user to the correct channel, and then the name of an individual or business is entered with the remote control.

The primary purpose of the telephone directory is to provide lists of those who have telephones, their telephone numbers, and in most cases their addresses. In addition, the directory is an aid in checking the spelling of names and in locating certain types of businesses through the yellow pages. Some directories are color coded, with residence listings on white pages, business numbers on pink pages, and business by categories and advertisements on yellow pages. Often, federal, state, county, and city government listings are included as blue pages. Directories usually are organized into three sections:

- Introductory pages
- Alphabetic pages (white pages)
- Yellow pages

The introductory pages sometimes are entirely overlooked by subscribers. This section precedes the white alphabetic pages and provides basic information concerning the telephone services in the area.

Some directories include ZIP code maps for the local area. Take a few moments to become familiar with the local directory, then use it frequently for getting information fast.

The white pages are an alphabetic listing of telephone subscribers with their telephone numbers and often their addresses.

The yellow pages directory, sometimes published separately, contains listings for businesses arranged by the product or services they sell. Physicians are listed alphabetically, usually under the heading Physicians and Surgeons, and have the option of another listing by type of practice.

In some metropolitan areas, a street address and telephone directory is published that is arranged by street address, followed by the name and telephone number of the person or business at that address.

Organizing a Personal Phone Directory

Organize telephone numbers in a tabbed 3 × 5-inch desktop file or a rotary file. Binders with clear sheet protectors also work well as personal phone directories. Emergency numbers might be typed on a colored card or flagged with a colored tab. A personal directory of telephone numbers should include all the numbers frequently called.

Identifying Community Resources

Patients often call the physician's office looking for information on various community resources. Those who are fighting cancer may be interested in programs offered by the American Red Cross. Those who are diabetic may wish to know the options for ordering blood glucose testing supplies through online services. Some patients may benefit from Meals on Wheels. The medical assistant should be concerned with providing good customer service to patients and visitors with whom they come in contact. Therefore, it is helpful to keep a list of the community resources that might be of assistance to patients. Often information can be found in the first few sections of the telephone book. The physician may want to keep a list of services most often used by the clinic's patients. Patients appreciate staff members who try to offer assistance and resources outside the physician's office.

CLOSING COMMENTS

A telephone is a tool; it can be used to build a physician's practice or to destroy it. Medical assistants must become proficient in good telephone technique and must make sure callers hear compassion and patience in their voices, even over the phone. A medical assistant must convey a genuine sense of caring for the patients who call the facility, just as if they were standing in the office. By keeping this in mind, the medical assistant plays a major role in patient satisfaction, and patients will find their medical care a pleasant process.

Patient Education

Today's telephone systems allow physicians to educate patients while they are on hold; recordings may be played that offer health information on subjects from A to Z. These messages can be professionally recorded and/or custom designed by the physician and staff. Special events may be announced, with the option to press a certain number for more information about the event.

Some phone directories offer listings of health information in the introductory pages. A patient may call a main number, then press a second number to reach the desired subject. Such features help address the needs of today's more information-oriented healthcare consumers, who are interested in healthy lifestyles and in gaining useful information immediately. Always be willing to teach and assist patients who must deal with these informational resources.

Legal and Ethical Issues

The guidelines for medical confidentiality apply equally to telephone conversations; therefore, take care that no one overhears sensitive information. Use discretion when mentioning the name of a caller or patient.

Do not place or receive personal phone calls during work hours. Time limitations for personal phone use should be described in the office policy manual. The telephone is a business line and should be reserved for patients and others conducting business with the office. The medical assistant should encourage friends and family to call at home so that all patient calls get through to the office.

Telephone and message records may be brought into court as evidence; make sure all messages are complete and legible. Most offices should keep these records for at least the same period as the statute of limitations in that state.

SUMMARY OF SCENARIO

Ashlynn is quickly becoming a part of the team at Dr. Frank's office and is developing into a well-liked asset to the staff. She has learned to slow down when speaking on the phone and to adjust her volume and pitch, depending on the patient with whom she is speaking. Although she tends to be quite talkative, she is balancing just the right amount of friendly chat with the business at hand. She does this by offering a friendly greeting to callers, getting to the business at hand, then being affable before ending the call. By expressing her concern and asking how she can be of help to the patients, Ashlynn shows them that she sincerely cares about their problems. She is careful about her tone of voice, realizing that patients may take her comments the wrong way if she does not treat them in a cordial manner. Dr. Frank is very pleased with her performance.

Ashlynn takes care when she speaks to patients and others on the phone so that she does not breach confidentiality in any way. She has become comfortable with the way she is to answer the telephone. The pace of her speech and the wording are now a habit. Ashlynn is determined to maintain a professional relationship with all the people related to her work environment. She is adept now at handling calls from angry patients and can maintain control with even the most aggressive callers. She leaves callers on hold for a minimum amount of time and reassures them frequently that she is attending to their situation. By treating callers as she would want to be treated, Ashlynn reduces frustration, and she feels that the office is more efficient at handling the large volume of calls that come in each day. She shows much promise for a long and rewarding career in the medical field and is satisfied with the current track of her career. As she continues to settle into her position, she looks forward to learning more about efficiency and time management. Her good attitude and desire to learn will only enhance her performance at work, making her a valuable employee and one worth promoting.

SUMMARY OF LEARNING OBJECTIVES

1. **Define, spell, and pronounce the terms listed in the vocabulary.**
   Spelling and pronouncing medical terms correctly bolster the medical assistant's credibility. Knowing the definition of these terms promotes confidence in communication with patients and co-workers.

2. **Determine and discuss the source of incoming and outgoing calls to a physician's office.**
   Incoming calls to a physician's office come from a wide variety of sources. Established or new patients may be calling to set appointments. Insurance companies may be seeking information about a claim. Hospitals, nursing facilities, or other healthcare units may need to report the progress of a patient. Laboratory results may be coming in for a patient who is very ill. Routine sales calls and telemarketing calls also come to the office, in addition to personal calls to the physician and staff members.

3. **Describe how to develop a pleasing telephone voice.**
   A pleasing telephone voice is one that is friendly and conveys a favorable impression of the physician's practice. Enunciate words and pronounce them clearly and distinctly. Vary the pitch of your voice, avoiding a monotonous or droning manner. Always be courteous and use tact. Both incoming and outgoing calls should be businesslike and handled in a professional manner.

4. **Demonstrate the correct way to hold a telephone handset.**
   The telephone handset should be held around the middle of the shaft, with the mouthpiece approximately 1 inch from the lips, in front of the teeth. Talk directly into the handset so that the caller can clearly hear what is said. Do not hold the mouthpiece beneath the chin, because the voice may not be heard clearly. To prevent sore muscles and neck problems, do not lean the head downward to hold the phone between the ear and the shoulder.

5. **Explain why courtesy is so important when speaking on the telephone.**
   Courtesy to patients and other callers is vital. First impressions are important, and a medical assistant's phone manner sets the tone for the caller's perception of the physician's practice. Customer service is important to today's physician, because many patients have choices among their healthcare providers, and the attitude of staff members may play a large part in such a decision. Patients who receive good customer care not only will continue to see the provider, they also will refer other patients to the physician. This is one of the best ways to help a practice grow.

6. **Demonstrate the correct way to answer the telephone in the office.**
   Medical assistants should answer the telephone promptly and professionally. The physician's image is affected by the way telephone calls are handled. Be courteous and polite to all callers.

7. **Discuss different ways to handle callers who want to speak to the physician.**
   The physician's time is valuable, but it also is centered on the patients. It is physically impossible for the physician to take all the calls each day. The medical assistant therefore must screen the calls and decide which ones should be put through to the physician. The medical assistant should offer to take a message and attempt to find out exactly what the caller's needs are and how they can be resolved. The patient should not feel that the physician is totally inaccessible but must also understand that patients in the office must have the physician's full attention.

8. **List the seven elements of a correctly handled telephone message.**
   The seven elements of a correctly handled phone message are (1) the name of the person to whom the call should be directed; (2) the name of the person calling; (3) the caller's telephone number; (4) the reason for the call; (5) the medical assistant's description of the action to be taken; (6) the date and time of the call; and (7) the initials of the

person taking the call, so that if any question arises, that person can be consulted.

9. **Demonstrate the correct way to record a message accurately and take a request for action.**

When taking a telephone message, strive for accuracy. Be sure to get all the information that the physician will need to act. Repeat any words or numbers that are not heard clearly.

10. **Demonstrate the most efficient way to call in a prescription or a prescription refill to a pharmacy.**

The medical assistant should follow the office policy and procedure manual when calling in new prescriptions or refills to a pharmacy. If a question ever arises as to what the physician meant, ask — do not guess. Mistakes with medications can cost the patient's life.

11. **Discuss how the medical assistant should handle callers who have a complaint.**

Callers who have a complaint should be handled in a manner similar to that for angry callers. Remain calm and offer to help. Take a serious interest in what the caller has to say. Let the caller know that his or her concerns are important to the staff and the physician. Find the source of the problem and determine exactly what the caller wants or expects as a resolution. Always follow up on complaints and make sure they were resolved as much to the caller's satisfaction as possible.

12. **Explain how angry callers might be handled.**

Never return anger when a caller is angry. Remain calm and speak in tones that are perhaps slightly quieter than those of the caller. This often prompts the caller to lower his or her tone of voice. Offer to help the angry person and ask questions to gain control of the conversation, moving it toward resolution. Do not argue with angry callers.

13. **List several questions to ask when handling an emergency call.**

First, ask for a phone number where the caller can be reached in case of a sudden disconnection. Ask about the chief symptoms and when they started. Find out whether the patient has had similar symptoms in the past and what happened in that situation. Determine whether the patient is alone, has transportation, or needs an ambulance. In severe cases, do not hang up the phone until the ambulance or police arrive.

14. **Discuss several useful sections of the introductory pages of the phone directory.**

Useful sections of the introductory pages include area codes, emergency service information, long distance calling information, time zones, government listings, and community service numbers. It may be helpful to tear these pages out, place them in clear sheet protectors, and add them to a binder for easy reference.

CONNECTIONS

📖 **Study Guide Connection:** Go to the Chapter 9 Study Guide. Read and complete the activities.

ⓔ **Evolve Connection:** Go to the Chapter 9 link at *evolve.elsevier.com/ kinn* to complete the Chapter Review and Chapter Quiz. Check out the other resources listed for this chapter to make the most of what you have learned from Telephone Techniques.

10

SCHEDULING APPOINTMENTS

Ramona West is the medical assistant in charge of scheduling appointments for Dr. Charlotte Brown. Ramona is an extremely organized person who thinks quickly and creatively. One of her professional goals is to ensure that the office remains on schedule throughout the day and that patient's waiting time is kept to an absolute minimum. She is fortunate that Dr. Brown is cooperative and time oriented, and they work well together to reach this common goal.

Ramona usually arrives at work at least 15 minutes early to begin her preparations for the day. She reviews the electronic medical record for each patient to make sure test results from previous visits are available to the physician and that the medical record is complete. She pays special attention to the

patients who arrive in the office as she completes her daily tasks, remembering the importance of providing patients with good customer service. Ramona greets each patient by name and carries on a brief but cordial conversation. Patients appreciate that she goes the extra mile to remember something about them, and this promotes excellent patient relations.

Ramona leaves a little time in the morning and afternoon for emergency appointments. The office uses an automatic call routing system to contact patients and confirm appointments in advance, which increases her show rate. Her friendly, caring attitude makes her a favorite among the patients, and Dr. Brown is pleased with the relationship-building skills Ramona has developed.

While studying this chapter, think about the following questions:

- How can the medical assistant contribute to an efficient daily routine?
- How does the medical assistant contribute to keeping the daily schedule on track?
- How can the schedule be put back on track when emergencies disrupt the day?
- How does the flexibility of the medical assistant contribute to office efficiency?

LEARNING OBJECTIVES

1. Define, spell, and pronounce the terms listed in the vocabulary.
2. Describe scheduling guidelines.
3. Discuss the advantages of computerized appointment scheduling.
4. Explain the features that should be considered when choosing an appointment book.
5. Explain how self-scheduling can reduce the number of calls to the medical office.
6. Discuss pros and cons of various types of appointment management systems.
7. Explain the importance of legible writing in the appointment book.
8. Explain the basic procedure to follow when the office is behind schedule.
9. Discuss the benefits of offering choices to patients when scheduling appointments.
10. Identify critical information required for scheduling patient admissions and/or procedures.
11. Discuss several methods of dealing with patients who consistently arrive late.
12. Name several reasons for failed appointments.
13. Recognize office policies and protocols for handling appointments.

VOCABULARY

automatic call routing A software system that answers phones automatically and routes calls to staff after the caller responds to prompts; also used to call a large number of patients to remind them of appointments or make announcements.

disruption An unexpected event that throws a plan into disorder; an interruption that prevents a system or process from continuing as usual or as expected.

established patients Patients who are returning to the office who have previously been seen by the physician.

expediency (ik-spe′-de-un-se) A means of achieving a particular end, as in a situation requiring haste or caution.

integral (in′-ti-grul) Essential; being an indispensable part of a whole.

interaction A two-way communication; mutual or reciprocal action or influence.

intermittent Coming and going at intervals; not continuous.

interval Space of time between events.

matrix Something in which a thing originates, develops, takes shape, or is contained; a base on which to build.

no-show A person who fails to keep an appointment without giving advance notice.

preauthorization A process required by some insurance carriers in which the provider obtains permission to perform certain procedures or services or refers a patient to a specialist.

precertification A process required by some insurance carriers in which the provider must prove medical necessity before performing a procedure.

prerequisite (pre-re′-kwe-zut) Something that is necessary to an end or to carry out a function.

proficiency (pruh-fi′-shun-se) Competency as a result of training or practice.

reimbursement Payment of benefits to the physician for services rendered according to the guidelines of the third-party payer.

screening A system for examining and separating into different groups; in the medical office, determining the severity of illness that patients experience and prioritizing appointments based on that severity.

socioeconomic Relating to a combination of social and economic factors.

template A predeveloped page layout used to make new pages with a similar design, pattern, or style; a standardized file type used in computer software as a preformatted example on which to base other files.

The physician's time is the most valuable asset of a medical practice. The person responsible for scheduling this time must understand the practice, be familiar with the working habits and preferences of the physician (or physicians), and have clear guidelines for time management in the practice.

Appointment scheduling is the process that determines which patients the physician sees, the dates and times of appointments, and how much time is allotted to each patient based on the complaint and the physician's availability. Time management involves the realization that unforeseen interruptions and delays always occur. Most medical care providers find that efficient appointment scheduling is one of the most important factors in the success of the practice. Scheduling can be done in a number of ways, and each facility must find the way that suits it best.

USING ESTABLISHED PRIORITIES FOR APPOINTMENT SCHEDULING

Patients often complain that the amount of money they pay to see the physician does not correspond with the amount of time the physician spends with the patient. A patient may say, "I only saw the doctor for 5 minutes and could not even remember all the questions I wanted to ask!" The patient must feel confident that the physician will take enough time to understand his or her concerns. Well-planned scheduling and adherence to that schedule allow the physician to do more than run in and out of examination rooms with little time for the patient to talk with the physician.

The person scheduling appointments must learn the physician's habits and desires. If the physician suggests scheduling patients every 15 minutes but always spends 20 to 25 minutes with a patient, the schedule must be adjusted. Talk with the physician and/or office manager and compromise so that the schedule is workable. Some physicians need prompting to end the patient visit and move to the next patient. The medical assistant assisting in the examination room can help the physician remain on schedule, because he or she teams with the scheduler and they work together for an efficient flow of patients through the office.

The scheduling system must be individualized to the specific practice. The following general guidelines can be applied to any practice, whether computer or paper based. Four factors must be considered in scheduling: the patient's needs, the physician's preferences and habits, the facilities available, and the duration of office visits.

Patient Needs

Consider the **socioeconomic** status of the area being served when determining office hours and appointment times. The office staff should answer the following questions:

- Is the office in a busy metropolitan area or a rural agricultural community?
- Are the patients young, middle aged, or retirement age?
- Is the area more industrial or residential?
- What type of patients are seen? Are they of a specific age or gender? Do they have common diagnoses? Is the physician a general practitioner?

- Are evening and weekend appointments essential for most of the patients served?

After these elements have been considered, the scheduler must allot time based on the patient's needs for each individual office visit. These needs can be assessed by determining the following:

- What is the purpose of this visit?
- What is the patient's age?
- Will the patient require the physician's time for the entire visit or will another staff member perform all or part of the service?
- Is the patient a parent who prefers to schedule appointments while the children are at school?
- Does the patient object to traveling after dark?
- Is the patient a day worker who cannot take time off from a job?
- Is the patient a child whose parents both work during the day?

The office should make every attempt to meet the patient's needs while balancing the physician's preferences and the available facilities.

Physician Preferences and Habits

Consider the preferences and habits of the physicians in the practice before establishing and implementing a scheduling plan. Ask the following questions:

- Does the physician become restless if the reception room is not packed with waiting patients?
- Does the physician worry if even one patient is kept waiting?
- Is the physician methodic and careful about being in the facility when patient appointments are scheduled to begin?
- Is the physician habitually late?
- Does the physician move easily from one patient to another?
- Does the physician require a "break time" after a few patients?
- Would the physician rather see fewer patients and spend more time with each one or schedule more patients each day?

All of these preferences and habits become an **integral** part of the scheduling process (Figure 10-1). Keep in mind that the physician cannot spend every moment of the day with patients. The physician also has telephone calls to make and receive, reports to examine and dictate, meetings to attend, mail to answer, and many other business responsibilities. An experienced staff can handle many but not all of these tasks.

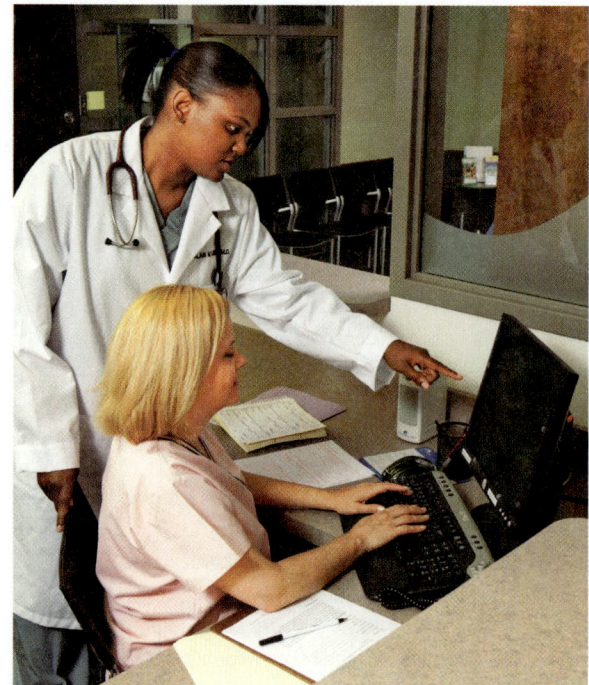

FIGURE 10-1 The habits and preferences of the physician must be considered when appointments are scheduled for patients.

minor surgery for the same time block, even if both doctors could be available. If the office has only one electrocardiograph, do not book two electrocardiographic procedures at the same time. As the medical assistant gains **proficiency** in scheduling, it becomes easier to pair patient needs with the available facilities according to the physician's preference. Major equipment frequently used or a certain room with such equipment may need its own scheduling column in the appointment book or software system.

Duration of Office Visits

The medical assistant who performs scheduling duties must know the amount of time required for various office visits and procedures. The office policy and procedure manual should have a list of the procedures performed in the physician's office with a notation of the time required for the procedure using established priorities. The time blocks are important, because the physician's **reimbursement** from insurance companies is based partly on the time requirements of the procedure or office visit. When scheduling, make sure to allow enough time to complete a procedure; for example, never schedule a Pap smear or minor surgery in a 10- or 15-minute time slot.

METHODS OF SCHEDULING APPOINTMENTS

The two most common methods of appointment scheduling are computerized scheduling and appointment book scheduling. Each has advantages and disadvantages, and the physician's office should weigh the benefits and choose the method that best suits the physician and the staff.

Computer Scheduling

The computer has replaced the appointment book in many practices. Software for appointment scheduling ranges from relatively simple

---

CRITICAL THINKING APPLICATION   10-1

- Ramona has noticed that Dr. Brown is taking a little longer with patients than normal and that she is running consistently behind schedule by approximately 5 to 15 minutes. How can Ramona help rectify this situation?
- Discuss ways of approaching the physician when he or she is the cause of the delays in the schedule. What opening remarks can the medical assistant use to start the discussion in a positive way?

Available Facilities

Getting a patient into the office at a time when no facilities are available for the services needed is pointless. For example, suppose that an office with two physicians has only one room that can be used for minor surgery. Do not schedule two patients requiring

programs that merely display available and scheduled times to more sophisticated systems that perform several other functions. Many programs can display such information as the length and type of appointment required and day or time preferences. The computer then can select the best appointment time based on the information entered into the computer.

The computer also can be used to keep track of future appointments. For example, when a patient calls and inquires about an appointment, the system can search by his or her name to find the time and date. Printouts also can be run to show the physician's daily schedule, including the patients' names and telephone numbers and the reason for the visit. Multiple copies of these schedules can be made, according to the needs of the practice.

Computer scheduling allows more than one person to access the system at once, and the information is available to all operators. The medical assistant can generate a hard copy of the next day's appointments before leaving each evening. In some facilities, employees keep an appointment book as a backup to computer scheduling.

Appointment Book Scheduling

Office suppliers carry a variety of appointment book styles. Some appointment books show an entire week at a glance, and many are color coded, with a special color used for each day of the week (Figure 10-2). This is very helpful when the physician asks the patient to return, for instance, in 2 weeks. If Wednesdays are colored yellow, the medical assistant can flip quickly to the correct day 2 weeks later and schedule the appointment. Multiple columns may be available to correspond with the number of doctors in a group practice, and the time can be divided according to their preferences.

Self-Scheduling

The future of appointment scheduling includes self-scheduling, which is a method by which a patient can log on to the Internet and view a facility's schedule, then select his or her own appointment time and make the appointment right then. The system should allow for patient confidentiality by showing only available times. Other patients' names should never be visible on an online system.

Software is available that allows the patient to self-schedule through secure links to the physician's appointment book. The software or Internet site for the physician's office should give the patient guidelines as to the amount of time needed for certain appointments or should allow only a certain length of time to be self-scheduled, such as 15 minutes. These systems will reduce the number of calls to the office and are available to the patient 24 hours a day. Some of these systems also send an automatic e-mail reminder to the patient the day before the appointment, requesting a reply to confirm. These systems are less frustrating to patients, who do not have to wait on hold to speak to the person who does scheduling for the office. Lengthy or complicated appointments should be scheduled through the office staff.

Although this type of system for making appointments appeals to most technologically savvy people, some patients stringently reject online scheduling because it requires at least minimal computer skills, which the patient may not have or be comfortable performing. If this method is used, some allowance must be made for patients who do not have computers. Other patients may object to online scheduling because they do not want their name anywhere on the Internet. This is a valid issue, and the office should allow these patients to schedule over the phone.

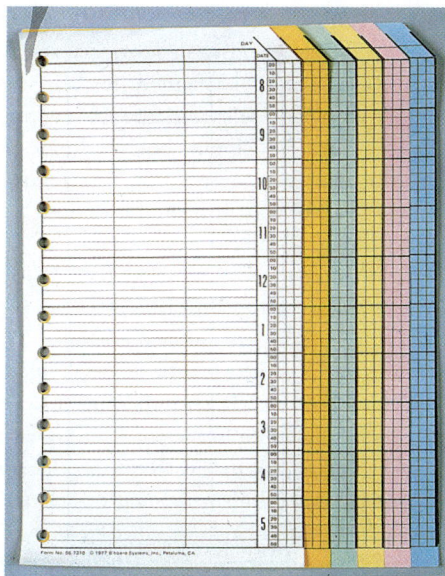

FIGURE 10-2 Color-coded appointment book pages help the medical assistant flip to the right day of the right week quickly. Appointments for multiple physicians can be color-coded in the book.

> ## CRITICAL THINKING APPLICATION 10-2
>
> The software used in Dr. Brown's office can allow patients to self-schedule. Ramona has heard about patient self-scheduling and would like to try this method in her office, but Dr. Brown is concerned that her patients enjoy personal contact and is not sold on the idea.
> - What can Ramona say to convince Dr. Brown to try this new, time-saving method of scheduling?
> - What challenges might the use of this system bring?

ADVANCE PREPARATION

After an appropriate method of setting appointments has been chosen, some advance preparation should be done. This is sometimes called establishing the **matrix** (Procedure 10-1). Block out time slots when the physician routinely is not available to see patients, such as days off, holidays, lunch or dinner breaks, time for hospital rounds, and meetings. In the space where a patient's name normally would appear, note the reason the time is blocked off. Most electronic scheduling software allows the user to create a **template** that can be used repeatedly when new appointment pages are needed. The template can be set to block time slots unavailable for appointments automatically, such as lunch hours and regular meeting times. Always try to account for every time period in each day.

Legality of the Appointment Book

Because the appointment book can be used as a legal record, it must be accurate and maintained so that it provides correct information about the patients at the office. Patients are expected to follow the physician's orders; this includes keeping appointments. If a patient

PROCEDURE 10-1

Manage Appointment Scheduling Using Established Procedures

GOAL: *To establish the matrix of the appointment page and enter information according to office policy.*

EQUIPMENT and SUPPLIES

- Appointment book or computer
- Office procedure manual
- Information about physician's office hours and availability
- Clerical supplies
- Calendar

PROCEDURAL STEPS

1. Determine the proper methods for scheduling an appointment by consulting the office procedure manual; make sure to follow established priorities when managing appointments.
   PURPOSE: To follow prescribed office policy and established priorities for appointment scheduling.

2. Become familiar with any software used for scheduling appointments.
   PURPOSE: To become proficient with the scheduling software used in the office.

3. Determine the hours the physician (or physicians) will not be available.
   PURPOSE: To make sure patients are not scheduled when the physician is unavailable and to prevent rescheduling issues.

4. Make a column in the appointment book or program for each provider.
   PURPOSE: Some medical facilities have multiple providers who maintain a schedule of patients. For example, many physicians employ physician assistants or nurse practitioners who also see patients.

5. Establish the matrix of the appointment book by blocking out the times the physician is unavailable or the office is closed.
   PURPOSE: To leave available only time slots that can be used for patient appointments.

6. Allow buffer time in the morning and afternoon.
   PURPOSE: To allow for emergencies and short rest or catch-up times for the staff and providers.

7. Determine the number of rooms available for patient examinations, treatments, and procedures.
   PURPOSE: The number of available rooms affects the number of patients that can be seen during a day.

8. Establish a list of procedures that details the amount of time needed for an appointment; use established priorities according to the office policy.
   PURPOSE: To better gauge how much time the physician will spend with patients, according to established priorities.

9. Put the appointment book in a convenient place for all employees who schedule appointments.
   PURPOSE: To make sure the appointment book is always readily available.

---

does not show up for an appointment or cancels it and does not reschedule, a notation of this fact should be placed in the patient's medical record. If a patient reschedules an appointment and subsequently keeps it, there is no need to document that it was rescheduled.

Pencil is used in the appointment book so that making changes is easier. The information in the book includes the patient's name and a phone number where the patient can be reached. Some offices list the reason for the appointment, but most note only the name and phone number. The reason for the visit is not necessary if the medical assistant references the time needed for the appointment and blocks off that amount of time. Although the appointment book can be used as a legal record, actual medical records are more likely to be used in matters of litigation. Because progress notes are dated, a copy of the medical record shows all pertinent information about the patient's adherence to the physician's orders, including the appointments with the physician. Pens are permanent, but the book can become illegible if a number of patients change or cancel their appointments. Because the appointment book could be produced in litigation as a legal record, it should be kept for the number of years that constitute the statute of limitations in that individual state. If the appointment book is discarded, its contents should be shredded to protect patient privacy.

TYPES OF APPOINTMENT SCHEDULING

Different types of appointment scheduling are used to meet the various needs of the medical facility, the providers, and the patients. Some offices use a combination of methods to create the right mix of activity during the day and to ensure that the day runs smoothly and efficiently. The medical assistant should become proficient at managing appointments (Procedure 10-2). The following section presents several methods of appointment scheduling.

Open Office Hours

With the open office hours method, the facility is open at given hours of the day or evening, and the patients are "scheduled" by the physician, who mentions to the patient that he or she should return "in a couple of weeks" for follow-up. The patients come in at **intermittent** times, knowing they will be seen in the order of their arrival. Physicians who use this method say that it eliminates the annoyance of broken appointments and an office running behind schedule. The open office hours method also has been called *tidal wave scheduling*. Some of these facilities allow online or telephone check-in, and patients are notified when it is close to their turn with the provider.

Few healthcare facilities in metropolitan areas have open office hours with no scheduled appointments, but this system still is found

PROCEDURE 10-2

Schedule and Monitor Appointments

GOAL: *To manage appointments as they are cancelled, not kept, or rescheduled throughout the business day.*

EQUIPMENT and SUPPLIES

- Appointment book or computer
- Office procedure manual
- Appointment cards
- Clerical supplies
- Telephone

PROCEDURAL STEPS

1. Determine the names of patients who have appointments either the day before or the morning of the appointment.
   PURPOSE: To prepare the medical records for the patients who have appointments.

2. Confirm the appointments if required.
   PURPOSE: To make sure the patient plans to keep the appointment and to provide an opportunity to reschedule or to call in a patient on the waiting list.

3. Make note of any patient arriving late in the appointment book. If this behavior has become a pattern, also note it in the medical record.
   PURPOSE: Repeated behavior that disrupts the clinic schedule should be documented.

4. Document failure to arrive for an appointment in the appointment book or scheduling program and in the patient's medical record.

5. Call the patient to attempt to reschedule the appointment and obtain a reason for the no-show.
   PURPOSE: To document failure to comply with physician's recommendation to return.

6. Reschedule missed appointments, if possible, after talking with the patient.
   PURPOSE: To keep the patient on schedule for medical care.

7. Write the new appointment time, date, and day on an appointment card or give the information to the patient over the telephone.
   PURPOSE: To ensure that the patient is aware of the new appointment time.

8. If the physician is running more than 15 minutes late, inform patients of the delay.
   PURPOSE: To offer the patients the opportunity to reschedule if necessary.

9. As patients arrive, place a check next to the name in the appointment book.

10. Offer the sign-in sheet to the patient for his or her signature.
    PURPOSE: To verify that the patient arrived in the clinic.

---

in some rural areas, where the way of life is governed not so much by the clock as by the needs of the people in the area. Open office hours scheduling is most commonly used at laboratories, imaging facilities, urgent care clinics, and emergency departments. Many emergency departments are open 24 hours a day. Although called *emergency departments,* many of these facilities deal with general practice cases.

The open office hours system can have many disadvantages. The office may already be crowded when the physician arrives, resulting in an extremely long wait for some patients. Patients may arrive in waves throughout the day, which causes parts of the day to be very busy and parts to be slow. This makes getting other office duties accomplished difficult. Without planning, the facilities and staff can be overburdened.

Scheduled Appointments

Studies have shown that practitioners can see more patients with less pressure when their appointments are scheduled. Unfortunately, the skill required for scheduling appointments often is not fully appreciated by the practitioner or office manager, and the responsibility is delegated to the least-qualified medical assistant. An efficient, bright individual proficient at multitasking should be assigned to the scheduling of duties. Although the skill and attitude of the assistant who manages the appointment schedule are very important, the ultimate success of the system lies in the cooperation of the physicians.

Different procedures require different amounts of time; the scheduler must understand how long it takes to draw blood, fill out new patient paperwork, and weigh and check the patient in; all procedures, even the simplest, must have an associated amount of time needed to complete the task. If the patient needs an average of 15 minutes to do new patient paperwork, this time must be included in the schedule. (This is why many offices ask new patients to arrive 15 minutes early for their appointment.) If an allergy shot takes only 20 minutes from check-in to checkout and does not require the patient to see the physician, the scheduler knows that other patients can see the physician while the medical assistant gives the allergy shot. The scheduler cannot efficiently set appointments without developing the skill of accurately assessing how long an office procedure takes.

Flexible Office Hours

Most scheduling practices are carryovers from the days when expectant mothers of families with young children relied on one wage earner. Today families commonly have two working parents. As a result, many healthcare providers are turning to extended day and flexible office hours. Staff hours are affected by these schedules, but this flexibility works to the advantage of the patient and the staff at the physician's office. Patients appreciate flexible office hours, because they can schedule an appointment after work or after children's school hours. Evening and weekend hours may increase the size of the practice because of the convenience offered to patients.

Wave Scheduling

Wave scheduling is an attempt to create short-term flexibility within each hour. Wave scheduling assumes that the actual time needed for all the patients seen will average out over the course of the day. Instead of scheduling patients at each 20-minute **interval**, wave scheduling places three patients in the office at the same time, and they are seen in the order of their arrival. This way, one person's late arrival does not disrupt the entire schedule.

Modified Wave Scheduling

The wave schedule can be modified in several ways. For example, one method is to have two patients scheduled to come in at 10 AM and a third at 10:30 AM. This hourly cycle is repeated throughout the day. In another version, patients are scheduled to arrive at given intervals during the first half of the hour, and none are scheduled to arrive during the second half of the hour.

Double-Booking

Booking two patients to come in at the same time, both of whom are to be seen by the physician, is poor practice. Of course, if each appointment is expected to take only 5 minutes, no harm is done by telling both to come at the same time and reserving a 15-minute period for the two. This is simply one method of wave scheduling. However, if each patient requires 15 minutes, two require 30 minutes. This must be reflected in the scheduling. It is not considered double-booking if a patient comes to the office to receive a treatment by someone other than the physician, such as a patient receiving physical therapy or an antiallergy injection.

Grouping Procedures

Grouping or categorizing of procedures is another method of scheduling that appeals to many practitioners. For instance, an internist might reserve all morning appointments for complete physical examinations, or a pediatrician might keep that time for well-baby visits. A surgeon might devote one day each week to seeing only referral patients. Obstetricians often schedule pregnant patients on different days from gynecology patients. The physician and staff can experiment with different groupings until the plan that works best for the practice eventually becomes evident. In applying a grouping system of appointments, the medical assistant may find it helpful to color-code the sections of the appointment book reserved for designated procedures.

Advance Booking

Often appointments are made months in advance. When any appointment is made, an appointment card should be completed and given to the patient. All appointment cards should mention that patients must give 24 hours' notice if they are unable to keep the time reserved for them. Most offices have some type of confirmation procedure by which patients are called the day before to verify that they intend to keep the appointment.

TIME PATTERNS

When booking appointments, a medical assistant should make it a policy to leave some open time during each day's schedule so that if a patient calls with a special problem that is not an immediate emergency, time will be available to book the patient for at least a brief visit. Mondays and Fridays generally are the most hectic days of the week. Keeping one time slot available in the morning and the afternoon specifically for emergencies also is a wise practice. A busy physician always fills these open slots, and having them in the schedule causes the least **disruption** during the day. If possible, set aside time in the morning and afternoon for a break. Even 15 minutes can give the physician time to return calls from patients, verify prescription calls, or answer questions.

PATIENT WAIT TIME

Be aware of the amount of time the patient sits in the reception area. Ideally, the patient's name is called to go to the examination room precisely at the scheduled appointment time (Figure 10-3). However, the scheduling process has failed if the patient then waits in the back office for 30 minutes to see the physician. Make it clear to the patient whether he or she is free to leave the office after the physician has finished the examination. Some patients mistakenly wait in the examination room until told they are free to leave. Always make sure the patient knows when to go where.

If a patient has waited longer than 15 minutes in the reception area, the medical assistant should briefly explain the delay and offer to reschedule the appointment. The longer patients sit and wait, the more anxious and frustrated they become. Remember, some patients are there to see the physician for test results or may be expecting a negative diagnosis. Do not make their visit more stressful by forcing them to wait for a long time. Briefly explain the situation and allow the patient to decide whether to wait or reschedule. If a delay is forthcoming, attempt to call patients who may be en route to the

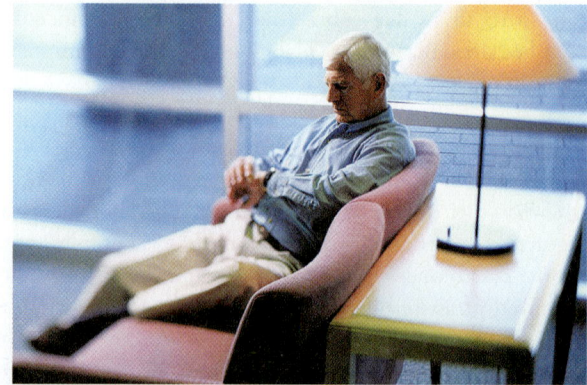

FIGURE 10-3 One of the most common patient complaints is the time spent in the reception area.

office and inform them that there will be a delay. Always ask for the patient's cell phone number for just such events.

CRITICAL THINKING APPLICATION   10-4

Ramona offers to reschedule patient appointments if the schedule ever falls more than 15 minutes behind. If a patient becomes belligerent about the delays, how can Ramona handle the situation in a professional manner?

TELEPHONE SCHEDULING

A pleasant manner and expressing a willingness to help are just as important on the telephone as when meeting patients face to face. This is especially true when making appointments, because the telephone contact may be the patient's first impression of the facility. Often the manner in which the booking is made makes more of an impact than the convenience of the appointment time.

Be especially considerate if the time requested for an appointment must be refused. Briefly explain why the time is not available and offer a substitute date and time. Comply with the patient's desires as much as possible, and do not show annoyance if the patient does not understand the scheduling process. Most people, however, understand the need for a well-managed office and are willing to cooperate.

Many offices offer the patient a choice when scheduling the appointment and let the patient decide which option is best for him or her. For example, the following dialog might take place during the scheduling call:

Medical assistant: *"Mrs. Thomas, Dr. Stern is available to see you in the office next Tuesday or Wednesday, January 6 or 7. Which day is better for you?"*

Patient: *"I will be working on Wednesday, so I would like to come in on Tuesday."*

Medical assistant: *"Do you prefer a morning or afternoon appointment?"*

Patient: *"The afternoon is best for me."*

Medical assistant: *"Great. Would 1:30 or 3:30 be a better time?"*

Patient: *"I can be there at 1:30. "*

Medical assistant: *"Then Dr. Stern will see you at 1:30 next Tuesday, January 6. Thank you for calling, Mrs. Thomas. We'll see you then!"*

These small courtesies give patients the feeling they control their time. Always repeat the time to reinforce the appointment and do not hesitate to ask the patient if he or she has a pen with which to jot down the time and date. While repeating the information to the patient, check the appointment book or computer screen to ensure that it was posted correctly.

Write legibly when using an appointment book. These records could be called into court, and the medical assistant must be able to read his or her own writing if asked to testify. Form the habit of entering the patient's daytime telephone number after every entry. The appointment may need to be canceled or the schedule rearranged in a hurry, and many precious minutes can be saved if

the telephone number is handy. Cell phone numbers also are quite useful for tracking down a patient quickly.

SCHEDULING APPOINTMENTS FOR NEW PATIENTS

Arranging the first appointment for a new patient requires time and attention to detail (Procedure 10-3). This first encounter provides the first impression of the office and may set the tone for all subsequent visits. Tact, courtesy, and professionalism are extremely important. During the conversation with the new patient, request preliminary information to help determine how much time to allot for the visit on the appointment schedule. The physician may also expect the medical assistant to give general instructions to patients seeking care for specific complaints. For example, the patient may be required to bring a urine specimen or to make sure laboratory tests are completed before the appointment. Some offices obtain enough information to build a patient medical record before the office visit; others wait until the patient actually arrives to construct the medical record.

After the necessary information has been recorded, offer the patient the first available appointment. Whenever possible, offer a choice between two dates and times. Ask the patient whether he or she knows the directions to the office or offer the physical address for those who want to obtain exact directions from one of the many Internet directions sites, such as MapQuest. Tell the patient whether any special parking conveniences are available and whether the office provides a token or parking validation. The patient's options for the first payment should also be discussed. If payment is expected immediately, inform the patient. The office staff should expect patient concerns about the amount of the first bill and should address this issue before the appointment so that there are no surprises or misunderstandings. Before ending the conversation, repeat the appointment date and time and then thank the patient for calling.

Some medical offices mail an information packet about their facility to new patients, especially if the appointment is several days away. With today's technology and the patient's e-mail address, such information can also be sent via the Internet. This information should inform the patient about the nature of the practice, introduce the medical staff, and explain appointment policies and financial arrangements.

If another physician has referred the patient, the medical assistant may need to call the referring physician's office to obtain additional information before the patient's appointment. This information should be printed out and given to the attending physician before the patient arrives. Remember to send a thank you note to anyone who refers a patient to the facility.

Many offices call each patient the day before the appointment as a reminder and a courtesy. This can be a time-consuming procedure, but most patients appreciate this service, and it may open appointments for others if the original patient cannot keep the scheduled time slot. E-mail and automatic dialers also can be programmed to call or send electronic reminders to patients about their appointments. This procedure can run automatically if the office has access to the proper equipment, which takes no time away from the medical assistant's other duties. Often, the medical assistant will need to conduct **preauthorization** or **precertification** to determine whether a patient is eligible for treatment or for certain procedures. The office

PROCEDURE 10-3

Schedule Appointments for New Patients

GOAL: *To schedule a new patient for a first office visit.*

EQUIPMENT and SUPPLIES

- Appointment book or computer
- Scheduling guidelines
- Appointment card
- Telephone

PROCEDURAL STEPS

1. Obtain the patient's full name, birth date, address, and telephone number.
   NOTE: Verify the spelling of the name.
2. Determine whether the patient was referred by another physician.
   PURPOSE: You may need to request additional information from the referring physician, and your physician will want to send a consultation report.
3. Determine the patient's chief complaint and when the first symptoms occurred.
   PURPOSE: To help gauge the time needed for the appointment and the degree of urgency.
4. Search the appointment book for the first suitable appointment time and an alternate time.

5. Offer the patient a choice of these dates and times to demonstrate sensitivity appropriate to the message being delivered.
   PURPOSE: Patients are better satisfied if they are given a choice.
6. Enter the mutually agreeable time in the appointment book, followed by the patient's telephone number.
   NOTE: Indicate that the patient is new by adding the letters NP.
7. If new patients are expected to pay at the time of the visit, explain this financial arrangement when the appointment is made.
   PURPOSE: The payment policy is explained to the patient, who can come prepared to pay.
8. Offer travel directions for reaching the office as well as parking instructions. E-mail or mail new patient paperwork.
   PURPOSE: To relieve any anxiety about being able to find the medical facility.
9. Analyze communications in providing appropriate responses and feedback by repeating the day, date, and time of the appointment before saying goodbye to the patient.
   PURPOSE: To verify that the patient understands the date and time of the appointment.

---

manager must make certain that these procedures are being done and assign these duties to a specific person(s). More about preauthorization and precertification is included in Chapter 20.

SCHEDULING APPOINTMENTS FOR ESTABLISHED PATIENTS

In Person

Most return appointments for **established patients** are arranged when the patient is leaving the office. A good policy is to have all patients stop by the front desk before leaving in case any information is needed from the patient or any outside scheduling must be done. The patient's medical record can be reviewed to see whether the physician ordered any laboratory tests or procedures, and these can be scheduled and discussed with the patient. When making a return appointment, follow the same procedures as for scheduling any appointment by phone, offering the patient choices in the day and time slots (Procedure 10-4). If a certain time the patient specifically requests is not available, offer two alternatives. Always give the patient an appointment card and any necessary instructions at this time, along with a bright smile (Procedure 10-5). Never forget to provide excellent customer service.

By Telephone

Usually the medical assistant needs only to determine when the patient must return and to find a suitable time in the schedule.

Established patients do not usually need directions and parking information unless the office has recently moved. If some time has passed since the patient's last visit, recheck certain information and enter any changes on the patient's medical record. Be sure to ask whether insurance companies or benefits have changed; also, verifying the patient's address and phone numbers is always a good idea. If an e-mail address is not on file, obtain one so as to have a quick, easy way to notify the patient of appointments and other events.

SCHEDULING OTHER TYPES OF APPOINTMENTS

The medical assistant also will make other types of appointments, and these will appear on the appointment schedule. They include surgeries the physician will perform at a hospital or other facility, hospital rounds and consultations, outside appointments and meetings, and even house calls if the physician makes them. The physician also must have time to get from one location to another, so driving time must be considered when arranging all appointments.

Some critical information is required when scheduling admission or treatments in other facilities. Always provide the scheduler with the patient's name, address, phone numbers (both home and cell), Social Security number, and insurance information and relay the procedures that are to be performed. Patient allergies should be mentioned if the patient is being admitted. Additionally, the facility may have forms that the patient needs to complete, so an e-mail address is helpful in such cases. Always send the admitting diagnosis and orders to the healthcare facility prior to admission time or with

PROCEDURE 10-4

Schedule Appointments for Established Patients or Visitors

GOAL: *To schedule a general appointment either by telephone or in person.*

EQUIPMENT and SUPPLIES

- Appointment book or computer
- Office procedure manual
- Clerical supplies
- Appointment cards
- Telephone

PROCEDURAL STEPS

1. Learn the proper methods for scheduling an appointment by consulting the office procedure manual.
   PURPOSE: To follow prescribed office policy for appointment scheduling.
2. Ask the name of the person wanting to make the appointment and obtain his or her phone number.
   PURPOSE: To be able to speak professionally with the individual and to identify the person in the patient database, if applicable. Ask for the phone number in case the line is disconnected or the appointment needs to be changed.
   SAY: *"To whom am I speaking, please?"*
3. Ask the reason for making the appointment.
   PURPOSE: To determine the time needed for the appointment.
   SAY: *"What is the reason for making this appointment?"*
4. Determine for whom the appointment is being made, if necessary.
   PURPOSE: To schedule the individual with the right provider or person.
   SAY: *"Mr. Adams, would you like to see Dr. Blake, or would you like to see our nurse practitioner, Mrs. Jackson?"*
5. Analyze communications in providing appropriate responses and feedback by giving the person a choice between 2 days of the week.
   PURPOSE: To allow the individual to choose a convenient time; this reduces the number of missed appointments. If the suggested days are not satisfactory, allow the person to suggest an alternate day.
   SAY: *"Would you prefer to come on Monday or Tuesday, Mr. Adams?"*

6. Give the person a choice between a morning or an afternoon appointment.
   PURPOSE: To allow the individual to choose a convenient time of day.
   SAY: *"Would morning or afternoon be better for you?"*
7. Give the person a choice between two specific times.
   PURPOSE: To allow the individual to choose the best time for his or her needs.
   SAY: *"Mr. Adams, would you prefer 9 AM or 11 AM?"*
8. Write the person's name and the phone number on the appropriate line of the appointment book or enter this information into the scheduling system.
   PURPOSE: To document the appointment and ensure that the time is reserved.
9. Analyze communications in providing appropriate responses and feedback by repeating the appointment day, date, and time back to the person.
   PURPOSE: Repeating the appointment time reduces errors and misunderstandings.
   SAY: *"I have you scheduled for 9 AM on Tuesday, March 14, Mr. Adams. If you are not able to keep your appointment, please let us know."*
10. If the person scheduling the appointment is in the office instead of on the phone, give the individual an appointment card.
    PURPOSE: Providing appointment cards reduces the number of missed appointments.

the patient. Some facilities require a history form prior to admission. The patient will be required to bring a form of picture identification, such as a state driver's license, and his or her insurance card.

Inpatient Surgeries

When scheduling a surgery, call the facility where the procedure will be performed as soon as the operation is planned. Most surgical departments and centers have a surgical secretary who makes these arrangements. Provide all necessary information and state any special requests the physician may have, such as the amount of blood to have available for the patient. The secretary may want all the patient's insurance information and certainly will want a phone number so that the patient can be contacted before the surgery if necessary. Make sure all this information is handy before placing the call.

Outpatient and Inpatient Procedure Appointments

A medical assistant often is asked to arrange laboratory or radiography appointments for patients. Before calling the facility to schedule the appointment, be sure all necessary information is handy. When the patient is informed of the time and place of the appointment, relay any special instructions, then note these arrangements in the patient's medical record. Some offices make a reminder call to the patient or send a reminder e-mail message.

Outpatient testing is common, because most physicians do not have extensive x-ray or laboratory equipment in their offices. Magnetic resonance imaging (MRI), computed tomography (CT) scans, numerous x-ray evaluations, ultrasonography, and simple blood tests all may need to be scheduled (Procedure 10-6). Provide the patient

PROCEDURE 10-5

Document Appropriately and Accurately

GOAL: *To document appropriately and accurately on all patient medical records and other office paperwork that concerns the patient.*

EQUIPMENT and SUPPLIES

- Any medical document
- Clerical supplies
- Computer or word processor
- Office policy and procedure manual

PROCEDURAL STEPS

1. Determine the information that needs to be added to the patient's medical record, appointment book, telephone message, or other office paperwork that concerns the patient.
   PURPOSE: To place pertinent, accurate information into the document.
2. Make sure the information is factual, timely, and accurate.
   PURPOSE: To ensure that the information is usable.
3. Document accurately in the medical record by writing or typing the information into the document.
4. Reread the information to make sure it is legible.
   PURPOSE: To be sure the information can be read even after several years by anyone who needs to access the information.
5. Date and sign the entry if necessary.
   PURPOSE: To authenticate the entry.

6. Make sure the entry meets any local, state, or federal guidelines that may apply to the information contained in the document.
   PURPOSE: To remain in compliance with local, state, and federal rules and regulations.
7. Make sure the entry is written in compliance with office policies and procedures.
   PURPOSE: To comply with office policy.
8. If the entry needs to be corrected, draw one line through it and make the new entry below or in the required place in the document.
   PURPOSE: To correct the document according to office policy and procedure guidelines.
9. Make sure the correction has not obliterated any part of the medical record or documentation that affects the patient.
   PURPOSE: No obliteration is acceptable in any part of the medical record.
10. Place the date and initial the corrected entry.
    PURPOSE: To authenticate the correction.

PROCEDURE 10-6

Schedule Outpatient Admissions and Procedures

GOAL: *To schedule a patient for outpatient admission or procedure within the time frame needed by the physician, confirm with the patient, and issue all required instructions.*

EQUIPMENT and SUPPLIES

- Diagnostic test order from physician
- Name, address, and telephone number of diagnostic facility
- Patient's demographic information
- Patient's medical record
- Test preparation instructions
- Telephone
- Consent form

PROCEDURAL STEPS

1. Obtain an oral or written order from the physician for the exact procedure to be performed.
   PURPOSE: To have a documented order for the procedure to be performed
2. Precertify the procedure with the patient's insurance company if necessary.
   PURPOSE: To make sure expected insurance benefits are valid and the procedure will be covered by the patient's insurance policy.

3. Determine the physician's and patient's availability.
   PURPOSE: To make sure the patient will be able to comply with the arrangements for the test and that the physician is available, if he or she must be present for the procedure. The urgency of the needed test results affects the time and date of the appointment needed.
4. Telephone the diagnostic facility and schedule the patient's procedure or test.
   - Order the specific test.
   - Provide the patient's diagnosis and orders.
   - Establish the date and time for the procedure.
   - Give the patient's name, age, address, and telephone number.
   - Provide the patient's demographic information, including identification and insurance policy numbers and addresses for filing claims.
   - Determine any special instructions for the patient or special anesthesia requirements.
   - Notify the facility of any urgency for test results.

PURPOSE: To schedule the procedure or admission and provide needed information.

5. Notify the patient of the arrangements:
   • Give the name, address, and telephone number of the diagnostic facility.
   • Specify the date and time to report for the test.
   • Give instructions on preparation for the test (e.g., eating restrictions, fluids, medications, enemas).
   • Explain any preadmission testing.
   • Remind the patient to take a form of picture identification and the insurance card.
   • Explain whether the patient needs to pick up orders or whether they will be forwarded to the facility in advance.
   • Ask the patient to repeat the instructions.

   PURPOSE: To make sure the patient understands the necessary preparations and the importance of keeping the appointment. If time permits, provide written instructions to the patient.

6. Have the physician review the consent form with the patient. The patient should sign the consent form, and a copy should be placed in the medical record. Note the arrangements on the patient's medical record.

   PURPOSE: To make sure the patient understands the risks, benefits, and alternatives to the procedure. To ensure follow-up on the diagnosis and/or treatment.

7. Implement time management principles to maintain effective office function by placing a reminder on the physician's tickler or desk calendar. Make sure the information is listed on the office schedule. Check the patient's postsurgical status. Follow up if results are not received in a timely manner.

   PURPOSE: To check whether the appointment was kept and a report was received from the testing facility.

---

with the name, address, and phone number of the facility where the tests will be done.

Some patients may require a series of appointments (e.g., at weekly intervals). Try to set up these appointments on the same day each week at the same time of day. This considerably reduces the risk of the patient forgetting an appointment.

In some cases the medical assistant may be responsible for scheduling inpatient admissions or inpatient surgical procedures (Procedures 10-7 and 10-8). This is similar to scheduling outpatient testing, but the medical assistant coordinates with a hospital rather than an outside facility.

Outside Visits

If the physician regularly makes house calls or visits patients in skilled nursing facilities, a special block of time must be reserved in the appointment schedule. The physician needs demographic information, such as addresses, room numbers, and the best route to each home or facility. Remember to allow for travel time. Most physicians do not make house calls, because seeing patients in the office is easier; however, such visits may be necessary in certain situations. The physician's medical bag should always be prepared and well stocked before he or she has to make any outside visits.

SPECIAL CIRCUMSTANCES

Late Patients

Probably every medical practice has a few patients who are habitually late for appointments. This seems to be a problem for which no cure has been found. Emergencies and small delays can happen to anyone, but a patient who constantly arrives late can put a strain on the practice. Such patients can be booked as the last appointment of the day. Then, if closing time arrives before the patient does, the staff

has no obligation to wait. Some medical assistants tell the patient to come in 30 minutes before the appointment time actually scheduled. Make an attempt to work with patients who have occasional difficulties arriving on time, but do not allow the schedule to be constantly disrupted by late patients.

> **CRITICAL THINKING APPLICATION   10-5**
> Seth Jones is always late for his appointments. How might Ramona approach him about this? What can Ramona do to assist Mr. Jones in arriving for appointments on time?

Rescheduling Canceled Appointments

Changes sometimes must be made in the appointment schedule. Unexpected conflicts might arise that force a patient to change the appointment time. When rescheduling an appointment, make sure the first appointment day and time is removed from the appointment book or database, then set the new appointment. Otherwise, the patient will be expected in the office on 2 days, and time will be wasted with calls and follow-up, only to discover that the appointment was rescheduled.

Emergency Calls

Periodically, emergency or urgent calls come into the office, and an appointment needs to be scheduled. To some extent, all calls that come in go through a **screening** process, and emergencies are prioritized to evaluate the urgency of the need to see the physician. Screening is an extremely important function that requires experience, a knowledge of signs and symptoms, and tact.

Emergencies may involve emotional crises in addition to the more obvious physical problems. Patients with emergencies and those who are acutely ill should be seen the same day. The urgency

PROCEDURE 10-7

Schedule Inpatient Admissions

GOAL: *To schedule a patient for inpatient admission within the time frame needed by the physician, confirm with the patient, and issue all required instructions.*

EQUIPMENT and SUPPLIES

- Admission orders from physician
- Name, address, and telephone number of inpatient facility
- Patient's demographic information
- Patient's medical record
- Any preparation instructions for the patient
- Telephone
- Admission packet

PROCEDURAL STEPS

1. Obtain an oral or written order from the physician for the admission.
   <u>PURPOSE:</u> To have a documented order for the admission.
2. Precertify the admission with the patient's insurance company if necessary.
   <u>PURPOSE:</u> To make sure expected insurance benefits are valid and the admission will be covered by the patient's insurance policy.
3. Determine the physician's and patient's availability if the admission is not an emergency.
   <u>PURPOSE:</u> To make sure the patient will be able to comply with the arrangements for the admission and that the physician is available to care for the patient during the admission. The urgency of the admission affects the time and date of the appointment needed.
4. Telephone the diagnostic facility and schedule the patient's admission.
   - Order any specific tests needed.
   - Provide the patient's admitting diagnosis.
   - Establish the date and time.
   - State the patient's room preferences.
   - Give the patient's name, age, address, and telephone number.

- Provide the patient's demographic information, including identification and insurance policy numbers and addresses for filing claims.
- Determine any special instructions for the patient.
- Notify the facility of any urgency for test results.
   <u>PURPOSE:</u> To schedule the admission and provide needed information.
5. Notify the patient of the arrangements:
   - Give the facility's name, address, and telephone number.
   - Specify the date and time to report for admission.
   - Provide any necessary instructions on preparation for the procedure (e.g., eating restrictions, fluids, medications, enemas).
   - Outline any preadmission testing.
   - Ask the patient to repeat the instructions.
   <u>PURPOSE:</u> To make sure the patient understands the preparation necessary and the importance of admittance. If it is the office policy, give the patient an admission packet that contains the orders and basic instructions for the admission.
6. Note the arrangements and the admission on the patient's medical record.
   <u>PURPOSE:</u> To ensure follow-up on the diagnosis and/or treatment.
7. Implement time management principles to maintain effective office function by placing a reminder on the physician's tickler or desk calendar. Make sure the information is listed on the office schedule. If the physician keeps a list of all inpatients, add the patient's name to that list.
   <u>PURPOSE:</u> To keep a record of the number of days the patient was seen in the hospital by the physician during rounds for insurance billing purposes.

PROCEDURE 10-8

Schedule Inpatient Procedures

GOAL: *To schedule a patient for inpatient surgery within the time frame needed by the physician, confirm with the patient, and issue all required instructions.*

EQUIPMENT and SUPPLIES

- Orders from the physician
- Inpatient facility's name, address, and telephone number
- Patient's demographic information
- Patient's medical record
- Any preparation instructions for the patient
- Telephone
- Consent form

PROCEDURAL STEPS

1. Obtain an oral or written order from the physician for the admission.
   <u>PURPOSE:</u> To have a documented order for the admission.
2. Precertify the admission with the patient's insurance company if necessary.
   <u>PURPOSE:</u> To make sure expected insurance benefits are valid and the admission will be covered by the patient's insurance policy.

PROCEDURE 10-8—cont'd

3. Determine the physician's availability if the surgery is not an emergency. Another physician may be the surgeon. If so, the surgery also must be coordinated with that office.
   PURPOSE: To make sure the physician is available to care for the patient during the admission and the surgery. The urgency of the surgery affects the time and date of the appointment needed.

4. Telephone the hospital surgical department and schedule the patient's procedure.
   - Order any specific tests needed.
   - Provide the patient's admitting diagnosis.
   - Establish the date and time.
   - Give the patient's name, age, address, and telephone number.
   - Provide the patient's demographic information, including identification and insurance policy numbers and addresses for filing claims.
   - Determine any special instructions for the patient.
   - Notify the facility of any urgency for the surgery.
   PURPOSE: To schedule the surgery and provide the facility with the needed information.

5. If the patient has not already been admitted to the hospital, notify him or her of the arrangements:
   - Give the facility's name, address, and telephone number.
   - Specify the date and time to report for admission.
   - Provide any necessary instructions on preparation for the procedure (e.g., eating restrictions, fluids, medications, enemas).
   - Explain any preadmission testing.
   - Ask the patient to repeat the instructions.
   PURPOSE: To make sure the patient understands the preparation necessary and the importance of surgery. If it is the office policy, give the patient an admission packet that contains the orders and basic instructions for the surgery.

6. The physician should review the consent form with the patient. Have the patient sign a consent for the surgical procedure. Keep the original consent in the patient's medical record and give the patient a copy.
   PURPOSE: To ensure that the patient understands the risks, benefits, and alternatives to the surgical procedure.

7. Note the arrangements on the patient's medical record.
   PURPOSE: To ensure follow-up on the diagnosis and/or treatment.

8. Implement time management principles to maintain effective office function by placing a reminder on the physician's tickler or desk calendar. Be sure the information is listed on the office schedule. If the physician keeps a list of all inpatients, add the patient's name to that list. After the procedure, follow up with the hospital on the patient's condition as required by the physician.
   PURPOSE: To check on the patient's status and keep a record of the number of days the patient was seen in the hospital by the physician during rounds for insurance billing purposes.

---

of the call initially can be determined by having a list of questions prepared for reference. The physician should help with this list; he or she should determine what is considered an emergency (life-threatening) or urgent (serious but not life-threatening). The patient may need to be referred directly to a hospital emergency department, or the physician may want to see the patient that day in the office. Remember to keep the patient on the phone until emergency medical technicians (EMTs) or other help arrives at the patient's location. Never place an emergency call on hold. Always obtain the name, phone number, and location at the start of the call so that the patient can be found if he or she loses consciousness or is disconnected.

Physician Referrals

If another physician telephones and requests that a patient be seen today, most offices honor that request if at all possible. It is important to keep a schedule that is not intolerant of this type of request.

Patients Without Appointments

The physician must agree to a policy for patients without appointments, and the medical assistants must carry it out. A patient who requires immediate attention most likely will be accommodated in the schedule somehow. If the patient does not need immediate care, a brief visit with the physician and a scheduled appointment at a later time may be the answer. Also, the medical assistant may simply have to turn down the request. Follow established office policy.

▌FAILED APPOINTMENTS

Why do patients fail to keep appointments? Some are simply forgetful. Once this tendency is detected in a patient, form the habit of telephoning or e-mailing a reminder the day before the appointment. **Automated call routing** offers the patient the option of canceling an appointment and can be programmed to keep calling until the patient responds and confirms or cancels the appointment.

A patient who has been pressed for payment may stay away because of an inability to pay for medical services. Do not make the mistake of classifying all such patients as "deadbeats." Many have every desire to pay, but they cannot afford to and feel embarrassed about their situation, so they avoid their appointments.

Patients also may fail to keep appointments because they are in a state of denial about their condition. For instance, if a patient recently tested positive for the human immunodeficiency virus (HIV), he or she may avoid appointments because going to see the physician forces the patient to face the reality of the disease. Take special care with such patients, and if denial is suspected, discuss this with the physician, who may want to refer the patient for counseling.

It is important to determine the reason for failed appointments and to do whatever is possible to remedy the situation. Telephone the patient to make sure no misunderstanding has occurred. If the patient's health is such that medical care must continue, write a letter and explain this to the patient. Send the letter by certified mail with return receipt requested. Keep the letter in the patient's medical record for legal protection.

NO-SHOW POLICY

Some patients may not realize the importance of keeping their appointments. The patient who does not arrive for a scheduled appointment or reschedule it is called a **no-show**. A busy practice must have a very specific policy on appointment no-shows and must enforce it effectively. The first time a patient fails to show, note the fact on the medical record and/or ledger card. The second time, warn the patient, and if a third no-show occurs, consider dropping the patient by using the customary methods that provide legal protection for the physician.

The physician may wish to charge patients for not showing up or for rescheduling the appointment. Be understanding whenever possible, but do not let a patient take advantage of the physician's time. The office policy manual must state that patients may be charged for missed appointments, especially if the time slot could not be filled with another patient. Because the time slot was scheduled and the physician was ready and available to treat the patient, it is ethical to charge the patient for missing an appointment, especially if he or she did not call to cancel or reschedule. Many physicians do not press this issue, but it is an available tool if needed.

Recording the Failed Appointment

When a patient fails to keep an appointment, a notation should be made in the patient's medical record and in the appointment book or database. If the patient is seriously ill, the physician should also be told about the failure to show.

INCREASING APPOINTMENT SHOW RATES

Everyone benefits from a full schedule of kept appointments. Appointment show rates can be increased in several ways.

Automated Call Routing

As mentioned earlier, automated call reminders can contact patients scheduled for appointments. The patient is asked to press a certain key on the phone to confirm the appointment and a different key to cancel the appointment. This same tool can be used to send messages to patients (e.g., a reminder that it is the time of year to get a flu vaccination), to introduce a new physician at the office, or announce the availability of a new procedure. The call can even be recorded by the physician so that it sounds more personal.

Appointment Cards

Most healthcare facilities use appointment cards to remind patients of scheduled appointments and to eliminate misunderstandings about dates and times (Figure 10-4). Make a habit of reaching for an appointment card while writing an entry in the appointment book. After the date and time have been written on the card, double-check with the book to make sure the entries agree.

Confirmation Calls

Patients who have made appointments in advance may appreciate a confirmation call to remind them they have a time set aside to see the physician. Always note the phone number the patient prefers the office to use for such calls. Many individuals now have home phone, cell phone, and work phone numbers; however, they may want calls from the physician to go only to their home phone. The preferred phone number can be highlighted in the medical record or on the computer. The office must use caution in making calls to patients because of the significance of privacy guidelines and standards. Some offices may want to prepare a release form in which the patient grants the office staff permission to contact the patient. Many physicians insist that messages left on voice mail not mention the term "doctor" or "doctor's office" for confidentiality reasons. The medical assistant might say, "This is Pam at Robert Welch's office confirming your appointment tomorrow at 2 PM. Please call us if you cannot make the appointment. Our number is 555-212-0909. Thank you!"

If the patient has signed the privacy policy and the policy states that messages from the physician's office may be left at certain numbers, the office certainly can leave messages at that number and mention that the call is from the physician's office. Still, it is a good idea to have an established policy on leaving messages that does not breach any patient's confidentiality.

E-Mail Reminders

Many computer scheduling programs can send an e-mail to patients the day before an appointment to remind them of it. This is a great timesaver for the office staff, because no time is taken to perform this duty other than the original scheduling of the appointment.

Mailed Reminders

The office staff may mail reminder cards to patients. This method is a bit time-consuming but worth the effort if the patients show up for their appointments.

A patient who is due for an appointment but has not yet arranged a date and time may be sent a reminder. A simple way of handling this is to have a supply of postcards on hand, and while patients are still in the office, have them write their name and address on the postcard. Then place the card in a tickler file under the date it is to be mailed.

HANDLING CANCELLATIONS AND DELAYS

When the Patient Cancels

Inevitably, cancellations occur. If a list is kept of patients with advance appointments who would like to come in sooner, the medical assistant can begin calling to try to get one of them in to fill the available opening. By keeping a list of patients willing to take the first cancelled appointment, the medical assistant can readily identify which patients to call to fill the vacancy. Each cancellation should be noted in the medical record, along with a reason for the cancellation if that information is available. If the patient simply reschedules an appointment, a notation need not be made in the medical record unless a pattern develops that might be significant to the patient's medical treatment.

When the Physician is Delayed

Some days the physician will be delayed in reaching the office. If advance notice of the delay is received, start calling patients with

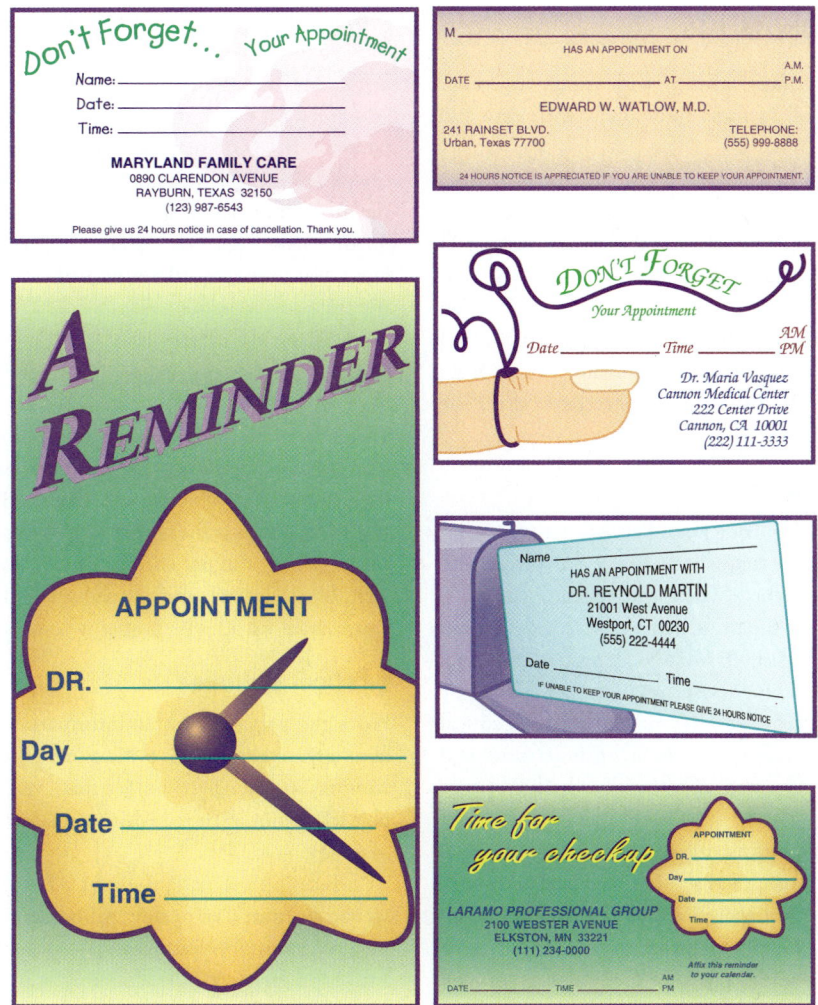

FIGURE 10-4 Examples of appointment cards.

early appointments and suggest that they come later. If some patients arrive before the office learns of the delay, explain that an emergency has detained the physician.

Show concern for the patient, but do not be overly apologetic, which might imply some degree of guilt. Most patients realize that a physician has certain priorities. The patient in the office may be inconvenienced, but it is not a "life or death" matter. If this kind of situation occurs frequently, however, consider devising a different scheduling system.

When the Physician Is Called to an Emergency

Physicians are conscious of their responsibilities for responding to medical emergencies, and most patients are understanding if the medical assistant takes time to explain what has happened. The medical assistant may say, "Dr. Wright has been called away to answer an emergency. She asked me to tell you she is very sorry to keep you waiting. There will be at least a 1-hour delay." The medical assistant should then ask the patient, "Do you want to wait? If that is inconvenient, I'll be glad to give you the first available appointment on another day. Or perhaps you'd like to have some coffee or do some shopping and return in an hour."

As quickly as possible, call the patients scheduled for a later hour. In many offices, especially those of obstetricians, surgeons, and general practitioners, a whole day's appointments sometimes must be cancelled. For this reason, it is particularly important to have the daytime telephone number of each patient available so that the appointment can be rescheduled. If at all possible, cancel appointments before the patient arrives in the office to find that the physician is not available. The **expediency** of the office staff in contacting patients who will be affected by an emergency is most appreciated.

When the Physician Is Ill or Out of Town

Physicians get ill, too, and patients scheduled to be seen during the course of the physician's recovery must be informed of this. They need not be told the nature of the illness.

When the physician is called out of town for personal or professional reasons, appointments must be canceled or rescheduled. Customarily, the patient is given the name of another physician, or possibly a choice of several, who will provide care during such absences. For security reasons, merely state that the doctor is unavailable. Stating over the telephone that the physician is out of town could lead to attempted burglary or other unauthorized intrusion on the premises.

OTHER TYPES OF APPOINTMENTS

The physician will need to meet with a wide range of other unscheduled callers. Handle all of these individuals with care and courtesy.

Physicians

Another physician dropping into the facility should be ushered in to see the physician as soon as possible, regardless of the appointment schedule. If the physician is seeing a patient, explain the situation and, if possible, take the visiting physician into a private room to wait. Then notify the physician as soon as possible. Visits from other physicians are usually brief and do not appreciably affect the schedule.

Pharmaceutical Representatives

Also known as *detail persons* or *reps,* representatives from pharmaceutical companies are frequent visitors to physicians' offices and generally are welcomed when the schedule permits. They are well trained and bring the physician valuable information on new drugs. The medical assistant often is expected to screen such visitors and turn away those whose products would not be used in that practice. If the representative or the pharmaceutical company is unknown to the office, ask for a business card and then check with the physician, who will decide whether to see the caller.

Specialists usually limit their conferences with pharmaceutical representatives to their line of practice. The medical assistant, together with the physician, can prepare a list of the representatives with whom the physician is willing to spend time; the list is the determining factor in future conferences. The medical assistant can say whether the physician will be available that day and give an estimate of the waiting time or suggest a later time at which the caller may return. The caller then can decide whether to wait or return later. The pharmaceutical representative usually is quite understanding and cooperative and willing to wait patiently a long while for just a brief visit with the physician. In turn, the medical assistant should treat the representative with courtesy, showing as much cooperation as possible.

Salespeople

Salespeople from medical, surgical, and office supply houses call regularly at physicians' offices. Sometimes they want to see the physician, but the office manager or the medical assistant in charge of ordering supplies usually can handle these calls.

Unsolicited salespeople sometimes can present a problem in the professional office. If the physician does not want to see such callers, the medical assistant must firmly but tactfully send them away. Suggest that they leave their literature and cards for the physician to study and say that the physician will contact them if further information is desired.

PLANNING FOR THE NEXT DAY

Before leaving at the end of the day, look over the appointments scheduled for the next day. Review the medical records for scheduled patients. If laboratory tests or other procedures were scheduled on the patient's last visit, determine whether the reports are available in the medical record. If the patient is scheduled for specific procedures on this visit, make sure everything needed for the procedure is on hand and available. Planning can save many precious moments at the time of the patient visit.

CLOSING COMMENTS

The person charged with the responsibility of scheduling appointments has a huge impact on the efficiency of the medical office. A friendly, helpful attitude is a **prerequisite** for cordial **interaction** with patients, as is the ability to make compromises that benefit both the physician and patient. An office that runs smoothly and stays on schedule indicates professionalism and competence and is greatly appreciated by all who come in contact with it.

Patient Education

Providing patients with an information booklet about the office can familiarize them with policies and procedures. Many physicians compile an extensive booklet that even provides tips as to when the physician should be called immediately, listing symptoms and signs of emergencies.

Educating the patient about office policies helps the facility run smoothly from day to day. All patients should be familiar with the policies about appointments. This leads to fewer misunderstandings and conflicts over bills that might include a charge for a missed appointment.

If the facility offers Internet-based appointment scheduling, patients must be taught how to use the system. A printed pamphlet or information sheet is helpful for providing instructions to the patient. A wise option is to have a special phone number patients can call if they have problems with the scheduling system. For best results, choose a program that is simple to use, easy to understand, and does not breach patient confidentiality.

Legal and Ethical Issues

The appointment schedule may be used as a legal record and could be brought by subpoena into a court of law. Make sure all handwriting in the book is completely legible and that information is routinely collected in a consistent manner for each entry. Do not fail to note a no-show both in the patient's medical record and the appointment schedule. This often is helpful when a physician must prove that the patient did not follow medical advice or that the patient contributed to his or her poor condition by missing appointments. Old appointment schedules should be kept for a time equal to that of the statute of limitations in the state where the practice is located.

SUMMARY OF SCENARIO

Ramona is an asset to the medical office, because her dedication and customer service skills help her interact with patients in a positive way. She genuinely cares about the patients and makes every effort to meet their needs while following Dr. Brown's preferences. She has found that her bright smile is a valuable aid when patients have been waiting and are growing restless.

Ramona cooperates with other staff members to get the patients seen as quickly as possible and to minimize wait time. She is flexible and can change the order of the patients seen, if needed, to maximize the use of time and facilities in the office. Because she is so cheerful and friendly, patients do not seem to mind when she asks for their cooperation. She keeps current phone numbers and cell phone information so that she can notify a patient quickly if Dr. Brown is running behind schedule. Ramona's proficiency on the computer also is an asset, and she makes frequent use of e-mail to take care of patient problems or rescheduling requests.

Because of the cooperation she receives from staff and patients alike, Ramona successfully runs an efficient office. She contributes to that efficiency by constantly refining her knowledge about her job. She pays attention to the times during the day that do not run as smoothly as others, evaluates the problems at those times, and then corrects them. Ramona also keeps the schedule moving by communicating with the clinical medical assistants, keeping them informed about arriving patients and those who have come early or are running late. She can quickly adjust and substitute a patient who already has arrived. Ramona has learned how to manipulate the schedule to accommodate an emergency. She knows that by making minor adjustments and keeping the waiting patients informed, the staff can handle any emergency.

All medical assistants need to develop skills in flexibility. Establishing a system that works, and using it correctly, makes patients and staff members more content with their experience in the physician's office.

SUMMARY OF LEARNING OBJECTIVES

1. **Define, spell, and pronounce the terms listed in the vocabulary.**
   Spelling and pronouncing medical terms correctly bolster the medical assistant's credibility. Knowing the definition of these terms promotes confidence in communication with patients and co-workers.

2. **Describe scheduling guidelines.**
   When appointments are scheduled, a medical assistant must consider (1) the patients' needs, (2) the physician's preferences, and (3) the available facilities. Make every attempt to schedule a patient at his or her most convenient time; this helps prevent no-shows. The physician will outline his or her preferences, which should be a high priority to the medical assistant. However, most physicians are flexible and make adjustments according to the needs of the office. The availability of facilities in the office is perhaps the most inflexible factor. If a certain room or piece of equipment is being used for one patient, it usually cannot be used for another.

3. **Discuss the advantages of computerized appointment scheduling.**
   Computerized scheduling programs are in demand, because they are easy to operate and simplify both the scheduling and changing of appointments. The computer can find the first available time much faster than a person scanning an appointment book. Most programs can prepare reports and even notify patients of the impending appointment automatically by e-mail. Web-based self-scheduling programs are becoming popular; these allow a patient to see the physician's available appointments and book his or her own date and time.

4. **Explain the features that should be considered when choosing an appointment book.**
   When an appointment book is chosen, all the needs of the office should be considered. If the practice has multiple physicians, the book should be arranged so that each physician is readily identified. Books that open flat on the desk surface are much easier to handle, but another style might be better if not enough space is available to open the book completely. The book also should provide enough space to write all the patient information needed in the various time slots, such as the name, phone number, and reason for the visit.

5. **Explain how self-scheduling can reduce the number of calls to the medical office.**
   Self-scheduling can vastly reduce the number of calls to the office, because a high number of everyday calls are requests to schedule appointments. Patients can even make an appointment at midnight if they desire.

6. **Discuss pros and cons of various types of appointment management systems.**
   Open office hours allow patients to come to the physician's office when it is convenient and wait their turn to see the physician. Scheduling of specific appointments is the most popular method of seeing patients. Flexible office hours allow patients to see the physician during the evening and often on weekends. Many of today's medical offices have some flexible scheduling, because most families now consist of two working parents. Wave scheduling brings two or three patients to the office at the same time, and they are seen in the order of their arrival. This type of scheduling can be modified in many ways to suit the needs of the facility. Other scheduling methods include double-booking and grouping of like procedures.

7. **Explain the importance of legible writing in the appointment book.**
   Because the appointment schedule might be called into a court of law, completely legible handwriting in the book is vital. Even if the book is 5 years old, the person charged with testifying in court should be able to read all entries clearly. Scribbled, messy handwriting implies incompetence and reflects on the practice.

8. **Explain the basic procedure to follow when the office is behind schedule.**

   When the office is running more than 15 minutes behind schedule, the medical assistant should briefly explain the delay to the waiting patients and then offer to reschedule their appointments. The patients should be kept informed of wait times until the schedule resumes.

9. **Discuss the benefits of offering choices to patients when scheduling appointments.**

   Giving a patient a choice in appointment times to better meet his or her needs is good customer service. Offering the patient a choice of 2 days, morning or afternoon, and two times helps ensure that the patient will keep the appointment.

10. **Identify critical information required for scheduling patient admissions and/or procedures.**

    Always provide the scheduler with the patient's name, address, phone numbers (both home and cell), Social Security number, insurance information, and relay the procedures that are to be performed. Patient allergies should be mentioned if the patient is being admitted. Additionally, the facility may have forms that the patient needs to complete, so an e-mail address is helpful in such cases. Always send admitting diagnosis and orders to the healthcare facility prior to admission time or with the patient. Some facilities require a history form prior to admission. The patient will be required to bring a form of picture identification, such as a state driver's license, and his or her insurance card.

11. **Discuss several methods of dealing with patients who consistently arrive late.**

    Patients who are habitually late for appointments might be told to arrive 15 minutes before the time written in the book. Some offices book these patients as the last appointment of the day, so that if they do not arrive promptly, they do not see the physician. Usually talking with the patient and gaining an understanding of why the patient arrives late improves the situation. The office can work with the patient to choose the best times that will result in a kept appointment.

12. **Name several reasons for failed appointments.**

    Some patients forget the appointment with the physician, and some are habitually careless about remembering their scheduled time. Small emergencies often come up, and in today's busy business world, some patients just cannot get away from their own offices or other obligations to visit the physician. In some cases patients do not keep appointments because they do not want to deal with a health issue confronting them.

13. **Recognize office policies and protocols for handling appointments.**

    Always follow written office policies and procedures when handling appointment setting. Each patient should be treated cordially, respectfully, and in the same manner as other patients. Follow these guidelines, but be flexible when a patient has a special problem or situation in scheduling. Whenever a question arises, discuss an action plan with a supervisor.

CONNECTIONS

📖   **Study Guide Connection:** Go to the Chapter 10 Study Guide. Read and complete the activities.

ⓔ   **Evolve Connection:** Go to the Chapter 10 link at *evolve.elsevier.com/ kinn* to complete the Chapter Review and Chapter Quiz. Check out the other resources listed for this chapter to make the most of what you have learned from Scheduling Appointments.

PATIENT RECEPTION AND PROCESSING

11

SCENARIO

Most people enter the healthcare field for very specific reasons. Georgina Robertson recalls being in a serious car accident when she was 6 years old. As a result, her vision was temporarily impaired. She remembers seeing a woman in a white uniform who offered words of comfort. The woman seemed to have a haze around her; combined with the hospital lights, it made her look as if she had wings. That vision of an "angel" never left Georgina, and it led to her decision to enter the medical field.

Today, Georgina works for Dr. Stuart Wade, a cardiologist in a large metropolitan area. Georgina is an experienced medical assistant, and she enjoys getting to know her patients. She makes notes on the medical record that remind her of special events in the lives of the patients who visit Dr. Wade's office. The patients feel that she truly cares about them, aside from her duties at the clinic. Although she is efficient and time conscious, she always has a moment to share a warm smile or hear about a new grandchild. Georgina is a valued member of the medical team in her office. She currently is attending a state college in the evening hours, gaining credits toward her bachelor's degree. She plans to continue her education and apply to medical school in the future.

While studying this chapter, think about the following questions:

- What are some ways to develop good rapport with patients?
- Why is the sign-in register a potential breach of patient confidentiality?
- What is the value of knowing some information about patients' personal lives?

LEARNING OBJECTIVES

1. Define, spell, and pronounce the terms listed in the vocabulary.
2. Explain the purpose of the office mission statement.
3. List several patient amenities and why these are important additions to the medical office.
4. Describe how to prepare for patient arrivals.
5. Explain why using the patient's name as often as possible is important.
6. Discuss how the medical assistant can help the patient prepare for an examination.
7. Discuss ways to make the patient feel at ease and comfortable in the medical office.
8. Explain how to place the medical record to prevent breach of confidentiality.
9. Discuss how the medical assistant might deal with talkative patients.

VOCABULARY

amenity (uh-me′-nuh-te) Something conducive to comfort, convenience, or enjoyment.

demographic (de-muh-gra′-fik) The statistical characteristics of human populations (as in age or income) used especially to identify markets.

fervent Exhibiting or marked by great intensity of feeling.

harmonious Marked by accord in sentiment or action; having the parts agreeably related.

incidental disclosure A secondary use or disclosure that cannot reasonably be prevented, is limited in nature, and occurs as a result of another use or disclosure that is permitted.

intercom A two-way communication system with a microphone and loudspeaker at each station for localized use.

perception A quick, acute, and intuitive cognition; a capacity for comprehension.

phonetic (fuh-ne′-tik) Constituting an alteration of ordinary spelling that better represents the spoken language, that uses only characters of the regular alphabet, and that is used in a context of conventional spelling.

progress notes Notes used in the medical record to track the patient's progress and condition.

sequentially (si-kwen′-shuh-le) Of, relating to, or arranged in a sequence.

The patient reception area should be an inviting place where patients feel comfortable. Visits to the physician can be times of great stress, and the office staff must do everything possible to make the experience pleasant for patients. A patient usually has a choice of healthcare providers and should be given excellent customer service. Good patient relations result in referrals to the physician, and this helps the practice grow. When patients have a good experience with a physician, they are likely to tell others. When the office staff is committed to making the patient feel welcome and the focus is on care of the patient, success of the practice is inevitable.

THE OFFICE MISSION STATEMENT

Healthcare providers often have a **fervent** reason for entering the medical field. For example, a physician remembers the heritage of her immigrant grandfather. She has fond memories of her grandfather's pride and is thankful for the opportunities he found in America after coming to the United States with nothing but the clothes on his back. The grandfather's dream was to see his granddaughter become a physician. On the most trying days, she can step into her office and look at a picture of her grandfather. Her memories help her find the strength and determination to care for her patients. This is the source of that physician's mission statement.

A mission statement defines the predominant goals of the organization in a succinct declaration consisting of a few sentences. The statement reflects the reasons that the practice exists. The physician develops the mission statement alone or may consult the office staff for input. Many offices display the mission statement prominently in the reception area and on printed material, such as patient information booklets. Whatever the contents, each employee of the facility should be familiar with the statement and have a personal commitment to promoting the physician's philosophy in everyday practice.

THE RECEPTION AREA

A first impression is lasting. Nowhere is this more important than in the healthcare facility, where the environment must appear orderly and faultlessly clean. The facility may be a physician's office, a hospital, a health maintenance organization, an insurance company, or one of the many other healthcare establishments. No matter the type of facility, the appearance of the reception room and the front desk, as well as a cordial greeting from the medical assistant, influence patients' **perception** of the entire facility and of the care they will receive.

The reception room is just that—a place to receive patients and visitors. The area should be planned for patients' comfort; it should be as attractive and cheerful as possible and kept clean and uncluttered. Some medical assistants have the opportunity to assist in the design and decoration of this very important area. Consider the traffic flow (the movement of patients from place to place in the reception room) and the flow of traffic through the rest of the office, so that it is unhindered and logical (Figure 11-1).

> ### CRITICAL THINKING APPLICATION   11-1
> Georgina believes that her patients enjoy a homey atmosphere, which is less intimidating than the sterile, clinical feel of some medical offices. How might she give her office this type of ambiance?

Fresh, **harmonious** colors and cleanliness are the foundation of an attractive room (Figure 11-2). Select comfortable furniture that can accommodate the peak load of patients seen each day and arrange it in conversational groups. Individual seating usually is the best choice for the physician's office. Provide good lighting, ventilation, and a regulated temperature. Reduce room clutter by providing a place to hang coats, rainwear, and umbrellas.

Most physicians' offices are well supplied with recent magazines, and some have various books. Publications with short items of popular interest are favorites, such as *Reader's Digest*. Any reading material placed in the reception room should be of interest to the general public; *Good Housekeeping, U.S. News and World Report, Real Simple, Oprah,* and *People* are examples of interesting magazines that most people enjoy reading. Some patients may donate magazines to the office; if there is a name in the subscription area, be sure to mark through it so that the patient's name cannot be read. The reception

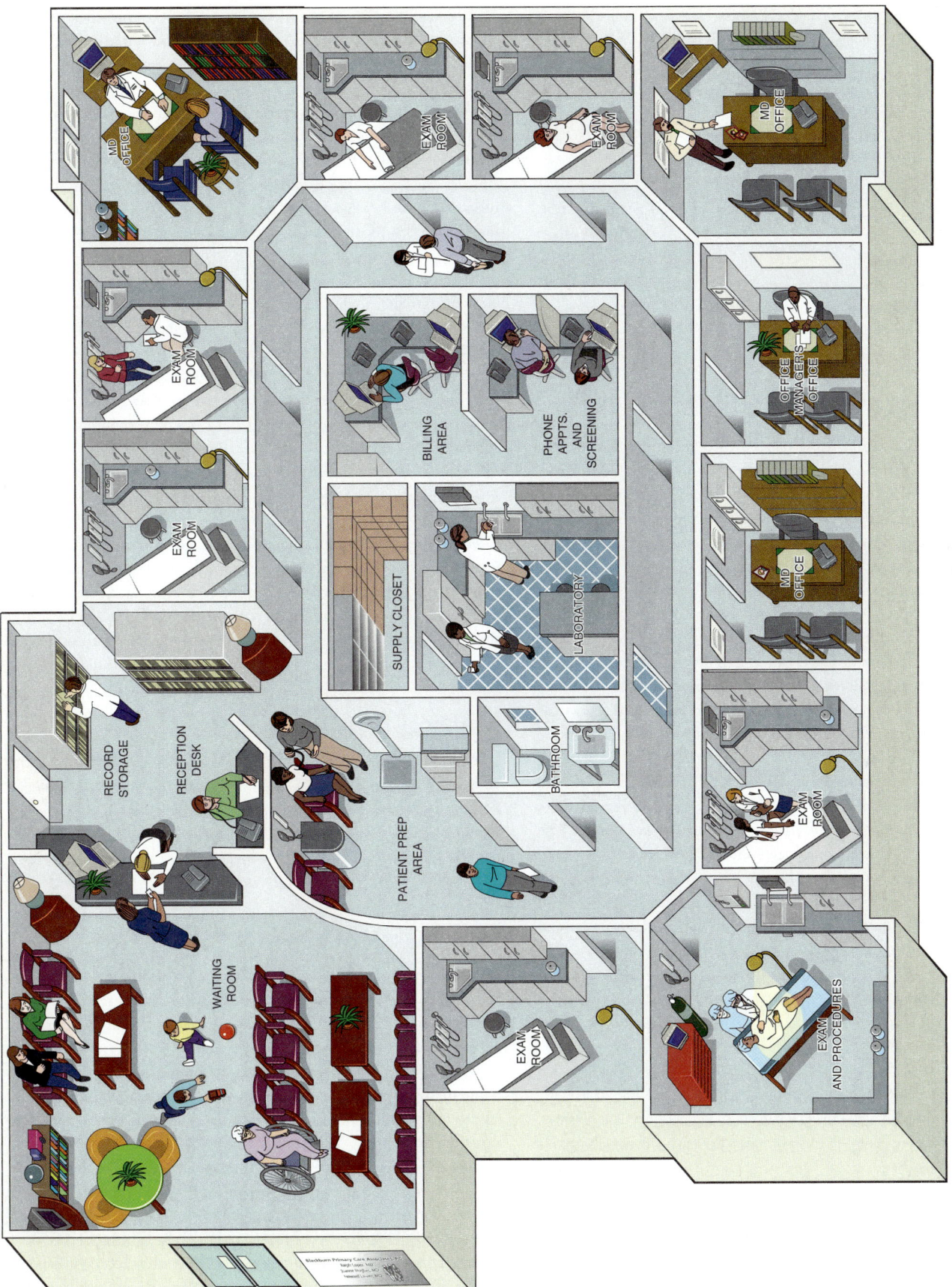

FIGURE 11-1 The medical office should be arranged so that the flow of traffic is conducive to the movement of patients throughout the office.

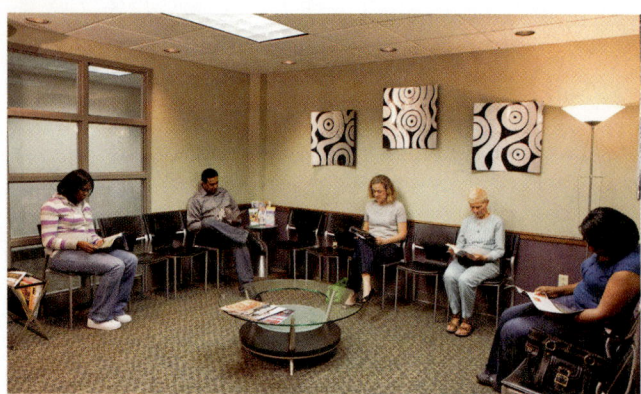

FIGURE 11-2 Patients appreciate cleanliness, restful colors, good ventilation, and light to read by when waiting in the reception area.

room, incidentally, is not the place for the physician's professional journals.

A writing desk with writing paper in the reception area for the convenience of patients is a nice touch, as is restful music from a concealed speaker. A lighted aquarium or an educational display of some sort enhances the attractiveness and individuality of the reception area in the professional practice. Patients often are interested in health-related brochures. The physician also may have a DVD or healthcare book library that allows patients to check out items of interest to them. A telephone in the reception area is an asset and can be programmed by the phone company not to allow long distance calls. A television or DVD player can help the time pass much faster, especially in pediatric offices. Children enjoy Disney movies and cartoon programs, and these hold their interest until it is time to see the physician. A children's corner equipped with small-scale furniture and some playthings works well. Youngsters who might otherwise get into mischief are kept pleasantly occupied. Toys should be easily cleanable; plastic washable items are especially good. Take extra care to ensure that no toy has sharp corners that could cause injury or small parts that could be swallowed. When selecting toys, make sure they will not stimulate the child toward noisy activity. Never place any type of ball in the reception area, because small children tend to throw them, and the balls can injure a patient or visitor.

CRITICAL THINKING APPLICATION   11-2

Georgina has a few patients who bring young children to their appointments. Sometimes the children are a bit disruptive and make other patients feel uncomfortable. How might Georgina handle this problem in the medical office? Some children misbehave in public, and the parents do not respond or correct them. How might Georgina deal with this situation if it arises?

Many modern offices offer a computer for patients to use while waiting to see the physician. This is a great **amenity**, because patients can make good use of their time in the reception area. Some patients may bring their personal laptop computers and use their wait time to complete projects. Providing Internet access for patients also is helpful; an amazing amount of work can be done just by checking

office e-mail. If patients are allowed to connect to the office network, the wise course is to provide one specific log-on name and password just for them so as to maintain control over access to private health information.

Periodically, take an objective look around the reception room. Could it use a little brightening or freshening up? Try to look at the room as if seeing it for the first time. The medical assistant is responsible for the appearance of the area by making sure the room remains neat and orderly throughout the day. Check the temperature and lighting for comfort. Scan the room at intervals during the day to ensure that it is in good order.

If the medical assistant's desk is in the reception area or in open view of patients, it should be free of clutter. In particular, patients' medical and financial records should not be in sight. Keep computer monitors out of view to protect patient confidentiality. Some offices use privacy screens that allow only the user to see the monitor, or they use a screen saver that activates after being idle for a few minutes. Medical assistants should not keep personal items on their desks.

PREPARING FOR PATIENT ARRIVAL

Advance preparation helps make the day go smoothly and contributes to a more relaxed atmosphere for all. Some offices prepare for the next day on the evening before, whereas others prepare each morning. The office should be consistent, and the same routine should always be performed so that important preparations are not left undone.

CRITICAL THINKING APPLICATION   11-3

Housekeeping chores will always be associated with preparing for each day in the physician's office. What are some ways Georgina can divide these tasks fairly among the staff members? How should Georgina handle the employee who feels that general housekeeping duties are not a part of the job description?

Preparing Medical Records

Review a list of patients who will visit the physician during the next appointment period. If an electronic medical record system is used, this task could be as simple as pulling up and printing a report. If a paper-based system is used, pull the medical records for the day (or the next day if this is done in the evenings) and check off the patient's name on a copy of the appointment schedule; this helps ensure that all the records have been located and are ready (Figure 11-3). Occasionally two or more patients may have the same or a similar name. Check the patient's Social Security number, date of birth, or other pertinent information to make sure the right medical record has been pulled. Review each record to verify that any recently received information (e.g., laboratory reports, radiograph readings) has been entered correctly and permanently attached to the record (Procedure 11-1); if a document is missing, attempt to obtain it prior to the patient's arrival using a fax or other electronic means. Arrange the medical records **sequentially** in the order in which the patients are scheduled to be seen. The medical assistant may be expected to place

PROCEDURE 11-1

Organize a Patient's Medical Record: Preparing the Medical Record for Use During Office Visits

GOAL: *To prepare patients' medical records for the daily appointment schedule and have them ready for the physician during the patient's office visit.*

EQUIPMENT and SUPPLIES

- Appointment schedule for current date
- Patient medical records
- Clerical supplies (e.g., pen, tape, stapler)

PROCEDURAL STEPS

1. Review the appointment schedule.
2. Identify the full name of each scheduled patient.
3. Pull the patients' medical records, checking each patient's name on your list as the record is pulled.
   PURPOSE: To determine that the correct medical records have been pulled and that no medical records have been omitted.
4. Review each medical record.
   PURPOSE: To reaffirm that:
   - The correct patient medical record has been pulled.
   - Any previously ordered tests have been performed.
   - The results of the tests have been posted or entered in the medical record.
   - Forms have been replenished inside the medical record (e.g., progress notes and others).
5. Annotate the appointment list with any special concerns.
   PURPOSE: To alert the physician about matters that should be checked or discussed with the patient.
6. Arrange the medical records sequentially according to each patient's appointment.
7. Place the medical records in the appropriate examination room or other specified location.

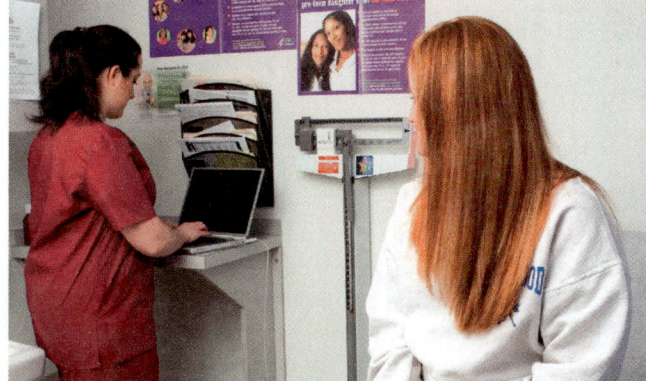

FIGURE 11-3 More physicians and their staff members are using electronic medical records to reduce paperwork and provide better, more efficient patient care. (From Bonewit-West K: *Today's medical assistant,* ed 2, St Louis, 2013, Saunders.)

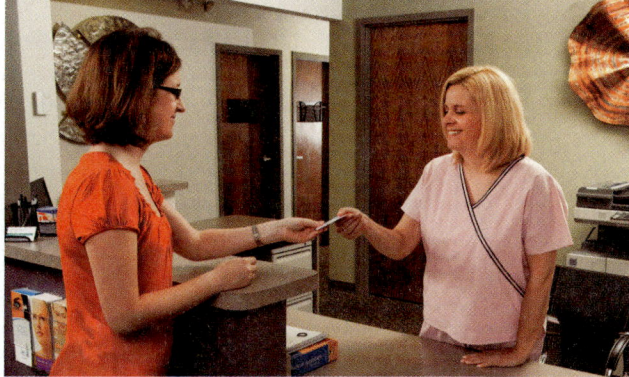

FIGURE 11-4 Greet all patients with a warm smile and assist them with forms they need to complete for the medical record.

the records of all the patients to be seen that day on the physician's desk, but the physician is more likely to prefer reviewing each record just before entering the examination room. Make sure enough space is available on the **progress notes** for the physician to write in the record. If not, place additional progress notes pages in the record.

GREETING THE PATIENT

Every patient has the right to expect courteous treatment in a physician's office. Regardless of the patient's economic or social status, each person who enters the reception room should receive a cordial, friendly greeting (Figure 11-4). A personal touch, such as greeting the patient by name, is an easy way to develop patient rapport. Use the patient's last name and title unless the patient insists on the use of his or her first name or prefers a nickname. For example, the medical assistant may say:

"How are you today, Mr. Roberts?"

"Ms. Nelson, the doctor will be in to see you shortly."

If the office has a policy of obtaining a copy of all patients' photo identification cards, such as the driver's license, these can be used to identify patients and greet them by name, even if they do not visit the office often. This practice also ensures that the person receiving benefits is actually the person covered by the insurance policy.

Patient Check-In

The reception desk should be in clear view of all visitors who come into the office. If only one medical assistant is present, welcoming each new visitor personally sometimes is impossible. Develop an announcement system that alerts the staff when people enter the office. Patients who enter an empty reception room do not know whether to sit down, knock on the glass partition, or try to announce themselves in some other way. Glass partitions are used to maintain some privacy; however, some physicians have eliminated them because they are so impersonal and they send the signal that the physician and staff are off limits to patients. If the partition is used, the office policy and procedure manual should dictate when the glass should remain open and when it should be closed.

A sign placed in the reception room that reads, "Please sign in and sit comfortably. We will be with you shortly," assures patients that their presence will be acknowledged. However, the best solution is to keep a staff member at the front desk at all times to greet patients and answer questions. Make sure no patient medical records are lying on the reception desk in view of patients signing in or approaching the desk when they arrive at the office. This prevents violation of the regulations established by the Health Insurance Portability and Accountability Act (HIPAA).

The medical assistant should check the reception room each time he or she has been away from the desk to see whether more patients have arrived. Greet these patients by name; if you do not know the person who has entered the reception area, ask the individual's name. Use a sign-in register that promotes patients' privacy. Although patients can read the names of others who are in the office to visit the physician, this is not considered a violation of HIPAA policy as long as the information disclosed is appropriately limited. This is one type of **incidental disclosure**, as described in Chapter 17. The sign-in sheet should have only the information needed to sign in, such as the patient's name, the provider's name, the arrival and appointment times, and a place to note that patients are new to the practice or that their address, insurance coverage, or other demographic information has changed (Figure 11-5). The best registers allow the staff to remove the patient's name and information after the person signs the document. Pressure-sensitive labels printed with lines for the patient's name, the appointment time, and a "yes" or "no" question about changes in insurance coverage are a practical, inexpensive solution for confidential patient registers. The signed label then can be placed in a separate log book or even inside the patient's medical record. The office can order custom registers that work like a pegboard, making the identifying information invisible to subsequent patients. Patients should not be expected to provide details of the reason for their visit in a public area.

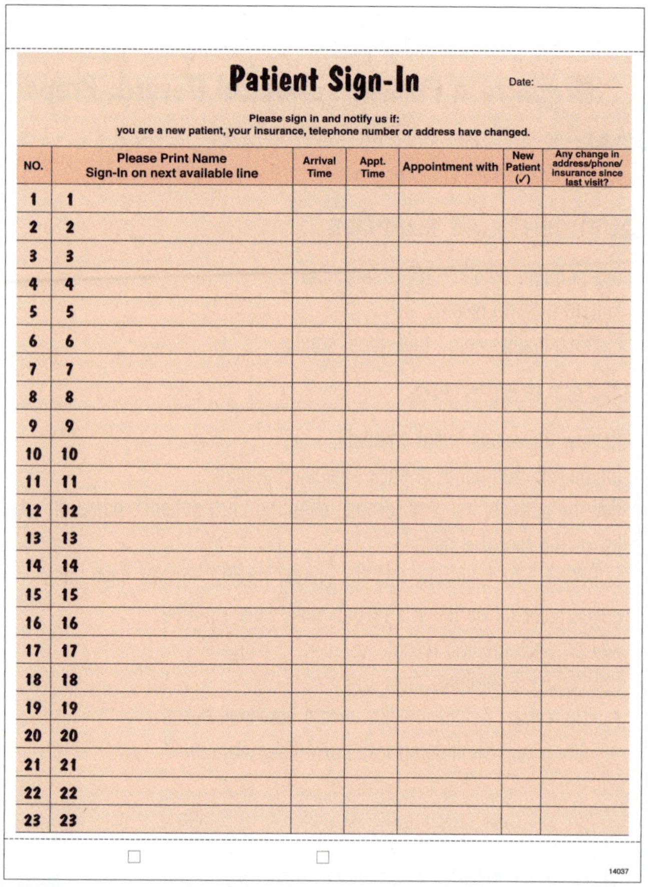

Patient Sign-In Date: ___________

Please sign in and notify us if:
you are a new patient, your insurance, telephone number or address have changed.

NO.	Please Print Name Sign-In on next available line	Arrival Time	Appt. Time	Appointment with	New Patient (✓)	Any change in address/phone/ insurance since last visit?
1	1					
2	2					
3	3					
4	4					
5	5					
6	6					
7	7					
8	8					
9	9					
10	10					
11	11					
12	12					
13	13					
14	14					
15	15					
16	16					
17	17					
18	18					
19	19					
20	20					
21	21					
22	22					
23	23					

14037

FIGURE 11-5 Sign-in sheets contain very basic information about the patient and provide information for the medical assistant about changes that need editing on the patient's demographic information.

Patient Interaction

Although the medical office can make patients feel jittery, the medical assistant should try to make everyone feel at ease and comfortable. Cultivate the habit of greeting each patient immediately in a friendly, self-assured manner. Establish eye contact and smile while introducing yourself to the patient. For example, "Good morning, I'm Elizabeth, Dr. Wade's medical assistant." Remember to ask about the patient before asking about insurance coverage; no patient wants to feel that the physician's main interest is the collection of an insurance check.

Patients like to be acknowledged when they arrive. All staff members should review the day's schedule in the morning to be prepared to greet patients by name and to know whether the patient is new or established. Learn how to pronounce each patient's name correctly; incorrect pronunciations may offend or irritate some people. If the name is unusual, write the **phonetic** spelling on the record for reference. Note if the patient prefers a nickname. Make notes on the medical record that help staff members remember names when talking to patients on the phone or in person. By using the patient's name often, the medical assistant also ensures that the correct patient is being treated.

Physicians and staff members sometimes make brief notes in the medical record about the current events in the patient's life. With this information, the medical assistant and the physician can read

CRITICAL THINKING APPLICATION 11-4

A patient passes Georgina in the hallway as she is leaving for lunch and stops to greet her. The patient's face is familiar, but Georgina cannot recall the patient's name. Occasionally, Georgina sees a patient outside of the office, such as in a grocery store, the library, and other places around town. Everyone forgets someone's name on occasion.

- How might Georgina and her staff members remember names?
- What special tips or techniques can help you remember names?
- What can Georgina do the next time she sees a patient and does not remember the person's name?

those notes before entering the examination room and share a short dialog with patients at the beginning of their visits. For example:

Medical assistant: *"Hello, Mrs. Williams, how are you today?"*
Mrs. Williams: *"I am doing very well, Georgina, how are you?"*
Medical assistant: *"I'm fine. How was the cruise you took with your husband last month?"*
Mrs. Williams: *"It was wonderful! The water was the bluest I have seen!"*
Medical assistant: *"You went to Cozumel, didn't you?"*
Mrs. Williams: *"Yes, we did! I'm surprised you remember, as many patients as you see each day!"*

This brief chat confirms that the staff members care about the individual patient, because they take an interest in their personal lives (Figure 11-6). Because the patient does not see the medical assistant or physician look at the notes before entering the patient room, the patient assumes that the information is recalled from memory. This is an impressive customer service technique. Most patients appreciate the physician's and staff's interest in their families, hobbies, and work. Computer-based medical records systems usually have a notes option where such information can be recorded.

Patients may feel somewhat anxious when visiting the physician's office, especially if they know they may be receiving bad news; perhaps a tumor has been discovered to be cancerous, or a family member may have been diagnosed with Alzheimer's disease. Watch the patient's body language. If a patient does not maintain good eye contact or seems otherwise uneasy, a gentle touch or a reassuring smile may be helpful as the office visit progresses. Remember to keep the patient's safety in mind and make certain that he or she has some type of support that will assure a safe arrival back home or at a family or friend's home after the office visit.

Some state regulations prohibit the placement of information other than health details in the medical record; however, most health professionals agree that a patient's mental and emotional health are connected to the person's physical health. Details about what is happening in patients' lives provide clues to their physical problems. As a simple example, a patient going through a divorce may experience depression that needs to be treated with medication. Without knowledge of the divorce, the physician does not have all the information needed to make a sound medical decision. Physicians can treat patients more effectively when such information is available in the medical record.

REGISTRATION PROCEDURES

On a patient's first visit to the physician's office, the staff performs certain registration procedures (Procedure 11-2). Most physicians use a patient information or registration form to gather **demographic** information about the patient. The form may be attached to a clipboard and handed to the patient with instructions to complete sections. The medical assistant must be ready and willing to answer any questions (Figure 11-7). The patient's name should appear prominently at the top of the form, followed by other pertinent facts in logical order. Most information sheets contain the following:

- Patient's full name and date of birth
- Responsible person's name and relationship to the patient
- Address and telephone number
- Name, address, and telephone number of spouse
- Occupation
- Place of employment
- Social Security number
- Driver's license number
- Nearest relative not living with the patient and his or her relationship
- Source of referral, if any

When the completed form is returned, check carefully to verify that all the necessary information has been provided.

Some practices place their registration paperwork on their Web site, and the patient can download, complete, and print the paperwork prior to their first office visit. If a good length of time will pass between making the appointment and arriving for the office visit,

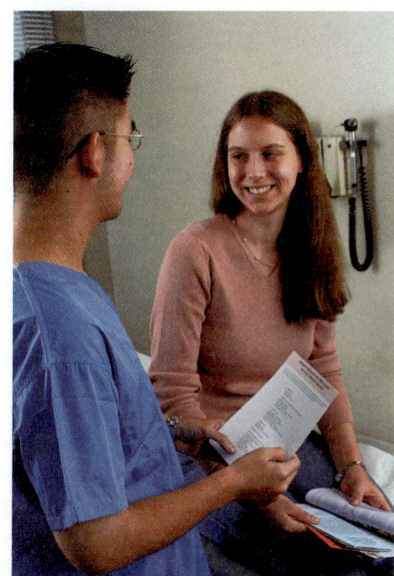

FIGURE 11-6 Patients appreciate being called by name and remembered from visit to visit. The medical assistant should develop a good relationship with the patient and be a caring advocate.

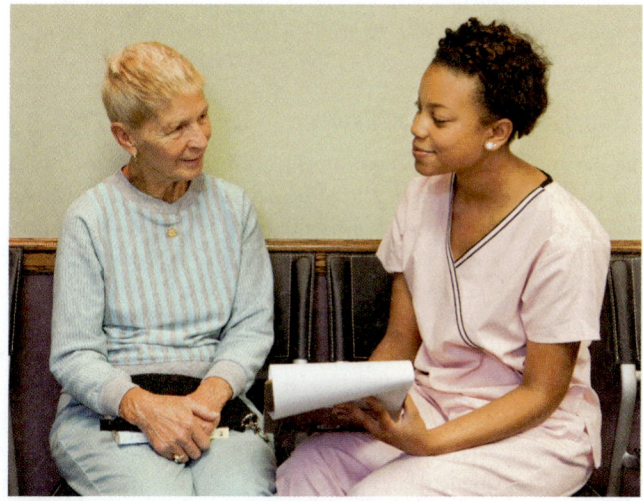

FIGURE 11-7 The medical assistant should take time to explain forms the patient does not understand and should always be willing to answer questions.

PROCEDURE 11-2

Register a New Patient

GOAL: *To complete a registration form for a new patient with information for credit and insurance claims and to inform and orient the patient to the facility.*

EQUIPMENT and SUPPLIES

- Registration form
- Clerical supplies (pen, clipboard)
- Private conference area

PROCEDURAL STEPS

1. Determine whether the patient is new to the practice.
2. Obtain and record the necessary information:
   - Patient's full name, birth date, and name of spouse (if married)
   - Home address, telephone number (include ZIP and area codes)
   - Occupation, name of employer, business address, telephone number
   - Social Security number and driver's license number, if any
   - Name of referring physician, if any
   - Name and address of person responsible for payment
   - Method of payment
   - Health insurance information (photocopy both sides of the insurance ID card)
   - Name of primary carrier
   - Type of coverage
   - Group policy number
   - Subscriber number
   - Assignment of benefits, if required
   PURPOSE: This information is necessary for credit and insurance claims.
3. Review the entire form and confirm the patient's eligibility for insurance coverage.
   PURPOSE: To verify that the given information is complete and legible.
4. Determine that required referrals have been received, if applicable.
   PURPOSE: Insurance coverage may not be valid without a referral.
5. Explain medical and financial procedures to patients.
   PURPOSE: To help the patient develop a comfort level and know what to expect.
6. Collect co-payments or balance payment charges.
   PURPOSE: To keep accounts current and prevent the need to mail statements.

---

the paperwork can be mailed to the patient, with instructions to bring the completed documents to the office visit. More information about patient forms used in the medical practice is found in Chapter 14; examples of many different forms are available on the Evolve Web site.

> ### CRITICAL THINKING APPLICATION   11-5
> Often some time is needed to complete forms when a new patient arrives in the office. How might Georgina keep the office on schedule when new patients arrive, requiring medical record construction and form completion? What are some ways to trim time from these activities?

Obtaining a Patient's History

The patient's personal history, medical history, and family history may be obtained by asking him or her to complete a questionnaire; the physician can augment this information during the patient interview. Some experienced medical assistants conduct the interview to obtain the patient's personal and medical history, family history, and chief complaint. This is a specialized procedure, and the medical assistant should be specifically trained to perform it for the individual practice.

When taking a patient history, talk with the patient in a private area or in the exam room. Follow the questionnaire and discuss the issues the patient relates as a past illness or injury, in addition to current health problems. Watch the patient's body language while listening. Use reflection, restatement, and clarification (see Chapter 5) when obtaining patient information. Discuss the patient's history thoroughly and make accurate notations in the medical record. Describe the current chief complaint, using the patient's own words whenever possible in documenting the problem. Remember that the medical assistant can never offer the patient any type of medical advice.

SHOWING CONSIDERATION FOR PATIENTS' TIME

The patient expects to see the physician or practitioner at the appointed time. The medical assistant should bring the patient to the examination room for treatment or consultation as close to the appointment time as possible or explain delays. All patients want to be kept informed about how long they should expect to wait to see the physician. Any delay longer than 10 to 15 minutes should be explained. A crowded reception room is not always an indication of a physician's popularity. It may simply mean that the physician or assistant is inefficient at scheduling patients. Always consider the patient's time and make every effort to streamline the office visit.

A solo or small practice should seldom have more than three to five patients in the reception room. Patients complain that the wait time in medical facilities is one of the most frustrating aspects of the medical profession. The patient who complains about medical fees or the care received may first have become agitated during a long wait to see the physician. Many patients are fearful and tense; long wait times intensify these feelings. The medical assistant can often put patients in a better frame of mind with just a friendly smile and a show of concern.

Patients with Special Needs

Some patients are physically challenged, some are very ill, and some are severely uncomfortable. Language or cultural barriers may exist. Observe the patient's appearance and behavior. Is the patient pale? Do the eyes or voice reflect pain or discomfort? Find out how the patient is feeling before suggesting that he or she be seated to wait for the physician. The patient may need to lie down in a cool room or perhaps be seen as an emergency case. Patients with disabilities, such as those who use a wheelchair, cane, walker, or crutches, may need extra attention. Some patients may need help disrobing even if a disability is not obvious. Ask if the patient needs assistance.

ESCORTING AND INSTRUCTING THE PATIENT

While in the physician's office, most patients prefer to be escorted rather than simply told where to go. This usually is the clinical medical assistant's responsibility, but the task may be assigned to an administrative medical assistant. Pronounce the patient's name correctly when calling the person to the clinical area (Figure 11-8). If unsure of the pronunciation, ask the patient. Write the name phonetically on the medical record for quick retrieval at the next appointment.

Some patients bring a family member or friend with them to their appointment. On occasion, several people want to accompany the patient when the person sees the physician. The office policy and procedure manual should address the maximum number of patients allowed in. If the patient insists on more visitors, explain that the exam rooms are small and have only one chair; suggest that the additional people may be uncomfortable standing in such a small room. If the patient still insists, make every attempt to satisfy the patient's needs.

Remember that to an employee of the practice, the office surroundings may become as familiar as home. A stranger to the practice's environment may be confused or disoriented by all the hallways, doors, and rooms. Uncertainty creates anxiety. Take the time to escort the patient personally to the appropriate examination or treatment room; do not point to the room and expect the patient to find the way. If a urine specimen is needed, direct the patient to the restroom and always explain what to do with the specimen.

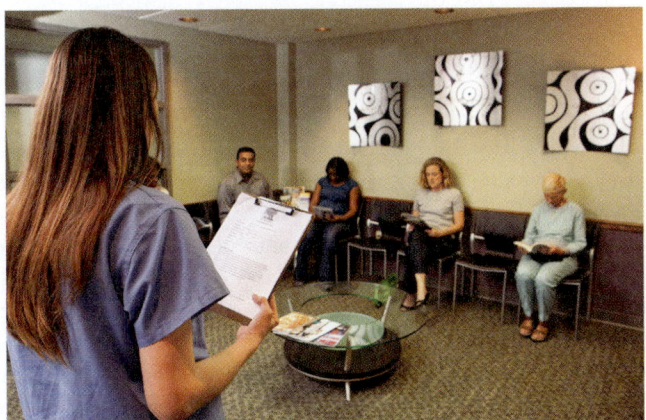

FIGURE 11-8 Pronounce the patient's name correctly and use it often. This promotes good customer service and pleases the patient. Announcing the patient's name does not violate HIPAA regulations.

On arrival in the examination room, tell the patient whether he or she needs to disrobe. Explain what garments, if any, can be left on, whether shoes are to be removed, whether jewelry needs to be removed, and any other necessary instructions. If a gown is to be worn, specify whether the opening should be in the front or back and tell the patient where he or she can hang up clothes if this is not obvious. An examination table should never be placed in such a position that the patient is exposed to passersby in the hallway if the door is opened. Imagine a patient ready for a Pap smear facing the door as the physician enters! Allow patients a sense of modesty at all times, and make all instructions completely clear. Be equally clear when the examination has been completed. Do not assume that patients know what is expected of them. Tell patients whether they should go to the physician's office for consultation or return to the reception area to wait, or whether they are free to check out with the front office and leave.

The medical assistant helps keep the schedule operating smoothly by immediately tidying each examination room and escorting the next patient in so that the physician has no idle moments waiting for a patient to be prepared. Try not to place a patient in an examination room just to clear out the reception area. Keeping the patient waiting after being gowned, draped, and positioned on the examining table is especially inconsiderate. Medical offices often are chilly or even cold, which makes a draped patient quite uncomfortable. A magazine rack on the wall of the treatment room is a welcome addition in some practices.

Remember that in today's litigious society, physicians prefer a second person in the room during examinations to avoid claims of sexual assault or harassment. The office may be equipped with a buzzer that alerts the medical assistant to enter the examination room after the physician has initially consulted with the patient. Be prompt in answering the buzzer and provide assistance during the examination. Patients may be uncomfortable and uneasy; offer words of encouragement, a smile, and a pat on the shoulder.

MEDICAL RECORD PLACEMENT

Medical records should never be left in the examination room to be picked up and read by a patient. This can cause misunderstandings, because patients rarely know medical terms and abbreviations. A number of methods are used to signal that a patient is ready to be seen. Often file holders are located on the doors of the examination rooms, and the medical record can be placed in the holder horizontally when the patient is ready to be seen. The physician can signal the medical assistant that he or she is finished examining the patient by placing the medical record in an upright position on leaving the exam room. Place the medical record so that the patient's name cannot be seen by other patients in the hallway. HIPAA considers names on medical records to be incidental disclosures; however, protecting patient privacy by simply turning the chart so that the name cannot be read is a good habit to cultivate.

Some offices have light call systems, by which a physician can press a button to call the medical assistant for help with the examination. Others have a visual item outside the door that signals what that particular patient needs next. Other offices place patients in examination rooms in a certain order, and the physician knows, for instance, that when he or she has finished with the patient in room

1, the next patient will be waiting in room 2. The office should develop a method that allows the most efficient use of time while providing high-quality care, and at the same time, protects patient confidentiality.

CHALLENGING SITUATIONS

Talkative Patients

Any professional office has problem patients. Talkative patients, for example, take up far more of the physician's time than is justified. An alert medical assistant usually can spot this tendency during the initial interview. The patient's history can be flagged with a symbol to alert the physician. The medical assistant can buzz the physician's **intercom** and remind him that the next patient is ready. Once the medical assistant has learned which patients take extra time, they can be booked for the end of the day, or more time can be allowed for them.

> ## CRITICAL THINKING APPLICATION   11-6
> Georgina has one patient who insists on sitting close to her desk and attempting to chat the entire time she is waiting to see the physician. Even worse, she comes to her appointments at least an hour early. How might Georgina subtly deal with this patient?

Children

Children frequently present special management challenges, whether they are patients or they accompany a patient. Usually, the parent or guardian accompanies the child into the exam room, but some exceptions exist, such as a case of suspected child abuse. Older children certainly can see the doctor without a parent, especially for routine visits, such as a school sports physical. However, minors still need a parent to consent to treatment in most cases. The physician cannot force the parent to leave the examination room by any means. Although this practice of separating children from their parents to treat their needs is not always feasible, it sometimes can be applied with great success.

Parents are responsible for their children's behavior while at the physician's office. If children are doing something that could harm themselves or other patients, quietly speak to the parents and allow them to handle the situation. When children behave badly, the medical assistant can go to the child, kneel down to his or her level, and offer a book or toy, leading the child away from any objects that could be broken or from other patients. The medical assistant can say, "Let's come over here and play next to your mom!" If the child continues to behave badly, call the parent to the exam room early, so that others in the reception area can relax and enjoy a pleasant office visit. The medical assistant should not discipline the child. Some patients may be anxious about receiving test results or have other issues, and an unruly child can make the situation even worse.

Angry Patients in the Reception Area

Every medical assistant eventually is confronted with an angry patient. The anger may simply reflect the patient's pain or fear of what the physician may discover during the examination. If possible, invite the patient into a room out of the reception area. Usually the best course is to let the patient talk out the anger. Pacify the patient using a calm attitude and speak in a low tone of voice. Under no circumstances should the medical assistant return the anger or become argumentative. Medical assistants must use good listening skills with angry people and must be empathetic.

Patient's Relatives and Friends

Patients sometimes are accompanied by a relative or well-meaning friend who may become restless waiting for the patient and attempt to discuss the patient's illness. The medical assistant should sidestep any discussion of a patient's medical care, except by direction of the physician. Avoid a too casual attitude, such as, "I'm sure there's nothing to worry about." A show of moderate concern and reassurance that "the patient is in good hands" usually takes care of the situation. Remember that health information cannot be released to anyone, including concerned friends and relatives, without the patient's consent.

THE FRIENDLY FAREWELL

As soon as the visit with the physician has been completed, the medical assistant should be ready to help the patient dress, if necessary, and make sure any questions the patient may have are answered. Answer questions if they can be addressed ethically and legally; otherwise, direct the patient to the physician. Some questions can be answered only by the physician; in such cases, the assistant can offer to get answers for the patient or bring the physician back to the examination room to answer the questions. Remember, patients view the medical assistant as an extension of the physician, and the medical assistant must be very careful to prevent accusations of practicing medicine without a license.

The medical assistant can help convey a sense of caring by terminating the visit cordially. If the patient will return for another visit, the assistant can say something like, "We'll see you next week." If this is the patient's last visit, a pleasant "I hope you'll be feeling better soon" is appropriate. Whatever words of goodbye are chosen, all patients should leave the facility feeling that they have received top-quality care and were treated with friendliness, respect, and courtesy.

PATIENT CHECKOUT

When the patient returns to the front office for checkout, greet him or her with a friendly smile and call the individual by name. Form the habit of asking patients whether they have any questions. Check the medical record to determine when the physician wants the patient to return. Most physicians note this information on the encounter form. Make the return appointment, remembering the technique of giving the patient choices for which day to come, morning or afternoon, and specific times. Then ask the patient for payment, using phrases such as, "Your co-pay today is $15, Mrs. Williams. Will you be writing a check or would you like to charge this visit to your Visa?"

Some offices insist that co-pays be collected before the office visit; this matter is handled according to the physician's discretion. Some

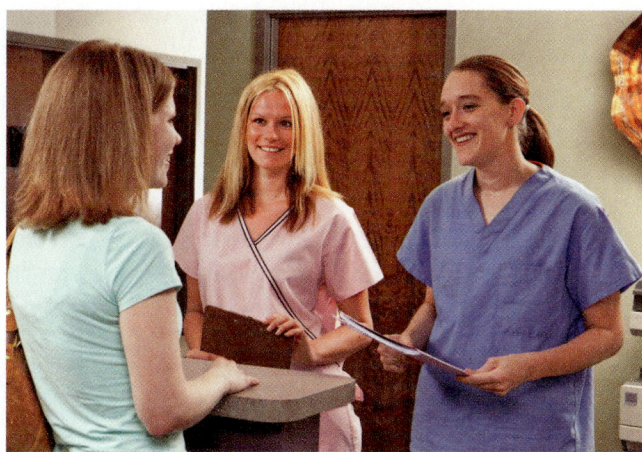

FIGURE 11-9 Always thank the patient for coming and wish him or her well.

patients do not believe they should have to pay before seeing the physician; they simply are not used to paying at the start of the visit. The medical assistant can say, "Mr. Thomas, would you like to go ahead and pay your co-pay now?" By giving the patient the option, it seems as if the medical assistant is helping the patient save time instead of insisting on collecting before seeing the physician. Follow the procedures outlined in the office policy and procedure manual for patient checkout.

Be sure to thank the patient for coming and wish the person well as he or she leaves the office (Figure 11-9).

CLOSING COMMENTS

A personal touch is vital to projecting a sense of care to the patients seen in the physician's office. Many medical offices are not concerned enough about the customer service aspect of the business. Patients talk about their experiences with their friends and relatives and may be an excellent source of referrals if they are treated with dignity and courtesy. If they have a good experience, they tell several people. If they have a poor experience, they tend to tell everyone they know. Make sure to play a part in having each patient feel a sense of satisfaction as he or she leaves the office. All patients should feel that their time and money have been well spent.

Patient Education

Offering a patient education center in the reception area is an effective way to provide patients with up-to-date information about healthcare issues. Brochures and information sheets can be displayed, and DVD programs that deal with health topics can be available for viewing while the patient is waiting to see the physician.

Both the physician and the medical assistants caring for patients should ask whether the patient has any questions during the office visit. Patients often complain that they did not get to speak to the physician long enough to get their questions answered completely.

Legal and Ethical Issues

A medical assistant must never offer medical advice to a patient unless specifically instructed to do so by the physician. The patient sees the medical assistant as an extension of the physician and tends to weigh advice and comments by the medical assistant with the same validity as if they came from the physician. Provide only information the physician has approved or that is included in the office policy and procedure manual.

When a patient complains, listen carefully and try to resolve the problem or assure the patient that the issue will be discussed with the appropriate staff member to find a solution. If someone other than the patient asks for information about the patient, refrain from discussion unless the patient or physician has authorized the release of information.

SUMMARY OF SCENARIO

Georgina is a person who truly makes a difference in the healthcare profession. She takes her role as a patient advocate seriously and strives to make her patients feel comfortable in Dr. Wade's office. She keeps the mission statement posted close to her desk and rereads it often to keep her focus clear. She shares the vision with the other staff members, who are supportive and in agreement with the purpose for which the office exists.

Dr. Wade promotes continuing medical education and encourages his staff members to participate in courses and seminars that will help them be more effective patient advocates. The office sends birthday and Christmas cards to the patients in the database, and at the annual holiday party, the staff hand-signs each Christmas card. Georgina sends a monthly newsletter to patients, some by mail and some by e-mail, to keep them up-to-date on office policies and interesting health information. All of these activities indicate a strong, caring attitude toward the patients. Georgina considers each one a customer of the clinic, and she is determined that they all receive excellent customer service.

Wait times are at a minimum in Dr. Wade's office. Cell phone numbers and e-mail addresses are gathered at registration and updated frequently so that the staff can quickly contact patients. Georgina offers new patients a form for evaluation of the office so that they can provide input about their experience as a new patient. All these efforts promote a trusting, caring relationship among physician, staff, and patients.

Medical assistants can develop a strong rapport with patients by treating them as they themselves would want to be treated. Patients enjoy hearing their own names and being recognized by staff members. Georgina remembers to greet each patient on his or her arrival at the clinic and always asks the names of patients she does not know. She knows that having a bit of personal knowledge about the patients will be of benefit to Dr. Wade, and the entire staff is cordial and friendly to all patients.

Georgina knows that she must keep the sign-in register confidential and uses a form that complies with HIPAA regulations. This prevents patients from obtaining private health information during check-in procedures. By protecting patient confidentiality, the office not only remains in compliance with federal regulations, but also puts the patients' interests first, ensuring that they can enter the office with confidence and trust.

SUMMARY OF LEARNING OBJECTIVES

1. **Define, spell, and pronounce the terms listed in the vocabulary.**
   Spelling and pronouncing medical terms correctly bolster the medical assistant's credibility. Knowing the definition of these terms promotes confidence in communication with patients and co-workers.

2. **Explain the purpose of the office mission statement.**
   The office mission statement is the philosophy of why the office exists. Often physicians themselves develop the mission statement, which outlines their vision and reasons for entering medical practice. Some physicians allow the office staff to assist in its development. All employees should become familiar with the mission statement and promote its ideas to all patients and visitors.

3. **List several patient amenities and why these are important additions to the medical office.**
   Patient amenities include such things as a VCR, television, computer, telephone, and a desk where patients can sit and balance a checkbook or review work while away from the office. These features turn the time spent in the physician's office into productive minutes instead of wasteful ones.

4. **Describe how to prepare for patient arrivals.**
   Some offices prepare for patient arrivals the evening before and some in the morning. Patients' medical records must be pulled; they should be checked for completed laboratory tests and posted results and to ensure that the progress notes for this visit are ample. Rooms should be checked and inventoried to make sure they are neat and clean and that sufficient supplies are on hand.

5. **Explain why using the patient's name as often as possible is important.**
   People like hearing their own names; a better relationship is built between the staff and patients when the names are used often. Patients feel that the office staff cares enough about them to acknowledge them, and this custom adds a personal touch.

6. **Discuss how the medical assistant can help the patient prepare for an examination.**
   The medical assistant should escort the patient to the examination rooms and other areas of the office. Always tell the patient when to disrobe and exactly what should be removed. Offer to assist with disrobing if the patient needs extra help. Take care that the patient's purse or wallet is in a secure place. Make sure doors do not open and expose the disrobed patient. Instruct the patient whether he or she may leave or should wait after seeing the physician. Ask whether the patient has any questions.

7. **Discuss ways to make the patient feel at ease and comfortable in the medical office.**
   The personal touch helps the patient feel at home and comfortable in the office. An attractive reception area with various patient amenities provides a warm atmosphere. Using the patient's name often and a gentle touch impart a sense of caring. Watch body language for clues and offer a reassuring smile when appropriate.

8. **Explain how to place the medical record to prevent breach of confidentiality.**

Some medical offices place patient medical records in a door file, which alerts the physician that the patient is ready to be seen. Other offices place the medical records in door files in a certain order. For example, if examination rooms 1, 2, and 3 are available, patients are seen in that order by the physician. Make every effort to place the medical record so that the patient's name is not visible to anyone passing by in the hallway.

9. **Discuss how the medical assistant might deal with talkative patients.** Talkative patients may be lonely and may enjoy the social interaction of their visits to the physician's office. Be as courteous as possible with talkative patients, letting them know when necessary that another patient is waiting or that the physician needs assistance. When this is said with a smile, most patients understand.

CONNECTIONS

Study Guide Connection: Go to the Chapter 11 Study Guide. Read and complete the activities.

Evolve Connection: Go to the Chapter 11 link at *evolve.elsevier.com/kinn* to complete the Chapter Review and Chapter Quiz. Check out the other resources listed for this chapter to make the most of what you have learned from Patient Reception and Processing.

12

OFFICE ENVIRONMENT AND DAILY OPERATIONS

Kayla Kemper performed her externship at Dr. Richard Tarago's office, a general practice clinic downtown that serves lower income patients, most of whom do not have medical insurance. Some patients have a co-payment of $5 to $25; others have no co-payment, depending on their income level. Kayla's family is quite wealthy, and working with patients whose lifestyle is very different from hers has been an eye-opening experience. On many days she wanted to leave the clinic, because she realized that a large number of patients were unable to seek medical care at the start of an illness, and when they finally came to the clinic, they were in worse condition.

Kayla is a caring person, and she saw the suffering many patients experienced daily. She found it tough to see people who had difficulty obtaining health care, yet she realized that a large number of Americans have no insurance coverage at all. Kayla discussed her feelings with the clinic manager, Elaine Mays, and expressed her concern for the patients in the clinic. Elaine asked whether Kayla would like to continue working with the patients, and Kayla admitted that she would, although it was not easy for her. Elaine then suggested that because Kayla's background is so different from the patients, she might want to stay at the clinic as a volunteer for a few months to add to her learning experience. She accepted the offer, and after 3 months as a volunteer, Elaine hired Kayla to work in the clinical area full time. The patients consistently commented on how compassionately and considerately Kayla treated them. Kayla truly learned the meaning of giving as it relates to the medical profession. Her externship was the start of her full-time career.

While studying this chapter, think about the following questions:

- What are some issues that might prevent a medical assistant from showing compassion to all patients? How can these issues be resolved?
- Why is it a good practice to allow the person who uses a certain supply to order it?
- Why might outsourcing be less expensive than doing testing or procedures in the office?
- How might an extensive list of community resources be helpful to patients?

LEARNING OBJECTIVES

1. Define, spell, and pronounce the terms listed in the vocabulary.
2. List five specific actions that must be taken to prepare for patients before the office opens in the morning.
3. Explain why patient traffic flow is an important consideration in the office design.
4. List some of the expenses involved in the operation of a medical practice.
5. Describe how prices can be compared for medical office supplies.
6. Discuss the importance of routine maintenance of office equipment.
7. List several ways to save money and prevent waste in the medical office.
8. Discuss fire safety issues in a healthcare environment.
9. Discuss critical elements of an emergency plan for response to a natural disaster or other emergency.
10. Identify emergency preparedness plans in the community.
11. Discuss potential roles of the medical assistant in emergency preparedness.
12. Describe the fundamental principles for evacuation of a healthcare setting.
13. Explain the difference between medical waste and regular waste.
14. Identify principles of body mechanics and ergonomics.

VOCABULARY

advance An amount of money or credit furnished in anticipation of repayment.

backorder An ordered item that is not delivered when promised or demanded but will be filled at a later date.

budget A plan for the coordination of resources and expenditures; the amount of money available or required for a particular purpose.

depleted Lessened markedly in quantity, content, power, or value.

discrepancies Differences between conflicting facts, claims, or opinions.

fiscal year An accounting period of 12 months during which a company determines earnings and profit; the fiscal year does not necessarily begin in January; the business determines the beginning of its fiscal year.

honorarium A payment in recognition of acts or professional services, usually on a special occasion.

incurred To become liable or subject to; to bring down upon oneself.

mitigating To cause to become less harsh or hostile; to make less severe or painful.

outsourcing The practice of subcontracting work to an outside company.

overhead The ongoing administrative expenses of a business that cannot be attributed to any specific business activity but are still necessary for the business to function (e.g., rent, utilities, insurance).

packing slip A list of items included in a shipment.

per diem By the day; per day. An allowance for daily expenses.

proactive Acting in anticipation of future problems, needs, or changes.

New medical assistants may have difficulty putting all their skills together and using them at the same time throughout the course of a day. Medical assistants must be multitaskers and must develop a good memory. They also must be efficient workers. While in school, medical assisting students spend several days learning a specific skill, such as phlebotomy. However, during the externship and on the job, the medical assistant may need to perform a phlebotomy, chart a procedure, and check out a patient, all within a matter of minutes.

Most of the general tasks in the physician's office are done daily, weekly, or monthly. Such tasks include preparing for the day, using the office policy manual, ordering and receiving supplies, cleaning, office budgeting, lunches and breaks, office security, travel arrangements, and ergonomics. The physician's office is a busy environment where the medical assistant encounters new challenges each day. This chapter details the general office environment and the daily operations that the medical assistant may perform in the physician's office. Multitasking is a critical skill that all medical assistants should strive toward; during a typical day, many duties will be carried out at one time and the medical assistant must keep track of the progress of each responsibility.

The more flexible the medical assistant, the more valuable he or she is to the physician. By learning and refining adaptation skills, medical assistants increase office efficiency, allowing the schedule to handle interruptions and emergencies. Remember that the patient is the reason the office exists and is of primary importance to the office staff. However, various tasks demand attention in the daily operation of the medical office.

THE OFFICE POLICY AND PROCEDURES MANUAL

Virtually all businesses have some type of policy and/or procedures manual, but it is especially important in the physician's office and other medical facilities. The manual should be easy to read, detailed, and logically organized. Besides providing administrative information, the manual also should provide procedural sheets that outline the steps of each procedure performed in the office. The manual should be a "living" document, constantly updated as technology advances and changed whenever regulations change. The manual must be reviewed annually for corrections and additions; this review must be documented as a step in the compliance with regulations established by the Occupational Safety and Health Administration (OSHA). Documentation can be a statement verifying that the manual has been reviewed; this statement should be dated and signed by the office manager or physician. One of OSHA's most common citations for noncompliance is having a policy manual but not following the stated policy in various areas. The medical assistant must form the habit of going to the office policy manual whenever in doubt about any procedure.

Using the Office Policy Manual

All employees should read the office policy manual when they begin working in the physician's office. Manuals and other office policy documents may be posted on the physician's Web site, often in the sections pertaining to employees. Some physicians make these and other employee-related documents available in pdf format. Reading the manual helps the medical assistant become informed about the expectations of supervisors. However, the office policy manual is not only used for new employees (Procedures 12-1 and 12-2). The manual should be a reference that all employees use whenever necessary. OSHA requires that the policy manual be reviewed at least annually to make sure all the information is accurate and up-to-date. Whenever revisions are made, insert a page in the manual giving the date the revisions become effective.

After the revised manual has been reviewed and accepted, a memo can be distributed detailing the changes made and where to look for them.

PROCEDURE 12-1

Explain General Office Policies

GOAL: *To communicate office policies and procedures effectively to employees, patients, and visitors in the office.*

EQUIPMENT and SUPPLIES

- Office policy manual
- Office procedure manual (if not included in policy manual)
- Patient information sheets (if needed)
- Patient information brochure (if needed)

PROCEDURAL STEPS

1. Design an office policy manual and a patient information brochure that provide general information for employees and patients. At a minimum, the information should include:
   - Philosophy statement
   - Goals
   - Description of the medical practice
   - Location and/or map
   - Phone numbers
   - Pager numbers
   - E-mail and Web site addresses
   - Staff names and credentials
   - Services offered
   - Hours of operation
   - Appointment system
   For employees:
   - Vacation, sick leave
   - Confidentiality
   - Grievances
   - Benefits
   - Payroll information
   - Other employee information

   <u>PURPOSE:</u> To give employees and patients a written document that details general information that can be used as a reference when needed.
2. Offer the brochure to new employees and patients or to any other employees and patients who do not have a current brochure.
3. Briefly discuss each section of the brochure with new employees and patients.
   <u>PURPOSE:</u> To acquaint employees and patients with the contents of the policy manual and answer questions that might arise about each section.
4. Watch for verification of understanding from the employee or patient, both verbally and nonverbally. Apply active listening skills.
   <u>PURPOSE:</u> By watching a patient's body language and listening to his or her questions, the medical assistant can determine whether the patient truly understands the information presented.
5. Demonstrate empathy in communicating with patients, family, and staff.
6. Ask the employee or patient if he or she has any questions.
   <u>PURPOSE:</u> To ensure understanding of the information presented.
7. If required, document in the medical record that the employee or patient received the information.
   <u>PURPOSE:</u> To help prove an employee or patient was given certain information about policies and procedures.

PROCEDURE 12-2

Explain the Physician's Instructions to Patients, Staff Members, and Visitors

GOAL: *To communicate office policies and procedures effectively to employees, patients, and visitors in the office so that they understand instructions from the physician.*

EQUIPMENT and SUPPLIES

- Office policy manual
- Office procedure manual (if not included in policy manual)
- Patient information sheets (if needed)
- Physician's orders, if applicable
- Patient information brochure

PROCEDURAL STEPS

1. Determine the communication needs of the employee, patient, or visitor.
   <u>PURPOSE:</u> To discover the best way to communicate information to a person who may have special needs.
2. Arrange for an interpreter, if needed, or involve a family member to assist the patient with the treatment procedures.
   <u>PURPOSE:</u> To make sure information is communicated and received accurately.
3. Provide instructions to the employee, patient, or visitor.
4. Watch for verification of understanding from the individual, both verbally and nonverbally. Apply active listening skills.
   <u>PURPOSE:</u> By watching body language and listening to questions, the medical assistant can determine whether the person truly understands the information presented.
5. Ask whether the person has any questions.
   <u>PURPOSE:</u> To ensure understanding of the information presented.
6. If required, document in the medical record that the employee, patient, or visitor (if necessary) received the instructions.
   <u>PURPOSE:</u> To help prove an employee or patient was given certain instructions about policies, procedures, and expectations or directions about treatment.

The office policy manual should include sections that deal with several topics, such as:

- Expected employee performance
- Tardy and absentee policy
- Sexual harassment
- Confidentiality
- Vacations, sick time, and paid time off
- Employee evaluation
- Continuing education
- Chain of command
- How to deal with certain patients and visitors

Some offices require employees to sign a document stating that they have read and understand the entire policy. The manual should be written clearly and concisely in language that is easily understood. It should be used if a question arises about policy matters and also when an employee is unsure of the reason for or way to proceed with a task. A procedures manual often is combined with the policy manual. Regardless of the setup, every office task should be detailed in one of the two documents.

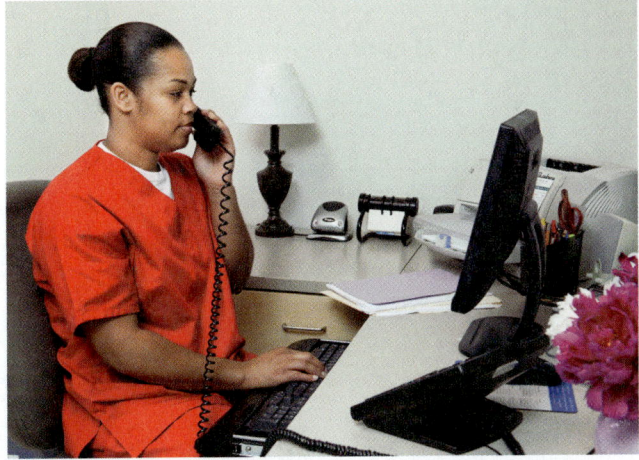

FIGURE 12-1 The telephone is the lifeline of a medical practice. The medical assistant will take several phone messages throughout the course of the day and must see that all of them are given proper attention and follow-up.

OPENING THE OFFICE

Employees arrive earlier than patients so that the office can be prepared for the day. Some office policies dictate that the office be readied for the next day the evening before, but for the purposes of this chapter, assume that the policy requires preparation in the morning.

Although the physician may trust the employees, office policy should demand that supervisors be **proactive** in preventing theft. Depending on the size of the clinic, a certain number of employees will have keys and will know the alarm codes for the facility. The best policy is to monitor this access and information strictly. When numerous keys are distributed, more employees have after-hours access to the office. By limiting this access, the physician may prevent some losses to theft. Two things in particular make the physician's office a target: money and drugs. Usually, only a limited amount of cash is kept in the office. However, most offices keep some medications, often narcotics, which can be addictive or sold for a profit on the street. If such items are used, they must be protected, not only for safety but also to remain in compliance with the law. Even during regular office hours, the staff should practice careful methods, such as keeping back doors locked securely, so that only those authorized are able to enter the building.

PREPARING FOR THE DAY AHEAD

Once the employees have arrived for work, all of them should begin preparing for patients and visitors. Each employee is responsible for his or her own work space, and the staff may work as a team to prepare common areas of the office, such as the reception area. When each person understands the duties required and when they are divided up among the staff, work can be completed quickly and efficiently.

Several duties are completed before the patients arrive. The voice mail or answering service should be checked to collect any messages left since the last time the staff was in the office (Figure 12-1). Some answering services send calls by e-mail or fax. Make sure a phone message book is handy when retrieving messages; write each one into the message book and include all information needed to respond to the message properly. This ensures that copies of the messages are available if one happens to get lost. Patients' records may need to be pulled so that the medical assistant can take action and follow up on the messages.

Print two copies of the day's appointments and place one copy on the physician's desk unless he or she chooses to view the appointments on a computer system. Use the other copy to pull medical records for the patients who will visit the office during the day if paper records are kept. If the office does not use electronic health records, keep the paper medical records in a convenient, central area so that staff members can find them easily once the patients begin to arrive. Make sure the physician has enough room in the progress notes section of the medical record to write the details of the office visit. If needed, add a new sheet of progress notes. Glance over the notes from the last visit to determine whether laboratory work or treatments were ordered and find out whether the results are available.

Patient exam rooms should be restocked with all the regular supplies used in the individual rooms. Items such as cotton balls, bandages, gauze pads, patient gowns, and drapes need to be replenished daily. The physician and patient should never be forced to wait in the examination room while the medical assistant searches for supplies. Check the restrooms to make sure adequate toilet paper, soap, and hand towels are available. If urine specimen cups and towelettes are kept in patient restrooms, make sure enough are available to last throughout the day.

Be sure prescription pads are available for the physician, although they should not be left in open areas or on counters in exam rooms (Figure 12-2). Many physicians keep one pad in their pocket and the extras stored in a locked cabinet. Physicians using electronic health records can print prescriptions directly from their computer system or have them sent to the pharmacy electronically. Patients should never have access to prescription pads, because they might try to forge a prescription; this is a breach of federal or state law

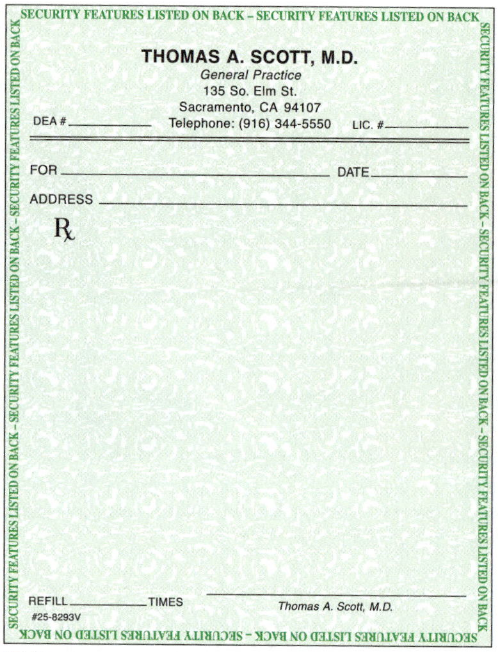

SECURITY FEATURES LISTED ON BACK – SECURITY FEATURES LISTED ON BACK

THOMAS A. SCOTT, M.D.
General Practice
135 So. Elm St.
Sacramento, CA 94107
DEA # _____ Telephone: (916) 344-5550   LIC. # _____

FOR _____   DATE _____

ADDRESS _____

Rx

REFILL _____ TIMES   _____
#25-8293V   Thomas A. Scott, M.D.

SECURITY FEATURES LISTED ON BACK – SECURITY FEATURES LISTED ON BACK

FIGURE 12-2 Keep a close watch on prescription pads, so that patients do not have access to them. Many electronic medical records (EMR) systems allow the physician to write prescriptions directly from the computer.

or both. Take extra care to keep prescription pads out of patients' sight.

Certain equipment may need to be turned on, such as computers, laboratory equipment, and copy machines. Lights should be turned on in all the examination rooms. If quality assurance tests need to be performed on any of the laboratory machines, run the tests and record the results.

Some specimens from previous days may need to be checked for results or additional testing, although many physicians today use outside laboratories. Always record test results in the patient's medical record. The medical assistant cannot decide whether a test result is abnormal; however, if that information is clearly indicated on the lab's report form, then act according to office policy. Some physicians only want to see the test results if they fall outside normal ranges. Most laboratories print test results so that abnormal results are emphasized; they may be printed in a different color ink or in a separate column labeled "Abnormal." If results are abnormal, the physician may need to do follow-up work or see the patient again. As mentioned, the medical assistant cannot judge whether a test result is abnormal, but if that information is clearly indicated, the medical assistant can file the document according to office policy.

CRITICAL THINKING APPLICATION   12-1
Kayla realizes that the office does not have a set method for letting the medical assistants know that laboratory results are ready to be filed. How might she handle this and what suggestions can Kayla make to Elaine?

The patient accounting system should be prepared for the day. Secure enough encounter forms for each patient in the appointment book. Stock the patient checkout area with plenty of appointment cards. If the office gives small gifts to patients, such as refrigerator magnets or coffee mugs, make sure they are available for use. Many offices place the physician's business card just outside the receptionist's window or in the patient reception area. Because patients often take one of the cards, this supply should also be checked.

Various specialty offices may need to prepare additional equipment; therefore, make sure everything necessary is available for the physician and staff members. The day runs smoother when the office is completely prepared for the patients. When all of these duties have been completed, the last task is to unlock the front door and begin welcoming patients to the practice.

PATIENT TRAFFIC FLOW

Ideally, the physician's office is located in an area of town that is easy to find, has ample parking, and does not force the patient to do any excess walking, especially upstairs. The medical assistant is usually not involved with designing the interior of the office; however, the placement of all furniture and equipment is an important factor in the efficient flow of traffic. Patients should be able to quickly determine the location of the patient waiting room. It is helpful if one room is designated as a "sick room" so that well patients will not be stricken with an illness just from visiting the office (when space is short, a face mask may be issued to patients with symptoms of communicable disease). Good traffic flow is important so that the patients and employees can maneuver through the office easily and avoid retracing their steps. Additionally, patients should be able to locate separate parts of the office, such as the lab or check-out areas. Neither patients nor employees should be subjected to dodging furniture or tripping over equipment cords. When moving through the hallways, guide the patient along the right side and leave the left for those traveling in the opposite direction.

CRITICAL THINKING APPLICATION   12-2
One of the older patients seems concerned that an ill child is coughing excessively in the waiting area. How can Kayla help alleviate the patient's concern? What can Kayla do to resolve the issue?

VISITORS TO THE OFFICE

Many people besides patients visit the physician's office. Some of these individuals have appointments; others stop by at random. The office policy manual should detail the procedure to follow in dealing with such individuals. Most physicians prefer to set aside a specific time for pharmaceutical representatives (also called *detail persons* or *drug reps*). These professionals usually are quite competent and knowledgeable about various drugs, and they should be treated with respect by all members of the office staff. In the past, pharmaceutical representatives were allowed to leave memo pads, pens, and other gift items for the physicians and staff that advertised a certain drug or treatment. Many states have laws that prevent pharmaceutical companies from providing these perks. However, some states may not have passed such laws, and physicians still can receive these items. Lawmakers are more concerned about perks such as an **honorarium** for serving as a guest speaker than about pens and notepads. However, many lawmakers believe that physicians' prescribing habits are directly related to pharmaceutical company perks. The company's goal is to educate the physician about their products so that the physician can better care for patients. Some states are developing laws that require reporting of any gifts of more than $25; in most states, this does not include the free samples of the actual drugs. In general, most physicians have decided not to accept these gifts so that no question arises of any breach of ethical conduct.

Pharmaceutical representatives are not the only salespersons who may visit the physician's office. Salespeople from office supply stores, medical equipment sellers, and others may stop by to make appointments or take orders for various items. The office manager usually can address the needs of salespeople and normally is authorized to place orders.

> **CRITICAL THINKING APPLICATION   12-3**
>
> One of the pharmaceutical representatives is extremely pushy. How can Kayla express that the physician cannot meet with the rep? What can Kayla do if the rep continues to be insistent about seeing the physician?

At times, other physicians stop by the office to see the doctor. They may not have an appointment, but the physician should be notified at once when another doctor is waiting in the reception area. If office policy allows, take the visiting physician to the doctor's office instead of forcing him or her to wait in the patient reception area. Because doctors understand busy schedules, most do not stop by another doctor's office without an important reason.

The physician's family members or friends may visit the medical office. Never send family members or friends away without notifying the physician of their presence and asking whether he or she has time to speak to them.

DAILY, WEEKLY, AND MONTHLY DUTIES

Develop a list of duties that are performed daily, weekly, and monthly. Checklists are helpful when staff members want to make sure all duties are completed. The lists help the supervisors divide work evenly among staff members. Be specific on the checklist and include every task that needs to be done, even the most insignificant ones. If a staff member is struggling to finish her daily duties, other staff members should assist so that all required jobs are completed for the day. Take the initiative and work as a team; the effort may be important when supervisors choose employees to promote or terminate.

Constant Cleaning

Patients expect the physician's office to be immaculate. Nothing should be or appear dirty in any part of the facility. Keeping the office truly clean helps curb the spread of germs and communicable diseases. Effective cleaning products should be used daily, especially

in high traffic areas. Countertops, sinks, door handles, and restrooms should be checked frequently and cleaned whenever necessary. When and if slow periods occur between patients or during lengthy office visits, take a cloth and use a disinfectant on nearby counters or around door handles. Look for things to clean in the office. By being conscientious about these things, the medical assistant becomes more valuable to the physician. Supervisors and physicians notice this productivity; good cleaning habits reflect positively on the medical assistant and are important factors in employee evaluations.

Cleaning Services

Many offices employ a cleaning service that performs more intensive chores. These professionals usually come to the facility during the evening, when patients and staff are gone. They clean and disinfect the bathrooms, vacuum, dust, and empty trash. They also may perform other specific tasks as required by the office staff. The office manager should establish some means of communicating with the head of the cleaning team. Many offices leave a notebook for the cleaning crew that details specific cleaning tasks to be performed in addition to regular cleaning tasks. The office manager should delegate a staff member to be the contact person for the service. If any task is not completed in a satisfactory manner, immediately contact the cleaning supervisor and resolve the problem. Make sure a log is kept so that tasks are listed and note whether they were completed or the reason they were not completed. Always inspect what is expected; the cleaning service must perform the jobs it is being paid to do. Do not allow situations to go unresolved. Be open and frank with services that do not meet expectations.

> **CRITICAL THINKING APPLICATION   12-4**
>
> Kayla has noticed that on the days after the cleaning crew has come, sodas, plastic ware, and other small items seem to be missing from the kitchen area. Today, she notices that an entire box of paper towels is gone from the office. Kayla knows the box was there the day before, because she personally checked in the shipment. How can Kayla handle this situation? How is the situation complicated if one of the people who cleans the office at night is a co-worker's sister?

Filing

The medical assistant rarely has a shortage of documents ready to be filed. Although this task sometimes is monotonous, filing is a critical job that must be completed accurately and in a timely manner (Figure 12-3). If a laboratory result is not placed in the right medical record, important information that may affect the patient's health could be lost.

SUPPLIES AND EQUIPMENT IN THE PHYSICIAN'S OFFICE

The medical assistant is responsible for stocking exam rooms and making sure all supplies and equipment are available and in good working order. The following sections describe the process of ordering and receiving medical supplies and equipment.

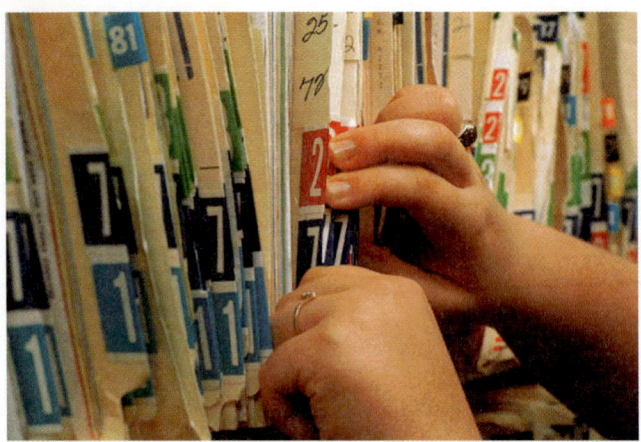

FIGURE 12-3 Filing is a critical job that must be done daily. Filing often is necessary even when an EMR system is used. Office administration files usually are kept in a manual system.

Identifying the Need for Specific Supplies

The medical assistant orders supplies periodically to ensure that the physician has everything needed to treat patients. The office policy and procedures manual details how employees should identify the need for certain supplies, order them, check them in, and place them in the office inventory for use. Nothing is more frustrating to the physician than reaching for an item during a procedure, only to find it is unavailable. Communication is the key to keeping supplies in stock.

Budgeting

Most offices use an annual **budget** to determine the amount of money to be spent on various categories of expenses (Figure 12-4). Some expenses involved in the operation of a medical practice include:

- Salaries
- Medical supplies
- Business equipment
- Medical equipment
- Utilities
- Rent or mortgage
- Insurance
- Maintenance
- Taxes
- Laboratory fees
- Office supplies

Expense categories are important, because most business expenses can be deducted on tax returns, and staff salaries are directly related to the physician's **overhead** costs. Always keep receipts for items to be used in the medical office and submit them in a timely manner to the office manager or other designated individual.

CRITICAL THINKING APPLICATION   12-5

Elaine has asked Kayla to prepare a budget for next year for her department. Kayla has never done this before. How can she prepare for this challenging task? What references can she use to develop an accurate budget for the coming year?

Businesses usually plan expenses for the year in advance, allocating expected income into various categories of expenses. Then, at least monthly, expenses are logged into a ledger or spreadsheet and separated into specific categories. This allows tracking of expenses to ensure that a category is not over budget. If a specific category of expenses is over budget, adjustments may need to be logged in, either to allot more funds to that category or to stop spending in that category until the next year. Exceeding the allowed amount in a budget is not necessarily uncommon; however, good business practice dictates that budgets come in very close to the estimations made at the beginning of the budget year. When a category goes over budget, money often must be taken from another budget category to cover the amount. This reduces the money available in the second category. Employees should not be allowed to spend money needlessly or wastefully. The physician should designate a minimum number of people to make purchases on behalf of the facility.

Comparing Prices

A good shopper is an asset to the physician's office. Compare prices when shopping for supplies and equipment. Tell salespeople that comparisons will be conducted and that price will be a strong consideration when the time comes to make a purchase. However, price should not be the only consideration. Warranties, bulk purchase opportunities, maintenance agreements, and other factors may influence the best deal available on a certain item. Quality is another important factor; the physician may be willing to pay more for an item based on its quality and durability. Personal preference also influences purchasing decisions. The clinical medical assistant may prefer one brand of needles over another, even though they are the same price. In most circumstances, those who regularly use a certain item should be allowed to decide the brand, model, or other specifics before the item is purchased.

Most companies produce a catalog, whether online or printed. When a need has been identified, compare the prices from at least three sources before placing an order. For instance, if 70% isopropyl alcohol is needed, and the stock must last 6 months, first determine how much is needed. Suppose that approximately one 16-ounce bottle is used per month in each of five treatment rooms. Further suppose that the following prices are listed:

Smith's Medical Supply	1 dozen bottles	$10. 53
Argosy Medical and Dental Supply	2 dozen bottles	$17. 44
Walgreens	1 bottle	$ .53
CVS Pharmacy	1 gallon	$ 6. 12

If these prices are compared, and assuming all other aspects of the products are equal, buying bottles of alcohol at Walgreens clearly is a better deal than buying one or two dozen at either Smith's Medical Supply or Argosy Medical and Dental Supply. The alcohol at Smith's costs approximately 87¢ per bottle; at Argosy, the cost is approximately 72¢ per bottle. Is the gallon a better buy? Let's work it out. The alcohol can always be poured into containers from the gallon bottle. A gallon has 128 ounces; it therefore can provide only 8 16-ounce bottles; the cost per bottle is approximately 76¢. Walgreens, at 53¢ per bottle, has the lowest price. Still, if Walgreens is 15 miles away, the gas used to get the alcohol may push the total

Chart of Accounts - Variance Analysis Template

	Budget	This month	Last month	This month last year	This year to date	Last year to date
ALL EXPENSES	100%					
Capital (IRS section 179) purchases						
Donations and contributions						
Dues						
Fees: Lab						
Fees: Retirement plan						
Insurance: Business						
Insurance: Malpractice						
Janitorial/maintenance						
Journals						
Lease payments: Equipment						
Legal, accounting and consultants						
Loan payments: Principal						
Loan payments: Interest						
Marketing: Ads, promotion and yellow pages						
Marketing: Meals and entertainment						
Meals: Business/staff meetings						
Miscellaneous						
Outside services						
Postage						
Rent and utilities						
Repairs and maintenance: Building						
Repairs and maintenance: Contracts						
Repairs and maintenance: Equipment						
Staff wages						
Staff benefits						
Staff retirement plan						
Staff continuing education						
Supplies: Clinical						
Supplies: Office						
Taxes and licenses						
Telephone/answering service/pager						
Travel and professional meetings						
Uniforms and laundry						
Doctor associate wages						
Doctor associate benefits						
Doctor associate retirement plan						
Doctor associate continuing education						
Ancillary provider wages						
Ancillary provider benefits						
Ancillary provider retirement plan						
Ancillary provider continuing education						
Owner's wages/draws						
Owner's benefits						
Owner's retirement plan						
Owner's auto						
Owner's dues						
Owner's individual and student loans						
Owner's insurances						
Owner's journals						
Owner's marketing: Meals and entertainment						
Owner's other						
Doctor-owner net income (practice profit)						

Adapted with permission from *Medical Practice Forms: Every Form You Need to Succeed.* Copyright © 2004 PMIC. Physicians may adapt for use in their own practices; all other rights reserved. "Three Steps to an Effective Practice Budget." Borglum K. *Family Practice Management.* January 2004:46-50, http://www.aafp.org/fpm/20040100/46thre.html.

FIGURE 12-4 Chart of accounts. Most physicians' offices operate on an annual budget to control expenditures and to make sure supplies and equipment are readily available.

cost higher than the total cost of driving 2 miles to Argosy to buy the product. Also consider delivery and shipping and handling charges, in addition to sales taxes, that might be added to the cost of the order. Some suppliers may cut the cost on certain items to get the order, either meeting or beating the deal offered by another supplier. Examine all costs before placing the order with a supplier.

Ordering Supplies

Responsibility for ordering supplies in the medical office should be assigned to one person. The medical assistant who assumes this task can use various methods to track the needed supplies and then place orders to replenish them. One simple method is to develop a spreadsheet that lists all the products and supplies that need to be ordered periodically (Procedure 12-3). Post the sheets in areas where supplies are stored. When staff members take supplies from storage, they should make a note on the spreadsheet. When it is time to place an order, the sheets are gathered and used to determine which supplies need to be replenished. Some offices use software programs to prepare orders, and others use a computer system to enter products taken from the supply area. Still others may use a sticker system, in which a coded sticker is removed when a product is used and placed on a card or form; that amount then is charged to the patient. Others use a note card system, in which a note card is prepared for each supply item, and after the inventory has been performed; orders are completed based on the needs reflected by the note cards. After determining the items that need to be ordered, browse medical or office supply catalogs to shop for the best prices (Procedure 12-4). The order may need to be divided and offered to two different suppliers if certain items can be obtained at a better rate.

The Internet is a valuable tool for shopping for supplies. Businesses often can find excellent prices and great discounts by ordering online (Figure 12-5). Some physicians and office managers may be hesitant to use credit card accounts online; however, if an account is established with an online supply company, they will hold payment information or perhaps extend credit, and the company credit card need not be used. Most physicians establish accounts with suppliers and pay the accounts monthly. Because credit card purchases involve fees and interest payments, the balance should be paid off monthly to prevent additional charges. These charges increase each month a balance is carried on the account, which makes the actual cost higher than just paying cash for the order.

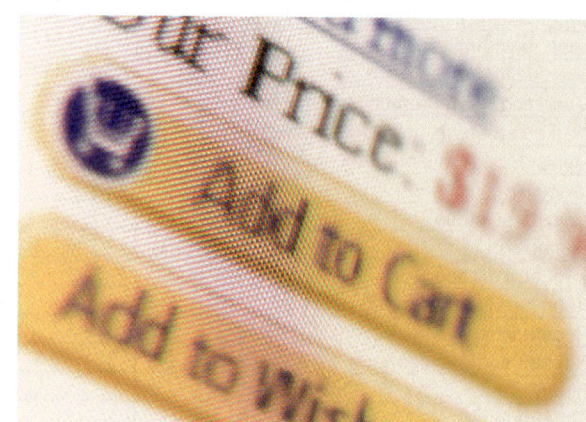

FIGURE 12-5 Competitive prices can be found using Internet research. Purchasing through the Internet is easy, safe, and convenient.

PROCEDURE 12-3

Inventory Office Supplies and Equipment

GOAL: To establish an inventory of all expendable supplies in the physician's office and follow an efficient plan or order control.

EQUIPMENT and SUPPLIES

- Computer
- Inventory and order control cards or stickers
- Computer spreadsheet or list of supplies on hand
- Pen or pencil

PROCEDURAL STEPS

1. Inventory all supplies on hand and enter this information into a computer spreadsheet.
   PURPOSE: To establish a record of all items in the current inventory.
2. Enter into the spreadsheet the name of the item, the number of items currently in stock, the usual price per item, and any bulk discounts.
   PURPOSE: To establish a beginning inventory.
3. Determine the point where the supply should be replenished and highlight or otherwise tag those items.
   PURPOSE: The notation or tag serves as an alert that supply is low.
4. Review the spreadsheet to determine which items are ready to be reordered.
5. When the order has been placed, note the date and quantity ordered on the spreadsheet.
6. When the order is received, note the date and quantity in the appropriate column, and add the new inventory to the spreadsheet.
   NOTE: If the order is only partially filled, make note of items that are backordered and monitor until the order is complete.
7. Repeat the inventory and ordering process each month.
   PURPOSE: To ensure that all supplies are available in the facility when needed.
8. Periodically ask for input from staff members about specific supplies purchased for use in the facility.
   PURPOSE: To provide the people who use the individual supply items an opportunity to suggest products they prefer and that are easy to use, reliable, and efficient.

PROCEDURE 12-4

Prepare a Purchase Order

GOAL: *To prepare an accurate purchase order for supplies or equipment.*

EQUIPMENT and SUPPLIES

- List of current inventory
- Phone
- Purchase order
- Fax machine
- Pen

PROCEDURAL STEPS

1. Review the current inventory and determine what items need to be ordered.
   PURPOSE: To determine what is needed so that the office will not be overstocked or understocked.
2. Complete the purchase order accurately, filling in all applicable spaces and blanks with the information requested.
   PURPOSE: To create an accurately completed purchase order, which helps eliminate mistakes in the order and in shipments.
3. List the items to be ordered, including quantity, item numbers, size, color, price, and extended price. Be sure all applicable information is included.
   PURPOSE: To help ensure accurate orders.

4. Provide the physician's signature, Drug Enforcement Administration (DEA) certificate, and medical license when needed.
   PURPOSE: Some items require these documents to verify that the physician is eligible to order them.
5. Call in, fax, mail, or electronically submit the order to the vendor. Keep a copy for your records. Keep any verification provided that the order was received, such as a fax receipt.
   PURPOSE: To document exactly what was ordered on what date and provide proof that the order was received.
6. Note on the inventory which items are on order.
   PURPOSE: To keep other staff members from preparing duplicate orders.
7. Keep a copy of the order in the appropriate place in the office filing system.
   PURPOSE: To reference the order if needed and have a copy of the items ordered to compare with the packing list once the items arrive at the office.

Replenishing Supplies

Replenish supplies at the reception desk regularly. Stationery, appointment cards, charge slips, sharpened pencils, pens, telephone message pads, and any items likely to be needed should be on hand when the day begins. Discovering that supplies are **depleted** during a busy day can seriously interrupt the flow of patient care. One person should be in charge of checking the inventory of supplies regularly and ordering as necessary. In a practice with several employees, a clinical assistant usually is responsible for checking clinical supplies and preparing the patient rooms; however, in a small practice, only one assistant may be available for all duties. Everything should be ready for the day before patients begin to arrive, so that the physician and medical assistant can give their undivided attention to the patients' needs.

Ordering Equipment

Ordering equipment is more involved than ordering simple supplies. Much of the equipment acquired for the physician's office is considered a capital purchase. Before purchasing this type of equipment, compare price, features, and benefits. The physician or office manager almost always is involved in the purchase of capital equipment. Different businesses use different monetary amounts to classify capital purchases; some use $1,000, whereas others may consider a capital purchase as one that exceeds $5,000. Physicians consult with accountants to determine the limits on capital purchase amounts. At least three estimates should be obtained before making a major equipment purchase.

The physician and staff members who will use the equipment will have questions about the features and benefits, in addition to the cost to purchase and the cost to use in the facility. Sometimes the cost of using certain equipment may exceed the cost of **outsourcing**. For instance, performing a complete blood count (CBC) in the office may cost $10. If the test can be outsourced by sending it to an outpatient laboratory and the resulting cost is $8, the physician could avoid equipment and maintenance costs. Also, if the physician continues to charge $10 for a CBC, he or she will make a profit of $2 on every test. Physicians should not order unnecessary tests; however, making a profit on procedures and treatments performed is certainly ethical. Remember, the physician's office is a business, and there is nothing unethical about making a profit.

CRITICAL THINKING APPLICATION   12-6
Kayla is talking with a patient who tells her husband that she doesn't know how they will afford lab tests. When Kayla walks by them, they stop talking. How can Kayla help the patient in this situation? Should Kayla mention to the patient that she overheard her concerns?

The medical assistant has numerous options when looking for equipment to purchase. Start the search on the Internet to get an idea of the price range of the equipment, both new and used. Local suppliers offer catalogs detailing the products and equipment available, and the suppliers' sales representatives can answer questions. Investigate whether used equipment might be for sale from the supplier. Physicians selling their practice or retiring might have equipment for sale. Obviously, some items should be purchased only from a medical supplier, but many great deals are available from various sources.

Receiving an Order

When an order arrives from a supplier, notify the person in charge of inventory. Boxes should be opened only if enough time is available to check them in properly. Carefully open the package and look for the **packing slip**, which is a list of items ordered and the items shipped. Occasionally an ordered item will not be included in the package because it has been placed on **backorder**. The item may be out of stock but will be sent to the physician as soon as it becomes available. Compare the items listed on the packing slip to the items found inside the box. If any **discrepancies** are found, bring them to the attention of the supplier immediately. Employees should never take items from the package before they have been checked against the packing slip. Once the order has been checked in, make a note on the packing slip that the package was received as expected and then place new stock in the proper place. Make sure stock is rotated, with the new items placed at the back and older items or those with earlier expiration dates placed at the front so that they are used first.

Warranty Information

Many purchased items include a warranty. Always mail warranty information to the manufacturer. Warranty cards usually resemble a postcard and have several questions about the purchaser. If the warranty card is completed and returned, the manufacturer can contact those who have purchased a certain product if defects are discovered or recalls are necessary. The warranty period begins on the date of purchase and usually lasts 1 year, but it can be longer, depending on the item purchased. Keep a copy of the completed warranty in a file with other information on the specific product or piece of equipment, such as the receipt for the purchase, expense records, owner's manuals, and maintenance records.

Invoices and Statements

An invoice is an itemized list of goods shipped that specifies the price and the terms of a sale. A statement is a summary of a financial account that shows the balance due and transactions that affect the account. Invoices precede statements. A medical supplier may send an invoice when a sale has been completed, and statements are mailed whenever an account has a balance. Some invoices request payment upon receipt, whereas others allow a certain period to make a payment (Figure 12-6). Read invoices and statements carefully and make sure they are free of errors before making a payment.

Troubleshooting Equipment Failure

When equipment fails to function properly, consult the owner's manual to determine the steps for troubleshooting. The owner's manual includes contact information so that the purchaser can reach the manufacturer if necessary. Today, purchasers have additional contact options, such as e-mail and live chat via the Internet; both offer fast access for problems that need to be solved quickly.

Equipment Maintenance

Medical office equipment must be maintained regularly, especially machines that perform testing procedures. The Clinical Laboratory

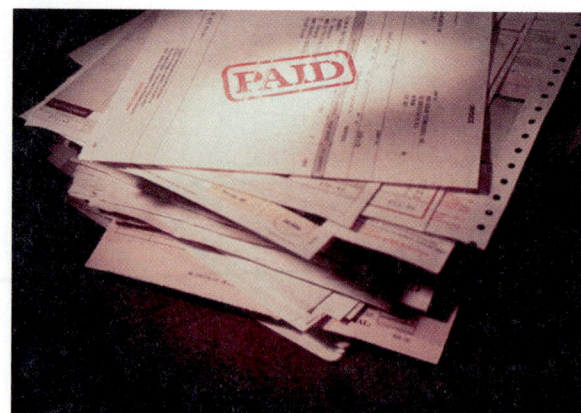

FIGURE 12-6 Invoices and statements must be compared carefully to orders actually received at the physician's office.

Improvement Amendments (CLIA) require that controls and calibrations be performed. All these requirements are designed to ensure that patient testing is accurate and that those results are reliable. Remember that the maintenance must be performed by an authorized user of the equipment; in general, if an employee is authorized to use the equipment, he or she also can take care of maintenance issues.

The maintenance process is similar to maintaining a car in good working condition. Periodically, the oil, filters, and tires must be changed, brake pads must be removed and replaced, and the engine must be kept clean. Similarly, medical office machines must be kept in good repair and working condition (Procedure 12-5).

Maintenance guidelines are included in the owner's manual, and they should be the basis of any maintenance plan. The medical assistant can develop a maintenance schedule to ensure that all office equipment receives proper, timely attention. Keep all information about each equipment item in a separate file and add maintenance records as they are produced. Routine maintenance is important for keeping equipment in top working order, so that patient care is not affected by the availability of equipment. Some machines may require proof of maintenance records to honor warranties. Some physicians prefer to lease equipment, such as copiers, that have a maintenance plan included in the monthly rate. This often proves to be more economical than purchasing expensive machines; the maintenance plan is usually in effect the entire time the equipment is leased, and better warranties are often attached to leased equipment. The medical assistant may be asked to perform comparative pricing on such items and help determine the most efficient direction the office should take with regard to leasing or making a purchase.

PREVENTING WASTE

Waste prevention reduces the production of waste or eliminates it entirely. Companies can reduce the cost of waste management, reduce long-term liability for the disposal of hazardous waste, and become more efficient to enhance profit margins. The key to successful waste management is the cooperation of employees; unless they are willing to participate in waste management efforts, most

PROCEDURE 12-5

Perform and Document Routine Maintenance of Office Equipment

GOAL: To ensure that all office equipment is in good working order at all times.

EQUIPMENT and SUPPLIES

- Spreadsheet with information on each piece of office equipment, including serial number and servicing schedule
- Pen or pencil
- Computer
- Access to all office equipment

PROCEDURAL STEPS

1. Gather information about each piece of equipment, including at least:
   - Name of equipment
   - Type of equipment
   - Manufacturer's or maker's name
   - Manufacturer's address
   - Contact phone numbers for technical support
   - Contact phone numbers for main office
   - Date purchased
   - Cost of product
   - Original receipt showing where the item was purchased
   - Date warranty begins and ends
   - Addresses to which equipment should be sent if under warranty
   - Number of times the equipment needs service in a year
   - Last date of service
   - Explanation of what was done during last servicing
   - Number assigned by the office manager to identify the equipment

   PURPOSE: To give the medical assistant all the information needed for maintenance and servicing of the equipment.

2. Place all the information about each piece of equipment into a spreadsheet.
   PURPOSE: To create a written record and documentation of all information about each piece of equipment.

3. Make a list of the months of the year. Note which equipment needs servicing in which months.
   PURPOSE: To create a calendar for equipment servicing.

4. Check the spreadsheet monthly to determine which equipment needs servicing that month.

5. Schedule equipment servicing and maintenance during the current month.
   PURPOSE: To establish a specific time the equipment will be available for servicing.

6. Check with co-workers to make sure servicing dates work with all schedules, especially if a piece of equipment will be out of service for any length of time.
   PURPOSE: To prevent scheduling conflicts during times the staff needs the equipment.

7. Schedule servicing appointments.

8. Oversee appointment scheduling to make sure the appointments are kept.

9. Record new information on the document or spreadsheet to reflect new times for servicing and any additional information.
   PURPOSE: To ensure that the most accurate information is on file about every piece of equipment in the office and that all maintenance records are documented.

---

efforts will be unsuccessful. Employees in a physician's office can reduce waste while saving money in the following ways:

- Use solar-powered calculators and battery rechargers
- Use refillable pens, pencils, and tape dispensers
- Use refillable calendars
- Use two-way billing envelopes
- Reuse file folders and binders
- Refurbish office equipment
- Use bulletin boards
- Reuse printer toner and ribbon cartridges
- Retrofit exit sign bulbs
- Convert to high-efficiency fluorescent lighting
- Reuse dishware
- Use reusable forced air filters
- Reuse single-sided paper

Avoiding waste and being conservative with products at the office save money and may result in an increase in employee wages and benefits. Always participate in efforts to preserve products and be open to trying new conservation methods.

LUNCH AND BREAK TIMES

Even though the physician's office is a busy place and often hectic, all staff members should take a morning and afternoon break and a lunch period. Many offices close between noon and 2 PM so that the staff can have lunch and use the time to rest and refocus (Figure 12-7). Often, office managers rotate lunches so that there is always someone at the front desk; some assistants go to lunch during the first hour and some during the second hour. Although many people run errands and try to complete personal tasks during lunch, health-care workers should make every effort actually to use breaks for their intended purpose so that they can serve patients to the best of their ability.

Be respectful of lunch hours and break times by leaving and returning at the appropriate time. Remember to clean any dishes used and put them away and to return food to the refrigerator that belongs there. If food produces a strong odor, close the lunchroom door and use ventilation if it is available in the room. Patients expect a clean, fresh smell in the office. Medical supplies that need to be refrigerated cannot be stored with food. Leftovers should be removed at least once a week. All employees should keep the lunch or break area clean. Always wash your hands or use hand sanitizer after lunch and all breaks and between patients.

SENDING AND RECEIVING E-MAIL

Electronic communications are sent and received frequently throughout the business day. E-mail used in the professional office should have a professional tone, good grammar, and accurate spelling. Never use Internet slang or abbreviations in any professional message. Treat e-mail information as confidential if it relates to a patient. Use the office e-mail system for work-related messages only. Use a separate, personal e-mail address for information that is not business related. The information on the company computer belongs to the company;

it does not belong to the user. If family and friends send jokes or off-color comics, the user can be held responsible for them and ultimately terminated for their content. Refrain from sending and receiving such messages on business computers. A good general rule to follow is to refrain from sending any e-mail at the workplace that supervisors should not read. Remember that the information services staff often can find e-mails and other improper files on computers, even if they have been deleted. Also, some computer systems can be monitored in real time, with every keystroke recorded and every Web site visited logged. Many businesses require employees to sign a statement that explains acceptable use of the Internet, e-mail, and computer systems policies. Employees may be terminated for noncompliance with these policies or improper use of the computer system.

INTERNET RESEARCH

The medical assistant may be asked to research various types of information using the Internet (Procedure 12-6). If a word or phrase is entered into a search engine, various Web sites containing the word or phrase appear on the results screen. Not all articles found on the Internet are reliable; some are completely false, and others are simply one person's or group's opinion. Look for information from sites that can be trusted, such as the American Heart Association or the American Medical Association. Once a good, informative site has been found, read through it carefully, because it may lead to more sites that provide additional information.

TRAVELING FOR BUSINESS PURPOSES

Throughout the course of a **fiscal year**, employees may attend seminars or workshops to gain additional information, learn new techniques or procedures, and obtain continuing education units (CEUs), which may be needed to maintain certification.

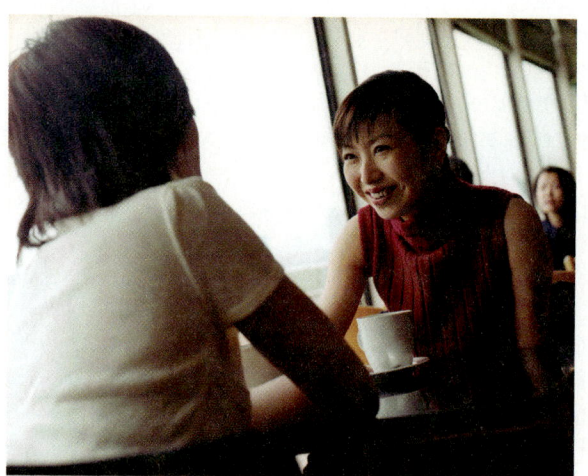

FIGURE 12-7 Use lunch periods and breaks to relax. Don't skip lunch or breaks, because this practice can lead to burnout.

PROCEDURE 12-6

Use the Internet to Access Information Related to the Medical Office

GOAL: *To use the Internet to research any topic related to the medical office.*

EQUIPMENT and SUPPLIES

- Computer
- Topic for research
- Printer

PROCEDURAL STEPS

1. Start the computer, if necessary.
2. Open a Web browser (e.g., Internet Explorer or Firefox).
   PURPOSE: The Web browser allows the user to access a home page, from where a search engine can be activated.
3. Open a search engine (e.g., Yahoo, Google, Dogpile, Alta Vista, WebCrawler).
4. Type the subject of the research in the Search box.

5. Review the results.
   PURPOSE: To make sure the search results contain valuable information on the subject.
6. Determine whether the search results are from a reliable source.
   PURPOSE: To obtain quality, accurate information from a source that can be trusted.
7. Decide what information is pertinent to the research project.
8. Print the information, if desired.
   PURPOSE: To make a hard copy of the information for later reference.
9. Create a file on the computer to store information about the research subject.
   PURPOSE: To allow referencing of the research information without repeating the search.

Seminars and Workshops

Both physicians and office staff members periodically attend seminars or workshops to participate in continuing education events or to learn new skills. Physicians are required to accumulate a certain number of continuing education credits each year, and a medical assistant also may need continuing education credits, depending on his or her type of certification. When planning to attend a seminar, consider not only the cost of the sessions, but also the cost of travel to and from the seminar and of lodgings, gas, and food. Invitations to attend seminars often arrive in the mail, although some arrive by e-mail. Watch for enrollment deadlines and make sure registration is done before the deadline date. Some seminars offer great discounts if registration is completed early.

Scheduling Travel, Hotel Rooms, and Car Rentals

The location of the event often dictates the type of travel arrangements that should be made (Procedure 12-7). Distant locations usually require an airline flight. A travel agent sometimes is used to book flights and hotel rooms, but more and more, companies are booking their own flights using the Internet. Other trips involve car travel. Staff members who travel by car are entitled to reimbursement for mileage expenses; in fact, the company should reimburse any reasonable business expense **incurred**.

Many organizations suggest hotels on the brochures for events. If the physician prefers a certain hotel, reservations should be made at that location if possible. However, do not hesitate to suggest a different hotel if one is closer to the event or offers a better price for the same amenities.

Renting a car may be necessary so that staff members can travel from place to place while attending the seminar. Take care when using a debit card to pay for rentals or deposits. Many establishments place a hold on the estimated total balance due, even if the balance may be paid in cash. This process could place a hold on available funds until the payment actually clears.

Travel Receipts

Travelers should keep all receipts obtained during the trip and turn them in to the office manager. Most business trip expenses are tax deductible. After the traveler returns to the office, a travel expense

---

PROCEDURE 12-7

Make Travel Arrangements

GOAL: *To make travel arrangements for the physician or another staff member.*

EQUIPMENT and SUPPLIES

- Travel plan
- Telephone
- Telephone directory
- Computer

PROCEDURAL STEPS

1. Verify the dates of the planned trip; consider:
   - Desired date and time of departure
   - Desired date and time of return
   - Preferred mode of transportation
   - Number in party
   - Preferred lodging and price range
   - Ticketing method
2. Telephone a trusted travel agency to arrange for transportation and lodging reservations or book the trip using Internet resources.
   PURPOSE: A travel agent might be better suited to answer questions about regulations for international travel. The Internet is an easy way to book trips and compare costs.
3. Arrange for traveler's checks, if desired.
   PURPOSE: Using traveler's checks is better than carrying large amounts of cash; they can be easily replaced if lost or stolen.
4. Print tickets or e-receipts from the computer.
5. Using the travel plan, check the tickets for errors.
   PURPOSE: To prevent errors resulting from misunderstanding and to verify compliance with travel requests.

6. Check to see that hotel and airline reservations have been confirmed and note the confirmation numbers.
7. Prepare an itinerary:
   - Date and time of departure
   - Flight numbers or identifying information for other modes of travel
   - Mode of transportation to hotel (or hotels)
   - Name, address, and telephone number of hotel and confirmation numbers if available
   - Name, address, and telephone number of travel agency
   - Date and time of return
   PURPOSE: The itinerary provides the details of the entire trip at a glance and is a more organized way to keep up with times, dates, confirmation numbers, and other details all in one document.
8. Keep one copy of the itinerary in the office files and e-mail or give one to the office manager and/or physician.
   PURPOSE: To help locate the traveler, if necessary, at every point of the trip.
9. E-mail or give several copies of the itinerary to the traveler.
   PURPOSE: To provide the traveler with extra copies for family or friends.
10. Collect all travel receipts when the traveler returns.
    PURPOSE: To prove all expenses during business travel, for tax purposes.

report should be completed, which details the expenses incurred and any repayment due the employee. Some businesses provide the traveler with **advance** money, which must be reconciled once all receipts have been collected. Remember that some businesses allow a set dollar amount for meals, such as $10 for breakfast, $20 for lunch, and $35 for dinner. This is called a **per diem**, which is an allowance for daily expenses. Account for each expense on the report and attach the receipts, then turn the report in to the designated person. Make a copy for personal records. Taxes should not be taken out of business expense reimbursements.

BASIC SAFETY AND SECURITY IN THE MEDICAL OFFICE

No one knows when the safety and the security individuals enjoy will be jeopardized. The saying "better safe than sorry" has never been truer than today. Never assume that any place of business is immune to crime.

Suspicious Persons

If a suspicious person enters the office, make every effort to keep a distance. Staff members should stay behind the counter or desk so that the person cannot grab or gain control of one of the employees. If you feel a serious concern about a suspicious individual, try to notify another employee early in the conversation. Pick up the telephone and dial the office manager's extension. Plan a code in advance for different emergency situations. For instance, use the phrase, "Norman is here to see you," which relates to Norman Bates of the movie *Psycho*, a frightening character. This alerts the office manager that a potential problem has arisen at the front desk and the police should be called. Even if the situation isn't life-threatening, the police would rather respond to a false alarm than arrive to find a crisis.

Robbery

Although physicians' offices rarely have an excess of cash on hand, thieves may assume that there is money to steal or, more likely, narcotics. Do not argue or fight with such people. Give them what they want; the object is to get them out of the office as quickly as possible. Once they are out, lock the doors and call the police. Do not touch any items the robber touched so that the crime scene is preserved. When such a situation occurs, employees clearly will be under duress; however, they should make every effort to remember basic identifying markers:

- Height
- Weight
- Hair color and length
- Clothing, especially the color
- Race
- Distinctive marks (e.g., scars, tattoos)

Make the observations as subtly as possible; criminals rarely react well to being sized up for later identification. If the criminal refuses to leave the office and the situation escalates, make every effort to find out what the person wants that will prompt him or her to leave. Remain as calm as possible throughout the ordeal. For more safety tips for employees, visit the Evolve site at *evolve.elsevier.com/ kinn*.

Office Security

Various valuable items can be found in the medical office. Narcotics are stored in a locked cabinet, and cash and checks are kept in the office. Prescription pads, cash, and checks must be locked up securely and kept out of sight. For these reasons, the office must always be secure. A thief does not know whether the office has narcotics or cash but will assume that they are available. Even if the office has neither, the staff must be prepared for office crime and be proactive in preventing such situations.

Alarm systems often are used to protect the medical office. Either the office is monitored, or an alarm sounds when tripped. Monitored alarms go off when a door or window is opened and the security code is not entered into the unit. When the alarm is tripped, an employee of the alarm company attempts to call the office to determine whether a true emergency exists. If no one answers, the alarm company sends the police to the facility. Occasionally a false alarm sounds, prompting the police to investigate. Many alarm companies charge the business a fee when the alarm is not a valid emergency.

Only a few staff members need to know the alarm code. The office manager and those who open and close the facility need to know the code, as does the physician. The fewer people who know the code, the better. A combination of letters and numbers is best for alarms, rather than a strictly numeric or alphabetic code.

The office manager should make daily bank deposits, putting all the cash and check payments from patients into the physician's checking account. The only cash that should remain in the office is a minimum amount of petty cash. Remember, a person who decides to rob the facility may assume that the physician has an abundance of cash on hand. Unless daily deposits are made, that assumption may be true. Never keep deposits in a purse or car, or put off going to the bank until the next day, or keep deposits at home overnight. Once the medical assistant takes the deposit out of the office to any location other than the bank, he or she is responsible for those funds.

Smoke Alarms and Fire Extinguishers

Smoke alarms should be installed in every physician's office. The two basic types of smoke alarms are photoelectric alarms and ionization alarms. If nuisance alarms continually sound (e.g., from making popcorn in the lounge area), changing the type of alarm may solve the problem. Smoke alarm batteries must be changed twice a year; the best time to do this is when daylight savings time occurs. Although the old batteries may not be dead, new ones will be fresh and certainly will last 6 months.

Fire extinguishers must be readily available and prominently mounted in a visible, convenient place. The extinguishers must be serviced annually by a fire professional certified to perform inspections. Also, staff members should be trained in the use of fire extinguishers; most fire departments offer this training for free or at a nominal charge. A multipurpose ABC fire extinguisher is appropriate for a small business. Staff members can remember the basic use of the fire extinguisher by memorizing the mnemonic device PASS:

P—Pull the pin
A—Aim the hose
S—Squeeze the handle
S—Sweep the nozzle

In addition, remember to "RACE":

R—Rescue

A—Alarm

C—Confine

E—Extinguish

To determine whether a physician's office is safe, answer the following questions:

- Are all exits accessible and unobstructed?
- Are all fire extinguishers operable and properly located?
- Are all emergency lighting units and exit signs operable?
- Are any extension cords or multiplug adaptors in use?
- Does an escape plan exist with two ways out and do employees know how to use it?
- Are fire alarms and the sprinkler system functioning correctly and easily accessible?
- Are all materials stored neatly and orderly without obstructing the sprinkler heads?
- Are all flammable liquids and materials stored away from heat sources?
- Are all plumbing, mechanical, and electrical systems functioning properly?

Fire Exits and Exit Routes

At least two exits in the medical facility must be designated fire exits. These exits must be clearly marked and easily accessible. The exit doors must remain unlocked during business hours so that people can get out in case of a fire or other emergency. For security reasons doors can be locked on the outside, but they must have an exit bar on the inside that allows people to leave by pushing on the exit bar. In case of a fire during office hours, remember to assist patients and visitors to exit the facility.

Employees should have regular drills that allow them to practice evacuating the building. An escape plan must be posted in every room of the facility showing the exit routes from that particular room. Two escape routes from each room should be posted, a primary route and a secondary route. Before leaving through a door, feel it; if it feels warm, exit by another route. If the facility is two stories tall, have ladders ready that attach to a window and unfold to allow escape. Buildings with two or more stories also should have stairwells that can be used in case of fire.

EMERGENCY PREPAREDNESS

According to the Federal Emergency Management Agency (FEMA), an emergency is any unplanned event that can cause death or significant injury to employees, patients, or the public. Emergencies can immediately shut down a business, disrupt operations, cause physical or environmental damage, or threaten a facility's financial standing or public image. All the following events are considered emergencies:

- Fire
- Hazardous materials spill
- Flood
- Hurricane
- Tornado
- Winter storm
- Earthquake
- Communications failure
- Terrorist act or attack
- Bioterrorism
- Civil disturbance
- Explosion

The event does not have to be a large-scale disaster to affect the medical community adversely.

Emergency management is the process of preparing for, **mitigating**, responding to, and recovering from an emergency (Procedure 12-8). Every medical office needs an emergency operations plan (EOP). The objectives of the plan should include:

1. Protecting the safety of patients, visitors, and staff
2. Providing prompt, efficient medical care
3. Establishing a clear chain of command
4. Maintaining and restoring essential services as quickly as possible
5. Protecting clinic property, facilities, and equipment

The first critical step in emergency preparedness planning is to determine what emergencies or disasters might happen in a single medical facility or in a general area. Kaiser Permanente has created a Hazard Vulnerability Assessment (HVA), which can be used by any medical facility to identify the hazards in a particular geographic area (Figure 12-8). After considering all the information gained by reviewing the HVA, outline an EOP that addresses each of the hazards that might affect the physician's office. Once those hazards have been identified, determine the steps that must be taken to enable the facility to respond properly to each hazard. Consider whether additional equipment and supplies must be purchased or whether the office list of community resources is up-to-date and can handle several referrals at once (Procedure 12-9). How would the office staff handle a mass influx of emergency patients, if need be, while still treating the patients scheduled on a particular day? What type of documentation would be necessary when caring for mass emergency patients? What medications are necessary to treat patients in an emergency? The HVA can help the physician and staff answer these and other questions, which will prepare them for many different types of emergencies.

The physician and staff should be ready to offer their services if disaster strikes, especially during a natural disaster such as a hurricane, flood, fire, or other emergency situation. Remember, the medical assistant can only perform duties for which he or she has been trained but can certainly assist a physician and take his or her direction as emergency care is given to a patient.

After the EOP has been written and reviewed, every employee on staff must be trained in how the plan should be followed. Written copies must be easily accessible. Employees should hold emergency drills once a quarter to practice their response. Without practice, the EOP will not work as smoothly as when employees know their roles and responsibilities during emergencies. One person should be designated the facility's safety officer. Make sure the chain of command is clear and all employees know to whom they should report for assignments during activation of the EOP. When additions are made to the EOP, make certain that they are dated so that users will know when the change became effective.

The medical assistant plays an important role in an emergency. All medical assistants must have current training in cardiopulmonary resuscitation (CPR) and first aid, and they must be able to

PROCEDURE 12-8

Develop a Personal (Patient and Employee) Safety Plan

GOAL: *To ensure patient and employee safety during any hazard or emergency situation.*

EQUIPMENT and SUPPLIES

- Hazard assessment for facility
- Office policy manual
- Community resource information
- List of contact information for all employees
- Clerical supplies for emergency action plan

PROCEDURAL STEPS

1. Complete a hazard vulnerability assessment for the facility.
   <u>PURPOSE:</u> To determine any potential hazards that could affect the facility and its patients and employees.
2. Consult the other health facilities in the area, in addition to emergency providers and law enforcement, to determine their roles in hazardous or emergency situations.
   <u>PURPOSE:</u> To determine the facility's role in a city or area-wide emergency and to gain an understanding of the services likely to be available or unavailable.
3. Review the hazard vulnerability assessment with the physician, supervisors, and employees.
   <u>PURPOSE:</u> To discuss the findings from the assessment and determine where action should be taken to plan for various potential safety issues.
4. Determine the method personnel will use to report their readiness for duty during any hazardous or emergency situation.
   <u>PURPOSE:</u> To account for each employee and evaluate additional personnel needs.
5. Develop an emergency operations plan (EOP) for each type of hazard that exists for the facility, based on its location, common weather issues, and disasters that might occur.
   <u>PURPOSE:</u> To be able to act quickly and efficiently if a hazard or disaster occurs.
6. Discuss and determine what hazards might exist both for patients and for employees and then make provisions for patient and employee safety and evacuation.
   <u>PURPOSE:</u> To protect patients and employees as a primary concern and to determine how best to care for both in a hazardous or emergency situation.

7. Determine what, if any, medical care can be given in the various hazards or emergencies that might affect the facility.
   <u>PURPOSE:</u> To be able to access and begin medical care quickly where needed during a hazardous situation or emergency.
8. Establish a clear chain of command for any hazard or emergency situation.
   <u>PURPOSE:</u> To make sure all employees know the chain of command so that the safety plan can be executed quickly and efficiently.
9. Make sure all employees remain within their scope of practice while carrying out the steps in the emergency action plan.
   <u>PURPOSE:</u> To continue to respect the scope of practice during emergency situations.
10. Act as a team and assist other workers as tasks are completed during the emergency. Relieve workers and allow for breaks and rest periods when necessary. Be compassionate toward all patients.
    <u>PURPOSE:</u> To recognize the effects of stress on all persons involved in emergency situations.
11. Continually evaluate personal stress and the need for breaks and rest during emergency situations.
    <u>PURPOSE:</u> To demonstrate self-awareness in responding to emergency situations.
12. Determine how resources will be restored for essential services and develop a list of contacts for every utility and service that affects the facility.
    <u>PURPOSE:</u> To maintain information to help the facility restore essential services (e.g., electricity) as quickly as possible.
13. Determine what areas of the facility might be vulnerable during an emergency and determine how those areas will be protected.
    <u>PURPOSE:</u> To protect vulnerable property and equipment against loss.
14. Conduct quarterly drills to practice initiating the emergency plan.
    <u>PURPOSE:</u> To be ready for hazardous situations and emergencies before the actual event and to make sure that each employee understands his or her role during an emergency.

perform the procedures for which they were trained in both capacities. Be willing to help wherever help is needed. Realize that stress compounds medical emergencies and can complicate other medical problems. Be aware of the personal need to step away for a few moments and collect your thoughts or to just take a few moments to breathe in and out slowly. Often only a few minutes away from the situation provides a new surge of energy to take back to the job at hand. The smallest acts are vital in an emergency; even the simple task of taking down names and injuries helps emergency

workers process patients faster and get them the care they need. Make it a habit to be a volunteer and put to use the valuable medical skills you have learned in class, during the externship, and on the job.

Before an emergency arises, the office must make contingency plans for information. All healthcare facilities need backup plans for the following:

- Communications
- Emergency power

Medical Center Hazard and Vulnerability Analysis

This document is a sample Hazard Vulnerability Analysis tool. It is not a substitute for a comprehensive emergency preparedness program. Individuals or organizations using this tool are solely responsible for any hazard assessment and compliance with applicable laws and regulations.

INSTRUCTIONS:

Evaluate potential for event and response among the following categories using the hazard specific scale. Assume each event incident occurs at the worst possible time (e.g., during peak patient loads).

Issues to consider for **probability** include, but are not limited to:
1 Known risk
2 Historical data
3 Manufacturer/vendor statistics

Issues to consider for **response** include, but are not limited to:
1 Time to marshal an on-scene response
2 Scope of response capability
3 Historical evaluation of response success

Issues to consider for **human impact** include, but are not limited to:
1 Potential for staff death or injury
2 Potential for patient death or injury

Issues to consider for **property impact** include, but are not limited to:
1 Cost to replace
2 Cost to set up temporary replacement
3 Cost to repair
4 Time to recover

Issues to consider for **business impact** include, but are not limited to:
1 Business interruption
2 Employees unable to report to work
3 Customers unable to reach facility
4 Company in violation of contractual agreements
5 Imposition of fines and penalties or legal costs
6 Interruption of critical supplies
7 Interruption of product distribution
8 Reputation and public image
9 Financial impact/burden

Issues to consider for **preparedness** include, but are not limited to:
1 Status of current plans
2 Frequency of drills
3 Training status
4 Insurance
5 Availability of alternate sources for critical supplies/services

Issues to consider for **internal resources** include, but are not limited to:
1 Types of supplies on hand/will they meet need?
2 Volume of supplies on hand/will they meet need?
3 Staff availability
4 Coordination with MOB's
5 Availability of back-up systems
6 Internal resources ability to withstand disasters/survivability

Issues to consider for **external resources** include, but are not limited to:
1 Types of agreements with community agencies/drills?
2 Coordination with local and state agencies
3 Coordination with proximal health care facilities
4 Coordination with treatment specific facilities
5 Community resources

FIGURE 12-8 Hazard and vulnerability analysis as an emergency preparedness tool for physicians' offices. (Modified from Kaiser Foundation Health Plan, Oakland, Calif.)

- Information systems support
- Electronic medical records
- Human resource information

Also, identify employees with special skills that might be useful in an emergency. For example, those who speak another language could help with patients of other cultures. All personnel at the medical facility need to know their role and where they should report in emergencies. By being prepared in advance, the physician's office team can execute its EOP efficiently and in a timely manner. Identify and learn as much as possible about the EOPs of other local and regional medical facilities and determine how the physician's office can assist if a larger scale emergency occurs. Remember that in a serious regional emergency, community emergency workers such as fire, police, and paramedic personnel focus their efforts where the need is greatest. Be prepared to support their efforts and to contribute to the emergency response.

Evacuating the Health Facility

An evacuation cannot commence until an order has been given by the safety officer. All lights should be on, and the exits must be clear, allowing for the unhindered evacuation of both patients and employees. Attempt the first exit route; if it is impossible, use the second exit route. Evacuate the people nearest the danger first, and then systematically evacuate all other persons, closing doors as they are passed. If traveling through smoke, keep low; do not allow anyone to run in smoke-filled areas. Do not enter doors that feel warm or those that emit smoke when opened slightly. Take everyone to the designated assembly area, leaving one staff member there to ensure that no one returns to the facility for any reason. Keep a count on all persons and notify the safety officer if someone is missing.

A fire in a medical facility can be devastating, not only because of the financial loss, but also because of the chemicals inside, which can make it much more intense. MSDS sheets are critical to the practice, since information about the flammability of each chemical is given. Additionally, the MSDS sheet provides information about other chemicals that can react with each other. Employees should immediately put the evacuation plan into action and get all patients out of the facility. Take first aid supplies only if an emergency kit has been assembled previously and can be reached safely. The patient sign-in sheet and an employee list will help to account for everyone who might have been in the office prior to evacuation. Make certain that each employee knows his or her duties during a fire, or in any emergency, in advance.

WASTE STORAGE AND DESTRUCTION

Two basic types of waste are found in physicians' offices: medical waste and regular waste. Medical waste includes anything that once was part of the human body. Not everything that originates in the human body is considered medical waste; the place where it is encountered makes the distinction. A used Kleenex in the trashcan in the reception area restroom is considered regular waste; however, that same tissue left in an exam room is considered medical waste. Most offices use a trash service to remove regular waste. Removing medical waste is slightly more complicated (Figure 12-9). OSHA requires records to prove that (1) medical waste was collected by the removal waste service, and (2) that the same waste was destroyed by the waste

PROCEDURE 12-9

Maintain a Current List of Community Resources for Emergency Preparedness

GOAL: *To help patients find organizations that can assist with their needs during an emergency and to establish a list of community resources that can be used for referral purposes during any type of emergency or for everyday use.*

EQUIPMENT and SUPPLIES

- Phone book
- Internet access
- Library access
- Newspapers
- Local volunteer guides
- Computer
- Pen or pencil
- Notepad

PROCEDURAL STEPS

1. Research the emergency resources available locally, regionally, and state-wide using the Internet, phone book, newspapers, and other guides.
   PURPOSE: To become familiar with various agencies that provide services in the local area.
2. Open a document on the computer in either a word processing program or a spreadsheet. Create a list of the resources in the document. Include the following information:
   - Name of agency
   - Purpose or mission of agency
   - Physical address
   - Mailing address, if different
   - Phone numbers
   - Web site address
   - Contact name and e-mail information
   - Hours of operation
   - Services offered or performed
   PURPOSE: To make information readily available before an emergency occurs.
3. Update the information whenever a change is needed.
   PURPOSE: To provide the most accurate information possible and shorten response time during an emergency.
4. Provide referrals to agencies when patients and their friends or families ask for it or when the physician recommends referral.
   PURPOSE: To get patients the help they need.
5. Ask patients for feedback, if possible, after they have used the agency's services.
   PURPOSE: To make sure the agencies are hospitable and provide the expected services.
6. Make note of those referred to the agencies and their experience, if applicable.
   PURPOSE: To provide a record of the referral.
7. When faced with an emergency, remain as calm as possible and keep the focus on the needs of the individuals who require assistance.
   PURPOSE: Emergencies can be extremely stressful for medical personnel, just as they are for patients. To be helpful, the medical assistant must remain calm and stay focused on the task at hand.
8. Step away from emergencies for brief breaks whenever possible.
   PURPOSE: To reduce stress and allow the medical assistant to regain a sharp focus on the tasks at hand.

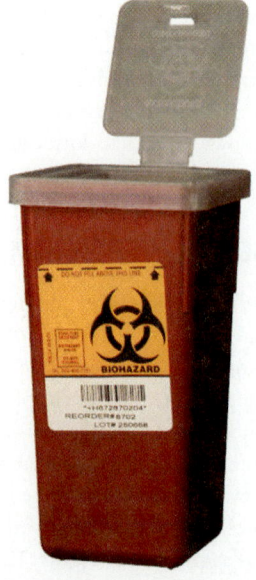

FIGURE 12-9 OSHA requires proper disposition of medical waste. The office must keep records of waste removal and incineration.

service. The medical waste service usually comes every few days, and the waste is picked up and then destroyed by incineration.

ERGONOMICS

Ergonomics is the applied science concerned with designing and arranging items so that they interact efficiently and safely. Most office injuries are caused by falls, repetitive movements, awkward postures, reaching, bending over, lifting heavy objects, or applying pressure or force (Figure 12-10). Most workplace injuries can be prevented by using proper body mechanics (Procedure 12-10). OSHA developed a four-pronged approach to addressing musculoskeletal disorders in the workplace. The approach includes a combination of industry-specific and task-specific guidelines, outreach, enforcement, and research. Since the implementation of these measures, OSHA has seen significant improvement in these problems. Plenty of information on ergonomics is available online, both through a general search and on the OSHA Web site. Most employers include information about ergonomics in the employee orientation and training and in handbooks.

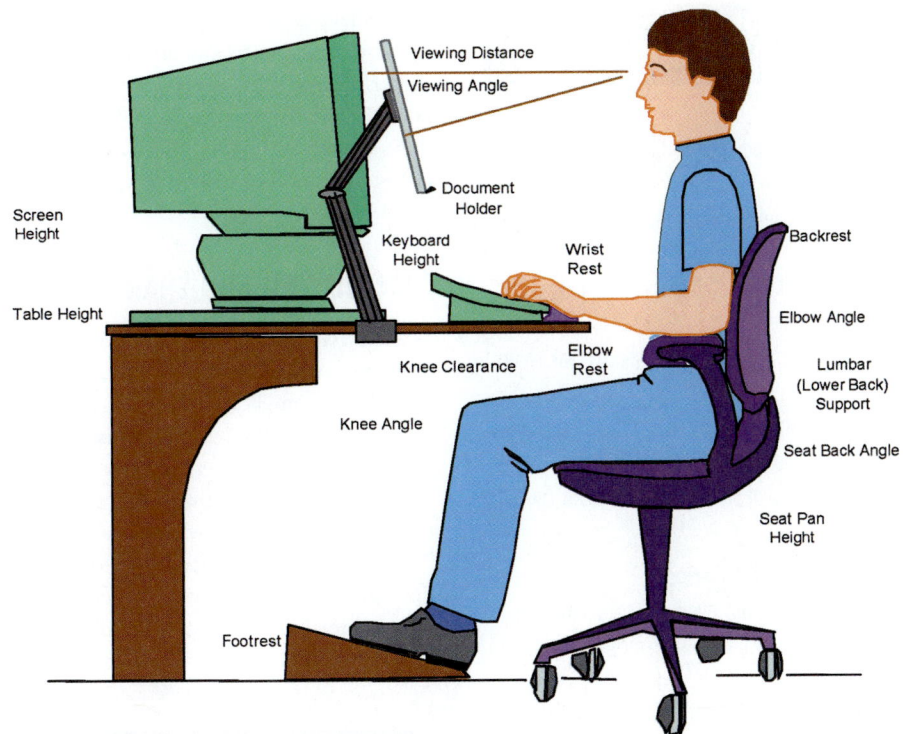

Figure 12-10 Medical assistants should use good body mechanics to prevent repetitive motion injuries. (Modified from Oregon Occupational Safety & Health Division [OR-OSHA]. Available at *www.orosha.org*).

PROCEDURE 12-10

Use Proper Body Mechanics

GOAL: *To prevent workplace injuries through the use of proper body mechanics.*

PROCEDURAL STEPS: LIFTING

1. Take a moment to evaluate the job and determine the best approach to the task.
   <u>PURPOSE:</u> To think before acting, so that proper body mechanics can be used to prevent injuries.
2. Test the weight of the load to lift and determine whether help is needed to move it safely.
   <u>PURPOSE:</u> To avoid lifting weight that is too heavy for one person.
3. Bow forward, then squat at the knees in front of the object.
   <u>PURPOSE:</u> To steady the body and prepare for the lift.
4. Lift the object, moving straight up, and steady the body before beginning to walk.
5. When placing the object, squat down and bend at the knees.
   <u>PURPOSE:</u> To avoid injury during the lifting and placing process.
6. Stand carefully, placing equal weight on both feet.

PROCEDURAL STEPS: COMPUTER USE

1. Sit directly in front of the computer monitor, avoiding a left or right placement, and use scroll bars on the screen to keep the working text in a comfortable position.
   <u>PURPOSE:</u> To eliminate neck twisting.

2. Adjust the monitor to a comfortable height, so that the user's eyes line up 2 to 3 inches below the top of the monitor casing.
   <u>PURPOSE:</u> To avoid neck and shoulder pain.
3. Adjust the viewing distance to approximately an arm's length.
   <u>PURPOSE:</u> At this distance, the user should be able to see the monitor clearly without making any bodily movements.
   <u>NOTE:</u> Remember that the text size can be adjusted in most software programs, which makes it easier to read and edit.
4. Keep the wrists straight and flat as they are placed on the keyboard.
   <u>PURPOSE:</u> To avoid repetitive motion injuries.
5. Keep the upper arms and elbows close to the body while typing and using a mouse.
6. Sit all the way to the back of the chair instead of leaving space between the chair and the body.
   <u>PURPOSE:</u> To prevent back and shoulder strain.
7. Keep the head and neck as straight as possible while working at the computer.
8. Place the feet flat on the floor or on a footrest.
9. Take a short break to stretch after 1 hour of steady work.
   <u>PURPOSE:</u> To allow the body to move and rest.

ERGONOMICS AND PREVENTING WORKPLACE INJURIES

Eye Strain

- Make sure the lighting is as even as possible in the office; check for glaring or flickering lights.
- Place the computer monitor at a comfortable horizontal distance for viewing.
- Reduce glare by using an antiglare filter or a liquid crystal display (LCD) display.
- Use a high-quality computer monitor; text characters should look sharp and clear.
- Set up the monitor to reduce eye strain; the monitor should be placed directly in front of the user, just below the straight ahead gaze.
- Take an eye break every 15 minutes or so to give the eyes a chance to relax and reduce strain.

Back, Neck, and Shoulder Pain and Injuries

- Take frequent breaks and change positions every 20 to 30 minutes.
- Warm up or stretch before starting activities that include repetitive movements or prolonged positions.
- Avoid twisting or bending movements.
- Position equipment directly in front of the user.
- Place the back and shoulders against the backrest of the chair.
- Avoid overstretching or overreaching; keep feet flat on the floor.
- Avoid bending the neck forward for prolonged periods.
- When lifting heavy objects, bend from the hips and not the waist.

Back Pain

- Refrain from twisting when lifting.
- Get close to the object.
- Bend the knees and grasp the object firmly.
- Lift straight up in one fluid movement.
- Hold the object close to the body.
- Move close to where the object is to be placed.
- Bend the knees when lowering the object.
- Avoid bad posture.
- Keep the feet slightly apart.
- Knees should be straight.
- Tuck the chin in slightly.
- Keep the shoulders back.
- Exercise and avoid a sedentary lifestyle.
- Never ignore pain.
- Stop smoking. Nicotine blocks the transport of oxygen and important nutrients to the spine's disks, and the lack of oxygen can impair the disks' ability to repair themselves. If the disks cannot repair themselves, the spine may suffer from degenerative disk disease.

Modified from articles on www.spineuniverse.com.

Guidelines are designed to educate individual workers about the ways ergonomics can affect them and how they can be injured in performing their everyday work duties. OSHA enforces ergonomic standards to ensure that employers take the necessary precautions to prevent ergonomic injuries and protect their employees. Ergonomic injuries must be reported annually on the appropriate OSHA forms.

IDENTIFYING AND SHARING COMMUNITY RESOURCES

Medical assistants must be able to identify community resources so that they can assist patients with needs that are not office-related and possibly not medical. At various times, patients need help with meals, rehabilitation, Medicare issues, exercise groups, and other services. Grocery stores that deliver are a great convenience for older patients. Get to know the people in the community, trade information, and refer patients when they need help with a particular issue. (See the following box, Community Resources, which lists organizations and services in which patients commonly are interested.) A phone directory can be created for a local community resource list (Procedure 12-11).

COMMUNITY RESOURCES

Check with these organizations for services available in the local area:

Alcoholics Anonymous
Alzheimer support organizations
American Cancer Society
American Heart Association
American Red Cross
Child Protective Services
Civic organizations
Council on Aging
Family services
Homeless organizations
Hospice services
Legal Aid societies
Mental health and mental retardation services
Public Health Department
United Way

To expand the knowledge base regarding resources available in the community, get involved in various organizations, especially health industry councils and organizations for medical assistants or other office staff members. Make introductions and be prepared to talk about the services the clinic offers. Ask questions about other facilities. Exchange business cards, if they are available; if so, send a thank you note to the contact and periodically get in touch. Patients appreciate that the office staff can refer them to local resources and help them gather information.

Emergency Phone Numbers

Every medical facility should keep a list of emergency and frequently called numbers close to each telephone in the office. The list

PROCEDURE 12-11

Develop and Maintain a Current List of Community Resources Related to Patients' Healthcare Needs

GOAL: *To help patients find organizations that can assist with their needs beyond the physician's office and to establish a list of community resources that can be used for referral purposes.*

EQUIPMENT and SUPPLIES

- Phone book
- Internet access
- Library access
- Newspapers
- Local volunteer guides
- Computer
- Pen or pencil
- Notepad

PROCEDURAL STEPS

1. Research the resources available in the local community using the Internet, phone book, newspapers, and other guides.
   PURPOSE: To become familiar with various agencies that provide services in the local area.
2. Open a document on the computer in either a word processing program or a spreadsheet. Create a list of the resources in the document. Include the following information:
   - Name of agency
   - Purpose or mission of agency
   - Physical address
   - Mailing address, if different
   - Phone numbers
   - Web site address
   - Contact name and e-mail information
   - Hours of operation
   - Services offered or performed
   PURPOSE: To make information readily available.
3. Update the information whenever a change is needed.
   PURPOSE: To provide the most accurate information possible.
4. Provide referrals to agencies when patients and their friends or families request it or when the physician recommends referral.
   PURPOSE: To get patients the help they need.
5. Ask patients for feedback, if possible, after they have used the agency's services.
   PURPOSE: To make sure the agencies are hospitable and provide the expected services.
6. Make note of those referred to the agencies and their experience, if applicable.
   PURPOSE: To provide a record of the referral.

---

should include 911, which summons police and fire departments in most areas of the country. Other numbers on the list might include:

- Local hospitals, including extensions that connect to the emergency department
- Local pharmacies
- Numbers of all physicians associated with the practice
- All employees' phone numbers
- Nonemergency police number
- Numbers of physicians periodically on call

Each office will have different numbers on the emergency phone list. The physician and office manager often provide input about the numbers included. The numbers must be updated periodically. If the list is kept on a computer, a new one can be printed out and distributed each time a phone number changes. Because the list is used in emergencies, it must always be current and accurate.

CLOSING THE OFFICE

When the day comes to an end, several duties must be performed before locking the doors and closing the office. First, check to see that all patients have left the facility. Walk through all exam rooms and treatment areas to make sure they are empty. At the same time, straighten the exam rooms so that they are ready for tomorrow's patients.

Other duties include locking file cabinets that contain patients' records, placing laboratory specimens in the outside lockbox for pick up, performing general housekeeping duties, running accounting reports, balancing the day sheet, and preparing the bank deposit. The phones must be turned over to the answering service or to voice mail.

CLOSING COMMENTS

Although the tasks discussed in this chapter include duties performed daily, the medical assistant should not be lazy about doing them. When the physician sees that the medical assistant is competent in completing small duties, he or she will consider the person competent at completing more difficult tasks. By consistently proving to be a skilled, dependable worker, the medical assistant will be promoted to higher levels of responsibility.

Always keep in mind that the patient is the primary concern in the physician's office. The medical assistant's efforts should be directed at making patients feel more at ease and encouraging them to follow the treatment plan devised by the physician. In this way, even the most unimportant office duties play a part in the patients' health and well-being.

Patient Education

Medical offices often use brochures and printed material to educate their patients. These materials must look professional and reflect a positive image of the physician and the facility. Make sure copied material is clean, without streaks, and attractively presented. If the information is written by an office staff member, make sure correct grammar is used and that several office members proofread the work for errors and proper use of the English language. Good first impressions are important, but every impression in the medical office molds public opinion about professionalism and competence.

Legal and Ethical Issues

Keep copies of all communications leaving the office that relate to patient care. If any information is handwritten, it must be completely legible to the patient. Because the appointment book and telephone messages also are considered a form of written communication, they must be clear and easy to read. Take enough time to write legibly so that no confusion arises if the document is referenced at a later date.

SUMMARY OF SCENARIO

Kayla learned much more during her externship than she had ever thought she would. She saw patients who had few belongings and no health insurance. Her experience helped her realize just how difficult obtaining medical care is without insurance. Kayla is happy that her clinic sees these patients and allows them to pay what they can to obtain medical care. She feels slightly guilty that she has had such an easy life as she listens to her patients' stories and their problems.

Kayla has developed a sense of caring for the people she helps in the clinic. She does not treat the patients disrespectfully; on the contrary, she treats them as individuals who are entitled to dignity. She understands that although she might not connect with all the patients, she can make a difference to the ones who enter the clinic by expressing an emotion she truly feels—compassion.

Elaine allowed Kayla to order many of the supplies she needs, because Kayla is the primary user of those items. This allows Kayla to use the items she has found perform best and with which she is most comfortable. Kayla suggested that the clinic outsource some of their laboratory tests because of the expense of buying the supplies to run the tests. This has allowed the clinic to keep prices lower, a great help to the patients.

Kayla found that most of the patients who come to the clinic need referrals, whether for food, clothing, other medical services, child care, or other needs. She designed a lengthy list of community resources, and she can tell patients where to go to receive help with various problems. The patients appreciate Kayla's willingness to help them. Even though Kayla comes from a completely different background, the patients have accepted her as a medical assistant who truly cares.

SUMMARY OF LEARNING OBJECTIVES

1. **Define, spell, and pronounce the terms listed in the vocabulary.**
   Spelling and pronouncing medical terms correctly bolster the medical assistant's credibility. Knowing the definition of these terms promotes confidence in communication with patients and co-workers.

2. **List five specific actions that must be taken to prepare for patients before the office opens in the morning.**
   The office should be cleaned, whether it is done the evening before or as one of the morning duties. Exam rooms should be checked for supplies and replenished, if necessary. The phone should be taken off of voice mail or the answering service should be called to inform them that the office staff has arrived for the day. Computers should be booted up and medical equipment turned on. Patients' records should be pulled for the patients who have appointments. Two copies of the appointment book should be made; one is placed on the physician's desk, and the other is used to pull the medical records. Individual offices may assign additional duties to the medical assistants who work in the office.

3. **Explain why patient traffic flow is an important consideration in the office design.**
   Patient traffic flow is important, because patients should not have to retrace their steps repeatedly as they move through the clinic. Furniture should be arranged so that getting from one place to another is easy and does not require dodging furniture and décor.

4. **List some of the expenses involved in the operation of a medical practice.**
   Operation of a physician's office involves many types of expenses. Lease or mortgage payments are among the largest expenses. Utilities, payroll, equipment and supplies, professional organization dues, insurance, maintenance, and taxes are examples of expenses that must be worked into the annual budget.

5. **Describe how prices can be compared for medical office supplies.**
   Compare unit prices by determining the cost of each individual item. If a bulk of 8 containers of White Out costs $9.99, then each individual bottle costs $1.25. If another company offers the same product at 10 for $12, then the individual cost is $1.20, which is the better buy of the two. However, the cost to buy the product, meaning the gas to get to the store or the shipping and handling costs, if any, may increase the price. Be aware of these factors and figure all possible costs before placing an order.

6. **Discuss the importance of routine maintenance of office equipment.**
   Office equipment must be periodically and regularly maintained to ensure proper working order and accurate testing results. The failure to perform regular maintenance may not only result in malfunction when the equipment is needed, but may also void warranties.

7. **List several ways to save money and prevent waste in the medical office.**

   Make sure trash bags are completely full before taking out the trash. Use refillable print cartridges and solar-powered calculators and adding machines. Print on both sides of the paper when possible. Monitor ordering to determine where budget cuts could be made. Watch carefully for areas where money could be saved or items could be bought in bulk.

8. **Discuss fire safety issues in a healthcare environment.**

   Fire prevention is critical in a healthcare facility, because fire and smoke are so dangerous. All healthcare facilities must have a fire safety plan in place, and both a primary and a secondary exit route must be posted in each room in case of fire or other emergency.

9. **Discuss critical elements of an emergency plan for response to a natural disaster or other emergency.**

   Emergency management is the process of preparing for, mitigating, responding to, and recovering from an emergency. Every medical office needs an emergency operations plan (EOP). The objectives of the plan should include protection of patients, visitors, and staff; provisions for prompt, efficient medical care; establishment of a clear chain of command; rapid maintenance and restoration of essential services; and protection of clinic property, facilities, and equipment.

10. **Identify emergency preparedness plans in the community.**

    Determine the emergency plans that exist in the local community by contacting large health facilities, regional hospitals, and fire/police stations. When establishing the physician's office emergency plan, consider these other facilities and agencies, incorporating them into the physician's plan where applicable.

11. **Discuss potential roles of the medical assistant in emergency preparedness.**

    The medical assistant must follow established office policies and procedures during any emergency. All employees should document that they have read the EOP, and this document should be displayed prominently and easily accessed.

12. **Describe the fundamental principles for evacuation of a healthcare setting.**

    An evacuation cannot commence until an order has been given by the safety officer. All lights should be on and the exits must be clear, allowing for the unhindered evacuation of both patients and employees. Attempt the first exit route, then use the second if the first route is impassible. Evacuate the people nearest the danger first, and then systematically evacuate all other persons, closing doors as they are passed. If traveling through smoke, keep low; do not allow anyone to run in smoke-filled areas. Do not enter doors that feel warm or those that emit smoke when opened slightly. Take everyone to the designated assembly area, leaving one staff member there to ensure that no one returns to the facility for any reason. Keep a count on all persons and notify the safety officer if someone is missing.

13. **Explain the difference between medical waste and regular waste.**

    Medical waste includes any disposed item that was once a part of the human body or used to clean up blood or body fluids. Regular waste is any other trash that does not have to go into a biohazard waste container.

14. **Identify principles of body mechanics and ergonomics.**

    OSHA developed a four-pronged approach to addressing musculoskeletal disorders in the workplace. The approach includes a combination of industry-specific and task-specific guidelines, outreach, enforcement, and research. Since the implementation of these measures, OSHA has seen significant improvement in these problems. Plenty of information on ergonomics is available online, and most employers include information about ergonomics in the employee orientation and training and in handbooks.

15. **Explain why keys and alarm codes should be shared with only a few people.**

    It is easier to keep track of alarm codes and keys if they are entrusted to only a few people. Also, if fewer people have the codes and keys, there is less chance someone will be able to use them to enter the office and steal equipment and supplies.

CONNECTIONS

Study Guide Connection: Go to the Chapter 12 Study Guide. Read and complete the activities.

Evolve Connection: Go to the Chapter 12 link at *evolve.elsevier.com/ kinn* to complete the Chapter Review and Chapter Quiz. Check out the other resources listed for this chapter to make the most of what you have learned from Office Environment and Daily Operations.

13

WRITTEN COMMUNICATIONS AND MAIL PROCESSING

Brandon Tipps is a medical assistant who works with his father, Dr. Rick Tipps. Brandon has considered continuing his education to become a doctor, but he is not sure whether he would like to be a medical doctor, an osteopathic physician, or a chiropractor. He decided to spend his summer off from college working in his father's family practice so that he can get a closer look at the inner workings of a physician's office.

Brandon has assisted with every procedure in the clinic, including the administrative skills required in the front office. The staff has been impressed with Brandon's ability to do any task, no matter how small, as if it were the most important task in the office. He continuously moves from employee to employee to ask what he can do to help. When the administrative medical assistant working in the front office, Darla Grover, was injured in a car accident and had to be off work for a while, Brandon stepped right in to do her job and quickly learned her duties. His help enabled the office to continue to run smoothly even with one employee absent for several weeks.

Brandon has an excellent command of the English language and types about 60 words per minute. Because he is organized and efficient, he can handle the enormous amount of incoming and outgoing mail with very little assistance from the office manager. He also is able to answer phones and schedule appointments. He speaks clearly and is an expert in customer service. Many of Dr. Tipps' patients have known Brandon since he was a small child, and they enjoy seeing him helping in his father's office. The patients and staff alike will certainly miss him once he returns to college.

While studying this chapter, think about the following questions:

- What types of difficulties can arise when a physician's family member works at the office?
- How do proofreader's marks help the medical assistant save time?
- What types of impressions could be formed by people who receive mail from a physician's office?
- Explain why any written communication discussed in this chapter should be worded in a professional manner.

LEARNING OBJECTIVES

1. Define, spell, and pronounce the terms listed in the vocabulary.
2. Recognize the elements of fundamental writing skills.
3. Explain the various parts of speech.
4. Name some essential references for the medical assistant's library.
5. Discuss applications of electronic technology in effective communication.
6. List the four common sizes of letterhead stationery.
7. Discuss the differences in the four letter styles.
8. Explain the four standard parts of a business letter.
9. Discuss the process of developing and the value of keeping a communications portfolio.
10. Discuss how to open, sort, and annotate incoming mail.
11. Explain how to save money when mailing.
12. Describe how to compose, proofread, and mail a business letter.
13. Organize technical information and summaries.
14. Describe the proper way to send a fax.
15. Explain how to process incoming mail.
16. Explain how to address an envelope according to the U.S. Postal Service's optical character reader guidelines.

VOCABULARY

academic degree A title conferred by a college, university, or professional school upon completion of a program of study.

amiable (a′-me-uh-buhl) Having qualities that make one liked and easy to deal with.

annotating Furnishing with notes that are usually critical or explanatory.

archived To have filed or collected records or documents.

bond A durable, formal paper used for documents.

categorically Placed in a specific division of a system of classification.

clauses Groups of words containing a subject and predicate and functioning as a member of a complex or compound sentence.

collect on delivery (COD) A method of payment used when an article or item is delivered and payment is expected before it is released.

concise (kun-sis′) Expressing much in brief form.

condescending Assuming an air of superiority.

continuation pages The second and following pages of a letter.

courier A messenger, especially one on official or diplomatic business; a service that provides delivery and transportation services for documents and/or packages.

curt Marked by rude or peremptory shortness.

disseminate (di-se′-muh-nat) To disperse throughout.

domestic mail Mail sent within the boundaries of the United States and its territories.

editing To prepare for publication or public presentation; to alter, adapt, or refine, especially to bring about conformity to a standard or to suit a particular purpose.

flush Directly abutting or immediately adjacent, as set even with an edge of a type page or column; having no indention.

girth A measure around a body or an item.

grammar The study of the classes of words, their inflections, and their functions and relations in the sentence; a study of what is preferred and what should be avoided in inflection and syntax.

international mail Mail that is sent outside the boundaries of the United States and its territories.

intrinsic (in-trin′-zik) Belonging to the essential nature or constitution of a thing; indwelling, inward.

phrases Groups of words with a specific grammatical function, such as a noun phrase or an adjective phrase.

portfolio A set of pictures, drawings, documents, or photographs either bound in book form or loose in a folder.

ream A quantity of paper weighing 20 lb or consisting of, variously, 480, 500, or 516 sheets.

recipient The receiver of some thing or item.

stationers (sta′-shuh-nerz) Sellers of stationery.

substance number A number based on the weight of a ream of paper containing 500 sheets.

superfluous (suh-puhr′-flu-uhs) Exceeding what is sufficient or necessary.

template Something that establishes or serves as a pattern.

watermark A marking in paper resulting from differences in thickness usually produced by the pressure of a projecting design in the mold or on a processing roll; it is visible when the paper is held up to the light.

Written correspondence and mail processing consume a large part of the day of the administrative medical assistant. When asked what skills they most want in an administrative assistant, many physicians specify the ability to spell accurately and to write a good letter. When a physician delegates the responsibility for composing letters or reports with the potential to reflect positively or negatively on the practice, he or she is expressing confidence in the medical assistant's abilities.

IMPORTANCE OF WRITTEN COMMUNICATIONS

Written communications offer the perfect opportunity for making a good impression on others. However, communications that make such an impression do not just happen; they require thought, preparation, skill, and a positive attitude. Written communications include original letters, memorandums, replies to inquiries, responses to requests for information, telephone messages, e-mail, transcriptions, orders for supplies, instructions for patients, and a variety of other forms. Communications that are courteous to the reader, correct in content, and **concise** without being **curt** are most appreciated. Remember that people may misjudge the "tone" of an e-mail and determine that the sender was rude or hateful, when the sender may have just been very direct and pointed. Communication truly is both

an art and a skill. The ability to communicate effectively is extremely important to the administrative medical assistant who wants to succeed and advance his or her career.

CRITICAL THINKING APPLICATION   13-1

Brandon has just found a small backlog of correspondence that accumulated during the first 3 days Darla was out of the office. A large amount of mail comes to the office each day. How can Brandon manage the daily mail and clear the pile of communications that accumulated over those 3 days?

Reflection on the Physician

Each member of the staff must be conscientious about the documents and materials in the office and those that leave it. An envelope addressed carelessly or a patient information sheet that has been photocopied over and over implies that the office staff is not concerned about the appearance of documents that leave the office. If the staff is careless in this respect, many patients assume the staff is careless with everything, including patient care.

Everything that happens in the medical office reflects on the physician or physicians who practice there. Letters with misspelled

TABLE 13-1 150 Frequently Misspelled or Misused English Words

absence	corroborate	inimitable	persistent	ridiculous
accede	definitely	inoculate	personal	sacrilegious
accessible	description	insistent	personnel	seize
accommodate	desirable	irrelevant	possession	separate
achieve	despair	irresistible	precede	siege
affect	development	irritable	precedent	similar
agglutinate	dilemma	judgment	predictable	sizable
all right	disappear	labeled	predominant	stationary
altogether	disappoint	led	predominate	stationery
analyses (pl.)	disastrous	leisure	prerogative	subpoena
analysis (s.)	discreet	license	prevalent	succeed
analyze	discrete	liquefy	principal	suddenness
anoint	discriminate	maintenance	principle	superintendent
argument	dissatisfaction	maneuver	privilege	supersede
assistant	dissipate	miscellaneous	procedure	surprise
auxiliary	drunkenness	mischievous	proceed	tariff
balloon	ecstasy	misspell	professor	technique
believe	effect	necessary	pronunciation	thorough
benefited	eligible	newsstand	psychiatry	tranquility
brochure	embarrass	noticeable	psychology	transferred
bulletin	exceed	occasion	pursue	truly
category	exhilaration	occurrence	questionnaire	tyrannize
changeable	existence	oscillate	rearrange	unnecessary
clientele	February	paid	recede	until
committee	forty	pamphlet	receive	vacillate
comparative	grammar	panicky	recommend	vacuum
concede	grievous	parallel	referring	vicious
conscientious	height	paralyze	repetition	warrant
conscious	incidentally	pastime	rheumatism	Wednesday
coolly	indispensable	perseverance	rhythmical	weird

words or errors give the reader a negative impression of the physician and the practice itself. Great care must be taken to ensure that each document in the office and sent from the office is well written and grammatically correct. Table 13-1 lists some frequently misspelled and misused words. For a list of more misspelled medical words, visit the Evolve site at *evolve.elsevier.com/kinn*.

WRITING SKILLS AND COMPOSING TIPS

All medical assistants must know the fundamental skills of proper business writing. Most business letters should be less than one

page long and carefully organized (Procedure 13-1). This takes practice and preparation. Everyone who writes letters develops a personal style.

The medical assistant should carefully read the letter to be answered. Make note of or underline any questions asked or materials requested. Decide on the answers to the questions and verify the information; this is called **annotating**. Draft a reply, proofread it, and then rewrite for clarity (Procedure 13-2). Keep most sentences short. Put only one idea in each sentence and eliminate **superfluous** words. Be careful about using medical terms in correspondence with patients. Instead, use language the reader can easily understand.

PROCEDURE 13-1

Compose Professional Business Letters

GOAL: *To compose a professional business letter that conveys accurate, helpful information that is easily understood, clearly written, and free of both spelling and grammatical errors.*

EQUIPMENT and SUPPLIES

- Computer
- Word processing software
- Draft paper
- Letterhead
- Printer
- Pen or pencil
- Highlighter
- Envelope
- Correspondence to be answered
- Other pertinent information needed to compose a letter
- Electronic or paper dictionary and thesaurus
- Writer's handbook
- Portfolio and/or templates

PROCEDURAL STEPS

1. Determine the reason for initiating a letter or other type of communication.
   PURPOSE: To ensure that the goals of the correspondence are fulfilled and that relevant information has been identified and included.
2. Make any necessary notes on the letter or a copy of the letter. A scrap sheet of paper may be used.
3. Prepare a draft of the letter, using good grammar, and save it in the computer.
   PURPOSE: To put the thoughts on paper for later revision and to make the letter easy to understand.
4. Proofread a printed copy of the letter, using proofreader's marks to make corrections.
   PURPOSE: To see the document as it will look once printed and to speed the process by using proofreader's marks.
5. Make any necessary corrections.
6. Allow the physician or other interested parties to proofread the letter, if the medical assistant is not the person whose signature will appear at the bottom.
   PURPOSE: To give the physician an opportunity to correct the letter and add thoughts, if desired.
7. Make any final changes, then print the letter on stationery. Allow the person whose name appears at the bottom to sign the letter.
8. Address the envelope using optical character reader (OCR) guidelines and place the letter and any supporting documents inside (see Procedure 13-5 for OCR guidelines).
9. Mail the letter using the correct postage.
   PURPOSE: Using incorrect postage or guessing can delay delivery of the document.

PROCEDURE 13-2

Organize Technical Information and Summaries

GOAL: *To compose information accurately and in an organized manner, using strong spelling and grammatical skills, so that it meets the goals of the writer and is usable by the receiver.*

EQUIPMENT and SUPPLIES

- Stationery
- Computer or typewriter
- Correspondence to be answered or notes
- Guide for proofreader's marks

PROCEDURAL STEPS

1. Scan the letter or memo to be answered or the notes about the correspondence to be written and highlight any questions that should be answered or points to be made.
   PURPOSE: To ensure that the goals of the correspondence are fulfilled and that relevant information has been identified and included.
2. Write the letter or memo using good grammar.
3. Print a draft copy of the letter or memo. Read it carefully and highlight changes to be made or note any additions to be made. Use proofreader's marks.
   PURPOSE: Reading a hard copy of a letter or memo is more conducive to finding errors and grammatical mistakes.
4. Revise the letter or memo using the notes and proofreader's marks.
5. Read the letter or memo once again on the screen. Perform spelling and grammar checks if those tools are available on the computer.
   PURPOSE: To locate any missed errors or misspelled words.
6. Print a final draft. Read the letter word for word and check once again for errors.
7. Have another person proofread correspondence that is especially important.
   PURPOSE: Often another person can find missed errors quickly.
8. Complete the final preparations for mailing the letter or distributing the memo. Address the letter using guidelines for optical character reader (OCR) and fast processing at the post office.

Most physicians use a highly professional and formal style in their dictation. The medical assistant responsible for composing correspondence for the office should strive for the same degree of formality the physician uses. It would be inappropriate for the assistant to write in a breezy, informal style when acting as the representative of an employer with a more formal approach. The principal point to remember is that every letter produced in your office should project the image of the physician, regardless of who composes or signs the letter.

Grammar Review

Good **grammar** is essential to the writing of effective, professional business letters. Medical assistants must understand the elements of acceptable grammar and writing skills.

Parts of Speech

Nouns. A noun is a person, place, or thing. Nouns can also be thoughts, ideas, or concepts, such as *freedom* or *courage*. Common nouns name general persons, places, or things (e.g., *teacher* and *city*). Proper nouns are specific (e.g., *Mrs. Adams* and *New York City*).

Pronouns. Pronouns replace nouns and provide the writer with shortcuts so that proper nouns do not have to be repeated constantly. Pronouns include words such as *it, you, he, she, her, his, them, mine, you, yours, its, ours,* and *theirs*.

Verbs. Action verbs are words that express movement, such as *run, drive,* or *type*. Linking verbs express a condition or state of being; they include *is, am, are, was, be,* and *been*. Linking verbs also express the senses, as in *smell, hear, taste, touch, feel,* and *look*.

Adjectives. Adjectives can describe nouns and pronouns, or they may show which one, how many, and what kind of. *A, an,* and *the* are special types of adjectives called *articles*. Examples of adjectives include a *golden* sunset, a *playful* dog, and a *crooked* nose.

Adverbs. Just as adjectives describe nouns, adverbs describe verbs, adjectives, or other adverbs. Adverbs specify when, where, to what extent, or how. Examples include *unusually* warm, *never* won, and *quite* cold.

Prepositions. Connecting words that show a relationship between nouns, pronouns, or other words in a sentence are called *prepositions*. Examples of prepositions include *by, from, of, to, in, at, with, into,* and *on*.

Conjunctions. Conjunctions join words or **phrases**. These helpful words include *and, or, nor,* and *but*.

Interjections. Interjections show strong feeling. They often are followed by an exclamation point and sometimes by a comma. *"Ouch! That really hurt!"* is a sentence that uses an interjection.

Making Sense of Sentences

Sentence structure is important when writing a professional letter or document. Medical assistants should know the basics of good sentence structure so that written documents make sense and represent the medical facility and staff in a positive way.

Types of Sentences. The four basic types of sentences are declarative, interrogatory, imperative, and exclamatory. Declarative sentences make a statement, whereas interrogatory sentences ask a question. Imperative sentences state a command or request. Exclamatory sentences express strong feeling.

Declarative:	*She was the last person here.*
Interrogatory:	*Are we going to the fair today?*
Imperative:	*Clean your room before dinner.*
Exclamatory:	*I am so excited for you!*

Sentence Structure. When written correctly, sentences follow certain patterns. Three very basic patterns are used to construct sentences:

- Subject—predicate
- Subject—object
- Subject—complement

The *subject* of a sentence usually is a noun; it is the word or group of words that acts, or that is acted on or described by the verb. The *predicate* is the part of the sentence that contains the verb; it tells what the subject is doing or experiencing, or what is being done to the subject. The *object* is a noun, pronoun, or group of words functioning as a noun or pronoun that receives the action of the verb. The complement is a word or group of words in the predicate that renames or describes a subject or object in the sentence.

Sentence Errors. Three main sentence errors plague most writers: the sentence fragment, the run-on sentence, and the comma splice.

A sentence fragment is an incomplete thought or a part of a sentence that is punctuated as though it were a complete sentence: *Although the doctor had seen the patient.*

A run-on sentence contains independent **clauses** that do not have a semicolon, a comma, or a conjunction between them. These are also called *run-together* or *fused* sentences: *The office was clean when the staff left on Friday the doors were locked.*

A comma splice is a sentence in which a comma alone joins independent clauses: *The storm grew worse, it began to snow.*

Personal Tools

Competent handling of written communications requires a basic knowledge of composition. A personal reference library that includes an up-to-date standard dictionary, a medical dictionary, a composition handbook, an English language reference manual, and a thesaurus is a tremendous help.

Those who have difficulty with spelling should keep a small, loose-leaf, indexed notebook or card index of troublesome words. If you need to look up the spelling of a word in the dictionary, record the word in the notebook or card index for quick reference. The physician or a medical assistant familiar with the practice might compile a basic list of frequently used medical terms and abbreviations as a reference.

EQUIPMENT AND SUPPLIES

To create a favorable impression with letters, the medical assistant must use good equipment and high-quality supplies. Regardless of the kind of equipment available, the medical assistant is responsible for knowing how to use it to the best advantage and how to keep it in good working condition. If the equipment manual is available, study it and keep it handy for reference when problems occur. Know how to maintain equipment so that the effort invested in composing correspondence has a high-quality appearance.

Equipment

Computers

Computer applications and electronic technology have made all types of communication easy, efficient, and effective. Various letters and documents can be saved and reused time after time by changing the name and the basic information in the text. Computers can add graphics to text, compute figures, and use multimedia in communications, all of which enhance the document's appearance and effectiveness.

Copiers

Maintain the copier so that copies are crisp and clear. The toner cartridge must be replaced or refilled when necessary, and this can be expensive. Multiple copies of documents usually are made on a copier rather than printed from the computer.

Scanners

Occasionally documents are scanned and sent by e-mail. Scanners provide high resolution and can produce images of written text and photos. Scanners often are used to create images so that older documents can be stored.

Printers

Machines that function only as printers are available and quite inexpensive; however, most medical offices can benefit from an all-in-one printer. These machines print, fax, copy, and scan laser-quality documents. Many all-in-one printers available today have advanced features, such as lab-quality photo printing, printing on both sides of the paper, and wireless connectivity.

Supplies

Stationery

Paper quality unquestionably affects the reader's overall impression of the communication. **Stationers** or printing companies are qualified to advise on the selection of paper, which can range from all sulfite (wood pulp) to all cotton fiber (sometimes called *rag*). Letterhead paper usually is **bond** paper that has a cotton fiber content of 25% or higher.

The weight of a type of paper is described by the **substance number**. This number is based on the weight of a **ream** that consists of 500 sheets of 17- × 22-inch paper. The higher the substance number, the heavier the paper. If the ream weighs 24 pounds (lb), the paper is referred to as *Sub 24* or *24-lb weight*. Letterhead stationery and matching envelopes are usually 16-, 20-, or 24-lb weight. This often is abbreviated as 16#, 20#, or 24#.

Sizes and Types of Letterhead Paper. Letterhead paper is available in four basic sizes:

Standard or letter	8½ × 11 inches
Monarch or executive	8½ × 10½ inches
Baronial	5½ × 8½ inches
Legal	8½ × 14 inches

Standard letterhead is used for general business and professional correspondence. Letterhead should be well designed and of a high-quality paper. The letter represents the sender and can help the receiver form an impression of the professionalism of the business.

Bond paper has a felt side and a wire side. When a sheet of letterhead is picked up and held to the light, a design or letters can be read from the printed side. This design, called a **watermark**, is an indication of quality. The side from which the watermark can be read is the felt side of the paper and the side on which printing or typing should be done. The watermark should always read across the page in the same direction as the typing.

> **CRITICAL THINKING APPLICATION   13-2**
>
> Brandon realizes that his father's office does not have a method of logging letters sent by certified mail. This forces the receptionist to dig through a patient's file to determine whether certified mail was actually sent and the notice of delivery received. How can this issue be resolved?

Continuation Pages. The second and continuing pages of a letter are placed on plain bond that matches the letterhead in weight and fiber content; these are called **continuation pages**. The stationery used for continuation pages should exactly match the letterhead but should not have the letterhead printing. Using different paper for the continuation pages is considered unprofessional.

Envelopes. Just as the continuation pages should be the same type of paper as the letterhead stationery, so should the envelopes. Envelopes are available in three basic sizes or types:

- No. 10
- No. 6¾
- Window

No. 10 envelopes are the general business size used for letter and legal stationery. No. 6¾ envelopes and window envelopes often are used for statements.

LETTER STYLES

A business letter usually is arranged in one of three styles: block, modified block or standard, or modified block indented. A fourth style, *simplified,* occasionally is used. The block and modified block styles are most commonly used in the physician's office.

Block Letter Style

When the block letter style is used, all lines start **flush** with the left margin (Figure 13-1). This style is considered the most efficient but is less attractive on the page.

Modified Block Letter Style

In the modified block style, the dateline, complimentary closing, and typed signature all begin at the center. All other lines begin at the left margin (Figure 13-2).

Modified Block Letter Style with Indented Paragraphs

The modified block letter style with indented paragraphs is identical to the block style except that the first line of each paragraph is indented five spaces (Figure 13-3).

Simplified Letter Style

In the simplified letter style, all lines begin flush with the left margin (Figure 13-4). The salutation is replaced with an all-capital subject

Elizabeth Blackwell, M.D.
223 Orange Avenue, N.W.
Cottonwood, UT 84121

January 26, 20—

Mr. Richard Fluege
3678 North Willow Avenue
Palm Beach, FL 33480

Dear Mr. Fluege:

Please send me full particulars on the professional suites you expect to offer for sale or rent in the Medical Arts Professional Annex.

In about six months, I will be ready to open my practice, and I am interested in locating in Florida. My preference is a street-level suite of approximately 2,000 square feet.

After I have had an opportunity to study the information you send me, I will write or telephone you if I have further questions.

Very truly yours,

Elizabeth Blackwell, M.D.

EB:mek

FIGURE 13-1 Block letter style.

MEDICAL ARTS PROFESSIONAL ANNEX
3678 North Willow Avenue
Palm Beach FL 33480

January 29, 20—

Elizabeth Blackwell, M.D.
223 Orange Avenue, N.W.
Cottonwood, UT 84121

Dear Doctor Blackwell:

We have two remaining street-level suites available for occupancy about July 1. These are marked on pages 3 and 4 of the enclosed descriptive brochure. If one of these suites appeals to you, we will be pleased to customize it for your practice.

Please feel free to call me collect at the number on the brochure for further discussion of your needs.

Sincerely yours,

Richard Fluege
Business Manager

RF:ab
Enclosure

FIGURE 13-2 Modified block letter style.

line on the third line below the inside address. The body of the letter begins on the third line below the subject line. The complimentary closing is omitted. An all-capital typed signature is entered on the fifth line below the body of the letter.

Types of Punctuation for Letter Styles

Traditionally the punctuation pattern used is based on the letter style. Normal punctuation is always used in the body of a business letter. In the other parts, either standard or open punctuation is used.

When standard punctuation is used, a colon is placed after the salutation, and a comma is placed after the complimentary closing. This is the punctuation pattern most often used, and it is appropriate with the block or modified block letter styles. When open punctuation is used, no punctuation is used at the end of any line outside the body of the letter unless that line ends with

WILLIAM OSLER, M.D.
1000 South West Street
Park Ridge, NJ 07656

January 26, 20—

Robert Koch, M.D.
398 Main Street
Park Ridge, NJ 07656

Dear Doctor Koch:

Mrs. Elaine Norris

Thank you for referring your patient, Mrs. Elaine Norris, for consultation and care. She was examined in my office today.

FINDINGS: The patient complained of pain in the left lower quadrant and some abdominal tenderness. She had a temperature of 100.2 degrees.

RECOMMENDATIONS: The patient was placed on a soft, low-residue, bland diet, antibiotics, and bed rest for a few days. Upper and lower gastrointestinal x-rays will be performed next week.

TENTATIVE DIAGNOSIS: Diverticulitis of large bowel.

Mrs. Norris has been asked to return here for reevaluation in about ten days.

Sincerely yours,

William Osler, M.D.

WO:gm

FIGURE 13-3 Modified block letter style with indented paragraphs.

ROBERT KOCH, M.D.
398 Main Street
Park Ridge, NJ 07656

January 30, 20—

William Osler, M.D.
1000 South West Street
Park Ridge, NJ 07656

ANNABELLE ANDERSON

You will be pleased to know, Bill, that Mrs. Anderson is progressing nicely. Her wound is healing. Her temperature has returned to normal, and she is beginning to resume her usual activities.

Mrs. Anderson has an appointment to return here for one more visit next week. At that time, I will ask her to return to you for any further care.

ROBERT KOCH, M.D.

RK:hb

FIGURE 13-4 Simplified letter style.

an abbreviation. This pattern is always used with the simplified letter style.

SPACING AND MARGINS

Generally, centering a letter on the page is the most attractive presentation. This is easily done with computer programs, such as Microsoft Word or WordPerfect. Business letters almost always are single spaced. If a letter consists of only a few lines, double-space both the inside address and the message and indent the first line of each paragraph five spaces.

The first typed entry, which is the date on the first page of the letter, usually is placed on the third line below the letterhead or on line 13 if the paper has no letterhead. The typing on continuation pages begins 1 inch from the top.

On standard letterhead, the side margins are usually 1 to 1½ inches on each side. If a letter is very short, making the margins wider creates a better appearance.

A 1-inch margin is the minimum at the bottom of the page. This can be increased if the letter will be carried over to a second page. Never use a second page to type only the complimentary closing and signature. Carry over a minimum of two lines of the body of the letter onto a continuation page. The heading of continuation pages is single spaced.

THE PARTS OF A LETTER

The structure of a letter and its placement on the page have been fairly well standardized into four main parts:

- Heading
- Opening
- Body
- Closing

Heading

The heading includes the letterhead and the dateline. The printed letterhead usually is centered at the top of the page and includes the name of the physician or group and the address. It may include the telephone number and the medical specialty or specialties. In a group or corporate practice, the names of the physicians may also be listed. Occasionally, the heading also includes the name of an office manager.

The dateline consists of the name of the month written in full, followed by the day and year. The date should not be abbreviated, nor should ordinal numbers (e.g., 1st, 2nd, 3rd) be used after the name of the month.

Opening

The opening consists of the inside address, the salutation, and the attention line, if one is used. The inside address has two or more lines, starts flush with the left margin, and contains at least the name of the individual or firm to whom the letter is addressed and the mailing address. When the letter is addressed to an individual, the name is preceded by a courtesy title, such as Dr., Mr., Mrs., Miss, or Ms. When addressing a letter to a physician, omit the courtesy title and type the physician's name, followed by his or her **academic degree**, such as *Rick P. Tipps, MD.* The name also could be written as *Dr. Rick P. Tipps.* However, do not use both a courtesy title and a degree that means the same thing, as in *Dr. Rick P. Tipps, MD.* Although this construction is often seen, even on the sign in front of physicians' offices, writing a doctor's name in this way is incorrect.

CRITICAL THINKING APPLICATION   13-3

Brandon has noticed that some of the correspondence leaving the office is signed incorrectly, with "Dr. Rick P. Tipps, MD" in the typed signature line. This is an uncomfortable situation, because Brandon realizes that the person who is typing the signature this way is the office manager.

- How might he approach her so that the mistake can be corrected?
- Is it wise to approach the office manager, or should Brandon go to his father? Why or why not?

The salutation is the letter writer's introductory greeting to the person being addressed; it is typed flush with the left margin on the second line below the last line of the address and is followed by a colon unless open punctuation is used. The words in the salutation vary, depending on the letter's degree of formality.

The attention line, if used, is placed on the second line below the inside address. If the medical assistant knows the name of the person for whom the letter is intended, that person's name is used in the inside address, and he or she is addressed personally. If the letter is addressed to a company or organization and directed to a division or department, the division or department name is placed on the attention line.

Body

The body of a letter includes the subject line, if one is used, and the message. In medical office correspondence, the subject of a letter frequently is a patient; in that case, the patient's name is used as the subject line or may be noted with the abbreviation "Re:". Because the subject line is considered part of the body of the letter, it is placed on the second line below the salutation. It may start flush with the left margin or at the point of indentation of indented paragraphs, or it may be centered. The word "Subject," followed by a colon, may be used or omitted entirely.

Begin typing the message on the second line below the subject line or on the second line below the salutation if no subject line is used. The first line of each paragraph may be indented five spaces, or it may start flush with the left margin, depending on the letter style chosen.

Closing

The closing includes the complimentary closing, the typed signature, the reference initials, and any special notations.

The complimentary closing is the writer's way of saying good-bye. This closing is placed on the second line below the last line of the body of the letter and is followed by a comma unless open punctuation is used. Only the first word is capitalized. The words used are determined by the degree of formality in the salutation. For example, if the salutation is *Dear Herb,* the closing might be *Cordially, Very truly yours,* or *Sincerely yours,* with consistent punctuation. If the letter is addressed to a business, the complimentary closing most often used is *Sincerely.*

A typed signature is a courtesy to the reader, especially if the name does not appear on the printed letterhead or if the personal signature is difficult or impossible to decipher. The typed signature is placed on the fourth line directly below the complimentary closing.

Reference initials that identify the writer and typist are placed flush with the left margin on the second line below the typed signature. If the writer's name is included on the signature line, the writer's initials need not be included in the reference block unless desired. The writer's initials, if used, should precede the typist's initials and are separated by a colon or diagonal line: GB:mek *(writer:typist)* and GB/mek *(writer/typist).*

Special notations sometimes are needed to indicate that enclosures are included with the letter or that copies of the letter are being distributed to others. If the letter has an enclosure, type the word *Enclosure* or *Enc.* on the first line below the reference initials. If more than one enclosure is involved, specify the number (e.g., *Enclosures 3*) or the name of the actual enclosure (e.g., *map* or *brochure*). If copies are to be sent to others, type this notation in the same manner as the enclosure notation or after it if both notations are needed. The copy notation usually is written as *c:* or *copy to:* followed by the name or names of those to whom a copy will be sent. If the person to whom the letter is addressed is not to know that copies are being distributed to others, use the notation *bc:* for "blind copy" on all copies except the original. Place this notation either in the upper left of the letter at the margin or below the last notation at the lower left margin.

Postscripts

Although a postscript sometimes may be used to express an afterthought, it often is used to emphasize an idea or statement. Begin the postscript on the second line below the last special notation. Follow the style of the letter, indenting the first line if paragraphs were indented in the body of the letter or starting at the margin if indentation was not used in the letter.

Continuation Pages

If the letter requires one or more continuation pages, the heading of the second and subsequent pages must have three items:

- Name of the addressee
- Page number
- Date

The heading should begin on the seventh line from the top of the page. Continuation of the body of the letter begins on the tenth line or the third line below the heading. The three accepted forms for the continuation page heading are:

RICK P. TIPPS, M.D.	Rick P. Tipps, M.D.	Rick P. Tipps, M.D.
Page 2	Page 2	-2-
July 5, 2010	July 5, 2010	July 5, 2010
	Subject: Susan Clemmons	

Signing the Letter

Some physicians prefer to compose and sign all letters that leave their offices. However, most are more than pleased to delegate the responsibility of composing and signing business letters to a competent assistant. Although not all authorities agree on the form to be followed, most recommend that a woman's typed signature include a courtesy title (Miss, Mrs., or Ms.) and that the title not be enclosed in parentheses. The courtesy title need not be included in the handwritten signature.

In general, the physician signs all of the following:

- Letters dealing with medical advice to patients
- Letters to officers or committees of the medical society
- Referral and consultation reports to colleagues
- Medical reports to insurance companies
- Personal letters

The medical assistant usually composes and signs letters concerning the following:

- Routine matters (e.g., arranging or rescheduling appointments)
- Orders for office supplies
- Notification to patients about surgery or hospital arrangements
- Collection of delinquent accounts
- Letters of solicitation

CRITICAL THINKING APPLICATION **13-4**

One of the employees has brought an urgent letter to Brandon that Brandon's father neglected to sign before leaving the office for the day. The letter is to another physician reporting his findings on a referred patient. The employee asks Brandon to sign the letter. What should he do? What are some ways to resolve this situation if the letter must leave in the mail today?

OTHER TYPES OF WRITTEN COMMUNICATION

The physician's office must deal with many types of written communications other than business letters. Remember, every piece of written communication that leaves the office reflects on the office. Make sure to follow the rules of grammar even when sending a simple business e-mail.

Telephone Messages

One of the most common types of written communication in the medical office is the telephone message. Seven items must be recorded when a phone message is taken:

- Name of the person to whom the call is directed
- Name of the person calling
- Caller's daytime or cell phone number (or both)
- Reason for the call
- Action to be taken
- Date and time of the call
- Initials of the person taking the call

E-Mail and Text Messages

E-mail and texting are popular ways to send written communications in today's computer-literate society. E-mail messages can be saved, printed for the patient's chart, and **archived** for storage. E-mails pertinent to the patient's care or a conflict situation should be printed, and a copy should be placed in the patient's medical record. E-mails that show a pattern of cancelled appointments should also be added to the patient's medical record. Any e-mail sent in a professional capacity from the physician's office or by a physician's representative should adhere to proper rules of grammar and should have accurate spelling. People tend to classify e-mail as casual communication, but because it is so frequently used in business, it should be written in the same professional manner as a mailed letter. Use of the proper letter format, including the inside addresses and date, is not necessary. However, the rest of the e-mail should read similarly to a letter. Never send e-mails or texts from the medical office that use abbreviations such as "r" for "are," or "u" for "you." Internet abbreviations of any kind are not acceptable in business communications. Use single spacing and do not use terms or sentences in all-capital letters (e.g., ARE THE TEST RESULTS AVAILABLE?); this implies shouting in e-language.

The medical assistant also should not immediately answer an e-mail that is derogatory, accusatory, or negative in some other way. Print the e-mail and go through it calmly, marking what needs to be addressed. Because attitude often is easily detectable in an e-mail, make sure the response has no hint of negativity. Once a professional response has been crafted, type and send it. In this situation, the best course often is to send a copy to the office manager, either openly or blindly, depending on the situation. This way, the medical assistant includes the supervisor in the conflict and keeps that individual aware of the brewing situation. The office manager can get involved if necessary or just monitor the situation and how the medical assistant handles it.

Realize that e-mails are not guaranteed to be a secure form of communication. Consider the alternatives before sending an e-mail containing privileged or confidential information. Many offices use a disclaimer with their e-mails, such as:

> This e-mail, including attachments, contains information that may be confidential, protected by attorney/client privilege, or exempt from disclosure under applicable law. This e-mail, including attachments, constitutes nonpublic information intended to be conveyed only to the designated recipient(s). If you are not an intended recipient of this communication, please be advised that any disclosure, dissemination, distribution, copying, or other use of this communication is strictly prohibited. If you have received this communication in error, please notify the sender immediately by reply e-mail and destroy all electronic and printed copies of the communication and any attached documents.

Text messages of a personal nature should not be sent during office hours. If the phone belongs to the office, it should never be used for personal texting. The office policy manual should address e-mailing and texting, and those policies should be strictly followed when communicating in this manner with patients or other business entities. Critical or confidential information may be e-mailed according to office policy but should never be sent via text or as an attachment to a text.

Patients must indicate their agreement to receive e-mail and text messages as outlined on the office privacy practices forms, which are usually given to the patients upon their first visit to the office. Some offices send appointment reminders through e-mail or texts, in addition to other types of information. The indications that the patient lists on the privacy practices forms can be changed whenever the patient wishes; if the patient wants to make a change, a new form must be signed. This document will contain information on sending e-mails and texts, so if a patient is willing to receive information from the physician's office via e-mail and text, he or she will indicate that on the privacy practices form. Texts may also be used throughout the business day from employee to employee, but patients should never be given the physician or other employees' cell phone numbers for texting purposes.

Faxed Messages

All faxes should have a cover sheet that states that the information in the fax is confidential and intended only for the person to whom the fax was sent (Procedure 13-3). Use correct grammar in all faxed messages. Use a fax only when absolutely necessary or when the information sent will not breach patient confidentiality. This helps prevent other individuals on the receiving end from reading faxed information. Most businesses use a disclosure statement similar to the example shown for e-mails on all faxed transmissions. Call ahead when faxing information to alert the person who is to receive the fax. This practice helps ensure that the fax goes to the right person, which promotes confidentiality.

Memorandums

Most offices **disseminate** various memorandums throughout the business week (Figure 13-5). These written documents also must be clear, concise, and grammatically correct. Remember that people reading memos, e-mails, faxes, and letters often can detect attitudes in written communications; therefore, make the document sound professional, even if the subject matter is frustrating or difficult.

When sending information to employees, make sure the important points are all included and presented in a way that does not sound **condescending**. Sometimes, it is wise to include a supervisor's initials on memos that might not receive a positive response so that employees realize the writer's supervisor is aware of and supports the information in the memo. Although e-mail is used on a daily basis in the medical office, memos are often necessary to denote policy changes and are often printed and added to the office policy manual. Some physicians and office managers require that employees initial memos to verify that they were read prior to filing them or adding them to policy manuals.

> ### CRITICAL THINKING APPLICATION 13-5
> - E-mail is used more and more often to communicate with employees. Brandon has noticed that very few printed memos circulate throughout the office. What are the advantages and disadvantages of communicating through e-mail with employees?
> - The office manager has given Brandon information to disseminate to all the employees of the clinic. She did not specify whether to give out the memo by hand or by e-mail, but she did state that the information was very important. Which would be the best method?

EDITING

All documents should go through an **editing** process before mailing or delivery. First proofread the document and then review it for accuracy in grammar and spelling. Table 13-2 shows proofreader's marks. Although these marks usually are used in copyediting, medical assistants who take the time to learn them will be able to process documents that need revision or need an answer twice as fast as those who make lengthy notes. Most software programs have spelling and grammar checks, as well as a dictionary and thesaurus. The programs also have a *Find* feature that allows the user to move through the document quickly and locate certain words or phrases that need to be changed. For instance, if a document uses the phrase "paper-based medical record," using the *Find* feature, each place that the word "paper" occurs can be edited to say "electronic." Editing also allows the user to track changes in a document and to compare the current version to a previous one.

Users can learn advanced features of the software program used in the medical office by taking courses online or at local community colleges. This extra effort can make editing documents go much faster. The more users know about the program, the more efficient they become in its use. Some programs offer free tutorials on their Web site. Also, textbooks available at local libraries or bookstores often include a tutorial CD that corresponds to lessons in the text.

PROCEDURE 13-3

Prepare a Fax for Transmission

GOAL: *To compose and transmit a clearly written, grammatically correct fax that is easily understood, free of spelling and grammatical errors, and sent in a manner that provides for patient confidentiality.*

EQUIPMENT and SUPPLIES

- Stationery
- Computer or typewriter
- Correspondence to be answered or notes
- Guide for proofreader's marks
- Fax machine or all-in-one device

PROCEDURAL STEPS

1. Determine the information and/or documents that need to be included in the fax transmission.
   PURPOSE: To ensure that the goals of the correspondence are fulfilled and that relevant information has been identified and included.

2. Complete a fax cover sheet to include as the first document to be faxed, using acceptable business grammar. Make certain that the fax cover sheet contains a disclosure statement.

3. Print a draft copy of the letter or memo. Read it carefully and highlight changes to be made or note any additions to be made. Use proofreader's marks.
   PURPOSE: Reading a hard copy of a fax is more conducive to finding errors and grammatical mistakes.

4. Revise the fax using the notes and proofreader's marks.

5. Read the fax once again on the screen. Perform spelling and grammar checks if those tools are available on the computer.
   PURPOSE: To locate any missed errors or misspelled words.

6. Prepare a final draft. Read the fax word for word and check once again for errors.

7. Have another person proofread a fax that is especially important.
   PURPOSE: Often another person can find missed errors quickly.

8. Scan any attachments that might need to be sent with the fax into the computer.

9. Make certain that the medical facility confidentiality statement is included on the bottom of the fax cover sheet.
   PURPOSE: To promote patient confidentiality once the fax arrives at its destination.

10. Send the fax.

11. Document that the fax was sent and received if required by office policy.
    PURPOSE: To have proof that the information was sent via fax and proof that the fax was received at its destination, if the fax machine has this capability.

12. When sending critical information via fax, call the receiving office to make certain that the fax was received. Document the person's name who verified that the fax and all attachments were received.
    PURPOSE: To provide documentation that information was sent and received.

13. If a fax is received in error, contact the sender immediately and inform him or her of the mistake. Do not read the fax any further than necessary to determine that it was sent in error.

Take advantage of these learning opportunities and show initiative and a willingness to learn.

DEVELOPING A PORTFOLIO

Letter composition can be made faster and easier by developing a **portfolio** of sample letters to suit the various situations that frequently arise. As the physician approves letters, add them to the office portfolio. For instance, suppose a letter is needed for a patient who wants to change an appointment. Compose a letter that is clear, concise, and courteous and make an extra copy to put in the portfolio. Alternatively, if a computer is used, store the letter on a disk or on the computer's hard drive. Do this each time a new kind of letter is written. Soon you will be able to select a letter from the portfolio and change it slightly to suit the current situation.

Templates also can help the medical assistant build a portfolio. A **template** is a guide or pattern that can be followed to create a new document. Microsoft keeps a wide array of templates on its Web site that can be downloaded to the user's computer and adapted for

individual use. New templates are added to the Web site often, and most are available at no cost to the user.

U.S. POSTAL SERVICE

The U.S. Postal Service (USPS) is an independent establishment of the executive branch of the U.S. government. The Postal Service has been transformed from messages sent to neighbors in colonial times to an agency dedicated to providing mail service to every single home and business in the United States. Today, many operations can be done online at *www.usps.com*.

MAIL PROCESSING

Incoming Mail

Each day a great variety of mail comes into the professional office and must be processed (Procedure 13-4). Common items in the daily mail include:

INTEROFFICE MEMORANDUM

TO	All Staff
FROM	Office Manager
DATE	December 1
SUBJECT	Holiday Schedule

Our entire facility will be closed on December 24, December 25, December 31, and January 1. The office will be on reduced staff during the days of December 26, 27, 28, 29, and 30. Assignments will be based on seniority of staff members. Please submit your preferences as soon as possible.

A

MEMO TO:	George Walker
FROM:	Stanley Barr
DATE:	February 8
SUBJECT:	Office rental

We are experiencing unexpectedly rapid growth in our business office and will soon need additional space for our increased number of employees. Do you have a larger facility available in this building? If so, I would like to hear from you regarding the location, square footage, and anticipated rental costs.

B

FIGURE 13-5 Examples of memorandums. Memos are intended to be short, specific, and to the point; memos can be delivered via e-mail if allowed by the office procedure manual.

TABLE 13-2 Proofreader's Marks

Symbol or Margin Notation	Meaning	Example
℘ or ↗ or ⅁	Delete	take it out
⌒	Close up	print as o ne word
⅁	Delete and close up	cloоse up
∧ or ⟩ or ⅄	Insert	insert here (something)
#	Insert a space	put onehere
ℰℊ#	Space evenly	space evenly where indicated
stet	Let stand	let marked text stand as set
tr	Transpose	change order the
[	Set farther to left	too far to the right
]	Set farther to right	too far to the left
¶	Begin a new paragraph	the same is true. In conclusion
(sp)	Spell out	set 5 lbs as five pounds
cap	Set in CAPITALS	set nato as NATO
lc	Set in lowercase	set South as south
ital	Set in italic	set oeuvre as oeuvre
bf	Set in boldface	set important as **important**
∨	Superscript or superior	as in πr2
∧	Subscript or inferior	as in H2O
⅄	Comma	red blue, and yellow
⅁	Apostrophe	Calvin's lizard was green.
⊙	Period	The end is near ⊙
; or j/	Semicolon	1, this 2, that
: or ⊡	Colon	is the following :
℘℘ or ⌣⌣	Quotation marks	He said, I did it.
( )	Parentheses	Run fast now.

- General correspondence
- Payments for service
- Bills for office purchases
- Insurance claim forms to be completed
- Laboratory reports
- Hospital reports
- Medical society mailings
- Professional journals
- Promotional literature and samples from pharmaceutical houses
- Advertisements
- Interoffice envelopes

In large clinics and medical centers, the mail is opened by specially designated people in a central department to speed up this daily task. In the average medical office, however, a medical assistant, often the receptionist, opens the mail using the ordinary letter-opening method.

Opening the Mail

Before any mail is opened, the physician and medical assistant should establish the procedure to follow for incoming mail; that is, what letters should be opened and what pieces, if any, the physician prefers to open personally. For example, the physician may prefer to open any communications from an attorney or accountant, even if they are not marked *Personal*. If you have any doubt about whether you should open an envelope, do not open the item; forward it to the person to whom it is addressed. Even a simple procedure such as opening the daily mail can be done more efficiently if a good system is followed.

Annotating

Annotating the mail is an additional service the medical assistant can perform. Read through each letter, underline the significant words

PROCEDURE 13-4

Receive, Organize, Prioritize, and Transmit Information Expediently

GOAL: *To efficiently sort through the mail that arrives daily in the medical office.*

EQUIPMENT and SUPPLIES

- Computer
- Draft paper
- Letterhead stationery
- Pen or pencil
- Highlighter
- Staple remover
- Paper clips
- Letter opener
- Stapler
- Transparent tape
- Date stamp

PROCEDURAL STEPS

1. Clear a working space on the desk or countertop.
2. Sort the mail according to importance and urgency:
   - Physician's personal mail
   - Ordinary first-class mail
   - Checks from insurance companies and patients
   - Periodicals and newspapers
   - All other pieces, including drug samples

   PURPOSE: To prioritize the mail for the physician so that the most important issues can be dealt with first.

3. Open the mail neatly and in an organized manner.
4. Stack the envelopes so that they all face in the same direction.
5. Pick up the top one and tap the envelope so that when you open it you will not cut the contents.

   PURPOSE: To avoid damaging the envelope's contents.
6. Open all envelopes along the top edge for easiest removal of contents.
7. Remove the contents of each envelope and hold the envelope to the light to make sure nothing remains inside.
8. Make a note of the postmark when this is important.
9. Discard the envelope after you have checked to see that the message inside has a return address. Some offices make it a policy to attach the envelope to each piece of correspondence until it has received attention.
10. Date-stamp the letter and attach any enclosures.

    PURPOSE: The date stamp identifies when the envelope and its contents were received at the office.
11. If an enclosure notation is present at the bottom of the letter, make sure the enclosure was included. If it is missing, indicate this on the notation by writing the word "No" and circling it.

    PURPOSE: To document that the enclosure or enclosures mentioned in the letter were not found inside the envelope.
12. Organize the mail for transmission to each person, and at the appropriate time, distribute it to the proper individuals.

and phrases, and note in the margin any action required; this makes taking action on the mail much easier. If the letter needs no reply, code it for filing at this time. A highlighter that does not photocopy may be used for annotating. When mail refers to previous correspondence, obtain this from the file and attach it or a copy. If the patient's chart is needed when replying to an inquiry, pull the chart and place it with the letter.

The medical office should have a specific place for the opened, annotated mail. After sorting, opening, and annotating the mail, place the items the physician will want to see in the established place, with the most important mail on top. Personal mail, of course, remains unopened. If a piece of personal mail addressed to the employer is opened by mistake, fold and replace it inside the envelope and write *Opened in error* across the outside, followed by the initials of the person who opened it. Use the same procedure with a piece of mail addressed to another office that may have been opened in error. In such cases, reseal the envelope with transparent tape and hand it to the mail carrier.

Responding to the Mail

In some offices the physician and medical assistant go over the mail together. Once the medical assistant has gained confidence, drafting a reply to most inquiries will be easy. Usually, the physician is very pleased to delegate this responsibility, especially for matters that do not relate to patient care.

Letters of referral from other physicians should be noted carefully so that an answer can be sent after the patient has been seen and the physician can give a report. If considerable time may pass before such information can be sent, a courteous gesture is to write a letter to the referring physician advising that a detailed report will follow. Some physicians send printed cards expressing thanks for referrals; others prefer to write thank you letters to professional colleagues.

Mail Requiring Special Handling

Payment Receipts

Payments from patients and insurance companies arrive at the office daily. All payments should be separated and recorded immediately in the day's receipts. A payment received on Monday should be recorded on Monday. Most patients consider their cancelled check a receipt; if the patient requests a receipt, one should be mailed. Otherwise, the receipt may be placed in the patient's chart for delivery on a future office visit.

CRITICAL THINKING APPLICATION   13-6

Brandon notices that Mrs. Attaway, a widow and long-time patient of his father, sent in a check for $125 for a bill. However, her insurance company had already paid $112 toward the bill. Brandon knows that Mrs. Attaway must be very careful with her money and has always paid her bills quickly. The policy of the office is to route the overpayment through the system, but refund checks are cut only once per month. What should Brandon do in this situation?

Insurance Information

Insurance information should be put in a predetermined place for handling by the billers. Documents relating to insurance should be passed to the appropriate person immediately to prevent delays and to comply with time limits that might result in the claim going unpaid.

Drug Samples

Sample drugs and related literature usually are delivered by pharmaceutical representatives, but they occasionally may arrive by mail. Determine from the physician what types of literature and samples should be saved. Most physicians keep pertinent new samples in a locked sample storage area, along with the accompanying literature for immediate reference. Other drug samples are **categorically** stored. Drugs should never be tossed into the trash.

Vacation Mail

When the physician is away from the office, a medical assistant generally is responsible for handling all mail. In this circumstance, all pieces should be examined carefully. The medical assistant then can decide how to handle each piece by asking the following questions:

- Is it important enough to warrant phoning or faxing the physician?
- Should it be forwarded for immediate attention?
- Should I answer it myself or send a brief note to the correspondent, explaining that the physician is out of the office and the reply will be delayed a bit?
- Can this wait for attention until the physician returns or would that give the appearance of negligence?

If the medical assistant is unable to contact the physician or forward important mail, he or she should always answer the sender immediately, explaining the delay and requesting cooperation. Instead of forwarding an original piece of mail and risking possible loss, make a copy for forwarding. Then, if the physician wants the letter answered, notations can be made on the copy and the copy can be returned to the office staff for answering, without defacement of the original letter.

When the physician is traveling from place to place, the envelopes for all communications sent to him or her should be numbered consecutively. This helps the physician to determine easily whether any mail has been lost or delayed. If a record is kept of each piece of mail sent out and its corresponding number, anything that might be lost can be identified and remailed if necessary.

Correspondence that does not require immediate action and that the medical assistant cannot answer until the physician returns should be placed in a special folder marked *Requires Attention;* this folder is placed on top of other accumulated mail. Mail the medical assistant can compose but that requires the physician's approval before mailing should be put into another special folder marked *For Approval.* When the physician returns, these letters can be rapidly checked and signed.

Any letters marked *Personal* may be acknowledged to the return address on the envelope. The brief acknowledgment should state that the physician is out of town for a certain length of time and will attend to the letter immediately on returning. This acknowledgment also should offer help in any way possible in the meantime.

Discard any mail that ordinarily would not be brought to the physician's attention. Some promotional literature falls into this category. Make sure mailings from professional organizations are saved.

In rare cases, the entire facility may be closed for a time. In such cases the post office can be contacted to hold mail until the facility reopens. The postal carrier cannot accept an oral request; a formal written request must be made. Never leave mail unattended to gather outside a mailbox or clutter up a doorway in a hall. Far too much money and mail of a confidential nature are sent to physicians' offices to run the risk of mail theft or destruction.

Outgoing Mail

Preparing outgoing mail is a daily duty and the medical assistant must stay on top of the mail so that it does not become outdated. Three basic envelopes are used for outgoing mail in the physician's office, including the No. 10, No. 6¾, and window envelopes.

Addressing the Envelope

Delivery Addresses. The USPS attempts to have all mail in standard-sized envelopes read, coded, sorted, and canceled automatically at regional sorting stations where mail can be processed at a rate of more than 30,000 letters per hour. The success of automatic sorting depends on the cooperation of mailers in preparing envelopes in a format that can be read by automatic equipment (Procedure 13-5).

The Postal Service provides three special sets of abbreviations: (1) state names; (2) long names of cities, towns, and places; and (3) names of streets and roads and general terms, such as *University* or *Institute.* The information can be obtained from the Postal Service, or a program can be purchased for the computer. When these abbreviations are used, it is possible to limit the last line of any **domestic mail** address to 27 strokes. The next-to-last line in the address block should have a street address or post office box number.

The address block should start no higher than 2¾ inches from the bottom. Leave a bottom margin of at least ⅜ inch and left and right margins of at least 1 inch. Nothing should be written or printed below the address block or to the right of it.

The regulations for addressing envelopes were developed mainly for volume mailers with computerized mailing lists (Figure 13-6). Some exceptions are acceptable to the Postal Service and its scanning equipment. For example, the traditional style of typing an address in lower case with initial capital letters can be read by the optical scanners. Also, if the ZIP code cannot fit on the line with the city and state, it can be placed on the line immediately below. When a suite number is used, most people place it after the delivery address,

PROCEDURE 13-5

Address an Envelope According to Postal Service Optical Character Reader Guidelines

GOAL: *To correctly address business correspondence so that the mail arrives at the post office and is processed by the U.S. Postal Service as efficiently as possible.*

EQUIPMENT and SUPPLIES

- Envelopes
- Computer or typewriter
- Correspondence

PROCEDURAL STEPS

1. Place the envelope in the printer.
2. Enter the word processing program, such as Microsoft Word, and check the *Tools* section for envelopes. The address block should start no higher than 2¾ inches from the bottom. Leave a bottom margin of at least ⅝ inch and left and right margins of at least 1 inch. Nothing should be written or printed below the address block or to the right of it.
   PURPOSE: To ensure correct placement of the address for accurate reading by the optical character reader (OCR).

3. Use dark type on a light background, no script or italics, and capitalize everything in the address.
   PURPOSE: To ensure that the OCR can read the address.
4. Type the address in block format using only approved abbreviations and eliminating all punctuation. If a suite number is to be included, type it above the delivery address on a separate line.
5. Type the city, state, and ZIP code on the last line of the address.
6. No line should have more than 27 total characters, including spaces.
7. Leave a ⅝- × 4¾-inch space blank in the bottom right corner of the envelope.
   PURPOSE: To allow for bar code scanning (BCS).
8. Mail addressed to other countries includes the city and postal code on the third line and the name of the country on a fourth line.

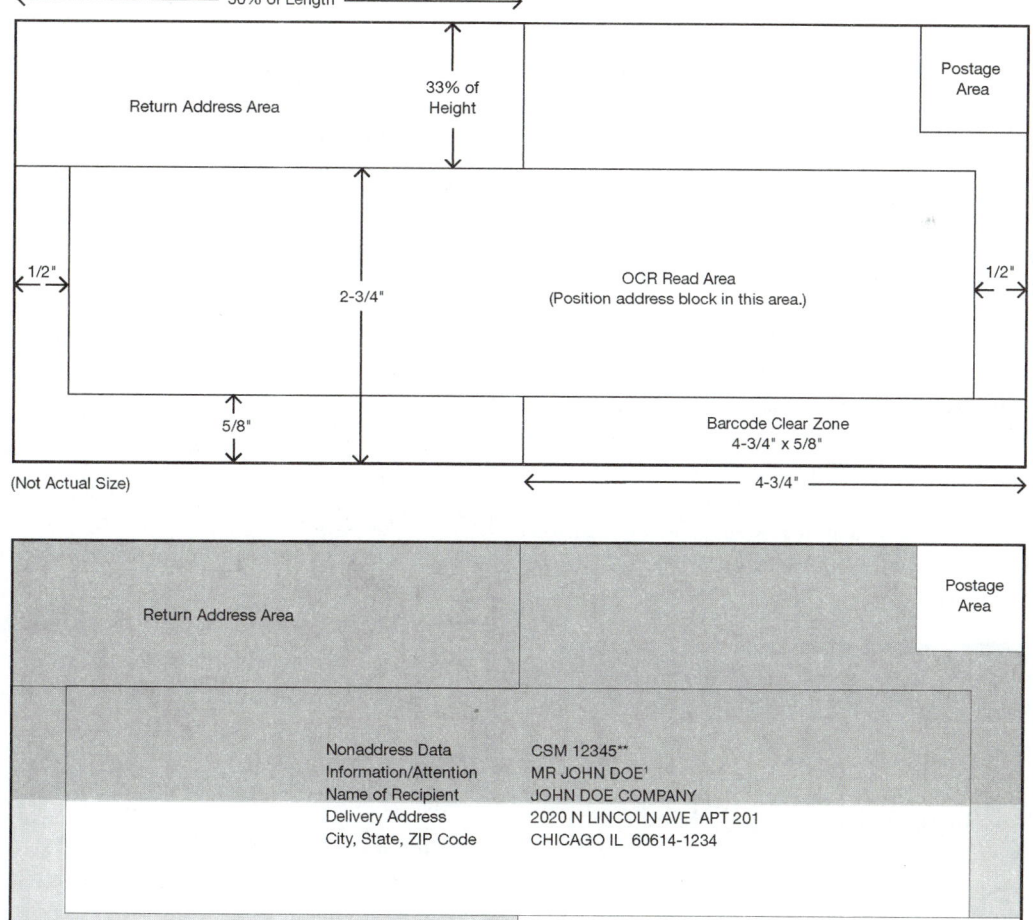

FIGURE 13-6 Addressing envelopes.

which is fine. However, if it does not fit in that space, it should be placed *above* the delivery address, not below it.

Return Addresses. Always place a complete return address on the envelope. If the envelope is mailed without a stamp or if the stamp falls off and the envelope has no return address, it will go to the dead letter office. There, postal employees open the mail to try to identify the sender, but huge delays may make the mail useless on delivery. If an address is found for the sender, the mail is returned in an official envelope with a notice of postage due. If an address is not found for the sender, the mail is destroyed.

Notations. Any notations on the envelope directed to the addressee (e.g., *Personal* or *Confidential*) should be typed and underlined on line 9 or on the third line below the return address, whichever is lower. Align it with the return address on the left edge of the envelope.

Any notations directed to the Postal Service (e.g., special delivery or certified mail), should be typed in all capital letters on the upper right side of the envelope immediately below the stamp area. If an address has an attention line, it should be typed above the organization line or on the line immediately above the street address or post office box number.

Sealing and Stamping Hints

When many envelopes need to go into the mail at one time (e.g., at statement time), the process can be speeded up by sealing several at a time:

- Fan out unsealed envelopes, address side down, in groups of six to 10.
- Draw a damp sponge over the flaps, and starting with the lower piece, turn down the flaps and seal each one.

Do not use too much moisture, because this may cause the glue to spread and several envelopes to stick together. A similar process simplifies stamping several letters at one time if a postage meter is not used. If possible, purchase stamps by the roll. Tear off about ten stamps from the roll. Fanfold the stamps on the perforations so that they separate easily. Fan the envelopes address side up. Starting at one end of the fanned envelopes, attach the stamp at the end of the strip, tear it off, and proceed to the next envelope. Automated sealers and stampers are also available to make this procedure easier and more efficient. Alternative stamping options are available on the Internet. Stamps can be purchased online and printed on the office printer. Personalized stamps are also available that allow the user to upload a photo or drawing to a stamp template and then print the stamps for use on office mail.

BASIC U.S. POSTAL SERVICE DELIVERY ADDRESS GUIDELINES

- Always put the address and the postage on the same side of the mail piece.
- On a letter, the address should be parallel to the longest side.
- Use the following:
  - All capital letters
  - No punctuation
  - At least 10-point type
  - One space between city and state

- Two spaces between state and ZIP code
- Simple type fonts
- Left-justified format
- Black ink on white or light paper
- No reverse type (white printing on a black background)
- If the address appears inside a window, make sure at least ⅛-inch clearance is present around the address. Sometimes parts of the address slip out of view behind the window, and the mail processing machines cannot read the address.
- If address labels are used, make sure no important information is cut off. Also make sure the labels are on straight. Mail processing machines have trouble reading crooked or slanted information.

More Tips

- Always put the attention line on top; never below the city and state or in the bottom corner of your mail piece.
- If the suite or apartment number cannot fit on the same line as the delivery address, put it on the line above the delivery address, not on the line below.
- Words such as "east" and "west" are called directionals, and they are very important. A missing or bad directional can prevent the mail from being delivered correctly.
- Use the free ZIP code lookup and the ZIP+4 code lookup on the Postal Service Web site to find the correct ZIP codes and ZIP+4 codes for the addresses.
- Almost 25% of all mail pieces have something wrong with the address, such as a missing apartment number or a wrong ZIP code. Some of those mail pieces may be delivered despite the incorrect address, but it costs the Postal Service time and money.
- If a first-class mail letter weighs 1 ounce or less and the address is parallel to the shortest side, the piece may be nonmailable or will be charged the nonmachineable surcharge.
- Sometimes it is not important that the mail piece reach a specific customer, just that it reach an address. One way to do this is to use a generic title such as "Postal Customer" or "Occupant" or "Resident," rather than a name, plus the complete address.
- Fancy fonts, such as those used on wedding invitations, do not read well on mail processing equipment. Fancy fonts look great on the envelopes, but they may slow down the mail.
- Use common sense. If you cannot read the address, the automated mail processing equipment cannot read the address, either.
- Some types of paper interfere with the machines that read addresses. The paper on the address side should be white or light in color. No patterns or prominent flecks, please! Also, the envelope shouldn't be too glossy; avoid shiny, coated paper stock.

Modified from the U.S. Postal Service Web site: www.usps.com. Accessed 9/25/12.

Cost-Saving Mailing Procedures

Using ZIP Codes. The ZIP code is a very important part of an address, just as the area code is a very important part of a telephone number. ZIP codes start with the number 0 on the East Coast and gradually become higher, up to number 9, on the West Coast and in Hawaii.

The five-digit ZIP code was introduced in 1961. The first three digits identify a major city or distribution point, and all five digits identify an individual post office, zone of a city, or other delivery unit. The Postal Service later developed the nine-digit ZIP code, consisting of the original five digits followed by a hyphen and four additional digits that further identify the addressee's street location. The ZIP code is transformed electronically into a bar code. The office computer may have this capability. The Postal Code claims that the ZIP+4 code, when used with the automated letter-sorting machinery, can eliminate 20 mail-handling steps and result in considerable savings. These savings are passed on to bulk mailers on mailings of 250 or more pieces that have typed addresses in machine-readable format along with the nine-digit ZIP+4 code.

Presorting. Bulk mailers can get a discount on postage for presorting their mail. A discounted presort rate is charged on each piece that is part of a group of 10 or more pieces sorted to the same five-digit code or a group of 50 or more pieces sorted to ZIP codes with the same first three digits. The USPS uses the words "presorting" and "bulk" interchangeably.

Using Correct Postage. Although mailing fees are still one of our better bargains, the mailing costs for even a small office are a sizable item in the annual budget, and carelessness can cause them to soar. If the facility does not have a postage meter that dispenses postage exactly, make sure you are not putting too many stamps on your outgoing mail. Use an accurate postage scale and remember that only the first ounce requires the base rate; additional ounces are charged at a lower rate. Also remember, the USPS does not deliver mail without postage.

Getting Faster Mail Service

Postage Meters. A postage meter is the most efficient way of stamping the mail in a large business office. It can print postage onto adhesive strips, which are placed on envelopes or packages, or it can print the postage directly onto an envelope. Metered mail does not have to be canceled or postmarked when it reaches the post office. This means that it can move on to its destination more quickly.

CRITICAL THINKING APPLICATION   13-7

- Brandon knows the mail processing would go much faster if the office invested in a postage meter. The office manager states that she has mentioned this to Brandon's father several times, but he did not purchase a meter. How might Brandon approach his father about this issue?
- What should Brandon do before discussing the postage meter with his father?

Mailing Practices. For large mailings, local letters should be separated from out-of-town letters. Letters or packages that need to be rushed should be taken directly to the post office for mailing. Others can be placed in street boxes or the building's mail chute for pickup. Packages should always be taken to a post office and weighed for proper postage. Place a letter tray on the desk or in some other convenient place so that all outgoing mail is kept together until it is ready to leave the office.

Classifications of Mail

Mail is classified according to type, weight, and destination. The ounce (oz) and the pound (lb) are the units of measurement. Domestic mail is sent to a destination within the United States and its territories; **international mail** is sent to a destination outside the United States. Letters to distant points of the globe are in almost all cases sent by air and can be expected to reach their destination within a few days. The rates for international mail are based on increments of ½ to 1 ounce. A table of mailing rates and current postage can be obtained from the post office or found online at *www.usps.com*.

Express Mail. Express mail is available 7 days a week, 365 days a year for items weighing up to 70 lb and measuring 108 inches in combined length and **girth**. This includes delivery on Sundays and holidays to most locations. It is the fastest mail service offered by the USPS. Service features include:

- Noon delivery between major business markets
- Merchandise and document reconstruction insurance
- Express mail shipping containers
- Shipment receipt
- Optional return receipt service
- Optional **collect on delivery (COD)** service
- Waiver of signature option
- Collection boxes
- Optional pickup service
- Automatic insurance up to $100 free of charge

First-Class Mail. First-class mail comprises sealed or unsealed handwritten or typed material, such as letters, postal cards, postcards, and business reply mail. Postage for letters weighing 13 oz or less is based on weight, in 1-oz increments. Envelopes larger than the standard No. 10 business envelope should have the green diamond border to expedite first-class delivery. The minimum quantity to mail at discount prices is 500 mail pieces. First-class mail over 13 oz automatically becomes Priority Mail. At the time of this publishing, first-class stamps cost 46¢. Postage rates usually are adjusted each May, although rates do not necessarily increase for all services annually.

The forever stamp, first issued by the USPS in 2007, is used as first-class postage on envelopes weighing 1 oz or less. Regardless of postal rate increases, and no matter the original purchase price, the forever stamp will always be valid for first-class mail.

Priority Mail. First-class mail weighing more than 13 oz is classified as priority mail, and the postage is calculated on the basis of destination and weight (maximum of 70 lb). Remember these tips about priority mail:

- If using an envelope or box not purchased from the USPS, make sure to mark it *Priority Mail*.
- Priority mail drop shipment is a special way to get mail delivered sooner. Sacks or trays of standard mail are sent to the post office nearest the zip code for delivery and then sent by standard mail.
- Priority mail parcels weighing more than 15 lb and larger than 84 inches in combined length and girth are charged a balloon rate.

Standard Mail. Standard mail consists of advertising, promotional, directory, or editorial material (or any combination of such material). It must be securely bound by permanent fastenings such as staples, spiral binding, glue, or stitching and cannot have the nature of personal correspondence. Loose-leaf binders and similar fastenings are not considered permanent. Mail in this class cannot weigh more than 15 lb.

Media Mail. Media mail is used for books, film, manuscripts, printed music, printed test materials, sound recordings, play scripts, printed educational charts, loose-leaf pages and binders consisting of medical information, videotapes, and computer-recorded media such as CD-ROMs and flash drives. Media mail cannot contain advertising or weigh more than 70 lb.

Business Mail. Businesses may want to consider the benefits of using business mail to acquire new customers and retain current customers and to develop new services for them, in addition to filling orders and completing transactions. Research business mail options on the USPS Web site.

Nonprofit Mail. Nonprofit organizations are eligible for additional mail discounts. Look for more information on the USPS Web site.

Special Services

Insured Mail. Insurance coverage against loss or damage is available for priority mail, first-class mail, and parcel post.

Registered Mail. Mail of all classes, particularly that of unusually high value, can be additionally protected by registering it. The sender may request evidence of its delivery. Registering a piece of mail also helps to trace delivery if necessary.

A registered letter is sent by going to the post office and completing the required forms. All articles to be registered must be thoroughly sealed with USPS tape; cellophane tape is not permitted. On receiving the item, the **recipient** must sign a form acknowledging delivery. A registered letter may be released to the person to whom it is addressed or to his or her agent. For an additional fee, a personal receipt may be requested (Figure 13-7, *A*). This ensures that the letter is released only to the individual to whom it is addressed. Such pieces bear the label *To Addressee Only.* Registered mail can be insured for up to $25,000.

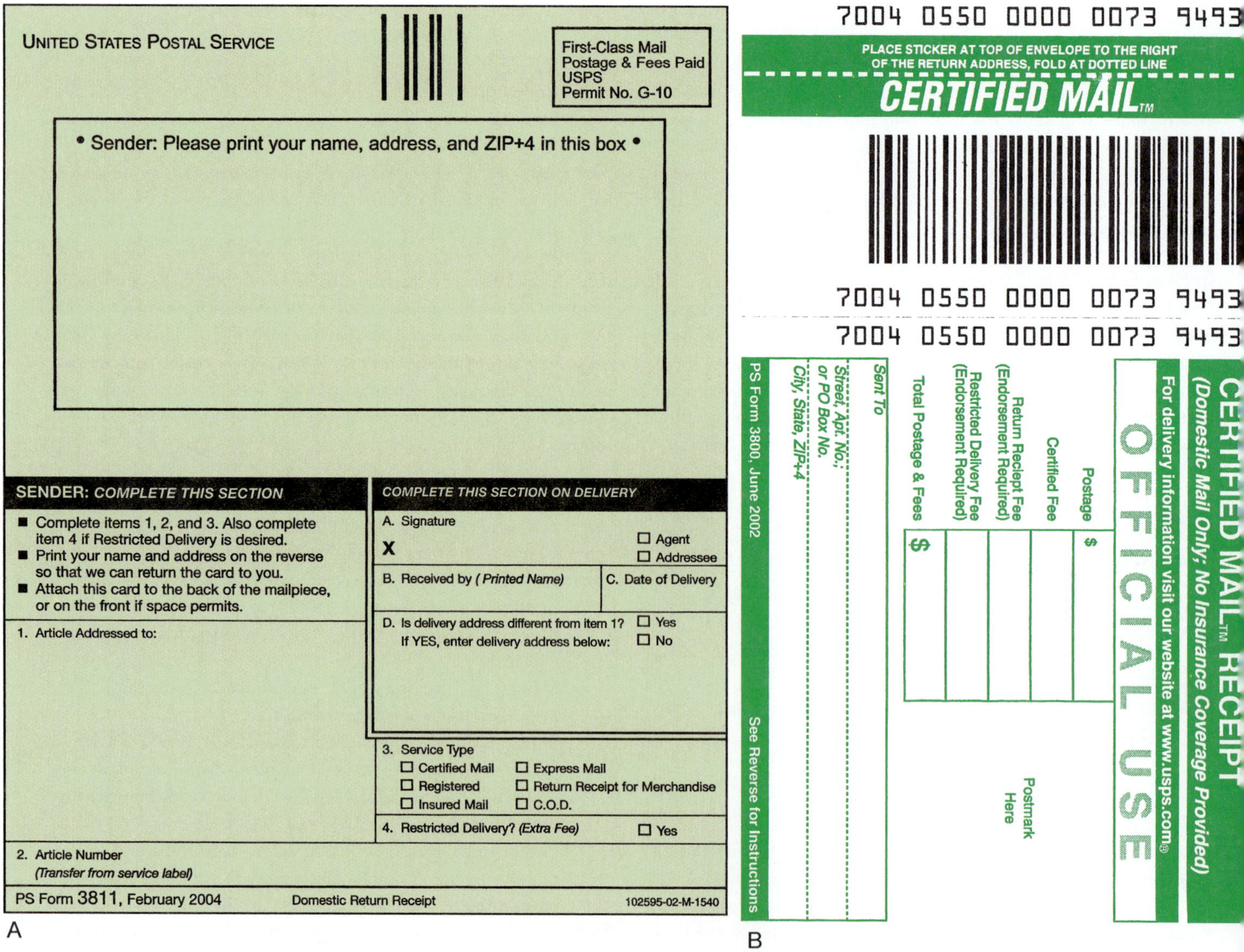

A

B

FIGURE 13-7 A, Delivery receipts for certified mail, registered mail, and insured mail. Attach to the back of the article and endorse the front with the phrase *Return Receipt Requested* adjacent to the article number. **B,** Receipt for certified mail. Attach the bottom portion of the receipt to the top of the envelope, just to the right of the return address.

Registered mail is tracked by number from the time of mailing until the time of delivery and is transported separately from other mail under a special lock. In case of loss or damage, the customer may be reimbursed up to certain limits, provided the value of the registered article was declared at the time of mailing and the appropriate fee was paid.

Postal Money Orders. Postal money orders are a convenient way to mail money, especially for a person who does not have a personal checking account. Domestic money orders may be purchased in amounts as high as $1,000.

Special Delivery. Mail of any class that has been marked *Special Delivery* is charged at the special delivery rate. Such pieces may be regular first- or second-class, registered, insured, or COD pieces. The *Special Delivery* designation generally does not speed up the normal travel time between two cities but does ensure immediate delivery of the item when it arrives at the designated post office.

Special Handling. Third- and fourth-class mail sent by special handling receives the fastest service and ground transportation practicable; about the same as for first-class mail. A special handling fee is charged in addition to the required postage and is determined by weight. This fee does not include insurance or special delivery at the destination; special delivery, if desired, is available at an added cost. If a parcel is sent by priority mail, special handling offers no additional advantage, because the mail already is traveling as quickly as possible.

Certified Mail. Any piece of mail without **intrinsic** value and on which postage is paid at the first-class rate will be accepted as certified mail. Items that should be certified include contracts, deeds, mortgages, bank books, checks, passports, insurance policies, money orders, and birth certificates; these are not themselves valuable but would be difficult to duplicate if lost. Certified mail often is used to aid debt collection.

Regular postage in addition to a certified mail fee must be affixed. For an additional fee, a receipt verifying delivery can be requested (see Figure 13-7, *B*). Certified mail can be sent special delivery if the prescribed fees are paid. A record of delivery of certified mail is kept for 2 years at the post office of delivery; however, no record is kept at the post office of origin. Furthermore, this type of mail does not provide insurance coverage unless it is purchased separately. In most offices, the office manager handles any mail that requires a signature for delivery. The liability for delivered items rests with supervisors or is designated by the office policy manual. The medical assistant should keep a supply of certified mail forms and return receipts on hand. These may be obtained at any post office. Full instructions are included on the forms. Fees and postage may be paid using ordinary postage stamps, meter stamps, or permit imprints. Certified mail can be mailed at any post office, station, or branch or can be deposited in mail drops or in street letter boxes if specific instructions are followed.

Certificate of Mailing. If a sender needs proof of mailing but is not especially concerned with proof of receipt of an item, the most economic method is to obtain a certificate of mailing. Obtain this form at the post office and fill in the required information. Attach a stamp for the current fee and hand the form to the postal clerk along with the piece of mail. The clerk will postmark the receipt, initial it, and hand it back as acknowledgment of having received the piece of mail at the post office. This is sometimes used when mailing tax reports or other items that must be postmarked by a certain date.

Private Delivery Services

Not all mail is delivered by the USPS. Actually, the USPS delivers only about 44% of the mail in the United States. Many private services pick up and deliver mail overnight. Among these are FedEx, United Parcel Service, Emery, Airborne Express, and DHL. These services are highly advertised and competitive. All large cities and many smaller communities have centralized points where packages can be dropped off for the service of the sender's choice. Pickup service also is available in many communities. Most moderately large cities have privately owned **courier** services that transfer mail and packages from place to place; the fees for courier services vary widely and often depend on the delivery times and distances that the items must travel.

CRITICAL THINKING APPLICATION   **13-8**

The office has always used FedEx for sending packages. However, Brandon wonders whether FedEx offers the best rates. How might he gather this information?

■ What should be considered in the choice of a private delivery service?

Handling Special Situations

Forwarding and Obtaining a Changed Address. If a piece of mail is marked *Forwarding Service Requested,* the post office will forward mail to the new address if it is sent within 12 months of the change or if the receiver has left a forwarding order with the post office. At that time, the forwarding order expires unless the receiver requests that it be continued. Between 12 and 18 months, the piece is returned to the sender with the new address noted. After 18 months, mail usually is returned with the reason for nondelivery noted. Forwarding is free when priority or first-class mail is used.

If the mailer wants to know an addressee's new address, this service can be obtained from the post office by placing the words *Address Correction Requested* beneath the return address on the envelope. This can be handwritten, stamped, typed, or printed. The new address is noted on a sticker and returned to the sender; this service has no charge if the item is sent priority or first-class mail. The post office charges a weighted fee for this service for standard mail and packages. If the envelope is marked *Change Service Requested,* the post office disposes of the piece of mail and returns a card to the sender showing the forwarding address of the addressee. If the piece was sent priority or first class, no charge is incurred for the service unless the notification is sent electronically, which involves a small charge.

Recalling Mail. If a letter has been dropped in the mailbox by mistake, do not ask the mail collector to give it to you; he or she is not permitted to do so. However, mail can be recalled by making written application at the post office, together with an envelope addressed identically to the one being recalled. If the letter has already left the local post office, the postmaster, at the sender's expense, can notify the postmaster at the destination post office to return the letter. However, there is no guarantee that the letter will be retrieved.

Returned Mail. If a letter is returned to the sender after an attempt has been made to deliver it, it cannot be mailed again without new postage. It is best simply to prepare a new envelope with the correct address, affix the proper postage, and place it in the mail.

When mail is returned to the medical office, be sure to correct the database, indicating that mail to a certain patient has been returned, so that postage is not wasted sending mail to that address again.

Tracing Lost Mail. Receipts issued by the post office, whether for money orders, registered mail, certified mail, or insured mail, should be retained until receipt of the item has been acknowledged. If no acknowledgment of receipt for such mailing arrives after an adequate interval, notify the post office to trace the letter or package. Regular first-class mail is not easily traced, but the post office makes every attempt to find it. In tracing a lost letter or package, the post office requires that a special form be filled out; information from any original receipt should be written on this form, along with any other identifying information.

USING MAIL MERGE

The *Mail Merge* feature in Microsoft Word is a useful way to create a group of documents that are similar in text but have unique identifying features. For instance, the physician wants to send a letter to all the patients informing them that the office is moving to a new address. However, the physician wants to personalize the letters rather than sending the same one with the greeting, "Dear Patients." *Mail Merge* can help the user create a set of letters, e-mails, and faxes; a set of labels and envelopes; or numbered items, such as tickets or coupons. Many assume that *Mail Merge* is very complicated, but easy-to-follow instructions can be found on the Internet at *www.microsoft.com.*

Closing Comments

Remember that every document sent from the medical office should project a professional image. Use neat handwriting when correspondence is not computer generated. All the office staff must be able to read items written years ago. It is worth the time and effort to brush up on English skills so that writing documents becomes as comfortable as setting an appointment or assisting in a procedure.

Patient Education

Medical offices often use brochures and printed material to educate their patients. It is critical that these materials look professional and reflect a positive image of the physician and the facility. Make sure copied material is clean, has no streaks, and is attractively presented. If the information was written by an office staff member, make sure correct grammar has been used and that several office members proofread the work for errors and proper use of the English language.

Legal and Ethical Issues

Keep copies of all communications leaving the office that relate to patient care. If any information is handwritten, it must be completely legible to the patient. As always, every document containing patient information must be treated as strictly confidential.

SUMMARY OF SCENARIO

Brandon has been a tremendous help to the office staff over the summer months. He has learned about every area of the medical clinic and has mastered several of the office procedures, both clinical and administrative. He has a greater understanding now of the business aspect of the medical office.

His duties as a temporary administrative medical assistant have opened his eyes to the value and importance of administrative personnel. He can easily see that everyone, from the receptionist to the scheduler to the insurance billers, plays a vital role in the smooth operation of the facility.

Toward the end of the summer, the office staff honors Brandon with a going-away party. He announces with a smile that he has decided he wants to become a pediatrician, based on his experience in his father's family practice. He tells the staff he plans to hire them all away from his father! Then, on a serious note, he thanks all the employees for their patience and for their willingness to let him learn from them. Everyone expects Brandon to be a complete success.

Sometimes, working with a member of the physician's family is difficult. Employees should understand that family members often have as much at stake in the success of the practice as the employee. Make every attempt to get along with family members, even if they are less than **amiable**.

Learning proofreader's marks helps the medical assistant work through a document needing revision or simple grammatical corrections much easier and faster. Once learned, the marks are simple to use, and they will be helpful throughout the medical assistant's career.

Every document makes an impression, and that impression can be positive or negative. Each document generated by the medical assistant needs to make a positive impression. Proofread everything, including e-mails and memos, and look for ways the wording can be made more accurate or more fitting to communicate the message. All documents must be professional — each one, each day, every single time — because they reflect on the physician and the medical office.

SUMMARY OF LEARNING OBJECTIVES

1. **Define, spell, and pronounce the terms listed in the vocabulary.**
Spelling and pronouncing medical terms correctly bolster the medical assistant's credibility. Knowing the definition of these terms promotes confidence in communication with patients and co-workers.

2. **Recognize the elements of fundamental writing skills.**
The medical assistant must be able to write general business letters, memos, meeting minutes, and various other documents necessary in the physician's office. The needed skills include spelling, grammar, basic sentence structure, and the parts of speech that make up a complete sentence. These fundamental writing skills apply not only to letters, but also to e-mails, reports, and all other documents.

3. **Explain the various parts of speech.**
The medical assistant should be familiar with the various parts of speech and the way to use them correctly in a sentence. *Nouns* name something, such as a person, place, or thing; *pronouns* are substitutes for nouns. Action *verbs* are words that express movement; linking verbs express a condition, a state of being, or the senses. *Adjectives* usually describe nouns, whereas *adverbs* usually describe verbs. *Prepositions* are connecting words, as are *conjunctions*. *Interjections* show strong feelings and are often followed by an exclamation point.

4. **Name some essential references for the medical assistant's library.**
Developing a personal tool collection that can assist the medical assistant with written communications in the medical office is very helpful. An up-to-date dictionary, a medical dictionary, a composition handbook, an English language reference manual, and a thesaurus are valuable additions to the references library.

5. **Discuss applications of electronic technology in effective communication**
Using electronic technology to communicate allows the medical assistant to complete tasks faster and more efficiently. Letters can be saved and used again by simply changing names and pertinent data. A portfolio of commonly used forms and letters can be stored electronically and used when needed.

6. **List the four common sizes of letterhead stationery.**
Standard (or letter) stationery, which is most commonly used for business purposes, is 8½ × 11 inches. Monarch (or executive) stationery is 8¼ × 10½ inches and is used for informal business correspondence. Baronial stationery is 5½ × 8½ inches, and legal stationery is 8½ × 14 inches.

7. **Discuss the differences in the four letter styles.**
Block is an efficient but less attractive letter style in which all lines begin flush with the left margin of the paper. Modified block is similar, but some lines begin at the center of the page instead of the left margin. Modified block with indented paragraphs is identical to block style, except for the indention of the paragraphs. Simplified letter style has lines that begin flush at the left margin, but other items, such as the salutation and complimentary closing, are omitted.

8. **Explain the four standard parts of a business letter.**
The four standard parts of a business letter are (1) the heading, (2) the opening, (3) the body, and (4) the closing. The heading includes the letterhead and dateline, and the opening includes the inside address and any attention or salutation line. The body is the message of the document, and the closing includes the signature, complimentary closing, reference initials, and special notations.

9. **Discuss the process of developing and the value of keeping a communications portfolio.**
Subsequent letters are much easier to draft if the medical assistant develops a portfolio that contains sample letters and other types of communications. Once a letter has been written, it can be saved on the computer hard drive, a CD, or a flash drive, or it can be printed and placed in a binder for easy viewing. If the letter is kept in a binder, the file name under which it is saved on the computer should be noted on each example so that the document can be easily found again. This is an excellent way to save time in the busy medical office.

10. **Discuss how to open, sort, and annotate incoming mail.**
Mail is one of the most common types of communication used in the physician's office and is handled according to the preferences of the physician, office manager, or office policy manual specifications The process for responding to and initiating written correspondence is outlined in Procedure 13-4.

11. **Explain how to save money when mailing.**
The medical assistant should consult the post office when mailing, checking for better rates, and using ZIP codes.

12. **Describe how to compose, proofread, and mail a business letter.**
Business letters must look professional and have sentences that are grammatically correct. The process for proofreading a business letter or publication for accuracy is outlined in Procedure 13-1.

13. **Organize technical information and summaries.**
Most written documents include the four standard parts of a basic business letter or memo — the heading, opening, body, and closing. If a list of questions is to be answered, address them in the same order as presented. When responding to any review of information, present it in the order that it was given. Follow office policies and procedures when organizing technical information and/or summaries.

14. **Describe the proper way to send a fax.**
Transmissions sent by fax must arrive at their destination in a confidential manner. The process for preparing a fax for transmission should be outlined in every office policy and procedure manual. Simply enter the phone number into the machine and place the document in the letter tray. If faxing from the computer, click on the fax icon and enter the number, then designate the document to send. Most fax machines provide a sender's receipt once the document has reached its destination.

15. **Explain how to process incoming mail.**

Most physicians' offices have a process for dealing with mail and other types of information that arrives at the facility. Fax transmissions are covered in Procedure 13-3, while the method for receiving, organizing, prioritizing, and transmitting information, including mail, is outlined in Procedure 13-4.

16. **Explain how to address an envelope according to the U.S. Postal Service's optical character reader guidelines.**

Addresses should be written in such a way that they are quickly and efficiently read by postal service machines. The process for addressing an envelope according to the Postal Service's optical character reader guidelines is outlined in Procedure 13-5.

CONNECTIONS

Study Guide Connection: Go to the Chapter 13 Study Guide. Read and complete the activities.

Evolve Connection: Go to the Chapter 13 link at *evolve.elsevier.com/kinn* to complete the Chapter Review and Chapter Quiz. Check out the other resources listed for this chapter to make the most of what you have learned from Written Communications and Mail Processing.

14

THE PAPER MEDICAL RECORD

SCENARIO

Susan Beezler has just begun her career in the medical assisting profession. She is attending medical assisting school in the morning and works part-time for a family practitioner in the afternoons as a clerical record assistant. Susan is eager to learn about medicine and looks forward to taking on more responsibility at the office.

The practice is growing swiftly and recently added a new physician, Dr. Alex Thomas. Dr. Thomas has enjoyed working with Susan and feels that her energy will be just what his patients need. He has taken a professional interest in Susan and often lets her assist him with patients when her other duties allow.

Susan knows that although she is a beginner in the office, she will gain trust from her supervisors and patients as long as she projects a teachable attitude. The office has not yet converted to an electronic records system, so

Susan uses the information she learned in school about paper medical records. She cheerfully performs filing and even does some transcription for Dr. Thomas. The other staff members are pleased with her willingness to perform the most mundane tasks.

Susan enjoys sharing her experiences with her classmates. She is the only one currently working in the medical field, and the other students ask her lots of questions about the "real world" of medicine. She is very careful not to breach patient confidentiality; she discusses situations only in general, never mentioning any patients' names.

Susan feels a great sense of pride that she is already a member of the healthcare team and able to contribute to the lives of her patients.

While studying this chapter, think about the following questions:

- How can the medical assistant earn the patient's trust so that the person is comfortable revealing the very private information required by a health history?
- Why is the simple task of filing such a critical duty in the physician's office?

- How can filing, often considered boring, be made more enjoyable?
- Why is it important that the medical record be legible?

LEARNING OBJECTIVES

1. Define, spell, and pronounce the terms listed in the vocabulary.
2. State several reasons accurate medical records are important.
3. Explain who owns the medical record.
4. Explain how to document appropriately and accurately.
5. Explain the difference between a traditional medical record and a problem-oriented medical record.
6. Explain how to establish and organize a patient's medical record.
7. Identify systems for organizing medical records.

8. Differentiate between subjective and objective information.
9. Describe various types of information kept in the medical record.
10. Explain how to make additions to a medical record.
11. Discuss correction of an entry in the patient's record.
12. Identify both equipment and supplies needed to file medical records.
13. Discuss filing procedures.
14. Describe indexing rules.
15. Discuss the pros and cons of various filing methods.
16. Identify types of records common to the healthcare setting.

VOCABULARY

alphabetic filing Any system that arranges names or topics according to the sequence of the letters in the alphabet.

alphanumeric Of or relating to systems made up of combinations of letters and numbers.

audit A formal examination of an organization's or individual's accounts or financial situation; a methodic examination and review.

augment To make greater, more numerous, larger, or more intense.

caption A heading, title, or subtitle under which records are filed.

chronologic order Of, relating to, or arranged in or according to the order of time.

continuity of care Continuation of care smoothly from one provider to another, so that the patient receives the most benefit and no interruption in care.

dictation (dik-tay'-shun) The act or manner of uttering words to be transcribed.

direct filing system A filing system in which materials can be located without consulting an intermediary source of reference.

gleaned Gathered bit by bit (e.g., information or material); picked over in search of relevant material.

indirect filing system A filing system in which an intermediary source of reference (e.g., a card file) must be consulted to locate specific files.

microfilm A film with a photographic record of printed or other graphic matter on a reduced scale.

numeric filing The filing of records, correspondence, or cards by number.

objective information Information gathered by watching or observing a patient.

obliteration (uh-bli-tuh-ra'-shun) The act of making undecipherable or imperceptible by obscuring or wearing away.

OUTfolder A folder used to provide space for the temporary filing of materials.

OUTguide A heavy guide used to replace a folder temporarily removed from the filing space.

power of attorney A legal instrument authorizing a person to act as the attorney or agent of the grantor.

pressboard A strong, highly glazed composition board resembling vulcanized fiber; heavy card stock.

procrastination (pruh-kras-tuh-na'-shun) Intentional postponement of doing something that should be done.

provisional diagnosis A temporary diagnosis made before all test results have been received.

purging The process of moving active files to inactive status.

quality control An aggregate of activities designed to ensure adequate quality, especially in manufactured products or in the service industries.

requisites (re'-kwuh-zuhts) Entities considered essential or necessary.

retention schedule A method or plan for retaining or keeping medical records and for their movement from active, to inactive, to closed filing.

reverse chronologic order Arranged in order so that the most recent item is on top and older items are filed further back.

shingling A method of filing in which a report is laid on top of the older report, resembling the shingles of a roof.

subjective information Information gained by questioning the patient or taking it from a form.

tickler file A chronologic file used as a reminder that something must be dealt with on a certain date.

transcription A written copy of something made either in longhand or by machine.

vested Granted or endowed with a particular authority, right, or property; to have a special interest in.

A medical records management system is only as good as the ease of retrieval of the data in the files. A fast pace is the norm in the medical office; therefore, staff members must be able to find patients' medical records quickly, and the records must be functional so that the needed information can be obtained easily.

Few things are more frustrating to the patient than being told, "We cannot locate your records." Patients have every right to question the competence of the medical care they are receiving if the office has problems simply finding a chart. Organization and adherence to set routines help ensure that medical records are accessible when needed.

In today's medical facilities, records are either paper based or computer based. The versatile medical assistant is knowledgeable about both systems and able to perform well with either.

THE IMPORTANCE OF ACCURATE MEDICAL RECORDS

Medical records are kept for four basic reasons. First, the medical record helps the physician provide the best possible medical care for the patient. The physician examines the patient and enters the findings in the patient's medical record. These findings are clues to the diagnosis. The physician may order many types of tests to confirm or **augment** the clinical findings. As the reports of these tests come in, the findings fall into place, much like the pieces of a jigsaw puzzle. Then, with the confirmation data to support the diagnosis, the physician can prescribe treatment and form an opinion about the patient's chances of recovery, assured that every resource has been used to arrive at a correct judgment. The medical record provides a complete history of all the care given to the patient.

The medical record also provides critical information for others. By reading through the record and discovering the methods used to treat the patient, healthcare professionals can provide **continuity of care**. Each person knows what the patient has experienced and can provide continuous care, even from one facility to another. For example, when a patient is transferred from a hospital to a skilled nursing facility, the information from the patient's hospital record helps the nursing facility staff to better care for the patient. When patients move from place to place or caregivers change, copies of the pertinent information should move with the patient to provide this continuity of care.

Second, medical records are kept as legal protection for those who provided care to the patient. A documented medical record is excellent proof that certain procedures were performed or that medical advice was given. An accurate record is the foundation for a legal defense in cases of medical professional liability. This is one reason writing legibly in the record and documenting exactly what happened to the patient, in addition to the provider's response, are critical. Remember: If it isn't charted, it didn't happen (Procedure 14-1).

Third, medical records provide statistical information that is helpful to researchers. The patient's record provides information about medications taken and the reactions to them. Medical records may be used to evaluate the effectiveness of certain kinds of treatment or to determine the incidence of a given disease. Physicians often take part in drug studies that track adverse reactions and side effects. The effects of various treatments and procedures also can be tracked and statistics **gleaned** from the information gathered from patients' records. Correlation of such statistical information may result in a new outlook on some phases of medicine and can lead to revised techniques and treatments. The statistical data from medical records also are valuable in the preparation of scientific papers, books, and lectures.

Fourth, medical records are vital for financial reimbursement. The information in the medical record supports claims for reimbursement and is required by most third-party payers.

OWNERSHIP OF THE MEDICAL RECORD

Who owns the medical record? Patients often assume that because the information in the medical record is about them, ownership of the record rightfully is theirs. However, the owner of the physical medical record is the physician or medical facility, often called the "maker," that initiated and developed the record. The patient has the right of access to the information within the record but does not own the physical chart or other documents pertaining to the record. The patient has a **vested** interest and therefore has the right to demand confidentiality of all information placed in the chart.

The actual medical record should never leave the medical facility where it originated. Even the physician should refrain from taking the record from the office to the hospital or nursing facility. If information from the record is needed, copies can be placed in a file, and progress notes can be written on site and inserted into the original record later. Patients' records should be kept in a locked room or locked filing cabinets when the office is closed.

Written medical records must be legible. Each record should be written as if the physician and staff expect it to eventually be involved in a lawsuit; therefore, every word must be legible to an average reader years after written. The record can help the physician prove that he or she treated a patient in a competent manner, or it can prove that the patient was not given competent care. Every person

---

PROCEDURE 14-1

Document Patient Care Accurately

GOAL: *To document appropriately and accurately on all medical records and other office paperwork that concerns the patient.*

EQUIPMENT and SUPPLIES

- Any medical document
- Clerical supplies
- Computer
- Office policy and procedures manual
- Progress notes

PROCEDURAL STEPS

1. Determine the information that needs to be added to the patient's medical record, appointment book, telephone message, or other office paperwork that concerns the patient.
   <u>PURPOSE:</u> To place pertinent, accurate information into the document or medical record.
2. Make sure the information is factual, timely, and accurate.
   <u>PURPOSE:</u> To ensure that the information is usable.
3. Write or type the information into the document.
4. Reread the information to make sure it is legible and makes grammatical sense.
   <u>PURPOSE:</u> To make certain that anyone who needs to access the information will be able to read it, even after several years.
5. Date and sign the entry, if necessary.
   <u>PURPOSE:</u> To authenticate the entry.

6. Make sure the entry meets any local, state, or federal guidelines that may apply to the information in the document.
   <u>PURPOSE:</u> To comply with local, state, and federal rules and regulations.
7. Make sure the entry is written so as to comply with office policies and procedures.
   <u>PURPOSE:</u> To meet the requirements of the facility's own office policy and procedures manual.
8. If the entry needs to be corrected, draw one line through it and make the new entry above it or directly after the information that needs to be corrected.
   <u>PURPOSE:</u> To correct the document according to the office policy and procedures guidelines.
9. Date and initial the corrected entry.
   <u>PURPOSE:</u> To authenticate the correction.
10. Make sure the correction has not obliterated any part of the medical record or documentation that affects the patient.
    <u>PURPOSE:</u> To comply with the rule that no obliteration is acceptable in any part of the medical record.
11. File the medical record in its proper place according to the facility's filing system.
    <u>PURPOSE:</u> To ensure that the medical record can be easily retrieved.

on staff at the physician's office is responsible for writing legibly in every medical record.

CREATING AN EFFICIENT MEDICAL RECORDS MANAGEMENT SYSTEM

The medical records management system should provide an easy method of retrieving information. The files should be organized in an orderly fashion The information also must be accurate, and corrections should be made and documented properly. The wording in the record should be easily understood and grammatically correct. An efficient method of adding documents to the chart must be established so that the physician or other provider always has the most up-to-date information.

Above all, the medical records management system must work for the individual facility.

Types of Records

The two major types of patient records are the paper medical record and the electronic medical record. As computer technology advances, the paper medical record seems more and more inefficient. It is difficult to use a paper-based record for multiple purposes. In most cases, only one person at a time can use the paper record. Misfiled information is common, and the entire record also can be misfiled. Data cannot be accessed easily for research and **quality control**, and in facilities with multiple departments, the information is difficult to share. The paper-based record is good evidence of patient care, but it is not nearly as useful in other capacities.

The electronic medical record (also called the *electronic health record*) is much more efficient than the paper record. Chapter 15 covers the electronic medical record in more detail.

ORGANIZATION OF THE MEDICAL RECORD

Source-Oriented Records

The traditional patient record is source oriented; that is, observations and data are cataloged according to their source—physician, laboratory, radiology department, nurse, technician—with no recording of a logical relationship among them. Forms and progress notes are filed in **reverse chronologic order** (most recent on top) and in separate sections of the record according to the type of form or service rendered (e.g., all laboratory reports together, all x-ray reports together, and so on). Some files are placed in **chronologic order**; that is, the items inside are filed according to the order of time. However, most patient files are in reverse chronologic order so that the physician and staff members do not have to search to the bottom of the chart to find a recent lab report on a test.

Problem-Oriented Medical Records

The problem-oriented medical record (POMR) is a departure from the traditional system of keeping patient records. It sometimes is referred to as the Weed system, because it was originated by Dr. Lawrence L. Weed, a professor of medicine at the University of Vermont College of Medicine.

The POMR is a record of clinical practice that divides medical action into four bases:

- The *database,* which includes the chief complaint, present illness, patient profile, review of systems, physical examination, and laboratory reports.
- The *problem list,* a numbered, titled list of every problem the patient has that requires management or workup. This may include social and demographic troubles in addition to strictly medical or surgical ones.
- The *treatment plan* includes management, additional workups needed, and therapy. Each plan is titled and numbered with respect to the problem.
- The *progress notes* include structured notes that are numbered to correspond with each problem number.

Several companies have developed file folders for organizing patient data according to the POMR (Figure 14-1). The problem list is entered on the divider cover for laboratory reports. Special sections are provided for current major and chronic problems and for inactive major or chronic problems. The divider cover for progress notes is a chart for listing medications and other therapeutic modalities. Progress notes follow the SOAP approach. SOAP is an acronym for the following:

- *S*ubjective impressions
- *O*bjective clinical evidence
- *A*ssessment or diagnosis
- *P*lans for further studies, treatment, or management

Some medical offices also use an *E* in the record to represent evaluation; others include *E* for education and *R* for response. The education notation documents that the patient was educated about his or her condition or given a patient information sheet. The response section is used to record an assessment of the patient's understanding of and possible compliance with the treatment plan.

The POMR has the advantage of imposing order and organization on the information added to a patient's medical record. The records are more easily reviewed, and the likelihood of overlooking a problem is greatly reduced. The SOAP method forces a rational approach to the patient's problems and assists the formulation of a logical, orderly plan of patient care (Figure 14-2). The POMR has continued to grow in popularity since its introduction in the 1970s. It is especially advantageous in clinics, group practices, and hospitals,

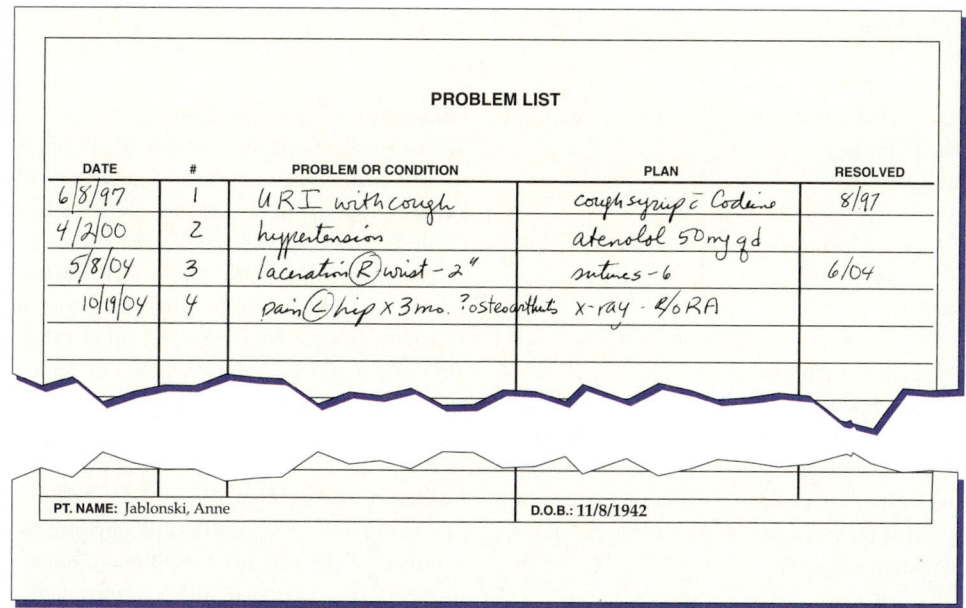

PROBLEM LIST

DATE	#	PROBLEM OR CONDITION	PLAN	RESOLVED
6/8/97	1	URI with cough	cough syrup c̄ Codeine	8/97
4/2/00	2	hypertension	atenolol 50 mg qd	
5/8/04	3	laceration (R) wrist - 2"	sutures - 6	6/04
10/19/04	4	pain (L) hip X 3 mo. ? osteoarthritis	x-ray - R/o RA	

PT. NAME: Jablonski, Anne   **D.O.B.:** 11/8/1942

FIGURE 14-1 A chart designed for a problem-oriented medical record (POMR). Some charts are specifically adapted to the POMR. (Courtesy Bibbero Systems, Petaluma, Calif.)

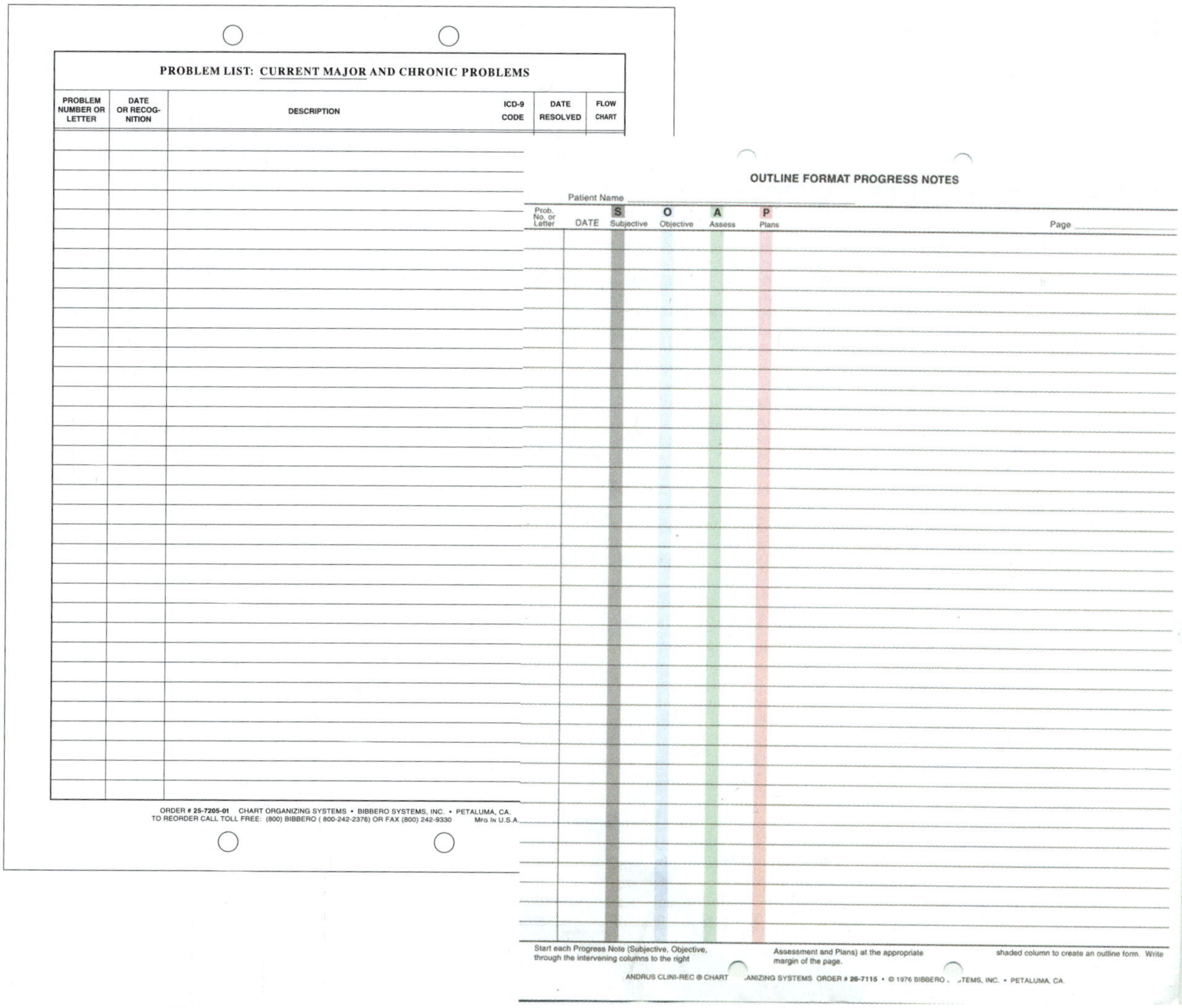

PROBLEM LIST: CURRENT MAJOR AND CHRONIC PROBLEMS

PROBLEM NUMBER OR LETTER	DATE OR RECOGNITION	DESCRIPTION	ICD-9 CODE	DATE RESOLVED	FLOW CHART

ORDER # 25-7205-01   CHART ORGANIZING SYSTEMS • BIBBERO SYSTEMS, INC. • PETALUMA, CA.
TO REORDER CALL TOLL FREE: (800) BIBBERO (800-242-2376) OR FAX (800) 242-9330   Mfrd. In U.S.A.

OUTLINE FORMAT PROGRESS NOTES

Patient Name

Prob. No. or Letter	DATE	**S** Subjective	**O** Objective	**A** Assess	**P** Plans	Page

Start each Progress Note (Subjective, Objective, Assessment and Plans) at the appropriate   shaded column to create an outline form. Write through the intervening columns to the right   margin of the page.

ANDRUS CLINI-REC ® CHART   ORGANIZING SYSTEMS ORDER # 26-7115 • © 1976 BIBBERO   STEMS, INC. • PETALUMA, CA

FIGURE 14-2 SOAP progress notes. The SOAP method keeps information organized and in a logical sequence. An actual progress note would include the physician's signature or initials after this entry. (Courtesy Bibbero Systems, Petaluma, Calif.)

where more than one person must be able to find essential information in the chart. Note that the SOAP method often is used in the POMR.

Some facilities use the CHEDDAR method in medical records. CHEDDAR signifies the following:

C—Chief complaint

H—History

E—Examination

D—Details (of problem and complaints)

D—Drugs and dosages

A—Assessment

R—Return visit information, if applicable

The physician decides which recording method he or she prefers, and the medical assistant must conform to that standard. The office policy and procedures manual provides specific instruction, if the standard used is different from one the medical assistant has used in the past. Never hesitate to ask the physician if you are unclear about any part of the documentation standard.

CRITICAL THINKING APPLICATION   14-3

Dr. Thomas wants Susan to thoroughly understand the SOAP method of charting, but she is more comfortable with the CHEDDAR method.

- How does the SOAP method differ from the CHEDDAR method?
- What are the pros and cons of each method?
- How can Susan adjust quickly to the new standard?

CONTENTS OF THE COMPLETE CASE HISTORY

The medical case history is the most important record in a physician's practice. For completeness, each patient's record should contain **subjective information** provided by the patient and **objective information** provided by the physician. If all entries are completed, the case history will stand the test of time. No branch of medicine is exempt from the need to keep patient history records.

Subjective Information

Personal Demographics

The patient's case history begins with routine personal data, which the patient usually supplies on the first visit when the medical record is established (Procedure 14-2). Most patients are required to complete a patient information form (Figure 14-3). The basic facts needed are:

- Patient's full name, spelled correctly
- Names of parents if the patient is a child
- Patient's gender
- Date of birth
- Marital status
- Name of spouse if married
- Number of children if any
- Home address, telephone number, and e-mail address
- Occupation
- Name of employer
- Business address and telephone number
- Employment information for spouse
- Healthcare insurance information

- Source of referral
- Social Security number

Personal and Medical History

The personal and medical history, which often is obtained by having the patient complete a questionnaire, provides information about any past illnesses or surgery the patient has had and about injuries or physical defects, whether congenital or acquired (Figure 14-4). It also includes information about the patient's daily health habits. Stickers can be used on the front of the medical record to indicate allergies, advance directives, and other information (Figure 14-5). These are useful for helping the health professional keep important facts about the patient in the forefront of the mind while treating the individual.

Patient's Family History

The family history comprises the physical condition of the various members of the patient's family, any illnesses or diseases individual members may have had, and a record of the causes of death. This information is important, because certain diseases may have a hereditary pattern. Most physicians are interested in the immediate family: children, parents, grandparents, and siblings.

Patient's Social History

The social history includes information about the patient's lifestyle. If the patient drinks, how many drinks per day or per week are consumed? If the patient smokes cigarettes, how many packs a day are smoked? Drug use and even marital information can be considered part of the social history.

CRITICAL THINKING APPLICATION   14-4

While taking a patient's medical history, Susan asks about his social history. She asks whether he drinks alcohol. The patient immediately becomes defensive and accuses Susan of getting too personal about his affairs.

- How might Susan explain her reasons for asking these questions? What options are available if the patient refuses to discuss his social history with Susan?
- Could this opposition to questions about the social history raise suspicion in Susan's mind? What might she suspect?

Patient's Chief Complaint

The patient's chief complaint is a concise account of the patient's symptoms, explained in the patient's own words. It should include the following:

- The nature and duration of pain, if any
- When the patient first noticed the symptoms
- The patient's opinion about the possible causes of the problem
- Remedies the patient may have applied before seeing the physician
- Whether the patient has had the same or a similar condition in the past
- Other medical treatment received for the same condition in the past

PROCEDURE 14-2

Organize a New Patient's Medical Record

GOAL: *To create a medical file for a new patient that will contain all the personal data necessary for a complete record and any other information required by the facility.*

EQUIPMENT and SUPPLIES

- Computer
- Clerical supplies (pen, clipboard)
- Registration form
- File folder
- Color-coded labels for folder
- Index label for folder tab
- Identification (ID) card (if using numeric system)
- Cross-reference card, if needed
- Financial ledger, if needed
- Routing slip
- Private conference area

PROCEDURAL STEPS

1. Determine that the patient is new to the office.
2. Obtain and record the required personal data.
   PURPOSE: To gather complete information for credit and insurance claim processing.
3. Write the information on the patient history form.
4. Review the entire form.
   PURPOSE: To make sure the information is complete and correct.
5. Select a label and folder for the record.
   PURPOSE: To choose the appropriate color for the patient's name if color coding is used.

6. Type the caption on the label and apply it to the folder.
   PURPOSE: To use the patient's name for alphabetic filing or an appropriate number for numeric filing.
7. For a numeric filing system, prepare a cross-reference card and a patient ID number.
   PURPOSE: To use numeric filing correctly. It is an indirect system that requires a cross-reference to a patient's name for locating the chart. The patient uses the number on the ID card when arranging appointments or making inquiries.
8. Prepare the financial card or put the patient's name in the computerized ledger.
9. Put the patient history form and all other forms required by the agency into the prepared folder as specified in the office policy and procedures manual.
10. Make a copy of the patient's health insurance identification card and driver's license.
    PURPOSE: To make a record of health insurance coverage and to keep the phone number and claims address on hand. The driver's license identifies the patient and ensures that the right person is receiving healthcare benefits.
11. Clip an encounter form on the outside of the patient's folder.

Most medical facilities use a pain scale to determine the severity of the patient's discomfort. The medical assistant might ask, "How bad is your pain on a scale of 1 to 10, with 1 being almost no pain, and 10 being the worst pain you've ever experienced?" The pain scale or wording used in individual facilities should be documented in the office policy and procedures manual and followed by the medical assistant.

Objective Information

Objective findings, sometimes referred to as *signs,* become evident from the physician's examination of the patient. These findings can be observed and measured.

Physical Examination Findings and Laboratory and Radiology Reports

After the physician has examined the patient, the physical findings are recorded in the history. The results of other tests or requests for these tests are then recorded or, if they appear on separate sheets, are attached to the history.

Diagnosis

Based on all the evidence provided in the patient's past history, the physician's examination, and any supplementary tests, the physician notes his or her diagnosis of the patient's condition in the medical record. If some doubt remains, this may be labeled a **provisional diagnosis**. A *differential diagnosis* is the process of weighing the probability of one disease causing the patient's illness against the probability that other diseases are causative. For example, the differential diagnosis of rhinitis, or a runny nose, could indicate allergic rhinitis (hay fever), the common cold, or even abuse of drugs or nasal decongestants.

Treatment Prescribed and Progress Notes

The physician's suggested treatment is listed after the diagnosis. Generally, instructions to the patient to return for follow-up treatment within a specific period also are noted here. If surgery or other treatment is needed, the patient must sign a consent form (Procedure 14-3).

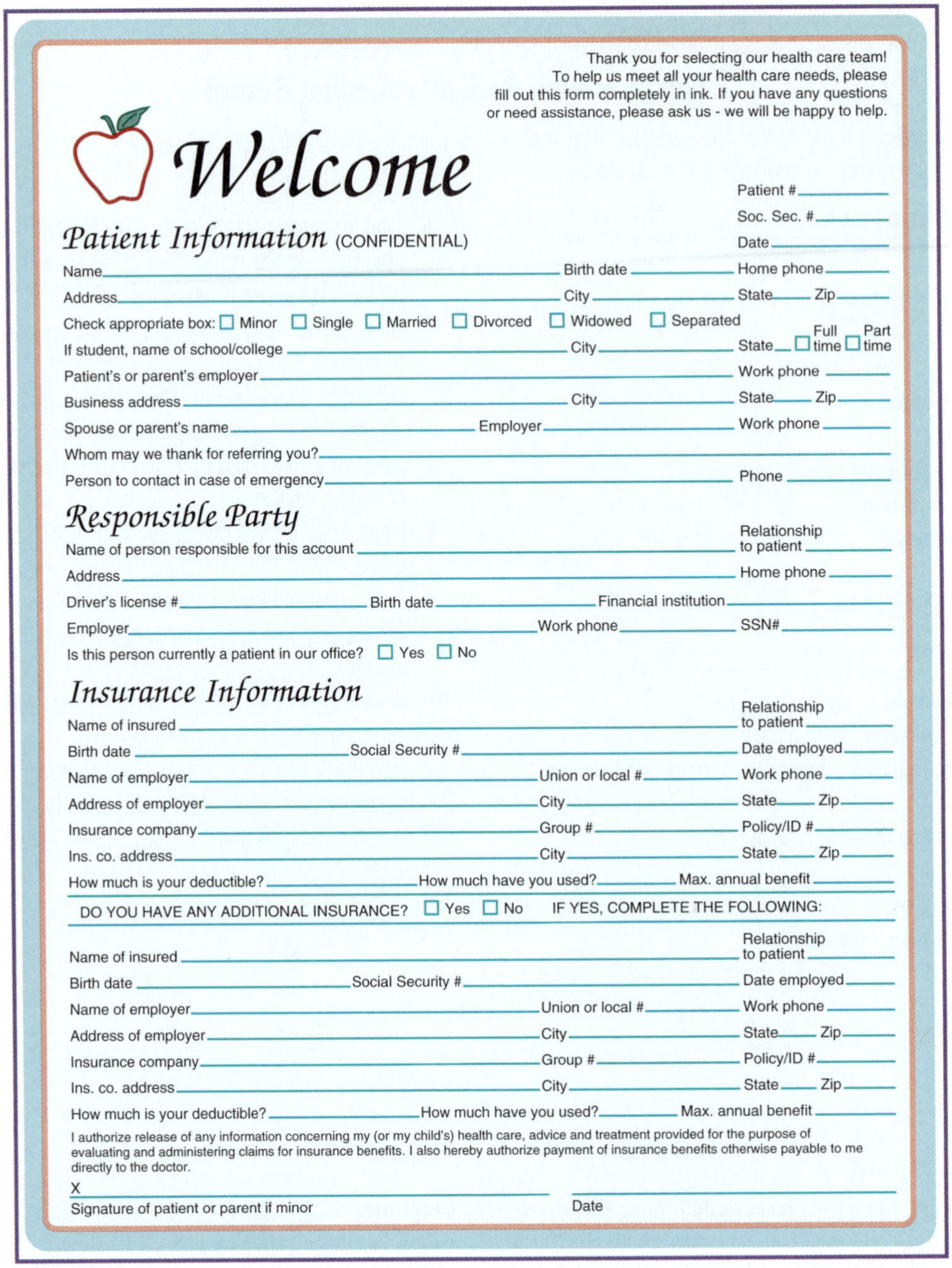

Thank you for selecting our health care team!
To help us meet all your health care needs, please
fill out this form completely in ink. If you have any questions
or need assistance, please ask us - we will be happy to help.

Welcome

Patient Information (CONFIDENTIAL)

Patient #_____
Soc. Sec. #_____
Date_____

Name_____ Birth date_____ Home phone_____
Address_____ City_____ State_____ Zip_____
Check appropriate box: ☐ Minor ☐ Single ☐ Married ☐ Divorced ☐ Widowed ☐ Separated
                                                                            Full ☐ time   Part ☐ time
If student, name of school/college_____ City_____ State_____
Patient's or parent's employer_____ Work phone_____
Business address_____ City_____ State_____ Zip_____
Spouse or parent's name_____ Employer_____ Work phone_____
Whom may we thank for referring you?_____
Person to contact in case of emergency_____ Phone_____

Responsible Party

Name of person responsible for this account_____ Relationship to patient_____
Address_____ Home phone_____
Driver's license #_____ Birth date_____ Financial institution_____
Employer_____ Work phone_____ SSN#_____
Is this person currently a patient in our office? ☐ Yes ☐ No

Insurance Information

Name of insured_____ Relationship to patient_____
Birth date_____ Social Security #_____ Date employed_____
Name of employer_____ Union or local #_____ Work phone_____
Address of employer_____ City_____ State_____ Zip_____
Insurance company_____ Group #_____ Policy/ID #_____
Ins. co. address_____ City_____ State_____ Zip_____
How much is your deductible?_____ How much have you used?_____ Max. annual benefit_____

DO YOU HAVE ANY ADDITIONAL INSURANCE? ☐ Yes ☐ No   IF YES, COMPLETE THE FOLLOWING:

Name of insured_____ Relationship to patient_____
Birth date_____ Social Security #_____ Date employed_____
Name of employer_____ Union or local #_____ Work phone_____
Address of employer_____ City_____ State_____ Zip_____
Insurance company_____ Group #_____ Policy/ID #_____
Ins. co. address_____ City_____ State_____ Zip_____
How much is your deductible?_____ How much have you used?_____ Max. annual benefit_____

I authorize release of any information concerning my (or my child's) health care, advice and treatment provided for the purpose of
evaluating and administering claims for insurance benefits. I also hereby authorize payment of insurance benefits otherwise payable to me
directly to the doctor.

X_____
Signature of patient or parent if minor   Date

FIGURE 14-3 The patient information form provides all the information the medical assistant needs to construct the patient's chart.

On each subsequent visit, the date must be entered on the chart, and information about the patient's condition and the results of treatment, based on the physician's observations, must be added to the history. Notations of all medications prescribed or instructions given, and the patient's own progress report, should be placed in the record. Any home visits are noted. If the patient is hospitalized, the name of the hospital, the reason for admission, and the dates of admission and discharge are recorded. Much of this information can be obtained from the hospital discharge summary.

Condition at the Time of Termination of Treatment

When the treatment is terminated, the physician records that information. For example: *August 18, 2013. Wound completely healed. Patient discharged.*

Obtaining the History

The medical assistant usually collects the routine personal data. The personal and medical history and the patient's family history may be obtained by asking the patient to complete a questionnaire, with the physician augmenting the information provided during the patient interview.

The Medical Assistant's Role

When the medical assistant is responsible for recording the patient's history, care must be taken to ensure that the patient's answers are not heard by others in the reception room. If privacy is not possible, the patient should be given a form to fill out, and the information should be transferred to the permanent record later. When privacy is available, the medical assistant may ask the patient questions and

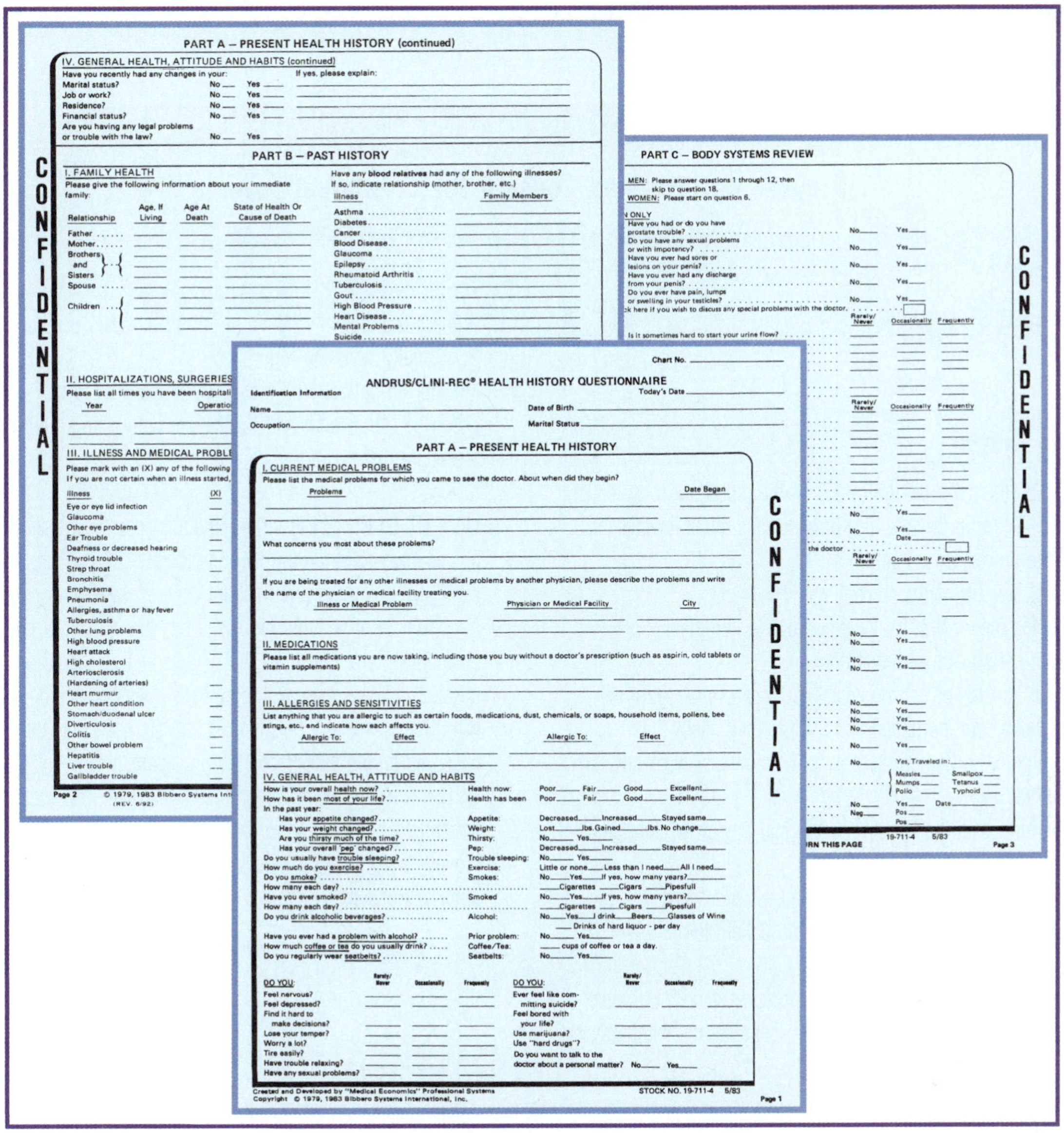

FIGURE 14-4 Database self-administered general health history questionnaire. Lengthy questionnaires should be completed by the patient before the individual is seen by the physician. Either mail the information to the patient in advance or ask the patient to come in early to complete the paperwork. (Courtesy Bibbero Systems, Petaluma, Calif.)

A
ALLERGIC: _____

B
CO-PAY
_____

C
ADVANCE DIRECTIVES
____ Durable Power of Attorney for Healthcare
____ Living Will
____ Healthcare Surrogate

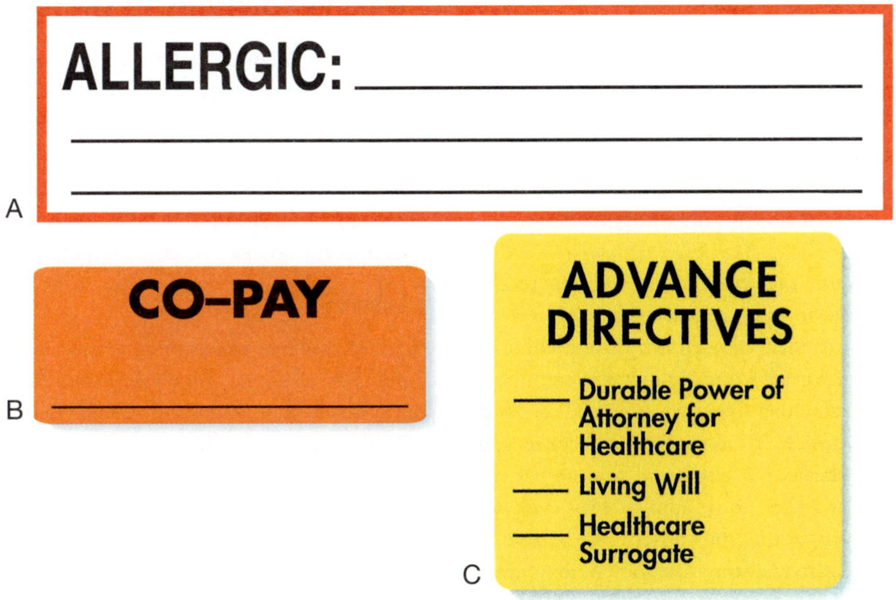

FIGURE 14-5 Chart stickers. Information on stickers on the outside of the chart allows the physician and medical staff to see important information about the patient quickly. (Courtesy Bibbero Systems, Petaluma, Calif.)

PROCEDURE 14-3

Prepare an Informed Consent for Treatment Form

GOAL: *To inform the patient adequately and completely about the treatment or procedure he or she is to receive and to provide legal protection for the facility and the provider.*

EQUIPMENT and SUPPLIES

- Pen
- Consent form

PROCEDURAL STEPS

1. After the physician has provided the details of the procedure to be done, prepare the consent form. Be sure the form includes the following:
   - Nature of the procedure or treatment
   - Risks and/or benefits of the procedure or treatment
   - Any reasonable alternatives to the procedure or treatment
   - Risks and/or benefits of each alternative
   - Risks and/or benefits of not receiving the procedure or treatment

   PURPOSE: To make sure the patient is fully informed about the procedure or treatment and the risks and/or benefits of having and not having it performed.

2. Personalize the form with the patient's name and any other demographic information the form lists.
   PURPOSE: To correctly identify the patient and the procedure.

3. Deliver the form to the physician for use as the patient is counseled about the procedure.
   PURPOSE: To prevent charges of practicing medicine without a license. The physician should explain procedures, risks, benefits, and alternatives and answer all the patient's questions.

4. Witness the patient's signature on the form, if necessary. The physician also usually signs the form.

5. Provide the patient with a copy of the consent form.
   PURPOSE: To ensure that the patient is fully informed about the procedure and has a copy of the information for his or her personal records.

6. Place the consent form in the patient's chart. The facility where the procedure is to be performed may require a copy.
   PURPOSE: To keep a permanent copy of the signed consent form.

7. Ask the patient whether he or she has any questions about the procedure. Refer questions that you cannot or should not answer to the physician. Make sure all the patient's questions are answered.
   PURPOSE: To make sure the patient has been fully informed by the physician before undergoing the procedure.
   NOTE: The medical assistant does not explain the consent form to the patient; this is the physician's responsibility.

8. Provide the patient with the date and time of the procedure and any other instructions required.

---

write or type the answers directly into the record. This method offers an opportunity to become better acquainted with the patient while completing the necessary records. If new patients must complete a lengthy questionnaire, the questionnaire may be mailed to the patient with a request that it be completed and returned to the physician before the appointment. If the record is to be computerized, requesting the information ahead of time gives the office staff the opportunity to transfer information to the computer before the new patient's visit.

The patient's chief complaint may have been indicated to the medical assistant, but the physician will question the patient in more detail. Many practitioners write their own entries on the chart in longhand. Some may type the findings directly into the computer. Others may dictate the material, either directly to the medical assistant or by using a recording device. If the material is dictated and typed, the physician should check each entry and then initial the entry to verify its accuracy. For a chart to be admissible as evidence in court, the person dictating or writing the entries must be able to attest that they were true and correct at the time they were written. The best indication of this is the physician's signature or initials on the typed entry.

MAKING ADDITIONS TO THE PATIENT'S RECORD

As long as a patient is under the physician's care, the medical history is building. Each laboratory report, radiology report, and progress note is added to the record, with the latest information always on top (Procedure 14-4). Although each item is important, the most recent usually is most significant to the patient's care. Again, the physician should read and initial each of these reports before it is placed in the record.

Laboratory Reports

Paper of different colors often is used for reporting different procedures. For example, urinalysis report forms may be yellow, blood count forms pink, and so on. When laboratory slips are smaller than the history form, they should be placed on a standard 8½- × 11-inch sheet of colored paper. Type or print the patient's name in the upper right corner, and then, with transparent tape, fasten the first report even with the bottom of the page. The second laboratory report is taped or glued in place on top of and approximately ½ inch above the first slip, allowing the date to show on the first report. With this method, called **shingling**, the latest report always appears on top

PROCEDURE 14-4

Add Supplementary Items to Patients' Records

GOAL: *To add supplementary documents and progress notes to patients' histories, observing standard steps in filing while creating an orderly file that facilitates ready reference to any item of information.*

EQUIPMENT and SUPPLIES

- Assorted correspondence, diagnostic reports, and progress notes
- Patients' files
- Computer
- Mending tape
- FILE stamp or pen
- Sorter
- Stapler

PROCEDURAL STEPS

1. Group all papers according to patients' names.
   PURPOSE: To expedite the filing process.
2. Remove any staples or paper clips.
   PURPOSE: Staples in the file folders are hazardous; paper clips are bulky and inadvertently may become attached to other materials.
3. Mend any damaged or torn records.
4. Attach any small items to standard-size paper.
   PURPOSE: Small items are easily lost or misplaced in files.
5. Group any related papers together.
6. Place your initials or stamp FILE in the upper left corner.
   PURPOSE: To indicate that the document has been released for filing.
7. Code the document by underlining or writing the patient's name in the upper right corner.
   PURPOSE: To indicate where the document is to be filed.
8. Continue steps 2 through 7 until all documents have been conditioned, released, indexed, and coded.
9. Place all documents in the sorter in filing sequence.
   PURPOSE: To allow the sorter to be taken to the file cabinet or shelf for insertion of documents into patients' folders.

(Figure 14-6). When checking previous reports, it is necessary only to run a finger down the slips until the desired date is found and then flip up the slips above.

Radiology Reports

Radiology reports usually are typed on standard letter-size stationery from the facility where the imaging was done. They are placed in the patient's history folder, with the most recent report on top. All radiology reports may be stapled together or kept behind a special divider in the chart.

Progress Notes

Reports on the patient's progress are continually added to the medical record. Each of the patient's visits should be entered into the chart, with the date preceding any notations about the visit. The medical assistant can type or stamp the date on the chart when readying the charts for the patient's visit. Every instruction, prescription, or telephone call for advice should be entered with the correct date. A wise course is to initial each entry, especially when several people are handling and making entries in a patient's record. This helps trace entries if some question arises.

MAKING CORRECTIONS AND ALTERATIONS TO MEDICAL RECORDS

Corrections sometimes must be made to medical records. The first step is to verify the proper procedure for making corrections in the facility's policy and procedures manual. Some physicians prefer a specific method for correcting errors in the medical record. Erasing, using correction fluid, or any other type of **obliteration** is never acceptable. To correct a handwritten entry:

1. Draw a line through the error.
2. Insert the correction above or immediately after the error, in a spot where it can be read clearly.
3. If indicated by the policy and procedures manual, write "Correction" or "Corr." in the margin.
4. The person making the correction should write his or her initials or signature below the correction and the date. Follow the format indicated in the policy and procedures manual (Figure 14-7).

Errors made while using the computer are corrected in the usual way. However, an error discovered in an entry at a later date is corrected in the same manner as for a handwritten entry. This is sometimes called an *addendum*. Never attempt to alter medical records without using this specific correction procedure, because this alteration of records may indicate a fraudulent attempt to cover up a mistake made by a staff member or the physician. Do not hide errors. If the error could in any way affect the patient's health and well-being, it must be brought to the physician's attention immediately.

CRITICAL THINKING APPLICATION   14-5

Susan has been using an incorrect abbreviation for several weeks and is having a difficult time remembering the right abbreviation. After taking a call from Mrs. Johnston, she remembers that she used the incorrect abbreviation in her chart last week. When Susan pulls the chart, she notices that entries have been made after the ones that Susan made on Mrs. Johnston's last visit. How does Susan correct her error?

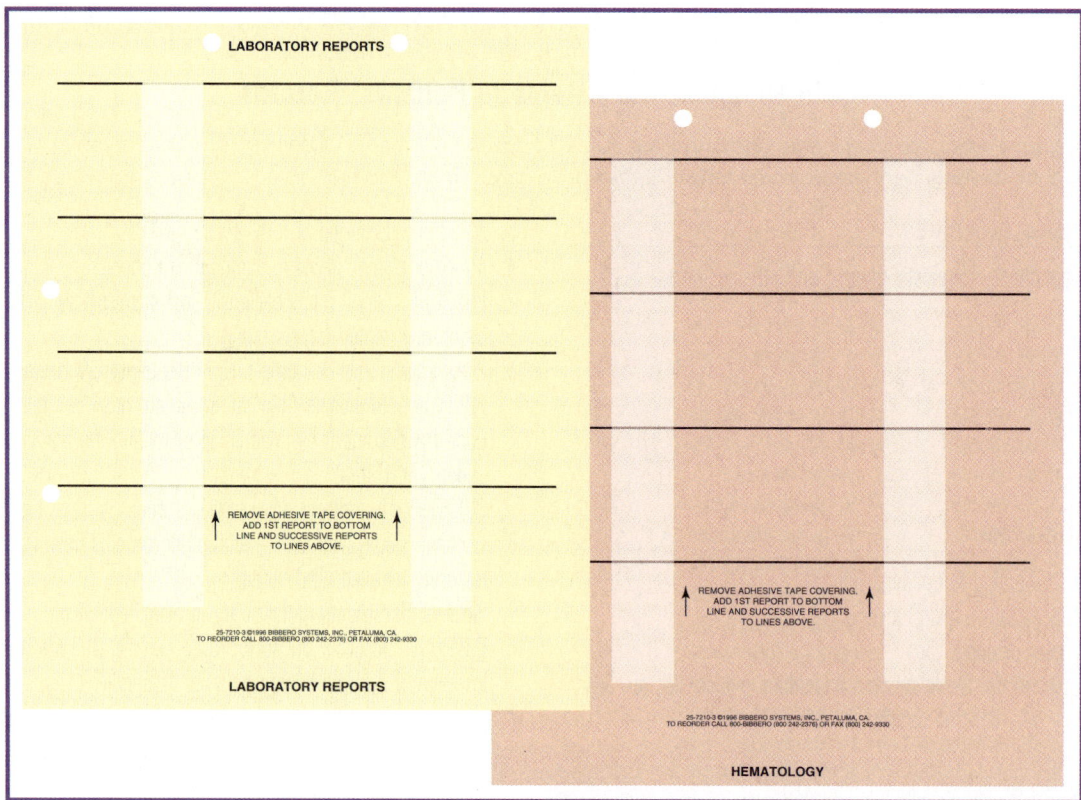

FIGURE 14-6 Shingled laboratory report forms. These forms make filing laboratory reports easy and provide a good adhesive so that the reports do not fall out of the chart if they are not standard size. (Courtesy Bibbero Systems, Petaluma, Calif.)

		error 10/15/XX ——— D. Bennett, CMA (AAMA)
10/15/XX	9:30 a.m. Tubersol Mantoux test: 9mm induration. ———————	
	12 ——— D. Bennett, CMA (AAMA)	

FIGURE 14-7 Corrections to medical records must be done in a legible manner and must be clearly understood. Always initial and date corrections to medical records. (From Bonewit-West K: *Today's medical assistant*, ed 2, St Louis, 2013, WB Saunders.)

KEEPING RECORDS CURRENT

One of the greatest dangers to good record keeping is **procrastination**. The record must be methodically kept current. The medical assistant is responsible for seeing that this is done.

Case histories and reports may accumulate on the physician's or the medical assistant's desk during the day. After the last patient has gone, check each history to make sure all necessary information has been recorded and that each entry is sufficiently clear for future understanding. Give the physician all abnormal reports to read and initial so that action can be taken and they can be filed in the patient's case history folder. Some physicians want to see every laboratory report, whether normal or abnormal; others prefer the abnormal results be circled or highlighted. Always adhere to written policy when reporting abnormal results and filing documents. If the medical assistant decides what the physician does and doesn't need to see, the assistant is practicing medicine without a license. Follow the requirements as set forth in the office policy and procedures manual.

While the physician is reviewing these reports, pull the histories of any patients seen outside the office that day and those of patients given special instructions by telephone or for whom prescriptions were ordered. These entries are made in the same manner as for an office visit, but the type of call is explained in parentheses after the date.

A prescription pad, printed on no-smear, carbonless paper, is available for a timesaving, write-it-once system. By placing the prescription blank over the patient's record, the prescription is automatically copied on the record as it is written. Prescription carriers with adhesive strips are also available for the physician who uses duplicate prescription blanks. Be very careful that prescription pads are not stolen by patients in an effort to obtain drugs illegally.

The patient's record should not leave the office. A physician's pocket call record can be used for outside calls, and the information can be transferred to the chart in the office. Notations should be made of any missed appointments or of refusals to cooperate with instructions as they occur.

After all records have been reviewed for the day, and if time is too short to file them, they should be placed in a file tray and locked away for the night. Do not leave histories out in view at night, especially if the facility has a cleaning service. On arrival the next morning, the medical assistant can index the histories for filing. Attach extra reports and information sheets. Always attach material to the chart permanently; do not simply drop forms into the folders. When this has been done, the records are ready for filing.

The physician may prefer to dictate progress notes rather than write them in longhand. Patient histories, physical examination findings, medications prescribed, follow-up findings, and summaries of telephone conversations all can be dictated. At the end of the day, the recorded information is either given to the medical assistant for transcribing into the records or prepared for an outside transcriber.

A great deal of time may be saved in transcribing these notes by using a continuous roll or pages of self-adhesive strips. After the **transcription** is complete, the physician may want to check the notes, underline important points, and initial each entry to verify that each is correct, in the event of an **audit** or litigation. The notes then are returned to the medical assistant for insertion into the charts. The use of self-adhesive strips saves the time and effort involved in removing the sheet from a chart that may be bound with metal fasteners, inserting the sheet into the typewriter, and putting the sheet back into the folder. It also simplifies the physician's part in checking and initialing the notes, because only the transcribed material is handled, rather than the bulky chart. These forms also are useful for shingling telephone message records kept in the patient's record (Figure 14-8).

TRANSFER, DESTRUCTION, AND RETENTION OF MEDICAL RECORDS

Regular Transfer of Files

In most medical offices, records are filed according to three classifications:

- *Active files,* which are the files of patients currently receiving treatment.
- *Inactive files,* which generally are the files of patients whom the doctor has not seen for 6 months or longer. When these individuals return for care, their folders are replaced among the active files.
- *Closed files,* which are the records of patients who have died, moved away, or otherwise terminated their relationship with the physician.

Some system must be established for regular transfer of files from active to inactive status or possibly destruction. The expansion of charts and the file space available can influence the transfer period. Charts for patients currently hospitalized may be kept in a special section for quick reference and then placed in the regular active file when the patient is discharged from the hospital. In a surgical practice, the chart frequently includes the specific date on which the patient is discharged from the physician's care, and the notation is made on the chart, "Return prn" (from the Latin *pro re nata,* "as the occasion arises" or "when needed"). This record may safely be placed in the inactive file. The process of moving a file from active to inactive status is called **purging**. In a general practice office, the outside

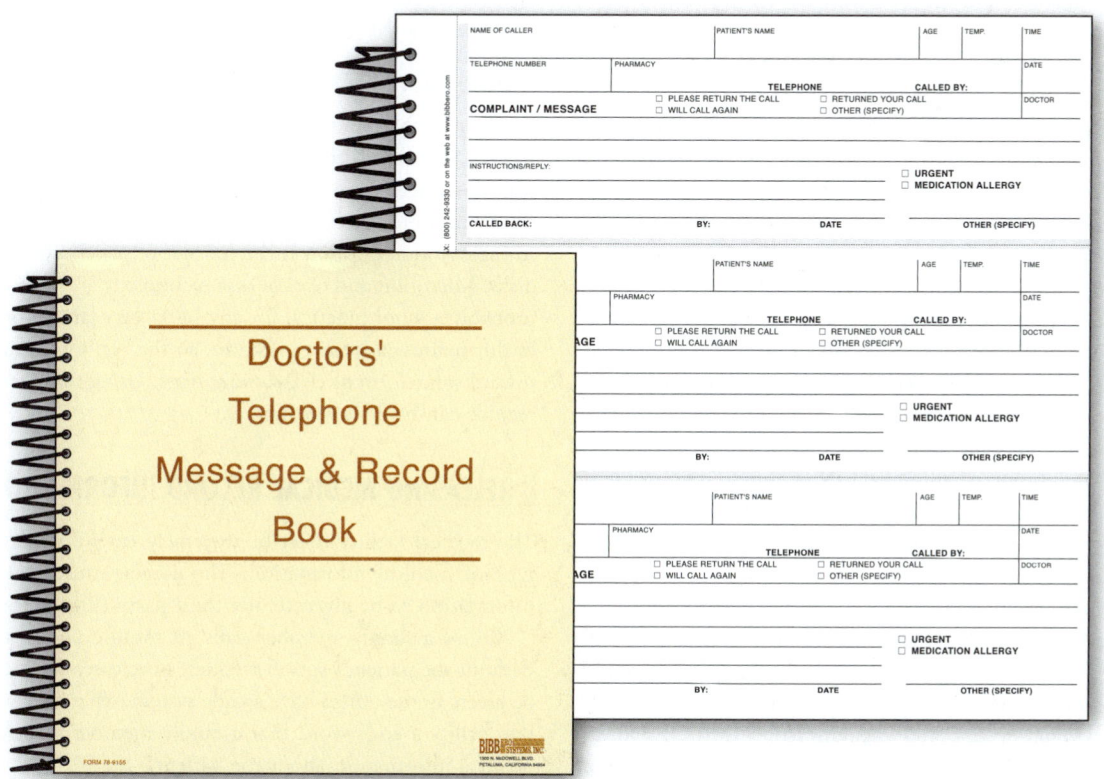

FIGURE 14-8 Shingled telephone message forms. These self-adhesive forms allow several telephone messages to be filed chronologically. (Courtesy Bibbero Systems, Petaluma, Calif.)

of the folder may be stamped with the date of the visit each time the patient is seen. It then is a simple matter to determine when the chart should be transferred to the inactive status; this is called the *perpetual transfer method.*

Most medical facilities use a year sticker on the file folder that indicates the last year the patient visited the clinic. If the file has a sticker showing that the patient's last visit was in 2011, and he or she presents to the clinic on January 5, 2013, a *2013* sticker should be placed over the one that indicates *2011*. These stickers often are included with color-coded filing systems. The medical assistant can easily look at a group of files and see which ones need to be changed to inactive or closed status.

Retention and Destruction

Physicians have an obligation to retain patient records that may reasonably be of value to a patient, according to the American Medical Association (AMA) Council on Ethical and Judicial Affairs. Currently, no standard, nationwide rule exists for establishing a records **retention schedule**.

Medical considerations are the primary basis for deciding how long to retain medical records. For example, operative notes and chemotherapy records should always be part of the patient's chart. The laws regarding the retention of medical records vary from state to state, and many governmental programs have their own guidelines for specific records retention. When no rules specify the retention of medical records, the best course is to keep the records for 10 years. However, for minors, the facility should keep the records until the minor reaches the age of majority plus 3 years.

If a particular record no longer needs to be kept for medical reasons, the physician should check the state law for any requirement that records be kept for a minimum time (most states do not have such a provision). The time is measured from the last professional contact with the patient. In all cases, medical records should be kept for at least the period of the statute of limitations for medical malpractice claims, which may be 3 years or longer, depending on state law. In the case of a minor, the statute of limitations may not apply until the patient reaches the age of majority. In summary, know the state requirements related to medical records retention and follow those guidelines; the office policy manual should address records retention pertaining to the state where the practice exists.

The records of any patient covered by Medicare or Medicaid must be kept at least 10 years. The Health Insurance Portability and Accountability Act (HIPAA) privacy rule does not include requirements for the retention of medical records. However, the privacy rule does require that appropriate administrative, technical, and physical safeguards be applied so that the privacy of medical records is maintained (Chapter 17 presents more detailed information about HIPAA).

Some physicians refuse to destroy or discard old records. The records should be stored somewhere other than the medical facility unless an abundance of storage space is available. The records should be kept in a facility where the temperature is controlled and the unit is locked. Always refer to state laws when discarding medical records, because state law varies with regard to medical record retention. For instance, some states require that pediatric records be kept 7 years after the patient turns 18; others require a 7-year retention period, to begin when the patient reaches his or her twenty-first birthday.

Before old records are discarded, patients should be given an opportunity to claim a copy of the records or have them sent to another physician. To preserve confidentiality when discarding old records, destroy the documents by shredding or through a professional document destruction service. HIPAA does not require any particular disposal method, but facilities must review their own circumstances to determine what steps are reasonable to safeguard patient information. The medical facility should keep a master list of all records that have been destroyed.

Protection of Records

Do not release original case histories to anyone outside the healthcare facility. Instead, prepare a summary or photocopy the materials needed for reference and retain the original in the physician's office. Because the facsimile machine is standard equipment in business offices, the transfer of information is simplified and the records remain in safekeeping. Often only certain aspects of the record are requested, and these can easily be supplied by faxing the required pages, observing precautions for confidentiality. Send only the information requested and make sure a release has been signed to provide the information. If possible, call before faxing confidential patient information and ask the person who is to receive it to retrieve it from the fax.

Occasions may arise when records are temporarily out of the office, although this should be an extremely rare occurrence. Some physicians release case histories to their colleagues, or an original record may be subpoenaed by a court. In such instances, a colored **OUTfolder** should be inserted into the file in place of the regular folder and a notation made of the name, date, and to whom the record was released. Interim papers may be placed in the OUTfolder until the original is returned.

Long-Term Storage

Large healthcare facilities may find it advisable to convert their records to **microfilm** for storage if the facility has not yet begun to scan documents into an electronic medical record system. If documents are stored electronically, they must be regularly backed up for storage. Another option is the transfer of paper records onto optical disks. Microfilm and optical disk technology are both expensive and probably are not practical for any but a very large group practice or health maintenance organization, so the facility should be moving toward some form of electronic storage. Using that method, medical records can be kept indefinitely.

RELEASING MEDICAL RECORD INFORMATION

The medical facility must be extremely careful when releasing any type of medical information. The patient must sign a release for information to be given to any third party (Procedure 14-5).

Often a family member calls to inquire about a patient, but without the patient's specific request or release, no information may be given. Some offices have a code system, whereby the patient gives the facility a code word that a family member must use to receive medical information about the patient.

Requests for medical information should be made in writing (Figure 14-9). Accepting a faxed request for medical information or a faxed release of information from a patient is unwise. Even requests

PROCEDURE 14-5

Prepare a Record Release Form

GOAL: *To provide a legal document indicating the patient's consent to the release of his or her medical records to another provider or healthcare facility.*

EQUIPMENT and SUPPLIES

- Medical record release form
- Pen
- Envelope

PROCEDURAL STEPS

1. Explain to the patient that a medical record release form is required to obtain records from another provider. If the patient is having records sent to another provider, a release also is required for that purpose.
   PURPOSE: To make sure the patient understands the record release procedure and purposes.

2. Review the record release form with the patient and ask whether the person understands the form or has any questions about it.
   PURPOSE: To provide the opportunity for questions and to make sure the patient understands the form.

3. Have the patient sign the form in the space indicated. If other demographic information is required (e.g., Social Security number or other names used), complete that information as well.

PURPOSE: The patient must sign the form for records to be released by any medical facility.

4. Make a copy of the form for the file, then mail it to the appropriate facility. Note the date the form was sent. Give the patient a copy if it is requested.
   PURPOSE: To have a record that the information or documents were actually requested on a certain date.

5. Check that the requested records arrived.
   PURPOSE: To make sure the records the physician needs to treat the patient accurately and competently are available in a timely manner.

6. Check the patient's medical record to determine whether a signed, current privacy policy document is on file. If not, have the patient sign one and place it in the record.
   PURPOSE: To ensure that all patients are notified of the office privacy policy.

RECORDS RELEASE AUTHORIZATION

TO _____
                    Doctor or Hospital

_____
                    Address

I HEREBY AUTHORIZE AND REQUEST YOU TO RELEASE TO:

ALL RECORDS IN YOUR POSSESION CONCERNING _____

_____ILLNESS AND/OR

TREATMENT DURING THE PERIOD FROM _____ TO _____.

NAME _____ TEL. _____

ADDRESS_____

SIGNATURE _____ DATE _____
              (If relative, state relationship)

WITNESS_____ DATE _____

25-8104 © 1973 BIBBERO SYSTEMS, INC., PETALUMA,, CA.

FIGURE 14-9 Authorization to release medical records. All requests for medical records should be made in writing, and the request should be kept in the patient's chart. (Courtesy Bibbero Systems, Petaluma, Calif.)

from the patient's attorney or third-party payers must be cleared by the patient for them to obtain information. Some attorneys may present a legal document called a **power of attorney** or a subpoena, which authorizes them to see the records. A durable power of attorney is used often in the medical field; it allows another person (usually an attorney) to make transactions during the time that the patient is suffering from an incapacitating medical condition. It may allow the attorney to pay a utility bill for a hospitalized patient, make bank transactions, cash a Social Security check, and perform other types of transactions that the patient is too ill to perform.

As both parties to a lawsuit begin to prepare their cases, they enter the discovery process. Each side must disclose the pertinent facts of the case that may influence the final outcome of that case. On each occasion that information is needed from the provider, a separate request must be sent. Because this request form is signed by the patient, it serves as a release.

Most offices charge a fee to copy medical records, whether it is a per-page charge or a per-chart fee. Before releasing medical records, make sure you have a written, up-to-date release that has been signed by the patient. Follow the steps in the policy and procedures manual. Some physicians designate the office manager to handle requests for records releases.

Pay particular attention to records release requests involving a minor. In most cases, the parent or legal guardian is entitled to read through the patient's medical records; however, according to the Department of Health and Human Services, there are three situations in which the parent may not be legally entitled to review the records of his or her minor child, including:

- When the minor is the one who consents to care and the parent is not required to also consent to care under state law
- When the minor obtains medical care at the direction of a court or a person authorized by the court
- When the minor, parent, and physician all agree that the doctor and minor patient can have a private, confidential relationship

If the physician believes that the minor might be in an abuse situation or that the parent or legal guardian may be harming the patient, the physician is required to act, both legally and ethically.

Remember that the patient ultimately decides whether a record can be released. If any question arises about what is to be released, consult the office manager or the physician.

CRITICAL THINKING APPLICATION 14-6

Susan has never seen a power of attorney and is curious about this type of document. How might she investigate and learn more about it? Whom should Susan approach first for this information? The physician has an attorney whom Susan has met once. Should she call her and ask about the document without notifying the physician? Why or why not?

The time may come when a patient decides that he or she no longer agrees to the release of medical information. In this case, the patient should sign a revocation form, and it must become part of the medical record (Figure 14-10).

Sometimes patients want to look at their own records. They certainly have a right to see this information, but some patients may

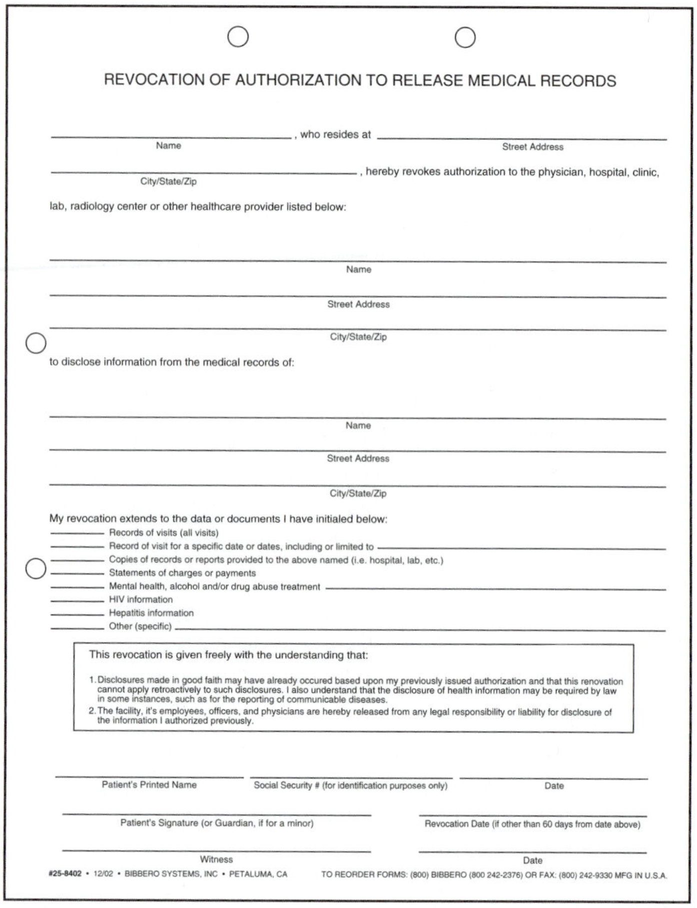

REVOCATION OF AUTHORIZATION TO RELEASE MEDICAL RECORDS

_______________ (Name), who resides at _______________ (Street Address)

_______________ (City/State/Zip), hereby revokes authorization to the physician, hospital, clinic, lab, radiology center or other healthcare provider listed below:

_______________ Name

_______________ Street Address

_______________ City/State/Zip

to disclose information from the medical records of:

_______________ Name

_______________ Street Address

_______________ City/State/Zip

My revocation extends to the data or documents I have initialed below:

- ______ Records of visits (all visits)
- ______ Record of visit for a specific date or dates, including or limited to ______
- ______ Copies of records or reports provided to the above named (i.e. hospital, lab, etc.)
- ______ Statements of charges or payments
- ______ Mental health, alcohol and/or drug abuse treatment ______
- ______ HIV information
- ______ Hepatitis information
- ______ Other (specific) ______

This revocation is given freely with the understanding that:

1. Disclosures made in good faith may have already occured based upon my previously issued authorization and that this renovation cannot apply retroactively to such disclosures. I also understand that the disclosure of health information may be required by law in some instances, such as for the reporting of communicable diseases.
2. The facility, it's employees, officers, and physicians are hereby released from any legal responsibility or liability for disclosure of the information I authorized previously.

Patient's Printed Name | Social Security # (for identification purposes only) | Date

Patient's Signature (or Guardian, if for a minor) | Revocation Date (if other than 60 days from date above)

Witness | Date

#25-8402 • 12/02 • BIBBERO SYSTEMS, INC • PETALUMA, CA TO REORDER FORMS: (800) BIBBERO (800 242-2376) OR FAX: (800) 242-9330 MFG IN U.S.A.

FIGURE 14-10 Revocation of release of medical records. (Courtesy Bibbero Systems, Petaluma, Calif.)

not understand the terminology used in the record. A staff member should always remain with a patient who is looking at his or her medical record. Remember, the original medical record should never leave the medical facility. The physician can ethically charge for any copies of the medical record, both in full or in part. Always follow office policy when releasing medical records.

When a release is presented to the office, copy only the records requested in the release. Do not provide additional information that is not requested. The person requesting the information can be charged reasonable copying fees.

DICTATION AND TRANSCRIPTION

Administrative medical assistants may find that transcribing **dictation** is a job they perform periodically. Transcription can be done from handwritten notes, such as those in shorthand, or from machine dictation. Smooth operation of the facility may depend on the timely, accurate performance of assigned responsibilities, such as record documentation and preparation of special reports. Accuracy and speed are primary **requisites**, as is a strong grasp of medical principles, especially anatomy and physiology.

Dictation may be done using a machine transcription unit or a portable transcription unit. Many healthcare facilities now use a system that is accessed by telephone; the physician calls the system using passwords or access codes and records the information for the medical record while speaking into the telephone. Later, employees transcribe the information into the medical record.

Voice Recognition Software

Some healthcare facilities use voice recognition software for transcription. These software systems are loaded onto an office computer and work through a USB port or the line-in jack of a telephone. When first installed, the software requires the user to say several sentences into the unit so that it "learns" to recognize the user's voice. The system can be used to dictate progress notes, letters, e-mails, and virtually any document in the medical office that needs to be created. Some systems have an authentication component that allows a type of electronic signature, such as those needed for hospital record dictation.

FILING EQUIPMENT

The vertical, four-drawer steel filing cabinet, used with manila folders with the patient's name on the tab, was the traditional system of choice for years. The most popular system today is color-coding on open shelves. Rotary, lateral, compactable, and automated files also are available. Some records are kept in card or tray files. Regardless of the type or style of equipment, the best quality is always an economy. Some factors that should be considered when selecting filing equipment are:

- Office space availability
- Structural considerations
- Cost of space and equipment
- Size, type, and volume of records
- Confidentiality requirements
- Retrieval speed
- Fire protection

Drawer Files

Drawer files should be full suspension; they should roll easily, close securely, and be equipped with a locking device. The best cabinets have a center trough at the bottom of each drawer with a rod for holding divider guides. A drawback of the vertical four-drawer files is that only one person can use a file cabinet at a time. Filing also is slower, because the drawer must be opened and closed each time a file is pulled or filed.

File cabinets are heavy and can tip over, causing serious damage or injury unless reasonable care is taken. Open only one file drawer at a time, and close it when the filing has been completed. A drawer left even slightly open can injure a passerby.

Shelf Files

Shelf files should have doors to protect the contents. A popular type of shelf file has doors that slide back into the cabinet; the door from a lower shelf may be pulled out and used for work space. Open shelf units hold files sideways and can go higher on the wall because no drawers need to be pulled out (Figure 14-11). File retrieval is faster, because several individuals can work simultaneously. Open shelf units without doors are the most economical, but they offer little protection or confidentiality for the records. They are susceptible to water and fire damage.

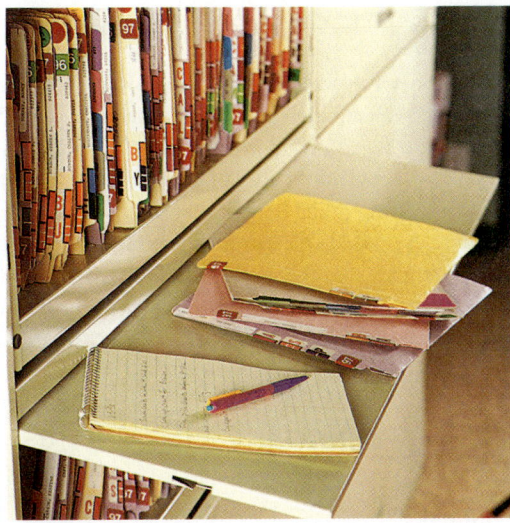

FIGURE 14-11 Open shelf filing is an efficient method, especially for color-coded filing systems. The shelf doors often can be used as workspace.

Rotary Circular Files

Rotary circular files can hold a large volume of records. They save space and clerical motion. The files revolve easily; some have push-button controls. Several people can work at one rotary file and use records at the same time. One disadvantage is that they afford less privacy and protection than files that can be closed and locked.

Lateral Files

Lateral files are good for personal files and are especially attractive for the physician's private office. They use more wall space than the vertical file but do not extend so far out into the room. The folders are filed sideways in the lateral file, left to right, instead of front to back as in a vertical file.

Compactable Files

An office with little space and a great volume of records might use compactable files, which are a variation of open shelf files. The files are mounted on tracks in the floor, and the units slide along the tracks so that access is gained to the needed records. One drawback is that not all records are available at the same time.

Automated Files

Automated files are very expensive initially and require more maintenance than other types of filing equipment. They are likely to be found only in very large facilities, such as clinics or hospitals. These files bring the record to the operator instead of the operator going to the record. When the operator presses a button indicating the appropriate shelf, the shelf automatically moves into position in front of the operator for record retrieval. The automated or power file is fast and can store large numbers of records in a small amount of space. However, only one person can use the unit at one time.

Card Files

Almost every office has some occasion to use a card file. This may be for patient ledgers, a patient index, a library index, an index of surgical tray setups, telephone numbers, or numerous other records. A good-quality steel box or tray is a sound investment.

Special Items

Metal framework is available that can convert a regular drawer file into suspension-folder equipment. The assistant with a great deal of filing may want to purchase a portable filing shelf that fits on the side of an opened drawer and can be moved from place to place as needed. Another special filing item is a sorting file, which can be a great time-saver. A portable file cart for temporary filing of unbilled insurance claims may be quite useful. It also may be used for preliminary sorting of charts to be refiled; this is sometimes called a *suspense file*.

FILING SUPPLIES

Divider Guides

Each file drawer or shelf should be equipped with plenty of dividers or guides. Some authorities recommend one guide for approximately each 1½ inches of material, or every eight to 10 folders. Guides should be of good-quality **pressboard** or strong plastic. Less well constructed guides soon become bent and frayed and have to be replaced. Divider guides have a protruding tab, which may be an integral part of the card or may be made of metal or plastic. The guides reduce the area of search and serve as supports for the folders. They are available in single, third, or fifth cut (one, three, or five different positions).

OUTguides

OUTguides are heavy guides used to replace a folder that has been removed temporarily (Figure 14-12). They should be of a distinctive color for quick detection. This makes refiling simpler and alerts the file clerk that a file is missing. Several colors may be used, each color designating the temporary location of the file. The OUTguide may have lines for recording information, or it may have a plastic pocket for inserting an information card.

File Folders

Most records to be filed are placed in covers or tabbed folders. The most commonly used is a general purpose, third-cut manila folder that may be expanded to ¾ inch. These are available with a double-thickness, reinforced tab, which greatly extends the life of the folder. Folders kept in drawers have tabs at the top; those kept on shelves have tabs at the side. Many folder styles are available for special purposes.

The vertical pocket, which is of heavier weight than the general purpose folder, has a front that folds down for easy access to contents and is available with up to a 3½-inch expansion. These are used for bulky histories or correspondence.

Hanging, or suspension, folders are made of heavy stock and hang on metal rods from side to side in a drawer. They can be used only with files equipped with suspension equipment.

Binder folders have fasteners that are used to bind papers in the folder. These offer some security for the papers, but filing the materials is time-consuming.

The number of papers that will fit in one folder depends on the thickness of the papers and the capacity of the folder. Near the bottom edge of most folders are one or more score marks, which should be used as the contents of the folders expand. Papers should never protrude from the folder edges, and they should always be inserted with their tops to the left. When papers start to ride up in any folder, the folder is overloaded.

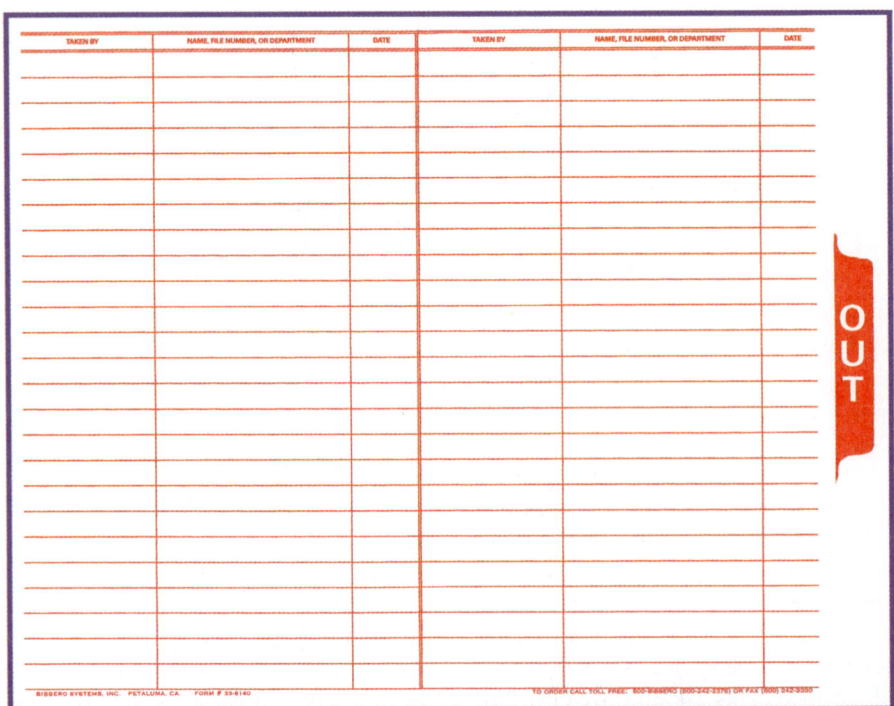

FIGURE 14-12 OUTguides allow tracking of a file not in its proper location by providing information on the location of the file. (Courtesy Bibbero Systems, Petaluma, Calif.)

Labels

The label is a necessary filing and finding device. Use labels to identify each shelf, drawer, divider guide, and folder. A label on the drawer or shelf identifies the nature of its contents. It should also indicate the range (alphabetic, numeric, or chronologic) of the material filed in that space.

The label on the divider guide identifies the range of folder headings following that divider guide up to the next divider (e.g., BaBo). The label on the folder identifies the contents of that folder only. This may be the name of the patient, subject matter of correspondence, a business topic, or anything at all that needs to be filed. Label a folder when a new patient is seen, existing folders are full, or materials need to be transferred within the filing system.

Labels are available in almost any size, shape, or color to meet the individual needs of any facility. Visit an office supply store and review the catalogs to find the best product to meet the needs of the facility.

A narrow label applied to the front of the folder tab is the easiest to use and satisfactory for folders kept in a drawer file. Labels for shelf filing should be identifiable from both front and back. Always type the label before separating it from the roll or protective sheet. Type the **caption** on the label in indexing order.

FILING PROCEDURES

Filing of all materials involves five basic steps: conditioning, releasing, indexing and coding, sorting, and storing and filing.

Conditioning

Conditioning of papers involves removing all pins, brads, and paper clips; stapling related papers together; attaching clippings or items smaller than page size to a regular sheet of paper with rubber cement or tape; and mending damaged records.

Releasing

The term *releasing* simply means that some mark is placed on the paper indicating that it is now ready for filing. This usually is either the medical assistant's initials or a FILE stamp placed in the upper left corner.

Indexing and Coding

Indexing means deciding where to file the letter or paper, and coding means placing some indication of this decision on the paper (Table 14-1). This may be done by underlining the name or subject, if it appears on the paper, or writing the indexing subject or name in some conspicuous place. If the paper logically could be filed in more

TABLE 14-1 Applying Indexing Rules

INDEXING RULE	NAME	UNIT 1	UNIT 2	UNIT 3
1	Robert F. Grinch	Grinch	Robert	F.
	R. Frank Grumman	Grumman	R.	Frank
2	J. Orville Smith	Smith	J.	Orville
	Jason O. Smith	Smith	Jason	O.
3	M. L. Saint-Vickery	Saint-Vickery	M.	L.
	Marie-Louise Taylor	Taylor	Marielouise	
4	Charles S. Anderson	Anderson	Charles	S.
	Anderson's Surgical Supply	Andersons	Surgical	Supply
5	Ah Hop Akee	Akee	Ah	Hop
6	Alice Delaney	Delaney	Alice	K.
	Chester K. DeLong	Delong	Chester	
7	Michael St. John	Stjohn	Michael	
8	Helen M. Maag	Maag	Helen	M.
	Frederick Mabry James	Mabry	Frederick	
	E. MacDonald	Macdonald	James	E.
9	Mrs. John L. Doe (Mary Jones)	Doe	Mary	Jones (Mrs. John L.)
10	Prof. John J. Breck	Breck	John	J. (Prof.)
	Madame Sylvia	Madame	Sylvia	
	Sister Mary Catherine	Sister	Mary	Catherine
	Theodore Wilson, M.D.	Wilson	Theodore (M. D.)	
11	Lawrence W. Sloan, Jr.	Sloan	Lawrence	W. (Jr.)
	Lawrence W. Sloan, Sr.	Sloan	Lawrence	W. (Sr.)
12	The Moore Clinic	Moore	Clinic (The)	

than one place, the original is coded for the main location and a cross-reference sheet is prepared, indicating this location, and coded for the second location. Every paper placed in a patient's chart should have the date and the patient's name on it, usually in the upper right corner. Include the chart number if a numeric system is used.

Sorting

Sorting is arranging the papers in filing sequence. Sort papers before going to the file cabinet or shelf. Do any necessary stapling of papers at the desk or filing table. Invest in a desktop sorter with a series of dividers, between which papers are placed in filing sequence. In the preliminary sorting, place the papers in the appropriate division in the sorter. It then is comparatively simple to arrange these groups into the proper sequence for filing.

Storing and Filing

When storing or filing papers in the folder, place items face up, top edge to the left, with the most recent date at the front of the folder. Lift the folder 1 or 2 inches out of the drawer before inserting new material, so that the sheets can drop down completely into the folder. However, the best course is to attach items to the file folder permanently so that they cannot fall out accidentally. When filing completed folders, arrange them in indexing order before going to the file cabinets.

Locating Misplaced Files

Unless files are promptly replaced after use, they may become lost. Papers may be misfiled, requiring a thorough search to find them, which wastes valuable time. After a methodic and complete search through the proper folder, check several places for the misplaced paper: (1) in the folder in front of and the one behind the correct folder; (2) between the folders; (3) at the bottom of the file under all the folders; (4) in a folder of a patient with a similar name; and (5) in the sorter.

INDEXING RULES

Indexing rules are fairly well standardized and based on current business practices. The Association of Records Managers and Administrators takes an active part in updating these rules. Some establishments adopt variations of these basic rules to accommodate their needs. In any case, the practices need to be consistent within the system.

1. Last names are considered first in filing; then the given name (first name), second; and the middle name or initial, third. Compare the names beginning with the first letter of the name. When a letter is different in the two names, that letter determines the order of filing.

abe
abi
abm
abx
acl
acm
ada
ade
adi

2. Initials precede a name beginning with the same letter. This illustrates the librarian's rule, "Nothing comes before something."

Smith, J.
Smith, Jason

3. With hyphenated personal names, the hyphenated elements, whether first name, middle name, or surname, are considered to be one unit.

Carlotta Freeman-Duque is filed as Freemanduque, Carlotta
Cindy-Jean Green is filed as Green, Cindyjean

4. The apostrophe is disregarded in filing.

Andersons' Surgical Supply
Andersons Surgical Supply

5. When indexing a foreign name in which you cannot distinguish between the first and last names, index each part of the name in the order in which it is written.

Cau Liu
Talluri Devi

If you can make the distinction, use the last name as the first indexing unit.

Liu, Jason

6. Names with prefixes are filed in the usual alphabetic order, with the prefix considered part of the name.

von Schmidt is filed as Vonschmidt
DeLong is filed as Delong
LaFrance is filed as Lafrance

7. Abbreviated parts of a name are indexed as written if that form generally is used by that person.

Ste. Marie is filed as Stemarie
St. John is filed as Stjohn
Wm. is filed as Wm
Edw. is filed as Edw
Jas. is filed as Jas

8. Mac and Mc are filed in their regular place in the alphabet.

Maag
Mabry
MacDonald
Machado
MacHale
Maville
McAulay
McWilliams
Meacham

If the files have a great many names beginning with Mac or Mc, some offices file them as a separate letter of the alphabet for convenience.

9. The name of a married woman is indexed by her legal name (her husband's surname, her given name, and her middle name or maiden surname).

> Doe, Mary Jones (Mrs. John L.)
> not Doe, Mrs. John L. (unless first name is unknown)

10. When followed by a complete name, titles may be used as the last filing unit if needed to distinguish the name from another, identical name.

> Mr. James D. Conley
> Conley James D Mr.
> Dr. James D. Conley
> Conley James D Dr.

Titles without complete names are considered the first indexing unit.

> Madame Sylvia
> Sister Theresa

11. Terms of seniority or professional or academic degrees are used only to distinguish the name from an identical name.

> Theodore Wilson, PhD
> Theodore Wilson, Sr.
> Theodore Wilson, Jr.
> Theodore Wilson, MD
> These examples would be filed in the following order:
> Theodore Wilson, Jr.
> Theodore Wilson, MD
> Theodore Wilson, PhD
> Theodore Wilson, Sr.

12. Articles (e.g., the, a) are disregarded in indexing.

> Moore Clinic (The)

FILING METHODS

The three basic filing methods used in healthcare facilities are:
- Alphabetic by name
- Numeric
- Subject

Patients' charts are filed either alphabetically by name or by one of several numeric methods. Subject filing is used for business records, correspondence, and topical materials.

Alphabetic Filing

Alphabetic filing by name is the oldest, simplest, and most commonly used system. It is the system of choice for filing patients' records in most physicians' offices.

The alphabetic system of filing is traditional and simple to set up, requiring only a file cabinet or shelf, folders, and some divider guides (Procedure 14-6). It is a **direct filing system** in that the person filing needs to know only the name to find the desired file. Alphabetic filing does have some drawbacks:
- The correct spelling of the name must be known.
- As the number of files increases, more space is needed for each section of the alphabet. This results in periodic shifting of folders to allow for expansion.
- As the files expand, more time is required for filing or retrieving each folder because of the greater number of folders involved in the search. The time can be greatly reduced by color-coding.

Numeric Filing

Some form of **numeric filing** combined with color and shelf filing is used by practically every large clinic or hospital. Management consultants differ in their recommendations; some recommend numeric filing only if more than 5,000 to 10,000 charts are involved. Others recommend nothing but numeric filing. Numeric filing is an **indirect filing system**, or one that requires use of an alphabetic cross-reference to find a given file. Some object to this added step and overlook the advantages of numeric filing, which are:
- It allows unlimited expansion without periodic shifting of folders, and shelves usually are filled evenly.
- It provides additional confidentiality to the chart.
- It saves time in retrieving and filing records quickly. One knows immediately that the number 978 falls between 977 and 979. By contrast, an alphabetic system, even with color-coding, requires a longer search for the exact spot.

Several types of numeric filing systems can be used. In the straight, or consecutive, numeric system, patients are given consecutive numbers as they visit the practice. This is the simplest numeric system and works well for files of up to 10,000 records. It is time-consuming, and the chance for error is greater, when documents with five or more digits are filed. Filing activity is greatest at the end of the numeric series.

In the terminal digit system, patients also are assigned consecutive numbers, but the digits in the number usually are separated into groups of twos or threes and are read in groups from right to left instead of from left to right. The records are filed backward in groups. For example, all files ending in 00 are grouped together first, then those ending in 01, and so on. Next the files are grouped by their middle digits so that the 00 22s come before the 01 22s. Finally, the files are arranged by their first digits, so that 01 00 22 precedes 02 00 22.

Middle-digit filing begins with the middle digits, followed by the first digit and finally by the terminal digits.

Some practices use the last four digits of each patient's Social Security number to file patient records. However, no law requires every U.S. resident to have a Social Security number; if a patient does not, a "pseudo number" would have to be issued.

Numeric filing requires more training, but once the system has been mastered, fewer errors occur than with alphabetic filing (Procedure 14-7).

PROCEDURE 14-6

File Medical Records Using an Alphabetic System

GOAL: *To file records efficiently using an alphabetic system and to ensure quick, easy retrieval of the records.*

EQUIPMENT and SUPPLIES

- Medical records
- Physical filing equipment
- Cart to carry records, if needed
- Alphabetic file guide
- Staple remover
- Stapler

PROCEDURAL STEPS

1. Using alphabetic guidelines, place the records to be filed in alphabetic order. If a stack of documents is to be filed, place them in alphabetic order inside an alphabetic file guide or sorter. Use rules for filing documents alphabetically.
   PURPOSE: To organize the filing process and file the record or document quickly without retracing steps and skipping from letter to letter.

2. Go to the filing storage equipment (shelves, cabinets, or drawers) and locate the correct spot in the alphabet for the first file.

3. Place the file in the cabinet or drawer in correct alphabetic order.

4. If adding a document to a file, place it on top so that the most recent information is seen first. This puts the information in the file in reverse chronologic order.
   PURPOSE: To provide access to the most pertinent and recent information.

5. Securely fasten documents to the chart. Do not just drop the documents inside the chart.
   PURPOSE: To keep vital information from falling out of the chart and being lost.

6. Refile the chart in its proper place.

PROCEDURE 14-7

File Medical Records Using a Numeric System

GOAL: *To file records efficiently using a numeric system and to ensure quick, easy retrieval of the records.*

EQUIPMENT and SUPPLIES

- Medical records
- Physical filing equipment
- Cart to carry records, if needed
- Numeric file guide
- Staple remover
- Stapler
- Paper clips

PROCEDURAL STEPS

1. Using numeric guidelines, place the records to be filed in numeric order. If a stack of documents is to be filed, write the chart number on the document. Use rules for filing documents numerically.
   PURPOSE: To organize the filing process and file the records or documents quickly without retracing steps and skipping from letter to letter.

2. Go to the filing storage equipment (shelves, cabinets, or drawers) and locate the numeric spot for the first file.

3. Place the file in the cabinet or drawer in correct numeric order.

4. If adding a document to a file, place it on top so that the most recent information is seen first. This puts the information in the file in reverse chronologic order.
   PURPOSE: To provide access to the most pertinent and recent information.

5. Securely fasten documents to the chart. Do not just drop the documents inside the chart.
   PURPOSE: To keep vital information from falling out of the chart and being lost.

6. Refile the chart in its proper place.

Subject Filing

Subject filing can be either alphabetic or **alphanumeric** (A 1-3, B 1-1, B 1-2, and so on) and is used for general correspondence. The main difficulty with subject filing is indexing, or classifying; that is, deciding where to file a document. Many papers require cross-referencing. All correspondence dealing with a particular subject is filed together. The papers in the folders are filed chronologically, the most recent on top. The subject headings are placed on the tabs of the folders and filed alphabetically.

Color-Coding

When a color-coding system is used, both filing and finding files is easier, and misfiling of folders is kept to a minimum. The use of color visually restricts the area of search for a specific record. A misfiled chart is easily spotted even from a distance of several feet. In color-coding, a specific color is selected to identify each letter of the alphabet. Any selection of colors may be used, and the division of the alphabet is determined by one's own needs. However, studies have shown that the frequency with which different letters occur varies widely.

Alphabetic Color-Coding

Files can be color-coded in several ways. One alphabetic system uses five different colored folders, with each color representing a segment of the alphabet. The second letter of the patient's last name determines the color.

As medicine continues to consolidate into larger facilities with more patients under one management, the filing of patients' charts becomes more complicated, and color-coding becomes more useful. Several color-coding systems use two sets of 13 colors: one set for letters A to M, and a second set of the same colors on a different background for letters N to Z.

Many ready-made systems are available for use. Self-adhesive, colored letter blocks with either two or three letters in the specific colors are supplied in rolls. The color blocks with the appropriate letter are placed on the index tab of the folder, along with the patient's full name. The letters are in pairs so that they can be seen from either side of the chart. Strong, easily differentiated colors are used, creating a band of color in the files that makes spotting out-of-place folders easy (Figure 14-13).

Numeric Color-Coding

Color-coding is also used in numeric filing. Numbers 0 through 9 are each assigned a different color. In a terminal digit filing system, the colors for the last two numbers are affixed to the tab. If the number 1 is red and 5 is yellow, all files with numbers ending in 15 form a red and yellow band. Usually a predetermined section of the number is color-coded.

Other Color-Coding Applications

Color can work in many other ways for the efficient medical office. Small tabs in a variety of colors can be used to identify certain types

FIGURE 14-13 With color-coding of patients' charts, a misplaced file is easily spotted. (Courtesy Bibbero Systems, Petaluma, Calif.)

of insured patients and other specific information. For example, a red tab over the edge of the folder may identify a patient on Medicaid; a blue tab may identify a Medicaid patient; a green tab may identify a workers' compensation patient; matching tabs may be attached to the insured's ledger card; research cases may be identified by a special color tab; and brightly colored labels on the outside of a patient's chart can indicate certain health conditions, such as drug allergies. In a partnership practice, a different color folder or label may identify each physician's patients. Color also can be used to differentiate dates; one color for each month or year.

The use of color in filing is limited only by the imagination. One word of caution: Every person in the facility who uses the files must know the key to the coding, and the key should also be written in the facility's policy and procedures manual.

ORGANIZATION OF FILES

Physicians find studying a disorganized history very difficult. Some systematic method must be followed in placing items in the patient folder. From the filing standpoint, it should be emphasized that when a patient record is not in actual use, it should be in only one place—the filing cabinet or on the shelf. Many precious hours can be lost searching for misplaced or lost records carelessly left unfiled (Procedure 14-8).

The patient's full name, in indexing order, should be typed on a label and the label attached to the folder tab. A strip of transparent tape can be placed on the label to prevent smudging. The patient's full name should also be typed on each sheet in the folder. Some of the types of records common to the healthcare setting, other than patient records, include health-related correspondence, general correspondence, practice management files, miscellaneous files, and tickler or follow-up files.

Health-Related Correspondence

Correspondence pertaining to patients' medical records should be filed with the case history. Other medical correspondence should be filed in a subject file.

PROCEDURE 14-8

Maintain Organization by Filing

GOAL: *To make sure various office filing systems are maintained and usable by all parties at the medical facility.*

EQUIPMENT and SUPPLIES

- Documents to be filed
- Various file folders
- Office filing systems (e.g., equipment maintenance, general office, and so on, if the facility's files are not kept in one general grouping)
- Clerical supplies

PROCEDURAL STEPS

1. Identify the correct filing system for the document. For example, equipment maintenance information may be placed in its own separate grouping of files, or it may be put in a general office filing system.
   PURPOSE: To determine the best place to put the document so that it can be easily retrieved.

2. Inspect the document to be added.
   PURPOSE: To condition, release, index, code, and/or sort the document if needed.

3. Add the document to the proper file in the correct filing system.
   PURPOSE: To make sure the forms the physician needs are available at all times.

4. Attach the document to the file permanently or according to office policy.
   PURPOSE: To keep information from falling out of the file and getting lost or misplaced.

5. Attach documents in the file with the most recent on top. Then place the record in the designated place in the filing system.
   PURPOSE: To allow easy access to the most recent data.

6. Continue the process until all documents have been filed in the filing system.

7. Consider staff needs and limitations when establishing a filing system.

General Correspondence

The physician's office operates as both a business and a professional service. Correspondence of a general nature pertaining to the operation of the office is part of the business side of the practice. Usually, a special drawer or shelf is set aside for the general correspondence. The correspondence is indexed according to subject matter or the names of the correspondents. The guides in a subject file may appear in one, two, or three positions, depending on the number of headings, subheadings, and subdivisions.

Practice Management Files

Of course, the most active financial record is the patient ledger. In facilities that still use a manual system, this is a card or vertical tray file, and the accounts are arranged alphabetically by name. At least two divisions are used: active accounts and paid accounts.

Miscellaneous Files

Papers that do not warrant an individual folder are placed in a miscellaneous folder. In that folder, all papers relating to one subject or with one correspondent are kept together in chronologic order, with the most recent on top, and then filed alphabetically with other miscellaneous material. Related materials may be stapled together. Never use paper clips for this purpose. When as many as five papers accumulate with one correspondent or subject, a separate folder should be prepared. Other business files include records of income and expenses, financial statements, income and payroll tax records, canceled checks, and insurance policies. These papers may be filed chronologically.

Tickler or Follow-Up Files

The most frequently used follow-up method is a **tickler file**, so called because it tickles the memory that something needs to be done or followed up on a particular date. The tickler file is always a chronologic arrangement. In its simplest form, it consists of notations on the daily calendar. If information, such as an x-ray report or laboratory report, is expected about a patient with an appointment to come in, the medical assistant might make a note on the calendar or tickler file a day ahead to check on whether the report has arrived.

The tickler file can be a part of a computerized medical record system or could be as simple as an e-mail sent to oneself. Many people put reminders on their cell phones using an application (app) specially designed for memos and reminders. The tickler file could also be a card file; 12 guides, one for each month, are placed at the front of the cabinet, container, or other object used to hold the folders. Notations of actions to be taken are placed behind the guides for specific days of the current month. Notations for future months are placed behind the guide for that month. To be effective, the tickler file must be checked the first thing each day.

> ### CRITICAL THINKING APPLICATION   14-8
> Susan is responsible for checking the tickler file daily. What types of documents and duties might she find inside these files?

The tickler file can be used in many ways. It is a useful reminder of recurring events, such as payments, meetings, and so forth. On the last day of each month, all the notations from behind the next month's guide are distributed among the daily numbered guides, and the guide for the month just completed is placed at the back of the file.

Transitory or Temporary File

Many papers are kept longer than necessary because no provision is made for segregating those with a limited usefulness. This situation can be prevented by having a transitory or temporary file. For example, if a medical assistant writes a letter requesting a reprint, the file copy is placed in the transitory folder. When the reprint is received, the file copy is destroyed. The transitory file is used for materials with no permanent value. The paper may be marked with a T and destroyed when the action is completed.

Temporary files also are useful when the physician sees patients who are physically transitory. For example, consider the patient who becomes ill while on vacation in New York City. She sees a physician there. However, the patient lives in Dallas and therefore is not likely to return to the physician in New York. Nevertheless, some documentation must exist that details the patient's treatment. A temporary file can be created and shredded after the state statute of limitations has expired. Some medical facilities keep all temporary or transient patient files in one expanded folder. Refer to the office policy and procedures manual to find the procedure for handling these patients' files.

CLOSING COMMENTS

Just as in every aspect of the medical profession, advances in medical records management are occurring rapidly, allowing physicians and other caregivers to perform their duties more efficiently and accurately. A medical assistant must constantly be willing to learn and to adapt to changes arising from legislation and technologic advances. Because many patients are computer literate, computers have become generally accepted as a means of recording medical information. This is a positive change, because many patients and providers were not in favor of computer-based medical records when the concept was first presented to the general public.

Patient Education

The medical assistant should always explain to the patient any paperwork the person may be required to complete or sign. Patients do not like simply to be told, "Sign here." Take the time to explain any form that needs completion or a signature so that the patient understands the reason for collecting the information and the medical staff's need to have it available.

Many forms are similar, and patients may complain about answering the same questions on multiple forms. Review and revise the forms used in the office often so that they are user friendly and nonrepetitive for the office staff and patient alike.

Patients may need reassurance that each staff member is committed to complete patient confidentiality. Always be open to answering questions about a patient's medical record.

Legal and Ethical Issues

The authority to release information from the medical record lies solely with the patient unless such a release is required by law through a subpoena. Ownership of the record often is a subject of controversy. The record belongs to the physician; the information belongs to the patient.

When a medical record is used as evidence in a court case, the person who entered information must be able to read it, no matter how long ago the entry was created.

Be sure to understand the laws governing records retention. Records should be kept through the period of the statute of limitations and possibly longer in certain situations. Take care with the medical chart, because it is the lifeline of patient care in the medical facility. When a chart is corrected, the proper method must be followed, and the record should never be obliterated (see steps 8 through 10 in Procedure 14-1).

SUMMARY OF SCENARIO

Susan looks forward to attending her medical assisting classes each day and works diligently to perform to the best of her ability in the classroom. She strives to do well on each procedure check-off and each examination she completes. Her instructors provide excellent feedback and appreciate her contributions to the class.

Susan has the attitude that everything she is allowed to do in the medical office is a learning tool. She regularly asks for additional responsibilities and is always ready to assist a co-worker. Dr. Thomas has recognized that she has the desire to learn, and he gives her many opportunities to glean more knowledge through the everyday activities in the office.

Although she is new to the medical profession, Susan learns quickly and thinks logically. She knows the rules and regulations on patient confidentiality and is always careful about the information she provides to those who request it. She is never hesitant about asking her office manager for guidance if she is unsure about any aspect of her duties. Susan is understanding and respectful when patients are concerned about their privacy. Her confidence and warm personality play a role in the trust she earns from the patients at the clinic.

Susan is willing to admit when she has made an error and has sought advice from Dr. Thomas and her office manager when an error needed correction.

Although filing is not one of her favorite duties, she can be counted on to do her best while completing this important task. She realizes that filing is critical, because the documents in the patient's medical record direct the care provided to the patient. An abnormal laboratory report that is missing can make a crucial difference in the patient's care. She takes pride in her work and is efficient and accurate where medical records are concerned. When she is faced with a task new to her, she considers it a learning experience and asks for help if she is not completely sure about the way to handle a situation.

Susan's co-workers are supportive and always willing to assist her as she learns to be the best medical assistant she can be. Her future as a professional medical assistant certainly holds opportunity and chances for advancement. Just as important, patients trust her. She has alleviated patients' concerns about electronic medical records by taking the time to explain privacy policies and exactly what information will be accessible to third parties. This trust also gives patients the confidence to reveal personal information and to know that it will be held in the strictest confidence, not just by Susan, but by each employee in the physician's office.

SUMMARY OF LEARNING OBJECTIVES

1. Define, spell, and pronounce the terms listed in the vocabulary.

Spelling and pronouncing medical terms correctly bolster the medical assistant's credibility. Knowing the definition of these terms promotes confidence in communication with patients and co-workers.

2. State several reasons accurate medical records are important.

Medical records must be accurate primarily so that the correct care can be given to the patient. The record also helps ensure continuity of care between providers so that no lapse in treatment occurs. The record serves as indication and proof in court that certain treatments and procedures were performed on the patient; therefore, it can be excellent legal support if it is well maintained and accurate. Medical records also aid researchers with statistical information.

3. Explain who owns the medical record.

The physician owns the physical medical record, but the patient owns the information contained in it.

4. Explain how to document appropriately and accurately.

All medical documentation must be correct, complete, and timely. Entries should be written in compliance with office policy and local, state, and federal law. Never obliterate any portion of the record. Re-read all entries to make certain that they are legible and that the entry makes grammatical sense (see Procedure 14-8).

5. Explain the difference between a traditional medical record and a problem-oriented medical record.

The POMR categorizes each of the patient's problems and elaborates on the findings and treatment plan for all concerns. Detailed progress notes are kept for each individual problem. This method addresses each of the patient's concerns separately, whereas a traditional record may address all problems and concerns at one time, usually covering one to three patient concerns per office visit. The POMR helps ensure that individual problems are all addressed.

6. Explain how to establish and organize a patient's medical record.

The patient's chart must be established and organized so that the components are easy to find (see Procedure 14-2). Use the data on the patient information forms to build the patient's medical record and to create a financial record. Follow office policy when creating new patient records.

7. Identify systems for organizing medical records.

Alphabetic filing is a simple, traditional filing system in which documents are filed in alphabetic order. Numeric filing systems use a number code to give order to the files. An alphanumeric system is a combination of the two.

8. Differentiate between subjective and objective information.

Very simply, subjective information is provided by the patient, whereas objective information is provided by the physician or provider. Examples of subjective information include the patient's address, Social Security number, insurance information, and description of what he or she is experiencing. Objective information is obtained through the physician's questions and observations made during the examination.

9. Describe various types of information kept in the medical record.

Both subjective and objective information are kept in the progress notes. Demographic information about the patient can be found, in addition to many types of reports, including consultations, lab reports, radiology and other imaging reports, and various types of correspondence.

10. Explain how to make additions to a medical record.

Items periodically must be added to patients' records, such as when test results arrive or new information becomes available. Determine where the document should be placed in the record, then condition, index, and code the documents, making sure that they have been released for filing. Sort them for easier filing, then place them in the correct medical record. (see Procedure 14-4).

11. Discuss correction of an entry in the patient's record.

The appropriate procedures must be followed to make corrections in a patient's chart. A single line should be drawn through the incorrect information and then initialed and dated. Some offices also require a notation of "Corr." or "Correction" on the chart. A medical assistant should never try to alter the medical record or cover up an error in charting.

12. Identify both equipment and supplies needed to file medical records.

Several types of equipment and supplies are needed to manage patients' records. A variety of shelving units and filing containers must be available. Open shelving allows maximum use of color-coded charts, which makes finding misfiles quick and easy. Many file folder styles are available, and several types of forms can be used in patients' charts. The preference of the physician and staff members who use these tools is important, as are concerns such as cost and availability. A medical assistant should be conservative when ordering supplies and purchasing equipment, ordering only the number needed to save on office supply costs.

13. Discuss filing procedures.

Some offices use an alphabetic filing system (see Procedure 14-6). Some offices use a numeric filing system (see Procedure 14-7). Review office policy to determine which system to use and the correct procedures to follow when filing documents.

14. Describe indexing rules.

Five basic steps are involved in document filing. (1) The papers are conditioned, which is the preparatory stage for filing. (2) The documents are released, which means they are ready to be filed because they have been reviewed or read and some type of mark has been placed on the document to indicate this. (3) The documents are indexed, which involves deciding where each document should be filed and coding it with some type of mark on the paper indicating that decision. (4) Sorting involves placing the files in filing sequence. (5) The actual filing and storing of the documents is the last step.

15. Discuss the pros and cons of various filing methods.

Both the alphabetic and numeric filing systems have advantages and disadvantages. Perhaps most important is the staff's preference. Some find it easier to retrieve files that are in standard alphabetic order, whereas others prefer a numeric system. The numeric system is more confidential than an alphabetic system. Some staff members prefer a combination of the two, the alphanumeric system. Both effectively keep medical records in good order and allow the medical assistant to spot a misfiled record quickly.

16. **Identify types of records common to the healthcare setting.**
Medical offices keep numerous files on hand for the administration and business aspects. For example, maintenance and supply records, personnel and human resources records, and budget and bill-paying records all are examples of files that help the staff conduct the facility's business. Some offices keep several different filing systems according to subject, whereas others keep one comprehensive system. The facility should use whatever system most benefits the employees and allows the fastest retrieval of files.

CONNECTIONS

📖 **Study Guide Connection:** Go to the Chapter 14 Study Guide. Read and complete the activities.

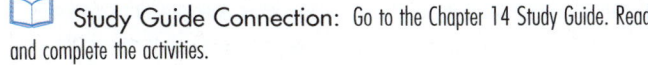 **Evolve Connection:** Go to the Chapter 14 link at *evolve.elsevier.com/kinn* to complete the Chapter Review and Chapter Quiz. Check out the other resources listed for this chapter to make the most of what you have learned from The Paper Medical Record.

15

THE ELECTRONIC MEDICAL RECORD

Sloan Swarten was hired as a medical assistant at the Southwest Family Medical Clinic in Tempe, Arizona, in October. Dr. Adkins and Dr. Brooks opened the practice 2 years ago. The clinic is fully electronic; no paper records are used at all. Sloan is more interested in the clinical aspect of medical assisting, but because she waited 6 months after finishing school to start looking for work, she had a difficult time finding a job. She accepted the position in medical records at Southwest, known to be a sizeable, busy practice, in the hope that she could soon transfer to the clinical side. Her supervisor, Jennifer Sanchez, stressed that the only available position was in the medical records department, but she also said she would consider moving Sloan to the clinical side after a few months if she performed well and if it proved to be a beneficial move for the clinic.

Sloan does not particularly like the medical records department, and she spends her breaks and lunch periods with the clinical medical assistants. She often remarks that she really would like to work on the clinical side. Sloan is computer literate, but she did not take the administrative classes at school very seriously, because she planned to do clinical work. Her probation period is 6 weeks, and she has decided to make the best of the medical records job until she is transferred. Sloan works with Alex, who supervises the electronic medical records aspect of the clinic. Since most of her previous experience was working with paper records, Alex had to learn the entire program when Southwest opened, and she has enjoyed becoming an expert, or **superuser**, on the system. Alex likes to learn new things and is able to find solutions to records issues quickly and efficiently. Sloan and Alex get along well, although Alex is concerned that Sloan doesn't really want to learn the electronic systems.

While studying this chapter, think about the following questions:

- Do you believe Sloan will make it to the clinical side of the office?
- Why is the medical records department one of the most important areas of the physician's office?
- From the information given in this scenario, what mistakes has Sloan already made, if any?
- Why is it important to know both administrative and clinical skills in the physician's office?

LEARNING OBJECTIVES

1. Define, spell, and pronounce the terms listed in the vocabulary.
2. Discuss the presidential Executive Order that led to the implementation of electronic medical record systems across the nation.
3. Discuss the principles of using the electronic medical record (EMR).
4. Distinguish between an electronic health record (EHR) and an electronic medical record (EMR).
5. Explain how the American Recovery and Reinvestment Act applies to the healthcare industry.
6. Define meaningful use.
7. List the three main components of meaningful use legislation.
8. Discuss the advantages and disadvantages of an electronic medical record system.
9. Explore the capabilities of an electronic medical record system.
10. Give several reasons patients are hesitant in accepting electronic health records.
11. Discuss the importance of nonverbal communication with patients when an EMR system is used.
12. Summarize the goals of the Nationwide Health Information Network (NHIN).
13. List the core capabilities of the NHIN.
14. Summarize the role of the medical assistant with regard to the changing technology in healthcare facilities and organizations.

VOCABULARY

alleviate To partly remove or correct; to relieve or lessen.

computerized physician/provider order entry (CPOE) A process of electronic data entry of medical practitioner or provider instructions for the treatment of patients.

culpability Meriting condemnation, responsibility, or blame, especially as wrong or harmful.

e-prescribing The use of electronic devices to communicate with pharmacies and send prescribing information, taking the place of writing a prescription by hand and physically giving it to a patient; new or refill prescriptions can be submitted electronically, cutting down on fraud and errors.

electronic health record (EHR) An electronic record of health-related information about a patient that conforms to nationally recognized interoperability standards and that can be created, managed, and consulted by authorized clinicians and staff from *more than one healthcare organization.*

electronic medical record (EMR) An electronic record of health-related information about an individual that can be created, gathered, managed, and consulted by authorized clinicians and staff *within a single healthcare organization.*

interoperable The capability of a system to work with or use the parts or equipment of another system.

parameters Any set of physical properties, the values of which determine characteristics or behavior.

personal health record (PHR) An electronic record of health-related information about an individual that conforms to nationally recognized interoperability standards and that *can be drawn from multiple sources but that is managed, shared, and controlled by the individual.*

prevalent Generally or widely accepted, favored, or practiced.

reasonable cause Circumstances that would make it unreasonable for the covered entity, despite the exercise of ordinary business care and prudence, to comply with the administrative simplification provision that was violated.

reasonable diligence The business care and prudence expected from a person seeking to satisfy a legal requirement under similar circumstances.

superuser A special account on a computer system that is used for system administration; also, a person in a facility who is able to make system-wide changes to a computer system.

willful neglect Conscious, intentional failure or reckless indifference to the obligation to comply with the administrative simplification provision violated.

With technology advancing at such a rapid pace, it is no surprise that the number of offices using an electronic medical record (EMR) system is growing steadily. Some physicians may not budge and will never change to electronic health records. However, because more and more hospitals are using electronic records, physicians, medical assistants, and other healthcare professionals must learn to communicate electronically about patients and to originate information by electronic means. For those who have worked in the healthcare industry for some time, this may present a challenge; however, today's medical students are being trained in the use of the EMR as a standard practice. In the not too distant future, the EMR will be the standard, and paper medical records will be much less common.

EXECUTIVE ORDER TO PROMOTE INTEROPERABILITY OF EMR SYSTEMS

On August 22, 2006, President George W. Bush issued an Executive Order designed to promote the interoperability of health records and the overall quality and efficiency of healthcare. He set a goal of establishing electronic health records for most Americans by 2014. The order took effect on January 1, 2007. It listed five requirements:

1. The agencies involved will implement **interoperable** systems as their current systems are upgraded (e.g., Centers for Medicare and Medicaid Services [CMS]).
2. Providers (e.g., a regional Veterans Affairs Hospital) and payers with whom the agencies do business also will implement interoperable systems as their current systems are upgraded. In other words, a hospital that receives federal funding, such as Medicare, must adopt electronic health record systems.
3. The prices paid by health insurance issuers will be available both to beneficiaries and enrollees in the health plan.
4. The agencies and providers will participate in the development of information about the overall cost of healthcare services and treatments.
5. The agencies and providers will develop and identify, for beneficiaries, enrollees, and providers, approaches that encourage the provision and receipt of high-quality, efficient healthcare.

An interoperable system sounds complicated; however, it simply is a system that is able to work with another system. For example, a physician could use his office EMR system to access the EMR system of a hospital to check the hospital's records on his patients. Although the language of the presidential order is complex and the technologic features such systems require are overwhelming to most medical assistants, keep the end goal in mind—providing high-quality, efficient care to patients.

The EMR is becoming the healthcare facility's most important business and legal record. The legal requirements are more intricate than those for a paper medical record. Just as a paper medical record is considered a legal record in court, so is the EMR.

TECHNOLOGIC TERMS IN HEALTH INFORMATION

Some confusion has arisen regarding the acronyms *EMR* and *EHR*. The National Alliance for Health Information Technology (NAHIT) identified 18 to 63 definitions for the five main terms that relate to the electronic medical record. To **alleviate** the confusion, NAHIT has established definitions for EMR and EHR that are easy to understand. The **electronic health record (EHR)** is an electronic record of health-related information about a patient that conforms to nationally recognized interoperability standards and that can be created, managed, and consulted by authorized clinicians and staff from *more than one healthcare organization.* The **electronic medical record (EMR)** is an electronic record of health-related information about an individual that can be created, gathered, managed, and consulted by authorized clinicians and staff *within a single healthcare organization.*

A **personal health record (PHR)** is defined by the NAHIT as an electronic record of health-related information about an individual that conforms to nationally recognized interoperability standards and that can be drawn from multiple sources but that is managed, shared, and controlled by the individual. Few PHRs currently exist, and most Americans do not know what a PHR is or how it can be of value to them.

The Health Insurance Portability and Accountability Act (HIPAA) uses the term *protected health information* (PHI), which is any information about health status, the provision of healthcare, or payment for healthcare that can be linked to an individual patient.

For the purposes of this chapter, *EMR* refers to the electronic system the physician uses in the ambulatory setting, because it is used within a single healthcare organization. To help yourself understand the difference between the EMR and the EHR, consider this scenario: If the Southwest Family Medical Clinic uses an EMR, their records are in electronic form, but the records are available electronically only inside the office or to staff members who log on to the system remotely. If the clinic were using an EHR, the physicians and staff would be able to see not only records generated in their clinic, but also records on their patients created at multiple other healthcare facilities, such as the local hospital, a regional imaging facility, or a freestanding laboratory. The clinic would have an interoperable access to the records created at other facilities. Healthcare professionals envision that the EHR eventually will provide a patient's medical records from birth to death.

In "Defining Key Health Information Technology Terms," a report published in 2008, NAHIT acknowledged the need to define three additional vital terms: health information exchange, health information organization, and regional health information organization. *Health information exchange* is the electronic movement of health-related information among organizations according to nationally recognized standards. *Health information organization* is an organization that oversees and governs the exchange of health-related information among organizations according to nationally recognized standards. A *regional health information organization* is a health organization that brings together healthcare stakeholders in a defined geographic area and governs health information exchange among them for the purpose of improving health and care in that community. The report stated that as multiple groups grappled with how to achieve the president's vision, these terms emerged to characterize some of the key building blocks of the envisioned health technologic infrastructure: electronic medical records and/or electronic health records for healthcare professionals; personal health records for individuals and healthcare consumers, and electronic health information exchange to enable efficient communication among these various records.

AMERICAN RECOVERY AND REINVESTMENT ACT (ARRA)

The American Recovery and Reinvestment Act of 2009 (ARRA), commonly known as the Economic Stimulus Package, was passed to promote economic recovery. This legislation was signed into law by President Barack Obama on February 17, 2009. The health information technology aspects of the bill provide slightly more than $31 billion for healthcare infrastructure and EHR investment. The sections of the ARRA that pertain to healthcare are collectively known as the Health Information Technology for Economic and Clinical Health Act, or HITECH Act.

HITECH ACT AND MEANINGFUL USE

The HITECH Act provides financial incentives for the meaningful use of certified EHR technology to achieve health and efficiency goals. It was incorporated into the ARRA to promote the adoption and meaningful use of health information technology. Remember, HIPAA was created in large part to simplify administrative processes using electronic devices. *Meaningful use,* defined simply, means that providers must show that they are using EHR technology in ways that can be measured significantly in quality and quantity. If providers meet the meaningful use requirements, they will qualify for incentive payments. Three main components of meaningful use can be identified, including:

- Use of certified EHR in a meaningful manner, such as **e-prescribing**
- Use of certified EHR technology for electronic exchange of health information to improve the quality of health care
- Use of certified EHR technology to submit clinical quality reports, procedure and diagnosis codes, surveys, and other measures

Criteria for meaningful use will be implemented in three stages:

- Stage 1 (2011 and 2012): Sets the baseline for electronic data capture and information sharing
- Stage 2 (expected to be implemented in 2013): Continues to expand on the baseline
- Stage 3 (expected to be implemented in 2015): Continues to expand on the baseline and will be further developed through future rule making

In Subtitle D of the HITECH Act, privacy and security concerns related to the electronic submission of health information are addressed. Several provisions strengthen the civil and criminal penalties of the HIPAA rules, most of which became effective in February, 2009. More of the provisions will become effective over the next few years, subject to future lawmaking.

Included in the February, 2009, modifications of HIPAA were:

- Establishment of categories of violations that reflect increasing levels of **culpability**
- Requirements that penalties be determined based on the nature and extent of the violation and the nature and extent of the harm resulting from the violation
- Establishment of tiers of increasing penalty amounts that determine the range of and authority to impose civil monetary penalties (Table 15-1)

TABLE 15-1 Categories of HIPAA Violations and Associated Penalties

CATEGORY: SECTION 1176(A)(1)	EACH VIOLATION	ALL SUCH VIOLATIONS OF AN IDENTICAL PROVISION IN A CALENDAR YEAR
(A) Did not know	$100 to $50,000	$1.5 million
(B) Reasonable cause	$1,000 to $50,000	$1.5 million
(C) (i) Willful neglect—corrected	$10,000 to $50,000	$1.5 million
(C) (ii) Willful neglect—not corrected	$50,000	$1.5 million

As indicated in Table 15-1, minimum and maximum penalty amounts are established and can be assessed by the Department of Health and Human Services (DHHS), depending on the nature of the violation. The DHHS determines the penalties on a case-by-case basis and may provide or continue to provide a waiver for violations that arise from a **reasonable cause** and are not **willful neglect** incidents that are not corrected in a timely manner. The DHHS will also consider whether the covered entity has provided **reasonable diligence** in its attempts to bring the facility into compliance with the law. Physicians can expect reductions in the amounts they are paid from Medicare and Medicaid if they are not in compliance by 2015. Remember, the computer system in the medical office must be more than a tool for data recall to be considered an EMR system; the physician must use the system for tasks, at a minimum, such as e-prescribing and **computerized physician/provider order entry (CPOE)**.

ADVANTAGES AND DISADVANTAGES OF THE EMR

According to a 2010 mail survey of 10,301 physicians done by the Centers for Disease Control and Prevention (CDC), 50.7% of physicians in office-based practices use full or partial EMR systems. The use of EMR systems in physicians' offices increased steadily from 2001 through 2010. The primary reason physicians have not yet adopted an EMR system is the expense. Other reasons include:

- Inability to find an EMR system that meets the practice's needs
- Uncertainty about a return on investment
- Physician resistance
- Loss of productivity or down time for installation and learning curve

The EMR has several advantages over a paper medical record. Most experts agree that the EMR can reduce medical errors by keeping prescriptions, allergies, and other information organized; it also can reduce costs by preventing duplicate tests. Staffing needs also may be reduced, because fewer personnel are needed to manage an EMR system. Because a computer keyboard is used to enter information into the record, the record is not nearly as likely to be illegible. Typed copy certainly is easier to read than handwriting, even if the record is several years old. EMR systems require individual user names and passwords, which secure the system from unauthorized users.

Compared to walls and file cabinets full of paper medical records, the EMR requires less storage space. One or two external hard drives with a terabyte of disk space each conceivably could hold all the medical records of all patients throughout the life of a physician's practice. This would eliminate the need to purge inactive files, and the resulting space requirement for the external hard drive may be no bigger than a large shoebox. The files may be duplicated regularly and placed off site as a backup.

Information can be accessed in a variety of locations, and more than one person can see the record at any given time. The patient database usually allows various types of statistical information to be recalled, which is a valuable tool. Patient information is available quickly in an emergency, even when the patient is not in his or her hometown. The physician and medical assistants can access progress notes, test results, and any other information about the patient, including patient education and appointment no-shows. The physician and medical assistants can access patient information using a smart phone or personal digital assistant (PDA).

Once the physician and staff become familiar with the system, they may find that they are able to see more patients in the course of a day than when paper records were used. All these advantages lead to cost savings and more efficient patient care.

However, the EMR system is not without disadvantages. Studies show that lack of capital is the most significant obstacle to adoption of the system; another stumbling block is the reluctance of employees in physicians' offices to make such substantial changes and to learn a new computer system. Employees may not be the only individuals resistant to a changeover to electronic records; patients often are fearful that their private health information will be available to unauthorized individuals, and they often assume that their records will be posted on the Internet. The startup costs of conversion to an EMR system usually are quite high, although most physicians realize that the system eventually will be worth the cost. "The Financial and Nonfinancial Costs of Implementing Electronic Health Records in Primary Care Practices," an article in the online journal *Health Affairs,* suggests that the startup cost for a five-physician practice is approximately $162,000, with $85,500 going toward maintenance costs during the first year (Fleming et al., 2011). The study also suggested that the implementation team would need an average of 611 hours to prepare for the implementation, and end-users, such as the physicians, medical assistants, and other staff members, would need about 134 hours of training to use the system. Both the physician and staff require extensive training in the EMR system and must be receptive to even more training to use the system to its full capacity. Training is time-consuming and takes the physician and staff away from treating patients for certain periods. Because not all computer systems are user friendly, care must be taken to choose a system that has technologic support, both live and online, that is available during the hours the healthcare facility is operating. Space for the equipment can be an issue, although usually less space is required than for a paper record system. Because healthcare facilities use different sets of abbreviations and terms, issues can arise with interaction of the office system with other systems. Finally, security and confidentiality are major concerns of both the healthcare professionals and the patients.

SUCCESSFUL CONVERSION TO AN EMR SYSTEM

- Get the entire facility "on board" with the change.
- Provide leadership to the staff.
- Encourage and praise the staff's hard work in making the conversion successful.
- As a medical assistant, be loyal and promote loyalty to the facility during the change.
- Use good people management skills, especially with those who are against the conversion. Many people who were initially averse to conversions later say they do not know how they ever worked without the EMR.
- Always give patients, visitors, and co-workers excellent customer service.
- Work as a team with other staff members.
- Use every employee's strong qualities where they are needed.
- Be willing to venture into a new system and keep a positive attitude.
- Remember that if medicine is anything, it is constant change.

CRITICAL THINKING APPLICATION   15-1

Some of the patients who visit Dr. Adkins and Dr. Brooks have expressed concern that electronic medical records may not be private enough and that their health information will be "floating around on the Internet." They are worried that unauthorized individuals could somehow access their information on the computer and do them harm.

- How might Sloan alleviate the patients' fears about their records being available on the Internet to so many people?
- What disadvantages with regard to confidentiality are associated with the EMR?
- Should a patient be allowed to decide whether his or her records will be kept on computer or on paper?

INCENTIVES FOR IMPLEMENTING EMR SYSTEMS

As mentioned earlier, the CMS has established an incentive program for health facilities that is based upon three specific stages and a set of objectives the facility must meet to receive the incentive payment. The incentive program includes stages and objectives with associated measures for determining whether the facility has met the objective. Stage 1 began in 2011, and Stages 2 and 3 will take effect in 2013 and 2015, respectively. To meet the requirements of Stage 1, Meaningful Use, eligible professionals must complete 15 core objectives, 5 of 10 objectives from the menu set, and 6 total clinical quality measures.

CAPABILITIES OF EMR SYSTEMS

The EMR system (also sometimes called a *practice management system*) can perform a multitude of tasks, saving time and money in the physician's office (Figure 15-1). As these systems become more

prevalent and technology advances, these capabilities will multiply. The following are some of the features of a typical EMR system.

- **Specialty software.** Patient data are captured and processed into a system that is specialty-specific, so that the terminology and patient care treatments are compatible with the physician's specialty. However, additional features can allow the physician to include terminology from other specialties.
- **Appointment scheduler.** The appointment scheduler allows the staff to track and schedule appointments, matrix the schedule, and account for recurring time blocks (Figure 15-2). The appointments can be merged into specific types with default times so that lengthy procedures are not scheduled in short appointment blocks. The scheduler features also allow various search **parameters**; if a patient calls because he or she cannot remember the appointment time, a search can be initiated using the date, physician's name, patient's name, or other search keywords.
- **Appointment reminder and confirmation.** The system can be programmed to initiate automatic reminder or confirmation calls to patients. The staff can record the reminders, and patients are prompted to choose options, such as "Press one," to confirm or reschedule appointments.
- **Prescription writer.** The EMR system can produce electronic prescriptions, which can be printed and given to patients or automatically submitted to a pharmacy. Lists can be created with the physician's most common drug choices and dosages. A patient allergies function can block the prescription of drugs the patient cannot take, and the system can generate a patient information sheet on new prescriptions.
- **Medical billing system.** The EMR billing system can manage all of the practice's billing and accounting systems. The system also can interface with clearinghouses for electronic claims submission and tracking. Reports can be generated that provide accurate details of the financial state of the practice at certain intervals or whenever requested.
- **Charge capture.** The charge capture functions can store lists of billing codes (e.g., International Classification of Diseases [ICD] and Current Procedural Terminology [CPT]) in addition to charges associated with procedures, supplies, and laboratory tests. Evaluation and Management (E/M) codes are used during office visits to obtain the highest possible reimbursement; these help the physician maximize profits while remaining in compliance with the law. Alerts can let the user know when a certain charge does not match a diagnosis code; for instance, a male patient would not undergo a gynecologic exam. In such cases, the software alerts the user and helps prevent errors that can lead to denial of insurance claims.
- **Eligibility verification.** EMR billing systems can perform online verification of insurance eligibility and can capture demographic data.
- **Referral management.** Current and referring physicians can be coordinated and automated, allowing the physician to share patient information with another physician. This reduces the patient's physical effort of transporting copies of records back and forth to referring physicians, eliminates the costs of such copies, and is faster and more efficient than copying and mailing patient records.

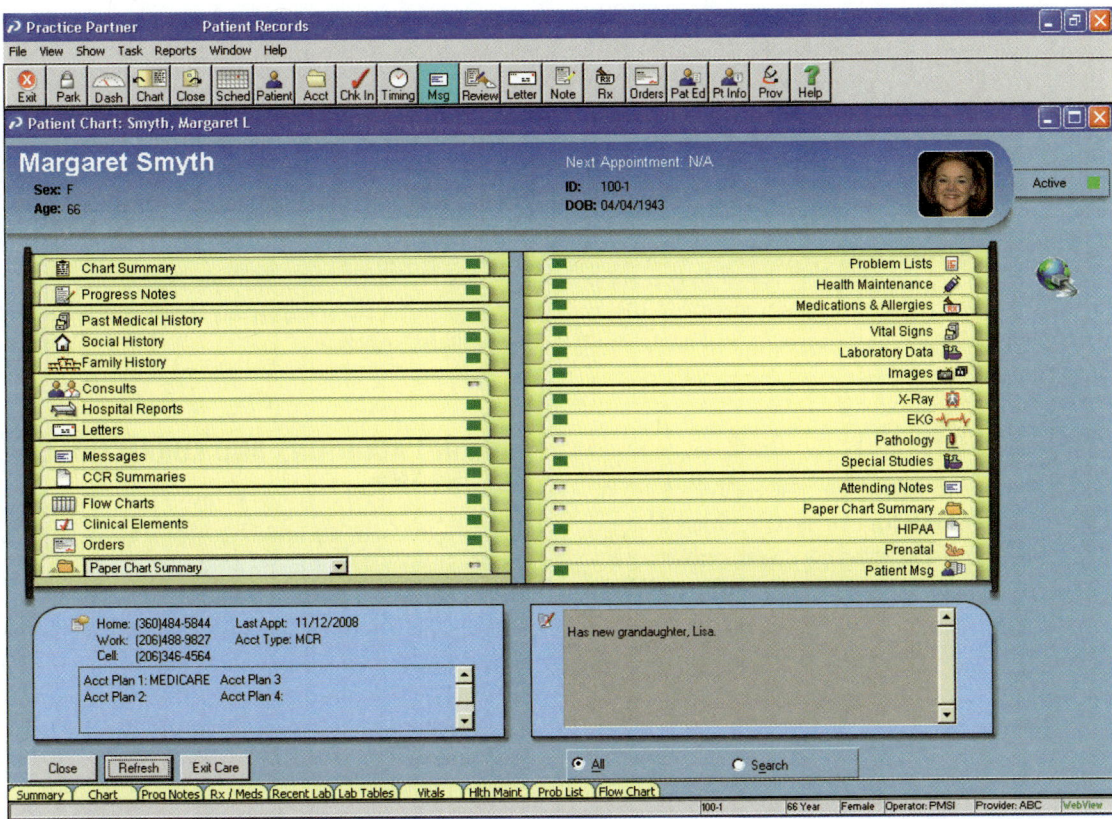

FIGURE 15-1 The electronic medical record (EMR) can perform numerous tasks in addition to displaying personal information about the patient. This allows the physician and medical assistants to interact with patients and provide better service. (Courtesy McKessan Corp., Alpharetta, Ga.)

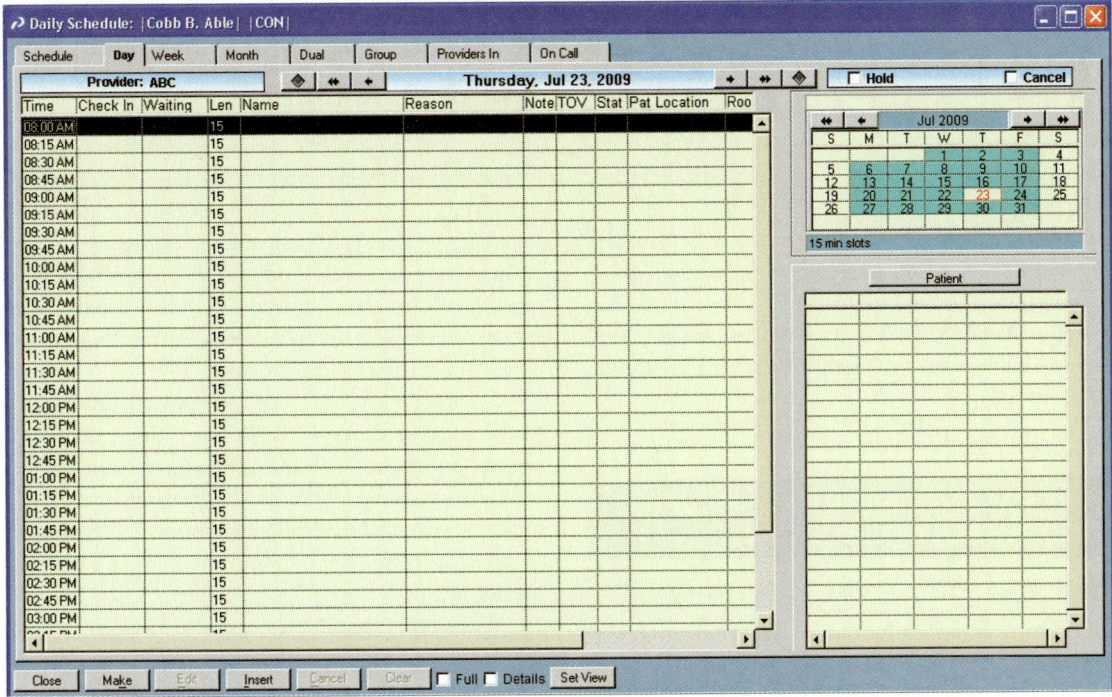

FIGURE 15-2 The EMR usually has a scheduling system that can be changed to manage the needs of the physician and office staff. (Courtesy McKessan Corp., Alpharetta, Ga.)

- **Laboratory order integration.** The laboratory order integration feature allows the user to interact with outside laboratories and to receive and post laboratory results to patients' records. Tests can be ordered from the physician's laptop, PDA, or smart phone. Results can be transmitted by fax, scan, or e-mail and uploaded directly into the patient's record.
- **Patient portal.** User-friendly patient portals can be added to the system that allow the patient to access medical records and perform other functions, such as setting an appointment, printing a child's immunization record, reviewing a statement, checking whether insurance has paid on the account, and completing new patient records online.

CRITICAL THINKING APPLICATION   15-2

Jennifer, the office manager, has noticed that Sloan seems frustrated in the training classes for the EMR system used by the clinic. During a break, Jennifer asks Sloan whether she is having any specific problems with the training classes. She also asks for Sloan's input on the system. Sloan says that she just prefers clinical work and that her typing skills are a little "rusty."
- How might Jennifer respond to Sloan's comments?
- Why might this be a warning sign that Sloan will not be a good match for the clinical side of the practice?

PATIENTS' CONCERNS ABOUT THE EMR

Patients worry about the security of their information, particularly about who can access it. Lawsuits often are filed when patients discover that an unauthorized person has accessed their protected health information. The medical assistant should listen to a patient's concerns and explain the safety procedures that apply to the EMR in language the patient can understand. Some facilities prepare a brochure to explain the conversion process to the patient and the advantages of the EMR system.

The medical assistant should expect hesitation and even reluctance from patients who are concerned about the privacy of their health information. Patients are concerned about lack of control over who views their records. Be prepared to answer their questions about the safety of their records as related to the EMR. The medical assistant must know how the EMR is protected and what security measures are in place to be able to reassure the patients that their records are protected at all times.

REASSURING PATIENTS ABOUT THE SECURITY AND CONFIDENTIALITY OF THE EMR

- Explain the conversion before the office changes and during the conversion.
- Never display a negative attitude about the change to an electronic medical record system; patients tend to reflect the attitude you show them.
- Prepare a pamphlet explaining the processes that will change in your particular office with use of the EMR.

- Take a moment to show the patient a little about the software once it has been implemented (using only their record). Most patients are interested in and perhaps even amazed by what the EMR can accomplish. Show the individual the log-in process (without revealing passwords) to reassure him or her that access to records is private and secure.
- Explain the records backup process to help alleviate patients' fears that their health information may be lost.
- Explain the office access policy regarding who can access and view patients' records.

MAKING ADDITIONS AND CORRECTIONS TO THE EMR

Additions to electronic health records must be made by making an additional entry. Never delete a previous entry or change it unless it is in the process of being entered. A good rule of thumb is to avoid changing any electronic entry after the initials of the maker have been added. This, of course, should take place immediately after the note is placed in the record. Once this has happened, a new entry must be made to correct information in a previous entry. Some EMR programs do not allow any changes to the record; in this case, the user must create a new entry to make corrections or add notes. Virtually all EMR systems place a date and time stamp on entries and log which employee has entered the record. This method also prevents another user from changing a record previously entered. Never share passwords to the EMR system with other employees; in some facilities, password infractions are grounds for immediate termination of employment.

NONVERBAL COMMUNICATION WITH THE PATIENT WHEN USING THE EMR

Although many patients are covered under a type of insurance that requires them to choose a primary care provider (PCP) and to have a referral to a specialist, remember that the patient has the option of changing that PCP or specialist, usually by making a phone call or sending a fax. Even if the change process takes a little longer, the patient still has the right to make a change. The patient may decide to change providers simply because he or she does not feel comfortable with that particular provider.

Because the change process is relatively easy, the physician wants to keep his or her patients (in most cases), because losing patients means loss of income. If the care begins to seem impersonal, patients may feel a strong desire to change providers, even though most offices and providers are moving toward an EMR system. Remember, patients are consumers of healthcare services, and they expect quality healthcare.

When using the EMR, the medical assistant must make sure his or her nonverbal communication sends the right message to the patient. Eye contact is absolutely essential (Figure 15-3). If the medical assistant constantly looks at the computer screen, the patient feels quite alienated from the information exchange process. Do not insinuate by physical action that the EMR is a "hidden entity"; for example, do not necessarily shield the computer screen from the patient's view when entering information. Although patients may not understand anything they see on the screen, they will feel more at ease if their information is not hidden from them. Also, modify your stance so that the patient feels like a part of the information process. Just as sitting in a chair across from a supervisor's desk can be intimidating, the patient may feel the same emotions sitting across from a medical assistant entering information into the EMR.

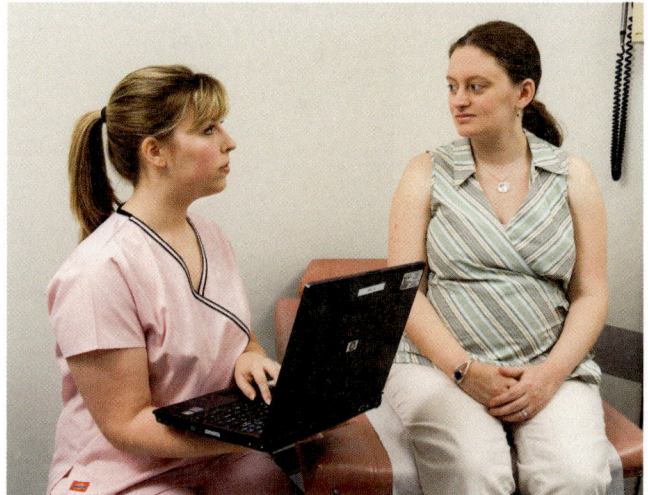

FIGURE 15-3 The medical assistant must make eye contact with the patient when using an EMR.

Take an open stance; sit next to or at an angle to the patient to support the impression that those in the healthcare facility and the patient are partners in the healthcare plan.

Remember that patients deserve to choose in most aspects of their healthcare plans; therefore, offer choices wherever possible. Never expect patients to make quick decisions about their care. They may want to consult family members or give some thought to important medical decisions. The medical assistant needs to promote time to think unless the patient is faced with a critical, time-sensitive decision. Physicians often assume that patients will automatically follow their instructions or orders; however, some patients prefer some time to think. Always follow up and make note of any wait time the patient requests, notify the physician, and enter that information into the EMR (Procedure 15-1). Make sure timely communication is kept with the patient and that any additional orders that need to be put in place are completed. The many features of the EMR allow the medical assistant to be efficient and highly competent if he or she is willing to make an extra effort to master the EMR system.

Also make sure patients understand all instructions given to them regarding test procedures or preparation for procedures. Most EMRs can print an instruction sheet, which the medical assistant can review with the patient. The customer service aspect of patient care is even more important when the facility uses an EMR system. Chapter 26 presents more customer service tips for the medical office.

PROCEDURE 15-1

Execute Data Management Using Electronic Healthcare Records such as the EMR

GOAL: *To obtain and enter patient data using the electronic health record (EHR) and/or electronic medical record (EMR).*

EQUIPMENT and SUPPLIES

- Patient's medical records
- Data to be included in medical records
- Computer

PROCEDURAL STEPS

1. Take a laptop computer or handheld device into the treatment room with the patient.
2. Welcome the patient warmly, maintaining eye contact.
   <u>PURPOSE:</u> To interact with the patient before opening the computer; the computer cannot become a barrier that blocks interpersonal interaction between the medical assistant and the patient.
3. Place the laptop on a secure, flat surface and open the patient's record. Do not place the device on a flimsy stand or try to operate it while holding the unit.
   <u>PURPOSE:</u> To avoid dropping and damaging the computer.
4. Stand so that the computer is more to the side rather than placed between you and the patient.
   <u>PURPOSE:</u> To keep the computer from becoming a barrier between patient and medical assistant.
5. Verify the patient's basic demographics (e.g., mailing address and phone number).

   <u>PURPOSE:</u> To make sure the computer has the most recent data needed to contact the patient.
6. Discuss the reason for the patient's visit to the office.
   <u>PURPOSE:</u> To record the chief complaint.
7. Enter data offered by the patient into the EMR. Follow office policy guidelines and enter the data as directed by the EMR instructional materials.
   <u>PURPOSE:</u> To comply with office policy and to enter data in the correct format.
8. Continue to maintain eye contact with the patient; do not constantly look down at the keyboard while entering data.
   <u>PURPOSE:</u> To maintain the human connection with the patient, so that the computer does not become a deterrent to interaction with the patient.
9. Use the proper technique for entering patient data (e.g. SOAP, CHEDDAR).
   <u>PURPOSE:</u> To follow the method of charting used in the facility.
10. After entering pertinent data, ask the patient whether he or she has any additional information or questions for the physician.
    <u>PURPOSE:</u> To make sure the data are complete and to document questions for the physician's attention.

11. Briefly read back to the patient the data about the chief complaint and symptoms.
    PURPOSE: To make sure all pertinent data have been entered and that the patient's explanations of symptoms and other issues were understood.
12. If data such as paper reports need to be entered, scan them into the computer and save them in the patient's EMR.
13. Electronically sign all entries.
    PURPOSE: To document who entered data into the record.

14. Save the data as indicated by the office policies and procedures manual and the EMR user manual.
    PURPOSE: To ensure that the data entered are retained in the EMR.
15. Follow the process specified in the EMR user manual for closing the EMR program and shutting off the computer.
    PURPOSE: To comply with instructions and to guard against loss of patient data.

CRITICAL THINKING APPLICATION   15-3

Jennifer walks behind Sloan's desk and notices that she is looking at the progress notes on a patient who was recently arrested and indicted for child abuse. The case has been in the newspaper and on television consistently for several weeks. Jennifer asks Sloan why she has accessed that record. Sloan hesitates and then says she must have entered the wrong patient ID number.
- Does Sloan's explanation sound convincing?
- Why is Jennifer concerned about Sloan looking at the patient's record?
- Just because the individual is a patient at the clinic, does that mean any employee has the right to look at the patient's EMR?

THE NATIONWIDE HEALTH INFORMATION NETWORK

The Nationwide Health Information Network (NHIN) was developed to provide a secure, national, interoperable health information infrastructure that will connect providers, consumers, and others involved in supporting healthcare. The organization is a critical part of the national information technology agenda. It will enable health information to follow the consumer, making it available for clinical decision making, and support appropriate use of healthcare information beyond direct patient care, so as to improve health. The goals of the organization are to:

- Develop capabilities for standards-based, secure data exchange nationwide
- Improve the coordination of care information among hospitals, laboratories, physicians' offices, pharmacies, and other providers
- Ensure that appropriate information is available at the time and place of care
- Ensure that consumers' health information is secure and confidential
- Give consumers new capabilities for managing and controlling their personal health records and provide access to their health information from electronic health records and other sources
- Reduce risks from medical errors and support the delivery of appropriate, evidence-based medical care
- Lower healthcare costs resulting from inefficiencies, medical errors, and incomplete patient information

NHIN has several core capabilities, including:
- Finding and retrieving healthcare information within and between health information exchanges and other organizations
- Delivering a summarized patient record to support patient care and the patient's health
- Supporting consumers' preferences regarding the exchange of their information, including the ability to choose not to participate in the NHIN
- Supporting secure information exchange
- Supporting a common trust agreement that establishes the obligations and assurances to which all NHIN participants agree; also, providing the ability to match patients to their data without a national patient identifier
- Supporting harmonized standards developed by voluntary consensus standards bodies for the exchange of health information among all such entities and networks

BACKUP SYSTEMS FOR THE EMR

Even the best or most expensive EMR system cannot function without power. If a natural disaster occurs and the physician's office is without electricity for several days or weeks, the physician must have a backup system for the EMR so that the office can function. HIPAA requires that the facility adopt a backup and recovery plan that includes daily off-site software backup for the EMR system. Several alternatives can be used for data preservation and backup.

- *External hard drive.* An external hard drive connects to the main computer and with fairly simple programming can copy the information in the EMR daily. Seven folders, one for each day of the week, can hold the information from the previous day; these folders are replaced with new, updated information at designated periods. CDs and DVDs can hold daily data, and some thumb drives have enough capacity to perform this task. Once a habit of a daily backup to the external hard drive has been established, the method is relatively simple and reliable.
- *Full server backup.* The physician may want to back up the EMR system on a dedicated server, which is a large-capacity computer set aside specifically for the EMR system. With these servers, a full backup should be performed monthly. Many large medical facilities and hospitals have one or more dedicated servers for the EMR system.

- *Online backup systems.* An online backup system can be used, usually for a subscription fee. Although the cost may be higher than for some other methods, online systems are easy to use, because there is no external drive to carry and no CD or thumb drive to put through the process of downloading data. However, a time investment is involved, because the process of contacting the company that offers the service and then downloading all the data takes several hours. Also, the initial download can take quite a while. Even so, an online system is very stable and reliable.

All these backup methods require an alternative power source in case of a disaster that interrupts electricity. Remember that backup systems are not effective if the data are stored at the medical facility, and the disaster happens at or affects that physical address. Information technology professionals usually recommend using two of these three methods for the best protection. The system must be protected from theft and unauthorized use, just as is the on-site system.

Medical assistants should keep their paper medical records skills sharp in case the EMR system is down for an extended period. Always have supplies available for alternative use in such instances.

THE MEDICAL ASSISTANT AND THE EMR

Once the medical assistant has trained on the EMR system and has had the opportunity to use it for a time, daily use should become second nature. In fact, it may be difficult to imagine a workday without the system! By being open to change and willing to learn, the medical assistant can set a good example for all employees and will be more receptive to the process of change. Be encouraging to other staff members while training on the system, and if technology comes easily to you, share your knowledge with others and assist wherever possible. Do not expect to master the system in a week; instead, realize that a new system has a learning curve and be patient with and receptive to the educational process. Keep technical support phone numbers handy and feel free to use them whenever a new or complicated issue arises. Work as a team, and if possible, help others who might find learning the system more of a struggle. Above all, while getting used to the new technology, make sure your attitude is one of enthusiasm, interest, and curiosity.

CLOSING COMMENTS

A primary goal of all healthcare facilities is to provide efficient, high-quality patient care. The EMR system can help the staff reach that goal. In the future, every physician's office, hospital, pharmacy, and other healthcare facilities may be able to access information in minutes, which will improve patient care and save lives. Stay abreast of news and articles related to EMR systems. Remember, the healthcare industry is one of constant growth and learning, and today's information technology provides the medical assistant with endless opportunities to make that growth personal and rewarding.

Patient Education

When educating patients about the EMR system, allow them to watch as their information is entered into the computer. Showing patients just a few of the system's capabilities may reassure them of its efficiency and possibilities. Always maintain eye contact with patients whose information is being entered into the computer. Physicians and medical assistants alike may have to relearn how to interact with patients in a natural way while using the laptop or PDA in the examination rooms. Realize that during the implementation period, processing and serving patients may take longer, because the staff is using new technology. Most patients are understanding about this if the medical assistant explains that a new system is in place and asks for patience. Because patients are not always technologically savvy, most will be supportive and interested in the EMR system.

Legal and Ethical Issues

Remember that the EMR system contains information that is confidential at all times. The patient must authorize the release of health information in electronic form, just as if it were a piece of paper. Electronic medical records systems must:

- Maintain the security and confidentiality of data
- Be easily retrievable
- Have safeguards against the loss of information
- Protect patients' rights to confidentiality and privacy
- Require identification and authentication for access

By supporting these requirements, the medical facility remains in compliance with applicable laws and gains the trust of patients, who are reassured that their health information is secure and safe.

SUMMARY OF SCENARIO

Jennifer has decided that Sloan is just not a good match for the practice. One week before Sloan's probationary period is up, Jennifer brings her into the office to talk. She reminds Sloan that she originally was hired to work in the administrative part of the office. She explains that, although Sloan's desire and enthusiasm for the clinical side were evident, Jennifer did not feel that Sloan was addressing her duties in a responsible way and that her work ethic needed improvement. Jennifer reminded Sloan of the patient's record she had accessed and explained that this was a breach of patient confidentiality and medical ethics.

Sloan was clearly affected by Jennifer's evaluation of her work. She opened up to Jennifer and expressed her remorse that she had waited so long after graduation to look for employment. She also said that she was beginning to feel desperate for a job and felt that she needed to take the administrative job in hopes of later getting the position she wanted. Sloan apologized for accessing the patient's record and said she understood that this breach alone was grounds for immediate termination.

Jennifer was impressed that Sloan was able to admit her mistakes and feel remorse for them. She agreed to allow Sloan to volunteer at the clinic in the back office two afternoons a week until she found permanent employment. Sloan was thankful that Jennifer was willing to help her reach her career goals. She said she would take the knowledge of her mistakes to heart and work very hard for Jennifer as a volunteer. Jennifer reiterated to Sloan that her breach of confidentiality would be a difficult issue to overcome in future employment.

SUMMARY OF LEARNING OBJECTIVES

1. **Define, spell, and pronounce the terms listed in the vocabulary.**
   Spelling and pronouncing medical terms correctly bolster the medical assistant's credibility. Knowing the definition of these terms promotes confidence in communication with co-workers and patients.

2. **Discuss the presidential Executive Order that led to the implementation of electronic medical record systems across the nation.**
   President George W. Bush issued an Executive Order in August, 2006, that presented the goal of having electronic health records for most Americans by the year 2014. The order included five requirements that outlined the relationship between the agencies involved in the initial implementation process and the beneficiaries they serve. In general, when computer upgrades were initiated, these agencies and beneficiaries agreed to implement interoperable systems that would lead to nationwide electronic medical record systems in the near future.

3. **Discuss the principles of using the electronic medical record (EMR).**
   Electronic medical records systems allow record sharing among various healthcare entities in a geographic area. This leads to better patient care, because healthcare professionals can put together a more detailed picture of the patient's health. Using the EMR or EHR, a physician can access hospital records on his or her patients, even if he or she was not the attending physician. Also, laboratory reports can be viewed on smart phones and PDAs without having to be mailed or faxed to the office. Having the whole picture about a patient's health enables the physician to make better treatment choices and provide the best care.

4. **Distinguish between an electronic health record (EHR) and an electronic medical record (EMR).**
   The electronic health record (EHR) is an electronic record of health-related information about an individual that conforms to nationally recognized interoperability standards and that can be created, managed, and consulted by authorized clinicians and staff from more than one healthcare organization The electronic medical record (EMR) is an electronic record of health-related information about an individual that can be created, gathered, managed, and consulted by authorized clinicians and staff within one healthcare organization.

5. **Explain how the American Recovery and Reinvestment Act applies to the healthcare industry.**
   The American Recovery and Reinvestment Act (ARRA) of 2009, commonly known as the Economic Stimulus Package, was meant to promote economic recovery. The health information technology aspects of the bill provide slightly more than $31 billion for healthcare infrastructure and EHR investment. The sections of the ARRA that pertain to healthcare are collectively known as the Health Information Technology for Economic and Clinical Health (HITECH) Act.

6. **Define meaningful use.**
   Meaningful use, defined simply, means that providers must show that they are using EHR technology in ways that can be measured significantly in quality and quantity. If providers meet the meaningful use requirements, they will qualify for incentive payments.

7. **List the three main components of meaningful use legislation.**
   The three main components of meaningful use are (1) use of certified EHR in a meaningful manner, such as e-prescribing; (2) use of certified EHR technology for electronic exchange of health information to improve quality of health care; and (3) use of certified EHR technology to submit clinical quality reports, procedure and diagnosis codes, surveys, and other measures.

8. **Discuss the advantages and disadvantages of an electronic medical record system.**
   Advantages of an EMR system include savings in time and money, reduced staffing needs, fewer medical errors, faster retrieval of information, and enormous technologic capabilities. Disadvantages include patient concerns about confidentiality, staff training, staff acceptance, and space and storage issues.

9. **Explore the capabilities of an electronic medical record system.**
   Some capabilities of an EMR system include specialty practice components, appointment scheduling features, prescription writers, medical billing systems, charge capture, eligibility verification, referral management, laboratory order integration, patient portals, and many other features that vary from system to system.

10. **Give several reasons patients are hesitant in accepting electronic health records.**
    The medical assistant should expect hesitation and even reluctance from patients with regard to the EMR system, because they are concerned about the privacy of their health information. Patients worry about lack of control over who views their records. Be prepared to answer their questions about the safety of their records as related to the EMR. Medical assistants must know how the EMR is protected and what security measures are in place so that they can reassure patients that their records are protected at all times.

11. **Discuss the importance of nonverbal communication with patients when an EMR system is used.**
    Eye contact is critical when an EMR system is used with patients. Body language must indicate that the medical assistant is open to and listening to the patient's concerns, not just concentrating on data entry. Physicians and medical assistants alike may have to relearn how to interact with patients in a natural way while using the laptop or PDA in the examination room. Realize that during the implementation period, processing and serving patients may take longer, because the staff is using new technology. Most patients are understanding about this if the medical assistant explains that a new system is in place and asks for patience. Because patients are not always technologically savvy, most will be supportive and interested in the EMR system.

12. **Summarize the goals of the Nationwide Health Information Network (NHIN).**
    The goals of the NHIN include developing capabilities for standards-based, secure data exchange nationwide; improving the coordination of care information among hospitals, laboratories, physicians' offices, pharmacies, and other providers; ensuring that appropriate information is available at the time and place of care; ensuring that consumers' health

information is secure and confidential; giving consumers new capabilities for managing and controlling their personal health records and providing access to their health information from electronic health records and other sources; reducing risks from medical errors and supporting the delivery of appropriate, evidence-based medical care; and lowering healthcare costs resulting from inefficiencies, medical errors, and incomplete patient information.

13. **List the core capabilities of the NHIN.**
The core capabilities of the NHIN are to find and retrieve healthcare information within and between health information exchanges and other organizations; to deliver a summarized patient record to support patient care and to support the patient's health; to support consumers' preferences regarding the exchange of their information, including the right to choose not to participate in the NHIN; to support secure information exchange; to support a common trust agreement that establishes the obligations and assurances to which all NHIN participants agree; to match patients to their data without a national patient identifier; and

to support harmonized standards developed by voluntary consensus standards bodies for the exchange of health information among all such entities and networks.

14. **Summarize the role of the medical assistant with regard to the changing technology in healthcare facilities and organizations.**
By being open to change and willing to learn, the medical assistant sets a good example for all employees and is more receptive to the process of change. Be encouraging to other staff members while training on the system, and if technology comes easily to you, share your knowledge with others and assist wherever possible. Do not expect to master the system in a week; realize that new systems have a learning curve and be patient with and receptive to the educational process. Keep technical support phone numbers handy and feel free to use them whenever a new or complicated issue arises. Work with others as a team, and if possible, offer to help those who might find learning the system more of a struggle. Above all, while getting used to the new technology, make sure your attitude is one of enthusiasm, interest, and curiosity.

CONNECTIONS

Study Guide Connection: Go to the Chapter 15 Study Guide. Read and complete the activities.

Evolve Connection: Go to the Chapter 15 link at *evolve.elsevier.com/kinn* to complete the Chapter Review and Chapter Quiz. Check out the other resources listed for this chapter to make the most of what you have learned from The Electronic Medical Record.

Reference

Fleming NS, Culler SD, McCorkle R, et al: The financial and nonfinancial costs of implementing electronic health records in primary care practices. *Health Affairs* Mar 1;30(3):481-489, 2011. Available at http://content.healthaffairs.org/content/30/3/481.abstract. Accessed November 12, 2011.

16

HEALTH INFORMATION MANAGEMENT

Laura Kelly graduated from her medical assistant training 1 year ago and is now employed at a freestanding urgent care center. She works with the quality assurance staff and also performs front office duties. She enjoys working with statistics, is very detail oriented, has excellent computer and coding skills, and is able to comprehend lengthy regulatory text, such as that used in the rules and guidelines established by the Health Insurance Portability and Accountability Act (HIPAA). She has proven to be a valuable employee, and her efforts help the center comply with privacy laws.

Laura thought that quality assurance involved only patient satisfaction when she began working for the center. She has learned that this is just a small part of the total quality picture of the facility. The center has developed a patient questionnaire to solicit input from patients, and she enjoys talking with them about their experiences. Laura rarely encounters complaints, and she is proud to work for a medical facility that employs individuals who are concerned about giving exceptional care to patients. She understands that providing quality in a healthcare facility has many aspects.

Laura also realizes that health information encompasses much more than the patient's medical record. She knows that health statistics are vital to research and that physicians rely on statistical information when prescribing drugs, giving treatments, planning for future growth, deciding on which services to offer, and performing other services. Providers frequently contact Laura to determine how many procedures of a certain type were done at the center during a given period. The facility's database is very sophisticated and allows her to access many types of statistics quickly. Her office also monitors people who enter the database and what information is accessed. Monitoring access is one method of ensuring that privacy is maintained.

Laura has attended continuing education workshops, which provided up-to-date information and enabled her to help the staff stay in compliance with the numerous regulations that govern the facility. She is eager to learn and assist her employers in keeping the center safe for all patients and visitors.

While studying this chapter, think about the following questions:

- How is health information used in today's medical facilities?
- What can the individual medical assistant do to improve the quality of care given in his or her employer's facility?
- Why is quality management an important aspect of today's healthcare industry?
- How do statistics affect healthcare?

LEARNING OBJECTIVES

1. Define, spell, and pronounce the terms listed in the vocabulary.
2. Describe several ways health information is used.
3. Explain the nine characteristics of quality health data.
4. Explain the four concerns of quality assurance.
5. Explain the functions of the National Center for Health Statistics (NCHS).
6. Give some types of statistics kept by the NCHS.
7. Define total quality management.
8. Explain the function of The Joint Commission (formerly the Joint Commission on Accreditation of Healthcare Organizations [JCAHO]).
9. Discuss the importance of healthcare standards in medical facilities.

VOCABULARY

adverse event An injury caused by medical management rather than the underlying condition of the patient.

authenticated Proved; with regard to medical records, it applies to a signature, initials, or computer keystroke by the maker of the record to verify that the record is correct.

benchmarks Items or factors that serve as standards against which other items or factors can be measured or judged.

circumvent (suhr-kuhm-vent′) To manage to get around, especially by ingenuity or strategy.

contraindications (kahn-truh-in-duh-ka′-shuns) Factors, such as symptoms or conditions, that make a particular treatment or procedure inadvisable.

disparities (di-spar′-uh-tez) Fundamentally different and often incongruous elements; elements that are markedly distinct in quality or character.

encrypted (in-kript′-ed) Encoded; converted from one system of communication to another.

erroneous (eh-ro′-ne-uhs) Containing or characterized by error or assumption.

gradients A change in parameters or the value of a quantity, such as temperature or pressure; a change in response with distance from the stimulus; a graded difference in physiological activity along an axis, as of the body or embryonic fluid.

near miss A situation in which an error is caught or corrected before it affects the patient.

nosocomial (no-suh-ko′-me-uhl) Originating or taking place in a hospital.

potentially compensable event (PCE) An adverse occurrence, usually involving a patient, that could result in a financial obligation for a business or organization.

quality assurance (QA) Activities designed to increase the quality of a product or service through process or system changes that increase efficiency or effectiveness.

sentinel events Unexpected occurrences involving death or serious physical or psychological injury, or the risk thereof.

standards Models or examples established by authority, custom, or general consent; something set up and established by authority as a rule for the measure of quantity, weight, extent, value, or quality.

transposed Altered in sequence; interchanged.

Before the 1990s, practitioners in the healthcare field were barely familiar with the term "health information management." Today, this well-respected profession employs thousands of individuals across the United States. As more medical facilities move toward computer-based medical records, more trained health information management professionals are needed. The medical assistant may want to pursue employment in this growing field.

The health information management profession is supported by a national organization, the American Health Information Management Association (AHIMA). In 1994 the association's House of Delegates developed the following statement:

> Health information management is the profession that focuses on healthcare data and the management of healthcare information resources. The profession addresses the nature, structure, and translation of data into usable forms of information for the advancement of health and healthcare of individuals and populations. Health information professionals collect, integrate, and analyze primary and secondary healthcare data; disseminate information; and manage information resources related to research, planning, provision, and evaluation of healthcare services.

EVOLUTION OF THE PROFESSION

In 1928 the American College of Surgeons realized that accurate medical records promoted good medical care. This desire for quality led to the establishment of the Association of Record Librarians of North America. In 1970 the organization changed its name to the American Medical Record Association. Medical records professionals found employment in hospitals, health clinics, insurance companies, and other organizations that used medical records. In 1991 the organization became known as the American Health Information Management Association. Advances in technology have brought the health information management profession from a paper-based environment into a highly sophisticated computer age, where physicians can access patient and statistical data in seconds.

HEALTH INFORMATION CERTIFICATIONS

AHIMA offers certifications in health information management, coding, and healthcare privacy and security. Because healthcare facilities are now provided financial incentives for converting to electronic medical records, the need for individuals in health information careers grows each year. Medical facilities need employees who can manipulate data and, at the same time, can keep patient records accurate and confidential. Health Information Technology certifications include:

- Registered Health Information Administrator (RHIA)
- Registered Health Information Technician (RHIT)
- Certified Coding Associate (CCA)
- Certified Coding Specialist (CCS)
- Certified Coding Specialist—Physician-based (CCS-P)
- Certified Health Data Analyst (CHDA)
- Certified in Healthcare Privacy & Security (CHPS)
- Certified Documentation Improvement Practitioner (CDIP)

Additional information about each certification and the eligibility requirements can be found in Table 16-1 and on the Evolve site at *evolve.elsevier.com/kinn.*

TABLE 16-1 Certifications in Healthcare Technology

CERTIFICATION INITIALS	CERTIFICATION NAME	OVERVIEW	ELIGIBILITY REQUIREMENTS
RHIA	Registered Health Information Administrator	Works as a manager in multiple healthcare settings as a critical link between providers, patients, providers, co-workers, and office visitors.	Complete the requirements of a baccalaureate program in Health Information Management accredited by the Commission on Accreditation for Health Informatics and Information Management Education (CAHIIME) or a comparable foreign program
RHIT	Registered Health Information Technologist	Works in multiple healthcare settings with solid potential for advancement into management, especially with a baccalaureate degree	Complete the requirements of an associate program in Health Information Management accredited by CAHIIME or a comparable foreign program
CCA	Certified Coding Associate	Exhibits a professional capability and competency in medical coding	U.S. high school diploma or equivalent; strongly recommended that candidate have 6 months of experience or have completed a program recommended by the American Health Information Management Association (AHIMA) or another formal coding training program
CCS	Certified Coding Specialist	Classifies medical data from patients' records into accurate diagnosis and procedure codes	U.S. high school diploma or equivalent; strongly recommended that candidate have at least 3 years of on-the-job experience in a hospital and have an academic background in anatomy and physiology, pathophysiology, and pharmacology
CCS-P	Certified Coding Specialist— Physician-based	Specializes in a physician-based setting	U.S. high school diploma or equivalent; strongly recommended that candidate have at least 4 years of on-the-job experience in multiple specialties for physician services and have an academic background in anatomy and physiology, pathophysiology, and pharmacology
CHDA	Certified Health Data Analyst	Develops an expertise in health data analysis and transforms data into accurate, consistent, and timely information	Associate's degree and 5 years of health data experience; RHIT credential or bachelor's degree and 3 years of experience; RHIA credential or master's degree and 1 year of experience
CHPS	Certified in Healthcare Privacy & Security	Develops competency in designing and implementing privacy and security systems in all types of healthcare organizations	Bachelor's degree and 4 years of experience in healthcare management; master's degree or higher, or RHIA or RHIT credential, with 2 years of experience
CDIP	Certified Documentation Improvement Practitioner	Captures and analyzes health information and can fluently translate the technoclinical language of the electronic medical record	RHIA, RHIT, CCS, CCS-P, registered nurse (RN), doctor of medicine (MD), or doctor of osteopathy (DO) credential and 2 years of experience in clinical documentation improvement; associate's degree or higher and 3 years of experience in clinical documentation improvement; must also have completed coursework in medical terminology and in anatomy and physiology

USES OF HEALTHCARE DATA

Healthcare data are used primarily to plan patient care, to plan for the future growth and development of the facility, and to ensure that patients receive continuity of care from one healthcare provider to another. However, the information provided by healthcare records can be useful in other ways.

Primary data are the information in the actual medical record; *secondary data* are generated from the information in the medical record. For example, when a drug is evaluated, statistics must be kept to help the manufacturers determine its effectiveness. Information on side effects and other **contraindications** is reviewed and used to make the drug safer and more marketable.

Healthcare organizations gather information on the number of patients who enter the facility with the same diagnosis. This and other information helps them plan the types of equipment required to meet the needs of this patient group. For instance, if the facility is located in a geographic area with a large number of patients with cardiac disease, the hospital may need to add a cardiac intensive care unit. Healthcare data and statistics guide planning for the needs of next week and the next decade.

The *Federal Register* (FR), which is published by the Office of the Federal Register, National Archives and Records Administration (NARA), provides daily access to rules, proposed rules, and notices of federal agencies and organizations, including those dealing with healthcare. Today's technology allows NARA to e-mail the FR's table of contents each day (Monday through Friday). Also, healthcare information can be accessed on the agency's Web site, which offers updated information about rules and regulations currently in effect, changes, new proposals, and final rulings. The FR is an excellent source of health data, and every medical facility should receive at least the daily table of contents e-mail, which can help the medical facility stay up-to-date on new regulations and changes in current ones.

CRITICAL THINKING APPLICATION 16-1

- Laura has noticed that the center keeps extensive records on the admitting diagnosis and the final diagnosis. Why is this information important to the center?
- If a certain physician is admitting numerous patients with the same diagnosis or for a certain procedure, what concerns might this raise for the facility? For what logical reason might this happen?

Third-party payers use healthcare information to determine whether claims should be paid. The data provide proof that a certain procedure or treatment was medically necessary and therefore its cost should be reimbursed. Government and regulatory agencies use data to ensure that healthcare facilities are in compliance with the various statutes and **standards** that govern them. Facilities use data to help determine whether they are providing high-quality healthcare to their patients.

WHAT ARE HIGH-QUALITY DATA?

The information in a database is only as reliable as the person who enters it into the computer. Nine characteristics of quality healthcare data have been identified: validity, reliability, completeness, recognizability, timeliness, relevance, accessibility, security, and legality.

- **Validity.** The validity of healthcare data is synonymous with accuracy. Accuracy is a primary characteristic of data, whether in paper-based or computer-based records. Great care must be taken that letters and numbers are not **transposed** when characters are typed on the keyboard.

- **Reliability.** The healthcare professional must be able to rely on the data. If a patient's medical chart indicates that he or she has no allergies, the medical assistant must be able to trust that information and give an injection, confident that the patient is not allergic to the medication. Reliability also pertains to the degree to which the information in the database can be trusted.

- **Completeness.** The information must be not only accurate, but complete. If the medical assistant gives an injection but fails to document it in the patient's chart, the record is incomplete. A court probably would rule that the injection could not be considered to have been given, because it was not documented in the patient's record. If a computer system is designed to upload new information into the database every night and the system malfunctions, the strong possibility exists that the records in the system are incomplete, possibly lacking vital information needed for the patient's care.

- **Recognizability.** All users of health information must be able to interpret the data in the health record. The facility should insist on consistent use of abbreviations to prevent misunderstandings when a patient's chart is reviewed. Some systems display charts to show an increase or a decline in basic vital signs (e.g., blood pressure, weight, and temperature). Such a system allows the physician to track symptoms over time without having to search through a paper record (Figure 16-1).

- **Timeliness.** Health information must be entered into the chart or database as soon as it is available. The medical assistant should never commit information to memory with the intention of entering it later. Reports from laboratories or medical testing centers also should be placed in the chart as soon as the physician has reviewed them so that patient care decisions are supported by the latest information. Whether paper or electronic, the medical record must be accurate, timely, complete, and accessible so that the patient receives optimum care from all providers.

- **Relevance.** The information in the database must be relevant to be useful. Needless and meaningless statistics about patient treatments or drug interactions do not benefit providers or users of health information.

- **Accessibility.** An advantage of a computer-based patient record is its accessibility; it can be viewed by more than one user at a time. The facility must take care to provide access only to individuals authorized to view the records. The computer system should have a log-in process that prompts for a password, and it should keep records of who accesses information by time and date. Paper-based patient records must be returned to their proper place when not in use so that they are accessible to all staff members.

- **Security.** Only certain employees should be allowed to access health information, and precautions must be taken to prevent access by intruders. Firewalls, which are similar to filters, allow

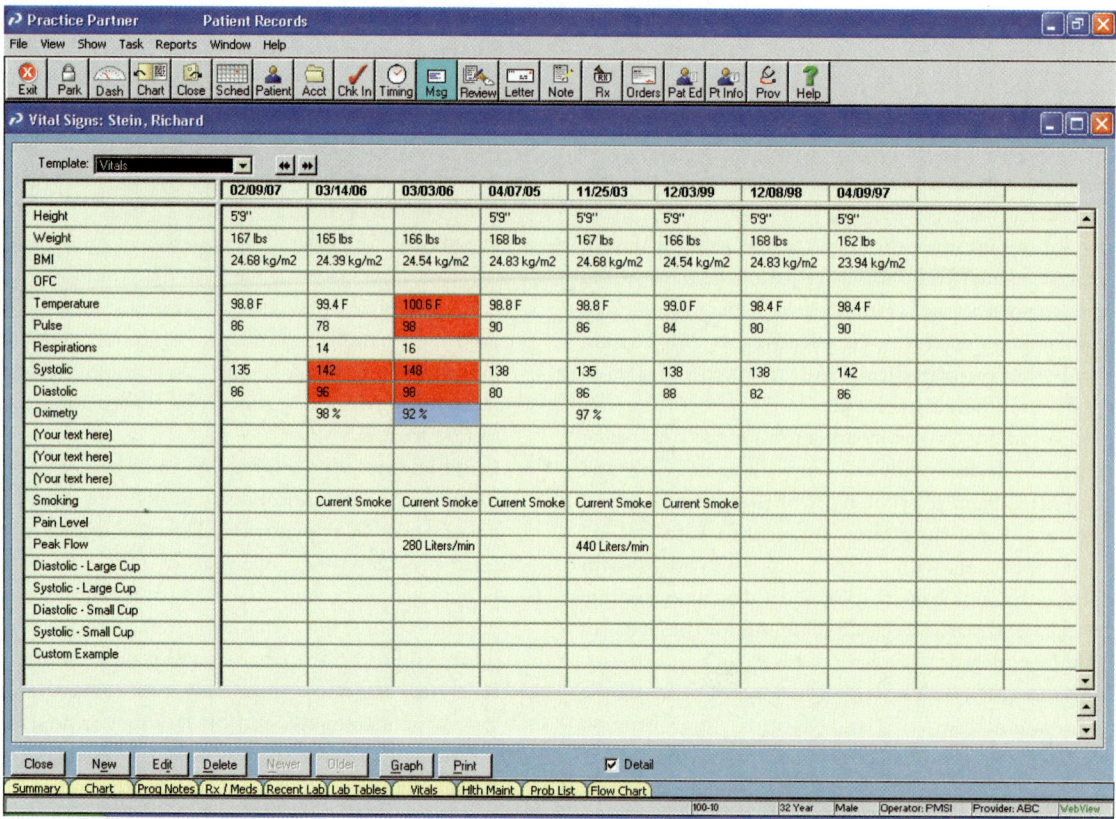

FIGURE 16-1 Electronic medical records allow the physician to determine whether changes in basic vital signs over time are significant. This type of data can help physicians determine the number of patients who have hypertension, and the information can then be used to contact patients with that diagnosis when a new hypertensive drug is available. (Courtesy McKessan Corp., Alpharetta, Ga.)

only certain types of data to enter or exit. Information can be **encrypted**, which means that it is changed into a code that can be read only after it has been unencrypted. These precautions are necessary because of the sensitivity of patient information. Also, care must be taken to ensure that no one can change the information already in the record.

- **Legality.** Medical records are regulated by many statutes. The laws on retention of records vary from state to state. Medical records cannot be altered, and they should be corrected according to accepted guidelines. The record must be completely legible and must be **authenticated** properly (Figure 16-2).

CRITICAL THINKING APPLICATION   16-2

- One of Laura's duties is to make sure medical records have been authenticated. Why is authentication of records important?
- One physician, Dr. Anthony, is consistently careless about record authentication. How can the center encourage him to complete this critical duty?

CHALLENGES OF QUALITY ASSURANCE PROBLEMS

Many larger medical facilities today have entire departments devoted to quality assurance. **Quality assurance (QA)** comprises activities designed to improve the quality of a product or service through process or system changes that increase efficiency or effectiveness. Although many people assume that quality is determined solely by

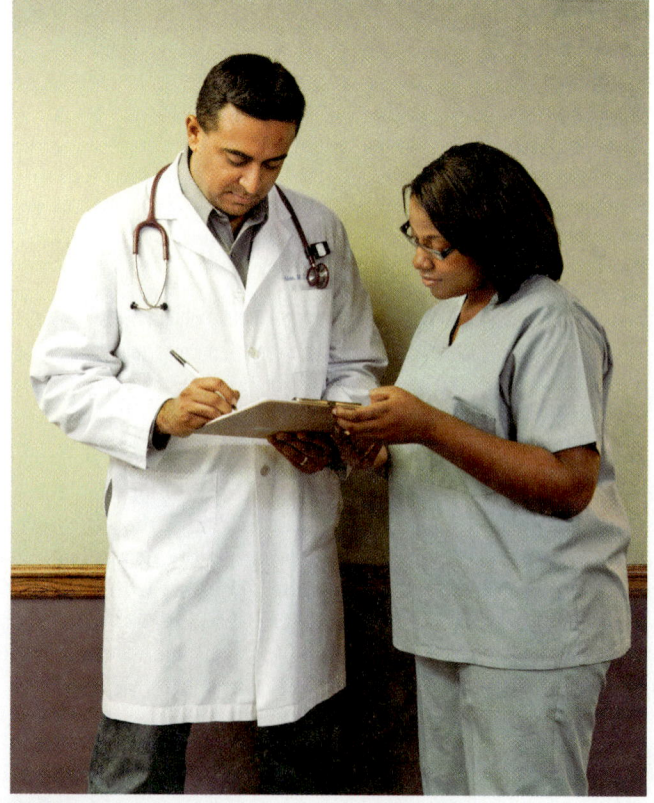

FIGURE 16-2 Physicians must authenticate medical records by initialing or signing their entries. Some computer systems automatically authenticate records.

the patient, much more is involved in quality assurance than just the patient's satisfaction with services rendered. The four concerns of quality assurance are overuse, underuse, misuse, and variations in the use of healthcare services. No medical assistant should attempt to **circumvent** any co-worker's attempts, especially in an attempts to make the co-worker look less competent. Instead, all of the staff members must work together toward the common goals set by the physician and office manager.

Costs rise when providers order excessive, unnecessary healthcare services. Overused treatments and services include hysterectomies, tympanostomy tubes, and antibiotics. Antibiotics are prescribed widely for common colds and acute bronchitis, but the drugs do not benefit patients with these illnesses.

Underuse of services and treatments can be equally costly. Mammograms and cervical cancer screening tests can detect medical problems early, yet many at-risk patients do not take advantage of these services (Figure 16-3). Beta blockers have been proved to reduce mortality in patients who have had heart attacks by as much as 43%, but they often are not prescribed for these patients. Patients with diabetes should have their eyes checked regularly, but many do not. All these are examples of underuse of services that can affect the quality of healthcare.

CRITICAL THINKING APPLICATION   16-3
- How might a medical assistant encourage patients to have screening tests done, such as mammograms and tests for cervical cancer?
- What marketing strategies could Laura help develop that would prompt more patients to take advantage of health screening opportunities?
- How do these services benefit the health facility?

Some healthcare services are misused. These errors can cause death, delay of correct diagnosis, unnecessary injuries, and increased healthcare costs. Laboratory tests that provide **erroneous** results are an example of misuse. Medication errors can be fatal to patients or can cause complications in a current illness. Hospital injuries and **nosocomial** infections promote further complications.

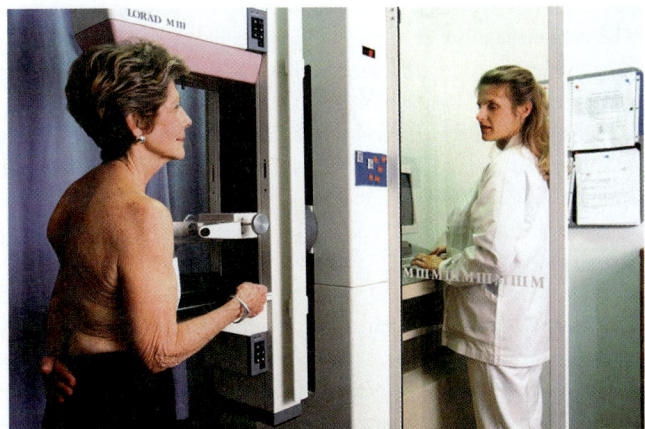

FIGURE 16-3 Healthcare professionals must encourage at-risk patients to have screening tests, such as those for breast and cervical cancer.

Services vary widely across the country. Live discharge rates (i.e., the number of patients who leave the hospital without expiring) are higher in some areas of the United States than in others. Individuals who seek medical care are more conscientious and are likely to seek health services in a different geographic area if they believe they will receive better care. All these issues contribute to the concept of high-quality healthcare.

CRITICAL THINKING APPLICATION   16-4
- Laura is concerned about the number of employees in her facility who are allowed to access patient information. For instance, all employees have access to all health information on all patients. Is this a good policy? Why or why not?
- Should all physicians have access to all patient records? Why or why not?

NATIONAL CENTER FOR HEALTH STATISTICS

The National Center for Health Statistics (NCHS), a division of the Centers for Disease Control and Prevention (CDC), is the primary provider of the health information statistics used to guide actions and policies affecting the health of the American public. The functions of the NCHS include:

- Documenting the health status of the U.S. population and important subgroups
- Identifying **disparities** in health status and the use of healthcare by race, ethnicity, socioeconomic status (SES), region, and other population **gradients** or **parameters**.
- Describing experiences with the healthcare system
- Monitoring trends in health status and healthcare delivery
- Identifying health problems
- Supporting biomedical and health services research
- Providing information to effect changes in public policies and programs
- Evaluating the impact of health policies and programs

Statistics are vital to many entities interested in the healthcare industry. Some statistics available through the NCHS are related to the following:

- Teenage pregnancy
- Incidence of infection with the human immunodeficiency virus (HIV)
- Alcohol and drug use
- Births
- Deaths
- Communicable diseases
- Infant health and mortality
- Leading causes of death
- Life expectancy
- Sexually transmitted diseases
- Suicide

TOTAL QUALITY MANAGEMENT

Total quality management is defined as management or control activities based on the leadership of top-level management and supported by the involvement of all employees and departments, from planning and development to sales and service. These management and control activities focus on quality assurance. Ideally, qualities that satisfy the customer are built into products and services as they are received from providers.

For total quality management practices to be effective, all employees must commit to providing patients with the best care possible. This includes both top-level management and the staff members who work directly with patients.

The Concept of Total Quality Management

Much of the thrust of today's interest in total quality management originated from the teachings of W. Edwards Deming, who earned a doctorate in mathematical physics from Yale University in 1928. Deming is perhaps best known for the work he did on quality management with Japanese managers and engineers. He developed 14 points for managers to institute that emphasize quality rather than quantity. By following these guidelines, medical assistants can help prevent medical liability claims.

1. Create constancy of purpose in improving the product or service, with the aims of becoming competitive, staying in business, and providing jobs.
2. Adopt a new philosophy. Western management must awaken to the challenge, learn their responsibilities, and take on leadership for change.
3. Stop depending on inspection to achieve quality. Eliminate the need for inspection on a mass basis by building quality into the product or service in the first place.
4. End the practice of awarding business on the basis of the price tag. Instead, minimize total cost. Move toward a single supplier for any one item, based on a long-term relationship of loyalty and trust.
5. Continually improve the system of production and service so as to improve quality and productivity and thus constantly reduce costs.
6. Institute training on the job.
7. Institute leadership. The aim of supervision should be to help people, machines, and gadgets to do a better job. Supervision of management is in need of overhaul, in addition to supervision of production workers.
8. Drive out fear so that everyone can work effectively for the company.
9. Break down barriers between departments. People must work as a team to foresee problems in production and in use that may be encountered.
10. Eliminate slogans, exhortations, and targets for the work force that ask for zero defects and new levels of productivity; these

only create adversarial relationships. Eliminate quotas and substitute leadership. Eliminate management by objective. Eliminate management by numbers and numeric goals. Substitute leadership.
11. Remove barriers that rob hourly workers of their right to pride in their workmanship. The responsibility of supervisors must be changed from sheer numbers to quality.
12. Remove barriers that rob people in management and engineering of their right to pride in their workmanship. This means abolishing the annual merit rating and management by objective.
13. Institute a vigorous program of education and self-improvement.
14. Put everybody in the company to work to accomplish the transformation. The transformation is everybody's job.

Deming believed that these points could help managers and employees achieve quality in their facility or business. They are widely used in countless business and service organizations today.

The Joint Commission

The Joint Commission is a nonprofit organization that provides accreditation services for healthcare facilities. Earning accreditation is a voluntary process, but more than 17,000 healthcare facilities in the United States are accredited by and comply with the standards of The Joint Commission. The organization sees its mission as one of continuously improving the safety and quality of care provided to the public by providing healthcare accreditation and related services, which help healthcare organizations improve their performance. Many think The Joint Commission deals only with hospitals; however, the organization has vastly expanded its services over the years to include ambulatory care, assisted living, behavioral healthcare, critical access hospitals, home care, laboratory services, long-term care, and office-based surgical centers. Administrative or clinical medical assistants may be employed in all of these; therefore, they should have some knowledge of The Joint Commission, its purpose, its regulations, and the types of facilities it serves.

Ambulatory care and office-based surgery centers, in addition to many other facilities, have found that competitive pressures in the healthcare market, combined with the rapidly changing healthcare field, have prompted them to seek accreditation. Providing high-quality patient care and continually striving for improved performance, both of which are proven by meeting accreditation standards, are **benchmarks** of success. For many years, healthcare facilities were interested in meeting the minimum standards that would reflect quality healthcare. Partly because of the fierce competition in the medical market, the goal recently has shifted from simply meeting minimum standards to exceeding standards and providing optimum healthcare (Figure 16-4).

RISK MANAGEMENT

A risk is any occurrence that could result in patient injury or any type of financial loss to the healthcare facility. Risk management is a program designed to identify, contain, reduce, or eliminate the potential for harm and financial loss to a facility if a compensable event occurs. In a healthcare facility, it usually involves the delivery system and actual workplace.

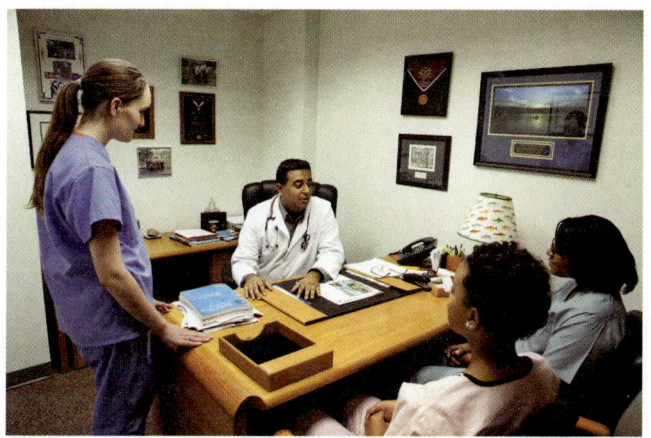

FIGURE 16-4 Accreditation of a healthcare facility takes teamwork and a commitment to quality assurance.

A facility's policies and procedures are designed to manage risk and prevent situations that could result in harm to people or property for which the healthcare facility could be held liable. Both the Occupational Safety and Health Administration (OSHA) and Clinical Laboratory Improvement Amendments (CLIA) have established regulations that promote risk management.

Effective risk management benefits the physician's office by cutting financial losses and improving the quality of healthcare provided by the staff. Risk management programs stress the prevention of financial loss and reduce the possibility of negative publicity resulting from **sentinel events**. The Joint Commission defines a sentinel event as an unexpected occurrence that involves death or serious physical or psychological injury or the risk of either. Sentinel events must be reported immediately and investigated thoroughly, and their contributing factors must be rectified to prevent recurrence of the problem. Records are kept of the sentinel events that happen in a facility, especially those involving a patient injury or death.

The Joint Commission defines sentinel events and monitors and investigates them in the facilities it accredits. A physician's office may have similar incidents, such as:

- Medication errors
- Delayed treatment
- Medical equipment failure
- Patient falls
- Fire
- Wrong-site surgery
- Unintended retention of foreign objects

Traditionally, hospitals are the facilities that have formed QA departments. However, numerous physicians' offices are appointing QA committees to help reduce risk and liability. Some physicians designate the office manager or another staff member as the site safety officer.

Risk and liability are synonymous with financial loss in the healthcare facility. For this reason, policies and procedures must be followed as specified in the office policy and procedures manuals. Attorneys are quite shrewd about using office policy and procedures manuals against the medical facility during a lawsuit. If the manual states that quality control procedures are to be performed daily, but no logs exist to prove they were, the attorney can surmise that the office does not follow its own policy; if this can be proved once, the

attorney will look for every other breach in office policy and will emphasize this during the court proceedings. If the office cannot follow its own policies, it likely will be judged as incompetent. This could result in a **potentially compensable event (PCE)**, creating a financial obligation for the healthcare facility. For the physician, a court award to a patient can mean that the physician will have to pay higher liability insurance premiums, which affects the overhead costs of running the facility and keeping it open. A higher overhead also may mean that the salaries of medical assistants and other employees must be frozen for a specified period or indefinitely.

All employees of healthcare facilities can help avoid liability by strictly following the office policy and procedures manual and by paying close attention to situations that might lead to office liability.

RISK MANAGEMENT: HELPING YOUR PHYSICIAN TO AVOID BEING SUED

1. Communication is the first step to preventing claims. Keep an open dialog with the patient and be sure to ask repeatedly whether the patient has any questions and whether he or she understands the physician's instructions.
2. Show that you care about patients. Form a professional but genuine relationship with them. Sincerely chat with them and express your hope that they will feel better soon. Never guarantee a cure or say that the doctor will "take care of everything." Patients who have a good relationship with the physician are much less likely to bring a medical liability claim to court.
3. Consider patients as active participants in their own healthcare. Explain their responsibility to follow instructions, take their medicine, and discuss questions with the physician whenever they arise. Without patients' cooperation, the physician cannot effectively help them overcome or deal with their illnesses.
4. Encourage patients to do research about their condition on reputable Web sites. Patients need to have a basic knowledge of their disease or condition. The more they know, the better they will be able to recognize serious symptoms or problems.
5. Suggest that patients write down questions and bring them to the office. Encourage them to take notes or provide them with information sheets on their disease or what to expect during a procedure.
6. Remember that if an event is not charted in the medical record, it didn't happen. Make sure comprehensive information about the patient, including attitude and compliance with orders, is included in the medical record.

ACKNOWLEDGING AND DISCLOSING MEDICAL ERRORS

One of a medical professional's most difficult tasks is dealing with a mistake that involves a patient. Most medical professionals do not intentionally make errors in any aspect of patient care, but unfortunately, mistakes happen from time to time in any business. Mistakes in the medical industry can cost patients their lives. Most errors are minor and easily rectified, but some lead to medical professional liability cases. All medical facilities need a plan for addressing errors when they occur, and they should use errors as an opportunity to learn. This allows supervisors to change procedures that led to the mishap and to train employees in ways to prevent mistakes.

The Institute of Medicine defines an error as "failure of a planned action or the use of a wrong plan" and an **adverse event** as "an injury caused by medical management rather than the underlying condition of the patient" (Table 16-2). However, patients often define errors much differently. A patient may consider rude attitudes or poor customer service as medical errors, although most physicians would not define these as errors. Earlier in this chapter, the term *sentinel event* was introduced, which is defined as an unexpected occurrence involving the death of or serious physical or psychological injury to a patient. Both an adverse event and a sentinel event can be considered errors; however, an adverse event is not necessarily a sentinel event. The least destructive type of medical error is a **near miss**, in which an error is caught or corrected before it affects the patient.

COMMON MEDICAL ERRORS

- Medication errors
- Documentation and follow-up on adverse drug reactions
- Lack of follow-up on abnormal test results
- Lack of follow-up on consultations
- Failure to educate the patient
- Lack of follow-up on no-show appointments

An intensive study by physicians Kathleen Mazor, Steven Simon, and Jerry Gurwitz reviewed information on the ways physicians deal with medical errors and how they inform patients and their families of those mistakes. The authors found that communication is the key to handling medical errors, and they concluded that physicians are ethically obligated to disclose such errors to the patient (Mazor et al., 2004). Likewise, medical assistants are ethically obligated to report every error they make directly to the physician responsible for the patient's care.

The most significant obstacle to disclosure usually is the fear of litigation. Some individuals will sue a physician for even the most insignificant mistakes. In Chapter 7, four elements were presented that must be offered as evidence to prove negligence: the physician must have the *duty* to care for the patient; proof of *dereliction of duty* must exist, meaning that the physician somehow failed to perform his or her duty as the patient's caregiver; the physician's action or lack of action must be the *direct cause* of the patient's condition; and the patient must prove that he or she suffered *damages* as a result of the physician's action or lack of action.

Medical assistants have important responsibilities when a medical error is made in the physician's office. They should never hide the error, especially when documenting the medical record. The error should be reported not only to the supervisor or office manager, but also to the physician, who can adjust the patient's course of care if necessary. The medical assistant also should allow the physician to be the person who talks with the patient about the error, because a medical assistant cannot answer the patient's questions about how the mistake will affect the person. Although many believe that an

TABLE 16-2   Preventable Adverse Events and Errors Identified by Family Physicians During Patient Visits

CLASSIFICATION	EXAMPLES	PATIENT VISITS WITH ERRORS (NUMBER/ PERCENT)
Office administration errors		57/16.5
Charting	Any part of record is not present, is in the wrong place, entire record is missing	37/10.5
General office administration	Staffing problems, missing or incorrect forms or paperwork, laboratory, x-ray, or imaging processing errors	21/6
Physician-related errors	Skill problems, time management problems (feeling rushed, interrupted)	28/8
Patient communication errors	Problems communicating with patient by physician, staff, or other physicians; appointment and screening errors	16/4.5
Preventable adverse events	Missed diagnosis, misdiagnosis, delayed treatment, incorrect treatment	15/4.3

From Elder NC, Vonder Meulen M, Cassedy A: The identification of medical errors by family physicians during outpatient visits, *Ann Fam Med* [online] 2(2):125-129, 2004. Accessed 9-21-2012.

apology is an admission of guilt, a sincere apology, when indicated, goes a long way in mending the relationship between the patient and physician or staff member and may even enhance the relationship, strengthening it and resulting in greater trust.

ACKNOWLEDGING AND REPORTING MEDICAL ERRORS MADE BY THE MEDICAL ASSISTANT

1. IMMEDIATELY inform the physician and supervisor when an error is discovered, no matter how insignificant the error.
2. Document the error in the medical record. Do not obliterate or change any part of the medical record as it stands; add an addendum or begin a new entry in the patient's progress notes.
3. Complete an incident report if indicated by the office policy and procedures manual.
4. Call the patient and ask him or her to come to the office. Use a phrase such as, "We'd like you to come into the office to discuss some things that have happened with your care. When would you like to come in?"

5. Do not disclose information prematurely. Allow the physician to make all the decisions about talking with the patient and make sure all the facts are available before the discussion with the patient.

6. Meet with the patient with the physician when the patient is told an error has been made. Conduct the meeting in a private area free of interruptions, preferably one that does not have a desk. The patient will be less intimidated if the physician sits next to him or her rather than behind a desk. Never relay information about a medical error via telephone or e-mail.

7. Use layman's terms when talking with the patient.

8. Offer a sincere apology for the error if appropriate.

9. A gentle touch on the patient's hand shows compassion and sincere sympathy.

10. Allow the patient to ask questions, both immediately and after the meeting has ended. The physician might say, "I know this is unexpected and upsetting news. If you think of other questions, I'd be happy to meet with you again or talk with you on the telephone. Here's the number where you can reach me."

11. Never make excuses for the mistake. The patient will receive the news much better if the blame is not placed on another person or facility.

12. Explain to the patient how the people involved will learn from the mistake. Explain any policy changes that the error may have prompted to assure the patient that supervisors or the physician have corrected the processes that led to the mishap.

13. Assure the patient that the staff and physician care about him or her and want the best for those who receive medical care at the facility. Patients need to feel that the physician and staff are sympathetic to their concerns.

14. Document all communication with the patient regarding the medical error.

Common sense must prevail in dealing with a medical error. To encourage admissions of error, some states now prevent the use of apologies as evidence of guilt in court in medical professional liability cases. Although many believe that apologies should be avoided so that there is no admission of guilt or liability, the medical assistant must cope with the feelings that he or she has after making a mistake. The apology may help reconcile those feelings and help the medical assistant move past the adverse event. Remember to discuss any patient contact after an error with the supervisor and the physician and to document such encounters in the patient's medical record when indicated.

CLOSING COMMENTS

Health information management is a critical aspect of today's healthcare facility. Although the regulations may seem stringent, the value of protecting the patient's privacy is immeasurable. Patients have the right to be cared for in a professional manner and to expect their health information to be kept confidential. The medical assistant should focus on following office policies and procedures and privacy guidelines. Take care when working with medical records and information.

Patient Education

Patients today are more health conscious than ever before, largely because of the abundance of medical information available on the Internet. Most large healthcare facilities employ patient advocates, who work with other professionals (e.g., insurance companies, case managers, and lawyers) to ensure that the patient receives quality medical care. The patient advocate helps resolve various issues regarding the patient's medical condition.

In general, an **advocate** is a person who supports or promotes the interests of another person. Medical assistants can serve as patient advocates in the physician's office. The National Patient Safety

BREAKDOWN OF OUTPATIENT ERRORS

Where do community-based physicians make errors? The California Academy of Family Physicians analyzed errors made over the course of a year by a group of 50 family physicians. The following chart shows a breakdown of the outpatient errors.

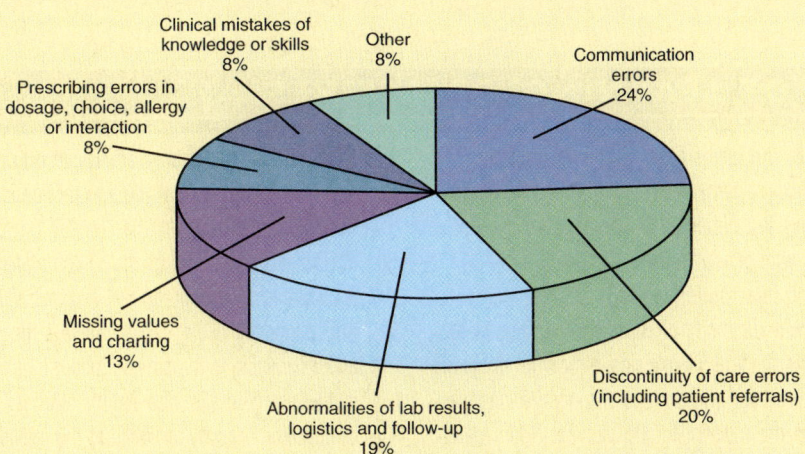

From Daftary AV: Diagnosing and treating medical errors in family practice, California Academy of Family Physicians, Monograph, March/April 2004.

Foundation (NPSF) encourages medical professionals to partner with patients and help them learn about the steps they can take to become more involved in their own healthcare.

The patient's good health is a team effort. Numerous professionals perform their duties to the best of their abilities toward a common goal—quality care. Communicating with the patient and working together build trust, reduce risk, and lessen liability in the medical facility. Each medical assistant must do his or her part to provide the patient with exceptional, first-rate care.

Legal and Ethical Issues

The medical assistant must be familiar with the laws affecting medical issues and must be able to guide patients as concerns arise. Be prepared to answer questions or direct such patients to the right source for information. Seminars that target compliance issues affecting the physician's office often are available to the medical assistant. Most employers are willing to pay for such seminars so that the office can remain in strict compliance with the law and regulations. Just as individuals practice defensive driving to keep a ticket off their driving record, physicians must practice some defensive medicine to prevent liability suits. Remember that the medical profession is one of constant change. The medical assistant must have a positive attitude about the learning process, especially when new rules and regulations take effect. When a problem arises, patients want their concerns to be acknowledged. They expect the medical professional to be truthful and empathetic and to apologize if necessary.

SUMMARY OF SCENARIO

Laura is learning more about health information management each day. She has earned the respect of her supervisors, who often give her lengthy, complicated documents on regulations and ask her to read and summarize them for the staff. She has a knack for picking out the actual requirements amid the excess of legalese.

Laura has developed good relationships with many of the staff physicians at the hospital. She has approached several of them about record authentication, and her bright personality helps foster a sense of cooperation between the medical staff and the center's staff. She has even received approval to give coupons good for one lunch at a popular nearby restaurant when physicians form the habit of authenticating their records in a timely manner. The physicians appreciate the recognition for completing their duties on schedule and definitely enjoy the lunch!

Laura has given thought to continuing her education in the health management field and possibly gaining certification in this area. She knows that this will lend credibility to the knowledge she has gained on the job. Her supervisors are pleased with her performance and know they can count on Laura to complete any task she is assigned on time and with accurate results. Laura looks forward to a long career at the center, serving both the patients and staff in the years to come.

Health information is used daily in medical facilities. The medical record probably is the most common source of health information that healthcare professionals use, but they also access databases that provide statistical and other information that affects patient care. Laura knows that she can contribute to quality healthcare by making sure records are accurate, complete, and reliable for the medical professionals who use them. Providing quality healthcare is mandatory in today's society, because physicians are susceptible to lawsuits and complaints when patients believe that they did not receive optimum care. Also, patients have the right to choose their healthcare providers, and they deserve and insist upon quality healthcare.

Laura has noticed that today's patients are more sophisticated and knowledgeable about health-related issues, primarily because of the ease of looking up their health issues on the Internet. Patients often tell the doctor what they think their diagnosis is, based on their own Internet research. This is proof that even patients are using healthcare information. Statistical information helps Laura's employers determine the diseases and disorders most likely to affect patients in their urgent care center. Computers are an invaluable tool that allows healthcare providers and facilities to share information so that they can better provide quality patient care.

SUMMARY OF LEARNING OBJECTIVES

1. **Define, spell, and pronounce the terms listed in the vocabulary.**
   Spelling and pronouncing medical terms correctly bolster the medical assistant's credibility. Knowing the definition of these terms promotes confidence in communication with patients and co-workers.

2. **Describe several ways health information is used.**
   Health information helps ensure continuity of care from provider to provider. It assists manufacturers in determining side effects of drugs. It provides statistical information about primary and secondary diagnoses. Health information also helps the medical facility plan for future needs and capital equipment.

3. **Explain the nine characteristics of quality health data.**
   (1) *Validity* means that the information is accurate; (2) *reliability* means that the information can be counted on to be accurate and that medical decisions can be based on it; (3) *completeness* means that the information is available in its entirety; (4) *recognizability* means that the data can be understood by users; (5) *timeliness* means that the information is the latest available to the provider about a patient or treatment; (6) *relevance* is the usefulness of the health data; (7) *accessibility* means that the information is easily available to the provider; (8) *security* involves efforts to keep unauthorized people from accessing the data; and (9) *legality*

refers to the correctness of the information and its authentication by the healthcare provider.

4. **Describe the four concerns of quality assurance.**

The four concerns of quality assurance are overuse, underuse, misuse, and variations in the use of healthcare services. Overuse (excessive use) of services raises costs (e.g., using the emergency department for nonemergencies). In underuse, patients do not take advantage of many services they should be using, especially if they are at-risk patients. Misuse of services often reflects errors, such as laboratory errors or misdiagnoses. Variations in services simply means that in different parts of the country, individuals use services in different ways, which can influence the quality of care overall in the United States.

5. **Explain the functions of the National Center for Health Statistics (NCHS).**

The NCHS, a division of the CDC, is the primary provider of health information statistics. Health statistics are important, because they enable providers to better treat their patients. For instance, if a certain area has a high number of outbreaks of a particular disease, physicians armed with this knowledge and with up-to-date information on the disease's treatment may be able to treat affected patients more quickly, promoting a full recovery. The NCHS also helps compile information such as the number of HIV infections, the number of teen pregnancies, and other vital health data useful to medical professionals.

6. **Give some types of statistics kept by the NCHS.**

The NCHS compiles statistics on alcohol and drug use, births, deaths, communicable diseases, infant health and mortality, and life expectancy.

7. **Define total quality management.**

Total quality management comprises management and control activities based on the leadership of top-level management and supported by the involvement of all employees and departments in an effort to provide quality assurance.

8. **Explain the function of The Joint Commission (formerly the Joint Commission on Accreditation of Healthcare Organizations [JCAHO]).**

The Joint Commission, a nonprofit organization, offers accreditation to facilities that want to excel in healthcare services. Accreditation is voluntary, but more than 17,000 healthcare facilities in the United States are accredited by the agency, including many that employ medical assistants and coders.

9. **Discuss the importance of healthcare standards in medical facilities.**

Without strong healthcare standards, quality cannot exist. The focus of quality assurance has shifted in recent years from just meeting the minimum standards to providing optimum quality. People expect high-quality healthcare. Organizations that seek accreditation or that focus their efforts on quality will exceed standards, not just meet them.

CONNECTIONS

Study Guide Connection: Go to the Chapter 16 Study Guide. Read and complete the activities.

Evolve Connection: Go to the Chapter 16 link at *evolve.elsevier.com/kinn* to complete the Chapter Review and Chapter Quiz. Check out the other resources listed for this chapter to make the most of what you have learned from Health Information Management.

Reference

Mazor KM, Simon SR, Gurwitz JH: Communicating with patients about medical errors: a review of the literature, *Arch Intern Med* 164:1690-1697, 2004.

Bibliography

Abdelhak M, Grostick S, Hanken MA, et al: *Health information: management of a strategic resource*, ed 3, St Louis, 2007, Mosby/Elsevier.

Institute of Medicine, Committee on Quality of Healthcare in America: *Crossing the quality chasm: a new health system for the 21st century*, Washington, DC, 2001, National Academy Press. Available at: www.nap.edu/catalog/10027.html

Maguire P: Strategies to tackle outpatient errors, *ACP-ASIM Observer* June 2002. Available at: www.acpinternist.org/archives/2002/06/errors.htm

Malaty W, Crane S: How might acknowledging a medical error promote patient safety? *J Fam Pract* 55:775-780, 2006.

Weiss GG: Medical errors: should you apologize? *Med Econ* 83:50-54, 2006.

17

PRIVACY IN THE PHYSICIAN'S OFFICE

Sabrina Ragland, a medical assistant with 12 years of experience, works for a gastroenterologist, Dr. Tim Taylor. Her mother-in-law, Elsa Ragland, has been a registered nurse (RN) for 40 years. For more than half of her career, Elsa has worked for a local internist, Dr. Royce Berry. A casual comment at a Ragland family picnic resulted in a medical professional liability lawsuit based on violation of patient privacy. Sabrina's and Elsa's careers were jeopardized by a simple exchange of what seemed to be innocent information.

Vivian Adams, a 42-year-old hospital insurance biller, saw Dr. Berry in his office for pain in the lower left quadrant. Ms. Adams was not a new patient, but she had not visited the office in approximately 2 years.

When she arrived for her appointment, she was presented with the office privacy policy and was asked to sign the document. Vivian glanced through it, signed it, and saw the doctor. He performed an examination and found that Vivian likely was suffering from irritable bowel syndrome (IBS); he then prescribed medication. Ms. Adams called the physician 1 week later, complaining that she was no better. Dr. Berry changed her medication without seeing her and did not hear from her again, other than her requests for refills of the IBS medication.

After 6 months with no improvement, Ms. Adams went to Dr. Taylor; he performed several diagnostic tests and told Ms. Adams that she had colon cancer. She was given a **bleak** prognosis. She told Dr. Taylor that she blamed Dr. Berry for not being more thorough in his testing. Sabrina was in the room and heard the comment.

That weekend at the picnic, Sabrina mentioned Ms. Adams to her mother-in-law and stated that the patient might sue Dr. Berry, although the patient never said those words. Elsa defended Dr. Berry and proclaimed that he was a good doctor, then expressed her hope that Ms. Adams would not sue her employer. One week later, Elsa was in a grocery store and saw Ms. Adams. Elsa immediately expressed her sympathy about the diagnosis and then asked whether there was anything she could do. Her intent was to be kind and to try to **avert** litigation against Dr. Berry. Her gesture might have been well received had Ms. Adams' daughter, Terri, not been with her. Terri was not yet aware that her mother had been diagnosed with cancer. Ms. Adams had told no one about her illness at that point. After the incident at the grocery store, the first person Ms. Adams called was her attorney.

While studying this chapter, think about the following questions:

- When can the medical assistant discuss a patient, with whom, and under what circumstances?
- What has the Health Insurance Portability and Accountability Act (HIPAA) done for the medical industry and the patients it serves?

- When new policies and procedures are implemented, how can the staff embrace the changes and ease the transition?
- What happens if the patient refuses to sign the privacy policy?

LEARNING OBJECTIVES

1. Define, spell, and pronounce the terms listed in the vocabulary.
2. Explain how the HIPAA Privacy Rule benefits the healthcare industry and patients.
3. Explain the difference between Title I and Title II of the Privacy Rule.
4. List the rights of patients under the Privacy Rule.
5. List the elements that must be included in a Notice of Privacy Practices.

6. Briefly explain what is expected of healthcare providers under the Privacy Rule.
7. Describe an incidental disclosure.
8. List the three instances when a parent is not considered the child's representative.
9. Explain the circumstances under which a provider may discuss protected health information with a patient's friends and family.
10. Discuss the role of the Notice of Privacy Practices in emergencies.

VOCABULARY

avert To see coming and ward off or avoid.

bleak Not hopeful or encouraging.

business associates Individuals or organizations that perform or assist a covered entity in the performance of a function or activity involving the use or disclosure of individually identifiable health information.

complainant (kuhm-pla′-nuhnt) The person making a complaint against another person and/or organization.

covered entities As defined by HIPAA, organizations that transmit information in an electronic form during a transaction.

divulge (duh-vuhlj′) To make known, as a confidence or secret.

due diligence The effort made by an ordinarily prudent or reasonable party to prevent harm to another party or oneself; doing everything possible to prevent something negative from happening; also called *due care*.

electronic fund transfer (EFT) The movement of funds between different accounts in the same or different banks using wire transfer, automated teller machines (ATMs), or computers, without the use of paper documents.

electronic media The means of electronic transmission, including the Internet, private networks, dial-up phone lines, and fax modems; includes information moved from one place to another while stored on an electronic device.

electronic remittance advice (ERA) An explanation that accompanies checks and relays details of the payment sent to the provider from the insurance company or other third-party provider.

healthcare providers Providers of medical or health services, individually or as organizations, that furnish, bill for, or are paid for services or products.

incidental disclosure A secondary use of health information that cannot reasonably be prevented, is limited in nature, and occurs as a result of another use or disclosure that is permitted.

individually identifiable health information Any part of a patient's health record that is created or received by a covered entity.

inferred Derived as a conclusion from facts and premises.

Office for Civil Rights (OCR) The division of the federal government that enforces privacy standards.

Office of the Inspector General (OIG) An office of the U.S. Department of Health and Human Services that conducts audits, investigations, and inspections involving laws pertaining to health and human services.

personal health information (PHI) The patient's own information that pertains to his or her health.

preclude To rule out in advance.

prevalent Generally or widely accepted, practiced, or favored.

privacy officer A person designated to ensure compliance with privacy standards for a covered entity.

protected health information (PHI) Any individually identifiable health information that may be transmitted and/or maintained in electronic form.

transactions As defined by HIPAA, transmissions of information between two parties to carry out financial or administrative activities related to healthcare.

verbiage A manner of expressing oneself in words.

The creation of privacy and security laws was a huge step toward more efficient healthcare and faster reimbursements. However, technology often forces organizations to move forward somewhat quickly. Healthcare facilities with already strapped budgets sometimes view such innovations as a hindrance. Compliance officers at larger facilities may wonder whether additional federal regulations are necessary.

Many healthcare workers believe that they can say nothing to anyone, about any patient, at any time. When employees of the physician's office gain an understanding of the compliance HIPAA requires, they can feel secure in their dealings with patients and other individuals.

HEALTH INSURANCE PORTABILITY AND ACCOUNTABILITY ACT

The Health Insurance Portability and Accountability Act, or HIPAA, was enacted in 1996. The act is a group of laws that affect employees of healthcare facilities, insurance companies, or other **covered entities** and the patients they serve. The federal government required all covered entities to be in compliance with HIPAA by April 14, 2003 (small healthcare plans received an extra year to comply). As technology advances and health records become computerized, legislation

dealing with privacy is imperative. HIPAA was developed partly to help ensure the confidentiality of medical records. The statute applies to records created or maintained by healthcare providers, health plans, and healthcare clearinghouses that engage in certain electronic transactions. The Office for Civil Rights, a division of the Department of Health and Human Services (DHHS), oversees the administration of HIPAA.

HIPAA's Privacy Rule includes the following requirements.

- Patients must give specific authorization before entities covered by the regulation can use or disclose protected information in most nonroutine circumstances, such as releasing information to an employer or for use in marketing activities. Doctors, health plans, and other covered entities must follow the rule's standards for the use and disclosure of personal health information.

- Covered entities generally must provide patients with written notice of their privacy practices and patients' privacy rights. The notice must include information that might be useful for patients choosing a health plan, physician, or other provider. Patients generally are asked to sign or otherwise acknowledge receipt of the privacy notice from direct treatment providers.

- Pharmacies, health plans, and other covered entities must obtain an individual's specific authorization before sending marketing materials. Pharmacies and other covered entities are explicitly forbidden to sell personal medical information to a business that would market its products or services under a business associate agreement. Physicians and other covered entities are allowed to communicate freely with patients about treatment options and other health-related information, including disease management programs.

- Ultimately, patients generally will be able to access their personal medical records and request changes to correct any errors. In addition, patients generally could request an accounting of non-routine uses and disclosures of their health information. Remind patients that they may be charged for copies of their medical record; this is an ethical practice for the physician's office.

Many healthcare organizations are concerned about the cost of implementing and maintaining measures for complying with the privacy regulations. However, the benefits of the Privacy Rule far outweigh the inconveniences of compliance.

Effect of the HIPAA Privacy Rule

The HIPAA Privacy Rule created national standards to protect individuals' medical records and other **personal health information (PHI)**. This group of laws was the first enacted to protect patients' privacy. The Privacy Rule benefits both patients and **healthcare providers**:

- Patients have more control over their medical records.
- Patients are able to make informed choices about the use of their PHI.
- Boundaries are set on the use and release of health records.
- Safeguards are established that healthcare providers must ensure to protect the privacy of health information.
- Violators are held accountable and face both civil and criminal penalties if patients' privacy rights are compromised.
- Public health is protected by the balance struck between public responsibility and disclosure of PHI.

Under the few laws that existed before the HIPAA Privacy Rule, personal health information could be distributed to others without notifying the patient or obtaining his or her authorization, even if the information exchange had nothing to do with the patient's medical treatment or healthcare reimbursement. A health plan could pass patient information to a financial lender, who might then deny the patient a home mortgage or credit card based on the health history. Employers could obtain health information and use it in personnel decisions. Because computers make information exchange so much easier, laws had to be enacted to protect patients' privacy.

Note that the abbreviation PHI has more than one meaning in medical terminology. PHI stands for both *personal* health information, which relates to the patient, and *protected* health information, which relates to information transmitted electronically. Always consider the context in which these abbreviations are used when interpreting information related to the electronic medical record.

Title I and Title II Provisions

HIPAA has two provisions, Title I and Title II. Title I covers insurance reform, and Title II deals with administrative simplification. Title I limits the use of pre-existing health conditions, which in the past prevented an employee from obtaining health insurance coverage or limited that coverage. If an individual left a job with insurance coverage and attempted to secure new coverage, a pre-existing health condition often would **preclude** that person from obtaining coverage for that illness. Many individuals were refused any coverage at all, especially if the condition was a serious one, such as a heart condition or high blood pressure. Today, because of HIPAA laws, discrimination against individuals in poor health now or in the past is prohibited. The regulations limit the use of pre-existing condition exclusions and guarantee that certain individuals can purchase healthcare insurance after leaving or losing a job.

The Consolidated Omnibus Budget Reconciliation Act (COBRA) was passed by Congress in 1986. COBRA provides certain former employees, retirees, spouses, former spouses, and dependent children with group health coverage. The premium usually is higher than that paid during employment but still usually lower than for individual health coverage. Most people who lose their job for any reason have difficulty paying for COBRA coverage.

Certain criteria must be met to qualify for COBRA coverage. The company must have at least 50 employees to be required to offer COBRA to its employees. The employees need not all be full-time workers; certain calculations allow part-time workers to be counted to reach the 50-employee benchmark. Also, the employee must be a "qualified beneficiary" to receive COBRA benefits. A *qualified beneficiary* is an individual who was covered under the healthcare plan the day before a qualifying event. A *qualifying event* is an incident that would cause an employee to lose healthcare coverage.

The goal of Title II is to reduce administrative costs in the healthcare industry. Often goals sound simple, but many steps must be taken to reach a goal. Many different objectives must be met to simplify the administrative costs involved in patient care. Several agencies must work together and agree on various regulations. They must share information and resources. Agencies must compromise and "give and take" when forming policies or working toward administrative goals.

CRITICAL THINKING APPLICATION 17-1
- How does information sharing help to cut patient healthcare costs?
- What other reasons might exist for sharing patient information?

Provisions of Administrative Simplification

Electronic media are used daily in modern physicians' offices and healthcare facilities. Because computer use has become **prevalent**, patients have begun to express concern about who sees **protected health information (PHI)** and what is done with that information.

Title II of HIPAA has two parts:

- Development and implementation of standardized electronic **transactions** using standard code sets
- Implementation of privacy and security procedures to prevent the misuse of health information by ensuring confidentiality

The second part of the administrative simplification provision deals with the privacy, confidentiality, and security of PHI and is the focus of this chapter.

Patients' Rights

Separate from the Patient's Bill of Rights, HIPAA provides for several patients' rights:

- The right to notice of a facility's privacy practices
- The right to have access to, view, and obtain a copy of their PHI
- The right to restrict certain parts or uses of their PHI
- The right to request that communications from the facility be kept confidential
- The right to request that the facility amend the PHI
- The right to receive notice of all disclosures of their PHI

These rights are the heart of the HIPAA Privacy Rule. They must be protected by all involved in the healthcare profession.

Right to Notice of Privacy Practices

Patients have the right to a copy of the Notice of Privacy Practices used in the physician's office (Figure 17-1). A copy of this document also must be prominently displayed in the office. These privacy practices are developed by the individual facility and must be written in language that patients will understand. Patients should be given a copy of the Notice of Privacy Practices and should sign an acknowledgment that they received it. If a patient refuses to sign the acknowledgment, the medical assistant can note that the document was offered to the patient and the person refused to sign. This proves **due diligence** on the part of the office and that a good faith effort was made to provide the patient with privacy information. Most patients sign the document. Be prepared to explain the Notice of Privacy Practices to patients. It must include:

- How PHI is used and disclosed by the facility
- The duties of the provider in protecting health information
- The patient's rights regarding PHI
- How complaints can be filed if patients believe their privacy has been violated
- Whom to contact at the facility for more information
- The effective date of the Notice of Privacy Practices

WALNUT HILL FAMILY AND PREVENTIVE MEDICINE CLINIC, PA
1701 W. Walnut Hill Lane, Suite 200
Dallas, Texas 75229
214-549-1111   214-549-1222 (FAX)
info@walnuthillclinic.com

NOTICE OF PRIVACY PRACTICES

THIS NOTICE DESCRIBES HOW MEDICAL INFORMATION ABOUT YOU MAY BE USED AND DISCLOSED AND HOW YOU CAN GET ACCESS TO THIS INFORMATION.
PLEASE REVIEW IT CAREFULLY.

YOUR MEDICAL RECORD (CHART) contains your symptoms, examination, and test results, diagnoses, treatment, and plan for follow-up. This is protected health information (PHI), and is used for many reasons. Your medical record serves as a:

- basis for planning your care and treatment (this includes scheduling and appointment reminders)
- means of communication among the many health professionals who contribute to your care
- legal document describing the care you received
- means by which you or a third-party payer can verify services billed
- tool in educating health professionals
- source of data for quality control programs and medical research
- source of information for public health officials (by law, certain illnesses must be reported)

YOUR HEALTH INFORMATION RIGHTS
Although your medical record (chart) is the physical property of the clinic, the information contained within the record belongs to you. You have the right to:

- request a restriction on certain uses and disclosures of your information
- obtain a paper copy of this notice
- inspect and obtain a copy of your medical record as provided in our office policy manual
- amend your health record (requests must be made in writing)
- request communications of your health information by alternative means or at alternative locations
- revoke your authorization to use or disclose health information except to the extent that action has already been taken
- obtain an accounting of any non-routine disclosures of your health information

OUR RESPONSIBILITIES
The Walnut Hill Family and Preventive Medicine Clinic is required to:

- maintain the privacy of your medical record (chart)
- abide by the terms of this notice
- notify you if we are unable to agree to a requested restriction
- accommodate reasonable requests you may have to communicate health information by alternative means or at alternative locations or phone numbers

We reserve the right to change our practices and to make new provisions effective for all protected health information we maintain. We will post a copy of our current notice in a visible location at all times. We will not use or disclose your protected health information without your authorization, except as described in this notice.

FOR MORE INFORMATION OR TO REPORT A PROBLEM
Please contact Sue Singer or Ron Rachels during regular office hours at 214-549-1111 or you can email or mail questions or complaints to Dr. Robbie Speasak at the above address. If you believe that your privacy rights have been violated, you can file a complaint with the Secretary of the Department of Health and Human Services. You will not be penalized in any way for filing a complaint.

FIGURE 17-1 HIPAA Notice of Privacy Practices.

Right to Access Protected Health Information

Patients must be allowed access to their personal health information (Procedure 17-1). The maker, not the patient, owns the record; however, the HIPAA Privacy Rule grants patients the right to access, inspect, and obtain a copy of their health information. Most physicians' offices require patients to request access in writing and to act on that request within 30 days (Figure 17-2). HIPAA restricts access to psychotherapy notes, information compiled for use in legal proceedings, and information exempted from disclosure by the Clinical Laboratory Improvement Amendments (CLIA).

CRITICAL THINKING APPLICATION   17-2

- Why is patients' access to protected health information important?
- When might the patient need access to his or her health records?

Right to Request Restrictions on Certain Uses and Disclosures of Protected Health Information

Patients can request restrictions on the use of their PHI. For instance, if a patient had an abortion many years ago and does not want that information released, she has the right to ask a provider not to **divulge** that information. The provider does not have to agree to the request but must review it and give a good reason for the restriction not to be honored. An appeal process should be in place for cases in which the provider does not agree with the restriction.

Right to Request Confidential Communications

Patients have the right to determine where they want to receive communications from the provider. The patient may prefer to be contacted on a cell phone instead of a home phone, or through e-mail. Providers must accommodate reasonable requests. Suppose a married female patient comes to the clinic for a pregnancy test. Further suppose that her husband has had a vasectomy. Clearly, a call to her home phone number with test results could initiate personal and private difficulties for the patient. Document the preferred method of communication in the patient's medical record and make certain that method is used for each contact until the patient dictates otherwise.

Right to Request Amendment of Protected Health Information

If patients inspect their medical record and find an error, they can request that changes be made to the record. This request should be made in writing. Providers must review the request and act on it in a timely manner, generally within 60 days. The request may be denied if the provider was not the creator of the record, as in the case of records provided by a consulting physician. Or, the provider may believe that the information is correct and complete. A review process must be in place by which such requests can be considered.

Right to Receive an Accounting of Disclosures of Protected Health Information

Patients may request that the physician provide an accounting of all disclosures of the patient's PHI that are nonroutine (as defined in the facility's Notice of Privacy Practices). Patients are entitled to receive this accounting annually without charge, but the provider can charge patients for additional accountings.

PROCEDURE 17-1

Apply HIPAA Rules in Regard to Privacy/Release of Information

GOAL: *To follow HIPAA guidelines so that the patient's confidentiality is kept and the patient's health information is protected.*

EQUIPMENT and SUPPLIES

- Copy of the HIPAA guidelines
- Office policy and procedures manual
- Release of information forms
- Notice of privacy policy

PROCEDURAL STEPS

1. Review the HIPAA law, office policy and procedures manual, and the facility's notice of privacy practices.
   PURPOSE: To make certain that all applicable laws and policies are followed when releasing medical information.
2. Examine the document requesting release of patient information.
   PURPOSE: To determine whether the document is valid and the information can be released to the requesting party. Most medical facilities require that all information requests be addressed in writing, and some require a specific time period for response, such as 1 week.
3. Compare the request to the facility's own information release form. Send the requestor a facility form, if necessary, by mail or fax.

PURPOSE: To obtain all of the information that the facility requires in releasing information. Some requests are not complete when received, and the medical assistant must make certain that all of the required information is provided before the release of a patient's information.

4. Determine what information is being requested.
   PURPOSE: The medical facility should not release any information other than what is specifically requested.
5. Make copies of the information for the requestor.
6. Mail or fax the information, depending upon the requested method of delivery. Make certain that fax submissions contain a confidentiality statement.
   PURPOSE: To ensure the patient's confidentiality.
7. Document the release of information in the patient's medical record, if required by office policy.
   PURPOSE: To provide a reference point for when the request was completed and mailed.

REQUEST TO ACCESS MEDICAL RECORD

Patients have the right to access their personal health information. We will be happy to accommodate any patient who wishes to exercise this access to inspect or obtain a copy of the record. Please provide the information requested on this form. This request will be acted upon within thirty (30) days. Standard copy charges will apply.

Patient Name _____

Date of Birth _____ Phone _____

Address _____

City _____ State _____ ZIP_____

Email Address _____

Date of Last Office Visit _____

Please note below what information should be copied or provided:

_____

_____

_____

Please note below the following change(s) that need to be addressed:

_____

_____

I wish to receive a regular accounting of non-routine disclosures of my protected health information.

☐ Yes   ☐ No

_____   _____

Patient Signature   Date

FOR OFFICE USE ONLY

Date Copied _____ Date Mailed _____

Certified Mail # _____

FIGURE 17-2 Request to access a medical record.

SEVEN COMPONENTS OF A HIPAA COMPLIANCE PROGRAM

The Office of the Inspector General (OIG) of the Department of Health and Human Services has developed seven components of an effective HIPAA compliance program:

1. Conducting internal monitoring and auditing
2. Implementing compliance and practice standards
3. Designating a compliance officer or contact
4. Conducting appropriate training and education
5. Responding appropriately to detected offenses and developing corrective action
6. Developing open lines of communication
7. Enforcing disciplinary standards through well-publicized guidelines

Responsibilities of Providers or Health Plans

The responsibilities placed on providers and health plans seems extensive when one reads the actual **verbiage** of the law. Do not be intimidated when reading a publication written by the federal government. These documents are rarely written for ease of understanding and may need to be reread several times before the reader grasps the meaning of a regulation.

In general, the HIPAA Privacy Rule requires that providers perform activities such as the following.

- Notifying patients of their privacy rights
- Explaining how their health information might be used
- Developing privacy procedures in the facility
- Implementing those privacy procedures
- Training employees so that they understand the procedures
- Designating an individual to be responsible for implementation
- Securing medical records so that they are not available to those who do not need them

HIPAA AND ELECTRONIC FUND TRANSFERS

As discussed earlier in this chapter, one of the main goals of HIPAA legislation is administrative simplification. After HIPAA was enacted, an amendment was added to place the **electronic fund transfer (EFT)** on the list of electronic health care transactions that are addressed in HIPAA.

Not only do EFTs cut costs, they help the provider to maintain patients' privacy, because checks and other written documents might be seen by other patients. By computerizing all of these transactions, privacy is maximized for the patient. The new legislation addresses both the EFT and **electronic remittance advice (ERA)**, the document that explains the payment being sent to the provider.

Because EFTs eliminate the need for paper, printing, and postage costs, using EFTs is more economical. Also, the facility saves staff time and expenses, because staff members are not required to manually process and deposit checks, According to the Centers for Medicare and Medicaid Services (CMS), the benefits of changing to an electronic system are obvious; however, many providers and health facilities have still not converted to electronic processing. This forces the physicians and employees to do paperwork instead of using that time to deliver health care to patients. Although all covered entities are required to comply with the adopted standards of HIPAA transactions, the health care EFT standards are expected to have the most substantial cost and benefit impacts on physician practices, hospitals, and commercial and government health plans. The CMS estimates that these entities will save $3 billion to $4.5 billion over the next 10 years. The EFT regulation became effective in January, 2012, and HIPAA-covered entities must be in compliance by January 1, 2014.

PERMISSION TO DISCLOSE PROTECTED HEALTH INFORMATION

Once the patient has signed the Notice of Privacy Practices, the physician may disclose PHI in the manner that is described in the policy. Virtually all the daily operations that involve PHI are covered under the privacy practices document.

Some offices ask patients to sign a receipt of the Notice of Privacy Practices annually. Others simply post the current policy prominently in the office and state where it can be found on the original notice that the patient signs. With either method, every current medical record should contain a signed Notice of Privacy Practices, an acknowledgement that the patient received the Notice of Privacy Practices, or a statement that the patient refused to sign it. Physicians also use separate release of information forms that detail exactly where to call a patient, whether the patient prefers e-mail communications, and/or specific releases for information related to human immunodeficiency virus (HIV) infection or psychotherapy (Figures 17-3 and 17-4).

At times, conflicting permissions may be an issue in the disclosure of PHI. Suppose a patient requests that a copy of his or her medical record be sent to a third party, such as an attorney. The patient signs the release at an office visit. Before the medical record is copied and sent, the attorney forwards a signed release for just the progress notes. Call the patient first and attempt to verify what he or she wants sent. Another option is to adhere to the most restrictive request; in this case, send only the progress notes. Always document any form of communication about the patient's preference in writing. The medical assistant may find it necessary to ask the patient to sign a new permission form. Do not hesitate to contact the patient if any question arises about what the person wants released.

New HIPAA legislation has been enacted that will require physicians to track any disclosure of a patient's medical information. Additionally, HIPAA will now affect the physician's **business associates**, such as clearinghouses, attorneys, accountants, and others who have access to protected health information. This is the first time the federal government has regulated the business associates of providers, and it means that business associates will have more culpability with regard to privacy violations. When a breach of privacy happens, the provider or business associate must provide notification to the patient in writing. Providers have until January 1, 2014, to comply with these regulations; however, patients will be able to request an accounting of disclosures back to 2011.

Identifying the Patient

Providers see numerous patients each day, and the medical assistant may not know each one by sight. Always insist on identification when releasing any type of health information to anyone. A state-issued driver's license or identification card is the best means of identification, but alternates may be necessary for those who do not have that particular document. The office policy and procedures manual should list acceptable forms of identification. When making any type of disclosure, make sure to note the reason the person has the authority to request and receive the PHI.

Patients' Names and Sign-In Sheets

A staff member in a physician's office may call out a patient's name when it is time to see the physician. Sign-in sheets that list patients' names may also be used. Covered entities are permitted to make such incidental disclosures if they comply with the minimum necessary requirements of HIPAA (Figure 17-5). An **incidental disclosure** is a secondary use that cannot reasonably be prevented, is limited in nature, and occurs as a result of another use or disclosure that is permitted.

The Privacy Rule is not intended to impede customary and necessary healthcare communications or practices or to require that all risk of incidental use or disclosure be eliminated to satisfy the rule's standards. Disclosures that could occur as a byproduct of engaging in healthcare communications or practices may be considered acceptable under the Privacy Rule. Incidental disclosures might include:

- Confidential conversations between providers or with patients, if a possibility exists that they may be overheard (e.g., by hearing the patient and physician talking through the wall when in an adjacent examination room)
- Seeing other patients' names when signing in
- A person not authorized to see PHI walks by medical equipment and sees material containing **individually identifiable health information** (e.g., sees a patient's name on an ultrasound screen)
- Physicians speaking with patients in semiprivate hospital rooms
- Healthcare staff orally coordinating patient care services at a nurses' station or central location in an office
- A pharmacist discussing a patient with a physician on the phone when another person is standing nearby

Most physicians' offices have implemented sign-in sheets that ideally allow only one patient to sign in at a time and that prevent the person from seeing other patients' names. Sign-in sheets that use pressure-sensitive stickers are a good example. The patient signs in on the form, then the sticker is removed and placed either in the patient's medical record or on a log sheet. Some offices are more technologically advanced and have a computer sign-in system. The patient arrives and goes to the computer screen, sees his or her name, and then presses "enter" to signify that he or she has arrived for the

**Patient Consent to the Use and Disclosure of Health Information
for Treatment, Payment, or Health Care Operations**

I understand that as part of my health care, the practice originates and maintains paper and/or electronic records describing my health history, symptoms, examination and test results, diagnoses, treatment, and any plans for future care or treatment. I understand that this information serves as:

- A basis for planning my care and treatment,
- A means of communication among professionals who contribute to my care,
- A source of information for applying my diagnosis and treatment information to my bill,
- A means by which a third-party payer can verify that services billed were actually provided,
- A tool for routine health care operations, such as assessing quality and reviewing the competence of staff.

I have been provided the opportunity to review the *"Notice of Patient Privacy Information Practices"* **that provides a more complete description of information uses and disclosures. I understand that I have the following rights:**

- The right to review the *"Notice"* prior to acknowledging this consent,
- The right to restrict or revoke the use or disclosure of my health information for other uses or purposes, and
- The right to request restrictions as to how my health information may be used or disclosed to carry out treatment, payment, or health care operations.

Restrictions:

I request the following restrictions to the use or disclosure of my health information:

_____

_____

May discuss treatment, payment, or health care operation with the following persons:

(Please check all that apply)   Spouse [   ]   Your Children [   ]   Relatives [   ]   Others [   ]   Parents [   ]

Please list the names and relationship, if you checked "Relatives" or "Others" above

_____

_____

Messages or Appointment Reminders: (Please check all that apply)

May we leave a message on your answering machine at home [   ] or at work [   ]? **Do not leave a message** [   ]
May we leave a message with someone at your **home** using the doctor's name or the practice name? Yes [   ] No [   ]
May we leave a message with someone at your **work** using the doctor's name or the practice name? Yes [   ] No [   ]
Messages will be of a nonsensitive nature, such as appointment reminders.

I understand that as part of treatment, payment, or health care operations, it may become necessary to disclose health information to another entity, i.e., referrals to other health care providers, labs, and/or other individuals or agencies as permitted or required by state or federal law.

I fully understand and accept the information provided by this consent.

_____   _____   _____
Signature   Print name of person signing   Date

*If other than patient is signing, are you the parent, legal guardian, custodian, or have Power of Attorney for this patient for treatment, payment, or health care operations? Yes [   ] No [   ]

_____

FOR OFFICE USE ONLY
[   ] Patient refused to sign the consent form.
[   ] Restrictions were added by the patient (see restrictions listed above)
[   ] "Consent form" received and reviewed by _____ on (date) _____
[   ] "Consent form" placed in the patient's medical record on (date) _____

FIGURE 17-3 Example of a HIPAA-compliant patient disclosure form. (From Klieger DM: *Saunders essentials of medical assisting,* ed 2, St Louis, 2010, WB Saunders.)

appointment. The patient's name appears only for 15 minutes or so before the appointment and for 15 minutes after. If the name is not on the screen, the patient is directed to see the office staff. This subtly teaches the patient to be on time for appointments. These devices save time, although the patient must receive brief training in how to use the system. The short time the patient's name is on the screen is an incidental exposure, but it is acceptable according to HIPAA guidelines, as explained previously.

Placement of Patient Medical Records

Many physicians' offices place medical records inside a wall folder just outside the examination room. By turning the record so that the name cannot be seen by someone passing in the hallway, the facility meets the minimum necessary requirement to protect patient privacy. The hallway area should be supervised, and nonemployees should be escorted when in the clinical area of the office.

CRITICAL THINKING APPLICATION   **17-3**

- Why is it important to safeguard the names of patients in hallways?
- How might Patient A be affected if Patient B sees Patient A's name on a chart in the medical facility?

GENERAL MEDICAL HEALTH CARE

AUTHORIZATION FOR RELEASE OF MEDICAL INFORMATION

I, _____ ____/____/____ _____ hereby authorize
       Print Patient's Name   Date of Birth   Social Security Number

General Medical Health Care 1234 Riverview Road, Anytown, FL 33333

to release medical, including HIV Antibody Testing, Psychiatric/Psychological, Alcohol and/or Drug Abuse, information records to:

To: _____

Address _____
       (Street)   (City)   (State)   (ZIP)

For the purpose of: 1. Drs. appointment on: _____

                    2. Other: _____

                  _____
                       Please Specify Reason for Disclosure

I understand that if I consent to the release of any of my medical records, the results of any HIV Antibody Testing, Psychiatric/Psychological, Alcohol and/or Drug Abuse information will be released.

I understand this consent may be cancelled upon written notice to the hospital, except that action by the hospital has been taken in reliance on this authorization, and that this authorization shall remain in force for a 90-day period in order to effect the purpose for which it is given. Alcohol and drug abuse information, if present, has been disclosed from records whose confidentiality is protected by Federal Law. FEDERAL REGULATIONS (42CFR, part II) prohibit making any further disclosure of records without the specific written authorization of the undersigned, or as otherwise permitted by such regulations. The confidentiality of HIV antibody test results is protected by Florida Law [Fla. Stat.ANN. 381.609 (2) (F)], which prohibits any further disclosure by a person to whom this information has been disclosed, without specific written consent of the undersigned or as otherwise permitted by state law.

_____   From: _____   To: _____
      (Date of Authorization)   (Dates to be Released)

_____
       Patient's Signature

_____
  Parent, Legal Guardian, or Authorized
       Representative Signature

_____
      Relationship to Patient

_____
          Witness

FIGURE 17-4 Example of a HIPAA-compliant patient disclosure form that includes permission for release of human immunodeficiency virus (HIV) and psychological information. (From Klieger DM: *Saunders essentials of medical assisting,* ed 2, St Louis, 2010, WB Saunders.)

Children's Health Records

The Privacy Rule does allow parents to see the medical records of their children as long as this is not inconsistent with state law. In most cases the parent is the child's personal representative under the Privacy Rule (Figure 17-6). However, under some circumstances, the parent is not considered the child's personal representative, such as:

- When the minor is the one who consents to care and the parent's consent is not required under state or other applicable law (e.g., an emancipated minor)
- When the minor obtains care at the direction of a court or a person appointed by the court
- When the parent agrees that the minor and healthcare provider may have a confidential relationship

A minor may need treatment for a sexually transmitted disease, pregnancy, or other issue that may best be treated with discretion, without involving the parent. The office manager may wish to identify such patients or individual office visits in a manner different from their normal record to ensure their privacy. Always be certain

HIPAA MINIMUM NECESSARY STANDARD
[45 CFR 164.502(b), 164.514(d)]

Background

The minimum necessary standard, a key protection of the HIPAA Privacy Rule, is derived from confidentiality codes and practices in common use today. It is based on sound current practice that protected health information should not be used or disclosed when it is not necessary to satisfy a particular purpose or carry out a function. The minimum necessary standard requires covered entities to evaluate their practices and enhance safeguards as needed to limit unnecessary or inappropriate access to and disclosure of protected health information. The Privacy Rule's requirements for minimum necessary standards are designed to be sufficiently flexible to accommodate the various circumstances of any covered entity.

How the Rule Works

The Privacy Rule generally requires covered entities to take reasonable steps to limit the use or disclosure of, and requests for, protected health information to the minimum necessary to accomplish the intended purpose. The minimum necessary standard does not apply to the following:

- Disclosures to or requests by a health care provider for treatment purposes.
- Disclosures to the individual who is the subject of the information.
- Uses or disclosures made pursuant to an individual's authorization.
- Uses or disclosures required for compliance with the Health Insurance Portability and Accountability Act (HIPAA) Administrative Simplification Rules.
- Disclosures to the Department of Health and Human Services (HHS) when disclosure of information is required under the Privacy Rule for enforcement purposes.
- Uses or disclosures that are required by other law.

The implementation specifications for this provision require a covered entity to develop and implement policies and procedures appropriate for its own organization, reflecting the entity's business practices and workforce. While guidance cannot anticipate every question or factual application of the minimum necessary standard to each specific industry context, where it would be generally helpful we will seek to provide additional clarification on this issue in the future. In addition, the Department will continue to monitor the workability of the minimum necessary standard and consider proposing revisions, where appropriate, to ensure that the Rule does not hinder timely access to quality health care.

http://www.hhs.gov/ocr/hipaa/

FIGURE 17-5 Overview for HIPAA's minimum necessary standard.

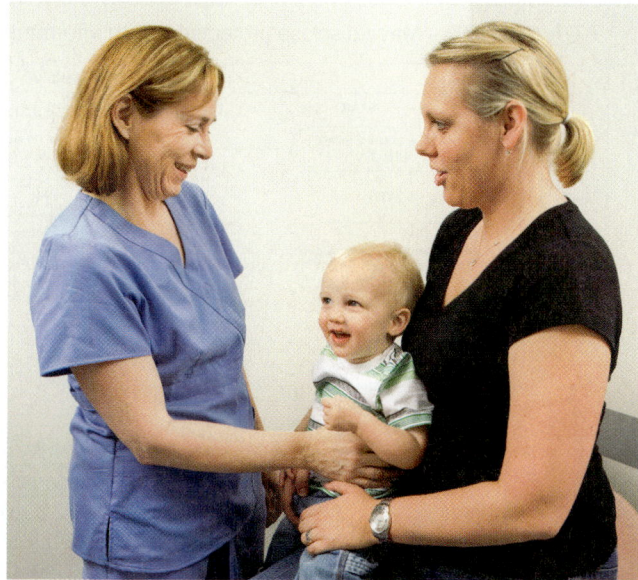

FIGURE 17-6 In most cases the parent is considered the child's representative and is allowed to see the child's medical records.

members, friends, or other individuals identified by the patient. The covered entity also may share relevant information with the family and these other people if it can reasonably be **inferred**, based on professional judgment, that the patient does not object or that the action is in the patient's best interest. Remember that if the patient has requested that such information not be shared with others, the provider must honor that request unless it is deemed unreasonable.

Both covered entities and business associates can discuss a patient's bill with a person other than the patient to obtain reimbursement. No limit is placed on those to whom such a disclosure may be made. However, the Privacy Rule does require a covered entity or business associate to reasonably limit the amount of information disclosed for such purposes to the minimum necessary and to abide by any reasonable requests by the patient for confidential communications and restrictions.

Telephone Messages and Faxes

Medical assistants must communicate with patients, and that communication often is initiated with a telephone call. At times the patient is not at home or available, and the medical assistant must use professional judgment about leaving a message and how much information to disclose to the person who answers the telephone. Even leaving a message on an answering machine can be questionable, because no one is sure who will hear a message containing PHI.

If the patient has requested that the provider or provider's employees communicate only in a confidential manner, such as by alternative means or at an alternative location, the provider must honor that request if it is reasonable. For instance, requests to receive calls at work instead of at home are reasonable requests, unless there are extenuating circumstances.

A fax can be sent containing PHI to another healthcare provider for treatment purposes or to another individual as requested by the patient. Use reasonable care in sending a fax, such as verifying the correct numbers, directing the fax to a certain person, and using

that state and national laws are not being broken when dealing with patients who are minors.

Discussing Information with Family and Friends

The Privacy Rule specifically permits covered entities to share information directly relevant to the patient's care with a spouse, family

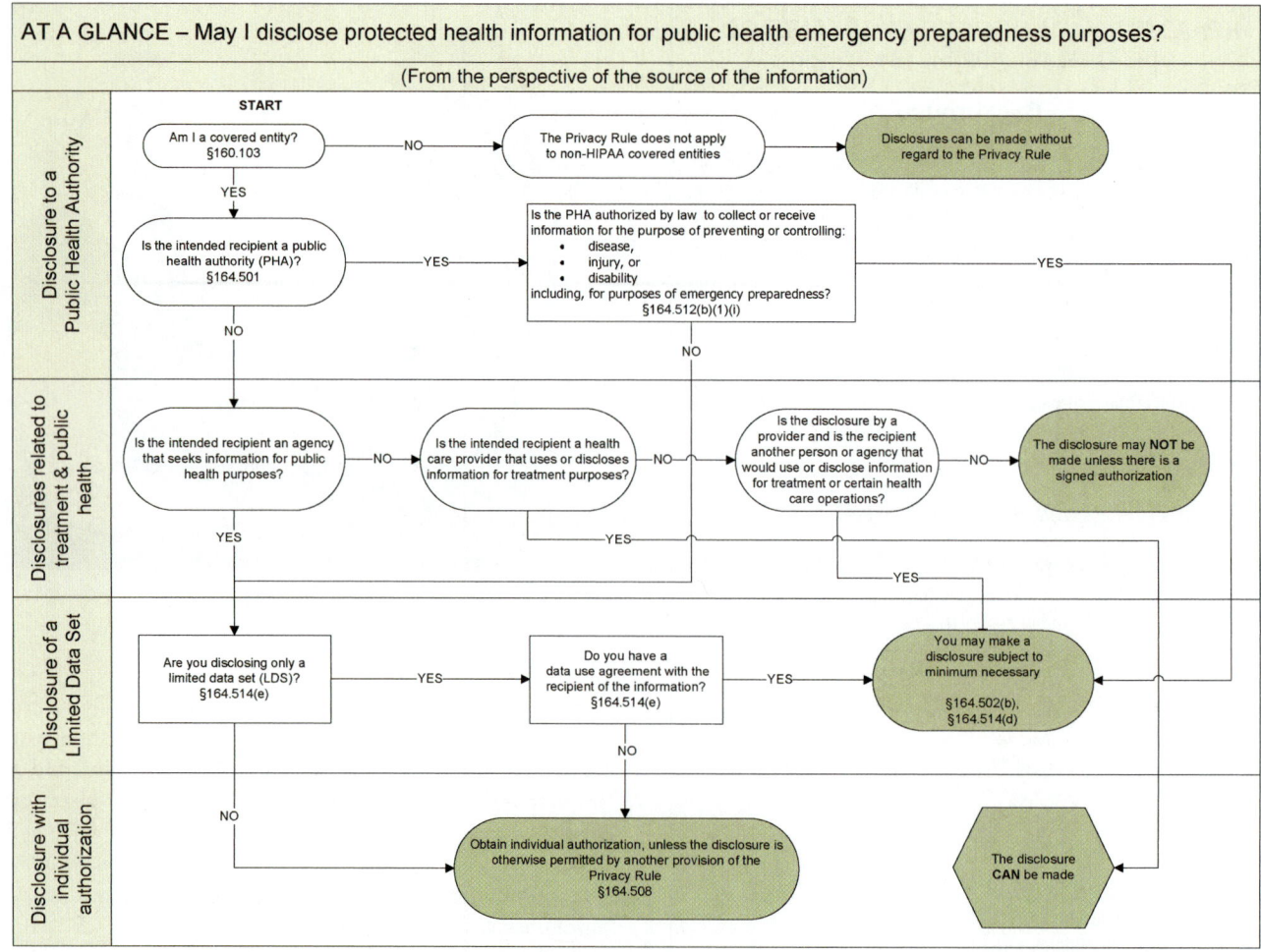

FIGURE 17-7 Guidelines for compliance with HIPAA's privacy regulations. (From Burton B: *Quick guide to HIPAA for the physician's office,* St Louis, 2003, WB Saunders.)

cover sheets that stress confidentiality. All fax machines should be located in secure areas to prevent unauthorized access to PHI. Information used for treatment purposes can be shared by fax, e-mail, or telephone with other healthcare providers.

Emergencies

Healthcare providers and facilities, such as hospitals, with a direct treatment relationship with individuals are not required to provide their Notice of Privacy Practices to patients at the time they are providing emergency treatment (Figure 17-7). In such situations, the HIPAA Privacy Rule requires only that providers give patients a notice when it is practical to do so after the emergency situation has resolved. In addition, the Privacy Rule does not require that providers make a good faith effort to obtain the patient's written acknowledgment of receipt of the notice.

Complaints About Privacy Violations

When a patient has a complaint about a violation of the privacy of his or her information, the first person he or she should talk to is the **privacy officer** at the facility where the incident occurred. If the complaint is not resolved, the patient should be directed to the office manager or physician. In the event the patient's issue has still not been resolved, he or she may file a written complaint, either on paper or electronically, with the **Office for Civil Rights (OCR)**. The

complaint must be filed within 180 days of when the **complainant** knew or should have known that the act had occurred. The OCR may waive the 180-day time limit if good cause is shown. Complaints must meet the following criteria:

- They must be filed in writing, either on paper or electronically.
- They must name the entity that is the subject of the complaint.
- They must describe the acts or omissions believed to be in violation of the Privacy Rule.
- They must be filed within 180 days of the incident.
- They must apply to an incident that occurred after April 14, 2003 (2004 for small health plans).

The OCR has 10 regional offices, each covering certain states. Complaints must be filed with the regional office that has jurisdiction over the state in which the incident occurred. A complaint form is available on the OCR Web site. The **Office of the Inspector General (OIG)** conducts investigations and audits when a question arises regarding privacy laws.

HIPAA AND EMERGENCY PREPAREDNESS

During major catastrophes and evacuations, healthcare providers face significant challenges in keeping their patients and staff members

PROCEDURE 17-2

Perform Risk Management Procedures

GOAL: *To prevent risk and liability in the physician's office.*

EQUIPMENT and SUPPLIES

- Copy of laws affecting the physician's practice
- Computer with Internet access
- Office policy and procedure manual

PROCEDURAL STEPS

1. Research laws that affect the medical office on the Internet. Make certain that the sites used for research are reliable.
   PURPOSE: To determine the laws that will influence the operations of a medical office and how they affect the role of the medical assistant.
2. Research your individual state on the Internet and look for patient confidentiality and disclosure laws.
3. Become familiar with office policies and procedures.
   PURPOSE: To make certain that policies and procedures are followed when carrying out daily operations at the medical facility.
4. Determine common risks that occur in the medical facility.
   PURPOSE: To learn what issues or situations might result in losses at a medical facility and determine ways to avoid such risks.
5. Perform a risk assessment at the medical facility.
   PURPOSE: To determine specific risks that are present at a medical facility.
6. Discuss the risks with office management or in a staff meeting.
7. Determine ways to eliminate the risks found during the assessment.
   PURPOSE: To work as a team to eliminate possible risks.
8. Devise a plan to eliminate or reduce risk in the medical office based upon the risk assessment.
   PURPOSE: To take specific steps toward the reduction of risk in the facility.
9. Document all risk assessments and management efforts.
   PURPOSE: To provide proof that risks were addressed and managed as required by regulatory and/or compliance agencies.

---

safe while providing continuity of their healthcare plans. Also, individuals with disabilities make the process more difficult; sometimes the healthcare provider and the patient are the only two resources available to find a safe place for themselves.

Medical offices must have a safety evacuation plan that covers major disasters and allows healthcare professionals to be available in case they are needed at a disaster site. The best plans are developed by the actual site that will use them, so that they are customized for that particular facility, area, and its resources. For instance, if the medical office is next door to the hospital where the physician has staff privileges, transporting patients would be easier than if the hospital were several blocks away. For this reason, the office staff should discuss the problems they would face in an emergency and plan for the individual needs of both the staff members and the patients. The patients' privacy is a primary factor during any emergency, so the plan must include contingencies for maintaining that privacy. By pre-planning, the medical facility performs one type of risk management; planning efforts and the subsequent use of the plan helps the physician and employees to avoid new or additional injuries and/or illnesses (Procedure 17-2).

The office staff must be aware of the acceptable times to communicate with others about patient care, especially in emergency situations. Just because an emergency exists does not mean that the medical assistant is automatically free to release health information about the facility's patients.

CLOSING COMMENTS

Every employee of the physician's office must read the policy and procedures manual to make sure he or she clearly understands the

CIRCUMSTANCES IN WHICH HEALTHCARE PROVIDERS MAY COMMUNICATE WITH FAMILY, FRIENDS, OR OTHERS INVOLVED IN A PATIENT'S CARE

- If the patient does not object and office policy is followed, healthcare providers can communicate with family, friends, and others involved in the patient's care. This should be indicated on the appropriate form and placed into the patient's medical record.
- If the patient is unconscious, healthcare providers may communicate with others if they believe it is in the patient's best interests; however, they may not share with any person information about a past condition unrelated to the current incident.
- The provider should obtain written permission from the patient to share information; however, this is not always mandatory and not always practical, especially during emergencies.
- Healthcare providers must set their own rules for verifying requests for information (e.g., a driver's license must be shown before copies of a patient's records are discussed or provided) and for determining whether the individual is entitled to the information.
- Other people designated by the patient can pick up medical supplies, x-ray films, or prescriptions. Most facilities and offices insist on some type of identification in these instances.
- Healthcare providers can discuss information with an interpreter, who then communicates with family and friends about the patient's healthcare.
- Through the healthcare facility's privacy policy, patients should designate in advance the individuals who can access and discuss their health information.

Guidelines for HIPAA Privacy Compliance

1. Consider that conversations occurring throughout the office could be overheard. The reception area and waiting room are often linked, and it is easy to hear the scheduling of appointments and exchange of confidential information. It is necessary to observe areas and maximize efforts to avoid unauthorized disclosures. Simple and affordable precautions include using privacy glass at the front desk and having conversations away from settings where other patients or visitors are present. Health care providers can move their dictation stations away from patient areas or wait until no patients are present before dictating. Phone conversations by providers in front of patients, even in emergency situations, should be avoided. Providers and staff must use their best professional judgment.

2. Be sure to check in the patient medical record and in the computer system to see if there are any special instructions for contacting the patient regarding scheduling or reporting test results. Follow these requests as agreed by the office.

3. Patient sign-in sheets are permissible, but limit the information requested when a patient signs in, and change it periodically during the day. A sign-in sheet must not contain information such as reason for visit because some providers specialize in treating patients with sensitive issues. Showing that a particular individual has an appointment with the physician may pose a breach of confidentiality.

4. Make sure patients sign a form acknowledging receipt of the NPP. The NPP allows the physician to release the patient's confidential information for billing and other purposes. If the practice has other confidentiality statements and policies besides HIPAA mandates, these must be reviewed to ensure they meet HIPAA requirements.

5. Format policies for transferring and accepting outside PHI must address how the office keeps this information confidential. When using courier services, billing services, transcription services, or email, ensure that transferring PHI is done in a secure and compliant manner.

6. Computers are used for a variety of administrative functions, including scheduling, billing, and managing medical records. Computers typically are present at the reception area. Keep the computer screen turned so that viewing is restricted to authorized staff. Screensavers should be used to prevent unauthorized viewing or access. The computer should automatically log off the user after a period of being idle, requiring the staff member to reenter their password.

7. Keep usernames and passwords confidential, and change them often. Do not share this information. An authorized staff member such as the PO will have administrative access to reset passwords if they are lost or if someone discovers the password. Also, practice management software can track users and follow their activity. Do not ever give out a password. Safeguards include password protection for electronic data and storing paper records securely.

8. Safeguard the work area; do not place notes with confidential information in areas that are easy to view by nonstaff. Cleaning services will access the building, usually after business hours; ensure that PHI is protected.

9. Place medical record charts face down at reception areas so the patient's name is not exposed to other patients or visitors to the office. Also, when placing medical records on the door of an examination room, turn the chart so that the identifying information faces the door. If medical record are kept on countertops or in receptacles, ensure that non-staff persons will not access the records. Handling and storing medical records will certainly change because of HIPAA guidelines.

10. Do not post the health care provider's schedule in areas viewable by non-staff individuals. The schedules are often posted for professional staff convenience, but this may be a breach in patient confidentiality.

11. Fax machines should not be placed in patient examination rooms or in any reception area where non-staff persons may view incoming or sent documents. Only staff members should have access to the faxes.

12. Direct mail and phone calls only to the appropriate staff members.

13. Recognize, learn, and use HIPAA TCS if involved in coding and billing.

14. Send all privacy-related questions or concerns to the appropriate staff member.

15. Immediately report any suspected or known improper behavior to supervisors or the PO so that the issue may be documented and investigated.

16. Direct all questions to the supervisors or PO.

FIGURE 17-8 Guidelines for HIPAA Privacy Rule compliance.

HIPAA Privacy Rule and how it relates to the individual office. Medical assistants are responsible for learning and following the guidelines set forth by HIPAA (Figure 17-8). If they are uncertain about any situation, they should contact the office's privacy officer for direction, or they should research the question on the HIPAA Web site. Never assume that a patient will not mind if certain information is disclosed. Always check the medical record to determine the patient's preferences. Keep current on changes in HIPAA regulations. Embrace changes designed to improve patient care and treatment.

Patient Education

HIPAA regulations can be confusing to even seasoned medical professionals, so imagine the confusion patients might feel in attempting to understand privacy regulations. Be patient when explaining the uses of health information in the medical facility. Take the time to review the information with the patient and to use terms the person understands. The medical assistant should stress that the privacy regulations put the patient more in control of his or her health information. Remember to tell patients that they can change expressed preferences, if necessary, by completing a new privacy notification.

Legal and Ethical Issues

Any government regulation takes several readings to understand. One of the facility's primary goals must be to remain in strict compliance, not only with HIPAA, but also with all laws and regulations that affect the medical office. The medical assistant may have to devote some study time to federal regulations to understand them adequately and to be able to act on the provisions.

Patient confidentiality is one of the most important facets of medical practice, but some medical professionals believe that the information about the patient belongs only to the physician or the facility. The information about the patient belongs to the patient and must be disclosed, according to office policies, when the patient requests it. Never release medical information without a written release signed by the patient.

SUMMARY OF SCENARIO

Sabrina and Elsa will experience many challenges as a result of the information exchange they shared at the family picnic. Their conversation probably began like any other, but once Sabrina told Elsa the details of Ms. Adams' visit, they violated patient privacy laws. Their future in the medical field is now uncertain.

Ms. Adams suffered emotionally after the breach of privacy. Her daughter, Terri, does not understand why her mother did not tell her about the illness. The relationship between the mother and daughter is now stressful, an interference with their normal bond during this critical time. The family questions whether to pursue the matter legally or spend the time they have left together in more productive ways. They have many decisions to make.

Dr. Taylor placed Sabrina on probation for 3 months. Before this incident, she had never received any type of disciplinary action. Elsa was not formally disciplined, largely because of her long-standing relationship with Dr. Berry. Still, there is sharp tension between them in the office now, as he faces a possible medical professional liability lawsuit and complaints about the privacy of Ms. Adams' PHI. Neither Sabrina nor Elsa will look at her job the same as before the incident; everything is different. They both feel that they have disappointed their employers, their patients, and themselves.

The medical assistant must remember that patients should be discussed only with others who are directly involved in the patient's medical care. The HIPAA Privacy Rule has made great strides in protecting patient privacy and in simplifying administrative processes. However, the rule is effective only if office policies are established and practiced. New policies may be difficult to implement, but gaining an understanding of the reason for the policy and its major goals can help the medical assistant embrace changes more readily.

SUMMARY OF LEARNING OBJECTIVES

1. **Define, spell, and pronounce the terms listed in the vocabulary.**
   Spelling and pronouncing medical terms correctly bolster the medical assistant's credibility. Knowing the definition of these terms promotes confidence in communication with patients and co-workers.

2. **Explain how the HIPAA Privacy Rule benefits the healthcare industry and patients.**
   HIPAA's Privacy Rule gave patients more control over their medical records. They are able to make informed choices on how their personal health information is used, and boundaries are set on the use and release of health records. Safeguards are established that healthcare providers must ensure to protect the privacy of health information. Violators are held accountable and face both civil and criminal penalties if a patient's privacy rights are compromised. The Privacy Rule also protects public health by striking a balance when public responsibility supports disclosure of personal health information.

3. **Explain the difference between Title I and Title II of the Privacy Rule.**
   Title I of the Privacy Rule covers the insurance industry. It limits the use of pre-existing health conditions that in the past would have either prevented an employee from obtaining health insurance coverage or limited the coverage. Title II deals with administrative simplification. This section is the source of the privacy and security laws that affect the patient. The goal of Title II is to reduce administrative costs in the healthcare industry.

4. **List the rights of patients under the Privacy Rule.**
   Patients have several rights under the Privacy Rule, including the right to notice of a facility's privacy practices; the right to have access to, view, and obtain a copy of their personal health information; the right to restrict certain parts or uses of their PHI; the right to request that communications from the facility be kept confidential; the right to ask the facility to amend the PHI; and the right to receive notice of all disclosures of their PHI.

5. **List the elements that must be included in a Notice of Privacy Practices.**
   A Notice of Privacy Practices must include details on how PHI is used and disclosed by the facility; the duties of the provider to protect health information; the patient's rights regarding PHI; how complaints can be filed if patients believe their privacy has been violated; whom to contact at the facility for more information; and the effective date of the Notice of Privacy Practices.

6. **Briefly explain what is expected of healthcare providers under the Privacy Rule.**
   Healthcare providers are expected to notify patients of their privacy rights; explain how their health information might be used; develop privacy procedures in the facility; implement those privacy procedures; train employees so that they understand the procedures in place; designate an individual to be responsible for implementation; and secure medical records so that they are not available to those who do not need them.

7. **Describe an incidental disclosure.**
   An incidental disclosure is a secondary use or disclosure that cannot reasonably be prevented, is limited in nature, and occurs as a result of another use or disclosure that is permitted.

8. **List the three instances when a parent is not considered the child's representative.**

   A parent is not considered the child's representative if (1) the minor consents to care and the parent's consent is not required under state or other applicable law (e.g., in the case of an emancipated minor); (2) the minor obtains care at the direction of a court or a person appointed by the court; or (3) the parent agrees to confidentiality between the minor and healthcare provider.

9. **Explain the circumstances under which a provider may discuss protected health information with a patient's friends and family.**

   A provider may discuss PHI with a patient's family or friends unless the patient has limited disclosure and has requested that he or she receive only confidential communication with the provider. Unless the patient makes this request, which should be in writing, the provider may discuss the patient with others as long as good judgment is used and the communication is related to the patient's treatment.

10. **Discuss the role of the Notice of Privacy Practices in emergencies.**

    Healthcare providers and facilities (e.g., hospitals) with a direct treatment relationship with individuals are not required to provide their notices of privacy practices to patients at the time they provide emergency treatment. The HIPAA Privacy Rule requires only that providers give patients a privacy notice when it is practical to do so after the emergency situation has resolved.

CONNECTIONS

📖 **Study Guide Connection:** Go to the Chapter 17 Study Guide. Read and complete the activities.

ℯ **Evolve Connection:** Go to the Chapter 17 link at *evolve.elsevier.com/kinn* to complete the Chapter Review and Chapter Quiz. Check out the other resources listed for this chapter to make the most of what you have learned from Privacy in the Physician's Office.

18

BASICS OF DIAGNOSTIC CODING

Sharon Oliver

SCENARIO

Mike Simeone has been employed by Dr. Buckner and Dr. Walker in their gastroenterology practice for the past 2 years. He works as an administrative assistant in medical records and simultaneously has been enrolled in the medical assisting program at his local college. As he has become more knowledgeable, Mike has been given more responsibility in tasks related to diagnostic coding, such as abstracting a diagnostic statement and selecting the most accurate diagnostic code for billing and reimbursement. To perform diagnostic coding, Mike uses a manual called the *International Classification of Diseases, Ninth Revision, Clinical Modification,* or ICD-9-CM.

Mike's experience working in medical records gives him an understanding of the importance of correct, thorough documentation. His strong skills in reading and understanding physicians' orders, treatment plans, chart notes, diagnostic statements, and other medical records will prove invaluable as Mike learns more about diagnostic coding and refines his coding skills.

Mike is aware of the legalities and importance of proper billing as it affects reimbursement. He knows that the practice is committed to compliance with all the regulations affecting the operation of the facility, and he knows the patients' charts are well documented, which makes his new tasks easier to accomplish. Mike is a conscientious worker and looks forward to using his experience to advance his position in the practice and in the medical assisting profession.

While studying this chapter, think about the following questions:

- How do the format, layout, and conventions of the ICD-9-CM manual help the medical assistant search for the most accurate and specific diagnostic code?
- Why is medical record documentation critical with regard to diagnostic coding?
- Why does the medical assistant need to know the steps for performing diagnostic coding?
- What are the benefits of using the diagnostic codes found in the ICD-9-CM?

LEARNING OBJECTIVES

1. Define, spell, and pronounce the terms listed in the vocabulary.
2. Identify three purposes of the most current diagnostic coding system.
3. Describe how to use the most current diagnostic coding system.
4. Explain and apply the basic coding rules in the use of the ICD-9-CM.
5. Explain where diagnostic information can be found and demonstrate how to abstract the diagnostic statement from the medical record.
6. Demonstrate the use of the Alphabetic Index in the selection of main and modifying terms and the appropriate code (or codes) or code ranges.
7. Explain the importance of the Tabular Index.
8. Correctly use instructional terms and symbols as defined in the ICD-9-CM.
9. Explain the use of V and E codes.
10. Perform diagnostic coding.

VOCABULARY

abstract An outline or summary of the diagnostic statement and/or procedures and services performed. In procedural coding, the outline or summary helps ensure that all procedures and services are included in an insurance claim submission and that nothing is omitted from or added to the encounter form or charge ticket; as a verb form, *abstract* means to compile this outline or summary for use in procedural coding.

Alphabetic Index Volume 2 of the ICD-9-CM coding manual; it lists conditions, injuries, illnesses, and diseases in alphabetical order by main terms, modifying terms, and subterms. It also contains the Classification of Factors Influencing Health Status and Contact with Health Service (V Codes) and the index for Supplemental Classification of External Causes of Injury and Poisoning (E Codes).

ancillary diagnostic services Services that support patient diagnoses (e.g., laboratory or radiologic services).

and In the context of the ICD-9-CM, *and* should be interpreted as *and/or.*

assessment The physician's determination of what is or may be wrong with the patient based on the findings from the history and physical examination (H&P). The assessment includes a preliminary, interim, or final diagnosis.

chief complaint (CC) The reason the patient has sought medical care, usually taken down in the patient's own words. It is recorded in the history documentation in the medical record, preceded by the abbreviation CC.

code first When more than one code is necessary to identify a given condition, *code first* or *use additional code* is used. A *code first* note is found at a manifestation code. A *use additional code* note is found at the etiology code when the underlying condition is sequenced first followed by the manifestation.

coding Converting verbal or written descriptions into numeric and alphanumeric designations.

conventions Abbreviations, punctuation, symbols, instructional notations, and related entities that help guide the medical assistant or coder in the selection of an accurate, specific code.

diagnosis The concise, technical description of the cause, nature, or manifestations of a condition or problem. *Initial diagnosis:* The physician's temporary impression, sometimes called a *working diagnosis. Differentiated diagnosis:* A comparison of two or more diseases with similar signs and symptoms. *Clinical diagnosis:* The conclusion the physician reaches after evaluating all findings, including laboratory and other test results.

diagnostic statement Information about a patient's diagnosis or diagnoses that has been extracted from the medical documentation.

etiology The science and study of the causes of disease. The cause of a disorder; a claim may be classified according to the etiology.

excludes Exclusion terms are always written in italics, and the word *excludes* often is enclosed in a box to draw particular attention to these instructions. Exclusion terms may apply to a chapter, a section, a category, or a subcategory. The applicable code number usually follows the exclusion term. An *excludes* note under a code indicates that the terms excluded from the code are to be coded elsewhere. The term *Excludes* means "DO NOT CODE HERE."

history and physical examination (H&P, HPE) At the patient's first visit with a new physician or an established provider or upon admission to a hospital, the history and physical examination (H&P) are documented. The H&P normally includes the chief complaint, a review of systems (ROS), the patient's personal and family medical history, a physical examination, an assessment of the findings from the history and physical exam, and a treatment plan for the patient, also referred to as Medical Decision Making (MDM).

includes When this term appears under a subdivision, such as a category (three-digit code) or two-digit procedure code title, it indicates that the code and title include these terms. Other terms also classified to that particular code and title are listed in the Alphabetic Index.

***International Classification of Diseases, Ninth Revision, Clinical Modification* (ICD-9-CM)** The manual that establishes the system for classifying disease to facilitate collection of uniform and comparable health information for statistical purposes, for indexing medical records for data storage and retrieval, and to facilitate payment.

***International Statistical Classifications of Diseases and Related Health Problems, Tenth Revision, Clinical Modification* (ICD-10-CM)** The current ICM rules manual, which contains the greatest number of changes in the ICD-CM system in ICD history. To allow more specific reporting of diseases and newly recognized conditions, the ICD-10-CM contains approximately 55,000 more codes than the ICD-9-CM.

manifestation An indication of the existence, reality, or presence of something, especially an illness.

notations Found in both the Alphabetic Index and the Tabular Index, notations are instructions or guides in classification assignments, defining category content or the use of subdivision codes; also called *instructional notations.*

notes Used to define codes and give coding instructions; often they are used to list the fifth-digit subclassification (or subclassifications) for certain categories.

principal diagnosis The initial identification of the condition or complaint the patient expresses in the outpatient medical setting based on the physician's assessment as documented in the medical record.

see A direction to the coder to look in another place; this instruction must always be followed. It is found in the Alphabetic Index, volumes 2 and 3.

see also A direction to the coder to look elsewhere if the main term or subterm (or subterms) for that entry are not sufficient for coding the information. If a code number follows, *see also* is enclosed in parentheses. If there is no code number, *see also* is preceded by a dash.

see category A direction to the coder to see a specific category (three-digit code); this instruction must always be followed.

SOAP notes A system of charting comprising the *s*ubjective findings, *o*bjective findings, *a*ssessment, and *p*lan for treatment.

Tabular Index Volume 1 of the ICD-9-CM coding manual; it contains all the diagnostic codes in numeric order, which are grouped into 17 chapters of diseases and injuries.

use additional code A *use additional code* note is found at the etiology code when the underlying condition is sequenced first, followed by the manifestation. A term that appears only in the Tabular Index (Volume 1) in subdivisions in which the user should add further information, by means of an additional code, to give a more complete picture of the diagnosis. In some cases, *if desired* follows the term. For the purpose of coding, the *if desired* phrase will not be used. When the term *use additional code if desired* appears, disregard "if desired" and assign the appropriate additional code.

with In the context of the ICD-9-CM, the terms *with, with mention of,* and *associated with* in a title dictate that both parts of the title must be present in the diagnostic statement to allow assignment of the particular code.

Accurate medical record keeping and efficient claims processing are possible only if *each and every* procedure and service provided during an office visit or encounter is identified. An encounter is any contact between a patient and a provider of service. The term *encounter* is used for all settings, including hospital admissions.

The physician or provider also must provide diagnostic information that demonstrates the need for the procedures and services. A **diagnosis** is the determination of the nature of a condition, illness, disease, injury, or congenital defect. In medical **coding**, the terms **assessment** and **diagnostic statement** are synonymous with diagnosis.

Both components (i.e., the diagnostic findings and the procedures and services) are used to determine the charges for an encounter and to generate an insurance claim. This chapter focuses on teaching the medical assistant how to gather diagnostic information and translate it into a diagnostic code. The *International Classification of Diseases, Ninth Revision, Clinical Modification* (**ICD-9-CM**) coding manual is used for this purpose. Two main parts of the ICD-9-CM are the Tabular Index (Volume 1) and the Alphabetic Index (Volume 2). The **Tabular Index** describes conditions, illnesses, diseases, and injuries; it also includes the sections Classification of Factors Influencing Health Status and Contact with Health Service (V Codes), and an index for Supplemental Classification of External Causes of Injury and Poisoning (E Codes). The **Alphabetic Index** is used to locate the codes in the Tabular Index based on the diagnosis provided in the medical record.

The ICD-9-CM manual is used to assign a standardized numeric or alphanumeric code to the diagnostic statement written by the provider. Diagnostic statements are found in operative reports, discharge summaries, history and physical (H&P) reports, and reports on ancillary diagnostic services that support the patient's diagnosis or diagnoses. **Ancillary diagnostic services** include radiology, pathology, and laboratory service reports. These reports are used by healthcare providers to code and report clinical information, as required for participation in Medicare and Medicaid insurance programs, and by most third-party payers and insurance carriers. The ICD-9-CM also is used to track healthcare statistics. Practice management software, clearinghouses, and third-party payers recognize these codes, which simplify the reimbursement process and speed payment to healthcare providers.

GETTING TO KNOW THE ICD-9-CM

What Is Diagnostic Coding?

Diagnostic coding is the translation or transformation of written descriptions of diseases, illnesses, or injuries into numeric or alphanumeric codes. Use of the ICD-9-CM facilitates accurate medical record keeping and efficient claims processing. The manual identifies the disease or injury for which a patient was treated as a three-, four-, or five-digit code. ICD-9-CM codes are used in the claims submission process to request reimbursement from payers, to track the diagnoses treated by the physician to provide statistical data for research, and for other purposes.

The CMS publication *"Avoiding Medicare Fraud and Abuse: A Roadmap for Physicians"* maintains that the five most important federal fraud and abuse laws that apply to physicians include the:

- False Claims Act (FCA)
- Anti-Kickback statute
- Physician Self-Referral Law (Stark Law)
- Social Security Act
- United States

Violations of these laws may result in non-payment of claims, Civil Monetary Penalties (CMPs), exclusion from the payor program, criminal and civil liability, and in extreme cases, jail time. These laws may be changed or updated, so the person who is responsible for coding must pay close attention to detail and act as a sort of "medical detective" to build a case against a physician or clinic. Both the ICD-9-CM and the CPT coding manuals are updated annually. The Federal Register announces most changes and new coding manuals often have a few pages dedicated to the updates for that particular year. Accurate use of the ICD-9-CM manual is essential for correct translation of the diagnostic statements in the medical record into numeric or alphanumeric codes.

Why Use ICD-9-CM Codes?

The ICD-9-CM codes are important for several reasons. They are used to:

- Standardize a system of diagnostic coding accepted and understood by all parties in the reimbursement cycle
- Create a more convenient method of data storage and retrieval

- Help maximize reimbursement to the provider
- Shortening the claims processing time
- Facilitate and assess regulatory compliance through the use of guidelines and other instructions
- Help evaluate the appropriateness and timeliness of medical care

Evolution of ICD Coding

Classification systems are used by healthcare organizations to organize healthcare data and make retrieval meaningful. The early Greeks were the first to group data by disease processes. Captain John Graunt of London was the first to publish mortality and morbidity statistics, in the London Bills of Mortality (1662), which was the first real attempt to study disease processes from a statistical viewpoint. Later, in the 1830s, William Farr introduced uniformity in the use of statistics. His work helped classify diseases by anatomic site. He published the International List of Causes of Death and provided the foundation for current vital statistics.

In 1893 Dr. Jacques Bertillon developed the Bertillon Classification of Causes of Death. The American Public Health Association (APHA) recommended adoption of this classification system for Canada, Mexico, and the United States and further recommended that the system be revised every 10 years. Subsequent revisions were called the International Classification System of Causes of Death. Revisions were completed in 1900, 1910, 1920, 1929, and 1938.

In the 1950s the U.S. Public Health Service published the International Classification of Diseases, which was adapted for indexing hospital records by diseases and operations. This became the International Classification of Diseases, Adapted (ICDA). Subsequent modifications in 1962 provided greater detail and introduced a classification for surgical procedures. In 1968, because of the need for even greater detail and specificity, the eighth revision of the ICDA was adapted for use in the United States (ICDA-8). ICDA-8 provided the basis for coding morbidity and mortality statistics in the United States and served as a method of indexing all diagnoses and operative procedures in hospital records.

In 1975 the ICDA was renamed the *International Classification of Diseases, Ninth Revision* (ICD-9). In 1979 the National Center for Health Statistics (NCHS) developed a modification of the ICD-9 for use in the United States. That modification, the ICD-9-CM, has been used in the United States ever since.

Legislation has been passed to formally adopt the tenth revision, or modification, of the diagnostic and procedural coding manuals (ICD-10) for use in the United States. ICD-10 is a significant upgrade and improvement to the coding manual currently in use. (See Appendix B for more information about the ***International Statistical Classifications of Diseases, Tenth Revision, Clinical Modification*** (**ICD-10-CM**) and the Procedural Coding System (ICD-10-PCS).) The effective date for these publications is October 1, 2014.

ICD-9-CM Codes

ICD-9-CM codes are listed in the Tabular Index (Volume 1) of the ICD-9-CM coding manual. The coding system consists of a three-digit category code that represents a specific disease, illness, condition, or injury within a general disease category. For example, 250 is the disease classification, or category, for diabetes mellitus. Up to two digits can be added for further definition and specificity. The two additional digits are the fourth digit, or subcategory, and the fifth digit, or subclassification.

Consider the example of diabetes category code 250 (Figure 18-1). Using this code and the conventions and guidelines (discussed later) in the ICD-9-CM manual, it can be determined that a fourth digit must be added that describes whether any disease manifestation is present that was caused by the diabetes, such as kidney disease or diabetic retinopathy. A fifth digit must also be added that describes the type of diabetes (e.g., type 1 controlled or type 2 uncontrolled).

The ICD-9-CM conventions, notes, and guidelines, combined with the diagnostic statement or statements from the medical record, provide the details needed to select the most accurate three-digit category code and, if applicable, a fourth digit (subcategory) and fifth digit (subclassification) code.

STRUCTURE OF THE ICD-9-CM

The ICD-9-CM is published in various media, including book, CD, and downloadable file. Every year the ICD-9-CM manual is reviewed for changes. Additions, revisions, and deletions are made to many of the diagnostic codes, code descriptions, and guidelines. The medical assistant must always use the current year's coding manual to ensure correct coding and billing and to comply with regulatory guidelines.

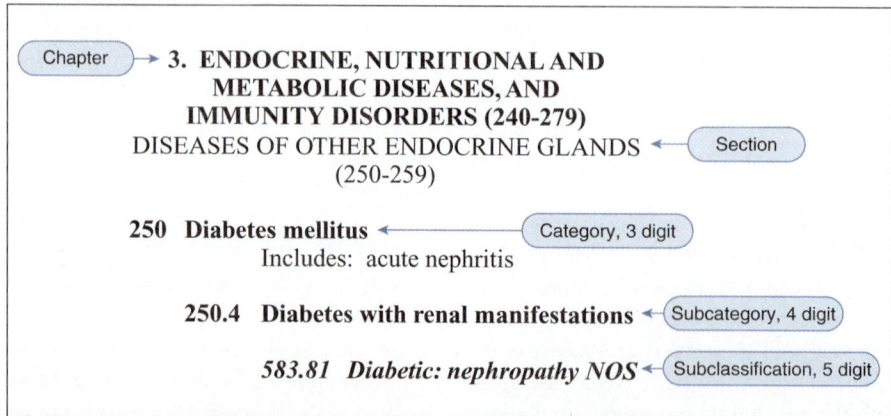

FIGURE 18-1 Example of category, subcategory, and subclassification.

Depending on the publisher, the layout, symbols, color coding, and some other features vary somewhat; however, the format, conventions, tables, appendixes, content, and basic structure are the same. The basic ICD-9-CM manual is made up of three volumes.

- Volumes 1 and 2, mentioned earlier, are used for diagnostic coding by hospitals, physicians, and all other providers of service. Volume 1, the Tabular Index, contains all the diagnostic codes, which are grouped into 17 *chapters* of disease and injury. Chapters are broad sections of the ICD-9-CM coding manual grouped by disease or illness (e.g., Chapter 10 contains diagnostic codes for diseases of the genitourinary system).
- Volume 2, the Alphabetic Index, is used the same way as an alphabetic index in any textbook, except that it refers the user back to the category codes in the Tabular Index rather than to page numbers.
- Volume 3 is used by hospitals to code inpatient procedures and services performed in the hospital environment. Most physician providers do not use Volume 3.

Most coding manuals, depending on the publisher, have an Introduction that provides the historical background. The ICD-9-CM coding manual also contains other useful information. In the ICD-9-CM, the coder will find the format and conventions of the coding manual; anatomic illustrations; special coding instructions for many conditions, illnesses, and injuries; and the current year's ICD-9-CM Official Coding Guidelines for using ICD-9-CM codes. The Centers for Medicare and Medicaid Services (CMS) prepares the guidelines for using the ICD-9-CM codes and instructions on how to report them on claim forms. The guidelines are a set of rules that have been developed to accompany and complement the official conventions and instructions provided in the ICD-9-CM manual.

Annual modifications are made to the ICD-9-CM through the ICD-9-CM Coordination and Maintenance Committee. The committee holds meetings twice a year, at which time modification proposals are submitted to the committee. Modification proposals that are approved are incorporated into the official government version of the ICD-9-CM and become effective for use October 1 of the year after their presentation.

Tabular Index (Volume 1)

The Tabular Index is a numeric listing of diagnosis codes and detailed descriptions. As mentioned earlier, a diagnosis is the determination of the nature of a disease, injury, condition, or congenital defect. The Tabular Index consists of the following:

- Seventeen chapters that classify diseases and injuries
- Two sections containing supplementary classification codes (V and E codes)
- Four appendixes (Appendix B, Glossary of Mental Disorders, was deleted October 1, 2004)

A chapter is a group of three-digit code numbers that describes a general category. For example, the code range 240-279 comprises Chapter 3: Endocrine, Nutritional and Metabolic Diseases, and Immunity Disorders.

Each of the 17 chapters is subdivided into four levels (see Figure 18-1):

- *Section*: A group of three-digit categories that represent a group of conditions or related conditions.

- *Category*: A three-digit code that represents a specific disease, illness, condition, or injury within a chapter (e.g., in Figure 18-1, Category 250 represents diabetes mellitus). A three-digit code is used only if it is not further subdivided.
- *Subcategory:* A fourth digit that adds information or description to the category code. For example, in Figure 18-1, under Category 250, a fourth digit is used to describe whether any disease process or manifestation exists that was caused by the diabetes mellitus. Category 250 has 10 fourth-digit subcategory codes. Fourth digits sometimes describe the location of the illness (e.g., code 410.2 indicates *of inferolateral wall*).
- *Subclassification:* A fifth digit which, when used appropriately, adds the highest level of detail to the illness or injury. In Figure 18-1, under Category 250, fifth digits are used to describe the type of diabetes mellitus (e.g., type 1 controlled or type 2 uncontrolled). Fifth digits sometimes describe the episode of care (e.g., code 410.21 indicates *MI* [myocardial infarction] *of inferolateral wall, initial*).

Supplemental Classifications

The two supplementary chapters in the Tabular Index contain V codes, which describe factors that influence health status and contact with health services that cannot be classified elsewhere, and E codes, which describe external causes of injury or poisoning.

V Codes. V codes are used either when the patient is not currently ill or to explain problems that influence a patient's current illness, condition, or injury. The Supplementary Classification of Factors Influencing Health Status and Contact with Health Service (V01-V89) is used in cases such as preventive vaccination or when a patient encounter is only for administration of a treatment, such as dialysis, chemotherapy, or screening.

E Codes. The E code chapter, the Supplemental Classification of External Causes of Injuries and Poisoning (E800-E999), classifies environmental or external causes of injury, poisoning, or other adverse effects on the body. For example, an E code would be used to describe the details of an automobile accident to explain how a patient's injuries occurred. E codes also identify the place of occurrence (i.e., where the event happened) and not the patient's activity at the time of the event.

Appendixes

The Tabular Index currently has the following four appendixes (as mentioned, Appendix B, Glossary of Mental Disorders, was deleted October 1, 2004).

- *Appendix A: Morphology of Neoplasms.* The term *morphology* means the form or structure, and *neoplasms* means new growth. Morphology code numbers consist of the letter M followed by five digits. The first four digits identify the histologic (tissue) type of the neoplasm, and the fifth digit indicates the neoplasm's behavior. M codes are used for statistical data only and are not used in physician billing. This appendix is used primarily by inpatient coders and morbidity and morphology statisticians.
- *Appendix C: Classification of Drugs.* The adverse effects of drugs are coded according to the American Hospital Formulary Service (AHFS) list. This section is used almost exclusively by pharmacies.

> **Example**
> **NEC**
> Diagnosis: Pneumonia due to gram-negative bacteria
> Index: Pneumonia
>   gram-negative bacteria NEC 482.83
> Tabular: 482.8 Pneumonia due to other specified bacteria
>   482.83 Other gram-negative bacteria
> Code: 482.83 Pneumonia due to gram-negative bacteria

Code 482.83 identifies gram-negative bacterial pneumonia that cannot be classified more specifically. The other subclassifications within 482.8 are for anaerobes (482.81), Escherichia coli [E. coli] (482.82), other than gram-negative bacteria (482.83), Legionnaire's disease (482.84), and other specified bacteria (482.89). None of these other subclassifications can be assigned to the diagnostic statement; therefore, 482.83 is the most appropriate code assignment.

> **NOS**
> Diagnosis: Bronchitis
> Index: **Bronchitis** 490
> Tabular: **490 Bronchitis, not specified as acute or chronic**
>   Bronchitis NOS
> Assign: 490 Bronchitis

The diagnosis was not specified by the physician as acute or chronic; therefore, the "not otherwise specified" code 490 must be assigned. In this situation, it would be appropriate for the coder to query the physician for more specific information.

FIGURE 18-2 Example of NEC and NOS abbreviations. (Modified from Buck CJ: *Step-by-step medical coding: 2012 edition,* St Louis, 2012, WB Saunders.)

- *Appendix D: Classification of Industrial Accidents.* This appendix concerns the Statistics of Employment Injuries categorized by the type of industry in which the accident occurred. This section usually is used by government organizations, such as the Occupational Safety and Health Administration (OSHA). It is seldom used by physician providers.
- *Appendix E: List of Three-Digit Categories.* All the three-digit category codes from the Tabular Index are listed in order, by chapter.

Conventions Used in the Tabular Index

Conventions are abbreviations, punctuation, symbols, instructional notations, and related entities that help the medical assistant or coder select an accurate, specific code. Conventions are found in the Tabular Index. Understanding their meaning and using them as guides are crucial to accurate coding. Each publisher offers its version of the ICD-9-CM, and some differences may be seen in the symbols, notations, colors, or other reference marks used. The most common conventions are described here.

Abbreviations. Two primary abbreviations are used in the Tabular Index: NOS and NEC (Figure 18-2).

- *NOS (not otherwise specified).* This abbreviation is the equivalent of "unspecified" and means that the diagnostic statement does not provide more specificity or definition. An NOS code typically is used when an illness has not been fully diagnosed (e.g., the physician documents a diagnosis as flu, with no other documentation). Because no additional documentation is available, the medical assistant can use a code with a description of "flu, NOS."

> | [ ] | Brackets enclose synonyms, alternative wording, or explanatory phrases. |
> |---|---|
> | ( ) | Parentheses are used to enclose supplementary words, which may be present or absent in the statement of a disease or procedure. These supplementary words do not usually affect the code number selected, but instead provide further definition or specificity to the code description. |
> | : | Colons are used in the Tabular Index after an incomplete term that needs one or more of the modifiers or adjectives that follow to make it assignable to a given category. |
> | { } | Braces enclose a series of terms, each of which is modified by the statement appearing to the right of the brace. |

FIGURE 18-3 Example of punctuation usage in the ICD-9-CM.

- *NEC (not elsewhere classifiable).* The category number for the term including NEC is used only when the coder lacks the information necessary to code the term to a more specific category. NEC means that the diagnostic statement contains specific wording but no specific classification exists to match the wording.

Punctuation. Four basic forms of punctuation are used in the Tabular Index: brackets, parentheses, colon, and braces (Figure 18-3). Each form serves a different purpose for reading and understanding the code descriptions.

Symbols. Symbols are used to designate the requirement of a fourth or fifth digit (or both), new entries, and revised text or codes. Other symbols may be included, depending on the publisher. Regardless of publisher, all symbols or other changes are described completely in the Introduction to the ICD-9-CM,. The most commonly used symbols are shown in Figure 18-4.

Other Conventions. Two other conventions used in both the Alphabetic Index and the Tabular Index are bold and italic fonts.

- **See category**: an instruction to the coder to see a specific category (three-digit code), and this instruction must always be used when it is present.
- **Bold:** Bold type is used for all codes and titles in the Tabular Index.
- *Italics:* Italic type is used for exclusion notes and to identify any diagnosis that should not be used as the **principal diagnosis**.

Instructional Notations. Instructional **notations** are critical to correct coding practices. The instructional notations appear in red type in the Tabular Index (Figure 18-5). The instructional notations include the following:

- **Includes:** A notation indicating that under a chapter, subchapter, category, subcategory or subclassification, separate terms can be found that further define, give examples of, or provide modifying adjectives, in addition to sites or conditions.
- **Excludes:** Exclusion terms are enclosed within a box and are printed in italics. The terms after the word *Excludes* are not classified to the chapter, subchapter, category, subcategory, or specific subclassification code under which they are found.

- **Notes:** Notes are used to define terms and give coding instructions. They often are used to list the fifth-digit subclassification (or subclassifications) for certain categories.
- **See:** The *See* instruction follows a main term and indicates that another term should be referenced. It is necessary to go to the main term referenced with the *See* note to locate the correct code.
- **See also:** The *See also* instruction is found after a main term in the Alphabetic Index. *See also* indicates that another main term may be referenced that may provide additional useful index entries. It is not necessary to follow the *See also* note when the original main term provides the necessary code.
- **See category:** This notation directs the coder to see a specific category (three-digit code). This instruction must always be followed.
- **Code first:** *Code first* notes are found under certain codes that are not specifically manifestation codes but that may indicate an underlying cause to the patient's problem. When a *Code first* note is present, and the patient has an underlying condition, the underlying condition should be sequenced first.
- **Use additional code:** According to an ICD-9-CM coding convention, an underlying condition must be sequenced first, followed by the manifestation. Wherever such a combination exists, a *Use additional code* note is found with the etiology code, and a *Code first* note is found with the manifestation code.

Related Terms

- **And:** In the context of the ICD-9-CM, *and* should be interpreted as *and/or.*
- **With:** The word *with* should be interpreted to mean *associated with* or *due to* when it appears in a code title, the Alphabetic Index, or an instructional note in the Tabular Index. The word *with* in the Alphabetic Index is sequenced immediately after the main term, not in alphabetical order.

Alphabetic Index (Volume 2)

The Alphabetic Index consists of an alphabetic list of diagnostic terms and related codes; three supplementary sections (the Hypertension Table, Neoplasm Table, and Table of Drugs and Chemicals), and a separate Alphabetic Index for E Codes (Index to External Causes). In most published versions of volumes 1 and 2, a Summary

□ or ○	The lozenge or circle symbol is found to the left of a disease code. The symbol will contain the number 4 or 5 and indicates that use of a fourth or fifth digit is required.
§	The section mark symbol is only used in the Tabular Index of Diseases and precedes a code denoting a footnote on the page.
•	The bullet symbol indicates a new entry.
△	The triangle symbol indicates a revision in the Tabular Index and a code change in the Alphabetic Index.

FIGURE 18-4 Symbols in the ICD-9-CM.

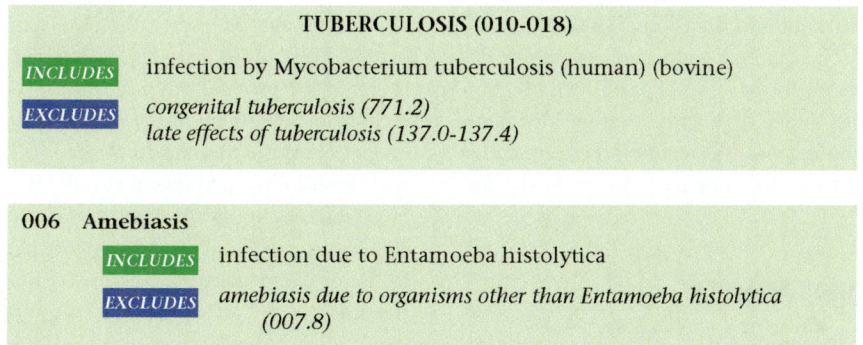

TUBERCULOSIS (010-018)

INCLUDES   infection by Mycobacterium tuberculosis (human) (bovine)

EXCLUDES   *congenital tuberculosis (771.2)*
late effects of tuberculosis (137.0-137.4)

006 Amebiasis

INCLUDES   infection due to Entamoeba histolytica

EXCLUDES   *amebiasis due to organisms other than Entamoeba histolytica (007.8)*

FIGURE 18-5 Example of instructional notations. (Modified from Buck CJ: *Step-by-step medical coding: 2012 edition,* St Louis, 2012, WB Saunders.)

of the Additions, Deletions, and Revisions to the Tabular Index for the current year is included and typically is found at the end of the main Alphabetic Index (Volume 2).

The Alphabetic Index includes main terms, nonessential modifiers, modifying terms, and subterms.

- *Main terms:* These terms appear in bold type.
- *Nonessential modifiers:* These terms are enclosed in parentheses and appear after the main term. They are supplementary words or explanatory information; they do not affect the code assignment.
- *Modifying terms:* These terms are indented two spaces to the right under the main term. They are called *essential modifiers,* because they change the description of the diagnosis in bold type.
- *Subterms:* These terms are indented two spaces under the level of the preceding line. These diagnoses are used when all conditions exist.

A diagnostic statement from the physician may contain many medical terms, but typically only one main term describes the patient's illness or injury.

Supplementary Sections of the Alphabetic Index

The Alphabetic Index includes three tables and one supplementary index (these are discussed in detail later in the chapter):

- *Hypertension Table:* Lists the types of hypertension and the manifestations and causes of hypertension.
- *Neoplasm Table:* Lists neoplasms by anatomic location. Neoplasms are further classified into four categories: malignant, benign, in-situ, and uncertain histologic behavior.
- *Table of Drugs and Chemicals:* Presents a classification of drugs and other chemical substances to identify poisonings and external causes of adverse effects.
- *Index to External Causes of Injuries and Poisoning (E Codes):* A supplementary index that lists E codes, which classify environmental events, circumstances, and other conditions as the cause of injury; the place of occurrence; and other adverse effects.

Procedures (Volume 3)

Volume 3 of the ICD-9-CM contains a Tabular Index and an Alphabetic Index of procedures. Unlike volumes 1 and 2, it is not used by physicians or providers. It is used primarily in hospitals and other facilities to code the inpatient procedures performed in those settings. The procedure codes consist of two digits followed by a decimal and then one or two additional digits. The Tabular Index of Volume 3 has 17 chapters, which contain codes and descriptions for surgical, diagnostic, and therapeutic procedures performed in a hospital setting. The Alphabetic Index of Volume 3 is an alphabetic listing of the surgical, diagnostic, and therapeutic procedure codes; it is used as a guide to find a specific code or codes in the Tabular Index of Volume 3.

BEGINNING THE CODING PROCESS

Medical Documentation

The steps for using the ICD-9-CM manual actually begin with interpreting and abstracting the medical documentation.

Information pertinent to code selection is culled from a variety of medical documents. Sources of diagnostic statements include the encounter form; treatment notes; discharge summary; operative report; and radiology, pathology, and laboratory reports.

Encounter Form

The encounter form is also known as a *superbill, fee slip,* or *charge ticket* (see Chapter 22).

In the physician's practice, the encounter form generally is a preprinted form. It also is the form the medical assistant uses most often to obtain the charges and diagnosis when performing charge and payment data entry and insurance billing. Although it is a convenience for the physician and medical staff, the encounter form can also be a source of errors that can reduce or delay reimbursement. It is vital that the preprinted form be reviewed annually to ensure that any diagnosis or procedure codes used on it have been updated, revised, or deleted according to the latest information from the *Current Procedural Terminology* (CPT) and ICD-9-CM coding manuals. If the preprinted encounter form is not updated annually, a code that has been revised or even deleted may be used for a diagnosis or procedure in data entry or insurance billing, and this will cause problems with reimbursement.

Treatment or Progress Notes

Treatment notes are the second most common medical document from which diagnostic information can be obtained. Chapter 14 discussed treatment notes and finding the assessment (or diagnosis) using SOAP notes. **SOAP notes** are a system of charting in which information is divided into the *s*ubjective findings, *o*bjective findings, *a*ssessment, and *p*lan for treatment.

History and Physical Exam

The **history and physical examination (H&P, HPE)** are the starting point of the patient's "story" regarding the reason the person sought or is receiving medical attention. The H&P begins with a statement in the patient's own words that describes the reason for seeking medical attention. This statement is called the **chief complaint (CC)** and is often abbreviated CC in the history documentation in the medical record. After the chief complaint, the physician documents any other pertinent history about medical, behavioral, and social factors, such as smoking, drinking, drug use, family history, previous surgeries, and hospitalizations. (To see an example of an H&P report, visit the Evolve site at *evolve.elsevier.com/kinn.*)

After taking the history, the physician performs a physical examination (PE). This includes both objective and subjective assessments of the patient's physical status. The final sections of an H&P include an assessment and a plan. The assessment is the physician's evaluation of the findings from the H&P, and it includes a preliminary, interim, or final diagnosis. The plan is the plan for treatment (also referred to as *Medical Decision Making* [MDM]) for the conditions noted in the assessment; it may include x-ray studies, laboratory tests, surgery, administration of medications, or other treatments.

Discharge Summary

The discharge summary is used primarily for extracting procedure and diagnostic information for patients who were hospitalized rather than seen in the physician's office. The main elements of a discharge summary are the patient's demographic information, admission date, date of discharge, H&P findings, clinical course, condition on discharge, discharge diagnosis, and aftercare plan. Diagnostic statements are obtained from the discharge diagnosis section. (To see an example of a discharge summary, visit the Evolve site at *evolve.elsevier.com/kinn.*)

Operative Report

For patients who underwent surgery as an outpatient or inpatient, the operative report also is used to extract procedure and diagnostic information. An operative report includes the preliminary diagnosis and procedure, the final diagnosis and procedure, and a detailed description of the operative procedure from start to finish. The medical assistant uses the final diagnosis when searching for and selecting a diagnosis code. (To see an example of an operative report, visit the Evolve site at *evolve.elsevier.com/kinn.*)

Radiology, Laboratory, or Pathology Report

Radiology, laboratory, and pathology reports are used to support and/or establish the diagnostic statement or statements. Any findings from these reports must be documented in the treatment notes in the medical record to be used for diagnostic coding, charge entry, or insurance billing purposes.

Extracting Diagnostic Statements

The basic steps in diagnostic coding are to analyze and abstract the diagnosis or assessment documented in the medical record. Then, in the ICD-9-CM manual, the medical assistant uses the Alphabetic Index, the Tabular Index, and the conventions and guidelines to select the most accurate and applicable diagnostic code. As a verb form, **abstract** means to create an outline or summary of information from a text or record. In diagnostic coding, an abstract is created to find all the diagnostic statements recorded during a patient encounter. The abstracted diagnostic statements then are broken down into the main term (or terms) and any modifying terms or subterms.

Main and Modifying Terms

The Alphabetic Index is organized by main terms, modifying terms (nonessential and essential), and subterms. Main terms indicate the condition, disease, illness, or injury. Modifying terms, as described earlier, modify (i.e., act as adjectives for) main terms. Modifying terms are indented two spaces below the main term. Subterms are indented two spaces below the modifying term and add more detail or information to the modifying term. Modifying terms and subterms further describe or add information or definition needed to narrow the search for an appropriate diagnostic code. Modifying terms and subterms affect the selection of appropriate codes; therefore, when selecting a code or code range, it is important to review the Alphabetic Index carefully, not only for main terms, but also for modifying terms and subterms.

As mentioned, a main term typically is the primary condition, disease, or injury. Modifying terms provide further specificity, or detail, such as the anatomic site or additional manifestations of the condition. For example, in the diagnostic statement "atherosclerotic heart disease," the condition (and thus the main term) is *disease*. The modifying term *heart* adds the anatomic location, and the subterm *atherosclerotic* adds the type of heart disease.

Main terms also can be found by eponym, synonym, or acronym. An *eponym* describes a disease, condition, or injury named after a person (e.g., Hodgkin's disease). *Acronyms* are abbreviations of words that create a new word; for example, the acronym for gastroesophageal reflux disease is GERD. GERD and gastroesophageal reflux disease both are medical terms. *Abbreviations* are slightly different; they are "shorthand" for common medical terms. For example, the abbreviation for upper respiratory infection is URI. *Synonyms* are words that are similar in meaning and can be used interchangeably. It is important that medical coders keep reference books on hand, including a medical dictionary that lists abbreviations, so that they can clearly understand the diagnostic statement.

Figure 18-6 shows diagnostic statements taken from various documents, including encounter forms, treatment notes, discharge

Diagnostic Statement	Main Terms	Modifying or Sub-Terms
Methicillin-resistant *Staphylococcus aureus* (MRSA)	*Staphylococcus*	*Aureus*
	Staphylococcus aureus	Methicillin-resistant Resistant Medication resistant
	MRSA	
Cerebrovascular accident (CVA)	accident	Cerebrovascular
	CVA	
Arteriosclerotic heart disease (ASHD)	Disease	Heart Arteriosclerotic
	Heart	Arteriosclerotic
	ASHD	
Varicosities, left leg	Varicose, Varicosity	Leg, veins
GERD	GERD	
Gastroesophageal reflux	Reflux	Gastroesophageal
URI	Infection	Respiratory, upper
	Respiratory	Infection, upper
Upper riratory infection	Infection	Respiratory, upper
	Respiratory	Infection, upper

FIGURE 18-6 Extracting main and modifying terms from a diagnostic statement.

summaries, and operative reports. The first column contains the diagnostic statement, including any related acronym or abbreviation. The second column lists the main term (or terms) which can be extracted from the diagnostic statement. The last column lists modifying and subterms that further define the main term.

In addition to using the conventions, notes, punctuation, and guidelines when choosing the diagnostic code or codes from the ICD-9-CM, the medical assistant must keep in mind two important considerations:

1. Nothing can be omitted from or added to the diagnostic statement that is not documented in the patient's medical record.
2. When the diagnostic statements are compared with any code description, the description of that code must match, in accordance with the conventions and guidelines, with no essential element of the statement added or missing.

CRITICAL THINKING APPLICATION   18-1

Mike sometimes is confused as to which term is the main term and which are modifying terms. What documents or references can help him determine the main term? Whom can he consult in the practice to make sure he understands the main term? What can happen if he selects a modifying or subterm instead of a main term?

STEPS IN ICD-9-CM CODING

Ten basic steps are required for accurate ICD-9-CM coding. The first step involves abstracting the diagnostic statement from the medical record and determining the main and modifying terms. The next four steps are performed using the Alphabetic Index to search for the code, codes, or code ranges that best fit the diagnostic statement. The remaining five steps are performed using the Tabular Index to verify and confirm that the code (or codes) located in the Alphabetic Index fully matches the diagnostic statement and is the most specific and accurate diagnostic code. Procedure 18-1 describes the basic coding steps and explains the purpose of each step.

Using the Alphabetic Index (Volume 2)

Once the medical assistant has abstracted the diagnostic statement from the medical record and identified the main terms, he or she begins searching for the best code in the Alphabetic Index. As mentioned previously, the Alphabetic Index is a comprehensive, alphabetic listing of all diagnoses, conditions, illnesses, diseases, and injuries in the ICD-9-CM manual. The most important thing to remember about the Alphabetic Index is that it should be used only as an aid to locating possible code matches. The Tabular Index, with its conventions, punctuation, notes, and guidelines, must always be used to confirm that the code (or codes) selected is accurate and specific and that no contraindications exist to use of the code found in the Alphabetic Index.

Never code directly from the Alphabetic Index. Even if only one code is found in the Alphabetic Index, it may be used only if a thorough review of the conventions and instructional notations in the Tabular Index does not contraindicate it. The Alphabetic Index does not tell you whether there are instructional notes for any possible additional coding rules.

Figure 18-7 presents an excerpt from the Alphabetic Index that includes cysts. Note first the nonessential modifiers in parentheses beside the bolded main term **cyst**. Nonessential modifiers add detail, but they do not have to be present in the diagnostic statement for the code to be acceptable for use. The nonessential modifiers are *mucus, retention, serous,* and *simple.* Directly below the main term **cyst** is a notation that provides guidance on the proper selection of codes in this category. The first modifying term indented under the main term **cyst** is *accessory, fallopian tube.* Directly under this modifying term, not indented, is another modifying term, *adenoid (infected),* for the main term **cyst**. Because there is additional indention, these are two separate modifying terms for the main term **cyst**. The third description indented under cyst is *adrenal gland.* Note that directly below *adrenal gland* is a second indention. This is a subterm that directly modifies *adrenal gland,* not the main term **cyst**.

Using the Tabular Index (Volume 1)

Figure 18-8 presents an excerpt from the Tabular Index that uses the category code for **cyst** (see Figure 18-7). Note that category code 364 refers to disorders of the iris and ciliary body. Indented below category code 364 are the subcategories 364.0 through 364.9. The code selected for the diagnosis of exudative cyst of the anterior chamber of the eye was 364.62. Look at 364.6. The description of subcategory 364.6 is *cyst of the iris, ciliary body, and anterior chamber.* Remember, *and* can mean either *and* or *or.* To the left of code 364.6 is a convention indicating that a fifth digit must be used. At this point, most but not all of the diagnostic statement has been included in the description of code 364.6; all except for the term *exudative.*

Knowing that the convention requires a fifth digit and that an essential word is missing from the diagnostic statement, the medical

Cyst *(Continued)*
  breast (benign) (blue dome)
      (pedunculated) (solitary)
      (traumatic) 610.0
    involution 610.4
    sebaceous 610.8
  broad ligament (benign) 620.8
    embryonic 752.11
  bronchogenic (mediastinal)
      (sequestration) 518.89
    congenital 748.4
  buccal 528.4
  bulbourethral gland (Cowper's) 599.89
  bursa, bursal 727.49
    pharyngeal 478.26
  calcifying odontogenic (M9301/0) 213.1
    upper jaw (bone) 213.0
  canal of Nuck (acquired) (serous) 629.1
    congenital 752.41
  canthus 372.75
  carcinomatous (M8010/3) - *see*
      Neoplasm, by site, malignant
  cartilage (joint) - *see* Derangement, joint
  cauda equina 336.8
  cavum septi pellucidi NEC 348.0
  celomic (pericardium) 746.89
  cerebellopontine (angle) - *see* Cyst,
      brain
  cerebellum - *see* Cyst, brain
  cerebral - *see* Cyst, brain
  cervical lateral 744.42

FIGURE 18-7 Excerpt from the Alphabetic Index illustrating main and modifying terms for a cyst.

PROCEDURE 18-1

Performing ICD-9-CM Coding

GOAL: *To perform accurate diagnosis coding using the ICD-9-CM manual.*

EQUIPMENT and SUPPLIES

- ICD-9-CM manual (volumes 1 and 2, current year)
- Encounter form or charge ticket
- Medical record
- Paper
- Pen or pencil

PROCEDURAL STEPS

Preparation

1. Abstract the diagnostic statement or statements from the encounter form and/or the patient's medical record.
   a. Determine the main terms in the diagnostic statement that describe the patient's condition.
   b. Determine what modifying words describe the main term in the diagnostic statement.
   PURPOSE: To extract all diagnoses or diagnostic statements from the medical record and to ensure that all parts of the diagnostic statement are included in the encounter form or medical record, with nothing missing or added. To identify the main, modifying, and subterms to be used to search the Alphabetic Index.

Alphabetic Index (Volume 2)

1. Locate the main terms taken from the diagnostic statement in the Alphabetic Index (Volume 2) of the ICD-9-CM manual.
   PURPOSE: To provide a starting point for searching the Alphabetic Index.
2. Locate the modifying words listed under the main term in the Alphabetic Index.
   PURPOSE: To ensure further specificity of the codes found in the Alphabetic Index.
3. Review the conventions, punctuation, and notes in the Alphabetic Index.
   PURPOSE: To ensure that no additional searches, exclusions, or similar terms are needed to complete the search in the Alphabetic Index
4. Choose a tentative code, codes, or code range from the Alphabetic Index that matches the diagnostic statement as closely as possible.
   PURPOSE: To prevent backtracking and repeated searches in the Alphabetic Index.

Tabular Index (Volume 1)

1. Look up the codes chosen from the Alphabetic Index in the Tabular Index (Volume 1).
   PURPOSE: To begin the process of determining whether the codes selected from the Alphabetic Index are appropriate and accurate.
2. Review notes, conventions, and the ICD-9-CM Official Coding Guidelines associated with the code and code description in the Tabular Index.
   a. Review conventions and punctuation.
   b. Review instructional notations:
      - Includes or excludes statements
      - Code first, code also, and code additional statements
      - and, or, and/or with statements
   PURPOSE: To ensure that the code or codes selected are appropriate for use and to determine whether they require additional codes, further specificity, or are excluded from use.
3. Verify the accuracy of the tentative code in the Tabular Index.
   a. Make sure all elements of the diagnostic statement are included in the codes selected.
   b. Make sure the code description does not include anything not documented in the diagnostic statement.
   PURPOSE: To ensure that the most accurate and specific code is selected and that no contraindication exists to use of the code or codes selected.
4. Carry the codes to their highest level of specificity (fourth and fifth digits if they are available).
   PURPOSE: To ensure further specificity of the codes found in the Alphabetic Index.
5. Assign the code (or codes) selected from the Tabular Index as the appropriate code for the patient's condition by documenting it in the patient's medical record.
   PURPOSE: To ensure that the medical record or encounter form contains documentation of the code or codes selected.

---

assistant must next review possible fifth digits available for code 364.6. The fifth-digit codes in Figure 18-8 range from 364.60 to 364.64. The code description for 364.62 contains the missing essential word: *exudative*. A review of the punctuation, instructional notes, *excludes* comments, and conventions does not contraindicate the use of code 364.62; therefore, it can be selected as the most specific and accurate code. *Note:* Beneath the codes requiring a fifth digit, brackets show which fifth digit is appropriate to use with the respective code.

CRITICAL THINKING APPLICATION   18-2

Mike found a tentative code in the Alphabetic Index for a diagnostic statement for one of his patients. When he turned to the Tabular Index, he found an instruction in the code description that stated that the diagnostic statement was excluded from use of the code he had selected. What steps might Mike have taken when searching in the Alphabetic Index that led him to the wrong code in the Tabular Index? What steps can he take to restart his search and find the appropriate code?

ICD-9-CM

● **364   Disorders of iris and ciliary body**

  ● **364.0 Acute and subacute iridocyclitis**

    Anterior uveitis, acute, subacute
    Cyclitis, acute, subacute
    Iridocyclitis, acute, subacute
    Iritis, acute, subacute

    Excludes *gonococcal (098.41)*
        herpes simplex (054.44)
        herpes zoster (053.22)

    ■**364.00 Acute and subacute iridocyclitis, unspecified**

    364.01 Primary iridocyclitis

    364.02 Recurrent iridocyclitis

    364.03 Secondary iridocyclitis, infectious

    364.04 Secondary iridocyclitis, noninfectious
      Aqueous:
        cells
        fibrin
        flare

    364.05 Hypopyon

  ● **364.1 Chronic iridocyclitis**

    Excludes *posterior cyclitis (363.21)*

    ■**364.10 Chronic iridocyclitis, unspecified**

    ● **364.11 *Chronic iridocyclitis in diseases classified elsewhere***

      Code first underlying disease, as:
        sarcoidosis (135)
        tuberculosis (017.3)

      Excludes *syphilitic iridocyclitis (091.52)*

  ● **364.2 Certain types of iridocyclitis**

    Excludes *posterior cyclitis (363.21)*
        sympathetic uveitis (360.11)

    364.21 Fuchs' heterochromic cyclitis

    364.22 Glaucomatocyclitic crises

    364.23 Lens-induced iridocyclitis

    364.24 Vogt-Koyanagi syndrome

  ■**364.3 Unspecified iridocyclitis**
    Uveitis NOS

● **364.4 Vascular disorders of iris and ciliary body**

  364.41 Hyphema
    Hemorrhage of iris or ciliary body

  364.42 Rubeosis iridis
    Neovascularization of iris or ciliary body

● **364.5 Degenerations of iris and ciliary body**

  364.51 Essential or progressive iris atrophy

  364.52 Iridoschisis

  364.53 Pigmentary iris degeneration
    Acquired heterochromia of iris
    Pigment dispersion syndrome of iris
    Translucency of iris

  364.54 Degeneration of pupillary margin
    Atrophy of sphincter of iris
    Ectropion of pigment epithelium of iris

  364.55 Miotic cysts of pupillary margin

  364.56 Degenerative changes of chamber angle

  364.57 Degenerative changes of ciliary body

  ■**364.59 Other iris atrophy**
    Iris atrophy (generalized) (sector shaped)

● **364.6 Cysts of iris, ciliary body, and anterior chamber**

  Excludes *miotic pupillary cyst (364.55)*
      parasitic cyst (360.13)

  364.60 Idiopathic cysts

  364.61 Implantation cysts
    Epithelial down-growth, anterior chamber
    Implantation cysts (surgical) (traumatic)

  364.62 Exudative cysts of iris or anterior chamber

  364.63 Primary cyst of pars plana

  364.64 Exudative cyst of pars plana

◄ New	◄▥ Revised	~~deleted~~ Deleted	● Use Additional Digit(s)	■ Nonspecific Code
● Not first-listed DX	**OGCR** Official Guidelines	**Coding Clinic**	Excludes	Includes	Use additional	Code first	Omit code

FIGURE 18-8 Excerpt from the Tabular Index illustrating codes 364 through 364.64.

Diagnostic Coding Decision Tree

A series of questions, called a *decision tree*, can help the medical assistant navigate the Alphabetic Index and Tabular Index in performing the steps for diagnostic coding. The decision tree for the main text is designed to guide the selection of the appropriate ICD-9-CM diagnostic code (Figure 18-9). (To see an example of the use of a diagnostic coding decision tree, visit the Evolve site at *evolve.elsevier.com/kinn*.)

EXAMPLES OF STEPS IN DIAGNOSTIC CODING

1. The diagnostic statement is *cholecystitis*. There is only one main term: *Cholecystitis*. In the Alphabetic Index, the main term, **Cholecystitis**, has a single code, 575.10. Turning to the Tabular Index, 575.10 states, *Cholecystitis, unspecified*. The surrounding codes all add information that is not contained in the diagnostic statement; for example, 575.1 states, *Cholecystitis*, but a symbol convention to the left of

the code contains the number 5, which means a fifth digit must be used for this diagnosis. Code 575.0 states, *Acute cholecystitis.* The diagnostic statement does not specify acute; therefore, 575.0 adds inaccurate information. In the same way, codes 575.11, 575.12, and 575.2 add information that is not contained in the diagnostic statement. Therefore, the final and most accurate code for the diagnostic statement, *Cholecystitis,* is 575.10.

2. Changing the diagnostic statement, *cholecystitis,* only slightly by adding *with calculus (cholelithiasis)* changes the Alphabetic Index search and also the code. The main term remains **Cholecystitis,** although **Cholelithiasis** also could be used as the main term. The choice of either as a main term guides the coder to the same place in the Tabular Index. Using **Cholecystitis** again as a main term guides the coder to 575.10; however, indented below the main term is the subterm *with calculus,* followed by *See Cholelithiasis.* The code for cholelithiasis is 574.2, but again, indented below *cholelithiasis* is the subterm *with cholecystitis* and the code 574.1. In the Tabular Index, code 574.2 refers only to the cholelithiasis, code 574.1; however, it is a combination code that includes cholelithiasis with cholecystitis. There is one more step, according to the symbol convention to the left of the code, which indicates that a fifth digit must be added. At the beginning of the subcategory for cholelithiasis (574), an instructional note provides the fifth digit definitions: 0 means *without mention of obstruction* and 1 means *with obstruction.* Because the diagnostic statement did not mention an obstruction, the most specific and accurate code to choose from the Tabular Index is 574.10.

CRITICAL THINKING APPLICATION   18-3

Mike is working with a medical record that has the terms "cholelithiasis" and "acute cholecystitis with calculus." How will the coding steps and decision tree questions affect or change the selection of a diagnosis code?

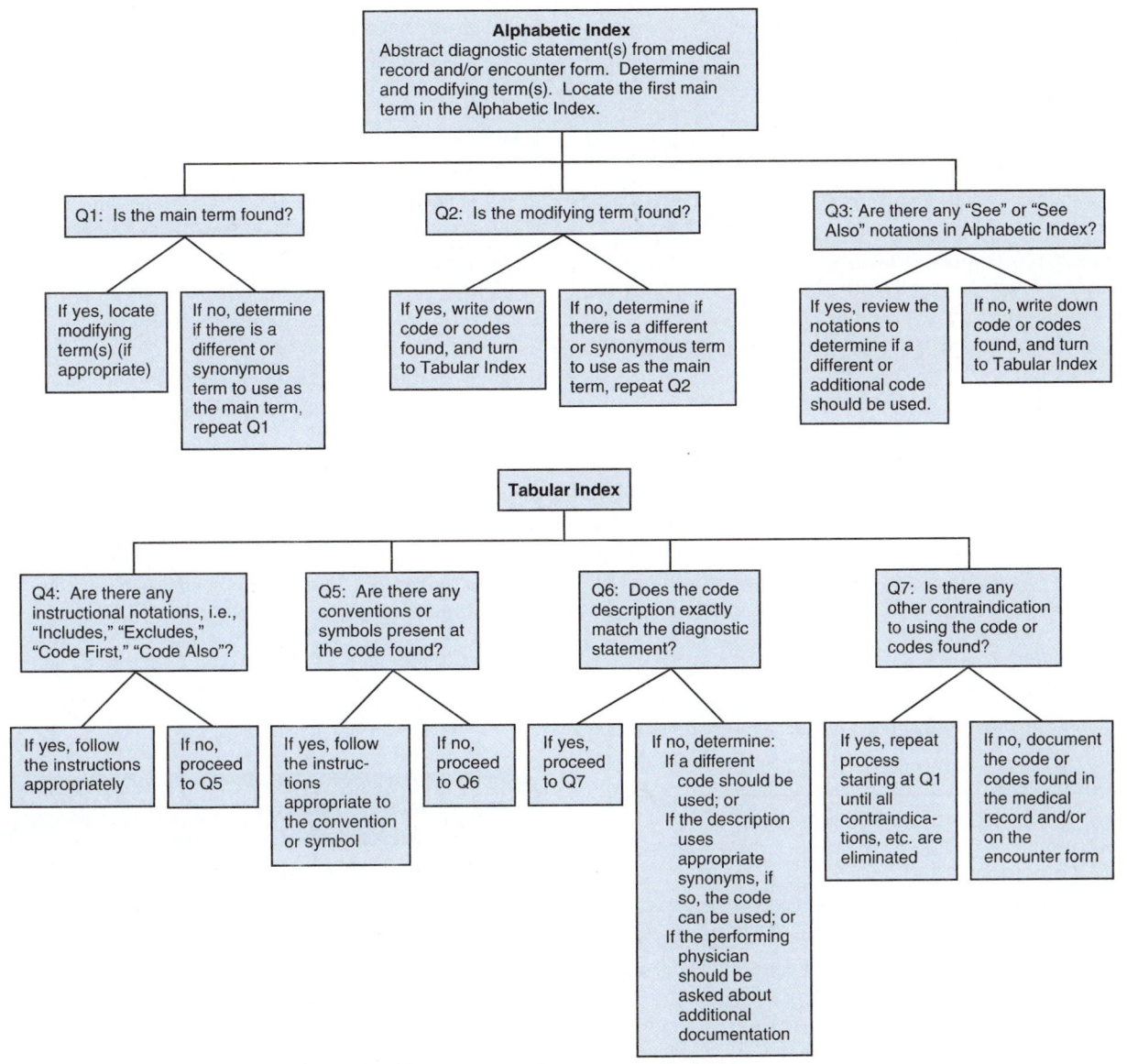

FIGURE 18-9 Decision tree for ICD-9-CM diagnostic coding.

SPECIAL CODING INSTRUCTIONS

Remember that all ICD-9-CM coding manuals, regardless of the publisher, have comprehensive instructional notes and conventions to help the coder select the most accurate diagnostic code or codes. When any discrepancy occurs between reference sources, including this text, the current year's ICD-9-CM coding manual is the final authority. This fact cannot be overemphasized. The medical assistant must always thoroughly review and refer to the conventions, instructional notations, code definitions, and other guidelines in the Alphabetic Index and Tabular Index when coding.

The following instructions are designed to provide some additional guidance in selecting diagnostic codes from various chapters in the ICD-9-CM; however, they are not to be considered a replacement for the ICD-9-CM manual, nor do they provide all the coding information, definitions, or explanations found in the manual. The steps for diagnosis coding in Procedure 18-1 are the same for all chapters of the ICD-9-CM, but special rules and considerations apply to some chapters that affect the code selection process.

Coding of Signs and Symptoms

Signs and symptoms are coded only if the physician has not yet reached a determination of the final diagnosis. If the physician's notes contain terminology such as "rule out" or "suspected," for example, the medical coder should use the patient's documented signs and symptoms, including subjective and objective findings. Subjective findings include the patient's chief complaint (CC) or statements regarding why the patient is seeing the physician. Objective findings are any measurable indicators found during the physical examination. Ill-defined conditions, signs, and symptoms are found in Chapter 16 of the Tabular Index (Volume 1). Figure 18-10 presents an illustration of the Signs and Symptoms section in Chapter 16.

Coding Suspected Conditions

When a diagnosis is stated as "questionable," "probable," "likely," or "rule out," code the patient's documented symptoms, signs, or CC. For outpatients, do not code the suspected condition if no final assessment or diagnosis has been made. If a patient is asymptomatic or has a family or personal history of a condition, a screening code from the Supplementary Classification of V Codes should be used.

Multiple Coding

Some conditions require the use of more than one code. In the Tabular Index, the instructional notation *Use additional code* means to use another code in conjunction with the one selected; *Code first* means that if more than one code is used, the code with the notation *Code first* should be the first or primary diagnosis. Multiple codes may be needed for late effects, complication codes, and obstetric codes to describe a condition more fully. Always review the ICD-9-CM manual guidelines, instructional notes, and conventions to determine when the use of multiple codes is appropriate. A patient diagnosed with diabetic retinopathy with type 1 diabetes requires multiple codes. The first code, 250.51, represents diabetes with ophthalmic manifestations; code 362.01 represents the diabetic retinopathy. The subclassification 1 designates type 1 diabetes. Figure 18-11 shows an example of multiple coding. Manifestation codes are ALWAYS a secondary code.

Using Combination Codes

A combination code is used to identify two diagnoses or a diagnosis with a secondary process (manifestation) or complication. A combination code contains descriptions of both conditions in the code definition in the Tabular Index. Combination codes are identified by referring to the subterms in the Alphabetic Index or by looking for *inclusion* and *exclusion* terms in the Tabular Index. An example of a combination code from the ICD-9-CM is shown in Figure 18-12.

Coding Late Effects and the Past Medical History

A *late effect* is a problem that remains after the acute phase of an illness or injury has ended. There is no time limit on when a late effect code can be used. Coding of late effects generally requires two codes: the condition or nature of the late effect is coded first (e.g., hemiplegia); then, the condition or nature of the effect is coded as a late effect. A late effect sometimes is described in the medical documentation as "old" or "residual" or as a "sequela," or some other phrase is used that indicates the passage of time since the onset of the original condition. A personal history of a condition more often is described as "history of …".

Be sure to distinguish between a late effect and a historical statement in a diagnosis. Whenever the diagnosis includes the term "effects of old …", "sequela of …", or "residuals of …", "due to …", the condition should be coded as a late effect. If the diagnosis is expressed in terms of "history of …", a V code is used to indicate a personal history of the condition.

Coding Impending or Threatened Conditions

Code any condition described at the time of discharge as "impending" or "threatened" as shown in the box.

- Use only if there is no final or determining diagnosis
- Use if "rule out" or "suspected" are included in the assessment or diagnostic statement.
- Signs and symptoms can be subjective and/or objective findings
  - Subjective: Chief complaint (CC) or patient's verbal statements
  - Objective: Any measurable indicators found during the physical examination
- Signs and Symptoms are found in Chapter 16, Ill-Defined Conditions, Signs and Symptoms, Volume 1 of the ICD-9-CM.

FIGURE 18-10 Rules for coding signs and symptoms.

RULES FOR CODING IMPENDING OR THREATENED CONDITIONS

1. If it did occur, code as a confirmed diagnosis.
2. If it did not occur, reference the Alphabetic Index to determine whether the condition has a subentry term for *impending* or *threatened;* also reference main term entries for *Impending* and *Threatened.*
3. If the subterms are listed, assign the given code.
4. If the subterms are not found, code the existing underlying condition or conditions, signs, or symptoms and not the condition described as "threatened" or "impending."

MULTIPLE CODING (ALSO KNOWN AS DUAL CODING)

Diagnosis: Diabetic retinopathy with type I diabetes

(Note: Retinopathy is the manifestation and diabetes is the etiology (cause) of the retinopathy or retinal hemorrhage.)

Diagnosis: Index: **Retinopathy,** diabetic 250.5 *[362.01]*
                                    diabetic 250.5 *[362.01]*

The Index subterm "diabetic" located under "Retinopathy" identifies the code for the etiology as 250.5 and directs you to the code for the manifestation of *[362.01]* retinopathy. The italicized code is never sequenced first as the first-listed diagnosis but is assigned to identify a manifestation.

Tabular: **250 Diabetes mellitus**

              250.5 Diabetes with ophthalmic manifestations
                        Use additional code to identify manifestation
                    250.51 Type I, not stated as uncontrolled

Note that the diagnosis of diabetes mellitus will always be reported with a five-digit code because the fifth digit indicates the type of diabetes. See the fifth-digit codes listed after code 250 in the Tabular of your ICD-9-CM.

    Code 250.51 is the correct code to describe the diabetes (etiology). The statement "Use additional code to identify manifestation..." in the Tabular at 250.5 directs you to assign a code that identifies the manifestation (retinopathy).

Tabular: **362 Other retinal disorders**
              362.0 Diabetic retinopathy
                        Code first diabetes (250.5)
                    362.01 Background diabetic retinopathy

Note that the "*Code first diabetes 250.5*" directs you to the etiology code (diabetes).

Codes: 250.51, 362.01 Diabetic retinopathy with type I diabetes

The multiple codes fully describe the diagnostic statement. The Guideline directs you to place the etiology code first, followed by the manifestation code.

FIGURE 18-11 Example of multiple coding. (Modified from Buck CJ: *Step-by-step medical coding: 2012 edition,* St Louis, 2012, WB Saunders.)

COMBINATION CODES

Diagnosis: Acute cholecystitis with cholelithiasis

Index: **Cholecystitis** with calculus (stones in the gallbladder) directs you to
              See Cholelithiasis

Index: **Cholelithiasis** with, cholecystitis, acute 574.0

Tabular: **574 Cholelithiasis**
              574.0 Calculus of gallbladder with acute cholecystitis

A fifth-digit subclassification is indicated as 0 for a case without mention of obstruction and as 1 when there is obstruction. There was no mention of obstruction in this case, so assign the fifth digit 0.

Code: 574.00 Acute cholecystitis with cholelithiasis

The single code 574.00 fully describes the diagnosis of acute cholecystitis with cholelithiasis.

FIGURE 18-12 Example of combination codes. (Modified from Buck CJ: *Step-by-step medical coding: 2012 edition,* St Louis, 2012, WB Saunders.)

Coding Infectious and Parasitic Diseases

Most often, multiple codes are needed to code infectious or parasitic diseases. The first code identifies the disease or condition (e.g., bacterial infection), and the second code identifies the organism causing the disease (e.g., streptococcal bacteria). The basic coding principles for the use of either combination or multiple codes apply throughout this section of the ICD-9-CM.

Coding Organism-Caused Diseases

Two categories for identifying the organism that causes a disease are found in other sections or categories. These codes, 041 and 079, may be used either as additional codes or as solo codes, depending on the diagnostic statement. For example, for a urinary tract infection (UTI) caused by *Escherichia coli*, the UTI is coded first (599.0) and the *E. coli* is coded second (041.4X).

Human Immunodeficiency Virus (HIV) Infection and Acquired Immunodeficiency Syndrome (AIDS)

For coding of HIV infection and AIDS, it is essential first to understand the descriptions of the codes available. The key is whether the patient has symptoms.

- Human immunodeficiency virus (HIV): This indicates only that the virus is present.
- Acquired immunodeficiency syndrome (AIDS): AIDS is a syndrome; a *syndrome* is defined as a "group of symptoms occurring together." AIDS is the manifestation (or manifestations) of and/or symptoms that can occur as a result of HIV infection.

Never code a patient as having HIV unless it is clearly documented as confirmed. Probable and suspected cases are never coded; instead, the signs and symptoms present should be coded. The code for a confirmed diagnosis of HIV infection is 042. The codes for illnesses and symptoms associated with AIDS are found primarily in Chapter 3 of the ICD-9-CM manual. Remember that stringent restrictions are placed on the disclosure of medical information regarding patients with HIV infection and/or AIDS. Make sure the patient has signed the appropriate release of medical information form before any disclosures are made to third parties.

Coding Complications of Care

A complication of medical or surgical care generally results in additional procedures or services for a patient, but often the complication is not mentioned as part of the diagnostic statement, which results in reduced reimbursement. It is important to review the medical documentation to determine whether a complication exists and to code the complication in addition to the diagnostic statement.

- Postoperative complications that affect a specific anatomic site or body system are classified according to the appropriate chapter (1 through 16) of the Tabular Index.
- Postoperative complications that affect more than one anatomic site or body system are classified according to Chapter 17 (Injury and Poisoning) of the Tabular Index.
- If the Alphabetic Index does not provide a specific main term and/or subterm to identify a postoperative complication, classify the complication to categories 996 through 999, Complications of Surgical and Medical Care, Not Elsewhere Classified.

Coding the Etiology and Manifestation

Etiology refers to the underlying cause or origin of a disease. **Manifestation** describes the signs and symptoms of the disease. In the Alphabetic Index, the etiology and manifestation codes are listed together. The etiology code is listed first, with the manifestation listed beside it in italicized brackets. These italicized codes are always listed secondary to the etiology code.

Coding Neoplasms

A neoplasm, or new growth, is coded by the site or location of the neoplasm and its behavior. The Neoplasm Table (Figure 18-13) is located in the Alphabetic Index under the main term **Neoplasms**. This table gives the code numbers for neoplasms by anatomic site in alphabetic order. Six possible code numbers exist for each anatomic site, depending on whether the neoplasm is malignant or benign, exhibits uncertain behavior, or is of an unspecified nature. Malignant

	Malignant					
	Primary	Secondary	Ca in situ	Benign	Uncertain Behavior	Unspecified
Neoplasm *(continued)*						
bone (periosteum)	170.9	198.5	—	213.9	238.0	239.2
Note—Carcinomas and adenocarcinomas, of any type other than intraosseous or odontogenic, of the sites listed under "Neoplasm, bone," should be considered as constituting metastatic spread from an unspecified primary site and coded to 198.5 for morbidity coding and to 199.1 for underlying cause of death coding.						
acetabulum	170.6	198.5	—	213.6	238.0	239.2
acromion (process)	170.4	198.5	—	213.4	238.0	239.2
ankle	170.8	198.5	—	213.8	238.0	239.2
arm NEC	170.4	198.5	—	213.4	238.0	239.2
astragalus	170.8	198.5	—	213.8	238.0	239.2
atlas	170.2	198.5	—	213.2	238.0	239.2
axis	170.2	198.5	—	213.2	238.0	239.2
back NEC	170.2	198.5	—	213.2	238.0	239.2
calcaneus	170.8	198.5	—	213.8	238.0	239.2

FIGURE 18-13 Neoplasm Table from the ICD-9-CM manual. (Modified from Diamond MS: *Mastering medical coding*, St Louis, 2006, WB Saunders.)

neoplasms are categorized into three separate subclassifications: primary, secondary, and in situ.

Terms Defining Malignant Neoplasm Sites

- *Primary:* Identifies the originating anatomic site of the neoplasm. A primary malignancy is defined as the original site or sites of the cancer.
- *Secondary:* Identifies sites to which the primary neoplasm has metastasized (spread). A secondary malignancy is defined as a second location to which the cancer has spread from the primary location.
- *In situ:* Carcinoma in situ is defined as the absence of invasion of surrounding tissues. Tumor cells are undergoing malignant changes but are still confined to the point of origin, without invasion of surrounding normal tissue. The In Situ column is used only if the physician uses that precise terminology.

Definitions of Benign, Uncertain Behavior, and Unspecified Nature Neoplasms

- *Benign:* The growth is noncancerous, nonmalignant, and has not invaded adjacent structures or spread to distant sites.
- *Uncertain behavior:* The pathologist is unable to determine whether the neoplasm is benign or malignant.
- *Unspecified nature:* Neither the behavior nor the histologic type of neoplasm is specified in the diagnostic statement.

The ICD-9-CM instructional notes state that the behavior of the neoplasm should be determined first when coding.

- Most coding decisions for malignant neoplasms are between primary and secondary.
- *In situ* is used only when the diagnostic statement contains that exact phrase.
- *Unspecified* is used only when no pathology study has been done and the neoplasm is still described with a term such as "tumor" or "growth."
- *Uncertain* is used only when the neoplasm's behavior is not malignant, the tumor is not in situ, or the behavior is unpredictable.

Note that there is also a code beginning with M that is called the *morphology code*. The morphology code is not typically used by physicians or providers when coding diagnoses.

Five Steps for Coding Neoplasms

The following steps can help the medical assistant determine the most specific and accurate diagnostic code for a neoplasm. These steps should be considered in addition to the basic diagnostic steps.

1. Using the Neoplasm Table in the Alphabetic Index, determine the site (anatomic location) of the neoplasm and select the row in the Neoplasm Table in which it appears.
2. Determine the neoplasm behavior and select the Neoplasm Table column that best defines the behavior: *Malignant, Benign, In-situ, Uncertain Behavior,* or *Unspecified Nature.*
3. If the neoplasm is malignant, determine whether the malignancy is primary, secondary, or in situ.
4. Link the appropriate Neoplasm Table column to the appropriate row.
5. Check the code in the Tabular Index to make sure the code complies with the guidelines, conventions, and instructional notations in the Tabular Index.

The ICD-9-CM manual also always provides additional information, definitions, and guidelines for coding neoplasms, just as it does for all other diseases, illnesses, and injuries.

Coding for the Circulatory System

Physicians use a wide variety of terms and phrases to identify components of the circulatory system. To code disorders of the circulatory system accurately, the coder must carefully review all inclusions, exclusions, conventions, guidelines, and instructional notations associated with each potential code selected.

Myocardial Infarction

A myocardial infarction (MI) is coded as follows:

- As *acute* if it is documented as such in the diagnostic statement or has a stated duration of 8 weeks or less.
- As *chronic* if it is so stated in the diagnostic statement or if symptoms persist after 8 weeks.

Other MI coding considerations include the following:

- If an MI is specified as "old" or "healed" without any current or presenting symptoms, it should be coded using category 412.
- A history of an MI uses code 412, which describes an *Old myocardial infarct.* This code is used only if the patient has no symptoms and only if the old MI was diagnosed by means of an electrocardiogram.
- If the patient is symptomatic, code the underlying condition or symptoms only if the underlying condition is not known.

Arteriosclerotic Cardiovascular Disease

Arteriosclerotic cardiovascular disease (ASCVD) is classified to subcategory 429.2, with an additional code used to identify whether arteriosclerosis is present. For example, the diagnostic statement "generalized arteriosclerotic cardiovascular disease" should be coded using 429.2 followed by 440.9, *generalized and unspecified atherosclerosis.*

Hypertensive Disease

A distinction is made in the ICD-9-CM between "elevated" and "high" blood pressure. High blood pressure is defined as hypertension. If a diagnostic statement does not contain the word *hypertension* or the phrase *high blood pressure,* the condition is coded as elevated blood pressure, not hypertension.

The Alphabetic Index contains a Hypertension Table (Figure 18-14) under the main term **Hypertension**. The table contains subterms that identify different types of hypertension and any complications caused by the hypertension. Hypertension is classified three ways: malignant, benign, and unspecified.

- *Malignant* hypertension usually is considered acute and life-threatening.
- *Benign* hypertension, although considered dangerous, is not considered acute or life-threatening.
- Unless the diagnostic statement specifically states "malignant" or "benign" hypertension, hypertension should be classified as *unspecified.*

Hypertension frequently is the cause of various forms of heart and vascular disease; however, the mention of hypertension in the diagnostic statement does not mean that a combination code for

	Malignant	Benign	Unspecified
Hypertension, hypertensive (arterial) (arteriolar) (disease) (essential) (fluctuating) (idiopathic) (intermittent) (labile) (low rennin) (orthostatic) (paroxysmal) (primary) (systemic) (uncontrolled) (vascular)	401.0	401.1	401.9
with			
heart involvement (conditions classifiable to 428, 429.0-429.3, 429.8, 429.9 due to hypertension) (*see also* Hypertension, heart)	402.00	402.10	401.90
with kidney involvement – *see* Hypertension, cardiorenal			
renal involvement (only conditions classifiable to 585, 586, 587) (excludes conditions classifiable as 584) (*see also* Hypertension, kidney)	403.00	403.10	403.90
with heart involvement – *see* Hypertension, cardiorenal			
failure (and sclerosis) (*see also* Hypertension, kidney)	403.01	403.11	403.91
sclerosis without failure (*see also* Hypertension, kidney)	403.00	403.10	403.90
accelerated (*see also* Hypertension, by type, malignant)	401.0	—	—
antepartum – *see* Hypertension, complicating pregnancy, childbirth, or the puerperium			

FIGURE 18-14 Hypertension Table from the ICD-9-CM manual. (Modified from Diamond MS: *Mastering medical coding*, St Louis, 2006, WB Saunders.)

hypertensive heart disease should be used. If a cause-and-effect relationship exists between the hypertension and the heart disease, it should be clearly documented in the clinical record or diagnostic statement.

Coding for Complications of Pregnancy, Childbirth, and the Puerperium

Coding for the obstetric patient is like using a specialty codebook within the main codebook. This is challenging for those who do not code obstetrics often. Some important terms regarding pregnancy are:

- *Antepartum*—meaning pregnancy (applies as soon as a pregnancy test result is positive)
- *Childbirth*—meaning delivery
- *Peripartum*—the period from the last month of pregnancy to 5 months' postpartum
- *Postpartum*—the puerperium (6 weeks after delivery)

Obstetric Coding Guidelines

To begin searching for obstetric codes, start at either of the main terms **Pregnancy** or **Delivery**. Look for a subterm regarding the condition, or start at the main term for the condition and look for a subterm that states *affecting pregnancy* or *during pregnancy.*

- Normal, uncomplicated prenatal and postpartum care for the mother and routine visits for the baby are coded with V codes as long as no current problem exists.
- Some mothers have conditions that put them at high risk; these situations are also coded with V codes unless a problem manifests itself during the pregnancy.
- Normal, uncomplicated delivery for the mother is coded using category 650, and a V code is used to describe the outcome of the delivery.

USE OF CATEGORY 650 AND V CODES IN PREGNANCY CODING

- In the ICD-9-CM manual, use codes from the Tabular Index (Volume 1), Chapter 11, in the 630-677 range. If the pregnancy is documented as a normal pregnancy or is unrelated to the reason for the physician encounter, use a V code (V22.2) in place of any Chapter 11 code.
- Chapter 11 codes are used only on the maternal record, not on the newborn record.
- Categories 640-648 and 651-676 require a fifth digit. The fifth digit indicates whether the encounter is antepartum or postpartum or whether the delivery occurred.

A normal, uncomplicated delivery is described as one in which no problem or complication occurred during the entire encounter and no procedures were performed other than those deemed normal. The available V codes used to describe the outcome of delivery are V27.0-V27.9. If the mother delivered a single baby, born live, without complication, the code would be V27.0.

In obstetric care, fifth digits are used only for obstetric patients with complications. In Figure 18-15, note that the fifth digits divide the pregnancy into three different "time zones," which are described in the ICD-9-CM as episodes of care:

- Before delivery (antepartum)
- Delivery (the episode of care when the delivery occurs)
- After delivery (postpartum)

The fifth-digit codes for the episode of care are:

0—Unspecified as to episode of care or not applicable
1—Delivered, with or without mention of antepartum condition
2—Delivered, with mention of postpartum complication
3—Antepartum condition or complication
4—Postpartum condition or complication

637 Unspecified abortion
  Requires following fifth digit to identify stage:
  Coding Clinic: 1994, Q2, P14

> 0 unspecified
> 1 incomplete
> 2 complete

Includes abortion NOS
  retained products of conception following
  abortion, not classifiable elsewhere

637.0 Complicated by genital tract and pelvic
[0-2] **infection** ♀   M

637.1 Complicated by delayed or excessive hemorrhage ♀ M
[0-2]

637.2 Complicated by damage to pelvic organs or
[0-2] **tissues** ♀   M

637.3 Complicated by renal failure ♀   M
[0-2]

637.4 Complicated by metabolic disorder ♀   M
[0-2]

637.5 Complicated by shock ♀   M
[0-2]

637.6 Complicated by embolism ♀   M
[0-2]

637.7 With other specified complications ♀   M
[0-2]

637.8 With unspecified complication ♀   M
[0-2]

637.9 Without mention of complication ♀   M
[0-2]

FIGURE 18-15 Excerpt from ICD-9-CM: pregnancy codes and use of fourth and fifth digits.

If the baby has a problem while the mother is still pregnant, code it only if it affects the mother's condition or management. Code the baby's problem on the mother's chart only if it creates a medical concern or a medical need for the mother to undergo testing or treatment. When it is appropriate to code a fetal condition that affects the mother's management, use codes for pregnant patients, not codes for babies.

Cesarean Delivery

Cesarean codes only define the reasons a cesarean delivery was performed; they do not describe cesarean deliveries as separate from vaginal births. A cesarean delivery is considered the treatment for a problem or condition that exists at the time of delivery.

Outcome of Delivery and Liveborn Infant Codes

- Outcome of Delivery codes (V27) are reported on the mother's health record after the delivery.
- A Liveborn Infant code or codes (V30-V39) describe the condition of the baby at delivery (e.g., liveborn or stillborn) and are reported on the newborn's record.

Newborn Coding

Babies are considered newborn or perinatal for the first 28 days. The code range used for these patients, 760-779, is found in Chapter 15 of the Tabular Index. After the twenty-eighth day of life, do not use codes specific to perinatal patients. Newborn codes should never be used on the maternal record. If a newborn is healthy, a code from the V code category 30 should be used in addition to any other Chapter 15 code.

Liveborn Infant Category

A fifth digit from the Liveborn Infant category is used only when a fourth digit of 0 is assigned. A fourth digit of 0 means that the baby was born in the hospital; the fifth digit then specifies whether the birth was cesarean. The other fourth digits (i.e., 1 and 2) represent births that occurred other than in the hospital. Cesarean deliveries are presumed to occur only in the hospital; therefore, no fifth digit is provided.

Coding Injuries

Injuries constitute a major section of the ICD-9-CM. They are classified first according to the type of injury and then by anatomic site.

- When coding injuries, separate codes should be assigned for each individual injury unless a combination code is provided.
- If a patient has multiple injuries, the most severe injury should be coded first.
- Superficial injuries, such as abrasions or contusions, are not coded when associated with more severe injuries at the same site.
- If an injury results in minor or major damage to peripheral nerves or blood vessels, the injury is coded first, with additional codes from categories 950-957, Injury to Nerves and Spinal Cord, and/or 900-904, Injury to Blood Vessels.

Coding Fractures

Fractures are coded first by anatomic site and then by type of fracture. The category code range for fractures, 800-829, is found in Chapter 17 (Injury and Poisoning) in the Tabular Index. Fractures can be classified as open or closed. A fracture is said to be *open* if the skin has been broken and the bone protrudes through the skin surface, or when a wound, such as a puncture, allows the bone to be seen. In a *closed* fracture, the bone is not exposed to the outside of the body. If no indication is given whether the fracture was open or closed, it should be coded as if it were closed.

Burns

The same principles for combination and multiple coding apply to burns. Code each burn separately unless specific combination codes are given in the Tabular Index. There are many combination codes. Because burns are coded by site and degree and by the extent of body surface involvement, all burn cases should have at least two codes, and a third if the wound is infected. Other types of wounds, lacerations, punctures, and so on use a different fifth digit to show that they are infected and therefore complicated. Because burn codes use the fifth digit for other information, an additional code is necessary to indicate infection.

Table 18-1 presents the Lund-Browder Chart for Determining Burn Percentages in Children. First, determine the child's age and then the body part or parts burned. Next, add the percentage listed in the Age column for each body area burned. The sum represents the percentage of the body burned. For example, if the entire left leg of a 10-year-old child were burned, the burn percentage would be calculated as follows:

$$\tfrac{1}{2} \text{ of thigh: } (4.25\%) \times 2 = 8.5\%$$

$$\tfrac{1}{2} \text{ of lower leg: } (3\%) \times 2 = 6\%$$

$$8.5\% + 6\% = 14.5\% \text{ of the body burned}$$

TABLE 18-1 Lund-Browder Chart for Determining Burn Percentages in Children

	UP TO 1 YEAR	1 YEAR	5 YEARS	10 YEARS	15 YEARS
½ of head	9.5%	8.5%	6.5%	5.5%	4.5%
½ of 1 thigh	2.75%	3.25%	4%	4.25%	4.25%
½ of lower leg	2.5%	2.5%	2.75%	3%	3.25%

http://medical-dictionary.thefreedictionary.com/rule+of+nines

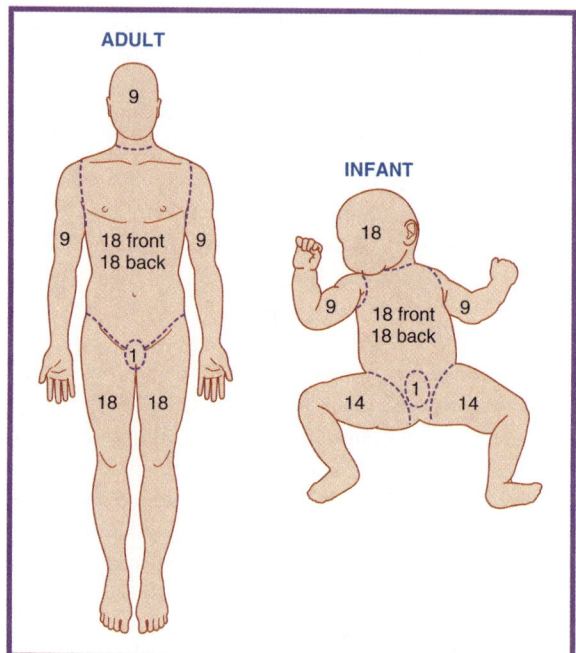

FIGURE 18-16 Rule of Nines for determining burn percentages in adults and infants.

Figure 18-16 presents the Rule of Nines, which is used to determine burn percentages in adults. Using the Rule of Nines, add the percentage listed for each body area burned. The sum is the percentage of the body burned. For example, the burn percentage for burns on the entire head and front and back torso in an adult would be calculated as follows:

Front and back of head: 4.5% × 2 = 9%

Front and back of torso: 9% × 2 = 18%

9% + 18% = 27% of the body burned

When evaluating burns on growing children, providers may find it necessary to change the percentage assignments to accommodate proportionally larger heads than adults. The percentages may also be changed if a patient has large buttocks, thighs, or a large abdomen that is involved in the burn.

Steps for Coding Burns

1. Code the burn to the site by degree. Under the main term **Burn**, find the subterm for the site and then the subterm for the degree. If the burn is stated to be at the same site but of a different degree, code to the highest degree. Omit the code for the lower level burn at the same site.
2. Determine the percentage of the body burned using category 948 (Chapter 17 in the Tabular Index). The fourth digit describes the total burned surface; the fifth digit describes the percentage of only third-degree burns; for example, 50% of total body surface burned with 15% third-degree burns.
3. If the burn is said to be infected, use code 958.3 as a third code to identify the infection.

Using E Codes

The ICD-9-CM uses E codes to describe the circumstances of an accident or injury. E codes are listed in a separate Tabular Index and Alphabetic Index (Figure 18-17). E codes describe the following:

- Nature of an event (e.g., fire, fall, collision, abuse)
- Place of occurrence
- Late effect of an injury
- Intent (e.g., self-inflicted, assault, accident)
- Drugs and chemicals that caused the injury or disease

E codes are never principal codes or listed first, because they are only supplementary information. They most often are used with injury codes, but they may be used with any condition that is the result of an external cause, such as a respiratory problem caused by smoke inhalation. The E code describing the initial incident is used only once, the first time the patient is treated for the condition. Some major categories of E codes include the following:

- Transport accidents
- Poisoning and adverse effects of drugs, medicinal substances, and biologics
- Accidents and falls
- Accidents caused by fire and flames
- Accidents caused by natural and environmental factors
- Late effects of accidents, assaults, or self-injury
- Assaults or purposely inflicted injury
- Suicide or self-inflicted injury

It is correct to use as many E codes as necessary to describe all the information provided by the record. It is acceptable to use nonphysician documentation to support these codes if it does not conflict with the physician's documentation. This is the only exception to the rule that diagnoses and diagnostic statements must be documented in the medical record by physicians if the information is to be used for code selection or billing purposes.

Table of Drugs and Chemicals

The ICD-9-CM's Table of Drugs and Chemicals contains a classification of drugs and other chemicals. It is used to identify poisoning states and external causes of adverse effects. Each of the substances is assigned a code, which is used based on the type of poisoning (e.g., overdose, wrong substance given or taken, or a prescription drug taken with alcohol). The table also contains a list of external causes of adverse effects caused by the ingestion or exposure to a drug or chemical.

The poisoning codes in the first column of the Table of Drugs and Chemicals should be determined and listed first, followed by the external cause (E code). The Table of Drugs and Chemicals has five E code headings: *Accidental Poisoning, Therapeutic Use, Suicide Attempt, Assault,* and *Undetermined Cause.*

E CODE INDEX

Railway Accidents	E800-E807
Motor Vehicle Traffic Accidents	E810-E819
Motor Vehicle Nontraffic Accidents	E820-E825
Other Road Vehicle Accidents	E826-E829
Water Transport Accidents	E830-E838
Air and Space Accidents	E840-E845
Vehicle Accidents Not Classified Elsewhere	E846-E848
Place of Occurrence	E849
Accidental Poisoning by Drugs, Medicinal Substances, Biologicals	E850-E858
Accidental Poisoning by Other Solid and Liquid Substances, Gases, Vapors	E860-E869
Misadventure to Patients During Surgical/ Medical Care	E870-E876
Surgical/Medical Procedures Cause of Abnormal Reaction of Patient or Later Complication, Without Mention of Misadventure at Time of Procedure	E878-E879
Accidental Falls	E880-E888
Accidents by Fire and Flames	E890-E898
Accidents Due to Natural/Environmental Factors	E900-E909
Accidents Caused by Submersion, Suffocation and Foreign Bodies	E910-E915
Other Accidents	E916-E928
Late Effects of Accidental Injury	E929
Drugs, Medicinal and Biological Substances Causing Adverse Effects in Therapeutic Use	E930-E949
Suicide and Self-Inflicted Injury	E950-E959
Homicide and Injury Purposely Inflicted by Other Persons	E960-E969
Legal Intervention	E970-E978
Injury Undetermined Whether Accidentally or Purposely Inflicted	E980-E989
Injury Resulting from Operations of War	E990-E999

FIGURE 18-17 Example of E codes. (Modified from Diamond MS: *Mastering medical coding*, St Louis, 2006, WB Saunders.)

EXTERNAL CAUSE CODES (E CODES) USED WITH THE TABLE OF DRUGS AND CHEMICALS

- *Accidental poisoning (E850-E869):* Accidental overdose of a drug; wrong substance given or taken, taken inadvertently; accidents in the use of drugs in medical and surgical procedures; and to show external causes of poisonings coded with the Tabular Index (Volume 1), Chapter 19, Injury and Poisoning, category codes 980-989.
- *Therapeutic use (E930-E949):* An adverse effect caused by proper administration of the correct substance in the proper dosage.
- *Suicide attempt (E962):* Self-inflicted injury or poisoning. Never code Suicide Attempt without documentation from the physician.
- *Assault (E961-E962):* Injury or poisoning inflicted by another person with the intent to injure or kill.
- *Undetermined (E980-E982):* Used only when neither accidental nor intentional circumstances can be determined.

E Codes Used with the Table of Drugs and Chemicals

An E code to identify a drug or chemical may be added to clarify the patient's circumstance whenever a drug or chemical is identified in the medical record as a causative substance. In addition to the E codes that identify the causative substances, the Table of Drugs and Chemicals includes a column for poisoning associated with each substance. These codes can be used with an E code from the other columns with one exception: a Poisoning code cannot be used with a Therapeutic Use code. Problems caused by correct substances properly used are considered adverse effects, not poisoning.

V Codes: Classification of Factors Influencing Health Status and Contact with Health Service

V codes are used to describe circumstances or encounters with a physician or healthcare provider when no current illness or injury exists. V codes may stand alone or may be principal or secondary. Some codes have a notation that they cannot be principal or stand-alone.

V Code Index for History Codes

In the Alphabetic Index, under the main term **History**, is the subterm *personal*. This means that the subterms are considered the patient's personal history. The subterm *family* indented two spaces under **History** describes the family history rather than personal history. Watch the subterm indentations closely to ensure that the code selected is the proper history code.

Diabetes Mellitus

Diabetes mellitus codes always require a fourth and fifth digit. The fourth digit describes any manifestations of the diabetes that may be present; the fifth digit describes the type of diabetes. The fourth-digit subcategories for category 250, diabetes mellitus, are divided by the presence or absence of complications and the nature of the complication. Figure 18-18 presents the fourth-digit subcategories 250.0-50.9.

The fifth digit is required to code the type of diabetes mellitus (DM). Determining the type of diabetes is critical to proper code assignment. The two types of DM are type 1, which includes both juvenile-onset DM and insulin-dependent diabetes mellitus (IDDM), and type 2, which sometimes is called adult-onset DM. Type 2 DM is not always treated with insulin and therefore is also called *non-insulin-dependent DM.*

Four fifth digits are used to specify the type of diabetes and whether it is under control:

0—Type II or unspecified type, not stated as uncontrolled. This fifth digit is used for patients with type 2 DM even if the patient requires insulin.

1—Type I (juvenile type), not stated as uncontrolled.

2—Type II or unspecified type, uncontrolled. This fifth digit is used for patients with type 2 DM even if the patient requires insulin.

3—Type I (juvenile type), uncontrolled.

MAXIMIZING THIRD-PARTY REIMBURSEMENT

The most important thing to remember in using the ICD-9-CM is to code the diagnosis to the highest level of specificity, linking the

Fourth Digit Subcategories for Diabetes Mellitus

- 250.0 Diabetes mellitus without mention of complication
- 250.1 Diabetes mellitus with ketoacidosis (defined as a life-threatening condition in which ketones, which result from the breakdown of fat for energy, accumulate in the bloodstream and the pH of the blood decreases)
- 250.2 Diabetes with hyperosmolarity (defined as a concentration of the body fluids that is abnormally increased)
- 250.3 Diabetes with other coma
- 250.4 Diabetes with renal manifestations
- 250.5 Diabetes with ophthalmic manifestations
- 250.6 Diabetes with neurological manifestations.
- 250.7 Diabetes with peripheral circulatory disorders
- 250.8 Diabetes with other specified manifestations
- 250.9 Diabetes with unspecified complication

FIGURE 18-18 Excerpt from ICD-9-CM: fourth-digit subcategories 250.0 through 250.9.

ICD-9-CM code to the *Current Procedural Terminology,* fourth edition (CPT-4) code. Obtaining the correct reimbursement is important to the practice's cash flow and depends on proper coding and billing techniques. Some other crucial points to remember when submitting diagnostic codes for claims include:

- Use the current year ICD-9-CM manual and stay informed of all changes, revisions, and additions published for that year to both the codes and the official coding guidelines.
- Code accurately from documented information, making sure the appropriate code or codes are assigned for all parts of the diagnostic statement, with no additions or omissions.
- Be sure the diagnosis corresponds to the symptoms and treatment. Many codes are specific to age and gender.
- Review data entry to make sure no digits have been transposed.
- Know the insurance carrier's rules and requirements for completion and submission of claims.
- Incomplete or inaccurate codes may result in delay or denial of reimbursement. An inaccurate diagnosis may have a lifelong negative effect on the patient.

CLOSING COMMENTS

Medical assistants have the trust of the physician and practice that employ them. Therefore, a medical assistant must be responsible and knowledgeable to ensure that no fraud takes place in the coding and claims submission process. Medical assistants are expected to adhere to ethical standards, assigning and reporting only codes clearly supported by concise documentation in the patient's chart. When in doubt, a medical assistant should consult the attending healthcare provider for clarification. Maintaining and continually enhancing coding skills and keeping informed of changes in codes, guidelines, and regulations are necessary responsibilities for a coding professional.

Patient Education

Since most patients are uneducated about medical billing and coding, they may not understand how the codes on their encounter forms relate to their diagnosis. If the patient approaches with questions, explain that the codes represent his or her diagnosis to the most specific and accurate level. The system of diagnostic coding standardized the way medical billing is handled by all parties in the reimbursement cycle. Since the coding system is much like a foreign language, be patient when explaining this process and answering questions; otherwise, those who are unfamiliar with its dialogue will have difficulty understanding the billing process.

Legal and Ethical Issues

By using the billing and coding system, providers are able to express the simplicity or complexity of a medical treatment or procedure. This specificity leads to the maximum reimbursement to the provider. The medical assistant must perform coding procedures accurately so that they reflect exactly what happened during the treatment. Codes must not be exaggerated to increase the reimbursement to the provider.

In the next chapter, procedure codes will be introduced; the procedure codes must "match" the diagnosis code – meaning that the procedure code must be a logical treatment for the diagnosis (more than one diagnosis may be listed on the claim form). For example, patients who are diabetic may be checked for a blood glucose level at each visit. Medical assistants should become familiar with the laws and regulations within their state regarding the billing and coding process. Medical assistants who are eager to learn will become successful and valuable employees.

SUMMARY OF SCENARIO

Mike is enthusiastic about his position and enjoys learning more about the coding process. He knows that as he gains experience and earns his certificate, he will be even more valuable as an employee. As Mike progresses with diagnostic coding, he also will be able to help the physicians and nursing staff be attentive to details when documenting a patient's chart.

Although using the superbill to enter the codes for billing is an easy tool, Mike has learned that knowing how to use the ICD-9-CM volumes is a necessary asset to ensure accurate coding. He also knows it is important when coding a diagnosis to make sure the medical documentation matches the encounter form and that all elements of the diagnostic statement must be included.

Furthermore, he must ensure that the diagnosis listed on the encounter form is fully documented in the patient's medical record. In addition, Mike has learned that the layout and structure of volumes 1 and 2 of the ICD-9-CM manual are designed to aid the selection of the most specific and accurate diagnosis code. Every feature of the manual provides guidance in choosing and confirming a diagnostic code that matches the diagnostic statement on the encounter form and in the medical record. The steps and decision tree for diagnostic coding ensure that Mike will be coding to the highest level of specificity and accuracy.

SUMMARY OF LEARNING OBJECTIVES

1. **Define, spell, and pronounce the terms listed in the vocabulary.**
   Spelling and pronouncing medical terms correctly bolster the credibility of the medical assistant. Knowing the definition of these terms promotes confidence in communication with patients and co-workers. Also, understanding the medical terms found in the diagnostic statement is essential for identifying and selecting the most accurate and appropriate diagnostic code or codes.

2. **Identify three purposes of the most current diagnostic coding system.**
   The ICD-9-CM is used to track healthcare statistics and to facilitate accurate medical record keeping and ease in processing claims. Use of the ICD-9-CM is mandatory for participation in many federal, state, and private insurance programs.

3. **Describe how to use the most current diagnostic coding system.**
   Each of the volumes of the ICD-9-CM has a specific use. The Alphabetic Index (Volume 2) is used to look for the disease or diseases documented in the clinical record. The coder then proceeds to the Tabular Index (Volume 1) to find and assign a code. The coder must follow guidelines provided in the specific manual used for coding in the medical facility.

4. **Explain and apply the basic coding rules in using the ICD-9-CM.**
   Several basic rules can assist the medical assistant in coding: (1) Make sure to use the most recent ICD-9-CM manual; (2) keep a medical dictionary handy; (3) proofread the claim and make sure it makes good sense; (4) do not use nonspecific codes; and (5) take care in coding pre-existing conditions.

5. **Explain where diagnostic information can be found and demonstrate how to abstract the diagnostic statement from the medical record.**
   Diagnostic information is found in the medical record and typically also on the encounter form or charge ticket. It can be located in the history and physical examination (H&P), treatment notes and discharge summary and also in various reports from the radiology and pathology departments and the laboratory. Information about the patient's diagnosis is extracted from the medical record; this information becomes the diagnostic statement.

6. **Demonstrate the use of the Alphabetic Index in selection of main and modifying terms, and appropriate code (or codes) or code ranges.**
   Main terms are selected from the diagnostic statement to begin the search for the best code or code ranges. A main term typically is the primary condition, disease, or injury. Modifying terms provide further specificity, or detail, such as the anatomic site or additional manifestations of the condition.

7. **Explain the importance of the Tabular Index.**
   Never code directly from the Alphabetic Index. The Tabular Index contains the most specific information. Check and recheck the codes to make sure the documentation supports the codes used on the claim.

8. **Correctly use instructional terms and symbols as defined in the ICD-9-CM.**
   The medical assistant should become familiar with all the symbols used in the ICD-9-CM. Instructional notations should be read thoroughly and all directions followed when coding a claim.

9. **Explain the use of V and E codes.**
   V or E codes may help clarify or further explain a code. V codes are used when the patient is not currently ill but is being seen by health service professionals. E codes are used to explain that some external cause contributed to an adverse effect in the body.

10. **Perform diagnostic coding.**
    The medical assistant's knowledge of accurate diagnostic coding contributes to the legal and financial health of the practice. In most cases ICD-9-CM codes are found on the provider's encounter form (or superbill) and/or in the practice management software. However, with literally thousands of current diagnostic codes, it may be necessary to code from the ICD-9-CM manual. Because these codes are updated yearly, they are an asset in coding compliance. The process for diagnosis coding is outlined in Procedure 18-1.

CONNECTIONS

Study Guide Connection: Go to the Chapter 18 Study Guide. Read and complete the activities.

Evolve Connection: Go to the Chapter 18 link at *evolve.elsevier.com/kinn* to complete the Chapter Review and Chapter Quiz. Check out the other resources listed for this chapter to make the most of what you have learned from Basics of Diagnostic Coding.

19

BASICS OF PROCEDURAL CODING

Carline A. Dalgleish, Sharon Oliver, and Alexandra Patricia Adams

SCENARIO

Sherald Vogt excelled on her diagnostic coding examinations, and she now looks forward to learning procedural coding. The process for coding procedures and services will prove to be similar to that of ICD-9-CM and diagnostic coding, except she will use a different coding manual, the *Current Procedural Terminology* (CPT), for most procedural and services rendered coding. She will also use the *Healthcare Common Procedural Coding System*, or HCPCS (pronounced "hic-pix") manual. As with the ICD-9-CM, accurate coding begins with the proper analysis of clinical information to abstract the correct data and accurately assign a procedure or service code. In the ICD-9-CM, she learned about coding conventions and guidelines. The CPT also has conventions, symbols, guidelines, and formal steps specific to procedural coding that Sherald will use to correctly assign procedure codes. Sherald is beginning to fully understand the impact diagnostic and procedural coding has on reimbursement, and her responsibility to uphold ethical standards when coding to keep her employers, Dr. Shuman, Dr. Taylor, and Dr. Caddell, in compliance with federal and state guidelines. She is excited to begin this new phase of her education and to have the opportunity to learn more skills, which will help her reach her goal of becoming an even more valuable asset to the practice.

While studying this chapter, think about the following questions:

- What will Sherald find similar to what she learned with the ICD-9-CM as she performs procedural coding?
- What will help Sherald in selecting the most specific and accurate CPT code?
- What are the differences between coding for the CPT and coding for HCPCS?
- What will Sherald learn about the legal and compliance implications of improper coding?

LEARNING OBJECTIVES

1. Define, spell, and pronounce the terms listed in the vocabulary.
2. Describe the steps for abstracting procedural data from clinical documentation.
3. Identify four purposes of the CPT.
4. List the six main sections of the CPT and describe their content.
5. Describe the coding conventions, guidelines, and layout of the CPT manual and their importance.
6. Describe the process and steps for selecting the most accurate code based on clinical documentation.
7. Explain the importance of correctly assigning Evaluation and Management (E/M) codes.
8. Discuss the importance of modifiers.
9. Define upcoding and explain why it must be avoided.
10. Explain the process for selecting the correct procedure codes.
11. Explain the process for selecting main and modifying terms.
12. Explain how to find codes in the Alphabetic Index of the CPT manual.
13. Explain how to analyze and select codes using the CPT Main Text.

VOCABULARY

abstract An outline or summary of the diagnostic statement and/or procedures and services performed. In procedural coding, the outline or summary assists in ensuring that all procedures and services are included in an insurance claim submission and that nothing is omitted or added to the encounter form or charge ticket; as a verb form, *abstract* also means to compile this outline or summary for use in procedural coding.

acronyms Abbreviations, such as ECG for electrocardiography.

add-on codes Codes that indicate additional or supplemental procedures carried out along with the primary procedure.

Alphabetic Index The reference section of the CPT manual; it is used to help find a code or code range.

bundled codes CPT codes designating procedures or services that are grouped together and paid for as one procedure or service, according to the National Correct Coding Initiative (NCCI) edits, established by the Centers for Medicare and Medicaid Services (CMS).

category In the CPT manual, the element indented one level below a subsection; it usually refers to a specific anatomic site or to procedures and/or services.

Category I codes Five-digit primary procedure or service codes, found in the Tabular Index, that are selected when performing insurance billing or statistical research.

Category II codes Special codes that can help providers track revenue and reimbursement; these codes are alphanumeric and end in the letter F.

Category III codes Codes for a new or experimental procedure or service, otherwise referred to as "Emerging Technology"; these codes are alphanumeric and end in the letter T.

crosswalked With regard to the coding process, a crosswalk is the reference from a deleted or changed code to its new code location in the manual.

downcoding A change in a code or codes for entries submitted for reimbursement. This change usually is made by the insurance company, generally because the code submitted in some way does not match the company's specifications.

eponym A name or term for something that is based on the name of a person (or occasionally a place or thing). Traditionally in medicine, discoveries often are named after the person or people who made the discovery.

established patient (EP) A patient who has received professional services (face to face) from the physician, or from another physician of the *exact* same specialty *and subspecialty* who belongs to the same group practice, within the past 3 years.

guidelines Found at the beginning of each section of the coding manual, guidelines are the specific definitions of items that must be read to appropriately interpret and report the procedures and services contained in that section.

HCPCS *Health Care Common Procedural Coding System;* also called *Level II codes,* HCPCS codes were created by the CMS to report supplies, materials, injections, and certain procedures and services not defined in the CPT manual.

main term The primary or key word or words abstracted from a medical record that are used to begin the code search in the Alphabetic Index. A main term can identify a procedure or service performed; an organ or anatomic site; a condition, illness, or injury; or an eponym, abbreviation, or acronym.

Main Text See Tabular Index.

modifiers Terms that serve as the means to report or indicate that a service or procedure performed has been altered by some specific circumstance but not changed in its definition or code.

modifying terms Key words selected after the main term has been chosen to help further define or describe the procedure or service performed.

new patient (NP) A patient who has *not* received any professional services (face to face) from the physician or another physician of the *exact* same specialty *and subspecialty* who belongs to the same group practice, within the past 3 years.

patient status (PS) The state of a patient as either new or established; appears in the Evaluation and Management section of the CPT.

physical status The physical condition of the patient.

place of service (POS) codes Codes used on professional claims to specify the facility or location where the service or services were rendered.

providers Individuals qualified by education, training, licensure or regulation, and facility privileging who perform a professional service within their scope of practice and independently report that professional service.

section One of the six primary divisions of the main body of the CPT.

subcategory In the CPT manual, the element indented one level below a category, usually a procedure or service unique to a specific category.

subsection In the CPT manual, the element indented one level below a section; it usually describes an anatomic site or organ system (e.g., Integumentary, Cardiology).

Tabular Index The Main Text of the CPT manual; it contains the alphanumeric listing of all Category I procedure and service codes and their respective descriptions.

unbundled codes Codes in which the components of a major procedure are separated and reported separately.

upcoding A deliberate increase in a CPT code, despite the lack of documentation, to the next highest reimbursable code so as to obtain higher reimbursements.

Procedural coding is defined as the transformation of verbal descriptions of medical services and procedures into numeric or alphanumeric designations. As with diagnostic coding and use of the ICD-9-CM manual, the medical assistant must develop meticulous accuracy when using the *Current Procedural Terminology* (CPT) manual, developed by the American Medical Association (AMA), and the *Healthcare Common Procedural Coding System* (HCPCS), developed by the Centers for Medicare and Medicaid Services (CMS). The medical assistant facilitates accurate medical recordkeeping and efficient processing of insurance claims by using the CPT and HCPCS, which identify appropriate procedures and services common to the physician's office. CPT and HCPCS (discussed later in the chapter) are used in the claims submission process to obtain reimbursement from payers, to track physicians' productivity, and to provide statistical data for research and other purposes.

GETTING TO KNOW THE CPT

The Evolution of CPT Coding

The CPT manual is a list of descriptive terms and identifying codes for reporting medical services and procedures performed by physicians. The CPT provides a uniform, or standard, language that accurately describes medical, surgical, and diagnostic services and enhances reliable communication among physicians, patients, and third parties. The manual was developed after the AMA recognized a need for a standardized description of services that would be universally understood by physicians, hospitals, insurance companies, and all involved in the reimbursement or statistical data collection process.

The second edition of the CPT, published in 1970, presented an expanded system of terms and codes to designate diagnostic and therapeutic procedures in surgery, medicine, radiology, laboratory, pathology, and medical specialties. At that time, the four-digit classification was replaced with the current five-digit coding system. The fourth edition was published in 1977 and included significant updates in medical technology. At the same time, a system of periodic annual updating was introduced to keep pace with the rapidly changing environment. The fourth edition is still in use today; however, at this writing, the AMA is in the process of developing the fifth edition of the CPT, the first major revision since 1977.

Purpose of CPT Procedural Coding

The CPT uses a five-digit classification system that is designed to do the following:
- Encourage the use of standard terms and descriptors to document procedures in the medical record
- Help communicate accurate information on procedures and services to agencies concerned with insurance claims
- Provide the basis for a computer-oriented system to evaluate operative procedures
- Contribute basic information for actuarial and statistical purposes

Before continuing, consider this important fact: there are roughly 150,000 procedure and service codes in the CPT manual and thousands more in the HCPCS manual. Memorizing the codes for each specific procedure and service would be impractical, if not impossible. Instead, the key to success is learning how to use the coding manuals to find the most specific and accurate code based on interpretation of the medical record. This requires a solid understanding of medical terminology, anatomy, and physiology and a knowledge of how to use the CPT manual and its symbols, conventions, guidelines, and notes. The goal of this chapter is to teach the skills, processes, and decisions required to use the CPT and HCPCS manuals. Remember, the CPT and HCPCS manuals for the current year are always the final authority. The symbols, guidelines, conventions, and other instructions found in the CPT manual contain all the information needed to select the correct code for the procedure or service documented in the medical record.

THE CPT CODE

Category I Codes

The CPT code is a five-digit code also known as a **Category I code**. Category I codes are located in the Tabular Index (also called the *Main Text*) of the CPT manual and arranged by sections. For example, codes beginning with 7 (e.g., 70100—a radiologic examination of the mandible, partial, with less than four views) are located in the Radiology section of the manual. Each code has a description of the service or procedure performed. Some CPT codes (e.g., Category II and Category III codes, discussed later) are alphanumeric.

Product Pending U.S. Food and Drug Administration Approval

Occasionally, a new vaccine is assigned a Category I code before the Food and Drug Administration (FDA) has approved the vaccine for use. These vaccines are listed in Appendix K and are identified in the Tabular Index of the CPT in various ways by different publishers. Some publishers use the letter P (approval pending); others use a lightning bolt symbol (⚡) in various colors to designate the pending FDA approval. These codes are tracked by the AMA to monitor FDA approval status. When the FDA status changes to approval, the lightning bolt symbol (⚡) or other "pending" identifier is removed.

Bundled Codes

Bundled codes indicate procedures or services that are grouped together and paid for as one procedure or service, as designated by the NCCI edits. If bundled codes are separated and used individually, a special report should be used to describe the circumstances that made the unbundling necessary.

Unbundled Codes

Unbundled codes are used when the components of a major procedure are separated and reported separately.

Category II

Category II codes are a set of supplemental tracking codes that can be used for performance measurement. Category II codes are optional; they cannot be used as a substitute for Category I codes, and they are not reported as part of the billing process. **Providers** can use Category II codes to help measure performance and outcomes. These codes describe clinical components that may be typically included in Evaluation and Management services or clinical services. No relative value is associated with them. In a Category II code, the fifth digit is the letter F.

Category II codes are described and listed in Appendix H of the CPT manual. They are listed in alphabetic order by condition instead of numerically. Category II codes are reviewed by the Performance Measures Advisory Group, which is composed of members from various medical organizations and government agencies. In some publisher's editions of the CPT manual, Category II codes are also listed in their own section immediately after the Medicine section and before the appendixes.

Category III

Category III codes are temporary codes assigned for emerging and new technology, services, and procedures that have not been officially added to the Main Text of the CPT manual. In a Category III code, the fifth digit is the letter T. Category III codes may be used in billing and reporting if no code in the Main Text accurately describes the technology, service, or procedure performed, and no Category I code matches the medical documentation. Category III codes have no reimbursement value. In most publisher's editions of the CPT manual, Category III codes are also listed in their own section immediately after the Medicine section and before the appendixes.

Modifiers

Modifiers (Table 19-1) give providers a means of indicating that a service or procedure performed was altered by some specific circumstance but was not changed in its definition. Two- or five-digit alphanumeric modifiers, included with the five-digit CPT code, can be used to supply additional information or to describe extenuating circumstances that affect the rendered procedure or service. For instance, modifier -50 adds the detail that a procedure was performed bilaterally, or on both sides of the body. For example, the code 99050 is used to describe care provided after normal business hours. To describe a situation in which an assistant surgeon is needed for a surgical procedure, modifier -80 can be used to allow the assistant surgeon to submit charges for his or her time and services (code 99080 describes a special report).

The modifiers for HCPCS are codes composed of two alphanumeric characters. Like the modifiers for CPT Category I codes, the HCPCS modifiers do not change the description of the code, but rather provide additional information or describe extenuating circumstances.

FORMAT OF THE CPT CODING MANUAL

In the CPT manual, each procedure or service is represented by a five-digit numeric code (Figure 19-1), a type of medical shorthand that saves enormous amounts of time and effort and helps to ensure accuracy of information. Just imagine, for example, if a billing department had to describe, in writing, every single one of the medical procedures and services represented by the codes in the CPT manual. Preparing one bill for one patient could take an hour or longer, and problems with reimbursement still would arise if the health insurance or third-party payer had additional questions or, worse, reduced or even denied payment based on its interpretation of the written narrative. In most instances, using the five-digit CPT codes eliminates the need for written descriptions, thus assuring clear communication, and the standardization of codes ensures that everyone in the reimbursement cycle understands exactly what procedure or service was provided to the patient. In addition, these codes enable automated computer processing of claims, which also saves time and effort.

CPT CONTENT

The CPT manual generally includes the following content, depending on the publisher:

- Comprehensive instructions for use of the manual, including steps for coding
- A complete Alphabetic Index

TABLE 19-1 Commonly Used CPT Code Modifiers	
MODIFIER	**DESCRIPTION**
-50	Bilateral procedure. If procedure was performed on both sides of the body (e.g., both knees, both eyes) and code description does not indicate that the procedure or service was performed bilaterally, modifier -50 is used.
-62	Two surgeons. When two surgeons work together as primary surgeons performing distinct parts of a procedure, each surgeon should report the procedure he or she performed to the insurance carrier and use modifier -62. (This prevents the insurance carrier from possibly rejecting a surgical charge as a duplicate.)

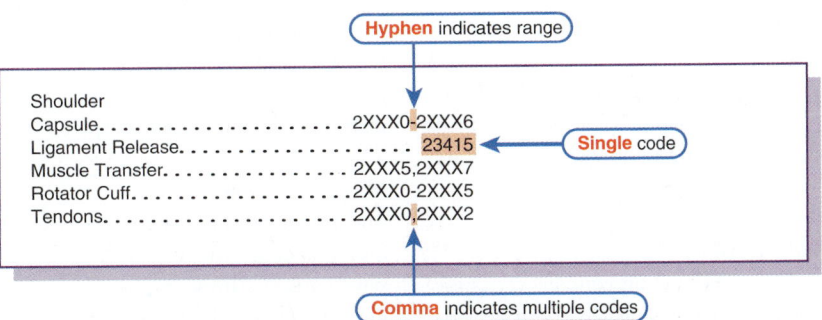

FIGURE 19-1 CPT code example. (From Buck CJ: *Step-by-step medical coding, 2012 edition,* St Louis, 2012, WB Saunders.)

- The Main Text (Tabular Index), composed of:
  - Six sections
  - Guidelines and notes
  - Conventions
  - Fourteen appendixes

The Indexes

The CPT has two primary divisions, the Alphabetic Index and the Main Text (Tabular Index). The **Alphabetic Index** is like any other index in a textbook; it is simply a guide to finding data in the body of the textbook. However, instead of providing the page numbers where the information is located, as a typical index does, the CPT's Alphabetic Index lists the code or code ranges, which are arranged in numeric order in each section of the Main Text.

Main Text

The **Tabular Index (Main Text)** is divided into six broad categories, or **sections,** with codes listed in numeric order in each section. Like the ICD-9-CM, the codes in the Tabular Index include definitions, guidelines and notes, which enable the coder to select the most specific code or codes based on the procedures and services descriptions documented in the medical record. The six sections of the Tabular Index include:

- Evaluation and Management
- Anesthesia
- Surgery (all body systems)
- Radiology
- Pathology and Laboratory
- Medicine

Each of the six sections reflect the general type of service. Sections are subdivided into subsections; subsections are further divided into categories; and categories can be subdivided into subcategories. Each level of a section provides more specificity regarding the procedure or service performed and the anatomic site or organ system involved (Table 19-2). In most instances, all four levels are found, although this is not a hard and fast rule.

In the CPT manual, the **subsection** is listed below the section and indented two spaces. The subsection usually describes an anatomic site or an organ system, as in the following examples:

- Anatomic site: heart, femur, or skull
- Organ system: digestive, integumentary, or cardiology

A **category** is listed below the subsection and indented two spaces. It generally refers to a specific procedure or service, but it can also indicate a more specific anatomic site:

- Procedures: esophagoscopy, incision and drainage, or cardiac catheterization
- Specific anatomic site: mitral valve, distal femur, or occipital bone

Subcategory is the lowest level of code description. The subcategory is listed below the category and indented two spaces. It provides even more specificity about an anatomic site or the procedure or service performed.

Evaluation and Management Section

The Evaluation and Management (E/M) section contains codes for the different types of encounters or visits patients have with providers; these encounters may include office, hospital, and emergency

TABLE 19-2 Section, Subsection, Category, and Subcategory Examples

SECTION	SUBSECTION	CATEGORY	SUBCATEGORY
Surgery	Musculoskeletal System	Application of Casts and Strapping	Body and Upper Extremity
Surgery	Cardiovascular System	Arteries and Veins	Embolectomy/ Thrombectomy
Medicine	Physical Medicine and Rehabilitation	Modalities	
Medicine	Neurology and Neuromuscular Procedures	Sleep Testing	
Radiology	Diagnostic Radiology	Head and Neck	
Radiology	Vascular Procedures	Aorta and Arteries	

department visits; consultations; and physician contact with patients in intensive care units, skilled nursing facilities, nursing homes, and other facilities. The code range in the E/M section is 99201 to 99499. The E/M section is further divided into subsections that include different types of services (e.g., office visits, hospital visits, consultations, skilled nursing facility, or nursing home visits). The subcategories of E/M services are further classified into levels of E/M services that are identified by specific codes. This classification is important, because the nature of a physician's work varies by type of service, place of service, and the patient status. The subsections, categories, and subcategories are written to further modify or describe the service or procedure performed.

Anesthesia Section

The Anesthesia section includes codes for anesthesia services rendered by anesthesiologists and anesthetists before, during, and after surgery. The code ranges in the Anesthesia section are 00100 to 01999 and 99100 to 99140. Codes are included for the types of anesthesia administered (e.g., general, local, and sedation anesthesia); other support services, including the anesthesiologist's preoperative and postoperative encounters with the patient, evaluation of the patient's physical status, and the administration of anesthesia, fluids, and/or blood; and monitoring services, such as blood pressure, temperature, and electrocardiography (ECG). Unusual forms of monitoring (e.g., intra-arterial, central venous, and Swan-Ganz) are not included and can be billed separately.

Surgery Section

The Surgery section, the largest section of the CPT, includes standardized codes for all invasive surgical procedures performed by physicians. An invasive procedure is defined as any medical procedure in which a bodily orifice or the skin must be penetrated by cutting, puncture, or other method. This section is divided into subsections typically identifying specific body systems, beginning with the integumentary (skin) system and ending with the ophthalmologic (eye) and otologic (ear) systems. In most instances, each subsection is further divided into categories and subcategories, which describe procedures and services unique to that anatomic subsection.

Radiology Section

The Radiology section includes codes for diagnostic imaging, including x-ray studies and scans, and for therapy used in the treatment of cancer. The code range in the Radiology section is 70000 to 79999.

Pathology and Laboratory Section

Codes are included for all diagnostic tests performed on bodily fluids and tissue, including urine, blood, sputum, and feces, as well as excised or biopsied cells, tissue, or body organs; and for evaluation of those fluids and tissues to identify any pathology or disease present. The code ranges for the Pathology and Laboratory section are 80047 to 80076 for Organ or Disease–Oriented Panels and 80100 to 89999 for all other tests.

Medicine Section

The codes for the Medicine section range from 90281 to 99199 and 99500 to 99607 (excluding the anesthesia code ranges described in the Anesthesia section). The Medicine section includes many and varied subsections, categories, and subcategories. This section can be considered a catchall section in that it includes codes for services and procedures that do not fit into any of the other sections of the CPT manual. Medical specialties, such as ophthalmology, otolaryngology, and allergy, which involve procedures and services that vary greatly from the traditional office encounter, are grouped in the Medicine section rather than the E/M section. Noninvasive diagnostic tests are included in the Medicine section rather than in the Surgery section, which typically includes only invasive procedures.

Conventions of the CPT Main Text

Conventions (Figure19-2) are special symbols used to provide additional information about certain codes. Examples of conventions include triangular and round symbols, which indicate that a code or description was revised, removed, or added. A plus sign (+) indicates an **add-on code**. Codes with a plus sign are additional codes that must be used with certain Category I codes. For example, one of the codes in the Surgery section, Integumentary subsection, is +15401. Code 15401 describes "each additional 100 sq. cm...." Just above code 15401 is code 15400, which describes a "xenograft of the skin… the first 100 sq. cm. or less…" If the medical documentation states that a "200 sq. cm. xenograft of the skin" was performed, the medical assistant would code the first 100 sq. cm. using code 15400, and the second 100 sq. cm. by using add-on code 15401 (+15401).

Another example of a symbol convention is a circle with a small round dot in the center. This symbol indicates that conscious sedation, rather than a general anesthetic, was used during a surgical procedure.

In most CPT manuals, the legend explaining the meanings of the convention symbols is found at the bottom of each page of the Tabular Index.

⊘ **Modifier -51 exempt.** This symbol is used to specify when a code is exempt from use of the modifier -51. Modifier -51 allows coders to specify that one procedure was performed multiple times. Normally, in the instance when the same procedure has been performed more than once, reporting of modifier -51 would be required to indicate that the same procedure (with the same definition and code) was performed two or more times; however, when this symbol appears in front of the code, the code description already indicates the procedure was performed more than once, and therefore modifier -51 is not required.

✚ **Add-on code.** An add-on code is used when more than one code must be used to completely describe a specific procedure or service. Some medical procedures are commonly carried out at the same time a primary procedure is being performed and are described as procedures performed by the same physician to include an additional treatment or procedure done at the same time or in conjunction with the main procedure being performed. Add-on codes can be readily identified by specific words used in the code description, such as additional digit(s), lesions(s), neurorrhaphy, etc. Add-on codes are always used in addition to the primary service or procedure and must never be reported as a stand-alone code.

• **New code.** In healthcare, scientific research results in new emerging technology procedures and services. Once a new procedure or service is approved for use or judged to be effective, a temporary **Category III** code is assigned. If the procedure or service is then adopted, and statistics bear out the integration of the new procedure with the more mainstream or traditional codes, then a permanent CPT-4 code is assigned, and the code is added to the main text of the CPT-4 manual.

▲ **Revised code.** In addition to the new codes added to the CPT-4 each year, many code descriptions are revised as well. The change may be only to clarify or improve the wording of the description, or, as is the case in most instances, it may be revised to add or remove terminology or information.

▶◀ **New or revised text.** Text within the guidelines is often revised to add or remove information, correct grammar, or further clarify the content.

⊙ **Conscious sedation.** This is a new convention, added in 2005, to describe CPT-4 codes that include conscious sedation use. Codes with this convention do not require the use of separate Conscious Sedation codes from the Medicine Section of the CPT-4.

✗ **FDA approval pending.** A symbol indicating that a CPT-4 category I code has been assigned to a vaccine product in anticipation of approval for use from the Food and Drug Administration (FDA).

FIGURE 19-2 *CPT Main Text conventions.*

Guidelines

Guidelines, which are found at the beginning of each section and some subsections of the CPT manual , add definitions and descriptions necessary to appropriately interpret and report the procedures and services in that section or subsection. For example, in the Medicine section, specific instructions are provided for handling unlisted services or procedures, special reports, and supplies and materials provided to the insurance company or the patient (Figure 19-3). Guidelines are written to assist in understanding when and under what circumstances codes may be used. It is important to thoroughly read and understand the guidelines provided throughout the Main Text. This is especially important when first learning to code, or working in a section of the CPT that is rarely used. It is also important to reread the guidelines after the CPT annual revisions, additions, and deletions, are effective January of each year. Selecting a code without reading the guidelines will usually lead to selection of the wrong code. Not only will this result in the potential for delayed or denied reimbursement, but continued inappropriate code selection can be considered fraud or abuse and can result in serious civil or criminal penalties.

Notes

Notes are typically found only in the category, subcategory, or code description area of the CPT. They apply only to the designated group of codes following the note and (unlike guidelines) not to the whole

---

99000—99116 Medicine

Miscellaneous Services

99000 Handling and/or conveyance of specimen for transfer from the physician's office to a laboratory

99001 Handling and/or conveyance of specimen for transfer from the patient in other than a physician's office to a laboratory (distance may be indicated)

99002 Handling, conveyance, and/or any other service in connection with the implementation of an order involving devices (e.g., designing, fitting, packaging, handling, delivery or mailing) when devices such as orthotics, protectives, prosthetics are fabricated by an outside laboratory or shop but which items have been designed, and are to be fitted and adjusted by the attending physician

(For routine collection of venous blood, use 36415)

99024 Postoperative follow-up visit, normally included in the surgical package, to indicate that an evaluation and management service was performed during a postoperative period for a reason(s) related to the original procedure

(As a component of a surgical "package," see **Surgery Guidelines**)

(99025 has been deleted)

FIGURE 19-3 Example of Miscellaneous Services in the Medicine section.

section. As do guidelines, notes provide additional information to assist in the selection of specific codes.

Unlisted Procedure or Service Code

Occasionally, even with the best documentation and the coder's best efforts, an accurate, specific code to match the procedure or service performed cannot be found in the CPT manual . In each section (and sometimes in subsections, categories, and/or subcategories), nonspecific codes have been provided. These codes are called Unlisted Procedures and Services. For example, code 29999 is found in the Surgery section, Musculoskeletal subsection. It describes an "unlisted procedure, arthroscopy." Unlisted codes can be used only when no Category I or Category III code provides an exact match to the medical documentation. When an unlisted code is used, a Special Report must be sent with the insurance claim that describes the procedure or service thoroughly.

Special Reports

When bills are submitted for services rendered or procedures performed, most insurance carriers or third-party payers require no additional information on the insurance claim form other than the procedure or service CPT code. When a bill is submitted for a service that is unlisted, unusual, or newly adopted, the third-party carrier requires a special report so that the company can determine whether provision of that service or procedure was medically appropriate.

Appendixes

The following appendixes are found in the CPT manual.

- Appendix A: *Modifiers:* Lists all the two-digit numeric or alphanumeric codes used to increase specificity and provide additional information about certain procedures and services.
- Appendix B: *Summary of Additions, Deletions, and Revisions:* For easy reference, at each annual update of the CPT, this appendix lists all changes made from the previous year.
- Appendix C: *Clinical Examples:* Provides helpful narrative examples that aid selection of the correct and most specific level of E/M codes.
- Appendix D: *Summary of CPT Add-on Codes:* Lists codes needed when more than one code is required to fully describe the service or procedure rendered or to identify a procedure performed concurrently with another procedure.
- Appendix E: *Summary of CPT Codes Exempt from Modifier -51:* Lists all procedures and services exempt from the use of modifier -51. Modifier -51 (99051) is the multiple procedures modifier. When multiple procedures are performed at the same session by the same provider, the primary procedure is reported, and the additional procedure or service is identified by appending modifier -51 to the procedure or service code. This is done only when the primary procedure code does not include the additional procedure in its description.
- Appendix F: *Summary of CPT Codes Exempt from Modifier -63:* Lists all procedures exempt from the use of modifier -63. Modifier -63 is used to report procedures performed on infants weighing less than 4 kg to identify the increased complexity common with these patients. Category I codes that state specifically "Exempt from modifier -63" do not require use of this modifier.

- Appendix G: *Summary of CPT Codes that Include Moderate (Conscious) Sedation:* Lists all procedure codes that include conscious sedation as part of the code description; this eliminates the need to code the sedation separately.
- Appendix H: *Alphabetic Index of Performance Measures by Clinical Condition or Topic:* Lists Category II codes used by providers tracking and measuring performance and outcomes.
- Appendix I: *Genetic Testing Code Modifiers:* Lists all modifiers, and their descriptions, unique to genetic testing.
- Appendix J: *Electrodiagnostic Medicine Listing of Sensory, Motor, and Mixed Nerves:* Lists each sensory, motor, and mixed nerve conduction study code. This appendix aids the accurate use of codes 95900, 95903, and 95904.
- Appendix K: *Product Pending FDA Approval:* Lists vaccine products for which FDA approval is pending and those that have been assigned Category I codes before approval.
- Appendix L: *Vascular Families:* Lists the elements of the vascular system, grouped by families, beginning at the aorta and ending at the termination point of each vessel. This appendix is designed to assist coding for the Cardiology subsection of the Surgery and Medicine sections.
- Appendix M: *Deleted CPT Codes:* Provides a summary of **crosswalked**, deleted and renumbered codes and descriptors.
- Appendix N: *Summary of Resequenced CPT Codes:* Provides a summary of CPT codes that do not appear in numeric sequence in the listing of CPT codes. Resequencing allows existing codes to be relocated to an appropriate location for the code concept, regardless of the numeric sequence.

BEGINNING THE CODING PROCESS

Medical Documentation

The steps for using the CPT manual actually begin not in the CPT coding manual but in the medical documentation. Information pertinent to code selection is taken from a variety of medical documents. Sources of information include the following:

- Encounter form (also called a *superbill, fee slip,* or *charge ticket*)
- History and physical report (H&P)
- Discharge summary
- Operative report
- Pathology report
- Radiology report

These documents were discussed in earlier chapters, and examples were given. Although these same forms are used for CPT coding, the information abstracted is different (as shown later in the chapter). As in ICD-9-CM coding, when the medical documentation is compared against any code description, all the elements of that code must substantially match, with nothing added or missing.

Many providers have CPT and ICD-9-CM codes preprinted on their encounter forms or charge tickets. However, it is important also to review the medical record carefully and compile an abstract of all the procedures and services rendered during an encounter. For example, on the encounter form, a provider checks off the procedure for a esophagogastroduodenoscopy (EGD); however, when the medical assistant reviews the medical record, he discovers that the operative report states that an EGD with biopsy was performed.

If the medical assistant had not reviewed the medical record, a code with a lower reimbursement amount for the procedure would have been submitted to the insurance carrier, and the provider would have lost revenue. Update encounter forms annually to ensure that code additions, changes, and revisions appear on the preprinted forms.

The coding steps and process outlined in this chapter, including use of the Alphabetic Index and the Main Text of the CPT, apply to all sections of the CPT manual. Some special considerations and differences apply to the E/M and Anesthesia sections.

The basic steps in medical coding are to (1) read, analyze, and abstract the procedure or service documented in the medical record and (2) compare it with the encounter form, operative report, or other documentation to ensure that all services and procedures have been recorded. The term **abstract**, used as a verb in this context, means to create an outline or summary of information from a text or record.

In procedural coding, an abstract is created to find all the procedures and services performed during a patient encounter and also to ensure that nothing has been omitted from or added to the encounter form or charge ticket that is not documented in the medical record. The abstracted data are then broken down into main terms and modifying terms. A **main term** is usually the primary procedure or service performed, and a **modifying term** further defines or adds information to the main term. Next, the main and modifying terms are used to find the code or code ranges in the Alphabetic Index. Last, the code selected is confirmed by reviewing the guidelines, notes, and conventions in the Main Text to verify that the most accurate code has been chosen.

USING THE ALPHABETIC INDEX

The Alphabetic Index is a comprehensive, alphabetic listing of all procedures and services in the CPT manual. Medical assistants must keep in mind the most important fact about the Alphabetic Index: it should be used only as an aid to finding the area in the Main Text to evaluate for selecting the proper code. The Alphabetic Index is not a substitute for the Main Text. Even if only one code is assigned, the Main Text must be used to ensure that the code selection is accurate.

The Alphabetic Index is used as a guide to search for one or more codes or code ranges. The index is similar to that found in any textbook; it is an alphabetic list of main and modifying terms found in the Main Text of the coding manual. In a typical index, the term or concept listed in the index is followed by a reference page or pages, where detailed information is presented in the body of the book. The Alphabetic Index in the CPT is used in the same way, except that it references codes or code ranges rather than pages. As discussed earlier, the Main Text is divided into sections, and the procedures and services are listed in numeric order by the Category I code.

The Alphabetic Index is organized by main terms that can stand alone. The CPT code set has been developed as stand-alone descriptions of medical procedures. Some of the procedures in the CPT are not printed in their entirety but refer back to a common portion of the procedure listed in a preceding entry. This is evident when an entry is followed by one or more indentations. This is the part before the semicolon (;) in the description. Do not confuse the two-digit modifiers discussed earlier in the chapter with modifying terms. *Modifiers* are numeric supplements to a Category I code, whereas *modifying terms* are words that add to or modify the meaning of the main term.

Modifying terms are indented two spaces below the main term. They further describe or add information or a definition needed to narrow the search for an appropriate procedure or service code. A main term might be a procedure, such as an excision, and each modifying term could provide further information about the anatomic location or the organ excised, the type of instrument used, or a special technique, or whether other procedures were performed at the same time as the excision, such as obtaining biopsy tissue for examination. Modifying terms affect the selection of appropriate codes; therefore, it is important to review the list of modifying terms when selecting a code or code range.

Consider the examples presented in Table 19-3. If the medical documentation contains the narrative description of a procedure as a "diagnostic cystoscopy," the main term is *Cystoscopy;* the modifying term is *diagnostic,* because it describes the type of cystoscopy performed. Another example is "esophagogastroscopy with biopsy and fulguration of lesions." In this example, the main term is *Gastroscopy* (the procedure performed), and the modifying terms are *esophago-* (which adds another anatomic site scoped at the same time as the gastroscopy); *with biopsy* and *fulguration* (two additional procedures performed during the gastroscopy); and *lesions* (describes the object of the biopsy and fulguration).

Two rules should be followed when coding any procedure or service:

- Be as specific as possible in code selection and use all pertinent words in the description given in your documentation.

- Never add any words, modifying terms, or descriptors to the procedure or service code description that change the definition of the procedure or service or that are not documented.

Once the medical documentation has been abstracted to determine the procedures and services performed and the main and modifying term or terms have been identified, the next step is to look for the terms in the Alphabetic Index. Use the Alphabetic Index to search for one or more codes or a code range that best describes the procedure or service documented in the medical record. Using the code or codes found in the Alphabetic Index search, locate each in the appropriate section, subsection, category, or subcategory of the Main Text and select the most specific code that best matches the medical record documentation.

Searching the Alphabetic Index

Begin the search by using one or all of the four primary classifications (or types) of main and modifying term entries:

- Procedure or service (e.g., examination, excision, scope, revision, repair, drainage)
- Organ or anatomic site (e.g., clavicle, mandible, humerus, liver, colon, uterus)
- Condition, illness, or injury (e.g., cholelithiasis, ulcer, fracture, pregnancy, fever)
- Eponym, synonym, abbreviation, or **acronym** (e.g., MRI [magnetic resonance imaging], Naffziger operation, Mosenthal test, GERD [gastroesophageal reflux disease])

As described previously, the CPT manual is divided into six sections (i.e., E/M, Anesthesia, Surgery, Radiology, Pathology and Laboratory, and Medicine). The sections may first list the procedure (e.g., excision, incision, repair), the organ or anatomic site (e.g., clavicle, liver), or a condition (e.g., a fracture or laceration).

TABLE 19-3 Identification of Main and Modifying Terms in the Alphabetic Index

CODE	MAIN TERM(S)	MODIFYING TERMS			
		FIRST	SECOND	THIRD	FOURTH
	Cystoscopy	Diagnostic			
	Gastroscopy	Esophago-	With biopsy	With fulguration	Of lesions
492000	**Cyst**	Abdomen			
		Ankle			
		Bartholin's gland			
		Bile duct			
21030	**Excision**	Cheekbone			
23140		**Clavicle**			
23146				**With allograft**	
23147				With autograft	
27355-27758			Femur		
Cyst excision: 49200					
Cyst excision of clavicle: 23140					
Cyst excision of clavicle with allograft: 23146					

TABLE 19-4 Comparing Codes in the Range 52234 to 52250

| CODE | MAIN TERM(S) | MODIFYING TERM | | | |
		FIRST	SECOND	THIRD	FOURTH
52234	Cystourethroscopy	Treatment or fulgurations	Of a lesion or lesions	Using either cryosurgery or laser surgery	With or without a biopsy
52235/52240	Same	Same	Same except for size of lesions	Same	Same
52204	Cystourethroscopy	with biopsy			
52214	Cystourethroscopy	with fulguration	Of bladder, urethra or glands		
52224	Cystourethroscopy	with fulguration	No mention of specific urinary system structure or organ		

Use the name of the performed procedure or service (anastomosis, splint, repair, stress test, therapy, vaccination); the organ or other anatomic site of the procedure (tibia, colon, salivary gland, aorta); the condition, illness, or injury (abscess, fracture, cholelithiasis, strabismus); or, if applicable, synonyms, **eponyms**, or abbreviations (ECG [electrocardiography], Stookey-Scarff procedure, Mohs' micrographic surgery).

Using *See* and *See Also* in the Alphabetic Index

The *see* statement in the Alphabetic Index points to another location in the Alphabetic Index to find the code or code range. The *see also* statement points to additional codes or code ranges in the Alphabetic Index that may be useful to the code found in the original search.

Use of the Semicolon

A semicolon at the end of a main description indicates that modifying terms and descriptions follow. Every indented description below a stand-alone code is related to that stand-alone code. If a main term has no additional modifying terms, the next entry is a stand-alone description of a different procedure, which is positioned flush left, without indentation.

Stand-Alone Codes and Code Ranges

In the Alphabetic Index, a procedure or service may list a single code, called a *stand-alone code,* or a range of possible codes that may match the medical documentation. Remember that the Alphabetic Index is an index; it is designed as a guide to the most suitable codes that match the documentation. It does not provide specificity; that is the purpose of the Main Text. At this point, the search is only for the closest match or matches to the medical documentation.

Because some medical procedures and diagnostic tests can be quite complex, there may be a single (stand-alone) code or a code range that may include one main term but several variations (or modifying terms) of the main procedure or service. For example, the code for *Craterization, phalanges, toe* is 28124, a stand-alone code. However, using the same main term, *Craterization,* but adding *any of the phalanges* (toes or fingers) yields a range of codes: 26235-29236. The code range is shown with a hyphen to indicate that all codes within that range could be appropriate.

In some cases a stand-alone code and a range of codes are listed for the same service or procedure. For example, *Craterization, femur,* lists both the stand-alone code 27360 and the code range 27070-27071. Once a stand-alone code or code range has been found in the Alphabetic Index, the next step is to look up each of those in the Main Text and select the code or codes that most closely match the medical documentation (Table 19-4).

Steps for Using the Alphabetic Index

1. Abstract the procedures and/or services performed from the medical documentation.
2. Determine the main and modifying terms from the abstracted information.
3. Select the most appropriate main term to begin searching in the Alphabetic Index.
4. Once the main term has been located, select one or more modifying terms, if needed, to narrow the search.
5. If no main or modifying term produces an appropriate code or code range, repeat steps 2, 3, and 4 using a different main term.
6. Find the code or code ranges that include all or most of the description of the procedure or service found in the medical record.
7. Disregard any code or code range containing additional descriptions or modifying terms that are not found in the abstracted information or the medical documentation.
8. Write down the code or code ranges that best match the medical documentation.

CRITICAL THINKING APPLICATION   19-1
Sherald is having trouble finding a procedure in the Alphabetic Index. What are some options and alternative ways she can perform an Alphabetic Index search?

USING THE TABULAR INDEX (MAIN TEXT)

Once the code or codes have been selected from the Alphabetic Index, the next stop is the Tabular Index (Main Text), where the final decision is made regarding the choice of code. In the Main Text, the conventions, symbols, guidelines, notes, and even the punctuation all play a part in choosing the most accurate code possible.

In the Main Text, look up each code or code range found in the Alphabetic Index. Read the description of the code thoroughly to ensure that the main elements abstracted from the medical documentation are all included in the code description, with nothing substantial omitted or added. Read the section guidelines and notes to determine whether additional codes should be used, add-on codes or modifiers are required, or use of the code is contraindicated.

Steps for Using the Main Text (Tabular Index)

Except for the special considerations required for coding from the Evaluation and Management (E/M) and Anesthesia sections, the following steps apply to all sections of the CPT manual (Procedure 19-1). The numbering of these steps is continuous with the numbering of the steps for the Alphabetic Index search.

9. Turn to the Main Text and find the first code or code range noted from the Alphabetic Index search.
10. Compare the description of the code with the medical documentation. Verify that all or most of the medical record documentation matches the code description and that there is no additional element or information in the code description that is not found in the documentation.

11. Read the guidelines and notes for the section, subsection, and code to ensure that there are no contraindications to the use of the code.
12. Evaluate the conventions, especially add-on codes (+) and exemption from modifier -51.
13. Determine whether any special circumstances require the use of a modifier.
14. Determine whether a Special Report is required.
15. Record the CPT code selected in the medical record documentation next to the procedure or service performed and in the appropriate block of the insurance claim form.

Coding Decision Tree

A series of questions, sometimes called a *decision tree,* can assist the medical assistant in navigating the Alphabetic Index and Main Text of the CPT. The decision tree for the Main Text is designed to guide the selection of the appropriate CPT Category I code or code range (Figure 19-4). (Visit the Evolve site at *evolve.elsevier.com/kinn* for an example of how to use the decision tree.)

Abstracting the procedure and service information from the patient's medical record or the encounter form is only the first step in the coding decision process. Procedure 19-1 illustrates the steps for using the Alphabetic Index and Main Text to guide the medical

---

PROCEDURE 19-1

Perform Procedural Coding: CPT Coding

CAAHEP COMPETENCIES: IV.C.IV.6., IV.P.IV.3., V.P.V.6., VII.P.VII.1., IX.A.IX.2.

ABHES COMPETENCIES: 3.v

GOAL: *Use the steps for procedure and service coding to find the most accurate and specific CPT Category I code.*

EQUIPMENT and SUPPLIES

- CPT coding manual (current year)
- Encounter form (charge ticket)
- Medical record
- Paper
- Pen or pencil
- Medical dictionary or medical terminology reference book

PROCEDURAL STEPS

1. Abstract the procedures and/or services performed from the medical documentation.
   PURPOSE: To ensure that all procedures and/or services are listed on the encounter form; that all procedures and services on the encounter form match the medical record; and that nothing documented in the medical record is missing from the encounter form.
2. Select the most appropriate main term to begin the search in the Alphabetic Index.
   PURPOSE: To have a starting point for the Alphabetic Index search.
3. Determine the main and modifying terms from the abstracted information.
   PURPOSE: To identify the term or terms to begin the search in the Alphabetic Index.

4. Once the main term has been located, select modifying term or terms if needed.
   PURPOSE: To provide additional specificity and help narrow the search for the code or code range in the Alphabetic Index.
5. If no modifying term produces an appropriate code or code range, repeat steps 2 and 3 using a different main term classification.
   PURPOSE: To aid in finding the most appropriate code or code range by using alternative methods of searching the Alphabetic Index.
6. Find code or code ranges that include all or most of the medical record procedure or service description.
   PURPOSE: To assist in directing the medical assistant to the proper section, subsection, category or subcategory of the Main Text of the CPT.
7. Disregard any code or code range containing additional descriptions or modifying terms not found in the medical record.
   PURPOSE: To prevent upcoding or downcoding errors and other compliance issues.
8. Write down the code or code ranges that best match medical documentation.
   PURPOSE: To prevent repeated reference to the Alphabetic Index by recording all possible matches to the code or code range being sought. This saves time and prevents redundant effort.

9. Turn to the Main Text and find the first code or code range found while searching the Alphabetic Index.
   <u>PURPOSE:</u> To begin the process of finding the most specific and accurate code.
10. Compare the description of the code with the medical documentation. Verify that all or most of the medical record documentation matches the code description and that there is no additional element or information in the code description that is not found in the documentation.
    <u>PURPOSE:</u> To avoid upcoding and downcoding errors and to ensure there are no contraindications to use of the code selected.
11. Read the guidelines and notes for the section, subsection, and code to ensure that there are no contraindications to the use of the code.
    <u>PURPOSE:</u> To ensure there are no instructions that would prevent the use of the code selected.
12. Evaluate the conventions, especially add-on codes (+) and exemption from modifier -51.

<u>PURPOSE:</u> To ensure there are no instructions that would prevent the use of the code selected.
13. Determine whether special circumstances require the use of a modifier.
    <u>PURPOSE:</u> To select, if appropriate, modifiers that provide additional information for the chosen code to explain certain circumstances or provide additional detail.
14. Determine whether a Special Report is required
    <u>PURPOSE:</u> To clarify and add additional detail when an unusual or extenuating circumstance exists or if a Category III or unlisted procedure Category I code is used.
15. Record the CPT code selected in the medical record documentation next to the procedure or service performed and in the appropriate block of the insurance claim form.
    <u>PURPOSE:</u> To complete the documentation and recording requirements.

---

assistant to the selection of the most specific and accurate procedure or service code from the CPT coding manual.

> **CRITICAL THINKING APPLICATION   19-2**
>
> If a patient were referred for epigastric pain and Dr. Shuman performed an ultrasound examination of the gallbladder, what would Sherald need to consider to properly code this encounter for the ultrasound examination?

SURGERY CODING

The steps for performing Surgery coding were outlined earlier in this chapter and are detailed in Procedure 19-1. Some guidelines and notes related to surgery coding must be considered when researching and selecting a procedure or service code. Always review the current year's guidelines for the Surgery section for the most up-to-date information. The following sections discuss a few of the more common guidelines. When coding procedures and services, be sure to read the guidelines and notes thoroughly; they always provide all the answers needed when determining the most accurate code.

General

Surgical Package Definition

The CPT code descriptions of surgical procedures typically include the following services:

- Local infiltration, digital block, and/or topical anesthesia
- Subsequent to the decision for surgery, one related E/M encounter on the day of, or the day before, the date of the procedure
- Immediate postoperative care, including documentation in the patient's medical record and talking with family and/or other physicians
- Writing orders for postsurgical care

- Evaluating the patient in the postanesthesia recovery area
- Typical postoperative follow-up care (see the list below for follow-up care)
- Typical postoperative follow-up care (includes care for approximately 6-8 weeks after surgery and usually done at the physician's office)

Integumentary System

Excision of Lesions—Benign or Malignant

Excision of benign lesions includes a simple closure and anesthesia. If an incision, excision, or trauma requires intermediate or complex closure, the repair by intermediate or complex closure is coded and reported separately.

Repair (Closure)

- *Simple repair:* Performed when the wound is superficial (epidermis, dermis, or subcutaneous) without significant involvement of deeper structures. This includes local anesthesia and chemical or electrocauterization of wounds not closed.
- *Intermediate repair:* Includes simple repair with a need for a layered closure of one or more of the deeper layers of subcutaneous tissue and superficial fascia in addition to the skin closure. Single-layer closure of heavily contaminated wounds that required extensive cleaning or removal of particulate matter also constitutes intermediate repair.
- *Complex repair:* Includes wounds that require more than layered closure (e.g., scar revision, extensive undermining, or stents or retention sutures). Necessary preparation includes creation of a limited defect for repairs or debridement of complicated lacerations or avulsions. Complex repair does not include excision of benign or malignant lesions, excisional preparation of a wound bed, or debridement of an open fracture or open dislocation.

Instructions for Listing Services for Wound Repair

- The repaired wound or wounds should be measured and recorded in centimeters whether curved, angular, or stellate.

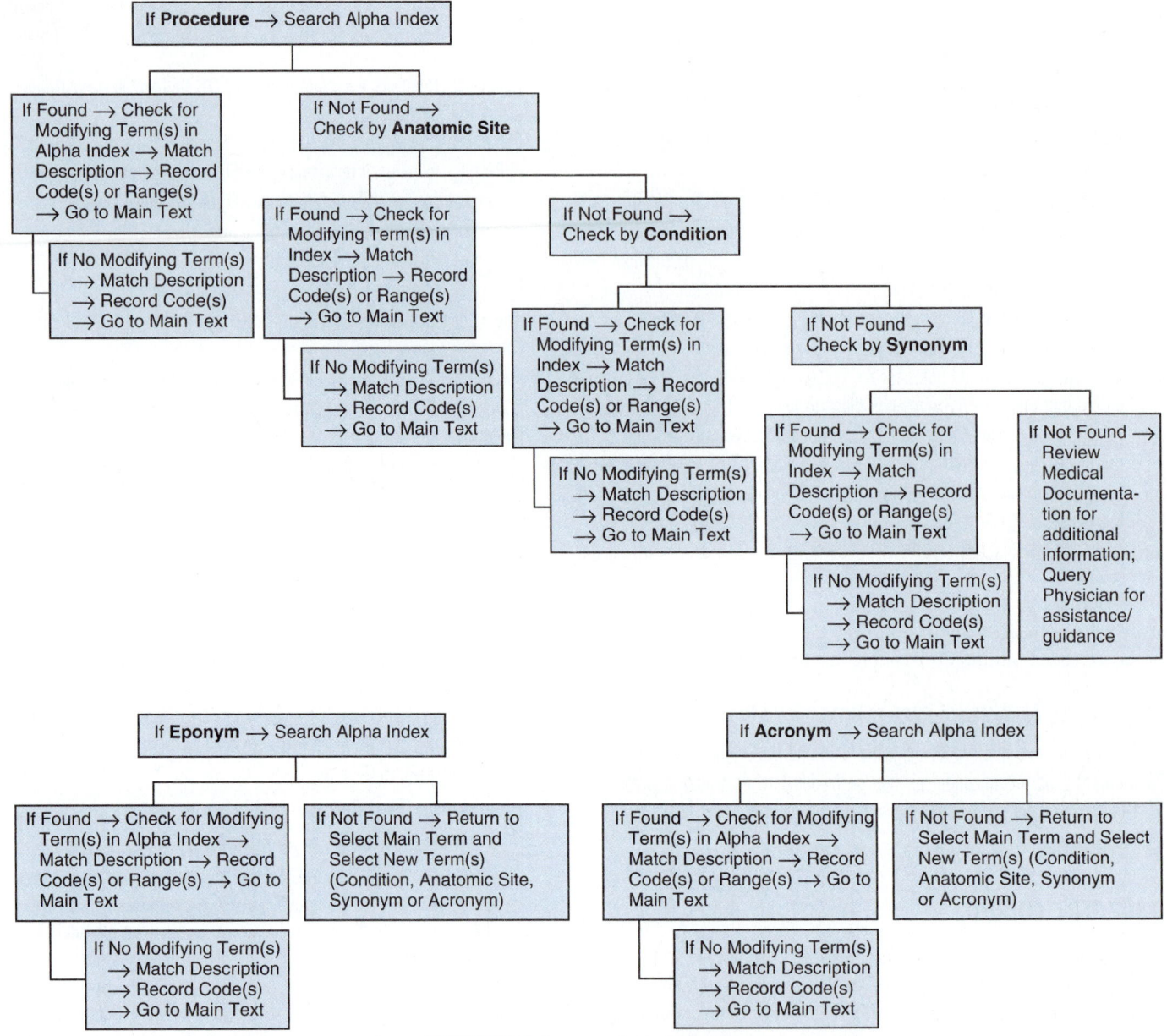

FIGURE 19-4 Decision tree for the CPT Main Text.

- When multiple wounds are repaired, add together the lengths of those in the same classification (simple, intermediate, or complex) and from all anatomic sites that are grouped together into the same code descriptor. Do not add lengths of repairs from different groupings of anatomic sites (e.g., face and extremities, or of different classifications (intermediate and complex).
- When wounds of more than one classification are repaired, list the more complicated repair as the primary procedure and the less complicated repair as the secondary procedure, using modifier -59.
- Debridement is considered a separate procedure only when gross contamination requires prolonged cleansing, when large amounts of dead or contaminated tissue must be removed, or when debridement is carried out separately without immediate primary closure.

- Wound repair that involves nerves, blood vessels, and/or tendons should be reported under the appropriate system for repair of those structures. The repair of these associated wounds is included in the primary procedure unless it qualifies as a complex repair, in which case modifier -59 applies.

Musculoskeletal System

Fractures

- *Closed fracture:* The fractured bone does not protrude through the dermis or epidermis.
- *Open fracture:* The fractured bone cuts through the skin layers and can be directly visualized.
- *Closed treatment:* The fracture site is not surgically opened (exposed to the external environment and directly visualized). The three methods of closed treatment of fractures are (1) without

manipulation, (2) with manipulation, and (3) with or without traction.

- *Manipulation:* Attempted reduction or restoration of a fracture or dislocated joint into its normal anatomic alignment by manually applied forces.
- *Open treatment:* Used when (1) the fractured bone is surgically opened or (2) an opening is made remote from the fracture site to insert an intramedullary nail across the fracture site.
- *Percutaneous skeletal fixation:* Fracture treatment that is neither open nor closed. The fracture fragments are not visualized, but a fixation device (e.g., pins) is placed across the fracture site, usually under x-ray imaging.

Cardiovascular System

Grafting for Coronary Bypass

Venous Grafts

- Venous grafting codes cannot be used as stand-alone codes if arterial grafts are also used during the performance of a bypass graft.
- Procurement of the saphenous vein graft is included in most venous grafting codes and should not be reported as a separate service.
- Procurement of upper extremity or femoropopliteal veins uses the harvesting code, which should be reported in addition to the bypass procedure.

Arterial Grafts

- To report combined arterial-venous grafts, two codes must be used: the arterial graft code and the appropriate combined arterial-venous graft code.
- Procurement of the artery for grafting is included in most venous grafting codes and should not be reported as a separate service, with the following exception: an additional code should be reported for an upper extremity artery or vein or a femoropopliteal vein.

Maternity Care and Delivery

The services normally provided in uncomplicated maternity cases include antepartum care, delivery, and postpartum care.

- *Antepartum care* includes the initial and subsequent history; physical examinations; recording of weight, blood pressure, and fetal heart tones; routine chemical urinalysis; monthly visits up to 28 weeks' gestation; biweekly visits to 36 weeks' gestation; and weekly visits until delivery. Any other visits or services provided within this period should be coded separately.
- *Delivery* includes admission to the hospital, the admission history and physical examination, management of uncomplicated labor, vaginal delivery (with or without forceps or episiotomy), or cesarean delivery. Medical problems complicating labor and delivery should be identified by using the codes in the Medicine and E/M sections in addition to codes for maternity care.
- *Postpartum care* includes hospital and office visits after vaginal or cesarean section delivery.

UNDERSTANDING EVALUATION AND MANAGEMENT

To properly code E/M services, the medical assistant must understand important differences, or variations, from the basic steps outlined earlier. The steps for finding a Category I code for E/M services are quite different from those discussed earlier in this chapter (Procedure 19-2). The instructions include identifying the section, subsection, category, and subcategory of the procedure or service; reviewing the reporting instructions and guidelines for the code chosen; reviewing the level of E/M service; determining the extent of history obtained and examination performed; and determining the complexity of medical decision making.

The E/M section is divided into broad subsections (Figure 19-5), such as *office visit, emergency room visit, hospital visit,* and *consultation.* These subsections are further divided into subcategories, which include the place where the services were rendered (e.g., the provider's office, a hospital emergency department, a skilled nursing facility, or the patient's home) and the **patient status (PS)** (i.e., whether the patient is new or established).

The first two steps in choosing an E/M code are:
1. Identify the place of service (POS)
2. Identify the patient status

Identifying the Place of Service

The "place of service" is the facility where the encounter between the patient and the provider occurred. The two most common places of service are "office" and "hospital." Refer to the Evolve site at *evolve.elsevier.com/kinn* for a complete list of POS locations and their two-digit identifying numbers, or **place of service (POS) codes**.

Identifying the Patient Status

The patient status choices are *new* or *established* patient. A **new patient (NP)** is one who has not received any professional services (face to face) from the physician or another physician of the exact same specialty and subspecialty, who belongs to the same group practice, within the past 3 years. An **established patient (EP)** is one who has received professional services from the physician or another physician of the exact same specialty and subspecialty, who belongs to the same group practice, within the past 3 years.

Once the POS and patient status have been established, the next step in selection of an E/M code is to determine the level of service provided.

Determining the Level of Service Provided

Key Components and Contributing Factors

The three key components for determining the level of service for E/M coding are: history, examination, and medical decision making. The four contributing factors are: counseling, nature of presenting problem, coordination of care, and time. The history, examination, and medical decision making components are considered primary key; that is, they are typically the three most important components for deciding the level of service. Counseling, nature of presenting problem, coordination of care, and time are secondary considerations.

History. To understand the levels of the history, it is important to know the definition and components of the patient history. The history relates to the patient's clinical picture and depends on the patient for answers to specific questions. The patient history is discussed in greater detail in Chapter 14 and later in Chapter 28.

Perform Procedural Coding: Evaluation and Management Coding

CAAHEP COMPETENCIES: IV.C.IV.6., IV.P.IV.3., V.P.V.6., VII.P.VII.1., IX.A.IX.2.

ABHES COMPETENCIES: 3.v

GOAL: *Use the steps for Evaluation and Management coding to find the most accurate and specific CPT Category I E/M section code.*

EQUIPMENT and SUPPLIES

- CPT coding manual (current year)
- Encounter form (charge ticket)
- Medical record
- Paper
- Pen or pencil
- Medical dictionary or medical terminology reference book

PROCEDURAL STEPS

1. Determine the place of service.
   PURPOSE: To determine where the procedure or service was performed.
2. Determine the patient status.
   PURPOSE: To determine whether the patient is a new or an established patient.
3. Review the guidelines and notes for the selected subsection, category, or subcategory.
   PURPOSE: To determine whether there are any contraindications for use of the code selected.
4. Identify the subsection, category, or subcategory of service in the E/M section.

PURPOSE: To ensure that the correct place of service and patient status are used and the appropriate level of service is selected.

5. Review the level of E/M service descriptions for each code in the subsection, category, or subcategory chosen.
   PURPOSE: To assist in the selection of the appropriate level of service.
6. Determine the level of service
   a. Determine the extent of the history obtained.
   b. Determine the extent of the examination performed.
   c. Determine the complexity of medical decision making.
   PURPOSE: To ensure that the correct level is chosen for the history, examination, and medical decision making.
7. If necessary, compare the medical documentation against examples in Appendix C, Clinical Examples, of the CPT manual.
   PURPOSE: To compare the medical documentation to the examples in Appendix C for assistance in selection of the appropriate level of service.
8. Select the appropriate level of E/M service code, and document it on the medical record or encounter form.
   PURPOSE: To complete the documentation and reporting requirements.

Levels of History

- *Problem-focused history:* A problem-focused history concentrates on the chief complaint; it looks at the symptoms, severity, and duration of the problem. It usually does not include a review of systems (ROS) or the family and social histories.
- *Expanded problem-focused history:* The physician proceeds as in the problem-focused history but includes a review of the systems that relate to the chief complaint. Usually past, family, and social histories are not included.
- *Detailed history:* The detailed history consists of the chief complaint; extended history of present illness; problem-pertinent system review extended to include a review of a limited number of additional systems; and the pertinent past, family, and/or social histories directly related to the patient's problems.
- *Comprehensive history:* A comprehensive history includes the chief complaint; extended history of present illness; review of systems that is directly related to the problem or problems identified in the history of the present illness plus a review of all additional body systems; and complete past, family, and social histories.

Examination. The examination is the objective part of the patient's visit. The physician examines the patient, obtains measurable findings, and makes notes referring to body areas and/or organ systems, as follows:

- Body areas: Head, including face and neck; chest, including breasts and axillae; abdomen; genitalia, groin, and buttocks; and back, including spine and extremities
- Organs and organ systems: Constitutional (e.g., vital signs, general appearance); eyes; ears, nose, throat, and mouth; cardiovascular; respiratory; gastrointestinal (GI); genitourinary; musculoskeletal; skin; neurologic; psychiatric; and hematologic, lymphatic, and immunologic

Levels of Examination. The examination is divided into the following levels:

- *Problem-focused examination:* The examination is limited to the single body area or single system mentioned in the chief complaint.
- *Expanded problem-focused examination:* In addition to the limited body area or system, related body areas or organ systems are examined.
- *Detailed examination:* An extended examination is performed on the related body areas or organ systems.
- *Comprehensive examination:* A complete multisystem examination is performed or a complete examination of a single organ system.

Medical Decision Making. When a physician makes medical decisions, the decisions are based on many years of education and

►Initial Nursing Facility Care◄

New or Established Patient

When the patient is admitted to the nursing facility in the course of an encounter in another site of service (e.g., hospital emergency department, physician's office), all evaluation and management services provided by that physician in conjunction with that admission are considered part of the initial nursing facility care when performed on the same date as the admission or readmission. The nursing facility care level of service reported by the admitting physician should include the services related to the admission he/she provided in the other sites of service as well as in the nursing facility setting.

Hospital discharge or observation discharge services performed on the same date of nursing facility admission or readmission may be reported separately. For a patient discharged from inpatient status on the same date of nursing facility admission or readmission, the hospital discharge services should be reported with codes 99238, 99239 as appropriate. For a patient discharged from observation status on the same date of nursing facility admission or readmission, the observation care discharge services should be reported with code 99217. For a patient admitted and discharged from observation or inpatient status on the same date, see codes 99234-99236.

(For nursing facility care discharge, see 99315, 99316)

►Typical unit times have not been established for 99304-99306.◄

►(99301-99303 have been deleted)◄

● **99304** Initial nursing facility care, per day, for the evaluation and management of a patient which requires these three key components:

- a detailed or comprehensive history;
- a detailed or comprehensive examination; and
- medical decision making that is straightforward or of low complexity.

Counseling and/or coordination of care with other providers or agencies are provided consistent with the nature of the problem(s) and the patient's and/or family's needs.

Usually, the problem(s) requiring admission are of low severity.

Subsequent Nursing Facility Care

►All levels of subsequent nursing facility care include reviewing the medical record and reviewing the results of diagnostic studies and changes in the patient's status (i.e., changes in history, physical condition, and response to management) since the last assessment by the physician.◄

● **99307** Subsequent nursing facility care, per day, for the evaluation and management of a patient, which requires at least two of these three key components:

- a problem-focused interval history;
- a problem-focused examination;
- straightforward medical decision making.

Counseling and/or coordination of care with other providers or agencies are provided consistent with the nature of the problem(s) and the patient's and/or family's needs.

Usually, the patient is stable, recovering, or improving.

● **99308** Subsequent nursing facility care, per day, for the evaluation and management of a patient, which requires at least two of these three key components:

- an expanded problem-focused interval history;
- an expanded problem-focused examination;
- medical decision making of low complexity.

Counseling and/or coordination of care with other providers or agencies are provided consistent with the nature of the problem(s) and the patient's and/or family's needs.

Usually, the patient is responding inadequately to therapy or has developed a minor complication.

● **99309** Subsequent nursing facility care, per day, for the evaluation and management of a patient, which requires at least two of these three key components:

- a detailed interval history;
- a detailed examination;
- medical decision making of moderate complexity.

Counseling and/or coordination of care with other providers or agencies are provided consistent with the nature of the problem(s) and the patient's and/or family's needs.

Usually, the patient has developed a significant complication or a significant new problem.

FIGURE 19-5 Example of Evaluation and Management (E/M) coding: new or established patient and place of service.

experience. Three elements comprise the medical decision making process:

1. The number of diagnoses and/or management options
2. The amount and/or complexity of data obtained, reviewed, and analyzed
3. The risk of significant complications and/or morbidity and/or mortality

Number of Diagnoses and Management Options. The physician's notes during the history and examination should help identify whether the patient's problem is minor, acute, stable, or worsening. The medical documentation should also identify whether a new problem exists or whether the physician plans to order any diagnostic tests to further investigate the patient's illness or injury.

Amount and Complexity of Data Reviewed. The medical documentation should also identify what laboratory tests, x-ray diagnostic procedures, and other tests have been ordered or reviewed.

Risk of Complications and Morbidity or Mortality. Risk is often involved in medical care, either from the treatment given to the patient or from the lack of treatment and professional care. *Morbidity,* the relative incidence of disease, and *mortality,* which relates to the number of deaths from a given disease, is an integral part of the assessment of risks made by the physician.

Medical Decision Making Complexity Levels. The four levels of complexity in medical decision making are: straightforward, low complexity, moderate complexity, and high complexity (Table 19-5).

Contributing Factors

Counseling. Counseling is a discussion with a patient and/or family regarding diagnostic results, impressions, recommended diagnostic studies, prognosis, risks and benefits of management or treatment options, and instructions for management, treatment, and/or follow-up. Almost all E/M services contain a degree of counseling with the patient and/or the family. This is factored into the E/M code, and as long as this factor does not exceed 50% of the time spent with the patient, it is included in the E/M code. It can be considered a contributing factor when the counseling exceeds 50% of the encounter.

Nature of Presenting Problem. The presenting problem is usually explained in the chief complaint. It can range from something as simple as a cold in an otherwise healthy patient to a life-threatening problem. Unless dealing with the nature of the presenting problem exceeds half of the patient encounter, it is included in the E/M code description and is not a factor in selecting the level of service.

Coordination of Care. Some patients need assistance in arranging for care beyond the visit or hospitalization. Some will need care in

a skilled nursing facility or home health care. Others will need hospice care. The primary physician usually coordinates this care. Coordination of care is also factored into the E/M code and is a consideration for determining the level of service only when it exceeds 50% of the patient encounter.

Time. Time is included in the E/M code descriptions only to assist physicians in selecting the most appropriate level of E/M service. The times expressed in the code descriptions are averages, and time is not a determining factor in code selection unless counseling exceeds more than 50% of the encounter. Only then can time be used as a determining component to code level selection.

At first, E/M coding is difficult to understand and put into practice. The steps for E/M coding provided here can serve as a guide to medical assistants in determining the place of service, patient status, and level of care provided, so that they can select the most accurate E/M code. Using the clinical examples in Appendix C of the CPT manual and comparing them to the medical documentation also can help medical assistants acquire a better understanding of E/M coding.

> **CRITICAL THINKING APPLICATION   19-3**
> Dr. Caddell performed a colonoscopy at the hospital on Cecil Matthews, who has been Dr. Caddell's patient for several years. Mr. Matthews came to the office with left lower quadrant pain and a history of colon cancer. What other factors or information would Sherald need to know to properly code Mr. Matthews' office visit (encounter)? What other factors or information would Sherald need to know to properly code Mr. Matthews' colonoscopy?

ANESTHESIA CODING

The codes for anesthesia are listed primarily in the Anesthesia section of the CPT manual, although codes for conscious sedation are found in the Medicine section. The codes selected are based typically on the anatomic location of the surgery performed; for example, code 00402 is used for anesthesia during a reconstructive procedure on the breast in the integumentary system.

Anesthesia coding differs from any other form of coding in the way anesthesia services are billed (Procedure 19-3). A standard formula has been established for payment of anesthesia services: Basic unit values + Time units + Modifying units (B + T + M). This formula is affected by two factors: the patient's **physical status** (PS) and any qualifying circumstances.

TABLE 19-5 Complexity of Medical Decision Making

NUMBER OF DIAGNOSES OR MANAGEMENT OPTIONS	AMOUNT AND/OR COMPLEXITY OF DATA TO BE REVIEWED	RISK OF COMPLICATIONS AND/OR MORBIDITY OR MORTALITY	TYPE OF MEDICAL DECISION MAKING
Minimal	Minimal or none	Minimal	Straightforward
Limited	Limited	Low	Low complexity
Multiple	Moderate	Moderate	Moderate complexity
Extensive	Extensive	High	High complexity

PROCEDURE 19-3

Perform Procedural Coding: Anesthesia Coding

CAAHEP COMPETENCIES: IV.C.IV.6., IV.P.IV.3., V.P.V.6., VII.P.VII.1., IX.A.IX.2.

ABHES COMPETENCIES: 3.v

GOAL: *Use the steps for anesthesia coding to select the most accurate and specific anesthesia code and to perform the anesthesia formula calculation to determine the charge for the service.*

EQUIPMENT and SUPPLIES

- CPT coding manual (current year)
- Encounter form (charge ticket)
- Medical record
- Conversion factor list (issued by an insurance carrier: for the purposes of this exercise, use the example in Figure 19-5)
- Paper
- Pen or pencil
- Calculator

PROCEDURAL STEPS

1. Read the medical documentation to determine what procedure or service was provided.
   PURPOSE: To ensure all procedures and/or services are listed on the encounter form; that all procedures and services on the encounter form are documented in the medical record; and that nothing documented in the medical record was omitted from the charge ticket.
2. Determine the anatomic site or organ system involved.
   PURPOSE: Anesthesia service codes use the anatomic site and organ system as a category.
3. In the Alphabetic Index, go to the heading Anesthesia and find the code or code range that includes all or most of the medical record procedure or service.
   PURPOSE: To avoid selecting a surgery or other type of procedure or service code other than anesthesia-related codes.
4. Write down the code or code range found in the Alphabetic Index, under the Anesthesia heading, that best matches the medical documentation.
   PURPOSE: To prevent repeated references to the Alphabetic Index by recording all possible matches to the code or code range being sought. This saves time and prevents redundant effort.
5. Turn to the Main Text, Anesthesia section, and find the code or code range found while searching the Alphabetic Index.
   PURPOSE: To verify and select the most specific anesthesia code.
6. Read the guidelines and notes for the section, subsection, category, or subcategory.

PURPOSE: To ensure the correct code is chosen and no instructions prevent the use of the code selected.

7. Evaluate the conventions, especially add-on codes (+) and exemptions from modifier -51.
   PURPOSE: To ensure the correct code is chosen and there are no contraindications to use of the code.
8. Document the code selected.
   PURPOSE: To determine the basic unit value and perform the anesthesia calculation to determine the charge.
9. Determine the basic unit value from the Relative Value Guide.
   PURPOSE: To perform the anesthesia calculation to determine the charge for the anesthesia service.
10. Determine the patient's physical status and document the appropriate modifier.
    PURPOSE: To perform the anesthesia calculation to determine the charge for the anesthesia service.
11. Determine whether any qualifying circumstance modifier should be used. If yes, document the modifier.
    PURPOSE: To perform the anesthesia calculation to determine the charge for the anesthesia service.
12. Determine the total anesthesia time, divide by 15 (minutes), and document the time.
    PURPOSE: To perform the anesthesia calculation to determine the charge for the anesthesia service.
13. Select the appropriate geographic conversion factor.
    PURPOSE: To perform the anesthesia calculation to determine the charge for the anesthesia service.
14. Calculate the charge for the anesthesia service using the anesthesia formula.
    PURPOSE: To determine the charge for the anesthesia service or procedure.
15. Document the anesthesia charge and the code in the medical record and on the encounter form or charge ticket.
    PURPOSE: To complete the documentation and recording requirements.

Anesthesia Formula

Basic Unit Value (B)

The Anesthesia Society of America (ASA) publishes a Relative Value Guide (RVG), which lists the codes for anesthesia services. The RVG compares anesthesia services and assigns a numeric value to each service based on the level of complexity; this numeric value is called the *basic unit value*.

Time Unit (T)

Anesthesia services are provided based on the time during which the anesthesia was administered, in hours and minutes. Typically 15 minutes equals 1 time unit, although this can vary because insurance carriers make that determination independently. The time starts when the anesthesiologist begins preparing the patient to receive anesthesia, continues through the procedure, and ends when the patient is no longer under the personal care of the anesthesiologist. The hours and minutes during which anesthesia was administered are recorded in the patient's record.

Modifying Unit (M)

Modifying units reflect circumstances or conditions that change or modify the environment in which the anesthesia service is provided. The two modifying characteristics for anesthesia services are qualifying circumstances and physical status modifiers. Table 19-6 presents

TABLE 19-6   Anesthesia Physical Status and Qualifying Circumstances Modifiers

MODIFIER	DESCRIPTION
Physical Status Modifiers*	
P1	A normal healthy patient
P2	A patient with mild systemic disease
P3	A patient with severe systemic disease
P4	A person with severe systemic disease that is a constant threat to life
P5	A moribund patient who is not expected to survive without the procedure
P6	A declared brain-dead patient whose organs are being removed for donor purposes
Qualifying Circumstances Modifiers†	
99100	Anesthesia for patient of extreme age, under 1 year or over 70
99116	Anesthesia complicated by utilization of total body hypothermia
99135	Anesthesia complicated by utilization of controlled hypothermia

*A physical status modifier is required for use in performing anesthesia calculations.
†Use a qualifying circumstances modifier code, if appropriate, in addition to the primary CPT Category I Anesthesia code.

a list of these modifiers and their descriptions; a list also can be found in the Anesthesia section of the CPT manual.

Qualifying Circumstances (QC). Sometimes anesthesia is provided in situations that make administration more difficult. These types of cases include provision of anesthesia in emergency situations, to patients of extreme age, during the use of controlled hypotension, and with hypothermia. There are four qualifying circumstances (QC) codes. Each of the five-digit codes is preceded by a plus sign symbol (+), indicating that it is an add-on code; these codes are used in addition to the Category I anesthesia code.

Physical Status Modifiers. The second type of modifying unit used in anesthesia coding is the physical status modifier. These modifiers are used to indicate the patient's physical condition at the time anesthesia was provided. There are five physical status modifiers, each composed of two characters: first the letter P, followed by a ranking of 1 to 6 (e.g., P1, P2, P3, and so on). P1 represents a normal healthy patient, and P6 represents a brain-dead patient whose organs are being harvested.

Conversion Factors

A conversion factor is the dollar value of each basic unit value. Each third-party payer issues a list of conversion factors. The conversion factor for any given geographic location (Figure 19-6) is multiplied by the number of basic unit values assigned to each procedure.

Calculating Anesthesia Services

Using the basic unit value (B), modifying unit (M), time unit (T), and conversion factor, the fee for anesthesia services is calculated according to the anesthesia billing formula (Figure 19-7):

$$(B + M + T) \times \text{Conversion factor}$$

RADIOLOGY CODING

The Radiology section (Figure 19-8) contains all diagnostic imaging codes, including not just x-ray studies, but also ultrasound, magnetic resonance imaging (MRI), and nuclear medicine procedures, in addition to radiation oncology and several other types of diagnostic imaging procedures, services, and therapies. The Radiology section is further subdivided into subsections, such as head and neck, then chest, spine, and pelvis, upper and lower extremities, abdomen, gastrointestinal and urinary tracts, gynecologic, obstetric, heart, and vascular procedures. The next subdivision, categories, defines the types or function of various procedures (e.g., diagnostic ultrasound, radiation oncology, hyperthermia, and so on) that are unique to the

Locality Name	Anesthesia Conversion Factor
Manhattan, NY	22.65
NYC suburbs/Long I., NY	22.74
Queens, NY	22.28
Rest of New York	19.91
North Carolina	20.23
North Dakota	19.70

FIGURE 19-6 Anesthesia conversion factors. (From Buck CJ: *Step-by-step medical coding, 2012 edition,* St Louis, 2012, WB Saunders.)

anatomic site subsection. In addition to the radiology procedure codes, codes are included for physician supervision and interpretation of diagnostic imaging data and for clinical and radiation treatment planning and administration of contrast materials during radiologic procedures.

The coding steps for radiologic procedures are the same as for other Category I codes. When searching by main term in the Alphabetic Index, using *Radiology* as the main term; a *See* note directs the coder to the more specific subcategories of nuclear medicine, ultrasound, radiation therapy, and x-ray studies. As always, a thorough review of the conventions, guidelines, and notes in the Main Text is essential to accurate coding.

PATHOLOGY AND LABORATORY SECTION

The subcategories for the Pathology and Laboratory section include organ panels (Figure 19-9) and disease panels, drug testing, therapeutic drug assays, evocative or suppression testing, consultations, urinalysis, chemistry, molecular diagnostics, infectious agents, microbiology, anatomic pathology, cytopathology, cytogenetic studies, and surgical pathology.

Organ or disease panels are groupings of numerous tests performed to diagnose the health or disease status of specific organ systems. To use a panel code, all the tests listed under the code selected must have been performed. Otherwise, the individual tests should be billed using a separate code for each. The codes for drug testing are *qualitative;* that is, they are based on the type of drug found. *Quantitative* assays, on the other hand, are performed to determine the amount of drug present.

CODING FOR THE MEDICINE SECTION

Immune Globulins

When coding administration of immune globulins, identify the immune globulin product administered and the method of administration using the codes in the *hydration, therapeutic, prophylactic, and diagnostic injections and infusions* subsection (Figure 19-10).

Immunization Administration for Vaccines or Toxoids

These codes are for the administration of vaccines and toxoids only and should be reported in conjunction with the appropriate codes in the *immunization administration for vaccine/toxoids* subsection (Figure 19-11).

Vaccines/Toxoids

These codes identify the vaccine product only. Codes in the *immunization administration for vaccines/toxoids* subsection must be used in addition to the vaccine or toxoid product codes. To meet the reporting requirements of immunization registries, vaccine distribution programs, and reporting systems, the exact vaccine product administered must be reported on the insurance claim.

Hydration, Therapeutic, Prophylactic, and Diagnostic Injections and Infusion

Hydration codes are intended to report a hydration intravenous (IV) infusion consisting of prepackaged fluid and electrolytes; they are

---

Medical Narrative

A 25-year-old female patient in good physical condition has anesthesia services while undergoing laparoscopy (CPT-4 Code 00840). The time for the anesthesia administration was 2 hours. For the purposes of this example the RBV basic unit value will be 4.

Basic Unit Value	= 4
+ Modifying Units: PS	= 0
+ QC	= 0
+ Time Units	= 8
= 12 Total Units	

The total units value of 12 is then multiplied by the conversion factor for the geographic location of the anesthesiologist's office. For the purposes of this exercise, the conversion factor for Manhattan, NY, will be $20.48, and for North Carolina, $15.77. For the office located in Manhattan, NY, multiply $20.48 by 12. The fee for the anesthesia services would be $245.76. For the office located in North Carolina, multiply 12 times $15.77, for a fee of $189.24.

FIGURE 19-7 Anesthesia formula and calculation example.

Radiology

Diagnostic Radiology (Diagnostic Imaging)

Head and Neck

70010	Myelography, posterior fossa, radiological supervision and interpretation
70015	Cisternography, positive contrast, radiological supervision and interpretation
70030	Radiologic examination, eye, for detection of foreign body
70100	Radiologic examination, mandible; partial, less than four views
70110	complete, minimum of four views
70120	Radiologic examination, mastoids; less than three views per side
70130	complete, minimum of three views per side
70134	Radiologic examination, internal auditory meati, complete
70140	Radiologic examination, facial bones; less than three views

FIGURE 19-8 Radiology section of CPT.

Pathology and Laboratory

Organ or Disease Oriented Panels

These panels were developed for coding purposes only and should not be interpreted as clinical parameters. The tests listed with each panel identify the defined components of that panel.

These panel components are not intended to limit the performance of other tests. If one performs tests in addition to those specifically indicated for a particular panel, those tests should be reported separately in addition to the panel code.

80048   Basic metabolic panel

This panel must include the following:

Calcium (82310)

Carbon dioxide (82374)

Chloride (82435)

Creatinine (82565)

Glucose (82947)

Potassium (84132)

Sodium (84295)

Urea nitrogen (BUN) (84520)

(Do not use 80048 in addition to 80053)

80050   General health panel

This panel must include the following:

Comprehensive metabolic panel (80053)

Blood count, complete (CBC), automated and automated differential WBC count (85025 or 85027 and 85004)

FIGURE 19-9 Pathology and Laboratory section of CPT.

Medicine

Immune Globulins

►Codes 90281-90399 identify the immune globulin product only and must be reported in addition to the administration codes 90765-90768, 90772, 90774, 90775 as appropriate. Immune globulin products listed here include broad-spectrum and anti-infective immune globulins, antitoxins, and various isoantibodies.◄

⊘ **90281**   Immune globulin (Ig), human, for intramuscular use

⊘ **90283**   Immune globulin (IgIV), human, for intravenous use

⊘ **90287**   Botulinum antitoxin, equine, any route

⊘ **90288**   Botulism immune globulin, human, for intravenous use

⊘ **90291**   Cytomegalovirus immune globulin (CMV-IgIV), human, for intravenous use

⊘ **90296**   Diphtheria antitoxin, equine, any route

⊘ **90371**   Hepatitis B immune globulin (HBIg), human, for intramuscular use

⊘ **90375**   Rabies immune globulin (RIg), human, for intramuscular and/or subcutaneous use

⊘ **90376**   Rabies immune globulin, heat-treated (RIg-HT), human, for intramuscular and/or subcutaneous use

FIGURE 19-10 Relationship of immune globulins and infusions in CPT.

(Figure 19-12). HCPCS codes, like CPT codes, are updated annually. They are designed to promote standardized reporting and collection of statistical data on medical supplies, products, services, and procedures.

CODING LEVELS: CPT AND HCPCS

Currently, two levels of procedure and services codes are used:
- Level I codes: These are the CPT codes, developed by the AMA and published in the current CPT manual.
- Level II: These are the HCPCS codes, developed by the CMS to describe medical services and supplies not covered in the CPT manual.

HCPCS Codes

The HCPCS (Level II) codes have five alphanumeric digits, beginning with one letter followed by four numerals. HCPCS also uses two alphabetic or alphanumeric character modifiers to add information or to supplement the Level II codes. HCPCS uses five conventions (Figure 19-13).

HCPCS Manual

Like the CPT manual, the HCPCS manual is divided into two parts: the Alphabetic Index and the Tabular Index. As with the CPT, procedures and services can be looked up in the Alphabetic Index and then confirmed as the most accurate and appropriate code by using the Tabular Index. The HCPCS manual has no subsections, categories, or subcategories; it has only sections, as outlined earlier.

not used to report the infusion of drugs or other substances. When multiple drugs are administered, report the service or services and the specific materials or drugs for each.

Home Health Procedures and Services

These codes are used by nonphysician health care professionals only. They are used to report services provided in a patient's residence (including assisted-living apartments, group homes, nontraditional private homes, custodial care facilities, and schools).

HEALTHCARE COMMON PROCEDURE CODING SYSTEM (HCPCS)

As mentioned previously, **HCPCS** is a collection of codes and descriptions that represent procedures, supplies, products, and services not covered by or included in the CPT coding system

An appendix contains all the HCPCS modifiers and their descriptions.

The coding steps for HCPCS are almost identical to those for CPT Category I codes (Procedure 19-4). A main term is determined and used to help find the procedure or service in the Alphabetic Index. The Alphabetic Index lists a code, codes, or code range. These codes or code ranges are then reviewed in the Tabular Index for specificity and accuracy. As with the CPT codes, the clinical documentation is the starting point, and the final code selected should add nothing to or omit anything from the description in the medical documentation. The final step is determining whether the code selected can stand alone or requires a modifier to further define or add needed information.

Coding using the HCPCS manual is essentially the same as coding for a CPT procedure or service. The conventions, layout, and format of the HCPCS manual are different, and the manual has only sections and subsections. The HCPCS codes can be used when a specific procedure or service is not found in the CPT coding manual.

CLOSING COMMENTS

Remember that new coding manuals are published each year and should be ordered in the early fall so that they arrive in a timely manner, allowing the medical assistant to review them. Always use the current years' manual so that the codes used are accurate and specific. The front of new manuals usually contains an introductory section that highlights changes and/or new regulations. If the office uses coding software, the publisher should offer annual updates that can be loaded to the computer. This helps to insure that all codes used are up-to-date for the current year.

Although the billing and coding process can be intimidating and overwhelming, approach it with a good attitude. No provider will

---

Immunization Administration for Vaccines/Toxoids

Codes 90465-90474 must be reported in addition to the vaccine and toxoid code(s) 90476-90749.

Report codes 90465-90468 only when the physician provides face-to-face counseling of the patient and family during the administration of a vaccine. For immunization administration of any vaccine that is not accompanied by face-to-face physician counseling to the patient/family, report codes 90471-90474.

If a significant separately identifiable Evaluation and Management service (e.g., office or other outpatient services, preventive medicine services) is performed, the appropriate E/M service code should be reported in addition to the vaccine and toxoid administration codes.

  (For allergy testing, see 95004 et seq)

  (For skin testing of bacterial, viral, fungal extracts, see 86485-86586)

  ▶(For therapeutic or diagnostic injections, see 90772-90779)◀

90465 Immunization administration under 8 years of age (includes percutaneous, intradermal, subcutaneous, or intramuscular injections) when the physician counsels the patient/family; first injection (single or combination vaccine/toxoid), per day

  (Do not report 90465 in conjunction with 90467)

+ 90466 each additional injection (single or combination vaccine/toxoid), per day (List separately in addition to code for primary procedure)

  (Use 90466 in conjunction with 90465 or 90467)

FIGURE 19-11 Relationship of immune vaccines/toxoids and administration codes in CPT.

⊙ **Special coverage instructions.** Indicates that there are instructions provided regarding circumstances in which the code might be included for reimbursement.

◆ **Not covered by or valid for Medicare.** These codes might result in reimbursement by private health insurance payors but not by Medicare. Their value may be only for statistical data collection but not for reimbursement.

✳ **Carrier discretion.** These codes may or may not be paid by health insurance carrier including Medicare.

▶ **New.**

⇒ **Revised.** The revised symbol is placed in front of codes with any data, payment, or miscellaneous change from the prior year.

FIGURE 19-13 HCPCS conventions.

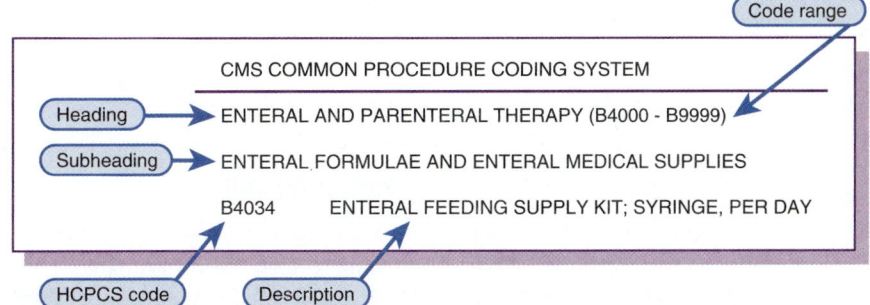

FIGURE 19-12 *Healthcare Common Procedure Coding System* (HCPCS) national codes, established by the Centers for Medicare and Medicaid Services. (Courtesy U.S. Department of Health and Human Services, Centers for Medicare and Medicaid Services, Atlanta, Ga.)

PROCEDURE 19-4

Perform Procedural Coding: HCPCS Coding

CAAHEP COMPETENCIES: IV.C.IV.6., IV.P.IV.3., V.P.V.6., VII.P.VII.1., IX.A.IX.2.

ABHES COMPETENCIES: 3.v

GOAL: *Use the steps for procedure and service coding to find the most accurate and specific HCPCS code.*

EQUIPMENT and SUPPLIES

- HCPCS coding manual (current year)
- Medical record
- Encounter form (charge ticket)
- Paper
- Pen or pencil

PROCEDURAL STEPS

1. Read the medical documentation to determine what procedures or services were provided.
   PURPOSE: To ensure that all procedures and/or services are listed on the encounter form; that all procedures and services on the encounter form match the medical record; and that nothing documented in the medical record is missing from the encounter form.

2. Determine the main and modifying terms from the abstracted information.
   PURPOSE: To identify the term or terms to begin the search in the Alphabetic Index.

3. After the main term has been located, select modifying term or terms if needed.
   PURPOSE: To provide additional specificity and help narrow the search for the code or code range in the Alphabetic Index.

4. Select the most appropriate main term to begin a search in the Alphabetic Index.
   PURPOSE: To start the search for the best code or codes in the Alphabetic Index.

5. If no modifying term produces an appropriate code or code range, repeat steps 2 and 3 using a different main term classification.
   PURPOSE: To aid in finding the most appropriate code or code range by using alternative methods of searching the Alphabetic Index.

6. Find the code or code ranges that include all or most of the medical record procedure or service description.
   PURPOSE: To assist in directing the medical assistant to the proper section, subsection, category, or subcategory of the Main Text of the HCPCS manual.

7. Disregard any code or code range containing additional descriptions or modifying terms not found in the medical record.
   PURPOSE: To prevent upcoding or downcoding errors and other compliance issues.

8. Write down the code or code ranges that best match the medical documentation.
   PURPOSE: To prevent repeated references to the Alphabetic Index by recording all possible matches to the code or code range being sought. This saves time and prevents redundant effort.

9. Turn to the Main Text, and find the first code or code range found while searching the Alphabetic Index.
   PURPOSE: To begin the process of finding the most specific and accurate code.

10. Compare the description of the code with the medical documentation. Verify that all or most of the medical record documentation matches the code description and that there is no additional element or information in the code description that is not found in the documentation.
    PURPOSE: To avoid upcoding and downcoding errors and to ensure there are no contraindications to use of the code selected.

11. Read the guidelines for the section and subsection and code to ensure there are no contraindications to the use of the code.
    PURPOSE: To ensure there are no instructions that would prevent use of the code selected.

12. Evaluate the HCPCS manual conventions.
    PURPOSE: To ensure there are no instructions that would prevent use of the code selected.

13. Determine whether any special circumstances require the use of a modifier.
    PURPOSE: To select, if appropriate, modifiers that provide additional information for the code selected to explain certain circumstances or provide additional detail.

14. Record the HCPCS code selected in the medical record documentation next to the procedure or service performed and in the appropriate block of the insurance claim form.
    PURPOSE: To complete the documentation and reporting requirements.

have confidence in the medical assistant who complains about the changing nature of the work he or she is assigned to complete. Look for opportunities to learn more about the process; many of the larger hospitals periodically offer free workshops about specific sections of coding manuals. Publishers of coding manuals will often bring authors to a hospital or clinic to conduct a seminar. Additionally, there are numerous online seminars or workshops that can be completed and physicians will often cover the costs of such programs if they are not free. A medical assistant who is eager to learn and takes

advantages of such opportunities will be much more valuable to his or her employer.

Patient Education

Like the diagnosis codes, procedure codes must be specific and accurate to ensure the maximum reimbursement for the provider. When patients have questions about items on their bills related to procedure codes, answer them or refer them to the person designated as the biller/coder in the provider's office. Patients who have surgery or other complicated procedures may receive bills from more than one provider. Even if they are confused and frustrated, take the time to educate them as to why they may have received separate bills from, for instance, a radiologist who completed x-ray reports or a pathologist who inspected specimens from surgical procedures. Patient questions are never insignificant and deserve courteous attention from the medical assistant.

Legal and Ethical Issues

Medical assistants must be responsible and remain knowledgeable about CPT to ensure that no fraud takes place in the coding and claims submission process. Medical assistants should also ensure that proper precautions are taken to avoid incorrect coding, data entry errors, and false claims submissions.

Codes or narratives in patient chart documentation should not be altered to increase insurance reimbursement or to accommodate policy coverage requirements. Deliberate misrepresentation, such as **downcoding** or **upcoding**, may carry criminal and/or civil penalties.

Downcoding, in which lower level codes are used even when the diagnostic statement indicates a higher level procedure or service, usually affects reimbursement only by lowering the amount received. However, it may have civil and criminal penalty implications if it is done to skirt insurance policy restrictions or pre-existing condition clauses. It is also common for insurance claims examiners to change the procedure code on a health insurance claim form to a procedure code with a lesser value. This happens most often when there is a mismatch of the official CPT description and the description written on the insurance claim form. It is important to review the explanation sent from the insurance carrier when payment is received to determine whether downcoding occurred and to refile or challenge the lowered code by providing additional information that will result in approval of the higher code used, if appropriate.

Upcoding, in which a higher level procedure or service code is used than is supported by the medical documentation, can result in civil and criminal penalties, including fines, loss of privileges as a participating provider, and even prison time. Stay familiar with laws that affect billing and coding procedures so that the provider receives the highest legal and accurate reimbursement possible for the procedures and treatments performed.

SUMMARY OF SCENARIO

Sherald has learned that procedural coding using the CPT is similar in many ways to ICD-9-CM diagnostic coding. The two coding manuals have unique but similar steps, conventions, and guidelines. She has also learned that proper abstracting of procedural data from the medical record is equally important in the ICD-9-CM and the CPT. In addition, Sherald discovered that HCPCS codes describe procedures and services not found in the CPT, such as medicines, ambulance services, and durable medical equipment. Sherald now knows the legal implications of coding compliance errors, such as upcoding and downcoding.

Sherald enjoys working toward becoming a medical assistant. As she progresses with learning procedural coding, she envisions herself as becoming more well rounded in her knowledge of the practice's administrative operations. The encounter form is a common document used to enter the procedure when a patient checks out, but knowing how to use the CPT manual is essential when notes must be coded from procedures or services performed by Dr. Shuman or Dr. Taylor. As with diagnostic coding, Sherald can pull the patient's chart for research and documentation if any questions arise about a claim. Sherald knows that coding to the highest level of specificity helps ensure accuracy and aids the practice in obtaining maximum reimbursement. Sherald continues to use the Internet to network and research. She stays informed of the changes in procedural coding by ordering the updated CPT manual each year.

SUMMARY OF LEARNING OBJECTIVES

1. **Define, spell, and pronounce the terms listed in the vocabulary.**
   Spelling and pronouncing medical terms correctly bolster the medical assistant's credibility. Knowing the definition of these terms promotes confidence in communication with patients and co-workers.

2. **Describe the steps for abstracting procedural data from clinical documentation.**
   The medical assistant must thoroughly read clinical documentation and look for all of the procedures that were performed and should be charged to the patient. Most physician offices use the encounter form to document procedures and services, but there are instances when the medical assistant will need to read through the medical record to determine what was done to the patient and what charges should be made.

3. **Identify four purposes of the CPT.**
   The CPT is designed to encourage the use of standard terms and descriptors to document procedures in the medical record; to communicate accurate information on procedures and services to agencies concerned with insurance claims; to provide the basis for a computer-oriented system to evaluate operative procedures, and to contribute basic information for statistical purposes.

4. **List the six main sections of the CPT and describe their content.**
   The Main Text has six sections: Evaluation and Management (E/M), Anesthesia, Surgery, Radiology, Pathology and Laboratory, and Medicine. Each section contains subsections, categories, and subcategories that further define, modify, and describe the procedure or service codes.

5. **Describe the coding conventions, guidelines, and layout of the CPT manual and their importance.**

The CPT guidelines, symbols, conventions, notes, and steps are designed to guide a medical coder through the process of analyzing and translating clinical documentation and selecting the most accurate code for the procedure performed or the services rendered. The CPT contains a comprehensive Alphabetic Index, a Main Text listing of the CPT Category I codes, and several appendixes and addenda. The Alphabetic Index is composed of main and modifying terms that help provide specificity in selecting code or code ranges to evaluate in the Main Text. The Main Text numerically lists all the CPT procedure and service codes and provides guidelines and conventions in selecting the most specific and most accurate code for insurance billing, reimbursement, and statistical data collection. The appendixes and addenda provide lists of deletions, additions, and changes to the previous year's CPT, modifiers, Category II and III codes, clinical examples for use of the E/M codes, add-on codes, exempt codes, codes that include conscious sedation, and drugs awaiting U.S. Food and Drug Administration (FDA) approval.

6. **Describe the process and steps for selecting the most accurate code based on clinical documentation.**

To use the CPT properly, the coder begins by reading and abstracting the medical documentation, then follows several specific steps using the CPT Alphabetic Index to find a numeric, Category I, CPT procedure or service code, codes, or range of codes. The steps for using the Alphabetic Index are (1) read the medical documentation; (2) select the main term classification to begin the search; (3) after locating the main term, select the modifying term or terms; (4) if no modifying term produces an appropriate code or code range, repeat steps 2 and 3 using a different main term classification; (5) find the code or code ranges that include all or most of the medical record procedure or service description; (6) disregard any code or code range containing additional descriptions or modifying terms not found in the medical record; (7) write down the code or code ranges that best match the medical documentation. Once the coder has found the code, codes, or code range in the Alphabetic Index, he or she moves to the CPT Main Text to refine the search and find the appropriate code.

7. **Explain the importance of correctly assigning evaluation and management (E/M) codes.**

The physician can only bill for services that are actually rendered to patients and must use the E/M guidelines to determine the correct codes for each patient. The amount of time spent with the patient and the level of medical decision making, in addition to the length and complexity of the history and examination process, all affect the code choice that applies to a particular patient encounter.

8. **Discuss the importance of modifiers.**

Modifiers enable the physician to indicate that a service or procedure was altered in some way but not changed in definition. Modifiers also allow the physician to provide additional information or to describe extenuating circumstances that affect the rendered procedure or service.

9. **Define upcoding and explain why it must be avoided.**

If a code is selected that not only matches the procedure or service performed but also adds modifying information that is not in the medical documentation, the information is considered "upcoded." Consistent upcoding can result in legal charges of fraud or abuse.

10. **Explain the process for selecting the correct procedure codes.**

The medical assistant must understand the process for selecting the correct procedure codes used for billing purposes. The selection directly influences the physician's total reimbursements. The process for code selection is outlined in Procedure 19-1.

11. **Explain the process for selecting main and modifying terms.**

The Alphabetic Index is organized by main terms that can stand alone or can be further detailed by using modifying terms that are indented under the main terms. The medical assistant should be as specific as possible in code selections, using all pertinent words in the description as found in the medical documentation.

12. **Explain how to find codes in the Alphabetic Index of the CPT manual.**

First, analyze the medical documentation to determine what services or procedures were performed. Select the main term from the documentation and search for it in the Alphabetic Index. Modifying terms help the coder find the appropriate code, which should then be located in the Main Text. Determine which code is the most accurate description for the procedure or service provided.

13. **Explain how to analyze and select codes using the CPT Main Text.**

After searching the Alphabetic Index, turn to the appropriate codes in the Main Text to perform the final coding steps. Read the section thoroughly to determine the most accurate code to assign to the procedure or service rendered to the patient. Code the procedure or service. The process for using the Alphabetic Index and Main Texts of the CPT manual are detailed in Procedures 19-2 to 19-4.

CONNECTIONS

Study Guide Connection: Go to Chapter 19 Study Guide. Read the Case Study and Workplace Applications and complete the assignments. Do online research for answers to the questions in the Internet Activities associated with basics of procedural coding.

Evolve Connection: For more information related to basics of procedural coding, go to evolve.elsevier.com/kinn and visit related Web links for Chapter 19. Click on the Medical Assisting Exam Review and answer the practice questions to sharpen your test-taking skills.

20

BASICS OF HEALTH INSURANCE

Carline A. Dalgleish, Sharon Oliver, and Alexandra Patricia Adams

SCENARIO

The instructor in Ann Snyder's administrative medical assistant class, Grant Wilson, knows that working with medical insurance can be quite rewarding, and experienced billers also find the field financially rewarding. Mr. Wilson works with Ann and her classmates, answering their questions and helping them to see that medical insurance is not as complicated as it seems.

The medical assistant who is able to pay attention to detail and likes paperwork will usually enjoy billing and coding activities. The person who performs these duties in the physician's office is a critical staff member, because the tasks that are done related to billing influence the physician's income. That income is used to pay clinic expenses and payroll, so all of the employees of the facility indirectly count on accurate and timely billing. The individual who contributes billing and coding skills, in addition to an understanding of health insurance and reimbursement guidelines, will be an asset to the practice and can look forward to a long and rewarding career.

Ann will learn that when insurance billing is broken down into manageable segments of information and applied to real-life situations, it becomes an interesting task. She will learn about the importance of verifying insurance eligibility and the steps for obtaining authorization for referrals and procedures; she also will learn that those benefits differ among insurance carriers, whether private, commercial, federal, or state insurance payers.

While studying this chapter, think about the following questions:

- How will Ann be able to remember all the benefits, exclusions, authorizations, and other required information for the multiple insurance carriers and third-party administrators?
- Why is it important to verify insurance eligibility and benefits before the patient is seen in a provider's office?
- Why is it important to understand the procedures for obtaining referrals and authorizations?
- What will Ann need to know to perform insurance deductible and co-insurance calculations?

LEARNING OBJECTIVES

1. Define, spell, and pronounce the terms listed in the vocabulary.
2. Discuss the purpose of health insurance.
3. Differentiate among the various types of insurance policies.
4. Explain the numerous classifications of insurance benefits available.
5. Explain how insurance benefits are determined.
6. Differentiate among the different types of managed care options.
7. List and discuss other major third-party payers.
8. Explain the procedure for verifying insurance benefits.
9. Discuss the different types of fee schedules.
10. Explain how to make managed care referrals and obtain precertifications.
11. Perform eligibility and verification of benefits procedures.
12. Perform a preauthorization procedure.
13. Demonstrate how insurance benefits are determined by calculating deductible and co-insurance payments.

VOCABULARY

allowed charge (allowable amount) The maximum amount of money that many third-party payers allow for a specific procedure or service.

authorization An alphanumeric/number given by the insurance company authorizing approval of a procedure or service. This does not guarantee payment.

beneficiary The individual entitled to receive benefits from an insurance policy or program or a governmental entitlement program offering healthcare benefits. Also called a *participant, subscriber, dependent, enrollee,* or *member.*

benefits The amount payable by an insurance company for a monetary loss to an individual insured by that company, under each coverage.

birthday rule An insurance rule that applies as follows: when an individual is covered under two insurance policies, the insurance plan of the policyholder whose birthday comes first in the calendar year (month and day, not year) becomes the primary insurance.

capitation A payment method used by many managed care organizations in which a fixed amount of money is reimbursed to the provider for patients enrolled during a specific period of time, no matter what services were received or how many visits were made.

carriers In insurance terms, companies that assume the risk of an insurance policy.

Civilian Health and Medical Program of the Uniformed Services (CHAMPUS) See TRICARE.

Civilian Health and Medical Program of the Department of Veterans Affairs (CHAMPVA) A comprehensive health care program in which the VA pays the cost of covered health care services and supplies for eligible beneficiaries; to be eligible, the individual cannot be eligible for TRICARE, but can be the spouse or child of a disabled veteran, as well as the surviving spouse or child of a veteran who died from a service-connected disability; a veteran who died while suffering a service disability; or a military member who died in the line of duty.

co-insurance A policy provision frequently found in medical insurance whereby the policyholder and the insurance company share the cost of covered losses in a specified ratio (e.g., 80/20 means that 80% is covered by the insurer and 20% by the insured).

commercial insurance plans Plans that reimburse the insured for expenses resulting from illness or injury according to a specific fee schedule as outlined in the insurance policy and on a fee-for-service basis. Sometimes called *private insurance.*

co-payment A sum of money that is paid at the time of medical service; a form of co-insurance.

deductibles Specific amounts of money a patient must pay out of pocket before the insurance carrier begins paying. Usually this amount ranges from $100 to $500. This deductible amount is met on a yearly or per-incident basis.

dependents The spouse, children, and sometimes domestic partner or other individuals designated by the insured who are covered under a healthcare plan.

disability income insurance Insurance that provides periodic payments to replace income when an insured person is unable to work as a result of illness, injury, or disease.

effective date The date on which an insurance policy or plan takes effect so that benefits are payable.

eligibility A term that describes whether a patient's insurance coverage is in effect and eligible for payment of insurance benefits.

exclusions Limitations on an insurance contract for which benefits are not payable.

explanation of benefits (EOB) A letter or statement from the insurance carrier describing what was paid, denied, or reduced in payment. It also contains information about amounts applied to the deductible, the patient's co-insurance, and the allowed amounts.

explanation of Medicare benefits (EOMB) An explanation of benefits from Medicare (see *explanation of benefits* [EOB]).

fee for service An established schedule of fees set for services performed by providers and paid by the patient.

fiscal intermediary An organization that contracts with the government to handle and mediate insurance claims from medical facilities, home health agencies, or providers of medical services or supplies.

government plans Entitlement programs or healthcare plans that are sponsored and/or subsidized by the state or federal government, such as Medicaid and Medicare.

grandfathered A legislative provision that allows the exception based on a preexisting condition.

group policy Insurance written under a policy that covers a number of people under a single master contract issued to their employer or to an association with which they are affiliated.

guarantor The person responsible for paying a medical bill.

health insurance Insurance protection, provided in return for periodic premium payments, that provides reimbursement of expenses resulting from illness or injury. It includes accident, disability income, medical expense, and accidental death and dismemberment insurance. Also known as *accident and health insurance* or *disability income insurance.*

Health Insurance Portability and Accountability Act (HIPAA) A law enacted in 1996 to improve the portability and continuity of health insurance coverage; to combat waste, fraud, and abuse in health insurance and healthcare delivery; to promote the use of medical savings accounts; to improve access to long-term care services and coverage; to simplify the administration of health insurance; and to serve other purposes. As a result, standards have been created for electronic health information transactions and for the privacy of health information. Also known as the Kassebaum-Kennedy Act.

health maintenance organization (HMO) An organization that provides a wide range of comprehensive healthcare services for a specified group at a fixed periodic payment. HMOs can be sponsored by the government, medical schools, hospitals, employers, labor unions, consumer groups, insurance companies, and hospital-medical plans.

indemnity plans Traditional health insurance plans that pay for all or a share of the cost of covered services, regardless of which physician, hospital, or other licensed healthcare provider is used. Policyholders of indemnity plans and their dependents choose when and where to get healthcare services.

individual policy An insurance policy designed specifically for the use of one person and his or her dependents. An individual policy generally does not offer some of the amenities of a group policy (e.g., lower premiums). Often called *personal insurance.*

insured An individual or organization covered by an insurance policy according to the policy terms; usually, the individual or group that pays the premiums. Blue Cross/Blue Shield refers to this person or group as the *subscriber.*

managed care plans An umbrella term for all healthcare plans that provide healthcare in return for preset monthly payments and coordinated care through a defined network of primary care physicians and hospitals.

medical savings accounts (MSAs) Tax-deferred bank or savings accounts that are combined with a low-premium, high-deductible insurance policy; they are designed for individuals or families who choose to fund their own healthcare expenses and medical insurance.

Medicaid A federal- and state-sponsored health insurance program for the medically indigent.

Medicare A federally sponsored health insurance program for those over age 65 and for individuals under age 65 who are disabled.

Medigap A term sometimes applied to private insurance products that supplement Medicare insurance benefits.

participating provider (PAR) A physician or other healthcare provider who enters into a contract with a specific insurance company or program and by doing so agrees to abide by certain rules and regulations set forth by that particular third-party payer.

policyholder A person who pays a premium to an insurance company and in whose name the policy is written in exchange for the insurance protection provided by a policy of insurance.

preauthorization A process required by some insurance carriers in which the provider obtains permission to perform certain procedures or services or refer a patient to a specialist.

premium The periodic (monthly, quarterly, or annual) payment of a specific sum of money to an insurance company, for which the insurer in return agrees to provide certain benefits.

primary care provider (PCP) A general practice or nonspecialist provider or physician responsible for the care of a patient for some health maintenance organizations. Also called a *gatekeeper.*

referral An insurance term used when a primary care provider wants to send a patient to a specialist. Typically, the provider must obtain authorization from the insurance carrier in advance to refer a patient.

remittance advice (RA) An explanation of benefits from Medicaid (see *explanation of benefits* [EOB]).

resource-based relative value scale (RBRVS) A fee schedule designed to provide national uniform payment of Medicare benefits after adjustment to reflect the differences in practice costs across geographic areas.

rider A special provision or group of provisions that may be added to a policy to expand or limit the benefits otherwise payable. It may increase or decrease benefits, waive a condition or coverage, or in any other way amend the original contract.

self-insured (or self-funded) plan An insurance plan funded by an organization having a large enough employee base that it can afford to fund its own insurance program.

self-referral Occurs when a patient or an insured individual refers himself or herself to a specialist without requesting the referral from the primary provider (e.g., a woman seeking an annual gynecologic examination). Managed care guidelines may require the patient to report the self-referral.

service benefit plans Plans that provide benefits in the form of certain surgical and medical services rendered rather than cash. A service benefit plan is not restricted to a fee schedule.

third-party administrator (TPA) An organization that processes claims and performs other business-related functions for a health plan.

third-party payers Entities that make payment on an obligation or debt but are not parties to the contract that created the debt.

TRICARE A government-sponsored program under which authorized dependents of military personnel receive medical care. Originally called *CHAMPUS.*

utilization review A review of individual cases by a committee to make sure that services are medically necessary and to study how providers use medical care resources.

workers' compensation A system of laws that protects employees against the loss of wages and the cost of medical care resulting from an occupational accident, disease, or death, unless the employee is proven negligent.

THE PURPOSE OF HEALTH INSURANCE

The purpose of health insurance is to help individuals and families offset the costs of medical care. **Health insurance** is defined as a contract for protection against financial losses resulting from illness or injury. This protection provides payment of monetary **benefits** for covered sickness or injury, depending on the insurance policy purchased. There are various types of health insurance, such as accident insurance, disability income insurance, hospitalization, medical expense insurance, and accidental death and dismemberment insurance.

Health insurance typically covers services and procedures considered medically necessary. Most insurance policies do not cover "elective" procedures, such as certain cosmetic surgeries that are not considered medically necessary. More and more of today's health insurance policies cover "preventive" care, which includes services provided to help prevent certain illnesses or that lead to an early diagnosis.

IMPACT OF INSURANCE BILLING ON THE MEDICAL OFFICE

Nearly all of the physician's income is derived from the insurance payments received for services rendered. Regular expenses, such as rent, salaries, medical and office supplies, equipment, and so on, depend on the practice's cash flow, which arises from proper and timely filing of insurance claims to meet the financial needs of the medical office. This is the most important job function of the coder/biller.

CYCLE OF HEALTH INSURANCE

The information that follows describes common types of insurance coverage and insurance carriers, the steps for obtaining insurance coverage information, and some of the terminology associated with obtaining insurance coverage and insurance billing. The **insured** or **policyholder**, defined as an individual, group, or employer, pays a set amount called a premium. A **premium** is the periodic (monthly, quarterly, or annual) payment of a specific sum of money to an insurance company for which the insurer agrees to provide certain benefits. This premium, in return, pays for an insurance policy that covers the insured for a specific type (or types) of coverage, such as basic and major medical coverage, accidental death or disability, and so on. When an insured or a covered beneficiary or dependent of the insurance policy becomes ill or suffers an injury, treatment is provided by a physician or other provider of service in a doctor's office, emergency department, or hospital, and the fee is paid by the insurance company when medical necessity and covered benefits are met.

Tasks Related to the Cycle of Health Insurance

The medical assistant's tasks are initiated when the patient encounters the provider, either by appointment, as a walk-in, or in the emergency department or hospital. Insurance billing and coding tasks typically completed by the medical assistant include:

- Obtaining information from the patient and the insured, including demographic, employment, and insurance data.
- Verifying the patient's **eligibility** for insurance payment by the insurance carrier or carriers, in addition to the benefits available and exclusions, and determining whether special authorizations are needed to refer the patient to specialists or for the performance of certain services or procedures (e.g., surgery or diagnostic tests).
- Performing diagnostic and procedural coding and reviewing the encounter form or charge ticket for completeness once the patient has been seen by the provider.
- Calculating insurance deductibles and co-insurance amounts and providing the patient with a statement showing the out-of-pocket amount he or she owes.
- Obtaining preauthorization for referral of the patient to a specialist or for special services or procedures that require advance permission.
- Completing an insurance claim form and submitting it to the insurance company for reimbursement for services and procedures performed.
- Posting payments and adjustments on the patient ledger or account and examining the **explanation of benefits (EOB)**, **explanation of Medicare benefits (EOMB)**, or **remittance advice (RA)** from the insurance company to identify what was paid, reduced, or denied and also the deductible, co-insurance, and allowed charges (also called *allowable amounts*).

- Adjusting the account to reflect an allowable amount, which is either written off (adjusted) or passed on to the patient for payment, and also any courtesy, professional, or other type of adjustment.
- Billing the patient for any outstanding balance or, if the patient has a secondary insurance, completing the secondary insurance claim form and submitting it to the insurance company with a copy of the EOB showing payment from the primary insurance carrier.
- Following up on any rejected or unpaid claims, making sure that any requests from the insurance carrier for more information about specific claims are answered as soon as possible.
- Meeting the timely filing requirements of each of the medical office's participating insurance carriers. Failure to do this results in zero payment from the insurance company and inability to bill the patient for the nonpayable amount.

Determining Primary and Secondary Coverage

When the patient is the insured, the patient becomes the guarantor, and the patient's insurance is primary. If the patient also is covered by another policy, that policy becomes the secondary insurance.

The only exception to this convention arises when the patient is not the insurance policy holder, such as when a child is insured by each parent. In such cases, the **birthday rule** applies; that is, under law, the insurance plan of the policyholder whose birthday comes first in the calendar year (month and day, not year) becomes the primary insurance.

Cost of Coverage

In this age of rising healthcare costs, most insurance carriers do not reimburse the full amount for services and procedures rendered. A **carrier** is an insurance company or third party that pays for medical care. The insured, or **beneficiary**, in most instances is required to pay certain out-of-pocket expenses, such as deductibles, co-payment or co-insurance charges, and costs for noncovered services.

A **deductible** is an amount a policyholder agrees to pay per claim or per accident toward the total amount of an insured loss before the insurance company begins payment of benefits. A deductible amount is stated in the insurance contract and normally ranges from $100 to $500. Under most circumstances the deductible must be paid only one time per calendar year; however, some policies have a deductible per occurrence.

The medical assistant should always verify the **effective date**, or date the insurance coverage began, on the patient's insurance card. An excellent policy for any provider's office is to call the insurance company to verify insurance eligibility, benefits, and **exclusions** before the patient's appointment or encounter with the provider. This verification is done by phone or fax and ensures that the insurance is in effect and the patient is eligible for benefits. Most major insurance carriers have a Web site dedicated to verifying eligibility and claims payments. (Verification of benefits is discussed in more detail later in the chapter.)

Co-insurance is a policy provision frequently found in medical insurance. Under this provision, the policyholder and the insurance company share the cost of covered losses in a specified ratio, such as 80/20 (i.e., 80% of services are paid by the insurance carrier and 20% by the insured).

Many plans now require a **co-payment**, which is a type of co-insurance that is collected at the time of service. Co-payments usually range from $10 to $25 for office visits but can vary according to the services rendered. Most managed care plans require a co-payment. In addition, any services or procedures that are not covered under the terms of an insurance policy are the responsibility of the policyholder or insured.

TYPES OF HEALTH INSURANCE

Health insurance is available to most people in this country through group or individual plans. In addition, many people are covered by government plans or entitlement programs. However, although health insurance might be available, it is not always affordable. A recent survey revealed that more than 40 million Americans have no regular source for obtaining medical care, and lack of health insurance was a major obstacle.

The types of health insurance available include group insurance, individual insurance, government-sponsored insurance, self-insured plans, and medical savings accounts. Government plans can be federal and/or state sponsored; they include Medicare, Medicaid, TRICARE, the **Civilian Health and Medical Program of the Department of Veterans Affairs (CHAMPVA)**, and workers' compensation.

Group Policies

Insurance written under a **group policy** covers a number of people under a single master contract (subsidized by employers) that is issued to their employer or to an association with which they are affiliated. Group coverage usually provides greater benefits at lower premiums because of the large pool of people from whom premiums are collected. Physical examinations are normally not required, and pre-existing conditions are often waived. Often the employee shares the cost of coverage through payroll deductions.

Individual Policies

Individuals who do not qualify for inclusion in a group or government-sponsored plan may apply to companies that offer **individual policies**, often called *personal insurance*. The applicant is normally required to fill out an extended health questionnaire and undergo a physical examination before acceptance. Unlike with group policies, with personal insurance there is a risk that coverage may be denied, or the individual may have to accept a **rider**, or limitation, on benefits the policy will cover. Premiums are almost always higher with individual policies, and often the benefits are less.

Government Plans

Many large groups of people are covered by **government plans** or entitlement programs. A patient who is age 65 or older is covered by Part A and Part B of Medicare. A medically indigent patient may be eligible for Medicaid, with or without Medicare. **Dependents** of military personnel are covered by TRICARE (formerly the **Civilian Health and Medical Program of the Uniformed Services [CHAMPUS]**); surviving spouses and dependent children of veterans who died as a result of service-related disabilities are covered by CHAMPVA.

Some wage earners are protected against the loss of wages and the cost of medical care resulting from an occupational accident, disease, or disability through workers' compensation insurance. An individual may collect benefits for health expenses from an automobile policy if the injury is related to a car accident or other such loss.

TRICARE

The federal government first became responsible for insuring a large group of people in 1956 with passage of Public Law 569. This law authorized dependents of military personnel to receive treatment from civilian physicians at the expense of the government. The program administering these benefits became CHAMPUS, which today is known as **TRICARE** (discussed in detail later in this chapter).

Medicaid

In 1965 the federal government provided for the medically indigent through a program known as **Medicaid**. Title XIX of Public Law 89-97, under the Social Security Amendments of 1965, provided for agreements involving cost sharing between federal and state governments to provide medical care for people meeting specific eligibility criteria.

Medicare

Established in 1965, **Medicare** is a federal health insurance program that provides healthcare coverage for individuals age 65 and older. The program also covers certain individuals under age 65 who have disabilities or end-stage renal disease (ESRD). The Medicare program was developed by the Healthcare Financing Administration (HCFA) as part of Title XVIII of the Social Security Act. The HCFA now is known as the *Centers for Medicare and Medicaid Services* (CMS).

Workers' Compensation

All state legislatures have passed workers' compensation laws to protect wage earners against the loss of wages and the cost of medical care resulting from occupational accident or disease, as long as the employee was not proven negligent. State laws differ as to the classes of employees included and the benefits provided by **workers' compensation** insurance.

Self-Insured Plans

Many large companies or organizations have a big enough employee base that they choose to fund their own insurance program. This is called a **self-insured** (or **self-funded) plan**. Technically, a self-funded plan is not insurance by true definition. The employer pays employee healthcare costs from the firm's own funds. Usually the costs of benefits and premiums for self-insured plans are similar to those for group plans. Self-funded plans tend to work best for companies that are large enough to offer good coverage and reasonable premium rates and are able to pay large claims for expensive medical services. Often a **third-party administrator (TPA)** or **fiscal intermediary** handles paperwork and claim payments for a self-insured group.

Self-funded healthcare or self-insurance is an arrangement in which an employer provides health or disability benefits to employees with its own funds or employees for health coverage with their personal funds. This is different from fully insured plans, in which the employer contracts an insurance company to cover the employees and dependents. In self-funded healthcare, the employer assumes the direct risk for payment of the claims for benefits. The terms of eligibility and coverage are set forth in a plan document, which includes provisions similar to those found in a typical group health insurance policy. Unless exempted, such plans create rights and obligations under the Employee Retirement Income Security Act of 1974 (ERISA).

Medical Savings Account

In 1996 Congress made tax-free **medical savings accounts (MSAs)** available to 750,000 American workers and their families. This is a type of self-insurance. Under a provision of the Kassebaum-Kennedy health insurance reform bill, small companies (50 or fewer employees), self-employed individuals, and the uninsured can purchase health insurance policies and make tax-free deposits to an MSA. They can use their MSA money to pay small and routine healthcare expenses, reserving a high-deductible medical insurance policy to pay large, catastrophic expenses. Money that remains in the account at year's end earns tax-free interest. People can also elect to use MSA money to pay their health insurance premiums during a job change, which should reduce *job lock,* a situation in which people do not change jobs for fear of losing their health insurance.

In an MSA program, generally associated with self-employed individuals, tax-deferred deposits can be made for medical expenses. Withdrawals from the MSA are tax free if used to pay for qualified medical expenses. The MSA must be coupled with a high-deductible health plan (HDHP). Withdrawals from MSA go toward paying the deductible expenses in a given year. MSA funds can cover expenses related to most forms of healthcare, disability, dental care, vision care, and long-term care, whether the expenses are billed through the qualifying insurance or otherwise.

Once the plan deductible has been met in a given year, the HDHP pays any remaining covered medical expenses in that year. If there are funds remaining in the MSA at the end of the year, the funds can either roll over for the following year or can be withdrawn as taxable income.

MSAs have been superseded by health savings accounts (HSAs), which were established as part of the Medicare Prescription Drug, Improvement, and Modernization Act of 2003. Existing MSAs were **grandfathered**.

CRITICAL THINKING APPLICATION   20-1

Ann understands how medical assistants can easily become intimidated by all the regulations that affect insurance coverage. Discuss differences and similarities between the different types of insurance companies and insurance coverage. How can the medical assistant effectively keep up with all of the rules pertaining to policies that are frequently presented in the office?

TYPES OF INSURANCE BENEFITS

An insurance package is tailored to the needs of each individual or group policy, and the combinations of benefits are limitless. This is also called "cafeteria style," in which employers can choose the benefits they want for their employees. A policy may contain one or any combination of the benefits described in the following sections (Table 20-1).

Hospitalization

Hospital coverage pays the cost of all or part of the insured person's hospital room and board and specific hospital services, such as the costs involved in having surgery in a hospital. Hospital insurance policies frequently set a maximum amount payable per day and a maximum number of days of hospital care, per the diagnosis-related group (DRG). Some insurance companies require that the hospital be accredited or licensed.

Surgical

Surgical coverage pays all or part of a surgeon's fee; some plans also pay for an assistant surgeon. Surgery includes any incision or excision, removal of foreign bodies, aspiration, suturing, and reduction of fractures. Surgery may be performed in a hospital, physician's office, or elsewhere. The insurer frequently provides the subscriber with a surgical fee schedule that establishes the amount the insurer will pay for commonly performed procedures.

Basic Medical

Basic medical coverage pays all or part of a physician's fee for nonsurgical services, including hospital, home, and office visits. Usually there is a deductible that the patient pays, in addition to a co-payment or co-insurance payment each time service is received. The insurance plan may include a provision for diagnostic laboratory, radiology, and pathology fees. Some medical plans do not cover routine physical examinations or preventive health checkups, such as mammograms or prostate examinations, if the patient does not have a specific complaint or illness.

The Affordable Care Act brings major changes to the healthcare industry, and several of its provisions have already taken effect. Beginning on January 1, 2014, all Americans will have access to affordable health insurance options, according to the HHS website. Some of the key provisions include:

- Prohibiting discrimination due to preexisting conditions based on gender or sex
- Eliminating annual limits on insurance coverage
- Ensuring coverage for individuals who are participating in clinical trials
- Making care more affordable through tax credits that will become available to people with income levels between 100% and 400% of the poverty line who are not eligible for other affordable coverage
- Increasing access to Medicaid, making the federal funding to states payable at 100% for the first 3 years, and 90% thereafter
- Promoting individual responsibility by making coverage mandatory or by charging a fee to those who do not have coverage, both of which will help to offset the costs of coverage

The four core categories of the Act include benefits for hospitalization and ER services, physician and midlevel practitioners care, pharmacy benefits, and laboratory and imaging services. In 2015 and beyond, additional provisions will go into effect, such as paying physicians based upon value and not volume.

TABLE 20-1 Types of Health Insurance and Plan Benefits

BENEFIT	COVERED	PAYS
Hospitalization	Cost of all or part of the hospital room and board; and specific hospital services (i.e., costs involved in having surgery in a hospital)	Maximum amount per day and maximum number of days
Surgical	Any surgical procedure, including but not limited to incision or excision; removal of foreign bodies; aspiration; suturing; reduction of fractures	Surgeon's fee Assistant surgeon's fee
Basic medical	Outpatient and/or physician office procedures and services	Physician's fees diagnostic, radiologic, laboratory, and pathology fees
Major medical	Catastrophic or prolonged illness or injury	Takes over when basic medical, hospitalization, and surgical benefits end
Disability	Accident or illness resulting in an inability for patient to work; can be paid whether work-related or not work related.	Cash benefits paid in lieu of salary while patient is unable to earn an income
Dental care	Preventive care and/or treatment and repair of teeth and gums	Typically pays 100% for preventive care, 50% for repair and treatment
Vision care	Eye exam and glasses	Set benefit amount, depending on vision care policy for examination and/or glasses
Medicare supplement	Deductible and co-insurance amounts unpaid by Medicare	Deductible and co-insurance amounts unpaid by Medicare
Special risk	Certain specific illnesses (cancer, heart failure) or accidents (automobile, airplane)	Typically pays a maximum benefit
Life insurance	Loss of life	Usually a lump sum payment of the life insurance benefit
Long-term care	Long-term skilled nursing or rehabilitation care	Set amount determined by policy benefits

To be in compliance with the Act, insurance plans must consist of 10 essential health benefits (EHBs), including the following provisions:

- Ambulatory patient services
- Emergency services
- Hospitalization
- Maternity and newborn care
- Mental health and substance abuse disorder services, including behavior health services
- Prescription drugs
- Rehabilitative and habilitative services and devices
- Laboratory services
- Preventative services and wellness services, as well as chronic disease management
- Pediatric services, including oral and vision care

Disability (Loss of Income) Protection

Disability insurance is a form of insurance that insures the beneficiary's earned income against the risk that a disability will make working uncomfortable (as with psychological disorders), painful (as with back pain), or impossible (as with coma). It encompasses paid sick leave, short-term disability benefits, and long-term disability benefits.

Weekly or monthly cash benefits are provided to employed policyholders who become unable to work as a result of an accident or illness. Many disability policies do not start payment until after a specified number of days or until a certain number of sick leave days have been used. Payment is made directly to the individual and is intended to replace lost income resulting from an illness or other disability. It is not intended for payment of specific medical bills, and it should not be confused with a regular insurance plan, entitlement program, or workers' compensation, in which compensation is provided for an employee who is injured on the job or cannot work as a result of a job-related illness or other disability.

Dental Care

Dental benefits programs offer a variety of options in the form of either fee-for-service or managed care plans that reimburse a portion of a patient's dental expenses and may exclude certain treatments.

Dental coverage is included in many fringe benefit packages. Some policies are based on a co-payment and incentive program, in which preventive dental care (e.g., cleaning and x-ray films) is covered 100%, with most other coverage paid at 50%.

Vision Care

Vision care insurance may include reimbursement for all or a percentage of the cost for refraction, lenses, and frames. Some vision plans also pay for corrective procedures, such as laser eye surgery.

Medicare Supplement

Many Medicare beneficiaries purchase a supplemental health insurance policy to help defray medical costs not covered or only partially covered by Medicare. Federal regulations now require Medicare supplement contracts to be uniform in benefits to avoid confusion for the purchaser. Medicare supplements that cover Medicare recipients' out-of-pocket expenses, including the deductible and co-insurance payments, are called **Medigap** policies.

Special Risk Insurance

Special risk insurance protects a person in the event of a certain type of accident, such as an automobile or airplane crash, or for certain diseases, such as tuberculosis or cancer. There is usually a maximum benefit.

Liability Insurance

Liability insurance covers losses to a third party caused by the insured. There are many types of liability insurance, including automobile, business, and homeowners' policies. Liability policies often include benefits for medical expenses resulting from traumatic injuries, lost wages, and sometimes pain and suffering payable to individuals who are injured in the insured person's home or car, without regard to the insured person's actual legal liability for the accident.

Life Insurance

Life insurance provides payment of a specified amount on the insured's death, either to his or her estate or to a designated beneficiary or, in the case of an endowment policy, to the policyholder at a specified date. Life insurance policies sometimes provide monthly cash benefits if the policyholder becomes permanently and totally disabled. Sometimes the proceeds from life insurance are used to meet the expenses of the insured person's last illness.

Long-Term Care Insurance

Long-term care insurance is a relatively new type of insurance that covers a broad range of maintenance and health services for chronically ill, disabled, or mentally retarded individuals. Services may be provided on an inpatient basis (at a rehabilitation facility, nursing home, or mental hospital), on an outpatient basis, or at home. The **Health Insurance Portability and Accountability Act (HIPAA)** of 1996 improved access to long-term care services and coverage.

HOW BENEFITS ARE DETERMINED

Insurance benefits may be determined and paid in one of several ways:

- Indemnity schedules
- Service benefit plans
- Resource-based relative value scale (RBRVS)
- Determination of the usual, customary, and reasonable (UCR) fees

Indemnity Schedules

An indemnity health insurance plan, also known as *major medical,* is a more flexible yet more costly option. Many people refer to this as a traditional plan, because it preceded the advent of managed care (e.g., health maintenance organizations, preferred provider organizations, and point of service [POS] plans).

Indemnity plans, or schedules, are traditional health insurance plans that pay for all or a share of the cost of covered services, regardless of which physician, hospital, or other licensed healthcare provider is used. Because physicians and other providers are paid for each office visit, test, procedure, or other service they deliver, indemnity plans are often called fee for service plans.

Policyholders of indemnity plans and their dependents choose when and where to get healthcare services. In exchange for premiums that members pay, the indemnity plan reimburses members or the provider when claims are filed. When the policy is purchased, the subscriber is often given a schedule of indemnities (i.e., a fee schedule), which explains the benefit payment amounts. Indemnity benefits are usually paid to the person insured unless that person has authorized payment directly to the provider, which is a common practice.

Service Benefit Plans

In **service benefit plans**, the insuring company agrees to pay for certain surgical or medical services without additional cost to the person insured. There is no set fee schedule. In a service benefit plan, surgery with complications would warrant a higher fee than an uncomplicated procedure. Premiums are sometimes higher for this type of coverage, but often payments are larger. Frequently payment of benefits is sent directly to the physician and is considered full payment for services rendered. Consider this example: the service benefit plan states that it will pay $900 for a cholecystectomy. If Dr. Jones charges $1,500 for this procedure, he has the right either to accept the $900 as payment in full and write off the balance due, or to request payment of the remaining $600 balance from the patient or the **guarantor** (i.e., the individual or group responsible for payment).

Resource-Based Relative Value Scale

The CMS annually publishes physician fee schedule information on its Web site, in addition to the formula for calculating physician fee schedule payment amounts. Physician fee schedule amounts vary, depending on *facility* or *nonfacility*. Physicians who own their own facility (e.g., office) would not use the facility columns on the Medicare Fee Service Schedule. Entities such as hospitals, skilled nursing centers, nursing homes, and rehabilitation hospitals should all be classified as facilities. Facility rates are almost always lower than nonfacility rates, but when the physician treats the patient at a facility, he or she should receive facility rates. The amount of resources required to perform a service is determined through the use of *relative value units* (RVUs), which the CMS assigns to the *Current Procedural Terminology* (CPT) codes (see Chapter 19). This system was implemented to standardize payment while providing an adjustment for overhead costs in different geographic areas. The formula for calculating payment takes into consideration these elements: physician expense, malpractice, geographic practice cost index, and the conversion factor. Since Medicare introduced the **resource-based relative value scale (RBRVS)** in 1992, most third-party payers have adopted similar approaches in developing their fees.

Usual, Customary, and Reasonable Fee

Some insurance companies agree to pay on the basis of all or a percentage of a usual, customary, and reasonable (UCR) fee. Charges for a specific service are compared with a database showing (1) charges to other patients for the same service by the same type of physician and (2) charges to patients by other physicians performing the same or similar services in the same geographic area. The insurance company determines whether the provider's charge is UCR, and any amount over the allowed charge is not paid. Sometimes *UCR* is used synonymously with *fee allowance schedule* when that schedule is set relatively high.

HEALTH INSURANCE PROVIDERS

Health insurance providers include managed care plans, Blue Cross/Blue Shield (BC/BS), **commercial insurance** companies, and federal and state government programs, including Medicare, Medicaid, TRICARE, workers' compensation, and disability insurance.

Managed Care

Managed care is an umbrella term for all healthcare plans that provide healthcare in return for preset scheduled payments and coordinated care through a defined network of physicians and hospitals. **Managed care plans** are healthcare plans that provide healthcare in return for scheduled payments and that coordinate healthcare through a defined network of **primary care providers (PCPs)**, hospitals, and other providers. The passage of the Health Maintenance Organization Act in 1973 provided for federal aid to health insurance prepayment plans that met certain criteria. This brought about a rapid growth in **health maintenance organizations (HMOs)**; an HMO provides comprehensive healthcare to an enrolled group for a fixed periodic payment. Some of these plans pay by **capitation**, which means that the provider is paid a fixed amount for each individual enrolled in the plan during a specified period (usually 1 year), regardless of the expenses or number of services provided to the patient.

It is important for the medical assistant to be familiar with individual managed care contract benefits and with the procedures and processes for filing insurance claims. Reviewing a managed care plan's specific handbook, contracts, and required forms should always be part of a medical assistant's routine. This familiarizes the medical assistant with that plan's benefits and preauthorization and referral requirements, which enables him or her to discuss those requirements with the patient and to prepare the required forms and insurance claims properly. Procedure 20-1 describes the process for properly applying managed care policies and procedures.

PROCEDURE 20-1

Apply Managed Care Policies and Procedures

CAAHEP COMPETENCIES: II.C.II. 1., IV.C.IV.6., IV.P.IV.3., V. P.V.6., VII.P.VII.1., IX.A.IX.2.

ABHES COMPETENCIES: 3.t

GOAL: *To act within the guidelines of the managed care contracts that the physician and/or medical facility has partnered.*

EQUIPMENT and SUPPLIES

- Managed care contracts
- Managed care handbooks
- Forms from managed care organizations

PROCEDURAL STEPS

1. Determine which managed care organization the patient belongs to.
   PURPOSE: To make certain the right information is applied to the right patient.

2. Read and study the policies and procedures that are set forth by the managed care organization.
   PURPOSE: To understand and abide by the regulations that apply to a specific patient.

3. Make certain that a signature is on file for the patient.
   PURPOSE: The signature authorizes the provider to release medical information to the insurance carrier and authorizes the carrier to pay the provider directly.

4. Determine the procedures and services to be billed on the claim.
   PURPOSE: To ensure that all procedures and services are included in the review of the managed care plan.

5. Determine whether all procedures and services to be billed are covered by the managed care plan.

   PURPOSE: To understand which services are covered, which are noncovered, and which require special forms for billing. This also helps the medical assistant explain to patients the benefits covered and the steps that must be taken for procedures and services requiring preapproval.

6. Obtain any forms that are needed to process patient claims.
   PURPOSE: To submit the correct forms to the managed care organization.

7. Become familiar with the information in managed care policy manuals and handbooks.
   PURPOSE: By becoming familiar with handbooks and guidelines, the medical assistant will be able to assist patients in finding needed information.

8. Determine whom to contact in case of questions about the various managed care organizations.
   PURPOSE: To be able to refer patients to the best source of information when they have questions or concerns.

9. Attend seminars and workshops when offered by the managed care organizations.
   PURPOSE: To stay up-to-date on information and policies.

10. Use information gained on a daily basis when working with managed care organizations.

TABLE 20-2 Comparison of HMO Models

MODEL	STRUCTURE	BILLING MODEL
IPA	General or family practice physician or physician group that practices independently and may contract with several IPAs	Capitation or fee for service
Staff	One or more physicians hired by an HMO	Salaried
Group	Multispecialty group with or without a PCP (gatekeeper); may contract with several IPAs	Capitation or fee for service

HMO, Health maintenance organization; *IPA,* Independent practice association; *PCP,* primary care provider.

Managed Care Policies and Procedures

Managed care has been met with considerable controversy, and it has pros and cons that must be considered. It is important that medical assistants be well versed in the various types of managed care plans to fully understand their impact on healthcare costs.

Advantages of managed care include the following:

- Healthcare costs are usually contained.
- Established fee schedules are used.
- Authorized services are usually paid for.
- Most preventive medical treatment is covered.
- Patients' out-of-pocket expenses tend to be less than with traditional insurance.

Disadvantages of managed care include the following:

- Access to specialized care and referrals can be limited.
- Physicians' choices in the treatment of patients can be limited.
- More paperwork may be required.
- Treatment may be delayed because of preauthorization requirements.
- Reimbursement historically is less than with traditional insurance.

Models of Managed Care

The two basic models of managed care are the HMO and the preferred provider organization (PPO). The HMO can be structured as an independent practice association (IPA), a staff model, or a group model or as an exclusive provider organization (EPO) (Table 20-2).
Health Maintenance Organization. As mentioned, an HMO is a plan that contracts with a medical center or group of physicians to provide both preventive and acute care for the insured. HMOs are state-licensed health plans that are regulated by HMO laws, which require them to include preventive care, such as routine physical examinations and other services, as part of their benefits package. HMOs always require referrals to specialists, precertification, and preauthorization for hospital admissions, outpatient procedures, and treatments.

An HMO member is typically enrolled for a specified period (month, quarter, or year). If the HMO is a capitation plan, it receives a "per member per month" (pmpm) fee for each enrollee.

Providers receive payment according to various structures. The two most common structures are capitation and **fee for service.**

Capitation is payment in advance to the provider by the HMO for a contracted group of patients, regardless of how often the patients are seen and even if the patients are never seen by the provider. If the physician provides services that cost less than the capitation amount, the physician makes a profit. Conversely, if the physician's services cost more than the capitation amount, the physician takes a loss. Fees charged for services to group members may be billed directly to the IPA rather than to the patient. Fees for services to nonmember patients are handled in the same manner as any other fee for service. The payment structure is based on the type of HMO model and the contract negotiated between the HMO and the provider or providers. The most common HMO models are the IPA, staff model, group model, and EPO.

Independent Practice Association. An IPA is an independent group of physicians and other healthcare providers who are under contract to provide services to members of different HMOs, in addition to other insurance plans, usually at a fixed fee per patient. The physicians in the IPA, who have separately owned practices, formally organize a physician association and continue to practice in their own offices. A physician may be contracted with several IPAs. Payments to providers by an IPA can be structured either as a capitation or fee for service.

Staff Model. A staff model HMO hires physicians and pays them a salary. Rather than contracting with physicians to create a network, the HMO owns the network. Medical care is given or authorized by the patient's PCP. No capitation or fee for service payment structure is used with the staff model; however, the physicians may receive bonuses biannually or annually based on the number of patients treated and/or the cost savings.

Group Model. A group model HMO contracts with a multispecialty medical group to deliver care to its members. The HMO reimburses the physicians' group, which is responsible for reimbursing physician members and contracted healthcare facilities. This arrangement is similar to an IPA in that the multispecialty group may organize a physician association; however, the group members typically practice together in one facility. The payment structure to the providers can be either capitation or fee for service.

Exclusive Provider Organization. An EPO combines features of an HMO (e.g., an enrolled group or population, primary care providers, and an authorization system) and a PPO (e.g., flexible benefit design, and fee-for-service payments). The plan is referred to as "exclusive" because employers agree not to contract with any other plan. Members must choose medical care from network providers, with certain exceptions for emergency or out-of-area services. If a patient decides to seek care outside the network, he or she generally is not reimbursed for the cost of treatment. Technically, many HMOs can be considered EPOs; however, EPOs are regulated under insurance statutes rather than federal and state HMO regulations.
Preferred Provider Organizations. Sometimes called a *participating provider organization,* a PPO is a managed care network of physicians and hospitals that have joined to contract with insurance companies, employers, or other organizations to provide healthcare to subscribers for a discounted fee. The PPO model of managed healthcare preserves the fee-for-service concept that many physicians prefer. An insurer representing its clients contracts with a group of providers; the providers agree on a predetermined list of charges for all services, including those for both normal and complex

procedures. Unlike HMOs, PPOs have no capitation or prepaid care. Typically the patient pays deductibles or co-insurance payments of 20% to 25% of the predetermined charge, and the insurer pays the balance. A provider who joins a PPO does not need to alter the manner of providing care and continues to treat and bill the patients on a fee-for-service basis. When a patient covered under a PPO plan comes for treatment, the physician treats the patient and bills the PPO.

Technically PPOs are not HMOs, but they do have more patient care management than regular indemnity insurance plans. PPOs furnish their subscribers with a list of member-providers from which subscribers can receive healthcare at PPO rates. Rates are quite often lower than those charged to non-PPO patients. If a patient goes to a physician who is not in the PPO network, the out-of-pocket cost is higher.

CRITICAL THINKING APPLICATION   20-2

The physicians in the practice where Ann works are not members of a PPO that is often used in their geographic area. Many patients are confused when they have to pay a larger out-of-pocket fee for their medical services. How can Ann explain the reason for these higher fees to patients?

Blue Cross/Blue Shield

Blue Cross/Blue Shield is America's oldest and largest system of independent health insurers. It began in 1929 when an executive at Baylor University in Dallas came up with a plan for teachers to budget for their future hospital bills.

BC/BS offers incentive contracts to healthcare providers. If the provider chooses to sign a member contract, he or she becomes a **participating provider (PAR)**. Participating providers agree to write off the difference or balance between the amount charged by the provider and the approved fee established by the insurer. They also agree to bill the patient only for the deductible and co-pay/co-insurance amounts that are based on BC/BS-allowed fees and the full charge fee for any uncovered service. In turn, BC/BS agrees to reimburse providers directly and in a shorter time.

BC/BS identification (ID) cards (Figure 20-1) carry the subscriber's name and ID number with a three-character alphabetic prefix (or a single alphabetic prefix if it is a government policy). The letters are an important part of the number and must be included on the claim form.

Most BC/BS benefits are based on the fee-for-service or UCR schedules for payment, although certain types of managed care contracts also are available, primarily to group employers.

Medicaid

As mentioned, Title XIX of Public Law 89-97 under the Social Security Amendments of 1965 provided for agreements with states for assistance from the federal government in providing healthcare for the medically indigent. All states and the District of Columbia have Medicaid programs, but these programs vary widely. A person eligible for Medicaid in one state may not be eligible in another state, and the services may differ.

The federal government provides basic funding to the state, after which the states individually elect whether to provide funds for extension of benefits. The state determines the type and extent of medical care that will be covered within the minimum requirements established by the federal government. Some local areas and states are developing HMOs that serve only patients who qualify for Medicaid.

A physician may accept or decline to treat Medicaid patients. The physician who does accept Medicaid patients automatically agrees to accept Medicaid payment as payment in full for covered services. The patient cannot be billed for the difference between the Medicaid fee and the physician's normal fee. The patient can be billed for any services that are not covered by Medicaid. Eligibility for benefits is determined by the respective states.

Examples of those who qualify for benefits include the following:

- Individuals who are medically needy
- Recipients of Aid to Families with Dependent Children (AFDC)
- Individuals who receive Supplemental Security Income (SSI)
- Individuals who receive certain types of federal and state aid
- Individuals who are qualified Medicare beneficiaries (QMBs)—Medicaid pays for Medicare Part B premiums, deductibles, and co-insurance for qualified low-income elderly
- Individuals in institutions or receiving long-term care in nursing facilities and intermediate-care facilities

Depending on the state in which Medicaid is administered, Medicaid recipients are identified with a Benefits ID Card (BIC), a monthly sticker, a label, or a letter showing proof of eligibility. A BIC looks like a white credit card (Figure 20-2) and is verified by a

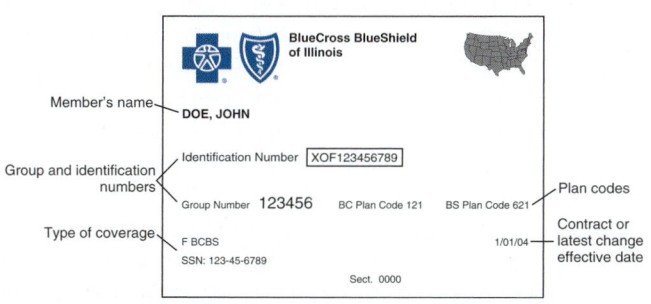

FIGURE 20-1 Blue Cross/Blue Shield identification card.

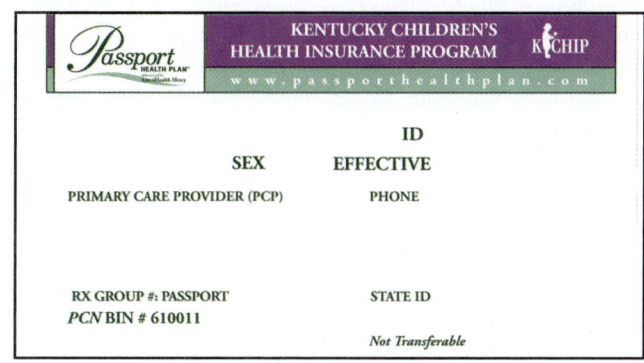

FIGURE 20-2 Medicaid Benefits ID Card.

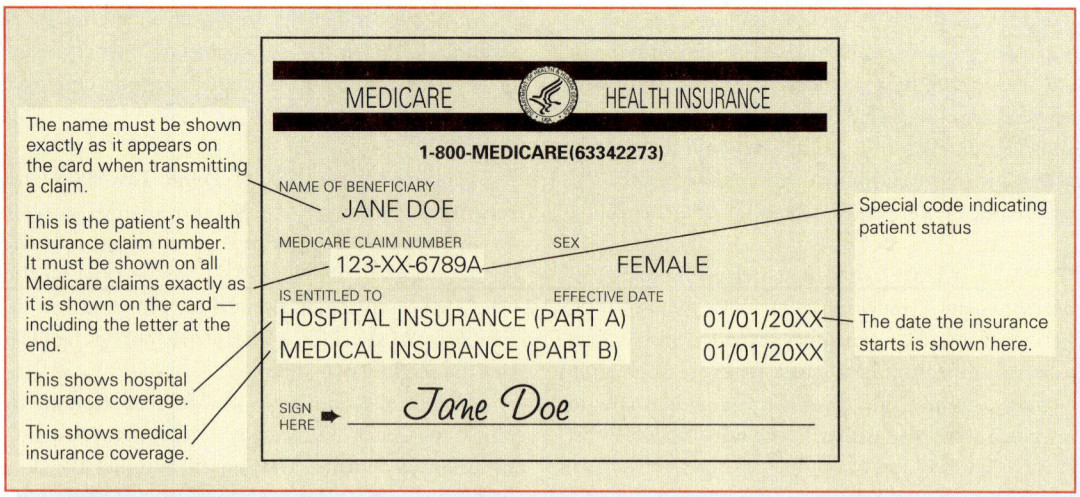

FIGURE 20-3 Medicare health identification card. (From Fordney MT: *Insurance handbook for the medical office,* ed 12, St Louis, 2012, WB Saunders.)

point of service (POS) device similar to a credit or debit card verification machine. The medical assistant must verify coverage each time the patient comes into the office, regardless of the type of ID the recipient is issued.

Medicare

Medicare is a federal health insurance program for the following:
- People age 65 years or older
- People who are permanently disabled or blind
- People receiving dialysis for permanent kidney failure or who have undergone kidney transplantation

Medicare was established July 1, 1966, under the Social Security Administration as a national health insurance program for those age 65 or older. Before Medicare was created, only 50% of the nation's elderly had any health insurance. Today Medicare is the world's largest insurance program. It serves more than 38 million older and disabled Americans. The scope of coverage increased in 1973 to include disabled persons younger than age 65 receiving Social Security benefits, railroad retirees, and civil service retirees. It also included disabled workers of any age, disabled widows, disabled dependent widowers, adults disabled before age 18 whose parents are eligible or are retired on Social Security benefits, children and adults with end-stage renal disease, and living kidney donors (including all expenses related to the kidney transplantation).

Medicare is administered by the CMS, which is a division of the Department of Health and Human Services (DHHS). The Medicare program is regulated by laws enacted by Congress. Medicare has two parts that cover healthcare services, Part A and Part B.

Medicare Part A

Part A is hospital insurance. Retired people 65 years of age or older and people who receive monthly Social Security or railroad retirement checks are automatically enrolled for hospital insurance benefits and pay no premiums for this insurance. Part A covers the following:
- Inpatient hospital care
- Skilled nursing facilities

- Home healthcare
- Hospice services

Part A is financed with special contributions deducted from employed individuals' salaries, with matching contributions from their employers. These sums are collected, along with regular Social Security contributions, from wages and self-employment income earned during a person's working years. A hospitalized patient on Medicare must pay a deductible toward hospital expenses. Typically the deductible amount changes annually by congressional enactment.

Medicare Part B

Part B is medical insurance. Those eligible for Part A are also eligible for Part B, but they must apply for this coverage and pay a monthly premium. Some federal employees and former federal employees who are not eligible for Social Security benefits and Part A may enroll in Part B. Certain disabled people younger than age 65 are also eligible. Part B covers the following:
- Outpatient hospital care
- Durable medical equipment
- Physicians' services
- Other medical services

A patient with Medicare Part B must meet an annual deductible before benefits become available, after which Medicare pays 80% of the covered, or allowed, benefits. Usually the physician accepts assignment of benefits for Medicare patients and is paid directly. In these cases the physician must accept the payment that Medicare allows and bills the patient only for 20% of the charge allowed by Medicare. If the physician does not accept assignment, the patient must pay the entire bill (which cannot be greater than the limit set by Medicare for nonparticipating physicians), and the patient receives a reimbursement check directly from Medicare.

Medicare health insurance cards (Figure 20-3) typically show nine numbers with a suffix of one or two alphabetic characters that denote the patient's status, such as wage earner (A), spouse of a wage earner (B), widow (D), or other designations. The health insurance claim number (HICN) or health identification card number (HIC#)

also identifies whether a person has Part A alone or both Part A and Part B insurance. If a patient's Medicare card has a claim number ending in the letter A, the HICN is the same as the person's Social Security number. If a patient's Medicare card has a claim number ending in B or D, the person's Social Security number is different from his or her issued HICN.

Many Medicare enrollees also carry private supplemental insurance that pays the deductible and the 20% co-payment not covered by Medicare. As mentioned, if the supplemental policy pays the deductible and the 20% co-payment, it is called a *Medigap policy*.

Medicare Advantage (formerly Medicare + Choice)

The Medicare Advantage program is commonly referred to as Part C, although Medicare does not label it as such. Medicare Advantage offers expanded benefits for a fee through private health insurance programs such as HMOs and PPOs that have contracts with Medicare. Patients must have a referral from their PCP before seeking treatment from another entity.

Medicare Part D

In 2006, drug and prescription benefits were added to Medicare, creating Part D. Medicare Part D gives Medicare recipients the option to choose, at a reduced cost, a prescription drug plan that pays for prescription drugs with just a small co-payment by the patient. Everyone with Medicare can get this coverage, which may help lower prescription drug costs and protect against higher costs in the future.

Private companies provide the Medicare prescription drug plans. Beneficiaries choose the drug plan and pay a monthly premium. As with other insurance, beneficiaries who decide not to enroll in a drug plan when they are first eligible may pay a penalty if they choose to join later.

TRICARE

TRICARE is the comprehensive healthcare program for family members of active duty personnel, military retirees and their eligible family members under the age of 65, and survivors of all uniformed services. (Before January, 1994, this program was known as CHAMPUS, created in 1966 under Public Law 89-614.)

The TRICARE program is managed by the military in partnership with civilian hospitals and clinics. It is designed to expand access to healthcare, ensure high-quality care, and promote medical readiness. All military hospitals and clinics are part of the TRICARE program and offer high-quality healthcare at low costs to plan users.

To be eligible for TRICARE, an individual must be a TRICARE or CHAMPVA recipient; must be entitled to retired, retainer, or equivalent pay; and must be listed in the Defense Department's Defense Enrollment Eligible Reporting System (DEERS), a computerized database that lists all active and retired service members. Coverage is also available for a TRICARE-eligible spouse under age 65 and dependent, unmarried children under age 21, or age 23 if in college full-time. Eligible spouses and children of active duty service members may enroll, as may TRICARE-eligible widows, widowers, and certain former spouses (those who have not remarried).

TRICARE offers three types of plans. More information about TRICARE eligibility requirements and the benefits of the three plans is available on the Evolve Web site *(evolve.elsevier.com/kinn)*.
- TRICARE Prime: The Department of Defense's managed care plan, similar to a civilian HMO
- TRICARE Extra: A preferred provider network plan
- TRICARE Standard: A traditional fee-for-service plan (formerly CHAMPUS)

CHAMPVA

CHAMPVA, a health benefits program similar to TRICARE, was established in 1973 for the spouses and dependent children of veterans suffering total, permanent, service-connected disabilities and for surviving spouses and dependent children of veterans who had died as a result of service-related disabilities. The Department of Veterans Affairs (VA) shares with eligible beneficiaries the cost of certain healthcare services and supplies. After eligibility for CHAMPVA has been determined and ID cards issued, the insured may obtain covered services and supplies from any provider who is appropriately licensed or certified to perform the services offered. Exceptions include certain mental health categories and freestanding ambulatory surgical centers.

Workers' Compensation

Federal and all state legislatures require employers to maintain workers' compensation coverage to meet minimum standards, covering a majority of employees, for work-related illnesses and injuries, as long as the employee was not negligent in performing the assigned duties. The law also protects wage earners against the loss of wages and the cost of medical care resulting from occupational accident or disease. State laws differ as to the classes of employees included and the benefits provided.

No state's workers' compensation laws cover all employees. However, if a patient says that he or she was injured in the workplace or is suffering from a work-associated illness, the medical assistant should check with the patient's employer to verify the insurance coverage.

Compensation benefits include medical care benefits, weekly income replacement benefits for temporary disability, permanent disability settlements, and survivor benefits when applicable. The provider of service (e.g., doctor, hospital, therapist) accepts the workers' compensation payment as payment in full and does not bill the patient. Time limitations are set for the prompt reporting of workers' compensation cases. The employee is obligated to promptly notify the employer; the employer, in turn, must notify the insurance company and must refer the employee to a source of medical care.

The purpose of workers' compensation laws is to provide prompt medical care to an injured or ill worker so that the person may be restored to health and return to full earning capacity in as short a time as possible.

Disability Programs

Disability income insurance is a form of health insurance that provides periodic payments to an individual to replace income (actual or presumed) when a sickness, injury, or disability that is not a work-related condition results in the insured being unable to work.

PROCEDURE 20-2

Apply Third-Party Guidelines

CAAHEP COMPETENCIES: II.C.II. 1., IV.C.IV.6., IV.P.IV.3., V. P.V.6., VII.P.VII.2., IX.A.IX.2.

ABHES COMPETENCIES: 8.c

GOAL: *To ensure that claims are processed quickly and result in the highest allowable reimbursement.*

EQUIPMENT and SUPPLIES

- Insurance carrier contracts (sample provided in student workbook)
- Insurance carrier handbooks (sample provided in student workbook)
- Clerical supplies
- Forms from insurance carrier
- Insurance claim forms (CMS-1500)

PROCEDURAL STEPS

1. Determine the patient's health insurance plan.
   PURPOSE: To bill the correct health insurance plan for services rendered.
2. Review the rules and regulations that govern that particular organization.
   PURPOSE: To be sure that the claim is accurate according to the guidelines in place for the patient's policy.
3. Make certain that a signature is on file for the patient.
   PURPOSE: The signature authorizes the provider to release medical information to the insurance carrier and authorizes the carrier to pay the provider directly.
4. Determine the procedures and services that are to be billed on the claim.
   PURPOSE: To ensure that all procedures and services are included in the review of the managed care plan.

5. Determine whether all procedures and services to be billed are covered by the health insurance plan.
   PURPOSE: To understand which services are covered, which are not covered, and which require special forms for billing. This also assists the medical assistant in explaining to patients the benefits covered and the steps that must be taken for procedures and services requiring preapproval. Procedures and services that are not covered should not be billed on the health insurance claim form; the patient must pay for those services.
6. Make sure that the patient is aware of any procedures that will not be covered by the health insurance plan.
   PURPOSE: To ensure that the patient understands what is covered or not covered, what the patient's financial obligation is, and what special procedures (e.g., preauthorization) must be performed, when applicable.
7. Pay close attention to the blocks on the insurance claim form that are designated "for local use."
   PURPOSE: These blocks are designed to include information particular to certain policies. The carrier manual (for that insurance company) will provide instruction as to what information should be included in that block.
8. Submit the claim to the correct insurance company address or clearinghouse.

A disability insurance policy can be obtained through employer-sponsored and/or government-funded programs, or private policies can be purchased through a commercial insurance company.

COMMERCIAL INSURANCE

Many people are covered by health insurance issued by private (commercial) insurance companies (e.g., Aetna, Connecticut General, Metropolitan, and Prudential). Physicians and medical societies control neither the premiums paid nor the benefits received from such policies. For traditional types of policies, payment is normally made to the subscriber unless the subscriber or insured has authorized that payment be made directly to the physician.

UNDERSTANDING INSURANCE PLAN REQUIREMENTS

It is important for the medical assistant to be familiar with the particular procedures and processes for filing insurance claims set by individual insurance carriers, third-party payers, and government programs. The medical assistant also must be familiar with the handling of other tasks associated with an individual insurance plan or policy. Medical assistants should make it part of their routine to review the carrier's handbook, contracts, and required forms to familiarize themselves with the plan's benefits and preauthorization

and referral requirements. This equips the medical assistant to discuss those requirements with the patient and to prepare the required forms and insurance claims properly. Procedure 20-2 describes the process for properly applying third-party payer policies and procedures.

CRITICAL THINKING APPLICATION   20-3

Ann has been working with Mike Holland, who is having coronary bypass surgery in 1 week. Discuss the possible differences in Mike's coverage if he has Medicare, Medicaid, or commercial insurance. Should the medical assistant explain other bills, such as those to the hospital and anesthesiologist?

UTILIZATION MANAGEMENT/UTILIZATION REVIEW

Utilization management is a form of patient care review by health-care professionals who do not provide the care. It is a necessary component of managed care to control costs. A **utilization review** committee reviews individual cases to make certain that medical care services are medically necessary (the specificity of diagnosis coding is critical) and to study how providers use medical care resources. This committee also reviews all physician referrals and cases

Verification of Eligibility & Benefits Form

Today's Date: _____ Patient Name: _____

Date of Birth: _____ Social Security Number: _____

Primary Insurance: _____ Phone Number: _____

Plan Identification Number: _____ Group Number: _____

Insured's Name: _____ Insured's SS# _____

Is This Plan a: ☐ PPO In Network ☐ PPO Out of Network ☐ Commercial/Indemnity

If out of network:

What is the benefit for surgery? _____% of the doctor's fee or, $_____ for

procedure. Is the copay for office visits different? ☐ Yes ☐ No _____

Insurance Effective Date: _____ Deductible Amt: $_____

Has the deductible been met this year? ☐ Yes ☐ No If no, amount remaining: $_____

Is it a calendar year (if no, note renewal date) ☐ Yes ☐ No _____

Copay for Office Visits: $_____ Can we collect copay during post op period? ☐ Yes ☐ No

Do we bill separately for x-rays during the post op period (example: hands)? ☐ Yes ☐ No

Pre-Existing Conditions? _____

	Approved Facilities	Pre-Authorization Needed (Y/N)	Separate Deductible? Note $ and Max.	Dollar Out of Pocket Max Per Year?
Laboratory				
Diagnostic Tests				
Surgery				

Where Do We Send the Claim?_____

_____

I Spoke With: _____ Direct Line: _____

Employee Initials: _____

FIGURE 20-4 Sample Verification of Insurance Benefits form.

of emergency department visits and urgent care. For referrals, the committee reviews the referral and either approves or denies it, so it is important to submit exact documentation and precise statements. The medical assistant should contact the utilization review department directly; it should never be left to the patient or covered member to contact this department.

VERIFICATION OF INSURANCE BENEFITS

It is important to verify insurance benefits before providing services to patients. Verifying benefits is necessary to ensure that the patient is covered by insurance and to determine what benefits will be paid for routine and special procedures and services. Verification protects the physician and the patient against unexpected medical care costs. An example of a Verification of Insurance Benefits form is shown in Figure 20-4. To verify benefits, the following steps should be taken (Procedure 20-3):

1. When a patient calls for an appointment, identify the type of insurance the patient has or the managed care organization to which the patient belongs.
2. When the patient arrives for the appointment, photocopy both sides of the patient's ID card. This is done to ensure the

Perform Verification of Eligibility and Benefits

CAAHEP COMPETENCIES: II.C.II. 1., IV.C.IV.6., IV.P.IV.3., V. P.V.6., VII.P.VII.6., IX.A.IX.2.

ABHES COMPETENCIES: 3.t

GOAL: *To confirm that the patient's insurance is in effect; to determine the benefits covered, exclusions, and noncovered procedures and services; and to determine whether precertifications are included or required.*

EQUIPMENT and SUPPLIES

- Patient record
- Verification of eligibility and benefits form
- Patient's insurance information
- Telephone and fax machine
- Pen

PROCEDURAL STEPS

1. When a patient calls for an appointment, identify the patient's insurance plan or managed care organization.
   PURPOSE: To prepare for and begin gathering required information to perform both insurance verification and insurance claim completion procedures.
2. At the time of the appointment, obtain and photocopy both sides of the patient's insurance ID card or cards.
   PURPOSE: To ensure that the correct ID, group, and policy numbers are obtained, in addition to the name, address, and phone number of the insurance carrier or carriers.
3. Complete the patient portion of the Verification of Eligibility and Benefits form, including demographic and insurance information for the patient and the contact information for the insurance plan. Complete one form for each of the patient's insurance plans.

PURPOSE: To document the information needed to perform the verification of eligibility and benefits. This form will later be filed in the patient's insurance record.

4. Contact the insurance carrier or carriers by phone to:
   - Verify that the patient is eligible for benefits and the insurance is in effect.
   - Determine the basic benefits, exclusions, and noncovered services of the insurance plan.
   - Determine whether there are deductibles, co-payments, or any other out-of-pocket expenses the patient is responsible for paying.
   - Determine whether preauthorization is required for referrals to specialists or for any procedures and/or services.
   PURPOSE: To confirm that the insurance is in effect and to determine benefits, preauthorizations, deductibles, and/or out-of-pocket expenses for which the patient is responsible.
5. Obtain the name, title, and phone number of the person to contact.
   PURPOSE: To identify and document the name of the individual providing the benefits and eligibility information and to serve as a reference if additional questions arise.
6. Document the information collected in the patient's medical record and on the Verification of Eligibility and Benefits form.

information obtained is correct, and because co-payments or amounts to be paid may appear on the back for hospital, office, and emergency department visits.

3. Contact the insurance carrier to verify that the patient is eligible for benefits and determine the basic benefits, exclusions or noncovered services; also find out whether preauthorization is required for referrals to specialists or for specific types of procedures and services.
4. Obtain the name, title, and phone number of the person contacted.
5. Document the information collected in the patient's medical record and on a verification of benefits form.
6. Give the patient a letter to read and sign that outlines his or her insurance plan's requirements and possible restrictions or noncovered items. This letter can also outline the patient's responsibility in helping with this process (Figure 20-5).
7. When referrals are required, explain the procedure to the patient; make sure he or she understands that without the referral, the patient is responsible for paying for the physician's services.
8. Collect any co-payments or deductibles.

PRECERTIFICATION AND PREAUTHORIZATION

Many insurance companies require precertification or **preauthorization**, usually within 24 hours, if a patient is to be hospitalized or undergo certain procedures. In addition, most managed care systems require preauthorization for a patient to be referred to a specialist or even for certain laboratory tests or other procedures. Insurance claims for payment will be denied if proper authorization is not obtained.

When a new patient makes an appointment, it is standard procedure to ask what type of insurance the patient has and to collect the patient's and insured's personal, employment, and insurance information on a patient registration form. If the patient belongs to an HMO, the medical assistant should check that plan contract for precertification or preauthorization requirements. This information may be obtained verbally, but it should also be documented in writing or in the electronic medical record and should be obtained before any procedures or treatments are begun. The following information should be obtained and recorded on the preauthorization form (Figure 20-6) before the insurance carrier is contacted:

- Patient's name, address, phone number, and identification number or numbers

Doctor Sample, M.D.

1234 Any Street

Any Town, USA 12345

123-456-7890

Notice to Patients:

Due to multiple policy changes for the different insurance companies, this office is unable to keep up with the requirements for each patient's individual policy. There are multiple requirements stated in your policy; some of which are on the back of your insurance card and some of which are not.

Some of the most common requirements are:
- Referrals to or from Primary Care Physicians
- Prior Authorizations for some Procedures and Services
    o Hospital Admission
    o Pre-Admission Testing
    o Surgery
    o Outpatient Procedures: Laboratory, Radiology, etc.
- Co-pay amounts
    o Primary Care Physicians
    o Specialists
    o Testing: Laboratory, X-ray, etc.
- Pre-Admission Testing
- Second Opinions

Our office checks on these particular requirements for our patients. But if you do not ask the insurance company about a particular requirement, <u>point blank</u>, they will not volunteer any information.

IT IS YOUR RESPONSIBILITY TO BE AWARE OF AND FULFILL ALL THE REQUIREMENTS OF YOUR INSURANCE POLICY.

Our office will be happy to assist you in any matter in accomplishing this task — **but you are responsible for informing us of your insurance company requirements.**

I understand that should the insurance information I have provided be incorrect, and a claim is denied, I will be responsible for the bill.

Patient's Signature: _____ Date: _____

FIGURE 20-5 Sample Patient Responsibility Notification.

- Provider's name, address, phone number, and provider identification number (PIN)
- Insurance plan's name, address, and contact person
- Telephone number (or numbers) of the contact person and the fax number
- Preliminary diagnosis
- Planned surgery, diagnostic test, or reason for referring the patient to a specialist
- Name, address, and phone number of the facility or specialist

- Co-payment amount or deductible
- Hospital benefits for inpatient and outpatient surgery
- Participating hospitals, radiology service providers, laboratories, and physicians

Once the information has been collected, it should be faxed to the insurance company. In case of an emergency, the authorization may be obtained by phone; however, the form should be faxed as soon as possible afterward. The form is faxed back to the provider by the insurance carrier with the authorization number and other vital information.

Mary Jo Smith
College Clinic
4567 Broad Avenue, WH
Telephone No.: (555) 486-9002
Fax No.:(555) 487-8976

MANAGED CARE PLAN AUTHORIZATION REQUEST

**TO BE COMPLETED BY PRIMARY CARE PHYSICIAN
OR OUTSIDE PROVIDER**

☐ Health Net   ☐ Met Life
☐ Pacificare   ☐ Travelers
☐ Secure Horizons ☐ Pru Care
☐ Other

Member/Group No.: 54098XX

Patient Name: Louann Campbell   Date: 7-14-20XX

☐ Male   ☐ Female   Birthdate: 4-7-1952   Home Telephone Number: (555) 450-1666

Address: 2516 Encina Avenue, Woodland Hills, XY 12345-0439

Primary Care Physician: Gerald Practon, MD   Provider ID #: TC 14021

Referring Physician: Gerald Practon, MD   Provider ID #: TC 14021

Referred to: Raymond Skeleton, MD   Office Telephone Number: (555) 486-9002

Address: 4567 Broad Avenue, Woodland Hills, XY 12345

Diagnosis Code: 724.2   Diagnosis Low back pain

Diagnosis Code: 722.10   Diagnosis Sciatica

Treatment Plan: Orthopedic consultation and evaluation of lumbar spine; R/O herniated disc L4-5

Authorization requested for: ☐ Consult Only   ☐ Treatment Only   ☐ Consult/Treatment
                               ☐ Consult/Procedure/Surgery   ☐ Diagnostic Tests

Procedure Code: 99244   Description: New patient consultation

Procedure Code: ___   Description: ___

Place of service: ☒ Office ☐ Outpatient ☐ Inpatient ☐ Other   Number of Visits: 1

Facility: ___   Length of Stay: ___

List of potential future consultants (i.e., anesthetists, surgical assistants or medical/surgical):

Physician's Signature: Gerald Practon, MD

TO BE COMPLETED BY PRIMARY CARE PHYSICIAN

PCP Recommendations: See above   PCP Initials: GP

Date eligibility checked: 7-14-20XX   Effective Date: 1-15-20XX

TO BE COMPLETED BY UTILIZATION MANAGEMENT

Authorized: ___ Auth. No. ___   Not Authorized ___

Deferred: ___   Modified: ___

Comments: ___

FIGURE 20-6 Sample preauthorization and/or referral form.

Obtaining preauthorization for referrals or certain procedures and services is required. Typically, the PCP, or "gatekeeper," is responsible for obtaining the authorization. A gatekeeper can be a PCP, a general or family practitioner, an internist, a pediatrician, and in some instances an obstetrician or a gynecologist.

Referral is a term used in managed care when a patient is referred from a PCP to a specialist. When completing a referral form, it is imperative that all necessary information be included (Procedure 20-4). Approval or denial of a referral can take anywhere from a few minutes to a few days. The three types of referral are as follows:

- A *regular referral* usually takes 3 to 10 working days for review and approval. This type of referral is used when the physician believes that the patient must see a specialist to continue treatment.

- An *urgent referral* usually takes about 24 hours for approval. This type of referral is used when an urgent situation occurs but is not life-threatening.

- A *STAT referral* can be approved by telephone immediately after it is faxed to the utilization review department. A STAT referral is used in an emergency situation as indicated by the physician.

A regular referral is the most common type and can be inconvenient for the patient. With most managed care plans, the member services department must be contacted to check the status of a referral. Remember this cardinal rule: never tell the patient the referral has been approved unless you have a hard copy of the authorization. **Authorization** is a term used in managed care for an approved referral. A referral becomes an authorization after it is reviewed by

PROCEDURE 20-4

Perform Preauthorization (Precertification) and/or Referral Procedures

CAAHEP COMPETENCIES: II.C.II. 1., IV.C.IV.6., IV.P.IV.3., V. P.V.6., VII.P.VII.4., VII.P.VII.5., IX.A.IX.2.

ABHES COMPETENCIES: 3.u

GOAL: *Using the information in the case study (found in the Study Guide), to obtain precertification from a patient's HMO for requested services or procedures.*

EQUIPMENT and SUPPLIES

- Patient record
- Precertification/preauthorization form
- Referral form
- Patient's insurance information, including telephone and fax numbers of insurance carrier
- Telephone and fax machine
- Pen

PROCEDURAL STEPS

1. Assemble the necessary documents and equipment.
   PURPOSE: To avoid wasting time searching for information or equipment needed to perform the task.
2. Examine the patient's record and determine the service or procedure for which preauthorization is being requested, including, if applicable, the specialist's name and phone number and the reason for the request.
   PURPOSE: To correctly complete the required form for gaining authorization from the patient's insurance carrier for the specified treatment.
3. Complete the preauthorization and/or referral form, providing all pertinent information requested.
   PURPOSE: To document the required information for the insurance carrier, including:

- The patient's demographic and insurance information
- The physician's identification information, including the National Provider Identification (NPI) and/or group ID number or numbers
- The diagnosis and planned procedure or treatment, or the name and contact information of the physician to whom the patient is being referred.

4. Proofread the completed form.
   PURPOSE: To ensure the accuracy of the information.
5. Fax the completed form to the patient's insurance carrier.
   PURPOSE: To inform the insurance carrier of the patient's medical condition and to request the following:

- Preauthorization for the specified treatment
- A verification or authorization number
- Confirmation of the specific number of procedures, services, or treatment sessions allowed and/or authorization for referral of the patient to a specialist

6. Place a copy of the returned, completed approval form in the patient's medical record.
   PURPOSE: To ensure that the approved procedure and service (or procedures and services) and/or the referral is properly filed for future reference.

---

utilization management and/or the medical director and has been approved. If a referral is approved, the PCP's office receives a copy of the authorization by mail or fax. Always review the authorization thoroughly. The patient will receive a letter with an authorization number and the approved services. The patient must bring the authorization to the specialist's office on the day the services will be provided. An authorization provides the following information to both the referring PCP and the specialist:

- An authorization code, which may be alphabetic, numeric, or alphanumeric
- The date on which the referral request was received by the utilization review department
- The date on which the referral was approved and its expiration date
  - An authorization is typically good for 60 days.
  - If the authorization expires and services have not been provided, an extension may be requested. Utilization management will change the expiration date and fax a copy to the PCP and specialist or will generate a new authorization with a new number.

- If services are provided after the expiration date, the claim will be denied. If this happens, contact utilization management or member services, ask for an extension, and answer a few questions. Sometimes the patient, the specialist's office, or both must be involved in this process.
- A diagnosis code
- The name, address, and telephone number of the contracted specialist where services will be provided
  - Sometimes the PCP refers the patient to a specialist but does not receive approval for that specialist and must get approval for another.
  - Always be sure that any specialist to whom the physician refers a patient is contracted with the same managed care plan as the PCP.
- The Comments section: this is the most critical area of a referral, because this area designates the services that have been approved.
  - It includes the specified number of authorized visits to the specialist.

○ An authorization may be issued for (1) evaluation only, (2) evaluation and treatment plan, (3) evaluation and biopsy, (4) evaluation and one injection, and so on.

○ When authorization for only an evaluation and/or treatment plan is given, the medical assistant must inform the patient that no treatment will be given; only an evaluation and/or treatment plan will be provided.

The PCP's office is notified if a referral is denied because of insufficient information or lack of medical necessity. Some medical groups notify both the PCP and the patient. When the PCP's office provides the utilization management committee with the necessary information, the referral is reviewed again.

Managed care changes on a day-to-day basis. To compete in this market, some insurance companies have added a benefit that allows a member or patient to self-refer (meaning an authorization is not required to see a specialist). Many plans for senior citizens now have a **self-referral** and a co-payment, in addition to some other insurance coverage. The procedure for obtaining a self-referral is essentially the same as for a provider of service. An authorization form is completed by the patient or with the assistance of the referred provider and faxed to the insurance company for approval.

CRITICAL THINKING APPLICATION   20-4

Ann has obtained precertification and knows the benefits that will be paid toward Jeff England's bill. Discuss how Ann can best explain insurance benefits, exclusions, co-insurance, deductibles, and allowable amounts to Jeff. How can she explain the reasons for and the process of preauthorization to patients?

FEE SCHEDULES

A healthcare practitioner has three commodities to sell: time, judgment (expertise), and services. In every case the healthcare practitioner must place an estimate on the value of these services. Fees for medical procedures and services differ from office to office based on the type of practice and the needs of the facility. The physician or physicians establishing the practice normally set the fees for procedures and services. In the past, most physicians worked on a fee-for-service basis; that is, patients were charged for the provider's service based on each individual service performed.

In recent years, **third-party payers**, particularly government and managed healthcare organizations, have greatly influenced what healthcare providers can charge by establishing the allowable charge. The **allowable charge** (or **allowable amount**) is the maximum that third-party payers will pay for a particular procedure or service (see Procedure 20-4). When healthcare providers establish a fee schedule, other factors influence what the charge for a particular procedure or service can be; these factors include the RBRVS and the lesser used RVS.

As discussed earlier in this chapter, the CMS developed the first comprehensive RBRVS-based fee schedule, which was adopted by Medicare in 1992. The RBRVS-based fee schedule adjusts fees for differences in resources used to provide each service. The amount of resources required to perform a service is determined through the use of RVUs, which are assigned to the CPT codes developed by the

AMA with an adjustment for overhead costs in different geographic areas. Since Medicare's introduction of RBRVS, most third-party payers have adopted similar approaches in developing their fees.

Resource-Based Relative Value Scale

The RBRVS is one of the outcomes of the Medicare Physician Payment Reform that was enacted in the Omnibus Budget Reconciliation Act of 1989 (usually called *OBRA '89*). Originally, Medicare Part B had paid physicians using a fee-for-service system based on UCR charges. However, implementation of the RBRVS in 1992 changed this system to a fee scale consisting of three parts:

- Physician work
- Charge-based professional liability expenses
- Charge-based overhead

The physician work component includes the degree of effort invested by a physician in a particular service or procedure and the time it consumed. The professional liability and overhead components are computed by the CMS.

The RBRVS fee schedule is designed to provide national uniform payments, after adjustment to reflect the differences in practice costs across geographic areas. The fee schedule includes a conversion factor, which is a single national number applied to all services paid under the fee schedule. Conversion factors are changed by Congress, usually annually, at the request of the CMS.

Depending on the contract between the provider and the insurance carrier (especially Medicare, Medicaid, and other government programs), the provider either writes off the difference between the RBRVS schedule and his or her fee or passes on the nonallowed portion of the charge to the guarantor for payment.

Contracts between the provider of service and the insurance payer vary greatly, depending on the insurance or third-party payer. It is important for the medical assistant to know the contract terms for each different third-party payer and, upon receipt of payment, to examine the EOB from the insurance carrier closely to ensure that all benefits have been reimbursed appropriately and correctly.

DEDUCTIBLES AND CO-INSURANCE

Many types of health insurance plans (e.g., indemnity, managed care, and Medicare) require a deductible and co-insurance amount that the patient must pay out of pocket. These plans typically have an annual deductible amount the patient must pay before the plan pays anything. In addition, members usually must also pay a percentage of each charge (co-insurance payment). Most indemnity plans have an annual out-of-pocket limit on the amount members must pay for co-insurance payments. This type of plan takes the major expense out of medical bills and helps keep premium costs down.

Consider this example, Mrs. Jones' plan has a $500 deductible, after which the insurance company pays 95% of all charges; this leaves Mrs. Jones with a 5% co-insurance expense in addition to the deductible. She also is responsible for a $1,000 out-of-pocket expense maximum, which means that once Mrs. Jones has paid $1,000 total, the insurance company pays 100% of any balance remaining. Mrs. Jones has incurred a $10,000 charge for cardiac surgery performed by her physician.

- In Figure 20-7, Column A shows that Mrs. Jones' total out-of-pocket expense is $1,000. She paid the $500 deductible,

	Column A	Column B
Total charge	$10,000	$20,000
Deductible (paid by Mrs. Jones)	(500)	(500)
5% (Mrs. Jones' portion)	(500)	(500)
Total amount paid by Mrs. Jones	$1000	$1000
Total amount paid by insurance	$9000	$19,000

FIGURE 20-7 Calculation of deductible and co-insurance.

	Column A	Column B
Total charge	$10,000	$20,000
Deductible (paid by Mrs. Jones)	(500)	(500)
5% (Mrs. Jones' portion)	(500)	(500)
Allowable amount $8500	(1500)	
Allowable amount $8500 with write off		(1500)
Total amount paid by Mrs. Jones	$2500	$1000
Total amount paid by insurance	$7500	$17,500

FIGURE 20-8 Calculation of allowable amount.

and 5% of $10,000, or an additional $500. The insurance company then paid the remaining balance of $9,000.

- In Figure 20-8, Column B shows that the cardiac surgery in this instance cost $20,000. Mrs. Jones' total out-of-pocket expense remains $1,000; therefore, in this case the insurance company is responsible for payment of the balance of $19,000. Because her maximum out-of-pocket expense, according to the plan described, is $1,000, even though the charges were doubled, she still pays only the $1,000 total out-of-pocket expense.

With Medicare and some other plans, a limit is placed on the amount that will be reimbursed for any procedure or service. This limit is called an *allowable amount*. The allowable amount can be all or part of a charge for a service or procedure. For example, a provider typically charges $80 for a Level I office visit; however, the insurance company benefit's allowable amount is only $60. Depending on the contract between the provider and the insurance carrier, the provider will either write off the $20 difference or pass on the nonallowed portion of the charge to the guarantor for payment. Because contracts between carriers and providers vary greatly, it is important for the medical assistant to examine the EOB from the insurance carrier closely and to be knowledgeable about the contract provisions between the provider of service and all insurance carriers the provider uses.

Deductibles and co-insurance are generally deducted from the total charge for services rendered; however, depending on the policies and procedures of the provider, they can be calculated for each individual charge. Allowable amounts are almost always deducted from an individual charge.

The steps for calculating deductible, co-insurance, and allowable amounts are presented in Procedure 20-5. Calculating deductibles, co-insurance, and allowable amounts is relatively simple. The

deductible and co-insurance are subtracted from the total charge for the services and procedures. The sum becomes the patient's responsibility or, if the patient has a secondary insurance, it can be billed to the secondary insurance carrier. Deductibles and co-insurance are generally deducted from the total charge for services rendered; however, depending on the policies and procedures of the provider, they can be calculated for each individual charge. Allowable amounts are almost always deducted from an individual charge.

Using the example in Figure 20-7, if the allowable amount for Mrs. Jones' $10,000 cardiac surgery is $8,500, the $1,500 difference between the physician's charge and the allowed amount would be either written off or passed on to the patient as an out-of-pocket expense. In Figure 20-8, Column A, a line has been added to show the $8,500 allowable amount and that $1,500 has been billed to the patient. In Column B, the amount has been written off, or absorbed as a cost, by the provider. Notice, too, that the insurance carrier pays $1,500 less for the cardiac surgery charge in Figure 20-8 than in Figure 20-7.

> ## CRITICAL THINKING APPLICATION   20-5
> An elderly patient comes to the office complaining that Medicare did not pay her bill in full. "Medicare is supposed to pay 80% of all of my bills, and I have already paid my portion," she insists. What information does Ann need to get to the bottom of this problem? How can she explain situations like this to patients?

Patient Education

Understanding how insurance plans handle reimbursement of benefits is challenging both for patients and for medical assistants. However, it is important that patients understand how their insurance works. Many people, especially elderly individuals, believe that if they have health insurance, all charges for their healthcare will be covered. They do not always understand the intricacies of deductibles, co-payments, medical necessity, and allowable charges.

The responsibilities of a medical assistant include keeping the patient informed and answering questions as they arise. Often medical facilities provide their patients with informational brochures that explain how health insurance and reimbursement work and give definitions of some of the more common terms used in the insurance claims process. If patients are well advised and comfortable with insurance facts before treatment begins, the medical experience will go more smoothly, and collection of fees not covered by the carrier will be easier. The medical assistant must use good communication skills, patience, and tact when discussing third-party reimbursement issues with patients.

Legal and Ethical Issues

Throughout their careers, medical assistants must remember that an individual's medical record is personal and private. Conversations between patients and their healthcare providers (and staff) are considered privileged communication. Nearly every day a medical assistant is in a position to read and hear information of a private medical nature, and both the caregiver and the patient expect that this information will not leave the medical office.

PROCEDURE 20-5

Perform Deductible, Co-insurance, and Allowable Amount Calculations

CAAHEP COMPETENCIES: I.F.3., II.C.II. 1., IV.C.IV.6., IV.P.IV.3., V. P.V.6., VII.P.VII.1.2., IX.A.IX.2.

ABHES COMPETENCIES: 3.t

GOAL: *To calculate the patient's out-of-pocket expense or the amount to be billed to a secondary insurance carrier and to determine the amounts to be written off or passed on to the patient for payment.*

EQUIPMENT and SUPPLIES

- Explanation of benefits (EOB) form; *or* explanation of Medicare benefits [EOMB]) form, remittance advice (RA) form, or verification of eligibility and benefits form
- Patient accounts receivable ledger
- Calculator
- Pen
- Paper

PROCEDURAL STEPS

1. Assemble the required materials and equipment.
   <u>PURPOSE:</u> To save time looking for the information needed to properly perform the procedure.
2. Using the EOB, EOMB, and/or the RA form and/or the Verification of Eligibility and Benefits form, in addition to the patient accounts receivable ledger, perform the following:
   - Write down the total charge from the EOB and/or the patient accounts receivable ledger.
   - Subtract the deductible amount from the total charge. If the deductible exceeds the total amount, subtract only that amount of the deductible that equals the total charge, and stop — do not continue with the other steps. Proceed to the other steps only after all of the patient's deductible has been paid.
   <u>PURPOSE:</u> To calculate and record the appropriate amount of deductible that must be paid by the patient according to the terms of his or her insurance policy.
3. If it is determined that all of the patient's deductible has been met, identify the co-insurance amount that the patient must pay (e.g., 20%).
   - Multiply this amount (e.g., 20%) by the total charge.
   - Subtract the sum from the total charge balance.

<u>PURPOSE:</u> To calculate and record the appropriate amount of co-insurance that must be met (and paid) by the patient according to the terms of his or her insurance policy.

4. Record the deductible and, if applicable, co-insurance amount or amounts on separate lines in the patient balance due column of the patient's account receivable ledger.
   - The sum becomes the patient's responsibility.
   - If the patient has a secondary insurance carrier, the sum can be billed to the secondary insurance carrier.

<u>PURPOSE:</u> To maintain a current balance and audit trail on the patient accounts receivable ledger and, when appropriate, to submit a statement to the patient for payment and/or submit a claim to a secondary insurance company.

<u>NOTE:</u> If an allowable amount is shown on the EOB, EOMB, or RA and is less than the amount of either the total charge or the individual charge for the date of service, proceed to steps 5 and 6. Otherwise, stop here.

5. Subtract the allowable amount of each individual charge from the actual (billed) charge.
6. Record the difference either in the adjustments or patient balance column.
   - If the provider of service writes off the difference as a courtesy, hardship adjustment, or as part of the contract the provider has with the insurance company, the amount is recorded in the adjustments column.
   - If the patient is responsible for paying the difference between the actual charge and the allowable amount, the amount is recorded in the patient balance column.

<u>PURPOSE:</u> To adjust and reconcile the patient accounts receivable ledger and deduct the appropriate allowable amounts from the patient ledger; or, to pass those amounts on to the patient for payment.

Unauthorized release of medical information carries over into the insurance claims processing area. Even though the patient expects the insurance form to be filled out and submitted for payment, this cannot be done without proper written release. This medical release form should be kept in the patient's chart, and it should be updated on a regular basis.

CLOSING COMMENTS

Managed care has often been criticized by the news media. Some types of managed care can create a physician-patient barrier that did not exist during the fee-for-service era. An extra effort in human relations by the medical assistant can help to overcome this barrier and put the patient at ease.

SUMMARY OF SCENARIO

There is still a lot of information on health insurance to digest, but Ann is now much more comfortable with its concepts and no longer feels that understanding the various topics is impossible. Ann understands that there are many different types of insurance carriers, including federal and state programs, commercial carriers, health maintenance organizations, and preferred provider organizations, and that each of these programs offers different benefits and has different requirements. She also understands that the best way to remember all the carriers and the benefits offered is to keep an up-to-date manual or computer record that keeps track of addresses, phone numbers, and benefits information for each carrier. In addition, she has learned that failure to verify benefits and eligibility or authorization for referrals, treatments, or procedures can result in a denial of payment for services rendered.

Understanding how to calculate the deductibles, co-insurance, and allowed amounts for procedures and services benefits both the provider and patient. The provider's productivity, income, and losses can be easily tracked, and the patient can be educated as to the exact amounts he or she is responsible for paying.

Now that Ann understands the basics of health insurance, she can look forward to learning the procedure for completing insurance claim forms for various insurance carriers for reimbursement.

SUMMARY OF LEARNING OBJECTIVES

1. **Define, spell, and pronounce the terms listed in the vocabulary.**
Spelling and pronouncing medical terms correctly bolster the medical assistant's credibility. Knowing the definition of these terms promotes confidence in communication with patients and co-workers.

2. **Discuss the purpose of health insurance.**
Medical assistants should have an understanding of the purpose of health insurance. This will help in the workplace not only by facilitating their knowledge of the subject, but also in helping them educate patients. The trend for insurance policies to encourage preventive medicine can be appreciated.

3. **Differentiate among the various types of insurance policies.**
Insurance policies fall into many different categories and are available in many different forms. The ability to differentiate among the various types of insurance policies gives medical assistants a solid background in what is available on the market, what is included in each policy category, and the function of each. It is also important for medical assistants to understand and appreciate that there are still many people in this country who cannot afford and do not receive high-quality healthcare.

4. **Explain the numerous classifications of insurance benefits available.**
Insurance packages are often tailored to the needs of each individual or group, and the ways to combine benefits are limitless. Health insurance policies normally contain a combination of the different benefits, such as surgical, medical, hospitalization, and major medical.

5. **Explain how insurance benefits are determined.**
Benefits are determined and paid in one of several ways: indemnity schedules, service benefit plans, UCR fees, and resource-based relative value scales. Medical assistants should become familiar with each of these methods and be able to differentiate the types of schedules, fees, and scales to determine which insurance payer uses them and how they affect reimbursement to the physician.

6. **Differentiate among the different types of managed care options.**
"Managed care" is a broad term used to describe a variety of health plans developed to provide healthcare services at lower costs. When the medical assistant is employed in a medical facility, he or she will undoubtedly be working with many types of managed care plans. Therefore, it is important to know the various types (e.g., HMO, IPA, and PPO) and understand how each one functions. The medical assistant should be well informed about the managed care policies most frequently seen in the practice.

7. **List and discuss other major third-party payers.**
Other major third-party payers the medical assistant should become familiar with are BC/BS, Medicaid, Medicare, CHAMPVA, TRICARE, and workers' compensation. Medicare is the largest third-party insurer in the country, making high-quality healthcare affordable for the elderly and select other groups. Medicaid is another government-sponsored healthcare plan for individuals who qualify for these benefits. Workers' compensation covers employees who are injured or who become ill as a result of accidents or adverse conditions in the workplace. Disability programs reimburse individuals for monetary losses incurred as a result of an inability to work for reasons other than those covered under workers' compensation. The medical assistant should be familiar with the major plans that are presented in the practice.

8. **Explain the procedure for verifying insurance benefits.**
Many problems for both the patient and the medical office can be prevented if the medical assistant develops and follows a procedure for verifying insurance benefits before services are rendered. This procedure includes gathering as much information as possible about the demographics of the patient and his or her insurance coverage. A pragmatic and tactful discussion with all new patients, to explain the medical office's established policy on insurance claims processing and the collection of fees not covered by the patient's policy, will pay off in the end.

9. **Discuss the different types of fee schedules.**
It is important for both the medical assistant and patients to realize that fees for medical procedures and services differ from office to office based on the type of practice and the needs of the facility. Until the advent of managed care, most physicians operated on a fee-for-service basis in which the provider would render his or her services and charge accordingly. In recent years, government and managed care organizations have

greatly influenced what healthcare providers can charge. Many third-party payers base reimbursements on what is referred to as the allowable charge. Other fee schedule types include the RVS and the RBRVS.

10. **Explain how to make managed care referrals and obtain precertifications.**

    Obtaining precertification, also known as *preauthorization,* and making referrals must be done according to the guidelines of the individual insurance companies. If the medical assistant is uncertain about the procedure, he or she should always refer to the company's insurance manual or check the process online, if possible.

11. **Perform eligibility and verification of benefits procedures.**

    Verification of insurance benefits is done to make certain that physicians are reimbursed for the services they provide for patients and also so that patients know their financial responsibility in advance. The process for verifying insurance benefits is outlined in Procedure 20-3.

12. **Perform a preauthorization procedure.**

    Preauthorization helps the medical assistant to ensure that the physician will be paid for the procedures and services provided to the patient. The process for obtaining preauthorization (precertification) is outlined in Procedure 20-4.

13. **Demonstrate how insurance benefits are determined by calculating deductible and co-insurance payments.**

    Medical assistants should become proficient at calculating the amounts due to the physician, considering deductibles, co-payments, and co-insurance amounts. The process for calculating insurance payments is outlined in Procedure 20-5.

CONNECTIONS

Study Guide Connection: Go to Chapter 20 Study Guide. Read the Case Study and Workplace Applications and complete the assignments. Do online research for answers to the questions in the Internet Activities associated with third-party reimbursement.

Evolve Connection: For more information on third-party reimbursement, go to *evolve.elsevier.com/kinn* and visit related Web links for Chapter 20. Click on the Medical Assisting Exam Review and do the practice questions to sharpen your test-taking skills. To learn more about office software, do the exercises for the AltaPoint demonstration found on the CD.

THE HEALTH INSURANCE CLAIM FORM

21

Carline A. Dalgleish, Sharon Oliver, and Alexandra Patricia Adams

SCENARIO

The school where Machelle Van Cleve receives her medical assistant training offers an optional job-shadowing module. For her assignment she chose a nearby health center, where she observed the administrative responsibilities of the medical assistants employed in this multispecialty practice. Machelle found that some of the offices were organized and efficient, whereas others lacked a structured routine, especially in the insurance department. Machelle, a detail-oriented person who enjoyed her studies related to billing and coding, heard numerous comments from employees in the administrative area related to the volumes of work in the billing offices. Her office manager explained that the mountainous paperwork was created as a result of managed care requirements, rejected claims needing further research, and inconsistencies in the demands of the various insurance companies.

Machelle agreed that keeping up with the requirements and regulations of the many third-party payers and government entitlement programs must be an overwhelming task. She concluded that billing and reimbursement are at the heart of the medical facility, and the correct completion of insurance claim forms is central to the success of the practice. She realized that becoming familiar with the complexities of the insurance claims process would be challenging, but she was convinced that through education, organization, and dedication she could become a valuable employee and an advocate for the patients who needed her assistance in resolving issues related to their claims for reimbursement.

While studying this chapter, think about the following questions:

- What will Machelle find is one of the most important, and basic, tasks that must be done properly before even beginning the insurance claim preparation?
- Why is it important for Machelle to learn the specific insurance billing requirements of different insurance companies and third-party payers?
- What has Machelle learned about the importance of auditing claims before they are sent to the insurance carrier for reimbursement?
- What does Machelle know about reimbursement and insurance claims follow-up?

LEARNING OBJECTIVES

1. Define, spell, and pronounce the terms listed in the vocabulary.
2. Discuss the differences between paper claims and electronic claims.
3. Understand the guidelines for completing the CMS-1500 Health Insurance Claim Form.
4. Explain how to complete each of the blocks of the CMS-1500 claim form.
5. Gather information for use on insurance claim forms.
6. Complete a CMS-1500 claim form appropriately for various federal, state, and commercial third-party payers.
7. Differentiate between "clean" and "dirty" claims.
8. Discuss methods of preventing claims rejections.
9. Describe ways of checking the status of claims.

VOCABULARY

assignment of benefits The transfer of the patient's legal right to collect benefits for medical expenses to the provider of those services, authorizing the payment to be sent directly to the provider.

audit A process done prior to claims submission to examine claims for accuracy and completeness. An audit can be performed manually or, if computer billing software is used, electronically.

audit trail The path left by a transaction when it has been completed; often referred to when tracking medical services used by patients or researching claims.

clean claims Insurance claim forms that have been completed correctly (no errors or omissions) and can be processed and paid promptly if they meet the restrictions on covered services and blocks.

clearinghouse A centralized facility to which insurance claims are transmitted. Clearinghouses separate, check, and redistribute claims electronically to various insurance carriers and may offer additional services to the physician.

direct billing A method of electronic claims submission that uses computer software to allow a provider to submit an insurance claim directly to an insurance carrier for payment.

dirty claims Claims that contain errors or omissions; such claims must be corrected and resubmitted to an insurance carrier to obtain reimbursement.

electronic claims Claims that are submitted to insurance processing facilities using a computerized medium, such as direct data entry, direct wire, dial-in telephone digital fax, or personal computer download or upload.

electronic data interchange (EDI) The transfer of data back and forth between two or more entities using an electronic medium.

electronic (or digital) signature A scanned signature or other such mark that is accepted as proof of approval of and/or responsibility for the content of an electronic document.

Employer Identification Number (EIN) The number used by the Internal Revenue Service that identifies a business or individual functioning as a business entity for income tax reporting.

incomplete claim A claim that is missing information and is returned to the provider for correction and resubmission. Also called an *invalid claim.*

intelligent character recognition (ICR) The electronic scanning of printed blocks as images and the use of special software to recognize these images (or characters) as ASCII text for uploading into a computer database.

National Provider Identifier (NPI) A lifetime number consisting of 10 digits that Medicare used to replace the Provider Identification Number (PIN) and the Unique Provider Identification Number (UPIN). CMS met the compliance requirement of using the NPI on all claims in May 2008; most insurance carriers have followed the CMS and now also use the NPI.

paper (hard copy) claims Insurance claims that have been completed manually, on paper, and sent by surface mail.

provider Any company, individual, or group that provides medical, diagnostic, or treatment services to a patient.

provider identification number (PIN) Numbers assigned to providers by a carrier for use in the submission of claims.

rejected claims Claims returned unpaid to the provider for clarification of any question; these claims must be corrected before resubmission.

Unique Provider Identification Number (UPIN) A number assigned by fiscal intermediaries to identify providers on claims for services.

universal claim form The form developed by the Health Care Financing Administration (HCFA; now the Centers for Medicare and Medicaid Services [CMS]) and approved by the American Medical Association (AMA) for use in submitting all government-sponsored claims. Also known as the *CMS-1500 Health Insurance Claim Form.*

Medical insurance means many things to many people. To some, it is a mound of paperwork. To others, it is a mass of confusion and regulations that seem to constantly change. To a patient with an illness or injury, health insurance helps defray the high costs associated with healthcare.

The **universal claim form**, originally called the HCFA-1500, was first developed in 1988 by the Health Care Financing Administration (HCFA) and approved for use by physicians and providers of outpatient services when submitting Medicare Part B claims for reimbursement. In 2001 the HCFA was renamed the Centers for Medicare and Medicaid Services (CMS), and the claim form was renamed the CMS-1500 Health Insurance Claim Form, commonly known as the CMS-1500. The form was subsequently adopted by almost all health insurance companies and third-party payers for use in the submission of physicians' claims for reimbursement. The current version of the CMS-1500 was adopted in August, 2005. As of May, 2008, only the CMS-1500 (08-05) claim form may be used to submit insurance claims.

TYPES OF CLAIMS

A medical assistant may submit insurance claims to a third-party payer or an insurance carrier either on hard copy (paper) or electronically. Hard copy claims are insurance claims submitted manually, on paper, by surface mail (i.e., the U.S. Postal Service). Electronic claims are insurance claims that are submitted to an insurance carrier via electronic media, such as the Internet. Most of today's computer programs generate claims internally from the information entered into the database.

Hard Copy (Paper) Claims

Advantages and Disadvantages of Paper Claims

Paper (hard copy) claims have advantages and disadvantages. The advantages include minimal start-up costs (because the forms are readily available through many vendors) and the ability to attach documentation explaining unusual circumstances that might affect reimbursement. The cost in time, labor, and postage is higher with paper claim submission, and reimbursement is much slower. Paper claims also require a lot of storage space.

Intelligent Character Recognition

Insurance claims created on paper (hard copy) are processed at the insurance payer using **intelligent character recognition (ICR)**. ICR is a system that scans documents and captures claims information directly from the CMS-1500 form. Medicare, Medicaid, TRICARE (formerly CHAMPUS), and many other insurance carriers have adopted the ICR system. The ICR system has replaced the optical character recognition (OCR) process, which had been in use until the early twenty-first century.

At the insurance carrier, ICR scanners transfer the information on claim forms into computers. This transfer is done using a red bulb scanner, which causes the red preprinted portion of the CMS-1500 form to appear invisible to the computer. The scanner "captures" only characters printed in black ink on the form and transfers them to the computer's memory. The resulting image allows for "clean" recognition of the data entered on the CMS-1500 form; that is, the data characters are not obstructed by the lines and text of the form.

The benefits of ICR scanning include greater efficiency in processing claims, improved accuracy, more control over the data input, and reduced data entry cost for the insurance carrier.

The medical assistant should use the following rules to complete the paper CMS-1500 form correctly so that the insurance carrier can scan the claim:

- Entries should be clear and sharp; carbon copies are not acceptable.
- Use pica type (10 characters per inch). The equivalent computer font is Courier 10 or OCR 10.
- All uppercase letters should be used.
- All punctuation should be omitted.
- All birth dates should be in this format: MM DD YYYY (with a space between each set of digits).
- Each entry should be kept within its respective block; all characters (e.g., X, Y, N) must fall completely within the designated block.
- A blank space should be substituted for the following:
  - Dollar signs and decimal points in charges and in ICD-9-CM codes
  - Dashes preceding procedure code modifiers
  - Parentheses around telephone area codes
  - Hyphens in Social Security numbers
- Titles and other designations (e.g., Sr., Jr., II, or III) should be omitted unless they appear on the identification (ID) card.
- When the charge is expressed in whole dollars, two zeros should be used in the "cents" column.
- Do not enter the alpha character "O" for a zero (0).
- If a typewriter is used, do not use lift-off tape, correction tape, or correction fluid.
- Because photocopies of claims cannot be scanned, all resubmissions must be prepared using the original (red print) claim form.
- No handwritten data (other than signatures) may be included on the form.
- Nothing should be stapled to the form.

- The name and address of the insurance company should be inserted in the proper area in the top margin of the claim form.

Electronic Claims

As mentioned, **electronic claims** are insurance claims that are transmitted over the Internet from the provider to the health insurance company. Most claims-processing software is designed to permit electronic claims generation. A mandate included in the Health Insurance Portability and Accountability Act (HIPAA) required the development of "transaction and code sets" for all insurance-related information sent electronically, including claim form submissions, claim status requests, and remittance (payment) processing.

The transaction and code set for CMS-1500 electronic claims submission is the ASC X12N 837P (HIPAA 837 Health Care Claim: Professional [837P]). All insurance billing data entered into the computer software program (i.e., patient, provider, charge, diagnosis, and procedure) is reformatted by the software program to conform with the transaction and code sets format and guidelines. For more information on implementation guides for transaction and code sets, refer to the Evolve site at *evolve.elsevier.com/kinn*).

HIPAA 837 HEALTH CARE CLAIM: PROFESSIONAL (837P) OVERVIEW

As part of the Health Insurance Portability and Accountability Act of 1996, standards were developed to protect patients' health information when it was transmitted electronically. These standards, known also as *transaction and code sets*, mandate the format of insurance claims, remittance information, claims attachments, and claims status submitted electronically. The insurance claim form for physician and provider services is called the HIPAA 837 Health Care Claim: Professional, or 837P. This standard contains the format and establishes the data contents of the Health Care Claim Transaction Set (837) for use in the context of an **electronic data interchange (EDI)**; that is, data that are transmitted electronically via the Internet. This transaction set can be used to submit healthcare claim billing information, encounter information, or both from providers of healthcare services to payers, either directly or via intermediary billers and claims clearinghouses.

Since 2003, all insurance claims submitted electronically, regardless of whether the claim is submitted directly to the payer or to a clearinghouse, have had to be submitted using the 837P standard, to comply with the HIPAA mandates. Any provider, payer, employer, or other entity that does not use these standards can be removed from participation in federal programs such as Medicaid, Medicare, and TRICARE and also may face stiff civil and/or criminal fines and imprisonment. All vendors, providers, clearinghouses, employers, and health insurance carriers that transmit protected health information electronically must have updated software that conforms to the HIPAA standards, including but not limited to the 837P. These software upgrades will be transparent to the medical assistant entering data into the computer for insurance claims processing; in other words, the format, screens, steps, and processes for entering data into the computer for the purpose of generating insurance claim forms, whether on paper to be mailed or to be transmitted electronically, should look and feel the same as before the transaction and code sets were implemented.

The CMS Web site *(cms.gov)* provides more information about the Transaction and Code Sets for the HIPAA 837 Health Care Claim: Professional, and the standards for other electronically submitted data, such as the Claims Payment and Remittance Advice (835), Healthcare Claims Status (276/277), Coordination of Benefits (837), and Referral Certification and Authorization (278).

Electronic Claims Submission

Electronic claims can be submitted in several ways. Claims can be transmitted directly to the insurance carrier, also known as *direct billing,* or to a claims clearinghouse, which then submits the claims to the insurance carrier.

Direct Billing. **Direct billing** is the process by which an insurance carrier allows a **provider** to submit insurance claims directly to the carrier electronically. Most major insurance carriers, including Medicare and Medicaid, provide small computer programs to providers that are used to enter patient and insured information, charges, and provider detail directly into the program. These data are then transmitted electronically directly to the insurance carrier. Many carrier-direct systems are supplied free of charge to the provider, but the direct system can transmit only to specific carriers.

Clearinghouse Submission. A **clearinghouse** is a vendor that allows a provider to submit all the insurance claims generated by the provider to the clearinghouse using special software. The clearinghouse then **audits** and sorts the claims and sends them in batches electronically to each of the different insurance carriers. A clearinghouse charges the healthcare provider a small fee for the service of receiving claim transmissions, checking and preparing the claims for processing, consolidating claims so that one transmission can be sent to each carrier, and submitting claims in correct data format to the applicable insurance payer. Other services that clearinghouses typically provide include:

- Auditing claims to make sure all required fields are completed and the data are correct
- Reporting the number of claims submitted and the number of errors and their specifics
- Forwarding claims to insurance carriers that accept electronic claims (e.g., Medicare, Medicaid, Blue Cross/Blue Shield, and others) or to another clearinghouse that may hold the contracts with specific payers
- Keeping provider offices updated as new carriers are added to the database
- Generating informative statistical reports

Clearinghouses are also called *third-party administrators* (TPAs), and they are designed to receive electronic claims from any provider.

Advantages of Electronic Submission

Typically, with electronic claims processing, payments are received in less than half the time required for turnaround of paper claims. Very soon after claims have been transmitted, the clearinghouse sends the provider tracking reports that describe which claims were received, audited, and forwarded to the insurance carrier. These

tracking reports also provide information regarding rejected claims and those needing additional information.

Electronic claims processing reduces payment turnaround time by shortening the payment cycle and can reduce average error rates to less than 1% or 2%. Some insurance companies even waive the attachment requirements for many procedures when claims are submitted electronically. For additional information on advantages and disadvantages, visit the Evolve site at *evolve.elsevier.com/kinn).*

CRITICAL THINKING APPLICATION   21-1

Machelle is interested in learning more about filing claims electronically. In the medical facility where she is doing her externship, she has asked to work with Frank Hern, who performs this procedure in the office. How can working closely with Mr. Hern benefit Machelle with regard to this subject?

DATA GATHERING GUIDELINES

When the first appointment is made for a patient, it is routine to ask the patient for all pertinent insurance information. Much of this information is on the Patient Registration form that is completed when the patient comes to the medical office for the initial visit; it is inserted into the medical chart and entered into the computer's patient database. This information should always be collected from every new patient seen by the provider. Returning or established patients should be asked during each visit whether their insurance information is complete and current. Many offices use a form that allows the patient to provide address and phone number updates, in addition to new insurance information.

The information needed to complete an insurance form (Table 21-1) is gathered from several sources: (1) the Patient Registration form, (2) the completed Verification of Eligibility and Benefits form, (3) referral and authorization information (when required by the insurance carrier), (4) the patient's medical record, (5) the encounter form or charge ticket, and (6) a photocopy of the patient's insurance card or cards, driver's license or state-issued ID card, and student ID (if applicable and available). The *Current Procedural Terminology* (CPT), *Health Care Common Procedural Coding System* (HCPCS), and *International Classification of Diseases, Ninth Revision, Clinical Modification* (ICD-9-CM) coding manuals and the individual insurance payer's claims processing manual or guidelines are also necessary resources for preparing insurance claims. Procedure 21-1 presents the steps for gathering patient and other information needed prior to completing the insurance claim form.

Verification of Eligibility and Benefits

Once the patient's and the insured's demographic and insurance information has been collected, the next step is to verify the patient's eligibility and benefits. This usually is done by phone, by calling the insurance carrier or carriers for the patient and confirming that the patient is covered by the insurance; this also provides an overview of the benefits available for the patient from the insurance policy. The information obtained over the phone should be verified by either fax or e-mail confirmation from the insurance carrier. For more information about verification of benefits and to see

TABLE 21-1 Information Required for Completion of CMS-1500 Form

BLOCK	INFORMATION NEEDED
	Completed Patient Registration form
	Photocopy of insurance card or cards—front and back
	Pertinent information from Verification of Eligibility and Benefits form
	Preauthorization and/or referral number (when applicable)
Section 1: Carrier Block	
Carrier Block	Insurance carrier's address
Section 2: Patient/Insured	
1	Type of insurance If patient's condition or illness is related to employment, auto accident, or some other type of accident, provide: • Date of onset of condition or accident • Responsible party's name, address, and phone number • Insurance carrier of responsible party, including address and phone number • Insurance ID number, policy, and/or group number
1a	Insured's identification (ID) number (primary insurance)
2	Patient's full name
3	Patient's date of birth and gender
4	Insured's name (primary insurance)
5	Patient's information • Permanent address (including apartment number if appropriate) • City, state, ZIP code • Telephone number
6	Patient's relationship to insured
7	Insured's information • Permanent address (including apartment number if appropriate) • City, state, ZIP code • Telephone number
8	Patient status • Employed? • Full- or part-time student?
9	Secondary (other) insured's name*
9a	Policy or group number of secondary insurance*
9b	Secondary insured's date of birth and gender*
9c	Secondary insured's employer or school name*
9d	Secondary insured's insurance plan or program name*
10a-c	If patient's condition or illness is related to employment, auto accident, or some other type of accident, make sure information is obtained as outlined in Block 1
11	Insurance policy, group, or FECA number of primary insurance
11a	Primary insured's date of birth and gender
11b	Primary insured's employer or school name
11c	Primary insured's insurance plan or program name

Continued

TABLE 21-1 Information Required for Completion of CMS-1500 Form—cont'd

BLOCK	INFORMATION NEEDED
11d	Determine whether the patient also is covered by a secondary health insurance plan
12	Confirm that the patient's release of information form has been signed and dated and is in the patient's record
13	Confirm that the insured's authorization of benefits form has been signed and dated and is in the patient's record
Section 3: Physician/Supplier	
14	Date illness, injury, or pregnancy began
15	Determine whether patient has had same or similar symptoms
16	From-To dates if patient was unable to work at current occupation
17	Name of ordering or referring provider
17a	Not required
17b	Ordering or referring provider's NPI number
18	From-To dates if patient encounter included an inpatient hospital stay
19	Determine whether insurance carrier in carrier block and Block 1 require any information entered in this field
20	Determine whether an outside lab was used; if so, enter charges billed to provider for outside lab services
21	ICD-9-CM code or codes for patient's condition, illness, or injury (maximum of four per claim)
22	Is Medicaid claim being resubmitted? If yes, provide reference number from original Medicaid claim submitted
23	If prior authorization and/or referral is required, provide authorization (approval) number from insurance payer
24A	From-To dates of service for current encounter
24B	POS code
24C	If an emergency, put a Y in this box
24D	CPT and/or HCPCS code CPT and/or HCPCS modifier(s) (maximum of four per charge line)
24E	Block 21 field or reference number (1, 2, 3 and/or 4)
24F	Total charge for CPT- or HCPCS-coded services listed in 24D. • If more than 1 day or unit is indicated in Block 24G, multiply the charge for the service(s) coded in Block 24D by the number of days/units in Block 24G; enter the result in Block 24F.
24G	Total number of days or units
24H	EPSDT or Family Plan code (Medicaid or AFDC)
24I	Qualifier ID code (if no NPI number is available)
24J	Rendering (treating) provider's NPI number—unshaded field PIN (if no NPI number is available)—shaded field
25	Rendering provider's federal tax ID number (EIN or SSN)
26	Patient's account number with rendering provider
27	Determine whether contract or agreement between provider and insurance carrier allows provider to accept assignment
28	Total charges from Block 24F, lines 1-6
29	Amount paid by patient, insured, or other insurance

TABLE 21-1 Information Required for Completion of CMS-1500 Form—cont'd

BLOCK	INFORMATION NEEDED
30	Balance due, if any amount paid is shown in Block 29
31	Signature of provider performing service or procedure
32	Address of facility where services were rendered
32a	NPI number of service facility in Block 32
32b	Qualifier ID number and PIN of facility in Block 32 (if no NPI is available)
33	Name, address, and phone number of performing (rendering) provider
33a	NPI number of provider in Block 33
33b	Qualifier ID number and PIN of provider in Block 33 (if no NPI is available)

*Only required if a secondary insurance exists and is to be submitted to the insurance carrier.
AFDC, Aid to Families with Dependent Children; *CPT*, *Current Procedural Terminology* coding method; *EIN*, Employer's Identification Number; *EPSDT*, Early and Periodic Screening, Diagnosis, and Treatment; *FECA*, Federal Employees Compensation Act; *HCPCS*, *Health Care Common Procedural Coding System* coding method ; *ICD-9-CM*, *International Classification of Diseases, Ninth Revision, Clinical Modification* coding method; *NPI*, National Provider Identifier; *PIN*, personal identification number; *POS*, place of service.

PROCEDURE 21-1

Gather Data to Complete CMS-1500 Form

CAAHEP COMPETENCIES: II.C.II.1., IV.C.IV.6., IV.P.IV.3., V. P.V.6., VII.P.VII.1., VII.P.VII. 2., VII.P.VII.3., IX.A.IX.2.

ABHES COMPETENCIES: 3.x

GOAL: *To gather all information and documentation required for completing an insurance claim.*

EQUIPMENT and SUPPLIES

- Patient Registration form
- Photocopy of patient's insurance card or cards, driver's license or state-issued identification card, and student ID (if applicable).
- Verification of Eligibility and Benefits form
- Preauthorization and/or Referral form
- Encounter form (charge ticket or superbill)
- ICD-9-CM coding manual
- CPT coding manual
- HCPCS coding manual

PROCEDURAL STEPS

1. Have the patient or patient's guardian complete the Patient Registration, Release of Information, and Authorization of Benefits form or forms in full and return them to the medical assistant.
   PURPOSE: To gather the required information to enter into the computer, so that the documents and files needed to ultimately receive the maximum reimbursement from the carrier. This process creates the record and allows the physician to begin documentation that will be used to complete the insurance claim form.

2. Ask for the patient's and the insured's driver's license and insurance card or cards. If the patient is a student, ask whether he or she has a student identification (ID) card; if so, request it from the patient. If a patient has more than one insurance policy, it is important to get the name, address, group, and policy number for each company.
   PURPOSE: To obtain state-issued identification of the patient so that the physician verifies that he or she is treating the right patient (who is eligible for benefits).

3. Photocopy the back and front of the patient's insurance card and place the photocopy in the medical record and/or the patient's insurance file. Most medical offices also photocopy the patient's and insured guarantor's driver's license or other state-issued ID card (and, when applicable, a student ID card) for verification of the patient's and insured's identity.

4. Confirm the patient's and insured's full name, address, phone number, date of birth, gender, and insurance information by comparing the Patient Registration form, insurance ID card, and state-issued ID card.

5. Determine whether someone other than the patient is the guarantor. The *guarantor* is the person or entity responsible for payment. The guarantor may be the patient, the insured, or a third party. If neither the patient nor the insured is the guarantor, obtain the guarantor's address, date of birth, and employer information, in addition to the guarantor's relationship to the patient (e.g., spouse, parent, self, or other).

6. Call the employer and confirm employment (optional). If the patient is insured under a group health plan, workers' compensation, TRICARE, or some other types of insurance, this information can be confirmed when verifying eligibility and benefits.

7. Confirm that the patient has signed and dated the Release of Information form.
   PURPOSE: To prove that the patient has agreed to allow the physician to release information to the insurance company or other third-party payor so that payment can be made on the claim.

8. Confirm that the insured has signed the Authorization of Benefits form. Signatures to authorize insurance billing, supplying of information to insurance companies, and acceptance of assignments of benefits

(if appropriate) should be obtained from all new patients and at the beginning of each new calendar year.

9. Contact the insurance carrier and perform a verification of benefits and insurance coverage.

10. Obtain any precertification or referral authorization or authorizations required by the insurance carrier or payer.

11. Code the diagnosis or diagnoses for the encounter using the ICD-9-CM coding manual.

12. Select any qualifying circumstance, physical or patient status, or other modifiers as appropriate.

13. Code the procedures and services rendered during the encounter using the CPT and/or HCPCS coding manual.

14. Select any CPT and/or HCPCS modifiers as appropriate.

15. Using Table 21-1 or a similar list of information to gather in preparation for insurance claim submission, confirm all information needed is available.

---

an example of a verification form, visit the Evolve site at *evolve.elsevier.com/kinn.*

Preauthorization and/or Referral

If any diagnostic or therapeutic services or procedures are to be rendered by the provider that require preauthorization approval, perform a preauthorization to obtain an authorization number. The authorization number, which confirms that precertification was performed, is placed in Block 23 on the CMS-1500 form. For more information about preauthorization and to see an example of the form, refer to the Evolve site at *evolve.elsevier.com/kinn.*

COMPLETING THE CMS-1500 FORM

The CMS-1500 Health Insurance Claim Form (Figure 21-1) is used by most health insurance payers for claims submitted by physicians and suppliers. The information needed to complete an insurance claim form includes the patient's and the guarantor's demographic and insurance information; the name, address, and phone number of the insurance company; the diagnostic, treatment, and procedures and services information; and the provider's billing information, including name, address, phone number, place of service, and the tax and provider identification numbers.

There are 33 blocks, or items, on the CMS-1500 form. These blocks are divided into three sections:

- **Section 1:** Carrier Block. The first section contains the address of the insurance carrier and is located at the top of the form (Figure 21-2).
- **Section 2:** Patient/Insured Section. The second section contains information about the patient and the insured; it includes Boxes 1 through 13.
- **Section 3:** Physician/Supplier Section. The third section contains information about the physician or supplier; it includes Boxes 14 through 33.

In the following guidelines, each of the 33 blocks contains the block title, description, and instructions for completing that block. Where applicable, special instructions are given for Medicare, Medicaid, TRICARE, group health plan, Federal Employees Compensation Act (FECA) and black lung (FECA/Black Lung) insurance, and other types of insurance. Procedure 21-2 provides detailed instructions on completing each section and block of the CMS-1500 claim form. (For hints on creating a work-friendly routine for completing insurance claims, refer to the Evolve site at *evolve.elsevier.com/kinn*).

Section 1: Carrier Block

The name and address of the payer is entered in this block. The payer is the carrier, health plan, third-party administrator, or other payer who will process the claim. Use the format shown in Figure 21-2.

Section 2: Patient/Insured Section—Blocks 1 to 8
(Figure 21-3)

Block 1: Type of Insurance. This block indicates the type of insurance the patient has. Indicate the type of health insurance coverage applicable to this claim by putting an X in the appropriate box (e.g., if a Medicare claim is being filed, mark the Medicare box). This information directs the claim to the correct payer and may establish primary liability. For example, if the claim is primary for Medicare, put an X in the Medicare box; if Medicare is secondary, put an X in the box for Other.

    Block 1a: Insured's ID Number. The ID number of the person who holds the policy.

    Block 2: Patient's Name. The name of the patient is the person who received treatment or supplies. The patient's last name should be entered first, then first name, and middle initial (e.g., Doe, John A.)

    Block 3: Patient's Birth Date and Sex. The patient's birth date and sex help identify the patient and distinguishes patients with similar names.

    Block 4: Insured's Name. The name of the person who holds the policy.

Primary and Secondary Insurance Determination. Generally, if the patient is insured, the patient's insurance is primary; any insurance carried by a spouse or other guarantor is considered secondary.

Determination of Primary and Secondary Insurance for a Child or Minor. In the case of a child whose mother and father both carry the child as a dependent on their insurance policies, primary and secondary insurance is determined by the birthday rule; that is, whichever parent's birth month and birth date falls first in a calendar year is considered primary. The year of the parent's birth is not used. Therefore, if the mother's birth month and day are February 20 and the father's are May 1, the mother's insurance is the primary insurance and the father's insurance is the secondary insurance.

    Block 5: Patient's Address. The patient's permanent address and telephone number are entered here. Do not use a temporary or school address.

Text continued on p. 389

1500

HEALTH INSURANCE CLAIM FORM

APPROVED BY NATIONAL UNIFORM CLAIM COMMITTEE 08/05

PICA | PICA | CARRIER

1. MEDICARE (Medicare #) MEDICAID (Medicaid #) TRICARE CHAMPUS (Sponsor's SSN) CHAMPVA (Member ID#) GROUP HEALTH PLAN (SSN or ID) FECA BLK LUNG (SSN) OTHER (ID)

1a. INSURED'S I.D. NUMBER (For Program in Item 1)

2. PATIENT'S NAME (Last Name, First Name, Middle Initial)

3. PATIENT'S BIRTH DATE MM DD YY SEX M F

4. INSURED'S NAME (Last Name, First Name, Middle Initial)

5. PATIENT'S ADDRESS (No., Street)

6. PATIENT RELATIONSHIP TO INSURED Self Spouse Child Other

7. INSURED'S ADDRESS (No., Street)

CITY STATE

8. PATIENT STATUS Single Married Other

CITY STATE

ZIP CODE TELEPHONE (Include Area Code) ( )

Employed Full-Time Student Part-Time Student

ZIP CODE TELEPHONE (Include Area Code) ( )

9. OTHER INSURED'S NAME (Last Name, First Name, Middle Initial)

10. IS PATIENT'S CONDITION RELATED TO:

11. INSURED'S POLICY GROUP OR FECA NUMBER

a. OTHER INSURED'S POLICY OR GROUP NUMBER

a. EMPLOYMENT? (Current or Previous) YES NO

a. INSURED'S DATE OF BIRTH MM DD YY SEX M F

b. OTHER INSURED'S DATE OF BIRTH MM DD YY SEX M F

b. AUTO ACCIDENT? YES NO PLACE (State)

b. EMPLOYER'S NAME OR SCHOOL NAME

c. EMPLOYER'S NAME OR SCHOOL NAME

c. OTHER ACCIDENT? YES NO

c. INSURANCE PLAN NAME OR PROGRAM NAME

d. INSURANCE PLAN NAME OR PROGRAM NAME

10d. RESERVED FOR LOCAL USE

d. IS THERE ANOTHER HEALTH BENEFIT PLAN? YES NO *If yes*, return to and complete item 9 a-d.

READ BACK OF FORM BEFORE COMPLETING & SIGNING THIS FORM.

12. PATIENT'S OR AUTHORIZED PERSON'S SIGNATURE I authorize the release of any medical or other information necessary to process this claim. I also request payment of government benefits either to myself or to the party who accepts assignment below.

SIGNED ______ DATE ______

13. INSURED'S OR AUTHORIZED PERSON'S SIGNATURE I authorize payment of medical benefits to the undersigned physician or supplier for services described below.

SIGNED ______

PATIENT AND INSURED INFORMATION

14. DATE OF CURRENT: MM DD YY ILLNESS (First symptom) OR INJURY (Accident) OR PREGNANCY(LMP)

15. IF PATIENT HAS HAD SAME OR SIMILAR ILLNESS. GIVE FIRST DATE MM DD YY

16. DATES PATIENT UNABLE TO WORK IN CURRENT OCCUPATION FROM MM DD YY TO MM DD YY

17. NAME OF REFERRING PROVIDER OR OTHER SOURCE 17a. 17b. NPI

18. HOSPITALIZATION DATES RELATED TO CURRENT SERVICES FROM MM DD YY TO MM DD YY

19. RESERVED FOR LOCAL USE

20. OUTSIDE LAB? YES NO $ CHARGES

21. DIAGNOSIS OR NATURE OF ILLNESS OR INJURY (Relate Items 1, 2, 3 or 4 to Item 24E by Line)

1. ___ . ___ 3. ___ . ___

2. ___ . ___ 4. ___ . ___

22. MEDICAID RESUBMISSION CODE ORIGINAL REF. NO.

23. PRIOR AUTHORIZATION NUMBER

24. A. DATE(S) OF SERVICE From MM DD YY To MM DD YY	B. PLACE OF SERVICE	C. EMG	D. PROCEDURES, SERVICES, OR SUPPLIES (Explain Unusual Circumstances) CPT/HCPCS MODIFIER	E. DIAGNOSIS POINTER	F. $ CHARGES	G. DAYS OR UNITS	H. EPSDT Family Plan	I. ID. QUAL.	J. RENDERING PROVIDER ID. #
1								NPI	
2								NPI	
3								NPI	
4								NPI	
5								NPI	
6								NPI	

25. FEDERAL TAX I.D. NUMBER SSN EIN

26. PATIENT'S ACCOUNT NO.

27. ACCEPT ASSIGNMENT? (For govt. claims, see back) YES NO

28. TOTAL CHARGE $

29. AMOUNT PAID $

30. BALANCE DUE $

31. SIGNATURE OF PHYSICIAN OR SUPPLIER INCLUDING DEGREES OR CREDENTIALS (I certify that the statements on the reverse apply to this bill and are made a part thereof.)

SIGNED DATE

32. SERVICE FACILITY LOCATION INFORMATION a. NPI b.

33. BILLING PROVIDER INFO & PH # ( ) a. NPI b.

PHYSICIAN OR SUPPLIER INFORMATION

NUCC Instruction Manual available at: www.nucc.org

APPROVED OMB-0938-0999 FORM CMS-1500 (08/05)

FIGURE 21-1 CMS-1500 Health Insurance Claim Form.

1500

HEALTH INSURANCE CLAIM FORM

APPROVED BY NATIONAL UNIFORM CLAIM COMMITTEE 08/05

XYZ INSURANCE COMPANY
102 MAIN STREET
ANYTOWN, MO 63030

CARRIER

PICA | PICA

FIGURE 21-2 CMS-1500 claim form: Carrier Block.

PROCEDURE 21-2

Complete an Insurance Claim Form

CAAHEP COMPETENCIES: II.C.II. 1., IV.C.IV.6., IV.P.IV.3., V. P.V.6., VII.P.VII.1., VII.P.VII.2., VII.P.VII.3., IX.A.IX.2.

ABHES COMPETENCIES: 3.x

GOAL: *To accurately complete a CMS-1500 (formerly HCFA-1500) claim form.*

EQUIPMENT and SUPPLIES

- Patient Registration form
- Photocopy of patient's insurance ID card or cards
- Encounter form (charge ticket or superbill)
- Copy of the completed Verification of Eligibility and Benefits form
- Copy of the completed Preauthorization and/or Referral form (when applicable)
- Claims processing manual or guidelines for the insurance payer for which the insurance claim is being completed
- Patient's medical record
- Patient's ledger
- CMS-1500 Health Insurance Claim Form
- Typewriter or computer

PROCEDURAL STEPS

1. Determine the type of insurance (e.g., Medicare, Medicaid, TRICARE, CHAMPVA, group health plan, FECA/Black Lung, health maintenance organization [HMO], automobile or other liability policy, workers' compensation).
2. Review the Patient Registration form, medical record, financial ledger, Verification of Eligibility and Benefits form, and Preauthorization and/or Referral form to ensure that all the information needed to perform the procedure has been assembled. Table 21-1 lists the required information for completing the CMS-1500 form.
3. Refer to the claims processing manual or guidelines for the type of insurance to be submitted.
4. Complete each block (as appropriate) of the CMS-1500 form

SECTION 1: CARRIER BLOCK

- Enter the name and address of the payer to whom this claim is being sent in the following format:
  - First line: Name of carrier
  - Second line: First line of address
  - Third line: Second line of address, if needed
  - Fourth line: City, state, and ZIP code

SECTION 2: PATIENT/INSURED INFORMATION

- **Block 1** Put an X in the appropriate box to indicate the type of healthcare coverage that applies to this claim. Mark only one box.
  NOTE: One (1) character may be entered in any box in the field. Only one box can be marked.
  - Medicare—Put an X in this box when filing a Medicare claim.
  - Medicaid—Put an X in this box when filing a Medicaid claim.
  - TRICARE (CHAMPUS)—Put an X in this box when filing a TRICARE claim.

- CHAMPVA—Put an X in this box when filing a CHAMPVA claim.
- Group Health Plan—Put an X in this box when filing any type of group health insurance claim.
- FECA/Black Lung—Put an X in this box only when filing a claim for a patient who qualifies for these programs, which should be shown clearly on the insurance card.
- Other—Put an X in this box if the insurance type is:
  - HMO
  - Commercial insurance
  - Automobile accident
  - Liability
  - Workers' compensation
- **Block 1a** Enter the insured's ID number as shown on the health insurance ID card for the specific payer this claim addresses.
  NOTE: A total of twenty-nine (29) characters may be entered in this block.
  - Medicare—Use the Health Identification Card (HIC) number.
  - Medicaid—Use the Medicaid ID number.
  - TRICARE/CHAMPVA—Use the ID number on the card.
  - Group Health Plan—Use the ID number on the card.
  - FECA/Black Lung—Use the FECA/Black Lung ID number.
  - Other: Follow instructions in the carriers' instruction manual.
- **Block 2** Enter the patient's full last name, first name, and middle initial. Suffixes should be entered after the last name. Do not include titles or professional suffixes. Use commas to separate each name. Do not use periods. Use a hyphen for hyphenated names.
  NOTE: A total of twenty-eight (28) characters may be entered in this block.
- **Block 3** Enter the patient's birth date in eight (8)–digit format (MM/DD/YYYY). Enter an X in the correct box to indicate the gender of the patient. Only one box can be marked. Leave blank if the gender is for some reason unknown.
  NOTE: Two (2) characters may be entered for month and date, and four (4) characters may be entered for the year. One (1) character may be entered in the box denoting gender.
- **Block 4** Enter the insured's full last name, first name, and middle initial. Suffixes should be entered after the last name. Do not include titles or professional suffixes. Use commas to separate each name. Do not use periods. Use a hyphen for hyphenated names.
  NOTE: Twenty-nine (29) characters may be entered in this box.
  - Medicare—Enter the insured's name if the patient is not the insured individual. Leave blank if the patient is the insured.
  - Medicaid—Leave blank. The patient is considered the insured, because each patient is assigned his or her own Medicaid ID number.

PROCEDURE 21-2—cont'd

- TRICARE/CHAMPVA—Enter the insured's name if the patient is not the insured individual. Leave blank if the patient is the insured.
- Group Health Plan—For employee-sponsored plans, the insured is the employee. Enter the insured's name if the patient is not the insured individual. Leave blank if the patient is the insured.
- FECA/Black Lung—Leave blank. The patient is considered the insured, because each patient is assigned his or her own FECA/Black Lung ID number.
- Other: Follow the carrier manual for the specific insurance being filed to accurately complete this section.

- **Block 5** Enter the patient's mailing address and phone number. The first line is for the address number and street; the second line is for the city and state; and the third line is for the ZIP code and phone number. Do not use punctuation in the address, other than a hyphen in a nine-digit ZIP code. Do not use hyphens in the phone number.
  NOTE: Twenty-eight (28) characters are allowed for the street address; twenty-four (24) for the city; and three (3) for the state. Twelve (12) characters are allowed for the ZIP code; three (3) for the area code; and ten (10) for the phone number.

- **Block 6** Put an X in the box that indicates the relationship of the patient to the insured. Mark only one box.
  NOTE: One (1) character may be entered in any box. Only one box should be marked.

- **Block 7** Enter the insured's address. The first line is for the address number and street; the second line is for the city and state; and the third line is for the ZIP code and phone number. Do not use punctuation in the address, other than a hyphen in a nine-digit ZIP code. Do not use hyphens in the phone number.
  NOTE: Twenty-nine (29) characters are allowed for the street address; twenty-three (23) for the city; and four (4) for the state. Twelve (12) characters are allowed for the ZIP code; three (3) for the area code; and ten (10) for the phone number.
  - Medicare—Leave blank; the patient is the insured.
  - Medicaid—Leave blank; the patient is the insured.
  - Group Health Plan—Leave blank if the patient is the insured; otherwise, enter the insured's address and phone number.
  - FECA/Black Lung—Leave blank; the patient is the insured.
  - Other: Follow instructions in the carriers' instruction manual.

- **Block 8** Put an X in the appropriate box indicating marital status and employment status; also student status (if applicable). Mark only one box on each line.
  NOTE: Only one (1) character may be marked in the boxes, and only one box per line should be marked.

- **Block 9** (Complete Blocks 9 and 9a-d only if YES is marked in Block 11d.) Use Blocks 9 and 9a-d when other group health coverage exists. Enter the last name, first name, and middle initial of the other insured if these are different from those shown in Block 2. Suffixes should be entered after the last name. Do not include titles or professional suffixes.

Use commas to separate each name. Do not use periods. Use a hyphen for hyphenated names.
NOTE: Twenty-eight (28) characters may be entered in this block.

- **Block 9a** Enter the group number or policy of the other insured.
  NOTE: Twenty-eight (28) characters can be entered in this field.

- **Block 9b** Enter the other insured's birth date in an eight (8)–digit format (MM/DD/YYYY). Put an X in the correct box to indicate the gender of the other insured. Only one box can be marked. Leave blank if the gender is for some reason unknown.
  NOTE: Two (2) characters may be entered for month and date, and four (4) characters may be entered for the year. One (1) character may be entered in the box denoting gender.

- **Block 9c** Enter the name of the other insured's employer or school.
  NOTE: Twenty-eight (28) characters may be entered in this field.

- **Block 9d** Enter the name of the other insured's insurance plan or program.
  NOTE: Twenty-eight (28) characters may be entered in this field.

- **Block 10a-c** Enter an X in the correct box to indicate whether one or more of the services described in Block 24 are for a condition or injury that occurred on the job or as a result of an automobile or other accident. Only one box on each line can be marked. Place the state postal code in the blank next to auto accident if the YES box is marked in that line.
  NOTE: One (1) character may be entered per line in either box, and two (2) characters may be entered in the place/state field.
  - 10a: If the patient's condition is related to employment injury or illness, put an X in the YES box.
  - 10b: If the patient's condition is related to an automobile accident, put an X in the YES box and enter the two-letter state designation in the PLACE (State) field.
  - 10c: If the patient's condition is related to some other type of accident, put an X in the YES box.

- **Block 10d** Refer to the most recent instructions from the applicable public or private payer regarding the use of this field.
  NOTE: Nineteen (19) characters may be entered in this field.

- **Block 11** Enter the insured's policy, group, or FECA number as it appears on the healthcare ID card. If Block 4 was completed, this block also must be completed.
  NOTE: Twenty-nine (29) characters may be entered in this field.
  - Medicare—Use the HIC number.
  - Medicaid—Use the Medicaid ID number.
  - TRICARE/CHAMPVA—Use the ID number on the card.
  - Group Health Plan—Use the ID number on the card (usually the Social Security number).
  - FECA/Black Lung—Use the FECA/Black Lung ID number.
  - Other: Follow the carrier manual for the specific insurance being filed to accurately complete this section.

PROCEDURE 21-2—cont'd

- **Block 11a** Enter the insured's birth date in an eight (8)-digit format (MM/DD/YYYY). Put an X in the box that indicates the gender of the insured.
  NOTE: Two (2) characters are allowed in the month and day spaces, and four (4) in the year space. One entry is allowed in the block to indicate gender.
- **Block 11b** Enter the name of the insured's employer or school.
  NOTE: Twenty-nine (29) characters are allowed in this block.
- **Block 11c** Enter the insurance plan or program name in this block. Some payers prefer an ID number of the primary insurer instead of a name in this block.
  NOTE: Twenty-nine (29) characters are allowed in this field.
- **Block 11d** Mark the appropriate box. If there is another health plan, Blocks 9 and 9a-d must be completed.
  NOTE: One (1) character may be entered in either box.
- **Block 12** Enter "Signature on File," "SOF," or the actual legal signature of the patient or an authorized person. When using a legal signature, enter the date signed in six (6)—digit (MMDDYY) or eight (8)—digit (MMDDYYYY) format.
  NOTE: Use the space available to enter the signature and date.
- **Block 13** Enter "Signature on File," "SOF," or the actual legal signature of the insured or an authorized person. When using a legal signature, enter the date signed in six (6)—digit (MMDDYY) or eight (8)—digit (MMDDYYYY) format.
  NOTE: Use the space available to enter the signature.

SECTION 3: PROVIDER/SUPPLIER INFORMATION

- **Block 14** Enter the date of the first time the present illness, injury, or pregnancy began in six (6)—digit (MMDDYY) or eight (8)—digit (MMDDYYYY) format. In the case of pregnancy, use the date of the last menstrual period (LMP).
  NOTE: Two (2) characters may be entered under MM and DD, and four (4) characters may be entered under the YYYY.
- **Block 15** Enter the first date the patient experienced the same or a similar illness in either six (6)—digit (MMDDYY) or eight (8)—digit (MMDDYYYY) format. Do not indicate previous pregnancies. Leave blank if unknown.
  NOTE: Two (2) characters may be entered under MM and DD, and four (4) characters may be entered under the YYYY.
- **Block 16** If the patient is employed and is unable to work in his or her current occupation, enter a six (6)—digit (MMDDYY) or eight (8)—digit (MMDDYYYY) date in the FROM and TO fields to explain the period in which the patient has been unable to work in his or her current occupation.
  NOTE: Two (2) characters may be entered under MM and DD, and four (4) characters may be entered under the YYYY.
- **Block 17** Enter the name (first name, middle initial, last name) and credentials of the professional who referred or ordered the service (or services) or supplies on the claim. Do not use a period or commas in the name. A hyphen can be used for hyphenated names.
  NOTE: Twenty-six (26) characters may be entered in this field.

For Medicare claims, the following services/situations require submission of the referring/ordering provider's information:

- ○ Medicare-covered services and items that are the result of a physician's order or referral
- ○ Parenteral and enteral nutrition
- ○ Immunosuppressive drug claims
- ○ Hepatitis B claims
- ○ Diagnostic laboratory services
- ○ Diagnostic radiology services
- ○ Portable x-ray services
- ○ Consultative services
- ○ Durable medical equipment
- ○ When the ordering physician is also the performing physician (as often is the case with in-office clinical laboratory tests)

- **Block 17a** If the referring provider, ordering provider, or other source does not have a National Provider Identifier (NPI) number, enter the qualifying ID number and the applicable personal identification number (PIN).
  NOTE: Two (2) characters may be entered in the qualifier field and seventeen (17) characters in the Other ID Number field.
- **Block 17b** Enter the NPI number of the referring provider, ordering provider, or other source, if available.
  NOTE: This field allows for entry of a ten (10)—digit NPI number.
- **Block 18** Enter the FROM and TO dates between which the patient was in the hospital, beginning with the admission date and ending with the discharge date; provide these dates in six (6)—digit (MMDDYY) or eight (8)—digit (MMDDYYYY) format. If the patient has not yet been discharged, leave the TO field blank. This block is used only when the hospitalization is related to the current illness or injury.
  NOTE: This field allows for entry of the following in each of the date fields: Two (2) characters may be entered under MM and DD, and four (4) characters under the YYYY.
- **Block 19** Refer to the most current instructions from the applicable public or private payer regarding the use of this field. Some payers ask for certain identifiers in this field. If identifiers are reported in this field, enter the appropriate qualifiers describing the identifier. Do not enter a space, hyphen, or other separator between the qualifier code and the number (see Table 21-3 for the list of qualifiers).
  NOTE: Eighty-three (83) characters are allowed in this field.
- **Block 20** Use this field when billing for purchased services. Put an X in the YES box if the reported services were performed by an entity other than the billing provider. Then enter the purchase price of those services. Marking the YES box indicates that an entity other than the one billing for the services performed the purchased services. Putting an X in the NO box indicates that no purchased services are included on the claim. When the YES box is marked, Block 32 must be completed. When billing for multiple purchased services, each service should be submitted on a separate claim form. Only one box can be marked. When entering the charge amount, enter the amount in the field to the left of the vertical line. Enter the number right justified to the left of the vertical line. Do not

use commas or a decimal point when reporting amounts. Negative dollar amounts are not allowed. Dollar signs should not be entered. Use "00" for the cents if the amount is a whole number. Leave the right-hand field blank.

NOTE: One (1) character may be entered in either box in the Outside Lab area, and eight (8) characters may be entered to the left of the vertical line and in the charges area.

- **Block 21** Enter the code(s) for the patient's diagnosis or condition. Up to four ICD-9-CM diagnosis codes can be listed. Relate lines 1, 2, 3, and/or 4 to the lines of service in Block 24E by line number. For the codes, use the highest level of specificity. Do not provide narrative descriptions in this field. When entering the code number, include a space (accommodated by the period) between the two sets of numbers. If entering a code with more than three beginning digits (e.g., E codes), enter the fourth digit on top of the period.

   NOTE: This field allows for entry of three (3) characters before the period; one (1) character above or on the period; and four (4) characters after the period in each of the four line areas.

- **Block 22** List the original reference number for resubmitted Medicaid claims. Refer to the most current instructions from the applicable public or private payer regarding the use of this field.

   NOTE: This field allows for entry of eleven (11) characters in the code area and eighteen (18) characters in the original reference number area.

- **Block 23** Enter any of the following: prior authorization number, referral number, mammography precertification number, or Clinical Laboratory Improvement Amendments (CLIA) number, as assigned by the payer for the current service. Do not enter hyphens or spaces in the number.

   NOTE: Twenty-nine (29) characters are allowed in this field.

- **Block 24** The six service lines in Block 24 have been divided horizontally to accommodate submission of the NPI number and of supplemental information to support the billed service. The top area of the six service lines is shaded; this is the location for reporting supplemental information. It is NOT intended to allow billing for 12 blocks.

   NOTE: The shaded area of lines 1 through 6 allows for entry of sixty-one (61) characters from the beginning of Block 24A to the end of Block 24G.

- **Block 24A** Enter the dates of service, both FROM and TO. If there is only one date of service, enter that date under FROM and leave TO blank, or re-enter the date placed in FROM.

   NOTE: Two (2) characters are allowed for each section of month, day, and year.

   ○ Enter the first date the service was provided, and the last date.
   ○ If services were provided on the same day, enter the same date in the FROM and TO fields in Block 24A.
   ○ Enter a date for each procedure, service, or supply in six (6)–digit (MMDDYY) or eight (8)–digit (MMDDYYYY) format.
   ○ When FROM and TO dates are shown for a series of identical services, enter the number of days or units in column G.

- **Block 24B** Enter the appropriate two (2)–digit code from the Place of Service code list for each block used or service performed.

   NOTE: Two (2) characters are allowed in the unshaded area.

- **Block 24C** Determine whether the services provided were an emergency. If required, enter Y for yes or N for no in the bottom, unshaded section of the field. An emergency is defined by federal or state regulations or programs, payer contracts, or as stated in the electronic 837P implementation guide.

   NOTE: Two (2) characters may be entered in the unshaded area.

- **Block 24D** Enter the *Current Procedural Terminology* (CPT) or *Health Care Common Procedural Coding System* (HCPCS) code or codes and modifiers (if applicable) from the appropriate code set in effect on the date of service. This field accommodates entry of up to four (4) 2-digit modifiers. The procedure code must be shown without a narrative description.

   NOTE: Six (6) characters may be entered in the unshaded area of the CPT/HCPCS field, and four sets of two (2) characters may be entered in the modifier area.

   ○ The CPT or HCPCS code for the procedure or service is entered in the first section of Block 24D.
   ○ The CPT or HCPCS modifier for the procedure or service (when applicable) is entered in the second section of Block 24D.
   ○ Any additional CPT or HCPCS modifiers are entered in the remaining sections of Block 24D.

- **Block 24E** Enter the diagnosis code reference number (pointer), as shown in Block 21, to relate the date of service and the procedures performed to the primary diagnosis. When multiple services have been performed, the primary reference number for each service should be listed first and other applicable services should follow. The reference numbers should be 1, 2, 3, or 4, or multiple numbers as explained. ICD-9-CM diagnosis codes should be entered in Block 21 only. Do NOT enter them in Block 24E. Enter the numbers justified to the left. Do not use commas between the numbers.

   NOTE: Four (4) characters may be entered in the unshaded area.

- **Block 24F** Enter the charge for the listed service or procedure. Enter the number right justified in the dollar area of the field. Do not use commas when reporting dollar amounts. Negative dollar amounts are not allowed. Dollar signs should not be entered. Enter "00" in the cents column area if the amount is a whole number.

   NOTE: Six (6) characters may be entered to the left of the vertical line, and two (2) characters may be entered to the right of the vertical line in the unshaded area.

- **Block 24G** Enter the number of days or units. This is usually used for multiple visits, units of supplies, anesthesia units or minutes, or oxygen volume. If only one service is performed, enter 1. Enter numbers right justified in the field. No leading zeros are required. If reporting a fraction of a unit, use the decimal point (see Table 21-3 for a description of qualifiers).

   NOTE: This field allows for entry of three (3) characters in the unshaded area.

PROCEDURE 21-2—cont'd

○ Enter the number of days or units. If there is only 1 day or unit, the numeral 1 must be entered.
○ Some services require that the actual number or quantity billed be clearly indicated on the claim form (e.g., multiple ostomy or urinary supplies, medication dosages, or allergy testing procedures). When multiple services are provided, enter the actual number provided.
○ For anesthesia, show the elapsed time (minutes) in Block 24G.

• **Block 24H** If the claim is Early and Periodic Screening, Diagnosis, and Treatment (EPSDT) or Aid to Families with Dependent Children (AFDC) related, enter Y for yes or N for no in the unshaded area of the field. If the claim is family planning, enter Y, or leave blank if N is in the unshaded area of the field.
NOTE: One (1) character is allowed in this field.

• **Block 24I** Leave blank if the rendering provider has an NPI number. If the provider of service does not have an NPI number, enter the qualifier number in the shaded area.
NOTE: This field allows for entry of two (2) characters in the shaded area.

• **Block 24J** If the rendering provider has an NPI number, enter it in the unshaded area. If the provider of service does not have an NPI number, enter the provider's PIN number or other ID number in the shaded area.
NOTE: Eleven (11) characters can be entered in the shaded area, and ten (10) characters for the NPI number are allowed in the unshaded area.

• **Block 25** Enter the provider's federal tax ID number or Social Security number. Put an X in the appropriate box (SSN or EIN) to show which was provided. Do not enter hyphens with numbers. Enter numbers left justified in the field.
NOTE: Fifteen (15) characters may be entered for the federal tax ID number or Social Security number, and one (1) character may be entered for the description of which number is provided.

• **Block 26** Enter the patient account number, if desired.
NOTE: This field allows for fourteen (14) characters.

• **Block 27** Put an X in the correct box (YES or NO) for accepting assignment. Only one box can be marked.
NOTE: One (1) character is allowed per box.

• **Block 28** Enter the total charges for the services in Block 24F.
NOTE: Seven (7) characters may be entered to the left of the vertical line, and two (2) characters may be entered to the right of the vertical line.

• **Block 29** Enter the total amount that was paid toward this claim by the patient or guarantor.
NOTE: Six (6) characters may be entered to the left of the vertical line, and two (2) characters may be entered to the right of the vertical line.

• **Block 30** Enter the total amount due. (This information does not exist in the electronic 837P implementation guide.)
NOTE: Six (6) characters may be entered to the left of the vertical line, and two (2) characters may be entered to the right of the vertical line.

• **Block 31** Enter "Signature on File," "SOF," or the actual legal signature of the practitioner or supplier. Enter the date the claim was signed in a six (6)–digit (MMDDYY) or an eight (8)–digit format.

• **Block 32** Enter the name, address, city, state, and ZIP code of the location where the services were rendered.
NOTE: Seventy-eight (78) characters may be used in this block. Enter the name and address in the following format:
○ First line: Name
○ Second line: Address
○ Third line: City, state, and ZIP code

• **Block 32a** Enter the NPI number of the service facility location.
NOTE: Ten (10) characters may be entered in this space. If the service facility does not have an NPI number, leave Block 32a blank.

• **Block 32b** If the service facility does not have an NPI number, enter the two (2)–digit non-NPI number qualifier, followed by the PIN or other ID number. Do not enter a space, hyphen, or other separator between the qualifier and number.
NOTE: Fourteen (14) characters may be entered in Block 32b.

• **Block 33** Identifies the provider requesting to be paid and should always be completed.
NOTE: Three (3) characters are available for the area code; nine (9) characters for the phone number; and eighty-seven (87) characters for billing provider information. Enter the provider's or supplier's billing name and address using the following format:
○ First line: Name
○ Second line: Address
○ Third line: City, state, and ZIP code

• **Block 33a** Enter the NPI number of the billing provider.
NOTE: Ten (10) characters are allowed. If the billing provider does not have an NPI number, leave blank.

• **Block 33b** If the billing provider does not have an NPI number, enter the two (2)–digit non-NPI qualifier and PIN or other ID number.
NOTE: Thirty-three (33) characters may be entered in this space. Do not put a space between the qualifier and ID number.

FINAL STEPS

1. Review the claim for accuracy and completeness.
PURPOSE: To double-check that no blocks or fields are inaccurate or missing required information.

2. Run or prepare an insurance claims log for all claims completed. For paper claims, make a copy of the claim and place it in the tickler file.
PURPOSE: To provide an audit trail of claims submitted.

3. For paper claims:
a. Use a paper clip to add any attachments to be sent with the claim.
b. Group all claims going to the same carrier and mail together in one large envelope.
c. Address the envelope, weigh the contents, attach postage, and mail.

4. For claims to be submitted electronically, follow the computer software instructions for the software used.
PURPOSE: To submit all claims electronically or by surface mail to the appropriate insurance carrier.

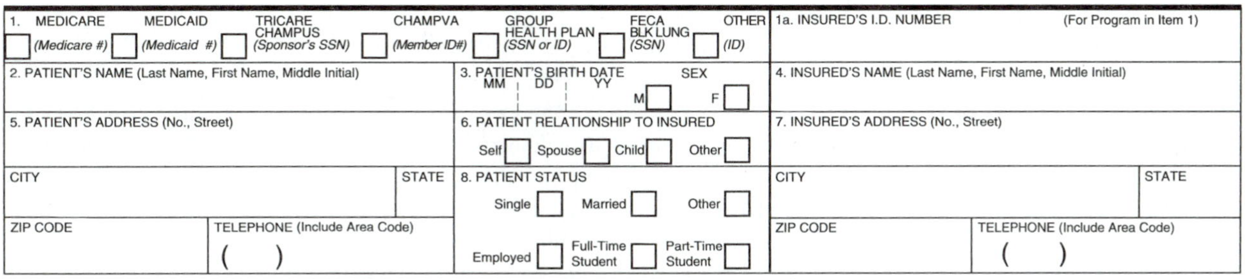
1. MEDICARE (Medicare #) MEDICAID (Medicaid #) TRICARE CHAMPUS (Sponsor's SSN) CHAMPVA (Member ID#) GROUP HEALTH PLAN (SSN or ID) FECA BLK LUNG (SSN) OTHER (ID)
1a. INSURED'S I.D. NUMBER (For Program in Item 1)
2. PATIENT'S NAME (Last Name, First Name, Middle Initial)
3. PATIENT'S BIRTH DATE MM DD YY SEX M F
4. INSURED'S NAME (Last Name, First Name, Middle Initial)
5. PATIENT'S ADDRESS (No., Street)
6. PATIENT RELATIONSHIP TO INSURED Self Spouse Child Other
7. INSURED'S ADDRESS (No., Street)
CITY STATE
8. PATIENT STATUS Single Married Other
CITY STATE
ZIP CODE TELEPHONE (Include Area Code) ( )
Employed Full-Time Student Part-Time Student
ZIP CODE TELEPHONE (Include Area Code) ( )

FIGURE 21-3 CMS-1500 claim form: patient and insured information, Blocks 1 to 8.

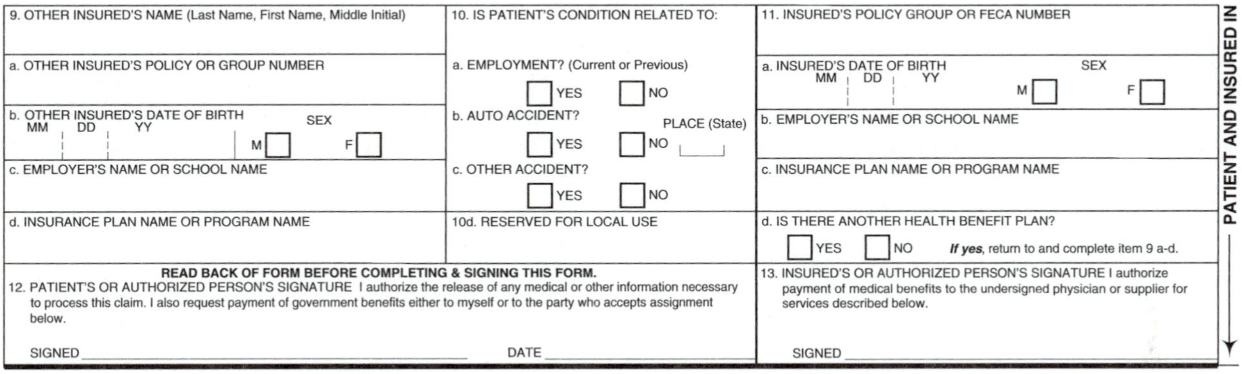
9. OTHER INSURED'S NAME (Last Name, First Name, Middle Initial)
10. IS PATIENT'S CONDITION RELATED TO:
11. INSURED'S POLICY GROUP OR FECA NUMBER
a. OTHER INSURED'S POLICY OR GROUP NUMBER
a. EMPLOYMENT? (Current or Previous) YES NO
a. INSURED'S DATE OF BIRTH MM DD YY SEX M F
b. OTHER INSURED'S DATE OF BIRTH MM DD YY SEX M F
b. AUTO ACCIDENT? YES NO PLACE (State)
b. EMPLOYER'S NAME OR SCHOOL NAME
c. EMPLOYER'S NAME OR SCHOOL NAME
c. OTHER ACCIDENT? YES NO
c. INSURANCE PLAN NAME OR PROGRAM NAME
d. INSURANCE PLAN NAME OR PROGRAM NAME
10d. RESERVED FOR LOCAL USE
d. IS THERE ANOTHER HEALTH BENEFIT PLAN? YES NO *If yes,* return to and complete item 9 a-d.
READ BACK OF FORM BEFORE COMPLETING & SIGNING THIS FORM.
12. PATIENT'S OR AUTHORIZED PERSON'S SIGNATURE I authorize the release of any medical or other information necessary to process this claim. I also request payment of government benefits either to myself or to the party who accepts assignment below.
SIGNED DATE
13. INSURED'S OR AUTHORIZED PERSON'S SIGNATURE I authorize payment of medical benefits to the undersigned physician or supplier for services described below.
SIGNED
PATIENT AND INSURED IN

FIGURE 21-4 CMS-1500 claim form: patient and insured information, Blocks 9 to 13.

Block 6: Patient Relationship to Insured.

- Self: Indicates that the patient is the insured.
- Spouse: Indicates that the patient is married to the insured.
- Child: Means that the patient is the insured's minor dependent.
- Other: May mean that the patient is an employee, that workers' compensation is the insurer, or that the patient is a ward or other dependent as defined by the insured's plan.

Block 7: Insured's Address. The insured's permanent address and telephone number are entered here. This address may be different from the patient's address in Block 5.

Block 8: Patient Status. These boxes are important for determining liability and for coordinating benefits.

- Single
- Married
- Other
- Employed: Put an X in this box if the patient is employed, whether full-time or part-time.
- Full-time student or part-time student: Put an X in the appropriate box, depending on the school's definition of full-time and part-time status. Generally, if the student is taking 6 or fewer credit hours, he or she is considered a part-time student.

Section 3: Patient/Insured Section—Blocks 9 to 13 (Figure 21-4)

NOTE: Blocks 11a-d are completed for the primary insurance. Blocks 9a-d are completed only if a secondary insurance claim is being submitted.

Block 9: Other Insured's Name. The name of the person who holds another policy on the patient. Block 9 is completed only if there is a secondary insurance policy and if that secondary policy is to be billed.

Block 9a: Other Insured's Policy or Group Number. The policy number of the insured in Block 9. See Block 1a for guidelines for Medicare, Medicaid, Group Health Plan, FECA/Black Lung, and Other ID numbers.

Block 9b: Other Insured's Date of Birth and Sex. The other insured's birth date and gender help identify the birth date and gender of the insured as indicated in Block 9. Block 9b is completed only if there is a secondary insurance policy and if that secondary policy is to be billed.

Block 9c: Employer's Name or School Name. This block identifies the other insured's employer or school name as indicated in Block 9. Block 9c is completed only if there is a secondary insurance policy and if that secondary policy is to be billed.

Block 9d: Insurance Plan Name or Program Name. The insurance plan name or program name identifies the name of the plan or program of the other insured as indicated in Block 9. Block 9d is completed only if there is a secondary insurance policy and if that secondary policy is to be billed.

Blocks 10a-c: Is Patient's Condition Related to: This block indicates whether the patient's condition is the result of an employment injury or illness, auto accident, or other accident.

Block 10d: Reserved for Local Use. Some third-party payers require that this box be used. Refer to the applicable third-party payer's instructions.

Block 11: Insured's Policy, Group, or FECA Number. Block 11 is completed for the primary insurance claim. The policy, group, or FECA number is the alphanumeric identifier for the insurance plan coverage. Workers' compensation claims use the carrier's alphanumeric identifier. The FECA number is the nine-digit alpha-numeric identifier assigned to the patient claiming a work-related condition under FECA.

Block 11a: Insured's Date of Birth and Sex. Block 11a is completed for the primary insurance claim. This information applies to the person identified in Block 1a.

Block 11b: Insured's Employer's Name or School Name. Block 11b is completed for the primary insurance claim. This refers to the name of the employer or school attended by the insured as indicated in Box 1a.

Block 11c: Insured's Insurance Plan Name or Program Name. Block 11c is completed for the primary insurance claim. The insurance plan name or program name refers to the name of the plan or program of the insured, as indicated in the Carrier Block (Section 1).

Block 11d: Is There Another Health Benefit Plan? This block indicates whether the patient has insurance coverage other than that indicated in Block 1. If there is a secondary coverage, put an X in the YES box; if not, or if no claim is being submitted using the secondary coverage, put an X in the NO box.

Block 12: Patient's or Authorized Person's Signature. The signature is an authorization for the release of any medical or other information necessary to process or adjudicate the claim. The signature of the patient or the patient's representative is required. In the case of computer-generated claims, an authorization form with the patient's signature must be kept in the patient's record authorizing the release of medical information. The phrase "Signature on File" may be entered in this field.

Block 13: Insured's or Authorized Person's Signature. The insured's or authorized person's signature indicates that there is a signature on file authorizing payment of medical benefits directly to the provider who appears in Blocks 31 and 32 of the claim. The signature of the patient or the patient's representative is required. In the case of computer-generated claims, an authorization form with the insured's signature must be kept in the patient's record authorizing the release of medical information. The phrase "Signature on File" may be entered in this field.

CRITICAL THINKING APPLICATION   21-2

It is office policy to request that patients assign benefits (payment) to the provider directly if the patient does not pay for services at the time of the encounter. One of the patients, Mr. Palmer, seems hesitant to sign Block 13 of the CMS-1500 form. How should Machelle explain the office policy to Mr. Palmer?

Physician/Supplier Section—Blocks 14 to 23 (Figure 21-5)

Block 14: Date of Current Illness, Injury, or Pregnancy. The date should be the date when the current illness or condition began, the date the injury happened or, in cases of pregnancy, the date of the last menstrual period (LMP).

Block 15: Same or Similar Illness. If the patient has had the same or a similar illness or condition, enter the onset date of the earlier condition. This block is used by the insurance carrier to determine whether any pre-existing condition existed, which might affect reimbursement.

Block 16: Dates Patient Unable to Work in Current Occupation. This section refers to the FROM and TO dates between which the patient was unable to work in his or her current occupation. If the patient has not returned to work, leave the TO field blank. This block is used to help determine an employee's long- or short-term disability payments.

Block 17: Name of Referring Provider or Other Source. The name of the referring provider, ordering provider, or other source that referred or ordered the service or procedure on the claim is entered in this block.

> A *referring physician* is a physician who requests an item or service for the beneficiary for which payment may be made.
>
> An *ordering physician* is a physician or, when appropriate, a non-physician practitioner who orders non-physician services for the patient.

Block 17a: Other ID. Block 17a currently is not reported (as of May 23, 2008); however, Block 17b must be reported when a service was ordered or referred by a physician.

Block 17b: NPI. The NPI refers to the individual national ID number (**National Provider Identifier**) that HIPAA assigns to each healthcare provider of services.

In the past, each insurance carrier, including government programs, assigned an identifier to each provider of service. Since 2007, as part of HIPAA, all allied healthcare providers of services have been assigned one individual NPI number that the provider can use regardless of which insurance carrier is billed for reimbursement. The NPI is a uniform, national ID number that has replaced Medicare's **Unique Provider Identification Number (UPIN)** and almost all other federal, state, and private insurance carriers' **provider identification numbers (PINs)**. However, the NPI does *not* replace the Social Security number (SSN), **Employer Identification Number (EIN)**, or federal Tax Identification Number (TIN) used by a

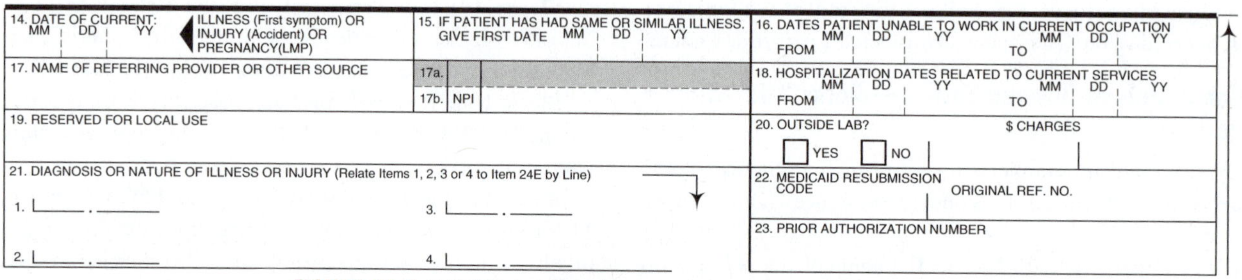

FIGURE 21-5 CMS-1500 claim form: physician or supplier information, Blocks 14 to 23.

provider of service. The SSN, EIN, and TIN are used for income and tax purposes and for reporting to the Internal Revenue Service.

Block 18: Hospitalization Dates Related to Current Services. These dates are the admission and discharge dates of the inpatient stay related to the services listed on the claim.

Block 19: Reserved for Local Use. Some payers ask for certain identifiers in this field. Refer to the applicable third-party payer's instructions. (To see a list of the identifiers that may still be used in some instances in this block, refer to the Evolve site at *evolve.elsevier.com/kinn*). Medicare has specific uses for this block if services were rendered by certain providers, or for certain services, drugs, or diagnostic tests. Refer to the *Medicare Claims Processing Manual* for instructions.

Block 20: Outside Lab?/Charges. This field refers to diagnostic laboratory services that have been rendered by an independent or separate provider as indicated in Block 32. Put an X in the YES box to indicate that an entity other than the provider billing for the service performed the diagnostic test and the provider in Block 33 paid the laboratory directly. Put an X in the NO box to indicate that no purchased tests are included on the claim. When the YES box is marked, the amount the provider was charged by the diagnostic laboratory is entered, and Block 32 should be completed with the name and address of the diagnostic laboratory or other entity.

Block 21: Diagnosis or Nature of Illness or Injury. This title refers to the signs, symptoms, complaint, or condition of the patient relating to the services on the claim. The diagnosis (ICD-9-CM) code or codes should be entered in this block. Enter one code for each of the four fields in the block. No more than four diagnosis codes should be used on one claim form.

Block 22: Medicaid Resubmission. The code and original reference number assigned by the insurance payer should be entered in this block if a Medicaid claim previously submitted has not been reimbursed; this also is done to resubmit the claim to Medicaid or its intermediary for payment.

Block 23: Prior Authorization Number. This is the payer-assigned number authorizing the service or services, procedure or procedures, and/or referral.

Physician/Supplier Section—Blocks 24 to 33
(Figure 21-6)

Block 24A: Date(s) of Service (lines 1-6). This date (or dates) is the actual month, day, and year that the service was provided.

Block 24B: Place of Service (lines 1-6). This block identifies where the services were provided. Enter the two-digit place of service (POS) code in Block 24B. Table 21-2 shows the two-digit place of service codes.

Block 24C: EMG (lines 1-6). This field is used to indicate whether the services provided involved an emergency. Enter a Y in this block if the services were provided in emergency circumstances. Medicare providers are not required to complete this item.

Block 24D: Procedures, Services, or Supplies (lines 1-6). In this field, identifying codes for reporting medical services and procedures are listed.

Block 24E: Diagnosis Pointer (lines 1-6). Enter the diagnosis code, or reference number, as shown in Block 21 to relate the date of service and the procedures performed to the primary diagnosis. Enter only one reference number per line item. When multiple services have been performed, enter the primary field number for each service (either a 1, a 2, a 3, or a 4). This is a required field. If two or more diagnoses are required for a procedure code (e.g., a Pap smear), the provider should reference only one of the diagnoses in Block 21.

Block 24F: $ Charges (lines 1-6). This is the total billed amount for each service line. If a series of services was performed on any one line, multiply the number of days or units (Block 24G) by the charge for one procedure or service and enter the total amount for all days or units.

Block 24G: Days or Units (lines 1-6). This title refers to the number of days that correspond to the dates entered in Block 24A, or to units, as defined in the CPT or HCPCS coding manual.

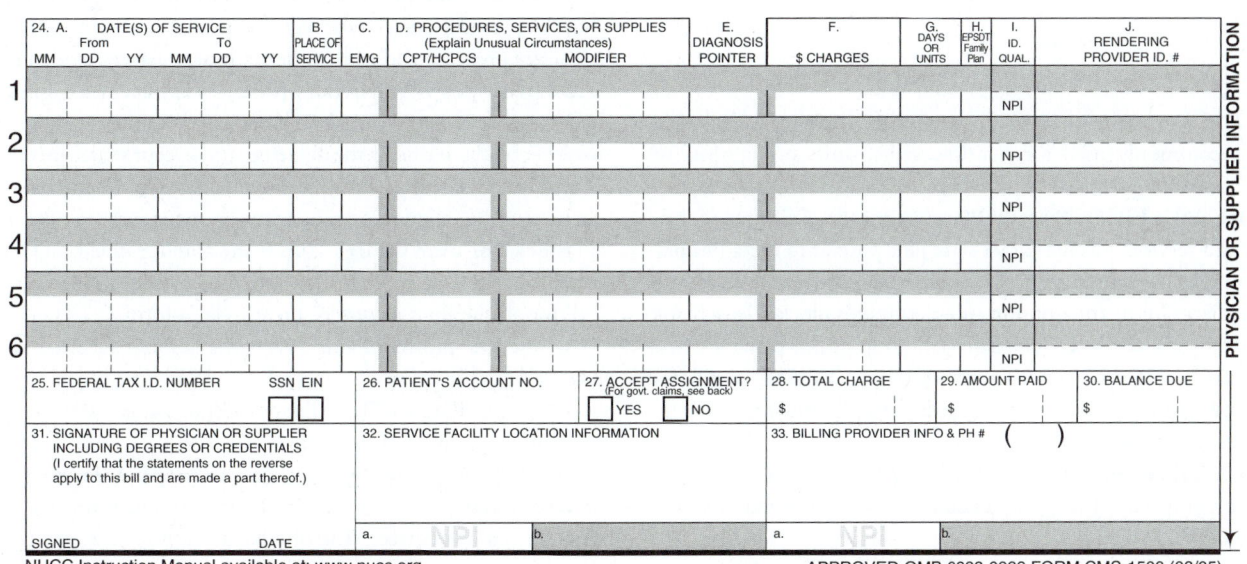

FIGURE 21-6 CMS-1500 claim form: physician or supplier information, Blocks 24 to 33.

TABLE 21-2 Place of Service Codes

CODE	DESCRIPTION	CODE	DESCRIPTION
11	Doctor's office	50	Federally qualified health center
12	Patient's home	51	Inpatient psychiatry facility
21	Inpatient hospital	52	Psychiatric facility—partial hospitalization
22	Outpatient hospital	53	Community mental health care (outpatient, 24-hour/day services, admission screening, consultation, and educational services)
23	Emergency department—hospital	54	Intermediate care facility/mentally retarded
24	Ambulatory surgical center	55	Residential substance abuse treatment facility
25	Birthing center	56	Psychiatric residential treatment center
26	Military treatment facility/uniformed service treatment facility	60	Mass immunization center
31	Skilled nursing facility (swing bed visits)	61	Comprehensive inpatient rehabilitation facility
32	Nursing facility (intermediate/long-term care facilities)	62	Comprehensive outpatient rehabilitation facility
33	Custodial care facility (domiciliary or rest home services)	65	End-stage renal disease treatment facility
34	Hospice (domiciliary or rest home services)	71	State or local public health clinic
35	Adult living care facilities (residential care facility)	72	Rural health clinic
41	Ambulance—land	81	Independent laboratory
42	Ambulance—air or water	99	Other unlisted facility

TABLE 21-3 Qualifiers Used to Report National Drug Code (NDC) Units

QUALIFIER	DESCRIPTION
F2	International unit
GR	gram
ML	milliliter
UN	unit

Table 21-3 shows the qualifiers to be used in this block. This field is most commonly used for multiple visits, units of supplies, or anesthesia minutes.

Block 24H: EPSDT/Family Plan (lines 1-6). This field identifies certain services covered under state plans. Refer to the appropriate insurance payer's guidelines (typically Medicaid or the Medicaid intermediary) for instructions on completing this block. Leave blank for Medicare, TRICARE, CHAMPVA, group health plans, FECA/Black Lung, and most other insurance types. (EPSDT stands for Early and Periodic Screening, Diagnosis, and Treatment, the child health program under Medicaid.)

Block 24I: Rendering Provider ID Qualifier (lines 1-6). The rendering provider is the person or company that rendered or supervised the care.

Block 24J: Rendering Provider ID Number (lines 1-6). Enter the NPI number of the individual performing/rendering the service in the shaded portion of Block 24J. If there is no NPI number, enter the provider's PIN and the appropriate two-character qualifier.

Block 25: Federal Tax ID Number. This is the unique tax identifier assigned to the provider by the Internal Revenue Service. It may be either the provider's Social Security number or an EIN.

Block 26: Patient's Account Number. This is the account number assigned to the patient by the provider of service. The account number assists the provider in locating the patient's financial information and record.

Block 27: Accept Assignment? "Accepting assignment" means that the provider agrees to accept assignment under the terms of the Medicare program and some other insurance payers. Put an X in the YES box in this block if the provider will **accept assignment** of benefits; that is, that he or she is a participating physician and agrees to abide by the terms of the agreement to accept what the insurance company pays and write off the difference between the original charge and the allowable amount set by the insurance carrier.

Block 28: Total Charge. This is the amount billed on this claim form for all services rendered. Add the charges reported in Block 24F for all the lines of service on the claim form.

Block 29: Amount Paid. This is the amount received from the patient or other payers.

Block 30: Balance Due. This is the amount left after the patient has paid a co-pay or co-insurance.

Block 31: Signature of Physician or Supplier (include degrees or credentials). The signature is the verification from the provider that the claim is correct. The physician can place his **electronic (or digital) signature** on the claim by typing his or her name or initials (if allowed by the insurance carrier) in the block.

Block 32: Service Facility Location Information. Enter the name, address, city, state, and ZIP code for the site where services were rendered.

Block 32a [service facility NPI number]. Enter the NPI number of the service facility.

Block 32b [service facility's non-NPI identifier]. If the service facility does not have an NPI, enter the payer-assigned unique identifier of the facility and the qualifier number.

Block 33: Billing Provider Info & PH. Enter the address and phone number of the provider that wishes to be paid on this claim.

Block 33a [billing provider's NPI]. Enter the billing provider's NPI number.

Box 33b [billing provider's non-NPI identifier]. If the billing provider does not have an NPI number, enter the professional's payer-assigned unique identifier. The two-character qualifier for the non-NPI identifier is also entered here.

GUIDELINES FOR CLAIMS REVIEW BEFORE SUBMISSION

The following guidelines can help ensure that a clean claim is submitted.

- Proofread the form carefully for accuracy and completeness.
- Make certain any necessary attachments are included with the completed form.
- Follow office policies and guidelines for claim review and signatures.
- Forward the original claim to the proper insurance carrier either by mail or electronically.
- If creating a paper claim, make a copy of the completed and signed claim form for the office records.
- If a non-computer-generated insurance log is maintained, enter the appropriate information in the insurance log and record the insurance submission information on the patient's ledger.
- The patient's and/or insured's name, address, and ID, group, and/or policy number should be identical to the information printed on the insurance card.
- The patient's birth date and gender should correspond with the medical record.
- The word NONE should be entered in Block 11 if Medicare is the primary payer.
- The referring, consulting, or ordering provider's name and NPI number should be entered in Blocks 17 and 17a, if applicable.
- In Block 27 (Accept Assignment?), put an X in the YES box if the physician is a participating provider (PAR) or has an agreement with the insurance carrier or payer to accept assignment.
- Make sure the diagnosis is not missing or incomplete.
- The diagnosis must be coded accurately, according to the ICD-9-CM coding manual, and must correspond to the treatment.
- The patient must have authorized the release of information, and Block 12 should contain a handwritten signature, the words "Signature on File," or the acronym SOF.
- Section 2, the Patient/Insured Section (Blocks 1 through 13), should be completed accurately according to the guidelines of the insurance carrier.

- Fees for each charge must be listed individually, or they must be correctly computed if more than 1 day or unit is entered in Block 24G.
- All required fields of the diagnosis and procedure section of the claim form (Blocks 14 through 24J) should be accurate and completed according to the guidelines of the third-party payer or insurance company.
- The physician's signature must be on the form.
- The provider's federal TIN, EIN, or SSN should be double-checked to ensure accuracy.
- The physician's NPI number, corresponding to the insurance carrier being billed, should be entered in Block 24J and again in Block 33a. The provider's PIN, when applicable, should be entered in Block 33b, with the qualifying number, when applicable.

PREVENTING CLAIM REJECTION

It is important for the medical assistant to understand and comply with the guidelines specific to completion of a CMS-1500 form for each third-party payer and insurance company to prevent delays in reimbursement—or worse, denial of payment. The guidelines for Medicare, Medicaid, TRICARE, and workers' compensation can be found online at any of the fiscal intermediaries (e.g., Medicare billing guidelines are on the CMS Web site). Most computer software billing systems have built-in "claim scrubbers" that help in the process, and if claims are sent electronically through a clearinghouse, claims auditing is done before the clearinghouse submits the claim to the third-party payer. Claims without significant errors of any type are called *clean claims*. Claims with incorrect, missing, or insufficient data are called *dirty claims*.

Denied or Rejected Claims

The two main reasons for denial of payment are technical errors and insurance policy coverage issues. Technical errors include incorrect or incomplete information or typographic or mathematical errors. A common reason for insurance coverage rejection is that a procedure listed on the claim is not a covered service or is considered a pre-existing condition by the insurance payer.

Explanation of Benefits

The reason for a claim denial or reduction in reimbursement is listed on the explanation of benefits (EOB; Figure 21-7) of commercial carriers, the remittance advice (RA) for commercial carriers and on Medicaid claims, and the explanation of Medicare benefits (EOMB) on Medicare claims. The EOMB, EOB, and RA are hard copy or electronic forms that list the amount paid by the insurance company, in addition to information about any noncovered services, denied claims (and the reason), deductible and/or co-insurance amounts, and other information about the claim or claims submitted.

Some descriptive terms for claims include the following:
- **Clean claim**. A complete, accurate claim.
- Dingy or **dirty claim**. An inaccurate or **incomplete claim** returned for more information or correction.
- **Rejected claim**. A claim for which payment has been denied for any reason (e.g., non-covered service, pre-existing condition, or ineligibility).

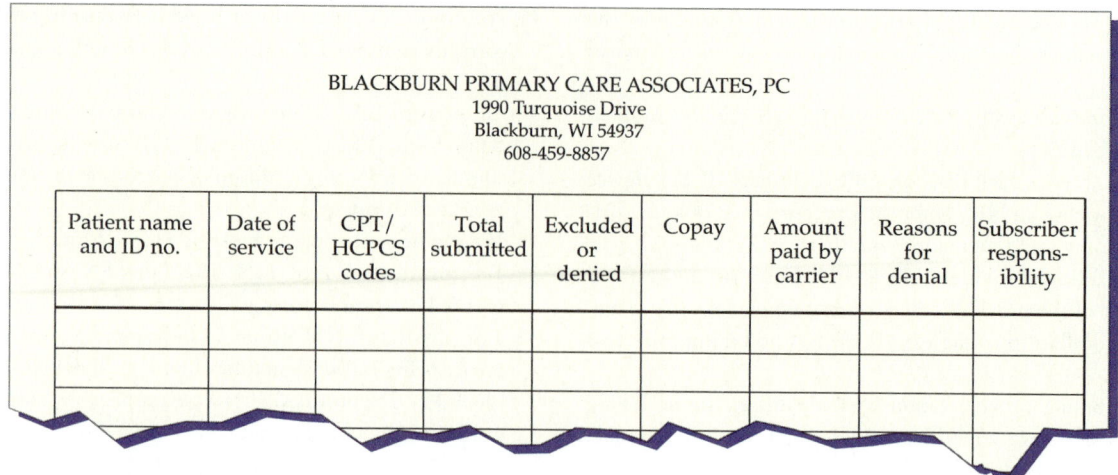

BLACKBURN PRIMARY CARE ASSOCIATES, PC
1990 Turquoise Drive
Blackburn, WI 54937
608-459-8857

Patient name and ID no.	Date of service	CPT/ HCPCS codes	Total submitted	Excluded or denied	Copay	Amount paid by carrier	Reasons for denial	Subscriber responsibility

FIGURE 21-7 Example of an explanation of benefits (EOB) form. (From Hunt SA: *Saunders fundamentals of medical assisting*, Philadelphia, 2002, WB Saunders.)

At times, a denied claim may involve policy issues beyond the control of the medical assistant. When this happens, he or she should contact the patient and discuss the problem. Normally, it is the patient's responsibility to resolve disputes regarding payment with the payer. The insurance policy is a contract between the company and the insured. However, the provider and those involved with the billing process in the medical facility should have a good understanding of the guidelines and requirements for the types of claims and various insurers handled most often in the facility and be willing to assist the patient wherever possible to ensure reimbursement.

> ### CRITICAL THINKING APPLICATION 21-3
> During her externship at the women's health center, Machelle sees a file containing a number of rejected claims. On closer examination, she notices that similar errors in certain blocks are repeatedly the cause for rejection. Discuss common errors on the CMS-1500 claim form and what can be done to prevent these mistakes and/or omissions.

CHECKING A CLAIM'S STATUS

It is often necessary to send a "tracer" to an insurance company to determine the status of a delinquent insurance claim. The accepted practice is to submit the tracer a day or two after the usual turn-around time of the payer, generally 30 to 60 days (10 to 14 days for an electronic submission). A tracer is typically a form letter asking the insurance company about the status of an unpaid insurance claim. An example of a tracer letter is shown in Figure 21-8. A claim's status can also be checked electronically using the ASC X12N transaction and code sets for the request and the response.

- ASC X12N 276 Health Care Claim Status Request
- ASC X12N 277 Health Care Claim Status Response

A duplicate copy of all submitted claims should be retained either in paper form or in the computer billing software. A structured routine for following up on claims unpaid within a specific time frame should be created to prevent overlooking a claim that should be filed or that has not been paid. The Insurance Claim Register, tickler files, and reports from the insurance database all help to keep track of paid and pending claims. If software is used to file claims, an insurance pending report and an insurance aging report (among others) can be generated.

The insurance aging report (Figure 21-9) can be sorted by the age of the claim, typically 30, 60, 90, and 120 days (or more), and by the payer (e.g., Medicare, Medicaid, and so on). Any of these methods is useful for following up on claims that have yet to be paid.

If claims are submitted electronically, either directly or through a clearinghouse, the medical assistant might allow 10 business days for claim turnaround before expecting reimbursement. For paper claims, allow an additional week or two to account for the necessary manual processing and mailing time. The length of time between a claim's submission and its payment varies from payer to payer; an experienced medical assistant soon becomes familiar with the individual payment patterns of third-party payers and their claim turnaround times. Most states have laws that require payment within 45 days for clean claims.

Audit Trails

Electronic transactions leave behind a path or trail as they are processed, and this trail can be tracked or audited to provide a record. This record, called an **audit trail**, can be used to verify that the information was processed correctly or to locate the source of an error. If an office uses a computerized accounting program and submits claims electronically, the software is capable of printing out an insurance aging report by date, by patient name, or by carrier name. If paper claims are used, however, the medical assistant should establish a follow-up procedure for tracking insurance claims. This can be accomplished by using an insurance claims register or log (Figure 21-10). This document can be developed and updated with little effort using a spreadsheet computer program, such as Microsoft Excel, if the provider's office is computerized. If the provider uses physician financial management and billing

INSURANCE CLAIM TRACER

INSURANCE COMPANY NAME _____ DATE _____

ADDRESS: _____

PATIENT NAME _____ INSURED: _____

POLICY/CERTIFICATE NUMBER _____ GROUP NAME/NUMBER _____

EMPLOYER NAME AND ADDRESS: _____

DATE OF INITIAL CLAIM SUBMISSION _____ AMOUNT: _____

An inordinate amount of time has passed since submission of our original claim as described above. We have not received a request for additional information and still await payment of this assigned claim. Please review the attached duplicate and process for payment within seven (7) days.

If there is any difficulty with this claim, please check one of these below and return this letter to our office.

Claim pending because: _____
Payment of claim in process: _____
Payment made on claim: Date: _____ To whom: _____
Claim denied: (Reason) _____
Patient notified: Yes _____ No _____
Remarks: _____

Thank you for your assistance in this important matter. Please contact _____ in our office if you have any questions regarding this claim.

Office of: _____ M.D.

Address: _____

_____ TELEPHONE NUMBER: _____

FIGURE 21-8 Example of an insurance claim tracer. (From Fordney MT: *Insurance handbook for the medical office*, ed 12, St Louis, 2012, WB Saunders.)

Blackburn Primary Care Associates
Patient Aging

NAME	CURRENT 0 - 30	PAST 31 - 60	PAST 61 - 90	PAST 91 - 120	PAST over 120	Total Balance
Mary Smith Last Payment on 08/08/XX	$120.00					$120.00
John Payne Last Payment on 07/06/XX		$250.00				$250.00
Jack Desmonde Last Payment on 05/25/XX			$500.00			$500.00
Jill Jayne Last Payment on 04/02/XX		$80.00		$100.00		$180.00
Report Aging Totals Percent of Total Aging	$120.00 11.4%	$330.00 31.4%	$330.00 47.6%	$100.00 9.5%		$1,050.00 100.0%

FIGURE 21-9 Example of an accounts aging record. (From Hunt SA: *Saunders fundamentals of medical assisting*, Philadelphia, 2002, WB Saunders.)

Patient's Name Group/Policy No.	Name of Insurance Company	Claim Submitted Date	Claim Submitted Amount	Follow-Up Date	Follow-Up Date	Claim Paid Date	Claim Paid Amt	Difference
Jones, Bob	BC/BS	1-7-03	319.37			2/28/03	294.82	24.55
Carson, David	BC	1-8-03	268.08	2-10-03	3-10-03			
Linden, Jan	Medicaid	1-9-03	146.15	2-10-03				
Paul, Emma	Medicare	1-10-03	96.28	2-10-03				
Cortez, Jose	Unicare	1-10-03	647.09	2-10-03				
Dimico, Joe	Tricare	2-1-03	134.78	3-10-03				
Coldman, Billy	Aetna	2-4-03	607.67	3-10-03				
Fritz, Renee	Travelers	2-10-03	564.55	3-10-03				
Wong, Chang	Prudential	2-15-03	1515.79					
Billings, Harry	Allstate	2-21-03	121.21					
Green, James	BC	2-24-03	124.99					

INSURANCE CLAIMS REGISTER   Page No._____

FIGURE 21-10 Example of an insurance claims register.

software, an audit trail report can be generated automatically from the software program.

Another method of tracking claims is a tickler file (Figure 21-11), also called a *suspense* or *follow-up file*. With this method, a copy of each insurance claim is filed chronologically, and the file is checked periodically for unprocessed (delinquent) claims. When the claim is paid, the copy is removed and the information is posted on the patient's ledger card. Delinquent claims remaining in the file after the normal contract time limits are pulled and then traced. If the claim has been denied, a letter may be sent to the insurance carrier's appeals department, with a copy to the patient.

Patient Education

The medical assistant should be able to explain confusing technical issues to patients in simple, understandable terms. Patients, especially elderly ones, quickly become confused and frustrated by insurance issues, especially Medicare rules and regulations, which change nearly every year. The medical assistant should attempt to keep patients fully informed of changes in insurance guidelines and patiently explain why some procedures and services are paid for and others are not.

Legal and Ethical Issues

The practice of medicine and the responsibilities of the medical assistant are greatly affected by the legislative process. It is extremely important to stay current on the laws that affect medicine, federal and state insurance programs (e.g., Medicare, Medicaid, workers' compensation, and TRICARE) and the completion of the CMS-1500 claim form.

HIPAA is responsible for implementation of various laws that protect individuals' health insurance and privacy standards. Medical assistants should familiarize themselves with this important insurance law.

Because of the emphasis on compliance in medical practices today, every medical office must create and implement a plan to identify potential compliance problems and correct them before a liability risk is incurred. All providers are required to avoid fraud and abuse charges by following the regulations and guidelines provided by government entities and third-party payers.

CLOSING COMMENTS

Accurate completion of the CMS-1500 claim form begins with gathering the patient's and the insured's demographic and insurance information, the diagnoses and procedures and services performed, and the provider's identifying information. The Patient Registration form is used to collect the patient's and insured's information, and confirmation of all collected information is an important task that should not be neglected. Confirmation of the information can be obtained through photocopies of the patient's and insured's insurance cards, driver's licenses; verification of eligibility and benefits; and, where applicable, securing approval for procedures, services, and referrals from the insurance payer in advance. It is wise to have a checklist of all the information the medical assistant will need to complete an insurance claim correctly.

The CMS-1500 claim form (version 08-05) is generally accepted by all insurance payers. The requirements for completing each block of the CMS-1500 form vary slightly, depending on the type of insurance carrier (e.g., Medicare, Medicaid, group health plan). When completing an insurance claim for a specific insurance payer, it is important that the medical assistant use the claims processing manual or guidelines for *that* insurance carrier, to make certain the claim is completed according to the payer's specific requirements.

As mentioned, accurate and complete insurance claim forms submitted for payment are called *clean claims*. Clean claims result in reimbursement without delay, as long as no insurance policy limitations prevent or reduce payments. Insurance claims submitted with incorrect or missing information are called *dingy* or *dirty claims* and can be returned for additional information by the payer. This delays reimbursement for services rendered, and if the additional information is not forwarded quickly to the payer, can result in denial of payment. It is essential that procedures be in place to review all claims before submission to ensure that the claim is complete and the information is accurate. Unpaid claims result in a loss of revenue for the provider. Audit trails, insurance aging reports, tickler files, and/or insurance claims registers are valuable tools in insurance claims follow-up.

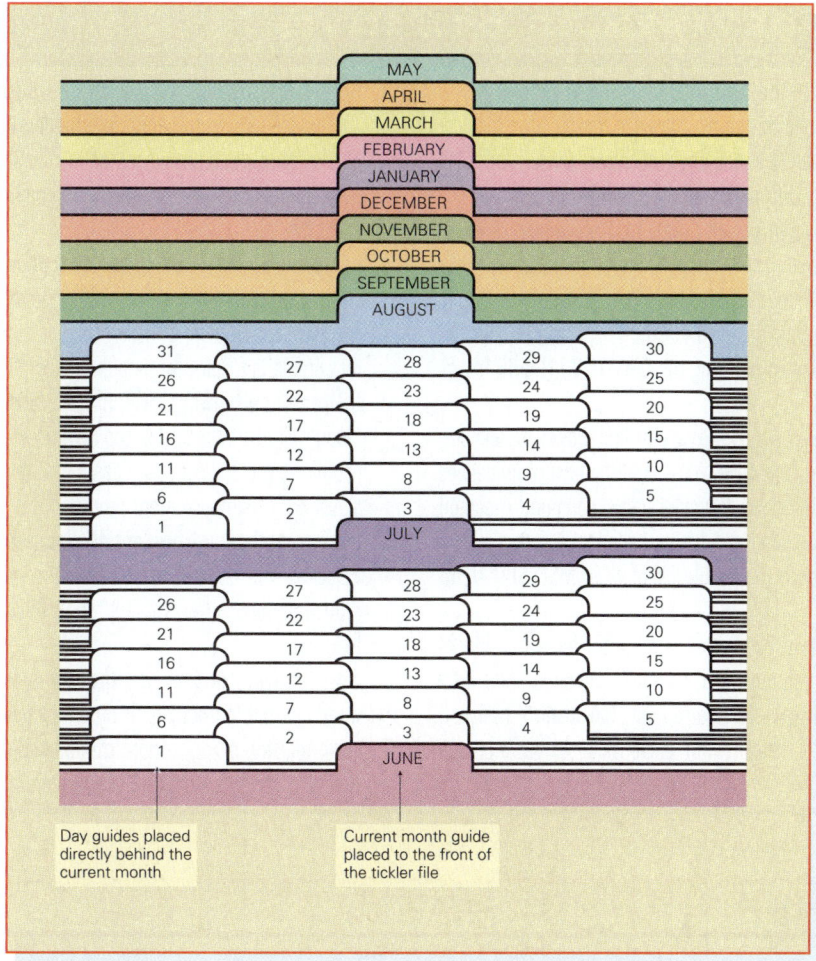

FIGURE 21-11 Example of an insurance claims tickler file. (From Fordney MT: *Insurance handbook for the medical office,* ed 12, St Louis, 2012, WB Saunders.)

SUMMARY OF SCENARIO

Machelle believes that she now has a better understanding of the insurance claims process. Before becoming a medical assisting student, she did not give much thought to what went on behind the scenes when she visited a medical office for her own personal healthcare. She now understands why all of the information is collected at the time of her visits to the doctor, including the patient registration form listing her demographic and insurance information.

Machelle has learned that the gathering of accurate data and verification of eligibility and benefits are some of the most important tasks performed, before she even begins to complete an insurance claim form. This information and the procedure to verify eligibility and benefits greatly reduce the chance of insurance claim denials or requests for additional information. No matter where

she works and regardless of whether the office is computerized, organization, communication, dedication, and attention to detail head the list of requirements for becoming successful.

Machelle has asked for her instructor's help in developing a reference manual for the various third-party payers common to her area; this will help her understand the requirements of the insurance carriers when submitting an insurance claim form. It also will greatly reduce the number of claims that are returned for more information, which delays reimbursement for services rendered.

Machelle is looking forward to more hands-on experience in the medical office where she is doing her externship so that she can gain as much knowledge as possible in every facet of medical assisting.

SUMMARY OF LEARNING OBJECTIVES

1. **Define, spell, and pronounce the terms listed in the vocabulary.**
   Spelling and pronouncing medical terms correctly bolster the medical assistant's credibility. Knowing the definition of these terms promotes confidence in communication with patients and co-workers.

2. **Discuss the differences between paper claims and electronic claims.**
   Insurance claims can be submitted in two forms: paper or electronic. Both have advantages and disadvantages; however, electronic claims normally have fewer errors and historically are paid faster.

3. **Understand the guidelines for completing the CMS-1500 Health Insurance Claim Form.**
   The insurance claim cycle begins when the patient first makes an appointment. The medical assistant should follow an established list of guidelines for completing the CMS-1500 claim form, including obtaining a signed authorization to release information and assign benefits, if applicable.

4. **Explain how to complete each of the blocks of the CMS-1500 claim form.**
   The CMS-1500 claim form had 33 blocks, and except for a few blocks that ask for standard information, completion requirements vary from payer to payer. To maximize reimbursement, the medical assistant should familiarize himself or herself with each major payer's unique requirements.

5. **Gather information for use on insurance claim forms.**
   The guidelines for gathering information needed to complete and submit an insurance claim are presented in Procedure 21-1. The medical assistant must have accurate, complete information to complete a claim form correctly.

6. **Complete a CMS-1500 claim form appropriately for various federal, state, and commercial third-party payers.**
   Accuracy in completing insurance claim forms is mandatory. The process for completing claim forms appropriately is outlined in Procedure 21-2.

7. **Differentiate between "clean" and "dirty" claims.**
   Clean claims are those that can be processed and paid quickly; dirty claims contain errors and/or omissions that often result in rejection, thus greatly slowing the reimbursement process.

8. **Discuss methods of preventing claims rejections.**
   Rejection and delay of claims cost the medical facility time and money. Proven methods of preventing claims rejections should be established and followed.

9. **Describe ways of checking the status of claims.**
   It is important to track claims once they have been submitted. An insurance claim register, or log, can be created and used as one method of tracking claims. A routine should be established for claims follow-up.

CONNECTIONS

Study Guide Connection: Go to the Chapter 21 Study Guide. Read the Case Study and Workplace Applications and complete the assignments. Do online research for answers to the questions in the Internet Activities associated with the health insurance claim form.

Evolve Connection: For more information related to the health insurance claim form, go to *evolve.elsevier.com/kinn* and visit related Web links for Chapter 21. Click on the Medical Assisting Exam Review and do the practice questions to sharpen your test-taking skills. To learn more about office software, do the exercises for the AltaPoint demonstration on the CD.

PROFESSIONAL FEES, BILLING, AND COLLECTING

22

SCENARIO

Jodie Bimmell, a registered medical assistant (RMA), has worked for Dr. Ted Crawford, an endocrinologist, for 3 years. She began as a receptionist, but she is proficient in mathematics and enjoys working with numbers. Because of Dr. Crawford's confidence in her abilities, he placed her in charge of the accounting functions for the practice 2 years ago. When patients are ready to leave, Jodie totals their bill and enters the charges and payments into the computerized billing system, which also allows her to schedule return appointments. Because Jodie also has learned quite a bit about medical insurance, she can answer most of the patients' questions about their coverage and the benefits or exclusions of their policies. She knows where to direct patients who have more complicated questions and how to follow up to ensure that they received an answer — one of the most important duties of a professional medical assistant. Jodie is able to decipher confusing explanations of benefits (EOBs) from insurance carriers and explain reimbursements to the patients. She has a great attitude about assisting patients with insurance questions and does not hesitate to call the insurance company or third-party payer on the patient's behalf. She provides patients with exceptional customer service.

Jodie knows to be careful when dealing with numeric transactions. Her handwriting is neat and legible, and she writes numbers the same way each time to prevent confusion and errors. She can work with a manual pegboard system in a pinch, but she uses the computerized billing system on a day-to-day basis. Jodie has some accounting background, which enables her to find errors easily and correct them. She is responsible for making sure the accounts balance on a daily, weekly, and monthly basis and considers errors a puzzle to solve and an opportunity to learn. She has never encountered an error she was unable to resolve by the end of the day.

Jodie provides a valuable service to Dr. Crawford's patients. She can be counted on to follow up on any detail that needs attention. When patients call her for assistance, she responds within 24 hours (often within 1 hour) with answers to their questions or a resource to help them. Jodie is willing to help any staff member with other duties when necessary and prides herself on being a patient advocate. She is an enthusiastic team player who puts the patients first.

While studying this chapter, think about the following questions:

- Why do the provider's usual fees influence the amount of reimbursement received from third-party payers?
- Why is professional courtesy used less frequently than in the past?
- How does the medical assistant effectively explain fees to patients?
- How can the medical assistant be a valuable patient advocate?

LEARNING OBJECTIVES

1. Define, spell, and pronounce the terms listed in the vocabulary.
2. List three values that are considered in determining professional fees.
3. Differentiate the terms *usual*, *customary*, and *reasonable*.
4. Discuss the value of fee estimates for patient treatment.
5. Explain basic bookkeeping computations.
6. Differentiate between bookkeeping and accounting.
7. Compare the manual and computerized bookkeeping systems used in ambulatory healthcare.
8. Identify procedures for preparing patient accounts.
9. Discuss the types of adjustments that may be made to a patient's account.
10. Explain both billing and payment options.
11. Describe the impact of both the Fair Debt Collection Practices Act and the Truth in Lending Act as they apply to collections.
12. Discuss procedures for collecting outstanding accounts.

VOCABULARY

account A statement of transactions during a fiscal period and the resulting balance.

account balance The amount owed on an account.

accounts receivable ledger A record of the charges and payments posted on an account.

credit An entry on an account constituting an addition to a revenue, net worth, or liability account; the balance in a person's favor.

credit cards Devices issued by a bank or other financial institution, retail stores, and other businesses that allow the card holder to make purchases prior to paying for them; the card holder is then billed, usually after interest has been added.

debit cards Cards that look like credit cards and by which money can be withdrawn, bills paid, or purchases made directly from the holder's bank account without the payment of interest.

debit An entry on an account representing an addition to an expense or asset account or a deduction from a revenue, a net worth, or a liability account.

decedent a person who is deceased.

disbursements Funds paid out.

fee profile A compilation or average of physician fees over a given period.

fee schedule A compilation of pre-established fee allowances for given services or procedures.

fiscal agent An organization under contract to the government (as well as some private plans) to act as financial representatives in handling insurance claims from providers of healthcare; also referred to as a fiscal intermediary.

instigate To goad or urge forward; to provoke.

intangible not made of physical substance; not able to be held or touched.

medically indigent Able to take care of ordinary living expenses but unable to afford medical care.

payables Balances due to a creditor on an account.

pegboard system An older method of tracking patient accounts that allows the figures to be proved accurate through mathematical formulas. It is still used in some small to medium practices; also called the write-it-once system.

posting Entering figures in an accounting system; transferring or carrying from a book of original entry to a ledger.

preponderance A superiority or excess in number or quantity; a majority.

professional courtesy Reduction or absence of fees to professional associates.

receipts Amounts paid on patient accounts.

receivables Total monies received on accounts.

secured A loan or line of credit that is backed by a pledge of payment and usually obtained using collateral.

transaction An exchange or transfer of goods, services, or funds.

trustee A person to whom property is legally committed to be administered for the benefit of a beneficiary or held by an administrator to be distributed to multiple individuals or businesses.

unsecured A debt that is not protected by collateral.

The practice of medicine is both a business and a profession, and the details of conducting the business aspects of the practice often are the responsibility of the medical assistant. Although service to the patient is the primary concern of the medical profession, a physician must charge and collect a fee for such services to continue providing medical care to patients. Many factors contribute to the determination of fees for the services and treatment rendered to the patient. The medical assistant is responsible for informing the patient about financial matters, for billing insurance companies or other third-party payers, and in some cases for making payment arrangements.

HOW FEES ARE DETERMINED

Setting fees is no simple matter. The physician has three commodities or values to sell: time, judgment, and services. Yet the value of these commodities is never exactly the same to any two individuals. Medical care has little value except to the patient receiving the care, and the value may not be consistent with the person's ability to pay. In every case, the physician must place an estimate on the value of the services. This estimated figure is known as the physician's *fee for service*. The value may then be modified by other considerations, such as an excessive length of time spent with the patient or an especially complicated group of illnesses suffered by one patient.

Impact of Managed Care

The **preponderance** of patients enrolled in health maintenance organizations (HMOs) and preferred provider organizations (PPOs) is an important consideration for the physician. Under managed care contracts, the physician agrees to accept predetermined fees for specific procedures and services instead of the fee-for-service method. The patient may have to make a co-payment, which is determined by the insurance contract and is collected at the time of service. A base capitation plan pays the provider a set amount for each patient enrolled in a group, and this amount is meant to cover all the patient's healthcare expenses in a given period. However, if one or two people in the group become very ill, the physician may actually lose money, because those patients may use all the groups' pooled money for that period.

Prevailing Rate in the Community

The economic level of the community plays a significant role in determining a physician's fees. Different communities have multiple cost-of-living scales, and this affects medical fees. The prevailing rate in the community must be taken into consideration by each physician. Interestingly, fees that are too low drive patients away just as quickly as fees that are too high, because the average person tends to judge the worth of a product by its cost, and low cost can be translated as low value.

Usual, Customary, and Reasonable Fees

Most insurance plans base their payments on a usual, customary, and reasonable (UCR) fee for a particular procedure.

- *Usual*—The physician's usual fee for a given service; the fee most frequently charged for the service.
- *Customary*—A range of the usual fees charged for the same service by physicians with similar training and experience who practice in the same geographic and socioeconomic area.
- *Reasonable*—The fee for an exceptionally difficult or complicated service or procedure that requires extraordinary time or effort by the physician.

For example, suppose Dr. Crawford's usual fee for new patients is $100. The customary charge for a first visit by other physicians in the same community with similar training and experience ranges from $75 to $125. Dr. Crawford's fee of $100 is within the customary range and would be paid by an insurance plan that pays on a usual and customary basis. However, if the range of usual fees in the community is $60 to $85, the insurance plan would allow only the maximum within the range, or $85. If Dr. Crawford spent 2 hours on a lengthy history and physical examination for a patient with a terminal illness, his charge of $175 might be considered reasonable, as long as he had documentation in the patient's chart to justify the charges. The Evaluation and Management (E/M) section of procedural coding manuals is carefully written to allow physicians to indicate the appropriate level, or extent, of the patient history, physical examination, and complexity of medical decision making.

> ### CRITICAL THINKING APPLICATION   22-1
> Jodie realizes that many of Dr. Crawford's patients are confused about insurance policies and managed care and that they are frustrated when payments are not as high as they expected. How can Jodie help patients better understand their policies? Is this duty truly a part of Jodie's job? Why or why not?

Fee Setting by Third-Party Payers

The physician does not act alone in determining fees. A third-party payer may provide a schedule of predetermined fees. Some require preapproval of the fee before service is rendered, and some require precertification before paying for certain services. Government programs, such as Medicare and Medicaid, have strict guidelines for reimbursement. The physician may have to adjust part of the fees to meet contractual obligations with the third-party payer.

Physician's Fee Profile

The **fiscal agent** (or *fiscal intermediary*) for government-sponsored insurance programs and some private plans keeps a continuous record of the usual charges submitted for specific services by each physician. When these fees have been compiled and averaged over a given period, usually a year, the physician's **fee profile** is established. The fee profile is used in determining the amount of third-party liability for services under the program. Physicians often object to the lag between a private fee increase and the point when it is reflected in payments by an insurance carrier. This interval can be as long as 2 to 3 years.

Insurance Allowance

In some individual cases, the physician may not want to charge the patient more than the person's insurance allows. This sometimes is a professional courtesy (which may be extended to healthcare professionals); in other cases, it is applied as the physician sees fit. Always charge the full fee first, with the understanding that after the insurance allowance has been received, the balance may be discounted or adjusted. If a smaller fee is quoted and charged at a discount, several things can happen:

- The lower fee can alter the physician's fee profile.
- Only the reduced fee can be recovered if it is necessary to bring litigation for payment.
- The insurance allowance may be reduced.
- The insurance company may take the position that the reduced fee is the physician's usual and customary fee and base its payment accordingly.
- Reducing fees and adjustments for professional courtesy may violate the physician's agreement with the third-party payer and could be considered fraudulent.

EXPLAINING FEES TO PATIENTS

Patients, especially new ones, naturally wonder how much their office visits and treatments will cost, but they often are reluctant to voice their concern. The first step in discussing financial issues is to make sure the conversation is held out of the hearing range of other patients. If the discussion is to be held during the checkout process, make sure this is done in a private area or that other patients are out of earshot. Patients are hesitant to discuss financial issues with strangers lingering.

Do not wait for the patient to ask about fees. The physician or the medical assistant should approach the subject if the patient does not do so. Be prepared to discuss costs with all patients and ask whether they have questions about the fees. The medical assistant might open the conversation by saying, "Mr. Conn, do you have any questions about the costs of your operation? If you do, I'll be glad to review them with you."

Never sidestep payment issues by saying, "Don't worry about the bill; let's just get you well first." The patient may later complain about the bill because he or she misunderstood the complexity of the service.

Even when the physician quotes a fee, the medical assistant often is responsible for explaining the physician's fees to the patient. Know how fees are determined and why charges vary. Develop a thorough knowledge of the physician's practice and policies so that handling perplexing situations involving fees becomes routine. Educate patients that the money spent for medical care is an excellent investment in the future. It is the rare patient who understands the intricate procedures involved in diagnosis and treatment, especially when third-party payers are involved, so be patient and understanding when questions arise about fees.

Explain that compliance with the physician's orders may actually save the patient money over time. Each patient should control and manage his or her current diseases and prevent symptoms from worsening or new disorders from developing; this ultimately reduces the patient's healthcare costs.

Discussion of Fees in Advance

Patients can better plan for medical expenses when fees are discussed before treatment. Most patients want to meet their financial obligations but rightfully insist on an accurate estimate of those costs before they commit to paying them. Misconceptions and complaints about overcharging and fee discrepancies often are eliminated when fees are explained to the patient before a procedure or surgery is scheduled, even to the point of describing how a fee is established. Some physicians offer a discount if a patient has no insurance and pays cash. Although some physicians will allow fee negotiation in special circumstances, most managed care contracts require the physician to charge the correct co-payment and do not allow further discounts.

Explanation of Additional Fees

When discussing patients' fees, remember to explain additional costs that extend beyond the physician's own charges. For example, if a patient is to undergo surgery, the person should know the costs of the operation, the anesthesiologist's and radiologist's charges, the laboratory fees, and the approximate hospital bill. If consultation becomes necessary, inform the patient that a separate bill will be sent by the consulting physician and that the consultation is for the benefit of the patient and the referring physician.

Fee Estimates

Most physicians give patients an estimate of medical expenses before hospitalization; these estimates often are developed in cooperation with local hospitals or surgery centers. Individual physicians occasionally work up their own estimate forms while in the treatment room with the patient. Patients must usually budget their money for medical procedures, and most physicians are willing to work with the patient to make payment arrangements, especially for expensive treatments or procedures, or when responding to emergency situations.

Estimates also are helpful when the patient is faced with long-term treatment. Always emphasize that the information is only an estimate and that the actual cost may vary somewhat. Estimate slips should be prepared in duplicate so that the patient has a copy. Retain the original in the patient's medical record. Using estimates (1) documents that a fee was quoted; (2) helps to eliminate the possibility of misquoting the fee later; and (3) simplifies collections by clarifying expected payments, which prevent misunderstanding and confusion over charges.

The Guarantor's Ultimate Responsibility

Patients must understand that the *guarantor* is the person ultimately responsible for the entire bill. The insurance policy is a contract between the policyholder or between a group of people (e.g., an employer) and an insurance company or managed care organization. The physician is not a party to this contract. Therefore, physicians and their staff are not responsible for pursuing insurance payment for the benefit of the patient. However, it is in the best interest of the staff to actively assist the patient if problems occur securing payment. This is true for two reasons.

First, the staff is almost always more knowledgeable about the insurance business than the patient. Many patients do not even read their insurance policies and have no idea what is and is not covered. Some patients expect insurance to pay all costs simply because they are paying a high premium or payment. The medical assistant may need to educate these patients about their policies and offer advice on how patients can effectively work with the insurance company to get answers to questions and make sure they are receiving all the benefits to which they are entitled.

Second, helping the patient secure payment means that the physician will be compensated for his or her services. If the medical assistant acts as a patient advocate with the insurance company, these efforts usually result in payment of the contracted amount of the bill. Make sure the proper co-payments are received and credited to patients' accounts.

Medical assistants gain knowledge about the insurance industry when they actively assist patients with their concerns. The more experience a medical assistant has in working with insurance and third-party payers, the more helpful he or she can be to patients. The medical assistant should keep a notebook with specific information about each type of policy the office handles; this will be a source of excellent guidance and suggestions when working with a particular payer.

Always be sure to secure guarantors in writing. Most patient information sheets have a section referring to the guarantor. A statement may be included that the guarantor signs, indicating an agreement to pay the costs of medical care. States have varying statutes that deal with guarantors, so be sure the office's policies reflect compliance with those laws. It is especially important to secure a written agreement to pay for services when the care will be long term or when a costly treatment or surgical procedure must be done.

Charging the Patient for Medical Services and Procedures

The slips attached to charts while the patient is in the office are called *encounter forms* (Figure 22-1; additional examples of encounter forms are available on the Evolve Web site). The encounter form provides information about the patient, such as the name, account

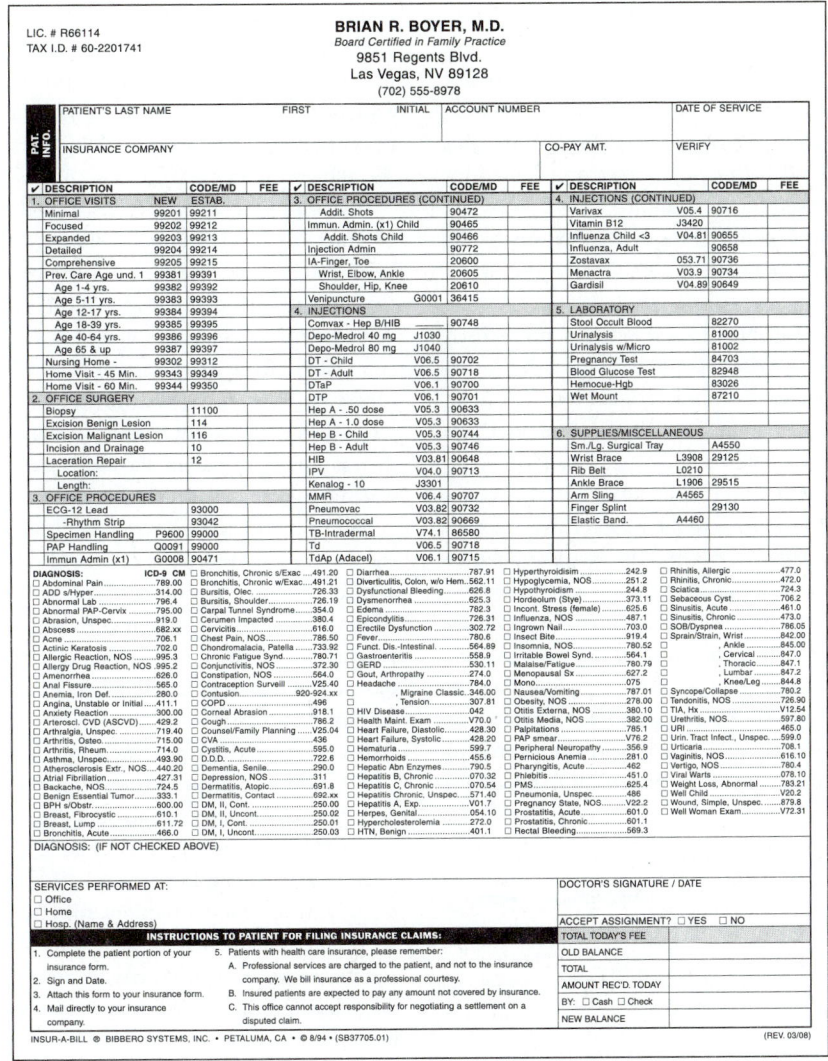

FIGURE 22-1 The encounter form is used by the physician and staff to document what was done to the patient during an office visit and to indicate when the physician wants the patient to return. The copies of the form may be used to bill third-party payers. (Courtesy Bibbero Systems, Petaluma, Calif.)

number, and previous balance. Current charges and payments for the visit are added after the physician sees the patient. The physician can indicate on the encounter form when the patient should return to the clinic. The medical assistant then schedules a return appointment and can even use the patient's copy of the encounter form to note the next appointment date and time.

The encounter form normally consists of three parts: a white top sheet, a yellow sheet, and a pink sheet. The colors can vary, but the white copy usually is kept as a permanent record by the office, and the yellow and pink copies are given to the patient. The patient uses the yellow copy for insurance billing (if it is not done by the office), and the pink copy is a receipt for the patient. Encounter forms sometimes are designed to work with a **pegboard system**, or they may be available in continuous forms that can be placed in the printer for computer use. Encounter forms have been known by many other names throughout the years, including *superbills, charge slips,* and *multipurpose billing forms.* Modern computer systems allow receipts to be printed directly from the computer.

COMPUTATIONS USED ON PATIENT ACCOUNTS

A business **transaction** is the occurrence of an event or of a condition that must be recorded. For example, when a service is performed for which a charge is made, when a debtor makes a payment on an account, when a piece of equipment is purchased, or when the monthly rent is paid, a business transaction has been completed. Each of these examples is a transaction that must be recorded in the accounting system. Medical assistants need to understand the difference between bookkeeping and accounting. Accounting is a four-stage process of recording, classifying, summarizing, and interpreting financial statements. The physician may have an accountant who provides periodic summaries and handles tax planning and payment for the physician. Bookkeeping is the recording stage of accounting. The medical assistant performs bookkeeping functions when posting a payment to a patient's account.

A patient's financial record is called an **account**. All of the patients' accounts together (in the entire practice) constitute the

accounts receivable ledger. Account (or ledger) cards vary in design (Figure 22-2), but all have at least three columns for entering figures:

- **Debit** column—located on the left; this column is used for entering charges and sometimes is called the *charge column.*
- **Credit** column—located to the right of the debit column; this column sometimes is headed *Paid* or *Payments* and is used for entering payments received on an account.
- Balance column—located on the far right; this column is used to record the difference between the debit and the credit columns.

An adjustment column is available in some systems and is used to enter professional discounts, write-offs, disallowances by insurance companies, and any other adjustments. In a computer system, when a patient is called up by name or identification number, the patient's balance appears. This is the individual patient's ledger.

Posting is the transfer of information from one record to another. Transactions are posted from the journal to the ledger; this is accomplished in one writing on the pegboard system. The **account balance** normally is a debit balance, which means that the charges exceed the payments on the account. A debit balance is entered simply by writing the correct figure in the balance column. A credit balance exists when payments exceed charges (e.g., when a patient pays in advance). This is common in obstetric practices. If a payment is made, that amount is entered and subtracted from the charge to arrive at the patient's account balance. If the patient or the patient's

insurance company pays more than the charge, the patient has a credit balance. Occasionally, an adjustment may be made to the patient's account; for instance, if the insurance company pays only $80 of a $100 charge, the physician may adjust $20 from the patient's account, especially if the physician is contracted to accept the allowed amount.

Discounts are also credit entries and are entered in the adjustment column; if there is no such column, the discount is entered in the debit column and enclosed in parentheses. When the entry is made this way, it is recognized as a subtraction from the charges. When columns are totaled, any figure in red or in parentheses is always subtracted. **Receipts** are cash and checks taken in payment for professional services. **Receivables** are charges for which payment has not been received; that is, amounts owed. **Disbursements** are cash amounts paid out. **Payables** are amounts owed to others but not yet paid.

All charges and payments for professional services are posted to the patient's account card or record daily. The record then becomes a reliable source of information for answering all inquiries from patients about their accounts. A separate account card or record is prepared for each patient at the time of the first visit or service. The record should include all information pertinent to collecting the account, such as:

- Name and address of the guarantor
- Insurance identification
- Social Security number
- Home and business telephone numbers
- Name of employer
- Any special instructions for billing

Billing statements to the patient and the patient's insurance carrier are prepared from the record. The patient's name, date, and diagnosis and the procedures performed are posted when the patient is leaving the office.

COMPARISON OF MANUAL AND COMPUTERIZED BOOKKEEPING SYSTEMS

Computerized Bookkeeping Systems

Computerized bookkeeping systems for medical offices vary in cost and capability. A computerized system reduces the time needed to balance the day sheet and the totals for monthly and year-to-date balances (Procedure 22-1). The software for these programs may need to be updated periodically. Several staff members can access the information in the computer at the same time, and output is legible over the long term compared to some handwritten information. Because computers are multiuse devices, several types of software programs can be housed on one computer. Manual systems are designed to do one thing and cannot provide information other than what has been posted on the system by hand.

Although most physicians have converted to an electronic billing system, some still use the pegboard for a number of reasons. Many rural physicians, those in practice for many years, and those that run small practices believe that conversion to an electronic system would not be worth the high cost involved in implementation. Although it is certainly the physician's choice as to the system the office uses, electronic medical records are more efficient. Nonetheless, the

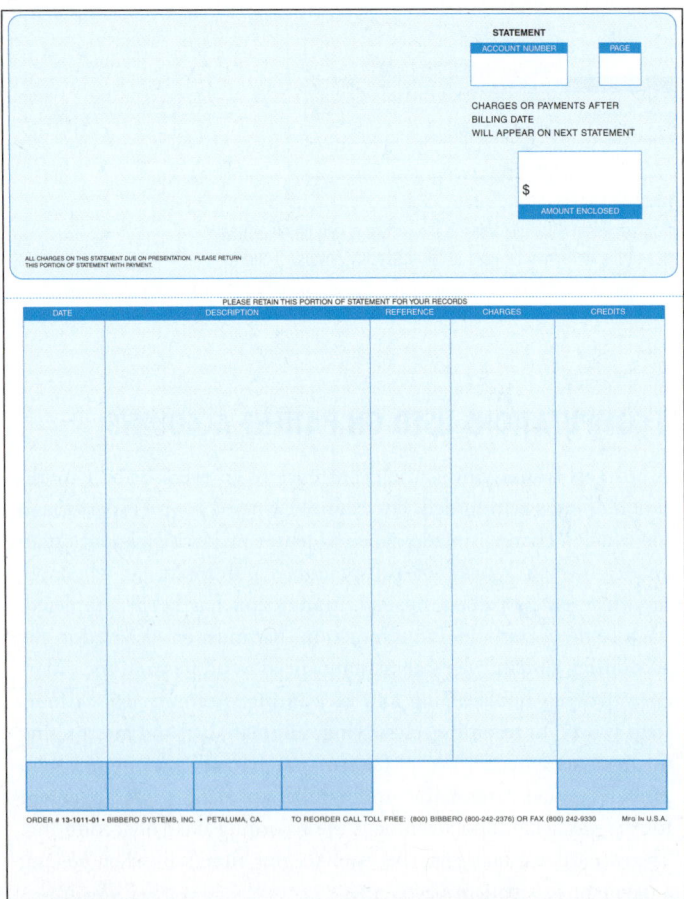

FIGURE 22-2 Patient account card used for computerized billing. (Courtesy Colwell Systems, Champaign, Ill.)

PROCEDURE 22-1

Use Computerized Office Billing Systems

GOAL: To use the computer to perform office billing functions efficiently, accurately, and in a timely manner.

EQUIPMENT and SUPPLIES

- Computer with billing software installed that contains a database of patients
- Physician's fee schedule
- Encounter forms
- Calculator

PROCEDURAL STEPS

1. Turn on the computer and open the applicable billing software program.
2. Generate a report that ages the accounts according to the last time a payment was made.
   PURPOSE: To determine the accounts that are 30, 60, 90, and 120 days old.
3. Review the accounts and determine whether any should be submitted to a collection agency.
   PURPOSE: To categorize accounts that are current and those that need outside collection action.
4. Run the software and print billing statements for all patients with a balance on their account.
   PURPOSE: To determine which patients need to be sent a statement. Some offices do not send bills to patients with less than $5 on their accounts to save postage and paperwork costs.

5. Review any notations in the computer billing system that relate to payment on the account.
   PURPOSE: To determine whether a patient has made payment arrangements on the account.
6. Determine whether any of the accounts need special handling.
   PURPOSE: To make sure that any follow-up activities have been done (e.g., calling the insurance company about denials, getting additional information from the physician).
7. Demonstrate sensitivity and professionalism in handling accounts receivable activities with patients.
   PURPOSE: To treat all patients fairly, to keep the billing information confidential, and to handle billing activities professionally.
8. Prepare the printed statements for mailing according to the billing cycle used by the clinic.
   PURPOSE: To mail a bill to a patient at the correct address in each month the person carries a balance.
9. Figure the best postage rate and use U.S. Postal Service (USPS) guidelines for mailing in bulk.
   PURPOSE: To save money on postage costs and send bulk mail in the most economical way.
10. Take the statements to the post office and mail.
    PURPOSE: To make sure the mail has been prepared according to USPS guidelines.

---

medical assistant benefits by learning how the manual pegboard system works. The bookkeeping concepts taught in using a manual system help the student understand the way a computerized system works. Whether manual or electronic, the physician's billing system must be accurate and cost effective and must allow quick retrieval of information.

Manual Bookkeeping Systems

Although we live in a technology-savvy world, there are many physicians who still use manual pegboard systems. Often, physicians who have been in practice for many years do not want to invest in a computerized billing system, because they may not plan to be in practice long enough to justify the cost. Usually, these doctors also still use a manual, written charting system. Additionally, some certifying exams still contain questions about manual systems. If the office experiences a power outage, the employees will have to use a manual system for the period in which patients are seen while the power is out. The medical assistant needs to be familiar with both manual and computerized bookkeeping systems. The pegboard is the most popular manual system for this purpose. The initial cost of materials for the pegboard system is slightly more than that for other manual accounting systems but is still less than the cost of most

billing management computer software systems. The pegboard is simple to operate, and once a medical assistant learns the pegboard system, computer systems are much easier to understand.

The system gets its name from the lightweight aluminum or Masonite board that is used. This board has a row of pegs along the side or top that holds the forms in place. The accounting forms are perforated for alignment on the pegs. All the forms used in any system must be compatible so that they can be aligned perfectly on the board. The pegboard system generates all the necessary financial records for each transaction in one writing, as follows:

- Encounter form
- Receipt
- Account (or ledger) card
- Accounting entry

The system also may include a statement and bank deposit slip. It provides current accounts receivable totals and a daily record of bank deposits and cash on hand, in addition to the record of income and expenses. The need for separate posting to patient accounts is eliminated, and the chance for error is reduced.

The pegboard system allows the medical assistant to keep control over cash, collections, and receivables and ensures that every cent is accounted for and properly entered. It provides a record of every patient, every charge, and every payment, plus a daily recap of earnings—a running record of receivables and an audited summary of cash—and requires little time.

Preparing Patient Accounts for Daily Transactions

If the medical facility uses a computerized billing system, turn on the computer and open the accounting software. Some advanced systems allow patients to check in at a computer in the reception area. When such a system is used, the patient must be taught how to enter his or her information. Once the patient has seen the physician and is ready to leave the office, he or she brings the encounter form to the checkout area. The medical assistant reviews the encounter form for the charges noted by the physician, and those charges are entered into the computer. Payments are noted after the charges have been entered.

Make sure the system has a reliable backup so that the patient account information is not lost. Back up the system daily to prevent the loss of all or part of patients' account information.

If a pegboard system is used, place a new day sheet on the board daily, even if there is still room left on the previous day sheet. This is helpful if a specific transaction needs to be looked up. The medical assistant can refer to a specific day sheet, rather than scan through several sheets, if he or she knows the date of the transaction. Most systems use no carbon required (NCR) paper on both encounter forms and account cards. If the encounter forms are shingled, lay the entire bank of receipts over the pegs, with the top one aligned with the first open writing line on the day sheet. The account card is placed underneath the encounter form but on top of the day sheet. Therefore, when the entry is recorded, the medical assistant writes on the encounter form, and the entry shows on the account card and the day sheet. Encounter forms should be used in numeric order. Save time by pulling account cards for all scheduled patients during morning preparation time.

Entering and Posting Transactions

When a computerized billing system is used, charges are entered into the computer at the end of the visit and payment is collected from the patient unless other arrangements have been made. The encounter form is referenced at the end of the visit. When a pegboard system is used, transactions are initiated before the patient goes to the exam room. The patient's ledger card is inserted under the first or next available receipt, with the first available writing line of the card aligned with the carbonized strip on the receipt. Enter the receipt number and date, the account balance in the space labeled *previous balance,* and the patient's name. The information recorded on the receipt is posted automatically to the ledger and the day sheet. The charge slip then is detached and clipped to the patient's chart to be routed to the physician.

After the service has been performed, the physician enters it on the encounter form and the patient or the nurse returns it to the medical assistant at the checkout desk. Charges are coded in the computerized billing system, and the computer also generates billing forms for insurance purposes. Whether a computerized or manual system is used, the charges posted to the patient's account should be taken from the physician's **fee schedule**. Computerized systems can automatically display the fees when a certain procedure code is entered.

When checking out a patient using a pegboard system, the medical assistant should insert the ledger card under the proper receipt and check the number previously entered to make sure the correct card is being used. Record the service by procedure code, post the charge from the fee schedule, enter any payment made, and write in the current balance (Procedure 22-2). If there is no balance, place a zero or a straight line in the balance column.

The transaction has now been posted to the journal and the account, and if payment was made by the patient, a receipt has been generated. The service receipt is given to the patient; no other receipt is necessary. The account card is ready for refiling.

File the encounter forms in numeric order for any internal audit. At the end of the month, the total of the encounter forms should equal the total of the charges recorded on the day sheets for the month (Figure 22-3).

Posting Other Payments and Charges

Payments may be received in the mail or may be brought in by patients some time after a service was performed. With a computer system, payments are simply entered into the computer and credited to the patient's account. With a manual system, payments are entered on the day sheet and the account card as described previously. Payments sent by mail do not require a receipt unless the patient specifically requests one.

The physician may have daily charges for visits to patients in a hospital or convalescent facility. Enter these charges on the day sheet and ledger card only. Surgery fees usually are recorded as one entry that includes the surgery and aftercare. All these charges are easily entered into a computer billing system.

CRITICAL THINKING APPLICATION   22-4

- Dr. Crawford sometimes forgets to write down information for billing when he goes to the hospital to check on his patients. Jodie has a difficult time entering the charges for hospital visits, because Dr. Crawford's records for these visits are not completely reliable. How might Jodie rectify this situation?
- How can Jodie help Dr. Crawford be more reliable in this area?

Summarizing Accounting Transactions

Computer systems figure the summary of accounting transactions automatically. Almost all systems have some type of error notification so that the medical assistant sees an error immediately and is prompted to correct it. With a manual system, all columns of the pegboard must be totaled and proved at the end of the day. Although all bookkeeping is done in ink, it is a good idea to write the totals in pencil until they have been proved. If an error is discovered, correct the entry in which it occurred. Do not attempt to erase or write over the incorrect entry. Simply draw one line through it and make a new entry on the first open writing line. Remember to reinsert the account card for these corrections. Also, if the entry included a receipt for the patient, make a new receipt and notify the patient of the correction.

PROCEDURE 22-2

Post Entries on a Day Sheet

GOAL: *To post 1 day's charges and payments and compute the daily bookkeeping cycle using a pegboard.*

EQUIPMENT and SUPPLIES

- Pegboard
- Calculator
- Pen
- Day sheet (a blank copy of an actual day sheet will work if no pegboard system is available)
- Receipts
- Ledger cards
- Balances from previous day
- Computer

PROCEDURAL STEPS

1. Prepare the board.
   - Place a new day sheet on the board.
   - Place a bank of receipts over the pegs, aligning the top receipt with the first open writing line on the day sheet.
2. Carry forward balances from the previous day.
   **PURPOSE:** To keep all totals current.
3. Pull ledger cards for the patients being seen that day.
4. Insert the ledger card under the first receipt, aligning the first available writing line of the card with the carbonized strip on the receipt.
   PURPOSE: To ensure that the staff member using the card correctly posts the entry to the receipt, ledger, and day sheet.
5. Enter the patient's name, the date, the receipt number, and any existing balance from the ledger card.
6. Detach the charge slip from the receipt and clip it to the patient's chart.
   PURPOSE: To allow the physician to indicate the service performed on the charge slip and return it to you.

7. Accept the returned charge slip at the end of the visit. If using a computerized system, pull up the patient's account on the screen.
8. Enter the appropriate fee from the fee schedule.
9. Locate the receipt on the board with a number matching the charge slip.
   PURPOSE: To make sure it is the correct receipt.
10. Reinsert the patient's ledger card under the receipt.
11. Write the service code number and fee on the receipt.
12. Accept the patient's payment and record the amount of payment and the new balance. Enter the payment amount into the computerized system, if applicable.
    PURPOSE: To bring the patient's account up-to-date and provide a current statement for the patient.
13. Give the completed receipt to the patient. Print the receipt using the computer, if applicable.
14. Follow your agency's procedure for refiling the ledger card.
15. Repeat steps 4 to 14 for each service of the day.
16. Total all columns of the day sheet at the end of the day. Computer systems provide this information electronically. Print daily reports if required at the end of the day.
    PURPOSE: To determine the total amount of the charges, receipts, and resulting balances for the day.
17. Write preliminary totals in pencil.
    PURPOSE: To facilitate any necessary changes.
18. Complete proof of totals and enter totals in ink.
19. Enter figures for accounts receivable control.
    PURPOSE: To complete the daily accounting cycle.

SPECIAL BOOKKEEPING ENTRIES

The following special entries sometimes are necessary. They may be performed either with a pegboard or a computer accounting system:

- Adjustments
- Credit balances
- Refunds
- Insufficient funds checks

Adjustments

At times a credit adjustment must be entered. This could be for professional discounts, insurance disallowances, account write-offs, or payments that come to the office after the account has been placed for collection (Procedure 22-3). If a patient or guarantor files for bankruptcy, the charge usually must be adjusted off the books.

If the system has an adjustment column or feature, enter adjustments there. Otherwise, because the adjustment is actually a subtraction from the charge, enter it in the charge column with the figure enclosed in parentheses or circled and with an explanation of the entry in the description column. When the column of figures is totaled, the circled figure is subtracted rather than added. The learner has a tendency to ignore the circled figures. This is incorrect; they must be subtracted.

Credit Balances

A credit balance occurs when a patient has paid in advance or an overpayment or duplicate payment is made (Procedure 22-4). For example, an overpayment occurs if the patient makes a partial payment and later the insurance allowance is more than the remaining balance. The difference between the total amount of money received and the amount owed must be entered in the balance column and enclosed within parentheses or circled. This indicates a credit balance. Some credit balances are created when an error is made in posting.

The credit balance is money owed to the patient. If the patient has paid in advance or wants to leave the overpayment in the account

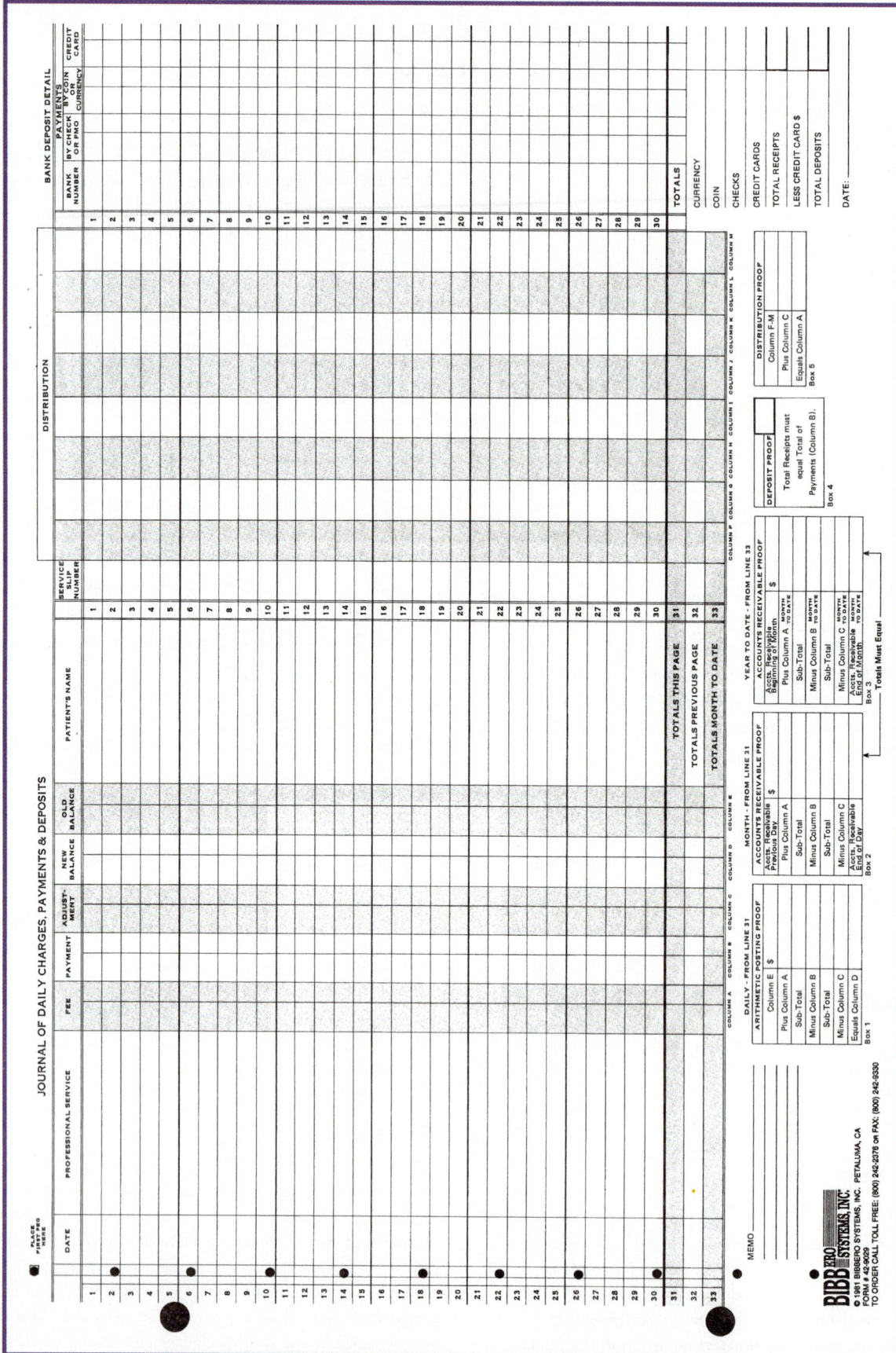

FIGURE 22-3 Sample day sheet used to log patient charges and receipts. (Courtesy Bibbero Systems, Petaluma, Calif.)

PROCEDURE 22-3

Post Adjustments

GOAL: *To process adjustments to patients' accounts accurately.*

EQUIPMENT and SUPPLIES

- Patient ledgers
- Office policy manual
- Explanation of benefits and remittance advice
- Bookkeeping system
- Clerical supplies
- Payments
- Calculator
- Computer

PROCEDURAL STEPS

1. Open checks that arrive in the mail as payment on patient accounts.
2. Paper-clip the check to the explanation of benefits (EOB) or remittance advice.
   <u>PURPOSE:</u> To keep the check with the EOB as payments are posted.
3. Post the payment to the patient's account using a computerized or manual system.
4. Determine whether an adjustment is necessary on the patient's account.
   <u>PURPOSE:</u> Adjustments may be necessary in cases of disallowed charges, noncovered services, and so on.
5. If necessary, review the office policy manual to ascertain the correct procedure for making adjustments to a patient's account.
   <u>PURPOSE:</u> To ensure that office policies are followed and are consistent with regard to patient accounts and adjustments.
6. If using a manual system, make sure the ledger card is aligned with the day sheet correctly.
7. Write the adjustment amount in the adjustment column of the ledger card.
8. Check the math to make sure the adjustment was posted correctly.

PROCEDURE 22-4

Process a Credit Balance

GOAL: *To return overpayments to patients in a timely manner.*

EQUIPMENT and SUPPLIES

- Patient ledgers
- Office policy manual
- Explanation of benefits and remittance advice
- Bookkeeping system
- Clerical supplies
- Payments
- Calculator
- Computer

PROCEDURAL STEPS

1. If necessary, review the office policy manual to determine the guidelines for credit balances.
   <u>PURPOSE:</u> To make sure office policy is followed.
2. Review the payment received and the explanation of benefits or remittance advice.
3. Post the payment to the patient's account using a computerized or manual system.
4. Determine whether an overpayment has been made.
5. Review the account to determine whether more insurance is expected on the account.
   <u>PURPOSE:</u> Some credit balances need not be made if more activity is expected on the account; only refund amounts that remain after the complete bill has been paid.
6. Adjust the credit balance off of the patient's account.
   <u>PURPOSE:</u> To refund the credit balance if it is due to the patient.

in anticipation of future charges, care must be taken in figuring the balance on future transactions. A charge increases the balance, but it reduces a credit balance.

Refunds

If a patient wants to have an overpayment refunded, write a check for the amount due and enter the transaction on the day sheet. In most cases, the refund results in a patient balance of zero (Procedure 22-5). Computer systems may automatically prompt a refund when the patient has a credit balance.

CRITICAL THINKING APPLICATION   22-5

Jodie receives a phone call from a patient who says that she is due a refund because her insurance company sent her an explanation of benefits for $654, and her balance was only $436. She demands an immediate refund, but Jodie has not yet received the check.

- What should Jodie do? Should she send the refund to the patient as requested?
- After investigating, Jodie suspects that the check sent to pay on the account was an error. What should she do in this situation?

PROCEDURE 22-5

Process Refunds

GOAL: *To process a patient's refund in a timely manner.*

EQUIPMENT and SUPPLIES

- Patient ledgers
- Office policy manual
- Explanation of benefits and remittance advice
- Bookkeeping system
- Clerical supplies
- Payments
- Calculator
- Computer

PROCEDURAL STEPS

1. Determine the amount of the refund to be processed.
   PURPOSE: To make sure the patient receives a refund in the correct amount.

2. Write a check for the amount of the refund using a computerized or manual system.
   PURPOSE: Always use a check to pay refunds so that the patient's name is on the back of the check as endorsement, proving the patient received the refund.

3. Give the check to the physician for a signature.
   PURPOSE: Most physicians prefer to sign their own checks.

4. Determine the correct mailing address for the patient.
   PURPOSE: To make sure the patient has not reported a change of address.

5. Make a copy of the check and put it in the patient's medical record.
   PURPOSE: To show that a check was mailed to the patient.

6. Mail the refund check to the patient.

PROCEDURE 22-6

Post Nonsufficient Funds Checks

GOAL: *To correctly note that a patient's check was returned because of insufficient funds.*

EQUIPMENT and SUPPLIES

- Patient ledgers
- Office policy manual
- Bookkeeping system
- Clerical supplies
- Calculator
- Computer

PROCEDURAL STEPS

1. Pull the ledger card for the patient who wrote the check or open the patient's account on the computer.
   PURPOSE: To post charges to the correct patient's account.

2. Determine the amount to be added back to the account as a result of the returned check.

PURPOSE: The physician's bank usually charges a fee for all checks returned by the bank because of insufficient funds.

3. Post the total amount on the patient's ledger card or on the patient's computerized account.
   PURPOSE: To account for the original check amount plus the fee for the returned check.

4. Send a certified letter to the patient notifying him or her of the returned check and demand fast payment.
   PURPOSE: Many states require that certified mail be used when notifying patients about nonsufficient funds checks.

5. Note this collection activity in the patient's medical record and keep a copy, noting the numbers on the certified letter for reference.

▌Insufficient Funds Checks

A patient may send in a check without having sufficient funds to cover it in the bank; this check is later deposited to the physician's account. The bank will return the check to the medical facility marked NSF (nonsufficient funds). Two accounting functions must be performed. First, deduct the amount of the check from the practice's checking account balance. Then add that amount back into the patient's account balance, including an NSF fee (if applicable) in the paid column. Place that amount in parentheses and increase the balance by the same amount. Write "NSF check" in the description column (Procedure 22-6). Some offices do not charge an NSF fee if the physician's bank does not charge the physician a fee; however, charging a fee does serve as a deterrent to writing NSF checks in the future.

BALANCING THE ACCOUNTS RECEIVABLE AND ACCOUNTS RECEIVABLE CONTROL

The accounts receivable control is a daily summary of what remains unpaid on the accounts. Most offices also complete an end of day summary. These summaries help the medical assistant determine the outstanding accounts receivable; that is, the amount patients owe the clinic. In collections, this information is used to send letters asking patients to pay their accounts based on the age of the account. (Aging accounts receivables is discussed later in this chapter.)

PAYMENT OPTIONS

Physicians allow patients to pay for medical services in different ways, often determined by the amount of the total service. Sizeable fees might be divided into several payments, but patients should pay for regular office visits when the service is rendered.

Payment for medical services is accomplished in the following four ways:

- Payment at the time of service
- Billing after making payment arrangements
- Insurance or other third-party billing
- Billing and collection assistance

Payment at the Time of Service

Most patients pay their co-pay, co-insurance, or total bill at the time medical services are provided. A large percentage of patients have some type of health insurance for at least major expenses. Every practice should encourage time-of-service collection. Many offices now collect co-pays or co-insurance before the patient sees the physician. This may offend some patients, because they are being asked to pay before receiving services. The medical assistant should explain that this practice is followed merely to save the patient time after seeing the physician, because co-pays usually are a set amount for each visit. Patients without health insurance should pay after the charges for the day have been totaled. If patients get into the habit of paying their current charges before they leave the office, no further billing and bookkeeping expenses are incurred. Inform patients making an appointment that payment is expected at the time of service so that they are not surprised when asked for payment at the end of the visit. The medical assistant may say, "Your charge for today is $25. Will that be cash, check, credit, or debit card?"

Many offices accept **credit cards** for the convenience of their patients. **Debit cards** now are also widely accepted for payment. Computers have made the electronic transfer of funds easy and convenient. If a patient asks to be billed, the medical assistant may say, "Our normal procedure is to pay at the time of service unless other arrangements are made in advance."

Many patients are hesitant to ask about charges and are unsure whether to offer to pay or to wait until asked. Make it easier for patients by offering to accept their payments, because most people are prepared to pay small bills on a cash basis.

The medical assistant must believe that the physician and the facility have a right to charge for the services provided. Do not be embarrassed to ask for payment for the valuable services the physician provides. Remember that the practice is a business, and the physician must meet the obligations necessary to keep it fiscally healthy, including salary expenses. When tact and good judgment are used in billing and collecting, patients appreciate the service they receive and the help the medical assistant provides. Give each patient individual attention and personal consideration; also, be courteous and show a sincere desire to help the patient with financial problems.

> ### CRITICAL THINKING APPLICATION   22-6
> Mr. Page comes to Jodie's desk to pay his account. His credit card is declined. How does Jodie handle this situation?
> - Mr. Page argues that he recently paid the balance of his account in full. What steps should Jodie take in this case?

Billing after Payment Arrangements

Most physicians prefer payment before or at the time of service. However, if fees for surgery or long-term care are involved, payment arrangements become necessary, and a regular system of billing must be established. The medical assistant therefore must explain to the patient the professional fees, the services the charges cover, and the office credit policies (Procedure 22-7). Most practices make payment arrangements with patients. The physician should decide what he or she expects of patients with regard to payments and how the patient will be informed. Although exceptions always occur to any rule, there must be a rule, which should be in writing and conveyed to the patient at the outset of the physician-patient relationship. Refer to the office policy and procedures manual for specific guidelines for payment arrangements in individual practices.

Using Credit for Medical Services

Because credit is so much a part of our economic system today, the physician's office usually accepts credit and debit cards for medical care. However, using a credit card can increase the total amount the patient will pay for the services. Suppose a patient uses a credit card to pay for minor surgery, and the physician's charge is $750. If the patient pays the balance in full during the next credit card billing cycle (which varies with every card), no charges above the $750 may be incurred. However, if the patient does not pay the entire bill, interest is charged on the account every month until the full bill is paid. In addition, late payment and over-the-limit fees can be astronomical, and the patient's credit card debt quickly can get out of control. Even small charges can multiply if the bill is not paid on time. In general, fees for routine office calls and small medical bills should be kept on a pay-as-you-go basis.

Some offices distribute information about credit cards or loans specifically for healthcare treatments. This is very popular for cosmetic surgeries, dental procedures, and laser eye surgeries. Offices that offer these types of procedures may want to investigate such alternative financing services. Although these options are valuable when used properly and repaid on time, they do create additional interest debt for the patient. Encourage patients to pay cash when obtaining medical services and to avoid using credit, because this saves them money in the long run. If the physician allows the patient to split large bills into two or three payments, the patient does not incur credit card interest charges.

Explain Professional Fees and Make Credit Arrangements with a Patient

GOAL: *To assist the patient in paying for services by making mutually beneficial credit arrangements according to established office policy.*

EQUIPMENT and SUPPLIES

- Patient's ledger
- Calendar
- Truth in Lending form
- Assignment of Benefits form
- Patient's insurance form
- Private area for interview

PROCEDURAL STEPS

1. Answer all questions about credit thoroughly and kindly.
2. Inform the patient of the office policy regarding credit.
   - Payment at the time of the first visit
   - Payment by bank card
   - Credit application

   PURPOSE: To ensure complete understanding of mutual responsibilities.
3. Have the patient complete the credit application.
   PURPOSE: To comply with office practices on the extension of credit.
4. Check the completed credit application.
   PURPOSE: To confirm that all the necessary information is included.

5. Discuss the possible arrangements with the patient and ask the person to decide which of them is most suitable.
   PURPOSE: To ensure better compliance. Patients usually keep a payment schedule if they have a voice in planning.
6. Prepare the Truth in Lending form and have the patient sign it if the agreement requires more than four installments.
   PURPOSE: To comply with legal requirements (Regulation Z of the Truth in Lending Act).
7. Be aware of the regulations of the Fair Debt Collection Act when working with patients on collections.
   PURPOSE: To abide by federal laws when collecting from patients.
8. Have the patient execute an assignment of insurance benefits.
   PURPOSE: To comply with credit policy.
9. Make a copy of the patient's insurance card and have the patient sign a consent for release of the information to the insurance company.
   PURPOSE: To ensure that a claim can be processed, because consent for the release of information is necessary on most insurance forms.
10. Keep credit information confidential.
    PURPOSE: To maintain patient confidentiality when performing billing and collection activities.

Truth in Lending Act

Regulation Z of the Truth in Lending Act (TILA), which is enforced by the Federal Trade Commission (FTC) and is part of the Consumer Credit Protection Act, requires that individuals be given certain information when credit is extended, such as the annual percentage rate (APR), the terms of the loan, and the total costs to the borrower. If an agreement exists between physician and patient that the physician will accept payment in more than four installments, the physician must provide a disclosure statement about finance charges (Figure 22-4), even if no finance charges are involved. The physician retains a copy of the form, and the original is given to the patient. Have the patient sign the agreement in your presence to document proof of signing. The disclosure statement must be kept on file for 2 years. Although the disclosure statement is designed as protection for the debtor, it can be a good collection tool for the creditor.

Although much less common than in the past, physicians occasionally permit their patients to pay in installments. As long as no specific agreement has been made for payment to the physician to be made in more than four installments and no finance charge is assessed, the account is not subject to TILA. In accepting such payments, the physician is not subject to the provisions of the regulation. However, the physician's office must make sure to send a statement for the full balance each billing cycle. If the statement is for only a partial payment, it becomes subject to TILA.

Helping patients budget their medical expenses is a fairly new aspect of the business side of medical practice. However, it is a real service to patients and demonstrates that the physician and the office staff are sincerely interested in helping patients; it also may prevent many collection problems. The physician can write an office policy that allows interest charges if the patient does not comply with the original payment arrangements. This provision could help the medical assistant collect payment, because patients will not want interest charges added to the account.

Fair Debt Collection Practices Act

The Fair Debt Collection Practices Act requires that debt collectors act fairly in their collection efforts; it also restricts how and when a person can be contacted about an outstanding debt. Collectors are strictly limited as to whom they may contact about a debt. The medical assistant must work within the framework of this act when collecting for the physician.

Obtaining Credit Information

Credit information is confidential. It should be guarded as carefully as a confidential medical history and should never be disclosed to unauthorized persons. If a call is received about a patient's credit history, follow office policy and only release information according to that policy and legal guidelines in your state. When asking for credit information from patients in the office, do so in a private area where others cannot overhear the conversation. Provide a desk or table away from the reception area where a patient can sit in total privacy and complete a credit application. Credit information is

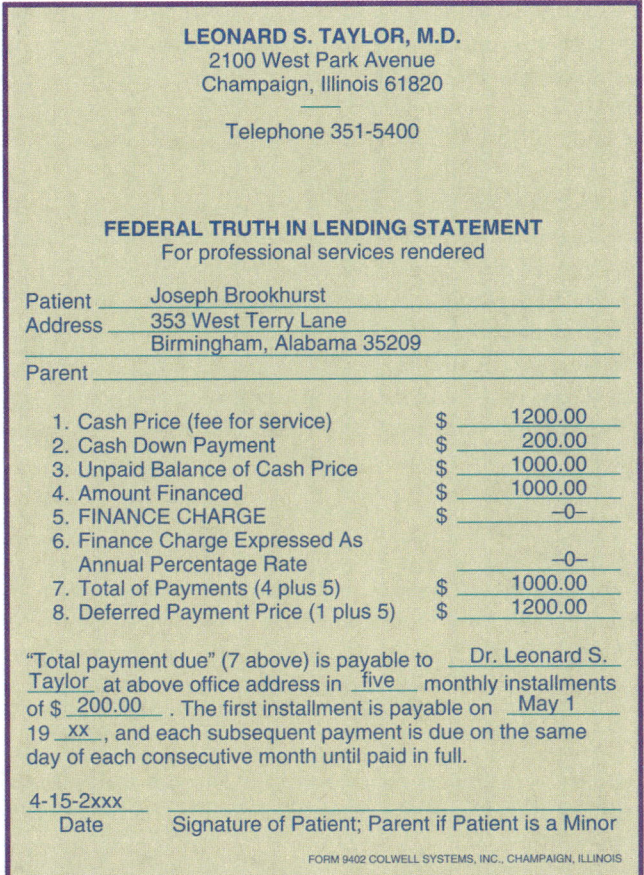

LEONARD S. TAYLOR, M.D.
2100 West Park Avenue
Champaign, Illinois 61820

Telephone 351-5400

FEDERAL TRUTH IN LENDING STATEMENT
For professional services rendered

Patient _____ Joseph Brookhurst _____
Address _____ 353 West Terry Lane _____
_____ Birmingham, Alabama 35209 _____
Parent _____

1. Cash Price (fee for service)	$	1200.00
2. Cash Down Payment	$	200.00
3. Unpaid Balance of Cash Price	$	1000.00
4. Amount Financed	$	1000.00
5. FINANCE CHARGE	$	–0–
6. Finance Charge Expressed As Annual Percentage Rate		–0–
7. Total of Payments (4 plus 5)	$	1000.00
8. Deferred Payment Price (1 plus 5)	$	1200.00

"Total payment due" (7 above) is payable to __Dr. Leonard S. Taylor__ at above office address in __five__ monthly installments of $ __200.00__ . The first installment is payable on __May 1__ 19 __xx__ , and each subsequent payment is due on the same day of each consecutive month until paid in full.

__4-15-2xxx__ _____
Date   Signature of Patient; Parent if Patient is a Minor

FORM 9402 COLWELL SYSTEMS, INC., CHAMPAIGN, ILLINOIS

FIGURE 22-4 Example of a disclosure statement used for compliance with the Truth in Lending Act. (Courtesy Colwell Systems, Champaign, Ill.)

personal, and great care must be taken to prevent misuse and identity theft. Never access a credit report on a patient unless it is necessary to process an application for credit privileges at the medical facility.

INSURANCE OR OTHER THIRD-PARTY PAYERS

Insurance billing in the medical office is a courtesy to patients. Often patients do not understand the policies and appreciate the assistance given by the medical office. Work diligently with patients to obtain the maximum reimbursement possible from insurance and third-party payers. Be a patient advocate by helping patients resolve issues with their policies so that patients obtain the benefits for which they pay.

Billing Procedures

Most physicians' offices and clinics send a billing statement to patients each month (Procedure 22-8). Billing can be accomplished using the following:

- Computer-generated statements
- Encounter forms
- Photocopied or scanned statements
- Online billing statements

The appearance of the statement makes a visual impact, just as a letter does; therefore, the statement heads should be printed or copied on clean, good-quality paper. Statements should be large enough to read easily and to allow itemization of charges. Envelopes should be imprinted with "Address Service Requested" in the appropriate place to maintain up-to-date mailing lists. A self-addressed return envelope included with the statement is convenient for the patient and encourages prompt payment.

PROCEDURE 22-8

Perform Billing Procedures

GOAL: *To bill insurance companies for patient procedures and services and obtain the maximum legal reimbursement.*

EQUIPMENT and SUPPLIES

- Patient ledgers
- Accounting system
- Calculator
- Claim forms
- Encounter forms
- Clerical supplies
- Computer

PROCEDURAL STEPS

1. Read the medical record or encounter form to determine the procedures and services to be billed.
   <u>PURPOSE:</u> To make sure all procedures and services performed by the provider are billed so that he or she can receive the correct reimbursement.

2. Determine the diagnosis code for each diagnosis noted by the provider.
   <u>PURPOSE:</u> To use the proper code to note each diagnosis.
3. Determine the procedure codes for all procedures noted by the provider.
   <u>PURPOSE:</u> To use the proper code to note each procedure.
4. Complete the claim form according to the directions for each block.
5. Determine the amount of money the provider is billing on the claim.
   <u>PURPOSE:</u> To bill for the correct amount in reimbursement.
6. Determine the address where the claim forms should be mailed.
   <u>PURPOSE:</u> To eliminate unnecessary delays in the carrier's receipt of the claim form.
7. Mail or electronically submit the claim form.
8. Note the date the claim should receive follow-up to make sure it is paid.
9. Bill the patient for the remaining balance, if any.
   <u>PURPOSE:</u> To clear the balance owed to the physician; to complete the claim form cycle accurately so that payment will not be delayed.

Computer-Generated Statements

Most statements now are computer generated. Patient accounts are established and stored in the computer so that a statement can be produced whenever needed. The statement provides information such as the service rendered on each date, the charge for each service, the date on which a claim was submitted to the insurance company, the date of payment, and the balance due from the patient. The computer may also be programmed to print messages on the statement, such as "Balance now 30 days past due."

Encounter Forms

Encounter forms usually are personalized for the practice. The form should have space for all the elements required to submit medical insurance claims, such as:

- Name and address of the patient
- Name of the insurance carrier
- Insurance identification number
- Procedure codes
- Fee for each service
- Diagnosis codes
- Place and date of service
- Physician's name and address
- Physician's signature

The encounter form often is used as a charge slip for office treatments. The physician checks or circles the services and procedures performed at the completion of the visit, and the form is taken to the checkout area. The medical assistant then totals the account and obtains payment from the patient.

Photocopied Statements

Some offices make a copy of the statements and mail them to patients each month as a bill. The copied statement should prominently display the balance due. Writing must be clear and legible. Usually, a window envelope is used for mailing, which means that the name and address on the ledger must be neat, correct, and positioned correctly for the envelope window. Office supply stores have stickers that can be attached to statements indicating that the bill is past due or close to collection action.

Online Billing Statements

If the medical facility uses a computer software system with e-billing capacity, patients can receive their statements by e-mail. Because of the security risk, the patient must agree to accept bills sent to them by e-mail. A computer hacker may be able to find information leading to identity theft when bills are sent and then paid using online systems. However, most facilities that accept online payments use a secure encrypted program to make the process safe for sensitive information. The patient could pay the bill using a credit card, debit card, or checking account. To use the checking account option, a patient usually is required to enter the bank's routing number and his or her checking account number. Some of these systems process the payment immediately; therefore, to avoid nonsufficient funds (NSF) charges, patients must take care that they have sufficient funds to cover the online payment before it is made.

Itemizing the First Statement

If the medical fee has been explained to the patient in advance, the monthly statement is merely a confirmation of what is owed, and

there should be no misunderstanding. However, it is good business practice and a courtesy to the patient to itemize the charges on the first statement. This is essential if the statement is to be used for billing the patient's insurance. Patients are entitled to an understanding of the physician's statement for medical services.

Time and Frequency of Billing

Patients expect to receive statements from their creditors monthly, and they plan their budgets around first-of-the-month bills received. Punctuality in billing encourages prompt payment.

Statements should be sent at least once each month. Some offices send bills immediately after treatment; others bill all patients on the same day each month. Mailing statements twice a month (e.g., half of the accounts on the tenth and the remaining half on the twenty-fifth) is also a common practice.

Once-a-Month Billing

If a monthly pattern is followed, bills should leave the office in time to reach the patient no later than the last day of each month and preferably before the twenty-fifth to encourage payment around the first of the month. Planning ahead for the preparation of statements can lighten the burden of once-a-month billing.

Cycle Billing

Many physicians prefer to use the cycle billing system, in which certain portions of the accounts receivable are billed at given times during the month, instead of preparation of all statements at the end of the month. Large businesses, such as credit card issuers and banks, also use cycle billing. Sending statements in cycles has many advantages; for example, it prevents once a month peak workloads and stabilizes cash flow. In a small office where billing is done only once a month, the unexpected illness or absence of the medical assistant who prepares the statements can leave the physician in a financial bind because of a delay in billing. Most patients wait for their statement to send in a payment.

When statements are prepared, accounts are separated into fairly equal divisions, the number of divisions depending on how many times billing is done during a month. For example, if the office expects to bill twice a month, divide the accounts into two equal groups; for weekly billing, divide into four groups; and for daily billing, divide into 20 groups. Small alphabetic groups can be combined to keep the divisions nearly equal in the number of statements to prepare on each billing day. If the files are color coded, the medical assistant may want to use the same alphabetic breakdown in billing. Regardless of constant changes in the individual accounts, the mailing dates for accounts in each section remain the same. A schedule for processing and mailing is established, and the workload is apportioned throughout the entire month.

Cycle billing allows the medical assistant to continue all routine duties each day, handling the statements on a day-to-day or weekly schedule rather than in one intensive period at the end of the month. This means that whole days need not be sacrificed from other duties to get statements in the mail. When the billing is spaced throughout the month, more time and consideration can be given to each statement, itemization of bills is less burdensome, and the likelihood of error is reduced.

Patients generally accept the cycle billing system quickly and often with enthusiasm. However, if your office decides to change from a once-a-month billing system to a cycle billing system, patients should be notified in advance and the new plan should be explained to them. To explain the new system to established patients, enclose a notice in each statement for 2 months before the transfer, describing the plan and indicating the future dates on which each patient will receive the bill. Before a physician adopts the cycle billing system, particularly in a small community, several factors should be taken into consideration:

- What is the general income level of the community and how and when does the average patient get paid?
- Do local companies pay employees at various times during the month or are most paychecks handed out at the beginning of the month?
- Would cycle billing benefit patients in addition to the overall operation of the office?

PROFESSIONAL COURTESY

In the past, many physicians did not charge professional colleagues or their close family members for medical care; this concept is called **professional courtesy**. In some cases, giving professional courtesy represents the loss of a large amount of potential income. If a substantial outlay in the cost of materials is involved, the professional colleague probably will want to reimburse the physician for the materials used. Most physicians today subscribe to a health insurance plan. If the care they receive is covered by insurance, it is entirely ethical for the attending physician to accept the insurance benefits in payment for services.

Professional courtesy often is extended beyond fellow physicians and their dependents. Many physicians treat their own medical assistants and often their families without charge and grant discounts to nurses and medical assistants not in their direct employ. Student externs should never expect to be treated while serving in an externship capacity. Professional courtesy is sometimes extended to others in the healthcare field (e.g., pharmacists and dentists). Before offering professional courtesy to anyone, the physician must determine whether doing so violates any of his or her contracts or agreements with managed care providers or third-party payers. Some may have restrictions on eliminating or writing off co-pays or co-insurance amounts. Make sure the extension of professional courtesy never jeopardizes any contracts. The physician or office manager is responsible for adhering to all legal agreements, but the medical assistant must follow through. Never offer any type of discount that is outside of established office policy or that has not been authorized by the physician.

BILLING MINORS

Minors cannot be held responsible for payment of a bill unless they are emancipated. Bills for minors are usually addressed to a parent or legal guardian. If a bill is addressed to a minor, the parent or parents could take the attitude that they are not responsible because they never received the bill.

If the parents are separated or divorced, the parent who brings the child in for treatment is responsible for payment. Whatever financial agreement exists between the parents is strictly their personal business and should not concern the medical office. The responsible parent should be so informed from the beginning.

If a minor appears in the office and requests treatment and you can ascertain that the person is legally emancipated, the minor is responsible for the bill. It may be wise to make a determination either with the business manager or with the physician as to whether your office wishes to treat an emancipated minor. Minors can be treated for certain conditions, such as sexually transmitted diseases (STDs), pregnancy, and birth control without parental consent. In these cases, the medical assistant must determine where the bill should be sent, if the minor carries a balance on his or her ledger card. Be sure that office policy is followed and that the policies line up with local, state, and national laws.

COLLECTION PROCEDURES

Most patients truly want to pay the bills they owe. However, sometimes a patient may have difficulty meeting his or her obligations. The patient may have lost a job or insurance coverage. An emergency could arise that depletes finances. When patients must choose between paying their medical bills and having electricity, the physician often is forced to wait for reimbursement. Although a few patients absolutely refuse to pay for their medical care, most are honest and willing to pay but may need help with a payment plan. Terms can be arranged for collecting payment in full when the office and the patient cooperate with each other. The medical assistant should attempt to work out a plan that the patient can abide by, and the patient should be expected to make promised payments.

Collection problems can arise if the medical assistant fails to get the necessary insurance information. In some instances, if the insurance forms are not completed correctly, the claim may be denied. Minor errors, such as failing to name the responsible party or omitting accurate numeric information, delay payment to the physician.

MEDICAL CARE FOR THOSE WHO CANNOT PAY

The medical profession traditionally has accepted the responsibility of providing occasional medical care for individuals unable to pay for these services. Despite the increased scope of government-sponsored care for the **medically indigent**, physicians still spend thousands of dollars each year providing services before securing some type of payment.

In many instances medical care of the indigent is available through social service agencies. Medical assistants should learn about local organizations and agencies that can aid patients in obtaining the necessary assistance. The physician can provide only medical services. Other agencies provide hospitalization, for example, or

---

CRITICAL THINKING APPLICATION **22-7**

Dr. Crawford has just finished seeing Dr. Franklin, who came to him as a patient. Dr. Franklin insists to Jodie that Dr. Crawford always extends him professional courtesy. This is not indicated on his account card, because several payments are shown on the record. Dr. Crawford has just left the office and is in an important meeting at the hospital.

- What should Jodie do?
- Does this event justify paging or calling the physician?

arrange for paying the costs of special therapy, rehabilitation, or medications. Unfortunately, there is still another segment of the population that consists of uninsured employees who are not eligible for public assistance, are not covered under a group policy, and cannot afford the high premiums for private medical insurance. Give special attention to helping these people arrange payment of their medical bills. If a physician accepts a case in advance for which a fee will not be paid, complete records must still be kept on the patient. The only deviation in procedure is that the financial record indicates no charge (n/c) in the debit column.

FEES IN HARDSHIP CASES

Sometimes a physician is faced with the problem of deciding whether to reduce or cancel a fee in a hardship case. Before adjusting or canceling a fee, the physician or medical assistant should have a frank discussion with the patient about his or her financial situation. Find out whether the patient is entitled to any funds for medical care or an insurance settlement of some kind. For instance, if the patient's injuries are the result of a car accident, there may be insurance through the automobile policy. Circumstances may qualify the patient for local or state public assistance, such as crime victim assistance. Keep information about such agencies that are available in the area and direct the patient to the appropriate one.

Discuss the fee in advance and make payment arrangements if the circumstances of hardship are known before services are rendered. The physician may suggest that a medically indigent patient seek care at a county hospital with public assistance. A physician should be free to choose his or her form of charity and should not feel obligated to substantially reduce or cancel a fee when the circumstances are known in advance.

After the physician and patient have agreed on a fee, special circumstances may arise that create a hardship after the fact. If the physician then agrees to reduce the fee, the patient should be told that the reduction will be effective only after the adjusted amount is paid in full. For instance, if a fee of $500 is reduced to $350, the full amount of the $500 charge should appear on the ledger, and when $350 has been received, the remainder can be written off as an adjustment.

Pitfalls of Fee Adjustments

Problems can arise when a physician begins to reduce his or her fees. Patients may begin to expect fees to be reduced in all circumstances. Patients may even doubt the competency of a physician who habitually reduces fees. Make fee reductions the exception rather than the norm.

Take great care in reducing the fee for care of a patient who dies. The physician's sympathy is with the family in such instances, but the physician's generosity in reducing a fee could be misinterpreted and result in a suit for malpractice. The family may suspect that the fee was reduced because the physician knows he or she made an error.

If the physician agrees to settle for a reduced fee in a situation in which the patient is disputing the cost, take care to make sure the negotiations are without prejudice. By taking this precaution, the physician protects his or her right to collect the original sum should the patient refuse to pay the lowered fee. The offer of a discount,

therefore, should be made in writing, with insertion of the words "without prejudice," and a definite time limit for making payment should be stated. Prepare two copies of the agreement and have the signatures witnessed by a staff member. Keep the original for the physician and give a copy to the patient.

A fee should never be reduced on the basis of a poor result or as a means of obtaining payment to avoid the use of a collection agency. A reduction for these reasons degrades the physician and the practice of medicine.

MEDICARE AND ADVANCE BENEFICIARY NOTICES

Occasionally, Medicare requires that the physician give the patient an Advance Beneficiary Notice (ABN). This form is given when the physician, healthcare provider, or supplier thinks that Medicare probably or certainly will not pay for services or items. The patient decides whether he or she still wants to receive the services from the provider and completes the information on the form (Figure 22-5).

PREPARING ACCOUNTS FOR COLLECTION ACTIVITY

Sometimes it becomes necessary to aggressively attempt to collect the balances that patients owe the physician. Persuasive collection procedures include telephone calls, collection reminders and letters, and personal interviews (Procedure 22-9).

Before beginning collection action, determine which accounts have a balance due and how old the account is. Some accounts are grouped together, or "aged," according to the dates of the last payment activity, whereas others are grouped according to the original date of service. Others are grouped by month, beginning with the month the bill was first charged. Common account aging categories are:

0-30 days
30-60 days
60-90 days
90-120 days

Computer accounting systems can age the accounts and indicate the type of activity needed. A bill less than 30 days old might need a friendly call or reminder letter, whereas one that is over 120 days may need a final letter to encourage payment before the account is turned over to a collection agency. Always allow the physician a final review of the names of patients being sent to a collection agency. This practice prevents the embarrassing situation of sending a relative who may have an unfamiliar name to collections. Once the accounts are aged, choose the most appropriate type of collection activity according to office policy.

COLLECTION TECHNIQUES

The medical assistant can use a variety of techniques to collect patient accounts. Often more than one technique must be used to obtain payment. Always be courteous and kind when using collection techniques.

Telephone Collection Calls

A telephone call at the right time, in the right manner, is more successful than notes, a statement, or a collection letter. The personal

A. Notifier: John Doe, MD, College Clinic, 4567 Broad Avenue, Woodland Hills, XY 12345 555-486-9002

B. Patient Name: Mary Judd   **C. Identification Number:** 0920XX7291

Advance Beneficiary Notice of Noncoverage (ABN)

NOTE: If Medicare doesn't pay for D. _B12 injections_ below, you may have to pay.
Medicare does not pay for everything, even some care that you or your health care provider have good reason to think you need. We expect Medicare may not pay for the D. _B12 injections_ below.

D.	E. Reason Medicare May Not Pay:	F. Estimated Cost
B12 injections	Medicare does not usually pay for this injection or this many injections	$35.00

WHAT YOU NEED TO DO NOW:
- Read this notice, so you can make an informed decision about your care.
- Ask us any questions that you may have after you finish reading.
- Choose an option below about whether to receive the D. _B12 injections_ listed above.
  Note: If you choose Option 1 or 2, we may help you to use any other insurance that you might have, but Medicare cannot require us to do this.

G. OPTIONS: Check only one box. We cannot choose a box for you.

☒ **OPTION 1.** I want the D. _B12 injections_ listed above. You may ask to be paid now, but I also want Medicare billed for an official decision on payment, which is sent to me on a Medicare Summary Notice (MSN). I understand that if Medicare doesn't pay, I am responsible for payment, but **I can appeal to Medicare** by following the directions on the MSN. If Medicare does pay, you will refund any payments I made to you, less co-pays or deductibles.

☐ **OPTION 2.** I want the D. _____ listed above, but do not bill Medicare. You may ask to be paid now as I am responsible for payment. **I cannot appeal if Medicare is not billed.**

☐ **OPTION 3.** I don't want the D. _____ listed above. I understand with this choice I am **not** responsible for payment, and **I cannot appeal to see if Medicare would pay.**

H. Additional Information:

This notice gives our opinion, not an official Medicare decision. If you have other questions on this notice or Medicare billing, call **1-800-MEDICARE** (1-800-633-4227/**TTY:** 1-877-486-2048).
Signing below means that you have received and understand this notice. You also receive a copy.

I. Signature: _Mary Judd_	J. Date: _March 20, 20XX_

According to the Paperwork Reduction Act of 1995, no persons are required to respond to a collection of information unless it displays a valid OMB control number. The valid OMB control number for this information collection is 0938-0566. The time required to complete this information collection is estimated to average 7 minutes per response, including the time to review instructions, search existing data resources, gather the data needed, and complete and review the information collection. If you have comments concerning the accuracy of the time estimate or suggestions for improving this form, please write to: CMS, 7500 Security Boulevard, Attn: PRA Reports Clearance Officer, Baltimore, Maryland 21244-1850.

Form CMS-R-131 (03/11)   Form Approved OMB No. 0938-0566

FIGURE 22-5 The Advance Beneficiary Notice (ABN) form is used to notify patients that Medicare may not pay for certain items and services. (From Fordney M: *Insurance handbook for the medical office,* ed 12, St Louis, 2012, WB Saunders.)

contact of a telephone call often prompts patients to mail in their payment. In the absence of time to make calls, the collection letter is the next best approach, but if collections are a serious problem, it may be worth an extra salary to hire a person to do the telephoning.

Always treat patients with the utmost respect on the telephone. Keep their financial record close by in case they have questions about their bill; also have their insurance company's phone number handy. Remember that some patients may not understand anything about insurance or third-party payers, so guide them to that understanding and be their advocate in getting as much reimbursement as possible so that the patient's share is smaller. Never simply insist that insurance has paid and their balance is due. This puts the patient into a negative mindset. Try using phrases such as the following:

"Mrs. Diggs, it looks as if your insurance company paid late last month. I believe you have a co-pay for your surgery that amounts to $450. Is that what you were expecting? Would you

like to take care of the whole balance or split that into two payments?"

"Mr. Hildebrand, we're showing that you have a balance due from your surgery. Your insurance has paid, and it looks as if you owe $700. We would be happy to help you by splitting that into two or three payments. What would work for you?"

"Mrs. Crumley, it seems that you have a balance due of $450 from your surgery, and I called to see whether I could help you budget that. You could pay $50 this week and split the remaining $400 into two payments over the next 2 months? We would be happy to work with you on this balance."

Always abide by office policy when making payment arrangements in collection situations. Never be belligerent with a patient. If he or she becomes irate, simply state that the person can call back when ready to discuss a solution for paying the account, say goodbye, and gently hang up the phone. Never listen to explicatives or allow verbal abuse.

PROCEDURE 22-9

Perform Collection Procedures

GOAL: *To collect the maximum amount of funds on each account.*

EQUIPMENT and SUPPLIES

- Patient ledger
- Office policy manual
- Clerical supplies
- Scripts for telephone collections so that students can role play this activity
- Letters for collection efforts
- Telephone
- Letterhead and envelopes
- Copies of claim forms previously filed

PROCEDURAL STEPS

1. Become familiar with office policy regarding turning accounts over to collections.
   PURPOSE: To make sure the policy is followed when accounts are turned over to collection agencies.
2. Review the patient's ledger to determine whether it needs collection activity.

PURPOSE: Some accounts may be past due, but patients may have made arrangements to pay them; in this case, collection activities should not commence.

3. Determine the type of collection activity the account needs.
   PURPOSE: An account that is only slightly past due does not need a harsh collection letter; determine the best approach for each particular account.
4. Begin collection efforts with telephone calls or postcards.
   PURPOSE: Many patients only need a small reminder that their account is past due.
5. Progress to more stringent collection efforts if the patient does not pay the account as promised.
6. Once all collection efforts have been exhausted, report the account to the physician for further disposition.
   PURPOSE: The physician should decide which accounts are given to collection agencies and which are simply written off as bad debts.
7. Document the final collection activity on the ledger and/or in the patient's medical record.

Written notification is a must before making a final demand for payment indicating that legal or collection proceedings will be started. Each case should be handled individually on the basis of the experience with the person involved.

GENERAL RULES FOR TELEPHONE COLLECTIONS

What to Do

- Call the patient when it can be done with privacy.
- Call between 8 AM and 9 PM.
- Determine the identity of the person with whom you are speaking. If you ask, "Is this Mrs. Noble?" and she answers, "Yes," it could be the patient's mother-in-law or daughter-in-law, who is also "Mrs. Noble." Use the person's full name. Include suffixes, such as "Thomas Melborn, III." This may sound too formal, but it helps to ensure that the correct person is on the phone.
- Be dignified and respectful. One can be friendly and formal at the same time.
- Ask the patient whether it is a convenient time to talk. Unless you have the attention of the called party, there is little to be gained by continuing. If told that it is an inopportune time, ask for a specific time to call back or get a promise that the patient will call the office at a specified time.
- After a brief greeting, state the purpose of the call. Make no apology for calling, but state the reason in a friendly, businesslike way. The physician expects payment, and the medical assistant is interested in helping the patient meet the financial obligation. Open the call with a phrase such as, "This is Alice, Dr. Crawford's financial secretary. I'm calling about your account." A well-placed pause at this point in the call sometimes gets an immediate response from the debtor with regard to the nonpayment.
- Assume a positive attitude. For example, convey the impression that the patient intended to pay and it is only a matter of working out some suitable arrangements.
- Keep the conversation brief and to the point; do not make threats of any kind.
- Try to get a definite commitment—payment of a certain amount by a certain date.
- Follow up on promises made by the patient. This is best accomplished by using a tickler file or a note on the calendar. If the payment does not arrive by the promised date, remind the patient with another call. If the medical assistant fails to do this, the whole effort has been wasted.

What Not to Do

- Do not call between 9 PM and 8 AM. To do so may be considered harassment.
- Do not make repeated telephone calls.
- Do not call the debtor's place of work if the employer prohibits personal calls.
- If a call is placed to the debtor at work and the person cannot take the call, leave a message asking the debtor to "call Mrs. Black at 727-9238" without revealing the nature of the call; that is, do not state that the call is from "Dr. Crawford's office" or "Dr. Crawford's medical assistant."
- Do not show hostility. An angry patient is a poorly paying patient. Insulted patients often do not pay at all.

Collection Letters or Reminders

Some consultants believe that a printed collection letter or reminder enclosed with a statement is more effective than a personal letter. Their attitude is that a patient may be embarrassed by a personal letter and feel that he or she has been singled out for attention. An impersonal printed message will probably encourage the debtor to send a payment. The printed form is a time saver and is recommended if a lack of time contributes to poor collection follow-up. Standard printed forms are readily available, or the medical assistant can design an original form.

Letters that are friendly requests for an explanation of why payment has not been made are effective in most cases. These letters should indicate that the physician is sincerely interested in the patient and wants to help resolve the financial obligations. Invite the patient to the office to explain the reasons for nonpayment so that payment arrangements can be made. To lessen the patient's embarrassment, these letters can suggest that previous statements may have been overlooked.

On receipt of such a letter, most patients make some effort to explain their failure to make payment. If a patient really is having financial difficulties, he or she may be able to get public assistance. If it is a temporary financial problem, the physician and the patient may together be able to work out a satisfactory installment plan for payment.

The medical assistant often is given a free hand in designing collection patterns and composing collection letters. Many medical assistants compose a series of collection letters, using model letters they have found effective. Such a series usually includes at least five letters in varying degrees of forcefulness.

Sometimes even a person with poor paying habits pays the bill if treated with respect and consideration. The medical assistant should never go beyond the authority granted by the physician in pursuing collections. If questions arise about special collection problems, always check with the physician before proceeding. This is particularly important with patients whom you do not know personally (e.g., patients whom the physician has seen in the hospital or at home and patients with no credit history). It is difficult to say whether the effects of pressing collections too hard (which can result in loss of patient good will) are more detrimental than the effects of not pursuing collections diligently enough (which can result in loss of revenue). The physician and the medical assistant should agree on general collection policies as outlined earlier in this chapter, and the policies then should be followed. In all cases in which an account is to be assigned to a collection agency, make sure the physician is aware of this and approves.

In most medical offices, the medical assistant signs collection letters using his or her title, such as "Medical Assistant" or "Financial Secretary" below the typewritten signature. Do not list "Collections" below the name, because the patient may assume that the account has been placed with a collection agency. Some physicians want to sign these communications personally, but generally the medical assistant who handles the accounts also signs the collection letters.

Personal Interviews

Personal interviews with patients sometimes can be more effective than a whole series of collection letters. By talking to a patient face to face, the medical assistant can come to an understanding of the problem more quickly, and an agreement about future payment plans can be reached.

Occasionally a patient may undergo a long course of treatment and yet make no attempt to pay anything on the account. Perhaps such a patient is only waiting for the physician or the medical assistant to suggest that a payment be made. When it is known in advance that the patient requires extensive treatment, the matter of payment should be discussed early in the course of treatment, the credit policy should be explained, and some agreement should be reached on a payment plan.

Because medical services are far more **intangible** than any commercial service, collection efforts must not be delayed too long. Any responsible, sincere patient will call or write the physician's office after receiving a second statement and explain the delay in payment or ask for a payment plan. This is best accomplished in a private, personal interview.

If the account ultimately must be referred to a collector, find a good agency with a high recovery rate. The value of medical accounts diminishes in direct proportion to the length of time that has elapsed since service was provided. Do not fight the law of diminishing returns. All collection activity is costly. Know when to stop and call on the services of a professional agency.

Special Collection Situations

Tracing "Skips"

When a statement is returned marked "Moved—no forwarding address," you may consider this account as a "skip." This generally is accepted as an indication that the patient is attempting to avoid liability for debts, although some skips are innocent errors. The person may have been careless in not leaving a forwarding address, or the mistake may have occurred in the physician's office; the wrong name or address may have been placed on the statement. However, immediate action should be taken with regard to returned statements. Do not wait until the next billing time to attempt to trace the debtor. The Internet can be a valuable tool in tracing skips. Using a search engine, such as Yahoo or Google, enter the patient's name. Patients might even be found on social networking sites, such as Facebook, and that information may provide clues about the person's whereabouts. Investigate the search results carefully so that collection efforts are directed at the right person.

Address Change Service. Two versions of address change service (ACS) are offered by the U.S. Post Office: one uses the traditional alpha participant code, and the other uses an intelligent mail barcode encoded with a business entity identifier (BEI) code. Both versions notify mailers electronically of a change of address (COA) or a reason for nondelivery. ACS is available for all classes of mail but must be used with either an ancillary service endorsement and a participant code or an intelligent mail barcode containing a BEI. If the mailer uses an ancillary service endorsement for manual notifications and does not participate in ACS, the USPS charges a higher fee per mail piece. For the fee structure, see the *Mailing Standards of the United States Postal Service Domestic Mail Manual,* available on the USPS Web site *(www.usps.com).* Mailers who want to participate in ACS must acquire either an ACS participant code or a BEI code from the National Customer Support Center (NCSC) and apply it to their envelopes, address labels, or address blocks in the required format. The locations of the notation Address Service Requested are shown in Figure 22-6.

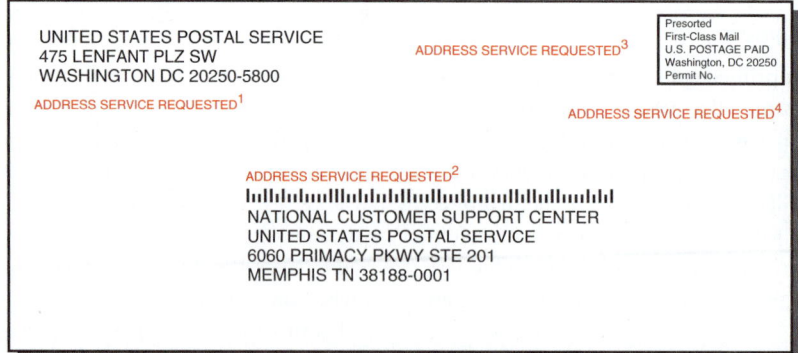

FIGURE 22-6 Address Service Requested envelope from the U.S. Postal Service.

If all attempts fail, turn the account over to a collection agency without delay. Do not keep a skip account too long, because the trail may become so cold as time elapses that even collection experts will be unable to follow it.

SUGGESTIONS FOR TRACING SKIPS

- Examine the patient's original office registration card.
- Call the telephone number listed on the card. Occasionally a patient may move without leaving a forwarding address but will transfer the old telephone number. The new telephone number may be given when you call the old number.
- If you are unable to contact the individual by telephone, make a few discreet calls to the references listed on the registration card to get leads.
- Check the Internet to secure the names and telephone numbers of neighbors or the landlord and contact these people to secure information about the debtor's whereabouts.
- Do not inform a third party that the person owes you money. Simply state that you are trying to locate or verify the location of the individual.
- Check the debtor's place of employment for information. If the person is a specialist in his or her field of work, the local union or similar organizations may be contacted. Although they may not give you the person's current address, they will relay the message that you are seeking to contact him or her. Often people are stirred to pay a bill if they think their employer may learn of their payment failure.
- Do not communicate with a third party more than once. This is specifically forbidden by law (Public Law 95-109, Sec. 804) unless the third party requests the collector to do so.

Claims Against Estates

A bill owed by a deceased patient may be handled a little differently from regular bills. Courtesy dictates that a bill not be sent during the initial period of bereavement, but do not delay longer than 30 days. The person responsible for settling the affairs of the estate, called an executor, is assembling outstanding accounts and expects to receive the medical bills along with all others. Use the following format to address the statement:

Estate of (name of patient)

c/o (spouse or next of kin, if known)

Patient's last known address

Do not address the statement to a relative unless you have a signed agreement that that person will be responsible. If for some reason the statement cannot be addressed as just suggested (e.g., if the patient was in an assisted-living facility or a skilled nursing facility and no relative's name is available), seek information from the county seat in the county where the estate is being settled.

A will generally is filed within 30 days of a death. The name of the executor or administrator usually can be obtained by sending a request to the Probate Department of the Superior Court, County Recorder's Office, in the county where the **decedent** lived. The time limits for filing an estate claim are determined by the state where the decedent resided.

After the name of the administrator or executor of the estate has been obtained, send a duplicate itemized statement of the account to that person by certified mail, return receipt requested. If no response is received in 10 days, contact the executor or the county clerk where the estate is being settled and obtain forms for filing a claim against the estate. (Some states do not have special claim forms and accept simple itemized statements.) This claim against the estate must be made within a certain time, which varies from 2 to 36 months, depending on the state where it is filed.

The executor of the estate either accepts or rejects the claim, and if it is accepted, sends an acknowledgment of the debt. Payment often is delayed because of the legal complications involved in settling an estate, but if the claim has been accepted, the physician eventually receives the money. If the claim is rejected and there is full justification for claiming the bill, file a claim against the executor within a limited time, according to state laws. The time limit in such cases starts with the date on the letter of rejection sent in response to the original claim.

Because states have different time limits and statutes with regard to these issues, the medical assistant should contact the physician's attorney or the local court for the exact procedure to follow; or, the physician may prefer to turn such matters over to his or her legal counsel immediately.

Bankruptcy

Bankruptcy laws were passed to secure equal distribution of the assets of an individual among the individual's creditors. These are federal laws that apply in all the states. When notified that a patient has declared bankruptcy, do not send statements or make any attempt to collect on the account from the patient.

Chapter 7 bankruptcy usually is a "no asset" situation. Because the physician's fee is an **unsecured** debt, there is little purpose in pursuing collection. Chapter 13 is known as *wage-earner bankruptcy*. Under Chapter 13, the patient-debtor pays a fixed amount to a **trustee** that is agreed upon by the court. This is then passed on to the creditors. During this period, none of the creditors can attach the debtor's wages or otherwise attempt to collect the debt. It sometimes is beneficial to file a claim under Chapter 13, because small payments may be made by the debtor under the supervision of the court over a period of 3 years. However, the debts are paid in order, **secured** debts first; consequently, the physician may never receive payment from a debtor who has filed bankruptcy.

USING OUTSIDE COLLECTION SERVICES

When everything possible has been done internally to follow up on an outstanding account and the office has not received payment, the question arises as to what step to take next, as follows:

- Should the facility sue for the payment?
- Should the account be sent to a collection agency?
- Should the account be written off as a bad debt?

Before forcing an account, first consider the time element: Has the patient been given a fair chance to pay this bill? Have statements been sent regularly and has a systematic method of following the account been used? Ask whether there might be a misunderstanding about the fee charged. Was the first statement fully itemized? A large, unexplained bill may frighten a patient into making no payments at all because the whole balance looks too large.

If the correct registration forms to secure advance credit information were used, the medical assistant should know the patient's financial ability to pay. However, illness may have caused a loss of salary and resulted in temporary inability to pay. Try to analyze the situation thoroughly. Could the patient have been dissatisfied with the care received? For some unknown reason, a patient may feel that he or she was not treated correctly. Perhaps the patient expected a complete cure too soon. Only an explanation of the condition, prognosis, and care can enlighten such patients, and this is best handled by the physician. If payment of a bill is pressed too hard and the patient is dissatisfied for some reason, a malpractice suit may be filed by the patient to seek retribution against the physician. The court can approve a period longer than 3 years in special cases but cannot approve a period longer than 5 years for collecting patient accounts.

Using a Collection Agency

The medical assistant should try every means possible to collect accounts before they become delinquent. As soon as the account is determined uncollectible through the office (i.e., the patient has failed to respond to the final letter or has failed to fulfill a second promise on payment), send the account to the collector without delay. Skips should be assigned immediately.

Even though collection by an agency means sacrificing 40% to 60% of the amount owed, further delay only reduces the chances of recovery by the professional collector. If the agency finds that the case deserves special consideration, it will ask the physician's advice before proceeding further.

Working with the Collection Agency

The collection agency needs certain data to enable it to begin collection procedures on overdue accounts:

- Full name of the debtor
- Name of the spouse
- Last known address
- Full amount of the debt
- Date of the last entry on account (debit or credit)
- Occupation of the debtor
- Business address
- Any other pertinent data

After an account has been released to a collection agency, the office makes no further collection attempts. Once the agency has begun its work, a number of guidelines and procedures should be followed:

- Send no more statements.
- Mark the patient's ledger or stamp it so that everyone knows it is now in the hands of the collector.
- Refer the patient to the collection agency if he or she contacts the office about the account.
- Promptly report any payments made directly to your office (a percentage of this payment is due the agency).
- Call the agency if any information is obtained that will be of value in tracing or collecting the account.
- Do not push the agency with frequent calls. The representatives of the agency will report regularly and will keep the office posted on collection progress.

Posting Collection Agency Payments

Collection agencies charge different percentages to collect delinquent accounts, but the agency with the cheapest fee is rarely the most effective. Agencies pay the net back, which is the amount of money paid to the facility after the agency has been paid its fee. The net back is the figure that should be considered when using a collection agency, not simply the fee percentage. If a patient sends a payment after the account has been turned over to a collection agency, the payment must be recorded on the account card. Because the agency charges a fee for collection efforts, the amount credited to the patient's account might be less than the actual payment amount. For instance, if the agency charges 25%, a $100 payment results in a $75 credit to the patient's account and the agency keeps $25. When posting the payment, place the amount to be credited in the adjustment column on the day sheet (Procedure 22-10). Some offices prefer the payment to go directly to the collection agency;

PROCEDURE 22-10

Post Collection Agency Payments

GOAL: *To post payments received on an account after it has been turned over to a collection agency.*

EQUIPMENT and SUPPLIES

- Patient ledgers
- Office policy manual
- Bookkeeping system
- Clerical supplies
- Calculator

PROCEDURAL STEPS

1. Determine that a payment has been received on an account that is now being serviced by a collection agency.
2. Notify the collection agency that the payment has been made.

PURPOSE: The collection agency is entitled to a portion of the money collected when a payment is sent to the medical office.

3. Send a notice to the patient, if necessary, to explain that the payment has been forwarded to the collection agency for credit.
4. Instruct patients to forward additional payments straight to the collection agency.
5. If office policy dictates, deposit the payment to the physician's account and then forward the fee due to the collection agency to its address.
   PURPOSE: To honor the contractual obligations with the collection agency.

---

either way, the adjustment eventually must be credited to the patient's account.

Making the Decision to Sue

The physician must decide whether he or she will benefit or suffer loss of good will by suing for a bill rather than writing it off as a loss. Some physicians believe it is unwise to resort to the court to collect medical bills unless extraordinary circumstances apply.

An account must be considered a 100% loss to the physician before legal proceedings are started. Remember never to threaten to **instigate** legal proceedings unless the physician is prepared to carry out the threat and has decided to pursue legal action. If the physician decides in favor of a lawsuit, investigate thoroughly and obtain as much information as possible for the proceedings. Litigation to collect a bill generally is in order when the following are true:

- The patient can afford to pay without hardship.
- The physician can produce office records that support the bill.
- The physician can justify the amount of the bill by comparing it with fee practices in the community.
- The patient's general condition after treatment is satisfactory.
- The persuasive powers of an ethical collection agency have been exhausted, and the agency advises suing.
- The patient can be given ample warning of the physician's intention to sue.
- The defendant (whether a patient or a parent or legal guardian) is legally liable for the services rendered to the patient.
- The statute of limitations has ruled out any possible malpractice action.
- The physician is neither indignant nor in a negative frame of mind.

Small Claims Court

Many medical practices find the small claims court a satisfactory, inexpensive means of collecting delinquent accounts. The law places

a limit on the amount of debt for which relief may be sought in small claims court. Because this varies from state to state (usually up to $10,000) and in some instances even within a state, this limit should be checked in local courts before recovery is sought in this manner.

Parties to small claims actions are not represented by an attorney at the hearing but may send another person to court on their behalf to produce records supporting the claim. Physicians often send their bookkeeper or medical assistant with records of unpaid accounts to show the judge.

If the court awards a judgment for the amount owed, the plaintiff in small claims court may also recover the costs of the suit. For a very small investment in time and money, the physician who uses this method saves the time of a regular court action and eliminates attorneys' fees.

After being awarded a judgment, the medical assistant still must collect the money. The only person in a small claims action who has the right of appeal is the defendant. An appeal by the defendant may have the judgment set aside. The plaintiff cannot file an appeal in a small claims action; the decision of the court is final.

The necessary papers for filing action and full instructions on the course to follow may be obtained from the clerk of the small claims court. A medical assistant who has never appeared in court probably would be wise to attend once as a spectator to preview the procedure; this should allow him or her to feel more at ease when appearing for the physician.

A collection agency to which an account may have been assigned may not file or handle a small claims action. It must either sue in the regular municipal or justice court or attempt to collect the debt in some other manner.

▌CLOSING COMMENTS

Billing and collecting are critical duties in the medical office, and a responsible medical assistant is a great asset in this important area.

Always maintain a positive attitude with patients and guarantors. Remember that those who are ill or facing challenges are not always at their best and may not respond in a positive way to calls about their accounts. Make every attempt to work with each patient to develop a workable plan to clear the account.

Patient Education

Most patients are unaware of the actual coverage they have through their insurance policies. The medical assistant should encourage patients to read the entire policy so that they become familiar with its limitations and exclusions. Tell patients that when calling the company with questions, they should always write down the date, time, and name of the person with whom they spoke. Using e-mail is helpful, because a record of the correspondence can easily be saved or printed. Making sure that patients have a general understanding of their health insurance coverage is well worth the effort.

Often patients do not dispute or question the company when a claim is rejected or not paid in the expected amount. Encourage them to call the company and question rejections if they do not understand why the claim was denied. Patients are paying for coverage, and they should receive all the benefits to which they are entitled.

Patients appreciate receiving an office policy brochure or booklet that informs them about payment and credit options. The patient can use the printed booklet as a reference whenever questions arise, and regular use of the booklet by most patients reduces the number of calls made to the office. Encourage patients to use the booklet. It should include helpful phone numbers or extensions and instructions on whom the patient should call at the medical facility for answers to questions.

Legal and Ethical Issues

A patient who has filed for bankruptcy cannot be contacted or billed further. A threat to take collection action must be fulfilled, or the creditor is in violation of the Fair Debt Collection Practices Act. Never say the physician intends to take action if he or she does not plan to follow through.

Because laws vary greatly from state to state, medical assistants should review the statutes pertaining to billing and collecting in the area where they live. Develop a good understanding of what is required of the small business, such as a physician's office, in collecting fees and billing for amounts due. Remember that laws change often, and constantly update policies to reflect current statutes.

SUMMARY OF SCENARIO

Jodie is a well-respected member of Dr. Crawford's office team. Her friendly attitude and flexibility attract patients, and she enjoys the interaction with them. She knows that there are only a few patients for whom she cannot work out some type of payment arrangement. She is professional in her dealings with those whom she contacts about outstanding accounts.

Dr. Crawford has noticed that more and more patients pay their accounts, and he attributes this to the care Jodie shows when working with them. She is never hesitant to ask for payment from patients, but at the same time, she is sensitive to their needs and struggles. She urges her patients to cooperate and to make a good attempt to pay their accounts; in return, Jodie arranges a payment schedule the patient can meet.

Although she initially was nervous about explaining fees to patients and asking for payment, Jodie has become more comfortable in doing this aspect of her job, since she understands the business aspect of the practice. The physician is operating the practice to make a profit and support his family, and the practice also is a source of support for the employees' families. Patients understand that physicians must charge for their services, and have become used to co-payments and co-insurance amounts. Many times, these fees are collected in advance, before the patient sees Dr. Crawford. This practice saves time on checkout, and most patients believe that the co-pay is a small cost compared to the entire fee that physicians charge to manage their care in one office visit.

Jodie has noticed that the usual, customary, and reasonable fees that Dr. Crawford charges his patients directly affect the reimbursements that are paid by various insurance and managed care companies. She has handled several claims in which the payer questioned the fee when it fell outside of the UCR ranges. Dr. Crawford commented that he uses professional courtesy much less frequently than in the past because of the many rules and regulations placed on providers by managed care companies. He still offers the occasional patient a professional discount when it does not violate the managed care contract that he holds with the insurer or managed care company.

Jodie's flexibility as an employee has paid off for Dr. Crawford several times. During a week-long period when the computer bookkeeping system was malfunctioning, Jodie was able to retrieve information from her backup disks and use a pegboard system until the system was repaired. Her preparation allowed the office to continue operations without skipping a beat. Most patients did not even notice that the computer was not in use for the week.

Many physicians still use the manual pegboard system out of habit and because it is a reliable method of keeping up with patient accounts. Some simply trust manual, written records more than computerized systems. This is a matter of personal choice; either system works in the physician's office.

Jodie has been able to fill in for other employees because of the versatility she gained from her medical assistant training. She has scheduled appointments and even assisted Dr. Crawford with minor office surgery. Jodie believes that performing other duties is a nice change periodically, and she keeps her skills sharp. She has proven herself to be a valuable and efficient employee.

SUMMARY OF LEARNING OBJECTIVES

1. **Define, spell, and pronounce the terms listed in the vocabulary.**
   Spelling and pronouncing medical terms correctly bolster the medical assistant's credibility. Knowing the definition of these terms promotes confidence in communication with patients and co-workers.

2. **List three values that are considered in determining professional fees.**
   Physicians offer the patient their time. They also make the most accurate judgments possible about the patient's medical condition. The services provided to the patient also figure into the fees set for various procedures.

3. **Differentiate the terms** *usual, customary,* **and** *reasonable.*
   Many third-party payers use the UCR method of determining fees for procedures. The *usual* fee is what the physician normally charges for a given service. The *customary* fee is the range of fees charged by physicians with similar experience in the same geographic area. Services or procedures that are exceptionally complicated and that require extra time deserve a *reasonable* fee that may be higher than the usual fee.

4. **Discuss the value of fee estimates for patient treatment.**
   Providing estimates for medical care helps patients plan their finances when an illness or injury occurs. Providing estimates prevents misquoting of the fee later. The office staff should keep a copy of the estimate in the patient's chart to help prevent misunderstanding and confusion over the charges.

5. **Explain basic bookkeeping computations.**
   Basic bookkeeping allows the physician to keep track of the amounts patients owe to the practice and the amounts the practice owes to others. Accounting is the four-stage process of recording, classifying, summarizing, and interpreting financial statements. By recording the day's charges and payments made on account, the physician can take a daily, monthly, and annual snapshot of the financial health of the practice. Adjustments are sometimes necessary on patients' accounts. Practice expenses are tracked and used to prove income tax deductions and equipment depreciation. Meticulous financial records must be kept so that the physician can keep the facility in operation and make a healthy business profit.

6. **Differentiate between bookkeeping and accounting.**
   Bookkeeping is the recording stage of accounting. The medical assistant performs bookkeeping functions when posting a payment to a patient's account. Accounting is a four-stage process of recording, classifying, summarizing, and interpreting financial statements. The physician may have an accountant who provides periodic summaries and handles tax planning and payment for the physician.

7. **Compare the manual and computerized bookkeeping systems used in ambulatory healthcare.**
   Most medical facilities now use a computerized bookkeeping system, which allows for regular backup so that vital information is not lost. Computerized systems allow fast record retrieval, and a patient's account can be found and adjusted quickly when posting charges and payments. Manual systems, although more time-consuming, can provide the same information and are valuable when the computer system is down or malfunctioning.

8. **Identify procedures for preparing patient accounts.**
   Computer medical accounting systems allow report-writing; this function can be used to create an accounts receivables list of all patients who owe money and to generate a bill. When using a manual system, the medical assistant must check each ledger to determine whether a billing statement should be sent. Use the office policy and procedures manual to determine billing parameters.

9. **Discuss the types of adjustments that may be made to a patient's account.**
   Adjustments are common on patient accounts and may be made to write off a disallowed balance, post a nonsufficient funds check, and correct errors, among other transactions.

10. **Explain both billing and payment options.**
    Physicians usually bill for payment in cycles, which allows a consistent flow of income to the office. A section of patient accounts is billed either weekly or biweekly, and patients send in their payments by mail, bring them in personally, or use an online payment system. Payment is usually requested at the time of service, especially if the patient uses a managed care system that requires a co-pay.

11. **Describe the impact of both the Fair Debt Collection Practices Act and the Truth in Lending Act as they apply to collections.**
    These laws provide the framework of rules that must be followed when collecting debts or extending credit. They affect office practices because they designate specific actions that are allowed when contacting patients about their bills. The office policy and procedures manual should provide guidelines for collecting patient accounts.

12. **Discuss procedures for collecting outstanding accounts.**
    Most of today's medical offices use computerized letters to prompt patients to pay overdue bills. Often, a message can be added to monthly statements that is increasingly more urgent, depending on the age of the account. Outstanding balances are also collected using telephone calls, e-mails, and personal discussions with the patient or guarantor.

CONNECTIONS

📖 **Study Guide Connection:** Go to the Chapter 22 Study Guide. Read and complete the activities.

🄴 **Evolve Connection:** Go to the Chapter 22 link at *evolve.elsevier.com/kinn* to complete the Chapter Review and Chapter Quiz. Check out the other resources listed for this chapter to make the most of what you have learned from Professional Fees, Billing, and Collecting.

BANKING SERVICES AND PROCEDURES

23

SCENARIO

Laura Anderson likes working with figures and has always been interested in bookkeeping. In high school she took all the bookkeeping and accounting courses offered, and during the summer months she helped out in the accounting department of the family business. She also worked part-time at City National Bank. Now, Laura wants to learn all she can about the financial transactions common to a medical practice. She is especially interested in electronic banking and all the possibilities it has to offer. Once her career in medical assisting is launched, Laura hopes to specialize in helping medical offices set up and run electronic medical record systems.

Although Laura has had considerable bookkeeping experience, she realizes that she still has a lot to learn about the daily financial duties in a medical office, including accounts payable, working with the business checkbook, making deposits, reconciling bank statements, and many other banking responsibilities.

Taking on the bookkeeping functions of a medical office involves not only responsibilities to the physician and employer, but also to patients and the vendors from whom the medical office purchases supplies. Laura realizes that to perform well in her upcoming career as a medical assistant, she must learn all she can about the topics pertinent to her special interest areas and stay current with the rapidly changing world of finance.

While studying this chapter, think about the following questions:

- How has banking changed over the years?
- How safe is Internet banking?
- How can an office manager know that an employee can be trusted with banking procedures?
- Why is making daily deposits a good idea?

LEARNING OBJECTIVES

1. Define, spell, and pronounce the terms listed in the vocabulary.
2. Describe banking procedures.
3. Explain how the Internet has changed traditional banking practices.
4. State the four requirements of a negotiable instrument.
5. Discuss the advantages of using debit cards.
6. Identify the three most common types of bank accounts.
7. Correctly write checks for bill payment.
8. Explain how to handle mistakes made in preparing a check.
9. Discuss precautions for accepting checks.
10. Discuss the actions necessary when a patient's check is returned.
11. Compare types of endorsements.
12. Prepare a bank deposit.
13. Accurately reconcile a bank statement for the office checking account.

VOCABULARY

disclaimer A denial of responsibility; a denial of a legal claim.

drawee A bank or facility on which a check is drawn or written.

drawer The person who writes a check.

e-banking Electronic banking via computer modem or over the Internet.

endorser The person who signs his or her name on the back of a check for the purpose of transferring title to another person.

holder The person who presents a check for payment.

maker Any individual, corporation, or legal party who signs a check or any type of negotiable instrument.

m-banking Banking through the use of mobile devices, such as cell phones and wireless Internet services.

negotiable Legally transferable to another party.

payee The person named on a draft or check as the recipient of the amount shown.

payer The person who writes a check in favor of the payee.

power of attorney A legal statement in which a person authorizes another person to act as his or her attorney or agent. The authority may be limited to the handling of specific procedures. The person authorized to act as the agent is known as the *attorney in fact.*

principal A capital sum of money due as a debt or used as a fund for which interest is either charged or paid.

reconciliation The process of proving that a bank statement and checkbook balance are in agreement.

Uniform Commercial Code (UCC) A unified set of rules covering many business transactions; it has been adopted in all 50 states, the District of Columbia, and most U.S. territories. It regulates the fields of sales of goods; commercial paper, such as checks; secured transactions in personal property; and particular aspects of banking, letters of credit, warehouse receipts, bills of lading, and investment securities.

Financial transactions in the professional office nearly always involve banking services and the use of checks. A medical assistant, therefore, must understand the responsibilities involved in accepting payments, endorsing and depositing checks, writing checks, and regularly reconciling bank statements. Payments received in the medical office should be deposited as soon as possible; ideally, on the same day. The medical assistant may very well be in charge of these financial responsibilities; therefore he or she must understand each transaction and its function.

BANKING IN TODAY'S BUSINESS WORLD

With the advent of the Internet, banking as we once knew it has changed. People once had to fight traffic and wait in line at crowded banks; today, they can sit in the comfort of their own homes and do their banking on the computer at any time of day. Banking transactions such as buying supplies, paying bills, and transferring funds between accounts can be done online. In addition, staff members have access to supply companies online and can review costs easily from the office instead of driving to numerous companies to compare prices.

Some banks have traded bricks and mortar to conduct all of their business online. The customers open their account online and deposits are made by using an application ("app") on a cell phone, tablet, or other electronic device. This type of banking service best fits the person who needs a simple account that can be accessed anytime and needs little maintenance.

In fact, people do not even have to sit in front of a computer terminal to conduct banking transactions. A physician may be sitting on a bus or a train or waiting for a flight and can carry out bank transactions. All this is possible just by turning on a laptop computer or using a mobile phone.

Online Banking

Online banking is a means of performing banking services electronically via the Internet. It also is called *personal computer (PC) banking, home banking, electronic banking,* **e-banking**, or *Internet banking.*

Many facilities have this capability, and most of them offer both basic and advanced services. With basic services, a customer usually can do the following:

- Check account balances
- Transfer funds between accounts
- Pay bills electronically
- Determine whether a check has cleared the bank
- Download account information
- View images of transactions (checks and deposits)

Online banking has advantages and disadvantages. One of the most obvious advantages is the ability to bank at one's own convenience in one's own home or office at any time. This can save considerable time and expense, especially if banking must be done daily. Many people find online banking a convenient and comprehensive method of money management. Other advantages include ease of use, portability, and availability.

Disadvantages of e-banking include learning to navigate the software. Service options are often more limited. In addition, some experts believe that there may be a slight increase in risk compared with conventional banking, although this has been debated by e-banking proponents. Despite the disadvantages, forecasts show that banking via the Internet is becoming more popular. The cost of online banking varies from bank to bank. Some charge a flat rate ($5 to $10 per month) with varying fees for additional transactions.

Online Convenience

Convenience probably is the number one reason people and businesses use the Internet for financial services. There is no frenzied drive to the bank during rush hour, waiting in line, or working around the confines of banking hours. Online banking is available 24 hours a day, 7 days a week. In addition to Internet banking services, clinic bills can be paid online, without the delay of mailing. Balance inquiries and various other transactions can be monitored easily. Costly fees for financial transactions left until the last minute can be avoided, because online transactions can be accomplished in a matter of seconds. Some banks now offer online transfers between banks, because many people have accounts at different banks.

Customer-Oriented Banking

Americans are becoming more and more mobile. They want to conduct business and take care of personal concerns on laptops or cell phones on their way to and from work. In addition, the rapid pace of life requires rapid or "instant" solutions; convenience has become a basic expectation of consumers where the banking industry is concerned.

Banks no longer consider customers as merely account numbers; to stay competitive, banks must look at the total customer picture. Many banks offer a type of interactive voice response system that operates through speech recognition, allowing customers to conduct business through a combination of talking into the telephone and using the telephone keypad. The call centers of some banks employ customer service personnel to answer questions and fulfill requests for all types of bank transactions.

Mobile banking, or **m-banking,** is a customer-oriented innovation that is emerging through the wireless technology market. Through the use of wireless devices, such as cell phones and wireless Internet services, customers can conduct a variety of financial transactions, set up alerts and notifications when bills are due, and make electronic transfers to pay these bills. Many banks offer applications (apps) that can be downloaded for free on smart phones and computers that will even let the user deposit checks from any location. Consider the services available through local banks when choosing the best banking facility for the physician's office.

ELECTRONIC FUNDS TRANSFERS

Electronic funds transfers (EFTs) are electronic payments of payroll, money owed to vendors or business establishments, and payments from government agencies. EFT payments are safe, secure, efficient, and less expensive than paper checks. The biggest advantage to using EFTs is the cost savings. The U.S. government pays $1.03 to issue each check payment, but only 10.5 ¢ to issue an EFT. Many EFTs are processed through an automated clearinghouse (ACH), which is an electronic network for financial transactions in the United States. An ACH processes large volumes of debit and credit transactions in batches. Rules and regulations that govern the ACH network have been established by the National Automated Clearing House Association (NACHA) and the Federal Reserve. The Federal Reserve banks, as a group, are the nation's largest clearinghouse operator. The Electronic Payments Network (EPN) is the only private-sector ACH in the country. Electronic processing becomes more prevalent each day, and business transactions are processed faster and more efficiently through electronic means. More information about clearinghouses can be found later in this chapter.

CRITICAL THINKING APPLICATION   23-1
Laura is excited about all the possibilities available with e-banking and m-banking. Where can Laura learn more about electronic banking and its advantages and disadvantages compared with conventional banking?

CHECKS

A check is a bank draft or order to pay a certain sum of money, payable on demand, to a specified person or entity. The concept of writing and depositing checks as a method of conducting financial transactions dates back as far as the Roman Empire. The word "check" was coined in England, where serial numbers were marked on these written orders of payment as a way to "check" on them. About 90% of all financial transactions in the United States are said to be accomplished by check.

A check is considered a **negotiable** instrument. For a check to be negotiable, it must:

- Be written and signed by a **maker**
- Contain a promise or order to pay a sum of money
- Be payable on demand or at a fixed future date
- Be payable to order or bearer

Debit Cards

The use of debit cards has vastly increased in the United States. Most debit cards are connected to a checking account. When the debit card is used, the amount of the transaction is immediately withdrawn from the available balance in the account. A pin number is assigned to the card for cash withdrawal and point of sale (POS) purchases. The cards usually have a MasterCard or Visa designation and can be used wherever those credit cards are accepted. The account can still be overdrawn, and in most situations, when there are not enough funds in the account to make a purchase, the card will be denied unless there is some type of overdraft protection on the account. Substantial fees may be charged if the bank elects to pay the debit when there are not enough available funds. Some banks now decline debit card charges at the point of sale when there are not sufficient funds in the account to pay the charge and do not charge any insufficient funds fees toward the attempted purchase. Stay abreast of recent banking legislation and always follow office policy when accepting debit cards as payment for medical services. The medical assistant may see various types of debit cards in the physician's office. Many states issue a debit card to individuals receiving child support payments or some types of state financial assistance.

ADVANTAGES OF USING DEBIT CARDS

Using debit cards to transfer funds has many advantages:
1. Debit cards are both safe and convenient, particularly for making payments online.
2. Transactions are completed quickly.
3. Expenditures are quickly calculated.
4. The cards can be used either as debit or credit cards. For debits, the user needs a personal identification number (PIN). For use as a credit card, the user often must provide identification.
5. Specific payments can be easily located online.
6. If stolen or lost, the debit card can be voided quickly with a minimum liability.
7. Receipts and statements provide a permanent, reliable record of disbursements for tax purposes.
8. The debit card statement provides a summary of receipts.
9. The cards usually can be used anywhere that accepts MasterCard or Visa.

Types of Checks

Medical assistants probably are familiar with the standard personal check, but many other types of checks also are used in business transactions.

Bank Draft

A bank draft is a check drawn by a bank against funds deposited to its account in another bank.

Cashier's Check

A cashier's check is a bank's own check drawn on itself and signed by the bank cashier or other authorized official. It is also known as an officer's or treasurer's check. A cashier's check is obtained by paying the bank cashier the amount of the check, in cash or by personal check. Many banks charge a fee for this service. Cashier's checks often are issued to accommodate a savings account customer who does not keep a checking account.

Limited Check

A check may be limited in the amount written on it and the time during which it may be presented for payment (e.g., 30, 60, or 90 days). A limited check often is used for payroll or insurance checks.

Money Order

Domestic money orders are sold by banks, some stores, and the U.S. Postal Service. Money orders often are used to pay bills by mail when a person does not have a checking account. The maximum face value varies, depending on the source. International money orders may be purchased for limited amounts, indicated in U.S. dollars, to send money abroad.

Traveler's Check

Traveler's checks, available at most banks, are designed for people who are traveling, because personal checks may not be accepted or carrying a large amount of cash might be inadvisable. Traveler's checks usually are printed in denominations of $10, $20, $50, and $100 and sometimes $500 and $1,000. They require two signatures from the purchaser, one at the time of purchase and the other at the time of use. The use of traveler's checks is becoming less common, because debit and credit cards are widely accepted throughout the world. However, the medical assistant may be presented with a traveler's check if a patient is on vacation or out of town and has a medical emergency. Follow office policy when determining whether this form of payment is acceptable.

Voucher Check

A voucher check has a detachable voucher form. The voucher portion is used to itemize or specify the purpose for which the check is drawn. It is used for the convenience of the **payer** and shows discounts and various other itemizations. This portion of the check, which is removed before the check is presented for payment, provides a record for the **payee** (Figure 23-1). Some government agencies use voucher checks to make various types of payments.

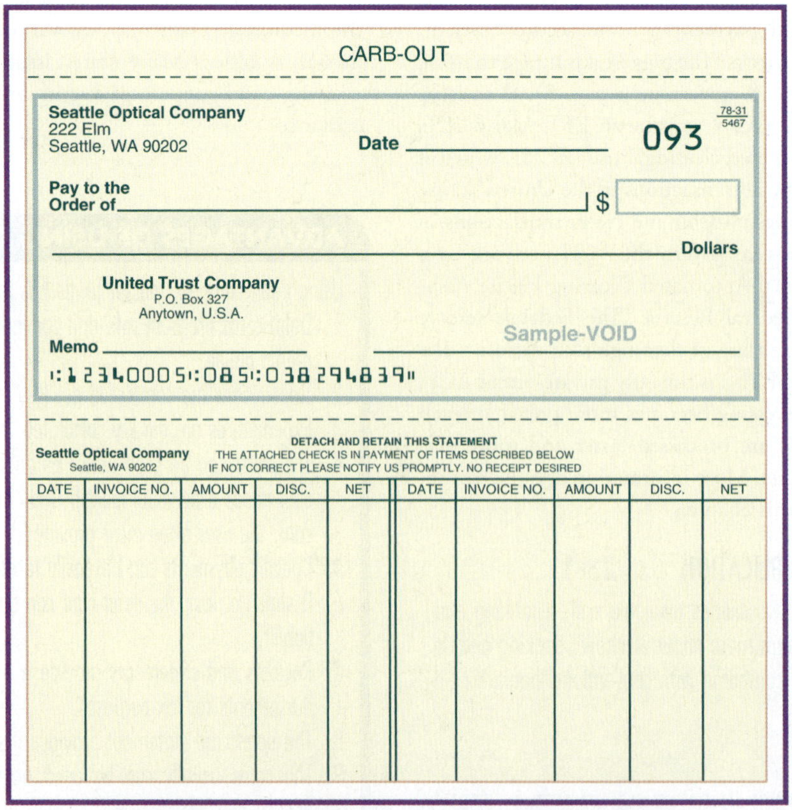

FIGURE 23-1 Page from a bank order book showing a sample voucher check.

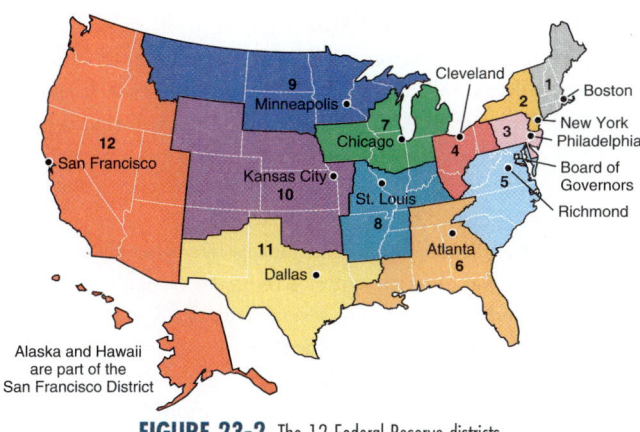

FIGURE 23-2 The 12 Federal Reserve districts.

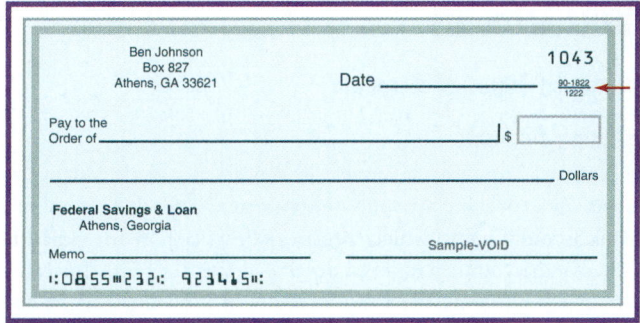

FIGURE 23-3 Sample check. The arrow indicates the American Bankers Association number. The numbers on the bottom left represent the bank's nine-digit routing number and the user's checking account number.

THE BANKING SYSTEM

The Federal Reserve

Wanting to provide the nation with a safer, more flexible, and stable monetary and financial system, Congress created the Federal Reserve in 1913 as the central bank of the United States. It consists of a seven-member Board of Governors with headquarters in Washington, D.C., and 12 Federal Reserve banks in major cities throughout the country (Figure 23-2). For additional information on the Federal Reserve System and its regional banks, visit its Web site at *www.federalreserve.gov.*

Routing and Account Numbers

A routing transit number (RTN) is a nine-digit code printed on the bottom left side of checks or other negotiable instruments. It identifies the bank upon which the check was drawn. Routing numbers also are used for direct deposits and bank wiring. The first two digits indicate the Federal Reserve district where the bank is located. The third digit indicates the particular district office, and the rest of the digits represent the individual bank identification number. Electronic payments can be made using the routing and account numbers and are processed at banks like regular checks.

American Bankers Association Number

The American Bankers Association (ABA) number appears in the upper right area of a printed check. The number is used as a simple means of identifying the area location of the bank on which the check is written and the particular bank in that area. The code number is expressed as a fraction (Figure 23-3):

$$\frac{90\text{-}1822}{1222}$$

In the top part of the fraction, before the hyphen, the numbers 1 to 49 designate cities in which Federal Reserve banks are located or other key cities; the numbers 50 to 99 refer to states or territories. The part of the number following the hyphen is a number issued to each bank for its own identification purposes. The bottom part of the fraction includes the number of the Federal Reserve district where the bank is located and other identifying information. The

ABA number is used to prepare deposit slips and to identify each check.

How Checks Are Processed

When a check is presented for payment, the **drawee** (the bank or facility on which the check is drawn or written) pays the specified sum of money written on the face of the check to the **holder** (the person presenting the check for payment). Checks received by the bank are turned over daily to a regional clearinghouse, which cancels each one by stamping, mechanically punching, or embossing them. The identifying code numbers, printed on the face of the check with magnetic ink, enable this "clearing" process to be accomplished quickly and efficiently. Checks due from and to all banks outside a specific region are settled by means of computerized entries. The cancelled check is either kept by the financial institution or returned to the **drawer** (the person who wrote the check). Many banks no longer provide cancelled checks on a regular basis. If the drawer needs proof of payment, a copy of the check can be requested from the bank if the checks are not returned in the monthly bank statement.

Clearinghouses

As the use of checks increased, the system became confusing, because so many different banks were involved. At first, messengers were used for collection; however, this involved a lot of traveling and carrying a lot of cash. Then, in a London coffee shop, a solution came about when two bank messengers who were discussing the shortcomings of the system realized they had checks for each other. They decided to exchange them and save some time and effort. This practice evolved into a system of check clearinghouses, or networks of banks that exchange checks, which is still in use. Banks in the United States can present checks to the Federal Reserve System or private clearinghouses for regional and national check collection.

Magnetic Ink Character Recognition

As mentioned, characters and numbers printed in magnetic ink are found at the bottom of checks. They represent a common machine language, readable both by machines and humans. When a check is deposited, the amount of the check also can be printed in magnetic ink below the signature. Magnetic ink character recognition (MICR) identification facilitates processing through a high-speed machine that reads the characters, sorts the checks, and does the bookkeeping.

BANK ACCOUNTS

Common Types of Accounts

Checking Accounts

By placing an amount of money on deposit in a bank, a depositor can set up a checking account. Simply stated, a checking account is a bank account against which checks can be written. Many variations in checking accounts have been developed over the years. Instead of a straight, non-interest-bearing account, an individual might have an insured money market checking account, which bears interest at the daily money market rate if a certain minimum balance is maintained. However, most banks do not offer interest-bearing checking accounts for businesses.

A physician often requires three different checking accounts:

- An account for personal and family expenses
- A separate checking account for office expenses
- A high-yield, interest-bearing account for funds reserved for paying insurance premiums, property taxes, and other seasonal expenses

The medical assistant most likely will deal only with the office checking account.

Savings Accounts

Money that is not needed for current expenses can be deposited in a savings account. In most cases, savings accounts earn interest on the amounts deposited; that is, the bank pays the depositor a certain percentage monthly or quarterly to use the money in the savings account. An ordinary savings account draws interest at the lowest prevailing rate and has no minimum balance requirement and no check-writing privileges. A physician may deposit a certain percentage of income into a savings account each month.

Interest-Bearing Accounts

Interest is a charge (or payment) in exchange for the use of money. It usually is figured as a percentage of the **principal**. Simple interest is computed annually; compound interest is figured on the principal and on any previous interest that has been added to the original sum of money and can be computed using a variety of time increments (e.g., daily, monthly, quarterly, and so on). Interest-bearing checking accounts draw a small amount of interest, usually 1% or 2%, on the average daily balance. Savings accounts normally pay a higher rate of interest than checking accounts (e.g., 2% to 3%). However, these rates fluctuate with the financial market.

Money Market Savings Account

An insured money market savings account requires a minimum balance, anywhere from $500 to $5,000; it draws interest at money market rates (usually a higher percentage rate than for a regular savings account); and it allows a specified number of checks (frequently three) to be written per month. A minimum fee may be charged for each transaction. Such checks usually are written to transfer funds to a checking account. Some businesses transfer excess funds from the business checking account to a money market account over the weekend or over an extended holiday period to draw interest on the funds (Figure 23-4).

Individual Retirement Accounts

Individual retirement accounts (IRAs) are a type of individual savings plan that are allowed special tax treatment at the federal and sometimes the state level. This tax-favored status distinguishes an IRA from an ordinary savings account; specific rules must be followed to qualify for the tax savings. IRA rules are stricter than those for ordinary savings accounts.

Physicians and healthcare organizations may offer their employees an IRA. Several different types of IRAs are available (e.g., traditional, Roth, and education). For several reasons, IRAs often are used as a means of preparing for retirement:

- Savings grows tax-deferred.
- Tax deductions are realized for contributions (with traditional IRAs).
- Interest earned may not be taxed at withdrawal (with Roth IRAs).

IRAs come in all shapes and sizes. Individuals considering an IRA must make sure to study the rules of each one before deciding which is best for their needs.

> ### CRITICAL THINKING APPLICATION 23-2
> The physician knows that Laura worked part-time in a local bank before coming to the clinic. He tells her that he is considering changing banks and asks Laura to research the interest rates on money market accounts at local banks. How does Laura accomplish this task?

The Business Account

A business bank account is used for business or company operations and managing cash related to day-to-day business functions. Many different types of accounts are available for businesses today, including checking, savings, and money market accounts, in addition to other types of financial elements. Before a business account is set up, careful consideration should be given to each of these elements to determine which best meets the particular needs of the business.

What to Look for in a Business Account

Most businesses want "the most bang for their buck." They want the most services possible for the least amount of money, just as individuals do with personal accounts. Some of the services available for business accounts are:

- Business checking with interest, accruing interest with either checking or savings accounts
- Free checks and deposits with a maintained minimum balance (which varies from bank to bank)
- Overdraft protection by linking the account to a savings account or to a bank-issued credit or debit card
- Online banking

Perks for Businesses

Many financial institutions offer perquisites ("perks") for businesses that open accounts. These may include:

- Business Express: A computerized cash management system that allows access to account information by telephone.
- "Sweep" account: An account in which excess funds over a minimum balance are "swept" into a higher yielding

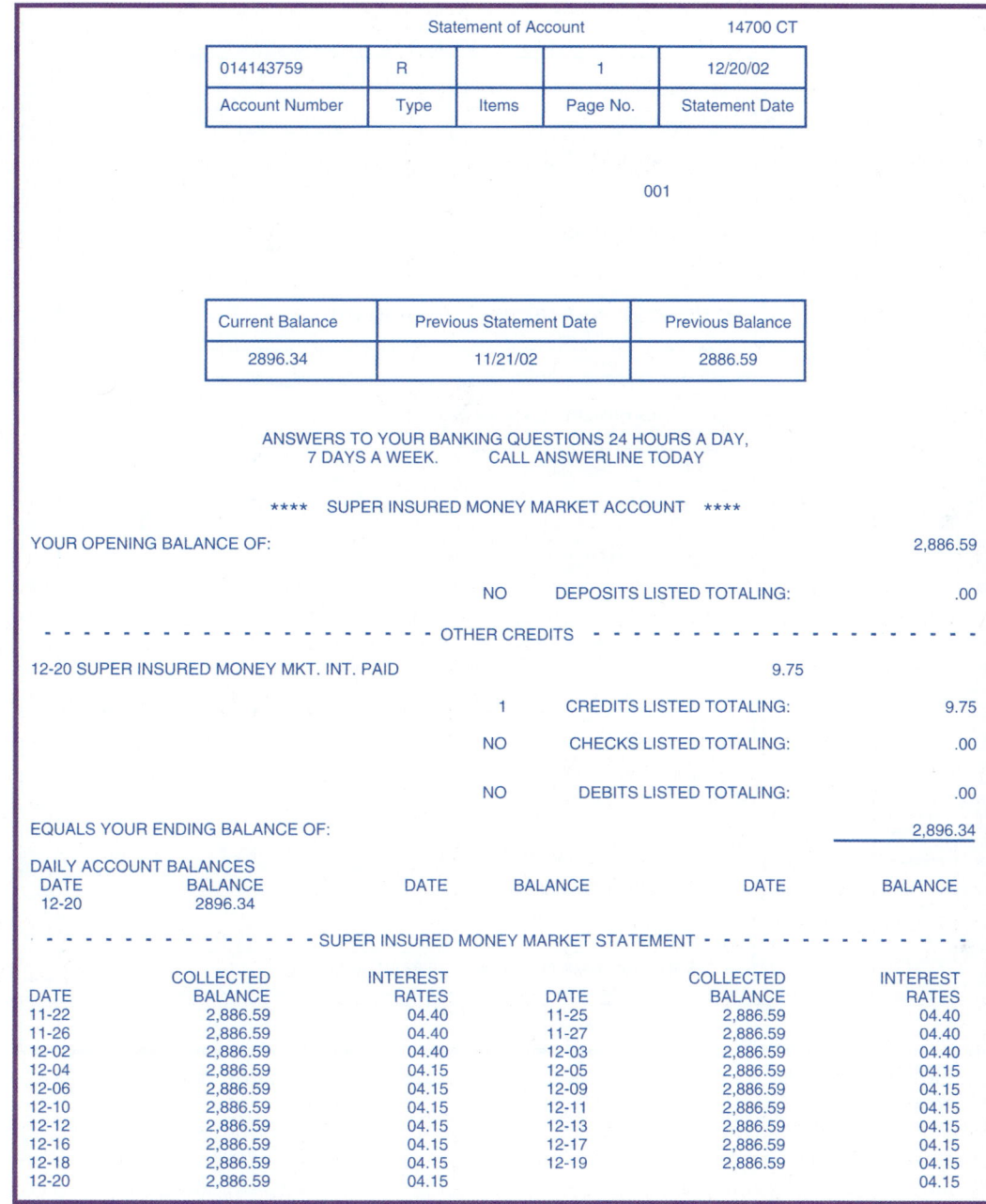

FIGURE 23-4 Example of a money market account statement. This type of check writing has limited privileges.

interest-bearing investment account. When the balance in the account drops below the minimum, funds are "swept" back into it automatically.

- Business checking with special features: A customized bank account designed for businesses with low to moderate transaction volumes and limited cash balances. This service helps business owners manage their day-to-day business and/or personal finances.
- Cash management account: Combines a checking account with a money market fund and a brokerage account. All cash activities are summarized on one monthly statement. This is ideal for business owners who do not have time to manage their money and/or investments.

- Other special features: Automatic bill paying, payroll preparation, smart phone applications, and timed business deposits.

Business Checks

The checkbook most widely used in the professional office is a ledger-type book with three checks per page and a perforated stub at the left side of the check (Figure 23-5). Checks may be bound in a soft cover or punched for a ring binder. The checks and matching stubs are numbered in sequence and preprinted with the depositor's name and account number, along with any additional information, such as address and telephone number. Numbered deposit slips in separately bound books are also supplied to the depositor.

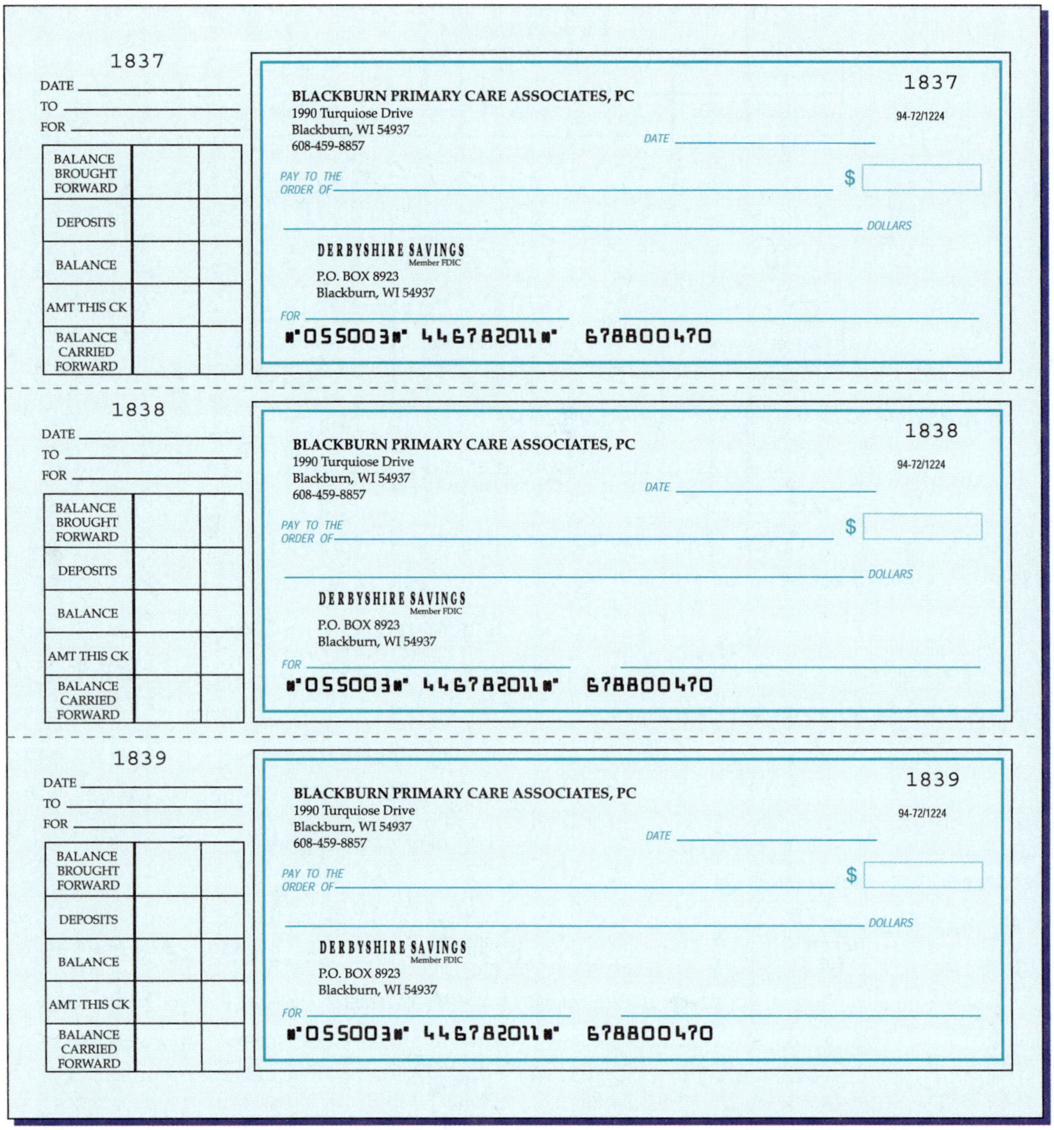
1837
DATE
TO
FOR
BALANCE BROUGHT FORWARD
DEPOSITS
BALANCE
AMT THIS CK
BALANCE CARRIED FORWARD

BLACKBURN PRIMARY CARE ASSOCIATES, PC
1990 Turquiose Drive
Blackburn, WI 54937
608-459-8857
1837
94-72/1224
DATE
PAY TO THE ORDER OF
$
DOLLARS
DERBYSHIRE SAVINGS
Member FDIC
P.O. BOX 8923
Blackburn, WI 54937
FOR
⑈055003⑈ 446782011⑈ 678800470

1838
DATE
TO
FOR
BALANCE BROUGHT FORWARD
DEPOSITS
BALANCE
AMT THIS CK
BALANCE CARRIED FORWARD

BLACKBURN PRIMARY CARE ASSOCIATES, PC
1990 Turquiose Drive
Blackburn, WI 54937
608-459-8857
1838
94-72/1224
DATE
PAY TO THE ORDER OF
$
DOLLARS
DERBYSHIRE SAVINGS
Member FDIC
P.O. BOX 8923
Blackburn, WI 54937
FOR
⑈055003⑈ 446782011⑈ 678800470

1839
DATE
TO
FOR
BALANCE BROUGHT FORWARD
DEPOSITS
BALANCE
AMT THIS CK
BALANCE CARRIED FORWARD

BLACKBURN PRIMARY CARE ASSOCIATES, PC
1990 Turquiose Drive
Blackburn, WI 54937
608-459-8857
1839
94-72/1224
DATE
PAY TO THE ORDER OF
$
DOLLARS
DERBYSHIRE SAVINGS
Member FDIC
P.O. BOX 8923
Blackburn, WI 54937
FOR
⑈055003⑈ 446782011⑈ 678800470

FIGURE 23-5 Example of business checks with stubs. (From Hunt SA: *Fundamentals of medical assisting,* Philadelphia, 2002, WB Saunders.)

Computer-Generated Checks. Instead of ordering checks printed by the bank, the physician may use personalized checks that can be ordered from printing houses to fit the office computer's financial software program (e.g., Quicken). The checks may have one or more copies that serve as the record of checks written.

One-Write Check Writing. A one-write system of writing checks can save time and minimize errors in medical office disbursements. An office with a pegboard bookkeeping system may want to include one-write check writing. By using a combination check writing system, one check and one record of checks drawn handle both bill paying and payroll check writing.

When the check is written, a permanent record is created through the carbonized line of the check onto the record of checks drawn and the employee's payroll record, including a record of all deductions. Space is provided for the payee's address so that the check can be mailed in a window envelope. This not only saves time but also ensures that the check goes to the correct address. Suppliers of basic pegboard systems also can provide a check writing system such as the one described.

BILL PAYING AND CHECK WRITING

Establishing a Bill-Paying System

Establish a systematic plan for writing checks and paying bills. Some offices have incorporated an online bill paying system and pay bills as soon as they are received. For those using manual systems, check writing usually is done on a specific day or days of each month. An exception sometimes arises when a good discount can be had if a bill is paid within a specified time, such as 10 days. Such discounts usually are indicated at the bottom of invoices or billing statements.

Before writing a check, fill in the information on the check stub. Make this a habit so that no check is missing without the notation as to its payee and amount. When writing a check in payment of a

PROCEDURE 23-1

Write Checks in Payment of Bills

GOAL: *To correctly write checks for payment of bills.*

EQUIPMENT and SUPPLIES

- Checkbook
- Bills to be paid

PROCEDURAL STEPS

1. Locate the first bill to be paid. Before writing the check, fill out the stub or the place designated for recording expenditures. Include the date, name of payee, amount of the check, the new balance to be carried forward, and usually the purpose of the check.
   <u>PURPOSE:</u> To prevent the possibility of delivering or mailing a check without entering the information in the checkbook.
2. Complete both the check and the stub with pen, computer, or typewriter.
   <u>PURPOSE:</u> To eliminate the danger of alteration for any reason.
3. Date the check the day it is written (do not postdate).
4. Write the name of the payee after the printed words, "Pay to the Order of" with the necessary information following. Do not use abbreviations unless so instructed.

5. Leave no space before the name, and follow it with three dashes if space remains.
6. Omit personal titles from the names of payees.
7. If a payee is receiving a check as an officer of an organization, the name of the office should follow the name (e.g., John F. Jones, Treasurer).
8. Start writing at the extreme left of each space. Leave no blank spaces. Keep the cents notation close to the dollars figure to prevent alteration.
9. Verify that the amount of the check has been recorded correctly on the stub, in the box for the dollar ($) amount, and on the line where the amount is written in words.
10. If a check is written for an amount less than 1 dollar, the figures by the $ sign may be circled or enclosed in parentheses ($0.65) to emphasize the amount.
11. Obtain signatures on the checks from the physician or other authorized person.

---

statement or invoice, it is a good practice to write on the invoice the number of the check, the amount that was paid, and the date it was paid. If any question arises about whether or when the bill was paid, the check stub can be easily referenced. Handling and writing checks must be done with extreme care (Procedure 23-1). Extra checks and deposit slips should be kept in a safe place so that the routing and account numbers cannot be used by unauthorized individuals.

Designated Times

Rather than haphazardly paying bills as they are received in the office, the medical assistant should establish a routine for paying bills at designated times, such as on the fifteenth and thirtieth days of each month. Most vendors allow a 30-day cycle to elapse before adding interest or late fees.

One method of handling accounts payable is to create a chronologic tickler file with dividers for each pay cycle (e.g., the tenth of the month, the twentieth, and the thirtieth). Behind each of the dividers, the invoices can be arranged alphabetically if desired. When the date arrives, the medical assistant can pull all the bills from that section and prepare the checks.

Paying Bills to Maximize Money

In establishing the procedure for accounts payable, a medical assistant should keep in mind that most vendors allow 30 days to pay. When each invoice is received, check the "terms," which usually are located at the top of the document. A few vendors offer a discount (normally 1% to 2%) if bills are paid within a shorter time. If the terms say "Net 30," this means the total amount of the bill is due within 30 days. Remember to allow a certain number of days for

mailing (2 to 5, depending on where payment is sent). If the business checking account is an interest-bearing one, do not pay bills before their due date. In this way, the funds in the account continue to draw interest until it is time to write the check. Also, if the practice has a weekly service (e.g., a laundry or cleaning service) that bills several times a month, accumulate the invoices and issue only one check per month. Checks are costly, and some banks charge businesses a fee for each transaction.

Automatic Withdrawals and Deductions

Some routine bills that are due monthly or on a regular billing cycle, such as insurance premiums, rent payments, and utility bills, can be set up to be paid automatically through prior arrangements with the bank.

Online Bill Paying

An online bill paying account can be established with a bank or other business entity. The bank pays bills by automatically debiting the customer's account and crediting the merchant's account. More banks are offering this service; however, not all vendors accept electronic transfers in payment of bills. If a business decides to take advantage of online bill paying, the options should be researched carefully for their advantages and disadvantages.

Writing Checks

Instructions

Writing checks is a routine and basically simple function; however, certain guidelines should be followed to prevent potential problems.

Figure 23-6 shows the correct method for writing a check for an amount less than a dollar (top). The check on the bottom shows an incorrect method of check writing. Note the incomplete name and the space available for altering the check (e.g., $ 6.00 could easily be changed to $26.00 or more, and 00 could be made into 88). When writing in the numeric amount of a check, begin as far to the left in the block as possible. When inserting the written amount of the check, again start as far to the left as possible, allowing no space for added or altered words. Writing checks for less than a dollar is not recommended.

Checkbook Stubs

The check stub (the part that remains in the book after the check has been written and removed) is the depositor's own record of checks written: the date, amount, payee, and purpose (Figure 23-7). It is important to complete the stub before writing the check. This prevents the possibility of a check being written without the stub being filled out. If the stub is not completed and the check is sent out, no record exists of the payee and the amount taken from the account until the cancelled check is returned at a later date. Consequently, the account cannot balance, nor can the amount on hand be determined until the cleared check shows up online or on the monthly bank statement.

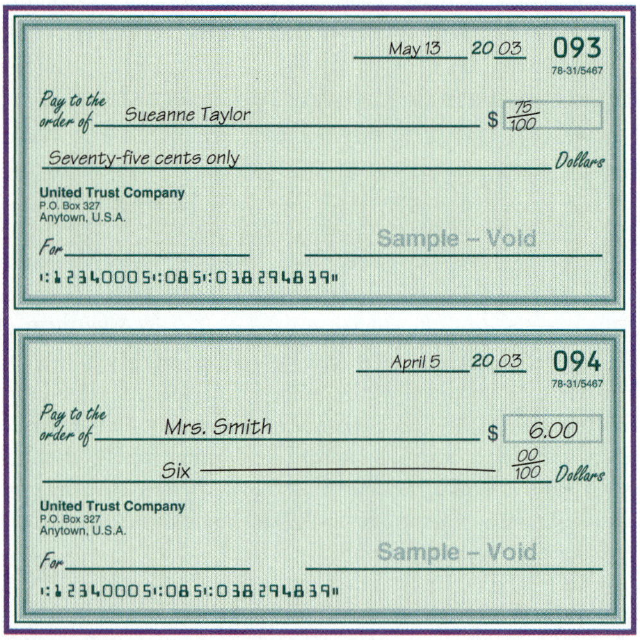

Signing Checks

After all checks have been written, place them on the physician's desk for signature, along with the invoices or other verifying information. In some practices the medical assistant in charge of financial matters is also allowed to sign the checks. To allow this, a **power of attorney** must be filed at the depositor's bank. The power of attorney may limit the check signing authorization to a certain amount or to a limited period. The medical assistant also is required to sign a signature card at the bank before writing any checks on the business account.

Handling Corrections

Do not cross out, erase, or change any part of a check. Checks are printed on sensitized paper so that erasures are easily noticeable, and the bank has the right to refuse to pay on any check that has been altered. (See Figures 23-6 and 23-7 for examples of correct and incorrect check writing.) If a mistake is made, write "VOID" on the stub and the check but do not throw out or destroy the check. It should be filed with the canceled checks so that it is available for auditing purposes.

Writing Cash Checks

A cash check is made payable to Cash or Bearer. Such checks are completely negotiable. Because these checks are easily cashed, it is poor policy to write cash checks until physically at the bank. These checks most often are used to replenish petty cash funds. Some bank personnel may require that the person receiving the cash endorse the check. Many experts in the banking business advise their customers not to endorse a check written for cash or petty cash; often, if a problem arises, the person who endorses the check is liable. A medical assistant should never endorse a check written for cash or petty cash, because he or she is not a party in the transaction.

FIGURE 23-6 *Top,* Correct method of writing a check. *Bottom,* Incorrect method of writing a check, with incomplete name and space for altering (e.g., 6.00 could be made into 26.00 or more, and 00 could be made into 88).

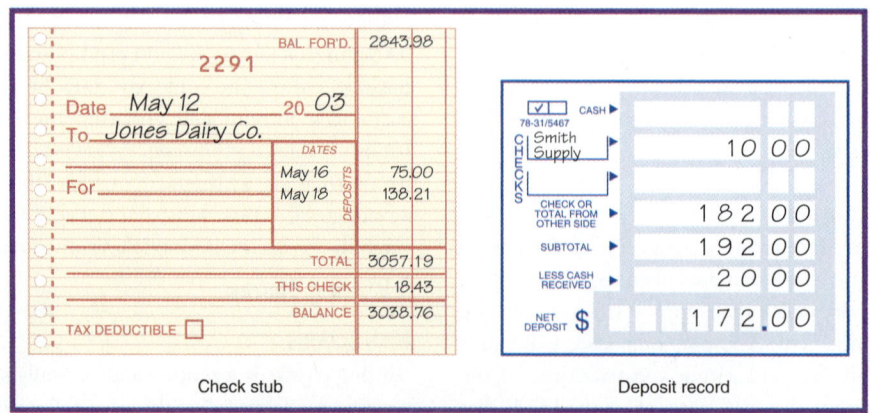

FIGURE 23-7 Methods of filling out a check stub.

Mailing Checks

When checks are sent through the mail, the check should not be visible through the envelope. Either place the check within a letter or fold it into a plain sheet of paper. Checks may be folded at the right end to conceal the amount of money written. Make sure the envelope is sealed before mailing. The medical assistant should personally mail all checks as soon as possible.

Special Problems with Checks

Special problems may arise when a check is written on nonexistent funds or when a payer, for a legitimate reason, wants to prevent the payee from cashing a check.

Overdraws or Overdrafts

When a depositor draws a check for more than the amount on deposit in the account, the account becomes overdrawn. In most states, issuing a check for more than the amount on deposit in the bank is illegal. Should this happen through error or oversight, the bank may refuse to honor the check and will return it to the bank that presented it for payment. Such a check is said to "bounce."

If a check is written by an established depositor, the bank may honor the check and notify the depositor that the account is overdrawn. If the bank thus pays or covers the check, it issues an overdraft on the depositor's account. Considerable fees ($10 to $35) normally are charged for an overdraft. The medical assistant should follow office policy regarding the charges for a returned check; some physicians may not charge the patient at all or will only charge the fee that the physician's bank charged to handle the patient's nonsufficient funds (NSF) check. Other physicians charge the highest fee allowed by law. States determine the maximum fee that can be charged for a returned check. Some accounts allow automatic withdrawals from savings accounts to cover overdrafts without additional charges.

If the check is returned to the physician's office unpaid, call the maker of the check immediately and ask him or her to forward the funds needed to cover the check and the fee. Most offices require that such payment be made in cash or through a money order. Legal remedies are available for the physician if the check remains unpaid.

Stop-Payments

A depositor or check writer who wants to rescind the check has the right to request that the bank stop payment on it. Stop-payment orders should be used only when absolutely necessary; as with overdrafts, most banks charge a fee for them. Reasons for stop-payment requests include:

- Loss of a check
- Disagreement about a purchase
- Disagreement about a payment

CRITICAL THINKING APPLICATION 23-3

When Laura arrives at the office on Monday morning, she discovers that a check is missing from the business checkbook and the stub is blank. What actions should Laura take to solve the problem?

PRECAUTIONS FOR ACCEPTING CHECKS

A medical assistant is presented with checks to pay for the physician's services every day. In most cases these are personal checks. Check fraud affects every financial institution and business throughout the United States. The best defense against check fraud is to train employees to detect some of the signs of a fraudulent check. The medical assistant can detect several signs of a phony check. If a check is not perforated on at least one side, it might be fraudulent. Also, the routing number and ABA number will be consistent with the physician's checking account numbers if the check is drawn on a local bank. Never accept a third-party check. For example, Mrs. Richards, a patient, receives a check written to her from her neighbor for $25. Mrs. Richards brings the check to her visit with the physician and presents it to the clinic to pay her co-pay. If the check is accepted and subsequently returned by the bank, obtaining reimbursement from the patient or the neighbor will be difficult.

Most patients who write checks to pay bills have no intention of committing fraud. However, checks should be examined while the patient is still in the office. Follow the guidelines in the office policy manual for accepting checks. The National Check Fraud Center suggests the following to minimize the chance of check fraud:

- Ask the bank to advise the office when new books of checks are ready, then either pick them up or use a parcel delivery service to have them delivered.
- Make sure cancelled checks and bank statements are in a secured area, such as a locking file cabinet. Do not throw them in the trash.
- Check bank statements immediately after receiving them. If check fraud is not reported within 30 days of receipt of a monthly statement, the bank does not have to reimburse the loss (**Uniform Commercial Code [UCC]** Code 4-406).
- Print a return address on an envelope or use printed stationery or return address stickers. If the return address is written in the maker's usual signature, it can be traced, duplicated, or forged.
- Do not discard credit card records or bills with trash. Instead, shred them.

For more information on how to prevent check fraud or what to do if fraud occurs, consult the National Check Fraud Center's Web site (*ckfraud.org*).

Acknowledging Payment in Full

If a patient presents a check to the office and the notation of "payment in full" appears on any part of the check, front or back, it may be best to refuse to accept the check unless insurance has paid its portion and the patient owes no more on the bill. This notation is a type of restrictive endorsement, and it can prevent the physician from ever collecting any balance due. If the check is taken, however, the following **disclaimer** should be written on the back of the check above the normal endorsement: "This check is deposited under protest, without prejudice, and with preservation of all rights of the payee against the drawer of this check, according to UCC §1-207."

Research state law to determine whether any further regulations apply to acceptance of a check with a payment in full endorsement. A check is considered to have been accepted if it is deposited and cashed. The office may have little recourse against a patient who still owes money unless the previously mentioned disclaimer is used.

PRECAUTIONS FOR ACCEPTING CREDIT AND DEBIT CARDS

Just as the medical assistant must take precautions when accepting checks, care must also be taken when accepting a credit or debit card as payment for medical services. The first precaution should be to make certain that the person presenting the card is the person to whom it was issued. Always ask for a driver's license and compare the name on the card to the name on the driver's license. Follow office policy when those names do not match. Sometimes, a married couple may use each other's cards, but if the office is strict about the card acceptance policy, then the spouse may need to be present in the office for the medical assistant to accept the card. Some patients may also use blank cards that are purchased with cash to pay on their accounts. If allowed by office policy, these cards are acceptable and will pay just like a normal credit card. If a patient becomes belligerent about card denial, refer him or her to the office manager.

CRITICAL THINKING APPLICATION   23-4

A new patient wants to pay for his services at the end of the office visit. The charge is $75. The patient writes the check for $100 and asks Laura for $25 in currency in return. How should Laura handle the situation?

GUIDELINES FOR ACCEPTING CHECKS

- Scan the check carefully for the correct date, amount, and signature.
- Do not accept a check with corrections on it.
- If you do not know the person presenting a personal check, ask for identification and compare the signatures.
- Accept an out-of-town check, government check, or payroll check only if you are well acquainted with the person presenting it and it does not exceed the amount of the payment.
- Acceptance of a third-party check generally is unwise. A third-party check is one made out to your patient by a party unknown to you. A check from the patient's health insurance carrier is an exception.
- When accepting a postal money order for payment, make sure it has only one endorsement. Postal money orders with more than two endorsements will not be honored.
- Do not accept a check marked "Payment in Full" unless it does pay the account in full up to and including the date on which it is received. If a check so marked is less than the amount due, you will be unable to collect the balance on the account once you have accepted and deposited such a check. It is illegal for you to scratch out the words "Payment in Full."
- Accepting checks written for more than the amount due and returning cash for the difference between the amount of the check and the amount owed is poor policy. If the check is not honored by the bank, your office suffers the loss not only of the amount of the check but also of the amount returned in cash.

Returned Checks

Occasionally the bank may return a deposited check because of some irregularity, such as a missing signature or missing endorsement. More often, it is returned because the payer has insufficient funds on deposit to cover the check. If a check is stamped "NSF," contact the maker immediately. If the person cannot be reached, waste no time in tracking down all leads, such as referrals, numbers obtained from credit cards, driver's license, and so forth. Add the amount of the check plus the NSF fee back to the patient's account balance.

Charging Fees

To cover their overhead costs, most banks currently charge both the payer and payee a fee of $10 to $35 for a check that has been returned because of insufficient funds. The medical assistant customarily notifies the person who wrote the check that it has been returned. Often the individual has a plausible excuse and simply requests that the check be "run through again." If this is the case, it is a wise practice first to call the bank and ask whether sufficient funds are available; this prevents additional delays and fees. Some offices add these charges to the patient's account in an attempt to recoup the expense.

Legal Options

Many NSF problems can be cleared up quickly and easily with courtesy and tact, assuming the situation was simply a mistake or an oversight. Bad checks may be reported to several organizations, and once the writer is in their database, the person will have difficulty writing a check to any business. Credit associations often are a great help when such problems arise. Turn the account over to a qualified collection agency if unable to collect on the account within a short time.

Before taking legal action to collect a returned check, make sure documentation exists proving that attempts were made to collect the check. The best evidence of this is a certified letter sent to the patient with a return receipt requested. The office is notified when the maker of the check has signed for the documents. Keep all this information so that copies can be attached to the claim.

After all reasonable options for collecting NSF checks have been exhausted, a medical assistant may use a collection method that involves the court system. Bad checks also can be reported to the district attorney's office. As mentioned, writing a check without sufficient funds to cover it is illegal and can lead to charges of "theft by check."

The medical assistant also can file against the maker of the check in small claims court. This is a special court in which disputes are resolved inexpensively and quickly; it is a commonly used method that avoids costly attorney fees. Filing fees are about $20 to $35, and there usually is a charge for having the papers served. Some restrictions apply, however. The amount for which the plaintiff (individual or company initiating the suit) can sue in a small claims lawsuit varies from state to state. Contact the local Clerk of the District Court for the necessary forms and instructions for completing a small claims suit. For more information on filing small claims, refer to the government legal department's Web site.

CRITICAL THINKING APPLICATION   23-5

When opening the mail, Laura notices a form from the bank with a check attached. It is a check from Elliott Benson, a new patient seen in the office the previous week, which is being returned for insufficient funds. How should Laura handle this problem?

The medical assistant must be "proactive" rather than "reactive" when it comes to problem patients. He or she should discuss fees with the patient on the first visit and gather all the financial and insurance information necessary to make a judgment as to whether the patient is able and willing to pay. An experienced medical assistant can often sense a "red flag" during this initial information-gathering process. If this happens, requesting payment in advance might be wise. This practice should not be abused, however, and the medical assistant should follow the established office policy or discuss the matter with the office manager or physician when necessary.

ENDORSEMENTS

An endorsement is a signature plus any other writing on the back of a check by which the **endorser** transfers all rights in the check to another party. Endorsements are made in ink, with either pen or rubber stamp, on the back of the check across the left (or perforated) end.

Why an Endorsement Is Necessary

The Uniform Negotiable Instrument Act, which applies in all states, explains the need for an endorsement as follows:

"An instrument is negotiated when it is transferred from one person to another in such a manner as to pass title to another party. If payable to bearer, it is negotiated by delivery. If payable to order, it is negotiated by the endorsement of the holder completed by delivery."

The name of the last endorser of the check shows who last received the money. If a check is cashed for someone who did not endorse it and is returned for some reason, the bank charges the check to the last endorser, not to the last person receiving the money. For this reason, it is not wise to cash a check made payable to another party without having the endorsement of the person who delivered the check to you for cashing.

Types of Endorsements

Four principal kinds of endorsements can be used: blank, restrictive, special, and qualified. Blank and restrictive endorsements are most commonly used.

Blank Endorsement

In a blank endorsement, the payee signs only his or her name. This makes the check payable to the bearer. It is the simplest and most common type of endorsement on personal checks but should be used only when the check is to be cashed or deposited immediately.

Restrictive Endorsement

A restrictive endorsement specifies the purpose of the endorsement (Figure 23-8). It is used in preparing checks for deposit to the physician's checking account.

Pay to the Order of
Midwest National Bank
Main Branch
For Deposit Only
CARLOS MACAULEY
301-012697

FIGURE 23-8 Example of a restrictive endorsement.

Special Endorsement

A special endorsement includes words specifying the person to whom the endorser makes the check payable. For instance, a check naming Helen Barker as the payee may be endorsed to the physician by writing on the back of the check as follows:

Pay to the order of
Theodore F. Wilson, M.D.
Helen Barker

The check is still negotiable but requires Dr. Wilson's signature or endorsement.

Qualified Endorsement

With a qualified endorsement, the effect of the endorsement is qualified by disclaiming or destroying any future liability of the endorser. Usually the words "without recourse" are written above by an attorney who accepts a check on behalf of a client but who has no personal claim in the transaction.

Methods of Endorsement

Stamp

As checks from patients and other sources arrive, they should be recorded in the ledger and immediately stamped with the restrictive endorsement "For Deposit Only." This is a safeguard against lost or stolen checks.

Any endorsement should agree exactly with the name on the face of the check. If the name of the payee is misspelled, the payee usually must endorse the check the way the name is spelled on the face, followed by the correctly spelled signature. Section 3-203 of the UCC states: "Where an instrument is made payable to a person under a misspelled name or one other than his own, he may endorse in that name or his own or both; but signature in both names may be required by a person paying or giving value for the instrument." Most banks accept routine stamp endorsement that is restricted to deposit only if the customer is well known and maintains an established account.

Signature

Some insurance checks or drafts require a personal signature endorsement; a stamped endorsement is not acceptable. This is stated on the back of the check. In such cases ask the payee to endorse the check, then stamp immediately below the signature the restrictive endorsement "For Deposit Only."

Making Deposits

The medical assistant's financial duties include depositing checks and reconciling the bank statements with the checkbook. Checks should be deposited promptly for these reasons:

Prepare a Bank Deposit

GOAL: *To prepare a bank deposit for the day's receipts and complete appropriate office records related to the deposit.*

EQUIPMENT and SUPPLIES

- Currency
- Checks for deposit
- Deposit slip
- Endorsement stamp (optional)
- Computer or typewriter
- Envelope

PROCEDURAL STEPS

1. Organize currency.
   PURPOSE: To arrange currency in the best order for speedy and accurate presentation to the teller.
2. Total the currency and record the amount on the deposit slip.
3. Place restrictive endorsements on the checks using an endorsement stamp.

PURPOSE: To transfer the title and protect checks from loss or theft.

4. List each check separately on the deposit slip with the American Banking Association (ABA) number and the amount.
5. Total the amount of currency and checks and enter on the deposit slip.
6. Enter the amount of the deposit in the checkbook.
   PURPOSE: To record the current balance in the account.
7. Prepare a copy of the deposit slip for the office record, including the names of the payers.
   PURPOSE: For verification of checks deposited, if necessary.
8. Place the currency, checks, and deposit slip in an envelope for transporting to the bank.

- A stop-payment order may be placed.
- The check may be lost, misplaced, or stolen.
- Delay may cause the check to be returned because of insufficient funds.
- The check may have a restricted time for cashing.
- It is a courtesy to the payer.

Preparing the Deposit

Deposit slips are itemized memoranda of cash or other funds a depositor presents to the bank with the money to be credited to the account. All deposits must be accompanied by a deposit slip. A carbon or photocopy of the deposit slip should be kept on file (Procedure 23-2).

Several types of deposit slips (sometimes called *deposit tickets*) are available. The commercial slip is used for the office checking account. The deposit slips are printed with the number of the account in magnetic ink characters to correspond to the checks. Preprinted deposit slips are ordered along with the checks.

Some write-it-once accounting systems include a deposit slip that the bank accepts as the itemization if it is attached to the customer's numbered deposit slip. The deposit slip should be prepared before the medical assistant goes to the bank, and the money should be organized and ready to present to the bank teller.

Payments on patients' accounts generally are made by check, but some are made in currency (paper money). Each type of payment is recorded separately on the deposit slip. The currency usually is listed first. Organize the currency so that all the bills face in the same direction (e.g., with the black ink [portrait] side up). Place the largest denomination bills on top.

Some banks prefer that checks be recorded individually by the ABA number; others use just the maker's name. If the checks are arranged alphabetically by the names of the patient accounts, with

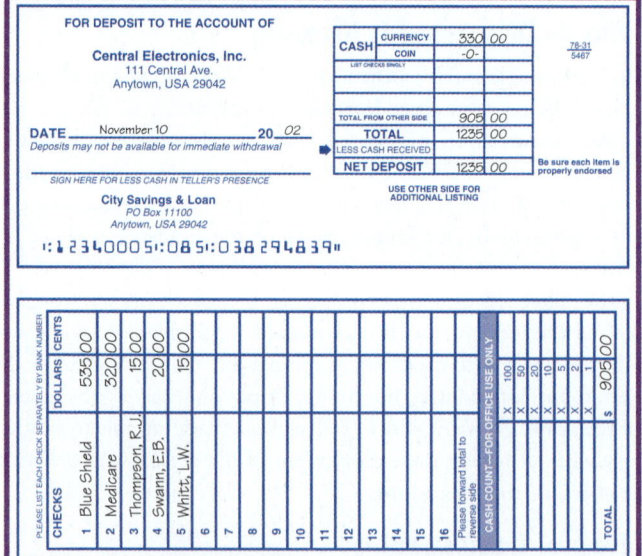

FIGURE 23-9 Front and back of a deposit slip.

these names included on your office copy of the deposit slip, you will have a ready reference of checks deposited should a question arise about a patient's payment. The following procedure should be used to prepare a deposit slip (Figure 23-9):

1. List all checks on the back of the deposit slip.
2. Transfer the total to the front of the slip.
3. Enter the amount of the total deposit on the deposit slip stub.

Money orders, whether postal, express, or others, are identified by "PO Money Order" or "Express MO." Remember that money orders cannot have more than two endorsements.

The deposit slip should be totaled carefully and the total entered in the checkbook. Any torn bills should be mended with transparent tape. Clip the currency together and clip the checks in a separate packet. Then place the entire amount in a heavy envelope for taking to the bank. A bank deposit should be made daily. Deposits can be made at any time during the business day. They can be made during the day or left in a drop box at night. Many banks require that deposits be made before 3 PM if the deposit is to be credited that business day.

Direct Deposits

Direct deposit is a plan in which payments are transferred, usually electronically, by a paying agency directly into the account of a recipient. Direct deposits are commonly used to pay salaries; paychecks are credited to employees' accounts (checking, savings, or any other type of account) at any financial institution.

Other Methods of Deposit

Advances in computer technology have allowed financial institutions to offer other methods of deposit to consumers and business customers. Some automated teller machines (ATMs) accept deposits, and checking accounts are available that allow the customer to conduct most banking services using the computer and ATMs. These types of accounts may limit the number of times the customer can use teller services without a fee.

Online banking allows customers to view their accounts, make transfers, order checks, pay bills, and perform numerous other transactions simply by logging onto the bank Web site and accessing the account with a password. Online banking also is an excellent way to research the checks that have cleared the bank and compute accurate bank balances.

BANK STATEMENTS AND RECONCILIATION

The bank periodically sends the customer a statement, which shows the status of the customer's account on a given date. This statement indicates the following:

- Beginning balance
- Deposits received
- Checks paid
- Bank charges
- Ending balance

Mailed Statements

Bank statements similar to the one in Figure 23-10 are prepared at regular intervals (usually once a month) and usually are mailed to the bank's customers. These statements may or may not include the accompanying cancelled checks, depending on the bank's policy and the type of account. The back of each page of the statement usually includes a reconciliation page so that the customer can determine what checks have still not cleared the bank, what deposits are not yet shown on the statement, and the accurate account balance.

Online Statements

Online statements, or e-statements, are an electronic version of a paper bank statement. Financial establishments that offer online banking services in an attempt to make banking easier for their customers claim that e-statements are a user-friendly way of viewing account balances and checking financial images online.

With e-statements, there is no need to continue receiving paper statements. The benefits include:

- The customer receives statements quickly and easily
- Statements can be saved in an electronic file for examination and printing at the customer's convenience.
- Fees are kept low, because paper and mailing costs are minimized.

Various banks offer different options, and fees vary. If the medical assistant has been authorized to set up an online banking account with the financial institution used by the medical facility, he or she should visit the bank to discuss the details of what is involved.

Reconciling the Bank Statement

The bank statement balance and the customer's checkbook balance usually differ, except in a relatively inactive account. The two balances must be reconciled. The **reconciliation** discloses any errors that may exist in the checkbook or, on rare occasions, in the bank statement (Figure 23-11).

The bank statement may include an entry for service charges that must be deducted from the checkbook balance. In all types of accounts, the bank may charge a fee for services. Usually in the case of an individual account, it is a flat fee; in a business account, the fee is based on services rendered. If the average or minimum balance is maintained at an established level, the bank may forego a service charge.

QUESTIONS TO ASK WHEN SEARCHING FOR A POSSIBLE ERROR

- Is your arithmetic correct?
- Did you forget to include one of the outstanding checks?
- Did you fail to record a deposit or did you record one twice?

Most banks ask to be notified within a reasonable time (e.g., 10 days) of any error found in the statement. The bank statement should be reconciled as soon as it is received. Most banks print a form for reconciliation on the back of the bank statement.

BANK STATEMENT RECONCILIATION FORMULA

Bank statement balance	$ _____
Less outstanding checks	$ _____
Plus deposits not shown	$ _____
Corrected bank statement balance	$ _____
Checkbook balance	$ _____
Less any bank charges	$ _____
Corrected checkbook balance	$ _____

If the two corrected balances agree, stop there. If they do not agree, subtract the lesser figure from the greater figure; the difference usually provides a clue to the error (Procedure 23-3). For instance, if the shortage is $35, examine all the transactions for $35 on the

0821-402054

#821

N
2

CALL (888) 555-2932
24 HOURS/DAY, 7 DAYS/WEEK
FOR ASSISTANCE WITH
YOUR ACCOUNT.

PAGE 1 OF 2   THIS STATEMENT COVERS: 6/22/02 THROUGH 7/22/02

INTEREST CHECKING
0821-402054

SUMMARY

PREVIOUS BALANCE	252.10	MINIMUM BALANCE	142.55
DEPOSITS	68.74 +	AVERAGE BALANCE	220.00
INTEREST EARNED	.18 +	ANNUAL PERCENTAGE	
WITHDRAWALS	109.55 −	YIELD EARNED	.96 %
CUSTOMER SERVICE CALLS	.00 −		
INTERLINK/PURCHASE FEE	.00 −	INTEREST EARNED 1994	2.23
MONTHLY CHECKING FEE AND OTHER CHARGES	.00 −		
▶ NEW BALANCE	211.47		

USE YOUR EXPRESS CARD TO MAKE UNLIMITED PURCHASES AT RETAILERS DISPLAYING
THE INTERLINK SYMBOL. (A $1 MONTHLY FEE MAY APPLY.)

TRY IT TODAY AT ARCO . . . MOBIL . . . LUCKY . . . RALPHS . . . SAFEWAY & MORE!

CHECKS AND WITHDRAWALS	CHECK	DATE PAID	AMOUNT	CHECK	DATE PAID	AMOUNT
	202	7/05	15.05	203	7/15	94.50

DEPOSITS				DATE POSTED	AMOUNT
	CUSTOMER DEPOSIT			7/22	68.74
	INTEREST PAYMENT THIS PERIOD			7/22	.18

BALANCE INFORMATION	DATE	BALANCE	DATE	BALANCE	DATE	BALANCE
	6/22	252.10	7/05	237.05	7/15	142.55
					7/22	211.47

24 HOUR CUSTOMER SERVICE

EACH ACCOUNT COMES WITH 3 COMPLIMENTARY CALLS PER STATEMENT PERIOD.

CALLS TO 24 HOUR CUSTOMER SERVICE THIS STATEMENT PERIOD: 0

INTEREST INFORMATION

FROM	THROUGH	INTEREST RATE	ANNUAL PERCENTAGE YIELD (APY)
6/22	7/22	1.00%	1.01%

INTEREST RATE/APY AS OF 7/22/02 IF YOUR BALANCE IS

$ 0 - 4,999 . . . . .1.00%	1.01%
$ 5,000 - 9,999 . . . . .1.00%	1.01%
$ 10,000 AND OVER 1.00%	1.01%

CALL 1-800-555-2932 IN CALIFORNIA ANYTIME FOR CURRENT RATES.

MEMBER FDIC

STATEMENT

FIGURE 23-10 Example of a regular checking account statement.

statement and checkbook register and determine whether one of them has a posting error. Check the math and make sure all figures were added and subtracted correctly. Look at each figure and make sure none has been transposed. These tips usually catch the mistake.

SIGNATURE CARDS

When an account is first opened at a banking facility, the depositor is required to affix his or her handwritten signature to a card, which is kept on file at the bank. If a check comes through and some suspicion arises that the depositor's signature has been forged, the bank personnel compare the signature on the check with the original on the signature card.

In a business situation, as in a medical office, the physician often delegates the responsibility of paying bills to the medical assistant or other office staff members. In this case, any staff member who has been authorized to sign the medical facility's checks must go to the bank and add his or her handwritten signature to the signature card. Only those whose names appear on the signature card are authorized to sign checks, and the bank is responsible for verifying any questionable signatures.

BONDING

To protect their business establishments from embezzlement or other financial loss caused by employees who handle large sums of money,

THIS WORKSHEET IS PROVIDED TO HELP YOU BALANCE YOUR ACCOUNT

1. Go through your register and mark each check, withdrawal, Express ATM transaction, payment, deposit or other credit listed on this statement. Be sure that your register shows any interest paid into your account, and any service charges, automatic payments, or Express Transfers withdrawn from your account during this statement period.

2. Using the chart below, list any outstanding checks, Express ATM withdrawals, payments or any other withdrawals (including any from previous months) that are listed in your register but are not shown on this statement.

3. Balance your account by filling in the spaces below.

ITEMS OUTSTANDING	
NUMBER	AMOUNT

ENTER

The NEW BALANCE shown on this statement _ _ _ _ _ _ _ _ _ _ _ _ _ _ _ _ _ $_____

ADD

Any deposits listed in your register $_____
or transfers into your account $_____
which are not shown on this $_____
statement. +$_____

TOTAL _ _ _ _ _ _ +$_____

CALCULATE THE SUBTOTAL _ _ _ _ _ _ _ $_____

SUBTRACT

The total outstanding checks and withdrawals from the chart at left _ _ _ _ _ _ _ −$_____

CALCULATE THE ENDING BALANCE

This amount should be the same as the current balance shown in your check register _ _ _ _ _ _ _ _ _ _ _ $_____

TOTAL $

IF YOU SUSPECT ERRORS OR HAVE QUESTIONS ABOUT ELECTRONIC TRANSFERS

If you believe there is an error on your statement or Express ATM receipt, or if you need more information about a transaction listed on this statement or an Express ATM receipt, please contact us immediately. We are available 24 hours a day, seven days a week to assist you. Please call the telephone number printed on the front of this statement. Or, you may write to us at United Trust Company, P.O. Box 327, Anytown, USA.

1) Tell us your name and account number or Express card number.

2) As clearly as you can, describe the error or the transfer you are unsure about, and explain why you believe there is an error or why you need more information.

3) Tell us the dollar amount of the suspected error.

You must report the suspected error to us no later than 60 days after we sent you the first statement on which the problem appeared. We will investigate your question and will correct any error promptly. If our investigation takes longer than 10 business days (or 20 days in the case of electronic purchases), we will temporarily credit your account for the amount you believe is in error, so that you may have use of the money until the investigation is completed.

FIGURE 23-11 Reverse side of a bank statement, which is used for reconciling a checking account.

physicians often purchase fidelity bonds. Fidelity bonds reimburse the physician for any monetary loss caused by employees. Bonding normally requires a personal background investigation. The three types of bonding are:

- *Position-schedule bonding,* which covers a specific position rather than an individual, such as a bookkeeper or receptionist
- *Blanket-position bonding,* which covers all employees
- *Personal bonding,* which covers specific individuals

CLOSING COMMENTS

Patient Education

Medical assistants might want to encourage patients to pay for professional services with a personal check because of the numerous benefits checks offer. If a patient attempts to pay for services with a third-party check (other than an insurance reimbursement), the medical assistant should tactfully explain why this is not a wise

PROCEDURE 23-3

Reconcile a Bank Statement

GOAL: *To reconcile a bank statement for a checking account.*

EQUIPMENT and SUPPLIES

- Ending balance of previous statement
- Current bank statement
- Canceled checks for current month
- Checkbook stubs
- Calculator
- Pen

PROCEDURAL STEPS

1. Compare the opening balance of the new statement with the closing balance of the previous statement.
   <u>PURPOSE:</u> To determine that the balances are in agreement.

2. Compare the canceled checks with the items on the statement.
   <u>PURPOSE:</u> To verify that they are your checks and that they are listed in the correct amount.

3. Arrange the canceled checks in numeric order and compare with the checkbook stubs.

4. Place a checkmark on each stub for which a canceled check has been returned.
   <u>PURPOSE:</u> To locate any outstanding checks.

5. List and total the outstanding checks.

6. Verify that all previous outstanding checks have cleared.

7. Subtract the total of the outstanding checks from the bank statement balance.
   <u>NOTE:</u> Do not include any certified checks as outstanding, because their amount has already been deducted from the account.

8. Add to the total in step 7 any deposits made but not included in the bank statement.
   <u>PURPOSE:</u> To correct the credits in the bank statement balance.

9. Total any bank charges that appear on the bank statement and subtract them from the checkbook balance. Such charges may include service charges, automatic withdrawals or payments, and nonsufficient funds (NSF) checks.
   <u>PURPOSE:</u> To correct the checkbook balance.

10. If the checkbook balance and the statement balance do not agree, match the bank statement entries with the checkbook entries. Review deposit slips and transactions against the day sheet and read all columns. Correct any errors that are found.

---

practice. In addition, if a patient makes a mistake when writing a check, the medical assistant is responsible for pointing it out and requesting a new check, because corrections on the face of a check often render it useless.

If a patient's check is returned from the bank marked "nonsufficient funds," or "NSF," the medical assistant should immediately call the patient and explain the problem, requesting that he or she correct the matter as soon as possible. It is important to remember, however, that most overdrafts are simply the result of mathematic errors or a delay in deposited funds being available for withdrawal. Therefore, the medical assistant should be patient and courteous when discussing NSF issues with patients. However, patients need to know that overdrafts are costly not only to them but also to the medical facility.

Legal and Ethical Issues

If a mistake is made in preparing a check, do not destroy the check. Rather, write "VOID" across the face of the check, make a note on the check stub, and file the check with the canceled checks for auditing purposes.

A stop-payment order may be placed with the bank in an emergency, such as when a check is lost or a disagreement occurs with regard to a purchase or payment.

Do not accept a check made payable to another party without the endorsement of the person who gives the check to you. If the check is returned by the bank for any reason, the check will be charged to the last endorser, not the last person to receive the money.

SUMMARY OF SCENARIO

Laura has gained considerable knowledge through her experiences and work with the various aspects of the banking world. The goals she set for completing the assignments and competencies were accomplished in the time frame allowed by the instructor. She is comfortable now that she can readily apply this knowledge to whatever medical facility in which she finds work.

Laura spent extra time outside of class exploring online banking and bill paying on the Internet, and she found a wealth of information available. Laura

now plans to visit several banks in her area to see what kind of e-banking services they offer.

The versatility of the medical assistant's role and the variety of the opportunities available reinforce to Laura that she has made the right career choice. The more that she studies and learns, the more she can contribute to the physician's office, using her knowledge to help develop office policies, teach the other staff members how to use the more advanced aspects of the computer system, and make wise decisions about the banking services that will most benefit the clinic.

SUMMARY OF LEARNING OBJECTIVES

1. **Define, spell, and pronounce the terms listed in the vocabulary.**
   Spelling and pronouncing medical terms correctly bolster the medical assistant's credibility. Knowing the definition of these terms promotes confidence in communication with patients and co-workers.

2. **Describe banking procedures.**
   Banking procedures include withdrawals, deposits, writing checks, reconciling bank statements, paying bills, and other transactions.

3. **Explain how the Internet has changed traditional banking practices.**
   The Internet allows many banking transactions to be done at home through a personal computer or cell phone. It also allows access to bank account information 24 hours a day, 7 days a week.

4. **State the four requirements of a negotiable instrument.**
   To be negotiable, an instrument (e.g., a check) must (1) be written and signed by a maker, (2) contain a promise or order to pay a sum of money, (3) be payable on demand or at a fixed future date, and (4) be payable to order or bearer.

5. **Discuss the advantages of using debit cards.**
   Advantages of debit cards include safety and convenience, quick calculation of expenditures, and a permanent record for tax purposes. They are faster to use than writing a check and can be used when a person is out of town or on trips, whereas checks rarely are accepted outside the user's home town area.

6. **Identify the three most common types of bank accounts.**
   The three most common types of bank accounts are checking accounts, savings accounts, and money market savings accounts.

7. **Correctly write checks for bill payment.**
   The medical assistant may be required to write checks on the practice account to pay bills. The process for writing a check is outlined in Procedure 23-1.

8. **Explain how to handle mistakes made in preparing a check.**
   Normally, when a mistake is made on a check, the check should be marked "VOID" and a new check should be written. Some banks accept minor errors if the maker initials the error. Erasures are not allowed, nor is the use of correction fluid.

9. **Discuss precautions for accepting checks.**
   Scan the check carefully for the correct date, amount, and signature. Make sure the check is perforated on at least one side. Do not accept a check with corrections on it. If you do not know the person presenting a personal check, ask for identification and compare signatures.
   a. Acceptance of a third-party check generally is unwise. A third-party check is one made out to your patient by a party unknown to you. A check from the patient's health insurance carrier is an exception.
   b. Do not accept a check marked "Payment in Full" unless it does pay the account in full up to and including the date on which it is received.
   c. Do not accept checks written for more than the amount due and return cash for the difference between the amount of the check and the amount owed

10. **Discuss the actions necessary when a patient's check is returned.**
    When a deposited check is returned, the maker should be contacted immediately, informed of the situation, and asked to remedy the situation either by immediately depositing funds in his or her account to cover the check or by paying the bill by alternative means, such as cash or a money order.

11. **Compare types of endorsements.**
    Endorsements include (1) a blank endorsement, in which the payee simply signs his or her name on the back of the check; (2) a restrictive endorsement, which specifies in which bank and which specific account the funds are to be deposited; (3) a special endorsement, which names a specific person on the back of the check as payee; and (4) a qualified endorsement, which disclaims future liability. This type of endorsement is used when the person who accepts the check has no personal claim in the transaction.

12. **Prepare a bank deposit.**
    Bank deposits should be made on a daily basis. The process for preparing a bank deposit is outlined in Procedure 23-2.

13. **Accurately reconcile a bank statement for the office checking account.**
    Bank statements should be reconciled as soon as they arrive at the physician's office or should be printed from the bank's Web site for reconciliation. The process for reconciling a bank statement is outlined in Procedure 23-3.

CONNECTIONS

Study Guide Connection: Go to the Chapter 23 Study Guide. Read and complete the activities.

Evolve Connection: Go to the Chapter 23 link at *evolve.elsevier.com/kinn* to complete the Chapter Review and Chapter Quiz.

24

FINANCIAL AND PRACTICE MANAGEMENT

Brenda Newman is the office manager for Dr. Susan Wilkins, a neurologist who is beginning her second year of practice. Dr. Wilkins is financially savvy and takes care with the money she has invested in her business. She encourages her employees to plan for the future and offers them a retirement plan, in addition to opportunities for investing in mutual funds through payroll deduction. Her accountant, Grant Schmidt, assists Dr. Wilkins with the financial aspects of her practice and is always willing to counsel the employees of the clinic about finances.

Mr. Schmidt has taught Brenda several methods of keeping track of the practice's finances. Brenda is interested in learning more about general accounting rules and bookkeeping. She is able to perform computerized accounting duties and is also able to use a pegboard system. She works with patients when they need to make payment arrangements and has an excellent collection ratio.

Dr. Wilkins is cost conscious and does not order random supplies and equipment. Instead, she and Brenda plan the inventory for a 6-month period and order supplies every 6 months. By ordering in precise amounts, Dr. Wilkins saves money and uses the extra funds for staff development events and seminars. Each month, the budget is printed and reviewed during a staff meeting to ensure that the office is on track with expenses.

The team effort involving Dr. Wilkins, Brenda, and Mr. Schmidt results in a balanced budget for the clinic, and subsequently the staff is able to enjoy more benefits and perks.

While studying this chapter, think about the following questions:

- Why is a constant flow of income preferable to a once-a-month influx for a physician's office?
- Why should the person entering numbers on a manual system make all numerals exactly alike all the time?
- How have computers affected the management of finances in the physician's office?
- How do a practice's finances affect the income of the medical assistant?

LEARNING OBJECTIVES

1. Define, spell, and pronounce the terms listed in the vocabulary.
2. List the four items all financial records should show at any given time.
3. Describe how to establish and maintain a petty cash fund.
4. Differentiate between accounts payable and accounts receivable.
5. Explain the difference between a single-entry and a double-entry accounting system.
6. Explain the importance of a trial balance.
7. Describe common periodic financial reports.
8. Explain how to process an employee payroll accurately.
9. Explain the purpose of Form W-4.
10. State the types of employment records required by the Internal Revenue Service (IRS).
11. Discuss the basis for the withholding amounts taken from employees' earnings.
12. Explain the requirements of the Federal Insurance Contributions Act (FICA).
13. Discuss the importance of setting a budget each fiscal year.

VOCABULARY

accounts payable Debts incurred and not yet paid.

accounts receivable Amounts owed to the physician.

accounts receivable trial balance A method of determining that the journal and the ledger are in balance.

accrual basis of accounting Method of accounting in which income is recorded when earned and expenses are recorded when incurred.

admonition Counsel or warning against fault or oversight.

assets The entire property of a person, association, corporation, or estate applicable or subject to the payment of debts.

balance sheet A financial statement for a specific date that shows the total assets, liabilities, and capital of the business.

bookkeeping The recording of business and accounting transactions.

cash basis of accounting A method of accounting in which income is recorded when received and expenses are recorded when paid.

cash flow statement A financial summary for a specific period that shows the beginning balance on hand, the receipts and disbursements during the period, and the balance on hand at the end of the period.

controls A standard of comparison to make sure answers obtained are accurate.

disbursements journal A summary of accounts paid out.

entry A record or notation of an occurrence, transaction, or proceeding.

equities The monetary value of a property or of an interest in a property in excess of claims or liens against it.

in balance The state in which the total ending balances of patient ledgers equals the total of accounts receivable.

invoice A paper describing a purchase and the amount due.

liabilities Things that are owed; debts.

packing slip An itemized list of articles included in a shipping package, giving the quantity and description of the package contents.

petty cash fund A fund maintained to pay small, unpredictable cash expenditures.

statement A request for payment.

statement of income and expense A summary of all income and expenses for a given period.

subsidiary Supporting other documents or records.

trial balance A method of checking the accuracy of accounts.

A physician's business records are the key to good management practice. Physicians need and appreciate medical assistants who can keep accurate financial records and can conduct the administrative side of the practice in a businesslike fashion. Financial records that are complete, correct, and current are essential for:

- Prompt billing and collection procedures
- Accurate budgeting
- Professional financial planning
- Accurate reporting of income to federal and state agencies

More than half of today's physicians run independent practices. According to CNNmoney, shrinking insurance reimbursements, changing regulations, rising business and drug costs are among the factors preventing many from keeping their practices afloat. But some experts counter that doctors' lack of business acumen is also to blame. Unless the physician and staff stay abreast of regulations affecting finances, the physician may find his or her practice failing.

WHAT IS ACCOUNTING?

Accounting is a system of recording, classifying, and summarizing financial transactions. **Bookkeeping** is the recording part of the accounting process. Bookkeeping must be done daily. In a small practice, it is the responsibility of the administrative medical assistant; in a larger practice, it is done by the office manager or financial manager. Summaries are prepared and personal and business tax returns are filed with the Internal Revenue Service (IRS).

Accounting Bases

Two general bases, or methods, of accounting are used: the cash basis and the accrual basis. Most physicians use the **cash basis of accounting**, which means that charges for services are entered as income when payment is received, and expenses are recorded when they are paid. Merchants, on the other hand, generally use an **accrual basis of accounting**. Income is considered earned when services have been performed or goods have been sold, even though payment may not have been received. Expenses are recognized and recorded when incurred, even though they have not been paid.

Financial Summaries

The financial records of any business should show the following at all times:

- How much was earned in a given period
- How much was collected
- How much is owed
- The distribution of expenses incurred

The accountant can prepare monthly and annual summaries from the daily entries that provide a basis of comparison for any given period with another, similar period. Periodic analyses of financial records result in improved business practices, better time management, curtailment or elimination of unprofitable services, and better budgeting of expenses. With the appropriate software, these analyses can be done on the computer. The medical assistant may see notations such as AR/AP, which stand for **accounts receivable** (Procedure 24-1) and **accounts payable** (Procedure 24-2).

PROCEDURE 24-1

Perform Accounts Receivable Procedures

GOAL: *To collect amounts due to the physician or medical facility.*

EQUIPMENT and SUPPLIES

- Patient ledgers
- Office policy manual
- Telephone
- Letterhead and envelopes
- Clerical supplies

PROCEDURAL STEPS

1. Determine the billing cycle for the medical facility according to the office policy manual.
   PURPOSE: To determine which groups of accounts are billed at different times of the month, as specified by the billing cycle.
2. Prompt the computer to compile a report on the age of accounts receivable. Many programs have this as an easily accessed report option.
   PURPOSE: To determine which accounts have a balance due.
3. Divide the accounts into the following categories:
   0-30 days old
   30-60 days old
   60-90 days old
   90-120 days old
   More than 120 days old
4. Determine the amounts due the physician and who owes these amounts.
   PURPOSE: To specify which accounts need to be billed.
5. Group accounts together when necessary.
   PURPOSE: Some physicians prefer to separate regular billings from past-due billings.
6. Print bills using the computer system or make copies of ledger cards.
7. Mail bills to patients.
8. Post payments to patients' accounts as they arrive at the office.
   PURPOSE: To credit payments to patients' accounts.
9. Demonstrate sensitivity and professionalism in handling accounts receivable activities.

CRITICAL THINKING APPLICATION   24-1

- Brenda has noticed several errors on encounter forms lately. These errors seem to be the result of a staff member not using a calculator to add up the charges when the patient is ready to check out. Brenda has approached the person who assists the patients in this area but has not seen any improvement. How might she convince the employee to follow precautions in adding charges? What are Brenda's options regarding the employee's job?
- How might Mr. Schmidt educate the staff about the importance of accurate financial records?

The Rules of Bookkeeping

Bookkeeping has many rules that the medical assistant must follow. First, use good penmanship so that the records are clearly legible, even years later. Use the same pen style and type of ink consistently. Keep columns of figures straight and write well-formed figures (a careless 9 may look like a 7; an open 0 may resemble a 6). Carry decimal points correctly. Ask the physician if any questions arise about bookkeeping issues (Figure 24-1).

Enter all charges and receipts immediately in the daily record or journal. Write a receipt in duplicate for any currency received. Writing receipts for checks is optional, but a consistent pattern should be followed. Post all charges and receipts to the patient ledger daily. Checks should be endorsed for deposit as soon as they are received. The **petty cash fund** should be used to pay for small, unpredictable expenses. Pay all other expenses by check. A cancelled check is the best proof of payment. Bills should be paid before their

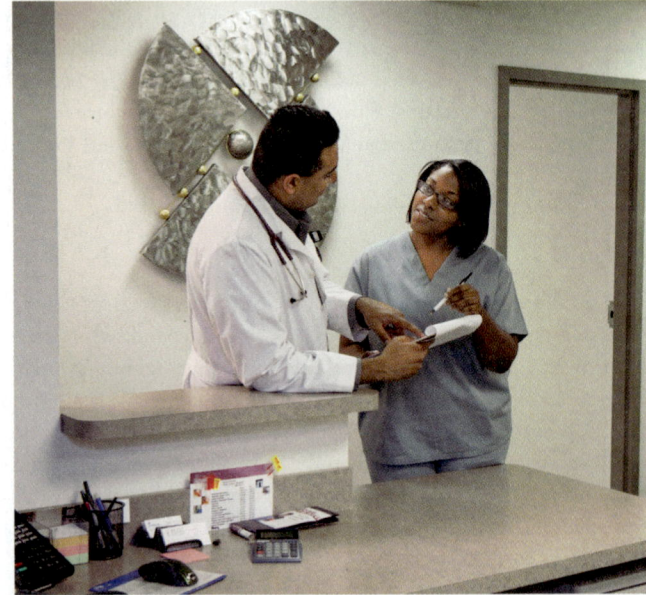

FIGURE 24-1 When the medical assistant is unsure about financial information, he or she should ask the physician. When an unfamiliar statement arrives, check with the physician to make sure it should be paid.

due date after they have been checked for accuracy. Place the date of payment and the check number on paid bills.

Do not erase, write over, or blot out figures. If an error is made, a straight line should be drawn through the incorrect figure and the correct figure written above it. Bookkeeping procedures are not

PROCEDURE 24-2

Perform Accounts Payable Procedures

GOAL: *To determine the age of accounts and decide what collection activity is needed.*

EQUIPMENT and SUPPLIES

- Patient ledger cards with a balance due
- Pen
- Computer
- Calculator

PROCEDURAL STEPS

1. Prompt the computer to compile a report on the age of accounts receivable. Many programs will have this feature as an easily accessed report option. Divide the accounts into categories as listed below:
   0-30 days old
   30-60 days old
   60-90 days old
   90-120 days old
   PURPOSE: To determine how old the various accounts are and place the accounts into categories as to when the last payment was made.

2. If the computer program does not perform this function, manually pull all ledger cards that have a balance due and divide them into the categories listed under step 1.

3. Examine the accounts to see which are awaiting an insurance payment. Action need not be taken if an insurance payment is expected and is not long overdue. Return those ledgers to the ledger tray.
   PURPOSE: To avoid collection activity on accounts for which a payment is expected.

4. Follow the office procedure for collections on the accounts left. Collection reminder stickers may be placed on the statements sent to the patient, or a collection letter may be sent. Make sure the stickers are inside the envelope, not on the outside.
   PURPOSE: To prompt the patient to make a payment by pointing out the age of the account.

5. Call patients whose accounts are more than 90 days old. Attempt to make payment arrangements with the patient.
   PURPOSE: To attempt to collect from the patient or determine why the patient has not yet paid the account.

6. Send a collection letter to patients whose accounts are more than 120 days old, if indicated, to encourage the patient to pay the bill. If it is the office policy, mention that the account is in danger of being sent to a collection agency.
   PURPOSE: To reach patients who are not available by telephone.

7. Add the total accounts receivable for each category and arrive at a figure outstanding for each. The physician may want a report weekly or monthly on these figures.
   PURPOSE: To have a current accounting of the amounts owed to the physician and to double-check the amount outstanding according to the pegboard system or software system.

8. Note in the chart and/or on the ledger any arrangements made with patients regarding payment of the accounts. Send a follow-up letter to remind the patients of their payment agreements.
   PURPOSE: To document arrangements made and remind the patients of their obligation and promise to pay.

---

complicated, but they do require concentration to prevent errors. There is no such thing as almost correct financial records. Either the books balance, or they do not balance. The bookkeeping is either right or wrong.

Kinds of Financial Records

Daily Journal

The daily journal is the chronologic record of the practice (i.e., the financial diary). The day sheet is the daily journal for practices that use a manual pegboard system. Although more practices use computerized systems, some still use a manual pegboard; however, using a manual system helps the medical assistant to understand the theory of accounting in the medical office. All information about services rendered, charges, and receipts first is recorded in the daily journal. It is important to record every transaction.

The practice may earn income from sources other than the professional services rendered in and out of the office. Such sources include rentals, royalties, interest, and so forth. If the physician owns the entire building and rents a few offices to other professionals, he will have to claim rental income on his tax returns. Additionally, if he has published any textbooks or has other royalty income, that will also need to be listed on his annual returns. Usually a special place is provided in the journal for such income. Any income that is not practice related should be recorded separately from patient receipts.

Checkbook

Receipts usually are deposited in the checking account, and a record of the deposit is entered in the journal and on the check register. A copy of each deposit slip should be kept with the financial records. Bills usually are paid by check or through online bill paying services, and a record of the payment is entered on the check stub and in the disbursements section of the daily journal.

CRITICAL THINKING APPLICATION   24-2

- Brenda has noticed two checks missing from the business checkbook. Dr. Wilkins is out of town for a week and cannot be contacted. How might Brenda determine where the checks are or to whom they were written?
- What steps can be taken to resolve the problem of not knowing the amount of a missing check?

Disbursements Journal

In simplified accounting systems in which manual posting is used, the **disbursements journal** usually consists of a section at the bottom of each day sheet and a check register page at the end of each month, plus monthly and annual summaries. It must show the following:

- Every amount paid out
- Date and check number
- Purpose of the payment

When a computer system is used to post disbursements, the cash or check payments screen is used. Payment information is entered, and the computer prints the check, or the information is entered after the check has been manually prepared.

Petty Cash Records

A petty cash fund and voucher system should be established to take care of minor unpredictable expenditures, such as postage due, parking fees, small contributions, emergency supplies, and miscellaneous small items. In the average facility, $25 to $50 is sufficient for the petty cash fund. If a larger sum is available, the tendency is to pay too many bills out of petty cash instead of writing a check.

When the check for this fund is exchanged at the bank for small bills and coins, the money is placed in a cashbox or drawer that can be locked or kept in the safe at night. Only one person should be in charge of the petty cash fund. This person must be able to account for the full amount of the fund at any time.

CRITICAL THINKING APPLICATION   **24-3**

- Brenda has noticed that on several occasions, employees have borrowed money from the petty cash fund. Is this an acceptable practice? Why or why not?
- How might Brenda keep an accounting of money taken from the petty cash drawer if she is not the person actually in control of it?

ACCOUNTING SYSTEMS

The basic principles of accounting are the same, no matter which system is in place. Remember that accounting and bookkeeping are separate functions; accounting is a four-stage process of recording, classifying, summarizing, and interpreting financial statements. Bookkeeping is the recording stage of accounting. The medical assistant performs bookkeeping functions when posting a payment to a patient's account. Most accounting for physician offices or medical clinics is performed by using either a single-entry or double-entry system.

The single-entry system is very basic and usually is used in small businesses, such as a one-physician office or a partnership that sees a relatively small number of patients. Single-entry systems are inexpensive, easy to use, and require little training. The system requires three basic records: the general journal, the cash payment journal, and the accounts receivable ledger. The general journal is a record (e.g., a day sheet) where transactions are entered. The cash payment journal in its simplest form is a record (e.g., a checkbook) that is used to make payments. The accounts receivable ledger provides information about the amounts owed the physician.

Double-entry bookkeeping is also inexpensive but requires a trained, experienced bookkeeper or the regular services of an accountant. The transactions may be recorded manually or by computer. In addition to the basic journals used in a single-entry system, numerous **subsidiary** journals may be used. The system is based on the following accounting equation:

Assets = Liabilities + Proprietorship (Capital)

Every transaction requires an **entry** on each side of the accounting equation, and the two sides must always be in balance. For this reason the system is called *double-entry bookkeeping,* and it is the most complete accounting system. An understanding of the basics of double-entry bookkeeping can help clarify the principles of all systems.

Assets are the properties owned by a business, such as bank accounts, accounts receivable, buildings, equipment, and furniture. The rights to these assets are called **equities**. The equity of the owner is called *capital, proprietorship,* or *owner's equity.* The equities of the creditors to whom money is owed are called **liabilities**. The owner's equity, or capital, is what remains of the value of the assets after the creditor's equities or liabilities have been subtracted.

For example, if the physician purchased equipment for $1,000, paid $250 down, and signed a promissory note for $750, the accounting equation would be as follows:

Assets	$1,000	=	Liabilities	$750
			+	
			Capital	250
	$1,000			$1,000

The total value of the asset is $1,000. The owner's equity is $250, and the creditor's equity is $750. The accounting terms *capital, proprietorship, owner's equity,* and *net worth* are used interchangeably.

Few medical assistants are trained in accounting. If a double-entry system is used, a practice management consultant or the accountant who does most of the actual bookwork and reports usually sets it up. The medical assistant in this instance generally maintains only the daily journal, from which the accountant takes the figures once a month. The double-entry system provides a more comprehensive picture of the practice and its effect on the physician's net worth. Errors show up readily, and the system has many built-in accuracy **controls**; however, because of the time and skill required, it is not frequently used in a small practice.

END OF DAY SUMMARIZING

Most computer accounting systems perform end of the day summarizing automatically. If the office uses the pegboard system, the bottom of the day sheet has three sections to be completed that will show that the accounts have balanced for the day; similar functions are calculated in computerized systems. The medical assistant may be responsible for making sure the transactions made during the day are entered correctly and that the summary is in balance. Computerized systems may use different titles for the transactions, but they perform the same functions.

The first part of the end of day summary is the proof of posting section, which deals with the transactions that occurred that day on the day sheet. The second section is the month-to-date accounts receivable proof; adding the day's totals to the month-to-date totals should result in a sum that balances to the penny. The last section is the year-to-date accounts receivable proof, which adds the accounts, including the day's totals, to the year-to-date total.

The totals at the bottom of the second and third sections must be identical. If the end of the day summarizing does not balance, the medical assistant first should check the addition of each column, both horizontally and vertically; in most cases this reveals the error. Make sure the instructions are followed to the letter. To prevent frustrating mistakes, it is best to use a calculator, even when adding small numbers.

These calculations are helpful because they allow the physician to see the financial health of his or her practice. The physician can look at the end of day summaries and see exactly how much money has been paid in, in addition to how much money is outstanding and due from patients, to the day. The information helps the physician to know whether the practice finances are on track for the month and/or the year.

TRIAL BALANCE OF ACCOUNTS RECEIVABLE

A **trial balance** should be done once a month after all posting has been completed and before the monthly statements are prepared. The purpose of a trial balance is to disclose any discrepancies between the journal and the ledger. It does not prove the accuracy of the accounts. For example, if a charge or payment was posted to the wrong account or if the wrong amount was entered in the journal and then posted to the ledger, the totals would still "balance," but the accounts would not be accurate.

To begin, pull all the account cards with a balance, enter each balance on the calculator, and total the figures. This should equal the accounts receivable balance figure on the control. If there is no daily control, total all the charges, all the payments, and all the adjustments for the month, then do the following computation:

Accounts receivable at first of month	$ _____
Plus total charges for month	$ _____
Subtotal	$ _____
Less total payments for month	$ _____
Subtotal	$ _____
Less total adjustments for month	$ _____
Accounts receivable at end of month	$ _____

The end of the month accounts receivable figure must agree with the figure arrived at by adding all the account card balances. The accounts are then said to be **in balance**. If the two totals do not agree, the error must be located.

Locating and Preventing Errors

After checking the adding machine tape and verifying that no error in calculation has been made, the first step in locating an error in the trial balance is to find the difference between the two totals. Then search the daily journal pages and the account cards for an entry for the identical amount. Check each one found and verify that it was posted correctly. Of course, more than one error may add up to this amount.

If only one error was made and the amount of the error is divisible by 9, a figure may have been transposed. For example, if the difference is $81 (a number divisible by 9), the person who posted to the account may have written $209 instead of $290. If the amount of the error is divisible by 2, the amount may have been posted to the wrong column, reversing a debit and a credit.

A common error is entering the wrong amount in the previous balance column or in figuring the new balance. This kind of error shows up on the pegboard daily proof but could easily go undetected in the single-entry system. Carrying forward the wrong amount results in another common error total from one day to the next (e.g., carrying forward the beginning accounts receivable total rather than the ending accounts receivable total). There is always a chance of sliding a number, which means writing the first digit in the wrong column, such as writing 400 for 40 or 60 instead of 600.

Many bookkeepers prevent errors in the cents column by using a line (—) instead of writing two zeros when only even dollars are involved. For example, instead of writing $12.00, the bookkeeper writes $12.—. This eliminates the possibility of misreading zeros as other numbers. It also speeds the adding process when columns must be totaled. Make sure the same type of pen is used for all entries and that figures are written the same way. Scan for errors in every column. Try to spot figures in which the numbers have been transposed or that are unclear, thus increasing the chance that the numbers will be read incorrectly when adding.

If the medical assistant is unable to locate any numeric error, an account card may have been lost, overlooked, or transferred as paid in full. As a last resort, pull each account card and review it for errors. Compare the card to the day sheet and check to make sure that everything has been entered accurately. Computer programs often have checks and balance reports that can help the user find errors, but remember that the computer works with the data that were entered. If a $152 charge was entered instead of $125, the computer may not catch such a mistake.

> ## CRITICAL THINKING APPLICATION   24-4
> What should Brenda do if she has repeatedly reviewed records in search of an error and is still unable to find it? To whom should this be reported?

ACCOUNTS PAYABLE PROCEDURES

Invoices and Statements

If an item is not paid for at the time of purchase, the vendor usually includes a **packing slip** with delivery of the merchandise. A packing slip describes the items enclosed. The vendor may also enclose an **invoice**. An invoice describes the items and shows the amount due. Always check to verify that the items listed on the packing slip and invoice are included in the delivery.

Invoices should be placed in a designated folder until paid. The facility may be making more than one purchase from the same vendor during the month. Some vendors request that payment be made from the invoice; others expect to send a statement later. A **statement** is a request for payment.

Paying for Purchases

At the time of payment, compare the statement with the invoice to verify its accuracy, fasten the statement and invoice together, write the date, the amount paid, and the check number on the statement, and place it in the paid file.

CRITICAL THINKING APPLICATION   24-5

- Brenda does not recall ordering a certain item from the office supply company. However, it was included in her last shipment and listed on the packing list. How can she determine whether the item was ordered?
- How would Brenda correct this problem if the item had not been ordered?

Recording Disbursements

Disbursements are funds paid out. Disbursements are distributed to specific expense accounts, such as:

- Auto expenses
- Dues and meetings
- Equipment
- Insurance
- Medical supplies
- Office expenses
- Printing, postage, and stationery
- Rent and maintenance
- Salaries
- Taxes and licenses
- Travel and entertainment
- Utilities
- Miscellaneous
- Personal withdrawals

Each check used to pay an expense should be entered on the disbursement page showing the date, the name of the company to which the check was written, the number and amount of the check, and the payment allocated to one or more of the expense accounts. Always separate personal expenditures from business expenses. Business expenses are tax deductible and are considered in determining net income from the practice, but personal expenditures are not. Although personal expenses are not deductible in determining net income from the practice, some qualify as personal deductions in computing personal income tax, so a careful accounting should be kept. Deductible expenses would include property taxes, interest paid out, contributions, and so on.

Accounting for Petty Cash

The petty cash fund is a revolving fund (Procedure 24-3). Petty cash can be used for a variety of items, such as expendable supplies, business meals, local transportation, photocopy service, and other items.

To establish the petty cash fund, a check is written payable to Cash or Petty Cash and entered in the disbursements journal under Miscellaneous. This is the only time the petty cash check is charged to Miscellaneous. Each time the fund is replenished, the amount of the check is spread among the various accounts for which the money was used. This is determined from a record of expenditures. The headings of the columns should correspond to headings in the disbursements journal to which they will be posted.

A pad of petty cash vouchers is kept in or near the cash box. For every disbursement from the fund, the person who handles the fund

---

PROCEDURE 24-3

Account for Petty Cash

GOAL: *To establish a petty cash fund, maintain an accurate record of expenditures for 1 month, and replenish the fund as necessary.*

EQUIPMENT and SUPPLIES

- Form for petty cash fund
- Pad of vouchers
- Disbursement journal
- Two checks
- List of petty cash expenditures

PROCEDURAL STEPS

1. Determine the amount needed in the petty cash fund.
2. Write a check in the determined amount.
   PURPOSE: To establish a fund.
3. Record the beginning balance in the petty cash fund.
4. Post the amount to Miscellaneous on the disbursement record.
   PURPOSE: To account for the original amount in the fund.

5. Prepare a petty cash voucher for each amount withdrawn from the fund.
   PURPOSE: The vouchers will be used for internal audit.
6. Record each voucher in the petty cash record and enter the new balance.
   PURPOSE: To record the current balance and determine the need to replenish the fund.
7. Write a check to replenish the fund as necessary.
   NOTE: The total of the vouchers plus the fund balance must equal the beginning amount.
8. Total the expense columns and post to the appropriate accounts in the disbursement record.
   PURPOSE: To record expenditures in the correct expense category.
9. Record the amount added to the fund.
10. Record the new balance in the petty cash fund.

should either have a receipt or prepare a voucher. The total of the petty cash vouchers and receipts plus the amount of cash in the box must always equal the original amount of the fund.

At the end of the month or sooner if the fund is depleted, a check is written to Cash to replenish the fund. However, instead of being charged to Miscellaneous, as was done when the fund was established, the amount of the check is divided among the various accounts affected.

Avoid the habit of borrowing from the petty cash fund. This **admonition** applies both to the physician and to the medical assistant. If the physician requests cash from the fund, request a personal check or an office check in exchange for cash from the fund when it is time to replenish the money. Although many offices use petty cash to make change, it is best to have a separate change fund to prevent errors. If the incorrect change is made and the petty cash drawer is shorted, the person responsible for petty cash will not be able to balance the fund.

COMMON PERIODIC FINANCIAL REPORTS

Financial summaries are compiled monthly and annually. They may be prepared either by the medical assistant manually or on the computer or by the accountant. Common summary reports include the following:

- Statement of income and expense
- Cash flow statement
- Trial balance
- Accounts receivable trial balance and aging analysis
- Balance sheet

The **statement of income and expense**, also known as the *profit and loss statement,* covers a specific period. It lists all the income received and all expenses paid during the period. The total income is called *gross income* or *earnings.* The income after deduction of all expenses is the *net income.*

A **cash flow statement** starts with the amount of cash on hand at the beginning of the month (or for any specified period). It then lists the cash income and the cash disbursement made throughout the period and concludes with a statement of the amount of cash remaining on hand at the end of the period.

A trial balance is necessary to determine that the books are in balance. All the columns in the disbursements journal must be totaled at the end of the month. The combined totals of all the expense columns must equal the total of the checks written. If the figures do not balance, recheck every entry until the error is found.

The **accounts receivable trial balance** is done before the monthly statements are sent out. First, record the total of the accounts receivable ledger at the end of the previous month; then add the charges for the current month and subtract the adjustments and the payments received. The remainder should equal the total of the accounts receivable ledger at the end of the current month.

The **balance sheet**, also known as a *statement of financial condition,* shows the financial picture of the practice on a specific date. Often it is done only once a year. The balance sheet is set up using the following accounting equation:

$$\text{Assets} = \text{Liabilities} + \text{Proprietorship}$$

The title of the statement had its origin in the equality of the elements: the balance between the sum of the assets and the sum of the liabilities and proprietorship. An aging analysis shows the amount of outstanding receipts in aging groups, such as current, 30 days, 60 days, 90 days, and 120 days.

At the end of the accounting year, it is very simple to combine the monthly reports to compile the annual summaries. The annual summaries simplify the reporting of income for tax returns.

RECENT LEGISLATION FOR SMALL BUSINESSES AND THEIR EXPENSES

Several new laws have been passed that relate to the small business and its financial accounting. First, as of January 1, 2013, the amount allowed for mileage is 56.5¢ for business miles driven. This rate fluctuates, depending on the cost of fuel, and has been changed midyear on some occasions. Employees are allowed 24¢ for driving when the purpose is medically related. Charitable organizations can claim 14 cents per mile when driving for business reasons.

PAYROLL RECORDS

Handling payroll records, whether for one employee or dozens of employees, involves frequent reporting activities (Procedure 24-4). Government regulations require the withholding of taxes from employees and payment of certain taxes by both employees and employers. To comply with government regulations, complete records must be kept for every employee. All records of employment taxes must be kept for at least 4 years. These should be available for review by the IRS. These records include:

- Social Security number of the employee
- Number of withholding allowances claimed
- Amount of gross salary
- All deductions for Social Security and Medicare taxes; federal, state, and city or other subdivision withholding taxes; state disability insurance; and state unemployment tax, where applicable

CRITICAL THINKING APPLICATION   24-6

On Friday Brenda hired a new employee, who reported to work on Monday. The new employee states that she cannot produce her Social Security card. Can Brenda allow the individual to work? How can Brenda verify a Social Security number?

Payroll Reporting Forms

Each employee and each employer must have a tax identification number. The Social Security number is the employee's tax identification number. Any person who does not have a Social Security number should apply for one, using Form SS-5, available online or from any Social Security Administration office.

The employer applies for a number for federal tax accounting purposes using Form SS-4, available at Social Security Administration offices. In states that require employer reports, a state employer number must also be obtained. This number is called the *employer identification number (*EIN) (formerly called the tax identification number).

PROCEDURE 24-4

Process an Employee Payroll

GOAL: *To process payroll to compensate employees and make accurate deductions.*

EQUIPMENT and SUPPLIES

- Checkbook
- Computer and payroll software, if applicable
- Pen
- Tax withholding tables
- Federal Employers Tax Guide

PROCEDURAL STEPS

1. Make sure all information and paperwork have been collected from the employees, including a copy of the Social Security card, a W-4 form, and an I-9 form.
   PURPOSE: To make sure the employee is eligible to work in the United States and to determine the withholding amounts to deduct from paychecks.
2. Review the time cards for all employees. Determine whether any employees need counseling because of late arrivals or habitual absences.
   PURPOSE: To address problems immediately and help correct habits that can lead to employee termination.

3. Figure the salary or hourly wages due the employee for the period worked.
   PURPOSE: To ascertain the amount owed to the employee.
4. Figure the deductions that must be taken from the paycheck. These usually include but are not limited to:
   - Federal, state, and local taxes
   - Social Security withholdings
   - Medicare withholdings
   - Other deductions (e.g., insurance, savings, and so on)
   - Donations to organizations, such as the United Way
   PURPOSE: To comply with federal, state, and local laws and deduct amounts for insurance, savings plans, and so on.
5. Write the check for the balance due the employee. Most software can print the checks and explanations of deductions.
6. Have employees sign for their paychecks if that is the office policy.
   NOTE: Make certain that the person is not an independent contractor, in which case a 1099 Form (IRS) should be issued.

Before the end of the first pay period, the employee should complete an Employee's Withholding Allowance Certificate (Form W-4) showing the number of withholding allowances claimed. Otherwise, the employer must indicate withholding on the basis of a single person with no exemptions.

The employee should complete a new form when changes occur in marital status or in the number of allowances claimed. Each employee is entitled to one personal allowance and one for each qualified dependent. Because employees can claim allowances based on their job situation, being the head of the household, and having dependent care expenses totaling more than $1,500, they may find that their allowances equal more than just a personal exemption and an exemption for their dependents. However, employees should be warned to take care in listing too many allowances, because this affects the amount of tax taken from their paycheck. If too little tax is taken out during the year, the employee may owe a significant amount of money to the IRS the following year.

The employee may elect to take fewer or no allowances, in which case the tax withheld will be greater and a refund may be due when the employee's annual tax report is filed. If an employee claims more than 10 withholding allowances or an exemption from withholding and his or her wages would normally be more than $200 per week, the employer is required to send copies of these W-4 forms to the IRS.

A supply of all the necessary forms for filing federal returns, preprinted with the employer's name, will be furnished to an employer who has applied for an employer identification number. Extra forms may be obtained from the IRS office.

> ### CRITICAL THINKING APPLICATION   24-7
> - Mr. Schmidt has explained to Brenda that the more withholding deductions an employee claims, the less tax is taken from the paycheck. If Brenda's new employee wants to claim seven deductions and she has only three children and is single, can she do so legally? Why or why not?
> - Why might it be risky to claim all the deductions to which a person is legally entitled?

Income Tax Withholding

Employers are required by law to withhold certain amounts from employees' earnings. These amounts must be reported and forwarded to the IRS to be applied toward payment of income tax. The amount to be withheld is based on:

- Total earnings of the employee
- Number of withholding allowances claimed
- Marital status of the employee
- Length of the pay period involved

The Federal Employer's Tax Guide includes tables to be used in determining the amount to be withheld. One table is for single people and unmarried heads of households and one is for married individuals. The tables cover monthly, semimonthly, biweekly, weekly, and daily or miscellaneous periods.

Employers Income Tax

A physician practicing as an individual is not subject to withholding tax but is expected to make an estimated tax payment four times a year. The accountant prepares four copies of Form 1040-S, Declaration of Estimated Tax for Individuals, for the ensuing year when the annual income tax return is prepared. The first form and the quarterly estimated tax for the next year are filed at the same time as the tax return. The remaining three forms, with the estimated tax due, must be filed on June 15, September 15, and January 15. It may be the business manager's responsibility to see that these returns are filed when due. The employer also contributes to Social Security and Medicare in the form of a self-employment tax.

Social Security, Medicare, and Income Tax Withholding

The Federal Insurance Contributions Act (FICA) provides for a federal system of old age, survivors, disability, and hospital insurance. The tax rate is reviewed frequently and is subject to change by Congress. As of 2009, the wage base for Social Security tax was $113,700 and the tax rate was 6.2% each for employers and employees. All wages are subject to the Medicare tax at a rate of 1.45% each for both employees and employers.

Quarterly Returns

Each quarter of the year, all employers subject to income tax withholding (including withholding on sick pay and supplemental unemployment benefits) of Social Security and Medicare taxes must file an Employer's Quarterly Federal Tax Return (Form 941) on or before the last day of the first month after the end of the quarter. Due dates for this return and full payment of the tax are April 30, July 31, October 31, and January 31. If deposits equaling full payment of taxes due have been made, the due date for the return is extended 10 days.

Annual Returns

The employer is required to furnish two copies of Form W-2, the Wage and Tax Statement, to each employee from whom income tax or Social Security tax has been withheld or from whom income tax would have been withheld if the employee had claimed no more than one withholding allowance. The forms should be given to employees by January 31. If employment ends before December 31, the employer may give the W-2 form to the terminated employee any time after employment ends. If the employee asks for Form W-2, the employer should give the employee the completed copies within 30 days of the request or the final wage payment, whichever is later.

Employers must file Form W-3, the Transmittal of Income and Tax Statement, annually to transmit wage and income tax withheld statements (Form W-2) to the Social Security Administration. These forms are processed by the Social Security Administration, which furnishes the IRS with the income tax data that it needs from those forms. Form W-3 and its attachments must be filed separately from Form 941 on or before the last day of February after the calendar year for which the W-2 forms are prepared.

Federal Unemployment Tax

Employers also contribute under the Federal Unemployment Tax Act (FUTA). Generally, credit can be taken against the FUTA tax for amounts paid into a state unemployment fund up to a certain percentage. Employers are responsible for paying the FUTA tax; it must not be deducted from employees' wages. For 2012 the FUTA tax was 6.2% of the first $7,000 in wages paid to each employee during the calendar year.

For deposit purposes, the FUTA tax is figured quarterly, and any amount due must be paid by the last day of the first month after the quarter ends. The formula for determining the amount due is set forth in the Federal Employer's Tax Guide.

An annual FUTA return must be filed on Form 940, Employer's Annual Federal Unemployment Tax Act (FUTA) Tax Return, on or before January 31 following the close of the calendar year for which the tax is due. Any tax still due is payable with the return. Form 940 may be filed on or before February 10 after the close of the year if all required deposits were made on time and if full payment of the tax due is deposited on or before January 31.

State Unemployment Taxes

All the states and the District of Columbia have unemployment compensation laws. In most states, the tax is imposed only on the employer, but a few states require employers to withhold a percentage of wages for unemployment compensation benefits. An employer may be subject to federal unemployment tax and not subject to state unemployment tax. In some states, for instance, an employer with fewer than four employees is not subject to the state unemployment tax. The regulations for a specific state should be checked.

State Disability Insurance

Some states require employees to be covered by disability or sick pay insurance. The employer may be required to withhold a certain amount from the employee's salary to pay for this insurance.

Budgets

Growing businesses must develop budgets that aid the planning of finances over a certain period. Medical offices should establish a new budget before the beginning of each fiscal year. The best way to begin a budget is to look at the expenses from the previous year (Figure 24-2). These expenses should be divided into categories, then a total should be derived for each category. Each month should represent

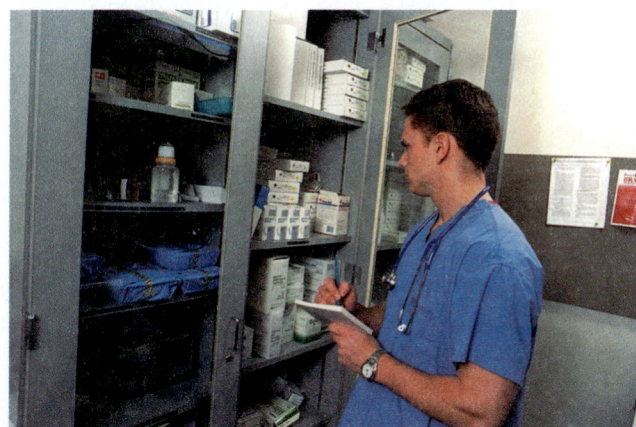

FIGURE 24-2 Inventory supplies and equipment before developing the annual budget. Once a good inventory has been completed, more accurate projections can be made for the expenses for the coming year.

approximately $\frac{1}{12}$ of the total budget, not including large capital expenses.

In the individual categories, examine expenses for those that could be eliminated or those that were under budget. For example, if $3,345 was spent on office supplies and the budget was $3,000, either more money needs to be allotted for this category or cuts in spending are necessary. If $3,345 was spent and the budget was $4,000, the excess may be placed in another category for the next year. Even quarterly and semiannual expenses should be annualized and then divided by 12 to obtain a monthly expense amount.

CRITICAL THINKING APPLICATION   24-8

- Brenda has developed a preliminary budget for next year. She realizes that several pieces of equipment need to be replaced. However, Dr. Wilkins has said she does not want to make any capital purchases over the next 2 years. How might Brenda approach Dr. Wilkins about the needed equipment?
- How might leasing equipment benefit the office? How can Brenda determine whether this would be more or less expensive than purchasing the equipment?

By monitoring expenses on a monthly basis, the physician can see whether the facility is over budget, under budget, or right on target. Categories in which overspending has occurred can be reconciled by taking funds from another category (e.g., category B) and adding them to the overspent category (category A). However, the amount taken must be subtracted from category B and added to category A. Those subtracted funds are no longer available in category B. Specific notes should be kept when categories are overspent so that an adjustment can be made for the next fiscal year.

The following categories should be considered for the physician's operating budget:

- Insurance
- Rent
- Depreciation
- Loan payments
- Advertising and promotions
- Legal and accounting
- Miscellaneous expenses
- Supplies
- Salaries and wages
- Utilities
- Dues, subscriptions, and fees
- Taxes
- Repairs and maintenance
- Medical equipment
- Administrative equipment
- Medication and pharmacy expenses

The physician should investigate whether leasing equipment might be a better option for the facility. Some leasing programs are very progressive and provide service contracts at no additional cost. Because depreciation costs are high, leasing might be the best answer to a new equipment need.

Insurance

Insurance coverage is one of the physician's major expenses. Almost every physician carries some type of malpractice insurance for protection against the cost of legal liabilities. Property and fire insurance are mandatory, and most physicians carry workers' compensation insurance to cover employee injuries and accidents. The medical assistant may be asked to shop for the best insurance rates at the time of renewals.

CLOSING COMMENTS

The physician comes to rely heavily on the person who manages the office's finances. It is important that this individual keep information confidential. The entire staff must be conscious of the costs involved in operating a medical office and should adhere to their respective budgets as closely as possible. The physician then may be willing to spend more money on pay increases and benefits to reward employees.

All office employees must attempt to save money and resources wherever possible. Medicare plays a pivotal role in a physician's income. For example, Medicare has recently cut costs for certain cardiovascular services, such as stress tests and echocardiograms, up to 35% to 40%. Private insurers usually follow Medicare's lead when determining their own costs, Medicare reimbursements are calculated according to a formula based on the current status of the economy; therefore, when the economy is poor, reimbursements to physicians go down, but medical equipment and supply costs continue to rise. Because reimbursements are critical to the physician's income, some doctors are forced out of medicine, leaving a gap in the availability of medical services to the community.

Patient Education

In some cases patients may not fully understand the costs involved in providing high-quality medical care. The medical assistant may need to educate the patient about the basic costs involved with the procedures performed in the office. Patients do not need a lengthy explanation but may be set more at ease by knowing that the physician does not set fees arbitrarily. The physician's office is a small business, like thousands of other small businesses, and should be able to pay its overhead and expenses.

Legal and Ethical Issues

A person who keeps financial records holds a position of great trust and responsibility. Some physicians require the person placed in charge of the office finances to be *bonded*. This means that the facility has done a security check on the individual and the person was found worthy to be placed in a position of responsibility. A bond is issued by an entity on behalf of a second party, guaranteeing that the second party will fulfill an obligation or series of obligations to a third party. In the event that the obligations are not met, the third party recovers its losses via the bond.

Records must be accurate and completed on a daily basis. Daily journals should be kept indefinitely to support tax returns.

SUMMARY OF SCENARIO

Brenda has learned much about the financial management of a physician's office. She is never hesitant to call the practice accountant, Mr. Schmidt, whenever a question arises. As she gains more experience, she comes to understand the budgeting process, cost management, and the various methods of accounting practice.

Many factors can affect the finances of a medical practice. However, a physician who is fairly conservative about spending and careful with investments likely will do well as a member of the community's healthcare professionals. Dr. Wilkins lives by this philosophy and also encourages her employees to manage money wisely. This attitude among the staff members promotes a sense of teamwork and cooperation for the benefit of all.

SUMMARY OF LEARNING OBJECTIVES

1. **Define, spell, and pronounce the terms listed in the vocabulary.**
   Spelling and pronouncing medical terms correctly bolster the medical assistant's credibility. Knowing the definition of these terms promotes confidence in communication with patients and co-workers.

2. **List the four items all financial records should show at any given time.**
   (1) How much was earned in a given period, (2) how much was collected, (3) how much is owed, and (4) the distribution of expenses incurred.

3. **Describe how to establish and maintain a petty cash fund.**
   Most offices pay for small, incidental expenses with petty cash. The process for maintaining a petty cash fund is outlined in Procedure 24-3.

4. **Differentiate between accounts payable and accounts receivable.**
   Accounts payable refers to the amounts of money owed by a business and not yet paid; *accounts receivable* refers to amounts owed to the business that are not yet paid.

5. **Explain the difference between a single-entry and a double-entry accounting system.**
   The single-entry accounting system uses three basic records: the general journal, the cash payment journal, and the accounts receivable ledger. The general journal is a record (e.g., a day sheet) in which transactions are recorded. The cash payment journal in its simplest form is a record (e.g., a checkbook) that is used to make payments. The accounts receivable ledger provides information about the amounts owed to the physician. The double-entry system, which is more difficult to use than the single-entry system, requires an entry on each side of the accounting equation, and each side must always balance.

6. **Explain the importance of a trial balance.**
   A trial balance reflects discrepancies between the journal and the ledger. It does not reveal errors in the individual accounts but shows errors in the overall balances of accounts.

7. **Describe common periodic financial reports.**
   Five common reports are used for accounting in the small business office: (1) the statement of income and expense (lists all the income received and all expenses paid during a set period), (2) the cash flow statement (lists cash income and cash disbursement made during a period, noting the beginning and ending balances on hand), (3) the trial balance (determines whether all of the books are in balance), (4) the accounts receivable trial balance (an equation that double checks the total of all A/R prior to sending monthly statements), and (5) the balance sheet (depicts the financial picture of the practice on a specific date).

8. **Explain how to process an employee payroll accurately.**
   Employee payroll is an essential function related to practice finances. The process for employee payrolls is outlined in Procedure 24-4.

9. **Explain the purpose of Form W-4.**
   The Employee's Withholding Allowance Certificate, or Form W-4, specifies the number of withholding allowances the employee is claiming. The more allowances claimed, the less money is taken from the employee's paycheck.

10. **State the types of employment records required by the Internal Revenue Service (IRS).**
    The IRS requires that several employment records be kept for at least 4 years: the employee's Social Security number; the number of withholding allowances claimed; the amount of gross salary; all deductions for Social Security and Medicare taxes; federal, state, and city or other subdivision withholding taxes; state disability insurance; and state unemployment tax.

11. **Discuss the basis for the withholding amounts taken from employees' earnings.**
    Several deductions are taken from the employee's wages as required by law. They are based on the employee's total earnings, the number of withholding allowances claimed, the employee's marital status, and the length of the pay period involved. The wage base for Social Security tax currently is $106,800.

12. **Explain the requirements of the Federal Insurance Contributions Act (FICA).**
    FICA requires that a certain amount be deducted from an employee's wages and designated for Medicare and Social Security programs. The current percentages are 1.45% for the Medicare contribution and 6.2% for Social Security. Both the employer and the employee contribute these amounts.

13. **Discuss the importance of setting a budget each fiscal year.**
    The physician's office must set a budget each fiscal year to prepare for all the expenses involved in running the office. Without a well-planned budget, the physician cannot control expenses. The expenditures from the past year should be evaluated when planning the new budget, paying particular attention to the expense categories that exceeded expected amounts.

CONNECTIONS

Study Guide Connection: Go to the Chapter 24 Study Guide. Read and complete the activities.

Evolve Connection: Go to the Chapter 24 link at *evolve.elsevier.com/kinn* to complete the Chapter Review and Chapter Quiz. Check out the other resources listed for this chapter to make the most of what you have learned from Financial and Practice Management.

25

MEDICAL PRACTICE MANAGEMENT AND HUMAN RESOURCES

SCENARIO

Katherine Martinson is the office manager for Dr. Michael Collins, a family practitioner in a group practice in a metropolitan area. The office usually carries a full schedule of patients each day. Katherine has been instrumental in the seamless operation of the facility. Before joining Dr. Collins, Katherine worked for a physician in the same group of doctors, Dr. Grant Bradley, who retired last year. She worked as an administrative medical assistant for 6 years before that. Her strength and ability to motivate employees led Dr. Collins to approach her about becoming his office manager once Dr. Bradley retired.

Katherine is a consummate professional, but she knows the importance of treating each employee as an individual. At weekly staff meetings, the employees offer input on the various procedures followed in the office. Katherine regularly consults with the staff members and always asks for input as to how the office can function more effectively. She implements many of the staff members' suggestions in the day-to-day activities of the office. She knows that employees need to feel a part of the team, and by trying the procedures others suggest, she validates them as an asset to the facility.

When a position is open, Katherine is careful about whom she hires, always checking at least three references per applicant and verifying each previous place of employment. She trains each employee in every aspect of the job and keeps checklists that reflect that the employee has been given instruction in certain skills.

Katherine makes sure each person has the tools needed to do his or her job. She also explains overhead costs to employees and helps them understand what is involved in the daily operation of the practice. With this information, the employees are more conservative about using supplies and more careful with equipment. Major changes are presented to the entire staff, and although Dr. Collins makes the final decision, he and Katherine seek the input of the employees. The cooperative attitude between management and the employees of the office provides a good atmosphere for teamwork, and Katherine and the physician are pleased with the results.

While studying this chapter, think about the following questions:

- How friendly should office managers become with the staff members?
- Why is checking references important when hiring a new staff member?
- How should negative employee evaluations be handled?
- How can the office manager promote an atmosphere of teamwork?

LEARNING OBJECTIVES

1. Define, spell, and pronounce the terms listed in the vocabulary.
2. Explain the importance of management in the medical office.
3. Discuss the desirable qualities of a medical office manager.
4. List and discuss the three types of leaders.
5. Discuss several types of power and whether power is a positive or negative entity.
6. Identify several ways in which employees are motivated.
7. Explain the difference between intrinsic and extrinsic motivation.
8. List several ways to prevent burnout.
9. Discuss what to look for when reviewing resumés and applications.
10. Explain why the telephone voice of an applicant is important.
11. List and discuss legal and illegal interview questions.
12. Identify the follow-up activities the office manager should perform after an interview.
13. Explain the importance of mentors for new employees in the medical office.
14. Describe how to conduct a performance review for an employee.
15. List the various types of staff meetings.
16. Explain how to arrange a group meeting.

VOCABULARY

advocate A person who defends or pleads the cause of another; one that supports or promotes the interests of another.

affable Pleasant and at ease in talking to others; characterized by ease and friendliness.

agenda (ah-jen'-duh) A list or outline of things to be considered or done.

ancillary (an'-suh-ler-e) Subordinate; auxiliary.

appraisal An expert judgment of the value or merit of; judgment as to quality.

blatant Completely obvious, conspicuous, or obtrusive, especially in a crass or offensive manner; brazen.

burnout Exhaustion of physical or emotional strength or motivation, usually as a result of prolonged stress or frustration.

chain of command A series of executive positions in order of authority.

cohesive Sticking together tightly; exhibiting or producing cohesion.

disparaging (dis-pahr'-uh-jing) Slighting; having a negative or degrading tone.

embezzlement Stealing from an employer; to appropriate goods, services, or funds for personal use without permission.

extrinsic (eks-trin'-zik) External to a thing, its essential nature, or its original character.

impenetrable Incapable of being penetrated or pierced; not capable of being damaged or harmed.

incentives Things that incite or spur to action; rewards or reasons for performing a task.

liaison A close bond or connection; a person with a connection, contract, link, or conspiracy with another person or group.

mentors Trusted counselors or guides.

meticulous (meh-tiku'-luhs) Marked by extreme or excessive care in the consideration or treatment of details.

micromanage To manage with great or excessive control or attention to details.

motivation The process of inciting a person to some action or behavior.

quackery practicing or pretending to have the ability to cure or treat a patient without qualifications to do so.

reprimands Criticisms for a fault; severe or formal reproofs.

retention The act of keeping in possession or use; keeping in one's pay or service.

subordinate Submissive to or controlled by authority; placed in or occupying a lower class, rank, or position.

targeted Directed or used toward a target; directed toward a specific desire or position.

The management of a professional medical office can greatly influence the success of the operation. Good management allows the physician to see and treat patients in a functional environment with the confidence that the business side of the facility is operating as it should be. A well-managed office is not something that just happens. Great effort and teamwork are necessary to ensure that the day-to-day activities are carried out efficiently and that the many details needing attention are handled expeditiously.

Although most medical assistants do not enter office management right after graduation, they certainly want to succeed and to advance their career. The information in this chapter can help the medical assistant understand what makes a good manager. Those traits can be developed as a new employee after graduation. Additionally, the medical assistant will learn the employment process from the office manager's point of view. This information also is valuable to a new medical assistant who is applying for a position. By studying office management, the medical assistant prepares for future management positions, but also learns to see both sides of the coin and understand why managers make certain decisions and enact policies.

TODAY'S OFFICE MANAGERS

The office manager in today's medical facilities must be versatile and able to perform several tasks at one time. The office manager is responsible for many more duties if the office is small and has a smaller patient load. These professionals must know how to complete almost all the tasks in the office and have good people management skills. In larger offices, human resources duties may be performed by a separate office, or an accountant may take care of all financial management issues. However, the more duties the office manager can perform, the more valuable he or she is to the clinic. Always be open to learning management duties, because taking on management positions usually results in an increase in salary and benefits. A sharp medical assistant who is ready to learn will advance quickly and find a variety of opportunities in the healthcare industry.

WHO'S IN CHARGE?

If the office has only one medical assistant, that person must be able to assume many management responsibilities with cooperation from the physician. When the office has two medical assistants, one administrative and one clinical, the administrative medical assistant often is expected to assume management duties. In an office with a larger staff, a **chain of command** must be established.

A facility with three or more employees should designate one person as supervisor or office manager. This individual needs management skills and the ability to deal with personnel matters. Other employees answer to the office manager, and the office manager answers to the physician or physicians. A chain of command allows the office staff to consult with the physician regarding administrative or clinical problems, complaints, or grievances; however, it prompts employees to allow individuals whom the physician has placed in charge to have the first opportunity to solve problems. It also allows the physician to check on the operation of the office, disseminate information on policy changes, and correct errors or grievances by dealing with one person instead of all employees.

QUALITIES OF AN EFFECTIVE MANAGER

- Uses good judgment
- Has good health
- Has the ability to organize
- Is willing to learn
- Possesses original ideas
- Has leadership ability
- Is fair with all employees
- Is flexible
- Has a sense of fairness
- Cares about employees
- Remains calm during crises
- Is open to constructive criticism
- Has good communication skills
- Uses good listening skills
- Is approachable

A medical assisting career is challenging and offers great opportunities for advancement. A recently graduated medical assistant, whose first position may have been as a receptionist, can be given more responsibilities based on good work and eventually may become the office manager of a large staff.

Management problems often can be prevented by defining carefully the areas of authority and the responsibilities of each employee. Many physicians say that friction among workers is their most common personnel problem. The importance of the chain of command cannot be overemphasized, and the physician must not undermine the office manager's authority by circumvention. When employees know what is expected of them, they can plan both their daily and long-term work more effectively.

Duties of the Medical Office Manager

The duties performed by medical office managers vary from place to place and practice to practice. Some physicians take a much more active role in office management than others. The best management plan for the physician is to hire a trustworthy, reliable office manager and then allow the person to run the business aspects of the office. This frees the physician to concentrate on taking care of patients.

Some of the tasks performed by the medical office manager include:

- Preparing and updating the policies and procedures manuals
- Making sure employees follow the policies and procedures manuals
- Developing job descriptions
- Recruiting new employees
- Performing orientation and training
- Conducting performance and salary reviews
- Dismissing employees
- Planning staff meetings
- Maintaining staff harmony
- Establishing work flow guidelines

- Ensuring compliance with all federal and state regulations
- Improving office efficiency
- Supervising the purchase and care of equipment
- Educating patients
- Eliminating time-wasting tasks for the physician
- Marketing the practice
- Performing customer service

Office management can best be accomplished by developing a thorough office policy and procedures manual and then enforcing its contents except in extraordinary circumstances. This is discussed later in the chapter.

The Power of Influence

Managers have a great deal of influence over the people they supervise. A successful manager must be interested in people and enjoy working with them on a daily basis. It is said that if one helps others get what they want in life, the individual usually also gets what he or she wants. An effective manager discovers the **motivation** behind employees' drives to be a part of the profession in which they are employed and then helps them achieve their individual goals. In turn, most employees are enthusiastic about working toward the facility's goals as a productive team member.

Successful managers know that their employees should be encouraged to perform at optimum levels, and they are confident enough in their own skills to give credit to employees who develop ideas and concepts for the team. These managers know how to let their employees help them "look good." A manager with a group of outstanding employees usually is looked on as an effective leader.

CRITICAL THINKING APPLICATION 25-1

When Katherine began as Dr. Collins' office manager, she found several supportive employees, but a few were concerned about their new boss. How can a new manager help employees be at ease during the first few weeks?

The Manager as a Leader

Leaders nurture other people. They take the time to discover what makes people tick and then give them opportunities that will help them rise to new levels of responsibility. Leaders have a strong belief in people, and they express confidence in their abilities, seeing them as successes rather than failures. Often this belief exists before people prove themselves, and that provides motivation for them to reach their potential.

Perhaps most important, leaders listen to their people. Few things are more frustrating than an employee attempting to talk to a manager who is working on some project or typing on the computer. Listening involves eye contact and questions to ensure that the employee is understood. Being willing to take the time to listen is a step toward success as a manager.

Instead of sitting across from employees at a desk, try sitting beside them in the chairs that are usually placed in front of a desk. When discussing issues with employees, this simple change in position places the office manager on an equal plane with the employee and implies more of a team effort. At times this positioning might be inappropriate, such as during discussions about disciplinary matters. Still, when attempting to get an employee to cooperate or come over to the office manager's way of thinking, position can play a large role in getting people "on the same page."

Types of Leaders

The three basic types of leaders are the charismatic leader, the transactional leader, and the transformational leader. Each has positive qualities, and all can be successful in business.

Charismatic leaders have a special way of inspiring an unswerving allegiance and devotion from their followers. They encourage people to overcome great obstacles and buy into their vision for the organization or business. They also tend to trust people in **subordinate** positions and earn trust in return.

Transactional leaders are structured and organized. They make sure their subordinates understand their duties and roles. These leaders are fair and provide rewards when they have been earned. The transactional leader is hardworking, a planner, and strict about budgets and time frames.

Transformational leaders are innovative and able to bring about change in an organization. These leaders are relationship builders. They stress shared values and strive to create a common ground among team members. Transformational leaders are the most effective when an organization is experiencing change and reorganization.

Styles of Management

Some managers are democratic and willing to listen to employees. These managers are fair-minded and ask the opinions of the staff when making decisions. In contrast, the autocratic manager is more of a dictator, making demands and insisting that tasks be done in a certain way—his or her way. The laissez-faire manager is easygoing and does not make a lot of demands on employees. This is a "go with the flow" manager who lets employees work on their own and does not **micromanage**.

Theories X, Y, and Z

Douglas McGregor, an American social psychologist, developed Theory X and Theory Y to distinguish two types of management. His book, *The Human Side of Enterprise,* published in 1960, explains these management types. In 1981, William Ouchi offered his own management theory, calling it Theory Z.

All these theories include several assumptions. Theory X, for example, suggests that humans dislike working and avoid it whenever possible. Because it is unpleasant, management must push, coerce, or threaten workers to do their jobs. Workers, according to Theory X, do not like responsibility and prefer to be directed than to lead. McGregor says that Theory X is applied best to large-scale employers, such as those involved in factories or manufacturing. Theory X is considered "hard" management.

Theory Y is virtually the opposite of Theory X. Theory Y holds that people enjoy work and that it is a normal component of life, as are rest and play. McGregor says that these humans, when motivated, work toward the goals of the organization. People seek and accept responsibility, enjoy job satisfaction, and are imaginative and creative. Theory Y applies to workers such as managers and other professionals. Theory Y is considered "soft" management.

Ouchi's Theory Z is a combination of American and Japanese management theories. Theory Z considers characteristics such as long-term employment, collective decision making, individual responsibility, and a holistic view of the employee and his or her family.

Maslow's Hierarchy of Needs

Maslow's hierarchy of needs, first discussed in the chapter on communications, also can be applied to management. The triangle of needs begins with physiologic needs (air, food, water, sleep) and safety needs. Moving upward, social needs and then esteem needs are addressed. The last need is self-actualization.

In the workplace, physiologic needs are met with lunch breaks, rest times, and days off. The worker's salary helps the person meet other physiologic needs, such as shelter. Safety needs are addressed in this theory as having a safe place to work and a sense of security through savings, health insurance, and retirement programs. Social needs are met through interaction with co-workers, working as a team, and enjoying the work family at events away from the office. Needs related to esteem include feeling appreciated, valued, and being recognized for good work. Continuing to set higher goals and working to reach them are steps toward self-actualization.

Frederick Herzberg believed that job enrichment had to exist for a worker to be motivated. He theorized that several factors affect job satisfaction, some negative and some positive. The six factors that can lead to job dissatisfaction include:

- Company policy
- Supervision
- Relationship with supervisors
- Work conditions
- Salary
- Relationship with co-workers

The six factors that lead to job satisfaction include:

- Achievement
- Recognition
- The work product
- Responsibility
- Advancement
- Growth

In his book, *The Motivation to Work,* Herzberg states three points:

1. Jobs must be satisfying and must motivate employees to grow and reach their full capabilities.
2. Employees who show greater ability should be given more responsibility.
3. If the job does not allow the employee to use his or her full ability, a different employee who can grow and find motivation in the work should be placed in that position.

These are only a few of the many theories about employment and management. The theory of management by objectives suggests that goal setting serves as a basis for greater job efficiency and better employee motivation and commitment and that it leads to planning for results instead of just planning to work. Some managers believe in the theory of management by walking around, which suggests that the more visible and engaged the manager is with his or her employees, the more productive they will be. Supervisors develop and modify their management style as they gain more experience. The medical assistant who understands the type of manager he or she has may find it easier to understand the manager's actions and preferences. This realization can lead to better job performance and promotions for the medical assistant.

Leading During Transitions and Change

Change is a part of the life of every person and every business. Most people initially are hesitant to face change, and many people try to avoid it completely. However, a business cannot experience growth without change. The manager who can lead subordinates through periods of change is a valuable asset to the organization. Employees need guidance on maintaining focus on the tasks at hand. The manager should remain visible to employees during times of change and communicate frequently through status reports and updates on policies and procedures.

The book *Who Moved My Cheese?* by Spencer Johnson, MD, is an innovative story that all managers should read. Any manager or employee experiencing a time of change should study this simple, short book. The opening quotes renowned author A.J. Cronin:

"Life is no straight and easy corridor along which we travel free and unhampered, but a maze of passages, through which we must seek our way, lost and confused, now and again checked in a blind alley. But always, if we have faith, a door will open for us, not perhaps one that we ourselves would ever have thought of, but one that will ultimately prove good for us."

Who Moved My Cheese? stresses several points about change that the good manager should remember:

- Change happens.
- Anticipate change.
- Monitor change.
- Adapt to change quickly.
- Move with the change.
- Enjoy change.
- Be ready to change again quickly and enjoy it again.

The simplicity of this advice does not diminish its truth. Change happens in everyone's job and personal life. Those who learn to adapt quickly and move forward do not become casualties of change.

The Role of Power

Power is the ability to influence employees so that they carry out their directives. Leaders use many types of power.

- *Coercive power* is manipulative, and the leader often makes threats or uses fear to accomplish goals. The fear of losing a job is a manipulation of power.
- *Granting rewards* is a more positive use of power. When the leader is able to give employees some type of reward for a job well done, most employees strive to reach their goals.
- *Expert power* is a factor when the leader is knowledgeable about a subject. Employees respect leaders who know their job and how things should be done. Most people look up to a person who has a high degree of knowledge about a given subject. Employees frequently are frustrated when they must work for someone who knows nothing about procedures or the service offered.
- *Legitimate power* is that of position or status. It does not really matter who the president of the United States is; the office itself carries the weight of power. Therefore, the individual who serves as president holds legitimate power.

- *Referent power* is granted from subordinates to those who lead by example. It is a power based on the admiration of the leader. Mentors, parents, and teachers often are the objects of referent power.

CRITICAL THINKING APPLICATION   **25-2**

- Katherine is a respected office manager in the office where she works, but several other managers in the office building are not as well liked. What makes a strong, effective office manager?
- Everyone has worked for at least one supervisor whom they did not like. What traits make a poor office manager?

Abuse of Power and Authority

Unfortunately, many managers may abuse the power they have. A manager who puts up barriers and erects emotional walls with employees has difficulty forming a **cohesive** team. Some managers use other people as tools to get what they want, and other managers stick to their own level or stature, relating only to the inner circle of decision makers in the facility.

When an organization has no checks and balances, power is easily abused. Working with a manager who cannot look inside himself or herself and see mistakes is difficult. Some managers stress rules and conformity, leaving no gray areas where subordinates are concerned. Some show a false humility and pretend to care, but most employees can see right through this half-effort at a relationship. Others only hire "yes" people, who agree with everything the manager says. All these are abuses of power and indications of a poor manager.

The Power of Motivation

A number of factors can motivate a person to reach a goal, including:

- A challenge
- Money
- Praise
- Satisfaction
- Freedom
- Fear
- Family
- Insecurity
- Competition
- Fulfillment
- Integrity
- Honor
- Reputation
- Responsibility
- Prestige
- Needs
- Love

Any of these motivators can prompt an employee to action. There are two general types of motivation. *Intrinsic motivation* is internal, or originates within a person. Intrinsic motivation is long term and can be focused toward a lifelong goal. **Extrinsic** *motivation* is external and more material in nature. Generally, extrinsic motivation is more short lived and less satisfying than intrinsic motivation.

CRITICAL THINKING APPLICATION 25-3

- Katherine knows that employees have different reasons and motivations for working. Some must work to help support their families, and others work simply because of a love for their field. How can Katherine discover her employees' motivations for working?
- How does this knowledge benefit the office manager?
- Can this knowledge help Katherine achieve her goals?

THE NEW OFFICE MANAGER

The medical assistant will encounter various reactions when entering a facility as the new office manager. Often, he or she will face negative reactions from employees. They may have felt an intense loyalty to the previous manager and may resent that the person was terminated, or they may have settled into a routine with an office manager they had had for many years. As mentioned earlier, most individuals resist change, and getting accustomed to a new supervisor can be extremely stressful. A new office manager wants to create a positive work environment; therefore, he or she must find ways to win the support of current employees.

The first thing a new office manager can do to begin garnering support is nothing. Never storm into an office and begin making radical changes in the first few days. Always observe for at least a few weeks and make notes about problem areas. Then, meet with the physician and share the information observed and present a plan for changes. Ask for the physician's input, because he or she may know the history of difficult situations and can provide guidance in moving forward with plans for change.

After discussing these plans with the physician, use strategy when attempting to move employees toward achieving office goals. Schedule individual meetings with employees and allow them to tell you three things they like about their jobs, three things they dislike, and three things they need to do their jobs more effectively. Surprisingly, the employee may need only a truly insignificant item, such as his or her own box of file folders or a stapler that works with larger stacks of paper.

Once all the meetings have been held, review the information the employees provided and create a plan of action. The information provides a preliminary road map for management, because the employees' responses give the new manager an excellent idea about what is important to them and where the problem areas are in the office. Also, choose one item from each employee's list of what they need to do their job more effectively and obtain it within 1 week of the interviews. Employees will be impressed that the new manager is interested in their opinions and wants to meet their needs for the good of the office.

Hold a staff meeting a week later, and wherever possible, move toward eliminating the issues the employees do not like about their jobs. Ask for input, and perhaps even more important, ask for their assistance in improving the work environment. If the new manager follows this process, the employees will realize that he or she can get things done, is interested in their input, and often acts based on their input. Do not change a slew of policies or procedures too quickly; remember that change is difficult for most people. However, indicate to the employees that their issues are important and will be addressed.

Distribute memos frequently that communicate with employees in a way that makes them feel like part of a team. Be willing to ask for input and try suggestions for dealing with problems in the flow of the workday.

Realize that some employees still will resist, which may make the new office manager feel frustrated. At some point staffing changes may be necessary, and this might include terminating employees who do not get onboard with the office moving in a positive direction. Although any terminations are stressful for the entire office, realize that this is a common situation when new managers begin their positions. This process is the first step in building a functional team.

CREATING A TEAM ATMOSPHERE

Teamwork is critical in the medical profession. In the physician's office, the manager must promote an atmosphere in which the employees are willing to work together toward common goals. Morale in the office may be low because of recent changes in policies or procedures, changes in staff or management, recent terminations of employees, lack of business, or any number of other reasons. The wise manager takes steps to improve employee morale constantly, including scheduling frequent meetings and keeping the employees abreast of changes and developments that affect them (Figure 25-1). Employees like to be kept "in the loop." Some managers try to shield employees from negative information, but this practice can cause rumors to circulate and worsen morale.

Managers can improve morale by scheduling activities that involve the families of employees and by making an obvious effort to include them in various events. One of the most effective ways to improve employee morale is to communicate. Regular staff meetings, e-mails, and memos are critical for good communication and smooth operation of the medical facility.

FIVE ESSENTIAL ELEMENTS OF TEAMWORK

1. *Mutual accountability:* Each person on the team holds the others accountable for the success of the organization.
2. *Common purpose and performance goals:* Short-term and intermediate goals must relate to the long-term goals of the group.
3. *Small size:* Most successful teams have a small number of members; fewer than 10 is optimum.
4. *Common approach:* All team members must learn to work together toward the goal.
5. *Complementary skills:* A variety of talents, skills, and abilities is needed for a successful team.

From Katzenbach JR, Smith DK: *Wisdom of teams: creating the high-performance organization,* Boston, 1992, Harvard Business School Publishing.

Use of Incentives and Employee Recognition

The staff of the physician's office should feel satisfaction with the working conditions and atmosphere in the facility. The office manager plays a part in ensuring that this happens.

Incentives give employees reason to perform over and above the level expected of them. If the staff meets or exceeds a goal that has

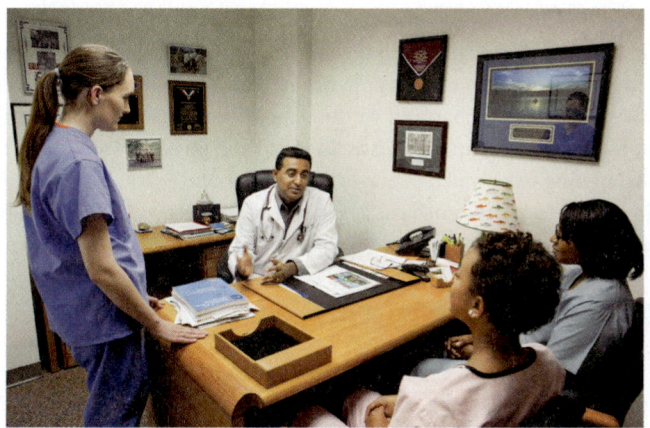

FIGURE 25-1 Communication is vital when building a team. Employees appreciate good communication with management. Sharing good and bad news openly with employees leads to fewer rumors and eases workers' concerns.

been set, the physician may elect to provide tickets to a sports or entertainment event for the entire staff. A paid day off is always a great incentive for accomplishing a goal. Some physicians have an incentive program that is related to collections for a given period. These ideas provide a goal for the employees to work toward and an opportunity to expand their efforts as a team.

Recognition is a strong method of improving employee morale and encouraging outstanding performance. Certificates for peak performance are a great way to motivate employees. For instance, the office manager may decide to award a certificate each month to the employee who provides the best customer service. Patients could even be involved by allowing them to nominate employees for this honor. When an award is at stake, most employees enjoy participating and striving to accomplish the goals that have been set.

CRITICAL THINKING APPLICATION   25-4

One of Katherine's employees, Jewel, is very sensitive about performing perfectly on the job. She is an excellent employee, but she has a few weaknesses. However, she has received a lot of recognition for the good things she has done at work. Katherine still feels that she needs to discuss with Jewel the areas where her performance is weak, but she knows it will upset her. How might Katherine deal with this sticky situation? How can Katherine reassure Jewel that she is pleased with her overall performance?

Problem Employees

Occasionally, problem employees disrupt the efficiency of the physician's office. Counseling these employees to find the source of their difficulties is the first step toward resolution. Many employees can be redirected to become productive staff members with a little patience and understanding on the manager's part. However, some employees have negative attitudes that seem **impenetrable**.

The manager must never hesitate to counsel the employee who is not performing at the expected level, and this includes employees with attitude problems. Establish a set regimen of counseling. Many offices allow one verbal warning before written reprimands go into

the employee's file. If the manager does not make a habit of writing formal **reprimands**, there may be insufficient documentation of problems with the employee once the manager is ready to terminate him or her. Even small offenses, such as being tardy, should at least be noted in the employee's file. The manager should never be in a position in which the termination of an employee cannot be justified by written documents.

Problem Patients

Patients can be quite challenging to the physician's staff and office manager. Most patients are genuinely concerned about their health and are cooperative with the physician's instructions. However, a few patients require extra understanding, which may lead to intervention by the office manager. Types of problem patients may include those who are:

- Complainers
- Angry
- Needy
- Demanding
- Violent
- Nonpaying
- Noncompliant
- Drug seeking
- Reschedulers

The office manager may act as a **liaison** between the patient and the physicians when issues arise that are somewhat complicated. Some patients may feel ignored or mistreated. Others may have a general lack of trust that makes complying with the physician's orders difficult for them. Cultural differences, social issues, and financial problems all can affect patient compliance and attitude. The rare patient may have a personality disorder or psychological problems that are frustrating as they receive medical treatment.

The time may come that the physician decides to discontinue care for a difficult patient. If that happens, the physician must notify the patient in writing and send the letter by certified mail, return receipt requested. Because some patients refuse to sign for mail, a copy of the same letter can be sent by regular mail. The physician must tell the patient that care is to be discontinued, inform the patient what day will be the final one the physician will provide care, and urge the patient to seek medical care from a new physician. The letter does not have to detail the reasons for the physician's decision, but those reasons should be explained in the patient's medical record. Always follow office policy in terminating patient care.

Preventing Burnout

Burnout is defined as exhaustion of physical or emotional strength or motivation, usually as a result of prolonged stress or frustration. Medical professionals are particularly susceptible to burnout because of the intensity of their jobs. Even small decisions could affect a patient's life. Therefore the office manager should take measures to help employees avoid burnout.

Some of the causes of burnout include a stressful, disorganized home or work environment; poor human relations skills; a feeling of being out of control of one's life; excessive expectations from supervisors or family members; long work hours or time away from family and friends; and not being able to relax either at home or in the work environment.

TIPS FOR PREVENTING BURNOUT

- Ask for help.
- Devote specific times to introspection or meditation.
- Understand what can be changed and what cannot be changed.
- Get some exercise.
- Organize and prioritize tasks.
- List tasks that are displeasing and delegate them to others, if possible.
- Understand personal limitations.
- Take short vacations at least twice a year.
- Identify goals and try to perform only tasks that lead to reaching them.
- Consider options, including changing jobs.
- Personalize work space with pictures and comforting items.
- Get a good understanding of a position and the stress involved before accepting it.

Keeping the Management Relationship Professional

When people work together for an extended period, they often become **affable**, and sometimes relationships develop into close friendships. This is a normal occurrence, but the office manager must be careful about becoming too close to his or her employees. When the relationship is friendly, reprimanding an employee when needed sometimes is difficult. Some employees take advantage of a good relationship with the office manager and may begin to arrive late or call in sick more than usual. A healthy respect for each other must be maintained. The manager can have a good rapport with employees without becoming overly friendly, and this is the best policy. Some facilities have strict rules about fraternization with subordinates outside the work facility. It is advisable to keep the relationship on a professional level at all times.

CRITICAL THINKING APPLICATION   25-5

- The clinical medical assistants usually celebrate payday by going out to eat after work every other Friday. After about 6 months on the job, they invite Katherine to join them. Should she go with the employees? Why or why not?
- Most offices plan parties for Christmas or at other times during the year. Are these good for employee morale, or should they be avoided?

The professional office manager serves as a liaison between the employees and the physician, but can also serve in the same capacity for the patients. Some patients have issues that, for whatever reason, they cannot seem to talk about with the physician; however, they may reveal this information to the medical assistant or the office manager. Employees may have similar situations.

Both the medical assistant and the office manager should serve as a patient **advocate**, but they can never hold back information the physician needs to know. For instance, if a patient tells the medical assistant or office manager that he has really been smoking, although he told the physician he had quit, the information must be given to the physician. Never suggest to or tell a patient that information can be withheld from the physician. If the patient asks the medical assistant to keep information from the physician, the medical assistant must refuse.

In the same manner, a medical assistant may have made a medication error and is afraid to tell the physician. The office manager must relay the information to the physician, who can determine whether the error could be harmful to the patient. Fortunately, most situations between the medical assistants and the physician are not life-threatening. The office manager who is fair and who also serves as an advocate for the medical assistant tries to rectify situations in a positive manner.

LAWS AFFECTING EMPLOYMENT

Numerous laws affect the way that employees are treated from the interview through the end of employment. The office manager should be familiar with these laws and how they affect the practice.
- Fair Labor Standards Act
  - Prescribes standards for wages and overtime pay
  - Requires that employees must be paid minimum wage and time and a half for overtime hours, as they apply
  - Prohibits those under age 18 from performing certain kinds of work and restricts the hours of workers under age 16
- Occupational Safety and Health Act
  - Regulates conditions affecting employees' safety and health in the workplace
- Workers' Compensation
  - Regulates the benefits of employees who have been injured on the job
  - Determines pay for employees who are not working because of an on-the-job injury
- Family and Medical Leave Act
  - Requires employers of 50 or more employees to offer up to 12 weeks of unpaid, job-protected leave to eligible employees for the birth of a child, an adoption, or a personal or family illness
- Pregnancy Discrimination Act
  - Forbids employers to refuse to hire a woman based upon pregnancy, childbirth, or related medical conditions
  - Requires employers to hold open a job for a pregnancy-related absence the same length of time that a job would be held open for employees on sick or disability leave
- Americans with Disabilities Act
  - Prohibits discrimination against individuals with disabilities (see Chapter 7)
- Age Discrimination Act
  - Prevents discrimination in hiring on the basis of age
  - Prevents discrimination in promoting, discharging, and compensating employees

Many more federal and state laws affect employers and employees. When a position is available at the medical office, the person conducting the interviews and making hiring decisions must be familiar with the laws that govern the practice.

SELECTING THE RIGHT STAFF MEMBERS

The most important asset to any medical facility is the staff that cares for the patients. From the physician to the receptionist, all play a vital role in the well-being of those who visit the office. Selecting staff members who can be molded into a cohesive team is not an easy task. Care should be taken to choose employees who have the necessary skills and the right personality for the office. Never try to select employees who are all alike. A variety of personality types works better than several similar personalities.

Understanding the Needs of the Office

The office manager should discuss with the physician the type of employee needed when an opening arises. Ask what qualities the physician desires in the person who occupies that particular position and the tasks for which the person will be responsible. Once the need has been established and the duties confirmed, the office manager can begin the recruiting process.

One of the most effective methods of finding new employees is through word of mouth. Ask other office managers, physicians, or medical professionals if they are aware of a person looking for employment who has the skills needed in the office. Keep a file of resumés that can be accessed when an opening occurs in the office. Often the physician or office manager may know of a person working in another area of the clinic or perhaps in a nearby hospital who may be interested in a job change. Be careful in approaching a person who is already employed. There is no harm in asking if a person is interested, but if the reply is negative, do not pursue the issue further.

Employment agencies can be used to find staff members, but they may charge a fee for their services. The office manager may want to contact a local medical assisting school to secure an extern. If the extern proves to be an asset to the office, he or she may be offered the permanent position. Online job postings and newspaper ads are another option for finding employees, but many resumés may be submitted from people who are not qualified, especially when the economy is not at its best. When creating an ad for the newspaper, list the basic requirements for the position. Briefly describe the office and location and the personality type sought. Some offices also list a few of the benefits offered to attract applicants and also may disclose a salary range.

Reviewing Resumés and Applications

Once several resumés or applications have been submitted, the office manager should set aside a quiet time to review the documents. Divide them into three stacks: stack one should contain resumés of individuals who will be called for an interview; stack two should consist of possible candidates but not the strongest; and stack three should contain applicants who will not be called.

During this preliminary review process, look for several items. First, make sure the documents are neatly prepared, free of error, and completely legible (Figure 25-2). The person hired probably will write in patients' charts, so this is a good opportunity to make sure the handwriting can be read easily. Second, look for gaps between positions. Make sure any lengthy time of unemployment is explained. The application should be filled out completely, and no notations of "see resume" should be included. The application provides important information, and an applicant who does not fill it out completely might be classified as lazy and prone to taking shortcuts. Watch for inconsistencies or oversights, including information that seems incomplete. Also look for resumés **targeted** toward the job opening available in the clinic. Targeted resumés are written specifically for a

certain position. With today's computer capabilities, job seekers can target their resumés for each job for which they apply, and this strategy tells the manager that the applicant has enough interest in the job to demonstrate that he or she meets their specific requirements.

Once the entire original stack of resumés has been reviewed and separated, return to the stack of potential interviews. Careful judgment and objectivity must be used in the search for an employee suitable for the practice. Before interviewing any applicant, the manager needs to know several details:

- What personal qualities and abilities must the applicant have?
- What responsibilities are involved with the position?
- What salary range is the physician willing to offer?
- How soon will the position be open?

Once these facts are clear, the manager should review the final resumés and applications with the following questions in mind:

- Do the applicant's handwriting and/or grammar meet the office's standards?
- Has the applicant been employed previously? What duties were performed?
- If previously employed, how long was the applicant in the last position? Why did the applicant leave?
- What are the applicant's skills? Do these meet the requirements for the position as set forth in the office procedures manual?
- Does the applicant seem to accept and enjoy responsibility?
- What is the applicant's formal education? Is he or she registered or certified? If not, is the applicant interested in taking the examination?
- Is the applicant a member of a professional organization? Does he or she attend meetings?

Arranging the Personal Interview

If the applicant sent a letter asking for an interview, note whether the letter was correctly typed and included essential contact information and whether the person also provided an attractive resume. Amazingly, some resumés do not include a contact telephone number! Managers can schedule interviews by e-mail, but speaking to applicants directly has its advantages. By conducting a prescreening interview with the applicant on the phone, the manager has an opportunity to judge the person's telephone voice, attitude, and communications skills. In addition, the manager may want to ask several questions about the person's education and experience. Because the employee probably will speak with patients on the telephone, clarity of speech is important. Those who perform well during the prescreening should be scheduled for an interview.

CRITICAL THINKING APPLICATION   **25-6**

- Katherine was impressed with Carol Limpken's resumé and application, but when scheduling an interview on the telephone, she noticed that Carol's grammar was not as professional as Katherine would like. Should this influence Katherine's decision to hire Carol?
- Why is speech such an important issue in the medical office?

APPLICATION FOR POSITION / Medical or Dental Office
AN EQUAL OPPORTUNITY EMPLOYER

(In answering questions, use extra blank sheet if necessary)

No employee, applicant, or candidate for promotion, training or other advantage shall be discriminated against (or given preference) because of race, color, religion, sex, age, physical handicap, veteran status, or national origin.

PLEASE READ CAREFULLY AND WRITE OR PRINT ANSWERS TO ALL QUESTIONS. DO NOT TYPE.

Date of Application

A. PERSONAL INFORMATION

| Name - Last | First | Middle | Social Security No. | Area Code/Phone No. ( ) |

| Present Address: - Street | (Apt #) | City | State | Zip | How Long At This Address?: |

| Previous Address: - Street | City | State | Zip | Person to notify in case of Emergency or Accident - Name: |
| From: | To: | | Address: | Telephone: |

B. EMPLOYMENT INFORMATION

| For What Position Are You Applying?: | ☐ Full-Time ☐ Part-Time ☐ Either | Date Available For Employment?: | Wage/Salary Expectations: |

| List Hrs./Days You Prefer To Work | List Any Hrs./Days You Are Not Available: (Except for times required for religious practices or observances) | Can You Work Overtime, If Necessary? ☐ Yes ☐ No |

Are You Employed Now?: ☐ Yes ☐ No

If So, May We Inquire Of Your Present Employer?: ☐ No ☐ Yes, If Yes:

Name Of Employer: Phone Number: ( )

Have You Ever Been Bonded? ☐ Yes ☐ No

If Required For Position, Are You Bondable? ☐ Yes ☐ No ☐ Uncertain

Have You Applied For A Position With This Office Before? ☐ No ☐ Yes   If Yes, When?:

Referred By / Or Where Did You Learn Of This Job?:

Can You, Upon Employment, Submit Verification Of Your Legal Right To Work In The United States?: ☐ Yes ☐ No
Submit Proof That You Meet Legal Age Requirement For Employment? ☐ Yes ☐ No

Language(s) Applicant Speaks or Writes (If Use Of A Language Other Than English Is Relevant To The Job For Which The Applicant Is Applying:

C. EDUCATIONAL HISTORY

Name & Address Of Schools Attended (Include Current)	Dates From	Dates Thru	Highest Grade/Level Completed	Diploma/Degree(s) Obtained/Areas of Study
High School				
College				Degree/Major
Post Graduate				Degree/Major
Other				Course/Diploma/License/Certificate

Specific Training, Education, Or Experiences Which Will Assist You In The Job For Which You Have Applied.

Future Educational Plans

D. SPECIAL SKILLS

CHECK BELOW THE KINDS OF WORK YOU HAVE DONE:

☐ BLOOD COUNTS	☐ DENTAL ASSISTANT	☐ MEDICAL INSURANCE FORMS	☐ RECEPTIONIST
☐ BOOKKEEPING	☐ DENTAL HYGIENIST	☐ MEDICAL TERMINOLOGY	☐ TELEPHONES
☐ COLLECTIONS	☐ FILING	☐ MEDICAL TRANSCRIPTION	☐ TYPING
☐ COMPOSING LETTERS	☐ INJECTIONS	☐ NURSING	☐ STENOGRAPHY
☐ COMPUTER INPUT	☐ INSTRUMENT STERILIZATION	☐ PHLEBOTOMY (Draw Blood)	☐ URINALYSIS
		☐ POSTING	☐ X-RAY

OFFICE EQUIPMENT USED: ☐ COMPUTER ☐ DICTATING EQUIPMENT ☐ WORD PROCESSOR ☐ OTHER:

| Other Kinds Of Tasks Performed Or Skills That May Be Applicable To Position: | Typing Speed | Shorthand Speed |

ORDER # 72-110 • © 1976 BIBBERO SYSTEMS, INC. • PETALUMA, CA. • (REV. 1/95)
TO REORDER CALL TOLL FREE: (800) BIBBERO (800-242-2376) OR FAX (800) 242-9330   MFG IN U.S.A.

(PLEASE COMPLETE OTHER SIDE)

FIGURE 25-2 Application for employment. Candidates for jobs in the medical office should complete applications accurately, leaving no blanks or unanswered questions. (Courtesy Bibbero Systems, Petaluma, Calif., *www.bibbero.com*.)

E. EMPLOYMENT RECORD

LIST MOST RECENT EMPLOYMENT FIRST   May We Contact Your Previous Employer(s) For A Reference? ☐ Yes ☐ No

1) Employer   Work Performed. Be Specific:

Address   Street   City   State   Zip Code

Phone Number
(   )

Type of Business   Dates   Mo. | Yr.   Mo. | Yr.
                          From   To

Your Position   Hourly Rate/Salary
                          Starting   Final

Supervisor's Name

Reason For Leaving

2) Employer   Worked Performed. Be Specific:

Address   Street   City   State   Zip Code

Phone Number
(   )

Type of Business   Dates   Mo. | Yr.   Mo. | Yr.
                          From   To

Your Position   Hourly Rate/Salary
                          Starting   Final

Supervisor's Name

Reason For Leaving

3) Employer   Worked Performed. Be Specific:

Address   Street   City   State   Zip Code

Phone Number
(   )

Type of Business   Dates   Mo. | Yr.   Mo. | Yr.
                          From   To

Your Position   Hourly Rate/Salary
                          Starting   Final

Supervisor's Name

Reason For Leaving

F. REFERENCES — FRIENDS / ACQUAINTANCES NON-RELATED

(1) _____
    Name   Address   Telephone Number   (☐ Work ☐ Home) Occupation   Years Acquainted

(1) _____
    Name   Address   Telephone Number   (☐ Work ☐ Home) Occupation   Years Acquainted

Please Feel Free To Add Any Information Which You Feel Will Help Us Consider You For Employment

READ THE FOLLOWING CAREFULLY, THEN SIGN AND DATE THE APPLICATION

"I certify that all answers given by me on this application are true, correct and complete to the best of my knowledge. I acknowledge notice that the information contained in this application is subject to check. I agree that, if hired, my continued employment may be contingent upon the accuracy of that information. If employed, I further agree to comply with Company/Office rules and regulations."

Signature: _____   Date: _____

FIGURE 25-2, cont'd

Set a time for the personal interview when the applicant can be given undivided attention. An applicant who is being considered for employment should have an opportunity to see the office during a period of a fairly normal amount of activity. The prospective employee who is interviewed in a peaceful, quiet office on the physician's day out may not be prepared for the activity on a normal working day.

Before interviewing any applicant, become thoroughly familiar with the federal, state, and local fair employment practice laws affecting hiring practices. Both men and women receive protection from on-the-job discrimination, sexual harassment, mandatory lie detector tests, and unfair discharge. Title VII of the Civil Rights Act of 1964, as amended by the Equal Employment Opportunity Act of 1972, prohibits inquiries into an applicant's race, color, gender, religion, and national origin. Inquiries about medical history, arrest records, or previous drug use also are illegal. Most states have laws designed to protect the rights of job applicants, and these laws may impose additional restrictions. Office managers must research the laws that pertain to employment in their own states.

If an actual application has not been submitted, have the applicant complete it at the time of the interview. The application form can serve as a check of the applicant's penmanship and thoroughness and becomes a permanent record if the individual is hired. Tell the candidate whether the form should be completed in the applicant's own handwriting and be sure to state this on the instructions. Check to see whether the applicant was **meticulous** about following instructions and filling in all the blanks. This serves as an indication of the individual's capacity for following directions.

The Interview

The manager's first priority is to make sure the applicant feels at ease (Figure 25-3). Shake his or her hand and ask a few social questions before starting the interview (Procedure 25-1). In general, use good manners and see that the person to be interviewed is comfortable. Most people feel some butterflies in the stomach when interviewing, but the manager will get a better idea of the person's capabilities if he or she is relaxed and able to discuss strengths and background openly.

Stress interviews usually are a waste of time. In a stress interview, the potential employee is placed in a difficult situation; for instance,

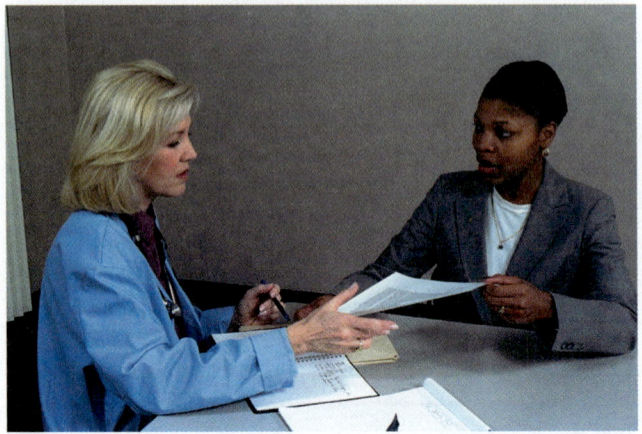

FIGURE 25-3 Put the job applicant at ease. Candidates perform at their peak when they are relaxed and calm.

the interviewer may call and invite the potential employee to the office for a "casual second interview." Upon arrival, he or she enters a room where several individuals are sitting at a table, prepared to grill the prospective employee. Although those who will be placed in higher management positions may be expected to survive such a situation and perform under that type of stress, the regular employee placed in such situations might assume that the employer will be highly demanding throughout the course of employment, and this might lead a great prospect to refuse opportunities at that particular office. The potential employee may not express his or her strengths and abilities as well when intentionally placed into a stress interview situation. Some interviewers make up nerve-wracking scenarios that might happen in the office and then ask the prospect, "How would you handle that?" Although the medical profession is certainly demanding, the interview should be a time for honest exchange of information and accurate evaluation of the potential employee.

Begin with a few open-ended questions that cannot be answered with a simple "yes" or "no," such as, "What were your duties during your last position?" When interviewing a recent graduate who does not have experience, ask questions such as, "What subject did you perform well in at school?" When speaking with the candidate, make a mental note of whether he or she displays essential personal qualities, such as the ability to converse easily, the capacity to listen, and a bright smile. The applicant should be interested enough in the position to ask intelligent questions and appear interested in the office and the physician's specialty.

Avoid inquiries that involve the applicant's privacy. The questions should be related to the available position and the applicant's ability to do the job. At all stages of the interview, the interviewer should avoid questions about age, race, marital status, and other discriminatory areas.

An interview is a two-way exchange of information between the applicant and the interviewer. If the applicant appears to be one who will receive serious consideration, explain what will be expected as an employee. Office policies regarding appearance, working hours, overtime, time off, and vacations may be discussed at this stage. Salary and other fringe benefits should be discussed once the manager is ready to offer the job. If the manager fails to mention these items, the applicant may be hesitant to inquire.

Some employers request a credit check before offering employment, especially if the individual will be handling practice finances. It can safely be assumed that one who is unable to handle personal financial affairs will be a poor risk in handling office finances. The medical assistant may also be required to submit to criminal background checks, drug screens, and even personality tests before or just after being offered a position. The medical assistant must be prepared to deal with the information obtained by such inquiries. If a long time has passed since the incident happened, be honest and explain that it was a mistake, it happened several years ago, and retribution has been made. Be prepared to answer questions about such events during the job interview.

Review the job description for the position being filled. The person being interviewed must understand the required duties and responsibilities of the job. Ask whether the applicant has any questions, and close the interview on a positive note. Let the candidate know when a decision will be made and what further contact the office will initiate.

PROCEDURE 25-1

Interview Job Candidates Effectively

GOAL: *To evaluate job candidates fairly and choose the best person to fill an available position in the medical facility.*

EQUIPMENT and SUPPLIES

- Candidate's completed job application
- Candidate's resumé
- Private area in the medical office
- Clerical supplies

PROCEDURAL STEPS

1. Review the job requirements the candidate will need to perform.
   PURPOSE: To evaluate candidates properly, the employer must determine the tasks the new employee will be expected to perform.
2. Match each job application with the corresponding resumé.
3. Separate strong candidates from moderate candidates and poor candidates.
   PURPOSE: To screen the best candidates and invite them to interview for the position.
4. Review each resumé and job application again and determine which candidates should be brought to the office for an interview.
5. Call each candidate and schedule an appointment for an interview.
6. Evaluate the applicant's speaking voice while making the appointment or the interview.
   PURPOSE: To determine the candidate's professionalism and ability to speak clearly and with clarity on the telephone.
7. Select several interview questions in advance to ask all of the applicants.
   PURPOSE: To avoid having to think of questions during the interview.
8. Note whether the applicant arrives on time for the interview.
   PURPOSE: If the candidate does not arrive on time for the interview, he or she may be a habitually late employee.
9. Introduce yourself to the applicant and proceed to a private area to conduct the interview.

10. Make the applicant feel as much at ease as possible.
    PURPOSE: Most individuals are a little nervous during job interviews, and if helped to relax, they are able to present their qualifications and skills confidently.
11. Ask the applicant the chosen questions.
12. Evaluate the answers and make notations about the candidate that are not demeaning or unprofessional.
    PURPOSE: Demeaning comments in an employee's file eventually may be seen if there is a subsequent lawsuit, and this can reflect poorly on the person who made the comments.
13. Ask the candidate whether he or she has any questions.
    PURPOSE: Evaluate the types of questions the employee asks; determine whether they are intelligent questions and whether they indicate a true interest in the position.
14. Offer strong candidates a brief tour of the facility.
15. State a date by which a hiring decision will be made and suggest that the candidate call the facility that day, if desired.
16. Evaluate all applicants fairly according to their experience and training.
17. Select the best three candidates and call them for a second interview, if desired.
18. Discuss the final hiring decisions with the physician or others with influence.
    PURPOSE: Some physicians want to make the final hiring decisions.
19. Make the final hiring decision.
20. Call the candidate to come to the office to discuss the position.
21. Negotiate salary and benefits.
22. Offer the position.
23. If the offer is declined, call the next candidate to the office to discuss the position until a satisfactory candidate accepts and agrees to a start date.

During the hiring process, the manager may want to invite serious prospects to lunch with the staff or for coffee in the more relaxed atmosphere of the employee lounge. This presents an opportunity to discover whether the applicant's personality will mesh with the atmosphere of the office. Employees appreciate being asked their opinion on those who are potential team members. An extensive list of interview questions can be found in Chapter 58.

Follow-Up Activities

When the interview is over, immediately take a few moments to rate the applicant while the interview is fresh in the memory. Jot down some notes so that the applicant will be remembered easily when the final decisions are being made as to who will be hired. Do not trust the impressions to memory, especially if several applicants have been interviewed. Never write harmful personal statements; instead, be objective and fair. Should the potential employee ever have cause to bring the physician to court for discrimination in hiring practices, there should be no **disparaging** information written down that would reflect negatively on the physician or office manager.

Always carefully check all references and follow through on any leads for information. Use the telephone in checking references, because people sometimes are less than candid in a letter; furthermore, letter writing is time-consuming, and a reply may never be sent. If the e-mail address for a reference is provided, this is an excellent way to check a reference, and the printed version may be added to the applicant's file.

Prepare a checklist before placing the call. When speaking with the person called, be sure to "listen between the lines." Note the tone of the replies to the questions. Do not ask questions that might incriminate the person answering them. The following questions are effective as an introduction:

- When did (the applicant) work for you?
- For how long?
- What were the duties and responsibilities?
- Did the employee assume responsibility well?

Some employers provide information only on the date of hire, job title, and date of termination of the employment. However, if the employer states, "She worked in our office from May, 2011, to July, 2012, and is NOT eligible for rehire," the reasonable assumption is that the employee did not perform well. The tone of voice and emphasis on the word "not" should be clues that this person is probably not right for the job. Still, if all other references are glowing, call and ask the applicant about the facility that gave the negative response. There could be a reasonable explanation for what might have been a bad experience. Respect the company's policy and do not press for further information.

Any person who is granted an interview should send a thank you letter to the person who interviewed him or her. Watch the mail to see whether any of the applicants perform this important follow-up task.

A second interview may be granted when the field is narrowed to two or three candidates. The physician may want to participate in these interviews. Some offices conduct a group interview with several staff members present. Remember that these interviews become more and more stressful for the candidate, and the manager should expect some nervousness. Do not "count off" in the interview for mild nervousness.

Making the Selection

Once the final interviews have been conducted, the best candidate must be chosen. Never rely strictly on a "gut instinct" about a potential employee. Base hiring decisions on logical conclusions drawn from all contacts with the applicant, including:

- Grammar and enunciation
- Appropriate manners
- Professional appearance
- Work history
- Match to required job skills
- Friendly, personable attitude

Some offices create a score sheet for interviews that lists the needs of the office and allows the office manager to assign points according to how the applicant fits.

When a decision has been reached to hire someone, it is best to bring the successful candidate back into the office to offer the position and negotiate the final details. The office manager may want to wait until the first-choice candidate has actually accepted the offer before notifying anyone else that the job has been filled. Do not expect the potential employee to answer the offer on the spot. Twenty-four hours is a reasonable time to consider the offer.

Remember to notify all final candidates for the position that it has been filled so that they can continue their job search. They may have hesitated to accept other interviews, and it is unfair to keep individuals who are seeking employment hoping for a telephone call from the physician's office. Good etiquette requires dropping them a note or calling to say that the position is filled. Although this is a rare practice in today's busy clinics, all of the applicants who interviewed were surely the manager's best candidates and professional individuals. Therefore, they deserve a brief call and a wish for success in their job search. Thank the individual for applying, and offer to keep his or her application on file, if the candidate was especially impressive.

PAPERWORK FOR NEW EMPLOYEES

The office manager should develop a checklist of the paperwork needed for newly hired staff and all of the information that should be covered with the new employee at the onset of the job. Basic new employee paperwork often includes:

- Job application
- Form I-9 (Employment Eligibility Verification)
- W-4 Form (Employee's Withholding Allowance Certificate)
- Notice of Workers' Compensation coverage
- Consent for background check, drug testing, and search (if applicable)
- Acknowledgement of receipt of company handbook or policy manual
- Agreements regarding pay, wage deductions, benefits, schedule, work location, and so on
- Notices of at-will employment status
- Acknowledgement of ethics statement
- Occupational Safety and Health Administration (OSHA) compliance acknowledgement or checklist

All of these forms, once signed, should be kept in the employee's personnel file. Other forms and paperwork may be necessary that vary from state to state and company to company. Make certain that Form I-9, Employment Eligibility Verification, is completed. Form I-9 is required by the federal government and used by the employer to make certain that the newly hired individual is eligible to work legally in the United States. A person who cannot provide the required documentation should not be allowed to remain as an employee. Employees should also understand the at-will employment status. Under the *at-will employment* principle, the employee or the employer can terminate employment for good cause, bad cause, or no cause, unless an express contract is signed for a specific term or the employee is a member of a collective bargaining group, such as a union.

ORIENTATION AND TRAINING: CRITICAL FACTORS FOR SUCCESSFUL EMPLOYEES

The hiring process does not end with hiring a new employee. Orientation and training help new employees to understand what is expected and to develop to their full potential (Figure 25-4). One of the most critical errors made when bringing new staff members aboard is not providing them with a fair orientation and training period.

Some managers assign a mentor to assist the new employee during the initial probationary period. A **mentor** is a guide whom the new staff member can approach with questions and concerns. Using this type of "buddy" system is a good practice, because the new person does not feel isolated and alone during the first few weeks on the job.

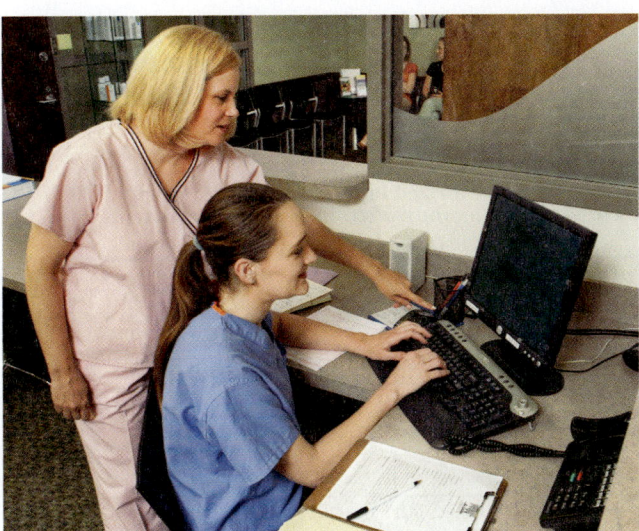

FIGURE 25-4 Training an employee well contributes greatly to the person's success.

Acquaint the new employee with the following:
- Staff members and their names
- Physical environment and layout of the office
- Nature of the practice and specialty
- Types of patients seen in the office
- Office policies
- Short- and long-range expectations

All new employees should be required to read the office policy and procedures manual. It is advisable for the manager to require the employee to sign a statement verifying that the manual (or manuals) have been read.

Make sure all federal and state regulations that apply to new employees are met. OSHA training must be provided to employees at risk for exposures *before they begin any duties.* Training required by the Health Insurance Portability and Accountability Act (HIPAA) also must be completed. Make certain that the employee's file is complete before allowing the employee to work even 1 hour. The manager must meet this federal requirement to prove that the employee is eligible to work in the United States (Figure 25-5).

CRITICAL THINKING APPLICATION   25-7

Katherine is bringing in a new employee who must begin work on the following Monday, because the staff has been short one person for approximately 2 weeks. However, Katherine will be going on vacation the same day. How can she ensure that the new employee is trained properly?

Job Description

The job description is a tool designed to inform employees about the duties they are expected to perform. Well-written job descriptions list the essential functions of the job and reveal the chain of command the employee should follow when questions or concerns arise. These documents provide a good guideline for employees so that they will understand exactly what is expected of them and their responsibilities at work.

The job description should include a statement that says the employee must perform any additional duties as assigned by the supervisor. With this statement in place, the employee cannot say, "That is not my job." All employees should be willing to pull together and assist with any tasks, but this statement gives added weight to assignments that are not specified in the written job description.

An effective manager understands the phrase "inspect what you expect." When duties are assigned, the manager should ensure that the tasks were completed correctly and in a timely manner. New employees should be monitored to make sure their delegated tasks are being done and done right. Without inspection, the manager cannot know whether the new employee is meeting expectations. Once employees have earned a degree of trust, inspecting their work is not as necessary as in the beginning. As mentioned earlier, many managers practice a skill called "management by walking around." By strolling through the areas where subordinates work, managers can observe and hear about issues that might be brewing, while at the same time improve morale by offering encouragement and praise.

Staff Development Training

Continuous training and staff development are vital aspects of any medical office. Constant advancements and technologic changes occur, and employees must be kept up-to-date on those changes. Meetings should be held at least quarterly to ensure that the staff is using the latest techniques and current regulations when dealing with issues that confront the medical facility. Watch the mail for seminar opportunities that will allow employees to earn continuing education units (CEUs) or learn new skills that will benefit the office. Get input from employees about what they would like to learn and look for those opportunities. Professional organizations, such as the American Association of Medical Assistants (AAMA) and the American Medical Technologists (AMT), offer CEUs on a regular basis; therefore, encourage all staff members to be certified and to join professional organizations. Most hospitals have numerous continuing education classes that they allow physician's office employees to attend.

Delegation of Duties

Delegating duties to subordinates allows managers to concentrate on the most critical aspects of their own jobs. Delegation also provides an opportunity for the employees to grow and learn new skills. Some managers are hesitant to assign duties to employees because they believe the tasks are too important not to be completed by the manager. This hesitation suggests either a refusal to release control or mistrust of the employees. However, this type of manager soon is overrun with tasks and unable to complete them. Managers should place trust in employees who have earned it and allow them to prove their abilities. Mistrust is a symptom of a poor hire. Discover the strengths of individual employees and then assign them tasks that will allow them to use those strengths. If a medical assistant was hired to do administrative duties but is good with phlebotomy, encourage and allow the employee to assist with venipunctures whenever needed.

OMB No. 1615-0047; Expires 08/31/12

Department of Homeland Security
U.S. Citizenship and Immigration Services

Form I-9, Employment Eligibility Verification

Read instructions carefully before completing this form. The instructions must be available during completion of this form.

ANTI-DISCRIMINATION NOTICE: It is illegal to discriminate against work-authorized individuals. Employers CANNOT specify which document(s) they will accept from an employee. The refusal to hire an individual because the documents have a future expiration date may also constitute illegal discrimination.

Section 1. Employee Information and Verification *(To be completed and signed by employee at the time employment begins.)*

Print Name: Last   First   Middle Initial | Maiden Name

Address *(Street Name and Number)*   Apt. # | Date of Birth *(month/day/year)*

City   State   Zip Code | Social Security #

I am aware that federal law provides for imprisonment and/or fines for false statements or use of false documents in connection with the completion of this form.

I attest, under penalty of perjury, that I am (check one of the following):

☐ A citizen of the United States
☐ A noncitizen national of the United States (see instructions)
☐ A lawful permanent resident (Alien #) _____
☐ An alien authorized to work (Alien # or Admission #) _____
until (expiration date, if applicable - *month/day/year*) _____

Employee's Signature   Date *(month/day/year)*

Preparer and/or Translator Certification *(To be completed and signed if Section 1 is prepared by a person other than the employee.) I attest, under penalty of perjury, that I have assisted in the completion of this form and that to the best of my knowledge the information is true and correct.*

Preparer's/Translator's Signature   Print Name

Address *(Street Name and Number, City, State, Zip Code)*   Date *(month/day/year)*

Section 2. Employer Review and Verification *(To be completed and signed by employer. Examine one document from List A OR examine one document from List B and one from List C, as listed on the reverse of this form, and record the title, number, and expiration date, if any, of the document(s).)*

List A	OR	**List B**	**AND**	**List C**
Document title:				
Issuing authority:				
Document #:				
Expiration Date *(if any)*:				
Document #:				
Expiration Date *(if any)*:				

CERTIFICATION: I attest, under penalty of perjury, that I have examined the document(s) presented by the above-named employee, that the above-listed document(s) appear to be genuine and to relate to the employee named, that the employee began employment on *(month/day/year)* _____ **and that to the best of my knowledge the employee is authorized to work in the United States.   (State employment agencies may omit the date the employee began employment.)**

Signature of Employer or Authorized Representative   Print Name   Title

Business or Organization Name and Address *(Street Name and Number, City, State, Zip Code)*   Date *(month/day/year)*

Section 3. Updating and Reverification *(To be completed and signed by employer.)*

A. New Name *(if applicable)*   B. Date of Rehire *(month/day/year) (if applicable)*

C. If employee's previous grant of work authorization has expired, provide the information below for the document that establishes current employment authorization.

Document Title: _____   Document #: _____   Expiration Date *(if any)*: _____

I attest, under penalty of perjury, that to the best of my knowledge, this employee is authorized to work in the United States, and if the employee presented document(s), the document(s) I have examined appear to be genuine and to relate to the individual.

Signature of Employer or Authorized Representative   Date *(month/day/year)*

Form I-9 (Rev. 08/07/09) Y Page 4

FIGURE 25-5 The I-9 Employment Eligibility Verification form is designed to help the employer gather the documents necessary to prove that an employee is eligible to work in the United States.

LISTS OF ACCEPTABLE DOCUMENTS
All documents must be unexpired

LIST A Documents that Establish Both Identity and Employment Authorization	LIST B Documents that Establish Identity	LIST C Documents that Establish Employment Authorization
OR		AND
1. U.S. Passport or U.S. Passport Card	1. Driver's license or ID card issued by a State or outlying possession of the United States provided it contains a photograph or information such as name, date of birth, gender, height, eye color, and address	1. Social Security Account Number card other than one that specifies on the face that the issuance of the card does not authorize employment in the United States
2. Permanent Resident Card or Alien Registration Receipt Card (Form I-551)		
3. Foreign passport that contains a temporary I-551 stamp or temporary I-551 printed notation on a machine-readable immigrant visa	2. ID card issued by federal, state or local government agencies or entities, provided it contains a photograph or information such as name, date of birth, gender, height, eye color, and address	2. Certification of Birth Abroad issued by the Department of State (Form FS-545)
		3. Certification of Report of Birth issued by the Department of State (Form DS-1350)
4. Employment Authorization Document that contains a photograph (Form I-766)	3. School ID card with a photograph	
	4. Voter's registration card	4. Original or certified copy of birth certificate issued by a State, county, municipal authority, or territory of the United States bearing an official seal
5. In the case of a nonimmigrant alien authorized to work for a specific employer incident to status, a foreign passport with Form I-94 or Form I-94A bearing the same name as the passport and containing an endorsement of the alien's nonimmigrant status, as long as the period of endorsement has not yet expired and the proposed employment is not in conflict with any restrictions or limitations identified on the form	5. U.S. Military card or draft record	
	6. Military dependent's ID card	5. Native American tribal document
	7. U.S. Coast Guard Merchant Mariner Card	
	8. Native American tribal document	6. U.S. Citizen ID Card (Form I-197)
	9. Driver's license issued by a Canadian government authority	
	For persons under age 18 who are unable to present a document listed above:	7. Identification Card for Use of Resident Citizen in the United States (Form I-179)
6. Passport from the Federated States of Micronesia (FSM) or the Republic of the Marshall Islands (RMI) with Form I-94 or Form I-94A indicating nonimmigrant admission under the Compact of Free Association Between the United States and the FSM or RMI	10. School record or report card	8. Employment authorization document issued by the Department of Homeland Security
	11. Clinic, doctor, or hospital record	
	12. Day-care or nursery school record	

Illustrations of many of these documents appear in Part 8 of the Handbook for Employers (M-274)

Form I-9 (Rev. 08/07/09) Y Page 5

FIGURE 25-5, cont'd

USING PERFORMANCE REVIEWS EFFECTIVELY

A new employee should be granted a probationary period. A period of 60 to 90 days has been traditional, but many employers believe that 2 weeks is sufficient to determine whether the employee will be able to learn and adapt to the position. Set a definite date for a performance review covering the probationary period at the time of initial employment. This review should not be squeezed in between patient visits or be given a token few minutes at the end of a day. Schedule a time that provides the opportunity to relax and talk. Tell the new employee how well expectations have been met and whether there are any deficiencies. Then give the employee an opportunity to ask questions. Sometimes an employee fails to perform because he or she was never told what was expected. Although the probationary period does not always allow time to train an individual fully for a specific position, it is fair to assume that the potential for being a satisfactory employee can be judged at this time. Now is the time to talk out any problems and make suggestions for improvement. Sometimes the employee is released after an unsuccessful probationary period.

The performance **appraisal** includes a judgment of both the quality and quantity of work, personal appearance, attitudes and team spirit, dependability, self-discipline, motivation, attendance, punctuality, and any other qualities essential to satisfactory performance of the job in question (Figure 25-6). The supervisor is responsible for ongoing performance appraisals of all employees, complimenting whenever possible and appropriate and offering helpful criticism when necessary. A formal performance appraisal at the end of the probationary period and at regular 6-month intervals thereafter, with a report to the physician-employer, is helpful for the employee's salary review (Procedure 25-2).

When negative information is to be relayed to the employee during a performance appraisal, sandwich the negative comment between two positive ones whenever possible. For instance, tell the employee, "Jewel, you are a pro at greeting patients and making them feel at home. I would like to see you improve your time management skills, however, because I feel you are spending too much time with each individual patient. I must confess that they feel a part of the clinic family. Just watch the time and keep making them feel so welcome!"

Managers also may use the "feel, felt, found" approach when talking with employees about their performance. For example, "Jewel, I feel the same way you do about the patients taking up a lot of our time. I know there are some that want to talk with us for hours, and I have felt the pressure of wanting to make them feel comfortable but having so much to do, too. I have found that if I

PROCEDURE 25-2

Conduct a Performance Review

GOAL: *To evaluate job performance fairly and determine the strengths and weaknesses of employees using accurate documentation.*

EQUIPMENT and SUPPLIES

- Employee's file
- Past evaluations of employee
- Notes and/or reports regarding employee behavior
- Private area in the medical office
- Clerical supplies

PROCEDURAL STEPS

1. Set an appointment with the employee to conduct the review.
2. Allow the employee to complete a self-evaluation of his or her own work.
   PURPOSE: To gain insight into how the employee sees his or her own work performance and to allow input as to how the employee feels that he or she has performed during the evaluation period.
3. Review the self-evaluation, then document additional information about the employee and his or her performance.
4. Share the information with any other supervisor or the physician, if dictated by office policy or if additional input is necessary.
   PURPOSE: To accommodate any additional input (e.g., by the physician) that needs to be documented and discussed during the review.
5. Complete the final written review and proofread it for accuracy and completeness.
6. Discuss the review with the employee during the evaluation appointment.
   PURPOSE: To promote an understanding of what is expected by the employer.
7. Progress through the interview and explain the results of the evaluation to the employee.
8. Allow the employee to respond to any of the points raised during the evaluation but do not allow an argumentative attitude.
   PURPOSE: To gain insight into the employee's reasons for any poor performance without allowing belligerence.
9. Allow the employee to respond in writing to the evaluation for a limited time (e.g., 5 days).
   PURPOSE: To give the employee a chance to insert his or her input into the performance report.
10. Ask the employee to sign the evaluation to document that it was reviewed with him or her. (The employee does not have to agree with the evaluation to sign it.)
11. Give a copy of the evaluation to the employee.
12. File the evaluation in the employee's file.

PERFORMANCE EVALUATION AND DEVELOPMENT PLAN (OFFICE AND CLERICAL)

NAME: _____ DATE OF EVALUATION: _____

DATE OF HIRE: _____ DEPARTMENT: _____

JOB TITLE: _____ SUPERVISOR: _____

DATE APPOINTED THIS JOB: _____ MANAGER: _____

LAST REVIEW DATE: _____ LAST REVIEW RATING: _____

NEXT REVIEW DATE: _____ CURRENT REVIEW RATING: _____

PURPOSE

The purpose of this evaluation is to:

1. SET GOALS WITHIN SCOPE OF PRESENT JOB.
2. COMMUNICATE OPENLY ABOUT PERFORMANCE.
3. EVALUATE PAST PERFORMANCE.
4. DISCUSS FUTURE DEVELOPMENT PLANS FOR GROWTH.

INSTRUCTIONS

1. Supervisor to review form prior to completion. If specific items are not applicable they should be left blank.

2. Supervisor and employee to review job description prior to review.

3. In "COMMENTS" section supervisor may indicate which factors should be more heavily weighted in this particular evaluation.

4. Comments should be specific and job-related. All appropriate evaluation factors should be commented on to some degree.

I. POSITION OBJECTIVES AND MAJOR RESPONSIBILITIES. Summarize specific responsibilities of the job.

_____

_____

_____

II. ACCOMPLISHMENTS AND/OR IMPROVEMENTS. What specific accomplishments and/or improvements has employee made since last review with respect to set goals?

_____

_____

_____

PLEASE CONSIDER THE EMPLOYEE'S DEMONSTRATED PERFORMANCE AND MARK THE CIRCLE WHICH MOST CLOSELY DESCRIBES THAT PERFORMANCE.

4 - Performance consistently far exceeds expectations and requirements.
3 - Performance consistently exceeds normal expectations and job requirements.
2 - Performance consistently meets expectations and job requirements
1 - Performance usually meets expectations and minimum job requirements.
0 - Performance does not meet job requirements.

– CONTINUED, NEXT PAGE –

FORM # 72-119 © 1987 BIBBERO SYSTEMS, INC. PETALUMA, CA

TO REORDER CALL TOLL FREE:
800-BIBBERO /(800 242-2376) OR
FAX: (800) 242-9330 MFG IN U.S.A.

FIGURE 25-6 Performance evaluation and development plan. Performance evaluations should be considered tools that help employees reach their personal goals and the goals of the organization. (Courtesy Bibbero Systems, Petaluma, Calif.)

Continued

7. DEPENDABILITY: CONSIDER ATTENDANCE, PUNCTUALITY, IDLE TIME AND RELIANCE WHICH CAN BE PLACED ON EMPLOYEE TO PERSEVERE AND CARRY THROUGH TO COMPLETION ALL ASSIGNED TASKS

○ 0   ○ 1   ○ 2   ○ 3   ○ 4

_____

_____

_____

8. COMPLIANCE WITH COMPANY POLICIES: DOES THE EMPLOYEE COMPLY WITH RULES AND REGULATIONS WHICH APPLY TO SAFETY, FAIR EMPLOYMENT PRACTICES AND GENERAL ADMINISTRATIVE PROCEDURE.

○ 0   ○ 1   ○ 2   ○ 3   ○ 4

_____

_____

_____

9. SPECIFIC PERFORMANCE	1	2	3	4	COMMENTS
A. Ability to handle scheduling:					
B. Willingness to work OT when necessary:					
C. Handling of calls and follow-up:					
D. Maintenance of equipment:					
E. Ability to handle patient complaints:					
F. Tact in dealing with patients:					
G. Speed (in specific technical procedures):					
H. Secretarial accuracy:					
I. Professional terminology:					
J. Assisting procedures:					
K. Laboratory techniques:					
L. X-ray techniques:					
M. Physical therapy:					
N. Collections:					
O. Medical Insurance:					
P. Bookkeeping:					

10. PERSONAL	1	2	3	4	COMMENTS
A. Grooming:					
B. Professional conduct:					
C. Energy, enthusiasm:					
D. Ability to handle stress:					

ADDITIONAL COMMENTS: _____

_____

_____

_____

_____

_____

FORM # 72-119 © 1987 BIBBERO SYSTEMS, INC. PETALUMA, CA

FIGURE 25-6, cont'd

explain that I have a meeting or another patient to assist, they are very understanding and not offended. Perhaps you can try that approach, too."

Peer Evaluations

Some innovative companies use peer evaluations of employees to get a different view of the work performed by a worker. Asking co-workers to assist in the evaluation process can promote teamwork and cooperation. The rare employee offers a poor evaluation because of a personal problem with another staff member, but for the most part, employees provide fair, unbiased evaluations, knowing that they also will be evaluated when it is their turn.

A process known as a *360-degree evaluation* is an excellent tool for evaluating any employee, including managers. Such evaluations usually consist of a questionnaire that is given to those who work closely with the employee, and they provide input about the employee's performance.

Poor Evaluations Made Easier

No supervisor enjoys giving an evaluation that is not a positive one. It is difficult to know where to begin when the employee has not performed as expected or hoped. Perhaps the best way to open the conversation is to say, "Rebecca, your review today is not going to be a positive one. It seems that we do not have a meeting of the minds about your duties and our expectations of you. Let's talk about your performance and discuss whether this position is a good match for you."

The manager should have good documentation of the problems that led to the poor evaluation. If so, these can be reviewed with the employee with specific times, dates, and descriptions of incidents. If the manager does not document these issues, the conversation can become an argument and grow quite heated. Firm dates and times leave little room for argument and place the manager on the offensive. The employee may be apprehensive or even defensive at this point, but the phrasing will certainly get his or her attention, and the discussion should produce either the motivation to improve or the clarity that termination is in order.

CRITICAL THINKING APPLICATION   25-8

While Katherine is explaining to a particularly poor employee why Katherine plans to terminate her, the employee begins screaming and accusing Katherine of discrimination and harassment. How should Katherine handle this situation? What are Katherine's options if the employee does not stop the inappropriate behavior?

Terminating Employees

Dismissing an employee is unpleasant at best, but if the ground rules are decided in advance, written into the policy manual, and explained to all employees, the problem is partially solved. The policies must be applied equally and impartially to all. The final decision for dismissal probably will be made by the physician, but it may be based on the recommendation of the office manager or supervisor. Unless there are mitigating factors that suggest otherwise, the person who does the hiring should do the firing.

A probationary employee who does not prove satisfactory should be dismissed at the end of the probationary period, with tact and a full explanation of the reasons for dismissal. In all fairness, an individual should be told why the employment is being ended and not be given weak excuses or untruths that do not help correct deficiencies. If the manager is not straightforward in giving the reason for dismissal, the employee will not have the opportunity to grow and improve his or her performance.

An employee who has been in service for some time and is offering unsatisfactory performance should be warned and given an explanation of the specific improvements expected (Figure 25-7). If a second chance does not produce improvement in performance or attitude, dismissal must follow. It should be done privately, with tact and consideration.

Most practice consultants believe that firing should come close to the end of the day, after all other employees have left, and that the break should be clean and immediate. If the office policy provides for 2 weeks' notice when an employee resigns, the physician may want to offer 2 weeks' pay unless the circumstances that led to the dismissal were extremely **blatant**. A dismissed employee should never be allowed to train or influence a replacement.

The exit meeting should be planned just as carefully as the employment interview. Be honest with the employee. Discuss both the employee's assets and liabilities and give the reasons for the termination. There is no need to dwell on the employee's deficiencies. These should have been thoroughly discussed at the warning interview, and the employee need only be told that the necessary improvements have not been made. Do listen to the employee's feedback, unless it becomes lengthy or abusive. This may reveal some important administrative problems that need correction.

After dismissing an employee, do not leave that person in the office unattended. Request and get the office keys and any other equipment in the employee's possession immediately before the dismissed employee leaves the building. Most states have strict payday laws that do not allow holding the final paycheck for any reason. Do not offer to give the employee a good reference unless it can be done sincerely. If there is any indication that an employee may become abusive or violent once told about the termination, the supervisor should bring a representative from the Human Resources Department or Security to the final interview. It is possible that an employee can "snap" and suddenly become violent; however, more often it is the warning flags raised by an employee's behavior before termination that justify care in the termination interview. This is why supervisors must always document any strange or suspicious behavior and any breach of policy or procedures in the employee's personnel file. Documenting everything creates a clear picture of the employee's actions throughout the time of employment. The supervisor must be willing to confront an employee about his or her actions at the workplace. Document employee behavior as instructed in the office policy manual.

Certain breaches of conduct, such as **embezzlement**, insubordination, and violation of patient confidentiality, are grounds for immediate dismissal without warning.

Occasionally an employee voluntarily terminates a job without giving a valid reason. The physician or office manager may want to follow up with a letter to the former employee to determine whether a problem prompted the resignation. The employee may reveal

TERMINATION / REHIRE EVALUATION FORM

Employee Name_____ Social Security No. _____

Department _____ Title _____

Termination Date _____

Reason for Termination: _____Resigned _____Laid Off_____Retired

Evaluation of Job Performance	Excellent	Very Good	Average	Poor	Unacceptable
Quality (accuracy, etc.)	☐	☐	☐	☐	☐
Quantity (productivity, consistency, etc.)	☐	☐	☐	☐	☐
Knowledge of Duties	☐	☐	☐	☐	☐
Reliability (absenteeism)	☐	☐	☐	☐	☐
Punctuality	☐	☐	☐	☐	☐
Ability to Cooperate with Co-workers	☐	☐	☐	☐	☐
Relationship with Patients	☐	☐	☐	☐	☐
Overall Attitude (willingness and commitment)	☐	☐	☐	☐	☐
Initiative	☐	☐	☐	☐	☐
Judgment	☐	☐	☐	☐	☐

Recommendation for Rehiring: _____

_____

_____

Comments:_____

_____

_____

_____

_____

_____

_____

_____

_____ Date _____
Supervisor's Signature

FORM # 72-123   PERSONNEL RECORDS ORGANIZING SYSTEMS • © 1987 BIBBERO SYSTEMS, INC. • PETALUMA, CA.
TO REORDER CALL TOLL FREE: (800) BIBBERO (800-242-2376) OR FAX (800) 242-9330   MFG IN U.S.A.

FIGURE 25-7 Termination form. Document the reasons for terminating an employee and make sure supporting documentation shows warnings and previous counseling efforts. (Courtesy Bibbero Systems, Petaluma, Calif.)

serious issues with other personnel or with the office that need to be addressed and corrected.

Fair Salaries and Raises

Medical office managers should recruit employees who will remain with the office for a long time. There are always situations when a part-time worker returns to college, or someone working during the summer months goes back to school. However, good employee **retention** is the goal.

To keep good employees, the practice must pay them a fair salary with regular raises if they perform as expected. The office manager can find information about salary comparisons on the Internet. Check the job duties and descriptions found on the Web and see whether the salary the medical facility offers is comparable to that for similar jobs in the area.

Merit raises are increases based on an employee's commendable performance. Cost of living increases are given when earned, usually after specific periods or annually, and are based on national statistics and trends. An employee who is promoted should also be awarded a salary increase. When the office pays a fair salary for work done, the physician retains happy employees.

STAFF MEETINGS

Some formal mechanism must be used to keep the office manager and other key employees current on the daily business affairs of the practice. One of the most common complaints from office personnel is that they are unable to discuss problems with the physician. The solution to this problem may be to hold regular staff meetings, which may be scheduled as frequently as weekly but should be held no less often than quarterly (Figure 25-8). Some of the best ideas on improvement come from the office staff; the expression and exchange of good ideas should be encouraged.

Set aside a specific time for regular meetings at an hour when the most people can attend with the least disruption (Procedure 25-3). The meetings need not be long or overly formal, but to be effective, they must be planned and organized. There must be a leader, and someone should be appointed to take notes. The effectiveness of the leader, a person who can balance firmness with fairness, is an important aspect of the meeting. This usually is either the physician or the office manager or supervisor. All members of the staff should be encouraged to submit ideas for discussion.

Draw up a simple **agenda** listing the issues to be discussed and prepare any supporting data needed for the meeting. There are many kinds of staff meetings. They may be purely informational,

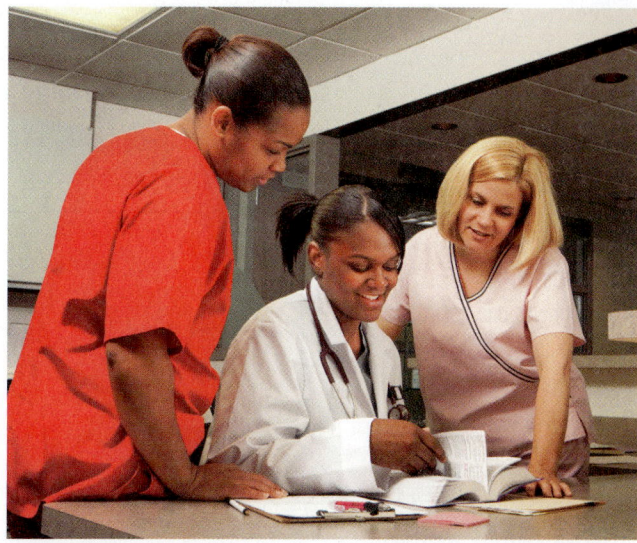

FIGURE 25-8 Periodic staff meetings are important tools for improving communication and resolving problems.

problem-solving, or brainstorming meetings. They may be work sessions for updating manuals, training seminars, or whatever is necessary to the individual practice. Meetings also may be scheduled to discuss new ideas and any changes in office procedures. Some meetings are held simply to resolve specific problems. The staff meeting must not be allowed to deteriorate into a gripe session. Individual complaints should be handled privately.

The meeting agenda might be similar to that of any business meeting:

1. Reading of the last meeting's minutes
2. Discussion of any unfinished business
3. Discussion of any problems in the clinical area
4. Discussion of any problems in the administrative area
5. Discussion of any problems in common areas
6. Adjournment

Some physicians like to combine the staff meeting with a breakfast or lunch. The time or place is not important as long as it is neutral and meets the needs of the practice. Meetings should be conducted regularly, democratically, and without interruption. Always follow up on the items discussed; otherwise, the only result will be frustration and a reluctance to discuss problems at future meetings.

SEEING THE WHOLE PICTURE

The office manager must keep a bird's-eye view on the office operations. He or she must look at the whole picture when difficulties arise. Remember, there are always two sides to every story, and there is usually truth intermingled with falsity. Do not form the habit of taking every word that an employee says as 100% accurate. This is not meant to suggest that all employees are not truthful, but rather to encourage the office manager to look at all sides before making critical decisions.

See issues from the employees' point of view. Try to understand their perspective when dealing with everyday situations in the medical facility. Do not become closed minded as a manager, unable to grasp what the employees see as important.

PROCEDURE 25-3

Arrange a Group Meeting

GOAL: *To plan and execute a productive meeting that will result in achieved goals and applied concepts for office procedures.*

EQUIPMENT and SUPPLIES

- Meeting room
- Agenda
- Visual aids and equipment
- Handouts
- Stopwatch or clock
- Computer or word processor
- Paper
- List of items for the agenda

PROCEDURAL STEPS

1. Determine the purpose of the meeting and draft a list of the items to be discussed. Include the desired results of the meeting.
   <u>PURPOSE:</u> To keep the focus on the issues at hand and make the meeting a productive one.

2. Determine where the meeting will be held, the time and date of the meeting, and the individuals who should attend.
   <u>PURPOSE:</u> To have the demographic information about the meeting on hand before posting a notice. Only necessary staff members should attend so that those not directly involved in the issues to be discussed can continue their regular duties.

3. Send a memo, e-mail, or letter at least 10 days in advance, if possible, to the individuals who should attend the meeting. Send a copy to any supervisors who should be kept informed about the issues to be raised in the meeting.
   <u>PURPOSE:</u> To allow for rescheduling if the key personnel cannot attend on the originally planned time and date; also to keep managers informed of important details in areas for which they are ultimately responsible.

4. Be sure that the notice includes the following information:
   - Date
   - Time
   - Place
   - Directions (if not held in a common meeting room or if held away from the office)

- Speakers and/or meeting topics
- Cost and registration information, if applicable
- List of items individuals should bring to the meeting
   <u>PURPOSE:</u> To fully inform those who should attend the meeting of the demographic information and their responsibilities.

5. Finalize the list of items to discuss and place them in priority order.
   <u>PURPOSE:</u> To keep the focus of the meeting on the issues at hand and to avoid discussion of nonrelated items; also to make sure the time spent in the meeting is productive for all involved.

6. Delegate any tasks that others can accomplish and follow up to be sure they fulfill their duties before the meeting.
   <u>PURPOSE:</u> To ensure that all needed information and items are available for the meeting.

7. Assign a staff member to take notes and keep time during the meeting.
   <u>PURPOSE:</u> To have notes so that a permanent record of what was discussed and the decisions made can be written after the meeting.

8. Make a list of all items that need to be taken to the meeting, including equipment such as microphones, projectors, screens, computers, disks containing presentations, and so on.
   <u>PURPOSE:</u> To be fully prepared and to have all needed items in place during the meeting.

9. Compile the final agenda for the meeting.

10. On the meeting day, transport all necessary items to the meeting room. Begin and end the meeting on time. Stay on track and follow the agenda.
    <u>PURPOSE:</u> Following the plan and showing consideration for the time staff members devote to meetings can promote a positive attitude for meetings and encourage group participation.

11. Follow up whenever necessary on items discussed in the meetings. Distribute a synopsis of the meeting to all the individuals who attended and keep a copy in a binder or folder.
    <u>PURPOSE:</u> To keep a permanent record of the meeting and the items discussed and decided.

OFFICE MANAGEMENT TOOLS

Patient Information Booklet

Only a very small percentage of practices have a booklet that explains the information basic to the operational and service aspects of the practice. Yet, the physician and staff can easily compile a patient information booklet cooperatively during a staff meeting. Experience has shown that if such a booklet is given to every new patient, the number of incoming telephone calls can be reduced by an average of 20% to 30%. It also can reduce misunderstandings and forgotten instructions. The booklet must be tailored to the specific practice.

The patient information booklet should be an introduction to the practice. If possible, it should be mailed to a new patient before the first visit. A supply also may be left with referring physicians' offices to be given to patients coming to your office. It should be designed to fit easily into a No. 10 business envelope. The cover should show the name of the practice, its location, and the practice logo, if there is one. Consider using a photograph of the medical building for easy identification by the new patient and a map to the office. Many offices save the booklet as a .pdf file so that it can be emailed to the patient.

A statement of philosophy frequently is included in the introduction, followed by a description of the practice. For example:

The doctors and staff would like to welcome you to our office. We work as a team with the goal of providing prompt and thorough care for your problems. We are always working to improve our care and service in any way possible. Our practice is limited exclusively to the musculoskeletal system and its disorders. Therefore, it is important for each patient to have a primary care physician, such as a pediatrician, a family physician, or an internist, to oversee the patient's primary medical care. Our role is most effective as a consultant to your primary care physician.

Describe the office policy regarding appointments and cancellations, telephone calls, and the function of the answering service. If a separate business telephone line is available, make sure to include this information. For example:

This office has two receptionists available to answer telephone calls during regular office hours. The office is very busy, and occasionally you will be asked to hold for a brief period. Please be patient with this. If you want to speak to a doctor, your call usually will be returned during the next available break period or at the end of the office day. We receive many calls during the day, and it is unfair to the patients who have scheduled appointments to interrupt the doctor continually for telephone calls. Therefore, the receptionist usually will take a message, and your call will be returned as soon as possible. Please inform the receptionist if your problem is urgent, and she will let the doctor know this.

Describe any **ancillary** or laboratory services provided, how test results are reported, and your policy on prescription renewals. Patients need to know the provisions for emergency procedures: What hospitals does the practice use regularly? What is the night and weekend coverage? Hospitalization procedures and postoperative care and follow-up may also be included:

One of the doctors in the group is always on call for emergencies. You may reach him or her by calling our office telephone number (714) 555-2323; the answering service will put you in touch with the doctor on call at that time. Our doctors are on staff at St. Joseph Hospital (714) 555-3333, and for children, Children's Hospital of Orange County (714) 555-4444. In case of emergency, call 911.

List all physicians in the practice; state their educational backgrounds, training, and board certifications; and define their specialties. List the names of key clinical and administrative staff members, such as registered nurses and nurse practitioners, medical assistants, the office manager, and the business manager. Provide the practice address, a map of how to get there, and information about the parking facilities.

Do not just stack these folders in the reception room for patients to pick up. Have the receptionist write the patient's name on the folder, hand it to the patient when he or she registers for the first appointment, and suggest that the patient keep it for future reference.

Financial Policy Folder

A separate, small folder covering the financial policies of the office can eliminate many questions and possible misunderstandings. Tailor the financial policy folder to the specific practice. Keep it small enough to fit into the billing envelope and send it out with the first monthly statement. If the practice sends out a welcome package before the patient's first visit, include the financial policy folder. Otherwise, present one at the first visit.

Spell out policies regarding billing and collection procedures and make it clear that patients are responsible for the uninsured portion of the fees. If payment is expected at the time of service, put this in the folder. Keep the language simple and straightforward so that the message is clear:

We ask that our services be paid for at the time they are rendered. You will be provided with an encounter form so that you may bill your insurance company and be reimbursed for services paid at the time of your visit. Simply attach the encounter form to your insurance form and mail it to the insurance company. The appropriate diagnoses and charges will be on the encounter form. There is usually a greater charge for the initial visit, because this involves more time than follow-up visits. If you are sent to an outside office for laboratory testing or special x-ray procedures, you will be billed separately by that office. We will be available to help if special circumstances arise involving difficulty with forms or receiving reimbursement. We will bill your insurance if you have a special situation such as surgery, prepaid health plans, Medicaid, or Senior Savers. We will complete disability papers as promptly as possible. However, you must obtain the necessary forms from your employer or the disability office.

The financial policy folder should also clearly state that the ultimate responsibility for payment lies with the patient.

Patient Instruction Sheets

In most medical offices, some patient procedures are performed over and over again. Instead of attempting to instruct a patient orally each time, why not develop clearly stated instruction sheets that can be reviewed with the patient and then give the patient the written instructions to take home? The following are some suggestions for patient instruction sheets:

- Preparation for an x-ray procedure or laboratory tests
- Preoperative and postoperative instructions
- Diet sheets
- Performing an enema
- Dressing a wound
- Taking medications
- Using a cane, crutches, walker, or wheelchair
- Care of casts
- Exercise therapy

MEDICAL PRACTICE ACTS

Medical practice acts existed as early as colonial days. However, these acts were later repealed, and in the mid-nineteenth century, practically none of the states had laws governing the practice of medicine. As one might expect, a rapid decline in professional standards followed. The general welfare of the people was endangered by medical **quackery** and inadequate care. By the beginning of the twentieth century, medical practice acts were established by statute and were again in effect in every state. The purpose of the medical practice acts is to:

- Define what is included in the practice of medicine in that state

- Govern the methods and requirements of licensure
- Establish the grounds for suspension or revocation of license

All physicians' offices must follow the laws and regulations set forth by the city and state where the practice is located (see Procedure 7-5). Medical assistants are required to report situations in which the law is being broken or that may lead to harm to another person, including the patient (see Procedure 7-6). However, before taking action that could do irreparable harm to another person's character, verify the facts and follow the facility's chain of command.

PHYSICIAN LICENSURE AND REGISTRATION

A graduate of a medical school must be licensed before beginning the practice of medicine. Licensure is regulated by state statutes through the Medical Practice Acts. It is important for a medical assistant to understand licensing and other laws and regulations intended to protect patients, physicians, medical assistants, and other healthcare workers.

Licensure

A Doctor of Medicine (MD), Doctor of Osteopathy (DO), or Doctor of Chiropractic (DC) degree is conferred upon graduation from a medical or chiropractic school. The license to practice medicine or chiropractic is granted by a state board, frequently known as the State Board of Medical Examiners or Board of Registration. Licensure may be accomplished by examination, reciprocity, or endorsement.

Examination

Every state requires medical doctors to pass a written examination. The Federation of State Medical Boards and the National Board of Medical Examiners agreed in 1990 to establish a single licensing examination, the Federation Licensing Examination (FLEX), for graduates of accredited medical schools. Medical graduates in the United States must pass the FLEX examination, the U.S. Medical Licensing Examination (USMLE), or the National Board of Medical Examiners' Examination (NBME). Osteopathic physicians pass the National Board of Osteopathic Medical Examiners' Comprehensive Osteopathic Medical Licensing Examination (COMLEX).

Reciprocity

Some states grant the license to practice medicine by *reciprocity*; that is, they automatically recognize that the requirements of the state in which the license was granted meet their standards.

Endorsement

Most graduates of medical schools in the United States have been licensed by endorsement of the National Board certificate. In simpler terms, a state offers a license to a physician based on the examinations taken to grant the license, not by virtue of the license granted from another state. Licensure by endorsement is granted on a case-by-case basis. Graduates who have not been licensed by endorsement are required to pass a state board examination.

In all states, graduates of foreign medical schools who are seeking licensure by endorsement must meet the same requirements as graduates of medical schools in the United States, in addition to various other qualifying factors.

Exemptions

Some graduates may not want to engage in the practice of medicine; their interests may lie in research, administration, or even in the practice of law with a special interest in medical liability. In such instances, licensure is not required. Licensed physicians in the Armed Forces, Public Health Service, and Veterans Affairs facilities need not be licensed in the state in which they are employed. However, the Department of Defense is encouraging states to require full licensure of military personnel.

Registration and Reregistration

After a license has been granted, reregistration is required annually or biennially. A physician can be *concurrently* registered in more than one state. The issuing body notifies the physician when reregistration is due. A medical assistant can aid the physician by being aware of when the registration fees are due, preventing a possible lapsing of the registration.

Many states require proof of continuing education in addition to payment of a registration fee. CEUs are granted to physicians for attending approved seminars, lectures, scientific meetings, and formal courses in accredited colleges and universities. A total of 50 hours per year is the average requirement for a license renewal. A medical assistant may be expected to help the physician arrange to complete the required units for license renewal.

Revocation or Suspension

Under certain conditions, the license to practice medicine may be revoked or suspended. Grounds for revocation or suspension of the license to practice medicine fall within one of three categories:

- *Conviction of a crime:* This may include felonies (e.g., murder, rape, larceny) and narcotics violations.
- *Unprofessional conduct:* Failure to uphold the ethical standards of the medical profession may be indicated by betrayal of patient confidence, giving or receiving rebates, and excessive use of narcotics or alcohol.
- *Personal or professional incapacity:* Such incapacity is difficult to label or prove. For example, advanced age or an injury may reduce the apparent capacity of some physicians. Certain illnesses can affect the memory or judgment necessary to practice medicine.

A physician studies many years to learn the profession before becoming licensed by the state to practice medicine. A medical assistant is not licensed to practice medicine and must never prescribe or attempt to diagnose a patient's ailment; this is the illegal practice of medicine. For this reason, a medical assistant must use great care in discussing patients' complaints and treatment with them, because patients identify the medical assistant's remarks as being the opinion of the physician.

CLOSING COMMENTS

Successful office managers care about their employees and the vision for the office. They must be strong promoters of the office mission statement. The areas of authority and responsibility must be clearly defined to prevent management problems. A solid office policy and procedures manual helps the office manager to run an efficient office.

Leadership is an important quality for any manager, and the medical office manager is no exception. The manager should develop good leadership skills, be fair and open minded, and treat employees and patients as he or she would want to be treated. These actions help ensure a pleasant, productive working environment.

Patient Education

Educate patients in the policies and procedures of the office by providing patient information folders or brochures. When these documents are prepared and given to patients formally, the patient is better informed and fewer calls come to the office.

Legal and Ethical Issues

Office managers must stay abreast of current employment laws and regulations for all the different agencies that govern the medical office. Joining an office manager's association helps the manager keep the office up-to-date and in compliance. Periodic checks on the Web sites of various organizations, such as OSHA, also help the manager stay aware of the most recent changes in policies and rules.

Documentation is a critical aspect of the office manager's duties. The manager should keep detailed notes on the performance of employees and always discuss poor performance with employees. Never allow bad habits to go unmentioned. To the extent that it is possible, treat employees in a similar fashion and extend fairness to all.

SUMMARY OF SCENARIO

Katherine has had an effect on all the staff members at Dr. Collins's office. She treats her employees well and is fair about office policies and procedures. Her subordinates appreciate her flexibility and professionalism as she deals with the many issues surrounding the operation of a medical office. Katherine treats the employees as team members, never speaking to them as if she were superior to them. She shares vital information with the staff so that they feel a part of the whole team, and she believes that even some negative information should be related to the staff so that everyone is aware of the challenges the office faces. She makes good hiring decisions and firmly believes in a good orientation and training program. Dr. Collins has placed a great deal of trust in Katherine, and she has performed well, proving to be reliable in her position as office manager.

Katherine knows that she should display a friendly attitude toward her staff members when appropriate to do so. She is kind and considerate and treats the staff as individuals. She does not fraternize with them but is open to having lunch with the staff at various times and participates in all casual office activities. She maintains a healthy distance so that she can be an effective manager, but she listens to those who are experiencing difficulty and is compassionate about helping whenever possible.

Katherine knows that she must be diligent in checking references so that she brings reliable, qualified individuals on board as staff members. Unless she receives acceptable references, she will not hire a medical assistant to become a part of her team. Once she hires someone, she conducts a thorough training program and takes special care to share the experience and skills of the new staff member with the rest of the team.

When Katherine must give a negative employee evaluation, she states that fact at the beginning of their meeting. Although she is compassionate, she is able to point out a staff member's shortcomings in a detailed, fair way. She usually is willing to give an employee time to improve, but if he or she fails to perform, Katherine does not hesitate to end the employment.

Katherine uses patient information folders as management tools. She has instructed her staff to explain the folders to patients fully and to tell them about the information in them. Because the staff takes the time to review the folders with patients, calls to the office have been reduced and the staff believes that patients are much more informed. They understand office policies much better, and the staff finds that they repeat basic information much less frequently. Katherine heads a cooperative team that functions well together every day, making the office efficient and the work environment a pleasant one of which to be a part.

SUMMARY OF LEARNING OBJECTIVES

1. **Define, spell, and pronounce the terms listed in the vocabulary.**
   Spelling and pronouncing medical terms correctly bolster the medical assistant's credibility. Knowing the definition of these terms promotes confidence in communication with patients and co-workers.
2. **Explain the importance of management in the medical office.**
   The physician counts on the office manager to run the business aspects of the office so that he or she can focus efforts on good patient care. A high degree of trust is placed in the office manager.
3. **Discuss the desirable qualities of a medical office manager.**
   A good office manager is fair and flexible. Good communications skills are necessary, as is attention to details. The manager should care about the employees and have a sense of fairness. The ability to remain calm in a crisis is important, as are the use of good judgment and the ability to multitask.
4. **List and discuss the three types of leaders.**
   Charismatic leaders inspire allegiance and dedication and encourage individuals to overcome great obstacles. *Transactional leaders* are structured, organized, hardworking, and planners. *Transformational leaders* are excellent during times of transition and effective at building relationships.
5. **Discuss several types of power and whether power is a positive or negative entity.**

Power can be both a positive and a negative entity. Power should not be used in a manipulative or coercive manner. *Expert power* is based on a high degree of knowledge about a certain subject. The use of rewards is a way of invoking power, and *legitimate power* is that of position or status. *Referent power* is granted from subordinates to those who lead by example.

6. **Identify several ways in which employees are motivated.**
Employees are motivated by various factors, including money, praise, insecurity, honor, prestige, needs, love, fear, satisfaction, and many others. An effective manager attempts to discover what motivates employees to do a good job.

7. **Explain the difference between intrinsic and extrinsic motivation.**
Intrinsic motivation comes from within the employee. Extrinsic motivation has an outside source.

8. **List several ways to prevent burnout.**
Asking for help, first and foremost, can prevent burnout. Managers often take on too many duties and do not delegate as much as they should. Exercise and rest help prevent burnout, as does understanding one's personal limitations. Focused goals are important and help keep the manager working toward the most critical tasks.

9. **Discuss what to look for when reviewing resumés and applications.**
Resumés and applications should be reviewed for accuracy and completeness. Gaps in employment dates should be explained fully, and the office manager should verify any references given. Documents should be legible, and the information should be consistent and without oversights.

10. **Explain why the telephone voice of an applicant is important.**
The telephone voice of an applicant is important because most employees have occasion to answer the telephone while at work. The employee's voice should be clear and easily understandable. Good grammar skills must be used to reflect a professional image.

11. **List and discuss legal and illegal interview questions.**
Title VII of the Civil Rights Act of 1964, as amended by the Equal Employment Opportunity Act of 1972, prohibits inquiries into an applicant's race, color, gender, religion, and national origin. Inquiries regarding medical history, arrest records, or previous drug use also are illegal. Most states have laws designed to protect the rights of job applicants, and these laws may impose additional restrictions. Office managers must research the laws that pertain to employment in their own states.

12. **Identify the follow-up activities the office manager should perform after an interview.**
After interviewing a prospective candidate, the office manager should verify the facts on the resumé and application and check several references. A comparison should be made between the candidates and the top two or three chosen for a possible second interview. It is wise to involve other staff members when choosing new employees for the office.

13. **Explain the importance of mentors for new employees in the medical office.**
Mentors help new employees by offering information about policies and procedures. The mentor can be an advocate that the new employee can approach when questions arise about any aspect of the medical office.

14. **Describe how to conduct a performance review for an employee.**
Performance reviews can be productive, positive experiences, or they can lead to termination of employment. The process for conducting a performance review is outlined in Procedure 25-2.

15. **List the various types of staff meetings.**
Staff meetings may be held to relay information, solve a problem, or brainstorm ideas. Some meetings are designed as work sessions, whereas others may be scheduled to discuss new policies or changes in procedures.

16. **Explain how to arrange a group meeting.**
Meetings will be held on at least a monthly basis in most physicians' offices. The process for arranging a group meeting is outlined in Procedure 25-3.

CONNECTIONS

Study Guide Connection: Go to the Chapter 25 Study Guide. Read and complete the activities.

Evolve Connection: Go to the Chapter 25 link at *evolve.elsevier.com/kinn* to complete the Chapter Review and Chapter Quiz. Check out the other resources listed for this chapter to make the most of what you have learned from Medical Practice Management and Human Resources.

MEDICAL PRACTICE MARKETING AND CUSTOMER SERVICE

26

SCENARIO

Monica Ray is a medical assistant who is also pursuing a bachelor's degree in marketing. She has worked for Dr. Julie Todd and Dr. Robert Todd for 2 years. Based on her career interests, the physicians have agreed to allow her to develop some new marketing strategies for their obstetrics and gynecology office. Because medical facilities are now so competitive, Monica knows that any physician who wants growth in the practice must market his or her services to the public. Also, physicians cannot depend only on insurance reimbursements to provide them a strong income through the life of the practice. Today, physicians must market themselves and their services to the public to ensure practice growth.

Monica is highly computer literate and can design Web pages. She plans to incorporate several ideas she found on other physicians' Web sites, including a method of online scheduling. She is also aware of the importance of social networking and wants to create a brand for the clinic using resources such as Facebook, Twitter, and YouTube. She is quite creative and is excited about the challenge of providing such a service to the patients of the clinic and about growing the patient base using social networking. Monica knows that planning is involved in any project, including creating the facility's Internet presence. She plans to speak to every employee of the office to get input regarding the design and content of the site. Patients will be able to provide her with additional suggestions on features they would like to see.

This new development for the office is just one way Monica hopes to incorporate more formal customer service techniques. She plans to share the information she is learning in the classroom with the physicians and staff at the clinic. Monica and the physicians are fortunate that the staff is enthusiastic and eager to try new methods of customer service; often employees are highly resistant to new techniques. The physicians will set specific goals with the help of the employees and devise a reward system for reaching them. An exciting few months are ahead for this innovative group of medical professionals!

While studying this chapter, think about the following questions:

- How important is an Internet presence to today's medical office?
- Why has "customer service" become a buzzword in the medical industry?
- How can social networking grow the practice patient base?
- Which is more important: the internal customer or the external customer?

LEARNING OBJECTIVES

1. Define, spell, and pronounce the terms listed in the vocabulary.
2. List the four steps to follow when preparing to implement a medical marketing strategy.
3. Explain the term *target market*.
4. Discuss how suggestion boxes might help the medical facility make improvements.
5. List and discuss the four Ps of marketing.
6. Explain the five steps for developing a plan in marketing.
7. Discuss how community involvement can make a difference in marketing efforts.
8. State the difference between advertising and public relations.
9. Determine ways to promote a new practice.
10. Prepare a presentation using PowerPoint.
11. Discuss applications of electronic technology in effective communication.
12. Organize technical information and summaries.
13. Discuss responses that help the medical assistant identify with the patient.
14. Explain the concept of the internal customer.
15. Design a presentation for a marketing event.
16. Locate resources and information for patients and employers.
17. Advocate on behalf of the patient and family and be able to deal and communicate with family members.

VOCABULARY

branding The process involved in creating a unique name and image in the customer's mind, mainly through advertising campaigns with a consistent theme.

marketing The process or technique of promoting, selling, and distributing a product or service.

objective Something toward which effort is directed; aim, goal, or purpose of action.

outreach The process of using marketing and education strategies to reach and involve diverse audiences through the use of key messages and effective programs.

prosthetic (prohs-thet′-ik) The surgical or dental specialty concerned with the design, construction, and fitting of prostheses, which are artificial devices that replace missing parts of the body.

tangible (tan′-juh-buhl) Capable of being appraised at an actual or approximate value; capable of being precisely identified or realized by the mind.

target market A specific group of individuals toward whom the marketing plan is focused.

Each medical office needs a mission statement that defines the reason for its existence. The physician's philosophy of medicine and reasons for pursing medicine as a career greatly influence the mission statement. With this statement in place, the staff can develop goals that will assist them in meeting the mission. The goals can be met through a **marketing** and **outreach** plan for the practice and by providing excellent customer service to patients and visitors to the facility.

DEVELOPING MARKETING STRATEGIES

If a business is to grow, marketing strategies are critical. A marketing strategy is designed to promote the services offered by the organization and encourage new business. Four steps are generally followed when preparing to implement or change medical marketing strategies:

1. Assess what has been done in the past.
2. Evaluate what is being done now to increase patient flow.
3. Decide what objectives are important and how meeting these objectives will be measured.
4. Develop a plan with various means of marketing the practice and a specific methodology for implementing each phase.

CRITICAL THINKING APPLICATION   26-1

Monica knows that the office has never attempted any formal marketing in the past. Because no one at her office is familiar with this task, who might she contact for advice and assistance?
- Even though her fellow staff members are not familiar with marketing, could they provide workable ideas?
- What are some ideas for marketing a medical practice?

Branding

The concept of **branding** is fairly new to the medical profession. Branding, applied to the physician's office, is the process involved in creating a unique concept or image that customers think of in association with the practice. Branding aims to establish a significant and differentiated presence in the market that attracts and retains loyal customers. This can be accomplished using a name, logo, tagline, catch-phrase, symbol, or design that makes your organization distinct and unique among others. A brand is a valuable element in a marketing campaign. The art of creating and maintaining a brand in the marketplace is called *brand management*. Global brands include Facebook, Apple, FedEx, and MasterCard; people all over the world recognize those brands. A local brand is one that is marketed in a small geographic area; for example, the Baylor Health Care System in Texas uses a distinct blue color on its Web sites, and its logo includes a flame symbol, easily identifying any Baylor facility throughout the area.

Branding helps the medical practice to stand out, ideally as a trusted authority in healthcare. Additionally, the physician can attract the types of cases that he or she is most interested in through branding; if the physician is interested in fibromyalgia, diabetes, or any other specific disease or condition, it may be incorporated into the practice through branding. The practice might use a tag line after the clinic name, such as:

Woodridge Clinic: The Diabetes Center

San Jose Family Practice: Caring for Each Family Member

The market climate has shifted to a highly competitive environment, and many physicians are forced to market their practice to gain any part of the local market share. Without a reasonably full schedule of patients, the physician cannot cover the costs of running the practice, and the business may not survive. The medical assistant can play a role in practice branding by following office procedures, treating patients with excellent customer service skills, and keeping a positive, enthusiastic attitude during every workday and with every patient.

SEVEN REASONS TO BRAND A MEDICAL PRACTICE

1. People prefer to buy brands, because they reduce perceived risk.
2. People buy brands for status.
3. People refer more often and more passionately to a brand that they like and trust.
4. You can build and accelerate your reputation through branding.
5. You can attract more of the cases you like through branding.
6. Branding will give you a competitive advantage.
7. A branded practice will be worth more than a nonbranded practice.

Knowing the Target Market

During the strategic phase of developing a marketing plan, the physician and office manager must identify the **target market** for the services provided by the clinic. The target market is the group or groups of individuals the office wants to reach. Reaching the target market means that the specific groups are made aware of the clinic and what it has to offer. With managed care restrictions and regulations, competition for patients has become keen among physicians, and a facility that does not pursue growth runs a great risk of not surviving.

Answer the following questions when considering the target market:

- What specific outcomes do we hope to accomplish?
- What are the needs and desires of our target market?
- What are the characteristics of a typical member of the target market?
- How can the target market be reached in the most cost-effective ways?

Staff meetings are excellent times to brainstorm about reaching target markets. The staff can explain the needs of the patients who are active at the medical office. If patients have made suggestions, they should be discussed and weighed with regard to which would benefit the patient population of the facility (Figure 26-1).

> ### CRITICAL THINKING APPLICATION 26-2
> What community resources could Monica seek as she is determining the target market of the practice? What information does she need to begin her search?

Suggestion boxes are a great way to solicit patient input. Ask patients for ideas about how the clinic could operate more smoothly and what additional services they would like to see introduced. Check the suggestion box frequently. If the patient leaves his or her name on the suggestion form, a good customer service tactic is to reward the patient for the suggestion. Mail the individual a coupon for a free lunch at a local restaurant or a free car wash at a local detailing shop. Involving other businesses in marketing efforts helps both attract new customers. Businesses in a central location, such as a strip mall, can work together to refer customers to each other.

Ethics, Marketing, and Public Relations

Not many years ago, advertising about the physician and his services was considered completely unethical. However, today's healthcare industry is highly competitive, and advertising is no longer considered unethical. Because competition for patients is so great, medical assistants who work in physicians' offices must use some marketing techniques to get new patients and keep the ones already coming to the clinic. This practice may not seem "right" to some employees, but the healthcare industry has changed over the past few decades, and physicians must invite change to be competitive. After all, the medical office is still a business. The goal of any business is to make money so that the owners can pay business costs and make a reasonable profit and employees can earn a healthy wage with which to support their own families.

The Four Ps

The four Ps of marketing are product, placement, price, and promotion. A physician's office offers medical services as a product. Some offices have **tangible** retail products that they also offer, such as vitamins, skin-sensitive cosmetics, or **prosthetic** devices. Placement involves the actual location of the medical office. The office may be located in an urban area close to large neighborhoods of young professionals or in a rural area with a few people living several miles apart. Placement can greatly influence the traffic to the facility. Placement also can refer to the setup of the office, the specific suite in a shopping strip where the office is located, or even the placement of retail objects on a shelf. Price is simply the amount of money charged for goods and services provided. Promotion refers to the methods used to get the product or services to the consumers (or, in the case of the medical office, to patients).

> ### CRITICAL THINKING APPLICATION 26-3
> - How can Monica investigate the charges for similar procedures at other clinics in her area?
> - Why is this information important to Monica?

Deciding What Services to Offer

Once the physician and office manager have identified the target market, decisions can be made about the services that should be offered to patients. For instance, suppose the office is situated in a neighborhood of young families. Both parents are very likely to work outside the home, so evening hours would be beneficial to these patients. The physician may decide to extend office hours to 8 PM twice a week and to open from 9 AM to noon on Saturdays. If several schools are in the area, particularly junior high and high schools, the physician may want to offer a special price on sports physicals during the fall. Because these physicals are required, if the physician offers them at a reasonable price, the entire family may decide to seek medical care from the physician.

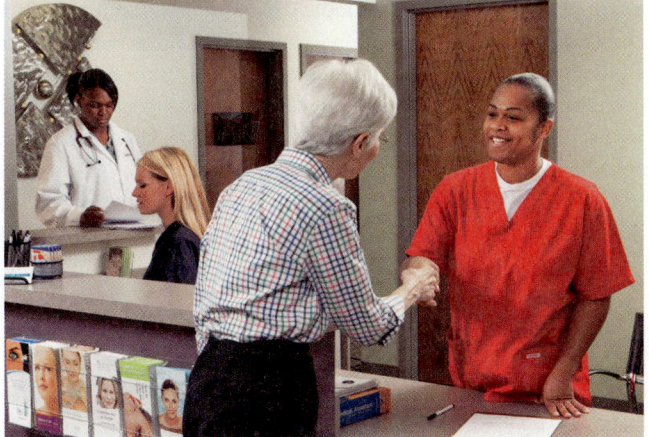

FIGURE 26-1 Friendly staff members are the best marketing tools. A smile is an excellent way to make patients feel welcome in the medical facility.

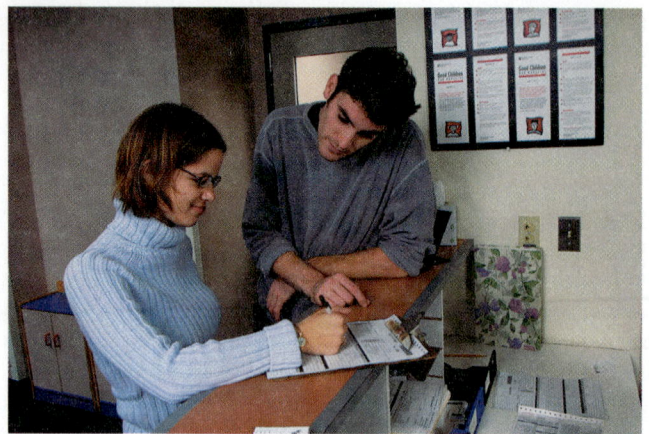

FIGURE 26-2 Offer services that are important in the geographic area of the office. College students may need to see a physician for minor illnesses, and they appreciate offices that provide short office visits for a reasonable fee.

If the office is located in a college town, the physician may want to offer a special student rate for short office visits (Figure 26-2). If a number of older adults live in the area, a senior citizen discount might be appropriate. Input from patients and staff members is valuable in determining what services to offer in the medical facility.

Developing a Plan for Marketing

The facility may use several specific planning steps for events, marketing strategies, and any number of other ideas the physician would like to implement. These steps are:

- Assessment
- Research
- Planning
- Execution
- Evaluation

Assessment is the phase of planning in which the problem or goals are reviewed. This is another excellent time for brainstorming. Research allows the physician or office manager to investigate the needs of the target market and then decide what the medical office can do to meet those needs. Planning of the concept follows, and once a firm plan is in place, it is executed, or carried out. Afterward, the participants evaluate what went well and what problems occurred so that future efforts will be even more successful.

Try this simple assessment tool, which will help clarify the patient population: Keep a log of all patients for a specific period; include the reason for the visit; the patient's age, ZIP code, gender, and marital status; and the number and ages of children. These simple demographics can provide a great base picture of the types of individuals using the physician's services.

PROMOTING THE PRACTICE

The physician and office manager should constantly watch for ways to promote the medical practice and keep its name in the public eye. Some of these methods are free, whereas others require detailed budgeting and planning.

The physician can allot a large portion of the practice budget to advertising and promotional costs. Some clinics publish a

health-related magazine and mail it or send it electronically to their patient base. Magazine and newspaper ads can be effective tools, but finding free sources to promote the practice eases the budget and will allow expansion in other areas.

Tapping into Free Community Resources

By becoming a member of various civic organizations, such as the Chamber of Commerce, the practice will receive notice of upcoming events and should plan to participate in them regularly. The more the public sees the physician in the community, the more likely this will affect the growth of the practice. Many good promotional activities are relatively free to the physician. Some newspapers offer an advice column in which different types of professionals give general medical advice to those who write in with questions. Physicians volunteer to answer these questions in print, and in return the office address, the office telephone number, and often the physicians' pictures are featured. This is an excellent way to generate patient calls and inform the public about the specialties and types of cases the physician handles.

CRITICAL THINKING APPLICATION   26-4

- Monica knows there are many opportunities and free resources in her area. Where should she begin to look?
- How might Monica's clinic partner with other businesses and services to provide excellent care to patients and to help one another at the same time?

Getting involved in the local community is another way to promote a medical practice. Some physicians sponsor Little League football teams, baseball teams, or bowling leagues. Sometimes entire staffs participate in charity events and marathons, wearing T-shirts with the clinic name printed on the back.

The physician or staff may have specific charities they support annually, or they may participate in United Way activities, which distribute funds to many different types of worthy organizations through payroll deductions. Some medical facilities have volunteer programs in which employees receive recognition for participation in various activities. A good example is blood donations. Many blood centers offer pins and recognition certificates for the number of pints of blood volunteers donate. The office staff may set a goal to reach a certain number of donated pints in a year, and as recognition certificates are collected, the staff may want to display them in a prominent place in the office. This is an indication to patients that the staff is concerned about the community and is volunteer minded. From a public relations standpoint, this is valuable to the medical office, because patients tend to expect medical professionals to be volunteer oriented.

Health fairs are a great way to promote the services offered by the clinic, resulting in name recognition and increasing public visibility. Some health fairs are huge, highly publicized events, whereas others are small, often held at a local shopping mall or grocery store. All these events could be worthy projects for the physician and the medical office.

CRITICAL THINKING APPLICATION   **26-5**
- What community organizations might help Monica in her efforts to make the office an integral part of the community?
- What resources and community organizations are available in your area that would be good avenues for practice marketing and community service?

Advertising Plans and Agencies

Most physicians' offices do not use advertising agencies to promote their practices, but occasionally an agency might be useful. If the practice schedules or sponsors a very special event that needs extensive planning, a public relations firm or advertising agency might be consulted. Unfortunately, the cost of these groups usually is high and beyond the reach of sole practitioners or small group practices. However, the money may be well spent if the event is critical and attendance is important to its success.

There is a difference between advertising and public relations. Advertising involves creating or changing attitudes, beliefs, and perceptions by influencing people with purchased broadcast time, print space, or other forms of written and visual media. Broadcast time could take the form of television commercials, radio broadcasts, or audiovisual aids. Print could be in a newspaper, magazine, or trade journal, and written and visual media may be a flier, brochure, or billboard. Public relations is a similar field but relies more on news broadcasts or reports, magazine or newspaper articles, and radio reports to reach the audience. Most public relations efforts are free, but often it is difficult to get others interested enough in the activities the medical office is planning to warrant coverage.

Communication as a Marketing Tool

Many medical offices use communications tools to market the practice and improve customer service. Sending out a monthly newsletter by mail or electronically provides health information and news about upcoming events. The newsletter can be personalized for the office and might even include news about patients and the medical staff, as long as permission is obtained.

Sending birthday cards is an excellent public relations tool. Some offices sign the greetings at staff meetings, and they are placed in a tickler file for the proper mailing date. Consider sending holiday greetings to wish patients well.

Automated call distribution is becoming a popular means of communicating with large numbers of people. A computer dials multiple numbers at the same time and plays a recorded message, which can be the actual physician with news about a new procedure or new associate joining the practice. Although many people block such calls to their homes and an equal number hang up, the success rate for automatic call distribution is actually quite good. Many individuals listen and respond to the calls, especially if they come from someone they know and the information is important. For instance, if a medical clinic were planning to move to another part of the city, a program could be initiated to notify all patients with telephone numbers that the office will be moving after a certain date. The message could include the address of the new location and even prompt patients to "press 1" if they need to schedule an appointment. The same principle could be applied to news about an upcoming health fair, a special seminar about a certain illness, or even an article that will be in the Sunday paper about the clinic.

Promoting a New Practice

Most physicians who open a new practice place an ad in local newspapers to announce the event. Usually a picture of the physician is included, and a map to the exact location may be available on the ad. Some physicians purchase clinics from others who are moving or retiring, but many open a freestanding clinic in a new building, and the word about the new facility must be spread for the business to be a success.

Providing business cards for all employees is a good way to increase public knowledge about the facility. Some offices offer incentives for patient referrals from the staff or other patients, but the physician must ensure that no state statutes or ethical standards prohibit this practice. The incentive could be a simple coffee cup with the clinic's logo on it or a book about a healthcare issue. Recognition is the important factor where referrals are concerned. A thank you card is the minimal acceptable "thanks" for patient referrals.

Some physicians hold an open house when the new facility opens. Often, those individuals who assisted with the business from its inception attend the open house to lend support to the owners. Bankers, attorneys, accountants, and other physicians often show their support by attending the open house. Place pictures from this event on the facility's Web site, in the local newspaper, or in the monthly newsletter. Choose an employee who is a proficient writer and assign him or her the task of writing and sending press releases to media outlets when the physician or practice is involved with a newsworthy event.

Developing and Giving Presentations

Today's medical assistant should be comfortable when speaking in front of individuals and groups. By developing additional skills, the medical assistant increases his or her value to the physician. Developing and giving presentations is not difficult, although one of the most prevalent fears in the United States is the fear of speaking in public (Procedures 26-1 and 26-2).

There are many different types of speeches, but remember that all public speaking is persuasive. The speaker is attempting to get the audience to do something, whether to buy a new medical product or convince people to participate in a clinical trial. The speaker always has a purpose and must be credible to persuade listeners to act. Credibility underlies all persuasion. When the speaker is proficient at this art, the audience's questions are answered, their concerns addressed, and their needs fulfilled, while at the same time the speaker's goals are met. If the speaker does a good job, the audience feels satisfied after hearing a persuasive speech. Persuasion should be nonadversarial and gentle so that the audience feels comfortable in making a decision.

In his book, *Presenting to Win: The Art of Telling Your Story,* Jerry Weissman calls persuasion "audience advocacy," by which he means the ability to view the self, a company, a story, or a presentation through the eyes of the audience. Answer the question, "What's in it for me?" which the audience is constantly thinking. To motivate the audience, the speaker must do the following:

PROCEDURE 26-1

Design a Presentation

GOAL: *To gain skill in designing presentations that can be used for a variety of projects in the medical facility.*

EQUIPMENT and SUPPLIES

- Information about the presentation's subject
- Software (e.g., PowerPoint), if needed
- Computer access
- Peripheral computer equipment, if needed

PROCEDURAL STEPS

1. Determine the goals of the presentation.
   <u>PURPOSE:</u> The goals and purpose of the presentation must be determined before beginning so that the presenter is sure to reach those goals.
2. Write an outline of the entire presentation.
   <u>PURPOSE:</u> The outline helps the presenter prepare so that no important points are left out of the presentation.
3. Build the presentation using software (e.g., PowerPoint), highlighting the major points of the presentation.
4. Evaluate the audience and adjust the presentation to appeal to that audience.
   <u>PURPOSE:</u> The presenter must know the audience to ensure a successful presentation.

5. Rehearse the presentation several times in front of a mirror.
   <u>PURPOSE:</u> Rehearsing in front of a mirror builds confidence.
6. Make a list of all equipment and materials to take to the presentation.
   <u>PURPOSE:</u> A list helps the presenter remember all items that need to be taken to the presentation.
7. Arrive for the presentation 15 to 30 minutes early, depending on the preparation and setup required.
   <u>PURPOSE:</u> Arriving early gives the presenter the opportunity to set up the presentation before the audience arrives.
8. Deliver the presentation within the prescribed period.
9. Ask the audience whether anyone has any questions about the information in the presentation.
   <u>PURPOSE:</u> A question and answer period allows the presenter to interact with the audience.
10. Thank the audience and remove all equipment and supplies when appropriate.
11. Send a thank you note to the organization for allowing the presentation, if appropriate.

- Know the audience
- Research the audience to know their needs, what they care about, and what they want to know
- Link all presentation information to the audience's needs
- Know the purpose of the presentation
- Rehearse the presentation repeatedly

When designing the content of the presentation, keep the audience in mind and nail down the most important points that must be conveyed to them.

Overcoming Anxiety

Because the fear of public speaking is so common, the speaker must develop ways to overcome it and make a successful presentation. Find the actions that promote relaxation and practice them before giving a speech. Look for a sympathetic face in the audience, and speak directly to that person. Never begin a presentation with an apology of any type, such as, "I didn't have much time to prepare," or "I'm not very good at presentations." This undermines the authority of the speaker. Greeting as many of the guests as possible before the presentation helps to develop a rapport and may reduce anxiety. In addition, the guests feel welcome and special because the speaker took the time to make introductions.

During the Presentation

Make sure the audience can hear everything that is said. The presentation cannot be effective if it cannot be heard. Make all movements purposeful; if a hand gesture is used, make it and then relax the arms. Do not wander around the room. If moving from place to place, go to a spot and then stop. Constant movement distracts from the message of the presentation.

Most individuals speak faster when making a presentation, so slow the pace just a little. Speak so that all the people in the back of the room can hear, but not so loudly that the people in the front rows have to cover their ears. Possibly most important, remember to relax. The physical reactions felt before speaking, such as an increase in pulse rate and a rush of adrenaline, are natural. Do not allow negative thoughts to enter your mind. Instead, deal with fear by knowing the topic and being confident about the message.

PREPARING A PRESENTATION

Answer these important questions when preparing a presentation:
- Who is the audience?
- What are the key points?
- When is the presentation?
- How long is the presentation?
- What will the physical surroundings be?
- Why should the audience listen?
- How will the presentation be done?

PROCEDURE 26-2

Prepare a Presentation Using PowerPoint

GOAL: *To enhance presentations using PowerPoint as a visual aid.*

EQUIPMENT and SUPPLIES

- Information about the presentation's subject
- Software (e.g., PowerPoint), if needed
- Computer access
- Peripheral computer equipment, if needed

PROCEDURAL STEPS

1. Open the PowerPoint program.
2. Have the outline of the presentation available.
3. Click on the "new slide" icon in the program.
4. Create the title slide using the slide layout section on the right side of the screen.
5. Create additional slides using the slide layout section or design the slides manually.
6. Limit the number of words on the slides so that a concise message results.
   PURPOSE: Too many words on one slide make the message difficult to understand.
7. Make sure the font is as large as possible on the slide, beginning with a size 18 font and increasing from there.
   PURPOSE: The font on a presentation must be easy to read from the back of the room.
8. Do not use more than three font types per slide.
   PURPOSE: More than three font types makes the presentation difficult to read.
9. Avoid using more than three text-only slides in a row.
   PURPOSE: Use clip art, photographs, graphs, and other items to enhance the presentation.
10. Insert photos or clip art into the presentation by clicking on "Insert," then clicking on "Picture," then choosing "Clip art" or "From file."
11. Format the background of each slide, or of all slides, by clicking on "Format," then "Background," and then choose a color or fill effects.

PURPOSE: A consistent background makes the presentation look more professional.

12. Click on "Slide show" and adjust the slide transitions so that the slides appear and disappear as desired and are timed correctly.
13. Click on "Custom animation" to change the entrance and exit of the slides to the effect that is desired.
14. Save the presentation frequently while working on it.
    PURPOSE: Saving the presentation frequently ensures that the work will not be lost.
15. Click on "View" on the task bar, then on "Slide sorter," which allows the slides to be moved around in the presentation.
16. To run the show continuously, click on "Slide show," then on "Set up show," then click the box labeled "Loop continuously until escape" in the "Show options" box.
    PURPOSE: Running the show continuously is helpful for situations in which the presentation can be watched while people are passing through an exhibit hall, and so on.
17. Make sure the presentation has been saved.
18. Practice giving the presentation several times to smooth all transitions and to become familiar with the content.
    PURPOSE: The more the presentation is practiced, the more comfortable the presenter will be.
19. Anticipate questions the audience may ask and have answers prepared.
    PURPOSE: Anticipating questions helps the presenter better prepare for the presentation and ensures that the presenter knows the material.
20. Offer other visual aids, such as handouts, if appropriate, when giving the presentation.
    PURPOSE: Visual aids help the audience remember the presentation and may prompt them to take any action the presenter wants them to take.

DESIGNING PRESENTATION CONTENT

Remember these points when designing a presentation:
- Use bulleted points consistently.
- Use white space between bullets.
- Align text systematically in one area of a slide and place graphics on the other side.
- Make sure visuals deal with the subject of the presentation and are necessary.
- Time the transition between slides.
- Make bulleted points appear in a systematic way so that readers see text as the speaker is talking and not before or after the points are mentioned.
- If a physical process is demonstrated, use visuals to enhance the demonstration.
- Choose the most readable font.
- Use hyperlinks effectively.
- Use midrange colors for backgrounds.
- Rehearse the narration.
- Use titles for charts and illustrations.
- Organize content well.

Building a Practice Web Site

One of the most popular and beneficial marketing tools for the physician is a professional Web site. If the physician or an office staff member has sufficient knowledge to construct a Web site, there is little or no cost to the doctor if free Web site services are used. Businesses that host Web sites on the Internet offer very reasonable costs, starting at around $25 a month.

Four basic steps are involved in building a Web site for a medical practice:

1. Define the objectives of the Web site.
2. Design the pages.
3. Locate a Web server to which the pages can be uploaded.
4. Upload the pages to the server.

Defining Objectives

When defining the **objectives** of the practice, consider the physician's goals. The physician and staff should discuss who the audience will be and what will be included on the site. Most Web Sites designed for physicians' offices and clinics are informational, developed for both patient and public use. Once the objectives have been clearly defined, specific content can be written to place on the Web Site. The practice website is a perfect example of the need to organize technical information and summarize activities in which patients might be interested. The objectives developed by the physician and staff need to be transformed into activities that will attract and interest the patients as well as the local community.

Designing Pages

When the objectives have been clarified, begin developing ideas about what the site will look like on the computer screen. Color choices, animation, and fonts enhance the look that is being created and make a strong statement about the medical facility. The menus should be designed so that viewers can navigate easily through the site. Most users appreciate a means to go back to the page previously viewed and grow frustrated with sites that have an excessive number of pop-up boxes. Consistency is important, so it is a good idea to keep the same design theme on each page of the Web site.

The most important part of the Web site is the text. It has been said that every word in a book must add to the story, and this is a good way to look at the text in a Web site. Avoid too much repetition and remain clear about what is being communicated on the site. Headings and titles help clarify the theme of each page. Use a spell-checker before uploading the message and making it available for public viewing.

Photographs, graphics, music, and video can add fun to the Web site, but be careful not to overdo them. Graphics often are large files that take time to download. Most people will not wait longer than about 10 seconds for a Web page to load before clicking elsewhere. When designing Web page graphics, remember that smaller is better. Graphics can be found by searching for "index of GIF files" or "GIF library." Once an appropriate file has been found, it should be copied onto the hard drive by right-clicking the graphic and selecting "Save picture as." Music can be found by searching for "mid" or "midi." The search can even specify a certain singer, song, or composer. Always respect any copyrights that are designated on any file used. Many Web sites offer these files for free.

For a more professional-looking Web site, consider purchasing Web development software, such as Macromedia's Dreamweaver or Microsoft's FrontPage. These feature-rich products are fairly inexpensive and can help the medical assistant create very attractive, easy to maintain Web sites. Most products integrate tutorial and "help" features that explain how to use them.

Hyperlinks are words or graphics on a Web page that take the viewer to another page or another Web site when clicked. To add a hyperlink, simply highlight the text field or graphic, select the hyperlink icon, and specify the destination address (uniform resource locator [URL]). Always specify the full URL to ensure that the link directs the user to the desired page.

The main page should always be assigned the file name "index.htm" or "default.htm." Other pages on the Web site can be assigned any name; however, keep the names short and do not use special characters.

Locating a Web Server

At this point, the design of the Web site is complete, but the files reside on the computer hard drive, not on the Internet. Now the pages are ready to be uploaded, or published, to a Web server that will allow them to be viewed on the Internet. The Internet service provider (ISP) that the office uses for e-mail and online services may offer free Web space to its customers. If not, a number of companies provide Web space at no charge, but the user usually is required to use banners on the site that advertise the ISP or other services. If no banner ads are desired, the medical facility may want to use a paid provider. Some Web hosting companies provide other services free of charge, such as simple Web page editors and e-mail addresses.

Uploading Pages

When a free Web server is used, instructions and passwords are sent to the users that describe how to upload files to the server. The password is necessary so that other people cannot alter the files. Copying the files from the local hard disk to the Web server is a simple process. The hosting site prompts the user for the name of the directory on the hard drive where the files are stored and for the names of the specific files to be uploaded. To avoid confusion, make sure the files saved on the server have the same file names used on the hard drive.

Once all the files have been uploaded, test the page on the Web server and make sure it functions properly and that all files have been uploaded correctly. It also is a good idea to test the page using a different computer to ensure that graphic files are being read from the server and not from the local hard drive.

Evaluating the Web Site

Include an e-mail address where viewers of the Web site can interact with the creator with comments. When viewers have this option, problems with the site can be readily identified and corrected. It also is advisable to check the site every few days to make sure it is functioning properly.

CRITICAL THINKING APPLICATION   26-6

Monica is considering a frequently asked questions (FAQ) section for the Web site. How might this help patients?
- What kinds of questions might be asked in this section?
- How might the inclusion of this section benefit employees?

Counters often can be added to the Web site that will indicate how many people viewed it. This helpful tool allows the medical facility to track how many people are viewing which pages.

Social Media and Networking

Social media can be considered a two-way street that allows a communication response to regular media, which is a one-way street, such as a newspaper article or a television report. Regular media allows only limited ability to give a response; one can write a letter to the editor of a newspaper, but the letter is not an immediate two-way response. Social media is sometimes called *consumer-generated media* (CGM) and is considered a blending of technology and social interaction that creates a thing of value. This technology has become important to businesses of all types and continues to evolve. Creative, tech-savvy people are producing innovative ideas for medical facilities to attract new patients.

Developing along with social media is another important concept, Web 2.0. This is the term used to describe the cumulative changes in the ways that end-users and software developers use the Web, resulting in application features that facilitate information sharing, interoperability, user-centered design, and collaboration. Instead of just reading content on the Web, users interact in a virtual community or social network. Many Web sites now contain icons representing Facebook, Twitter, YouTube, Pinterest, and other types of social media to promote interaction, with the hope of creating a loyal customer or user who will return to the site or business repeatedly.

Earlier in the chapter, we considered Baylor Health Care System in Texas with regard to its branding messages. The organization has incorporated social media to interact with those in need of the

services that the hospital system offers, but also uses games, craft ideas, health tips, and other interesting applications that a user may enjoy just for fun. Baylor uses Facebook as a resource, a platform to share medical news and health information, and to connect with its "fans." The system uses Twitter to announce classes on healthcare issues, present surveys, share news related to healthcare, and allow patients to comment on care received at Baylor facilities. For example, a tweet mentions an article about Baylor's Animal Therapy Program and points the user to Baylor's Pinterest board, where photos of the animals, procedures for obtaining therapy animals, and videos of patients using the therapy animals can be found. The Baylor YouTube Channel offers videos with instructions about making an emergency kit for a family, Ask the Expert videos cover subjects such as stress, cervical cancer, and anterior cruciate ligament (ACL) injuries and also presents healthy cooking demonstrations for cancer patients. Baylor uses all of these aspects of social media to their best advantage in an effort to meet its organizational goals, recruit new users to its services, and retain current users.

From just this one example, it is easy to understand how an aggressive, well-planned social media approach can positively affect the financial health of a facility. These processes put individuals "into" the Web, making the experience more interactive and responsive. The medical assistant who can use social media in a professional way will be a valuable asset to the medical practice.

SOCIAL NETWORKING SITES OF INTEREST TO MEDICAL ASSISTANTS

- Healthranker
- Organized Wisdom
- Peoples MD
- Trusera
- FitLink
- Limeade
- American Well
- Daily Strength
- Group Loop
- Health 2.0
- Mamaherb
- MDJunction
- Patients Like Me
- Real Mental Health
- Real Self
- Right Health
- Twit2Fit
- Vitals

HIGH-QUALITY CUSTOMER SERVICE IN THE MEDICAL PRACTICE

Treating the Patient as a Customer

The best way to increase the number of patients in a medical office is through word of mouth. When patients are satisfied with the treatment they receive, they refer other patients to the physician. However, if they are dissatisfied, they will tell everyone they know!

Because patients often have a choice about who provides their healthcare services, it is important that the physician's office become the patient's first choice. Some patients are so loyal to a certain physician that even if their healthcare coverage no longer pays for visits, they continue to see that doctor. This happens because of the attitude of the physician and his or her office staff.

Medical assistants, whether just out of school or already established in their careers, must provide patients with good customer service. Patients do not hesitate to tell the physician if the medical assistant is not cordial and helpful. Providing excellent customer service is mandatory for every employee of the practice.

Helpful Attitude

The physician and staff should project a helpful attitude in every contact with the patient. They should sincerely ask, "How may I help you?" and then take steps to assist the patient in whatever way possible. Instead of pointing in the general direction of the radiology department, a staff member should take the patient there and introduce him or her to the receptionist. Instead of telling a patient on the telephone, "Ann handles the insurance billing. I'll transfer you to her," say, "One moment, Mrs. Brown, let me see if Ann is at her desk." Place Mrs. Brown on hold, call Ann, and let her know that she has a call. Then return to Mrs. Brown, tell her that Ann is at her desk, and transfer the call at that time. Be courteous and kind to every patient and visitor to the office. Good customer relations must be one of the primary goals of the medical facility. Patients count on the staff members to be reliable and available to help them to the best of their abilities.

Phrases That Undermine Successful Customer Service

The following are some phrases that should never be used when relating to patients and visitors.

- "I don't know."
  Say instead: "Although I don't know the answer, I will find out for you." The medical assistant will not know the answer to every question but must be willing to find out the information.
- "I don't care."
  Say instead: "We do care about your concerns and want to help." If the medical assistant cannot honestly make this statement, he or she should consider another profession.
- "I can't be bothered."
  Say instead: "I truly want to give this matter my full attention. Where can I contact you once I have looked into the matter?" Some people may expect immediate attention and service, but they may have to be patient and wait their turn to receive assistance.
- "Ask someone else."
  Say instead: "I will be happy to find out who handles that for you." The medical assistant should never project the attitude that the patient's concerns are unimportant.
- "It's not my job."
  Say instead: "I am not one of the employees who files insurance, but I will be happy to ask Amanda, our insurance supervisor, to contact you and answer your questions." Do not ever tell the patient or a supervisor that a certain duty is not a responsibility. Find the right person to help the patient.
- "It's not my fault."
  Say instead: "I was not involved with that decision, but I know that our office manager would be happy to speak with you about it." Although blame should never be placed on another employee, any touchy issue should be referred to the office manager, especially if the medical assistant is not the final decision-making authority.

- "I didn't do it."
  Say instead: "I will see if I can get to the root of this issue." Be willing to assist the patient even if you are not involved in the situation at hand.
- "I know that."
  Say instead: "Yes, I understand. Let me try to help you." Do not use sarcasm and never make snippy remarks to patients.
- "I'm right, you're wrong."
  Say instead: "Our policy is clear about this matter, but let's see if we can come up with a compromise." Accusatory remarks should never be made to a patient.

All these alternate phrases give the patient or visitor a more positive view of both the office and those who work in the facility.

Identifying with Patients

Patients appreciate staff members who can identify with the problems they are facing. This is especially effective when a patient is upset or angry. For example, if a patient comes to the office complaining that charges were placed on his account for procedures that were not performed, the medical assistant may respond with a phrase such as, "Mr. Roberts, I understand that you're upset about these additional charges. I know I would be upset if I were billed for something I didn't receive. Let me help you by doing this …"

Identifying with the patient shows understanding on the part of the staff member, no matter how upset the patient may be. Always acknowledge and restate the patient's concern. It proves that the medical assistant was listening and is interested in resolving the problem.

Remember, it costs much more to find new customers than to keep existing customers happy. Providing helpful, personal service impresses even the most difficult patient. To patients and visitors to the clinic, the employees to whom they speak represent the whole company. Perceptions and opinions likely will be formed based on experiences with only one person. Each individual employee must be aware that to the patient, each employee is the healthcare facility.

What Do Patients Expect?

First, patients expect to be treated according to the Golden Rule. They expect their concerns to be met with responsiveness, which means that the medical assistant should have a caring attitude. They also expect the professionals in the medical office to be knowledgeable about their field or specialty. An insurance biller should know more than just the basics of insurance filing. The office manager should have a certain degree of authority to handle problems and complaints. Patients also expect confidentiality and trust from the staff of the medical office. They expect an organized office that runs on schedule. They also expect that if a staff member promises to do something, it is as good as done. Patients' expectations can be better assessed by using customer service evaluation forms. For an example of a customer service evaluation form, visit the Evolve site at *evolve.elsevier.com/kinn*.

Remembering the Internal Customer

Most of us do not have problems figuring out who the external customers are in a medical practice. Patients, their families and friends, and visitors to the office are external customers. But who is the internal customer?

Internal customers are employees and staff members of the facility. Although they work for the business, they also are served by the business. If they are not pleased with the atmosphere of the medical facility, they are sure to look elsewhere for employment. Keeping the internal customer is just as important as keeping the external customer.

CLOSING COMMENTS

Providing good customer service is a commitment that must be made by every employee of the medical facility, every single day. There will be times when the customer is not right, but he or she should be treated with dignity and respect at all times. In addition, an expert customer service provider has a knack for making the customer think he or she was right all along! The medical office is no exception to the requirements for providing good service to its patients, and doing so results in an excellent reputation for the clinic, built by those who matter most—the patients.

Patient Education

A practice's marketing and public relations efforts provide endless opportunities for patient education. Most physicians agree that part of the obligation of the medical profession is to educate patients about healthcare issues. The practice's public relations and marketing staffs can work together to provide information to patients of the facility and to the general public. Many physicians attend health fairs, where brochures and pamphlets can be distributed about

conditions such as diabetes, heart disease, hypertension, and other disorders. Screenings for cholesterol and blood pressure checks are good ways to market a practice and gain new patients.

The medical assistant who knows how to build and maintain a simple Web site can be of great value to the physician. The practice's Web site could provide opportunities for educating patients, in addition to special sections for upcoming events, an online newsletter, and appointment setting. The Web site address should be included on stationery, business cards, and other documents used to promote the facility. Using Facebook, Twitter, YouTube, and other types of social media will place the healthcare facility in strategic positions to thrive amid the fierce competition of today's healthcare industry.

Legal and Ethical Issues

The physician must take care that patients do not use the information in brochures or on the practice Web site as medical advice or as a substitute for the physician's counsel. When attaching links to other Web sites, be sure they are reputable. The patient may consider information on the practice's Web site to be an extension of the physician's advice, so make sure everything on the Web site is accurate.

The physician should carefully review all printed information used to promote the medical facility. Make sure no misleading statements are included. A disclaimer should be used to remind patients that the information given in brochures and on Web sites is only general information. Patients should discuss specific medical issues with the physician.

SUMMARY OF SCENARIO

Monica knows that without growth, many businesses eventually fail. She is confident that with a simple marketing plan, the clinic will experience steady, continuous expansion. She has spoken to all the office staff members and gained input from both employees and patients of the clinic. Many offered excellent suggestions that Monica can incorporate into her marketing plan.

One of her first activities was to develop an annual calendar of special events and outreach efforts. A monthly newsletter and the practice Web site will be the main thrusts of her marketing plan. The newsletter will be available both in print and online. The patients in the office database who have e-mail addresses will receive automatically a computer-generated e-mail message containing a link that will take them directly to the online newsletter. Inside, patients will find health information and details about upcoming events.

Monica also planned one special activity for each month of the year. She scheduled a blood drive, a Christmas toy drive, and mini–health fair. Because both Dr. Julie and Dr. Robert Todd are dedicated to students who want to pursue medicine, Monica even planned a career day for high school students interested in becoming physicians, inviting representatives from the medical school that the Todds attended. Because this is considered a public service, Monica was able to get press coverage on the local radio station and in the newspaper at no cost.

Monica visited a new restaurant close to the office that serves heart-healthy dishes, met with the manager, and discussed ways the two businesses could help each other. They decided to provide a "buy one entrée, get one free" coupon to patients who referred other patients to the clinic. In turn, Dr. Robert Todd agreed to hold his free nutrition seminars at the restaurant. This arrangement has proved to work well for both businesses. Monica obtained this new agreement by making an effective presentation to the restaurant manager. Her skills in putting an interesting, informative presentation together helped her secure the agreement.

An Internet presence is important to businesses that want to grow in today's society. Consumers often look on the Internet first when planning purchases, shopping, or looking for community resources. Monica plans to track responses to each event promoted on the practice Web site to determine what efforts were the most effective in promoting the clinic. The Web site will allow her to count the number of times it is accessed and which pages were the most popular. She will keep the physicians informed and be open to their suggestions throughout the year. Monica is anxious to see the results of her marketing efforts and feels confident of success. Social media enhances the Web site, offering patients several options to increase their knowledge about health-related subjects and find opportunities to participate in events that will promote good health.

SUMMARY OF SCENARIO—cont'd

The staff members understand that no matter what efforts are used to promote the facility and obtain new patients, it is their responsibility to provide exceptional customer service so that the patients will be happy with their experience. In the medical industry today, customer service has become as important as in the retail world. Patients have choices as to who provides their healthcare, so they must be treated cordially and fairly by medical professionals who truly want to serve their needs. The success and growth of the facility depends on customer service. Monica knows that the medical office has more than one type of customer, and that the internal customers (employees) are critical to the clinic's success. She includes other employees in marketing decisions and often asks for their input. The more involved employees feel in company decisions, the more they feel as if they are a part of the community that is created in the individual facility. Monica has helped to create a fun, exciting workplace, and she looks forward to going to work every single day.

SUMMARY OF LEARNING OBJECTIVES

1. **Define, spell, and pronounce the terms listed in the vocabulary.**
   Spelling and pronouncing medical terms correctly bolster the medical assistant's credibility. Knowing the definition of these terms promotes confidence in communication with patients and co-workers.

2. **List the four steps to follow when preparing to implement a medical marketing strategy.**
   When preparing to implement marketing strategies, first evaluate what currently is being done toward the marketing effort. Then decide on the objectives of the marketing plan and how they will be measured. Finally, develop a specific plan and timeline for implementing each phase.

3. **Explain the term *target market*.**
   A target market is a very specific group of people or individuals whom the medical facility wants to serve. Geography, lifestyle, and personality all are ways to classify individuals into specific target markets. When identifying a target market ask, "Who is our patient?" "What does our patient want?" and "Why is it wanted?" These questions can help the medical facility design a marketing plan to meet the needs of these individuals.

4. **Discuss how suggestion boxes might help the medical facility make improvements.**
   Suggestions from patients and employees should always be welcomed in the medical office. Often these people see the facility from a different point of view, and their suggestions can enhance the atmosphere and the services offered.

5. **List and discuss the four Ps of marketing.**
   The four Ps of marketing are product, placement, price, and promotion. The *product* in a medical office includes the services and any actual retail items that might be sold. *Placement* relates to the location of the office and its convenience for the patients and to the placement of retail items in the facility. *Price* represents the charges for goods and services, and *promotion* entails the ways in which the services are promoted to the general public and the target market.

6. **Explain the four steps for developing a plan in marketing.**
   The facility first should assess the efforts that have been made in the past, then research the results of those efforts. Next the plan is developed, which should include very specific steps for each aspect of the endeavor. After the plan has been executed, the staff must evaluate its effectiveness and determine whether the goals were met. The evaluation is important in planning future marketing strategies.

7. **Discuss how community involvement can make a difference in marketing efforts.**
   Involvement in the community is an excellent way to promote the medical profession and remain in the public eye. These efforts can result in new patients for the facility. The public sees medical professionals as caring and compassionate; volunteer activities reinforce this attitude and help meet patients' expectations.

8. **State the difference between advertising and public relations.**
   Advertising is a medium that attempts to create or change attitudes, beliefs, and perceptions through purchased broadcast time, printed material, or other forms of communication. Public relations is a similar field but relies more on news broadcasts or reports, magazine or newspaper articles, and radio reports to reach the audience.

9. **Determine ways to promote a new practice.**
   A new medical practice can be promoted by placing an announcement in the newspaper about its opening. Some physicians hold an open house, inviting the public to visit the office. A Web site is an excellent promotional tool and should be listed on business cards and stationery. Community service and volunteer activities that mention the practice also help spread the word about the services available.

10. **Prepare a presentation using PowerPoint.**
    PowerPoint is a user-friendly program that can produce effective presentations. The process for preparing a presentation using PowerPoint is outlined in Procedure 26-2.

11. **Discuss applications of electronic technology in effective communication.**
    The Internet is a form of communication, and the physician can make use of it by developing a Web site for the practice. The Web site might highlight a featured procedure, explaining it in detail. Space can be devoted to providing the background information on the physicians and medical assistants at the clinic. Directions with maps are popular additions to physician Web sites. In addition, many doctors place their new patient forms on their Web site so that the forms can be filled out before a patient's first visit. The physician's Web site is a valuable communications tool that can help employees provide patients with even better customer service.

12. **Organize technical information and summaries.**
    The clinic Web site is the perfect place to provide patients with technical information about the physician's specialty and the procedures and

treatments available at the clinic. The Web site might have a procedure tab along the top of the home page that leads to all the procedures done in the office, with a brief description of each. Graphics or photos make the pages more interesting. Summaries of estimated costs might be appropriate. The patient must be able to navigate the Web site easily and find information quickly.

13. **Discuss responses that help the medical assistant identify with the patient.**

Identifying with the patient is an effective customer service tool. The medical assistant should express his or her understanding of the patient's concerns and then tell the patient that the situation can be resolved and how it will be resolved. Four magic words in customer service are, "Let me help you."

14. **Explain the concept of the internal customer.**

External customers are those who visit the facility, such as patients. However, staff members and employees are *internal customers,* who want to derive a sense of satisfaction from working for the medical office. Internal customers are just as important as the external customers.

15. **Design a presentation for a marketing event.**

A sharp, effective presentation helps the medical assistant secure permission to hold or promote a marketing event. The process for designing a presentation is outlined in Procedure 26-1.

16. **Locate resources and information for patients and employers.**

Many physicians include a "links" page on their Web site that displays several other businesses and organizations that might be of interest to the patient. Examples of such organizations include the local blood bank; hospitals where the physician has staff privileges; local branches of national organizations, such as the American Heart Association or American Association of Retired Persons; various insurance Web sites; the Web site for the Centers for Medicare and Medicaid Services (CMS); and numerous others. Patients appreciate access to information on businesses and organizations.

17. **Advocate on behalf of the patient and family and be able to deal and communicate with family members.**

The professional medical assistant must be a patient advocate and must be willing to assist patients with their healthcare needs. Communicate with the patient and family members just as if they were your own family. Always follow up when referring patients to community resources. Medical assistants must want to help patients with reasonable tasks, and their attitude must reflect that helping is a pleasure, not an obligation.

CONNECTIONS

📖 **Study Guide Connection:** Go to the Chapter 26 Study Guide. Read and complete the activities.

ⓔ **Evolve Connection:** Go to the Chapter 26 link at *evolve.elsevier.com/kinn* to complete the Chapter Review and Chapter Quiz. Check out the other resources listed for this chapter to make the most of what you have learned from Medical Practice Marketing and Customer Service.

27

INFECTION CONTROL

Rosa Lucia is a certified medical assistant working in a multiphysician pediatric practice. She is quite concerned about contracting an infectious disease while caring for her patients. Rosa learned about Standard Precautions while enrolled in her medical assisting program and now must implement that knowledge in the workplace. Two important factors in preventing the spread of infection are understanding how to break the chain of infection and recognizing the importance of correct and frequent hand washing.

While studying this chapter, think about the following questions:

- How can Rosa achieve these goals?
- What is the significance of an Exposure Control Plan in Rosa's pediatric office?
- What are the important details of the office's compliance with the guidelines established by the Occupational Safety and Health Administration (OSHA)?
- How can Rosa implement required infection control procedures in the pediatric office?

LEARNING OBJECTIVES

1. Define, spell, and pronounce the terms listed in the vocabulary.
2. Apply critical thinking skills in performing patient assessment and care.
3. Describe the characteristics of pathogenic microorganisms and the diseases they cause.
4. Apply the chain-of-infection process to healthcare practice.
5. Compare viral and bacterial cell invasion.
6. Differentiate between humoral and cell-mediated immunity.
7. Summarize the impact of the inflammatory response on the body's ability to defend itself against infection.
8. Analyze the differences among acute, chronic, latent, and opportunistic infections.
9. Specify potentially infectious body fluids.
10. Integrate OSHA's requirement for a site-based Exposure Control Plan into office management procedures.
11. Explain the major areas included in the OSHA Compliance Guidelines.
12. Remove contaminated gloves while following Standard Precautions principles.
13. Perform an eye wash procedure to remove contaminated material.
14. Summarize the management of postexposure evaluation and follow-up.
15. Participate in a mock environmental exposure event with documentation of the steps taken.
16. Apply the concepts of medical and surgical asepsis to the healthcare setting.
17. Demonstrate the proper hand-washing technique for medical asepsis.
18. Differentiate among sanitization, disinfection, and sterilization procedures.
19. Demonstrate the correct procedure for sanitizing contaminated instruments.
20. Apply patient education concepts to infection control.
21. Discuss the legal and ethical concerns regarding medical asepsis and infection control.

VOCABULARY

anaphylaxis (an-uh-fuh-lak′-sis) An exaggerated hypersensitivity reaction that in severe cases leads to vascular collapse, bronchospasm, and shock.

antibodies (an′-ti-bah-dees) Immunoglobulins produced by the immune system in response to bacteria, viruses, or other antigenic substances.

antigen (an′-ti-juhn) A foreign substance that causes the production of a specific antibody.

antiseptics (an-ti-sep-tik) Substances that inhibit the growth of microorganisms on living tissue (e.g., alcohol and povidone-iodine solution [Betadine]).

autoimmune (o-to-im′-yuhn) Pertaining to a disturbance in the immune system in which the body reacts against its own tissue. Examples of autoimmune disorders include multiple sclerosis, rheumatoid arthritis, and systemic lupus erythematosus.

candidiasis (kan-duh-de-uh′-sis) An infection caused by a yeast that typically affects the vaginal mucosa and skin.

coagulate (ko-ag′-yuh-late) To form into clots.

contaminated Soiled with pathogens or infectious material; nonsterile.

disinfectant A liquid chemical that is capable of eliminating many or all pathogens but is not effective against bacterial spores.

fomites Contaminated, nonliving objects (e.g., examination room equipment) that can transmit infectious organisms.

germicides (jur′-muh-sids) Agents that destroy pathogenic organisms.

hereditary (huh-re′-duh-ter-e) Pertaining to a characteristic, condition, or disease transmitted from parent to offspring on the DNA chain.

interferon (in′-tuhr-fir-on) A protein formed when a cell is exposed to a virus; the protein blocks viral action on the cell and protects against viral invasion.

opportunistic infections Infections caused by a normally nonpathogenic organism in a host whose resistance has been decreased.

palliative A substance that relieves or alleviates the symptoms of a disease without curing the disease.

parenteral (puh-ren′-tuh-ruhl) The injection or introduction of substances into the body by any route other than the digestive tract (e.g., subcutaneous, intravenous, or intramuscular administration).

pathogenic (path′-o-jen-ik) Pertaining to a disease-causing microorganism.

permeable (pur′-me-uh-buhl) Allowing a substance to pass or soak through.

pyemia (pi-em′-e-uh) The presence of pus-forming organisms in the blood.

relapse The recurrence of the symptoms of a disease after apparent recovery.

remission The partial or complete disappearance of the clinical and subjective characteristics of a chronic or malignant disease.

resident bacteria Bacteria that live in or on a certain part of the body, such as the skin or mucosa.

rhinitis (rin-i′-tis) Inflammation of the mucous membranes of the nose.

spores A thick-walled, dormant form of bacteria that is very resistant to disinfection measures.

sterile (ster′-il) Free of all microorganisms, pathogenic and nonpathogenic.

tinea (tin′-e-uh) Any fungal skin disease that results in scaling, itching, and inflammation.

transient bacteria Bacteria temporarily living in or on a certain body part, such as the hands.

urticaria (uhr-tuh-kar′-e-uh) A skin eruption that creates inflamed wheals; hives.

vectors Animals or insects (e.g., ticks) that transmit the causative organisms of disease.

The concepts of disease transmission and the body's response to infection form the basis for understanding the importance of the first line of defense in preventing disease. Before we can assist in the prevention of disease, we have to look at methods we can use to minimize the chances of being a carrier of disease. One of the simplest ways to prevent the spread of disease is to wash your hands or use alcohol-based hand rubs. As you continue through the remainder of this textbook, you should refer to the fundamental concepts of this chapter when faced with an infection control issue. Because of the need for infection control and the impact on medical practice of the guidelines established by the Occupational Safety and Health Administration (OSHA), every procedure must begin and end with hand hygiene practices. The concepts in this chapter are basic to all clinical skills, and following them can reduce the transmission of disease organisms and lessen the severity of disease. They also may save a patient's or co-worker's life, or even your own.

DISEASE

Disease is defined as any sustained, harmful alteration of the normal structure, function, or metabolism of an organism or cell. This pathologic condition of the body presents a group of clinical signs, symptoms, and laboratory findings that set it apart as an abnormal entity, different from other normal and pathologic conditions. We recognize and categorize many types of diseases: **hereditary** (genetic), drug-induced, **autoimmune,** degenerative, communicable, and infectious, to name only a few. Sometimes a specific disease may fit two or more categories.

Any disease caused by the growth of **pathogenic** microorganisms in the body falls into the category of *infectious diseases.* The entrance of a living microbe into the body is not disease, because until the infected cell or individual shows a harmful alteration in structure, physiology, or biochemistry, disease either is not detected or is not considered present. In fact, a pathogen may be ingested, injected, or inhaled and never cause disease. However, an unaffected person still can transmit the infection to another person. In this case we call the unaffected person a *carrier*.

Microorganisms are almost everywhere. We carry them on our skin, in our bodies, and on our clothing. They can be in ice, boiling water, the soil, and the air. The only places free of microorganisms are certain internal body organs and tissues and sterilized medical equipment and supplies. In the normal state, organs and tissues that do not connect with the outside by means of mucus-lined membranes are free of all living microorganisms.

CONDITIONS REQUIRED FOR MICROBIAL GROWTH

To grow and flourish, microbes require certain conditions. To maintain a healthcare environment as free of pathogenic organisms as possible, the medical assistant must prevent or eliminate as many of these growth requirements as possible.

- Nutrients: Pathogens thrive on contaminated surfaces and equipment. Most microbes need the same nutrients we do: carbohydrates, proteins, and fats.
- Moisture: Microbes require moisture for cellular activities.
- Temperature: Most pathogenic microbes flourish at body temperature (98.6° F [37° C]).
- Oxygen: Some microbes, called *aerobes,* require oxygen to grow and multiply; others, called *anaerobes,* thrive in environments without oxygen.
- Neutral pH: pH refers to the acid-base level of a solution on a scale of 1 to 14, with 7 being neutral. Most pathogens prefer a neutral pH for optimum growth.

THE CHAIN OF INFECTION

Certain factors are required for an infectious disease to spread. These factors, or links, make up the chain of infection. Break the chain, and you break the infectious process (Figure 27-1).

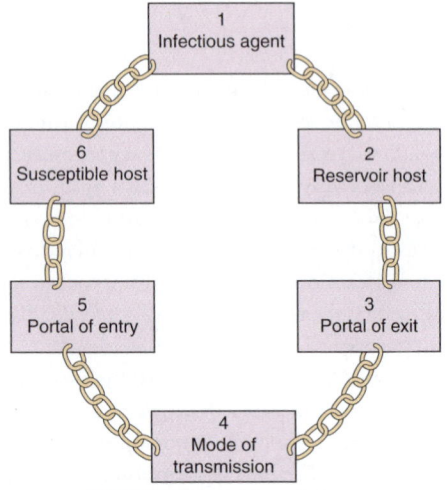

FIGURE 27-1 The chain of infection.

The chain of infection starts with the infectious agent. Five groups make up the potentially pathogenic agents or microorganisms: viruses, bacteria, protozoa, fungi, and rickettsiae. (Additional information about typical diseases caused by these pathogens is presented in Chapter 55.) Infection cannot occur without the presence of an infectious microorganism, so the best way for healthcare workers to prevent the spread of disease is to use adequate infection control procedures, such as consistent hand washing and proper use of **antiseptics**, in addition to effective disinfection and sterilization methods.

The smallest of all pathogens, viruses, lead the list of important disease-causing agents. Viral microorganisms are intracellular parasites that take over the deoxyribonucleic acid (DNA) or ribonucleic acid (RNA) of the invaded cell. Viral invasion may not cause significant immediate symptoms, because host cells infected with viruses can produce a substance called **interferon,** which protects nearby cells. Interferon leaves the infected cell and acts somewhat like a Paul Revere, warning neighboring cells that "a virus is coming!" The neighboring cells then produce antiviral proteins that may destroy the viruses once they enter. Antibiotics are unable to destroy viral invaders that enter a normal cell and multiply within the cell. The only way to destroy a viral invader is to destroy the host cell. Therefore, the treatment for viral infections typically focuses on relieving symptoms, or **palliative** treatment. To counteract and slow the rate of viral replication, interferon and the antiviral agents acyclovir (Zovirax), valacyclovir hydrochloride (Valtrex), adefovir dipivoxil (Adefovir), penciclovir (Denavir), and famciclovir (Famvir) may be prescribed, depending on the specific viral agent. Viral diseases include the common cold, influenza, herpes, infectious hepatitis, and acquired immunodeficiency syndrome (AIDS), which is caused by the human immunodeficiency virus (HIV).

Bacteria are tiny, simple cells that produce disease in a variety of ways. Pathogenic bacteria can secrete toxic substances that damage human tissues, act as parasites inside human cells, or grow on body surfaces, disrupting normal human functions. Bacteria are classified according to their shape, or morphology; they may be spherical (cocci), rod shaped (bacilli), or spiral shaped (spirilla) (see Chapter 55). Some bacteria can produce resistant internal structures, called **spores,** that make treatment difficult. When bacteria invade the body, the patient can be treated in a number of ways. The most common approach is to use antibiotics to destroy the invader or inhibit its growth. We all have nonpathogenic bacteria that reside in various body systems; for example, a harmless form of *Escherichia coli (E. coli)* lives in the large intestine. These bacteria protect against disease by competing for nutrients that pathogenic bacteria require to grow and multiply. Common diseases caused by bacteria include tuberculosis, urinary tract infections, pneumonia, and strep throat.

ANTIBIOTIC RESISTANCE

Antibiotic resistance is one of the world's most significant public health problems. Infectious microorganisms that once were easily treated with antibiotics are growing increasingly resistant to the actions of these drugs. Resistance occurs when an antibiotic is used inappropriately to treat an infection, resulting in a change or mutation of the pathologic organism that in some way reduces or eliminates the effectiveness of the drug.

If antibiotic medication is prescribed inappropriately (e.g., for a viral infection) or inaccurately (e.g., lower dosage, fewer days than recommended) or perhaps not taken by the patient as prescribed, some of the bacteria that survive the initial antibiotic treatment may mutate, allowing the microorganism to survive even in the presence of the antibiotic. Although mutations are rare, overuse of antibiotics provides more opportunity for them to occur. Antibiotics should be used to treat bacterial infections; however, they are not effective against viral infections, such as the common cold, most sore throats, and the flu. Cautious use of antibiotics is the key to preventing the spread of resistance. The Centers for Disease Control and Prevention (CDC) recommends that physicians:

- Prescribe antibiotic therapy only when it will benefit the patient.
- Treat the patient with an antibiotic that is specific to the infecting pathogen.
- Prescribe the recommended dose and treatment duration of the medication.

CRITICAL THINKING APPLICATION   27-1

Susie Chen, a 3-year-old patient, is being seen today because of complaints of a cough and nasal congestion. Susie's father does not understand why the pediatrician did not order an antibiotic for his daughter's viral infection. Rosa needs to reinforce the doctor's decision. How can she help the father understand the proper use of antibiotics?

Protozoa are unicellular parasites that can replicate and multiply rapidly once inside the host. Examples of diseases caused by protozoa include giardiasis, which typically is caused by the ingestion of water contaminated by feces, and malaria, in which *Plasmodium* organisms invade the blood system. Protozoal infections frequently are seen in tropical climates, which have large insect populations. These insects serve as **vectors** for many protozoal diseases. For example, the mosquito transmits the organisms that cause malaria.

Fungi may be unicellular or multicellular; they include such organisms as mushrooms, molds, and yeasts. Many forms are pathogenic and can cause disease, such as **candidiasis** and **tinea** infections. Fungi grow best in warm, moist environments. Treatment with antifungal agents includes application of topical preparations (e.g., Lotrimin) for tinea infections; vaginal suppositories (e.g., Monistat) for candidiasis; and oral medications, such as fluconazole (Diflucan), ketoconazole (Nizoral), and terbinafine (Lamisil). Fungal infections also are called *mycotic* infections.

Rickettsiae are microorganisms that have characteristics of both bacteria and viruses. Like viruses, they are obligate parasites that must live within a host cell for growth; however, they are larger than viruses, so they can be viewed with a microscope. Vectors such as fleas, ticks, and mites usually transmit pathogenic forms of rickettsiae. Diseases caused by rickettsiae can be treated with antibiotics; they include Rocky Mountain spotted fever, which is transmitted by a tick.

The second link in the chain of infection is the reservoir. Reservoirs may be people, insects, animals, water, food, or **contaminated** instruments. Most pathogens must gain entrance into a host or else they will die. The reservoir host supplies nutrition for the organism, allowing it to multiply. The pathogen either causes infection in the host or, in the case of vector-borne diseases, exits the host in great enough numbers to cause disease in another host.

The chain of infection continues with the means, or portal, of exit; that is, how the pathogen escapes the reservoir host. Exits include the mouth, nose, eyes, ears, intestines, urinary tract, reproductive tract, and open wounds. The use of Standard Precautions (e.g., latex gloves, masks, proper wound care, correct disposal of contaminated products, hand washing) helps control the ability of infectious material to spread from one host to another.

After exiting the reservoir host, organisms spread by transmission. Transmission either is direct or indirect. Direct transmission occurs from contact with an infected person or with discharges from an infected person, such as feces or urine. Indirect transmission occurs from droplets in the air expelled by coughing, speaking, or sneezing; vectors that harbor pathogens; contaminated food or drink; and/or contact with contaminated objects (called **fomites**). Proper sanitation of water and food; the use of sanitization, disinfection, and sterilization procedures; and the use of **germicides,** such as Wavicide and Cidex, help control the transmission of pathogens.

The next step in the chain of infection is the means, or portal, of entry. This is how the transmitted pathogen gains entry into a new host. Like the means of exit, the means of entry may be the mouth, nose, eyes, intestines, urinary tract, reproductive system, or an open wound. The first line of defense against pathogenic invasion is the intact *integumentary* system, or skin, which serves as a mechanical barrier to infection. Anatomic defense mechanisms also include tears, cilia, mucous membranes, and the pH of body fluids. The body's second line of defense includes the inflammatory process and immune system response. The immune system responds by producing **antibodies** specifically designed to combat the presence of a foreign substance, or **antigen.** This process is called *humoral immunity* and is the responsibility of the body's B cells. The immune system also reacts at the cellular level with T-cell activity in *cell-mediated immunity* by causing the destruction of pathogenic cells at the site of invasion. An example of cell-mediated immunity is *phagocytosis,* in which specialized immune system cells called *macrophages* actually ingest and destroy pathogenic microbes (see Chapter 54). If the host is susceptible (i.e., capable of supporting the growth of the infecting organism), the organism multiplies. Factors that affect a host's susceptibility include the location of entry, the dose of organisms, and the individual's state of health. If conditions are right, the organism reaches infectious levels, and the susceptible host can start the chain of infection all over.

Individuals who are effectively immunized against a disease, such as hepatitis B, are not susceptible to the disease even if they are exposed to the pathogen, because their immune system has created antibodies to protect them. In addition to immunization, other ways to reduce susceptibility to disease organisms are proper nutrition and a healthy lifestyle.

THE BODY'S NATURAL PROTECTIVE MECHANISMS

The body has multiple levels of protection against the invasion of pathogenic microorganisms. The following are some of these mechanisms:

- Intact skin serves as a natural barrier to disease.
- Mucous membranes lining the openings of the body help protect underlying tissues and trap foreign substances.
- Tiny, hairlike projections, called *cilia,* line the respiratory tract and move in a coordinated upward motion to expel trapped foreign substances.
- Trapped substances can be expelled with sneezing and coughing before the organisms invade underlying tissue.
- Some body secretions, such as tears, have antimicrobial properties that help destroy invading pathogens.
- The natural pH of many of the body's organs discourages the growth of microbes. The acidic pH of urine, the vaginal mucosa, and the stomach helps prevent pathogenic invasion. The body's resident microbes create and maintain this environment.

CRITICAL THINKING APPLICATION   27-2

Tommy Anderson, a 5-year-old patient, is seen in the office because of an outbreak of impetigo. Rosa must apply the concepts of the chain of infection and infection control methods to teach Tommy and his mother how to prevent the spread of the infection to other members of the family. What procedures should she follow after Tommy's visit to prevent the spread of the infection to other patients, other staff members, and herself?

THE INFLAMMATORY RESPONSE

When trauma occurs to the body or it is exposed to pathogens, protective mechanisms are alerted, and the body responds in a predictable manner, called the *inflammatory response* (Figure 27-2). To defend itself, the body initiates specific responses to destroy and remove pathogenic organisms and their byproducts; or, if this is not possible, to limit the extent of damage caused by the invading pathogen. This process results in the four classic symptoms of inflammation: *erythema* (redness), *edema* (swelling), pain, and heat.

When the body is exposed to an infectious agent or a foreign substance, cellular damage occurs at the site. Inflammation mediators (i.e., histamine, prostaglandins, and kinins) are released and cause three different responses at the cellular level. All three actions are designed to increase the number of white blood cells (WBCs) at the injury site.

First, blood vessels at the site dilate, causing an increase in local blood flow, which results in redness (inflammation) and heat. Blood vessel walls become more **permeable,** which assists in the release of WBCs to the site. The WBCs begin to form a fibrous capsule around the site to protect surrounding cells from damage or infection. Blood plasma also filters out of the more permeable vessel walls, resulting in edema, which puts pressure on the nerves and

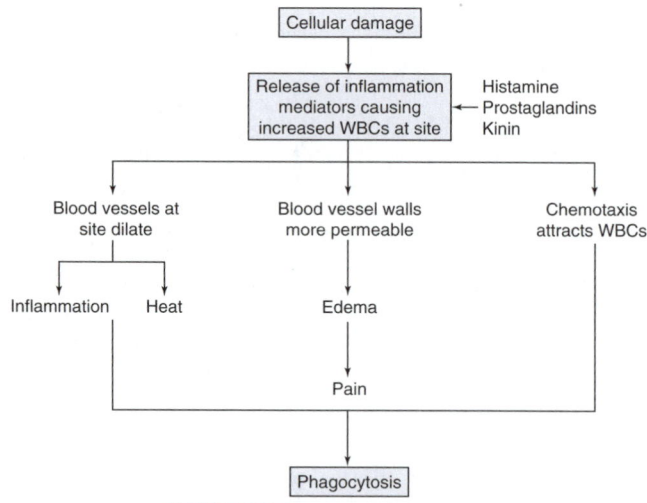

FIGURE 27-2 The inflammatory response.

causes pain. Finally, chemotaxis, or the release of chemical agents, occurs, attracting even more WBCs to the site. The increased number of WBCs at the site results in phagocytosis, or the engulfing and destruction of microorganisms and damaged cells. Destroyed pathogens, cells, and WBCs collect in the area and form a thick, white substance called *pus.* If the pathogenic invasion is too great for localized control, the infection may collect in the body's lymph nodes, where more WBCs are present to help fight the battle. This causes swollen glands, or *lymphadenopathy.* If the body is too weak or the number of pathogens is too great, the infection may spread to the bloodstream. A systemic infection, called *septicemia* or *blood poisoning,* may occur that ultimately could affect the entire body. Another term for septicemia is **pyemia.** Without appropriate medical intervention, death can occur.

CRITICAL THINKING APPLICATION   27-3

Rosa's next patient appears to have a localized inflammatory response to a splinter. What signs and symptoms should she expect the patient to show?

Rosa answers a telephone call from a patient who had surgery 3 days ago. The patient is concerned that the incision site is red, swollen, and hot. Is this a normal postoperative response? How might Rosa know whether the response is abnormal?

TYPES OF INFECTIONS

Acute Infection

An acute infection has a rapid onset of symptoms but lasts a relatively short time. The prodromal period is that time when the patient first shows vague, nonspecific symptoms of disease. In an acute viral infection, the host cell typically dies within hours or days. Symptoms appear after the tissue damage begins. In most acute infections, such as the common cold, the body's defense mechanisms eliminate the virus within 2 to 3 weeks.

Chronic Infection

An infection that persists for a long period, sometimes for life, is called a *chronic* infection. In the case of chronic viral hepatitis B, patients are *asymptomatic,* or without symptoms, but the virus is detectable with blood tests and remains transmissible throughout the person's life. Hepatitis B, or serum hepatitis, is transmitted by blood or blood products and by all body fluids. It is a serious health hazard to medical personnel. All individuals employed in a healthcare setting should be immunized against hepatitis B.

Latent Infection

A latent infection is a persistent infection in which the symptoms cycle through periods of **relapse** and **remission.** Cold sores and genital herpes are latent viral infections caused by the herpes simplex virus (HSV) types I and II, respectively. The virus enters the body and causes the original lesion. It then lies dormant, in nerve cells away from the surface, until a certain provocation (illness with fever, sunburn, or stress) causes it to leave the nerve cell and seek the surface again. Once the virus reaches the superficial tissues, it becomes detectable for a short time and causes a new outbreak at the site. Another herpes virus, varicella-zoster virus, causes chickenpox (varicella). This virus may lie dormant along a nerve pathway for years and later erupt as the painful disease shingles (zoster).

Opportunistic Infections

Opportunistic infections are caused by organisms that are not typically pathogenic but that occur in hosts with an impaired immune system response, such as individuals infected with HIV. Over time, the person's immune system becomes weakened, and diseases result that are not typically seen in patients with a healthy immune system, such as certain types of pneumonia and oral candidiasis.

OSHA STANDARDS FOR THE HEALTHCARE SETTING

Chapter 7 introduced the role of OSHA in protecting patients and healthcare personnel from potentially harmful substances in the medical facility. In 1987, in response to concern about the increasing prevalence of HIV and the hepatitis B virus (HBV), the Centers for Disease Control (now the CDC) recommended a new approach to potentially infectious materials called *Universal Precautions.* The underlying concept of Universal Precautions is that because healthcare workers cannot know whether a patient has an infectious disorder, all blood and certain body fluids must be treated as if known to be infectious for blood-borne pathogens. Therefore, precautions must be implemented for all patients, regardless of the information available about the person's individual health history. In turn, Universal Precautions protect patients from any blood-borne infection the healthcare worker may carry.

POTENTIALLY INFECTIOUS FLUIDS

Items contaminated with any of the following potentially infectious materials require special handling:

- Cerebrospinal fluid (CSF); mucus; and synovial, pleural, pericardial, peritoneal, and amniotic fluids
- Liquid or semiliquid blood
- Vaginal and seminal secretions
- Saliva in dental procedures
- Body fluid visibly contaminated with blood
- Unknown body fluid
- Wound drainage
- Human tissue, including tissue culture, cells, or exudates

The human immunodeficiency virus (HIV) has been isolated from CSF and synovial and amniotic fluids; hepatitis antigens have been detected in synovial, amniotic, and peritoneal fluids.

Exposure Control Plan

OSHA recognizes that healthcare employees face significant health risks as the result of occupational exposure to blood or other potentially infectious materials that may contain HBV, the hepatitis C virus (HCV), or HIV. In July 1992, OSHA began enforcing work practice controls to reduce or eliminate occupational exposure to blood-borne pathogens. Employers whose workers are at risk for occupational exposure to blood or other infectious materials must implement an Exposure Control Plan that details employee protection procedures. The Exposure Control Plan must identify job classifications and/or specific work-related tasks in which an employee potentially may be exposed to blood and/or body fluids. The plan must describe how an employer will use a combination of controls, including personal protective equipment (PPE), training, medical surveillance, hepatitis B immunizations, record keeping of occupational injuries, postexposure follow-up, and labeling of hazardous materials. Engineering controls, such as safer medical equipment, puncture-proof sharps containers, and shielded needle devices, in addition to PPE (e.g., gloves, gowns, and face shields), are recommended as the primary ways to reduce or eliminate employee exposure.

The plan must be reviewed and updated at least annually to incorporate the use of safer medical devices designed to eliminate or minimize occupational exposure to contaminated waste. In addition, the Exposure Control Plan must be readily available to all employees for review and training. It does not have to be a separate document and may be included as part of the facility's procedures manual or in the health and safety manual developed by the site.

CRITICAL THINKING APPLICATION   27-4

Based on what you have learned about OSHA requirements for environmental safety in a healthcare facility, evaluate your clinical laboratory at school. Does it meet all of OSHA's standards? Is an environmental safety plan in place? Develop an Exposure Control Plan for your facility and share it with your peers.

OSHA's Bloodborne Pathogens Standard

The CDC estimates that medical personnel annually experience almost 600,000 exposure incidents from contaminated sharps. In response to the CDC's concern about employee risk, Congress passed the Needlestick Safety and Prevention Act, which took effect in April, 2001. Employers are required to keep a confidential sharps injury log that describes the device involved in the incident and the details of how and where the incident occurred. Employers also must make available to employees effective sharps management devices, such as syringes with self-sheathing needles, needles that retract after use, and needleless intravenous (IV) systems that do not require sharps for **parenteral** administration. Parenteral exposure includes accidental needlesticks, occupation-related human bites, and exposure of nonintact skin (e.g., cuts and abrasions on the employee's hands) to potentially infectious material. An employer who fails to comply with OSHA's Bloodborne Pathogens Standard could face a maximum penalty of $7,000 for the first violation and up to $70,000 for repeated violations.

The Bloodborne Pathogens Standard also clarifies the use of washing or flushing of any exposed body area or mucous membrane immediately or as soon as possible after exposure to potentially infectious materials. This includes hand washing after the removal of gloves or other PPE.

The CDC recently published new recommendations regarding hand hygiene in healthcare facilities. Although hands should be washed with antimicrobial soap and warm running water when available, studies have shown that correct use of alcohol-based hand rubs significantly reduces the number of microorganisms on the skin, takes less time than traditional hand washing, and causes less irritation to the skin, especially if the solution is mixed with emollients. The CDC's recommendations for adequate hand hygiene are as follows:

- Visibly soiled hands should be washed for a minimum of 15 seconds with antimicrobial soap and warm running water.
- Gloves reduce hand contamination by 70% to 80%. Alcohol hand rubs should be used before and after contact with each patient, and also after removing gloves, to prevent cross-contamination among patients and healthcare workers.
- To use an alcohol hand rub properly, apply the label-recommended amount to the palm of one hand and rub the hands together, covering all surfaces until the hands are dry.
- Studies have shown that even after careful hand hygiene, healthcare workers with artificial nails have more pathogenic microbes under their nails and on their fingertips than workers with natural nails. Artificial nails also cause nail changes that contribute to the transmission of microbes.
- Natural nail tips should be no longer than ¼ inch to prevent microbial growth in the nail bed.

Allergic contact dermatitis from alcohol hand rubs is uncommon (Figure 27-3).

The best way to reduce the occupational risk of infection is to follow the Pathogen Standards. Healthcare workers must take adequate and consistent precautions to protect themselves and their patients. Figure 27-4 summarizes the Bloodborne Pathogens Standard. If an exposure incident occurs, such as an accidental needlestick, the facility must have specific policies and procedures in place for management of the employee who was exposed.

▌Compliance Guidelines

Because the Pathogen Standards are written to cover employees working in all health fields, only some of the regulations apply to the ambulatory care setting. Safety and infection control

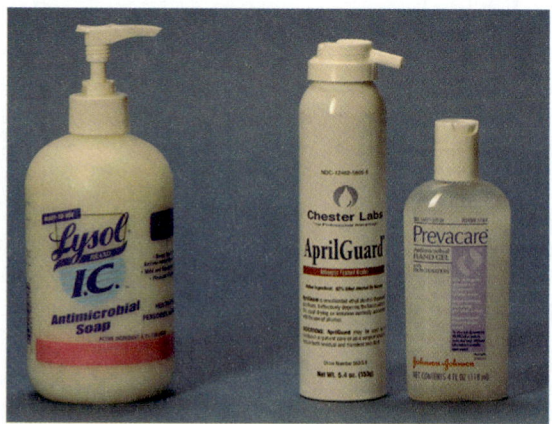

FIGURE 27-3 Antimicrobial soap and alcohol-based hand rubs. (From Bonewit-West K: *Clinical procedures for medical assistants,* ed 7, St Louis, 2008, WB Saunders.)

fundamentals go beyond hand washing and knowledge of the disease cycle. The information is presented here as it applies to the medical assisting profession.

Barrier Protection

Medical assistants routinely should use appropriate barrier precautions when contact with blood or other body fluids is expected. Barrier protection, or PPE, includes specialized clothing or equipment that prevents the healthcare worker from coming in contact with blood or other potentially infectious material, thereby preventing or minimizing the entry of infectious material into the body. Barrier devices include disposable gloves, face masks, face shields, protective glasses, shoe covers, laboratory coats, barrier gowns, mouthpieces, and resuscitation bags (Figure 27-5).

Since the implementation of Universal Precautions, the use of latex gloves has become commonplace in healthcare facilities. Unfortunately, allergic reactions associated with latex products also have increased. Hypersensitivity reactions to latex gloves or the powder that lines them may be localized, involving **urticaria,** dermatitis, conjunctivitis, and **rhinitis,** or they may be systemic, producing asthmatic reactions or **anaphylaxis.** If a healthcare worker or a patient shows signs of sensitivity to latex, the healthcare provider is required to provide gloves made of nonallergenic materials as a barrier device.

Gloves must be worn if the medical assistant is at all likely to be involved in any of the following activities (Procedure 27-1):

- Touching a patient's blood, body fluids, mucous membranes, or skin that is not intact.
- Handling items and surfaces contaminated with blood and body fluids.
- Performing venipuncture, finger sticks, injections, and other vascular procedures.
- Assisting with any surgical procedure. If a glove is torn during the procedure, the glove should be removed, the hands washed carefully, and a new glove put on as soon as possible.
- Handling, processing, and disposing of all specimens of blood and body fluids.
- Cleaning and decontaminating spills of blood or other body fluids.

Requirements of Employers: OSHA Bloodborne Pathogens Standard

EXPOSURE CONTROL PLAN

Each medical office must develop a written exposure control plan (ECP). The purpose of an ECP is to identify tasks where there is the potential for exposure to blood and other potentially infectious materials.

- A timetable must be published indicating when and how communication of potential hazards will occur.
- The employer must offer employees the hepatitis B vaccine within 10 working days of employment (at no cost to the employee). If employees sign a form to refuse the vaccine, they can change their mind at no cost to the employee.
- The employer must document the steps that should be taken in case of an exposure incident, including a postexposure evaluation and follow-up, strict record keeping, implementation of engineering controls, provision for personal protective equipment, and general housekeeping standards. This plan must be posted in the medical office.
- There must also be written procedures for evaluating the circumstances of an exposure incident.
- Training records must be kept for 3 years.

ENGINEERING CONTROLS AND WORK PRACTICES

The employer must provide engineering controls, or equipment and facilities that minimize the possibility of exposure. Examples of engineering controls include the following:

- Providing puncture-resistant containers for used sharps.
- Providing handwashing facilities that are readily accessible.
- Equipment for sanitizing, decontaminating, and sterilizing.

The employer must also enforce work practice controls. Work practice controls also minimize the possibility of exposure by making sure employees are using the proper techniques while working. Examples include the following:

- Enforcing proper handwashing or sanitizing procedures.
- Enforcing proper technique for using and handling needles to prevent needle sticks.
- Enforcing proper techniques to minimize the splashing of blood.

PERSONAL PROTECTIVE EQUIPMENT

Employers must provide, and employees must use, personal protective equipment (PPE) when the possibility exists of exposure to blood or contaminated body fluids. This equipment must not allow blood or potentially infectious material to pass through to the employee's clothes, skin, eyes, or mouth. Examples of PPE include the following:

- Gowns
- Face shields
- Goggles
- Gloves

If an employee has an allergy to powder or latex, the employer must provide hypoallergenic or powderless gloves. The employee cannot be charged for PPEs.

EXPOSURE INCIDENT MANAGEMENT

An exposure incident is contact with blood or biohazard infectious material that occurs when doing one's job. When an exposure incident is reported, the employer must arrange for an immediate and confidential medical evaluation. The information and actions required are as follows:

- Documenting how the exposure occurred.
- Identifying and testing the "source" individual, if possible.
- Testing the employee's blood, if consent is granted.
- Providing counseling.
- Evaluating, treating, and following up on any reported illness.

Medical records must be kept for each employee with occupational exposure for the duration of employment plus 30 years.

COMMUNICATION OF POTENTIAL HAZARDS TO EMPLOYEESS

A medical assistant will be exposed to hazardous chemicals on the job. Most chemicals handled by assistants are not any more dangerous than those used in the home. In the workplace, however, exposure is likely to be greater, concentrations higher, and exposure time longer.

The "right to-know" law, OSHA's hazard communication standard, states that each employee has a right to know what chemicals he or she is working with in the workplace. The right-to-know law is intended to make the workplace safer by making certain that all information regarding chemical hazards is known to the employee. This information is supplied in the material safety data sheet (MSDS), a fact sheet about a chemical that includes the following information:

- Identification of the chemical
- Listing of the physical and health hazards
- Precautions for handling
- Identification of the chemical as a carcinogen
- First-aid procedures
- Name, address, and telephone number of manufacturer

Many MSD information sheets can be obtained in repositories on the Internet. An MSDS should be updated at least every 3 years. Employers must ensure that all products have an up-to-date MSDS when they enter the workplace.

Potential hazards are also communicated with labels and color. Any containers with biohazard waste must be orange (or reddish orange) and must display the biohazard symbol. These labels and colors alert employees to the risk of possible exposure.

FIGURE 27-4 Requirements of employers: OSHA's Bloodborne Pathogens Standard. (From the Occupational Safety and Health Administration: Available at www.osha.gov)

SAFETY ALERT

Protective equipment contaminated with body fluids of any kind must be removed and placed in a designated area or biohazard container. The hands or any other exposed areas must be washed or flushed as soon as possible. Protective eyewear and/or face shields must be worn whenever splashes, sprays, or droplets are possible. Standard prescription eyeglasses are not considered effective. Utility gloves may be reused if they are intact (i.e., have no cracks, tears, or punctures). All PPE must be removed before leaving the medical facility (Figure 27-6).

CRITICAL THINKING APPLICATION 27-5

Rosa is caring for an injured 3-year-old child with an open wound on his right knee. She puts on disposable gloves to clean the wound, and the mother demands to know why. How can she explain her actions?

Environmental Protection

Environmental protection refers to minimizing the risk of occupational injury by isolating or removing any physical or mechanical health hazard in the medical workplace. Every medical assistant must adhere to these safety rules.

- Read warning labels on biohazard containers and equipment.
- Minimize splashing or spraying of potentially infectious materials. Blood that splatters onto open areas of the skin or mucous membranes is a proven mode of transmission of HBV.
- Bandage any breaks or lesions on your hands before gloving.
- If any body surface is exposed to potentially infectious material, scrub the area with antimicrobial soap and warm running water as soon as possible after the exposure.
- If your eyes come in contact with body fluids, continuously flush them with water as soon as possible for a minimum of 15 minutes using an eye wash unit. A stationary unit connected to warm running water is the best method for properly flushing potentially

infectious material out of the eyes (Figure 27-7 and Procedure 27-2).

- Contaminated needles and other sharps should never be recapped, bent, broken, or resheathed. Needle units are now required to have sliding shields or some other protective device for use after injection.
- Reusable sharps that are contaminated should not be processed in a way that requires employees to reach into containers to grasp them.
- Immediately after use, dispose of syringes and needles, scalpel blades, and other sharp items in a labeled, leakproof, puncture-resistant biohazard container. The container must be located as close as possible to the area where the instruments are used.
- All specimens must be placed in a container that prevents leakage during collection, handling, processing, storage, transport, and shipping. Avoid contaminating the outside of the container or the label with the specimen substance. If the outside is contaminated, the container should be disinfected. One method is to use a 1:10 dilution of sodium hypochlorite (household chlorine bleach and water) and place the container in a leakproof bag for transport. The container must have a biohazard label to alert others that it holds potentially infectious material. Gloves should be worn throughout this procedure.
- Mouth pipetting or the sucking of blood through tubing is prohibited.
- Contaminated test materials should be decontaminated before reprocessing or should be placed in impervious bags and disposed of according to policy.
- Equipment requiring repair that has been contaminated with blood or body fluids should be decontaminated before being repaired in the office or transported for repair. There is no documented evidence of HIV transmission from contaminated environmental surfaces, but surface contamination is a proven mode of transmission for HBV.
- Smoking, eating, drinking, applying cosmetics or lip balm, and handling contact lenses are prohibited in work areas where the reasonable likelihood of contamination from pathogens exists.

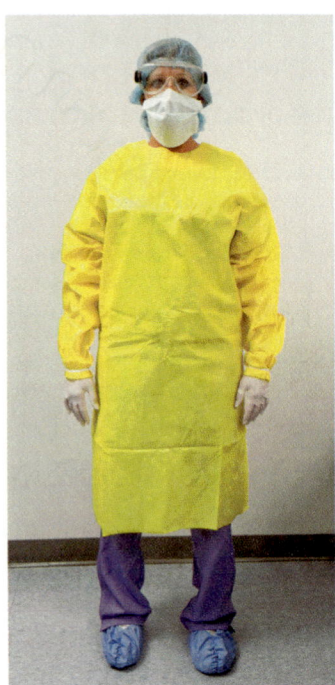

FIGURE 27-5 Personal protective equipment.

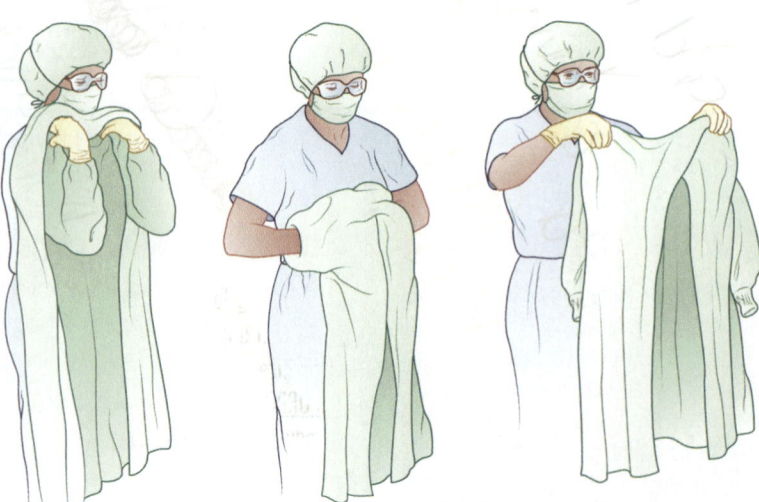

FIGURE 27-6 Removing a contaminated gown. (From Fuller JK: *Surgical technology: principles and practice*, ed 5, St Louis, 2010, WB Saunders.)

PROCEDURE 27-1

PROCEDURE 27-1

Train in and Practice Standard Precautions: Use Standard Precautions to Remove Contaminated Gloves and Discard Biohazardous Material

GOAL: *To minimize exposure to pathogens by aseptically removing and discarding contaminated gloves.*

EQUIPMENT and SUPPLIES

- Latex or alternative disposable examination gloves
- Biohazard waste container with labeled red biohazard bag

PROCEDURAL STEPS

1. With the dominant hand, grasp the glove of the opposite hand near the palm and begin removing the first glove (Figure 1). The arms should be held away from the body with the hands pointed down.

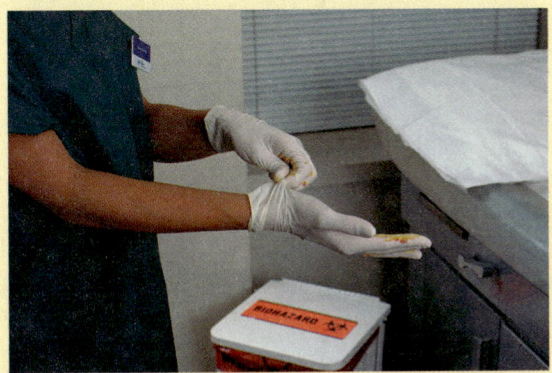

PURPOSE: Holding the hands down and away from the body helps prevent possible contamination.

2. Pull the glove inside out until you reach the fingers, holding the contaminated glove in the dominant gloved hand (Figure 2).

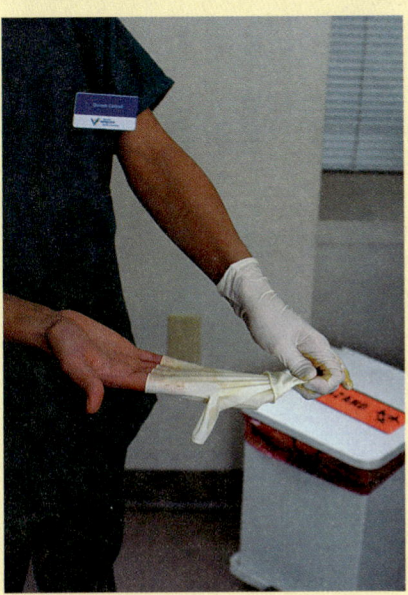

PURPOSE: Taking off the glove inside out prevents transmission of pathogens to another surface.

3. Insert the thumb of the ungloved hand inside the cuff of the other contaminated glove (Figure 3).

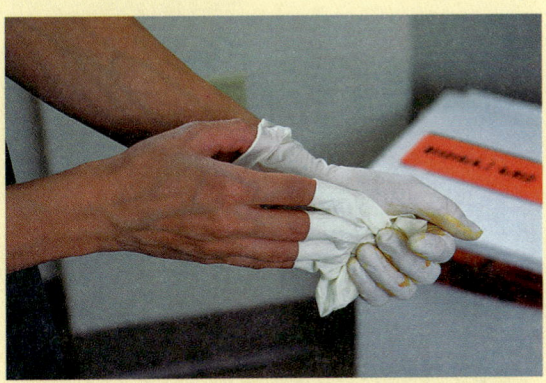

4. Pull the glove down the hand, inside out, over the contaminated glove being held, leaving the contaminated side of both gloves on the inside.
   PURPOSE: This technique protects the wearer from the contaminated surfaces of both gloves.

5. Properly dispose of the inside-out, contaminated gloves in a biohazard waste container (Figure 4).

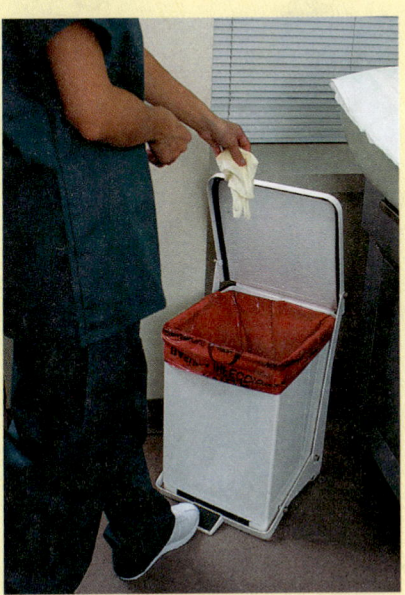

PURPOSE: To prevent the spread of infection.

6. Perform a medical aseptic hand wash as described in Procedure 27-4 or sanitize the hands.
   PURPOSE: To minimize the number of pathogens on the hands, thereby reducing the number of transient bacteria and the risk of transmission of pathogens.

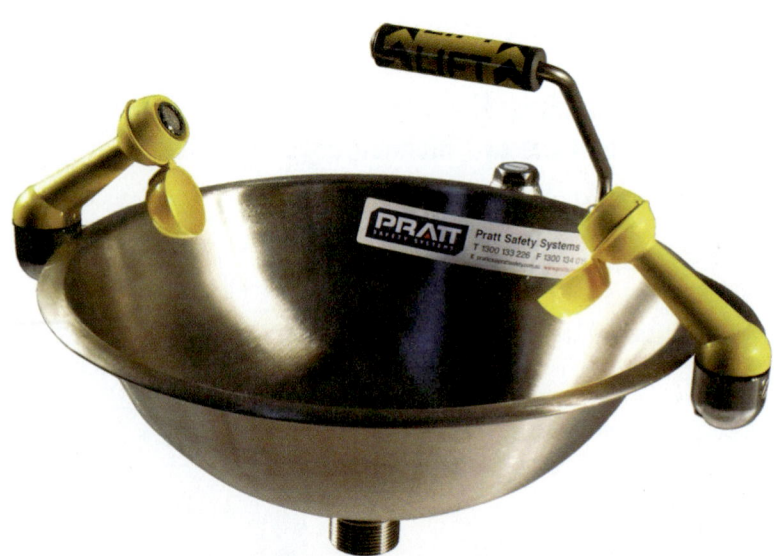

FIGURE 27-7 Eye washing unit.

PROCEDURE 27-2

Demonstrate the Proper Use of Eye Wash Equipment: Perform an Emergency Eye Wash

GOAL: *To minimize the risk of occupational exposure to pathogens if body fluids come in contact with the eyes.*

EQUIPMENT and SUPPLIES

- Plumbed or self-contained eye wash unit
- Disposable gloves

PROCEDURAL STEPS

1. Don gloves and remove contact lenses or glasses.
   <u>PURPOSE:</u> To ensure flushing of all material in the eyes.
2. Following the manufacturer's directions, turn on the eye wash unit. If it is a plumbed unit, the control valve should remain on until the unit is manually shut off.
   <u>PURPOSE:</u> The unit must be plumbed so that it can remain on until manually turned off.
3. Hold the eyelids open with the thumb and index finger to ensure adequate rinsing of the entire eye and eyelid surface (Figure 1).

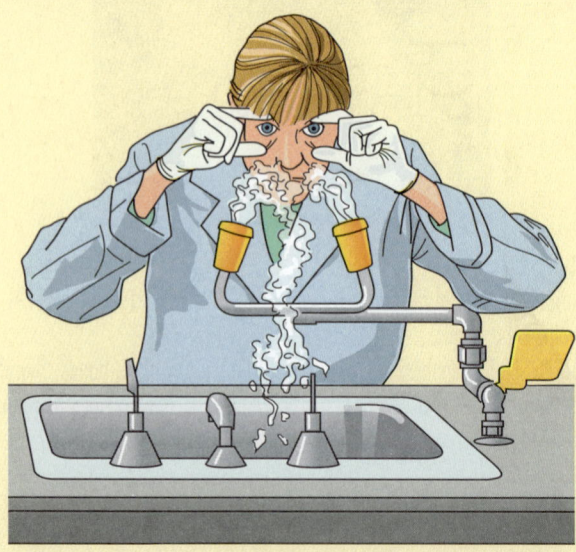

<u>PURPOSE:</u> The normal reflex is to close the eyes tightly, which prevents removal of all the contaminated material.
4. Avoid aiming the water stream directly onto the eyeball.
   <u>PURPOSE:</u> A direct water stream may cause discomfort and/or damage the eye.
5. Flush the eyes and eyelids for a minimum of 15 minutes, rolling the eyes periodically to ensure complete removal of the foreign material.
   <u>PURPOSE:</u> To completely remove the potentially dangerous substance from the eyes.
6. Sanitize your hands.
   <u>PURPOSE:</u> To prevent cross-contamination.
7. After completion of the eye wash, follow postexposure follow-up procedures.
   <u>PURPOSE:</u> The facility's policies may include physician follow-up and completion of an exposure incident form.

- Food and beverages cannot be kept in refrigerators, freezers, or cabinets or on countertops where infectious materials could be present.

Housekeeping Controls

The Bloodborne Pathogens Standard requires certain housekeeping measures to ensure a sanitary work area. Facilities must post a schedule for cleaning and decontaminating each work area where exposures could occur. This documentation must include information about the surface cleaned, the type of waste encountered, and procedures performed in the designated area.

- Work surfaces must be immediately decontaminated with a **disinfectant** (e.g., a 1:10 solution of sodium hypochlorite) after accidental spills of blood or body fluids, at the end of each procedure, and at the end of each shift.
- Disinfection and decontamination of all reusable containers must be done on a routine basis.
- Sharps containers must be as close as possible to the work area. Never attempt to reach inside a sharps container and do not overfill them. Replace containers on a routine basis, and be certain that the lid is closed securely before preparing them for biohazard waste disposal.
- Never pick up spilled material or broken glassware with the hands. Brooms, brushes, dustpans, and pickup tongs or forceps should be used, and the material should be placed immediately into an impervious biohazard bag or container at the spill site (Figure 27-8). Use an absorbent, professional biohazard spill preparation as directed to decontaminate the site.
- Handle soiled linen as little as possible and always wear gloves or other protective equipment during disposal. Linens soiled with blood or body fluids should be double bagged and transported in labeled, leakproof biohazard bags.
- Contaminated materials and/or infectious waste must be handled with extreme caution to prevent exposure. Biohazard waste must be collected in impermeable red polyethylene or polypropylene biohazard-labeled bags or containers and sealed (Figure 27-9). This waste must be disposed of in accordance with all federal, state, and local regulations. Disposal methods include treatment

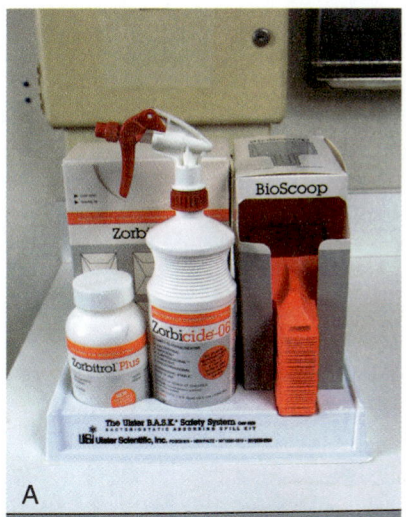
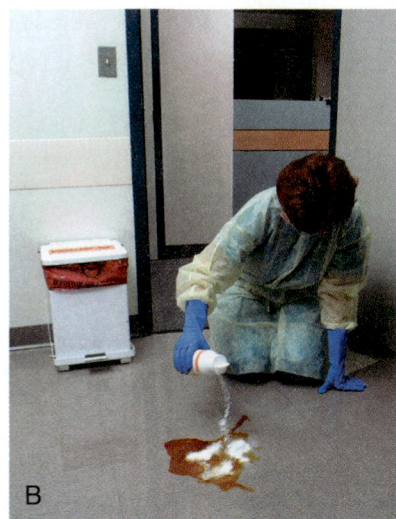
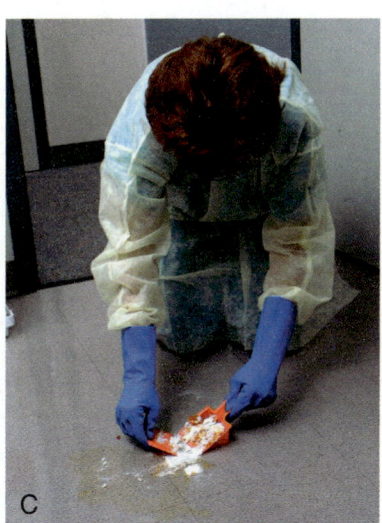
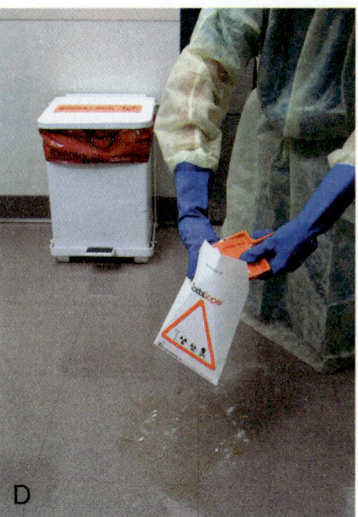
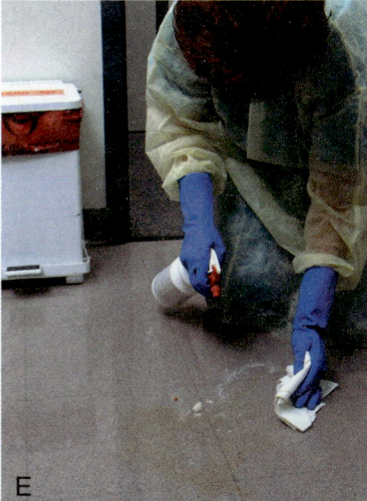
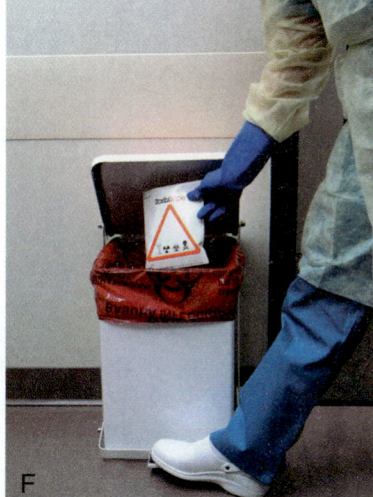

FIGURE 27-8 Cleaning up spilled material. **A,** Clean-up kit with printed instructions. **B,** Sprinkle congealing powder over the spill. **C,** Scoop up the spill. **D,** Place the contents in a biohazard bag. **E,** Wipe the area thoroughly with a germicide. **F,** Place all contaminated material in a biohazard bag or container.

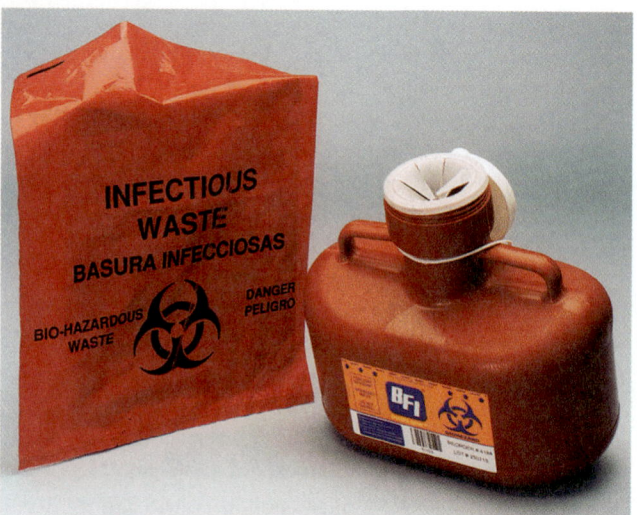

FIGURE 27-9 Biohazard bag and biohazard sharps container.

Hepatitis B Vaccine Declination

I understand that due to my occupational exposure to blood or other potentially infectious materials I may be at risk of acquiring hepatitis B virus (HBV) infection. I have been given the opportunity to be vaccinated with hepatitis B vaccine, at no charge to myself. However, I decline hepatitis B vaccination at this time. I understand that by declining this vaccine, I continue to be at risk of acquiring hepatitis B, a serious disease. If in the future I continue to have occupational exposure to blood or other potentially infectious materials and I want to be vaccinated with hepatitis B vaccine, I can receive the vaccination series at no charge to me.

Name: _____   Date: _____

FIGURE 27-10 Sample hepatitis B declination form. (From the Occupational Safety and Health Administration: Available at www.osha.gov.)

by heat, incineration, steam sterilization, chemical treatment, or other equivalent methods that renders the waste inactive before it is placed in a landfill.

> **CRITICAL THINKING APPLICATION   27-6**
> Using the techniques learned in Chapter 1, create a mind map that outlines the details of OSHA's Bloodborne Pathogens Standard.

Hepatitis B Vaccination

Hepatitis B vaccine must be available free of charge to all employees at risk for occupational exposure to blood-borne pathogens, whether they are full-time or part-time workers, within 10 days of starting employment. The vaccine is administered by intramuscular injection in three doses. The second injection is administered 4 weeks after the first, and the third injection 6 months after the first. The U.S. Public Health Service does not currently recommend routine boosters for hepatitis B immunization. However, if they are recommended in the future, boosters must be made available to eligible employees without cost.

Although vaccination is almost 96% effective, employees should have a blood titer drawn after completion of the injection cycle to determine whether they have created antibodies against the disease. If the employee did not respond to the first series or if the series was not completed, revaccination with a second three-dose series is recommended. If antibodies still do not develop, no further vaccination is given.

Employees have the right to decline hepatitis B immunization, but they are required to sign a declination form (Figure 27-10) that is kept on file as a record of the employee's refusal. An employee who changes his or her mind may receive the vaccine at a future date free of charge.

Postexposure Follow-Up

If a worker is exposed through an accidental needlestick, a human bite, exposure to broken skin, or from a splash or splatter onto mucous membranes, such as the eyes, certain procedures must be followed. Procedure 27-3 presents the specific steps to be taken for exposure to contaminated waste.

- Immediately, or as soon as possible after exposure, the worker should wash or flush the exposed area.
- The exposure incident must be immediately reported to the supervisor.
- The employee must immediately receive a confidential medical evaluation. The physician caring for the exposed employee must receive written details of the exposure incident, including the route and circumstances surrounding the incident. All documentation related to the exposure must remain confidential, may not be disclosed to any individual without the employee's express written permission, and must be kept for at least the duration of the worker's employment plus 30 years.
- An incident report must be filed that documents the details surrounding the exposure incident, the route or type of exposure, and the identity, if known, of the source individual. The source individual is the person, living or dead, whose blood or potentially infectious material was the source of the occupational exposure.
- The source individual is screened for HBV, HCV, and HIV. Depending on state regulations, consent may or may not be required from the source individual to perform the screening. If consent is required but not given, the employer must document that consent was not received from the source individual. If screening is done, OSHA requires that the employee be informed of the results of the source individual's tests.
- The exposed worker is tested for HBV, HCV, and HIV if consent is given. If the employee refuses the tests but blood is drawn, the sample must be stored 90 days for the worker to decide whether screening is wanted.
- If the employee has not been vaccinated against HBV, vaccination is offered.
- The injured employee must receive a copy of the healthcare provider's written opinion within 15 days of completion of the evaluation.
- The exposed worker must receive health counseling about the risk of illness or other adverse outcomes of exposure and the potential for and consequences of transmission of the disease to family, patients, and others.

PROCEDURE 27-3

Participate in a Mock Environmental Exposure Event with Documentation of Steps: Implement the Facility's Environmental Safety Plan

GOAL: *To manage an exposure incident according to OSHA standards.*

SCENARIO: *Rosa is administering a hepatitis B vaccine, and the patient suddenly jumps back. The contaminated needle becomes dislodged and jabs Rosa. What procedural steps must be taken to comply with OSHA standards?*

EQUIPMENT and SUPPLIES

- Antibacterial soap and warm running water
- Exposure incident report form

PROCEDURAL STEPS

1. Immediately wash the exposed site with antibacterial soap and warm running water.
   PURPOSE: To sanitize and disinfect the exposure site as quickly and thoroughly as possible.

2. Immediately report the exposure incident to the site supervisor.
   PURPOSE: The facility supervisor (e.g., office manager, practice manager, physician) is responsible for following through with the facility's Exposure Control Plan.

3. Complete an exposure incident report that details the type of injury, the details surrounding the incident, the equipment involved, and any other pertinent details.
   PURPOSE: The facility must report exposure incidents to OSHA. OSHA evaluates the incident based on required standards, including employee training, availability of current protective devices (e.g., needle covers and location of sharps containers) and the extent of employee injury. The incident report also serves as a written record of the incident, which establishes the need for employee healthcare.

4. After the incident report has been completed, the employee is immediately sent for a confidential medical evaluation. This may be in a related employee health office, local emergency department, or private physician's office. The employer must cover the costs of all related healthcare.
   PURPOSE: All employee records regarding the exposure incident must be kept completely confidential and separate from any other employee records.

5. A blood sample is taken from the "source" individual to test for hepatitis B and C and for the human immunodeficiency virus (HIV).
   PURPOSE: A blood sample from the source is tested to determine whether the person is positive for any of these infectious diseases.

6. A blood sample is taken from the employee to test for hepatitis B and C and for HIV; if the employee refuses testing, a blood sample is still taken and stored for 90 days; if the employee continues to refuse testing, the sample is destroyed after 90 days.
   PURPOSE: To determine whether the employee currently is infected with hepatitis B or C or HIV.

7. If the patient's blood tests negative, the employer must provide free education and counseling for the employee. If the patient's blood tests positive for hepatitis B, C, or HIV, the employee is offered free care and counseling.
   PURPOSE: If the patient's screening test is negative, it is still possible that the person may have been recently exposed and the screening did not detect the early stages of the disease. The employee must be offered follow-up testing for 6 months to ensure that he or she was not infected. If the patient tested positive for any of the three infectious diseases, the employee is offered treatment (appropriate medications, education, and counseling) and follow-up screening. According to the Centers for Disease Control and Prevention (CDC), if no indication of disease is seen within 6 months, it will not develop.

8. Confidential medical records of the exposure incident, blood work outcomes, and treatment must be kept for the duration of employment plus 30 years.

POSTEXPOSURE MANAGEMENT

Recommendations for HBV postexposure management include initiation of the hepatitis B vaccine series in any susceptible, unvaccinated person who sustains an occupational blood or body fluid exposure. Postexposure prophylaxis (PEP) with hepatitis B immune globulin (HBIG) and/or hepatitis B vaccine series should be considered for occupational exposures after evaluation of the hepatitis B surface antigen status of the source and the vaccination and vaccine-response status of the exposed person. Guidance is provided to clinicians and exposed HCP for selecting the appropriate HBV PEP.

Immune globulin and antiviral agents (e.g., interferon with or without ribavirin) are not recommended for PEP of hepatitis C. For HCV postexposure management, the HCV status of the source and the exposed person should be determined, and for a healthcare professional (HCP) exposed to an HCV-positive source, follow-up HCV testing should be performed to determine whether infection develops.

Recommendations for HIV PEP include a basic 4-week regimen of two drugs (zidovudine [ZDV] and lamivudine [3TC]; 3TC and stavudine [d4T]; or didanosine [ddI] and d4T) for most HIV exposures and an expanded regimen that includes the addition of a third drug for HIV exposures that pose an increased risk for transmission. When the source person's virus is known or suspected to be resistant to one or more of the drugs considered for the PEP regimen, the selection of drugs to which the source person's virus is unlikely to be resistant is recommended.

Healthcare students are at risk for blood-borne pathogen exposure and should follow all OSHA guidelines designed to protect individuals from exposure. A complete, unabridged copy of OSHA's Bloodborne Pathogens Standard may be obtained at the OSHA Web site (*www.osha.gov*).

CRITICAL THINKING APPLICATION   27-7

Rosa's office has been especially busy today. While administering an injection to a frightened 6-year-old child, a co-worker accidentally sticks herself with the needle. She tells Rosa about the incident, but she doesn't know what to do next. What steps should be taken to manage the situation?

ASEPTIC TECHNIQUES: PREVENTION OF DISEASE TRANSMISSION

Asepsis means freedom from infection or infectious material. *Medical asepsis* is defined as the destruction of disease-causing organisms after they leave the body. When we practice the principles of medical asepsis, we are directing our efforts at preventing reinfection of the patient or the cross-infection of other patients or ourselves. The goal is to eliminate or minimize pathogens by following OSHA's Bloodborne Pathogens Standard and disinfecting objects as soon as possible after contamination. This creates a healthcare environment as free of pathogens as possible.

Surgical asepsis is the destruction of organisms before they enter the body. This technique is used for any procedure that invades the body's skin or tissues, such as surgery or injections. Anytime the skin or a mucous membrane is punctured, pierced, or incised (or will be during a procedure), surgical aseptic techniques are practiced. Everything that comes in contact with the patient should be **sterile,** including gowns, drapes, instruments, and the gloved hands of the surgical team. Minor surgery, urinary catheterization, injections, and some specimen collections, such as blood collection and biopsies, are performed using surgical aseptic technique (see Chapter 57).

Because the hands themselves cannot be sterilized, the goal of hand washing is to reduce skin bacteria through the use of mechanical friction, antimicrobial soaps, and warm, running water. Normally, two types of bacteria are found on the skin: **transient bacteria,** which are surface bacteria that are introduced by fomites and remain a short time, and **resident bacteria,** which are found under fingernails, in hair follicles, in the openings of sebaceous glands, and in the deeper layers of the skin. The goal of thorough hand washing is to remove or reduce the numbers of transient bacteria on the surface of the skin, thus preventing them from becoming resident bacteria.

The most effective barrier against infection is the unbroken skin. If the skin and mucous membranes are intact, medical asepsis can be practiced for most noninvasive procedures (i.e., those that do not penetrate human tissues), such as pelvic and proctologic examinations. Instruments and objects used in medical aseptic procedures must be decontaminated or sterilized before use on another patient. Medical aseptic procedures may include the use of gowns and masks, but these are not sterile and are worn to protect the healthcare worker more than the patient.

Another practical application of aseptic technique is to set up work areas in the medical office's laboratory so that one side of the laboratory is the "clean" side, where only noninfectious procedures are performed, and the other is the "dirty" side, where potentially infectious materials are processed or cleaned.

Hand Washing

The hands must be washed, using the correct technique, before and after each patient is examined or treated and also when stipulated by the Bloodborne Pathogens Guidelines. A lengthy scrub is not necessary each time, but the first scrub in the morning should be extensive, lasting 2 to 4 minutes. Subsequent hand washing may be brief unless the hands are excessively contaminated. A good antimicrobial soap with chlorhexidine (e.g., Hibiclens), which has antiseptic residual action that lasts several hours, should be used. Each office sink should be equipped with a liquid soap dispenser. A water-soluble lotion may be rubbed into the hands after they have been washed and dried. Dry, cracked, chapped skin is no longer intact and can result in the transmission of disease.

Proper hand washing depends on two factors: running water and friction. The water should be warm, because water that is too hot or too cold causes the skin to become chapped. Friction is the firm rubbing of all surfaces of the hands and wrists. Remember that your fingers have four sides, and fingernails have two sides. For medical hand washing, all jewelry except a plain wedding band is removed. A wristwatch may be left on if it can be moved up on the forearm away from the wrist area. The hands are washed under running water with the fingertips pointing downward. Soap and friction are applied to the hands and wrists. The water is allowed to wash debris away from the wrists and down toward the fingertips (Procedure 27-4).

Remember, the goal of aseptic hand washing is to protect you from infection and prevent cross-contamination from one patient to another. Use this procedure after you finish with one patient and before you attend to another patient; after you finish handling one specimen and before you handle another specimen; before and after you use toilet facilities; whenever you touch something that causes your hands to become contaminated; when you arrive at work and before you leave the office; before and after eating; and at the end of the day.

As stated earlier, alcohol-based hand rubs may substitute for hand washing unless the hands are visibly contaminated. Evidence suggests that hand antisepsis with an alcohol-based hand rub is more effective at reducing nosocomial infections than plain hand washing. Using antimicrobial-impregnated wipes (e.g., towelettes) is not a substitute for using an alcohol-based hand rub or antimicrobial soap.

Sanitization

Instruments and other items used in office surgery, examination, or treatment must be carefully cleaned before proceeding with the steps of disinfection or sterilization. Sanitization is the cleansing process that reduces the number of microorganisms to a safe level, as dictated in public health guidelines. This cleansing process removes debris such as blood and other body fluids from instruments or equipment. Blood and debris must be removed so that later disinfection with chemicals or sterilization with steam, heat, or gases can penetrate to all the instrument's surfaces (Procedure 27-5).

Train and Practice Standard Precautions: Perform Medical Aseptic Hand Washing

GOAL: *To minimize the number of pathogens on the hands, thus reducing the risk of transmission of pathogens.*

EQUIPMENT and SUPPLIES

- Sink with warm running water
- Antimicrobial liquid soap in a dispenser (bar soap is not acceptable)
- Nail brush or orange stick
- Paper towels in a dispenser
- Water-based antimicrobial lotion
- Biohazard waste container with labeled red biohazard bag

PROCEDURAL STEPS

1. Remove all jewelry except your wristwatch if it can be pulled up above your wrist and a plain gold wedding ring.
   PURPOSE: Jewelry can harbor microorganisms.
2. Turn on the faucet with a paper towel and regulate the water temperature to lukewarm.
   PURPOSE: Use a paper towel to prevent touching of contaminated surfaces; water that is too hot can cause skin to become dry and chapped.
3. Wet your hands, apply soap, and lather using a circular motion with friction while holding your fingertips downward (Figure 1). Rub well between your fingers. If this is the first hand wash of the day, use a nail brush or an orange stick and clean under every fingernail. Inspect your nails thoroughly.

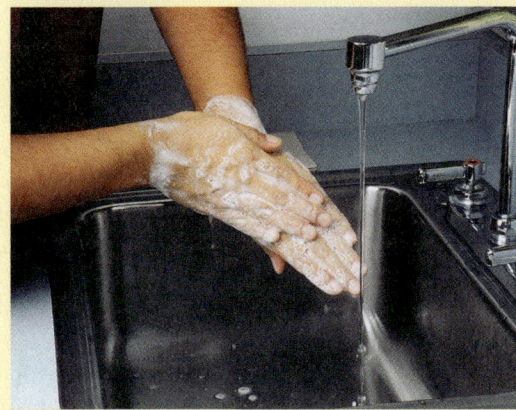

PURPOSE: Friction removes soil and contaminants from the hands and wrists.

4. Rinse well, holding your hands so that the water flows from your wrists downward to your fingertips (Figure 2).

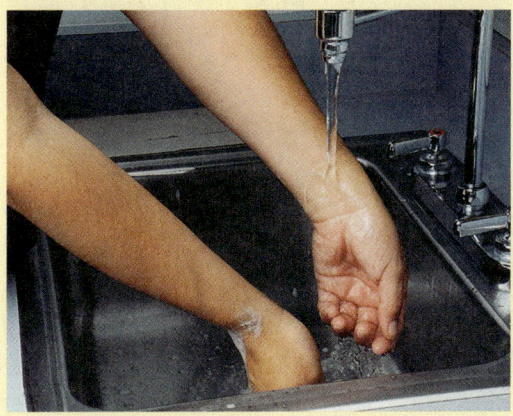

PURPOSE: Soil and contaminants will wash off the skin and down the drain.

5. If this is the first hand wash of the day or if your hands are obviously contaminated, wet your hands again and repeat the scrubbing procedure using a vigorous, circular motion over the wrists and hands for at least 1 to 2 minutes.
   PURPOSE: Time is required for friction and motion to eliminate all possible soil and contaminants.
6. Rinse your hands a second time, keeping the fingers lower than your wrists.
   PURPOSE: To ensure removal of all transient bacteria.
7. Dry your hands with paper towels. Do not touch the paper towel dispenser as you are obtaining towels (Figure 3).

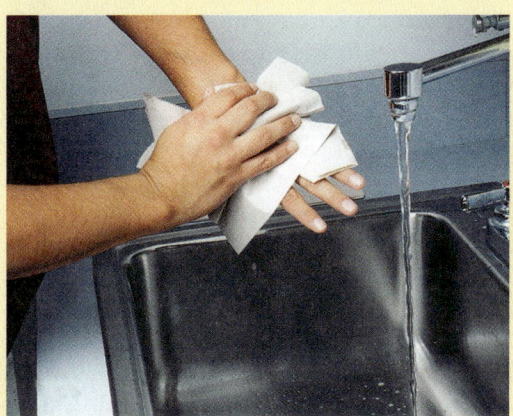

PURPOSE: Touching the dispenser contaminates your hands, and you will need to start over.

8. If the faucets are not foot operated, turn them off with a paper towel (Figure 4).

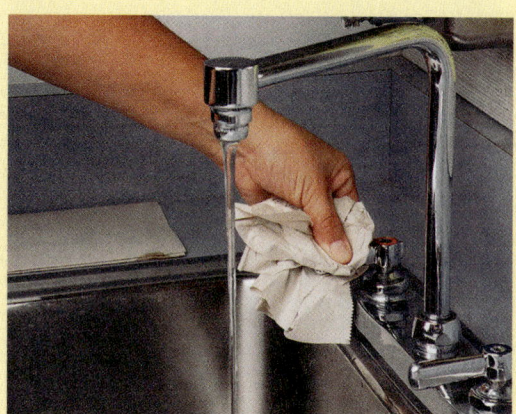

   <u>PURPOSE:</u> The faucet is dirty and will contaminate your clean hands.

9. After you finish drying your hands and turning off the faucets, place used towels into a biohazard waste container.
   <u>PURPOSE:</u> Always discard contaminated waste in a biohazard waste container immediately to eliminate the source of infection.

10. Apply a water-based antibacterial hand lotion to prevent chapped or dry skin.
    <u>PURPOSE:</u> Chapped skin eliminates the first line of defense against infectious organisms.

11. Repeat the procedure as indicated throughout the day.
    <u>PURPOSE:</u> To eliminate contaminants and prevent the transmission of pathogens to yourself and others.

The medical assistant should always wear gloves (thick utility gloves if the instruments have sharp or pointed edges) while performing sanitization to prevent possible personal contamination with potentially infectious body fluids that may be present on the articles being cleaned. The procedure should be completed immediately after use of the instruments in a separate workroom or area or on the "dirty" side of the utility room to prevent cross-contamination of clean instruments and equipment. If this is not possible, rinse the used items under cold water immediately after the procedure and place them in a low-sudsing, rust-inhibiting, enzyme-containing detergent solution. Never allow blood or other substances that can **coagulate** to dry on an instrument.

When you are ready to sanitize instruments, drain off the soaking solution and rinse each instrument in cold running water. Separate the sharp instruments from the others, because metal instruments may damage the cutting edges, and sharp instruments may damage other instruments or injure you. Clean all sharp instruments at one time, when you can concentrate on preventing injury to yourself. Open all hinges and scrub serrations and ratchets with a small scrub brush or toothbrush. Rinse the instruments in hot water and then check carefully that they are in proper working order before they are disinfected or sterilized. The items should be hand dried with a towel to prevent spotting.

Sanitization is a very important step, and it cannot be overlooked or done carelessly. The use of disposable instruments minimizes the need for sanitization, disinfection, and sterilization.

Ultrasonic Sanitization

Sound waves can be used to sanitize instruments. The instruments are placed in an ultrasonic bath of cleaner and water. Sound waves cause the solution to vibrate, which loosens the materials attached to the instruments. Ultrasonic cleaners are beneficial because they do not damage even the most delicate instruments, and workers do not run the risk of an accidental sharps injury.

Disinfection

Disinfection is the process of killing pathogenic organisms or of rendering them inactive. It is not always effective against spores, the tuberculosis bacilli, and certain viruses. Disinfectant chemicals may kill microbes within a short time, but they usually are very hard on instruments. Some chemicals, such as Cidex, are effective enough to kill all organisms, but the usual immersion time for these sterilants is 10 hours or longer. For equipment and countertop surfaces, the cheapest and most reliable method of disinfection is to use a 1:10 bleach solution. This is an effective and noncaustic disinfectant that can be used to wipe laboratory countertops where human blood and other body fluid samples are handled. It also can be used for soaking reusable rubber goods before sanitization. In addition, bleach solution is an effective disinfectant for surfaces that have come in contact with viruses, including HIV.

Many types of disinfecting agents are available and have varying degrees of effectiveness. It is important to follow the manufacturer's guidelines on how to use each product properly and to understand its advantages and disadvantages and the possible sources of error.

Disinfection is very difficult to verify, because no convenient indicators ensure destruction of organisms. Even when the manufacturer's directions for chemical strength and immersion times are followed, common errors can cause chemicals to lose their effectiveness:

- Instruments are not thoroughly sanitized, and attached organic matter inhibits or prevents the action of the disinfectant. No chemical can kill unless it reaches all instrument surfaces; therefore, complete sanitization is absolutely necessary.
- Sanitized instruments are not dried, and the moisture on the instruments dilutes the disinfectant solution beyond effective concentration levels.

PROCEDURE 27-5

Train in and Practice Standard Precautions: Use Standard Precautions for Sanitizing Instruments and Discarding Biohazardous Material

GOAL: *To follow Standard Precautions in removing all contaminated matter from instruments in preparation for disinfection or sterilization.*

EQUIPMENT and SUPPLIES

- Sink with cold and hot running water
- Sanitizing agent or low-sudsing soap with enzymatic action
- Utility gloves that are decontaminated and show no signs of deterioration
- Chin-length face shield or goggles and face mask if contamination with blood-borne pathogens is possible
- Disposable brush
- Disposable paper towels
- Disposable gloves
- Disinfectant cleaner prepared according to manufacturer's directions
- Biohazard waste container with labeled red biohazard bag

PROCEDURAL STEPS

1. Put on utility gloves.
   <u>PURPOSE:</u> To provide personal protection against potentially infectious matter and sharp instruments.
2. Put on a face shield or goggles and mask if potential for splashing of infectious material exists (Figure 1).

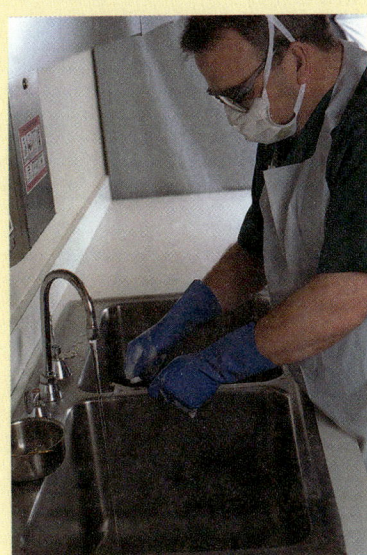

   <u>PURPOSE:</u> To provide personal protection against potentially infectious matter.
3. Separate the sharp instruments from other instruments to be sanitized.
   <u>PURPOSE:</u> To prevent possible self-injury and exposure to infectious matter.
4. Rinse the instruments under cold running water.
   <u>PURPOSE:</u> To help remove debris and prevent coagulation of body fluids.

5. Open hinged instruments and scrub all grooves, crevices, and serrations with a disposable brush (Figure 2).

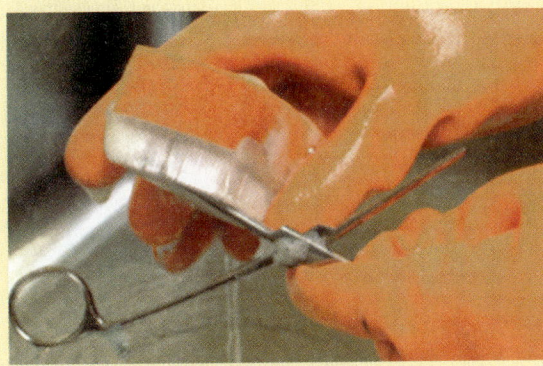

   <u>PURPOSE:</u> Microorganisms can hide under contaminants and may not be destroyed by the disinfection process.
6. Rinse well with hot water.
   <u>PURPOSE:</u> Hot water removes all soap and contaminant residue.
7. Towel dry all instruments thoroughly and dispose of contaminated towels and disposable brush in a biohazard waste container. Do not touch the paper towel dispenser as you are obtaining towels.
   <u>PURPOSE:</u> All contaminated material must be discarded in a labeled biohazard container and/or a labeled red biohazard bag. Touching the dispenser contaminates your hands. Wet instruments can rust or become dull and also dilute disinfectant or sterilizing chemicals.
8. Remove the utility gloves and wash your hands according to Procedure 27-4.
   <u>PURPOSE:</u> To remove any possible contaminants.
9. Towel dry your hands and put on disposable gloves. Decontaminate the utility gloves and work surfaces using disinfectant cleaner.
   <u>PURPOSE:</u> To prevent personal exposure to contaminants. All equipment and working surfaces should be cleaned and decontaminated with a disinfectant to prevent transmission of infectious organisms.
10. Dispose of the contaminated towels in a biohazard waste container.
    <u>PURPOSE:</u> All contaminated material must be disposed of in a labeled biohazard container and/or a labeled red biohazard bag.
11. Remove the disposable gloves according to Procedure 27-1. Dispose of the gloves in a biohazard waste container. Sanitize the hands.
    <u>PURPOSE:</u> To prevent the spread of infectious organisms and to remove any possible contaminants.
12. Towel dry your hands and place sanitized instruments in a designated area for disinfection or sterilization.
    <u>PURPOSE:</u> Sanitized instruments must be removed from the cleaning area to prevent possible cross-contamination.

- The disinfectant solution is left in an open container, and evaporation changes its concentration.
- Solutions are not changed after the recommended period for use has expired.
- Solutions are not prepared properly or are not mixed properly before use.
- The manufacturer's recommended temperature for use and storage is not maintained.

Alcohol is the most widely used antiseptic, but recent studies indicate that it is not as effective as other products in inhibiting the growth and reproduction of microorganisms on the skin's surface. Other antiseptic chemicals, such as povidone-iodine solution (Betadine), are effective antimicrobial agents that are safe to use on a patient's skin. Disinfection by boiling is both impractical and ineffective at killing many pathogens, including bacterial spores and viruses. In addition, an article must be immersed at a rolling boil for at least 15 minutes to be adequately disinfected.

CRITICAL THINKING APPLICATION   27-8

Rosa is responsible for orienting the new medical assistant in the office in sanitization and disinfection procedures. Outline the important concepts and methods of each.

Sterilization

Sterilization, or the destruction of all microorganisms, is essential for surgical asepsis. To ensure proper sterilization for aseptic procedures, an area should be set aside in each office for just this purpose. The area should be divided into two sections. One section is used for receiving contaminated materials. This area should have a sink, receiving basins, proper cleaning agents, brushes, autoclave wrapping paper, sterilizer envelopes and tape, sterilizer indicators, disposable gloves, and designated biohazard waste containers. The other section should be reserved for receiving the sterile items after removal from the autoclave. Clear, clean plastic bags in which to store sterile packs may be kept in the sterile area. Both areas should be spotlessly clean and well organized. Sterile technique is addressed in Chapter 57.

ROLE OF THE MEDICAL ASSISTANT IN ASEPSIS

Medical asepsis is one of the few procedures that directly affect the health of the patient, the physician, and the staff. The spread of pathogens in the ambulatory care setting can be controlled only through effective, consistent application of the Bloodborne Pathogens Standard and by proper sanitization, disinfection, and sterilization of supplies, equipment, and work surfaces.

The medical assistant must develop an inner sense for performing aseptic procedures properly. It is important that these techniques be done on such a routine basis that they become an unbreakable habit. The use of disposable items is highly recommended for infection control purposes. However, when disposable equipment is used, the assistant must follow recommended disposal guidelines.

CLOSING COMMENTS

Patient Education

The medical assistant should take every opportunity to educate patients about the infection process and about ways to prevent the transmission of disease. The best time to instruct a patient in aseptic techniques that can be used at home is while performing the aseptic procedure. For example:

- While washing your hands, explain to the patient that this routine is part of daily hygiene and is particularly important for patients who are very young or old or who seem to get sick frequently. Instruct the patient that the hands should be washed before and after meals; after sneezing, coughing, or blowing the nose; after using the restroom; before and after changing a dressing; and after changing an infant's diaper.
- Advise the patient to carry an alcohol-based hand rub and to use it as indicated throughout the day.
- Explain to the patient how using disposable tissues to cover the nose and mouth when coughing or sneezing reduces the chance of spreading illness among household members.
- Discuss proper ways of discarding used tissues, especially if a member of the household has or might have a communicable disease.
- Instruct the patient in the differences between sterile and clean dressings and bandages. Demonstrate each step in changing a dressing properly and explain how to dispose of contaminated items.

A medical assistant can help patients live healthier lives in many ways. For example, here are a few more suggestions for teaching the patient about asepsis and infection control:

- Set up an information table in the waiting room with take-home pamphlets and literature.
- Mail a periodic newsletter to patients about infection control, especially during flu season.
- Demonstrate and explain aseptic procedures to patients and family members, inviting them to participate.

Legal and Ethical Issues

Medical asepsis and infection control in the ambulatory care setting give rise to numerous legal and ethical concerns. Personal discipline is the primary concern in medical asepsis. Typically, the medical assistant is alone when performing a medical aseptic procedure; therefore, if contamination occurs, he or she is the only one who knows. If contamination should occur, the medical assistant must start over again with clean supplies.

One of the medical assistant's main responsibilities is to perform disinfection and sterilization procedures with precision and total effectiveness. There is no room for compromise. Patients should have absolute assurance that they are being treated in an aseptic atmosphere and under aseptic conditions. This assurance is just as important for the protection of the physician and staff as it is for the patient. Allowing the physician to assume that the correct aseptic techniques were used when preparing a procedure and allowing him or her to use contaminated equipment on a patient may result in a malpractice lawsuit. Honesty on the part of the medical assistant builds self-respect and contributes to professional achievement.

A primary reason for performing aseptic procedures completely and effectively is to prevent the development of nosocomial infections in susceptible patients. These infections, which are acquired in the healthcare environment, can be especially dangerous for elderly or debilitated patients. Ignorance of the various aseptic techniques or carelessness can be dangerous and is inexcusable before the law.

More than 48 states have adopted Good Samaritan legislation, which protects bystanders and first responders from liability when they perform lifesaving procedures at the scene of an accident. If the individual acts in good faith, is not compensated, and performs techniques to the best of his or her knowledge, the person is not liable for civil damages. However, because OSHA regulates employer responsibility for the management of blood-borne pathogens, exposure at the scene of an accident is not covered by employer postexposure incident policies. Therefore, healthcare workers who volunteer their assistance in an emergency must enact blood-borne precautions as much as possible without expecting medical follow-up at the workplace.

SUMMARY OF SCENARIO

Implementing Standard Precautions throughout daily practice is crucial to the welfare and protection both of the patient and the healthcare worker. Rosa must be sure to wash her hands routinely and/or to use an alcohol hand rub. She also must familiarize herself with the office's Exposure Control Plan; follow OSHA's Bloodborne Pathogens Standard; use PPE when needed; follow environmental protection guidelines; use appropriate procedures for cleaning up contaminated spills and other housekeeping controls; and understand postexposure follow-up if an accidental exposure occurs. In addition, Rosa must follow guidelines for sanitization, disinfection, and sterilization of appropriate instruments and equipment.

SUMMARY OF LEARNING OBJECTIVES

1. **Define, spell, and pronounce the terms listed in the vocabulary.**
   Spelling and pronouncing medical terms correctly bolster the medical assistant's credibility. Knowing the definitions of these terms promotes confidence in communication with patients and co-workers.

2. **Apply critical thinking skills in performing patient assessment and care.**
   Completing the Critical Thinking Application exercises throughout the chapter helps the student become more adept at critical analysis of real-life situations.

3. **Describe the characteristics of pathogenic microorganisms and the diseases they cause.**
   Pathogenic microorganisms include viruses, bacteria, protozoa, fungi, and rickettsiae.

4. **Apply the chain-of-infection process to healthcare practice.**
   The chain of infection is the way infectious disease is spread. It begins with the infectious agent and moves to the host, the means or portal of exit from the host, the mode of transmission, and the means or portal of entry into a new host. It ends with the presence of the infection in a susceptible host. At least one of these links must be broken to stop the spread of infection.

5. **Compare viral and bacterial cell invasion.**
   Bacterial infections can be treated with antibiotics, but viral infections, which involve viral takeover of cellular DNA or RNA material, cannot be treated with antibiotics, because viruses are not cells but parasites within a cell.

6. **Differentiate between humoral and cell-mediated immunity.**
   Humoral immunity creates specific antibodies to combat antigens. Cell-mediated immunity attacks the source of infection at the cellular level.

7. **Summarize the impact of the inflammatory response on the body's ability to defend itself against infection.**
   The inflammatory response is one aspect of the body's ability to defend itself against infection. It involves the body's reaction to the introduction of a foreign substance or antigen, an increase in blood flow to the site, and the release of inflammatory mediators that attract white blood cells to the site. WBCs isolate and destroy the source of inflammation.

8. **Analyze the differences among acute, chronic, latent, and opportunistic infections.**
   Acute diseases have a rapid onset and short duration. Chronic diseases are present over a long period, perhaps a lifetime. Latent diseases cycle through relapse and remission phases. Opportunistic infections are caused by organisms that are not typically pathogenic but that occur in hosts with an impaired or weakened immune system response, such as individuals with HIV.

9. **Specify potentially infectious body fluids.**
   Potentially infectious body fluids include CSF; mucus; synovial, pleural, pericardial, peritoneal, and amniotic fluids; blood; vaginal and seminal secretions; saliva; and human tissue.

10. **Integrate OSHA's requirement for a site-based Exposure Control Plan into office management procedures.**
    OSHA requires incorporation of a site-based Exposure Control Plan into office management procedures. The plan must be revised annually and must be available for employees to review. It must reflect current safety technology, identify employees at risk for exposure, and contain specifics about protection from blood-borne pathogens, including PPE, training, hepatitis B immunization, exposure, follow-up, record keeping, and the labeling and disposal of all biohazard waste.

11. **Explain the major areas included in the OSHA Compliance Guidelines.**

    The OSHA Compliance Guidelines include barrier protection devices, environment protection, housekeeping controls, hepatitis B immunization, and postexposure follow-up.

12. **Remove contaminated gloves while following Standard Precautions principles.**

    Refer to Procedure 27-1.

13. **Perform an eyewash procedure for the removal of contaminated material.**

    Refer to Procedure 27-2.

14. **Summarize the management of postexposure evaluation and follow-up.**

    Postexposure evaluation and follow-up are as follows: The site is cleaned and the exposed individual reports to the supervisor immediately. Medical assessment is performed immediately. Testing of the source individual's and worker's blood is performed if possible and if consent is given. Health counseling is provided. Strict confidentiality of all medical records is maintained.

15. **Participate in a mock environmental exposure event with documentation of the steps taken.**

    Procedure 27-3 summarizes the steps required for the management of a postexposure needlestick.

16. **Apply the concepts of medical and surgical asepsis to the healthcare setting.**

    Medical asepsis is the removal or destruction of pathogens. Medical aseptic techniques are used to create an environment that is as free of pathogens as possible. Surgical asepsis is destruction of all microorganisms. Surgical asepsis is used when the patient's skin or mucous membranes are disrupted.

17. **Demonstrate the proper hand-washing technique for medical asepsis.**

    Refer to Procedure 27-4.

18. **Differentiate among sanitization, disinfection, and sterilization procedures.**

    Sanitization is cleaning of contaminated articles or surfaces to reduce the number of microorganisms. *Disinfection* involves the use of physical or chemical means to destroy pathogens or their components on inanimate surfaces or objects. *Sterilization* removes all living microorganisms.

19. **Demonstrate the correct procedure for sanitizing contaminated instruments.**

    Refer to Procedure 27-5.

20. **Apply patient education concepts to infection control.**

    Take every opportunity to demonstrate aseptic techniques, to educate patients about proper management of infectious materials at home, and to emphasize the importance of frequent and consistent hand washing.

21. **Discuss the legal and ethical concerns regarding medical asepsis and infection control.**

    The medical assistant is responsible for applying infection control procedures in all situations at all times to prevent cross-contamination and the development of nosocomial infections in patients.

CONNECTIONS

Study Guide Connection: Go to the Chapter 27 Study Guide. Read and complete the activities.

Evolve Connection: Go to the Chapter 27 link at *evolve.elsevier.com/kinn* to complete the Chapter Review and Chapter Quiz. Check out the other resources listed for this chapter to make the most of what you have learned from Infection Control.

PATIENT ASSESSMENT

28

SCENARIO

Chris Isaccson, CMA (AAMA), works in an ambulatory care setting at the community hospital. He is responsible for initial patient interviews, taking medical histories, and documentation. Chris is having difficulty gathering the information needed from some of the patients. They do not always respond openly and honestly to him, and the attending physician is not satisfied with his work. His supervisor is responsible for helping him improve his interviewing skills.

While studying this chapter, think about the following questions:

- How can Chris learn to develop helping relationships so that the patient's medical history is as comprehensive as possible?
- Would it help if Chris displayed greater sensitivity to diverse populations?
- Would using active listening techniques and attending to the patient's nonverbal behaviors better enable Chris to develop therapeutic communications skills?

- How can Chris's supervisor help him become a better communicator and demonstrate comprehensive and accurate documentation in patients' charts?

LEARNING OBJECTIVES

1. Define, spell, and pronounce the terms listed in the vocabulary.
2. Apply critical thinking skills in performing patient assessment and care.
3. Employ the concept of holistic care in the patient assessment process.
4. Describe the components of the patient's medical history.
5. Define and apply the qualities of a helping relationship.
6. Display sensitivity to diverse patient populations.
7. Demonstrate therapeutic communications, including the use of the linear communication model and active listening techniques.
8. Recognize the importance of nonverbal communication when interacting with patients.
9. Identify barriers to communication and their impact on patient assessment.
10. Detect a patient's use of defense mechanisms and the resultant barriers to therapeutic communication.
11. Use therapeutic communication techniques with patients across the lifespan.
12. Demonstrate professional patient interviewing techniques.
13. Integrate detailed information about the chief complaint into concise, accurate documentation methods.
14. Differentiate among various medical records systems employed in the physician's office.
15. Describe the connection between the interview process and implementation of patient education practices.
16. Determine risk management strategies for the ambulatory care setting.
17. Use reflection, restatement, and clarification techniques to obtain a patient history.

VOCABULARY

biophysical (bi-o-fi'-zi-kuhl) The science of applying physical laws and theories to biologic problems.

cognitive (kog'-nuh-tiv) Pertaining to the operation of the mind; referring to the process by which we become aware of perceiving, thinking, and remembering.

congruence (kon-groo'-ents) Agreement; the state that occurs when the verbal expression of the message matches the sender's nonverbal body language.

familial Occurring in or affecting members of a family more than would be expected by chance.

holistic Considering the patient as a whole including the physical, emotional, social, economic, and spiritual needs of the person.

present illness The chief complaint, written in chronologic sequence, with dates of onset.

psychosocial Pertaining to a combination of psychological and social factors.

rapport (ra-por') A relationship of harmony and accord between the patient and the healthcare professional.

signs Objective findings determined by a clinician, such as a fever, hypertension, or rash.

symptoms Subjective complaints reported by the patient, such as pain or visual disturbances.

As medical professionals directly involved in gathering information from patients about their health status, medical assistants must remember that a healthy state is more than the absence of disease. The assessment process should be a reflection of the entire patient, not just a report about signs and symptoms. Individual lifestyles and environmental factors can create disease and therefore should be considered when we gather information about the patient's chief complaint. For example, if a patient smokes or works in a stressful occupation, he or she may be more prone to hypertension. As health professionals, we should consider all patient factors, including **cognitive**, **psychosocial**, and behavioral data, when gathering information about the patient's health status. Consider this: do you think a patient who does not have health insurance to help pay for medication can afford prescribed drugs? This method of analyzing the development of disease is based on a **holistic** perspective. Holistic patient care recognizes that illness is the result of many factors, not just physical ones.

Assessment factors are a list of **biophysical** signs and symptoms. As the first step in treating a disease process, the physician must determine the patient's medical diagnosis. The identification of disease begins with the physician's *working diagnosis,* which he or she has determined through the patient's history, the report of the chief complaint, and the physical examination. Next, the physician orders laboratory tests, diagnostic examinations, and/or a referral visit to another physician to substantiate or refute the working diagnosis. Once the test results have been received, the *clinical diagnosis* is established. The patient then is treated, and after a period of time is re-evaluated to see whether the clinical diagnosis has changed. If it has, the new diagnosis is called the *differentiated diagnosis.* The physician continues to evaluate the patient's progress, ordering tests and/or altering treatment as needed.

However, patient care does not start with the physical examination; it begins when the patient first makes contact with the office. Even before the examination, the medical assistant has the opportunity to interact with the patient to ensure that he or she feels comfortable during the process and that all the necessary information is obtained.

Interviewing patients, assisting with examinations, and documentation are important responsibilities for a medical assistant. You must know the components of a medical history and the techniques for securing, because these will help the physician diagnose and treat the patient. The more complete the medical history, the more efficient the physician's care and treatment will be.

MEDICAL HISTORY

Collecting the History Information

When a new patient calls or comes in for an appointment, the person is asked to complete a health history form. Besides being useful for diagnosing and treating the patient, the self-history allows the patient more participation in the process. The form may be mailed to the patient's home before the appointment or may be completed in the office during the first visit.

If you are responsible for taking a portion of the medical history, conduct the interview in a private area free of outside interference and beyond the hearing range of other patients. Patients will not talk freely where they may be overheard or interrupted. Legally and ethically, the patient has the right to privacy, and access to the patient's medical record is permitted only to healthcare workers directly involved in the patient's care or to individuals the patient has specified on his or her Health Insurance Portability and Accountability Act (HIPAA) release form.

Listen to the patient. Do not express surprise or displeasure at any of the patient's statements. Remember, you are there not to pass judgment but to gather medical data. Documentation of information gathered while taking the medical history is included in the progress notes section of the medical chart. The medical assistant records the information in an organized manner, exactly as given by the patient, without opinion or interpretation. The progress notes should include the purpose of the patient's visit, written as the chief complaint (CC), and the patient's vital signs (VS), including height and weight, if preferred by the physician; in addition, if the patient reports pain, it should be documented using a scale of 1 to 10, with 1 being the least amount of pain and 10 being the greatest amount.

In some facilities, the physician takes the medical history during the patient's initial visit. The physician correlates the physical findings in the examination with the information in the history. The complete medical history and the physical examination are the starting point and foundation of all patient-physician contacts.

Components of the Medical History

Medical history forms vary, depending on the physician's preference and the practice specialty (Figure 28-1). The most commonly used medical history forms include these components:

- *Database:* The record of the patient's name, address, date of birth, insurance information, personal data, history, physical examination, and initial laboratory findings. As new information is added, it becomes a part of this database.
- *Chief complaint (CC)* or **present illness**: The purpose of the patient's visit. The medical assistant should gather as much information about the health problem as possible and record it concisely using the patient's own words as often as possible.
- *Past history (PH)* or *past medical history (PMH):* A summary of the patient's previous health. It includes dates and details regarding the patient's usual childhood diseases (UCD or UCHD), major illnesses, surgeries, allergies, accidents, and immunization record. Each medical practice has a policy on how to document a patient's allergies; they typically are written in red ink or identified by a colored sticker so that all healthcare workers can easily take note of potential allergic reactions. Included in the patient's medication history should be a record of frequently used over-the-counter (OTC) medications, including supplements and currently prescribed drugs.
- *Family history (FH):* Details about the patient's parents and siblings and their health; if they are deceased, the age and cause of death. This information is important, because certain diseases and disorders have **familial** and/or hereditary tendencies.
- *Social history (SH):* This section includes information about the patient's lifestyle, hobbies, entertainment preferences, education, occupation, use of tobacco and alcohol, sleeping habits, level of exercise, diet, last menstrual period (LMP) for female patients, and method of birth control if the patient is sexually active. It may be important to note the patient's cultural and religious background, because these could influence certain lifestyle and dietary choices. This information helps the physician to plan treatment for the patient or to determine causative factors for disease. It also provides a holistic picture of the patient's health.
- *Systems review (SR)* or *review of systems (ROS):* These questions provide a guide to the patient's general health and help detect conditions other than those covered under the present illness. Often a patient may think certain health problems irrelevant and may fail to mention them. However, these problems may help the physician determine the cause of the disorder currently being explored. A systems review is obtained through a logical sequence of questions about the state of health of body systems, beginning with the head and proceeding downward. The physician typically completes this section of the medical history while conducting the physical examination.

UNDERSTANDING AND COMMUNICATING WITH PATIENTS

To provide high-quality patient care, we must communicate effectively with the patient and provide a warm, caring environment. Positive reactions and interactions with the patient are vital. Because medical care by nature is extremely personal, a medical assistant must always remember that each patient is an individual with certain anxieties. These anxieties often cause people to act and react in different ways; therefore, effective verbal and nonverbal communication with each patient is absolutely essential.

Healthcare professionals accept the responsibility of developing helping relationships with their patients. The interpersonal nature of the patient–medical assistant relationship carries with it a certain amount of responsibility to forget one's self-interest and focus on the patient's needs. A medical assistant can elicit either a positive or a negative response to patient care simply by the way he or she treats and interacts with patients. You usually are the first person with whom the patient communicates; therefore, you play a vital role in initiating therapeutic patient interactions (Procedure 28-1).

Sensitivity to Diversity

Practicing respectful patient care is extremely important when working with a diverse patient population. Empathy is the key to creating a caring, therapeutic environment. Empathy goes beyond sympathy. A medical assistant who is empathetic respects the individuality of the patient and attempts to see the person's health problem through his or her eyes, recognizing the effect of all holistic factors on the patient's well-being. Empathetic sensitivity to diversity first requires those interested in healthcare to examine their own values, beliefs, and actions; you cannot treat all patients with care and respect until you first recognize and evaluate personal biases. We think and act a certain way for many reasons. The first step in understanding the process is to evaluate your individual value system. Why do you have certain attitudes or beliefs about the worth of individuals or things?

> ### CRITICAL THINKING APPLICATION   28-1
> What do you value most in life? What is important to you? What influences you to act in a certain way? Make a list of five things you value the most and share them with the class. Try to determine why you feel so strongly about those particular things.

Many different factors influence the development of a value system. Value systems begin as learned beliefs and behaviors. Families and cultural influences shape the way we respond to a diverse society. Other factors that influence reactions include socioeconomic and educational backgrounds. To develop therapeutic relationships, you must recognize your own value system to determine whether it could affect your method of interaction. Preconceived ideas about people because of their race, religion, income level, ethnic origin, sexual orientation, or gender can act as barriers to the development of a therapeutic relationship. You will be unable to treat your patients empathetically unless you can connect with them in some way. Personal biases or prejudices are monumental barriers to the development of therapeutic relationships (Figure 28-2).

FORM 8184	MEDICAL RECORD				

NAME   AGE   SEX   S M D W

ADDRESS   PHONE   DATE

SPONSOR   ADDRESS

OCCUPATION   REF BY   ACKN

CHIEF COMPLAINT

PRESENT ILLNESS

FAMILY HISTORY		**URINARY TRACT**	
MOTHER	FATHER	NOCTURIA	FREQUENCY
BROTHERS		PAIN	BURNING
SISTERS		BLEEDING	INFECTION
TB	DIAB	MALIG	INCONTINENCE
HT DIS	NEPH	EPILEP	**GENITAL TRACT**
PSYCH		AGE AT MENST	TYPE PERIOD
PAST HISTORY — GENL HEALTH		INTERMEN BLEEDING	
		AMENORRHEA	DYSMENORRHEA
CHILDHOOD DISEASES		VAG DISCH	IRRITATION
SC FEV	RHEUM FEV	ALLERGY	PAINFUL PERIOD
OTHER		L M P	
USUAL WEIGHT		CHILDREN — L	D S B
ACCIDENTS		MARRIED YRS.	YOUNGEST CHILD

SOCIAL HISTORY   COFFEE   TOBACCO   ALCOHOL   **NEUROMUSCULAR**

REVIEW OF SYSTEMS		STRENGTH	NERVOUSNESS
E E N T — EYES		SLEEP	WORRY
EARS		MUSCULAR PAIN	
NOSE		JOINT PAIN	
THROAT		ABNORMAL SENSATIONS	
NECK		DEFORMITIES	
BREASTS			
HEART — LUNGS		**OPERATIONS**	
PAIN	COUGH		
BLEEDING	DYSPNEA		
IRREG	EDEMA		
GASTROINTESTINAL		**TREATMENTS**	
APPETITE	DIET		
INDIGESTION	PAIN		
NAUSEA	VOMITING		
JAUNDICE	BLEEDING	**COMMENTS**	
BOWEL HABITS			
HEMORRHOIDS			
PAIN WITH STOOL	ITCHING		
OTHER			
OTHER			

FORM 8184 COLWELL SYSTEMS, CHAMPAIGN, ILL.

FIGURE 28-1 A general medical history form. (From Klieger DM: *Saunders textbook of medical assisting,* St Louis, 2005, WB Saunders.)

Obtain and Record a Patient History

Complete this procedure with another student playing the role of the patient. To make the experience more realistic, choose a student about whom you know very little. To maintain the student's privacy, he or she does not have to share any confidential information.

GOAL: *To obtain an acceptable written background from the patient to help the physician determine the cause and effects of the present illness. This includes the chief complaint (CC), present illness (PI), past history (PH), family history (FH), and social history (SH).*

EQUIPMENT and SUPPLIES

- History form
- Two pens: a red pen for recording the patient's allergies and a black pen to meet legal documentation guidelines
- Quiet, private area

PROCEDURAL STEPS

1. Greet and identify the patient in a pleasant manner. Introduce yourself and explain your role.
   PURPOSE: To make the patient feel comfortable and at ease.
2. Take the patient to a quiet, private area for the interview and explain why the information is needed.
   PURPOSE: A quiet, private area is necessary to protect confidentiality and prevent interruptions. An informed patient is more cooperative and therefore more likely to provide useful information.
3. Complete the history form by using therapeutic communication techniques, including restatement, reflection, and clarification. Make sure all medical terminology is adequately explained. A self-history may have been mailed to the patient before the visit. If so, review the self-history for completeness.
   PURPOSE: Therapeutic communication techniques help the medical assistant gather complete information; the self-history is designed to save time and to involve the patient in the process.
4. Speak in a pleasant, distinct manner, remembering to maintain eye contact with your patient.
   PURPOSE: Positive nonverbal behaviors create a friendly, caring atmosphere.
5. Remain sensitive to the diverse needs of your patient throughout the interview process.
   PURPOSE: Incorporate awareness of your personal biases into treating all patients with respect despite their diverse backgrounds.
6. Record the following statistical information on the patient information form:
   - Patient's full name, including middle initial
   - Address, including apartment number and ZIP code
   - Marital status
   - Sex (gender)
   - Age and date of birth
   - Telephone numbers for home, cell, and work
   - Insurance information if not already available
   - Employer's name, address, and telephone number
7. Record the following medical history on the patient history form:
   - Chief complaint
   - Present illness

- Past history
- Family history
- Social history

PURPOSE: The physician needs this information to make an accurate assessment and diagnosis. The physician usually completes the review of systems (ROS) during the pre-examination interview.

8. Ask about allergies to drugs and any other substances and record any allergies in red ink on every page of the history form, on the front of the patient record, and on each progress note page. Some practices apply allergy alert labels to the front of each patient record or mark the record accordingly if using an EHR system.
   PURPOSE: The presence of an allergy may alter medication and treatment procedures.
9. Record all information legibly and neatly and spell words correctly. Print rather than writing in longhand. Do not erase, scribble, or use whiteout. Do not leave any blank spaces or skip lines between documentation entries. If you make an error, draw a single line through the error, write "error" above it, add the correction, and initial and date the entry.
   PURPOSE: To maintain a medical record that is understandable and defensible in a court of law.
10. Thank the patient for cooperating and direct him or her back to the reception area.
11. Review the record for errors before you pass it to the physician.
12. Use the information on the record to complete the patient's medical record. Keep the information confidential.
    PURPOSE: All information concerning the patient must remain in the office. This information may be legally and ethically discussed only with the physician.

DOCUMENTATION PRACTICE

Mr. Bonski is a new patient being seen today for the first time. His CC is dizziness for 2 weeks. He denies having headaches and has no previous Hx of ear infections or hypertension. He does not take any prescribed medications but uses Tylenol as needed for a headache. T 97.6, P 88, R 22, BP 172/94. Document pertinent patient findings using the SOAPE method.

S: _____

O: _____

A: _____

P: _____

E: _____

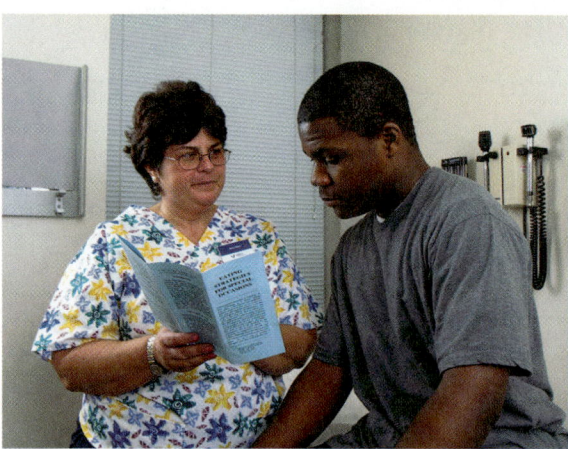

FIGURE 28-2 Respectful patient care.

CRITICAL THINKING APPLICATION   28-2

Honestly evaluate your personal biases. What do you find unacceptable in people? Do you prejudge an individual based on his or her affiliation with a particular group or because of a certain lifestyle decision? Do these biases create barriers to the development of therapeutic relationships? If so, how can you get beyond these barriers?

Consider the following scenarios and discuss them with your classmates:

- While you are conducting a patient interview, the patient informs you that he has tested positive for the human immunodeficiency virus (HIV). Do you think this will affect your therapeutic relationship?
- You are responsible for recording an in-depth interview on a homeless person with very poor hygiene. Will this cause a problem with your professional manner?
- You are told by your office manager that an inmate of the county prison is being brought in this afternoon for an examination. Do you think his status will affect your interaction with the patient?
- You are attempting to interview a 20-year-old patient who brought her two young children with her to the office today. She is a single mother who is pregnant with her third child and is on welfare. What do you think? Will you have difficulty being empathetic?

SENSITIVITY TO DIVERSITY

Regardless of the type of healthcare facility in which you work, you will care for a wide variety of patients. Some things to consider about diverse groups include:

- Patients of Asian backgrounds may have been raised in a culture that considers it extremely rude to establish eye contact. Americans view an unwillingness to establish eye contact as a sign of distrust or embarrassment, but for those from Japan or China, lack of eye contact may be a way of demonstrating respect.
- Personal space may be an issue for patients from diverse backgrounds. If a patient appears very uncomfortable with touch or lack

of personal space, attempt to accommodate him or her as much as possible during the office visit.
- Research has shown that older people face unique communications problems in the healthcare environment. When caring for an aging individual, it is important to focus patient teaching and information on the patient rather than the family member who may be present.
- Patients may use their religious beliefs and values to understand and cope with their health problems. However, using religion to guide healthcare decisions may result in a conflict with the physician's recommendations. Healthcare workers may need to find a balance between respect for a patient's beliefs and the delivery of high-quality healthcare.

Therapeutic Techniques

The linear communication model describes communication as an interactive process involving the sender of the message, the receiver, and the crucial component of feedback to confirm reception of the message. The message can be sent by a number of different methods, such as face-to-face communication, telephone, e-mail, and letter; however, there is no way to confirm that the message was actually received unless the patient provides feedback about what he or she interpreted from the message. Feedback completes the communication cycle by providing a means for us to know exactly what message the patient received and therefore whether it requires clarification.

For example, as a medical assistant, one of your responsibilities will be to provide patient education on how to prepare for diagnostic studies. Let's say you have to explain to an elderly patient how to prepare for a colonoscopy. Even though you provide a detailed explanation of the preparation procedure, in addition to a handout explaining the step-by-step process, how do you really know whether the patient understands? You ask the patient to provide feedback by explaining the process back to you. As a member of the healthcare team, you must become an effective communicator. You will play a vital role in collecting and documenting patient information. If your methods of collection or recording are faulty, the quality of patient care may be seriously impaired.

Active Listening Techniques

Active listeners go beyond hearing the patient's message to concentrating, understanding, and listening to the main points in the discussion. Active listening techniques encourage patients to expand on and clarify the content and meaning of their messages. They are very useful communication tools to implement when a patient is agitated or upset, because these methods help the medical assistant clarify the important details of the patient's chief complaint.

Three processes are involved in active listening: restatement, reflection, and clarification. Restatement is simply paraphrasing or repeating the patient's statements with phrases such as, "You are saying ..." or "You are telling me the problem is ..."

Reflection involves repeating the main idea of the conversation while also identifying the sender's *feelings*. For example, if the mother of a young patient is expressing frustration about her child's behavior, a reflective statement identifies that feeling with the response, "You sound frustrated about …" Or, if a patient who has been newly diagnosed with insulin-dependent diabetes shows anxiety about administering injections, an appropriate reflective statement recognizes the patient's feelings: "You appear anxious about …" Reflective statements clearly demonstrate to patients that you are not only listening to their words; you also are concerned and are attending to their feelings.

Clarification seeks to summarize or simplify the sender's thoughts and feelings and to resolve any confusion in the message. Questions or statements that begin with "Give me an example of …" or "Explain to me about …" or "So what you're saying is …" help patients focus on the chief complaint and give you the opportunity to clear up any misconceptions before documenting patient information.

Listening is not a passive role in the communication process; it is active and demanding. You cannot be preoccupied with your own needs, or you will miss something important. For the duration of the patient interview, no one is more important than this particular patient. Listen to the way things are said, the tone of the patient's voice, and even to what the patient may not be saying out loud but is saying very clearly with body language.

Nonverbal Communication

Much of what we communicate to our patients is conveyed through the use of conscious or unconscious body language. Our nonverbal actions, such as gestures, facial expressions, and mannerisms, are learned behaviors that are greatly influenced by our family and cultural backgrounds. The body naturally expresses our true feelings; in fact, experts say that more than 90% of communication is nonverbal.

Most of the negative messages communicated through body language are unintentional; therefore, it is important to remember while conducting patient interviews that nonverbal communication can seriously affect the therapeutic process.

The verbal messages you send are only part of the communication process. You have a specific context in mind when you send your words, but the receiver puts his or her own interpretations on them. The receiver attaches meaning determined by his or her past experiences, culture, self-concept, and current physical and emotional states. Sometimes these messages and interpretations do not coincide. Feedback from the patient is crucial in determining whether the patient understood the message. Successful communication requires mutual understanding by both the interviewer and the person being interviewed.

Observing your patient during the interview fosters mutual understanding. The purpose of observing nonverbal communication is to become sensitive to or aware of the feelings of others as conveyed by small bits of behavior rather than words. This sensitivity enables you to adapt your behavior to these feelings; to deliberately select your response, either verbal or nonverbal; and thereby to have a favorable effect on others. The favorable effect may consist of providing emotional support, conveying that you care, defusing the patient's fear or anger, or providing an invitation to release pent-up feelings by talking about the situation that aroused the feelings. Table 28-1 lists some nonverbal behaviors by patients that may indicate anxiety, frustration, or fear.

TABLE 28-1 Observation of Nonverbal Communication in Patients

AREA OBSERVED	OBSERVATION	INDICATION
Breathing patterns	Rapid respirations, sighing, shallow thoracic breathing	Anxiety, boredom, pain
Eye patterns	No eye contact, side-to-side movement, looking down at the hands	Anxiety, distrust, embarrassment
Hands	Tapping fingers, cracking knuckles, continuous movement, sweaty palms	Anxiety, worry, fear
Arm placement	Folded across chest, wrapped around abdomen	Anxiety, worry, fear, pain
Leg placement	Tension, crossed and/or tucked under, tapping foot, continuous movement	Frustration, anger

HELPFUL LISTENING GUIDELINES

- Listen to the main points in the discussion.
- Attend to both verbal and nonverbal messages.
- Be patient and nonjudgmental.
- Do not interrupt.
- Never intimidate your patient.
- Use active listening techniques: restatement, reflection, and clarification.

You can do much to put a patient at ease by the tone of your voice. Your facial expression and the ease and confidence of your movements demonstrate a sincere interest to the patient. Therapeutic use of space and touch also are important ways of sending nonverbal messages to your patients. You should establish eye contact, sit in a relaxed but attentive position, and avoid using furniture as a barrier between you and the patient. Give the patient your undivided attention and let your body language inform each patient that you are interested in his or her medical problems (Figure 28-3).

The key to successful patient interaction is **congruence** between verbal and nonverbal messages. Although choosing the correct words is very important, only 7% of the message received is verbal; therefore, to be seen as honest and sensitive to the needs of your patients, you must be aware of your nonverbal behavior patterns. The nonverbal message the patient receives from the medical assistant's listening behavior should be, "You are a person of worth, and I am interested in you as a unique individual."

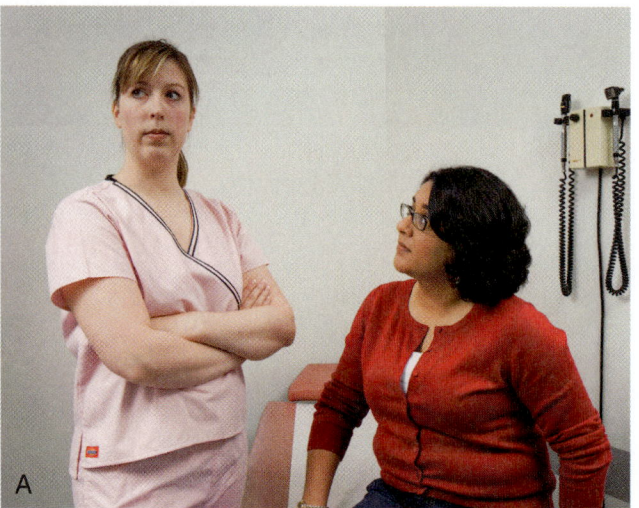
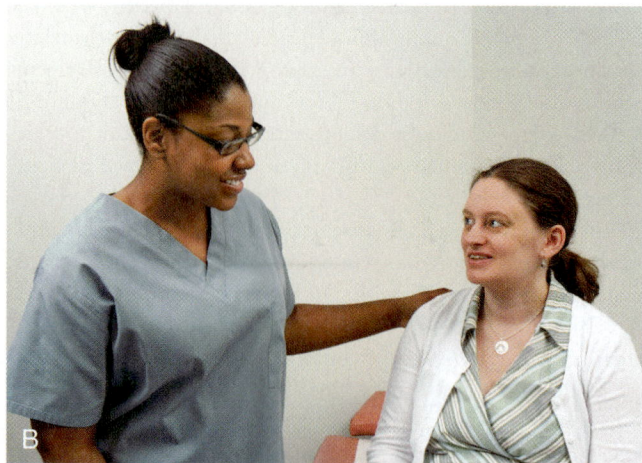

FIGURE 28-3 A, Ineffective nonverbal language. **B,** Therapeutic nonverbal language.

NONVERBAL LANGUAGE BEHAVIORS

Nonverbal behavior—your body language—can have either a positive or negative effect on patient interactions. Positive nonverbal behaviors enhance the patient's experience in the healthcare setting. Communication experts recommend the following:

- When gathering a health history, lean toward the patient to show interest.
- Face the patient squarely and at eye level to help make the process more comfortable and to demonstrate sensitivity and empathy.
- Eye contact is essential for therapeutic communication unless the patient is from a culture that discourages this.
- A closed posture (crossed arms or legs) may indicate disinterest.
- Be sensitive to the patient's personal space when possible. Maintain a comfortable distance from the patient, at least an arm's length, when conducting the interview.
- Be careful with body gestures such as hand and arm movements. Gestures, such as nodding your head when the patient talks, can display interest but too much body movement can be distracting.
- Your tone of voice should reflect your interest in the patient. Speaking too quietly or too loudly can detract from therapeutic communication.
- Continually observe the patient's body language during the interview; watch for signs of confusion, boredom, worry, and so on so that you can respond appropriately.

Environmental Factors

Before you meet with the patient, prepare the physical setting, which may be an examination room or an office. In any location, optimum conditions are important to achieving a smooth, productive interview.

Open-Ended Questions or Statements

An open-ended question or statement asks for general information or states the topic to be discussed but only in general terms. Use this communication tool to begin the interview, to introduce a new section of questions, or whenever the person introduces a new topic. It is a very effective method of gathering more details from the patient about the chief complaint or health history. Examples include:

"What brings you to the doctor?"

"How have you been getting along?"

"You mentioned having dizzy spells. Tell me more about that."

This type of question or statement encourages patients to respond in a manner they find comfortable. It allows patients to express themselves fully and provide comprehensive information about their chief complaint.

Closed Questions

Direct, or closed, questions ask for specific information. This form of questioning limits the answer to one or two words, a "yes" or "no" in many cases. Use this form of question when you need confirmation of specific facts, such as when asking about past health problems. For example:

"Do you have a headache?"

"What is your birth date?"

"Have you ever broken a bone?"

INTERVIEWING THE PATIENT

The interview, or gathering the patient's medical history, is the first and most important part of data collection. The medical history identifies the patient's health strengths and problems and is a bridge to the next step in data collection, the physical examination performed by the physician. At this point, the patient knows everything about his or her own health status and you know nothing. Your skill in interviewing helps glean the necessary information and builds **rapport** for a successful working relationship.

Consider the interview as a form of contract between you and your patient. The contract consists of spoken and unspoken language and addresses what the patient needs and expects from the healthcare visit. The patient interview consists of three stages: the initiation or introduction, the body, and the closing.

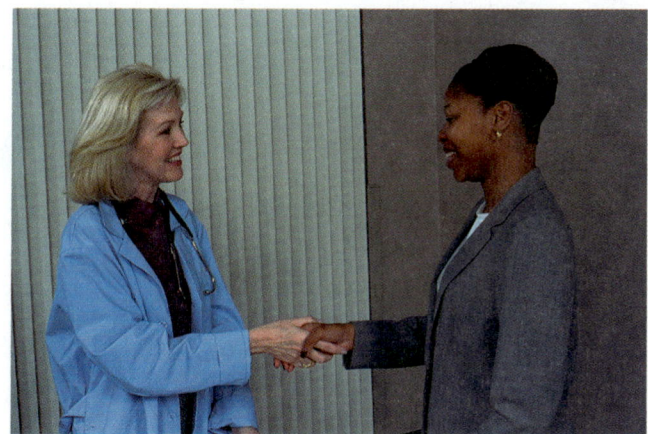

FIGURE 28-4 Greeting the patient.

The initiation of the interview is the time to introduce yourself, to identify the patient, and to determine the purpose of the interview (Figure 28-4). If you are nervous about how to begin, remember to keep it short. The patient probably is nervous, too, and is anxious to get started. Address the patient by his or her last name and give the reason for the interview. For example: "Mr. Coleman, my name is Stacey, and I am a certified medical assistant who works with Dr. Yang. I have some questions to ask you about your health history. Would you mind sharing this information with me?"

After the brief introduction, move on to the body of the interview. This is when you use various therapeutic communication techniques to determine the reason the patient is seeking healthcare, the patient's perception of the problem, the characteristics of the problem, and the patient's expectations of care. During this time, use active listening skills, meaningful silence, congruent verbal and nonverbal communication, and a combination of open-ended and closed statements and questions to gather the details of the patient's history and current health problem (Table 28-2).

Conclude the interview by summarizing the results of your interaction. The closing of the interview should clarify the patient's chief complaint, the purpose of the health visit, and the patient's expectations of care. This is the patient's opportunity to add any additional details or to explain further the characteristics of the health problem.

PREPARING THE APPROPRIATE ENVIRONMENT

Ensure Privacy
Make sure the room you use is unoccupied for the entire time allowed for the interview. The patient needs to feel sure that no one can overhear the conversation or interrupt.

Prevent Interruptions
Inform your co-workers of the interview and ask them not to interrupt you during this time. You need to concentrate on the patient and establish rapport. An interruption can destroy in seconds what you have spent many minutes building up.

Prepare Comfortable Surroundings
Conducting the interview in comfortable surroundings reduces the patient's anxiety. Keep the distance between you and the patient to 4 to 5 feet.

TABLE 28-2 Therapeutic Communication Techniques

TECHNIQUE	VALUE
Open-ended questions and statements	Encourage the patient to respond in more detail
Direct or closed questions	Ask for specific information; usual reply is a "yes" or "no" answer
Listening	Nonverbally communicates your interest in the patient
Silence	Nonverbally communicates your acceptance of the patient and willingness to wait until the patient is ready to answer
Establishing guidelines	Helps the patient know what to expect during the interview
Acknowledgment	Shows the importance of the patient's role and respect for autonomy
Restating	Checks your interpretation of the patient's message for validation
Reflecting	Shows the patient your acknowledgement of his or her feelings
Summarizing	Helps the patient separate relevant from irrelevant material; provides clarity to the interview

Arrange chairs so that you and the patient are comfortably seated at eye level, and the desk or table does not act as a barrier between you.

Take Judicious Notes
Note taking should be kept to a minimum while you try to focus your attention on the person. Note taking during the interview has disadvantages, such as breaking eye contact and shifting your attention away from the patient, which diminishes the patient's sense of importance. However, it is important to write down pertinent details as you are interviewing, because you may forget important facts if you do not note them at the time of the discussion. With experience you will develop a personal type of shorthand that you can use during the interview process.

Interview Barriers

Providing Unwarranted Assurance
Mrs. Miller says to you, "I know this lump is going to turn out to be cancer." The typical reply is almost automatic: "Don't worry, I'm sure everything will be fine." This type of answer indicates that her anxiety is insignificant and denies her the opportunity to discuss her fears further. A reflective response, such as, "You sound really worried about …" acknowledges her feelings and demonstrates empathy and a willingness to listen to her concerns.

Giving Advice

Mrs. Thompson has just finished talking to the doctor. She looks at you and says, "Dr. Rowe says I need surgery to get rid of these gallstones. I just don't know. What would you do?" If you tell her how you would handle the situation, you may have shifted the accountability for decision making from her to you, and she has not worked out her own solution. Does this woman really want to know what you would do? Probably not. You could respond to her question with, "Based on what the doctor told you, what do you think you should do?" or "Do you need further information to make your decision?" If the patient continues to question the physician's recommendations, the medical assistant should encourage further discussion with the physician.

Using Medical Terminology

You must adjust your vocabulary to fit the patient. The more the patient understands about what is happening and the management of the problem, the better the outcome. Misinterpreted communication is the most common error in patient care. One of the biggest problems for the patient is understanding medical terminology. Closely observe the patient's body language while he or she receives instructions or patient education. If the patient shows signs of not understanding the procedure, ask the patient to repeat back to you the information or instructions. This demonstration–return demonstration form of providing feedback ensures that the patient completely understands what is happening. It also gives the medical assistant the opportunity to clarify any misconceptions.

Leading Questions

During the interview, you ask the patient, "You don't smoke, do you?" By asking questions in this manner, you indicate the preferred answer. Telling you that he or she does smoke would surely meet with your disapproval. Keep your questions positive. A better way of asking would be, "Have you ever smoked?" or "Do you use tobacco?"

Talking Too Much

Some medical assistants associate helpfulness with verbal overload. The patient may let the interviewer talk at the expense of his or her own need to explain what is wrong. Always remember that when interviewing a patient, you should listen more than you talk. Pay close attention to the patient's body language to make sure you are giving the patient ample opportunity to discuss the health problem.

Defense Mechanisms

In Chapter 5 we discussed the impact of defense mechanisms on professional communications. Many individuals respond to anxiety-provoking situations by automatically relying on defense mechanisms. Because defense mechanisms are used consciously or [un]consciously to block an emotionally painful experience, it is [understa]ndable that patients facing a traumatic diagnosis or a dif[ficult treat]ment feel the need to protect themselves from the reality [of illness]. The problem is, how can we ensure compliance with [treatment if the] patient is in denial, projecting feelings onto the [family members o]r repressing the need for treatment or diagnostic [testing? The medic]al assistant must be sensitive to patients' use

of defense mechanisms and must consistently apply therapeutic communication techniques to interactions with patients.

DEFENSE MECHANISMS

Patients may use defense mechanisms to protect themselves from a situation or medical information that they cannot manage psychologically. Defense mechanisms may hide any of a variety of thoughts or feelings: anger, fear, sadness, despair, or helplessness. A patient who uses defense mechanisms can be very difficult to deal with; however, if the medical assistant is aware of the patient's need for psychological protection, he or she may be able to find a way to provide care for the patient while maintaining a therapeutic relationship. For example, Mrs. Alicia Simone, a 48-year-old patient, has just been told she has cancer of the breast. The following are defense mechanisms she might display to protect herself from the psychologic reality of her disease.

- *Denial:* The patient completely rejects the information.
  "I couldn't possibly have breast cancer. You must be mistaken."
- *Suppression:* The patient is consciously aware of the information or feeling but refuses to admit it.
  "I don't think the test is accurate. My mammograms are always normal."
- *Reaction formation:* The patient expresses her feelings as the opposite of what she really feels. For example, if she is angry at the medical assistant for insisting that a biopsy be scheduled, she may express the opposite emotion.
  "I appreciate your trying to help me, but I just can't come to the hospital that day."
- *Projection:* The patient accuses someone else of having the feelings that she has. For example, if the patient is angry about the diagnosis, she may say to the medical assistant, "You don't have to lose your temper about this," even though the medical assistant is acting completely professional.
- *Rationalization:* The patient comes up with various explanations to justify her response.
  "I think the results are wrong. I didn't follow the directions for the tests like I should have, and besides, there's no history of breast cancer in my family."
- *Undoing:* The patient tries to reverse a negative feeling by doing something that indicates the opposite feeling. For example, if the patient feels angry and violated about the diagnosis but she finds those feelings unacceptable, she may say, "Don't worry, dear, I'm not upset with you for telling me about this."
- *Regression:* The patient reverts to an old, usually immature behavior to ventilate her feelings. Perhaps instead of discussing the diagnosis and the need for treatment, she just storms out of the office. Or she may say, "I can't possibly schedule a procedure without discussing this with my mother."
- *Sublimation:* The patient redirects her negative feelings into a socially productive activity. For example, Mrs. Simone eventually becomes an active member of a local support group for women recovering from breast cancer.

CRITICAL THINKING APPLICATION   28-3

Mr. Gonzales, a 48-year-old patient recently diagnosed with hypertension, did not show up today for his follow-up appointment. Chris calls to find out why he failed to keep the appointment, and the patient tells Chris he forgot to come, even though an appointment reminder call was made yesterday. He also tells Chris he has not been taking his medicine and does not understand why it is so important for him and his wife to meet with the dietitian. Is this patient using defense mechanisms? How should Chris respond to the patient? What communications skills might be helpful to promote a therapeutic relationship?

Communication Across the Lifespan

The key to communicating effectively with patients is using an age-specific approach. Given the age and developmental level of your patient, how can you best interact with the person and with significant family members?

For example, Tasha, a 2-year-old patient, is scheduled for a physical examination. How can you best interact with her and her father to ensure that the history phase of the visit is complete and accurate? Therapeutic use of nonverbal language is essential to interacting with children of all ages. Getting down on the child's level, establishing eye contact, and using a gentle but firm voice are ways of gaining the child's confidence and cooperation. Children fear the unknown, so explaining all procedures with language the child understands is important. At the same time, the medical assistant must communicate with the child's caregiver so that he or she can contribute to the intake process (Figure 28-5). The following are some important guidelines for obtaining the health history of a child.

- Make sure the environment is safe and attractive.
- Do not keep children and their caregivers waiting any longer than necessary, because children become anxious and distracted quickly.
- Do not offer a choice unless the child can truly make one. If part of the treatment requires an injection, asking the child whether she'd like her shot now is most likely to get an automatic "No!" However, giving her a choice of stickers after the injection is appropriate.
- Praising the child during the examination helps reduce anxiety and increase self-esteem. When possible, direct questions to the child so that he or she feels like part of the process.
- Involving the child in the examination by permitting him or her to manipulate the equipment may help relieve anxiety. If possible, use your imagination and make a game of the assessment or the procedure.
- A typical defense mechanism seen in sick or anxious children is regression. The child may refuse to leave the mother's lap or may want to hold a favorite toy during the procedure as a comfort measure. Look for signs of anxiety, such as thumb-sucking or rocking during the assessment, and encourage caregivers to be involved in the process to help make the child feel as safe as possible.
- Listen to parents' concerns and respond truthfully to questions (Figure 28-6).

Older children may also have difficulty during the health visit (Figure 28-7). To help school-aged children gain a sense of control, give them the opportunity to make certain decisions about

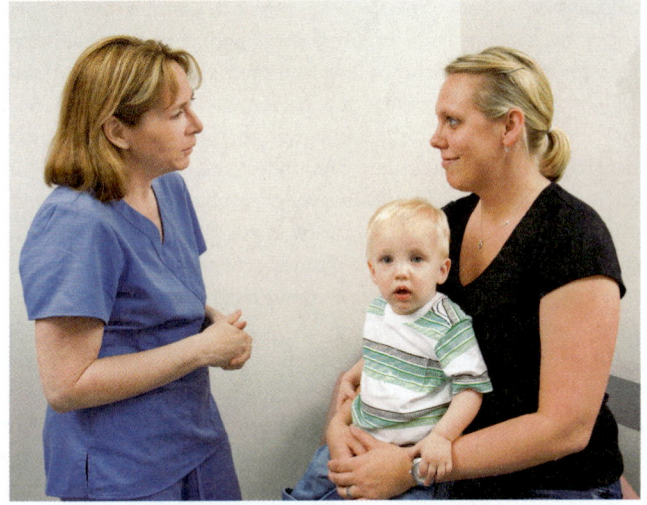

FIGURE 28-6 Responding to parental concerns.

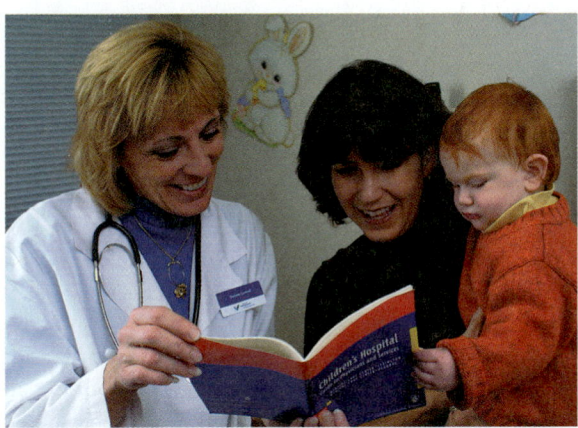

FIGURE 28-5 Interacting with a parent and child.

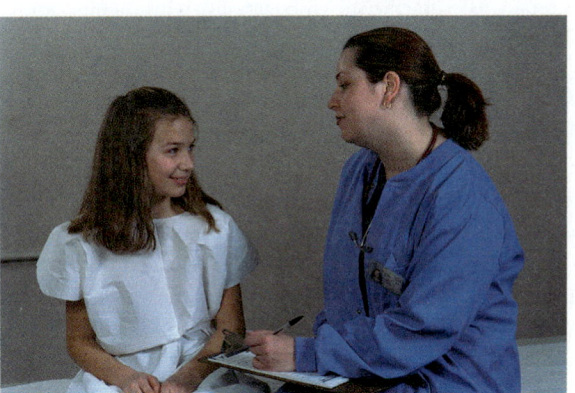

FIGURE 28-7 Interacting with a school-aged child.

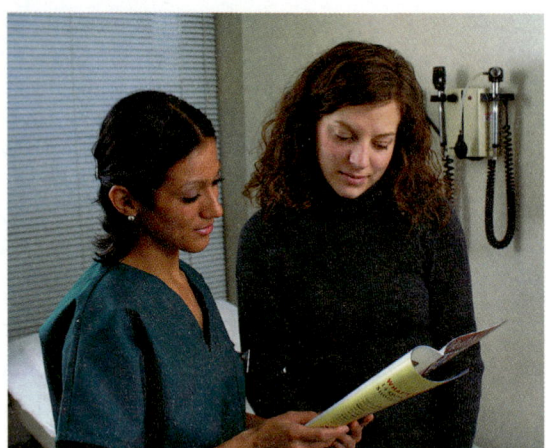

FIGURE 28-8 Interacting with an adolescent.

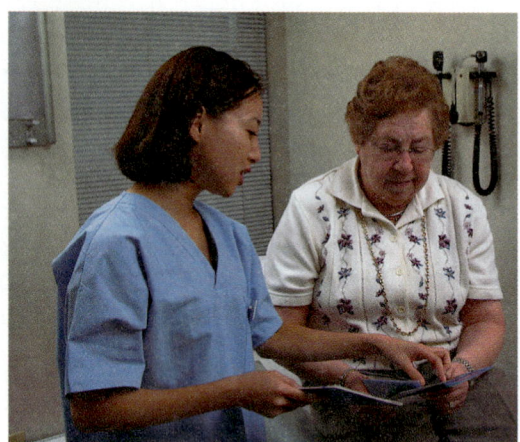

FIGURE 28-9 Adult patient education.

treatment. For example, Heather, a 13-year-old patient with diabetes, could be given the choice of having her father present during the visit. Or, if she requires an insulin injection, she could choose the site of the injection or perhaps administer the medication herself. This gives the medical assistant an opportunity to observe her technique and allows Heather to exert her independence.

Privacy is an important issue to consider with older children, especially adolescents. During the physical examination, respect privacy by keeping body exposure to a minimum and adequately preparing the child for procedures and positions. In addition, older children want to know what is going on during the examination, what to expect, and what the findings mean; therefore, keeping them informed in a language they can understand is important. Teen patients should always be encouraged to ask questions, which should be answered as completely and clearly as possible. Take every opportunity to teach your patients, regardless of their age, about their disease and to share information about significant wellness factors (Figure 28-8).

Patient education is extremely important when interacting with adult patients. Using language the adult patient understands and involving the patient in treatment decisions as much as possible are essential to developing a helping relationship with your older patients. Adults are bombarded by multiple responsibilities, which means that stress-related health problems are not unusual in these patients. Get to know your adult patients and emphasize preventive healthcare when possible (Figure 28-9). (Specific communication techniques for therapeutic interactions with aging adults are addressed in Chapter 48.)

Recognizing and Responding to Verbal and Nonverbal Communications

The medical assistant not only must implement therapeutic communication skills, but also must observe the patient to interpret the person's message and level of understanding. In the following critical thinking exercise, Chris, the medical assistant from the opening scenario, conducts a patient interview implementing the therapeutic communication skills discussed in this chapter, including active listening techniques, open and closed questions and statements, positive nonverbal interview skills, and effective observation of the patient's body language.

CRITICAL THINKING APPLICATION   28-4

Toby Anderson, a 48-year-old patient, was recently diagnosed with hypertension and prescribed Lotensin bid for treatment. He is being seen today for follow-up measurement of his blood pressure. Mr. Anderson is 45 pounds overweight and was given information about a reduced-calorie, low-sodium diet 1 month ago, but he has not lost any weight. He tells Chris that he has been having side effects from the medication. He is sitting with his arms across his chest, tapping his foot and occasionally cracking his knuckles.

Communication factors Chris should consider include the following:

- What nonverbal language is being used by Mr. Anderson and how should Chris interpret it?
- Mr. Anderson tells Chris he is not following that crazy diet and never will. What therapeutic communication skills can Chris use to get more information out of Mr. Anderson and to reinforce the physician's recommendations?
- During the discussion Mr. Anderson tells Chris he stopped taking the Lotensin because of the side effects. What communication techniques and therapeutic body language can Chris use to emphasize the need for Mr. Anderson to take his medicine as prescribed?

Document the patient interview using the CC method.

CC: _____

_____

_____

_____

ASSESSING THE PATIENT

After completion of the interview, the patient is escorted to an examination room and prepared for the physical examination, which is performed by the physician or a qualified healthcare professional, such as a physician assistant (PA) or nurse practitioner. During the examination, the healthcare provider methodically checks all the body's systems. As this examination proceeds, the provider mentally compares the system with established norms. If something deviates from the accepted normal range, it is documented in the patient's chart. The physical examination typically starts with the head and progresses downward to the feet. However, the order may vary, depending on the physician's specialty.

Signs and Symptoms

After completing the examination, the physician documents all the signs and symptoms gathered during the physical assessment process. To better understand the examination procedure, the medical assistant must know the difference between a sign and a symptom.

Subjective findings, or **symptoms**, are perceptible only to the patient; they are what the patient feels and can be interpreted only by the patient. For example, only the patient experiences and can define the quality of his or her discomfort, pain, nausea, or dizziness. Symptoms of the greatest significance in identifying a disease are called *cardinal symptoms*. For example, crushing chest pain and difficulty breathing are cardinal symptoms of a potential heart attack.

Objective findings, or **signs**, can be observed and/or measured by the physician or medical assistant. They are the indicators of health or disease that a physician detects when examining a patient. The physician feels, sees, hears, or measures the signs that often are associated with a certain disease or abnormal condition. For example, a mass that a physician palpates, or feels, in the patient's abdomen is an objective finding and a sign of an abnormal condition. In addition, objective data can be measured and recorded, and repeat measurements can be taken to confirm the presence of or changes in the sign. The patient's temperature, pulse, respirations, and blood pressure are objective signs the medical assistant measures and records regularly.

The medical assistant also needs to know the difference between a functional disorder and an organic (physical) disorder. When a condition or disease is *functional,* it is without an organic cause; that is, when inspected, the organ appears normal, without any evidence of disease, even though the patient's signs or symptoms indicate a problem. An example of a functional problem would be a patient who has repeated bouts of elevated urinary albumin, but all tests on the kidneys show normal, healthy organs. Or a patient is diagnosed with irritable bowel syndrome even though diagnostic studies have failed to show any evidence of intestinal disease. A functional disorder can be difficult for the patient to deal with, because even though the patient is suffering with certain health problems, all diagnostic tests fail to show that anything is wrong with the affected system.

An *organic* disease or condition is one in which the abnormality can be seen or felt or clinically proven through laboratory or other diagnostic tests. For example, an electrocardiogram (ECG) can confirm that a patient with chest pain is having a heart attack. A colonoscopy performed on a patient who complains of bloody stools can reveal evidence of ulcers in the colon.

ASSESSING PAIN

Pain is difficult to assess. We typically rely on the patient's report of symptoms to determine the individual's level of pain. Some questions you can ask to determine the patient's perception of pain include:

- Where is the pain located? Is it associated with any particular movement?
- Can you describe how it feels? Is it constant or intermittent? Does anything relieve the pain?
- When was the onset of the pain? Did something cause the pain to start?
- Are you taking any medication to relieve the pain? What is it and how often are you taking it? Is it effective? When was your last dose?
- Does pain affect your daily activities?
- On a scale of 1 to 10, with 10 being the highest level of pain, where would you rate your pain?

DOCUMENTATION

Various methods can be used for charting, depending on the healthcare provider's preference. However, certain charting procedures have been standardized to meet the legal requirements for maintaining medical records accurately and concisely. Complete, accurate documentation is one of the primary responsibilities of a medical assistant (Figure 28-10).

Professional Medical Offices
1722 E. North Avenue Suite 109
Aloha, HI 99751

Patient Name	Gastrin, Eleanor C.		DOB 8/15/62	Chart # 3361
	Last	First MI		Allergies Iodine

Date	Time	Progress Note
7/4/20XX	10 AM	C/O fever x 3 days. Productive cough. T-101, P-72,
		Error ~~R-6t~~ R-16 CI 7/4/XX C.Isaccson, CMA (AAMA)
7/4/20XX	10:20AM	Late entry
		Denies wheezing, SOB C.Isaccson, CMA (AAMA)

FIGURE 28-10 Documentation correction.

PHYSICIAN'S ASSESSMENT OF BODY SYSTEMS

Appearance
Body build, posture, and gait
Height and weight fluctuation
Nutritional status
Hygiene and grooming
Emotional state and mood

Head and Neck
Size, shape, and contour of head
Hair and scalp
Palpation of neck, thyroid, and trachea
Difficulty swallowing
Change in voice, hoarseness

Eyes
Visual acuity and field
Inspection of eyelids and eyeballs
Pupillary reaction and eye movement
Inspection of internal eye structures
Measurement of ocular pressure

Nose
Size, shape, and symmetry
Deviated septum, nasal congestion
Sense of smell

Ears
Hearing deficits
Inspection of size, symmetry, placement
Discharge, ringing in the ears, infection

Mouth and Throat
Inspection of gums, teeth, tongue, pharynx
Bad breath, changes in salivation
Sense of taste

Respiratory
Size and shape of chest
Breath sounds
Phlegm, cough, sneezing, wheezing
Coughing of blood, asthma, emphysema
Upper or lower respiratory tract infections

Cardiovascular
Shortness of breath, chest pain
Reflected pain in the jaw, arms, upper back
Heart murmur, palpitations, night sweats
Cold or bluish hands, leg cramps, varicose veins
Hypertension, valvular disease

Gastrointestinal
Symmetry, tenderness, pain
Changes in appetite, nausea, vomiting
Jaundice, ulcers, gallstones
Bowel sounds
Change in bowel habits: diarrhea, constipation, hemorrhoids, stool color

Urinary
Changes in urinary habits: hesitancy, urgency, frequency, night voiding, pain when voiding, loss of stream force
Kidney stones, urinary tract infections
Dribbling, incontinence
Indicators of infections

Genitalia (Male)
Infertility, sterility, impotence
Testicular pain or mass
Penile discharge or discomfort
Erections, hernias
Prostate or testicular enlargement

Genitalia (Female)
Menses regularity, flow, pain, duration
Premenstrual symptoms, menopause
Obstetric history, birth control method
Breast symmetry, discharge, masses
Estrogen therapy, reproductive surgeries
Pain during intercourse, sterility

Lymph Glands
Enlargement, tenderness

Neurologic
Level of consciousness, headaches
Reflex reactions, general weakness
Speech changes, memory loss, seizures
Changes in balance, lack of coordination

Endocrine
Weight change, fatigue, bulging eyes
Increased thirst or hunger, neck swelling
Excessive sweating, heat or cold intolerance

Skin
Color, turgor, and tone
Lesions or scars
Temperature, rashes, itching
Moles, sores, acne

Arms and Legs
General appearance and symmetry
Palpation of arm muscles
Range of motion, limitation of movement
Inspection of fingernails
Deformities, joint stiffness
Gait

Legs and Feet
Symmetry, scars, bruises, swelling, open areas
Broken bones, deformity, sprains, strains
Gout, arthritis, osteoporosis
Inspection of toenails

Correct Method of Charting

- Check the name on the record and make sure the information being charted is recorded on the correct form on the correct patient's chart. Confirm the patient's identity by checking his or her birth date.
- Do all charting in black ink; never use pencil.
- Write in a clear, legible manner.
- The month, day, and year must precede the entry; many facilities also require the time of the documentation.
- All unusual complaints, symptoms, or reactions must be noted in detail. Include complete information regarding the onset (when the problem started), duration (how long episodes last), and frequency (how often episodes occur) of each reported sign and symptom. *Example:* Pt reports night cough, which started 2 days ago, lasts approximately 10 minutes, and occurs 3-4 times per night.
- Describe objective data, such as the presence of a wound, using correct anatomic medical terminology. *Example:* Observed wound on left distal anterior tibia approximately 2 cm long and 1 cm wide.
- If the patient reports pain, record the quality and intensity of the pain using a pain scale of 1 to 10. *Example:* Pt c/o dull pain at wound site, a 4 on a scale of 1-10.
- If the patient's comments are entered in the patient's own words, enclose them in quotation marks. *Example:* Pt states, "I fell against a stone foundation while cutting the grass and slashed my leg."
- Document the complete medication history, including both prescription and over-the-counter (OTC) medications taken on a regular basis, the last dose taken of the medication, its effectiveness, and any other pertinent details. *Example:* Pt reports taking 2 ibuprofen tablets for pain with moderate relief; last dose taken 45 minutes ago.
- Record details about the previous history of the current chief complaint (CC). *Example:* Pt reports having a similar cough 3 weeks ago.
- When entering information in the medical record, sign the entry, including the appropriate initials after your name (e.g., CMA).
- Learn to be observant and to note anything that seems pertinent.
- Use accurate spelling, abbreviations, symbols, and terminology (Table 28-3).
- Review your documentation immediately after completion so that you can detect errors while the information is fresh in your mind.
- Do not leave any blank spaces on the record and do not skip lines between documentation entries.
- Never scribble, erase, or use whiteout on an error. For legal purposes, it is crucial that the corrected error be readable.
- Correct the error by drawing one line through it. Write "error" above the corrected word or words and date and initial the correction. Then write in the correction.
- If details are omitted, add information by documenting after the last entry. Record "late entry," include date and time of note, and document the omitted information (see Figure 28-10).

Medical Terminology

Medical terminology is a language system based on Latin. It addresses processes that occur in specific body systems, procedures, diagnostics, and diseases. The system depends on the use of a suffix, which

is defined first, a root word, and many times a prefix. The parts of the word are connected using a combining form "o" except in terms with a suffix that begins with a vowel. For example, osteitis is defined as inflammation (the suffix "-itis") of the bone (root word "oste"). The combining form "o" is not needed to connect the suffix and root word, because the suffix begins with an "i." In the term *osteopathic*, the suffix "-ic" means pertaining to, and the two root words "path" (disease condition of) and "oste" (bone) are connected with the combining form "o."

If a word is unfamiliar to you, it is important to learn the meaning, correct spelling, pronunciation, and proper use of the term. Consistent use of a good medical dictionary is essential. To aid your learning, some frequently used medical word parts and their definitions are presented in Table 28-4. In addition, a terminology glossary can be found in the back of this textbook, a vocabulary section appears at the beginning of each chapter, and an overview of understanding medical terms can be found on the Evolve Web site *(evolve.elsevier.com/kinn)*. Because the physician communicates using medical terminology and the medical assistant should use medical terms when documenting in the patient record, it is essential that you become comfortable and familiar with the medical language system and its correct use.

Charting Methods

Problem-Oriented Medical Record

The problem-oriented medical record (POMR) is a form of documentation that introduces a logical sequence to recording the information obtained from the patient. It is based on the scientific method and was designed to present the patient's health problem efficiently and record systematically how it was managed. The medical history and physical examination fit into a special format that clarifies the patient's health problems. Each patient problem, or diagnosis, is defined and documented on a problem list sheet at the beginning of the medical record. Each time the patient is diagnosed with a new health problem, that diagnosis is added to the problem list in numeric order. If the patient is successfully treated for the health problem and cured, the physician documents next to that diagnosis on the problem list "Problem resolved" and dates it accordingly. Because the patient's diagnoses are identified and numbered at the beginning of the medical record, the POMR is very helpful for record audits. In addition, the format is designed for and easily adapted to electronic health record (EHR) systems. The POMR system has four basic parts:

1. *Database:* This includes the patient's health history, the physical examination findings, and the results of baseline laboratory and diagnostic procedures. This information allows the physician to compile a health problem list for the patient.
2. *Problem list:* This list of the identified patient problems is kept in the front of the patient's chart. It serves as a table of contents or index for the record and defines the patient's health concerns, including diagnoses, treatments, and educational needs. The problem list takes a holistic approach by including both psychosocial and physical needs. Each problem entered is listed numerically and dated and is supported by the database. The problems then are identified and referred to throughout progress note documentation by their assigned number. If over time an additional problem is identified, it is added to the problem list. If the problem is resolved, the date

TABLE 28-3 Medical Abbreviations

ABBREVIATION	DEFINITION	ABBREVIATION	DEFINITION
ABD	abdomen	DM	diabetes mellitus
ABG	arterial blood gases	DNR	do not resuscitate
ac	before eating	DVT	deep vein thrombosis
ACLS	advanced cardiac life support	Dx	diagnosis
ad lib	as desired	ECG	electrocardiogram
AFP	alpha-fetoprotein	ENT	ears, nose, throat
AKA	above the knee amputation	FBS	fasting blood sugar
ASAP	as soon as possible	f/u	follow up
ASHD	atherosclerotic heart disease	FUO	fever of unknown origin
BE	barium enema	fx	fracture
bid	twice a day	GC	gonorrhea
BM	bowel movement	GI	gastrointestinal
BMR	basal metabolic rate	GTT	glucose tolerance test
BOM	bilateral otitis media	GU	genitourinary
BP	blood pressure	HCT	hematocrit
BUN	blood urea nitrogen	Hgb	hemoglobin
bx	biopsy	HIV	human immunodeficiency virus
$\bar{c}$	with	HPI	history of present illness
C&S	culture and sensitivity	HS	at bedtime or hour of sleep
CA	cancer	HTN	hypertension
CABG	coronary artery bypass graft	Hx	history
CAD	coronary artery disease	I&D	incision and drainage
CBC	complete blood count	I&O	intake and output
CC	chief complaint	IG	immunoglobulin
CHF	congestive heart failure	lytes	electrolytes
CHO	carbohydrate	MI	myocardial infarction
CNS	central nervous system	NG	nasogastric
c/o	complains of	NKA	no known allergies
COPD	chronic obstructive pulmonary disease	NPO	nothing by mouth
CPK	creatinine phosphokinase	N/V	nausea and vomiting
CPR	cardiopulmonary resuscitation	p	after
CSF	cerebrospinal fluid	PE	pulmonary embolism
CT	computed tomography	prn	as needed
CVA	cerebrovascular accident	pt	patient
CXR	chest x-ray	PE	physical examination
DAT	diet as tolerated	PT	physical therapy
dc	discontinue	q	every
D&C	dilation and curettage	RBC	red blood cells
DDx	differential diagnosis	R/O	rule out

TABLE 28-3 Medical Abbreviations—Cont'd

ABBREVIATION	DEFINITION	ABBREVIATION	DEFINITION
ROM	range of motion	Sx	symptoms
Rx	treatment	Tx	treatment
s̄	without	UA	urinalysis
SOB	shortness of breath	URI	upper respiratory infection
STD	sexually transmitted disease	UTI	urinary tract infection
stat	immediately	VS	vital signs

TABLE 28-4 Medical Word Parts

WORD PART	MEANING	WORD PART	MEANING	WORD PART	MEANING
a-	without	cephal/o	head	gest/o	pregnancy
-ac	pertaining to	-cide	killing	-globin	protein
aden/o	gland	-clast	to break	gloss/o	tongue
adip/o	fat	colp/o	vagina	gluc/o	glucose, sugar
-al	pertaining to	contra-	against	-gram	recording
-algesia	sensitivity to pain	crani/o	skull	hem/o	blood
-algia	pain	-crit	to separate	hemi-	half
angi/o	blood vessel	cyan/o	blue	hepat/o	liver
ankyl/o	stiff	cyst/o	urinary bladder	hist/o	tissue
ante-	before	cyt/o	cell	hydr/o	water
anter/o	front	-derma	skin	hyper-	above; excessive
anti-	against	dipl/o	double	hyp/o	deficient
arter/o	artery	dors/o	back	hyster/o	uterus
arthro	joint	-dynia	pain	-iasis	abnormal condition
articulo	joint	dys-	painful, abnormal	infra-	below
-ase	enzyme	-ectasia	dilation, stretching	inter-	between
ather/o	fatty plaque	-ectomy	excision	intra-	within
aur/o	ear	-emesis	vomiting	jaund/o	yellow
auto-	self	-emia	blood condition	kines/o	movement
axill/o	armpit	encephal/o	brain	lact/o	milk
bi-	two	endo-	within	-lapse	to sag
bi/o	life	enter/o	small intestine	later/o	side
-blast	immature	eosin/o	red	leuk/o	white
blephar/o	eyelid	epi-	above	lip/o	fat
brady-	slow	erythem/o	flushed; red	lith/o	stone
bucc/o	cheek	-esis	condition	-lithiasis	condition of stones
carcin/o	cancerous	eu-	good; normal	-logy	study of
cardi/o	heart	gastr/o	stomach	-lysis	to break down
-cele	hernia	-genesis	forming	macro-	large

Continued

TABLE 28-4 Medical Word Parts—Cont'd

WORD PART	MEANING	WORD PART	MEANING	WORD PART	MEANING
mal-	bad	-pepsia	digestion	-sclerosis	hardening
-malacia	softening	per-	through	-scope	instrument to visualize
mast/o	breast	peri-	surrounding	semi-	half
medi/o	middle	-pexy	fixation	somat/o	body
mega-	large	-phagia	eating	spl/o	spleen
-megaly	enlargement	-phasia	speech	-stasis	to stop
morph/o	shape	phleb/o	vein	-stenosis	tightening
my/o	muscle	-plasty	repair	stomat/o	mouth
necr/o	death	-plegia	paralysis	-stomy	new opening
neo-	new	-pnea	breathing	sub-	under
nephr/o	kidney	-poiesis	formation	supra-	above
neur/o	nerve	poly-	many	tachy-	fast
odyn/o	pain	post-	after	thorac/o	chest
olig/o	scanty	-prandial	meal	thromb/o	clot
-oma	tumor; mass	pre-	before	-tomy	cutting
onych/o	nail	proxim/o	near	tox/o	poison
oophor/o	ovary	prurit/o	itching	trans-	across; through
ophthalm/o	eye	pseudo/o	false	-tresia	opening
orch/o	testis	-ptosis	drooping; sagging	tri-	three
orth/o	straight	py/o	pus	-tripsy	to crush
oste/o	bone	pyel/o	renal pelvis	ur/o	urine
ot/o	ear	pyr/o	fever	varic/o	varicose veins
pan-	all	quadric-	four	vascul/o	vascular
para	near; beside	ren/o	kidney	ventr/o	front
path/o	disease	-rrhage	bursting forth	viscer/o	internal organs
-penia	deficiency	-rrhea	flow	vit/o	life

of problem resolution is entered next to the problem. For example, if Mrs. Xu is diagnosed with hypertension and that particular health problem is listed as diagnosis #3, every time Mrs. Xu comes to the office for follow-up of her blood pressure, the documentation piece begins by identifying the diagnosis by its number (#3). This system makes it very easy for the physician or medical assistant to scan the progress notes, review all documentation relating to diagnosis #3 (hypertension), and obtain a relatively quick and comprehensive history of how the patient's blood pressure is being managed and controlled.

3. *Plan:* This is a written plan for each problem identified on the problem list. It outlines further studies, treatments, and patient education (Figure 28-11).

4. *Progress notes:* Using the first letter of each part of the progress notes spells the acronym SOAP; therefore, this portion of the

POMR system is called the *SOAP notes* (or *SOAPE notes* when evaluation is included) (Figure 28-12). Each progress note uses the following format:

- **S** for *subjective* data: This information includes the purpose of the visit, with the patient's words in quotation marks, or a summary of the patient's statement about the chief complaint. For example, the subjective note may record exactly what the patient says, such as, "I feel horrible, exhausted, coughing all night long." If the patient's exact words are not documented in quotation marks, the subjective entry typically starts with "Patient states …," "Patient c/o …," or "Caregiver reports …" The medical assistant documents this information based on details gained from the patient interview.

- **O** for *objective* data: This is anything that is observed or measurable, including vital signs, the exact anatomic

PATIENT RECORD

Name Fiddteman, Fred D.

Number   Blood Type: A+

ALLERGIES/SENSITIVITY

Penicillin

Prob. No.	Date	PROBLEM DESCRIPTION	Date Resolved	Index	Prob. No.	Date	PROBLEM DESCRIPTION	Date Resolved	Index
1	10/2011	Hypertension - essential		✓					
2	10/2011	Diabetes mellitus (mild)		✓					
3	1/2011	Bilat. Grade II Retinopathy							
4	5/3/2012	L lower lobe pneumonia	5/2012						

Prob. No.	CONTINUING MEDICATIONS	Start	Stop	Prob. No.	CONTINUING MEDICATIONS	Start	Stop
1	Sinoserp 1 mg. b.i.d.	10/11	11/11				
2	Orinase 0.5 gm. daily	10/12	11/12				
1	Hydrodiuril 50 mg. A.M.	10/11					
2	1500 cal. diet low Na hi K	2/12					

Periodic Health Examination	Dates	1/10	3/11	3/11	6/12						

FIGURE 28-11 Initial plan for POMR progress notes.

location of an injury, difficulty with gait, and so on. Objective data can be measured repeatedly, which means that regardless of how many different healthcare workers observe the patient or document the sign, the same or very similar numbers or explanations would be given. The medical assistant is responsible for documenting complete and accurate objective data about all of the patient's signs. This information should be in such specific detail that even an individual who has not seen the patient can visualize the person's state of health. Typically the medical assistant charts only the subjective and objective data, leaving the remainder of the documentation to the physician.

* **A** for *assessment* of the problem: Usually this is the physician's preliminary diagnosis of the cause of the patient's chief complaint. The physician or healthcare provider makes a judgment about what is wrong with the patient and documents it in this section; the medical assistant is not involved in this piece.
* **P** for the *plan* of care: This is the physician's documentation of how the health problem will be managed,

including diagnostic studies, treatments, and patient education.

* **E** for *evaluation:* This is the assessment of the patient's understanding of the treatment or of the person's ability to comply with the treatment plan. It also may be used to document a follow-up on medication or treatments administered in the physician's office. For example, if a patient with asthma receives a breathing treatment during the office visit, a note is made regarding the effectiveness of the treatment.

CRITICAL THINKING APPLICATION   28-5

Document the following scenario using the POMR method:

The patient c/o a sore throat with pain of 5 on a 1-10 scale and fever for 2 days. He has been taking OTCs for relief of symptoms. His VS are T 100.4, P 88, R 20. He also has an erythemic, papular rash across his chest.

S: _____

O: _____

PROBLEM-ORIENTED PROGRESS NOTES			
Name Jessica Michaels		**DOB** 9/20/06	**Doctor** Frank Edwards, MD
DATE	**TIME**	**PROBLEM NUMBER**	**FORMAT:** Problem Number and TITLE: S = Subjective O = Objective A = Assessment P = Plan
10/15/12	9:30 AM	1	S: Mother states child has runny nose
			and sore throat x 2d. Taking Tylenol prn.
			O: Vital signs: T 98.8 (TA) P 96 R 24; Wt 42 lb.
			C. Isaccson, CMA (AAMA) _____
			A: Upper respiratory tract infection. _____
			P: 1. Prescribe Rondec DM, 1/2 tsp q6h prn
			cough and congestion. _____
			2. Mother to contact office if child does
			not improve. F. Edwards MD _____

FIGURE 28-12 Structured notes for the POMR system. (Courtesy Bibbero Systems, Petaluma, Calif.)

Source-Oriented Medical Record

The source-oriented medical record (SOMR) is the most common form of record keeping used by physicians practicing in medical offices. The data in the patient record are organized in divided sections, which include the History and Physical (H&P), Progress Notes, Laboratory Results, Consultations, and so on. All information is filed in reverse chronologic order, with the most recent report or progress note placed on top. Progress notes are made each time the patient is seen or contacted by telephone. Documentation in the Progress Notes section is based on details surrounding the patient's chief complaint or the treatment protocol. For example, if a patient is being seen today for the flu, the note may read, "CC flu-like symptoms, fever Xs 3 days, general discomfort, yellow nasal drainage, productive cough." The primary disadvantage of the SOMR system is that it can be very time-consuming to find a back entry about a particular problem or treatment.

Electronic Health Records

Many ambulatory care settings, especially multipractice facilities and health maintenance organizations (HMOs), use electronic systems to collect and file patient information and link offices. These EHR systems usually are designed for the particular needs of the practice. They are set up so that information is entered directly and downloaded into the patient's computerized file as the patient is interviewed or assessed. This is done using personal digital assistants (PDAs), laptop computers, or computer stations located throughout the facility (Figure 28-13).

Proponents of the EHR believe this type of record keeping reduces practice overhead and improves staff efficiency, cuts the cost of running the practice, and improves patient care. The EHR system can cut costs by reducing the physical resources needed to operate the practice (e.g., paper, chart material, copiers, and so on) and by drastically reducing the amount of space needed to store medical records. With the EHR, patients' charts are on computerized files

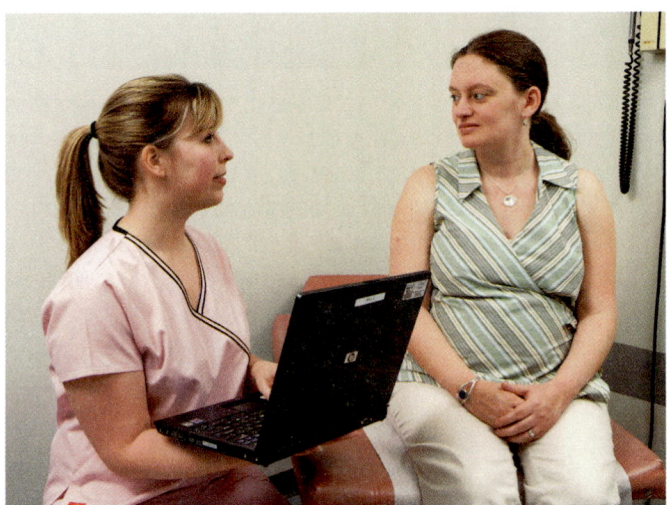

FIGURE 28-13 A medical assistant uses a laptop computer to conduct the patient interview.

and therefore are easily accessible, which saves time for the staff, and all documentation pieces are easily legible. In addition, the physician's office system can be linked to the hospital or laboratory so that diagnostic tests can be downloaded into a patient's file and be readily available for the physician to review and share with the patient.

The most significant problem with EHR systems is that if a major electrical or computer malfunction occurs, patient information cannot be accessed. Backup files must be maintained, and special attention must be paid to patient confidentiality to prevent accidental sharing of private information.

CLOSING COMMENTS

Patient Education

Finding time to conduct patient education in a busy healthcare practice can be challenging. Every opportunity to interact with patients should be considered a potential "teaching moment." The perfect time to begin the education process is during the initial patient interview, because this is when you first become aware of lifestyle factors or financial, social, or psychological problems that may negatively affect the patient's wellness. Your interactions with patients and implementation of therapeutic communications skills and interview techniques are crucial to the quality of care patients receive in your practice.

Legal and Ethical Issues

The medical history is a confidential record that can be shared only with healthcare personnel directly involved in the patient's care. Data provided to you by the patient or that you read in the patient's chart are confidential; you must not share any of this information with anyone. The consequences for disclosing private information to individuals not involved in the patient's care can be very serious and can result in the loss of your job, court-imposed fines, and even imprisonment.

In addition to maintaining patient confidentiality, consistently implementing correct documentation procedures is crucial for medical practices. The medical chart is considered a legal record, and court cases can be won or lost based on the clarity and completeness of staff documentation. It is absolutely essential that medical assistants document all patient information in a factual, nonjudgmental manner. Risk management practices focus on these problems as a way of reducing the chances of professional liability claims.

FACTORS THAT CONTRIBUTE TO SOUND RISK MANAGEMENT PRACTICES

- Periodic review or audit of patients' office records
- Consistent charting of accurate and complete clinical facts and test results
- Adequate office procedures for informing patients of test results and for documenting this communication
- Appropriate use of abbreviations and legible recording on the patient record; also, corrections made in the legally required manner
- Documentation that shows diagnostic test results were received, reviewed by the attending physician, and filed in a timely manner
- Documented evidence of appropriate discharge and continuing care instructions

Important Provisions of the Health Insurance Portability and Accountability Act

- The patient has the right to request that the physician's practice limit the disclosure of protected health information (PHI) for treatment, payment, and healthcare operations (TPO). For example, if the patient had an abortion 5 years ago, she may request that this information not be shared unless absolutely necessary.
- The facility is not required to comply with this request, but if agreement is reached, the restriction on sharing the information must be documented, and all employees must comply with the agreement. Therefore, if a physician referral includes sending the patient's chart to a consulting physician, the medical assistant must make sure the restricted information is not included in the material sent.
- The patient has the right to request that confidential information be sent in a manner that the patient decides is best. For example, some patients may request that all phone calls from the office be made to a work number rather than home, whereas others may give approval for messages to be left on the home answering machine or voice mail. Whatever the patient's preference, this information must be documented and followed each time the office attempts to contact the patient.
- The facility owns the patient record, but the patient owns the information included in the record. Patient confidentiality must be secured regardless of the type of documentation or record system used in the healthcare setting. Safeguards mandated by HIPAA include:
  - Using passwords to secure access to all electronic medical records (EMRs).
  - Using computer monitor shields to protect patient information if data are left on the screen.
  - Turning monitors away from patient traffic areas to prevent accidental release of information.
  - Securing all medical records; charts may not be left out in the office area nor placed on the back of examination doors.

SUMMARY OF SCENARIO

The office supervisor met with Chris and reviewed essential techniques for gathering patient information. Therapeutic communication includes demonstrating respectful patient care, using active listening skills, observing nonverbal behaviors, and using a combination of both open and closed questions to gather the best possible detail about the patient's chief complaint. The supervisor gave Chris a variety of information on meeting the needs of a diverse patient population and gave him suggestions on how to develop empathetic, helping relationships. One of the suggestions she made was that Chris develop a community resource file to which he can refer if a patient needs additional assistance outside the healthcare setting. Chris learned to identify the parts of the patient interview and became familiar with typical barriers to patient communication so that interviews would run more smoothly and he could gather more specific information from patients. Chris's workplace uses POMR documentation methods, so he reviewed the specifics of this type of record keeping with his supervisor. The significance of patient confidentiality was emphasized, and Chris agreed to work at implementing the techniques for therapeutic communication.

SUMMARY OF LEARNING OBJECTIVES

1. **Define, spell, and pronounce the terms listed in the vocabulary.**
    Spelling and pronouncing medical terms correctly bolster the medical assistant's credibility. Knowing the definition of these terms promotes confidence in communication with patients and co-workers.

2. **Apply critical thinking skills in performing patient assessment and care.**
    Completing the Critical Thinking Application exercises throughout the chapter can help the student medical assistant become more adept at critical analysis of real-life situations.

3. **Employ the concept of holistic care in the patient assessment process.**
    Holistic care involves assessing the patient's health status through the collection of physical, cognitive, psychosocial, and behavioral data. The medical assistant should consider all these factors when collecting data on the patient's health problems.

4. **Describe the components of the patient's medical history.**
    The medical history consists of the patient's database, past medical history, and family and social histories, in addition to the review of systems.

5. **Define and apply the qualities of a helping relationship.**
    Developing a professional helping relationship with patients is the responsibility of all healthcare workers. The helping relationship involves consistent application of respectful patient care that recognizes the impact of a patient's anxieties on interactions and responses to treatment.

6. **Display sensitivity to diverse patient populations.**
    Sensitivity to diverse populations includes the application of empathetic communications and an awareness of the impact of individual value systems and personal prejudices on patient interactions.

7. **Demonstrate therapeutic communications, including the use of the linear communication model and active listening techniques.**
    The linear communication model illustrates communication as an interactive process between the sender and the receiver of the message, with feedback as a crucial part of the process. Active listening techniques, which include restatement, reflection, and clarification, help the medical assistant go beyond hearing the message to actually listening and appropriately responding to the patient's main point.

8. **Recognize the importance of nonverbal communication when interacting with patients.**
    Approximately 90% of patient interactions occur through nonverbal language. The key to successful patient interaction is congruence between verbal and nonverbal messages.

9. **Identify barriers to communication and their impact on patient assessment.**
    Certain communication styles can be misleading or can restrict the patient's response. The medical assistant must be careful to avoid using such faulty techniques as inappropriately providing reassurance, giving advice, using medical terminology without clarification, asking leading questions, and talking too much. These behaviors interfere with the process of gathering complete data during the interview and are obstacles to developing rapport with the patient.

10. **Detect a patient's use of defense mechanisms and the resultant barriers to therapeutic communication.**
    Patients use defense mechanisms to protect themselves in emotionally challenging situations. A medical assistant must consistently apply nonjudgmental therapeutic communication skills to maintain professional relationships.

11. **Use therapeutic communication techniques with patients across the lifespan.**
    Therapeutic communication techniques vary according to the age and developmental level of the patient. A medical assistant should be aware of how to interact most effectively with various age groups, including young children, adolescents, adults, elderly patients, and family members. Age-specific application of interview styles enables clear communication between the health professional and the patient.

12. **Demonstrate professional patient interviewing techniques.**
    The patient interview is divided into the introduction, the body, and the summary, or closing. Throughout the interview, the medical assistant should use professional interviewing techniques, such as empathetic patient care, sensitivity to patient diversity, active listening skills, appropriate nonverbal communication, attention to the interview environment, avoidance of communication barriers, and the framing of questions and statements in an open or closed manner, depending

on the information needed and the patient's communication behaviors.

13. **Integrate detailed information about the chief complaint into concise, accurate documentation methods.**

   The ability to document accurately and completely is an essential skill for all medical assistants. Documentation should describe the patient's chief complaint, identify all pertinent signs and symptoms, and demonstrate correct use of medical terminology, with appropriate abbreviations. Any error in the medical record must be corrected according to legally approved methods.

14. **Differentiate among various medical records systems employed in the physician's office.**

   Three main forms of medical records systems are (1) the POMR method, which uses SOAPE charting to define the patient's health problems; (2) the SOMR method, the most frequently used form of medical record keeping, which organizes patient data into specific sections; and (3) the EMR system, which compiles computer records for patient data.

15. **Describe the connection between the interview process and implementation of patient education practices.**

   The perfect time to initiate patient education is during the initial patient interview. A medical assistant should take advantage of every "teaching moment" to get to know his or her patients and promote patient wellness.

16. **Determine risk management strategies for the ambulatory care setting.**

   Risk management practices focus on reducing the chances of professional liability claims and maintaining compliance with HIPAA standards. Accurate, complete documentation in the patient's medical record is crucial for successful risk management. In addition, maintaining strict confidentiality of patient information and factual, nonjudgmental, legible recording of patient data are essential to professional patient care.

17. **Use reflection, restatement, and clarification techniques to obtain a patient history.**

   Refer to Procedure 28-1.

CONNECTIONS

📖 **Study Guide Connection:** Go to the Chapter 28 Study Guide. Read and complete the activities.

📧 **Evolve Connection:** Go to the Chapter 28 link at *evolve.elsevier.com/kinn* to complete the Chapter Review and Chapter Quiz. Check out the other resources listed for this chapter to make the most of what you have learned from Patient Assessment.

29

PATIENT EDUCATION

SCENARIO

Taylor DiSalvo is a medical assistant in a busy family practice office. He currently is working with one of the patients, Sam Ignatio, who is 62 years old and has been married for 30 years. Mr. Ignatio has just been diagnosed with type 2 diabetes mellitus. Mr. Ignatio knows nothing about his disease or how to manage it; he has never seen a glucometer and never handled needles. In addition, his diet is high in fats and carbohydrates, and he does not exercise regularly. Mr. Ignatio is 50 pounds overweight, has functional deafness in his left ear and decreased sound quality in his right ear, and shows early signs of diabetic-related vision loss. Taylor is responsible for assisting with Mr. Ignatio's patient teaching plan.

Mr. Ignatio is faced with a serious illness, and his future health depends on compliance with a wide range of lifestyle changes. The methods Taylor chooses to teach this patient about his disease can have a significant impact on his eventual health outcome.

While studying this chapter, think about the following questions:

- How should Taylor begin Mr. Ignatio's patient education?
- What are some of Mr. Ignatio's individual characteristics that may affect his ability to learn all the information required to manage his disease?
- How can Taylor make sure Mr. Ignatio understands the importance of following treatment and disease-monitoring guidelines?
- What teaching approaches and materials would best meet the needs of this patient?
- Are any community resources available that could help Mr. Ignatio learn how to manage his disease?

LEARNING OBJECTIVES

1. Apply critical thinking skills in performing the patient assessment and patient care.
2. Recognize the implications of health and illness models for patient education.
3. Instruct patients according to their needs to promote health maintenance and disease prevention.
4. Define six patient factors that have an impact on learning.
5. List at least five guidelines for patient education that can affect the patient's overall wellness.
6. Demonstrate empathy in communicating with patients, family members, and staff.
7. Display respect for individual diversity.
8. Summarize educational approaches for patients with language barriers.
9. Determine potential barriers to patient learning.
10. Develop and maintain a current list of community resources related to patients' healthcare needs.
11. Implement a variety of teaching methods and strategies responsive to the individual patient's needs.
12. Demonstrate the ability to develop an appropriate and effective patient teaching plan.
13. Demonstrate recognition of the patient's level of understanding in communications.
14. Document patient education.
15. Describe the role of the medical assistant in patient education.
16. Integrate the legal and ethical elements of patient teaching into the ambulatory care setting.

This chapter focuses on helping students recognize the individual learning needs of patients, and it also provides guidelines for developing effective teaching approaches. The key to patient compliance with prescribed treatments is empowerment; that is, providing the patient with information and support that enable the person to take charge of his or her health problem. The concepts in this chapter are basic to all patient education interventions, and a medical assistant who follows them can positively affect a patient's understanding of the disease process and the person's willingness to comply with the disease management steps recommended by the physician.

PATIENT EDUCATION AND MODELS OF HEALTH AND ILLNESS

Patient education should begin with the first contact between the patient and the healthcare team. A well-informed patient is more likely to comply with treatment and adopt a healthy lifestyle. However, informing a patient about his or her disease is only part of the health teaching process. The key to successful health teaching is to empower the patient to accept the responsibility of his or her disease process and to become willing to implement teaching guidelines.

As a result of reductions in hospital admissions and shorter hospital stays, patients and families have had to assume responsibility for care that once was provided by the hospital staff. This means that those who work in ambulatory care settings have an even greater responsibility to meet the educational needs of their patients. To develop an effective teaching approach, we must implement a holistic model that considers not only the patient's physical state, but also his or her psychological, social, and spiritual needs (Figure 29-1). The holistic model suggests that we look at patients and determine their needs based on a complete view of their lives rather than just as an analysis of their specific diseases. It is our responsibility not only to teach patients about disease processes, but also to help them implement related skills and changes in lifestyle to promote recovery and improve function. In the case of Mr. Ignatio, diabetes mellitus is a complicated disease that requires an in-depth understanding of the disease process and significant lifestyle changes. When considering the impact of this diagnosis on the patient (in this case, Mr. Ignatio), the medical assistant should keep in mind the following factors, because they will affect the patient's response.

- *Emotional effect of the disease:* Is Mr. Ignatio in shock and denial? Is he angry or depressed? How will his emotional reaction to the diagnosis affect his response to patient education efforts?
- *Social impact:* How will his family and employer respond to the demands of the diagnosis? Does he have a support system that will assist him in making healthy lifestyle choices?
- *Intellectual impact:* Is Mr. Ignatio able to understand the complexities of the disease and treatment recommendations?
- *Economic impact:* Can he afford the treatment for diabetes? Does he have health insurance to cover the cost or will he need

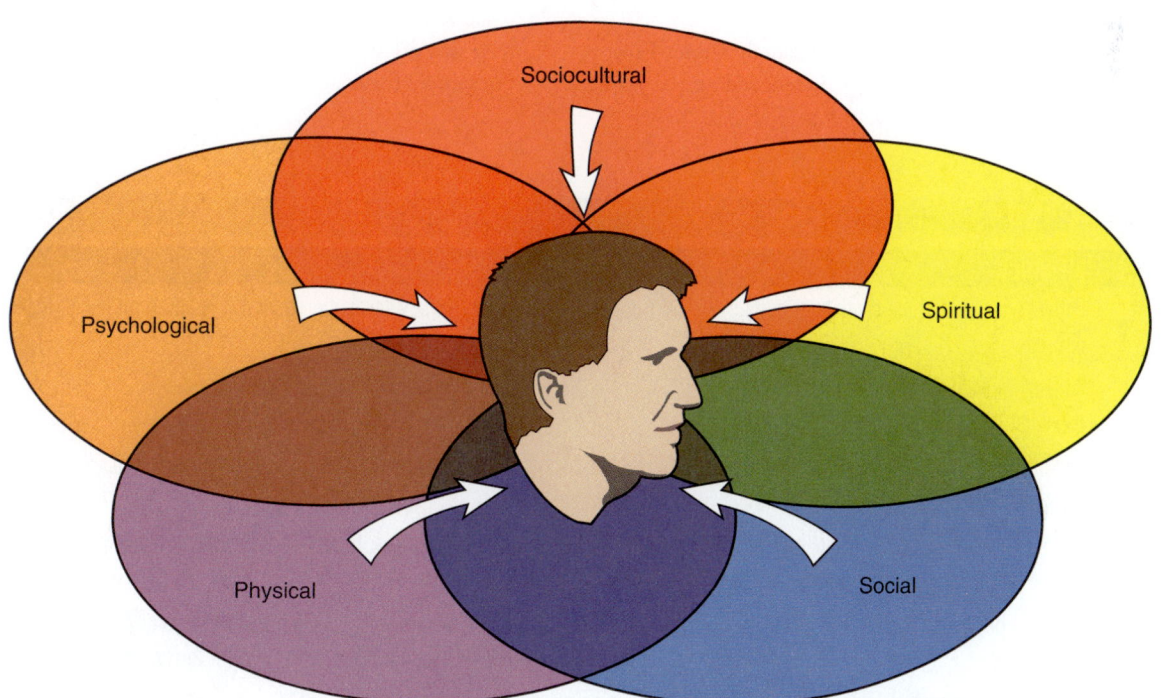

FIGURE 29-1 The holistic approach. (Modified from Sorrentino SA, Gorek B: *Mosby's essentials for nursing assistants,* ed 4, St Louis, 2010, Mosby.)

assistance in paying for ongoing diagnostic and treatment recommendations?

- *Spiritual impact:* What is Mr. Ignatio's spiritual response to his diagnosis?

The health belief model may help the medical assistant understand why some people do not follow recommended guidelines to maintain their health and prevent the development of disease.

This model focuses on individuals' attitudes toward and beliefs about themselves and their health. The model suggests that we first consider how the patient perceives his or her risk of developing a disease and the potential severity of the condition. For example, even though Mr. Ignatio's mother and sister developed type 2 diabetes in their sixties, he may believe he is not going to have the same problem. Therefore, even though wellness information encouraged him to lose weight, exercise, and eat a healthy diet, he didn't believe he was in danger of developing diabetes, so he didn't believe he needed to follow these disease prevention recommendations. He may also believe that even if he does develop diabetes, the consequences of the disease are not that serious, so why bother altering his lifestyle to prevent it?

Another factor considered in the health belief model is the patient's perceived benefits of action; that is, whether the patient believes altering health behaviors will prevent him from developing the disease. In this case, because Mr. Ignatio has a strong family history of the disease, he may have decided he was going to get diabetes anyway, so why should he bother exercising and watching his diet? He may have believed he was going to develop diabetes no matter what he did, so why bother trying to prevent it? Until the patient believes that teaching and health promotion guidelines affect him and are worth pursuing, he will not follow suggested health promotion tips or comply with treatment protocols.

Table 29-1 outlines the health belief model and presents suggested methods for applying the model in patient teaching efforts in the ambulatory care setting.

The five stages of grief, as defined by Dr. Elisabeth Kübler-Ross, are another model that may be helpful for understanding the way patients respond to health threats. When a patient faces a serious health threat, the grief process may delay the patient in adjusting to the disease and starting to take control of his or her health. For example, Mr. Ignatio may respond to the news of his diagnosis with what is commonly the first stage of the grief process—denial. Perhaps both his mother and sister suffered serious complications from diabetes, including blindness and leg amputation, and he may be using denial to deal psychologically with the burden of the diagnosis. Each individual goes through the stages of grief in his or her own way and at his or her own pace. This process can take weeks to months; however, until the patient reaches the point of accepting the diagnosis and the possible ramifications of the disease, compliance with patient education will be very difficult to achieve.

The five stages of grief are:

- *Denial and isolation.* The patient denies the existence of the disease, may be unwilling to accept the reality of the situation, and refuses to discuss the health problem or remember health teaching interventions. For example, Mr. Ignatio refuses to meet with the dietitian because he says his diet is fine and there is no need to change it.
- *Anger.* The patient may be very angry and hostile when forced to discuss the condition. Mr. Ignatio may say, "Why did this happen to me? I am a good person, why did I get diabetes?"
- *Bargaining.* The patient tries to bargain for privileges or time. Mr. Ignatio may say, "Look, I know I am supposed to start this new diet, but Christmas is coming, and I'll meet with the dietitian after the holidays."
- *Depression.* The patient grieves the loss of health. Mr. Ignatio may be very sad about the diagnosis. He doesn't want to have to deal with the complexities of the disease, he just wants it to go away so he can live his life without the fear of diabetic complications.
- *Acceptance.* The patient finally gets to the point where he or she accepts the diagnosis and is ready to make the best of it. At this point, Mr. Ignatio may be willing to use community resources for education and support.

TABLE 29-1 The Health Belief Model		
PRINCIPLES	**DEFINITION**	**PATIENT EDUCATION USE**
Perceived susceptibility	Patient's opinion on the chances of getting a disorder.	Supply information on the risk level; individual risk is based on health habits and family history.
Perceived severity	Patient's opinion on the seriousness of the condition and its health risks.	Outline the potential complications of the disease.
Perceived benefits	Patient's belief in the value of altering lifestyle factors and complying with treatment.	Emphasize the positive results that can occur if the patient complies with healthcare recommendations.
Perceived barriers	Patient's opinion on the financial and psychological costs of compliance.	Identify patient barriers and work to reduce them through patient education, family outreach, and use of community resources.
Cues to action	Methods developed to activate patient compliance.	One-on-one education interventions; detailed handouts; family involvement in education efforts; follow-up at subsequent office visits; referral to community resources.
Self-efficacy	Patient has the confidence to take action to achieve a healthier state.	Ongoing education and support.

SUGGESTIONS FOR THERAPEUTIC INTERACTIONS FOR PATIENTS IN GRIEF

- *Denial and isolation:* Reinforce each education intervention with handouts that explain the disease and treatment. Encourage the patient's family to attend visits to the physician's office and to become involved in the patient's care.
- *Anger:* Use therapeutic communication techniques, especially reflection, to acknowledge the patient's feelings about the diagnosis. Recognize the patient's need to use defense mechanisms as protection from the reality of the disease. Remember, the patient is not angry at you or the physician; he or she is angry about the diagnosis and its accompanying challenges.
- *Bargaining:* Rely on the physician's recommendations regarding postponing certain treatments. Discuss the patient's bargaining requests with the physician and other staff members to work out a solution that promotes patient compliance with healthcare recommendations.
- *Depression:* Use available community resources to provide support for the patient and family. The physician may recommend that the patient attend a support group, meet with a dietitian, or use professional counseling services to deal with depression.
- *Acceptance:* Take advantage of this time to renew education efforts by providing multiple methods for learning about the disease, such as CDs, DVDs, professional Web sites, and community support services.

Patient Factors that Affect Learning

Many factors or characteristics may affect the patient's ability to learn. Medical assistants must be aware of these factors to develop a patient education approach that best meets the needs of each patient.

GUIDELINES FOR PATIENT EDUCATION

- Provide knowledge and skills to promote recovery and health.
- Encourage patient ownership and participation in the teaching process.
- Include the family and significant others in education interventions, with the patient's approval.
- Promote safe, appropriate use of medications and treatments.
- Encourage patient adaptation to healthy behaviors,
- Provide information about accessing community resources.

Perception of Disease Versus Actual State of Disease

Patients respond to a particular diagnosis in many different ways. One predictor of how a patient will respond, and therefore how he or she will react to health education, is the patient's perception of the disease. Previous life experiences may greatly influence the patient's knowledge base and/or desire to learn about the disease. Does the patient recognize and accept the seriousness of the diagnosis? Or, perhaps, does the patient overreact to potential disease risks? Both of these responses affect the patient's willingness to learn about the disease and his or her compliance with treatment recommendations.

How do you think Taylor's patient education efforts will be affected if Mr. Ignatio does not consider diabetes a serious disease?

Patient's Need for Information

The patient's perception of the impact of the disease on his or her general health also determines the need for information about the disease. Does the patient express a desire to learn all he or she can about the disease, or does the patient resist or act indifferent to teaching efforts? A vital part of patient education is encouraging patient ownership of the learning process. To accomplish this, you first may have to persuade the patient that he or she needs to understand the disease before an improvement in overall wellness can be achieved.

Mr. Ignatio tells Taylor that his father was a diabetic and had to have both legs amputated because of the disease. Mr. Ignatio says that it doesn't matter whether he controls his blood sugar; he will still have major health complications. What is the appropriate response?

Patient's Age and Developmental Level

Depending on the patient's age and ability to understand information about the disease, you may have to adapt the teaching plan to meet specific learning needs. For example, educating a 9-year-old patient with type 1 diabetes about disease management requires a different approach from the one used for Mr. Ignatio. The medical assistant should be flexible and creative in providing learning opportunities that support the physician's attempt to educate the patient about disease prevention and health maintenance. Often the key to patient understanding and compliance is the involvement of family members.

During his assessment of Mr. Ignatio's diet, Taylor learns that his wife cooks all his meals and packs his lunch daily. What should Taylor do to make sure Mr. Ignatio's diet complies with diabetic recommendations?

Patient's Mental and Emotional State

Even a well-planned teaching intervention can be ineffective if the patient is unable to pay attention because of anxiety, stress, anger, or denial (Figure 29-2). Frequently patients use defense mechanisms to protect themselves from the reality of a serious illness. It is important that the medical assistant be sensitive to the patient's mental state and adapt teaching interventions as needed.

Mr. Ignatio has just been told about his disease. He already shared that his father died of diabetes. Do you think he is able to pay attention to patient teaching about how to give his insulin injections? What should Taylor do to manage this problem?

Influence of Multicultural and Diversity Factors on Patient Education

Culture, family background, and religious beliefs influence patients' actions. Working with patients from diverse backgrounds is an exciting challenge; however, for patient education to be successful, it is essential that the medical assistant be aware of and sensitive to the impact of these factors on patient learning (Figure 29-3). Some questions you should consider when teaching a patient from another background include:

- Is language an issue with your patient (Figure 29-4)? If the patient is unable to understand spoken English or to read it

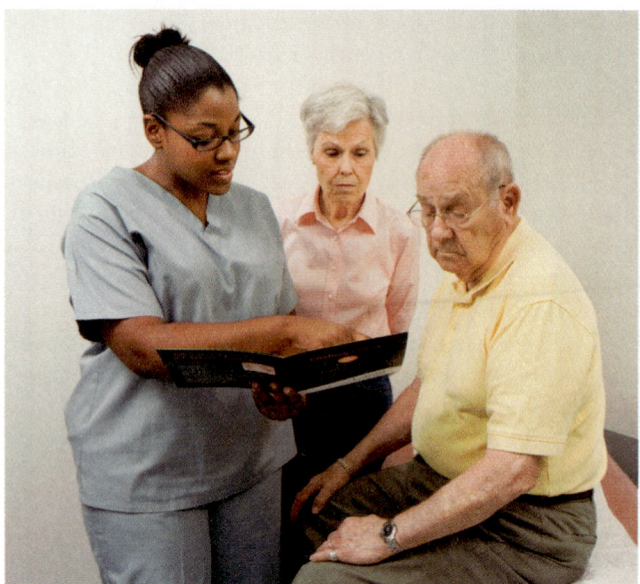

FIGURE 29-2 Demonstrating sensitivity to the patient's needs.

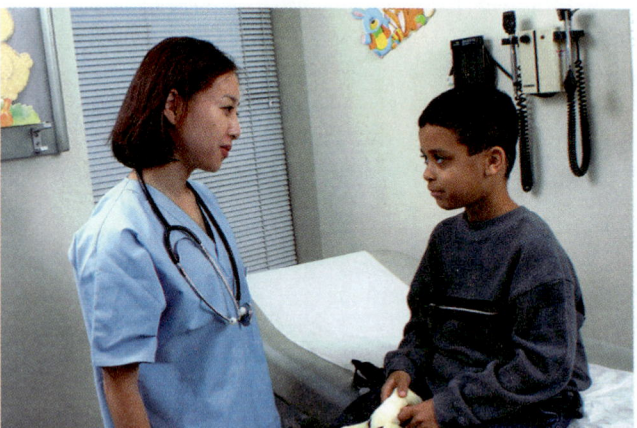

FIGURE 29-3 Considering diversity.

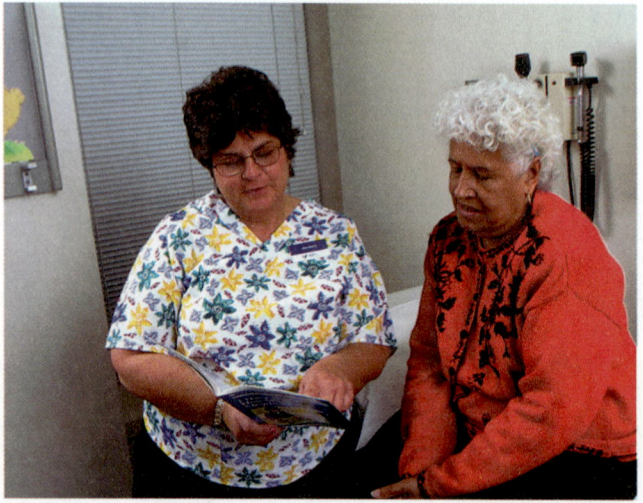

FIGURE 29-4 Managing language barriers.

correctly, do you have an alternative method for getting the information across?

- Do the patient's culture, ethnic background, or religious beliefs influence the way he or she perceives disease and the role of healthcare workers?
- What strategies or techniques might minimize patient education problems?
- Are community resources available that could facilitate patient learning?

APPROACHES FOR LANGUAGE BARRIERS

- Address the patient by his or her last name (e.g., Mrs. Martinez, Mr. Nugyen).
- Be courteous and use a formal approach to communication.
- Use gestures, tone of voice, facial expressions, and eye contact to emphasize appropriate parts of the discussion.
- Integrate pictures, handouts, models, and other aids that visually depict the material.
- Monitor the patient's body language, especially facial expression, for understanding or confusion.
- Use simple, everyday words as much as possible.
- Demonstrate all procedures and have the patient return the demonstration to check for understanding.
- Implement the teaching plan in small, manageable steps.
- Give the patient written instructions for all procedures and treatments.
- Use an interpreter when appropriate, if available.

Patient Learning Style

Chapter 1 presented information on individual learning styles that affect you as a student. These same factors have an impact on your patient's learning preference. Some patients learn best from discussion or lecture, whereas others must think or reflect about the material before understanding it. Some patients can learn from observing; others must act or do something with the material to learn it. Start your teaching intervention by asking your patient how he or she prefers to learn new material and pattern your teaching interventions along those lines.

Mr. Ignatio tells Taylor that he could never learn things by listening to someone tell him what to do. What approach to learning might best meet his needs?

Impact of Physical Disabilities

The patient first must be assessed to determine whether he or she can adequately hear instructions, see written material, and manipulate any required treatment equipment. All teaching efforts are lost if disabilities interfere with a patient's capacity to understand information or to handle equipment properly. A hearing or speech impairment may require the use of sign language with supplemental written instructions. If the patient is unable to manipulate equipment because of a physical disability or vision problem, family or community resources may be necessary for the patient to manage his or her care.

Mr. Ignatio's physical assessment revealed hearing and vision problems. Is he able to understand verbal instructions clearly? Will he be able to draw up the correct amount of insulin? What can be done to adapt the teaching intervention to meet his needs?

THERAPEUTIC COMMUNICATION WITH PATIENTS WITH SPECIAL NEEDS

Patients with Vision Loss

- Alert the patient that you are in the room and identify yourself; do not touch the patient without warning.
- The patient is unable to pick up your body language; use clear, concise language and a normal tone of voice.
- Provide all written material in a large font or print size; large-print educational materials often can be ordered.

Patients with Hearing Loss

- Stand in front of the patient or within the person's field of vision before you begin speaking; the patient may be able to lip-read.
- You may need to touch the patient lightly to get her or his attention.
- Use expanded speech; lower the tone of your voice and pronounce each syllable.
- Carefully observe the patient's body language for understanding or confusion.
- Use gestures or demonstration as needed to get the message across.
- Clearly print any information needed to clarify the patient teaching.
- If a patient is wearing a hearing aid, ask the person whether it is on and working before starting the conversation; the patient may turn a hearing aid off to prevent annoying background noise.
- Provide written handouts that review the material being taught.
- Request family assistance in verifying that the patient received and understood the material.

Patients with Language Barriers

- Determine whether the patient can read and/or understand English.
- If possible, have an interpreter present; if an interpreter is not available, a family member may be able to help with communication.
- If available, use a dictionary that translates as many words as possible for the patient.
- Use gestures or demonstration to get the message across.
- Carefully observe the patient's body language to determine the level of understanding.
- If available, order educational materials in the patient's native language; send materials home in English if a family member can interpret the material for the patient.

CRITICAL THINKING APPLICATION   29-1

Implement the holistic education model and the health belief model to determine and respond to Mr. Ignatio's individual learning needs.

THE TEACHING PLAN

What is it that patients need to know to manage a disease effectively? What is it about an individual patient that needs to be addressed for a teaching intervention to work? What are the immediate and long-term goals of patient education? What teaching materials or strategies should be used to meet the patient's learning needs and also effectively relay the information? How can the teaching plan be implemented successfully? How does the medical assistant manage the limited time available for patient teaching? How do you know the patient is learning and actually implementing this knowledge into disease management? A vital aspect of patient teaching is to be flexible and to provide information about what patients want to know when patients want to know it. These and other guidelines for developing an appropriate and effective teaching plan follow.

Assess the Patient's Learning Needs

Developing a teaching plan that works for a particular individual first requires an assessment of the patient as a learner and consideration of any characteristics that might affect the learning process. Many of these factors already have been addressed, such as the patient's learning preference, perception of the illness, age, background, multicultural influences, language barriers, and disabilities. The medical assistant also must consider what the patient already knows about the diagnosis and whether that knowledge includes misconceptions about the disease.

The goal of the assessment process is to create a teaching plan that meets the patient's needs for understanding and managing his or her illness. Therefore, in the learning assessment, the medical assistant should consider what the patient needs to know, what the patient wants to know, and what can be done in the time available for learning.

Before developing a specific approach to patient education, the medical assistant must consider potential barriers to learning other than those already presented, such as the presence of pain. A patient in acute distress is unable to concentrate on the information. In this case, the amount of material must be adjusted to meet the patient's immediate needs, and time should be planned in the future for a more in-depth teaching session.

Does Mr. Ignatio exhibit any potential barriers to learning about his disease?

POTENTIAL BARRIERS TO PATIENT LEARNING

- Individual learning style
- Age and developmental level
- Use of defense mechanisms
- Language
- Motivation to learn
- Physical limitations or disabilities
- Emotional or mental state
- Cultural or ethnic background
- Pain
- Time limitations

Determine the Teaching Priorities

Once you have done an adequate assessment of your patient as a learner and you understand your patient's learning needs, the next question is, "Where do I start?" A patient such as Mr. Ignatio has a significant amount of information to learn before he can manage his disease completely. The volume of information might seem overwhelming unless priorities are established. How do you figure out what material should be first? The first question to ask is, "What are the patient's immediate versus long-term needs?" What must this patient learn today to be able to take care of himself, and what does he need to know overall about his illness to promote healthy behaviors?

Because the patient learning assessment told you what your patient knows about his or her disease, that is a good place to start. Confirm what the patient knows about the problem and attempt to correct any potential misconceptions. If you start with something the patient knows and understands, he or she will feel more competent and capable of managing new material. You then should go on to the new material that is causing the patient the most anxiety. If the patient is nervous or afraid about a particular aspect, he or she will be unable to pay attention to any other new material until that anxiety has been addressed.

For example, if Mr. Ignatio is most concerned about giving himself injections, that is the first skill he should learn. Once he is confident about that particular part of treatment, he will be able to pay attention to diet and exercise recommendations. You should always begin with the basic details about the disease and add more information during each patient visit.

Every interaction with the patient is an opportunity for health education. A major problem with delivering high-quality patient education in an ambulatory healthcare setting is the lack of time you have to spend with each patient. Therefore, medical assistants must take advantage of every "teaching moment"; that is, every time you interact with a patient, use it as an opportunity to assess the patient's current education needs and provide as much information or guidance about that specific learning need as possible during the time available.

Use the waiting room as a place for learning by providing up-to-date educational materials on a wide variety of health issues. Many offices have DVD equipment in the waiting room for patient education while the patient is waiting to be seen. These can be specific to the type of physician practice or can provide general health information.

Decide on the Appropriate Teaching Materials

What teaching materials would best meet the needs of your patient? A wide variety of patient education materials is available, and deciding which materials best meet your patient's needs depends on the patient's learning preference, individual characteristics, and lifestyle factors. Individualized instruction is the key to understanding and patient compliance; however, additional materials can help reinforce the information.

When possible, all patient instruction should include a handout or some type of printed material that reinforces information and that the patient can use as a resource. Patient factors such as the use of defense mechanisms, emotional state, and language barriers can limit

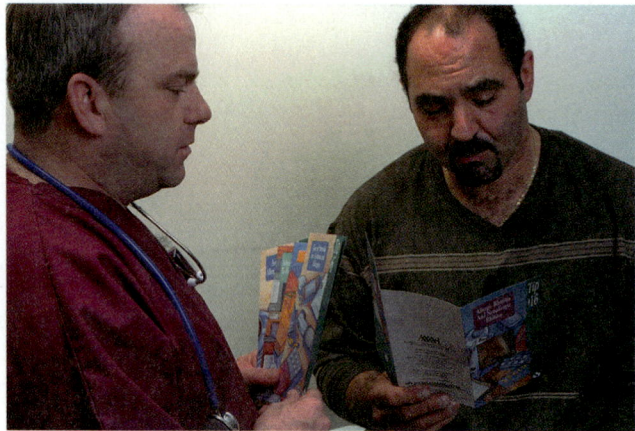

FIGURE 29-5 Reviewing printed information.

the patient's ability to comprehend and remember information. Printed information is needed to help the patient and the patient's family understand what is happening and what needs to be done to improve the patient's health (Figure 29-5). Informational flyers can be ordered from medical office suppliers, pharmaceutical company representatives, and health education companies. Many hospitals also offer free educational materials about diagnostic procedures, immunizations, and other disease-related topics. The ambulatory care setting where you are employed may develop its own educational materials. Some guidelines to follow if you are responsible for developing or ordering educational supplies include the following:

- The material should be written in lay language at a sixth to eighth grade level to promote general patient understanding.
- Information should be well organized and clearly described.
- All material should be checked for accuracy.
- Handouts should be attractive and professional.
- Copies should be available in other languages when possible and in large print for visually impaired clients.

IDENTIFYING COMMUNITY RESOURCES

One of the roles of the medical assistant in the ambulatory care setting is to assist patients and their families in finding and using community education and support services. The healthcare facility should keep an up-to-date file of area resources that identifies the name of the group and the services provided; the contact person; a telephone number and address; meeting times and location if applicable; and a related Web site if available. This information can be found in a number of different locations, such as the blue pages of the local phone book, through the community outreach or speakers bureau of area hospitals, or online by searching for area educational institutions at .edu sites or local chapters of national organizations at .org sites. For example, the American Cancer Society operates local branches throughout the United States, and information on local services can be found on the national home page (www.cancer.org).

An excellent comprehensive Internet site operated by the U.S. National Library of Medicine and the National Institutes of Health is MedlinePlus. Both health professionals and consumers can depend on it for accurate information that is updated frequently. The site provides a variety of information about health issues, an extensive list of diseases and conditions, a medical encyclopedia and dictionary, health information in Spanish, extensive details on prescription and nonprescription drugs, health information from the media, and links to thousands of clinical trials. It can be bookmarked at *medlineplus.gov.*

Other teaching materials include CDs, DVDs, and professional Internet sites to reinforce or expand knowledge. These learning aids promote self-directed and self-paced learning. They also permit the patient to access material in a nonstressful environment, which improves the patient's learning potential. Depending on the patient's age or access to the appropriate technology, using media resources or referring the patient to physician-approved healthcare sites on the Internet can help develop patient ownership of the learning process and provide excellent resources for patient referral. However, using the Internet as a resource for patient education information has its drawbacks. It is important that the patient understand that there is no oversight or control over information posted on the Web; therefore, some sites may offer information that is erroneous, out of date, or misleading. Provide patients with accurate, well-researched sites and/or keep informed about what sites patients are accessing to make sure online recommendations support the physician's treatment protocol.

Decide on the Appropriate Teaching Methods

A variety of methods may be used to get the message across to your patients. One of the best ways to manage a large amount of information within a short time is to use community resources to reinforce the message. Your local area provides a wide range of education services for your patients to help them better understand and manage their health problems, to promote wellness, and to provide support for treatment compliance. Hospitals and many community agencies and organizations provide patient education opportunities, support groups for specific problems or diseases, and learning materials. These same groups may help the patient by providing professional consultation for many topics, including diet, exercise, and emotional support. It is important that the medical assistant be aware of the various resources available in the community for patient education and referral.

Based on your evaluation of Mr. Ignatio's learning needs, what community resources would help him and his family better understand and manage his disease?

Teaching patients specific skills also is an important component of health education. The best way to teach a patient how to manipulate and operate medical equipment accurately is to use demonstration and return demonstration of the skill (Figure 29-6). Using the exact piece of equipment the patient will be using at home, the medical assistant first should demonstrate to the patient how to perform the skill, ask for questions and explain further as needed, and then have the patient return the demonstration before leaving the office. This gives the medical assistant the opportunity to observe the patient performing the task and correct any mistakes or clarify any misconceptions before the patient has to use the equipment at home alone.

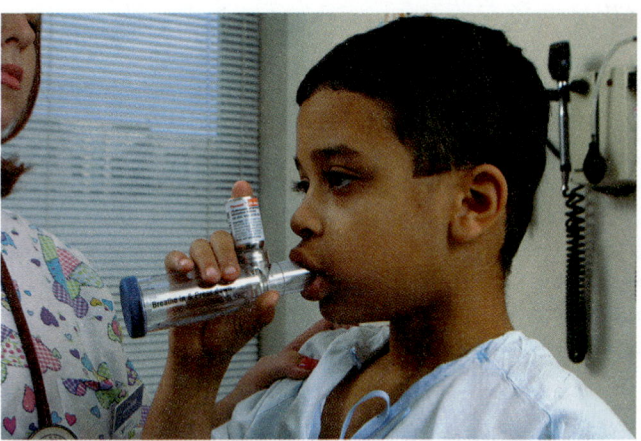

FIGURE 29-6 Demonstration and return demonstration.

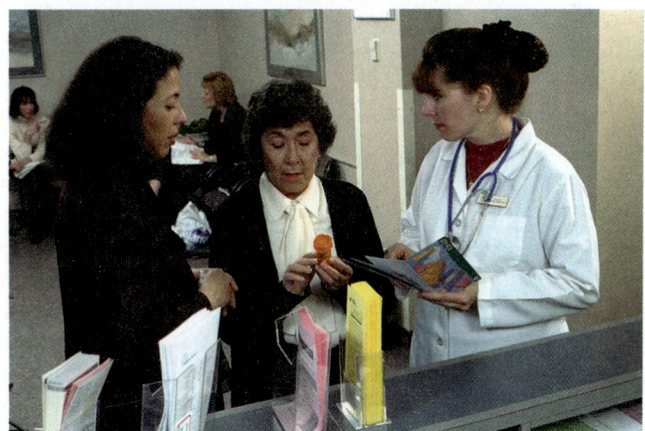

FIGURE 29-7 Family involvement in patient education.

For some patients, an effective method of monitoring health education is to have the patient keep a journal of his or her activities and response to treatment. For example, a patient trying to adapt to a new diet could record the daily intake to get a better idea of whether he or she is following through with dietary recommendations. In the case of Mr. Ignatio, recording blood glucose levels from routine glucometer readings would reinforce the results of compliance with medication and diet therapies.

Another vital link to the success of patient education is family involvement. If the patient is being treated holistically, the family plays an integral role in patient wellness. Involving family members in patient education efforts provides support and understanding for the patient while managing family concerns about the patient's welfare. An educated family member can be an excellent resource for patient concerns and a vigilant reinforcer of healthy behaviors (Figure 29-7).

CRITICAL THINKING APPLICATION   29-2

The physician recommends that Mr. Ignatio start a 1,200-calorie diabetic diet for weight reduction and blood glucose control; that he monitor his glucometer readings three times a day; and that he start with three injections of insulin daily. After you consider various teaching methods, which strategies do you think would be most useful in helping Mr. Ignatio to learn about his disease and to follow the doctor's recommendations?

Implement the Teaching Plan

After you have completed the patient assessment, decided on teaching materials and methods that match your patient's characteristics and learning needs, and adapted the material and your approach for any potential barriers to learning, it is time to implement the plan. Conduct the lesson in a quiet area away from distractions. Assemble the equipment the patient will need to follow through with treatment. The patient should learn to handle and practice on the same type of equipment that will be used at home so that no problem occurs in transferring the skill. Time is always an issue in the ambulatory care setting, so it is important to present only the material or skill it is possible for the patient to master before the end of the appointment. Throughout the lesson, remember to maintain an adequate pace for learning—not too fast and not too slow—to optimize the patient's understanding.

A crucial aspect of successful patient teaching is to consistently ask for feedback about the process (Figure 29-8). It also helps to restate, repeat, or rephrase the material to make sure the patient understands the process. As patients provide correct feedback about what they are learning or demonstrate skills correctly, it is important to be positive about their progress. It also helps to summarize the material learned or the skills mastered at the end of each teaching intervention as a way of reviewing the material and clarifying important concepts.

The medical assistant should continue to evaluate the teaching plan throughout the process to make sure the time was adequate for learning and that the patient understood the information needed to follow through with care at home. In addition, plans should be made for the education intervention during the patient's next visit. All of this information needs to be included in the progress note about the lesson. In addition, the medical assistant must document details about the material covered, the patient's competency or level of skill in learning treatment techniques, and any referrals made for community and hospital experts or education groups.

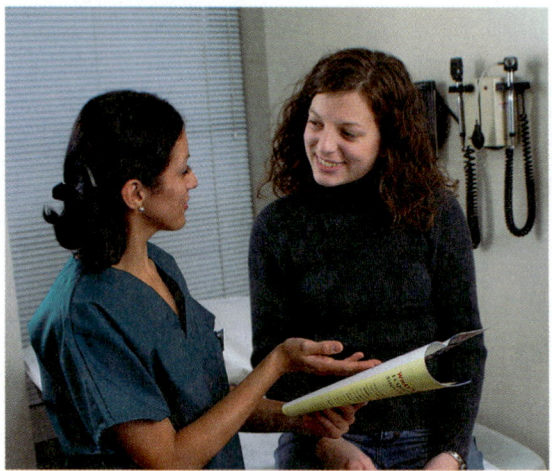

FIGURE 29-8 Patient feedback.

5. Summarize the material learned or skill mastered at the end of each teaching interaction.
6. Outline a plan for the next meeting.
7. Evaluate the teaching plan.
   - Was there enough time to complete the lesson?
   - Was the patient physically and psychologically ready for the information?
   - Were the goals for the session reached?
8. Document the teaching intervention.
   - Material covered
   - Patient response or level of skill performance
   - Plans for next session
   - Community referrals

Role of the Medical Assistant as Patient Educator

- Reinforce physician instructions and information
- Encourage patients to take an active role in their health
- Use each patient interaction as an opportunity for health teaching
- Keep information relevant to the patient's needs
- Establish and maintain rapport with the patient
- Communicate clearly
- Be sensitive to the patient's learning factors
- Modify the teaching plan as needed to best meet the patient's needs

---

SUMMARY OF THE PATIENT TEACHING PLAN

1. Perform an assessment.
   - Consider pertinent patient factors.
   - Identify barriers to learning.
   - Prioritize patient information.
2. Determine the patient's immediate and long-term needs.
   - Decide on the appropriate teaching materials and methods; prepare the teaching area and assemble the necessary equipment and materials.
   - Demonstrate techniques and procedures using the supplies the patient will use at home.
   - Provide positive feedback when the patient displays skills correctly.
3. Maintain an adequate pace while teaching (not too fast).
4. Repeatedly ask for patient feedback to confirm understanding.
   - Barriers to learning are eliminated.
   - Immediate learning needs can be addressed.
   - Repetition and rephrasing promote understanding.

CRITICAL THINKING APPLICATION   29-3

Taylor has just completed the initial patient education session with Mr. Ignatio and his wife. He used demonstration–return demonstration to teach Mr. Ignatio how to check his blood glucose levels properly with the glucometer he will be using at home. He also demonstrated how to draw up and administer an insulin injection. Taylor answered Mrs. Ignatio's questions about the diabetic diet, but he referred the couple to the dietitian at the hospital for further information on that topic. Taylor plans to review the skills practiced today at Mr. Ignatio's next appointment and to continue the teaching intervention, emphasizing the importance of checking the feet daily for open areas or any signs of infection.

Accurately and completely document Taylor's initial education intervention.

CLOSING COMMENTS

Legal and Ethical Issues

Providing adequate, correct, understandable information to patients is integral to the informed consent mandate in the Patient's Bill of Rights. All patients have the right to information before they agree to receive care. An extension of this concept is the right of patients to understand their disease process and to manage their health. Another consideration arising from the Patient's Bill of Rights is the issue of patient confidentiality as it relates to patient education. When developing and implementing the teaching plan, designing teaching interventions and strategies, and referring patients for community assistance, the medical assistant must protect the patient's confidentiality.

Essential factors in risk management for the ambulatory care setting include conducting adequate patient education and follow-up. Also integral to risk management is the importance of documenting each patient education intervention completely and accurately. The patient's chart should clearly describe the education intervention, methods and materials used, the patient's response to the intervention, the date of each session, and the individual who conducted each intervention. Each documentation entry should completely describe the material covered and the patient's feedback about the information so that no doubt exists that the patient understood the information and was able to perform any related skills properly and adequately.

Teaching interventions should demonstrate sensitivity to multicultural factors and diverse populations. Meeting the needs of all patients without evidence of prejudice is a key risk management step.

HIPAA Applications

The following applications relate to provisions of the Health Insurance Portability and Accountability Act (HIPAA).

- The patient has the right to restrict who can receive personal health information (PHI). At the first office visit, the patient should complete a release of information form that identifies, if the patient agrees, a particular family member, close friend, or any other individual who the patient states can receive disclosures of health information.

- Only the person or persons identified on the HIPAA release form completed by the patient have the right to the patient's personal information. Therefore, if an individual requests information about the patient, the medical assistant first must check the release form to determine whether the individual was approved by the patient before discussing the patient's condition. This holds true regardless of the individual's relationship to the patient.

- If the physician believes that it is in the patient's best interest that family members be involved in patient health education, the medical assistant can contact the family only if the patient has given approval. This permission should be included in the patient's HIPAA information and should be documented in the medical record so that all employees can read evidence of the patient's approval.

SUMMARY OF SCENARIO

After working with Mr. Ignatio, Taylor realizes the significance and complexity of educating patients in the ambulatory care setting. Despite the time constraints typical in this particular healthcare setting, patients still must learn how to manage their disease and follow treatment guidelines. Approaching each patient as an individual learner with particular needs and characteristics is crucial to the ultimate success of the teaching plan. By using a holistic approach and taking into account the health belief model, Taylor has considered the ramifications of diabetes mellitus for Mr. Ignatio's life and has made efforts to include family and community resources in the management of his disease.

SUMMARY OF LEARNING OBJECTIVES

1. Recognize the implications of health and illness models for patient education.

   The holistic model suggests that patient education should consider all aspects of the patient's life, including physical, emotional, social, intellectual, economic, and spiritual needs. The health belief model analyzes what people believe to be true about themselves and their health. This model suggests that healthcare practitioners consider how the patient perceives the risk of developing the disease and whether he or she believes that altering health behaviors will prevent the disease. Kübler-Ross's stages of grief may also help explain a patient's reaction to a particular diagnosis, especially if the disease requires a drastic change in lifestyle. Grief is an ongoing process, with patients moving through denial, anger, bargaining, depression, and finally resolution at their own pace and in their own way.

2. Apply critical thinking skills in performing the patient assessment and patient care.

   Completing the Critical Thinking Application exercises throughout the chapter will help the student medical assistant become more adept at critical analysis of real-life situations.

3. Instruct patients according to their needs to promote health maintenance and disease prevention.

   Many factors or patient characteristics may affect the patient's ability to learn. Medical assistants must be aware of these factors to develop a patient education approach that best meets the needs of each patient.

4. List at least five guidelines for patient education that can affect the patient's overall wellness.

   The guidelines for patient education include providing knowledge and skills that promote recovery and health; including family in education interventions; encouraging patient ownership of the education process; promoting safe use of medications and treatments; encouraging healthy behaviors; and providing information on how to access community resources.

5. **Define six patient factors that have an impact on learning.**

   Patient factors that have an impact on learning include the patient's perception of disease versus the actual state of disease; the need for information; age and developmental level; mental and emotional state; the influence of multicultural and diversity factors; individual learning style; and the impact of physical disabilities on the education process.

6. **Display respect for individual diversity.**

   Culture, family background, and religious beliefs influence a patient's actions. For patient education to be successful, it is essential that the medical assistant be aware of and sensitive to the impact of these factors on patient learning. Consider the patient's language, ability to understand English verbally or read it correctly, and cultural relationships to healthcare workers. Develop techniques to minimize the patient's education problems.

7. **Demonstrate empathy in communicating with patients and family members.**

   The medical assistant should encourage patient ownership and participation in the teaching process while including family and significant others in education interventions, with patient approval.

8. **Summarize educational approaches for patients with language barriers.**

   Educational approaches for patients with language barriers include addressing the patient formally and courteously; using nonverbal language to promote understanding; integrating pictures or models that illustrate the material; observing the patient for understanding or confusion; using simple lay language; demonstrating procedures; implementing teaching in small, manageable steps; providing written instructions; and using an interpreter when available.

9. **Demonstrate recognition of the patient's level of understanding in communications.**

   Some of the communication techniques that the medical assistant can use to assure patient understanding include repeatedly asking for patient feedback to confirm understanding; using repetition and rephrasing to promote understanding; and summarizing the material learned or skill mastered at the end of each teaching interaction.

10. **Determine potential barriers to patient learning.**

    Potential barriers to patient education include the patient's learning style, physical limitations, age, and developmental level; any emotional or mental state that interferes with learning; use of defense mechanisms; cultural or ethnic factors; language; the presence of pain; a patient's lack of motivation to learn; and limited time for teaching.

11. **Develop and maintain a current list of community resources related to patients' healthcare needs.**

The medical assistant should assist patients and their families in finding and using community education and support services when needed. The healthcare facility should maintain a current file of area resources that identifies the name of the group and the services provided; the contact person; a telephone number and address; meeting times and location if applicable; and a related Web site if available. Provide patients with accurate, well-researched sites and/or be informed about what sites patients are accessing to make certain that online recommendations support the physician's treatment protocol.

12. **Implement a variety of teaching methods and strategies responsive to the individual patient's needs.**

    Teaching materials and methods that are effective include the use of printed materials, DVDs, CDs, and approved Internet sites to gather information; referral to community resources and experts; demonstration and return demonstration of medical skills; patient journals of events; and involvement of family members in the education process.

13. **Demonstrate the ability to develop an appropriate and effective patient teaching plan.**

    The parts of the teaching plan include assessing learning needs; eliminating learning barriers; determining teaching priorities; using appropriate teaching materials and methods; gathering feedback repeatedly to ensure that the patient understands; summarizing the material at the end of each education session; planning for the next meeting; evaluating the effectiveness of the session; and completely and accurately documenting the details of the teaching intervention.

14. **Document patient education.**

    The medical assistant must document details regarding the material covered, the patient's competency or level of skill in learning treatment techniques, and any referral made for community and hospital experts or education groups.

15. **Describe the role of the medical assistant in patient education.**

    The role of the medical assistant in patient education is to reinforce the physician's instructions and information by encouraging patients to take an active part in their health; using teaching moments effectively; keeping information relevant to the patient; establishing and maintaining patient rapport; communicating clearly; remaining aware of learning factors; being flexible with the teaching plan; and using community resources for learning and support.

16. **Integrate the legal and ethical elements of patient teaching into the ambulatory care setting.**

    Appropriate patient education reflects the emphasis of the Patient's Bill of Rights on patient confidentiality and informed consent. Risk management practices related to patient education include accurate and complete documentation of patient education sessions, sensitivity to the diverse needs of the patient, and application of HIPAA practices.

CONNECTIONS

Study Guide Connection: Go to the Chapter 29 Study Guide. Read and complete the activities.

Evolve Connection: Go to the Chapter 29 link at *evolve.elsevier.com/kinn* to complete the Chapter Review and Chapter Quiz. Check out the other resources listed for this chapter to make the most of what you have learned from Patient Education.

30

NUTRITION AND HEALTH PROMOTION

SCENARIO

Marcia Schwartz, CMA (AAMA), is employed by an internal medicine practice in her hometown. She recognizes that many of the patients seen in the practice have diseases that are influenced by diet and lifestyle factors. She learned about the importance of good nutrition and wellness in her medical assisting program. In addition, Marcia has continued to attend workshops and read about current trends in nutrition, so she is prepared to provide assistance to her patients as directed by the physician.

While studying this chapter, think about the following questions:

- How can Marcia help her patients understand the importance of and suggested requirements for the primary nutrients?
- What should Marcia know about dietary guidelines for fat consumption?
- What is the importance of vitamins and nutrients and in what foods can they be found?
- How can Marcia educate patients using the new MyPlate Web site?
- Is Marcia able to teach patients the significance of the body mass index (BMI) and how it can be calculated?
- What are the general guidelines for therapeutic nutrition?
- Is it important that Marcia be able to teach patients how to read food labels?
- What factors contribute to a healthy lifestyle?

LEARNING OBJECTIVES

1. Define, spell, and pronounce the terms listed in the vocabulary.
2. Apply critical thinking skills in performing the patient assessment and patient care.
3. Analyze the relationship between poor diet and lifestyle choices and the risk of developing diet-related diseases.
4. Recognize the impact of cultural influences on dietary choices.
5. Classify the types and functions of dietary nutrients.
6. Describe the roles of carbohydrates, fats, protein, and fiber in the daily diet.
7. Explain the function of appropriate amounts of vitamins, minerals, and water in the diet.
8. Apply the 2010 Dietary Guidelines for Americans using the Choose MyPlate Web site developed by the U.S. Department of Agriculture (USDA).
9. Implement nutritional assessment techniques.
10. Correlate a patient's calculated body mass index (BMI) with the risk for diet-related disease.
11. Compare the concepts of therapeutic nutrition.
12. Interpret food labels and their application to a healthy diet.
13. Demonstrate to the patient how to understand nutrition labels on food products.
14. Summarize the causes of eating disorders and obesity and their impact on a patient's health.
15. Define the concepts of health promotion.
16. Describe the role of the medical assistant in nutrition and health promotion.

VOCABULARY

amino acids The organic compounds that form the chief constituents of protein and are used by the body to build and repair tissues.

cholesterol (kuh-les′-tuh-rol) A substance produced by the liver and found in animal fats that can produce fatty deposits or atherosclerotic plaques in blood vessels.

deficiencies (di-fi′-shun-sees) Conditions that result with below normal intake of particular substances.

diabetes mellitus type 1 A disease in which the beta cells in the pancreas no longer produce insulin. The individual must rely on daily insulin administration to use glucose for energy and prevent complications.

diabetes mellitus type 2 A disease in which the body is unable to use glucose for energy as a result either of inadequate insulin production in the pancreas or resistance to insulin on the cellular level.

digestion The process of converting food into chemical substances that can be used by the body.

diverticulosis (di-vuhr-ti-kyuh-lo′-suhs) The presence of pouch-like herniations through the muscular layer of the colon.

free radicals Compounds with at least one unpaired electron, which makes the compound unstable and highly reactive. Free radicals are believed to damage cell components, ultimately leading to cancer, heart disease, or other diseases.

hydrogenated (hi-drah′-juh-na-ted) Combined with, treated with, or exposed to hydrogen.

macular degeneration A progressive deterioration of the macula of the eye that causes loss of central vision.

neural tube defects Any of a group of congenital anomalies involving the brain and spinal column that are caused by failure of the neural tube to close during embryonic development.

obesity An excessive accumulation of body fat; defined as a body mass index (BMI) of 30 or higher.

osteoporosis (ah-ste-o-puh-ro′-ses) Loss of bone density; lack of calcium intake is a major factor in its development.

psyllium (si′-le-um) A grain found in some cereal products, in certain dietary supplements, and in certain bulk fiber laxatives; a water-soluble fiber.

registered dietitian (RD) An individual with a minimum of a bachelor's degree in food and nutrition who is concerned with the maintenance and promotion of health and the treatment of diseases through diet.

triglyceride (tri-gli′-suh-ride) A fatty acid and glycerol compound that combines with a protein molecule to form high- or low-density lipoprotein.

turgor A term referring to normal skin tension; it is the resistance of the skin to being grasped between the fingers and released. Turgor is decreased with dehydration and increased with edema.

vertigo Dizziness; a sensation of faintness or an inability to maintain normal balance.

Good health is a state of emotional and physical well-being that is determined to a large extent by diet and lifestyle factors. Health promotion and disease prevention practices focus on sound nutrition, regular exercise, avoidance of smoking and tobacco, limited alcohol intake, management of stress, and avoidance of environmental contaminants. We are what we eat, because the food we consume is used to build and repair every part of our bodies. A well-nourished person is also better able to ward off infections. Consequently, a poor diet and risky lifestyle behaviors are directly related to multiple health problems.

The physician, the medical assistant, and the **registered dietitian (RD)** are all closely involved in the nutritive care of a patient. The physician prescribes the diet, and ideally the dietitian instructs the patient in how to follow it. If professional aid is not available, the medical assistant may be asked to discuss the diet with the patient, answer questions, and explain certain aspects of the modifications involved. The patient may hesitate to ask the physician details about a recommended diet, or he or she may call with questions about how to implement the diet after leaving the office. The medical assistant, therefore, frequently is the person to whom the patient turns for answers. You should be able to answer basic questions on healthy nutrition and should have a fundamental knowledge of the diets physicians most often prescribe.

HEALTH PROBLEMS RELATED TO POOR NUTRITION AND LIFESTYLE FACTORS

- Anemia: Low iron or folate intake
- Cancers: High-fat, low-fiber, low-complex-carbohydrate diet; high alcohol and sodium intake; sedentary lifestyle; tobacco use
- Constipation: Low fiber, inadequate fluids; high-fat diet; sedentary lifestyle
- Diabetes mellitus type 2: High-calorie, high-fat, low-complex-carbohydrate diet; obesity; sedentary lifestyle
- Hypercholesterolemia and atherosclerosis: High-fat, low-fiber diet; high sugar and alcohol intake; tobacco use; sedentary lifestyle
- Hypertension: High-calorie, high-fat diet; high alcohol and sodium intake; tobacco use; sedentary lifestyle; obesity; stress
- Osteoporosis: Low calcium intake; inadequate vitamin D intake or lack of sun exposure; high alcohol intake; sedentary lifestyle; tobacco use
- Stroke: High-fat, low-fiber, low-complex-carbohydrate diet; high alcohol intake; tobacco use; stress

People eat the way they do for many reasons. When encouraging patients to make significant changes in their diets, the medical assistant must be sensitive to these reasons. The choices people make about what they eat are greatly influenced by their background and relationships. Every culture, religion, and ethnic group has its own beliefs and practices with regard to food. For example, according to the Hindu religion, eating beef is forbidden. Certain Jewish practices govern the types of foods that are eaten and how they are prepared. Food is more than sustenance; it represents family and celebrations and has an entire psychological component that the medical assistant must recognize in order to care for the individual patient most effectively.

REASONS FOR PEOPLE'S FOOD CHOICES

- *Convenience:* People choose what is easiest and quickest, including eating out and take-home meals.
- *Cost:* What a person can afford.
- *Emotional comfort:* "Feel good" foods are chosen based on cultural and psychological influences.
- *Routine:* People eat what they always eat out of habit, personal preference, and availability.
- *Positive experiences:* A food is associated with a fond memory, eaten by someone the person admires, or chosen because of the influence of marketing and advertising.
- *Ethnic or regional influences:* The person grew up with the food; it is associated with the individual's cultural background; or it is part of the regional diet where the person lives.
- *Health and weight:* People think a particular food is good for them or will help them maintain or lose weight.

CULTURAL EATING PATTERNS

- *Asian diets* emphasize whole grains in the form of millet, rice, and noodles and also fruits, vegetables, legumes, and nuts and seeds; fats are derived largely from vegetable oils, such as peanut or sesame oils. Dairy products are not traditionally eaten. Protein sources typically are broiled or stir-fried fish and seafood, egg whites, tofu, and nuts.
- *Latin American diets* emphasize food from plant sources at each meal, especially maize (corn) and potatoes, in addition to fruits, vegetables, whole grains, beans, and nuts. Poultry, fish, and dairy typically are consumed daily and meat and eggs weekly.
- *Mediterranean diets* emphasize whole grains, fresh fruits and vegetables, and all types of legumes, such as beans, lentils, and peas daily; olive oil replaces other fats and oils; fish, poultry, and eggs are consumed weekly and meat monthly.
- *Mexican diets* emphasize corn or flour tortillas, cabbage, legumes, squash, tomatoes, corn, and potatoes daily. Dairy is used in the form of cheeses, but milk is not regularly consumed. Protein sources typically are fish, beef, poultry, lamb, and many types of beans.

NUTRITION AND DIETETICS

The term *nutrition* refers to all the processes involved in the intake and use of nutrients. *Nutrients* are the organic and inorganic chemicals in food that supply the energy and raw materials for cellular activities. Nutrients include carbohydrate, fat, protein, vitamins, minerals, and water.

Metabolism is the process in which nutrients are used at the cellular level for growth and energy production and excretion of waste. Metabolism occurs in two phases, anabolism and catabolism. *Anabolism* is the building phase, in which smaller molecules, such as **amino acids**, are combined to form larger molecules, such as proteins. An example of anabolism is the creation by the liver of *glycogen,* a stored form of glucose. In this process, many units of glucose are combined to form a more complex glycogen molecule. *Catabolism* is the breaking-down phase, in which larger molecules are broken down and converted into smaller units, such as when stored glycogen is broken down into glucose molecules for energy.

Digestion is a combination of mechanical and chemical processes that occur in the mouth, stomach, and small intestine. These processes result in the breakdown of nutrients into absorbable forms, including amino acids, fatty acids, glycerol, and glucose. Most nutrients are absorbed in the small intestine and then carried by the bloodstream to all parts of the body.

The term *nutrition* also is used to indicate nutritional status, or the condition of the body resulting from the use of nutrients. *Dietetics* is the practical application of nutritional science to individuals. It is the combined science and art of feeding individuals or groups, given a wide range of economic factors and/or health conditions, according to the principles of nutrition and dietary management. A registered dietitian's role is the promotion of good health through proper diet and the therapeutic use of diet in the treatment of disease.

Nutrients

To nurture life, the nutrients in food must perform one or more of three basic functions in the body: (1) provide a source of fuel or energy, (2) supply material to build and repair tissues, and (3) regulate metabolic processes. Because no one food supplies all the nutrients required, a combination of different foods is necessary to promote health. With a little planning, all the body's needs can be met by a well-balanced diet. Dietary **deficiencies** result in undernourishment or malnourishment and may lead to a variety of diseases. Good nutrition is an important part of health promotion for all individuals but especially for pregnant women, young children, and the elderly.

The role of diet in supplying energy is crucial to body functions. Every action of the body, whether voluntary or involuntary, requires energy. Even when a person is asleep, the body still needs a source of energy to keep vital organs functioning. *Basal metabolism* is the amount of energy needed to maintain essential body functions. The *basal metabolic rate* (BMR) is the amount of energy used by a fasting, resting individual to maintain vital functions. The rate is determined by the amount of oxygen used and is defined in units of heat energy called *calories* (cal). Because this unit represents a relatively small amount of energy and because metabolism involves much larger amounts of energy, the large calorie (Cal), or kilocalorie (kcal), is commonly used. A kilocalorie is defined as the amount of heat required to raise the temperature of 1 kg of water 1°C.

Of the seven food constituents (carbohydrates, proteins, fats, water, minerals, vitamins, and fiber), only carbohydrates, proteins, and fats are capable of furnishing the body with energy. The amount of energy, or kilocalories, a person needs varies according to the individual's activity level, basal metabolic requirements, and whether disease is present. Most adults age 20 to 40 require 1,800 to 2,200 kcal/day. A patient generally is said to be overweight or underweight depending on how his or her current weight compares with nutritional assessment standards. **Obesity** is likely to result when more calories are consumed than are expended or because of certain endocrine imbalances.

Nutrients can be categorized as those that are a required part of the diet and those that can be anabolized in the body. An *essential* nutrient cannot be manufactured by the body and therefore must be included in the diet or a deficiency disease occurs. Certain amino acids are examples of essential nutrients. A *nonessential* nutrient can be created in the body and therefore does not need to be included in the diet; for example, both **cholesterol**, which is manufactured in the liver, and vitamin D, which is synthesized from exposure to the sun, are nonessential nutrients.

Nutrient Components

Carbohydrates

Carbohydrates (CHO) are chemical organic compounds composed of carbon, hydrogen, and oxygen that are primarily plant products. They are divided into three groups based on the complexity of their molecules: simple sugars (e.g., table sugar, molasses, syrup, honey, candy, baked goods, and milk); complex carbohydrates (starch) (e.g., whole-grain products, cereal, pasta, rice, potatoes, legumes, fruits, vegetables, and seeds); and dietary fiber, which is found in bran, oatmeal, whole-grain breads, beans, fruits, vegetables, seeds, and dried fruits. Each has a function in health and consists of many variations. With the exception of fiber, carbohydrates are easily digested and absorbed into the body. Simple sugars are quickly absorbed, whereas complex carbohydrates must be processed before they can be absorbed in the intestinal tract. Dietary fiber is indigestible and passes through the gastrointestinal tract unchanged.

HOW MANY TERMS CAN APPLY TO BREAD?

Dietary guidelines recommend that at least half of the grains consumed each day come from a whole-grain source.

Whole grains contain the entire grain kernel—the bran, germ, and endosperm. People who eat whole grains as part of a healthy diet have a reduced risk of some chronic diseases. However, labels can be confusing. How do you know which is a healthy choice? Understanding the following definitions associated with grain foods can help. Review the definitions and see what you think about the healthiest grain choices.

- *Bran*—The tough, fibrous covering of a grain that is the primary source of fiber in grain products.
- *Enriched* or *fortified bread*—Since 1942, and with legislation amended in 1996 to include folate, the U.S. government has required that thiamin, riboflavin, niacin, folate, and iron be added to refined grain products because the process of creating white flour destroys these nutrients.
- *Refined* or *white flour* or *bread*—Bread produced through a process that removes the coarse parts of the grain (the fiber and nutrients); the flour is bleached to create the white color.
- *Stone-ground flour*—A process used to grind the grain; may include white flour.
- *Unbleached flour*—Similar to white flour in nutritional value and nutrient content.
- *Wheat flour* or *brown bread*—Bread made from wheat (white bread also is made of wheat) or any other type of flour that contains molasses to color the bread brown.
- *Whole-grain* or *whole-wheat flour*—Flour for which the entire grain kernel is ground; unrefined flour.

The main function of carbohydrates is to supply fuel for energy and for all basic cellular activities. To meet energy needs, carbohydrate is metabolized at a rate of 4 cal/g. When digested, carbohydrate is converted into glucose, which is carried by the bloodstream to cells that need energy. A small amount of concentrated glucose is stored in the liver and muscles as glycogen. This stored glucose is available to supplement dietary supplies of carbohydrate. As with all nutrients, excess amounts of carbohydrate are converted into fat and stored in the body as *adipose* tissue. In addition to serving as the body's primary energy source, carbohydrate also is needed to regulate protein and fat metabolism. As long as sufficient amounts of dietary carbohydrate are available to meet the body's energy needs, protein and fat are not needed to supply energy. This *protein-sparing* effect allows protein to be used for its intended purpose—the repair and growth of tissues.

Carbohydrate is used for energy with limited production of waste materials, whereas protein and fat metabolism creates byproducts that are challenging for the body to process and excrete. For example, the metabolism of fat for energy results in the production of ketone bodies, which can cause an increase in the acidity of the blood and possibly kidney damage from the excretion of ketones. In addition, the central nervous system (CNS) requires a constant minute-to-minute supply of glucose to function properly. Neurons find it difficult to use fat or protein for energy.

Dietary fiber, commonly called *roughage*, is the portion of a plant that cannot be digested or absorbed. However, fiber's inability to be digested makes it an important dietary asset. Fiber adds bulk to the intestinal tract that stimulates peristalsis and promotes regular bowel movements. In addition, *soluble fiber*, which is found in oat bran, peas, beans, certain fruits, and **psyllium**, lowers blood cholesterol levels, reducing the risk of heart disease. Soluble fiber combines with cholesterol in the intestine and is excreted through the bowel, which prevents the absorption of cholesterol into the bloodstream. *Insoluble fiber*, which is found in whole grains and beans, promotes regular bowel movements, which prevents constipation and hemorrhoids. It also prevents **diverticulosis** by stimulating and toning the muscles lining the large intestine, and it is thought to help prevent colon cancer. The recommended daily fiber intake is 20 to 35 g, and 5 to 10 g of this should be soluble fiber. Table 30-1 identifies food sources of both soluble and insoluble

TABLE 30-1 Food Sources of Fiber

FOOD	SERVING SIZE	TOTAL FIBER (g)	SOLUBLE FIBER (g)	INSOLUBLE FIBER (g)
Spaghetti, cooked	1 cup	2	0.5	1.5
Whole-wheat bread	1 slice	2.5	0.5	2
White rice, cooked	½ cup	0.5	0	0.5
Bran flake cereal	¾ cup	5.5	0.5	5
Corn flake cereal	1 cup	1	0	1
Oatmeal, cooked	¾ cup	3	1	2
Banana	1 medium	2	0.5	1.5
Apple, with skin	1 medium	3	0.5	2.5
Orange	1 medium	2	0.5	1.5
Pear, with skin	1 medium	4.5	0.5	4
Strawberries	½ cup	1	0	1
Broccoli	½ cup	2	0	2
Corn	½ cup	1.5	0	1.5
Potato, baked with skin	1 medium	4	1	3
Spinach	½ cup	2	0.5	1.5
Kidney beans	½ cup	4.5	1	3.5
Popcorn	1 cup	1	0	1

From the American Dietetic Association: Accessed January 12, 2010. Available at www.eatright.org/cps/rde/xchg/SID-5303FFEA-A120B9BE/ada/hs.xsl/nutrition_5440_ENU_HTML.htm.

fiber. Eating fruit unpeeled and eating raw vegetables can greatly increase the fiber content of the diet.

Recommendations for Carbohydrate Consumption

- Carbohydrates should account for 55% to 57% of the total calories consumed each day (i.e., 271 to 288 g for a 2,000-calorie diet).
- Fiber-rich fruits, vegetables, and whole grains should be eaten as often as possible.
- People should consume 15 g of fiber for every 1,000 calories eaten.
- The intake of simple sugars, especially sugar-sweetened drinks, should be reduced, and snacking on foods high in sugars and starches should be limited.
- Fruits and vegetables: Based on the typical 2,000-calorie diet, 2 cups of fruit and 2½ cups of vegetables should be eaten daily; a variety of dark green, orange, and starchy vegetables and legumes should be consumed.
- Whole grains: At least three 1-ounce servings should be eaten each day. Whole grains should make up at least half of the daily grain consumption. One ounce is equal to one slice of bread, 1 cup of dry cereal, or ½ cup of cooked rice, pasta, or cereal.
- Dairy: Includes milk, yogurt, cheese, and fortified soymilk. These provide calcium, vitamin D, potassium, protein, and other nutrients. Choose low-fat or fat-free products to limit calories and saturated fat. By age, the requirements are: children 9 years or older, teens, and adults—3 cups/day; age 4 to 8 years—2½ cups/

day; and age 2 to 3 years—2 cups. One cup is equal to 1 cup of yogurt, 1½ ounces of natural cheese, or 2 ounces of processed cheese.

CRITICAL THINKING APPLICATION   30-1

A patient, George Hawthorne, recently was diagnosed with hypertension and hypercholesterolemia. He has a family history of colon cancer. The physician recommends a high-fiber diet. Describe how Marcia could reinforce the physician's information by explaining the purpose of dietary fiber, the difference between soluble and insoluble fibers, and the types of foods Mr. Hawthorne should include in his diet.

Fats

Fats are the storage form of fuel used to back up carbohydrates as an available energy source. Fat is a much more concentrated form of fuel, producing 9 cal of energy per gram when metabolized. Dietary fats, or *lipids,* provide essential fatty acids and are needed for the absorption of the fat-soluble vitamins, A, D, E, and K. Fat gives food flavor and creates a feeling of *satiety* or satisfaction after eating. *Adipose* tissue, the stored form of fat in the body, supports and protects vital organs, insulates the body to help in the regulation of body temperature, and plays an important role in protecting nerve fibers and relaying nerve impulses. Lipids are also crucial to cell membrane development.

Saturated and Unsaturated Fatty Acids. When digested, fats are broken down into fatty acids and glycerol. The main building blocks of fat are *fatty acids,* which can be either saturated or unsaturated. *Unsaturated* fatty acids can take on more hydrogen under the proper conditions and therefore are less heavy and less dense. If fatty acids have one unfilled hydrogen bond, the fat is called *monounsaturated.* Olives and olive oil, peanuts and peanut oil, canola oil, pecans, and avocados contain monounsaturated fats. *Polyunsaturated* fats, such as safflower, corn, cottonseed, and soy oils, have two or more unfilled hydrogen bonds. Unsaturated fats are found in plants and are usually liquid at room temperature. Monounsaturated fat should be used as frequently as possible to replace saturated fat in the diet. Research on olive oil indicates it may offer some protection against heart disease and breast cancer, and canola oil is another rich source of monounsaturated fatty acids.

The chemical structure of a *saturated* fatty acid contains all the hydrogen possible; these fats, therefore, are denser, heavier, and solid at room temperature. Saturated fats are found in whole milk dairy products, eggs, lard, meat, and **hydrogenated** fats, such as margarine. Some saturated fats, such as those in soft margarines, are partially hydrogenated. These fats usually are soft at room temperature. Most saturated fats come from animal sources. The main exceptions are coconut and palm oils, which are of plant origin but are exceptionally high in saturated fat. The primary dietary factor associated with high blood cholesterol levels is a high intake of foods high in saturated fat.

WHAT IS A TRANS FAT?

Trans-fatty acids are byproducts created when polyunsaturated oils are solidified by the addition of hydrogen. Manufacturers use this process to preserve food products, because they are much more resistant to rancidity after hydrogenation. This lengthens the shelf life of the processed food, and the product tastes better. Trans fats are found naturally in meat and dairy products, but Americans consume most of their trans fats in processed foods, such as margarine, crackers, cookies, doughnuts, biscuits, chips, frozen meals, french fries, and other items containing or fried in partially hydrogenated oils. Trans fats raise the level of low-density lipoprotein (LDL), the so-called bad cholesterol, and lower the level of high-density lipoprotein (HDL), or "good" cholesterol, in the blood. Scientific evidence indicates that saturated fat, trans fat, and dietary cholesterol combine to raise the LDL level, resulting in an increased risk of coronary heart disease (CHD). According to the National Institutes of Health, more than 12.5 million Americans have CHD, and more than 500,000 die from its complications each year. Since 1993, nutritional food labels have been required to list the amounts of saturated fat and dietary cholesterol in products. Since January, 2006, manufacturers also have had to include trans fats on the label if the amount exceeds 0.5 g per serving. Label readers should be cautious, however, because eating more than the designated serving size can drastically increase the amount of trans fats consumed.

BENEFITS OF OMEGA-3 FATTY ACIDS

The omega-3 fatty acids have a number of beneficial effects in the body:
- They are present in large amounts in the cerebral cortex.
- They help form the retina.
- They have antiinflammatory effects, including improving the immune response, protecting blood vessels (e.g., the coronary arteries), and inhibiting the formation of blood clots.

Omega-3 fatty acids are found in cold water fish, including mackerel, salmon, tuna, and trout; in certain oils, including canola, flaxseed, soybean, and wheat germ oil; and in walnuts, soybeans, and soybean kernels. The benefits of omega-3 fatty acids can be obtained by consuming two servings of cold water fish weekly.

Foods High in Saturated Fat. Even a fat-free food can become high in saturated fat, depending on how it is prepared (e.g., a fat-free potato cooked as french fries). Therefore, we not only need to lower our intake of foods with saturated fat, we also need to be cautious about how foods are prepared. Foods should be grilled, roasted, broiled, baked, or cooked in the microwave rather than fried. Only lean meats should be used, and visible fat should be cut off before eating. Low-fat or fat-free products should be substituted when possible. Some foods high in saturated fat include the following:

Whole-milk dairy products	Oil-packed fish
Whole-milk cheeses	Salad dressing
Butter	Mayonnaise
Cream	Meat (especially red meat)
Ice cream	Coconut and palm oils
Egg yolks	

A **triglyceride** molecule is created when three fatty acids attach to a molecule of glycerol. This structure is the main storage form of lipids. Triglyceride molecules are transported throughout the body via the bloodstream as lipoproteins. Dietary fats determine the saturation level of triglyceride chains. The total amount of triglycerides in the blood is used as a diagnostic tool for determining a patient's risk for hypertension and heart disease. The acceptable triglyceride range in men is 40 to 160 mg/dL; for women, it is 35 to 135 mg/dL.

Cholesterol. Cholesterol is a nonessential nutrient that plays a vital role in metabolic activities. It is synthesized only in animal tissue, so it is not found in plant foods. The primary food sources of cholesterol are egg yolks and organ meats, although all animal sources of food contain cholesterol. As a nonessential nutrient, cholesterol also is manufactured in the body, particularly in the liver.

The confusion between "good" and "bad" fat stems from the distinction between the fat in food and the fat in our bodies. The good fats in our diet are monounsaturated and polyunsaturated fats. The bad dietary fats are cholesterol, trans fats, and saturated fats. As mentioned, the fat in our bodies is divided into two lipoprotein categories. The good fats, or high-density lipoproteins, carry cholesterol from body tissues or the bloodstream to the liver for metabolism and excretion. The bad fats, or low-density lipoprotein and very-low-density lipoprotein (VLDL), carry cholesterol to the cells.

TABLE 30-2 Total and Low-Density Lipoprotein (LDL) Cholesterol Level Recommendations

AGE (yr)	TOTAL CHOLESTEROL (mg/dL)			LDL CHOLESTEROL (mg/dL)		
	ACCEPTABLE	BORDERLINE	HIGH	ACCEPTABLE	BORDERLINE	HIGH
2 to 20	<170	170-199	>200	<110	110-129	>130
>20	<200	200-239	>240	<130	130-159	>160

LDL and VLDL form atherosclerotic plaques on arterial walls, and these plaques frequently result in heart disease, hypertension, and strokes. However, serum LDL levels often can be successfully changed through diet. Using polyunsaturated and monounsaturated fat products reduces total serum cholesterol levels. In addition, using monounsaturated fats (olive, peanut, and canola oils) reduces LDL levels. Aerobic exercise is an important tool for lowering total serum cholesterol levels, increasing HDL levels, and reducing triglycerides. The higher the serum level of HDL, the greater the protection against cardiovascular disease. The normal HDL range is 30 to 80 mg/dL. A level below 40 is considered a major risk for heart disease, whereas a value of 60 or greater is thought to protect against heart disease. Heart experts recommend an LDL level below 100 mg/dL and an HDL level of 60 mg/dL or greater (Table 30-2).

Another potential health risk from a high-fat diet is obesity. Too much fat in the diet is deposited in the body as stored adipose tissue. Currently fats make up 35% to 40% of the total calories in the American diet. Nutritionists and epidemiologists believe that reducing dietary fat to 30%, with saturated fat and trans fat making up no more than 10% of calories, would reduce the risks of cancer, atherosclerosis, hypertension, and heart disease.

Recommendations for Fat Consumption

- Keep total fat intake to 20% to 35%, or approximately 17 g of fat per day for a 2,000-calorie diet.
- No more than 10% of daily calories should come from saturated and trans fats.
- Limit cholesterol to less than 300 mg/day.
- Use only lean cuts and smaller portions of meat; trim visible fat.
- Substitute poultry and fish for red meat; remove poultry skin before eating.
- Avoid adding fat in the cooking process.
- Limit intake of organ meats and egg yolks.
- With an elevated serum cholesterol, limit eggs to two or three per week or use egg substitutes or egg whites only.
- Use low-fat or fat-free milk and milk products.
- Use low-fat or fat-free products.
- Choose liquid monounsaturated oils, such as canola or olive oil.

CRITICAL THINKING APPLICATION   30-2

Mr. Hawthorne is attempting to control his hypercholesterolemia with diet and exercise. What recommendations about fat intake can Marcia make that will help him lower his total cholesterol and LDL levels and raise his HDL level?

Antioxidants. Cholesterol has been high on the list of dietary villains for years and is thought to be a serious contributor to the development of heart disease. Recent studies indicate that the problem may lie not with the cholesterol itself but with the way it reacts with oxygen, or the process of oxidation, in the bloodstream. The normal body process of using oxygen for energy, combined with environmental factors, such as pollution and tobacco smoke, creates **free radicals**, which can cause cellular damage. Our bodies have developed mechanisms to protect us against oxidizing free radicals through the use of antioxidant vitamins C, E, and beta-carotene, but their amounts are not always sufficient. When enough antioxidants are circulating in the blood, cholesterol is prevented from oxidizing. If the level of antioxidants is insufficient, the opposite is true, and damage to arteries begins. Therefore, in addition to lowering cholesterol, saturated fat, and trans fat intake, increasing dietary intake of antioxidants may prove beneficial in preventing cardiovascular disease. Research indicates that a diet rich in antioxidant vitamins also may be linked to protection against some cancers and **macular degeneration**. Naturally occurring antioxidants are found in many fruits and vegetables and certain seasonings.

FOODS THAT CONTAIN ANTIOXIDANTS

Vitamin C
Broccoli
Cabbage
Cauliflower
Grapefruit
Lemons
Oranges
Peppers
Strawberries
Tangerines

Cantaloupe
Carrots
Kale and spinach
Mustard greens
Pumpkin
Sweet potatoes
Winter squash

Vitamin E
Almonds
Chick peas
Oatmeal
Soy beans
Sunflower seeds
Wheat germ

Mixed Antioxidants
Cloves
Green tea
Oregano
Rice
Rosemary
Sesame
Thyme
Wheat bran
Wine

Beta-Carotene
Apricots
Broccoli

Proteins

Proteins are very large, complex molecules. They are composed of units known as *amino acids,* which are the materials the body uses to build and repair tissues. Twenty amino acids are necessary for normal growth and maintenance of tissues. Of these, eight are essential amino acids that must be included in the diet because humans do not have the enzymes necessary for their formation.

Proteins are classified according to whether they contain all essential amino acids in good proportion. *Complete proteins* come from animal sources and have a mixture of all eight essential amino acids. *Incomplete proteins* do not supply the body with all the essential amino acids. These are the vegetable proteins, which must be used in specific combinations because each is missing or extremely low in one or more of the essential amino acids.

To prevent the wasting of protein for energy and to permit the creation of needed amino acid compounds, dietary protein must be adequate, the diet must supply essential amino acids, and enough carbohydrate and fat must be consumed to prevent the burning of protein for energy. Fortunately, most foods have a mixture of proteins that supplement one another. Because little, if any, storage of amino acids occurs in the body, it is important that a source of protein be included at each meal. Patients with extensive burns or those with wound healing problems often are prescribed high-protein diets to encourage tissue regeneration. Healthy adult women need approximately 45 g of protein a day, and men need approximately 55 to 60 g. The average North American diet contains twice that amount. Excess protein is metabolized and either converted to glucose, burned as fuel, or stored as fat in adipose tissue.

FUNCTIONS OF PROTEIN

- Builds and repairs body tissue, including new tissue, blood, enzymes, and hormones
- Aids the body's defense mechanisms against disease by creating antibodies
- Regulates fluid and electrolyte balance
- Provides energy when carbohydrate and fat stores are depleted

FOOD SOURCES OF PROTEIN

- Complete proteins: Meat, fish, poultry, eggs, and dairy products
- Incomplete proteins: Whole grains (e.g., barley, bulgur, cornmeal, oats, rice, whole-grain breads), cashews, sesame seeds, sunflower seeds, walnuts; soy products, dried legumes, peanuts; broccoli, dark green, leafy vegetables

Recommendations for Protein Consumption

- Consume no more than 18% of daily calories from protein or approximately 91 g of protein per day for a 2,000-calorie diet.
- *2010 Dietary Guidelines for Americans,* from the U.S. Department of Agriculture (USDA), recommends eating 5½ to 6 ounces of cooked lean meat, poultry, or fish each day.
- One ounce of meat equals one egg, ¼ cup of dry beans, 1 tablespoon of peanut butter, ½ cup of cooked beans, or ½ cup of tofu.

If incomplete proteins are the only source of protein in the diet, a food that is protein deficient in one amino acid should be eaten with one that is high in the same amino acid to get the needed mix

of essential amino acids. Vegetarianism has become increasingly popular, and many different forms exist. Some vegetarians consume no red meat but eat fish and poultry. Lacto-ovovegetarians eat primarily vegetable foods but include eggs and/or dairy products in their diets. Lactovegetarians consume milk and milk products in addition to vegetables but no other animal sources of food. Vegans consume no animal proteins at all, relying solely on vegetable foods for protein.

Those who eat some animal protein in the form of fish, eggs, and milk generally are not at risk nutritionally. However, vegans must include a variety of vegetable foods to ensure the nutritional adequacy of their diets. To supply sufficient protein, vegetables that complement each other must be eaten together to get the correct proportion of amino acids. This is customarily done in the diets of different cultures. For example, in Mexico, beans are combined with rice, and in Middle Eastern countries, wheat bread is combined with cheese.

Tips for vegetarians from the USDA Web site *(www.mypyramid.gov)* include the following:

- Build meals around protein sources that are naturally low in fat, such as beans, lentils, and rice, rather than high-fat cheeses.
- Try calcium-fortified, soy-based beverages in place of milk.
- Try vegetarian products such as soy-based sausage patties or links and veggie burgers made from soybeans, vegetables, and/or rice.
- Add meat substitutes, such as tempeh (cultured soybeans with a chewy texture), tofu, or wheat gluten (seitan), to soups and stews to boost protein without adding saturated fat or cholesterol.

EXAMPLES OF NUTRITIONALLY BALANCED INCOMPLETE PROTEIN COMBINATIONS

Combining two or more sources of incomplete amino acids provides a complete protein. For example:
- Black beans and rice
- Peanut butter sandwich on whole-grain bread
- Split-pea soup with whole-grain bread
- Lentil soup and cornbread
- Walnuts, peanuts, and rice
- Whole-wheat pasta, broccoli, and spinach
- Sunflower seeds and navy bean soup

Vitamins (Micronutrients)

Vitamins are organic substances that occur in minute quantities in plant and animal tissues; they are needed for specific metabolic processes to proceed normally. Vitamins function as catalysts and help or allow metabolic reactions to proceed. Originally they were lettered or numbered as they were discovered. However, as they have been identified chemically, they have been given more specific names. In many cases their chemical names are as well known as their letter designations.

Vitamins are divided into two groups: *fat soluble* (A, D, E, and K) and *water soluble* (B complex and C). Some vitamins are nonessential, meaning they can be manufactured in the body. Vitamin A is produced from beta-carotene food sources such as carrots, pumpkin, and sweet potatoes. Ultraviolet light from the sun initiates the production of vitamin D in the skin. Vitamin K is created from intestinal bacteria.

FUNCTIONS OF VITAMINS

- Regulate the synthesis of bone, skin, glands, nerves, brain, and blood
- Aid in the metabolism of protein, carbohydrates, and fats
- Prevent nutritional deficiency diseases
- Support good health at all ages

Vitamins do not cure an illness other than a health problem that is caused by the lack of a specific vitamin. For example, adding vitamin C to a patient's diet does not cure bleeding gums unless the condition is specifically caused by a lack of ascorbic acid (the chemical name for vitamin C). It should also be noted that toxic symptoms from excessive ingestion of fat-soluble vitamins can occur, because these vitamins can be stored in adipose tissue. Water-soluble vitamins typically are excreted in the urine. However, a large intake of some water-soluble vitamins may cause adverse effects (Table 30-3). Nutrition experts agree that vitamins provide the greatest benefit when they are obtained through food as part of the diet rather than in supplement form. However, supplements may be needed in the following cases:

- Patients showing signs and symptoms of a vitamin or mineral deficiency
- Folate for women planning on becoming pregnant or in their childbearing years
- Iron and folate for pregnant and lactating women
- Calcium for lactose-intolerant individuals
- Daily vitamins for the elderly, who may have difficulty chewing, have malabsorption problems, live alone, or make poor food choices
- Postsurgical or burn patients, who require more protein and nutrients to grow and repair tissue
- Strict vegetarians, who may need vitamins B_{12} and D, along with iron and zinc
- Patients who have had gastric bypass surgery, who may require multiple nutrients, including vitamin B_{12}, protein, and iron

Extensive research is underway studying the role vitamins play in disease prevention and treatment. Research indicates that antioxidant vitamins (C, E, and A) may prevent cell membrane damage that leads to cancer and heart disease. Vitamins C and E also appear to protect against the development of cataracts. Vitamin E is recommended to help prevent blood clot formation and coronary heart disease (CHD). The B vitamins may help lower LDL levels, and folic acid is recommended for women planning a pregnancy to prevent **neural tube defects**.

Diet also can affect the action of prescribed medications. For example, vitamin K can interfere with the action of warfarin anticoagulants. Therefore, a sudden dietary increase or decrease in vitamin K–rich foods can alter how long it takes a clot to form in patients undergoing anticoagulant therapy. High levels of vitamin K are found in dark green, leafy vegetables such as kale, collards, Swiss chard, broccoli, and spinach; green tea; and lentils and soy beans. For stable anticoagulant treatment, patients should not increase or reduce their intake of vitamin K–rich foods without consulting their physician. They also should inform the physician if they are taking vitamin supplements that contain vitamin K.

Because vitamins and dietary supplements are categorized as food and not as drugs, no standards or regulatory mechanisms apply to their production. Therefore, various brands differ in the amount of substance available, its quality, and its level of absorption. The U.S. Pharmacopoeia (USP), an independent organization that sets standards for drugs, recently developed standards for vitamins. It is recommended that consumers look for the USP label for products that adhere to these standards.

Minerals (Electrolytes)

The human body requires minerals in relatively small amounts; nevertheless, they are absolutely essential for life (Table 30-4). Of the 19 or more minerals that form the mineral composition of the body, at least 13 are needed to maintain a healthy state. Minerals must be supplied by the diet or by supplements. Recommended daily intakes have been established for 12 minerals. Minerals contribute to the body's water-electrolyte balance and acid-base balance and are essential components of enzymes. Minerals also help regulate muscular and nervous activities, blood clotting, and normal heart rhythm.

Dietary recommendations for the daily intake of minerals, based on a 2,000-calorie diet, are:

- Potassium: 4,000 mg
- Sodium: 1,800 mg
- Calcium: 1,300 mg
- Magnesium: 400 mg
- Copper: 2 mg
- Iron: 18 mg
- Phosphorus: 1,800 mg
- Zinc: 14 mg

Minerals recommended in the largest amounts include sodium, potassium, calcium, chlorine, phosphorus, and magnesium. Those present in very small amounts, the trace elements, include iron, zinc, copper, selenium, chromium, manganese, iodine, and fluorine. The minerals needed only in trace amounts seem either to behave as part of a hormone or enzyme system or to work with vitamins in various metabolic reactions throughout the body. For example, iodine is part of the thyroid hormone thyroxine, and zinc is part of the hormone insulin. Cobalt is an essential part of vitamin B_{12}.

Calcium, iodine, and iron are the minerals most frequently missing in the American diet. Some of the leading causes of disease-related mineral deficiencies are **osteoporosis** from lack of vitamin D and/or calcium and iron-deficiency anemia. High sodium levels are associated with hypertension. Current dietary guidelines recommend that everyone, even children, reduce their sodium intake to less than 2,300 mg a day, which is about 1 teaspoon of salt per day. Adults age 51 or older, African-Americans of any age, and individuals with high blood pressure, diabetes, or chronic kidney disease should consume less than 1,500 mg of sodium a day.

TABLE 30-3 Vitamin Facts

VITAMIN	U.S. RDA*	BEST SOURCES	FUNCTIONS	DEFICIENCY SYMPTOMS†	TOXIC?	PROCESSING TIPS	DID YOU KNOW?
A (carotene)	5,000 IU/day	Yellow or orange fruits and vegetables; green, leafy vegetables; fortified oatmeal; liver; dairy products	Formation and maintenance of skin, hair, and mucous membranes; aids vision in dim light; bone and tooth growth	Night blindness; dry, scaly skin; frequent fatigue	Yes, in high doses, but beta-carotene is nontoxic	Serve fruits and vegetables raw and keep covered and refrigerated; steam vegetables; broil, bake, or braise meats.	Low-fat and skim milk often are fortified with vitamin A, which is removed with the fat.
B₁ (thiamine)	1.5 mg/day	Fortified cereals and oatmeal, meat, rice, pasta, whole grains, liver	Helps the body release energy from carbohydrates during metabolism; growth and muscle tone	Heart irregularity, fatigue, nerve disorders, mental confusion	No, high doses are excreted by the kidneys	Do not rinse rice or pasta before and after cooking. Cook in minimal water.	Pasta and breads made of refined flours have B₁ added because it is lost in the milling process.
B₂ (riboflavin)	1.7 mg/day	Whole grains; green, leafy vegetables; organ meats; milk; eggs	Helps the body release energy from protein, fat, and carbohydrates during metabolism	Cracks in the corners of the mouth, rash, anemia	No toxic effects reported	Store food in containers that light cannot penetrate; cook vegetables in minimal water; roast or broil meats.	Most ready-to-eat cereals are fortified with 25% of the U.S. RDA for vitamin B₂.
B₆ (pyridoxine)	2 mg/day	Fish, poultry, lean meats, bananas, prunes, dried beans, whole grains, avocados	Helps build body tissue and aids metabolism of protein	Convulsions, dermatitis, muscular weakness, skin cracks, anemia	Long-term megadoses may cause nerve damage in hands and feet	Serve fruits raw or cook for shortest time in little water; roast or broil meats.	Because vitamin B₆ aids in the use of protein in the body, the need for it increases with protein intake.
B₁₂ (cobalamin)	6 mcg/day	Meats, milk products, seafood	Aids cell development, functioning of the nervous system, and metabolism of protein and fat	Anemia, nervousness, fatigue, and in some cases, neuritis and brain degeneration	No toxic effects reported	Roast or broil meat and fish.	Vegetarians who do not eat any animal products may need a supplement.
Biotin	0.3 mg/day	Cereal/grain products, yeast, legumes, liver	Involved in the metabolism of protein, fats, and carbohydrates	Nausea; vomiting; depression; hair loss; dry, scaly skin	No toxic effects reported	Storage, processing, and cooking do not appear to affect this vitamin.	Biotin deficiency is extremely rare in the United States.
Folate (folacin, folic acid)	0.4 mg/day	Green, leafy vegetables; organ meats; dried peas, beans, and lentils	Aids in genetic material development and is involved in red blood cell production	Gastrointestinal disorders, anemia, cracks on the lips	Some evidence of toxicity in large doses	Store vegetables in refrigerator and steam, boil, or simmer in minimal water.	Deficiencies can occur in premature infants and pregnant women.

Continued

TABLE 30-3 Vitamin Facts—cont'd

VITAMIN	U.S. RDA*	BEST SOURCES	FUNCTIONS	DEFICIENCY SYMPTOMS†	TOXIC?	PROCESSING TIPS	DID YOU KNOW?
Niacin	20 mg/day	Meat, poultry, fish, enriched cereals, peanuts, potatoes, dairy products, eggs	Involved in carbohydrate, protein, and fat metabolism	Skin disorders, diarrhea, indigestion, general fatigue	Nicotinic acid form should be taken only under physician's care	Roast or broil beef, veal, lamb, and poultry. Cook potatoes in minimal water.	Niacin is formed in the body by converting an amino acid found in proteins.
Pantothenic acid	10 mg/day	Lean meats, whole grains, legumes, vegetables, fruits	Helps in the release of energy from fats and carbohydrates	Fatigue, vomiting, stomach stress, infections, muscle cramps	No toxic effects reported	Serve fruits and vegetables raw.	It is believed some pantothenic acid is produced in the gastrointestinal tract.
C (ascorbic acid)	60 mg/day	Citrus fruits, berries, and vegetables, especially peppers	Essential for structure of bones, cartilage, muscle, and blood vessels; also helps maintain capillaries and gums and aids in absorption of iron	Swollen or bleeding gums, slow wound healing, fatigue/depression, poor digestion	Intake of 1 g or more can cause nausea, cramps, and diarrhea	Do not store or soak fruits and vegetables in water; refrigerate juices and store only 2 to 3 days.	Smokers may benefit from an increased intake of vitamin C.
D	400 IU/day	Fortified milk, sunlight, fish, eggs, butter, fortified margarine	Aids bone and tooth formation; helps maintain heart action and nervous system	In children: rickets and other bone deformities In adults: calcium loss from bones	High intakes may cause diarrhea and weight loss	Storage, processing, and cooking do not appear to affect this vitamin.	Sunlight starts vitamin D production in the skin.
E	30 IU/day	Fortified and multigrain cereals; nuts; wheat germ; vegetable oils; green, leafy vegetables	Protects blood cells, body tissue, and essential fatty acids from harmful destruction in the body	Muscular wasting, nerve damage, anemia, reproductive failure	Relatively nontoxic	Store in air-tight containers away from light.	Most fortified cereals have 40% of RDA.
K	Not established‡	Green, leafy vegetables; fruit; dairy and grain products	Essential for blood clotting functions	Bleeding disorders in newborns and those on blood-thinning medications	Not toxic as found in food	Store in containers away from light.	Vitamin K is also formed by bacteria in the colon.

Information for this chart was obtained from the U.S. Food and Drug Administration, the American Institute for Cancer Research, and the U.S. Department of Agriculture/Human Nutrition Information Service.

IU, International units; mg, milligrams; mcg, micrograms; RDA, recommended dietary allowance.

* For adults and for children over 4 years of age.

†Many of these symptoms also can be attributed to conditions other than vitamin deficiency. If they persist, the patient should see the physician.

‡No official RDA has been established for vitamin K; however, the recommended amount is 1 mcg/kg of body weight.

TABLE 30-4 Functions of Minerals in the Body

FUNCTIONS	SOURCES	DEFICIENCY SYMPTOMS	TOXICITY SYMPTOMS
Calcium (Ca^{2+}) Helps muscles contract and relax, thereby helping to regulate the heartbeat Plays a role in normal functioning of the nervous system Aids blood coagulation and functioning of some enzymes Helps build strong bones and teeth May help prevent hypertension	Primarily found in milk and milk products; also found in dark green, leafy vegetables; tofu and other soy products; sardines; salmon with bones; and hard water	Poor bone growth and tooth development, leading to stunted growth and increased risk of dental caries, rickets (bowing of the legs) in children, osteomalacia (soft bones) and osteoporosis (brittle bones) in adults, poor blood clotting, and possible hypertension	Kidney stones
Chloride (Cl$^-$) Involved in the maintenance of fluid and acid-base balance Provides an acid medium, in the form of hydrochloric acid, for activation of gastric enzymes	Major source is table salt (sodium chloride); also found in fish and vegetables	Disturbances in acid-base balance, with possible growth retardation, psychomotor defects, and memory loss	Disturbances in acid-base balance
Magnesium (Mg^{2+}) Helps build strong bones and teeth Activates many enzymes Participates in protein synthesis and lipid metabolism Helps regulate heartbeat	Raw, dark green vegetables; nuts and soybeans; whole grains and wheat bran; bananas and apricots; seafood; coffee, tea, and cocoa; and hard water	Rare but in disease states may lead to central nervous system problems (confusion, apathy, hallucinations, poor memory) and neuromuscular problems (muscle weakness, cramps, tremor, cardiac arrhythmia)	Drowsiness, weakness, and lethargy Severe toxicity: skeletal paralysis, central nervous system depression, respiratory depression, and ultimately coma and death
Phosphorus (PO$_4$) Helps build strong bones and teeth Present in the nuclei of all cells Aids the oxidation of fats and carbohydrates (energy metabolism) Helps maintain acid-base balance	Milk and milk products, eggs, meats, legumes, whole grains, soft drinks (used to make the "fizz")	Rare but with malabsorption can cause anorexia, weakness, stiff joints, and fragile bones	Hypocalcemic tetany (muscle spasms)
Potassium (K$^+$) Plays a key role in fluid and acid-base balance Transmits nerve impulses, helps control muscle contractions, and promotes regular heartbeat Needed for enzyme reactions	Apricots, bananas, oranges, grapefruit, raisins, green beans, broccoli, carrots, greens, potatoes, meats, milk and milk products, peanut butter and legumes, molasses, coffee, tea, cocoa	Possibly impaired growth, hypertension, bone fragility, central nervous system changes, renal hypertrophy, diminished heart rate, and death	Hyperkalemia (excess potassium in the blood) with cardiac function disturbances

Continued

TABLE 30-4 Functions of Minerals in the Body—cont'd

FUNCTIONS	SOURCES	DEFICIENCY SYMPTOMS	TOXICITY SYMPTOMS
Sodium (Na⁺) Plays a key role in the maintenance of acid-base balance Transmits nerve impulses and helps control muscle contractions Regulates cell membrane permeability	Salt (sodium chloride) is the major dietary source; minor sources are foods such as milk and milk products and several vegetables	Hyponatremia (too little sodium in the blood)	May cause hypertension, which can lead to cardiovascular diseases and renal (kidney) disease; salt tablets can cause gastric irritation
Chromium (Cr³⁺) Activates several enzymes Enhances the removal of glucose from the blood	Liver and other meats, whole grains, cheese, legumes, and brewer's yeast	Weight loss, abnormalities of the central nervous system, and possible aggravation of diabetes mellitus	Inhibited insulin activity
Copper (Cu²⁺) Aids in the production and survival of red blood cells A component of many enzymes involved in respiration Plays a role in normal lipid metabolism	Shellfish (especially oysters), liver, nuts and seeds, raisins, whole grains, and chocolate	Anemia, central nervous system problems, abnormal electrocardiograms, bone fragility, impaired immune response; may be a factor in failure to thrive in premature infants	In Wilson's disease and Huntington's chorea (both hereditary diseases), copper accumulation causes neuron and liver cell damage
Fluorine (Fl⁻) Aids the formation of solid bones and teeth, thereby reducing the incidence of dental caries, and may help prevent osteoporosis	Fluoridated water (and foods cooked in fluoridated water), fish, tea, gelatin	Increased susceptibility to dental caries	Fluorosis and mottling of teeth
Iodine (I⁻) Helps regulate energy metabolism as part of thyroid hormones Essential for normal cell functioning, helps to keep skin, hair, and nails healthy	Primarily from iodized salt, also found in saltwater fish, seaweed products, and vegetables grown in iodine-rich soils	Goiter, cretinism in infants born to iodine-deficient mothers, with accompanying mental retardation and diffuse central nervous system abnormalities	Little toxic effect in individuals with normal thyroid gland functioning

Iron (Fe^{3+})

Essential to the formation of hemoglobin, which is important for tissue respiration and ultimately growth and development

A component of several enzymes and proteins in the body

Heme sources: organ meats, especially liver, red meats, and other meats
Nonheme sources: iron-fortified cereals; dark green, leafy vegetables; legumes; whole grains; blackstrap molasses; dried fruit; and foods cooked in iron pans

Iron-deficiency anemia and possible alterations that impair behavior

Idiopathic hemochromatosis, which can lead to cirrhosis, diabetes mellitus, skin pigmentation, arthralgias (joint pain), and cardiomyopathy

Manganese (Mn^{2+})

Needed for normal bone structure, reproduction, and normal functioning of cells and the central nervous system

A component of some enzymes

Nuts, whole grains, vegetables and fruits, coffee, tea, cocoa, and egg yolks

None observed in humans

Iron-deficiency anemia through inhibiting effect on iron absorption; pulmonary changes, anorexia, apathy, impotence, headaches, leg cramps, and speech impairment; in advanced stages of toxicity resembles Parkinson's disease

Selenium (Se)

Acts as an antioxidant with vitamin E to protect cells from oxidative damage

A component of an enzyme system

Protein-rich foods (meat, eggs; milk), whole grains, seafood, liver and other meats, egg yolks, and garlic

Keshan disease (a human cardiomyopathy) and Kashin-Bek disease (an endemic human osteoarthropathy)

Physical defects of the fingernails and toenails; also hair loss

Zinc (Zn^{2+})

Plays a role in protein synthesis

Essential for normal growth and sexual development, wound healing, immune function, cell division and differentiation, and smell acuity

Whole grains, wheat germ, crabmeat, oyster, liver and other meats, brewer's yeast

Depressed immune function, poor growth, dwarfism, impaired skeletal growth and delayed sexual maturation, acrodermatitis

Severe anemia, nausea, vomiting, abdominal cramps, diarrhea, fever, hypocupremia (low blood serum copper), malaise, fatigue

From Poleman CM, Peckenpaugh NJ: *Nutrition essentials and diet therapy*, ed 6, Philadelphia, 1991, Saunders; Garrison RH, Somer E: *The nutrition desk reference*, New Canaan, Conn, 1985, Keats Publishing; and Griffeth HW: *Complete guide to vitamins, minerals and supplements*, Tucson, 1988, Fisher Books.

SODIUM, BLOOD PRESSURE, AND THE DASH DIET

Research has proven that individuals with a sodium intake of more than 2,400 mg a day have a high risk of developing hypertension. On average, adults in the United States are estimated to consume 3,300 mg of sodium per day. A healthy body excretes excess sodium through the kidneys, but sodium's attraction for fluid can cause hypertension to develop. How can you cut down on salt intake? You should avoid pickles, olives, and sauerkraut; all processed meats (lunch meat) and processed fish, but especially those that are smoked; salty snacks; fast and processed foods; canned soups; and cheese, especially processed.

The Dietary Approaches to Stop Hypertension (DASH) diet has been recommended as a means of lowering blood pressure. Daily guidelines for the DASH diet include the following:

- Four to five servings of both fruits and vegetables
- Seven to eight servings of whole grains
- 6 ounces or less of meat, fish, and poultry
- Four to five servings per week of nuts, seeds, and dry beans
- 2 to 3 cups of milk
- 2 to 3 teaspoons of oils
- 5 tablespoons of added sugar per week
- 1,500 to 2,000 mg of sodium per day
- Total fat should not exceed 22% of calories

Water

Water is all too often overlooked when nutritional status is evaluated. The body is approximately 80% water and can survive longer without food than it can without water. Water is part of almost every vital body process.

Water is lost daily from the body in urine, feces, sweat, and expiration. Extensive water losses from diarrhea, vomiting, burns, or perspiration can lead to electrolyte losses that result in life-threatening imbalances. Water is contained in almost all foods; however, a healthy diet should include about eight glasses of water a day.

FUNCTIONS OF WATER

- Plays a key role in the maintenance of body temperature
- Acts as a solvent and the medium for most biochemical reactions
- Acts as the vehicle for transport of substances such as nutrients, hormones, antibodies, and metabolic waste
- Acts as a lubricant for joints and mucous membranes

CHOOSE MYPLATE

In 1992, to reflect dietary guidelines that called for more consumption of grains and less consumption of meat, sweets, and fats, the USDA introduced the Food Guide Pyramid. In 2011 the Pyramid design was changed to a dinner plate icon that represents how to

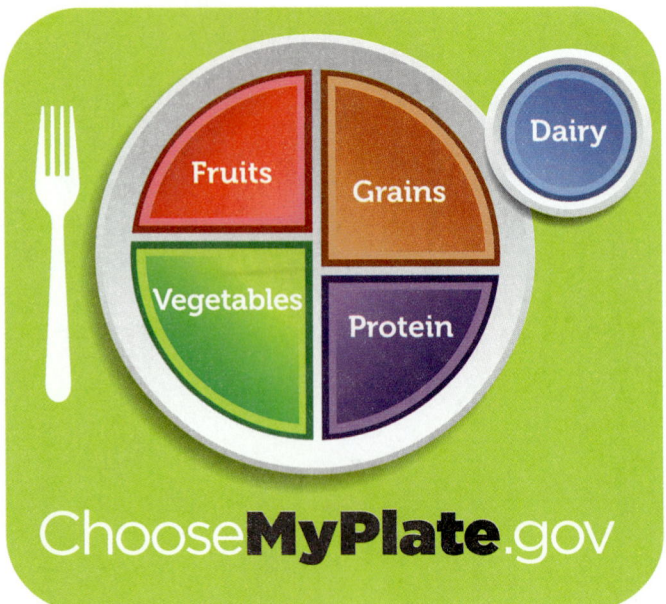

FIGURE 30-1 Choose MyPlate. (From US Department of Agriculture: Accessed September 10, 2011. Available at *www.choosemyplate.gov*).

build a healthy plate at mealtime. The plate includes choices from the five basic food groups, with recommendations based on the *2010 Dietary Guidelines for Americans* (Figure 30-1). At the ChooseMyPlate Web site *(www.choosemyplate.gov)*, consumers can determine individual dietary needs that match their particular age, health status, exercise level, and food preferences. Students should use the Web site to take advantage of the many learning opportunities. It is also an excellent source for patient education information on dietary guidelines.

Current recommendations include the following:

1. *Balance calorie intake*: Use the ChooseMyPlate Web site to determine how many calories are needed each day to manage your weight; include exercise to help balance calories; enjoy food but eat less; avoid oversized portions. Use a smaller plate, bowl, and glass. When eating out, choose a smaller size option, share a dish, or take home part of your meal.
2. *Foods to eat more often*: Increase your daily intake of vegetables, fruits, whole grains, and fat-free or 1% milk and dairy products. Make half your plate fruits and vegetables. Make half your grains whole grains.
3. *Foods to eat less often*: Cut back on foods high in solid fats, added sugars, and salt. Use food labels to compare sodium content and choose lower sodium versions.
4. *Drink water instead of sugary drinks.*

Many patients have never been educated in nutrition and do not know how to plan a healthy diet for themselves or their families. Good nutrition is a balance between carbohydrates, protein, vitamins, minerals, fiber, and water, with limited amounts of fat, sodium, sugar, and alcohol. Calorie intake must be balanced with energy output to maintain a healthy body weight.

HIGHLIGHTS OF THE U.S. DEPARTMENT OF AGRICULTURE'S DIETARY RECOMMENDATIONS

Adequate Nutrients within Caloric Needs

- Consume a variety of nutrient-dense foods while limiting saturated and trans fats, cholesterol, added sugars and salts, and alcohol.
- Meet dietary recommendations by adopting a balanced eating pattern.
- Most Americans need to increase consumption of vitamin E, calcium, potassium, and fiber.
- Childbearing women should increase their intake of iron-rich and folic acid–containing foods or take supplements.
- Individuals over age 50 should consume vitamin B_{12}-fortified foods.
- Aging individuals, those with dark skin, and people who are not exposed to sunlight should eat vitamin D–fortified foods or take a supplement.

Weight Management

- Balance the intake of calories with those expended.
- With aging, calories should be decreased and physical activity increased to prevent gradual weight gain over time.
- Those who need to lose weight should do so slowly.
- Reducing the caloric intake by 50 to 100 calories per day prevents weight gain; reducing it by 500 calories a day promotes weight loss.
- Control portion sizes and reduce the intake of saturated fats, added sugars, and alcohol.

Carbohydrates

- Choose fiber-rich fruits, vegetables, and whole grains.
- Limit the use of added sugar and sweeteners.
- Practice good dental hygiene and limit sugary snacks to reduce dental caries.

Sodium and Potassium

- Consume less than 2,300 mg of sodium per day (approximately 1 teaspoon of salt).
- Consume potassium-rich foods.

Alcoholic Beverages

- Use moderate consumption: one drink per day for women and two for men.
- Avoid alcohol if you are or may become pregnant or if lactating.

Food Safety

- Clean all fruits, vegetables, and cooking surfaces.
- Keep raw, cooked, and ready to eat foods separate.
- Cook foods to the recommended temperature to kill microbes.
- Chill perishable foods and defrost foods properly.
- Avoid unpasteurized milk products, raw eggs, and raw or undercooked meats.

Physical Activity

- Engage in 30 to 60 minutes of moderate physical activity per day to prevent weight gain; 60 to 90 minutes for weight loss.
- Children and adolescents should be physically active 60 minutes a day.

- Aging people should participate in regular exercise to maintain function.
- Include aerobic activity, stretching, and weight training.

Food Groups to Encourage

- For a 2,000-calorie diet, consume 2 cups of fruit and 2½ cups of vegetables a day.
- Eat dark green and orange vegetables, legumes, and starches several times a week.
- At least half of the grains consumed should be whole grains.
- Consume 3 cups of fat-free or low-fat milk or milk products a day; children age 2 to 8 years should consume 2 cups a day.

Fats

- Less than 10% of calories should come from saturated fats and less than 300 mg of cholesterol should be consumed each day; keep trans fats as low as possible.
- Consume less than 35% of calories from fat.
- Choose low-fat or fat-free milk products and lean meats.

NUTRITIONAL STATUS ASSESSMENT

During the physician's examination of the patient, he or she will assess the patient's nutritional status. The physician considers the patient's age; height and weight; body mass index (BMI); overall health status; any recent changes in weight; diet and exercise habits; and lifestyle, culture, and educational background. In addition to this information, the physician may check the patient's skin **turgor** to determine the level of hydration and perform various techniques to assess the percentage of body fat.

Body Fat Measurement

The location of body fat may be related to an increased risk of developing diabetes, stroke, hypertension, and coronary artery disease. Studies indicate that the body has two places to store fat: at the hips and in the abdomen. Fat at the hips is more common in women and is used to store energy for special purposes, such as during pregnancy and breastfeeding. Abdominal fat, or central obesity, seems to be more dangerous to overall health. Health risks related to weight range from no increased risk with normal weight to severe risk from central obesity, with the risk from other types of obesity falling somewhere in between.

To determine the patient's status, the waist and hips are measured and correlated with the waist to hip ratio (the bigger the belly, the higher the ratio). Normal ratios are less than 0.75 in women and 0.90 to 0.95 in men. Waist measurements also can predict the risk of developing a weight-related disease. Men at increased risk for disease have a waist measurement greater than 40 inches (102 cm); for women, the risk is increased with a waist measurement greater than 35 inches (88 cm).

At the physician's request, the medical assistant may perform body fat measurements on a patient. The percentage of body fat may be an indicator of overall health and of risk for cardiovascular disease. Body fat can be measured by several methods. A reliable method of

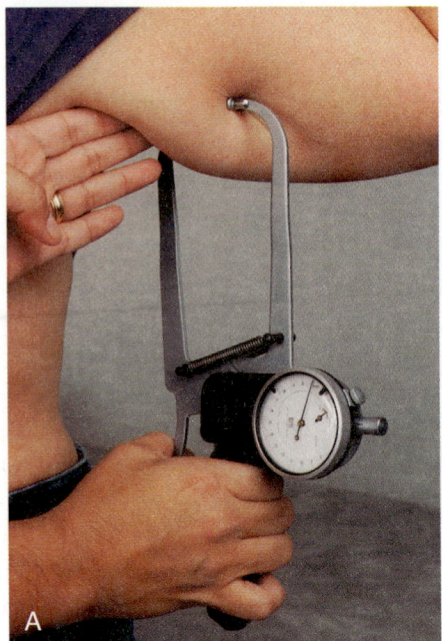 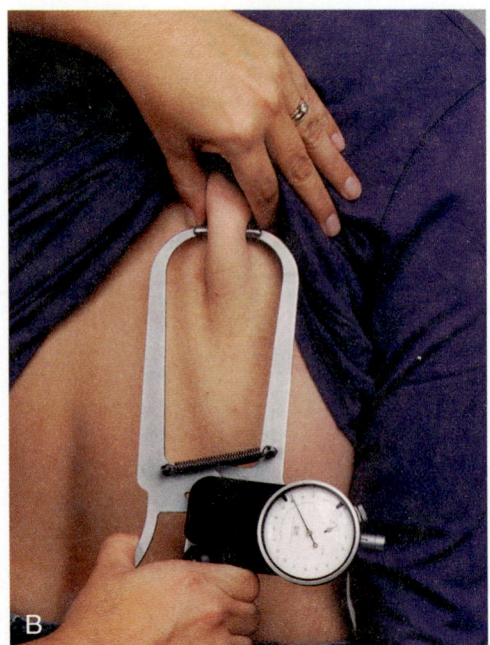

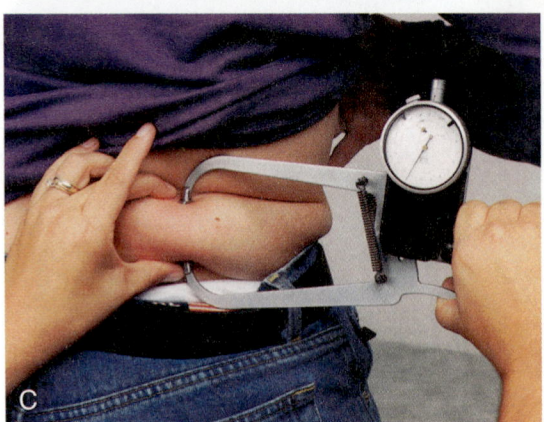

FIGURE 30-2 Determining fat fold measurements. **A**, Triceps. **B**, Subscapular. **C**, Suprailiac.

measuring body fat uses a specially designed caliper to measure the thickness of a fold of tissue in three areas: the triceps, the subscapular, and the suprailiac regions (Figure 30-2). However, an increasing number of patients have fat folds that are too large for calipers to measure. The physician may also order a dual energy x-ray absorptiometry (DEXA) scan, in which two x-ray beams are used to give accurate feedback on the body fat percentage, where the fat is distributed, and bone density.

Body Mass Index

To determine how healthy a patient's weight level is, the physician may ask the medical assistant to calculate the patient's BMI. The BMI is the relationship of weight to height that mathematically correlates the patient's measurements with health risks. It is a more accurate predictor of weight-related diseases than traditional height-weight charts because it provides a good estimate of the degree of body fat.

A patient's BMI can be determined by two methods. The nomogram in Figure 30-3 can be implemented using the patient's weight in kilograms or pounds and height in centimeters or inches. To practice using the nomogram, angle the edge of a piece of paper or a ruler from your weight (on the left) to your height (on the right). Then read the BMI based on your gender where the edge crosses the centerline. The BMI also can be calculated mathematically by dividing the weight in kilograms by the square of the height in meters (BMI = Weight [kg] | Height [m^2]). However, most physicians' offices have either a wheel device the medical assistant can use to determine the patient's BMI or a BMI chart (Table 30-5). Most physicians require the medical assistant to record the patient's BMI after the height and weight have been measured, because decisions on the patient's health status are based on the BMI. Table 30-6 correlates the BMI with risks for disease.

Individuals with a BMI of 19 to 22 are thought to live the longest. Death rates are significantly higher for people with a BMI of 25 or above. If the risk is anything other than acceptable, dietary modifications may be needed. The physician must make this decision when all the information on the patient has been evaluated.

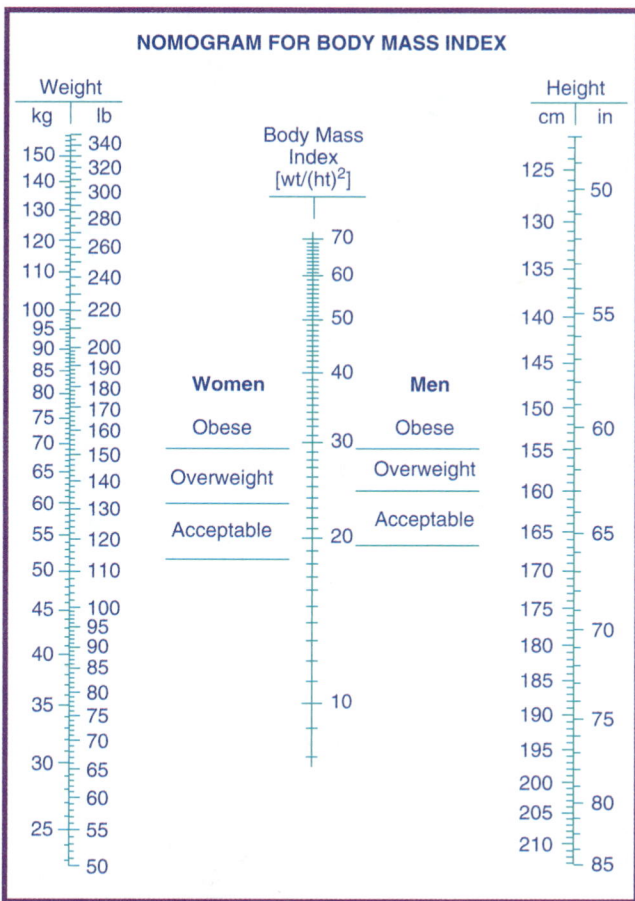

FIGURE 30-3 Nomogram for body mass index.

CRITICAL THINKING APPLICATION   30-3
The physician encourages Mr. Hawthorne to lose weight to lower his BMI of 29. Explain how Marcia should teach Mr. Hawthorne about the importance of his BMI, how it is measured, and how he can calculate this value at home.

THERAPEUTIC NUTRITION

Although most patients are treated medically, without a therapeutic diet, some illnesses and diseases can be cured and some patients' recovery can be facilitated by the use of special diets. For example, patients with hypertension, hypercholesterolemia, certain gastrointestinal diseases, and **diabetes mellitus type 1** and **type 2** all benefit from a therapeutically planned diet. It is important to take into consideration the patient's lifestyle, cultural influences, and background to ensure cooperation.

Modifying a Diet

The following features of a normal diet (or combinations of them) can be modified to create a therapeutic diet:

- Consistency
- Calorie level
- Amounts of one or more nutrients
- Degree of bulk or fiber
- Spiciness
- Levels of specific foods

In general, a normal diet is modified by restricting or increasing the foods that are sources of the nutrient involved in the disease process. Except for the nutrient in question, the recommended daily allowances usually can be met. However, if several restrictions are ordered for the same patient, a nutrient supplement may be necessary.

Liquid Diet

Two types of liquid diets are used. A clear liquid diet includes only transparent or translucent liquids, such as broth soups, tea, and gelatin. In some cases, apple juice and cranberry juice may be allowed. A full liquid diet includes all foods allowed on a clear liquid diet plus milk, custards, strained cream soups, refined cereals, eggnog, milkshakes, and all juices. This diet may be indicated as part of preparation for certain diagnostic tests (e.g., colonoscopy) or for the first several days after major surgery.

Soft or Light Diet

When a soft or light diet is prescribed, foods with roughage are eliminated (no raw fruits or vegetables). No strongly flavored or gas-forming vegetables are allowed (e.g., onions, beans, broccoli, and cauliflower), and spices also may be limited. This diet often is used after surgery to place less strain on the gastrointestinal system or for patients with certain gastrointestinal disorders.

Mechanical Soft Diet

A mechanical soft diet is a regular diet in which the food is chopped, ground, or pureed, depending on the degree of texture change required. No foods or spices are restricted. This diet may be used after dental or oral surgery or for patients who have difficulty chewing or swallowing.

Bland Diet

A bland diet restricts dietary components classified as gastrointestinal irritants. Such a diet limits any foods that are chemically irritating (e.g., caffeine, pepper, chili, nutmeg, and alcohol) or mechanically irritating (e.g., high-fiber foods). No fried foods or highly concentrated sweets are allowed. Gas-forming vegetables belonging to the onion and cabbage family also are eliminated. A bland diet commonly is used for problems of the gastrointestinal tract. Such a diet should supply sufficient nutrients for the individual to meet the recommended daily allowances, unless fruits and vegetables are eliminated.

Elimination Diet

Diets that modify the levels of specific foods most frequently are used to treat allergies of various kinds. Two basic elimination regimens are used. A simple elimination diet removes only one or two foods that are suspected of causing the allergy. The Rowe elimination diet involves a more extensive program. With this method, the basic diet consists of a few hypoallergenic foods, such as rice cereal, apples, pears, carrots, sweet potatoes, lamb, and milk substitutes. In children, if no allergic reaction is observed, single food-family groups are added slowly over about 10 days while the child is observed for the onset of allergic symptoms. The most common food allergies

TABLE 30-5 Body Mass Index Chart*

HEIGHT (in)	19	20	21	22	23	24	25	26	27	28	29	30	31	32	33	34	35
							BODY WEIGHT (lb)										
58	91	96	100	105	110	115	119	124	129	134	138	143	148	153	158	162	167
59	94	99	104	109	114	119	124	128	133	138	143	148	153	158	163	168	173
60	97	102	107	112	118	123	128	133	138	143	148	153	158	163	168	174	179
61	100	106	111	116	122	127	132	137	143	148	153	158	164	169	174	180	185
62	104	109	115	120	126	131	136	142	147	153	158	164	169	175	180	186	191
63	107	113	118	124	130	135	141	146	152	158	163	169	175	180	186	191	197
64	110	116	122	128	134	140	145	151	157	163	169	174	180	186	192	197	204
65	114	120	126	132	138	144	150	156	162	168	174	180	186	192	198	204	210
66	118	124	130	136	142	148	155	161	167	173	179	186	192	198	204	210	216
67	121	127	134	140	146	153	159	166	172	178	185	191	198	204	211	217	223
68	125	131	138	144	151	158	164	171	177	184	190	197	203	210	216	223	230
69	128	135	142	149	155	162	169	176	182	189	196	203	209	216	223	230	236
70	132	139	146	153	160	167	174	181	188	195	202	209	216	222	229	236	243
71	136	143	150	157	165	172	179	186	193	200	208	215	222	229	236	243	250
72	140	147	154	162	169	177	184	191	199	206	213	221	228	235	242	250	258
73	144	151	159	166	174	182	189	197	204	212	219	227	235	242	250	257	265
74	148	155	163	171	179	186	194	202	210	218	225	233	241	249	256	264	272
75	152	160	168	176	184	192	200	208	216	224	232	240	248	256	264	272	279
76	156	164	172	180	189	197	205	213	221	230	238	246	254	263	271	279	287

*To use the table, find the appropriate height in the left-hand column. Move across to a given weight. The number at the top of the column is the BMI at that height and weight. Pounds have been rounded off.

From the National Institutes of Health/National Heart, Lung, and Blood Institute: *Clinical guidelines on the identification, evaluation, and treatment of overweight and obesity in adults: the evidence report,* June 1998. Accessed January 12, 2010. Available at *www.nhlbi.nih.gov/guidelines/obesity/bmi_tbl.htm.*

TABLE 30-6 Body Mass Index and Disease Risk

BODY MASS INDEX	CLASSIFICATION	DISEASE RISK
18.5 or less	Underweight	Low
18.5-24.9	Normal weight	Low
25-29.9	Overweight	Increased
30-34.9	Obese	High
35-39.9	Obese	Very high
40 or greater	Extremely obese	Extremely high

bowel. In either case, foods high in cellulose are considered to be high in fiber, because the body does not digest this carbohydrate well, and a residue is left in the colon. In some instances, a low-residue diet is distinguished from a low-fiber diet. In this case, a low-fiber diet eliminates foods with high cellulose content, and a low-residue diet restricts milk in addition to fiber content. Either diet should supply all the nutrients needed; however, if milk is restricted drastically, the calcium level must be watched carefully. Low-fiber diets are prescribed for patients with certain gastrointestinal disorders such as diverticulitis. High-fiber diets are recommended for patients with hypercholesterolemia or diabetes mellitus and to prevent certain forms of cancer.

Diabetic Diet

The specific diet for a patient with diabetes is determined by the individual's health needs. The basic goal of managing the disease is to maintain consistent control of the blood glucose level. When developing a diabetic diet plan, the physician or dietitian must consider additional factors, such as the need for weight control, individual patient preferences, exercise patterns, and lifestyle factors.

seen in children are chocolate, wheat, eggs, and milk. With some children, meeting the recommended daily allowances for all nutrients may be difficult; in such cases, supplements should be ordered.

High- or Low-Fiber Diet

The amount of bulk or fiber in the diet is either increased or decreased, depending on the specific disorder of the colon or large

TABLE 30-7 Diabetic Diet Exchanges per Day

EXCHANGE GROUPS AND SERVING SIZES	NUMBER OF EXCHANGES OR SERVINGS IN EACH GROUP				
	1,200*	1,500*	1,800*	2,000*	2,200*
Starch or bread: One exchange equals 1 oz. bread and ½ cup cooked cereal, grain, or pasta	5	8	10	11	13
Meat and cheese: One exchange equals 1 oz.; high-fat exchanges should be used no more than three times per week	4	5	7	8	8
Vegetables: One exchange equals ½ cup cooked, 1 cup raw, and ½ cup juice	2	3	3	4	4
Fruits and sugar: No more than 10% of total daily carbohydrates; each exchange equals 15 g carbohydrate	3	3	3	3	3
Milk products: One exchange equals 1 cup (8 oz); skim and very-low-fat milk products are recommended	2	2	2	2	2
Fats: One exchange equals 1 teaspoon of fat	3	3	3	4	5

*Number of calories in the prescribed diabetic diet.

General guidelines for a healthy diabetic diet include the following:

- Five servings of dark-colored fruits and vegetables and six of whole grains each day
- Two weekly servings of fatty fish (salmon, cod, mackerel)
- Complex carbohydrates that are high in fiber (e.g., whole grains)
- Monounsaturated fats (olive and canola oil)
- Daily serving of nuts, seeds, or legumes
- Fish or soy over poultry or other meat
- Avoidance of fad diets, especially those with high-protein, low-carbohydrate foods
- Reduced salt intake
- Avoidance of saturated fats (animal fat) and trans fats

Traditionally, the diabetic diet has been based on exchange lists, which group foods according to similar calorie, carbohydrate, protein, and fat content. The objective of exchange lists is to achieve the proper balance of carbohydrates, proteins, and fats while maintaining healthy weight and blood glucose levels. Menus are developed based on the food groupings and the optimum number of daily calories needed to meet the patient's needs. Foods can be substituted for one another within an exchange list but not among lists. A copy of the exchange list can be obtained from the American Diabetes Association. Table 30-7 lists the number of exchanges per day allowed within certain calorie-restricted diabetic diets.

Diabetes educators agree, however, that the simplest way to teach patients about the relationship between diet and blood glucose levels is to focus on the total number of carbohydrates patients can consume daily while maintaining their recommended blood glucose level. Patients then can decide how they want to distribute carbohydrate intake throughout the day. The number of grams of carbohydrate a patient with diabetes can eat each day is determined by a combination of the following factors: the patient's weight and whether weight loss or maintenance is part of the treatment plan; the level of exercise, because physical activity lowers the blood glucose level; prescribed diabetic medications, including insulin; and other factors, such as age and blood lipid levels.

TABLE 30-8 Grams of Carbohydrate in Breakfast Foods

FOOD TYPE	SERVING SIZE	CARBOHYDRATE (g)
1% Reduced fat milk	1 cup	12
Bran Chex	⅔ cup	23
Frosted Flakes	¾ cup	26
Apples and cinnamon instant oatmeal	1 packet	27
Low-fat granola	½ cup	30
Toast	1 slice	15
White table sugar	1 teaspoon	4
Pancakes	2	15
Pancake syrup	2 tablespoons	30
Light pancake syrup	2 tablespoons	4
Fruit yogurt	1 cup	40
Fruit yogurt with NutraSweet	1 cup	19
Fruit juice	½ cup	15
Banana	½	15

Therefore, people with diabetes can eat sugary foods as long as they restrict themselves to the total number of carbohydrates allowed for that snack or meal and the decision to eat that food adheres to the rules of healthy nutrition. In other words, a patient with diabetes can have a whole-wheat raisin bagel for breakfast as long as the total carbohydrate grams for that food do not exceed the number of carbohydrates that should be eaten for that particular meal. Table 30-8 presents breakfast choices for a patient with diabetes restricted to a total of 50 g of carbohydrate.

All carbohydrates raise the blood glucose level to a similar degree. In general, 1 g of carbohydrate raises the blood sugar level of a person who weighs 150 pounds by 4 points; for a person who weighs 200 pounds, it raises the level by 3 points. However, not all carbohydrates raise the blood glucose level at the same rate. Choosing a carbohydrate that takes longer to affect the blood glucose level helps control hyperglycemic peaks, which are associated with the complications of diabetes mellitus. A rating system known as the Glycemic Index may help solve this problem. The Glycemic Index rates carbohydrate foods on a scale from slowest to fastest effects on blood glucose levels. The lower the Glycemic Index value of the food, the longer it takes to raise the patient's blood glucose level. One of the scales is based on 100 glycemic units, which is equivalent to the number of units in a glucose tablet. The Glycemic Index of foods helps diabetics understand the impact of different carbohydrates on the blood glucose level, but it can be a complicated tool to understand, and it must be used in conjunction with a dietary plan that considers the nutritional guidelines for all foods.

GLYCEMIC INDEX (GI) VALUES OF SOME FOODS

FOOD	GI VALUE (0-100 SCALE)
Honey	91
Puffed rice	90
White potato	87
Corn chips	72
White rice	72
Whole-wheat bread	72
Shredded wheat	70
Brown rice	66
Refined sugar	64
Rye bread	64
Oatmeal cookies	57
Potato chips	56
Oatmeal	53
Sweet potato	50
Spaghetti	38
Yogurt	38
Milk	34
Kidney beans	33
Fructose	22
Soybeans	14

CRITICAL THINKING APPLICATION   30-4

Samantha Rashad recently was diagnosed with diabetes mellitus type 2. She has met with the dietitian, but she has some questions about her 1,200-calorie diabetic diet. The goals of her dietary management are to maintain blood glucose levels within normal range while encouraging weight loss. Based on Marcia's knowledge of the components of a healthy diet, what recommendations can she make to Ms. Rashad?

Heart-Healthy Diet

The goals for a heart-healthy diet are to encourage the patient to eat foods that reduce the overall cholesterol levels and LDL, increase the HDL, and keep blood pressure within normal limits. Other factors that must be considered for patients at risk for heart disease are obesity and the patient's typical exercise patterns. Obesity is associated with elevated lipid levels; therefore, weight management must be part of the patient's dietary plan. In addition, researchers report that an aerobic exercise program must be included to maintain cholesterol at a healthy level.

AMERICAN HEART ASSOCIATION EATING PLAN FOR HEALTHY AMERICANS

- Eat at least 4.5 cups a day of a variety of fruits and vegetables.
- Eat six or more servings a day of a variety of grain products, with at least 3 servings a day of fiber-rich whole grains.
- Eat fish at least twice a week, particularly fatty fish (e.g., salmon).
- Include fat-free and low-fat milk products, legumes, skinless poultry, and lean meats.
- Choose fats and oils with 2 g or less of saturated fat per tablespoon (e.g., canola or olive oil).
- Limit the intake of foods high in calories or low in nutrition.
- Limit foods high in saturated fat, trans fat, and/or cholesterol.
- Eat less than 1,500 mg of sodium a day.
- Limit sugar-sweetened beverages to no more than 36 ounces a week.
- Eat at least 4 servings a week of nuts, legumes and seeds.
- Eat no more than 2 servings a week of processed meats.
- Women should limit their alcohol intake to one drink a day and men to two drinks a day.
- Balance calorie intake with the number of calories burned each day. If overweight or obese, multiply your ideal body weight by 15 (active) or 13 (not active) to find the number of calories you should eat to gradually achieve your ideal body weight.
- Get enough physical activity to keep fit. Exercise at least 30 minutes every day.

From the American Heart Association Nutrition Center: Accessed September 9, 2011. Available at www.heart.org/HEARTORG/GettingHealthy/NutritionCenter/HealthyDietGoals.

CROSS-CULTURAL TIPS FOR REDUCING SODIUM AND FAT

- Limit the use of soy or teriyaki sauce, even the low-sodium type.
- Eat fresh or frozen fruits and vegetables; choose canned products low in sodium or rinse them before eating.
- Bake or broil meats rather than frying; limit beef products; remove skin from chicken before cooking; increase the intake of unprocessed fish.
- Cook with olive or canola oil.
- Limit servings of cured foods, such as ham and bacon; avoid pickles and other foods prepared in brine; limit condiments such as mustard and ketchup.
- Cook rice and pasta without added salt; do not use instant versions, which are higher in sodium.
- Do not add salt to food; use substitute spices, such as lemon, lime, and herbs.

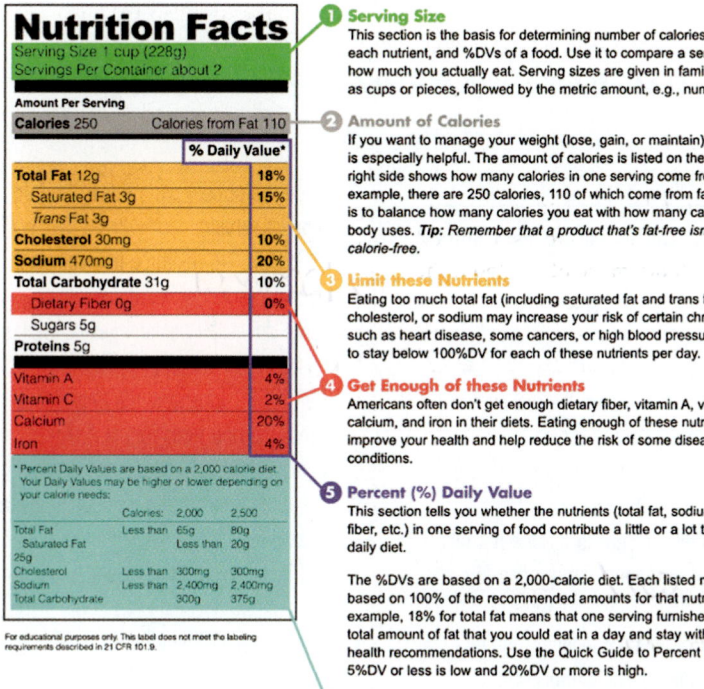

Nutrition Facts
Serving Size 1 cup (228g)
Servings Per Container about 2

Amount Per Serving

Calories 250   Calories from Fat 110

	% Daily Value*
Total Fat 12g	18%
Saturated Fat 3g	15%
Trans Fat 3g	
Cholesterol 30mg	10%
Sodium 470mg	20%
Total Carbohydrate 31g	10%
Dietary Fiber 0g	0%
Sugars 5g	
Proteins 5g	
Vitamin A	4%
Vitamin C	2%
Calcium	20%
Iron	4%

* Percent Daily Values are based on a 2,000 calorie diet. Your Daily Values may be higher or lower depending on your calorie needs:

	Calories:	2,000	2,500
Total Fat	Less than	65g	80g
Saturated Fat	Less than	20g	25g
Cholesterol	Less than	300mg	300mg
Sodium	Less than	2,400mg	2,400mg
Total Carbohydrate		300g	375g

For educational purposes only. This label does not meet the labeling requirements described in 21 CFR 101.9.

① Serving Size
This section is the basis for determining number of calories, amount of each nutrient, and %DVs of a food. Use it to compare a serving size to how much you actually eat. Serving sizes are given in familiar units, such as cups or pieces, followed by the metric amount, e.g., number of grams.

② Amount of Calories
If you want to manage your weight (lose, gain, or maintain), this section is especially helpful. The amount of calories is listed on the left side. The right side shows how many calories in one serving come from fat. In this example, there are 250 calories, 110 of which come from fat. The key is to balance how many calories you eat with how many calories your body uses. *Tip: Remember that a product that's fat-free isn't necessarily calorie-free.*

③ Limit these Nutrients
Eating too much total fat (including saturated fat and trans fat), cholesterol, or sodium may increase your risk of certain chronic diseases, such as heart disease, some cancers, or high blood pressure. The goal is to stay below 100%DV for each of these nutrients per day.

④ Get Enough of these Nutrients
Americans often don't get enough dietary fiber, vitamin A, vitamin C, calcium, and iron in their diets. Eating enough of these nutrients may improve your health and help reduce the risk of some diseases and conditions.

⑤ Percent (%) Daily Value
This section tells you whether the nutrients (total fat, sodium, dietary fiber, etc.) in one serving of food contribute a little or a lot to your total daily diet.

The %DVs are based on a 2,000-calorie diet. Each listed nutrient is based on 100% of the recommended amounts for that nutrient. For example, 18% for total fat means that one serving furnishes 18% of the total amount of fat that you could eat in a day and stay within public health recommendations. Use the Quick Guide to Percent DV (%DV): 5%DV or less is low and 20%DV or more is high.

⑥ Footnote with Daily Values (DVs)
The footnote provides information about the DVs for important nutrients, including fats, sodium and fiber. The DVs are listed for people who eat 2,000 or 2,500 calories each day.

— The amounts for total fat, saturated fat, cholesterol, and sodium are maximum amounts. That means you should try to stay below the amounts listed.

FIGURE 30-4 Nutritional facts label. (From US Food and Drug Administration: Accessed May 2, 2012. Available at *www.fda.gov/ Food/LabelingNutrition/PrintInformationMaterials/ucm114155.htm*).

CRITICAL THINKING APPLICATION   30-5

Ms. Rashad's blood pressure at this visit was 182/94. She is concerned about the risks of heart disease and wants to lower her blood pressure. What facts about a heart-healthy diet should Marcia share with her to help her understand the importance of nutrition in overall wellness?

READING FOOD LABELS

The USDA requires that all food products carry a nutritional facts label (Figure 30-4). These labels are a source of information about the nutrients in the product. When a designated diet is planned or implemented, the food label can be used as a valuable source of nutritional information (Procedure 30-1).

In the label's Nutrition Facts panel, manufacturers are required to provide information about certain nutrients. In the list below, the mandatory components of a food label are italicized, and the voluntary components are presented in the order in which they must appear:

- *Serving size*
- *Calories per serving*
- *Calories from fat in each serving*
- *Grams of total fat*
- *Grams of saturated fat*
- *Grams of trans fat*
  - Polyunsaturated fat
  - Monounsaturated fat
- *Milligrams of cholesterol*
- *Milligrams of sodium*
- *Milligrams of potassium*
- *Grams of total carbohydrate*
- *Grams of dietary fiber*
  - Soluble fiber
  - Insoluble fiber
- *Grams of sugars*
- Sugar alcohol (e.g., the sugar substitutes xylitol, mannitol, and sorbitol)
- Other carbohydrate (the difference between total carbohydrate and the sum of dietary fiber, sugars, and sugar alcohol if declared)
- *Grams of protein*
- *Percent of Daily Value of vitamin A*
  - Percent of vitamin A present as beta carotene
- *Percent of Daily Value of vitamin C*
- *Percent of Daily Value of calcium*
- *Percent of Daily Value of iron*
- Other essential vitamins and minerals

If a claim is made about any of the optional components or if a food is fortified or enriched with any of them, nutrition information for these components must be provided. These mandatory and voluntary components are the only ones allowed in the Nutrition Facts panel. The required nutrients were selected because they address today's health concerns. The order in which they must appear reflects the priority of current dietary recommendations.

PROCEDURE 30-1

Teach the Patient to Understand Food Labels

GOAL: *To explain to the patient the nutritional labeling of food products.*

EQUIPMENT and SUPPLIES

- One each of three bars: Snickers candy bar, granola bar, fat-free fruit bar
- Pencil and paper
- Patient medical record

PROCEDURAL STEPS

1. Using the patient's health and family histories, assess the individual to determine cultural influences that may affect dietary choices.
   PURPOSE: Cultural factors may influence the patient's dietary choices.

2. Introduce yourself and explain to the patient that you are going to teach him or her how to read a food label. Be sure to include reasons why food labels are a valuable source of nutritional information in diet planning.
   PURPOSE: Explaining the rationale for consistently reading food labels encourages the patient to participate in the education process.

3. Using the labels on each bar, point out the nutritional information according to the guidelines in the text.
   PURPOSE: Using actual labels assists learning and reinforces practical applications.

4. Give the patient the pencil and paper to write down the serving size of each type of bar.
   PURPOSE: Writing down information aids memory retention.

5. Compare the similarities and differences among the bars.
   PURPOSE: Comparing the results reinforces learning.

6. Have the patient write down the total number of calories for each product serving.
   PURPOSE: To reinforce the significant effect of high-calorie snacks on overall nutritional health.

7. Write down the percentages of total, saturated, trans, and unsaturated fats.
   PURPOSE: To review the importance of a low-fat diet and the role of saturated and trans fats in disease.

8. Compare the similarities and differences among the bars.

9. Together, analyze the nutritional level of each.

10. Discuss any new information learned.
    PURPOSE: To gather feedback about the learning experience so that the patient's learning needs are clarified.

11. Ask the patient whether he or she will use this information when shopping and how it will be implemented in nutritional planning.
    PURPOSE: Role-play implementation of the information to determine the patient's level of learning.

12. Document the education intervention, including the feedback received from the patient about his or her understanding of how to read food labels.
    PURPOSE: Documentation in the medical record provides proof of patient education and an assessment of the patient's ability to apply the knowledge to daily practice.

How to Use Label Information

When evaluating the nutritional value of a food product, begin with the serving size information, which is listed in both household and metric units. The amount of each nutrient in the food is expressed in two ways: in terms of weight per serving and as a percentage of the daily value. By using the percentage of daily value, you can determine whether a food contributes a lot or a little of a particular nutrient. However, if you eat more or less than the serving size on the label, you will need to adjust the amounts of nutrients and number of calories accordingly. Keep in mind that the percentage of daily value is based on the amount of food usually eaten in 1 day. The goal is to choose foods that total 100% of your daily nutrition needs.

The ingredient list also can help you learn more about the foods you eat. Ingredients are listed in descending order of weight. That helps you get an idea of the proportion of an ingredient in a food (Figure 30-5). Artificial colors have to be named in the ingredient list; they no longer can be stated as "color added." This is an important item for individuals with food allergies or certain specialized diets. In addition, the total percentage of juice in juice drinks must be declared so that you can see exactly how much juice is in the product.

INGREDIENT LABEL

INGREDIENTS: COOKED WHITE RICE, WATER, COOKED CHICKEN TENDERLOINS, GREEN BEANS, CARROTS, RED PEPPERS, BROWN SUGAR. CONTAINS LESS THAN 2% OF MODIFIED FOOD STARCH, MUSTARD (VINEGAR, MUSTARD SEED, SALT, SPICES, TURMERIC), DIJON MUSTARD (WATER, MUSTARD SEED, DISTILLED VINEGAR, SALT, WHITE WINE, CITRIC ACID, TARTARIC ACID, SPICES), HONEY, MALTODEXTRIN (FROM CORN), SALT, EGG YOLK SOLIDS, SODIUM PHOSPHATE, VINEGAR POWDER (MALTODEXTRIN, MODIFIED FOOD STARCH, VINEGAR SOLIDS), XANTHAN GUM FLAVORS, SPICES, LEMON JUICE CONCENTRATE

FIGURE 30-5 Ingredient label.

The front package label is where manufacturers often place statements describing the nutritional qualities of their product. The government has set strict conditions under which statements such as "low fat," "cholesterol free," and "good source of fiber" can be used as part of the front label. The Food and Drug Administration (FDA) permits claims linking a nutrient or food to the risk of a disease or health-related condition, but only claims supported by scientific evidence are allowed.

REGULATED NUTRITIONAL CLAIMS FOR FOOD LABELS

- **Light:** One-third fewer calories than in the regular product
- **Fresh:** Raw; never frozen, processed, or preserved
- **Calorie-free:** Less than 5 calories per serving
- **Sugar-free:** Less than 0.5 g of sugar per serving
- **Sodium-free:** Less than 5 mg of sodium per serving
- **Fat-free:** Less than 0.5 g of fat per serving
- **Saturated fat–free:** Less than 2 g of saturated fat per serving
- **High:** Provides more than 20% of the recommended daily consumption (per serving) of the nutrient (e.g., high-fiber)
- **Lean:** Cooked meat or poultry with less than 10.5 g of fat per serving, of which less than 3.5 g is saturated fat
- **Extra lean:** Cooked meat or poultry with less than 4.9 g of fat per serving, of which less than 1.8 g is saturated fat
- **Low-sodium:** Less than 140 mg of sodium per serving
- **Low-calorie:** Less than 40 calories per serving
- **Low-fat:** 3 g or less of fat per serving
- **Low saturated fat:** 1 g or less of saturated fat per serving and not more than 15% of calories from saturated fat
- **Low cholesterol:** 20 mg or less of cholesterol per serving and 2 g or less of saturated fat

From the U.S. Food and Drug Administration: Accessed January 12, 2010. Available at www.fda.gov/Food/GuidanceComplianceRegulatoryInformation/GuidanceDocuments/FoodLabelingNutrition/FoodLabelingGuide/ucm064911.htm.

Organic Foods Production Act

In 1990 the USDA initiated regulations for organically grown food, and in 2002 the agency revised the regulations governing the production and labeling of organic foods. Until then, organizations from state governments to trade and consumer groups contributed to the regulation of organic products, resulting in often conflicting standards about which products could be labeled organic. Under the new guidelines, foods labeled organic must have been produced without exposure to pesticides, chemical fertilizers, or sewage sludge. The food cannot have been irradiated to extend shelf life, nor can it contain any genetically modified ingredients. In addition, animals raised for organic meat, eggs, and milk cannot be given antibiotics or growth hormones, must be fed organic feed, and must have had access to the outdoors.

The 2002 regulations extended the rules to cover labeling for organic foods. Products with a "100 percent organic" label are limited to strictly organic ingredients. Products simply labeled "organic" identify the food as being made up of 95% organic materials. Products that fall into these two categories can display a "USDA Organic" seal. Foods containing at least 70% organic ingredients may be labeled "made with organic ingredients" and may list up to three of them on the package. Under the new regulations, any product containing less than 70% organic ingredients may not be marketed as an organic food.

FOOD-BORNE DISEASES

Eating or drinking contaminated food can result in a food-borne disease. Many different types of bacteria, viruses, and parasites can contaminate food, but the most common are *Escherichia coli* and *Salmonella* and *Campylobacter* organisms. Patients may experience a variety of symptoms, but the first typically are gastrointestinal: nausea, vomiting, stomach pain, and/or diarrhea. Usually a delay of several hours to days occurs after ingestion of the contaminated substance before symptoms begin. This is the *incubation period*, when the microbes are attaching to the intestinal wall and beginning to multiply. The diagnosis is confirmed with laboratory tests, of which the most common is a stool sample. However, more sophisticated tests may be needed to diagnose viral pathogens. Treatment depends on the patient's symptoms; if diarrhea and vomiting are severe, one of the biggest concerns is dehydration, especially in young children and older adults. In such cases, replacing fluid and electrolytes is the most important aspect of care. Other treatments include the use of antidiarrheal medications (e.g., Imodium) and drugs that coat the gastrointestinal tract (e.g., Pepto-Bismol).

When medical assistants are screening phone calls from patients experiencing gastrointestinal symptoms, some important factors are:

- Fever of 38.6°C (101.5°F) or higher
- Diarrhea lasting longer than 3 days
- Prolonged vomiting
- Blood in the stool
- Signs of dehydration (reduced urination, dry mouth, **vertigo**, and altered skin turgor)

For a list of food safety guidelines, visit the Evolve site at *evolve.elsevier.com/kinn*.

FOOD CONTAMINANTS

Environmental contamination of food can be a serious problem. The FDA regularly monitors the presence of contaminants in the food chain and issues warnings as needed to protect consumers from possible danger. Mercury is the most common heavy metal found in food, primarily fish. Other environmental contaminants include cadmium from industrial processing; lead found in old paint and old plumbing; and polychlorinated biphenyls (PCBs), which are part of discarded electrical equipment. Each of these can have serious toxic effects on humans. For example, mercury at toxic levels can poison the nervous system, especially that of a developing fetus. The FDA therefore recommends that pregnant women, women of childbearing age, nursing mothers, and young children not eat any fish known to have high mercury levels. These include king mackerel, swordfish, shark, and any fresh water fish from lakes or rivers known to be contaminated with mercury.

EATING DISORDERS

An eating disorder is any eating behavior pattern that can lead to a health problem. The two problems that cause the most serious health risks are anorexia nervosa and bulimia. These disorders can damage all the body systems and can cause death. Although 90% of reported cases occur in adolescent and young adult women, the incidence in males and middle-aged women is rising.

Anorexia nervosa is characterized by self-induced starvation. Anorexic individuals typically are adolescents when first diagnosed and tend to be perfectionists who are extremely sensitive to failure and any criticism. They use avoidance of food as a way of controlling their feelings and fear of becoming grossly overweight if they allow themselves to eat. As a result, they lose an excessive amount of weight, usually 15% to 60% of their normal body weight, resulting in extreme malnourishment. They can die without medical intervention. If necessary, patients are fed intravenously or by nasogastric tube feedings to establish an immediate level of nourishment to the body systems. Patients with anorexia nervosa have a significantly distorted body image and require psychotherapy to alleviate depression, to deal with their emotional issues, and for assistance in forming a positive self-image.

Bulimia is more common than anorexia and is characterized by cycles of binging and purging. This behavior pattern usually begins in adolescence when an individual who is slightly overweight diets but fails to achieve the expected results. Psychologically the person believes that self-worth is related to being thin. Usually the pattern begins with some form of stress that upsets the individual, who then turns to food for consolation. Intake during a binge period can reach as high as 20,000 calories. The eating binge is followed by self-induced punishment in the form of vomiting, using laxatives and enemas, excessive exercise, and food abstinence. Most individuals with bulimia have a normal or an above-normal body weight, but their weight can vary as much as 10 pounds during binging and purging cycles. Treatment programs are a combination of medication, psychotherapy, and nutritional counseling. The goal is to help the patient establish healthy eating patterns and develop an improved self-image.

CRITICAL THINKING APPLICATION   30-6

A close friend of Marcia's sister is visiting, and Marcia hears the friend tell her sister that she is using Ex-Lax after every meal and secretly exercising for 3 hours at night after the rest of the family is asleep. The young woman is 5 feet, 6 inches tall and determined not to weigh more than 100 pounds at graduation. What should Marcia do?

OBESITY

Overweight and obesity affect more than 60% of the American population. Obese individuals are at risk for a wide range of health problems, including hypertension, diabetes mellitus type 2, coronary artery disease, stroke, gallbladder disease, osteoarthritis, sleep apnea, and certain types of cancer. The physician's assessment of patients with weight problems includes an evaluation of the BMI and/or the patient's waist to hip ratio, in addition to the presence or risks of conditions associated with obesity. As the BMI rises, so do the risks for cardiovascular disease, hypertension, and hypercholesterolemia, and death.

Gastrointestinal surgery, or *bariatric* surgery, may be an option for people who are severely obese, have attempted unsuccessfully to lose weight by traditional means, and have been diagnosed with obesity-related health problems. The operation promotes weight loss by reducing the size of the stomach to the point that food intake is restricted and/or by interrupting the digestive process by surgically

circumventing part of the small intestine. Three different types of surgical procedures can be performed: restrictive surgery, which reduces the size of the stomach and slows the movement of food through it; malabsorptive surgery, which bypasses most of the small intestine, affecting nutrient digestion and absorption; and combined restrictive-malabsorptive surgery, which uses both techniques to reduce the amount of food ingested and the digestion and absorption of nutrients.

Patients seeking bariatric surgery must meet certain criteria, including a BMI of 40 or greater, or a BMI of 35 to 39.9 along with a diagnosed obesity-related health problem, such as diabetes mellitus type 2 or severe sleep apnea. The patient also must undergo counseling and psychiatric evaluation, because bariatric surgery requires a lifelong commitment to dietary change. The procedure is successful for long-term weight loss only if the individual is willing to commit to making drastic behavioral changes and undergoing regular medical checkups for the rest of his or her life. In addition, the cost of the procedure ($20,000 to $35,000) may be prohibitive, and insurance coverage varies by state and insurance provider.

The Harvard School of Public Health reports that 100,000 cases of cancer a year can be directly linked to obesity, according to the following distributions:

- Breast: 11%
- Colon: 14%
- Esophageal: 39%
- Kidney: 31%
- Non-Hodgkin's lymphoma: 20%
- Pancreatic: 14%

Medications for Obesity

Weight-loss medications fall into two categories: appetite suppressants and lipase inhibitors. Appetite-suppressant medications, such as phentermine (Adipex-P, Fastin, Ionamin, Oby-Trim, Pro-Fast, Zantryl) and sibutramine (Meridia), promote weight loss by reducing the appetite or increasing the feeling of being full. Orlistat (Xenical), a lipase inhibitor, blocks the release of the enzyme lipase, which metabolizes fat for absorption. If fat is not broken down, it cannot be absorbed, which results in a decrease in dietary fat absorption by about one third. Most weight-loss medications have been approved by the FDA for short-term use only, typically restricted to a few weeks. Meridia and Xenical are the only weight-loss medications that have been approved for use longer than 2 years. In early 2007, orlistat was approved for over-the-counter (OTC) sale for adults age 18. The OTC version of orlistat is sold under the brand name alli. Alli is meant to be taken with a reduced-calorie, low-fat diet, exercise, and a daily multivitamin. The response to medications for weight loss varies among patients, but the average weight loss is 5 to 22 pounds more than might have been lost without medication. Most of the weight is lost in the first 6 months of treatment, after which the patient's weight stabilizes or may even increase. The use of weight-loss medications must be combined with improvement in overall nutrition and exercise to have long-lasting effects and reduce weight-related health risks.

HEALTH PROMOTION

The concept of health promotion includes such aspects as adequate nutrition, a healthy environment, ongoing health education, and an overall attempt to prevent disease and maintain optimum wellness. Wellness goes beyond the absence of disease to a state of moving toward fitness, managing stress, and maximizing individual potential. Health promotion employs immunizations, appropriate personal hygiene, environmental sanitation standards, protection against occupational hazards, nutritious diets, and periodic health screenings and examinations to diagnose health problems early and promote wellness.

The medical assistant plays a key role in assisting the physician in many of these areas. In addition, the medical assistant can serve as a patient advocate by interacting with local social service agencies or insurance companies on the patient's behalf. The medical assistant also plays an important role in scheduling and in assisting the physician with health screenings, physical examinations, and health teaching. Components of wellness that all medical assistants should promote include exercise, stress management, and health screening.

Exercise

Exercise is defined as physical exertion for the maintenance or improvement of health or for the correction of a physical handicap. Exercise improves cardiorespiratory endurance; maintains musculoskeletal health by improving or maintaining strength, flexibility, and bone integrity; and relieves stress. Although most Americans say they know about the benefits of exercise, only 20% to 25% of adults exercise enough to gain significant health benefits. Twenty-five percent are not active at all, and more than half of all American youths 12 to 21 years of age are not vigorously active on a regular basis.

A well-balanced diet is only half of the fitness equation; to ensure good health, adequate exercise and sufficient rest form the other half of the equation. As with special diets, exercise programs must be approved for each individual by the physician. It is the physician who determines the patient's exercise needs and tolerance levels to safeguard the patient from overexertion and potential injury.

Many forms of exercise are available. Some patients may find that it is best to go to a gym and develop a formal program of physical fitness. Others may purchase home exercise equipment so they can exercise in privacy. Many feel just getting out in the fresh air and walking is the best form of exercise. Each individual should find the outlet that brings enjoyment and enrichment to his or her life. It is not the form of exercise that is important, but the participation in physical activity that promotes wellness.

If you are working with a patient who cannot engage in a full physical exercise program, you can suggest range-of-motion exercises. These exercise patterns are designed to improve circulation and promote muscle tone by putting each joint through its full range of motion. Patients with disabilities such as partial paralysis, arthritis, bursitis, and musculoskeletal deformities may be helped by these exercises. Range-of-motion exercises are presented in Chapter 43.

CRITICAL THINKING APPLICATION   30-7
The physician tells Mr. Hawthorne that he must exercise to maintain a healthy lifestyle. What can Marcia tell him about the benefits of exercise and possible methods that might help him follow through with the physician's recommendation?

Stress Management

Stress stimulates the fight-or-flight response that physically prepares us to either fight off a stressor or run away from it. Unfortunately, most of the stress we experience on a daily basis is not something we can either physically battle or effectively run away from. Therefore the stress response can lead to multiple health problems if it is not managed therapeutically. The stress response results in the release of epinephrine (adrenaline), which increases the heart and respiratory rates, slows peristalsis, increases blood supply to the skeletal muscles while reducing blood to the periphery, causes overall muscular tension, and raises the blood pressure. If stress is permitted to build without release, multiple health problems can occur, some of which can lead to chronic disorders. One of the best methods for reducing stress is exercise.

Health Screening

Routine physical examinations and health screenings are important components of health promotion. The patient scheduled for a physical examination should have a health history completed or updated and should be weighed; blood pressure, temperature, pulse, and respirations recorded; and any complaints documented on the chart. The physician may order the following studies as part of a health screening process:

- Tuberculin skin test
- Papanicolaou (Pap) smear
- Prostate-specific antigen (PSA) levels
- Hemoccult test after age 50
- Colonoscopy or sigmoidoscopy every 3 to 5 years after age 50
- Mammogram yearly after age 40
- Urinalysis
- Serum cholesterol
- Chest x-ray films
- Electrocardiogram (ECG)

CLOSING COMMENTS

Patient Education

Because medical assistants may be asked to discuss a diet plan with a patient, it is extremely important that they have a thorough knowledge of diet therapy. The patient must understand the prescribed diet and the rationale for using it. If the patient feels uneasy or if his or her questions go unanswered, the person may be less motivated to follow a diet plan. You can be a valuable asset to the physician, the dietitian, and the patient in the implementation of a specific diet.

When talking to patients about a diet, the medical assistant may find the following helpful:

- Use charts and diagrams to illustrate diets.
- Consider the patient's dietary likes and dislikes.
- Remember that ethnic and cultural foods are important.
- Encourage the patient to play an active role in the learning process.
- Suggest local support groups that can help in diet maintenance.

You also can play a vital role in health promotion by making sure patients are scheduled for annual examinations and that they follow up with the physician's recommendations for dietary changes, exercise programs, stress management approaches, and health screening procedures. The medical assistant is the link between the patient and the physician, and between the patient and available community resources.

Legal and Ethical Issues

Always remember that you are not a physician, nor are you a dietitian; follow the physician's instructions. If you are not sure of the answer to a question, always ask the physician. If your workplace employs a registered dietitian, refer questions about meal patterns and food selection changes to that individual. Direct patients seeking advice in the field of nutrition and exercise programs to someone who is a qualified expert. Use community resources as needed.

SUMMARY OF SCENARIO

As a certified medical assistant working in an internal medicine practice, Marcia must be familiar with the types and functions of dietary nutrients, the USDA dietary recommendations, including the chooseMyPlate.gov Web site, how nutritional assessments are conducted, the concepts of therapeutic nutrition, how to apply the interpretation of food labels to patient practice, and the concepts of health promotion. Recommendations for nutrition are constantly changing as research is done on the dietary needs of healthy people. Marcia can refer her patients to the USDA Web site (*www.choosemyplate.gov*) for updated information on dietary recommendations and for educational material on nutrition.

Physicians now rely on the BMI to determine a patient's risk for diet-related diseases, and medical assistants in a physician's office must be familiar with various therapeutic diets so that they can answer patients' questions about foods that should be included or avoided.

As a certified medical assistant, Marcia must make a commitment to lifelong learning so that she can provide her patients with up-to-date information on nutrition-related topics and can use community resources to support patient care.

SUMMARY OF LEARNING OBJECTIVES

1. **Define, spell, and pronounce the terms listed in the vocabulary.**
   Spelling and pronouncing medical terms correctly bolster the medical assistant's credibility. Knowing the definitions of these terms promotes confidence in communication with patients and co-workers.

2. **Apply critical thinking skills in performing the patient assessment and patient care.**
   Completing the Critical Thinking Application exercises throughout the chapter can help the student medical assistant become more adept at critical analysis of real-life situations.

3. **Analyze the relationship between poor diet and lifestyle choices and the risk of developing diet-related diseases.**
   Research has found that lifestyle and dietary habits directly correlate with the development of certain diseases and disorders. These include certain types of anemia, constipation, diabetes mellitus type 2, hypercholesterolemia, atherosclerosis, hypertension, osteoporosis, and cerebrovascular accidents.

4. **Recognize the impact of cultural influences on dietary choices.**
   People eat the way they do for many reasons. Encouraging patients to make significant lifestyle changes with regard to their diets requires sensitivity to these reasons. The choices people make about what they eat are greatly influenced by their background and relationships. Every culture, religion, and ethnic group has its own beliefs and practices with regard to food.

5. **Classify the types and functions of dietary nutrients.**
   Nutrients consist of carbohydrates, fats, proteins, vitamins, minerals, and water. Their primary functions are to provide the body with energy,

protection, and insulation; build and repair tissues; and regulate metabolic processes.

6. **Describe the roles of carbohydrates, fats, protein, and fiber in the daily diet.**
   The primary function of carbohydrates is to provide the body with a ready source of energy. Dietary fat provides essential fatty acids and is needed for the absorption of fat-soluble vitamins. Adipose tissue helps protect the organs of the body, insulates, and serves as a concentrated form of stored energy. Protein builds and repairs tissue and assists with metabolic functions. Dietary fiber plays an important role in maintaining regularity and helping to prevent cancer and heart disease.

7. **Explain the function of appropriate amounts of vitamins, minerals, and water in the diet.**
   Vitamins are essential for metabolic functions and are classified as either fat soluble or water soluble. They regulate the synthesis of body tissues and aid the metabolism of nutrients. Vitamins also play a vital role in disease prevention. Minerals help to maintain electrolytes and acid-base balance and to regulate muscular action and nervous activities throughout the body. Water is part of almost every vital body process.

8. **Apply the 2010 Dietary Guidelines for Americans using the Choose MyPlate Web site developed by the U.S. Department of Agriculture (USDA).**
   In 2011 the Pyramid design was changed to a dinner plate icon that represents how to build a healthy plate at mealtime. The plate includes choices from the five basic food groups, with recommendations based on the 2010 Dietary Guidelines for Americans. At the MyPlate Web site

(www.choosemyplate.gov) consumers can determine individual dietary needs that match their particular age, health status, exercise level, and food preferences.

9. **Implement nutritional assessment techniques.**

The physician's assessment of the patient's nutritional status includes an evaluation of the patient's current health and lifestyle habits and also body fat measurements. Body fat can be measured by using the waist to hip ratio, by using calipers to measure fat folds, or by calculating the BMI.

10. **Correlate a patient's calculated body mass index (BMI) with the risk for diet-related disease.**

The BMI is the relationship of weight to height, which correlates with health risks. The BMI is a more accurate predictor of weight-related diseases than traditional height-weight charts, because it provides a good estimate of the degree of body fat. Individuals with a BMI of 19 to 22 are thought to live longest. The incidence of diet-related disorders and the mortality rate are significantly higher for people with a BMI of 25 or higher.

11. **Compare the concepts of therapeutic nutrition.**

Therapeutic nutrition uses various diets to help treat or prevent disease. Diets can be modified in many ways; these may include changes in consistency and taste, monitoring of caloric levels, altering the amounts and types of specific nutrients, and managing the fiber content of foods. Two examples of diet therapies are the diabetic diet and the heart-healthy diet, both of which can have a significant impact on a patient's wellness.

12. **Interpret food labels and explain their application to a healthy diet.**

The federal government requires all food manufacturers to follow certain guidelines when labeling packages. Labels provide facts on the nutritional value of foods. The food label can be a valuable tool in patient compliance with specialized diets (see Figure 30-4).

13. **Demonstrate to the patient how to understand nutrition labels on food products.**

Refer to Procedure 30-1.

14. **Summarize the causes of eating disorders and obesity and their impact on a patient's health.**

An eating disorder is defined as any eating behavior pattern that can lead to a health problem. In anorexia nervosa, profound malnutrition occurs because of an individual's attempt to control his or her life by not eating. Bulimia is characterized by bingeing and purging episodes. Obesity has become a national health emergency. Obese individuals have a higher risk of a wide range of health problems, including hypertension, diabetes mellitus type 2, coronary artery disease, stroke, gallbladder disease, osteoarthritis, sleep apnea, and certain types of cancer.

15. **Define the concepts of health promotion.**

Health promotion considers all aspects of patient care, including the concepts of general wellness, adequate nutrition, environmental health and safety, health education needs, and disease prevention. The components of health promotion include exercise, stress management, regular physical examinations, and health screening.

16. **Describe the role of the medical assistant in nutrition and health promotion.**

The medical assistant plays a key role in promoting nutrition and health. He or she serves as a patient advocate and as a liaison between the patient and community resources. It is important that medical assistants understand the various implications of nutrition and specific diets, so that they can answer patients' questions, which promotes compliance with treatment.

CONNECTIONS

Study Guide Connection: Go to the Chapter 30 Study Guide. Read and complete the activities.

Evolve Connection: Go to the Chapter 30 link at *evolve.elsevier.com/kinn* to complete the Chapter Review and Chapter Quiz. Check out the other resources listed for this chapter to make the most of what you have learned from Nutrition and Health Promotion.

31

VITAL SIGNS

SCENARIO

Dr. Susan Xu is a member of a multiphysician primary care practice. Each physician in the practice has a medical assistant who works directly with him or her. Carlos Ricci, CMA (AAMA), is Dr. Xu's assistant. Carlos graduated from a medical assistant program 3 years ago and enjoys the variety of patients seen in Dr. Xu's practice. One of Carlos' primary responsibilities is to accurately measure and record each patient's vital signs before the patient is seen by Dr. Xu.

While studying this chapter, think about the following questions:

- What factors might alter a patient's vital signs?
- What methods can Carlos use to gather and record a patient's temperature, pulse, respirations, blood pressure, height, weight, and body mass index (BMI)?
- What are the most recent guidelines for diagnosing and treating hypertension?

LEARNING OBJECTIVES

1. Define, spell, and pronounce the terms listed in the vocabulary.
2. Apply critical thinking skills while performing patient assessment and patient care.
3. Cite the average body temperature, pulse rate, respiratory rate, and blood pressure for various age groups.
4. Describe emotional and physical factors that can cause the body temperature to rise or fall.
5. Convert temperature readings between the Fahrenheit and Celsius scales.
6. Obtain and record an accurate patient temperature using three different types of thermometers.
7. Describe pulse rate, rhythm, and volume.
8. Locate and record the pulse at multiple sites.
9. Demonstrate the best way to obtain an accurate respiratory count.
10. Specify physiologic factors that affect blood pressure.
11. Differentiate between essential and secondary hypertension.
12. Interpret revised hypertension guidelines and treatment.
13. Identify the different Korotkoff phases.
14. Accurately measure and document blood pressure.
15. Accurately measure and document height and weight.
16. Convert kilograms to pounds and pounds to kilograms.
17. Identify patient education opportunities when measuring vital signs.
18. Determine the medical assistant's legal and ethical responsibilities in obtaining vital signs.

VOCABULARY

apnea (ap'-nee-uh) Absence or cessation of breathing.

arrhythmia An abnormality or irregularity in the heart rhythm.

arteriosclerosis (ar-ter'-ee-o-scler-o-sis) Thickening, decreased elasticity, and calcification of arterial walls.

bounding Term used to describe a pulse that feels full because of increased power of cardiac contraction or as a result of increased blood volume.

bradycardia (brad-i-kahr'-dee-uh) A slow heartbeat; a pulse below 60 beats per minute.

bradypnea (brad-ip-nee'-uh) Respirations that are regular in rhythm but slower than normal in rate.

cerumen (see-room'-men) A waxy secretion in the ear canal; commonly called *ear wax.*

chronic obstructive pulmonary disease (COPD) A progressive, irreversible lung condition that results in diminished lung capacity.

diurnal (die-ur'-nl) **rhythm** Pattern of activity or behavior that follows a day-night cycle.

dyspnea (disp-nee'-uh) Difficult or painful breathing.

essential hypertension Elevated blood pressure of unknown cause that develops for no apparent reason; sometimes called *primary hypertension.*

febrile (feb'-ril) Pertaining to an elevated body temperature.

homeostasis Internal adaptation and change in response to environmental factors; multiple functions that attempt to keep the body's functions in balance.

hyperpnea (hahy-per-nee'-uh) An increase in the depth of breathing.

hypertension High blood pressure.

hyperventilation Abnormally prolonged and deep breathing, usually associated with acute anxiety or emotional tension.

hypotension Blood pressure that is below normal (systolic pressure below 90 mm Hg and diastolic pressure below 50 mm Hg).

intermittent pulse A pulse in which beats occasionally are skipped.

orthopnea (or-thop'-nee-uh) Condition in which an individual must sit or stand to breathe comfortably.

orthostatic (postural) hypotension A temporary fall in blood pressure when a person rapidly changes from a recumbent position to a standing position.

otitis externa Inflammation or infection of the external auditory canal (swimmer's ear).

peripheral (puh-rif'-er-uhl) Term that refers to an area outside of or away from an organ or structure.

pulse deficit Condition in which the radial pulse is less than the apical pulse; may indicate a peripheral vascular abnormality.

pulse pressure The difference between systolic and diastolic blood pressures (30 to 50 mm Hg is considered normal).

pyrexia (pi-rek'-see-uh) Febrile condition or fever.

rales Abnormal or crackling breath sounds during inspiration.

rhonchi (ron'-ki) Abnormal rumbling sounds on expiration that indicate airway obstruction by thick secretions or spasms.

secondary hypertension Elevated blood pressure resulting from another condition, typically kidney disease.

sinus arrhythmia Irregular heartbeat that originates in the sino-atrial node (pacemaker).

spirometer Instrument that measures the volume of air inhaled and exhaled.

stertorous (stuh-tuh'-rus) Term that describes a strenuous respiratory effort marked by a snoring sound.

syncope (sing'-kuh-pee) Fainting; a brief lapse in consciousness.

tachycardia (tak-i-kahr'-dee-uh) A rapid but regular heart rate; one that exceeds 100 beats per minute.

tachypnea (tak-ip-nee'-uh) Condition marked by rapid, shallow respirations.

thready Term that describes a pulse that is scarcely perceptible.

wheezing A high-pitched sound heard on expiration; indicates obstruction or narrowing of respiratory passages.

Measurement of vital signs is an important aspect of almost every patient visit to the medical office. These signs are the human body's indicators of internal **homeostasis** and the patient's general state of health. Because medical assistants are chiefly responsible for obtaining these measurements, it is imperative that they have confidence in the theoretic and practical applications of vital sign measurement. A medical assistant who understands the principles of and the reasons for these measurements becomes a valuable asset to any medical office.

Accuracy is essential. A change in one or more of the patient's vital signs may indicate a change in general health. Variations may suggest the presence or disappearance of a disease process and therefore may lead to alteration of the treatment plan. Although the medical assistant obtains vital signs routinely, it is a task that requires consistent attention to accuracy and detail. These findings are crucial to a correct diagnosis, and vital signs should never be measured with indifference or casualness. In addition to performing accurate

measurement, care must be taken when charting the findings on the patient's medical record.

Vital signs are the patient's temperature, pulse, respiration, and blood pressure. These four signs are abbreviated *TPR* and *BP* and may be referred to as *cardinal signs.* The medical assistant must understand the significance of the vital signs and must measure and record them accurately. *Anthropometric* measurements are not considered vital signs but usually are obtained at the same time as vital signs. These measurements include height, weight, body mass index (BMI), and other body measurements, such as fat composition and an infant's head circumference.

FACTORS THAT MAY INFLUENCE VITAL SIGNS

Vital signs are influenced by many factors, both physical and emotional. A patient may have drunk a hot or cold beverage just before the examination or may be angry or fearful about what the physician may find. For example, consider that a patient has been asked to return to have a repeat Papanicolaou (Pap) smear because the first one showed the presence of suspicious cells. The medical assistant measures the patient's blood pressure and finds it significantly elevated compared with previous readings. The patient may be anxious and apprehensive about the test results, and the elevated blood pressure readings reflect her anxiety.

What temperature reading might be expected in a patient who could not find a parking place and had to walk four blocks to the office, knowing he would be late for his appointment? If you said it would be elevated, you are right. Certainly, this patient's metabolism would increase because of the physical exercise, and as a result, his temperature would be elevated, along with his pulse, respirations, and blood pressure.

For one reason or another, many patients are apprehensive during an office visit. These emotions may alter vital signs, and the medical assistant must help the patient relax before taking any readings. Measurements sometimes must be obtained a second time, after the patient is calmer or more comfortable. For a better picture of the patient's vital signs, the medical assistant may be asked to record the vital signs twice: at the beginning of the visit and just before the patient leaves the office.

TEMPERATURE

Physiology

Body temperature is defined as the balance between heat lost and heat produced by the body. It is measured in degrees Fahrenheit (F) or degrees Celsius (C). The process of chemical and physical change in the body that produces heat is called *metabolism*. Body temperature is a result of this process. The core body temperature is maintained within a normal range by the thermoregulatory center in the hypothalamus. The average body temperature varies from person to person and is different in each person at different times throughout the day. In a healthy adult, this **diurnal rhythm** varies from 97.6°F to 99°F (36.4°C to 37.3°C); the average daily temperature is 98.6°F (36.8°C). Body temperature is lowest in the morning and highest in the late afternoon. Factors that may affect body temperature include the following:

- *Age:* The body temperature of infants and young children fluctuates more rapidly in response to external environmental temperatures. Teething may cause a slight elevation in temperature but should not be the cause of a fever. Aging adults lose their ability to respond therapeutically to environmental temperature extremes, making them more susceptible to hypothermic or hyperthermic reactions.
- *Stress and physical activity:* Both exercise and emotional stress can increase the metabolic rate, causing an elevation in temperature.
- *Gender:* Hormone secretions result in fluctuations of the core body temperature in women throughout the menstrual cycle.
- *External factors:* Smoking, drinking hot fluids, and chewing gum can temporarily elevate an oral temperature.

In illness, an individual's metabolic activity is increased; this causes an increase in internal heat production, which in turn raises the body temperature. The increase in body temperature is thought

to be the body's defensive reaction because heat inhibits the growth of some bacteria and viruses.

When a fever is present, superficial blood vessels (those near the surface of the skin) constrict. The small papillary muscles at the base of hair follicles also constrict, creating goose bumps. Chills and shivering may follow, producing internal heat. As this process repeats itself, more heat is produced, and the body temperature becomes elevated or rises above the normal range. When more heat is lost than is produced, the opposite effect occurs, and body temperature drops below normal range.

Fever

Infection, either bacterial or viral, is the most common cause of fever in both children and adults.

Infants do not usually develop **febrile** illnesses during the first 3 months of life; if one is present, it usually is very serious. However, fever, or **pyrexia**, is very common in young children and accounts for an estimated 26% of office visits. Fevers are classified according to the 24-hour pattern they follow. The three most common patterns are:

- *Continuous fever,* which rises and falls only slightly during a 24-hour period. The temperature consistently remains above the patient's average normal temperature range and fluctuates less than 3 degrees.
- *Intermittent fever,* which comes and goes, alternating between elevated and normal levels.
- *Remittent fever,* which fluctuates considerably (i.e., by more than 3 degrees) and never returns to the normal range.

Variation from the patient's average body temperature range may be the first warning of an illness or a change in the patient's current condition. Patients with fever usually have loss of appetite (*anorexia*), headache, thirst, flushed face, hot skin, and general malaise. Some patients experience an acute onset of chills and shivering followed by an increase in body temperature. A serious possible complication in young children with high fevers is a febrile seizure. Medication to reduce the fever, or *antipyretic* drugs (e.g., Tylenol), should be taken as instructed to prevent dangerous spikes in temperature. Age-related normal values for temperature readings are shown in Table 31-1.

TEMPERATURES CONSIDERED FEBRILE

- Rectal, temporal, or aural (ear) temperature over 100.4°F (38°C)
- Oral temperature over 99.5°F (37.5°C)
- Axillary temperature over 98.6°F (37°C)
- Fever of unknown origin (FUO): a temperature over 100.9°F (38.3°C) that lasts 3 weeks in adults and 1 week in children without a known related diagnosis

Temperature Readings

A clinical thermometer is used to measure body temperature. It is calibrated in the Fahrenheit or the Celsius scale. The Fahrenheit scale is used most often in the United States, but hospitals and many ambulatory care settings use the Celsius scale. The formulas for conversion from one system to the other are as follows:

TABLE 31-1 Age-Related Temperature Norms

AGE	FAHRENHEIT	CELSIUS
Newborn (axillary)	98.2°	36.8°
1 year	99.7°	37.6°
6 years to adult (oral)	98.6°	37°
Elderly over age 70 (oral)	96.8°	36°

TABLE 31-2 Average Adult Temperatures

SITE	FAHRENHEIT	CELSIUS
Oral	98.6°	37°
Axillary	97.6°	36.4°
Tympanic	98.6°	37°
Temporal artery	98.6°	37°

$$°C = (°F - 32) \times \frac{5}{9}$$

$$°F = \left(°C \times \frac{9}{5}\right) + 32$$

For example, if an infant's temperature is measured at 101° F, the Celsius conversion would be:

$$°C = (101°\,F - 32) \times \frac{5}{9}$$
$$= 69 \times \frac{5}{9}$$
$$= 345 \div 9$$
$$= 38.3°\,C$$

If the ambulatory care setting where you work uses a Celsius thermometer, patients may ask you what the temperature is in Fahrenheit degrees because that is the scale they understand. If the facility does not have a conversion chart available, you will need to convert the temperature mathematically. For example, if an infant's temperature is 39° C, what is the Fahrenheit reading?

$$°F = \left(°C \times \frac{9}{5}\right) + 32$$
$$= \left(39°\,C \times \frac{9}{5}\right) + 32$$
$$= (351 \div 5) + 32$$
$$= 70.2 + 32$$
$$= 102.2°\,F$$

CRITICAL THINKING APPLICATION   31-1

Using the correct formula, convert the following temperatures from one system to the other.

99° F = _____ °C   102° F = _____ °C

38° C = _____ °F   39.5° C = _____ °F

Several types of thermometers and several different methods can be used to take temperature readings. A digital thermometer is placed under the tongue, in the armpit, or rectally; a tympanic thermometer is inserted into the ear; and a temporal artery scanner is moved across the forehead. Average temperature values for adults at the four most common sites are shown in Table 31-2.

Axillary temperatures are approximately 1° F (0.6° C) lower than accurate oral readings because axillary readings are not taken in an enclosed body cavity. When taken correctly, the tympanic (ear) temperature is an accurate measure because it records the temperature of the blood closest to the hypothalamus. However, recent research on the newest device for obtaining temperature, the temporal artery (TA) thermometer, indicates that this method is more accurate than tympanic measurement for identifying elevated temperatures in infants. Pediatricians, therefore, may prefer TA temperatures in infants suspected of having a fever. The TA thermometer also records accurate temperature readings in all age groups of patients. The tympanic method still is considered a fast, accurate, and noninvasive way of recording temperatures for older children and adults.

When obtaining an oral temperature, you do not have to indicate the site when documenting the reading in the patient's chart. However, you should write (T) for tympanic, (A) for axillary, or (TA) for temporal artery readings after recording the temperature to clarify that an alternative site was used. Oral temperature cannot be measured accurately in young children because the technique requires patients to hold the thermometer under the tongue and keep the mouth closed. To take an infant's temperature rectally, lubricate the probe tip, hold the baby securely with the legs elevated, and insert the probe approximately ½ inch; hold the probe carefully throughout the procedure to prevent rectal damage. However, pediatricians may prefer that infants' temperatures be taken with a temporal thermometer because it is more comfortable for the baby, is less invasive, and eliminates the possible complication of a perforated rectum.

For patients older than 3 years and for those unable to hold a thermometer properly in their mouth during the procedure, a tympanic or temporal thermometer can be used; if not, a less accurate axillary temperature can be obtained.

CRITICAL THINKING APPLICATION   31-2

The mother of a 3-year-old calls the office to report that her child had an axillary temperature of 101° F at 9 o'clock this morning. The schedule is very full today, so Carlos has to decide whether the child should be seen today or first thing tomorrow. When should Carlos schedule the appointment?

Types of Thermometers and Their Uses

Digital Thermometer

Digital thermometers are battery operated and are available in both Fahrenheit and Celsius scales. Disposable covers fit snugly over the

PROCEDURE 31-1

Obtain Vital Signs: Obtain an Oral Temperature Using a Digital Thermometer

GOAL: *To accurately determine and record a patient's temperature using a digital thermometer.*

EQUIPMENT and SUPPLIES

- Digital thermometer
- Probe covers
- Biohazard waste container
- Disposable gloves as appropriate
- Patient record

PROCEDURAL STEPS

1. Sanitize your hands.
   PURPOSE: To ensure infection control.
2. Assemble the needed equipment and supplies.
3. Identify your patient and explain the procedure. Make sure the patient has not eaten, consumed any hot or cold fluids, smoked, or exercised during the 30 minutes before the temperature is measured.
   PURPOSE: Identification of the patient prevents errors, and explanations are a means of gaining implied consent and patient cooperation. The temperature will be inaccurate if hot or cold food or fluids have been ingested, or if the patient has exercised within 30 minutes.
4. Prepare the probe for use as described in the package directions (Figure 1). Make sure probe covers are always used.
   PURPOSE: To ensure infection control.

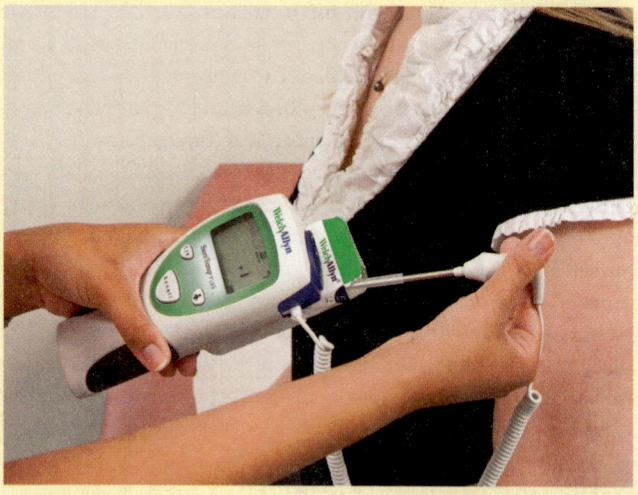

5. Place the probe under the patient's tongue (Figure 2) and instruct the patient to close the mouth tightly without biting down on the thermometer. Help the patient by holding the probe end.
   PURPOSE: Air seeping into the mouth interferes with an accurate body temperature reading.

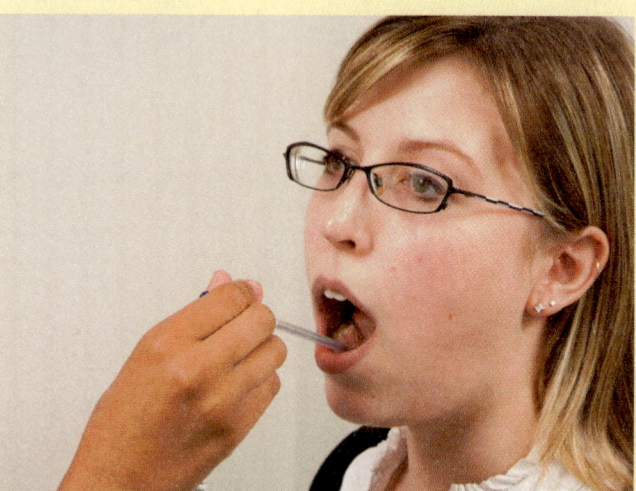

6. When a beep is heard, remove the probe from the patient's mouth and immediately eject the probe cover into an appropriate biohazard waste container.
   PURPOSE: The probe cover is contaminated and must be discarded in a biohazard waste container.
7. Note the reading in the LED window of the processing unit.
8. Record the reading in the patient's medical record (e.g., T = 97.7° F).
   PURPOSE: Procedures that are not recorded are considered not done.
9. Sanitize your hands and disinfect the equipment as indicated.
   PURPOSE: To observe infection control measures and Standard Precautions.

3/27/XX 10:05 AM T 97.7°F ————— **C. Ricci, CMA (AAMA)** _____

---

probes and are easily and quickly removed by pushing in the colored end of the probe. The instrument sounds a beep when the process is completed (10 to 60 seconds), and the reading appears on a light-emitting diode (LED) screen on the face of the instrument (Procedure 31-1). Because the only part of the instrument that comes in contact with the patient is the probe, which is sheathed, the risk of cross-infection is greatly reduced (Figure 31-1). Another type of digital thermometer resembles the old mercury thermometers that the Occupational Safety and Health Administration (OSHA) no longer allows clinicians to use in healthcare facilities. These thermometers have a digital screen on which the temperature is read and should always be covered by a disposable sheath.

Temperature should not be taken orally if the patient recently has had something hot or cold to eat or drink or has just smoked, because these factors may artificially alter the patient's temperature. In addition, the patient must be able to hold the thermometer under the tongue with the lips tightly sealed around the probe of an accurate oral reading is to be obtained.

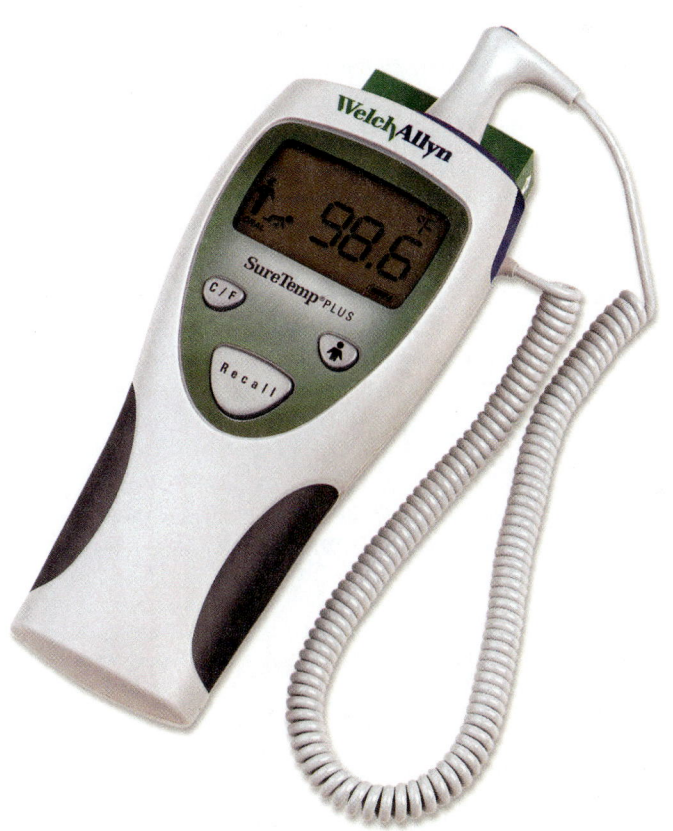

FIGURE 31-1 Digital thermometer. (Courtesy Welch Allyn.)

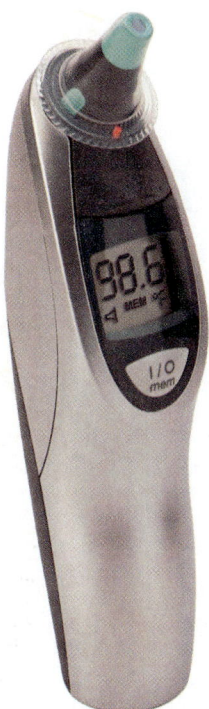

FIGURE 31-2 Tympanic thermometer. (Courtesy Welch Allyn.)

Tympanic Thermometer

The tympanic membrane of the ear can be used for quick, accurate, and safe assessment of a patient's temperature. It shares the blood supply that reaches the hypothalamus, which is the brain's temperature regulator. The ear canal is a protected cavity, so aural temperature is not affected by factors such as an open mouth, hot or cold drinks, or even a stuffy nose, which would prevent a patient from keeping the mouth closed during the procedure. In addition, the covered probe is designed to bounce an infrared signal off the eardrum without touching it, so the risk of spreading communicable diseases during temperature measurement is greatly reduced.

The tympanic measurement system consists of a handheld processor unit equipped with a tympanic probe, which is covered with a disposable speculum for use (Figure 31-2).

When the probe is placed into the ear canal, it gently seals the external opening of the canal, and the infrared energy emitted by the tympanic membrane is gathered. This signal is digitized by the processor unit and is shown on the display screen. Accurate readings are obtained in less than 2 seconds (Procedure 31-2). Both the speed of the tympanic thermometer and the comfort it affords the patient have greatly influenced its popularity. However, this unit should not be used (1) if the patient has bilateral **otitis externa**, because the procedure would be uncomfortable for the patient, and (2) if impacted **cerumen** is present in both ears, because the reading may be inaccurate.

Temporal Artery Scanner

The temporal artery scanner uses an infrared beam to assess the temperature of the blood flowing through the temporal artery of the lateral forehead, where the artery lies about 1 mm below the skin (Figure 31-3). Because the artery is so close to the skin, it provides good surface heat conduction, allowing the thermometer to obtain a fast, accurate, and noninvasive measurement of the body temperature.

To perform the procedure, place the probe in the center of the forehead, halfway between the eyebrows and the hairline. Bangs should be pushed back off the forehead (this method cannot be used if bandages cover the area). Depress the button on the scanner and gently stroke the probe across the forehead toward the hairline (at the temples), keeping the probe flat on the patient's skin. As the scanner moves across the forehead, repeated temperature measurements are taken and the highest measurement is recorded; keeping the button depressed, lift the scanner from the temporal area and lightly place the probe behind the earlobe. Release the button and remove the probe. Recording an accurate temperature takes about 3 seconds (Procedure 31-3).

Axillary Thermometer

Studies indicate that axillary temperatures are accurate when performed correctly. Axillary temperatures take more time to register the correct body temperature, but the method is safe, simple, and easy to perform (Procedure 31-4). Axillary temperatures are taken with a digital thermometer, which is placed into the axillary fold. If the digital thermometer has more than one probe, the oral (blue) probe with a disposable probe cover should be used. Because tympanic and temporal thermometers are relatively expensive, the axillary method may be a viable way for parents of young children to get accurate temperature readings at home. However, parents should be aware that the axillary temperature may be as much as one degree less than the child's actual core temperature.

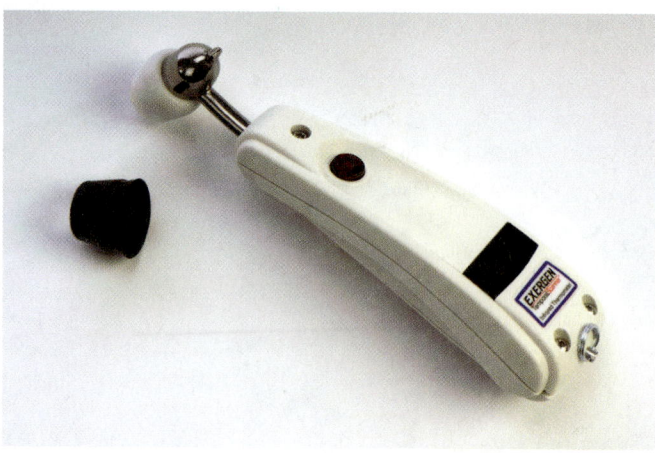

FIGURE 31-3 Temporal artery thermometer.

Disposable Thermometer

Disposable thermometers (those that are used only once) are frequently used on small children in the home. The reading is obtained by a heat-sensitive material that changes color according to the elevation of body temperature. Two types of disposable thermometers frequently are used by parents of young children. One type is placed under the child's tongue (Figure 31-4); the other is placed on the forehead. Although both types are fairly reliable, the temperature-sensing materials have expiration dates, which often are overlooked, and specific storage requirements may apply. Disposable thermometers are considered to be good screening devices but are not as accurate as other methods.

Cleaning Thermometers

Digital Thermometers

The digital unit or individual digital thermometers should be routinely cleaned with disinfectant. When ejecting the probe shield or

---

PROCEDURE 31-2

Obtain Vital Signs: Obtain an Aural Temperature Using the Tympanic Thermometer

GOAL: *To accurately determine and record a patient's temperature using a tympanic thermometer.*

EQUIPMENT and SUPPLIES

- Tympanic thermometer
- Disposable probe covers
- Biohazard waste container
- Disposable gloves as appropriate
- Patient record

PROCEDURAL STEPS

1. Sanitize your hands.
   <u>PURPOSE:</u> To ensure infection control.
2. Gather the necessary equipment and supplies.
3. Identify your patient and explain the procedure.
   <u>PURPOSE:</u> Identification of the patient prevents errors, and explanations are a means of gaining implied consent and patient cooperation.
4. Place a disposable cover on the probe (Figure 1).
   <u>PURPOSE:</u> To ensure a clean surface and prevent cross-contamination.

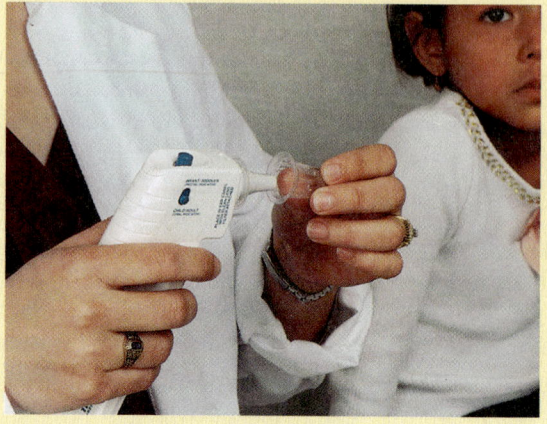

5. Follow the package directions to start the thermometer.
6. Insert the probe into the ear canal far enough to seal the opening. Do not apply pressure (Figure 2). For children younger than age 3, gently pull the earlobe down and back; for patients older than age 3, gently pull the top of the ear up and back.
   <u>PURPOSE:</u> The external ear must be pulled gently to open the external auditory canal and expose the tympanic membrane for an accurate reading.

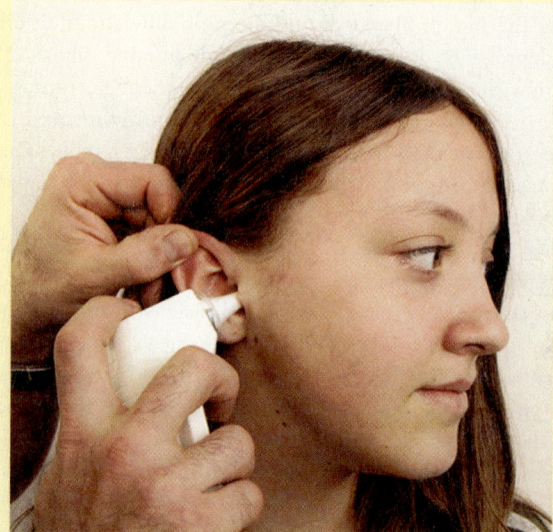

(From Bonewit-West K: *Clinical procedures for medical assistants,* ed 7, St Louis, 2008, Saunders.)

7. Press the button on the probe as directed. The temperature will appear on the display screen in 1 to 2 seconds.

PROCEDURE 31-2—cont'd

8. Remove the probe, note the reading (Figure 3), and discard the probe cover into a biohazard container without touching it.
   PURPOSE: The probe cover is contaminated and must be discarded in a biohazard waste container.

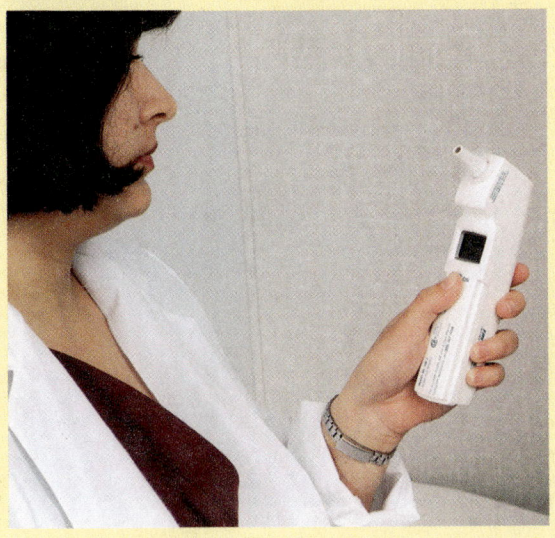

9. Sanitize your hands and disinfect the equipment if indicated.
   PURPOSE: To ensure infection control.
10. Record the temperature results (e.g., T = 98.6° F [T]) in the patient's medical record.
    PURPOSE: Procedures that are not recorded are considered not done.

3/30/XX   2:20 PM   T 101.2°F (T) — — — — — — —
C. Ricci, CMA (AAMA) _____

PROCEDURE 31-3

Obtain Vital Signs: Obtain a Temporal Artery Temperature

GOAL: *To accurately determine and record a patient's temperature using a temporal artery scanner.*

EQUIPMENT and SUPPLIES

- Temporal artery thermometer
- Patient record
- Alcohol swab

PROCEDURAL STEPS

1. Sanitize your hands.
   PURPOSE: To ensure infection control.
2. Gather the necessary equipment and supplies.
3. Introduce yourself, identify your patient, and explain the procedure.
   PURPOSE: Identification of the patient prevents errors, and explanations are a means of gaining implied consent and patient cooperation.
4. Remove the protective cap on the probe. The probe can be cleaned by lightly wiping the surface with an alcohol swab.
5. Push the patient's hair up off of the forehead to expose the site. Gently place the probe on the patient's forehead, halfway between the eyebrows and the hairline.
   PURPOSE: This places the probe directly over the temporal artery.

6. Depress and hold the SCAN button and lightly glide the probe sideways across the patient's forehead to the hairline just above the ear (Figure 1). As you move the sensor across the forehead, you will hear a beep, and a red light will flash.
   PURPOSE: This verifies that the scanner is recording temperatures as it moves across the surface of the temporal artery.

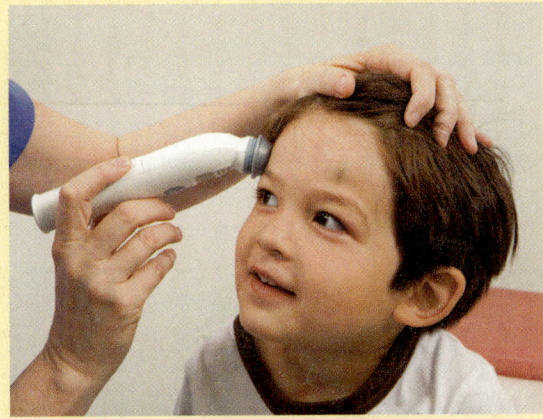

PROCEDURE 31-3—cont'd

7. Keep the button depressed, lift the thermometer, and place the probe on the upper neck behind the ear lobe (Figure 2). The thermometer may continue to beep, indicating that the temperature is rising.
   PURPOSE: To continue scanning of the temporal artery until the highest temperature is recorded on the thermometer.

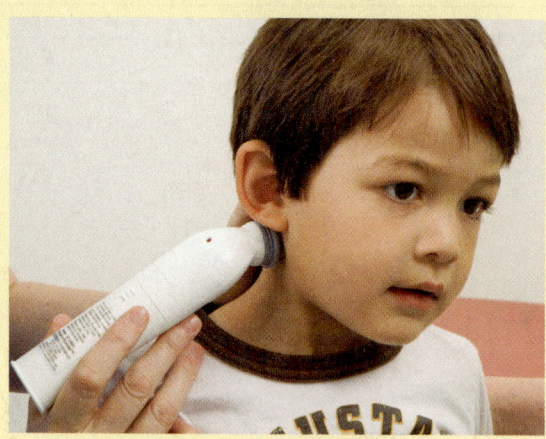

8. When scanning is complete, release the button and lift the probe. Note the temperature recorded on the digital display. The scanner automatically turns off 15 to 30 seconds after release of the button.
9. Disinfect the thermometer if indicated and replace the protective cap.
   PURPOSE: To ensure infection control.
10. Sanitize your hands.
11. Record the temperature results (e.g., T = 101.6° F [TA]) in the patient's medical record.
    PURPOSE: Procedures that are not recorded are considered not done.

PROCEDURE 31-4

Obtain Vital Signs: Obtain an Axillary Temperature

GOAL: *To accurately determine and record a patient's temperature using the axillary method.*

EQUIPMENT and SUPPLIES

- Digital unit
- Thermometer sheath or probe cover
- Supply of tissues
- Biohazard waste container
- Disposable gloves as appropriate
- Patient gown as needed
- Patient record

PROCEDURAL STEPS

1. Sanitize your hands.
   PURPOSE: To ensure infection control.
2. Gather the needed equipment and supplies.
3. Introduce yourself, identify your patient, and explain the procedure.
   PURPOSE: Identification of the patient prevents errors, and explanations are a means of gaining implied consent and patient cooperation.
4. Prepare the thermometer or digital unit in the same manner as for oral use.
5. Remove the patient's clothing and gown the patient as needed to access the axillary region.
6. Pat the patient's axillary area dry with tissues if needed.
   PURPOSE: To ensure an accurate reading. Do not rub the area, because this may cause an elevated reading.

7. Cover the thermometer or probe and place the tip into the center of the armpit, pointing the stem toward the upper chest, making sure the thermometer is touching only skin, not clothing.
   PURPOSE: To obtain the most accurate axillary reading; contact with clothing alters the reading.
8. Instruct the patient to hold the arm snugly across the chest or abdomen until the thermometer beeps.
   PURPOSE: To prevent air from leaking in and interfering with the temperature reading.
9. Remove the thermometer, note the digital reading, and dispose of the cover in the biohazard waste container.
10. Disinfect the thermometer if indicated.
11. Sanitize your hands.
12. Record the axillary temperature on the patient's medical record (e.g., T = 97.6° F [A]).
    PURPOSE: Procedures that are not recorded are considered not done.

4/2/XX 9:30 AM T 98.2°F (A) — — — — — C. Ricci, CMA (AAMA) _____

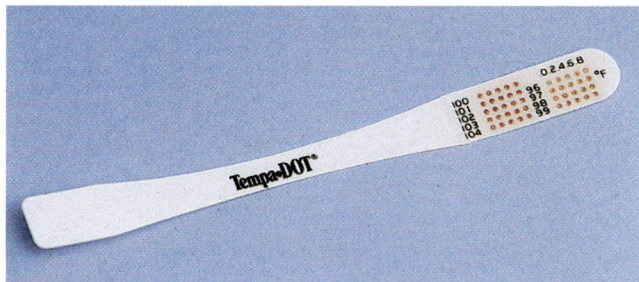

FIGURE 31-4 Tempa-Dot disposable oral strip thermometer. (Courtesy Tempa-Dot, Sommerville, NJ.)

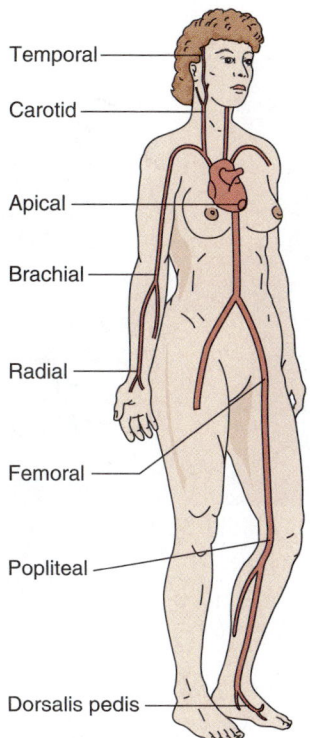

FIGURE 31-5 Pulse sites.

removing the sheath, be careful not to contaminate the probe or the processing unit. If a chance exists that a patient's body fluids touched the unit, wipe it with disinfectant before returning it to the storage area.

Tympanic Thermometers

The same guidelines for a digital unit are followed in the cleaning of a tympanic thermometer. When using the device on a small child, be conscious of what the child touches. If the processing unit is touched, be sure to wipe it with disinfectant after use. However, be careful not to get the tip of the probe surface wet, and always use probe covers, because disinfectant can ruin the probe surface.

CRITICAL THINKING APPLICATION   31-3

How should the medical assistant adapt temperature-taking techniques in the following scenarios?
- A patient who talks continuously with the thermometer in his mouth
- A 7-year-old patient with bilateral otitis externa
- A 3-month-old patient when a temporal artery thermometer is available
- A 46-year-old patient with a severe asthma attack
- A 72-year-old patient with bilateral impacted cerumen
- A 28-year-old patient who has just smoked a cigarette

Disposable Thermometers

Always discard a disposable thermometer in the appropriate waste container immediately after use to prevent contamination and the spread of pathogens to other patients. If you are instructing a parent in the use of a disposable thermometer at home, be sure to emphasize that it should be discarded immediately in a childproof container.

PULSE

A patient's pulse rate reflects the palpable beat of the arteries throughout the body as they expand in response to contraction of the heart. With every beat, the heart pumps an amount of blood, known as the *stroke volume*, into the aorta. Arteries branch off the aorta as it travels down through the center of the abdomen, transferring the pulse beat throughout the body. To measure the pulse, an artery is used that is close to the body surface and can be pushed against a bone. Palpating a **peripheral** pulse gives the rate and rhythm of

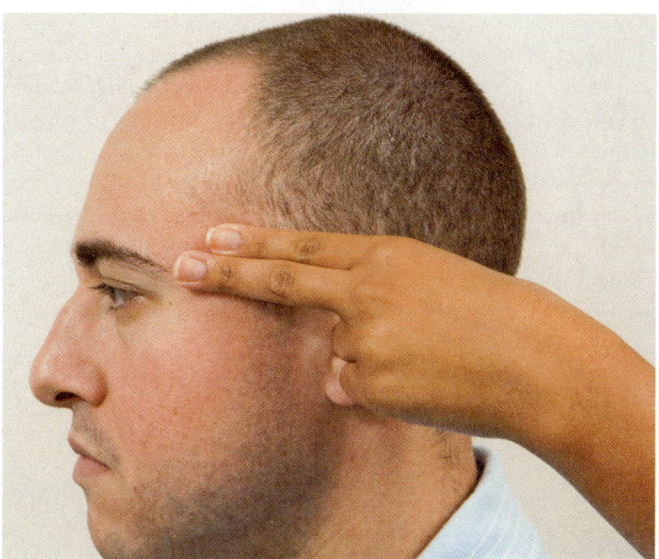

FIGURE 31-6 Temporal pulse.

the heartbeat and local information about the condition of the artery used.

Pulse Sites

A pulse rate may be counted any place where an artery is near the surface of the body and the vessel can be pressed against a bone. The most common sites used to feel this rhythmic throbbing are the temporal, carotid, apical, brachial, radial, femoral, popliteal, and dorsalis pedis arteries (Figure 31-5).

The *temporal* pulse is located in the temple area of the skull, parallel and lateral to the eyes (Figure 31-6). It is seldom used as a pulse

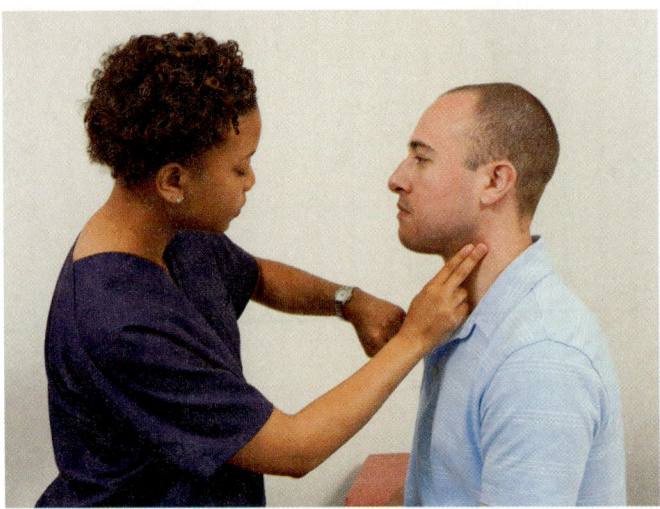

FIGURE 31-7 Carotid pulse.

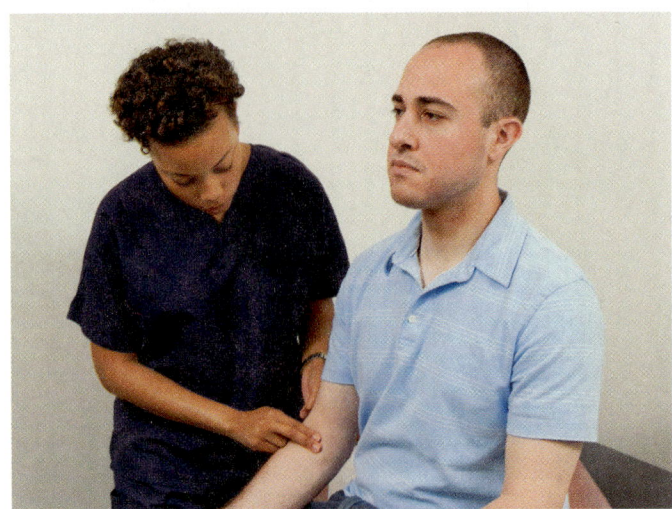

FIGURE 31-8 Brachial pulse.

site but may be used as a pressure point to help control bleeding from a head injury.

The *carotid* artery is located between the larynx and the sternocleidomastoid muscle in the front and to the side of the neck (Figure 31-7). It most frequently is used in emergencies and to check the pulse during cardiopulmonary resuscitation (CPR). It can be felt by pushing the muscle to the side and pressing against the larynx.

The *apical* heart rate, or the heartbeat at the apex of the heart, is heard with a stethoscope. It is used for infants and young children because the radial pulse is difficult to palpate in young patients or in adults if the radial pulse is difficult to feel or is irregular. An apical count may be requested if the patient is taking cardiac drugs or has **bradycardia** or **tachycardia**. To determine the presence of a **pulse deficit**, the physician may listen to the apical beat while the medical assistant counts the pulse at another site. The apex of the heart is located in the left fifth intercostal space on the midclavicular line,

that is, between the fifth and sixth ribs on a line with the midpoint of the left clavicle. The stethoscope is placed just below the left nipple between the fifth and sixth ribs. The pulse should be counted for 1 full minute and should be documented with (AP) beside the recorded count (Procedure 31-5).

The *brachial* pulse is felt at the inner *(antecubital)* aspect of the elbow. This is the artery that is felt and heard when blood pressure is measured (Figure 31-8). It also can be felt in the groove between the biceps and triceps muscles on the inner surface of the middle upper arm. This is the pulse that is checked on infants and young children receiving CPR.

The *radial* artery is the most frequently used site for counting the pulse rate. It is best found on the thumb side of the wrist, 1 inch below the base of the thumb (Figure 31-9).

The *femoral* pulse is located at the site where the femoral artery passes through the groin. The examiner must press deeply below the inguinal ligament to palpate this pulse.

PROCEDURE 31-5

Obtain Vital Signs: Obtain an Apical Pulse

GOAL: *To accurately determine and record the patient's apical heart rate.*

EQUIPMENT and SUPPLIES

- Watch with a second hand
- Patient gown as needed
- Stethoscope
- Patient record
- Alcohol wipes

PROCEDURAL STEPS

1. Sanitize your hands and clean the stethoscope earpieces and diaphragm with alcohol swabs.
   PURPOSE: To ensure infection control and to follow Standard Precautions.

2. Introduce yourself, identify your patient, and explain the procedure.
   PURPOSE: Identification of the patient prevents errors, and explanations are a means of gaining implied consent and patient cooperation.

3. If necessary, assist the patient in disrobing from the waist up and provide the patient with a gown that opens in the front.
   PURPOSE: To expose the chest and provide privacy and warmth.

4. Assist the patient into the sitting or supine position.
   PURPOSE: To allow easier access to the apical site at the apex of the heart.

PROCEDURE 31-5—cont'd

5. Hold the stethoscope's diaphragm against the palm of your hand for a few seconds.
   <u>PURPOSE:</u> To warm the diaphragm, promoting patient comfort.
6. Place the stethoscope just below the left nipple in the intercostal space between the fifth and sixth ribs over the apex of the heart (Figures 1 and 2).
   <u>PURPOSE:</u> This is the point of maximum contractile strength, where the heartbeat can be heard best.

7. Listen carefully for the heartbeat.
8. Count the pulse for 1 full minute. Note any irregularities in rhythm and volume.
   <u>PURPOSE:</u> The apical pulse is always measured for 1 full minute to obtain the most accurate reading.
9. Help the patient sit up and dress.
10. Sanitize your hands.
11. Record the pulse in the patient's chart (e.g., AP = 96) and record any arrhythmias.

4/22/XX 4:10 PM AP 92, irregular — — — — — —
C. Ricci, CMA (AAMA) _____

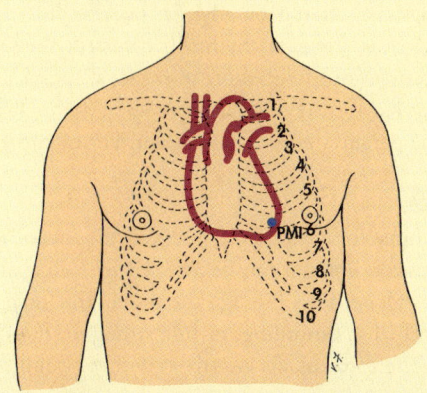

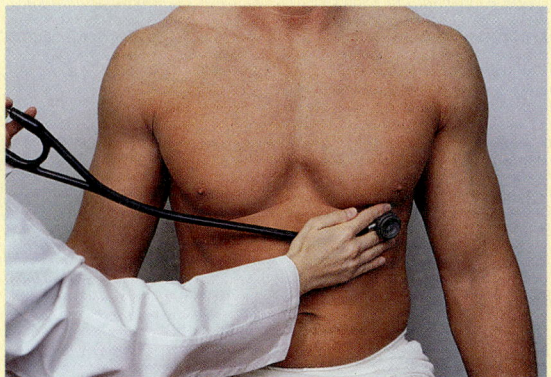

The *popliteal* pulse is found at the back of the leg behind the knee. Palpation of this pulse requires the patient to be in a recumbent position with the knee slightly flexed. The popliteal artery is deep and difficult to feel. It is palpated and also monitored with a stethoscope when a leg blood pressure reading is necessary. The physician checks blood flow through the popliteal artery if a circulatory system problem, such as a blood clot, is suspected in the lower leg.

The *dorsalis pedis* (pedal) artery is felt across the arch of the foot, just slightly lateral to the midline, beside the extensor tendon of the great toe. This pulse may be congenitally absent in some patients. Because a good pulse rate at this site is an indicator of normal lower limb circulation and arterial sufficiency, the physician checks the pedal pulses in patients with peripheral vascular problems (e.g., patients with diabetes mellitus).

Characteristics of a Pulse

When measuring a pulse, you must note three important characteristics: rate, rhythm, and volume. These characteristics vary with the size and elasticity of the artery and the strength and regularity of the heart's contractions. A patient's pulse may reveal valuable information about the cardiovascular system.

Rate

The pulse rate is a measure of the number of heartbeats felt from the movement of blood through an artery. When the heart contracts, pressure throughout the arteries is increased, and the arteries expand. When the heart relaxes, arterial pressure is decreased, and the arteries relax. Each contraction and relaxation of the heart muscle is a heartbeat, and each resulting expansion and relaxation of the arteries is

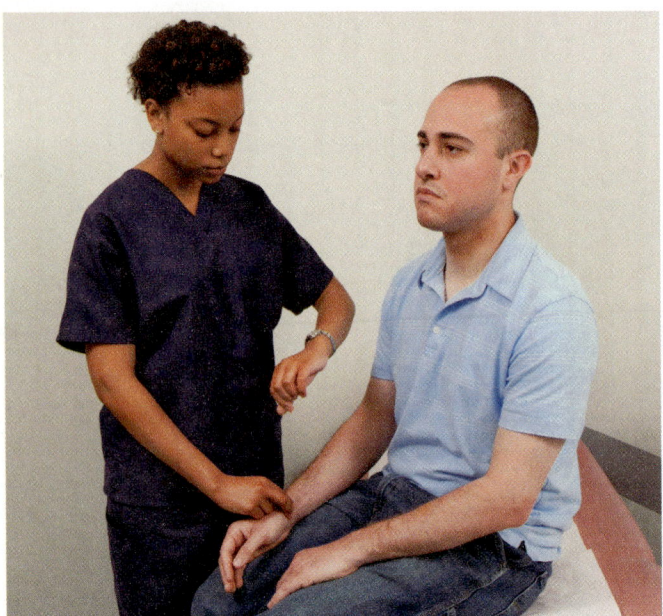

FIGURE 31-9 Radial pulse.

TABLE 31-3 Approximate Age-Related Pulse Ranges

AGE	RANGE (BREATHS PER MINUTE)	AVERAGE
Newborn	120-160	140
1-2 years	80-140	120
3-6 years	75-120	100
7-11 years	75-110	95
Adolescence to adulthood	60-100	80

the pulse rate. Normally, the heartbeat (rate) and the pulse rate are the same. The rate of the pulse is the number of heartbeats (pulsations) that occur in 1 minute. Because the body must balance heat loss by increasing circulation (a faster heart rate), the pulse rate is proportionate with the size of the heart. The smaller the body, the greater is the heat loss and the faster the heart must pump to compensate. Therefore, infants and children normally have a faster pulse than adults; as the aging process progresses, the pulse rate declines.

Pulse rates normally vary as a result of a person's age, body size, gender, and health status. The rate is affected by an individual's activities and psychological state, and by certain medications. It usually is faster in women (70 to 80 beats per minute) than in men (60 to 70 beats per minute). Children tend to have more rapid pulse rates than adults. The rate is more rapid when sitting than when lying down, and it increases when an individual stands, walks, or runs. During sleep or rest, the pulse rate may drop to as low as 45 to 50 beats per minute. Well-conditioned athletes tend to have pulse rates of 50 to 60 beats per minute, because consistent aerobic exercise strengthens the heart muscle (the myocardium) so that each heart contraction ejects an increased volume of blood into the arterial system. Table 31-3 lists the normal pulse ranges for various age groups of patients.

Rhythm

The pulse rhythm is the time between pulse beats. A normal rhythm pattern has an even tempo, which indicates that the intervals between the beats are of equal duration. An abnormal rhythm, or **arrhythmia**, is described according to the rhythm pattern detected. An **intermittent pulse** may occur in healthy individuals during exercise or after drinking a beverage containing caffeine. A common irregularity found in children and young adults is **sinus arrhythmia**, in which the heart rate varies with the respiratory cycle, speeding up at the peak of inspiration and slowing to normal with expiration. If beats are frequently skipped or if the beats are markedly irregular,

the physician should be advised, because this may indicate heart disease. If an irregular rhythm is detected, the apical pulse should be measured for a full minute to ensure accuracy, and the rate should be recorded for the physician's review. A note also should be made that the patient's pulse was irregular. For example: P-86 irregular.

Volume

The volume (pulse amplitude) reflects the strength of the heart when it contracts. Volume can be assessed by feeling the strength of the pulse as blood flows through the vessel. The force of each pulse beat is described as **bounding**, or full; strong, or normal; or **thready**, or weak. The force of the heartbeat and the condition of the arterial wall, whether hard or soft, influence the volume. The pulse may vary only in intensity and otherwise may be perfectly regular. This condition also can indicate heart disease. The pulse force is recorded using a three-point scale.

THREE-POINT SCALE FOR MEASURING PULSE VOLUME

3+	Full, bounding pulse	Pulsation is very strong and does not disappear with moderate pressure.
2+	Normal pulse	Pulsation is easily felt but disappears with moderate pressure.
1+	Weak, thready pulse	Pulsation is not easily felt and disappears with slight pressure.

Determining the Pulse Rate

Radial and Apical Pulse Rates

The patient should be in a comfortable position, with the artery to be used at the same level as or lower than the heart (Procedure 31-6). The limb should be well supported and relaxed. The patient may be lying down or sitting. As with all pulse readings, the pads of the first three fingers are placed over the artery. The thumb should never be used to determine the pulse rate, because the thumb has its own pulse, and the medical assistant's pulse rate may be confused with the patient's rate. Push the radial artery against the bone until the strongest pulsation is felt. The pulse should be counted for 1 full minute. The 15- or 30-second interval may be used once the medical assistant becomes proficient at performing the skill.

Variations from normal quality should be noted, such as an arrhythmia or a pulse that is thready or bounding. Some pulses are

Obtain Vital Signs: Assess the Patient's Radial Pulse

GOAL: *To accurately determine and record a patient's radial pulse rate, rhythm, and volume.*

EQUIPMENT and SUPPLIES

- Watch with a second hand
- Patient record

PROCEDURAL STEPS

1. Sanitize your hands.
   PURPOSE: To ensure infection control.
2. Introduce yourself, identify your patient, and explain the procedure.
   PURPOSE: Identification of the patient prevents errors, and explanations are a means of gaining implied consent and patient cooperation.
3. Place the patient's arm in a relaxed position, palm downward, at or below the level of the heart.
   PURPOSE: The patient's radial artery is more easily palpated when the patient is relaxed and in this position.
4. Gently grasp the palm side of the patient's wrist with your first three fingertips approximately 1 inch below the base of the thumb (Figure 1).
   PURPOSE: This position puts your fingertips directly over the radial artery. Press firmly (but do not press too hard, or you will occlude the artery and feel nothing).

5. Count the beats for 1 full minute using a watch with a second hand.
   PURPOSE: Counting for 1 full minute allows you to obtain an accurate count, including any irregularities in rhythm and volume.
6. Sanitize your hands.
   PURPOSE: To ensure infection control.
7. Record the count and any irregularities on the patient's medical record (e.g., P = 72). The pulse usually is recorded immediately after the temperature.
   PURPOSE: Procedures that are not recorded are considered not done.

5/6/XX 8:35 AM P 72, reg ———————
C. Ricci, CMA (AAMA) _____

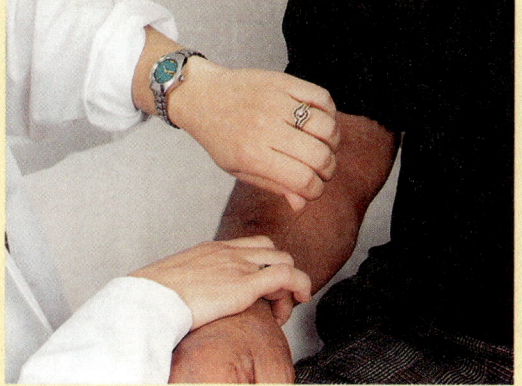

---

more difficult to feel than others, and finding the correct pressure to be used for each patient and site requires repeated practice and experience.

Both you and the patient should be in a relaxed position. The sensitivity in your counting fingers is greatly reduced if you are in an awkward position. Too much pressure obliterates the patient's pulse, and too little pressure prevents detection of irregularities or of all the beats. Record the number of beats in 1 minute. Assess the pulse, including rate, rhythm, and volume. If the pulse rate is counted at any site other than the radial artery, the rate should be recorded along with a notation of the site used. The apical pulse should always be auscultated for a full minute to detect any irregularities in rate and rhythm.

CRITICAL THINKING APPLICATION   31-4

Mrs. Arnez has a documented thready pulse. What site should Carlos use to measure the pulse?

Femoral, Popliteal, and Pedal Pulses

Pulses in the lower extremities may be difficult to find and equally difficult to hear. A Doppler unit, which is an ultrasound unit that magnifies the pulsation, may be used to locate and count these pulses accurately (Figure 31-10). This unit is battery operated and can be attached to a stethoscope so that only you hear the beat, or it can be set so that both you and your patient can hear the pulsations.

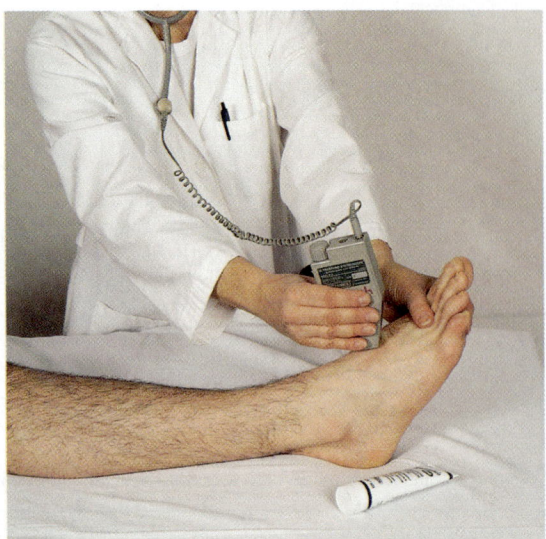

FIGURE 31-10 Doppler ultrasound unit measuring the pedal pulse. (From deWit S: *Fundamental concepts and skills for nursing*, ed 3, St Louis, 2009, Saunders.)

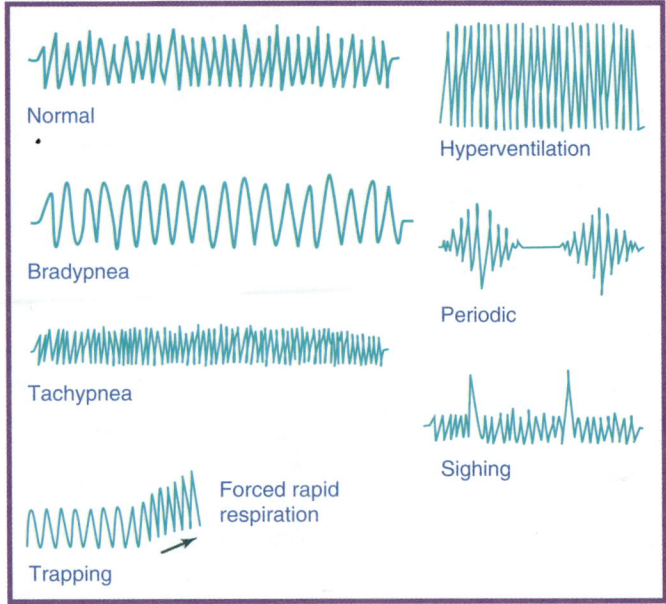

FIGURE 31-11 Respiratory rate patterns, called *spirograms*, are recorded using a spirometer.

RESPIRATION

Physiology

The purpose of respiration is to provide for the exchange of oxygen and carbon dioxide among the atmosphere, the blood, and the body cells. Oxygen is taken into the body to be used for life-sustaining body processes, and carbon dioxide is released as a waste product.

One complete inspiration and expiration is called a *respiration*. During the inspiratory phase, the diaphragm contracts and drops down while the intercostal muscles pull the ribs up and outward, causing the lungs to expand and fill with air. During the expiratory phase, the diaphragm returns to its normal elevated position and the intercostal muscles relax, causing the lungs to expel the waste air back into the atmosphere.

Respiration is both internal and external. *External respiration* is the exchange of oxygen and carbon dioxide in the lungs. *Internal respiration* occurs at the cellular level, when oxygen in the bloodstream is transferred into the cells for energy, and carbon dioxide is released as a waste product and transported back to the lungs for exhalation.

The respiratory center in the medulla oblongata, located in the brain between the top of the spine and the brainstem, is sensitive to changes in blood oxygen and carbon dioxide levels. When blood carbon dioxide levels become elevated, the respiratory control center sends a message to the respiratory system that triggers breathing. Respiration, therefore, is controlled by the involuntary nervous system; this means that we breathe automatically. Because a person can control respiration to a certain extent, it also is a voluntary body function. However, breathing ultimately is under the control of the medulla oblongata, which is why we can hold our breath only for a given length of time. Once the blood's carbon dioxide level rises to the point where cells become oxygen starved, a stimulus is sent to the respiratory muscles (the diaphragm and intercostal muscles) and breathing begins involuntarily.

TABLE 31-4 Approximate Age-Related Respiration Ranges

AGE	RANGE (BREATHS PER MINUTE)	AVERAGE
Newborn	30-50	40
1-3 years	20-30	25
4-6 years	18-26	22
7-11 years	16-22	19
Adolescence to adulthood	12-20	16

Characteristics of Respirations

Normally, a person's breathing is relaxed, automatic, and silent. When assessing a patient's respirations, you must note three important characteristics: rate, rhythm, and depth.

- *Rate:* The rate of respiration is the number of respirations per minute and is described as normal, rapid, or slow. Figure 31-11 shows sample rate patterns recorded with a **spirometer**. **Dyspnea** occurs in patients with pneumonia, asthma, or **chronic obstructive pulmonary disease (COPD)**. It also occurs after physical exertion or at very high altitudes. Other alterations in breathing are **bradypnea, apnea, tachypnea**, and **hyperpnea**. Hyperpnea usually is accompanied by **hyperventilation** and often is found when the patient is extremely anxious or in pain. **Orthopnea** frequently occurs in patients with congestive heart failure (CHF) and COPD. **Wheezing** signals difficulty breathing in patients with asthma. Typically, a ratio of four pulse beats to one respiration is seen. As a rule, both the pulse and respiratory rates respond to exercise or emotional upset. Table 31-4 lists normal respiratory ranges for patients in various age groups.
- *Rhythm:* The term *rhythm* refers to the breathing pattern. A regular breathing pattern is normal in adults; however, the

PROCEDURE 31-7

Obtain Vital Signs: Determine the Respiratory Rate

GOAL: *To accurately determine and record a patient's respirations. Remember that the respiratory count may be altered if the patient is aware that you are counting his or her breaths. Respirations typically are counted immediately after the pulse has been taken while the fingers are still at the radial site.*

EQUIPMENT and SUPPLIES

- Watch with a second hand
- Patient record

PROCEDURAL STEPS

1. Sanitize your hands.
   PURPOSE: To ensure infection control.
2. Introduce yourself and identify the patient.
   PURPOSE: Identification of the patient prevents errors.
3. The patient's arm is in the same position used to count the pulse. If you have difficulty noticing the patient's breathing, place the arm across the chest to detect movement.
   PURPOSE: This position allows you to feel or see the rise and fall of the chest wall.
4. Note the rise and fall of the patient's chest.
   PURPOSE: Inspiration and expiration make up one complete breathing cycle or respiration.

5. Count the respirations for 30 seconds, using a watch with a second hand, and multiply by 2.
   PURPOSE: Counting for 30 seconds allows you to obtain an accurate count and determine any irregularities in rhythm or depth or unusual breathing patterns. If respirations are abnormal in any way, count for 1 full minute.
6. Release the patient's wrist.
7. Sanitize your hands.
   PURPOSE: To ensure infection control.
8. Record the respirations on the patient's medical record after the pulse recording (e.g., R = 18).
   PURPOSE: Procedures that are not recorded are considered not done.

5/12/XX 1:15 PM R 18 — — — — — — — — C. Ricci, CMA (AAMA) _____

---

breathing pattern for infants varies. Automatic interruptions, such as sighing, are also considered normal.

- *Depth:* The *depth* of respiration is the amount of air inhaled and exhaled. When a patient is at rest, normal respirations have a consistent depth, which can be noted as you watch the rise and fall of the chest. Rapid, shallow breathing at rest occurs with some diseases, such as asthma and emphysema.

Normally, no noticeable breath sounds occur during the breathing process, except during snoring. Noticeable breath sounds are a sign of certain diseases, such as pneumonia, asthma, and pulmonary edema. After auscultating breath sounds with a stethoscope, the physician can describe the characteristics of breath sounds by using specific terminology (e.g., **rales, rhonchi, stertorous** breathing).

When an individual cannot inspire enough oxygen to supply all body cells with oxygenated blood, normal skin coloring, particularly around the mouth and the nail beds, changes to a bluish, dusky color. This coloration, which indicates an increased level of carbon dioxide in the blood, is called *cyanosis.* The patient also may have other signs and symptoms, such as vertigo, chest pain *(angina),* and numbness in the fingers and toes.

Counting Respirations

Because most people are unaware of their breathing, do not mention that you will be counting their respirations (Procedure 31-7). The respiratory rate is easily controlled, and patients self-consciously alter their breathing rate when they know they are being watched. Therefore, count the respirations while appearing to count the pulse. Keep your eyes alternately on the patient's chest and your watch while you

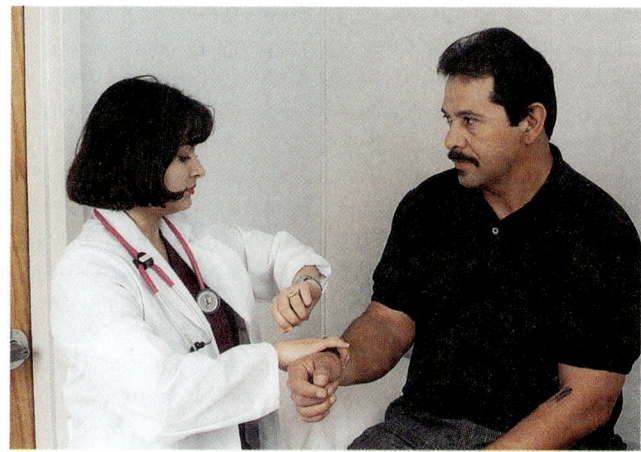

FIGURE 31-12 Hand position when counting respirations. The hands should be left in place as if still counting the patient's pulse.

count the pulse rate, and then, without removing your fingers from the pulse site, determine the respiratory rate. Counting respirations first may be easier, because that number is not as difficult to remember (Figure 31-12). If the patient is supine, the arm may be crossed over the chest so that respirations can be felt with the rise and fall of the chest. Another way of observing respirations is to watch the movement of the patient's shoulders with each inspiration. Count the respirations for 30 seconds and multiply the number by 2. Do not use the 15-second interval, because this count can vary by a factor of +4 or −4, which is significant when one is dealing with

TABLE 31-5 Approximate Age-Related Blood Pressure Ranges

AGE	RANGE
Newborn	60-96/30-62
1-3 years	78-112/48-78
4-6 years	78-112/50-79
7-11 years	85-114/52-79
Adolescent	94-119/58-79
Adult	100-119/60-79

TABLE 31-6 Hypertension Categories

BLOOD PRESSURE	NORMAL	PREHYPERTENSION	HYPERTENSION
Systolic, mm Hg	Less than 120	120-139	140 or higher
Diastolic, mm Hg	Less than 80	80-89	90 or higher

such a small number. Note any variation or irregularity in the rate. Record the respiratory count on the medical record.

CRITICAL THINKING APPLICATION   31-5

Tina Anderson, a 36-year-old patient who is obese, is wearing a heavy knit sweater, and Carlos needs to obtain a respiratory count. What could he do to obtain an accurate measurement of Tina's respiratory rate?

BLOOD PRESSURE

The blood pressure reading reflects the pressure of the blood against the walls of the arteries. Each time the ventricles contract, blood is pushed out of the heart and into the aorta, exerting pressure on the walls of the arteries. There are actually two blood pressure readings: the *systolic* pressure is the highest pressure level that occurs when the heart is contracting and the first pulse beat heard; the *diastolic* pressure is the lowest pressure level when the heart is relaxed and is the last sound heard. Systole (heart contraction) and diastole (heart relaxation) together make up the cardiac cycle. The difference between systolic and diastolic pressures is the **pulse pressure**.

Blood pressure is read in millimeters of mercury, abbreviated *mm Hg*. However, you need not include the abbreviation when documenting the reading on the patient's medical record. Blood pressure is recorded as a fraction, with the systolic reading the numerator (top) and the diastolic reading the denominator (bottom) (e.g., 130/80). Table 31-5 lists normal blood pressure ranges for patients of various age groups.

Factors That Affect Blood Pressure

Physiologic factors that determine blood pressure include blood volume, peripheral resistance created by blood viscosity (the thickness of the blood), vessel elasticity, and the condition of the heart muscle and arterial walls.

Volume is the amount of blood in the arteries. An increased blood volume raises blood pressure, and a decreased blood volume lowers blood pressure. Therefore, with extensive bleeding or hemorrhage, the blood volume drops, and so does the blood pressure.

The *peripheral resistance* of blood vessels refers to the relationship of the lumen (the diameter of the vessel) to the amount of blood flowing through it. The smaller the lumen, the greater is the resistance to blood flow. Blood pressure is higher with a small or reduced-size lumen and lower with a large lumen. Vessels affected by fatty

cholesterol deposits called *atherosclerotic plaques* become narrower over time, resulting in smaller vessel lumens and therefore higher blood pressure.

Vessel elasticity is the ability of an artery to expand and contract to supply the body with a steady flow of blood. With advancing age, certain lifestyle factors, or the presence of **arteriosclerosis**, vessel elasticity may decrease, causing the arterial walls to become firm and resistant; as a result, the blood pressure is increased.

The condition of the myocardium is a primary determinant of the volume of blood flowing through the body. A strong, forceful contraction empties the heart and tends to keep the blood pressure within normal limits. If the myocardium becomes weak, pressure in the vessels begins to increase in an attempt to maintain an adequate level of circulating blood to meet the oxygen and nutrient needs of the body.

Evaluating the Blood Pressure

When a patient's blood pressure is being tracked, frequent readings should be taken at about the same time of day and by the same person. **Secondary hypertension** is caused by another underlying pathologic condition, such as renal disease, complications of pregnancy, endocrine imbalance, arteriosclerosis, atherosclerosis, and brain injury. Temporary hypertension may occur with stress, pain, exercise, and exhaustion. Many patients experience "white coat hypertension," that is, their blood pressure becomes elevated in the medical environment, although it is normal when they are away from the healthcare facility. An adult is diagnosed with **essential hypertension** (primary hypertension) if the systolic pressure is 140 mm Hg or higher and/or the diastolic pressure is 90 mm Hg or higher. Essential hypertension is the most common type of hypertension. It has no single identified cause but is associated with obesity, a high blood level of sodium, elevated cholesterol levels, and family history.

In 2003, the American Heart Association (AHA) published new guidelines for the diagnosis and management of hypertension. A new category of blood pressure, prehypertension, was identified, and normal blood pressure levels were lowered to less than 120/80. Table 31-6 identifies the categories of normal, prehypertensive, and hypertensive blood pressures.

The goal of the new recommendations is to reduce the number of people who die each year from hypertension-related illnesses such as coronary artery disease, heart attack, heart failure, kidney disease, and stroke. Hypertension can occur in children or adults, but individuals of African-American descent, middle-aged and elderly people, patients with diabetes mellitus, and those with kidney disease are at greatest risk. Hypertension has been called *the silent killer*, because it frequently has no symptoms, and individuals may go for long periods without knowing they have a problem. Hypertension often is discovered during medical treatment for another problem. Signs and symptoms may include blurred vision, angina, vertigo, dyspnea, fatigue, headache, flushing, nosebleeds *(epistaxis)*, and palpitations.

The revised treatment guidelines for hypertension have four basic aspects:

1. Individuals with prehypertension should be diagnosed and encouraged to make lifestyle changes before they require medical treatment and/or move into the hypertensive category. The AHA recommends limiting intake of salt and eating a diet rich in potassium, calcium, magnesium, and protein while reducing total fat intake, especially saturated fat and cholesterol. Prehypertensive individuals also should restrict their alcohol intake, engage in regular physical activity, and lose weight if necessary to maintain a healthy BMI range. Many times, just losing weight lowers blood pressure.

2. In people older than 50 years of age, the systolic reading is more important than the diastolic reading. Individuals over 50 should be treated if they have a systolic pressure of 140 mm Hg or higher, regardless of their diastolic blood pressure. Medical treatment at this age can reduce the development of cardiac and kidney disease later in life.

3. Most patients with hypertension require two or more medications to achieve desired blood pressure levels. The goal of treatment is to maintain blood pressure below 140/90 mm Hg, or below 130/80 mm Hg in patients with diabetes or kidney disease. Patients should be treated with both a diuretic, to help the body excrete excess amounts of fluid and sodium, and an antihypertensive medication.

4. A patient-centered treatment approach should be implemented to motivate patients and to maintain compliance with hypertension management. The medical assistant can play an active role in establishing a therapeutic relationship with the patient by providing ongoing education and support to ensure compliance with physician-recommended treatment. Using community resources, such as local dietician referrals, may also help patients comply with treatment.

CRITICAL THINKING APPLICATION   31-6

Mr. Samuel Long, a 43-year-old patient, recently was diagnosed with essential hypertension. What should Carlos discuss with Mr. Long to emphasize the dangers of his disease and to teach him about possible lifestyle modifications that he must make to improve his health? Are any community resources available that might help Mr. Long and his family effectively manage his disease?

Hypotension is an abnormally low blood pressure, which may be caused by emotional or traumatic shock; hemorrhage; central nervous system disorders; and chronic wasting diseases. Persistent readings of 90/60 mm Hg or lower usually are considered hypotensive. **Orthostatic (postural) hypotension** can cause patients to experience vertigo or **syncope**. Some medications can cause orthostatic hypotension.

Measuring Blood Pressure

The instrument used to measure blood pressure is called the *sphygmomanometer.* The term *manometer* refers to an instrument used to measure the pressure of a liquid or a gas. *Sphygmo-* means pulse. Therefore, *sphygmomanometer* means an instrument used to measure blood pressure in the arteries. The instrument consists of an inflatable cuff, an inflation bulb with a control valve, and a pressure gauge. The blood pressure mechanism consists of an aneroid dial attached to an inflatable cuff (Figure 31-13, *A*) or a blood pressure floor model (Figure 31-13, *B*).

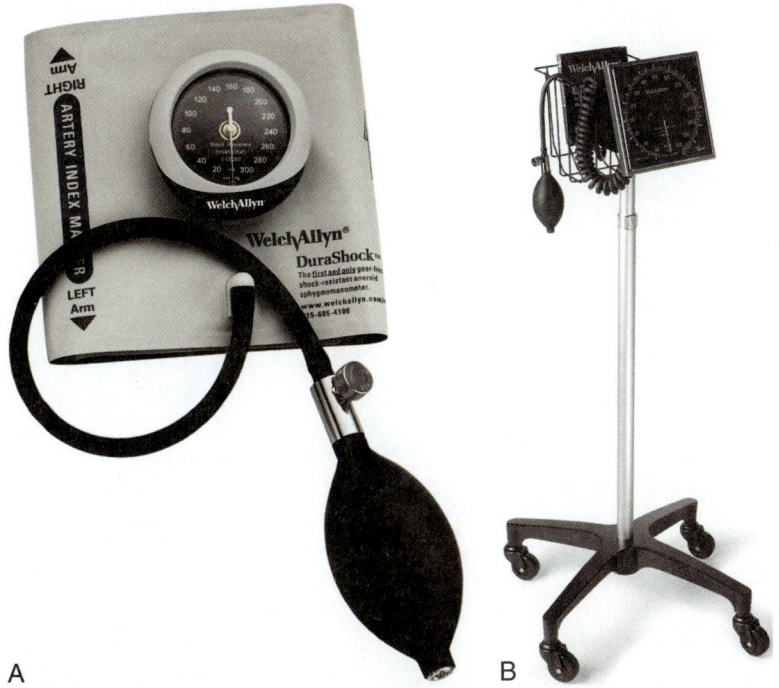

FIGURE 31-13 A, Aneroid dial system with an inflatable cuff. **B**, Aneroid floor model with a large, slanted face.

Sphygmomanometers are delicately calibrated instruments that must be handled carefully. They should be recalibrated regularly and checked for accuracy, by you or by a medical supply dealer. The needle on the aneroid dial sphygmomanometer should rest within the small square or circle at the bottom of the dial. The dial can be calibrated by connecting it to a calibrated manometer. Pump both manometers to 250 mm Hg and record readings on both machines at least four different times as the pressure is released. A correctly calibrated mechanism shows a difference of no more than 3 mm Hg between the two readings at any time during the deflation period. If the sphygmomanometer is not correctly calibrated, the patient's blood pressure reading will be inaccurate.

The sphygmomanometer must be used with a stethoscope. The objective of the procedure is to use the inflatable cuff to obliterate (cause to disappear) circulation through an artery. The stethoscope is placed over the artery just below the cuff, and the cuff is slowly deflated to allow the blood to flow again. As blood flow resumes, cardiac cycle sounds are heard through the stethoscope, and gauge readings are taken when the first (systolic) and last (diastolic) sounds are heard (Procedure 31-8).

Blood pressure cuffs and stethoscopes are available in drug and retail stores for patients to use to measure their own blood pressure at home. These units can be aneroid, electronic, or computerized sphygmomanometers (Figure 31-14). If you have patients who are monitoring their pressure at home, be sure that they understand the mechanics of obtaining a reading accurately. It is best to have the patient bring his or her equipment to the office and demonstrate its use. While the patient is showing you the home equipment, you will

PROCEDURE 31-8

Obtain Vital Signs: Determine a Patient's Blood Pressure

GOAL: *To perform a blood pressure measurement that is correct in technique, accurate, and comfortable for the patient.*

EQUIPMENT and SUPPLIES

- Sphygmomanometer
- Stethoscope
- Antiseptic wipes/alcohol swabs
- Patient record

PROCEDURAL STEPS

1. Sanitize your hands.
   <u>PURPOSE:</u> To ensure infection control.
2. Assemble the equipment and supplies needed. Clean the earpieces and diaphragm of the stethoscope with alcohol swabs.
   <u>PURPOSE:</u> To follow Standard Precautions.
3. Introduce yourself, identify the patient, and explain the procedure.
   <u>PURPOSE:</u> Identification of the patient prevents errors, and explanations are a means of gaining implied consent and patient cooperation.
4. Select the appropriate arm for application of the cuff (no mastectomy on that side, without injury or disease). If the patient has had a bilateral mastectomy, the blood pressure should be taken using a large thigh cuff with the stethoscope over the popliteal artery.
   <u>PURPOSE:</u> The pressure of the cuff temporarily interferes with circulation to the limb.
5. Seat the patient in a comfortable position with the legs uncrossed and the arm resting, palm up, at heart level on the lap or a table.
   <u>PURPOSE:</u> To expose the brachial artery; also, to promote patient relaxation and ensure a true reading. Crossed legs may increase the blood pressure, and positioning of the arm above heart level may cause an inaccurate reading.
6. Roll up the sleeve to about 5 inches above the elbow or have the patient remove the arm from the sleeve.
   <u>PURPOSE:</u> Tight clothing prevents an accurate reading.
7. Determine the correct cuff size.
   <u>PURPOSE:</u> An incorrect cuff size prevents accurate measurement of blood pressure. The cuff should fit comfortably around the patient's arm, and the bladder should be located over the brachial artery between the lines designated on the cuff. Pediatric, normal adult, and large adult cuff sizes should be available.
8. Palpate the brachial artery at the antecubital space in both arms. If one arm has a stronger pulse, use that arm. If the pulses are equal, select the right arm.
   <u>PURPOSE:</u> A stronger pulse is easier to measure; the right arm is the universal arm of choice.
   <u>CAUTION:</u> If a female patient has had a mastectomy, the blood pressure should never be taken on the affected side. Compressing the arm may cause complications. If she has had a bilateral mastectomy, another site such as the popliteal artery must be used, which requires use of a thigh cuff.
9. Center the cuff bladder over the brachial artery with the connecting tube away from the patient's body and the tube to the bulb close to the body (Figure 1).
   <u>PURPOSE:</u> Pressure must be applied directly over the artery for an accurate reading. The cuff and its tubing should not touch the stethoscope. Noise from the tubing can interfere with a correct reading.

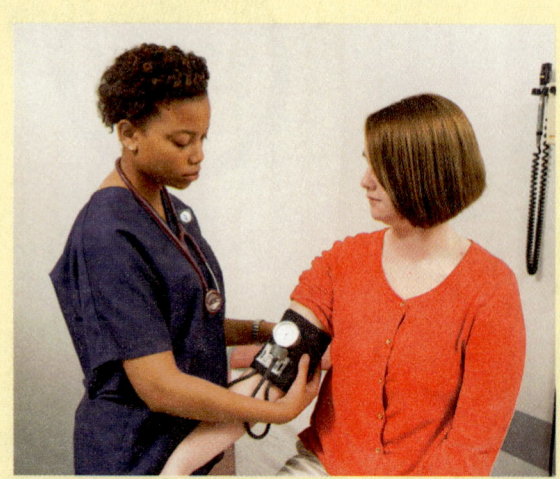

10. Place the lower edge of the cuff about 1 inch above the palpable brachial pulse, normally located in the natural crease of the inner elbow, and wrap it snugly and smoothly.
    PURPOSE: To help ensure an accurate reading. The cuff should be high enough on the arm that the stethoscope does not touch it, so that cuff sounds do not interfere with listening to the blood pressure sounds. A loose cuff results in an inaccurate reading.
11. Position the gauge of the sphygmomanometer so that it is easily seen.
    PURPOSE: An aneroid gauge should show the needle within the zero mark.
12. Palpate the brachial pulse, tighten the screw valve on the air pump, and inflate the cuff until the pulse can no longer be felt. Make a note at the point on the gauge where the pulse could no longer be felt. Mentally add 30 mm Hg to the reading. Deflate the cuff and wait 15 seconds (Figure 2).
    PURPOSE: The point where the brachial pulse is no longer felt provides an estimate of the systolic pressure. Pumping the cuff above that level ensures that phase I of the Korotkoff sounds will be heard.

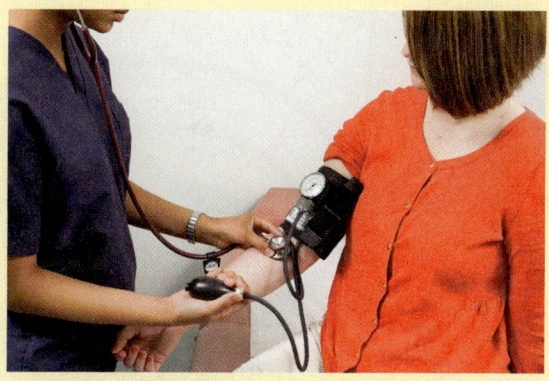

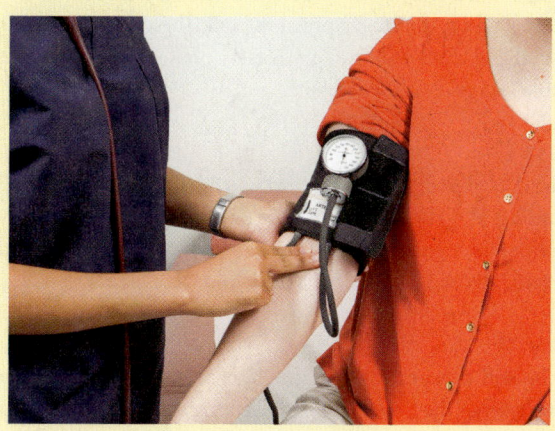

13. Insert the earpieces of the stethoscope turned forward into the ear canals.
    PURPOSE: With the earpieces in this position, the openings follow the anatomic line of the ear canal and the blood pressure will be accurately heard.
14. Place the stethoscope's diaphragm over the palpated brachial artery for an adult patient or the bell for a pediatric patient. Press firmly enough to obtain a seal but not so tightly that the artery is constricted.
    PURPOSE: Forming a seal around the head of the stethoscope aids listening for blood pressure sounds.
15. Close the valve and squeeze the bulb to inflate the cuff, rapidly but smoothly, to 30 mm above the palpated pulse level, which was previously determined (Figure 3).

16. Open the valve slightly and deflate the cuff at a constant rate of 2 to 3 mm Hg per heartbeat.
    PURPOSE: Careful, slow release allows you to listen to all sounds.
17. Listen throughout the entire deflation; note the point on the gauge at which you hear the first sound (systolic) and the last sound (diastolic) until the sounds have stopped for at least 10 mm Hg. Read the pressure to the closest even number.
18. Do not reinflate the cuff once the air has been released. Wait 30 to 60 seconds to repeat the procedure if needed.
    PURPOSE: Not allowing the blood to refill in the brachial artery results in inaccurate readings.
19. Remove the stethoscope from your ears and record the systolic and diastolic readings as BP systolic/diastolic (e.g., BP 120/80).
    NOTE: It is recommended that the blood pressure be checked and recorded in each arm during the initial assessment of the patient and then bilaterally periodically after that for patients with hypertension.
20. Remove the cuff from the patient's arm and return it to its proper storage area. Clean the earpieces of the stethoscope with alcohol and return it to storage.
21. Sanitize your hands.
    PURPOSE: To ensure infection control.
    ADDENDUM: The physician may direct the medical assistant to record the blood pressure with the patient in two different positions to determine whether orthostatic hypotension is a factor. To perform this skill:
    1. Measure and record the patient's blood pressure (as detailed earlier) while the patient is either supine or sitting.
    2. Leave the cuff in place.
    3. Have the patient stand, and immediately measure the blood pressure again.
    4. Record the second blood pressure, as well as any patient symptoms, such as complaints of (c/o) vertigo or lightheadedness.

    5/19/XX 11 AM BP 120/80 ℗ arm ——————
    C. Ricci, CMA (AAMA) _____

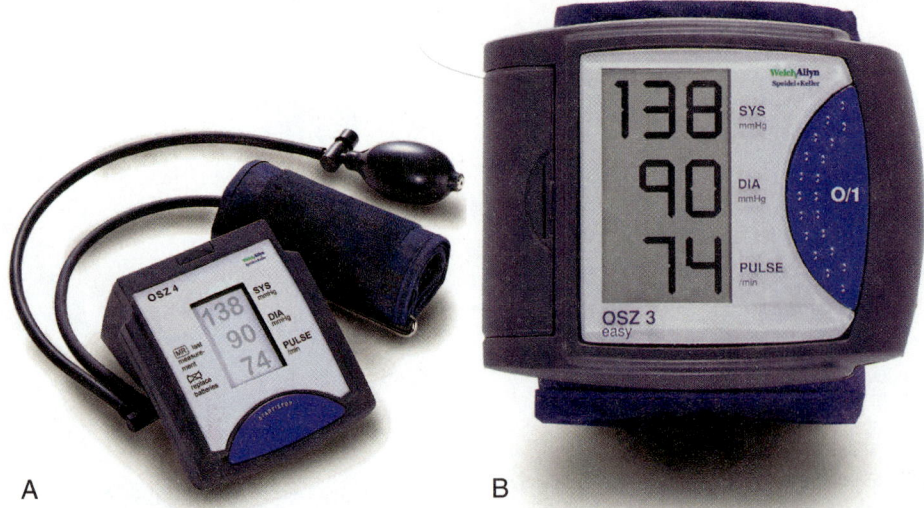

FIGURE 31-14 Personal blood pressure systems. **A,** Digital arm cuff. **B,** Digital wrist cuff.

have an ideal opportunity to check technique and calibration and to answer any questions the patient may have about use of the equipment. This is also a good opportunity to reinforce treatment plans, such as medication, diet, and exercise. It is helpful for a patient who is monitoring blood pressure readings at home to keep a log and review it with the physician during visits to help detect blood pressure variations during normal daily activities.

COMMON CAUSES OF ERROR IN BLOOD PRESSURE READINGS

- The limb used for measurement is above the level of the heart.
- The rubber bladder in the cuff is not completely deflated before a reading is started or retaken.
- The pressure in the cuff is released too rapidly.
- The patient is nervous, uncomfortable, or anxious, which may cause a reading higher than the patient's actual blood pressure.
- The patient drank coffee or smoked cigarettes within 30 minutes of the blood pressure measurement.
- The cuff is applied improperly.
- The cuff is too large, too small, too loose, or too tight.
- The cuff is not placed around the arm smoothly.
- The bladder is not centered over the artery, or the bladder bulges out from the cover.
- The practitioner fails to wait 1 to 2 minutes between measurements.
- Instruments are defective:
  - Air leaks in the valve
  - Air leaks in the bladder
  - Aneroid needle not calibrated to zero

Korotkoff Sounds

Two basic heart sounds are produced by the functioning of the heart during the cardiac cycle. The first sound, produced at systole (contraction), is dull, firm, and prolonged and is heard as a *lubb* sound. The second sound, produced at diastole (relaxation), is shorter and

sharper and is heard as a *dupp* sound. Therefore, *lubb-dupp* is the sound of one heartbeat.

Korotkoff sounds are the sounds heard during auscultation of blood pressure. These sounds are produced by vibrations of the arterial wall when the blood surges back into the vessel after it has been compressed by the blood pressure cuff. These sounds were first discovered and classified into five distinct phases by Russian neurologist Nikolai Sergeyevich Korotkoff.

Phase I

Phase I is the first sound heard as the cuff deflates. The blood is resurging into the patient's artery and can be heard quite clearly as a sharp, tapping sound. Note the gauge reading when this first sound is heard. Record this as the systolic blood pressure.

Phase II

As the cuff deflates, even more blood flows through the artery. The movement of the blood makes a swishing sound. If you do not follow proper procedure in inflating the cuff, you may not hear these sounds because of their soft quality. Occasionally, blood pressure sounds completely disappear during this phase. Loss of the sounds followed by their reappearance later is called the *auscultatory gap.* The silence may continue as the needle falls another 30 mm Hg. Auscultatory gaps occur particularly in hypertension and certain types of heart disease, so if you notice such a gap, make sure to report it to the physician.

Phase III

In phase III, a great deal of blood is pushing down into the artery. The distinct, sharp tapping sounds return and continue rhythmically. If you do not inflate the cuff enough, you will miss the first two phases completely and you will incorrectly interpret the beginning of phase III as the systolic blood pressure (phase I).

Phase IV

At this point, the blood is flowing easily. The sound changes to a soft tapping, which becomes muffled and begins to grow fainter. Occasionally, these sounds continue to zero. This may occur in children, in patients of any age after exercise or with a fever, or in a pregnant patient with anemia. The AHA recommends that the beginning of phase IV be recorded as the diastolic reading for a child. Some physicians call the change at phase IV the *fading sound* and want it recorded between systolic and diastolic recordings (e.g., 120/84/70, with 84 representing the gauge reading when the sounds of phase III have ended and those of phase IV are beginning). Other physicians consider phase IV the true diastolic pressure.

Phase V

All sounds disappear in this phase. Note the gauge reading when the last sound is heard. Record this as the diastolic pressure.

Palpatory Method

The systolic pressure may be checked by feeling the radial pulse rather than hearing it with the stethoscope. Place the cuff in the usual position and palpate the radial pulse, noting rate and rhythm. Inflate the cuff until the pulse disappears, and then add 30 mm Hg more of inflation to get above the systolic pressure. Do not remove your fingers from the pulse or change the pressure of your fingers. Slowly release the pressure in the cuff and wait for the pulse to be felt again. Note the reading on the gauge, and record the first pulse felt as the systolic pressure. For example, if you first felt the radial pulse at 52 mm Hg, the palpated blood pressure is recorded as 52/P, with P indicating that the systolic reading was palpated. The diastolic and Korotkoff phases cannot be determined by this method. This method can be very useful in times of a medical emergency, such as shock, when the patient's blood pressure cannot be auscultated.

CRITICAL THINKING APPLICATION   31-7

Vital signs are documented in this order: temperature (T), pulse (P), and respirations (R). Blood pressure is recorded after TPR. Correctly document the following vital signs:

1. Oral temperature 101.2°; apical pulse 90; respirations 22; and orthostatic blood pressure 138/88 supine and 110/70 standing
2. Tympanic temperature 36.8°; radial pulse 66; respirations 18; and bilateral blood pressure 128/76 in the left arm and 132/80 in the right arm
3. Temporal temperature 102.4°; apical pulse 102; and respirations 27
4. Axillary temperature 97.7°; carotid pulse 58; respirations 24; and palpated blood pressure 62

OSHA GUIDELINES FOR MEASURING VITAL SIGNS

Guidelines established by the Occupational Safety and Health Administration (OSHA) for the measurement of vital signs include the following:

- Wash hands before and after each procedure.
- Always use protective disposable sheaths on all forms of thermometers.
- Immediately disinfect any equipment that has become contaminated during the procedure.

- Wear gloves if the potential exists for contacting any open areas or body fluids.
- When caring for a patient with a known respiratory infectious disorder, such as tuberculosis, use protective clothing, including a face shield or mask as indicated.
- Dispose of all contaminated material, including thermometer covers, gloves, and disinfectant swabs, in the proper biohazard waste containers.

ANTHROPOMETRIC MEASUREMENT

Anthropometry is the science that deals with measurement of the size, weight, and proportions of the human body. These measurements often are included in the initial recording of vital signs and before the physician performs a physical examination or a well-baby check. Because they are indicators of the patient's state of health and well-being, height and weight measurements and the associated BMI are discussed as aspects of the vital signs. Other measurements are discussed when pertinent in the specialty chapters.

Measuring Weight and Height

A patient's weight and height can be helpful in diagnosis, and the medical assistant must obtain these readings with accuracy and empathy (Procedure 31-9). In many medical settings, weight and height are measured routinely as the patient is escorted to the examination room. If this is the patient's first visit, anthropometric measurements are written in the history database and are used as reference information during future visits as needed. Many physicians now use BMI to determine the risk for certain diseases, so the medical assistant may have to use accurately measured height and weight to determine the patient's BMI, as discussed in Chapter 30.

Certain medical specialties and specific medical problems may require continuous monitoring of weight. Hormone disorders (e.g., diabetes), growth patterns (seen in children), and eating disorders (e.g., obesity, bulimia) require accurate weight checks as part of every medical visit. In addition, maternity patients must have their weight monitored to make sure they are gaining weight but also as a precaution against too much weight gain, which may indicate fluid retention. Patients with cardiovascular disorders who tend to retain fluid should have their weight checked each time they are seen in the office. Some scales are calibrated in kilograms, others in pounds. When weight must be converted from one to the other, use the formulas shown later in the chapter.

Accurate height or length measurements are important when caring for children (see the chapter on pediatrics). The physician also may request routine height screening for patients diagnosed with osteoporosis, because these patients may lose height over time.

Weight

Some patients are sensitive or secretive about their body weight, so the scale should be located in an area that provides privacy from staff and other patients. Your manner and approach are very important in keeping patients from feeling embarrassed or shy. As explained in Chapter 30, healthcare specialists are depending more on BMI than on traditional height and weight tables, but accurate

PROCEDURE 31-9

Obtain Vital Signs: Measure a Patient's Weight and Height

GOAL: *To accurately weigh and measure a patient as part of the physical assessment procedure.*
NOTE: *Make sure the scale is located in an area away from traffic to maintain the patient's privacy.*

EQUIPMENT and SUPPLIES

- Balance scale with a measuring bar
- Paper towel
- Patient record

PROCEDURAL STEPS

1. Sanitize your hands.
   PURPOSE: To ensure infection control.
2. Introduce yourself, identify your patient, and explain the procedure.
   PURPOSE: Identification of the patient prevents errors, and explanations are a means of gaining implied consent and patient cooperation.
3. If the patient is to remove his or her shoes for weighing, place a paper towel on the scale platform. The patient may be given disposable slippers to wear.
4. Check to see that the balance bar pointer floats in the middle of the balance frame when all weights are at zero.
   PURPOSE: A floating pointer indicates that the scale is properly adjusted and in balance.
5. Help the patient onto the scale. Make sure a female patient is not holding a purse and that a male or female patient has removed any heavy objects from pockets.
6. Move the large weight into the groove closest to the patient's estimated weight. The grooves are calibrated in 50-lb increments. If you choose a groove that is more than the patient's weight, the pointer will immediately tilt to the bottom of the balance frame. You then must move it back one groove (Figure 1).

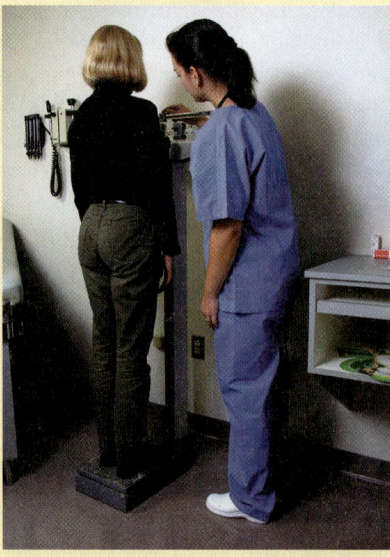

7. While the patient is standing still, slide the small upper weight to the right along the pound markers until the pointer balances in the middle of the balance frame.

PURPOSE: The pointer floats between the bottom and the top of the frame when both lower and upper weights together balance the scale with the patient's weight.

8. Leave the weights in place.
9. Ask the patient to stand up straight and to look straight ahead. On some scales, the patient may need to turn with the back to the scale.
10. Adjust the height bar so that it just touches the top of the patient's head (Figure 2).
11. Leave the elevation bar set but fold down the horizontal bar.
    PURPOSE: To maintain the height recording while protecting the patient from possible injury.

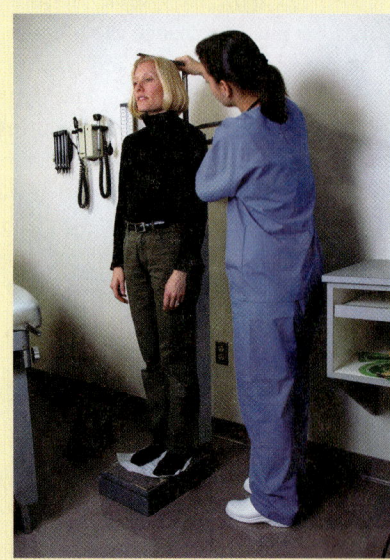

12. Assist the patient off the scale. Make sure all items that were removed for weighing are given back to the patient.
13. Read the weight scale. Add the numbers at the markers of the large and small weights and record the total to the nearest ¼ lb on the patient's medical record (e.g., Wt: 136½ lb).
14. Record the height. Read the marker at the movable point of the ruler and record the measurement to the nearest ¼ inch on the patient's medical record (e.g., Ht: 64¼ in).
15. Use the patient's weight and height to record the BMI if this is office procedure.
16. Return the weights and the measuring bar to zero.
17. Sanitize your hands.
18. Record the results on the patient's medical record.

5/26/XX 11:07 AM Wt 136½ lb, Ht 64¼ in — — —
C. Ricci, CMA (AAMA) _____

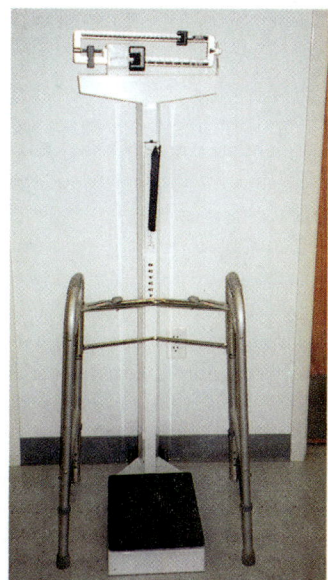

FIGURE 31-15 A walker is placed over the scale to aid the patient's balance.

measurements of height and weight are still required to accurately determine a patient's BMI. When patients are unstable, assist them onto the scale and help them balance themselves. A walker can be placed over the scale for the patient to use as hand support when getting on or off, or to maintain balance while on the scale (Figure 31-15).

If the physician prescribes weight measurement at home, make sure the patient understands the importance of weighing himself or herself each day at the same time in clothing of similar weight. Body weight may vary considerably from early morning to late afternoon. Teach the patient how to record weight on a graphic record and how to make any other important notations.

WEIGHT CONVERSION FORMULAS

To Convert Kilograms to Pounds
1 kg = 2.2 lb
Multiply the number of kilograms by 2.2.
Example
A patient weighs 68 kg: 68 × 2.2 = 149.6 lb.

To Convert Pounds to Kilograms
1 lb = 0.45 kg
Multiply the number of pounds by 0.45, or divide the number of pounds by 2.2 kg.
Example
A patient weighs 120 lb: 120 × 0.45 = 54 kg, or 120 ÷ 2.2 = 54.5 kg.

CRITICAL THINKING APPLICATION 31-8
- A patient weighs 87 kg; how many pounds does he weigh?
- A patient weighs 148 lb; how many kilograms does she weigh?

Height

Height can be measured in inches or centimeters. Measurement is easily accomplished by moving the parallel bar attached to a wall ruler or on the scale. Length measurements used in pediatrics are discussed in Chapter 42.

CRITICAL THINKING APPLICATION 31-9

Mrs. Johnson is being seen for the first time by Dr. Xu. In what order should Carlos take her vital signs and her anthropometric measurements? Should blood pressure be measured in both arms, with the patient both sitting and standing? If so, what is the rationale?

CLOSING COMMENTS

Patient Education

All patients should know how to use a thermometer safely and accurately, as well as the preferred site based on age and other patient factors. Because many types of temperature-reading equipment are available, ask the patient what type of equipment he or she uses at home to obtain temperature readings. Inexpensive digital models have greatly simplified home temperature taking.

In teaching how to assess the pulse rate, familiarize the patient with counting the beats and explain how to determine rate, rhythm, and regularity of the beat. Use diagrams to teach pulse points, and have the patient measure your pulse to assess the patient's accuracy and to provide any needed assistance.

If a patient is to keep track of respirations, a family member or helper must do this for the patient. The patient and all caregivers also should be taught self-assessment of impending complications, as well as how to perform preventive breathing exercises.

Monitoring blood pressure at home has become very common. Suggest that the patient bring his or her equipment to the office and practice with it. In this way, you can make sure the patient is using the equipment correctly and is recording the results accurately in a record book.

Weight management can be a trying and emotional experience for a patient. Understanding how weight is affected by time of day, by a particular activity, or by the type of scale used can help the patient maintain a positive attitude. Have an assortment of weight management literature available for the patient to take home, and use community resources when indicated to help the patient with weight-related issues (see Chapter 30 for further details).

RESPONSIBILITIES OF THE MEDICAL ASSISTANT IN OBTAINING VITAL SIGNS

- Monitoring vital signs is a key responsibility of the medical assistant.
- It is crucial to measure and describe all facets of each vital sign correctly.
- The information must be accurately and clearly documented.
- The medical assistant should take advantage of all opportunities to answer questions and to help the patient understand the significance of healthy vital signs.
- Patient privacy must be maintained throughout all procedures

- Family members or caregivers should be included in patient care and education as indicated.
- Community resources should be used to promote holistic patient care.
- The medical assistant should be sensitive to cultural and socioeconomic factors that may affect the patient's compliance with the physician's recommendations, such as diet, exercise, weight control, and the use of medication.

Legal and Ethical Issues

The medical assistant must remember that as the physician's agent, he or she plays an important role in preventing legal claims against the physician and the medical office. The medical assistant must always function within the legal boundaries of the profession. When obtaining vital signs, carefully select your response to a patient who asks about the results. Remember, medical assistants are not qualified to diagnose a patient problem, that is, never evaluate or give an opinion of what the results may mean. For example, if a patient asks, "Is my blood pressure better?" you might reply, "The reading is 160/90 today." You have not said that it is worse, the same, or better, but you have informed the patient of the current blood pressure reading.

Always be accurate in transcribing results into the patient's medical record. If results are incorrectly recorded, the patient may be incorrectly diagnosed or treated. This can result in legal action that may implicate you. A careless attitude toward assessment of vital signs and documentation can lead to possible legal entanglement. Every procedure in this chapter is accompanied by a reminder to record the test results. If no entry has been made, the assumption is that the procedure was not done. Develop sensitivity toward proper conduct and performance so that you can protect yourself and your physician-employer.

SUMMARY OF SCENARIO

Carlos recognizes the significance of measuring and recording each patient's vital signs and anthropometric measurements. Dr. Xu relies on Carlos to provide this information accurately. Carlos has never let these procedures become routine and has never done them without focusing on the task, because vital signs are an important reflection of a person's health status.

Carlos knows that a number of factors can alter a patient's vital signs, including the external environment, smoking, drinking hot beverages, exercise, and anxiety and pain. Carlos evaluates patient factors such as age, gender, level of compliance, and the presence of disease to determine the best method of accurately measuring vital signs. In addition, Carlos is sensitive to the need for safeguarding patient privacy. When he was first hired by Dr. Xu, he was concerned about privacy and confidentiality when he discovered that the patient scale was in the hall next to the waiting room. After he discussed this with the office manager, the scale was moved to an examination room, so that patients could be weighed in privacy.

Carlos attended a workshop last year on the revised AHA guidelines for the diagnosis and treatment of hypertension, and he is prepared to explain those recommendations to patients. He recognizes his role in motivating patients diagnosed with prehypertension to stick with recommended lifestyle changes and follow the physician's treatment protocol. Carlos continues to care for patients while providing valuable assistance to Dr. Xu in her busy primary care practice.

SUMMARY OF LEARNING OBJECTIVES

1. **Define, spell, and pronounce the terms listed in the vocabulary.**
   Spelling and pronouncing medical terms correctly bolsters the medical assistant's credibility. Knowing the definitions of these terms promotes confidence in communication with patients and co-workers.

2. **Apply critical thinking skills while performing patient assessment and patient care.**
   Completing the Critical Thinking Application exercises throughout the chapter can help the student medical assistant become more adept at critical analysis of real-life situations.

3. **Cite the average body temperature, pulse rate, respiratory rate, and blood pressure for various age groups.**
   Normal ranges for vital signs are summarized in Tables 31-1 through 31-5. The normal average pulse, respiratory rate, and blood pressure vary according to age, whereas temperature values vary according to age and the site used.

4. **Describe emotional and physical factors that can cause body temperature to rise or fall.**
   Multiple factors can affect body temperature, including the external environment, age, stress, physical exercise, gender, and illness.

5. **Convert temperature readings between Fahrenheit and Celsius scales.**
   Using the formulas presented in this chapter, perform correct calculations to convert temperatures between Fahrenheit and Celsius scales.

6. **Obtain and record an accurate patient temperature using three different types of thermometers.**
   The patient's temperature can be measured orally and in the axillary region with a digital thermometer, in the ear using an aural thermometer, and at the temporal artery using a temporal artery thermometer. Axillary temperature is approximately 1° F (0.6° C) lower than an accurate oral reading, because the reading is not taken in an enclosed body cavity. Tympanic temperature is accurate because it records the temperature of the blood that is closest to the hypothalamus. The temporal artery scanner is considered most accurate for infants. After documenting the temperature reading, record (T) for a tympanic reading, (A) for an

axillary reading, or (TA) for a temporal artery reading to clarify the site. Procedures 31-1 thru 31-4 explain how to take and record patient temperatures using a variety of thermometers.

7. **Describe pulse rate, volume, and rhythm.**
   Pulse *rate* reflects the number of times the heart contracts in 1 minute. Pulse *volume* is the amount of force placed on the arterial walls when the heart beats; the *rhythm* of the pulse is the length of time between beats. Monitor and record the pulse rate, noting whether the rhythm is regular or arrhythmic, and the volume is bounding, normal, or thready.

8. **Locate and record the pulse at multiple sites.**
   The most common sites used to feel the pulse are the temporal, carotid, apical, brachial, radial, femoral, popliteal, and dorsalis pedis arteries. Procedures 31-5 and 31-6 present the specifics on recording apical and radial pulses.

9. **Demonstrate the best way to obtain an accurate respiratory count.**
   Count the number of respirations for 30 seconds and then multiply by 2. This should be done immediately after taking the patient's pulse, while still holding the pulse point, and without warning the patient, because the patient may inadvertently alter the respiratory rate if he or she is aware that you are counting breaths. Refer to Procedure 31-7.

10. **Specify physiologic factors that affect blood pressure.**
    Physiologic factors that affect blood pressure include the amount or volume of blood in circulation; the condition of the blood vessels, including the presence of atherosclerosis and arteriosclerosis; the degree of blood viscosity; and the strength of the myocardium.

11. **Differentiate between essential and secondary hypertension.**
    The cause of essential hypertension is unknown; it is diagnosed when a patient has a systolic reading higher than 140 mm Hg and/or a diastolic reading higher than 90 mm Hg. Secondary hypertension is caused by an underlying condition, such as renal disease, pregnancy, or a congenital heart defect.

12. **Interpret revised hypertension guidelines and treatment.**
    AHA guidelines for the diagnosis and management of hypertension include a new category—prehypertension. Normal blood pressure is identified by readings below 120/80. Table 31-6 identifies the categories of normal, prehypertensive, and hypertensive blood pressures. The goal of the new recommendations is to reduce the number of people who die each year from hypertension-related illness. Treatment includes a combination of weight management, sodium reduction, lifestyle changes, and the use of two or more antihypertensive and diuretic medications.

13. **Identify the different Korotkoff phases.**
    The Korotkoff phases are the categories of sounds heard during blood pressure measurement. These sounds are produced by vibrations of the arterial wall when the blood surges back into the vessel after it has been compressed by the blood pressure cuff. Phase I is the first sound heard as the cuff deflates and is the systolic reading; phase II is the swishing sound made by the movement of blood through the artery, but you may have an auscultatory gap in which sounds completely disappear; phase III involves distinct, sharp tapping sounds made as the blood rushes through the artery; in phase IV, the sound changes to a soft tapping, which becomes muffled and begins to grow fainter; and in phase V, sound completely disappears. The last sound heard is the diastolic reading.

14. **Accurately measure and document blood pressure.**
    A sphygmomanometer is used with a stethoscope to hear the systolic over diastolic sounds. (Procedure 31-8 outlines the method for performing this skill.)

15. **Accurately measure and document height and weight.**
    A patient's height and weight are anthropometric measurements that are recorded during the initial patient visit and periodically after that, depending on the patient's needs and the physician's preference. The scale should be kept in a private location. Variations in weight may indicate physical or emotional disorders, including diabetes, CHF, hormone abnormalities, depression, and eating disorders. Procedure 31-9 describes the techniques involved. Determine the patient's BMI as indicated. Chapter 30 discusses the BMI in greater detail.

16. **Convert kilograms to pounds and pounds to kilograms.**
    To convert kilograms (kg) to pounds (lb), multiply the number of kilograms by 2.2. To convert pounds to kilograms, divide the number of pounds by 2.2 kg, or multiply the number of pounds by 0.45 kg.

17. **Identify patient education opportunities when measuring vital signs.**
    Patient education about vital signs includes confirming the patient's ability to monitor vital signs at home as needed, providing assistance in working home equipment systems, and confirming understanding of the need to comply with the physician's recommendations.

18. **Determine the medical assistant's legal and ethical responsibilities in obtaining vital signs.**
    Legal and ethical implications for the medical assistant include following the physician's guidelines with patient disclosure, monitoring and recording vital signs accurately, and being consistently alert to inaccurate readings or potential carelessness.

CONNECTIONS

Study Guide Connection: Go to the Chapter 31 Study Guide. Read and complete the activities.

Evolve Connection: Go to the Chapter 31 link at *evolve.elsevier.com/kinn* to complete the Chapter Review and the Chapter Quiz. Peruse other resources listed for this chapter to increase your knowledge of Vital Signs.

32

ASSISTING WITH THE PRIMARY PHYSICAL EXAMINATION

Felicia Grand, a newly hired certified medical assistant (CMA, AAMA), works for Dr. Anna Kosto, who is a member of a busy multi-physician primary care practice. One of Felicia's chief responsibilities is to assist Dr. Kosto with physical examinations. Her duties include preparing and maintaining the examination room and equipment; getting the patient ready for specific physical examinations; and gowning, draping, and positioning the patient as needed. Because Felicia will be assisting with examinations, she must become familiar with the physical examination procedure and the order in which the physician needs various pieces of medical equipment. It also is important that Felicia protect herself from possible injury by using appropriate body mechanics throughout her day in the office.

While studying this chapter, think about the following questions:

- What equipment does Felicia need to gather before the physician enters the examination room to make sure the examination goes smoothly and without interruption?
- With what examination and treatment positions should Felicia be familiar, and when should the various positions be used?
- What measures can Felicia take to protect herself from injury when lifting heavy items or assisting with the transfer of patients?

LEARNING OBJECTIVES

1. Define, spell, and pronounce the terms listed in the vocabulary.
2. Apply critical thinking skills in performing the patient assessment and patient care.
3. Describe the structural development of the human body.
4. Differentiate among the functions of the body systems and the major organs and structures of each system.
5. Outline the medical assistant's role in preparing for the physical examination.
6. Summarize the instruments and equipment the physician typically uses during a physical examination.
7. Describe the six methods of examination and give an example of each.
8. Outline the basic principles of properly gowning and draping a patient for examination.
9. Name the various positions that may be used during an examination and identify the purpose of each.
10. Position and drape a patient in six different examining positions while remaining mindful of the patient's privacy and comfort.
11. Demonstrate proper body mechanics in transferring a patient from a chair to the examination table and back.
12. Outline the sequence of a routine physical examination.
13. Prepare for and assist in the physical examination of a patient, correctly completing each step of the procedure in the proper sequence.
14. Summarize the role of the medical assistant in the physical examination process.
15. Determine the role of patient education during the physical examination.
16. Discuss the legal and ethical implications of the physical examination.

VOCABULARY

auscultation The act of listening to body sounds, typically with a stethoscope, to assess various organs throughout the body.

bruit (broo′-it) An abnormal sound or murmur heard on auscultation of an organ, vessel (such as a carotid artery), or gland.

clubbing Abnormal enlargement of the distal phalanges (fingers and toes) associated with cyanotic heart disease or advanced chronic pulmonary disease.

colonoscopy Procedure in which a fiberoptic scope is used to examine the large intestine.

electrocardiogram (i-lek-tro-kar′-de-uh-gram) A graphic record of electrical conduction through the heart.

emphysema (em-fuh-ze′-muh) Pathologic accumulation of air in the alveoli, which results in alveolar destruction and overall oxygen deprivation; in the lungs, the bronchioles become plugged with mucus and lose elasticity.

gait Manner or style of walking.

hematopoiesis (hi-ma-tuh-poi-e′-suhs) The formation and development of blood cells in the red bone marrow.

intercellular Term referring to the area between cells.

intracellular Term referring to the area within the cell membrane.

manipulation Movement or exercising of a body part by means of an externally applied force.

mastication (mas-tuh-ka′-shun) Chewing.

murmur Abnormal sound heard during auscultation of the heart that may or may not have a pathologic origin; it is associated with valve disease or a congenital heart defect.

nodules (nah′-juhls) Small lumps, lesions, or swellings that are felt when the skin is palpated.

palpation The use of touch during the physical examination to assess the size, consistency, and location of certain body parts.

peristalsis (per-uh-stahl′-suhs) Rhythmic contraction of involuntary muscles lining the gastrointestinal tract.

sclera The white part of the eye that forms the orbit.

transillumination Inspection of a cavity or organ by passing light through its walls.

trauma Physical injury or a wound caused by an external force or violence.

vasoconstriction (va-zo-kuhn-strik′-shun) Contraction of the muscles lining blood vessels, which narrows the lumen.

To promote health maintenance, healthcare professionals must understand the anatomy and physiology of the body, the role each part plays, how each component functions, and what happens to the body when disease occurs in body systems.

ANATOMY AND PHYSIOLOGY

Anatomy is the study of how the body is shaped and structured. It encompasses a wide range of subjects, including structural development, levels of organization, relationships among microscopic parts, and the interrelationship of structure and function.

Physiology is the study of body functions. This field is subdivided into areas of study; some physiologists spend their entire lives studying only one function, such as how cells work or how a single organ, such as the small intestine, is interrelated in function with the stomach and the large intestine.

Separating these two sciences is almost impossible, because one continuously influences the other. Function affects structure, and structure affects function; for example, an infant can suck effortlessly because of the lack of teeth in the mouth. Once teeth appear, sucking becomes more tiresome, and the child begins to chew and bite. Phenomena in structure and function affect the interrelationships of all body systems.

Structural Development

Cells

The basic unit of life is the cell. Cells determine the functional and structural characteristics of the entire body. Cells are microscopic in size, have a variety of shapes, and perform a vast array of functions. It is estimated that the human body is composed of approximately 100 trillion living, functioning cells. A cell is made up of three primary parts: the plasma membrane that surrounds the cell, creating an outer covering; the **intracellular** environment, which includes the cytoplasm that contains the living material that carries on the cell's function; and the nucleus of the cell, which contains the genetic code of the cell that determines the cell's function.

Tissues

When cells with similar structure and function are placed together, they form tissues. The study of tissues is known as *histology*. All of the body tissues are grouped into four types. The types of tissues distributed throughout the body and where they are located are as follows:

- *Epithelial tissue:* This type of tissue makes up the skin, glands, and linings of body cavities and organs; is packed closely together with little or no **intercellular** material; and is classified according to shape as *squamous* (flat), *cuboidal* (square), *columnar* (long and narrow), or *transitional* (varying shapes that can stretch). Epithelial cells may be arranged in a single layer of cells of the same shape, called *simple epithelium*, or in many layers of cells named according to the shape of the cells in the outer layer; this is called *stratified epithelium*.

- *Connective tissue:* This tissue supports and binds other body tissues. Types of connective tissue include collagen, bone, cartilage, adipose, ligaments, tendons, blood, and lymph. Connective tissue is the most frequently occurring tissue in the body and has the widest distribution.

- *Muscle tissue:* This tissue produces movement. It is classified as skeletal muscle (striated, voluntary), which is attached to bones and produces voluntary body movements when contracted; cardiac muscle (striated and involuntary), which forms the heart muscle wall; or smooth muscle (nonstriated and involuntary), which lines the walls of blood vessels and hollow organs and causes such actions as **peristalsis** and **vasoconstriction**.

- *Nervous tissue:* This type of tissue conducts nerve impulses between the periphery and the central nervous system. It also effects rapid communication between body structures and controls the body's functions to maintain homeostasis. Nervous tissue is made up of neurons and supportive structures called *neuroglial* cells.

Organs

An *organ* is composed of two or more types of tissue bound together to form a more complex structure for a common purpose or function. An organ may have one or many functions; for example, the pancreas has an endocrine function because it produces the hormone insulin, and a digestive function because it produces digestive enzymes. Organs also may be part of one or several systems. For example, in the male system, the urethra is part of both the urinary and the reproductive system.

Systems

A *body system* is composed of several organs and their associated structures. These structures work together to perform a specific function in the body. Each system has specific units in it, and each performs specific functions. Table 32-1 summarizes the body systems; their primary cells, organs, and structures; and the major functions of each.

PRIMARY CARE PHYSICIAN

Primary care physicians (PCPs) treat patients of all ages for a broad range of diseases and complaints. A PCP is qualified to provide continuing healthcare for the entire family, from birth to old age.

TABLE 32-1 Organization of Body Systems

BODY SYSTEM	CELLS, ORGANS, AND STRUCTURES	FUNCTIONS
Blood	Arteries, arterioles, veins, venules, white blood cells, red blood cells, platelets, plasma	Transports materials and collects wastes throughout the body; white blood cells fight infection; red blood cells carry oxygen; platelets help form clots; plasma carries dissolved nutrients and other materials
Cardiovascular	Heart, valves, arteries, arterioles, veins, venules	Circulatory system transports materials in the blood throughout the body; veins return deoxygenated blood to the heart, which pumps it into the lungs; oxygenated blood is pumped into the aorta and branching arteries to cells throughout the body
Endocrine	Pituitary, pineal gland, hypothalamus, thyroid, pancreas, adrenal cortex and medulla, parathyroid, thymus, ovaries, testes	Produces hormones that circulate in the blood to target tissue that stimulates a particular action
Integumentary	Skin, subcutaneous tissue, sweat and sebaceous glands, hair, nails, sense receptors	Protection, temperature regulation; senses organ activity
Gastrointestinal	Mouth, tongue, teeth, pharynx, esophagus, stomach, small intestine, large intestine, liver, gallbladder, pancreas, appendix	Mastication, swallowing, digestion, absorption of nutrients, excretion of waste materials
Lymphatic and immune	Lymph, lymph vessels, lymph nodes, thymus, tonsils, spleen, lymphocytes, antibodies	Maintains fluid balance; protects internal environment; defends against foreign cells and disease; provides immunity to some diseases
Musculoskeletal	Bones, joints, muscles, tendons, ligaments, cartilage	Movement, posture, heat production, support, protection, mineral storage, hematopoiesis
Nervous	Brain, spinal cord, neurons, neuroglial cells, peripheral nerves, autonomic nerves	Controls body structures to maintain homeostasis; higher-order thinking and reflex centers that control autonomic processes; carries sensory stimulus to the brain and motor impulses to the periphery
Reproductive	*Female:* Estrogen and progesterone, ovum, ovaries, fallopian tubes, uterus, vagina, vulva, mammary glands *Male:* testosterone, sperm, epididymis, vas deferens, prostate gland, testes, scrotum, penis, urethra	Produces hormones; reproduction

TABLE 32-1 Organization of Body Systems—Cont'd

BODY SYSTEM	CELLS, ORGANS, AND STRUCTURES	FUNCTIONS
Respiratory	Nose, sinuses, pharynx, larynx, trachea, bronchi, lungs, bronchioles, alveoli	Responsible for inhalation of oxygen and exhalation of carbon dioxide externally and exchange of oxygen and carbon dioxide internally at the cellular level; acid-base regulation
Sensory	Eyes, ears, taste buds, olfactory receptors, sensory receptors	Helps sense changes in the external and internal environments through vision, hearing, balance, taste, and smell
Urinary	Nephron unit, bilateral kidneys, ureters, urinary bladder, urethra	Filters waste material from the blood; reabsorbs fluid and electrolytes as needed; excretes waste in the urine; maintains electrolyte, water, and acid-base balances; regulates blood pressure; activates red blood cells

Most health insurance programs have converted to the primary care referral system. This means that most patients are required to have a PCP as the gatekeeper in personal healthcare. Therefore, the PCP must be contacted first, before the patient can be referred to specialty physicians for care.

The PCP evaluates the patient's total healthcare needs, provides personal medical care within one or more fields of medicine, and refers the patient to a specialist when an advanced or serious condition warrants additional expertise. The medical assistant's clinical responsibilities in a primary care office include assisting with patients who may have problems in any of the body systems and with procedures in all age groups. With such a diversified scope of practice, the physician and medical assistant must work as a team to use their time efficiently and still provide quality, patient-centered healthcare.

PHYSICAL EXAMINATION

The purpose of a physical examination is to determine the patient's overall state of well-being. All major organs and body systems are checked during a physical examination. As the physician examines the entire body, he or she interprets the findings, and by the time the examination has been completed, the physician has formed an initial diagnosis of the patient's condition. Often laboratory and other diagnostic tests are ordered to supplement the physician's initial diagnosis. The results of these tests are used to refine the patient's diagnosis, to help the physician plan or revise treatment for the patient, to evaluate and maintain current drug therapy, and/or to determine the patient's progress.

Preparing for the Physical Examination

Role of the Medical Assistant in the Physical Examination

Assessment of the patient begins with the first contact in the office. Before the examination, the medical assistant has the opportunity to make sure that the patient feels comfortable during the examination process and that all the necessary medical information has been obtained. As part of patient preparation, the medical assistant should verify the patient's insurance information and document current

medications and allergies. The medical assistant's duties include preparing and maintaining the examination room and equipment, preparing the patient, and assisting the physician during the physical examination.

Room Preparation. The medical assistant is responsible for making sure the examination room is ready for any procedure that might be performed during the physical examination. The area should be as comfortable as possible for the patient and free of any potential dangers (Procedure 32-1). The examination room is prepared as follows:

- The area should be checked at the beginning of each day and between patients to make sure it is completely stocked with equipment and supplies and that all equipment is functioning properly. The medical assistant must understand how to take care of and operate all equipment and instruments and should refer to operation manuals supplied by manufacturers as needed.
- Expiration dates must be checked regularly on all packages and supplies, and expired materials should be discarded.
- The room should be private, well lit, and at a comfortable temperature for the patient during the physical examination.
- The area should be cleaned and disinfected daily and between patients as needed to prevent the spread of infection and to ensure patients' comfort. All potentially contaminated surfaces, including the examination table, are disinfected between patients, with an appropriate disinfectant. After cleaning the table, change the examination paper by unrolling a new piece.
- Drapes, gowns, and all other patient supplies are arranged before the patient enters the room so that they are ready for use.
- To save time, the instruments and equipment needed for the examination are prepared and arranged for easy access before the physician enters the room.
- The examination room should contain all materials required for observing Standard Precautions, including disposable gloves, a sink with an antibacterial hand-washing agent, paper towels, biohazard waste containers, sharps containers, and impervious gowns and face guards. Sharps containers are replaced when they are two-thirds full, as indicated by Standard Precautions (see Chapter 27).

PROCEDURE 32-1

Prepare and Maintain the Examination and Treatment Areas

GOAL: *To prepare an examination room for a patient procedure, maintain equipment and supplies needed for the physical examination, and demonstrate maintenance of the room after a patient visit.*

EQUIPMENT and SUPPLIES

- Examination table
- Patient gown
- Drape
- Stethoscope
- Ophthalmoscope
- Scale with height measurement bar
- Tongue depressor
- Cotton balls
- Examination light
- Percussion hammer
- Lubricating gel
- Examination gloves
- Sphygmomanometer
- Otoscope with disposable speculum
- Tape measure
- Gauze sponges
- Pen light
- Nasal speculum
- Tuning fork
- Biohazard container
- Laboratory request forms
- Specimen bottles/lab requisitions
- Thermometer
- Cotton-tipped applicators
- Hemoccult supplies
- Table paper
- Spray disinfectant

PROCEDURAL STEPS

1. Check the examination room at the beginning of each day and between patients to make sure it is completely stocked with equipment and supplies and that the equipment functions properly.
   <u>PURPOSE:</u> The room must be ready for patient services.
2. Check all equipment and instruments to make sure they are operational; refer to manuals supplied by the manufacturers as needed.
3. Check expiration dates on all packages and supplies regularly and discard expired materials.
   <u>PURPOSE:</u> To maintain the patient's safety.
4. The room should be private, well lit, and at a comfortable temperature for the patient during the physical examination.
   <u>PURPOSE:</u> To maintain confidentiality and the patient's safety and comfort.
5. Prepare the examination room before and between patients according to acceptable medical rules of asepsis.
   <u>PURPOSE:</u> The room must be aseptically clean to prevent the spread of infection.
6. After each patient use: Don disposable examination gloves, spray the table and any other contaminated surface with a disinfectant, and clean the area with disposable towels; discard waste and the gloves in an appropriate biohazard container and put clean paper on the table.
7. Sanitize your hands.
   <u>PURPOSE:</u> To ensure infection control and to prevent the transmission of pathogens from one patient to another.
8. Inventory the supplies needed after each patient visit and restock as needed.
   <u>PURPOSE:</u> The room must be maintained and ready for each examination.

Patient Preparation. Getting the patient ready for the examination includes taking care of paperwork before the patient enters the examination room and performing related clinical skills.

- Make sure the medical record is complete and that any needed consent forms have been signed. The medical assistant is not responsible for obtaining informed consent, but he or she should review the paperwork to make sure that informed consent forms were reviewed by the physician and that the patient signed the forms.
- Introduce yourself and address the patient by his or her preferred name, making sure to maintain respect at all times. Pay close attention to the patient's nonverbal language to make sure the patient understands what to expect.
- Verify the accuracy of the insurance information according to office policy. In most facilities, the policy is to make a copy of the patient's insurance card when the patient first enters the office or, if the patient has been to the office recently, to ask whether any of the insurance information has changed.

- Obtain specimens (e.g., urine, blood) if they have been preordered by the physician, or if this practice is part of the office policy.
- Measure and record the patient's height, weight, body mass index (BMI), and vital signs.
- Conduct the initial investigation into the reason for the visit and explain the examination procedure to the patient. Be prepared to answer the patient's questions and allay any fears.
- Ask the patient whether he or she needs to empty the bladder before the examination, because a full bladder may interfere with the examination and may be uncomfortable for the patient.
- Help the patient physically prepare for the examination. Explain to the patient what clothing should be removed and in what direction to put on the gown (open to the front or to the back, depending on the type of examination), and provide a drape to ensure the patient's privacy. Offer assistance as needed.
- Assist the patient into and out of various examination positions as needed.

- Throughout this entire sequence of events, explain what is happening, and consistently maintain the patient's privacy and confidentiality.
- Document patient data in the medical record, completing all forms required.
- Place the patient's medical record in the designated area for the physician, usually in a chart holder on the examination room door; make sure that no identifiable patient information is visible, in accordance with regulations established by the Health Insurance Portability and Accountability Act (HIPAA).
- Help the patient with dressing as needed after the examination.

Assisting the Physician. The medical assistant should be prepared to help the physician complete the physical examination as comprehensively and efficiently as possible. You have already prepared the room, so all equipment and supplies are available and in good working order; you also have prepared the patient by gathering the needed information and measuring and recording vital signs. During the examination, the physician may expect the medical assistant to do the following:

- Hand him or her instruments and equipment as requested and provide supplies as needed.
- Alter the position of a gooseneck lamp to better illuminate the area being examined and turn lights off and on during specific phases of the examination.
- Position and drape the patient during different phases of the examination.
- Assist in collecting and properly labeling specimens such as urine, Pap smear specimens, and throat cultures.
- Conduct follow-up diagnostic procedures as ordered, including an **electrocardiogram** (ECG), eye or ear screening, urinalysis, and phlebotomy.
- Schedule postexamination diagnostic procedures such as mammography, x-ray examination, or **colonoscopy**.

Supplies and Instruments Needed for the Physical Examination

The instruments typically used during the physical examination are shown in Figure 32-1. They enable the physician to see, feel, inspect, and listen to parts of the body. All equipment must be in good working order, properly disinfected, and readily available for the physician's use during the examination. The instruments most frequently used for a physical examination are described in the following paragraphs. Physical examinations typically are performed from the head to the feet; the instruments are listed in the order in which the physician typically would request them.

Ophthalmoscope. An ophthalmoscope is used to inspect the inner structures of the eye. It consists of a stainless-steel handle containing batteries and an attached head, which has a light, magnifying lenses, and an opening through which the eye is viewed. Examination rooms usually are equipped with wall-mounted electrical units for the ophthalmoscope and otoscope, a dispenser for disposable speculums, and a wall-mounted sphygmomanometer.

Tongue Depressor. A tongue depressor is a flat, wooden blade used to hold down the tongue when the throat is examined.

Otoscope. An otoscope is used to examine the external auditory canal and tympanic membrane. It has a stainless-steel handle containing batteries or is part of a wall-mounted electrical unit. The head of the otoscope has a light that is focused through a magnifying

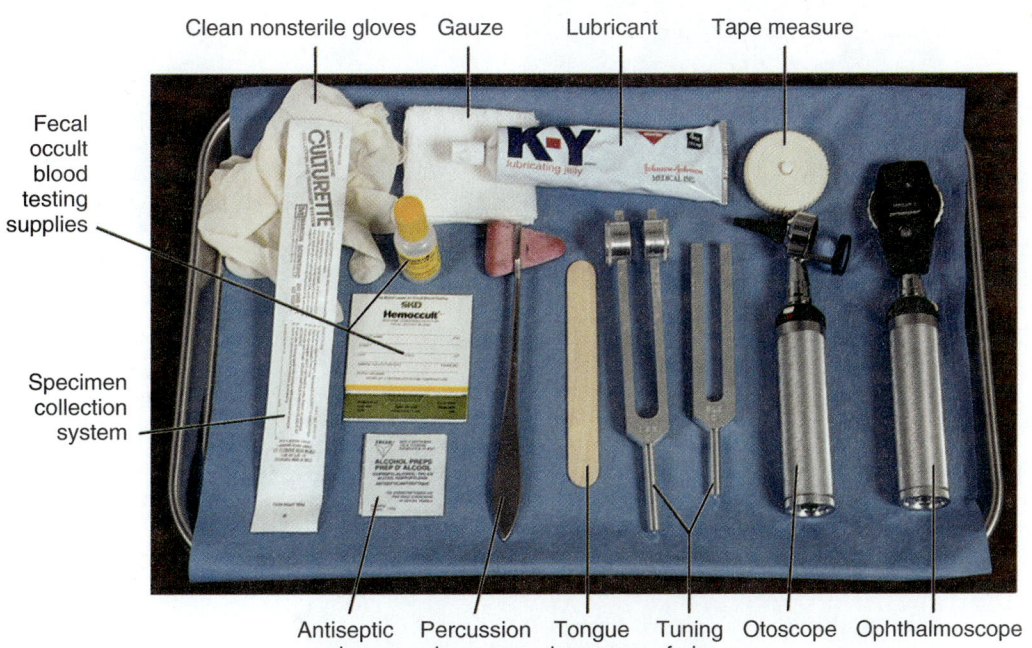

FIGURE 32-1 Instruments for the physical examination. (From Bonewit-West K: *Clinical procedures for medical assistants,* ed 7, St Louis, 2008, Saunders.)

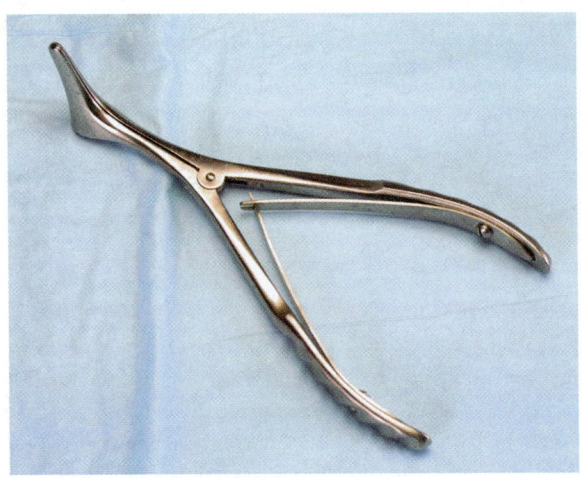

FIGURE 32-2 Nasal speculum.

lens and should be covered with a disposable ear speculum. The light also may be used to illuminate the nasal passages and throat.

Nasal Speculum. A nasal speculum is a stainless-steel instrument used to inspect the lining of the nose, nasal membranes, and internal septum (Figure 32-2). When the handles of the nasal speculum are squeezed, the tips spread apart to dilate the nostrils, allowing the physician to visualize the internal aspects. An otoscope with a special attachment may also be used for nasal visualization.

Tuning Fork. Tuning forks are aluminum fork-shaped instruments that consist of a handle and two prongs (Figure 32-3, *A*). The prongs produce a humming sound when the physician strikes them against his or her hand. Tuning forks are available in different sizes, and each size produces a different pitch level. A tuning fork is used to check the patient's auditory acuity (Figure 32-3, *B*) and to test bone vibration (Figure 32-3, *C*). This aluminum instrument consists of a handle and two prongs that produce a humming sound when the physician strikes the prongs against his or her hand.

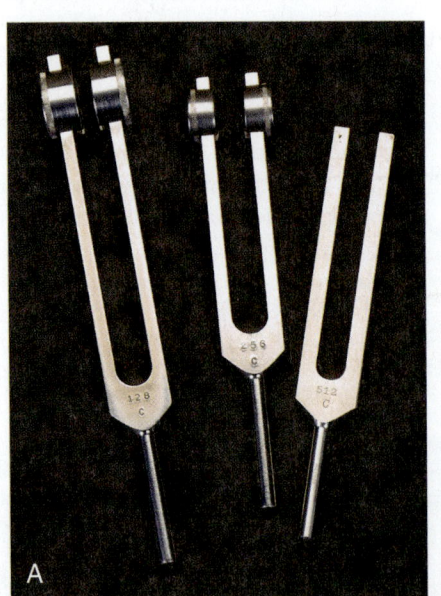
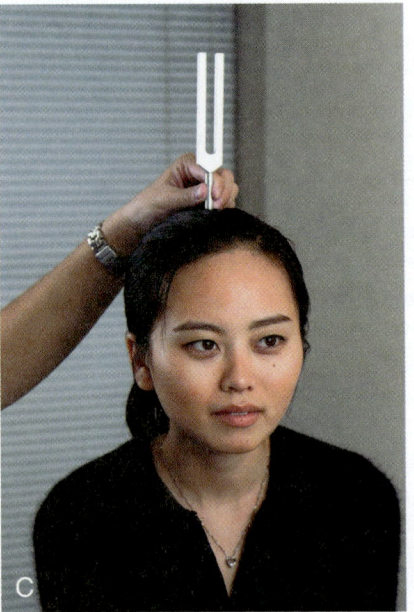
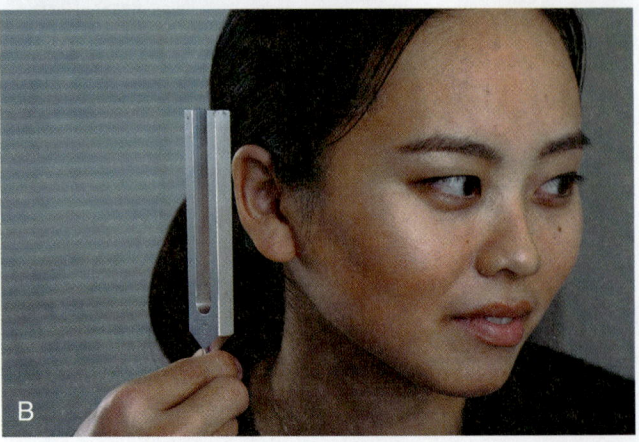

FIGURE 32-3 **A**, Tuning forks. **B**, Sound vibration test. **C**, Bone vibration test.

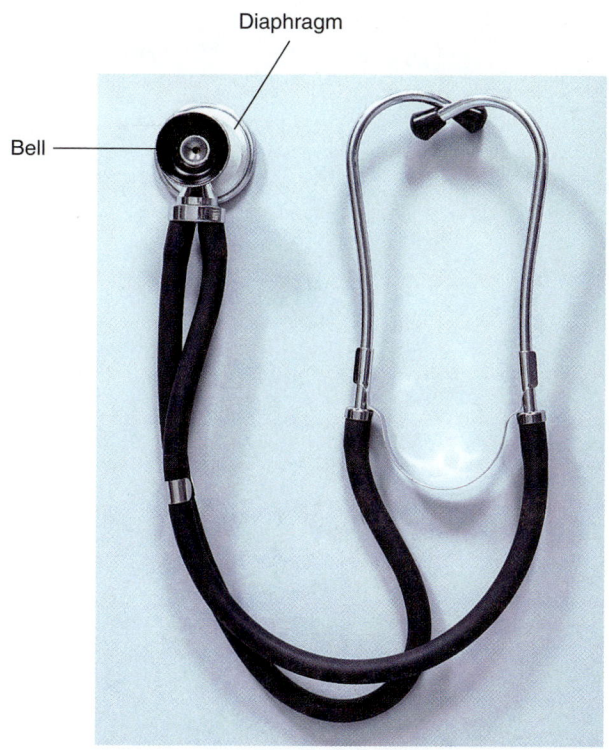

FIGURE 32-4 Stethoscope. (Modified from Seidel HM: *Mosby's guide to physical examination,* ed 6, St Louis, 2006, Mosby.)

Tape Measure. A tape measure is a flexible ribbon ruler that is usually printed in inches and feet on one side and in centimeters and meters on the opposite side. Measurements may be used to assess length and head circumference in infants, wound size, and so on.

Stethoscope. A stethoscope is a listening device used when certain areas of the body are auscultated, particularly the heart and lungs. This instrument is available in many shapes and sizes. All have two earpieces that are connected to flexible rubber or vinyl tubing (Figure 32-4). At the distal end of the tubing is a diaphragm or bell (many have both), which, when placed securely on the patient's skin, enables the physician to hear internal body sounds.

Reflex Hammer. A reflex hammer is sometimes called a *percussion hammer.* This stainless-steel instrument has a hard rubber head that is used to strike the tendons of the knee and elbow to test the neurologic reflexes.

Gloves. Disposable examination gloves protect the healthcare worker and the patient from microorganisms. According to Standard Precautions, gloves must be worn whenever the potential exists for contact with any body fluid, broken skin or wounds, or contaminated items.

Additional Supplies. Gauze squares, cotton balls, cotton-tipped applicators, specimen containers, hemoccult packets, Pap smear supplies for female patients, lubricating jelly for vaginal and rectal examinations, and laboratory request forms should be easily accessible during the examination.

Assisting With the Physical Examination

Methods of Examination

Examinations are performed as both a routine confirmation of the absence of illness and a means of diagnosing disease. Healthcare providers use six methods to examine the human body. All six are part of a complete physical examination.

Inspection. During inspection, the examiner uses observation to detect significant physical features or objective data. This method of examination ranges from focusing on the patient's general appearance (general state of health, including posture, mannerisms, and grooming) to more detailed observations, including body contour, **gait**, symmetry, visible injuries and deformities, tremors, rashes, and color changes.

Palpation. In **palpation**, the examiner uses the sense of touch (Figure 32-5, *A*). A part of the body is felt with the hand to determine its condition or the condition of an underlying organ. Palpation may involve touching the skin or performing a firmer exploration of the abdomen for underlying masses. This technique involves a wide range of perceptions, including temperature, vibration, consistency, form, size, rigidity, elasticity, moisture, texture, position, and contour. Palpation is performed with one hand, both hands (bimanual), one finger (digital), the fingertips, or the palmar aspect of the hand. A pelvic examination is done bimanually, whereas an anal examination is performed digitally. Do not confuse palpation with *palpitation*, which is a throbbing pulsation felt in the chest.

Percussion. Percussion involves tapping or striking the body, usually with the fingers or a small hammer, to elicit sounds or vibratory sensations. Percussion aids determination of the position, size, and density of an underlying organ or cavity. The effect of percussion is both heard and felt by the examiner; it is helpful in determining the amount of air or solid matter in an underlying organ or cavity. The two basic methods of percussion are *direct percussion* and *indirect percussion.* Direct (immediate) percussion is performed by striking the body with a finger. With indirect (mediate) percussion, which is used more frequently, the physician places his or her hand on the area and then strikes the placed hand with a finger of the other hand (Figure 32-5, *B*). Both a sound and a sense of vibration are evident. The examiner quantifies the sound in terms of pitch, quality, duration, and resonance.

Auscultation. For **auscultation**, the physician uses a stethoscope to listen to sounds arising from the body (not the sound produced by the physician, as in percussion, but sounds that originate within the patient's body). Auscultation is a difficult method of examination, because the physician must distinguish between a normal sound and an abnormal sound (Figure 32-5, *C*). It is particularly useful for evaluating sounds originating in the lungs, heart, and abdomen, such as a **murmur**, a **bruit**, and bowel sounds.

Mensuration. Mensuration is the process of measuring. Measurements that are recorded include the patient's height and weight, the length and diameter of an extremity, the extent of flexion or extension of an extremity, the size of the uterus during pregnancy, the size and depth of a wound, and the pressure of a grip. Measurements are taken with a flexible tape measure, a circular wound measurement device (Figure 32-6), or a specialized piece of equipment (e.g., a goniometer, which is used to measure joint angles) and usually are recorded in centimeters.

Manipulation. **Manipulation** is the passive movement of a joint to determine the range of extension or flexion of a part of the body. Manipulation may or may not be grouped with palpation. It usually is considered separate from the four standard methods of

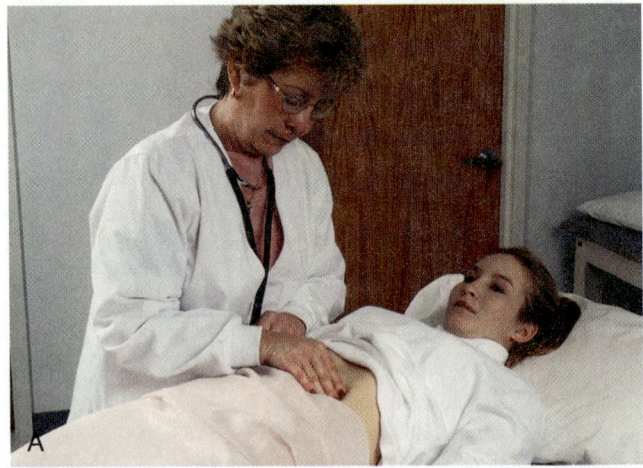

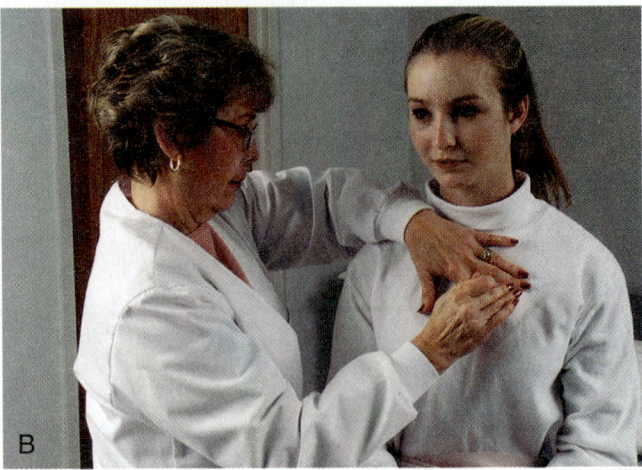

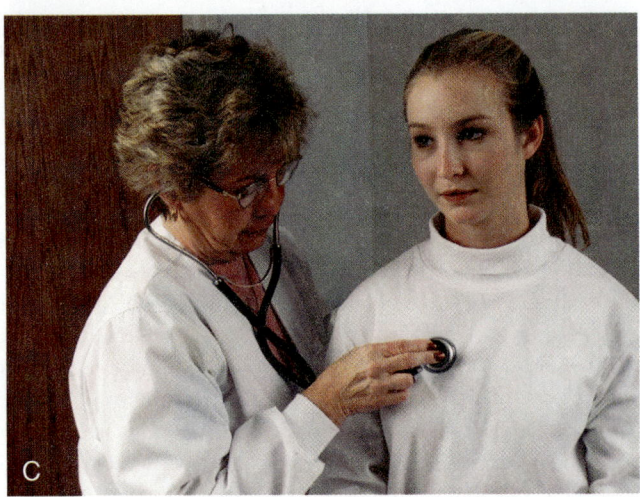

FIGURE 32-5 A, Demonstration of palpation. **B**, Demonstration of percussion. **C**, Demonstration of auscultation. (From Zakus SM: *Mosby's clinical skills for medical assistants,* ed 4, St Louis, 2001, Mosby.)

examination (inspection, palpation, percussion, and auscultation) and is grouped with mensuration, especially by an orthopedist or a neurologist. Insurance and industrial reports often request this information in detail. For example, a patient involved in a work-related accident that caused joint damage may have to perform assisted range-of-motion (ROM) exercises to the joint, with subsequent measurements of joint flexion and extension.

Positioning and Draping the Patient for the Physical Examination

Various patient positions are used to facilitate a physical examination. The medical assistant instructs the patient about and assists the patient into these positions, ensuring as much ease and modesty as possible, and helps the patient maintain the position during the examination with as little discomfort as possible. Do not place a patient into a position that is uncomfortable or that compromises the patient's privacy until it is necessary to complete that part of the examination. Never leave the patient's side if he or she is in a position that could result in a fall.

Draping the patient with an examination sheet protects the individual from embarrassment and keeps the patient warm. However, the sheet must be positioned so that it allows complete visibility for

the examiner and does not interfere with the examination. During the general examination, each part of the body is exposed one portion at a time. For gynecologic and rectal examinations, the sheet is positioned on the diagonal across the patient, or in a diamond shape, to provide maximum comfort for the patient while allowing the physician to perform the examination (Procedure 32-2, 32-3, Figure 2).

A number of positions are used for medical examinations.

Fowler's Position. In Fowler's position, the patient sits on the examination table with the head of the table elevated 90 degrees, or simply sits at the edge of the table. This position is useful for examinations and treatments of the head, neck, and chest, and for patients with orthopnea who have difficulty breathing while lying down. Drape placement varies, depending on the type of physical examination done and the need to maintain the patient's privacy (see Procedure 32-2, Figure 1).

Semi-Fowler's Position. Semi-Fowler's position is a modification of Fowler's position. The head of the table is positioned at a 45-degree angle instead of at a full 90-degree angle. This position is useful for postoperative examination, for patients with breathing disorders, and for patients who have an elevated temperature or are suffering from head **trauma** or pain (see Procedure 32-2, Figure 2).

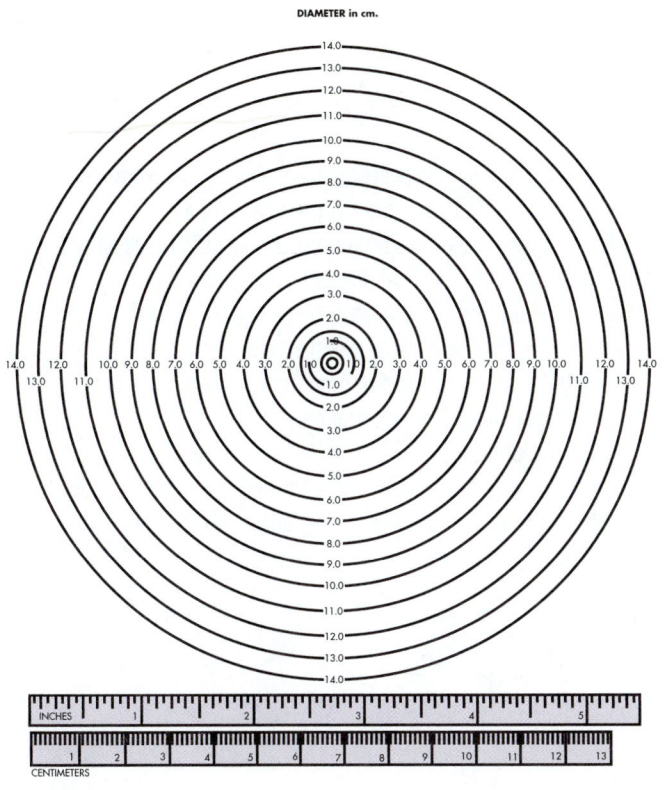

DIAMETER in cm.

DISCARD AFTER USE

FIGURE 32-6 Circular wound measurement device. (From Perry AG, Potter P: *Clinical nursing skills and techniques*, ed 7, St Louis, 2010, Mosby.)

The drape and/or gown should cover the entire patient from the nipple line down.

Supine (Horizontal Recumbent) Position. In the supine position, the patient lies flat with the face upward and the lower legs supported by the table extension (see Procedure 32-3, Figure 1). This position is used for examination of the front of the body, including the heart, breasts, and abdominal organs. The patient's gown should open down the front, and the drape should be placed over any exposed area that is not being examined.

Dorsal Recumbent Position. In the dorsal recumbent position, the patient lies face upward, with the weight distributed primarily to the surface of the back. This is accomplished by flexing the knees so that the feet are flat on the table. This position relieves muscle tension in the abdomen and may be used for examination and/or inspection of the rectal, vaginal, and perineal areas, or it may be used if the patient experiences back discomfort when lying supine. This position can be used for digital examination of the vagina and rectum, but it is not used if an instrument such as a speculum is needed. To ensure the patient's privacy, it is important to keep the patient completely draped, with the drape in a diamond shape, until the physician is present (see Procedure 32-3, Figure 2).

Lithotomy Position. The patient should not be placed in the lithotomy position until the physician is in the examination room and is ready for this part of the examination. Place the patient on his or her back with the knees sharply flexed and the arms at the sides or folded over the chest; have the patient slide the buttocks down to the bottom edge of the table. Support the feet in stirrups placed wide

---

PROCEDURE 32-2

Prepare the Patient for and Assist With Routine and Specialty Examinations: the Fowler's and Semi-Fowler's Positions

GOAL: *To position and drape the patient for examinations of the head, neck, and chest, or patients who have difficulty breathing when lying flat.*

EQUIPMENT and SUPPLIES

- Examination table
- Table paper
- Patient gown
- Drape
- Spray disinfectant
- Examination gloves

PROCEDURAL STEPS

1. Prepare the examination room according to acceptable medical rules of asepsis.
   <u>PURPOSE:</u> The room must be aseptically clean to prevent the spread of infection.

2. Sanitize your hands.
   <u>PURPOSE:</u> To ensure infection control.

3. Greet and identify the patient, introduce yourself, and determine whether the patient understands the procedure. If the patient does not, explain what to expect.
   <u>PURPOSE:</u> To promote the patient's understanding and cooperation during the examination.

4. Give the patient a gown. Explain the clothing that must be removed for the particular examination being done and whether the gown should open in the front or in the back. Provide assistance as needed. Give the patient privacy while changing. Knock on the examination room door before re-entering to make sure the patient has completed undressing and gowning.

5. For Fowler's position, either elevate the head of the bed 90 degrees or instruct the patient to sit at the end of the table (Figure 1). Extend the foot rest as needed for patient comfort. The patient may be more comfortable in semi-Fowler's position. In this modification of Fowler's

PROCEDURE 32-2—cont'd

position, the head of the table is elevated 45 degrees. Semi-Fowler's position may be used for postoperative follow-up or for patients with a fever, head injury, or pain. It also is a comfortable, supportive position for patients with breathing disorders (Figure 2).

6. Drape the patient according to the type of examination and the required patient exposure.
   PURPOSE: Draping the patient provides warmth and privacy while giving the physician access to the examination site.
7. After the examination has been completed, assist the patient as needed to get off the table and get dressed.
8. Clean and disinfect the examination room according to Standard Precautions. Roll clean paper over the table.
   PURPOSE: To ensure infection control and to prevent the transmission of pathogens from one patient to another.
9. Sanitize your hands.
10. Follow up with the physician's orders regarding scheduling of diagnostic studies, collection of specimens, and/or scheduling of future appointments.

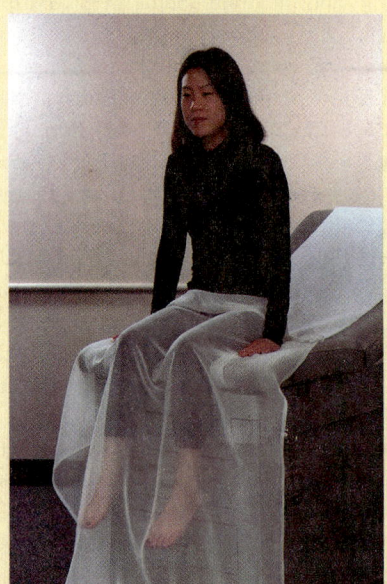

1

fowler's (handwritten)

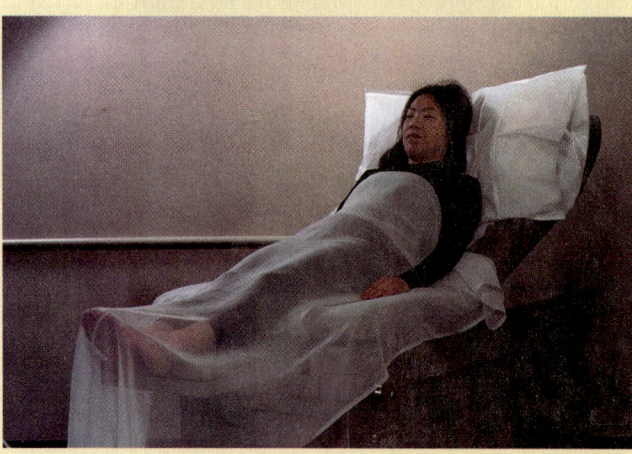

2

Semifitter fowler's (handwritten)
45 degree angle (handwritten)

PROCEDURE 32-3

Prepare the Patient for and Assist With Routine and Specialty Examinations: the Horizontal Recumbent and Dorsal Recumbent Positions

GOAL: *To position and drape the patient for examinations of the abdomen, heart, and breasts in the horizontal recumbent (supine) position and of rectal, vaginal, and perineal areas in the dorsal recumbent position.*

EQUIPMENT and SUPPLIES

- Examination table
- Table paper
- Patient gown
- Drape
- Spray disinfectant
- Examination gloves

PROCEDURAL STEPS

1. Prepare the examination room according to acceptable medical rules of asepsis.

PURPOSE: The room must be aseptically clean to prevent the spread of infection.

2. Sanitize your hands.
   PURPOSE: To ensure infection control.

3. Greet and identify the patient, introduce yourself, and determine whether the patient understands the procedure. If the patient does not, explain what to expect.
   PURPOSE: To promote the patient's understanding and cooperation during the examination.

4. Give the patient a gown. Explain the clothing that must be removed for the particular examination being done and whether the gown should open in the front or in the back. Provide assistance as needed. For the horizontal recumbent position, the gown should be open in the front. Give the patient privacy while changing. Knock on the examination room door before re-entering to make sure the patient has completed undressing and gowning.

5. Do not place the patient in these positions until the physician is ready for that part of the examination.
   PURPOSE: To ensure the patient's privacy, comfort, and modesty.

6. Pull out the table extension that supports the patient's legs. For the horizontal recumbent (supine) position, help the patient lie flat on the table with the face upward (Figure 3). For the dorsal recumbent position, have the patient lie flat on the back and flex the knees so the feet are flat on the table (Figure 4). If needed, help the patient move down toward the foot of the table for the examination.

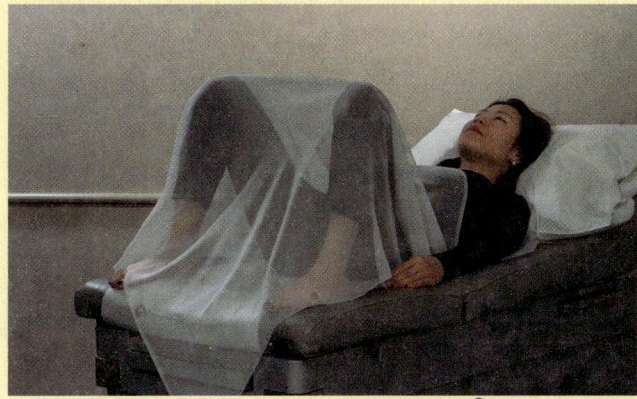

4

dorsal recumbent

7. Drape the patient from nipple line to feet in the supine position, and diagonally with the point of the drape between the feet for the dorsal recumbent position.
   PURPOSE: Draping the patient provides warmth and privacy while giving the physician access to the examination site.

8. After the examination has been completed, assist the patient as needed to get off the table and get dressed.

9. Clean and disinfect the examination room according to Standard Precautions. Roll clean paper over the table.
   PURPOSE: To ensure infection control and to prevent the transmission of pathogens from one patient to another.

10. Sanitize your hands.

11. Follow up with the physician's orders regarding scheduling of diagnostic studies, collection of specimens, and/or scheduling of future appointments.

supine

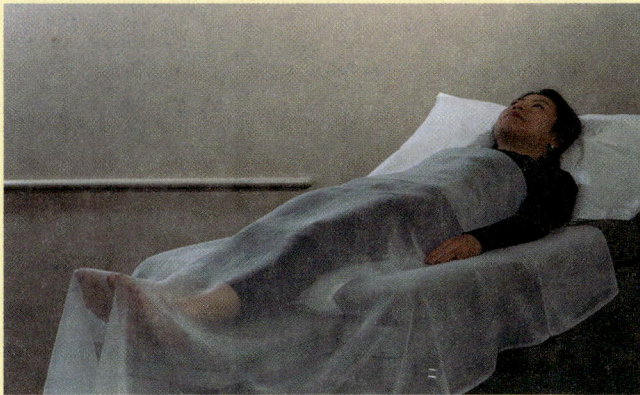

3

apart and somewhat away from the table, with the stirrup arms extended to match the length of the patient's legs. If the heels are too close to the buttocks, the possibility of leg cramps increases, and it is more difficult for the patient to relax the abdominal muscles. Make sure the stirrups are locked in place. Place a drape diagonally over the patient's abdomen and knees. The drape must be long enough to cover the knees and touch the ankles and wide enough to prevent the sides of the thighs from being exposed. The physician lifts the drape away from the pubic area when the examination begins (Procedure 32-4, Figure 1). The lithotomy position is used

primarily for vaginal examinations that require the use of a speculum and for Pap smears.

Sims' Position. Sims' position is sometimes called the *lateral position.* The patient is placed on the left side; the left arm and shoulder are drawn back behind the body so that the body's weight is predominantly on the chest. The right arm is flexed upward for support. The left leg is slightly flexed, and the buttocks are pulled to the edge of the table. The right leg is sharply flexed upward. The drape extends diagonally from under the arms to below the knees. The physician can raise a small portion of the sheet from the back of the patient

PROCEDURE 32-4

Prepare the Patient for and Assist With Routine and Specialty Examinations: the Lithotomy Position

GOAL: *To position and drape the patient primarily for vaginal and pelvic examinations and Pap smears.*

EQUIPMENT and SUPPLIES

- Examination table
- Table paper
- Patient gown
- Drape
- Spray disinfectant
- Examination gloves

PROCEDURAL STEPS

1. Prepare the examination room according to acceptable medical rules of asepsis.
   PURPOSE: The room must be aseptically clean to prevent the spread of infection.
2. Sanitize your hands.
   PURPOSE: To ensure infection control.
3. Greet and identify the patient, introduce yourself, and determine whether the patient understands the procedure. If the patient does not, explain what to expect.
   PURPOSE: To promote the patient's understanding and cooperation during the examination.
4. Give the patient a gown. Instruct the patient to undress from the waist down with the gown open in the back. If the physician also will be doing a breast examination, the patient should undress completely and put on the gown so that it opens in the front. Provide assistance as needed. Give the patient privacy while changing. Knock on the examination room door before re-entering to make sure the patient has completed undressing and gowning.
5. Do not place the patient in this position until the physician is ready for that part of the examination.
   PURPOSE: To promote the patient's privacy, comfort, and safety.
6. Pull out the table extension that supports the patient's legs and help the patient lie face upward on the table. Pull out the stirrups, adjust their extension length for the patient's comfort, and lock them in place.
7. Reinsert the table extension and have the patient move toward the foot of the table with her buttocks on the bottom table edge. Gently place

the patient's legs in the stirrups, checking for comfort. Some offices may stock cloth or paper stirrup covers to protect the patient and make the position more comfortable. The patient's arms can be placed alongside the body or across the chest (Figure 1).

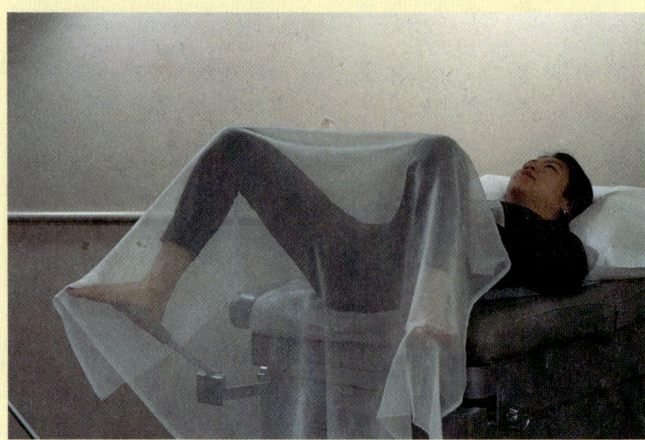

8. Drape the patient diagonally with the point of the drape between the feet. The drape should be large enough to cover the patient from the nipple line to the ankles and wide enough so the patient's thighs are not exposed.
   PURPOSE: To provide warmth and privacy for the patient while giving the physician access to the examination site.
9. After the examination has been completed, assist the patient as needed to get off the table and get dressed.
10. Clean and disinfect the examination room according to Standard Precautions. Roll clean paper over the table.
    PURPOSE: To ensure infection control and to prevent the transmission of pathogens from one patient to another.
11. Sanitize your hands.
12. Follow up with the physician's orders regarding scheduling of diagnostic studies, collection of specimens, and/or scheduling of future appointments.

---

to expose the rectum sufficiently. The remaining portion of the sheet covers the patient's chest area and thighs. This position is used for rectal examination, for instillation of rectal medication, and for some perineal and pelvic examinations (Procedure 32-5, Figure 1).

Prone Position. In the prone position, the patient lies face down on the table on the ventral surface of the body. This is the opposite of the supine position and is another of the recumbent positions. The drape should cover from the middle of the back to below the knees, with the gown opening in the back. On a female patient, the drape should extend high enough to cover the breasts if the patient

is to be turned over to the dorsal recumbent position during the examination (Procedure 32-6, Figure 1). This position is used for examination of the back and for certain surgical procedures.

Knee-Chest Position. For the knee-chest position, the patient rests on the knees and the chest with the head turned to one side. The arms can be placed under the head for support and comfort, or they can be bent and placed at the sides of the table near the head. The thighs are perpendicular to the table and slightly separated. The buttocks extend up into the air, and the back should be straight. The patient needs assistance to do the knee-chest position

PROCEDURE 32-5

Prepare the Patient for and Assist With Routine and Specialty Examinations: the Sims' Position

GOAL: *To position and drape the patient for examination of the rectum, instillation of rectal medication, perineal examination, and some pelvic examinations.*

EQUIPMENT and SUPPLIES

- Examination table
- Patient gown
- Table paper
- Drape
- Spray disinfectant
- Examination gloves

PROCEDURAL STEPS

1. Prepare the examination room according to acceptable medical rules of asepsis.
   PURPLE: The room must be aseptically clean to prevent the spread of infection.
2. Sanitize your hands.
   PURPOSE: To ensure infection control.
3. Greet and identify the patient, introduce yourself, and determine whether the patient understands the procedure. If the patient does not, explain what to expect.
   PURPOSE: To promote the patient's understanding and cooperation during the examination.
4. Give the patient a gown and explain the clothing that must be removed for the particular examination being done. Tell the patient that the gown should open in the back. Provide assistance as needed. Give the patient privacy while changing. Knock on the examination room door before re-entering to make sure the patient has completed undressing and gowning.
5. Do not place the patient in this position until the physician is ready for that part of the examination.
   PURPOSE: To promote the patient's privacy, comfort, and safety.
6. Help the patient turn onto the left side; the left arm and shoulder should be drawn back behind the body so that the patient is tilted onto the chest. Flex the right arm upward for support, slightly flex the left

leg, and sharply flex the right leg upward. Help the patient move the buttocks to the side edge of the table (Figure 1).

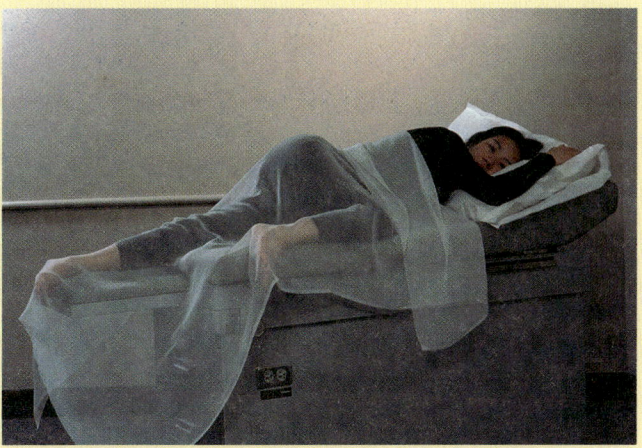

7. Drape the patient diagonally in a diamond shape, with the point of the diamond dropping below the buttocks. Make sure the drape is large enough to prevent exposure of the patient.
   PURPOSE: Draping the patient provides warmth and privacy while giving the physician access to the examination site.
8. After the examination has been completed, assist the patient as needed to get off the table and get dressed.
9. Clean and disinfect the examination room according to Standard Precautions. Roll clean paper over the table.
   PURPOSE: To ensure infection control and prevent the transmission of pathogens from one patient to another.
10. Sanitize your hands.
11. Follow up with the physician's orders regarding scheduling of diagnostic studies, collection of specimens, and/or scheduling of future appointments.

PROCEDURE 32-6

Prepare the Patient for and Assist With Routine and Specialty Examinations: the Prone Position

GOAL: *To position and drape the patient for examination of the back and certain surgical procedures.*

EQUIPMENT and SUPPLIES

- Examination table
- Patient gown
- Table paper
- Drape
- Spray disinfectant
- Examination gloves

PROCEDURAL STEPS

1. Prepare the examination room according to acceptable medical rules of asepsis.
   PURPOSE: The room must be aseptically clean to prevent the spread of infection.
2. Sanitize your hands.
   PURPOSE: To ensure infection control.

PROCEDURE 32-6—cont'd

3. Greet and identify the patient, introduce yourself, and determine whether the patient understands the procedure. If the patient does not, explain what to expect.
   PURPOSE: To promote the patient's understanding and cooperation during the examination.
4. Give the patient a gown and explain the clothing that must be removed for the particular examination being done. Tell the patient that the gown should open in the back. Provide assistance as needed. Give the patient privacy while changing. Knock on the examination room door before re-entering to make sure the patient has completed undressing and gowning.
5. Do not place the patient in this position until the physician is ready for that part of the examination.
   PURPOSE: To promote the patient's privacy, comfort, and safety.
6. Pull out the table extension and help the patient lie down on his or her stomach (Figure 1).

7. Drape the patient over any exposed area that is not included in the examination. For female patients, the drape should be large enough to cover from the breasts to the feet so that the patient is not exposed accidentally if she is asked to roll over.
   PURPOSE: Draping the patient provides warmth and privacy while giving the physician access to the examination site.
8. After the examination has been completed, assist the patient as needed to get off the table and get dressed.
9. Clean and disinfect the examination room according to Standard Precautions. Roll clean paper over the table.
   PURPOSE: To ensure infection control and to prevent the transmission of pathogens from one patient to another.
10. Sanitize your hands.
11. Follow up with the physician's orders regarding scheduling of diagnostic studies, collection of specimens, and/or scheduling of future appointments.

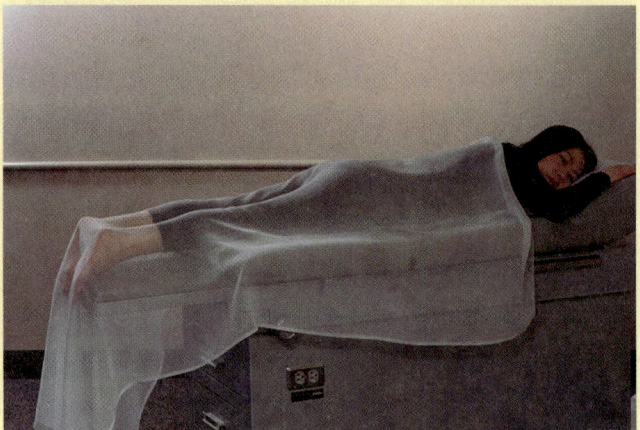

Prone

correctly. Most patients have difficulty maintaining this position, so they should not be placed into it until it is required. The medical assistant must remain next to the patient for assistance and support the entire time the knee-chest position is needed. If the correct knee-chest position cannot be obtained, the patient may have to be placed in a knee-elbow position. This position puts less strain on the patient and is easier to maintain. These positions are used for proctologic examination and for sigmoid, rectal, and occasionally vaginal examinations. The patient's gown should open in the back, and a fenestrated (opening) drape or a single sheet should be draped diagonally over the patient's back at the sacral area (Procedure 32-7, Figure 1).

Trendelenburg's Position. Trendelenburg's position is rarely used in the ambulatory care setting, but it may be needed if a patient has severe hypotension or is going into shock. This position can be achieved only if the examination table separates so that the head can be tilted lower than the legs (Figure 32-7).

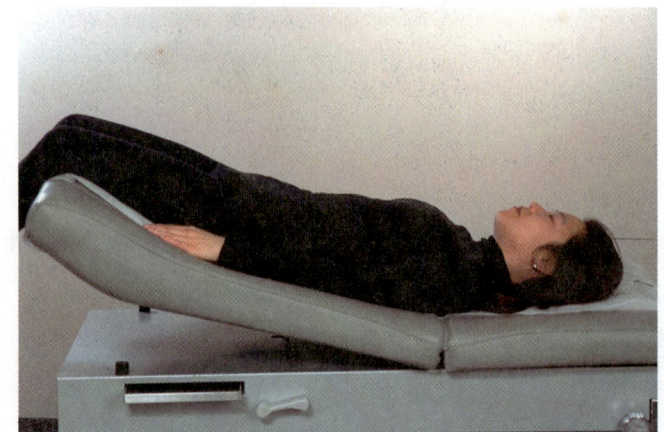

FIGURE 32-7 Trendelenburg's position.

Recovery position

PROCEDURE 32-7

Prepare the Patient for and Assist With Routine and Specialty Examinations: the Knee-Chest Position

GOAL: *To position and drape the patient for examinations of the back and rectum and for certain surgical procedures.*

EQUIPMENT and SUPPLIES

- Examination table
- Table paper
- Patient gown
- Drape
- Spray disinfectant
- Examination gloves

PROCEDURAL STEPS

1. Prepare the examination room according to acceptable medical rules of asepsis.
   PURPOSE: The room must be aseptically clean to prevent the spread of infection.
2. Sanitize your hands.
   PURPOSE: To ensure infection control.
3. Greet and identify the patient, introduce yourself, and determine whether the patient understands the procedure. If the patient does not, explain what to expect.
   PURPOSE: To promote the patient's understanding and cooperation during the examination.
4. Give the patient a gown and explain the clothing that must be removed for the particular examination being done. Tell the patient that the gown should open in the back. Provide assistance as needed. Give the patient privacy while changing. Knock on the examination room door before re-entering to make sure the patient has completed undressing and gowning.
5. Do not place the patient in this position until the physician is ready for that part of the examination.
   PURPOSE: To promote the patient's privacy, comfort, and safety.
6. Pull out the table extension if necessary. Help the patient lie down on his or her back and then turn over into the prone position. Ask the patient to move up onto the knees, spread the knees apart, and lean forward onto the head so that the buttocks are raised. Tell the patient

to keep the back straight and turn the face to either side. The patient should rest his or her weight on the chest and shoulders (Figure 1).

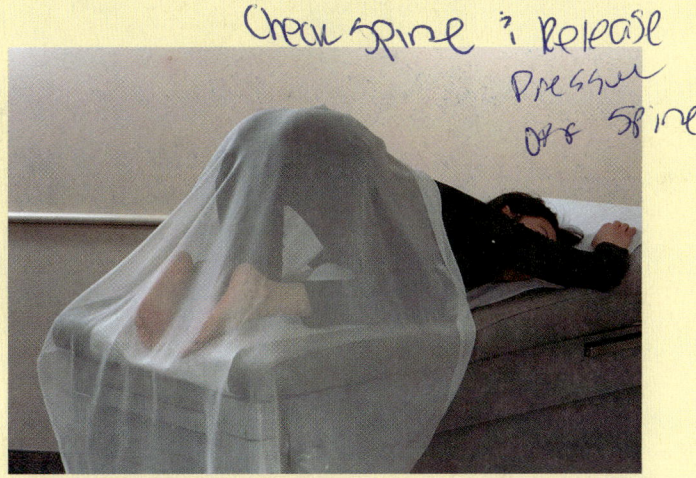

Check spine ? Release Pressure off spine (handwritten)

7. If the patient has difficulty maintaining this position, an alternative is to place weight on bent elbows with the head off of the table.
8. Drape the patient diagonally so that the point of the drape is on the table between the legs.
   PURPOSE: Draping the patient provides warmth and privacy while giving the physician access to the examination site.
9. After the examination has been completed, assist the patient as needed to get off the table and get dressed.
10. Clean and disinfect the examination room according to Standard Precautions. Roll clean paper over the table.
    PURPOSE: To ensure infection control and to prevent the transmission of pathogens from one patient to another.
11. Sanitize your hands.
12. Follow up with the physician's orders regarding scheduling of diagnostic studies, collection of specimens, and/or scheduling of future appointments.

Left Lateral Position - Recovery Position i having problem breathing (handwritten)

CRITICAL THINKING APPLICATION 32-2

Determine the correct patient position and method of gowning and draping for the following examinations:
- Insertion of a rectal suppository
- Annual Papanicolaou (Pap) smear
- Examination of the back
- Patient with dyspnea
- Breast examination

PRINCIPLES OF BODY MECHANICS

Proper body mechanics should be used consistently throughout the work environment when sitting or standing, lifting or carrying objects, pushing or pulling, or transferring patients. Without consistent application of correct anatomic alignment, injuries, especially lower back injuries, easily occur.

Proper body alignment begins with good posture. Maintaining posture requires a combination of muscle efforts. Good posture keeps the spine balanced and aligned while a person is sitting or

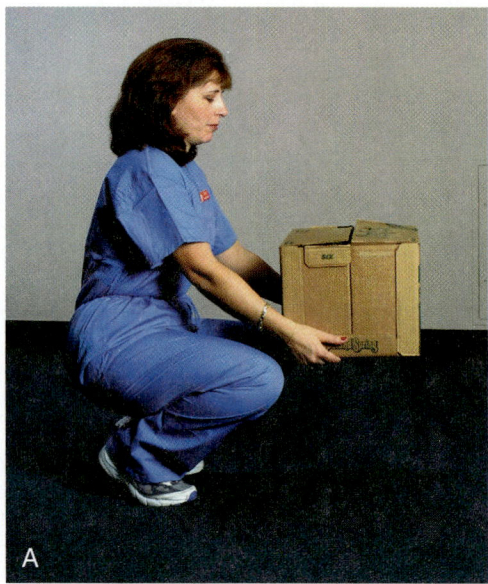
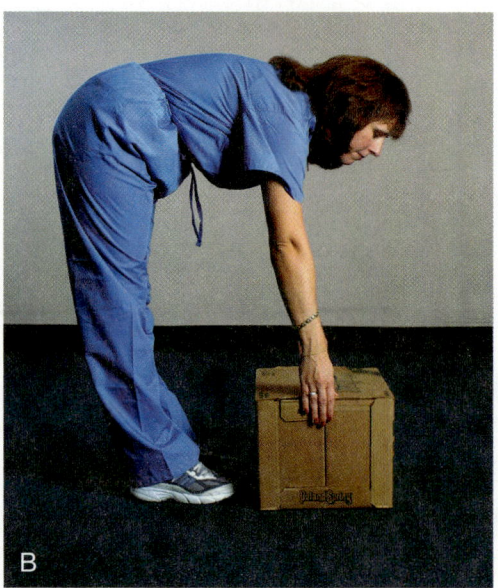

FIGURE 32-8 A, Proper lifting technique. **B,** Improper lifting technique.

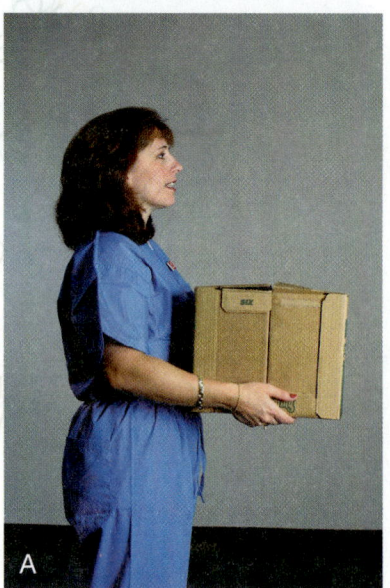
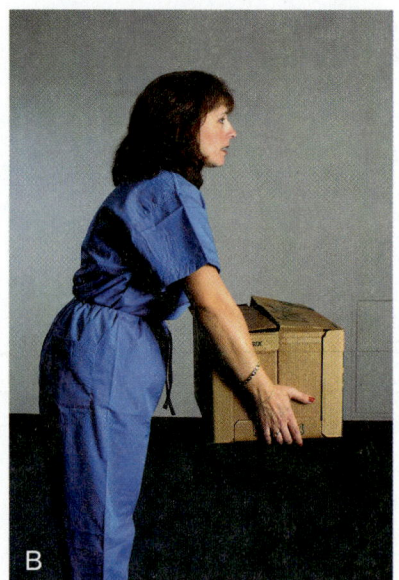

FIGURE 32-9 A, Carrying an item close to the body. **B,** Improper carrying technique.

standing. A person in good body alignment can maintain balance without undue strain on the musculoskeletal system.

When reaching for an object, avoid twisting or turning; instead, move the feet to face the object needed. This prevents undue strain on the lumbar region. Do not cross the legs while sitting, because this interferes with circulation to the legs and feet. When sitting, keep the popliteal area (behind the knees) free of the edge of the chair. Pressure in this area interferes with circulation and may damage nerves behind the knees. Do a mental check of your posture regularly. Hold the head erect, the face forward and the chin slightly up, the abdominal muscles contracted up and in, the shoulders relaxed and back, the feet pointed forward and slightly apart, and the weight evenly distributed to both legs, with the knees slightly bent. Always be on the alert for poor body mechanics that may cause injury (Figures 32-8 and 32-9).

SAFE LIFTING TECHNIQUES

- Always get help if the load is too heavy.
- Maintain correct body alignment with the legs spread apart for a broad base of support.
- Do not reach for items. Clear barriers out of the way and get as close as possible to what needs to be lifted.
- Bend at the knees with the feet shoulder width apart and keep the back straight. Use the major muscle groups of the arms and legs rather than the weaker ones of the back to help lift a heavy item (see Figure 32-8).
- When carrying a heavy item, keep the weight as close to the body as possible (see Figure 32-9).

- Move the feet in the direction of the lift. Do not twist or turn on fixed feet.
- Bend the knees while keeping the back straight when lowering an item at the completion of a lift.
- If possible, slide, roll, or push a heavy item rather than lifting or pulling it.

Transferring a Patient

Frequently, patients need assistance in moving from a chair to the examination table or back again. Patients can be transferred in multiple ways, but all should focus on correct body mechanics. If the patient is in a wheelchair, move the chair close to the examination table, lock the wheels, and lift the foot rests of the wheelchair out of the way (Figure 32-10). Explain the procedure to the patient and ask for his or her assistance.

If one side of the patient is stronger than the other, always provide support on the strong side. Place a step stool in front of the wheelchair next to the side of the examination table. Support the patient close to your body on the strong side, with one hand under the axillary region and the other either grasping the patient's hand or holding the forearm. When bending, always bend at the knees and maintain the back's three natural curves, allowing the leg muscles to help in lifting. Give the patient a signal and lift as the patient assists. Anchor the step stool with one foot, and help the patient step up onto the stool with the strong leg, then pivot (Figure 32-11). Ease the patient down onto the table, bending your knees while keeping your back aligned. Make sure the patient is comfortable and is safely positioned on the table (Figure 32-12). You may need to remain with the patient until the examination has been completed to ensure the patient's safety. If the physician prefers that the patient be in a supine position, place one arm across the patient's shoulders and the other under the knees, and smoothly lower the patient's upper body to the table while raising the legs. Use the same pivoting techniques with proper body mechanics to help transfer the patient from the exami-

nation table back to the locked wheelchair. If the patient must hold onto you, have the person hold your waist or shoulders, not your neck.

EXAMINATION SEQUENCE

The physical examination sequence is fairly standard; however, variations may occur, depending on the physician's specialty, the medical necessity for the examination, and the physician's preference. Patients are more cooperative and less anxious if they understand what is expected of them; therefore, you should start by giving the patient a brief explanation of the examination process. Assemble all supplies and instruments needed for the examination before the physician enters the room. As the physician proceeds with the examination,

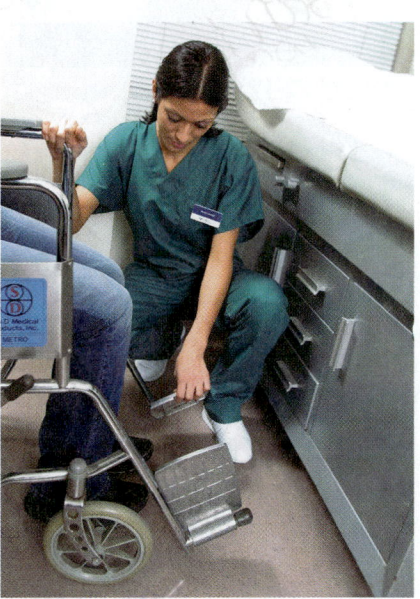

FIGURE 32-10 Wheels locked and foot rests elevated.

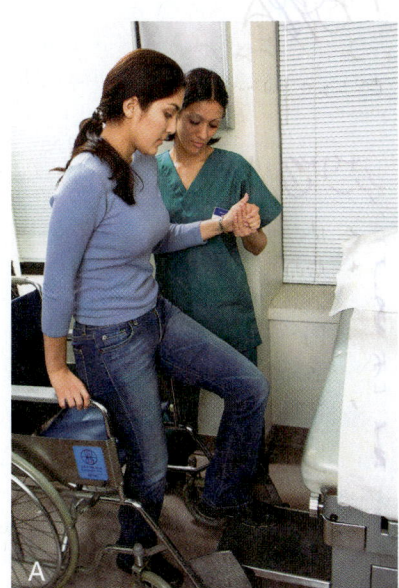
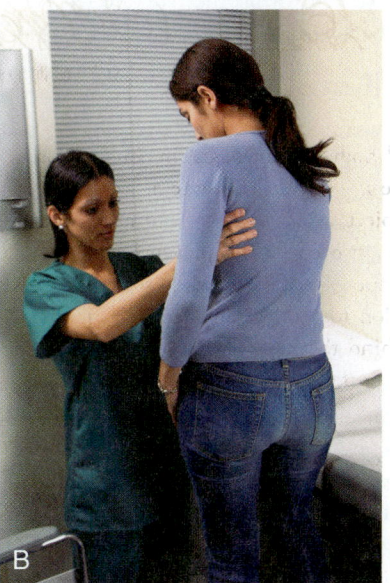

FIGURE 32-11 **A,** Strong side support. **B,** Pivot with support.

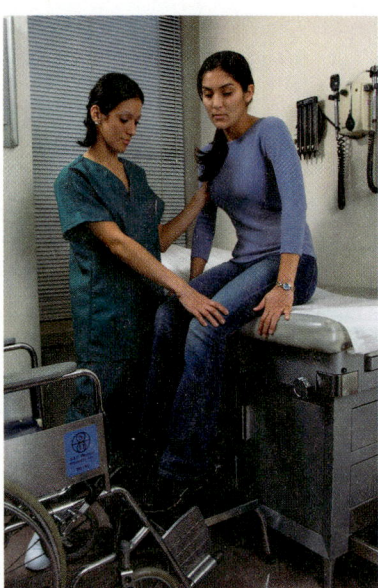

FIGURE 32-12 Sitting on a table with support.

make sure the patient remains unexposed by adjusting the drape and gown as needed. In every examination, the medical assistant assists the physician by handing him or her the correct instruments and needed supplies.

Having a female assistant in the room during the examination of a female patient can help prevent lawsuits. If the physician is male, a female medical assistant must remain with a female patient throughout the examination unless the physician excuses the medical assistant from the room.

When the physician begins the examination, the medical assistant should keep conversation to a minimum and remain inconspicuous. The examination usually starts with the patient seated on the examining table in Fowler's position. If the physician uses reflected light, the light source should be behind the patient's right shoulder. If illuminated instruments are used, standard overhead lights are sufficient. Take care not to shine a light directly into the patient's eyes; this can be done by turning on lights while they are directed away from the patient and carefully moving the light toward the area.

Presenting Appearance (General Appearance)

The physician starts the physical examination by observing the patient's appearance. Either *presenting appearance* or *general appearance* may be used on the medical record. These terms note whether the patient appears well and in good health (e.g., the patient appears disoriented or in distress; well nourished or undernourished; and answers questions with ease or confusion).

The patient's gait often provides important information. The patient may limp, walk with the feet wide apart, have a shuffle step, or have difficulty maintaining his or her balance. In addition to gait, all the patient's body movements are observed for possible muscle actions that the physician deems unusual. Posture also is checked for indications of pain, stiffness, or difficulty with limb movement. If the medical assistant notes any of these observations or the patient reports any complaints, these should be recorded in the patient's medical record along with the vital signs before the physician begins the examination.

Nutrition and Stature

The medical assistant measures the patient's height and weight before the examination begins, and these measurements are recorded in the patient record, along with the BMI. During the examination, the physician notes the body build and proportions. Any *gross* (immediately obvious) deformities are recorded. Sometimes abnormalities in height or body proportion may be caused by hormonal imbalances.

Speech

Speech may reveal a pathologic condition. Some basic speech defects include *aphonia*, the inability to speak because of loss of the voice, which is commonly seen with severe laryngitis or overuse of the voice; *aphasia*, the loss of expression by speech or writing because of an injury or disease of the brain; and *dysphasia*, lack of coordination and failure to arrange words in proper order, usually caused by a brain lesion. With *motor aphasia*, the patient knows what he or she wants to say but cannot use muscles properly to speak, perhaps seen as slurred or incoherent speech that might occur after a cerebrovascular accident (CVA). In *sensory aphasia*, the patient pronounces words easily but uses them inaccurately, as in jumbled speech.

Breath Odors

Breath odors may or may not be diagnostic, although they often are associated with poor oral hygiene or dental care. Acidosis produces a strong odor of acetone, which is sweet and fruity, and may result from diabetes mellitus, starvation, or renal disease. A musty odor usually is associated with liver disease, and the odor of ammonia may be noted in cases of uremia.

Skin

The condition of the skin can be a good reflection of the patient's nutritional status and hydration level. If dehydration is suspected, skin *turgor* is checked by pinching the skin on the posterior surface of the hands. The tissue is observed to see how quickly it returns to the normal location. A delay indicates a decrease in tissue fluid, confirming the diagnosis of dehydration. Extreme dryness, scaling, extended time for wound healing, or frequent breaks in the skin may indicate systemic disease.

Fingernails and toenails often give some indication of a person's health. Brittle, grooved, or lined nails may indicate local infection or systemic disease. Clubbing of the fingertips is associated with some congenital heart or lung diseases. *Spooning* of the nail is seen in some patients with severe iron-deficiency anemia. *Beau's lines* appear after an acute illness but grow out and disappear. The PCP may refer a patient with skin disorders to a dermatologist for diagnosis and treatment.

Head

Once the physician makes the overall observations of the patient's general condition, physical examination typically begins with the head and face and moves downward to the feet. The face reflects the patient's state and tells the physician a great deal about how the patient handles stress and illness. The skull, scalp, and face are palpated for size, shape, and symmetry. The distribution or lack of hair and the hair texture may indicate hormonal changes. Excessive hair, especially facial hair in females, indicates a hormonal imbalance. As the head is palpated, the physician assesses possible **nodules**, masses, or signs of trauma.

Eyes

The pupils are checked for reaction by shining a light into one eye at a time. If the pupils constrict equally and smoothly to a light stimulus, the physician documents "PERRLA" (which means the pupils are equal, round, respond to light, and adjust and focus on objects). The **sclera** is checked for color, which ranges from white to pale yellow. If the eye is inflamed, it will be evident in the sclera. A sclera with a yellow tone indicates liver disease. Movements of the eyes are tested by having the patient follow the physician's finger. If eye movement is within average range, the note "extraocular movement (EOM) intact" is written. The physician uses the ophthalmoscope to examine the interior of the eye, including the retina and the intraocular vessels. Some diseases, such as diabetes mellitus or hypertension, damage the blood vessels of the retina.

Ears

The ears are examined with an otoscope. The external ear is checked first for inflammation of the external auditory canal or for earwax *(cerumen)*. The tympanic membrane (eardrum) is examined and should appear pearly gray. Scars on the eardrum frequently are the result of earlier, chronic ear infections or perforations. The color of the eardrum is important to the diagnosis, because it may indicate fluids such as blood or pus behind the eardrum in the middle ear. The patient may be asked to swallow several times to allow observation of movement of the tympanic membrane, which occurs because of pressure changes in the eustachian tube. The eustachian tube equalizes air pressure between the middle ear and the throat. The ability of the tympanic membrane to move is crucial to the hearing process.

Nose and Sinuses

The mucosa of the nasal cavity is examined for color and texture. The sinuses cannot be seen, but the frontal and maxillary sinuses may be examined by firm palpation over the area and by **transillumination**. When disorders of the eyes, ears, nose, and throat are observed, and the physician believes that the condition warrants the attention of a specialist, the patient is referred to an ophthalmologist or an otorhinolaryngologist (ear, nose, and throat specialist).

Mouth and Throat

The mouth, or oral cavity, usually is thought of in terms of oral hygiene and dental care. Dental hygiene includes the condition of the teeth, how the patient cares for the teeth and gums, and whether the teeth of the upper and lower jaws meet properly (occlude) for chewing. Healthy gums are pale pink, glossy, and smooth and do not bleed when pressure from a tongue depressor is applied. The palatine tonsils usually are visible. The physician may use a tongue depressor and a piece of gauze to grasp the tongue to examine it carefully. The floor of the mouth is examined by both inspection and palpation for enlarged lymph nodes, salivary gland function, and ulcerations. The insides of the cheeks and the gumline are also examined for any abnormal marks or color.

Neck

The neck is examined for ROM by having the patient move the head in various directions. The thyroid gland is given special attention for symmetry, size, and texture. The physician manually palpates the thyroid area, and the patient is asked to swallow several times. The carotid artery is palpated and auscultated for possible bruits. The lymph nodes are palpated. *Lymphadenopathy* (enlargement of the lymph nodes) occurs if the patient has an infection of the face, head, or neck.

Reflexes

The patient's reflexes are checked with the patient in high Fowler's and supine positions. While the patient is sitting, the biceps are checked with the patient's arm flexed and supported by the examiner. The knee jerk (patellar reflex) and the ankle jerk (Achilles reflex) are checked using *tapotement* (a tapping or percussing movement) with either the fingers or the reflex hammer. The plantar reflexes (Babinski and Chaddock reflexes) are tested with the patient in an upright or supine position.

Chest

While the patient is still in the sitting position, the chest, heart, and lungs are examined. The chest is examined for symmetric expansion. A tape measure may be used, especially if variation exists between the upper and lower chest expansion. A patient with a history of **emphysema** may have a barrel-shaped chest. The physician may use percussion to determine the density of lung tissues.

With the stethoscope to the patient's back, the examiner auscultates lung sounds. The patient is asked to take deep, regular breaths. This may produce slight dizziness, but the patient should be assured that it is only the result of the deep respirations and will rapidly pass. The physician notes the types of respirations and the presence of lung sounds in all lobes.

Because considerable concentration is required to interpret heart sounds, the physician must have complete silence when listening to the patient's heart. The heart is examined with a stethoscope from both anterior and posterior approaches to the patient. Further examination may include auscultation on the left lateral side. In patients with heart disease, the physician may spend an extended time listening to heart sounds. If chest or heart abnormalities are found, the physician typically orders further diagnostic tests, including blood analysis, x-ray evaluation, and an ECG. Once the results of these studies have been analyzed, the physician may refer the patient to a cardiologist for treatment of a heart condition, or a pulmonologist or a respiratory care specialist for treatment of a breathing disorder.

Abdomen

For the abdominal part of the examination, the patient is lowered to the dorsal recumbent position and the drape is lowered to the pubic hair line. The gown is raised to just under the breasts. The physician stands to the patient's right side if at all possible. The patient's arms may be placed at the side, or the hands may be crossed over the chest or under the head. Relaxation of the abdominal muscles is absolutely essential for the abdominal examination. To assist in this and to promote patient comfort, a small pillow can be placed under the head and knees. The physician auscultates the abdomen in all quadrants to confirm the presence of complete bowel sounds and palpates the abdomen for any abnormalities. The physician also may use percussion to determine the density, position, and size of underlying abdominal organs.

Breast and Testicles

Careful breast examination is part of the physical examination for every female, regardless of whether she is symptomatic. The breasts are examined both visually and by palpation with the patient in high Fowler's position and then again in the supine position. Breast cancer is the most common malignancy in women, and early detection is the key to successful treatment. This is a good opportunity to discuss and reinforce the consistent use of monthly self-breast examination (SBE) (the technique is presented in Chapter 41). For male patients who have reached puberty or are 15 years of age or older, the physician will perform a testicular examination. This is an important self-examination for all males to perform each month, because testicular carcinoma is a major health risk (the technique is presented in Chapter 40).

Rectum

The rectal examination usually follows the abdominal examination or may be part of the examination of the male or female genitalia.

Preserving the patient's comfort and dignity is vital. For this part of the examination, the physician needs examination gloves and lubricating jelly. The examination light should be directed at the perineal area during the examination.

Hemoccult test specimens often are collected at the time of the digital rectal examination. If this is a procedure the physician performs, be sure to include the necessary collection folder with the examination equipment. Patients diagnosed with gastrointestinal (GI) disorders may be referred to a gastroenterologist (see Chapter 39). Procedure 32-8 presents the steps for assisting with the physical examination.

ROLE OF THE MEDICAL ASSISTANT

The physical examination establishes a baseline from which a patient's healthcare needs are determined. The examination should never be considered routine. Each patient's needs are special, and the medical assistant must be prepared to assist when needed. Throughout the procedure, the medical assistant must treat the patient with respect and guard the individual's privacy as much as possible.

The primary role of the medical assistant is to have the room, equipment, and supplies stocked and ready; the patient prepared, with vital signs, height, weight, and BMI measured and recorded;

PROCEDURE 32-8

Prepare the Patient for and Assist With Routine and Specialty Examinations: the Physical Examination

GOAL: To aid the physician in the examination of a patient by preparing the patient and the necessary equipment and ensuring the patient's safety and comfort during the examination.

EQUIPMENT and SUPPLIES

- Stethoscope
- Gauze sponges
- Ophthalmoscope
- Pen light
- Scale with height measurement bar
- Nasal speculum
- Tuning fork
- Tongue depressor
- Biohazard container
- Cotton balls
- Examination light
- Laboratory request forms
- Percussion hammer
- Specimen bottles and laboratory requisitions
- Lubricating gel
- Examination gloves
- Patient gown
- Sphygmomanometer
- Drapes
- Otoscope with disposable speculum
- Thermometer
- Cotton-tipped applicators
- Tape measure
- Hemoccult supplies
- Spray disinfectant
- Table paper

PROCEDURAL STEPS

1. Prepare the examining room according to acceptable medical rules or asepsis.
   PURPOSE: The room must be aseptically clean to prevent the spread of infection.
2. Sanitize your hands.
   PURPOSE: To ensure infection control.
3. Locate the instruments for the procedure. Set them out in order of use within reach of the physician and cover them until the physician enters the examination room.
   PURPOSE: To promote time management and ensure that all needed equipment and supplies are ready.
4. Greet and identify the patient, introduce yourself, and determine whether the patient understands the procedure. If the patient does not, explain what to expect.
   PURPOSE: To promote the patient's cooperation during the examination.
5. Review the medical history with the patient and investigate the purpose of the visit. Record the interview results.
   PURPOSE: To verify that all information is current and complete.

6. Measure and record the patient's vital signs, height, weight, and body mass index (BMI).
   <u>PURPOSE:</u> To gather data needed before the examination begins.

7. Instruct the patient on how to collect a urine specimen, if ordered, and hand the patient a properly labeled specimen container (see Chapter 52). Obtain blood samples for any tests ordered (see Chapter 53). Obtain a resting electrocardiogram (ECG) if ordered (see Chapter 49).
   <u>PURPOSE:</u> To obtain all specimens and perform all tests as ordered by the physician before the physical examination.

8. Hand the patient a gown and drape. Instruct the patient about clothes that should be removed for the examination and whether the gown should open in the front or in the back. Help the patient with undressing as needed (most patients prefer to undress in privacy). Knock on the door before re-entering the room to protect the patient's privacy.
   <u>PURPOSE:</u> To assist the patient in preparing for the examination and to safeguard the patient's privacy, comfort, and safety.

9. Assist the patient as needed in sitting at the foot of the examination table; place the drape over the patient's lap and legs. If the patient is elderly, confused, or feeling faint or dizzy, do not leave him or her alone.
   <u>PURPOSE:</u> To provide for the patient's warmth and privacy and to prevent a fall or injury.

10. Place the patient's medical record in the designated area or inform the physician that the patient is ready. Be careful to place information showing the person's identity out of sight to protect the patient's privacy.

11. Assist during the examination by handing the physician each instrument as it is needed and by positioning and draping the patient.

12. When the physician has completed the examination, allow the patient to rest for a moment, then help the patient from the table. Assist with dressing, if necessary. Use proper body mechanics if assistance in transfer is needed.
    <u>PURPOSE:</u> To ensure the patient's stability and safety and to protect yourself from injury.

13. Return to the patient and ask whether he or she has any questions. Give the patient any final instructions, and schedule tests as ordered by the physician and/or the next appointment.
    <u>PURPOSE:</u> To clarify instructions, eliminate any misunderstandings, and allow the patient to discuss any concerns. If the patient's misunderstandings or concerns are beyond your scope of experience or skill, arrange for the physician to speak with the patient again.

14. Put on gloves and dispose of used supplies and linens in designated biohazard waste containers. Clean surfaces with disinfectant. Disinfect all equipment.
    <u>PURPOSE:</u> To prevent cross-contamination with any potential infectious materials.

15. Remove the gloves, discard them in the biohazard waste container, and sanitize your hands.
    <u>PURPOSE:</u> To ensure infection control.

16. Replace used supplies and prepare the room for the next patient.

---

documentation completed regarding the patient's chief complaint or reported data; and the patient properly gowned and in position for the examination. During the examination, the medical assistant should be prepared to hand the physician needed equipment or to assist in any other way necessary. After the examination has been completed, the medical assistant should assist the patient as needed; complete any diagnostic procedures ordered by the physician; assist in the patient's discharge; answer the patient's questions or complete patient education; and disinfect and restock the room in preparation for the next patient.

CRITICAL THINKING APPLICATION   32-3

Alice Greenbaum, a 68-year-old patient of Dr. Kosto, is scheduled for an annual physical examination, including a breast check and a Pap smear. Mrs. Greenbaum appears anxious about the examination and asks Felicia whether the gynecologic examination is necessary. How should Felicia answer this patient? What might be helpful in easing the patient's fears and preparing her for the examination?

CLOSING COMMENTS

Patient Education

The physical examination process is an excellent time for the medical assistant to assess the need for patient education. This assessment should be performed to identify the best way to meet the patient's needs. When identifying these needs, consider the following:

- The information the patient needs to know
- How to convey the information so that the patient understands it
- How the patient will use the information
- Whether any community resources are available that might help the patient understand and learn more about health problems or treatment protocols

Develop a plan to teach the patient. Think about the different modalities available, such as pamphlets, pictures, DVDs, demonstrations, and community resources. The more interesting the information, the more fun it is to teach the patient and the more enjoyment the patient will get out of learning. Many facilities keep patient education files that contain handouts on a wide range of health issues. The medical assistant should always review teaching plans with the physician and follow the physician's direction in patient education.

CRITICAL THINKING APPLICATION   32-4

Dr. Kosto serves as the PCP in the area for residents of group homes for the developmentally delayed. Jimmy Cosgrove, a 38-year-old patient who is severely retarded, is being seen today for an annual physical examination. Felicia is responsible for preparing the patient for the examination. Describe how Felicia should prepare the examination room and the patient.

Legal and Ethical Issues

The medical assistant must recognize that a legal and ethical contract exists between the patient and the physician. As the physician's employee, the medical assistant is part of that contract. Information gained during the physical examination is confidential and must remain that way. The medical assistant must uphold ethical responsibilities as written in the Code of Ethics of the American Association of Medical Assistants (AAMA): to render service, respect confidential information, and uphold the honor and high principles of the profession.

HIPAA Applications

- Remember that conversations in the healthcare facility may be overheard. Guard patient confidentiality when gathering information about the chief complaint, scheduling diagnostic tests, or processing samples. If the front desk has a privacy glass, make sure it remains closed; turn away from the waiting room when talking on the phone; and avoid any conversations about the patient that may be overheard.
- Place medical records on the examination room door with identifying information facing the door to prevent those passing by from recognizing the patient's name. If electronic medical records (EMRs) are used, safeguard patient information by closing patient files and locking computers when you will be out of the room.
- Place the physician's schedule away from patient areas and maintain patient confidentiality during the admissions procedure in the facility. Many facilities no longer use sign-in sheets, but if they are used, the staff must completely block the names of previous patients from sight to maintain confidentiality.

SUMMARY OF SCENARIO

As a new medical assistant, Felicia has a great deal of responsibility when it comes to assisting with physical examinations. She must prepare the room for the particular examination ordered and must prepare and care for the patient during the procedure. Preparing the room includes making sure appropriate supplies and equipment are readily available and planning for the patient's privacy during the examination. Each examination is different, just as each patient has his or her own set of needs. Felicia helps the patient into a variety of positions, depending on the examination, and properly gowns and drapes the patient to safeguard privacy. Felicia is responsible for making sure the examination runs smoothly for the physician and for supporting the patient throughout the process. To protect herself against injury, Felicia uses proper posture and body alignment, remembering to bend at the knees and use her arm and leg muscles, rather than her back, to lift heavy items.

She always asks for help if a load is too heavy, and she pushes a heavy item rather than lifting it.

SUMMARY OF LEARNING OBJECTIVES

1. **Define, spell, and pronounce the terms listed in the vocabulary.**
   Spelling and pronouncing medical terms correctly bolsters the medical assistant's credibility. Knowing the definitions of these terms promotes confidence in communication with patients and co-workers.
2. **Apply critical thinking skills in performing the patient assessment and patient care.**
   Completing the Critical Thinking Application exercises throughout the chapter can help the student medical assistant become more adept at critical analysis of real-life situations.
3. **Describe the structural development of the human body.**
   The human body is made up of trillions of microscopic cells that determine the functional and structural characteristics of the entire body. A cell is made up of three primary parts: the plasma membrane, the cytoplasm, and the nucleus. When cells with similar structures and functions combine, tissues are formed. The body has four types of tissue: epithelial, connective, muscular, and nervous tissue. A combination of two or more types of tissues creates an organ, and a number of organs joined together form a body system.
4. **Differentiate among the functions of the body systems and the major organs and structures of each system.**
   A body system is composed of several organs and their associated structures. These structures work together to perform a specific function in the body. Each of the body's systems has specific units within it, and each performs specific functions. Table 32-1 summarizes the body systems; their primary cells, organs, and structures; and the major functions of each.
5. **Outline the medical assistant's role in preparing for the physical examination.**

Before the examination, the medical assistant has the opportunity to interact with the patient to ensure that he or she feels comfortable during the examination process, and that all necessary medical information has been obtained. The medical assistant's duties include preparing and maintaining the examination room and equipment; preparing the patient by conducting the initial interview and measuring vital signs; assisting the physician with positioning and draping; and providing instruments and supplies as needed during the physical examination.

6. **Summarize the instruments and equipment the physician typically uses during a physical examination.**

Instruments and supplies typically used in a physical examination include nasal speculum, ophthalmoscope, otoscope, tongue depressor, reflex hammer, various tuning forks, stethoscope, sphygmomanometer, thermometer, examination gloves, tape measure, scale, examination light, disposable gloves, biohazard container, specimen bottles, laboratory requisitions, hemoccult test supplies, patient gown, drapes, and lubricating gel.

7. **Describe the six methods of examination and give an example of each.**

The examiner uses *inspection* to detect significant physical features, such as the patient's general appearance. With *palpation*, the sense of touch is used to feel the brachial pulse before a blood pressure reading is taken. *Percussion* involves tapping or striking the body to elicit sounds or vibratory sensations, as in percussion of the chest to detect fluid in the lungs. A stethoscope is used to *auscultate* or listen to the lungs and heart. *Mensuration* is the process of measuring the patient's height and weight. *Manipulation* is the passive, assisted movement of a joint to determine the range of extension or flexion.

8. **Outline the basic principles of properly gowning and draping a patient for examination.**

The patient should be instructed on whether to wear the gown open in the front or open in the back, depending on the type of examination to be done. Draping requires constant attention to maintaining the patient's privacy throughout the examination while assisting the physician with exposure of the area being examined. The general rule is to cover all exposed body parts until the point in the examination when the physician must evaluate that particular area.

9. **Name the various positions that may be used during an examination and identify the purpose of each.**

The position assumed by the patient during the examination depends on the part of the body to be examined or the procedure to be done. Possible patient positions include the sitting positions of *Fowler's position*, in which the patient sits straight up, and *semi-Fowler's position*, in which the patient's torso is elevated 45 degrees; the *dorsal recumbent position*, in which the patient lies on the back with the legs bent; the *supine position*, in which the patient lies flat on the back; the *lithotomy position*, in which the patient's buttocks are at the bottom of the table and the legs are positioned in stirrups; the *prone position*, in which the patient lies on the stomach; *Sims' position*, in which the patient lies on the left side with the limbs flexed so that the weight of the body is tilted forward; and the *knee-chest position*, in which the patient is on the knees with the buttocks elevated and the weight of the body tilted downward toward the chest (see Procedures 32-2 through 32-7). Trendelenburg's position, in which the patient's head is lower than the legs, is not typically used in the ambulatory care setting.

10. **Position and drape a patient in six different examining positions while remaining mindful of the patient's privacy and comfort.**

Procedures 32-2 through 32-7 outline the steps for positioning and draping patients.

11. **Demonstrate proper body mechanics in transferring a patient from a chair to the examination table and back.**

Good body mechanics principles include maintaining balanced posture, bending the knees while maintaining the back's three natural curves, and using leg muscles to help lift. Move the wheelchair close to the examination table, lock the wheels, and lift the foot rests of the wheelchair out of the way. Provide patient support close to your body on the patient's strong side. Place a step stool in front of the wheelchair next to the side of the examination table, and with one hand under the axillary region and the other grasping the patient, anchor the step stool with one foot and help the patient step up onto the stool with the strong leg; then help the patient pivot into a sitting position on the table.

12. **Outline the sequence of a routine physical examination.**

The examination sequence depends on the type of examination and the physician's preference. The physician typically begins the examination by noting the patient's general health appearance, nutrition status, speech, breath odor, skin condition, and reflexes. The physician then begins the physical examination, starting at the head and working down through the body to the rectum. Any abnormalities are noted and may be further investigated with diagnostic tools after the examination has been completed.

13. **Prepare for and assist in the physical examination of a patient, correctly completing each step of the procedure in the proper sequence.**

Prepare the examination room and the patient; complete the initial patient interview and measure and record vital signs; gather the needed equipment and place it in the order of use; gown and drape the patient as needed; provide patient instruction and check for understanding throughout the process; assist during the examination by handing the physician instruments, managing changes in light, collecting samples as ordered, and conducting diagnostic procedures as ordered; assist the patient when the examination is done, including helping the patient dress, scheduling further diagnostic tests as ordered, and answering the patient's questions. Complete the documentation, disinfect the examination room and equipment, and restock supplies to ready the room for the next patient (see Procedure 32-8).

14. **Summarize the role of the medical assistant in the physical examination process.**

The medical assistant must pay attention to the patient's needs and assist the physician with the procedure. This includes preparing the room and supplies, preparing the patient, documenting pertinent patient information, and assisting the physician throughout the process. After the examination has been completed, the medical assistant should help the patient as needed, complete diagnostic procedures as ordered, and disinfect and restock the examination room for the next patient.

15. **Determine the role of patient education during the physical examination.**

Before, during, and after the physical examination are excellent times to provide appropriate patient education. The medical assistant should clarify or reinforce any information provided by the physician and should take advantage of "teaching moments" to promote patient well-being.

16. **Discuss the legal and ethical implications of the physical examination.**

The medical assistant is part of the legal contract established between the patient and the physician. This contract begins at the time of the first visit to the ambulatory care facility. Maintaining confidentiality and providing respectful service are crucial to the integrity of that patient contract.

CONNECTIONS

Study Guide Connection: Go to the Chapter 32 Study Guide. Read and complete the activities.

Evolve Connection: Go to the Chapter 32 link at *evolve.elsevier.com/ kinn* to complete the Chapter Review and the Chapter Quiz. Peruse other resources listed for this chapter to increase your knowledge of Assisting With the Primary Physical Examination.

PRINCIPLES OF PHARMACOLOGY

33

SCENARIO

Kathy Augustino, CMA (AAMA), was hired recently to work for a primary care physician in her hometown. Her responsibilities include administering medications to a wide range of patients. To give patients medications correctly and safely in the ambulatory setting, she must understand the basic principles of pharmacology.

While studying this chapter, think about the following questions:

- What should Kathy know about the management of controlled substances in the ambulatory care setting?
- If Kathy is not familiar with a medication, how can she learn about the properties of the drug?
- Is it important that Kathy understand the clinical uses of prescribed drugs as well as over-the-counter (OTC) drugs?
- One of Kathy's responsibilities is phoning in drug orders to the pharmacy. What parts of the prescription should she recognize?
- A primary care practice has patients of all ages. What factors related to age might affect the action of medications on Kathy's patients?

LEARNING OBJECTIVES

1. Define, spell, and pronounce the terms listed in the vocabulary.
2. Apply critical thinking skills in performing patient assessment and care.
3. Distinguish among the government agencies that regulate drugs in the United States.
4. Cite the areas covered in the regulations established by the Drug Enforcement Administration (DEA) for the management of controlled or regulated substances.
5. List the DEA regulations for prescription drugs for each of the five schedules of the Controlled Substance Act.
6. Explain the medical assistant's role in preventing drug abuse.
7. Differentiate among a drug's chemical, generic, and trade names.
8. Describe the use of drug reference materials.
9. Explain the five pregnancy risk categories for drugs.
10. Define the five medical terms used to describe the clinical use of drugs.
11. Cite safety measures for the use of over-the-counter (OTC) drugs.
12. Diagram the parts of a prescription.
13. Demonstrate the ability to transcribe a prescription accurately.
14. Relate the principles of pharmacokinetics to drug use.
15. Describe factors that affect the action of a drug.
16. Compare the therapeutic classifications of medications.
17. Differentiate among commonly used herbal remedies and alternative therapies.
18. Examine the role of the medical assistant in drug therapy education.
19. Identify the medical assistant's legal responsibilities in medication management in an ambulatory care setting.

VOCABULARY

angina pectoris (an-ji'-nuh/pek'-tuh-ruhs) Spasmlike pain in the chest caused by myocardial anoxia.

bronchodilator (brahn-ko-di'-la-tuhr) Drug that relaxes contractions of the smooth muscle of the bronchioles to improve lung ventilation.

cirrhosis (suh-ro'-suhs) Chronic, degenerative disease of the liver that interferes with normal liver function.

colloidal (kah-loid'-uhl) Pertaining to a gluelike substance.

enteric-coated Term that refers to an oral medication that is coated to protect the drug against the stomach juices; this design is used to ensure that the medicine is absorbed in the small intestine.

formulary List of drugs compiled by a health insurance company that identifies the drugs the insurance company will cover under benefits.

generic Medication that is not protected by trademark.

hypercholesterolemia (hi-per-kuh-les-tuh-ruh-le'-me-uh) Elevated blood levels of cholesterol.

lumen An open space, such as within a blood vessel or the intestine, or in the inside of a needle or an examining instrument.

metabolic alkalosis Condition characterized by significant loss of acid in the body or an increased amount of bicarbonate; severe metabolic alkalosis can lead to coma and death.

over-the-counter (OTC) drugs Medications sold without a prescription.

spermicide (spuhr'-muh-side) Chemical substance that kills sperms cells.

therapeutic range The blood concentration of a drug that produces the desired effect without toxicity.

tinnitus A noise sensation of ringing heard in one or both ears.

Pharmacology is the broad science of the origin, nature, chemistry, effects, and uses of drugs. *Clinical pharmacology* is the study of the biologic effects of a drug used as a medical treatment and the actions of a drug in the body over time, including the rate at which it is absorbed by body tissues; where it is distributed or localized in the tissues; the route by which it is excreted; and its toxicity, or poisonous effect.

Medical assistants must have a general understanding of the types of drugs available and their uses. For every medication administered, a medical assistant must understand the drug's action, typical side effects, route of administration, and recommended dose, as well as the individual patient factors that can alter the drug's effect and elimination. Drugs are constantly being developed and released for patient treatment; therefore, medical assistants must continually update their knowledge of specific drugs used in the ambulatory care setting. Correct management of drug administration and patient education are crucial factors in providing safe drug therapy for all patients.

GOVERNMENT REGULATION

Several federal agencies combine forces to regulate, safeguard, and manage the development and use of medications in the United States. The Food and Drug Administration (FDA), a division of the Department of Health and Human Services, regulates the development and sale of all prescription and **over-the-counter (OTC) drugs**. Pharmaceutical companies developing new medications must gain FDA approval before the drugs can be sold to consumers. The approval process begins with chemical testing in the laboratory and progresses to toxicity testing in laboratory animals, and finally to human clinical trials, which involve volunteers who participate in controlled drug studies. Only one of 10 new drugs ever reaches the clinical testing phase. If the drug is found to have an acceptable benefit-to-risk ratio (i.e., it is effective without causing an unacceptable degree of harm to the user), the FDA approves the medication for release.

The original manufacturer of the drug is awarded copyright protection on that particular chemical compound for 17 years; this means that during the 17-year period, other pharmaceutical companies cannot produce **generic** copies of the drug. Besides approving new drugs for the marketplace, the FDA establishes manufacturing standards for drug purity and strength and ensures that generic brands are effective and safe.

STANDARDS FOR GENERIC DRUG MANUFACTURERS

The Food and Drug Administration (FDA) has found no difference in the rates of reported side effects between brand name and generic drugs. Generic drugs must meet the following standards:

- The generic version must have the same active ingredients, labeled strength, route of administration, and dosage form (tablets, patches, and so on).
- Generics do not have to replicate the human clinical trials of the brand-name drugs, but applicants must prove that the product performs exactly as the brand-name version does.
- Generic versions must act in the same period of time as the brand-name version, delivering the same amount of active ingredient into the bloodstream in the same amount of time.
- The label of the generic drug must contain the same information for patient education.
- The generic manufacturing process must ensure comparable quality and production standards. Brand-name firms produce approximately 50% of the generic drugs on the market, making generic versions of their own products or other brand-name products.

OTHER FEDERAL AGENCIES INVOLVED IN THE REGULATION OF DRUGS

Besides the Food and Drug Administration, two other agencies are involved in the regulation of drugs in the United States:
- Drug Enforcement Administration (DEA): The DEA is the federal law enforcement agency responsible for controlling narcotics, investigating the illegal sale of dangerous substances, and preventing drug abuse through public education.
- Federal Trade Commission (FTC): The FTC regulates the advertising of over-the-counter drug preparations.

Controlled Substances

The Drug Enforcement Administration (DEA) was established in 1973 as part of the Department of Justice to enforce federal laws regarding the use of illegal drugs. According to the Controlled Substances Act (CSA), which was passed in 1970, a drug or other substance that has the potential for illegal use and abuse must be placed on the controlled substance list. Any new medication with an action similar to a drug already on the controlled substance list also is considered to have the potential for abuse.

Most controlled drugs provide significant assistance to patients in need of their particular actions, such as pain relief or anesthesia for surgery. However, certain guidelines must be followed to comply with the storage of controlled substances, their record keeping, and security requirements. In addition, federal law requires that all medical personnel, including medical assistants, share the responsibility for managing controlled substances on site. Precautions must be taken to monitor patients' drug use, protect prescription pads, maintain the records required by law, and report any known or suspected drug diversion or theft.

According to the guidelines set forth in the CSA, controlled substances are divided into five sections, or *schedules,* depending on their addictive abilities and likely degree of abuse. The classifications range from Schedule I drugs, which are illegal and cannot be prescribed, to Schedule V medications, which have the least potential for addiction and abuse (Table 33-1).

Every medical practice that stores and administers medications that fall into any of the schedule categories should have a copy of the controlled substances regulations. This list can be obtained from the regional DEA office. It is also important to ensure that the office is included on the DEA's mailing list, so that the practice receives updates as drugs are added, deleted, or moved from one schedule to another.

Regulation of Controlled Substances

Specific CSA regulations govern the record keeping, physician registration, and inventory of controlled substances. Complete, accurate records on the purchase and management of scheduled drugs in the ambulatory care setting must be maintained. These records must be kept separate from the patient's medical record for 2 years and must be readily available for inspection by the DEA at all times. Each time a controlled substance is dispensed and administered in the office, documentation of that process includes the number of doses of the

drug on site both before and after the medication is dispensed. Medical practices that dispense and administer controlled substances on site use forms developed for this purpose. Any discrepancy in the count of the medication available must be documented and co-signed by two employees.

Every physician who prescribes or has controlled substances on site must register with the DEA for a Controlled Substance Registration Certificate. The physician receives a specific DEA registration number that must be included on all controlled substance prescriptions. The certificate is renewable every 3 years and is specific to a particular site of practice. Therefore, if the physician dispenses or prescribes scheduled drugs at more than one site, a DEA registration number must be obtained for each site.

All controlled substances must be stored in a safe or immovable locked cabinet, and the keys must be kept in a secure location. Prescription forms should be kept out of areas used by patients and preferably secured in an area that prohibits unauthorized or illegal use. All DEA forms used by the facility to order controlled substances also must be kept in a locked area.

Many ambulatory practices no longer keep controlled substances on site. However, if drugs are lost or stolen, the incident must be reported immediately to the regional DEA office and to local law enforcement authorities. If a controlled substance is damaged or must be discarded (e.g., a pill falls to the floor during dispensing), two employees must be present to witness the medication being flushed down the sink or toilet, and both must document the procedure on the controlled substance inventory form used by that office. If a large quantity of scheduled drugs must be discarded, the local DEA office should be contacted for guidance.

CRITICAL THINKING APPLICATION   33-1

Kathy is responsible for maintaining the inventory of controlled substances in the office. While checking the supply of meperidine, she notices that the expiration date on the medication is today. She must dispose of the remaining two pills. According to DEA regulations, how should she dispose of the medication?

Individual states also may regulate controlled substances; therefore, it is essential that medical assistants know their state's legal requirements.

Specific guidelines apply to prescription orders for controlled substances:
- The prescription must be written in ink or typed.
- It must include the date prescribed; the name and address of the patient; and the name, address, and DEA number of the physician.
- The amount prescribed must be written out ("ten" rather than "10"); the prescription usually is written for small amounts of the drug.
- The physician must manually sign all prescriptions for controlled substances, although the medical assistant can prepare the prescriptions for the physician's signature.
- Drugs in Schedules II, III, and IV must include this label when dispensed by the pharmacy: *Federal law prohibits the transfer of*

TABLE 33-1 Classification of Controlled Substances

SCHEDULE	GUIDELINES	DRUG EXAMPLES
I	• No accepted medical use • Never prescribed for use • High potential for abuse • Possession of these drugs is illegal	Heroin, lysergic acid diethylamide (LSD), marijuana, methaqualone (Quaalude), mescaline (peyote), amphetamine variations, phencyclidine (PCP), Ecstasy, GHB acetylcodone, Dipipan
II	• Accepted for medical use but with severe restrictions • High potential for abuse • May cause severe psychological or physical dependence	Opium extracts, morphine, methadone, cocaine precursors, amphetamine, barbiturates, methylphenidate (Ritalin), oxycodone (Percocet or OxyContin), hydromorphone HCl (Dilaudid), meperidine HCl (Demerol), codeine, alfentanil (Alfenta), alphaprodine (Nisentil), Burgodin, secobarbital (Seconal), fentanyl
III	• Accepted for medical use • Potential for abuse less than with Schedule I or II drugs • May cause moderate to low physical dependence or high psychological dependence • Includes combination drugs that contain limited amounts of narcotics or stimulants	Paregoric, acetaminophen and codeine (Tylenol with codeine), benzphetamine, suppositories with barbiturates, anabolic steroids, testosterone, butabarbital (Butisol), Fiorinal, Voranil, Empirin, hydrocodone (Vicodin), buprenorphine
IV	• Accepted for medical use • Low potential for abuse • May cause limited physical or psychological dependence compared with Schedule III drugs • Includes minor tranquilizers and hypnotics	Meprobamate (Equanil), chlordiazepoxide (Librium), diazepam (Valium), flurazepam (Dalmane), chloral hydrate, propoxyphene napsylate (Darvon), Rohypnol ("date rape" drug), pentazocine lactate (Talwin), alprazolam (Xanax), triazolam (Halcion), temazepam (Restoril), chlorazepate dipotassium (Tranxene), lorazepam, Klonopin, (Ativan), zolpidem tartrate (Ambien), barbital, Lexatin, Urbanyl, clonazepam (Klonopin), diethylpropion (Tenuate), Motofen, Capla, midazolam (Versed), Donnatal, Meridia, zolpidem tartrate (Ambien), eszopiclone (Lunesta)
V	• Accepted for medical use • Low potential for abuse • May cause limited physical or psychological dependence compared with Schedule IV drugs • Includes drug mixtures containing limited amounts of narcotics	Cough medicines containing limited quantity of codeine (Robitussin A-C), alkaloids, kaolin and pectin belladonna (Donnagel), diphenoxylate with atropine (Lomotil) May be sold by a pharmacist in some states; buyer must be 18 years old and must show identification

this drug to any person other than the patient for whom it is prescribed.

Other specific rules may apply, depending on the schedule to which the prescribed controlled substance is assigned. The symbols C-II, C-III, C-IV, and C-V are used to indicate the specific schedule:

- Schedule II (C-II) prescriptions:
  - Must be written unless an absolute emergency exists that requires a telephone prescription order. The amount in the phone order is limited to that needed during the emergency, and the physician must deliver a written prescription to the pharmacy within 72 hours.
  - Cannot be refilled
  - In certain states, must be provided as multiple-copy prescription order forms
- Schedule III (C-III) and IV (C-IV) prescriptions:
  - May be ordered orally or in writing
  - May be refilled up to five times within 6 months of the original order

- Schedule V (C-V) prescriptions:
  - May be ordered orally or in writing
  - May be refilled up to five times within 6 months of the original order
  - Depending on the state, may be dispensed by the pharmacist without a prescription

CRITICAL THINKING APPLICATION   33-2

Kathy is responsible for the orientation of a new medical assistant in the practice. Summarize the important points about government regulation of controlled substance prescriptions that she should include in the orientation.

DRUG ABUSE

Any drug, from aspirin to alcohol, can be misused or abused. The use of illegal and legal drugs has increased tremendously. Treatment programs for drug abuse are available throughout the United States for people from all walks of life. Programs include detoxification, rehabilitation, and long-term rehabilitation maintenance.

Medical assistants may encounter patients who are misusing or abusing drugs. It is important to be alert to the symptoms of drug dependence and to notify the physician when you suspect that a patient, or a co-worker, may have a problem with drug or alcohol dependency.

Drug *misuse* is the improper use of common drugs that can lead to dependence or toxicity. Examples of people with chronic dependencies include those who cannot have a bowel movement unless they take a laxative; those who have used nasal decongestants for so long that they cannot breathe without the use of nasal sprays; and those who take so many antacids that they suffer systemic **metabolic alkalosis**.

Drug *abuse* is the continuous or periodic self-administration of a drug that could result in addiction (physical dependence). Drug *dependency* is the inability to function unless under the influence of a substance; it may be psychological or physical. *Psychological dependency* is the compulsive craving for the effects of a substance. *Habituation* is a mild form of psychological dependency, such as the need for caffeine. *Physical dependency*, or addiction, is a person's need to use a substance continuously so that the body can function, and also to prevent physical discomfort. This type of dependency occurs when abused substances produce biochemical changes in cells and tissues, most commonly in the nervous system. When a substance that causes physical dependency is discontinued, withdrawal symptoms occur. Withdrawal symptoms may be mild or serious, leading to convulsions and possibly death.

Regardless of the type of drug abused, it will have two effects on the person: acute and chronic. The acute effect is what the person feels when intoxicated, or directly under the influence of a particular substance. Chronic effects include the temporary or permanent physical and mental changes that result from long-term abuse.

Medical assistants often must answer patients' questions about drug abuse. The medical assistant should read and keep up to date on drug-related issues. Pamphlets and agency referral names should be available for patients. In addition, patients' concerns and questions about drug abuse should be conveyed to the physician.

THE MEDICAL ASSISTANT'S ROLE IN PREVENTING DRUG ABUSE

By following these guidelines, the medical assistant can help prevent drug abuse:

- Carefully monitor patients who repeatedly call for prescription refills of controlled substances.
- Request medical records for patients who report previous prescriptions for scheduled drugs.
- Keep prescription blanks in a safe place away from patient treatment areas, and minimize the number of prescription pads in use at any given time.
- Never use prescription pads for notepads, and never use preprinted or presigned forms.
- Secure computers used for electronic health record (EHR) documentation to prevent patient access to prescription generation.

- Keep only a limited supply of controlled substances on hand.
- Keep accurate, complete records of controlled substances dispensed on site and those prescribed. Include specific documentation in the patient's chart for all prescribed controlled substances.

DRUG NAMES

A single drug may have up to three names: a chemical name, a generic name, and a trade name. The chemical name represents the drug's exact formula. For example, the chemical name of the analgesic acetaminophen is *N*-(4-hydroxyphenyl). *Acetaminophen* is the generic name, and the trade name is *Tylenol*. All drugs are assigned a generic, or nonproprietary (official), name. This name is much simpler than the chemical name, and it is not protected by copyright. The trade, or brand, name is assigned by the manufacturer and is protected by copyright. To prevent confusion, the use of generic names rather than trade names is encouraged. Drugs also are classified by their use. For example, Advil is a brand name for the generic drug ibuprofen, which is classified as an analgesic and an anti-inflammatory agent.

APPROACHES TO STUDYING PHARMACOLOGY

A pharmaceutical glossary could be a book in itself. Many terms are combinations of the condition to be treated plus the prefix *anti-* (e.g., antianginal, antianxiety, antiarrhythmic, anticoagulant, anticonvulsant, antidiarrheal). Notice how these names emphasize the drug's effect (use) rather than its action in the body. More recent classifications, such as parasympathomimetic and cholinesterase inhibitor, describe the pharmacologic action rather than the therapeutic use. Both viewpoints are necessary for a more complete understanding of drugs and their action in the human body. No one can remember all there is to know about clinical pharmacology. The number of new drugs introduced into use far exceeds the number of older drugs replaced or discontinued. The number of drugs available for clinical use grows beyond the ability to learn all there is to know about each medication. Therefore, it is essential that a medical assistant understand how to use pharmacology resource books as references.

Drug Reference Materials

Reference books that are updated annually or periodically should be available for easy reference at all medical facilities. Most references list drug information in the following sequence:

1. *Action:* How the drug provides therapeutic results in the body, or the use of the drug.
2. *Indication:* The conditions for which the drug is used.
3. *Contraindications:* Conditions that make administration of the drug improper or undesirable.
4. *Precautions:* Necessary actions that must be taken because of special conditions of the patient, the drug, or the environment; they need to be considered if the drug is to be successful or not harmful. The drug's pregnancy risk category is included in this section, as are precautions for nursing mothers (Table 33-2).
5. *Adverse reactions:* Commonly observed side effects on a tissue or organ system other than the one targeted by the medication.

TABLE 33-2 Pregnancy Risk Drug Categories

DRUG CATEGORY	RISK/DESCRIPTION
A	Remote risk. Controlled studies in women have failed to demonstrate risk to fetus.
B	Slightly more risk than A. Animal studies show no risk, but controlled human studies have not been done; *or* animal studies show risk, but controlled studies in women have shown no risk.
C	Greater risk than B. Animal studies have shown risk, but no controlled human studies have been done; *or* no studies have been done in animals or women.
D	Proven risk of fetal harm. Human studies show proof of fetal damage, but the potential benefits of use during pregnancy may make its use acceptable.
X	Proven risk of fetal harm. Studies in women or animals show definite risk of fetal abnormality. Risks outweigh any possible benefit.

Adverse reactions include *hypersensitivity*, which causes an allergic reaction to the drug; *idiosyncrasy*, or an unexplained, unusual response to the drug; psychological dependence or habituation to the drug; and physical dependence on the compound, causing signs and symptoms of withdrawal in the patient if the medication is removed. For example, patients prescribed certain diuretics (e.g., Lasix) are at risk for potassium depletion, so they must take a potassium supplement or must eat a daily dietary source of potassium (bananas are a common source) to prevent complications.

6. *Dosage and administration:* Usual route, dosage, and timing for administering the drug.
7. *How supplied:* Description of how the medication is packaged and specifics on how it should be administered.

Package Inserts

Every drug package contains an insert describing all the significant aspects of using the drug, including information on the chemical formulation of the drug and clinical studies. The information in the insert is controlled by the FDA and serves as an excellent quick reference on new medications in the ambulatory setting.

Physicians' Desk Reference

The *Physicians' Desk Reference* (PDR) is published annually by Thomson Medical Economics Company (Oradell, New Jersey). The PDR is provided free to physicians who subscribe to *Medical Economics* magazine. Copies can be purchased through the publisher or in local bookstores. Supplements are published quarterly throughout the year. The PDR contains information on approximately 2,500 drugs and includes product descriptions that are identical to the information provided in package inserts. The drug manufacturers pay for this space, so the PDR could be considered the Yellow Pages of the drug industry. The PDR is the most commonly used drug reference book and should be available in all healthcare facilities.

The book's sections are color-coded and cross-referenced for easy use. The various sections allow you to begin searching for information about a drug from any starting point. You can start with the usage, classification, generic name, manufacturer's name, or trade name of a drug or what the drug looks like. A special photographic section enables visual identification of products. Once you know which drug you want to study, the product information section lists the actual package insert information alphabetically, first by the manufacturer, then by the brand name. A separate PDR volume, the *Physicians' Desk Reference for Nonprescription Drugs*, is published annually for OTC drugs and dietary supplements. The six sections of the PDR are color-coded as follows:

- *Manufacturer's index (white):* Alphabetical listing of pharmaceutical companies that includes the drugs manufactured by each company; it also provides contact information for each manufacturer
- *Brand and generic section (pink):* Alphabetical listing of all drugs included in the PDR volume, with complete information for each
- *Product category index (blue):* Alphabetical listing compiled according to drug category; drugs with similar actions are listed alphabetically in each category
- *Product identification section (gray):* Illustrated section that shows actual-size photographs of the tablets and capsules listed in the PDR
- *General and diagnostic product information area (white):* Alphabetical listing of diagnostic product information and the uses of these products

U.S. Pharmacopeia/National Formulary

The *U.S. Pharmacopeia/National Formulary* (USP/NF) is the official source of drug standards for the United States. The *Pharmacopeia* was combined with the *National Formulary*, which lists the chemical formulas for all accepted drugs. This combined reference lists and describes all approved medications in the United States considered useful and therapeutic in the practice of medicine. Single drugs rather than combined products (compound mixtures) are listed. If a drug name is the same as the official name in this volume, the drug is followed by the initials USP (e.g., digitoxin, USP).

Learning About Drugs

The study of pharmacology is difficult at best. However, a few tips can help make it easier:

- First, take advantage of opportunities to observe the use of drugs in patient care. Studying about atorvastatin calcium (Lipitor) becomes more meaningful when you see how its lipid-lowering action actually affects a patient's blood cholesterol level.
- Second, concentrate on the most important drugs in each classification. As you expand your knowledge to other drugs in each category, you will easily understand new drugs by noting the similarities and differences between them and the basic, important drugs you studied first.

- Third, learn about a drug's primary action and use, then expand your knowledge to its other actions and uses. Soon you will be able to name the drug that is usually indicated for a particular condition. By knowing a drug's secondary effects, you will be able to understand what side effects are likely to occur during use of the drug. More important, you will be aware of contraindications to use of the drug. Knowledge of the drug's actions will enable you to predict what toxic reactions might occur from an overdose.

TERMINOLOGY DESCRIBING DRUG USES

diagnostic	Helps to determine the cause of a particular health problem (e.g., injecting antigen serum for allergy testing).
palliative	Indicates that the drug does not cure but provides relief from pain or symptoms related to the disorder (e.g., the use of an antihistamine for allergy symptoms or narcotics for pain relief).
prophylactic	Prevents the occurrence of a condition (e.g., vaccines prevent the occurrence of specific infectious diseases).
replacement	Provides the patient with a substance needed to maintain health (e.g., insulin for patients with diabetes, levothyroxine sodium [Synthroid] for patients with hypothyroidism).
therapeutic	Treats a disorder and cures it (e.g., antibiotics cure bacterial infections).

Dispensing Drugs

Drugs are dispensed in two ways: over the counter and by prescription. OTC drugs are available to the public for self-medication without a prescription. These drugs have been approved by the FDA for general consumer use, but patients taking prescription drugs should keep their healthcare providers informed about their OTC drug use.

A medical assistant directly involved in patient care should have an understanding of some basic facts about OTC drugs. Today patients are better informed about their personal healthcare, and many want to be active participants in healthcare decisions. They need facts to make informed choices when using OTC preparations. Most OTC preparations are safe if used as directed on the package; however, patient education contributes greatly to the safe and correct use of OTCs. Patients should be encouraged to do the following when choosing or using an OTC:

- Carefully read the package label and insert for use guidelines.
- Take only the recommended dose.
- Monitor the expiration date and discard the medication when appropriate.
- Never combine an OTC with a prescription drug without the physician's knowledge.
- Recognize that many OTC drugs are contraindicated in pregnancy, for nursing mothers, and for young children, and if certain diseases are present.
- Check with the pharmacist if questions or concerns arise.

The number of prescription drugs that have been granted OTC status is constantly increasing, and as the list of OTC drugs increases, so does the need for consumer education. Many OTC medications influence the safety and effectiveness of prescription drugs; therefore, gathering information to discern a complete and accurate pattern of the patient's use of OTC drugs should be part of every visit to the physician.

Prescription Drugs

Federal law makes drugs that are dangerous, powerful, or habit-forming illegal to use except under a physician's order. A *prescription* is an order written by the physician for the dispensing of a particular medication by the pharmacist and its administration to the patient. Sometimes an order may be written by the physician on the patient's medical record; however, most often it is an order written on a prescription blank for the pharmacist to fill (Figure 33-1). The prescription must be signed by the physician, or the order cannot be carried out (Procedure 33-1). If the physician requests that the medical assistant phone in a prescription to the pharmacy, all pertinent information for the medication order must be written down and reviewed by the physician for accuracy before the call is made. A note is made in the patient's chart that a medication order was phoned into the pharmacy, with all of the pertinent information about the order included.

Appropriate medical terminology and abbreviations must be used to complete the prescription. The more common terms and abbreviations are listed in Table 33-3. In an attempt to reduce the number of medication errors caused by incorrect use of medical terminology, the Joint Commission (formerly known as The Joint Commission on Accreditation of Healthcare Organizations [JCAHO]) recently developed a "Do Not Use" list of abbreviations, acronyms, and symbols that should not be used for documentation purposes in accredited institutions. The Joint Commission also created an ancillary list of possible future inclusions. Both of these lists are presented in Table 33-4. In addition to the Joint Commission lists, facilities

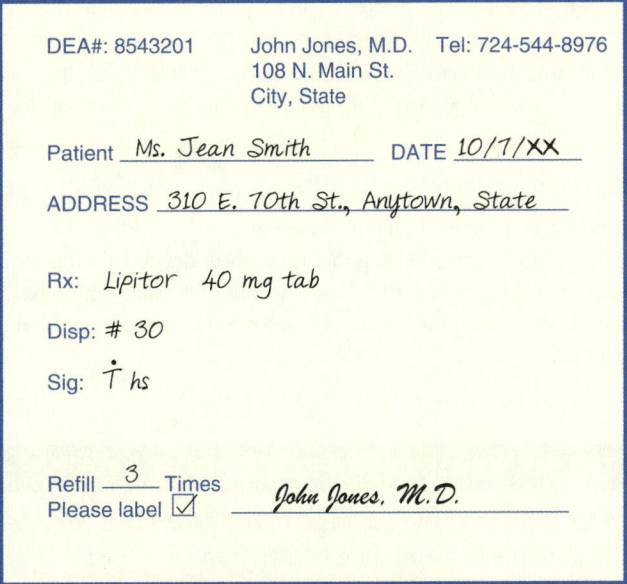

FIGURE 33-1 Sample prescription.

PROCEDURE 33-1

Maintain Medication and Immunization Records: Prepare a Prescription for the Physician's Signature

GOAL: *To accurately prepare a prescription for the physician's signature using the appropriate abbreviations and prescription format.*

EQUIPMENT and SUPPLIES

- Prescription pad
- Drug reference materials if needed
- Black pen
- Patient chart

PROCEDURAL STEPS

1. Refer to the physician's written order for the prescription. If the physician gives a verbal order to write a prescription, write down the order and review it with the physician for accuracy.
   PURPOSE: To ensure accuracy in writing the ordered medication.
2. If you are unfamiliar with the medication, look it up in a drug reference book (e.g., the *Physicians' Desk Reference* [PDR]).
   PURPOSE: The medical assistant should be familiar with the details of the drug, including the correct spelling, form in which it is dispensed, strength, recommended dose, storage guidelines, drug-drug interactions, and possible side effects, to make sure the transcription is correct and to be prepared to answer the patient's questions about the medication.
3. Ask the patient about drug allergies.
   PURPOSE: The patient should be asked about drug allergies each time a medication is prescribed or dispensed, because these can change over time.
4. Using a prescription pad that has the physician's name, address, telephone number, and DEA registration number preprinted on the slip, begin to transcribe the physician's order (refer to Figure 33-1).
5. Record the patient's name and address and the date on which the prescription is being written.
6. Next to the Rx, write in legible handwriting the name of the drug (correctly spelled), the dosage form (e.g., tablet, capsule, or other, using correct abbreviations), and the strength ordered. This is the inscription. For example, if the physician orders Lipitor, 40-mg tablets,

by mouth, one tablet at bedtime, the first line of the prescription should read: Lipitor 40 mg tabs.
7. On the next line, write *Disp.* This is the subscription, which includes directions to the pharmacist on the amount to be dispensed and the form of the drug. For the Lipitor order, the subscription would read: Disp: #30.
8. Next comes the signature. This includes directions for the patient, such as how and when to take the medicine; it usually is preceded by the abbreviation *Sig:* For the Lipitor order, the signature would read: Sig: ī tab po hs.
9. The physician has told you that the patient can get three refills of the prescription, so this information should be added at the bottom of the prescription on the designated line.
10. The physician must review and sign the prescription before it is given to the patient.
11. Document in the patient's medical record the medication order and any pertinent details, including patient education and refill information.
    PURPOSE: All patient education should be documented for future reference, and the details about the prescription, as well as refill information, must be included for future prescriptions and/or refill orders.

TELEPHONING A PRESCRIPTION INTO THE PHARMACY

Using the steps outlined above, complete the prescription including the patient's full name and address; the practitioner's full name and address; the DEA number if the prescription is for a controlled substance (Schedule II drugs must be filled with a written prescription and/or an EHR program that is authorized to fill scheduled drugs); and the drug name, strength, dosage form, quantity prescribed, direction for use, and the number of refills (if any) authorized. The physician must review the prescription for accuracy before the medical assistant telephones the pharmacy. Document the telephoned pharmacy order in the patient's medical record as you would for any prescribed drug.

---

have the option of creating their own list of problematic abbreviations that employees should avoid using.

Table 33-5 lists the top 50 prescribed drugs by retail sales in 2010, along with their classifications. Review this list to become familiar with some of the most commonly prescribed medications.

THE SIX PARTS OF A PRESCRIPTION

- *Superscription*: Patient's name and address, the date, and the symbol Rx (for the Latin word *recipe*, meaning "take")
- *Inscription*: Main part of the prescription; name of the drug, dosage form, and strength

- *Subscription*: Directions for the pharmacist; size of each dose, amount to be dispensed, and the form of the drug ordered (tablets, capsules, or some other form)
- *Signature*: Directions for the patient; usually preceded by the symbol Sig (for the Latin word *signa*, meaning "mark"); the place where the physician indicates the instructions to be put on the label to tell the patient how, when, and in what quantities to use the medication
- *Refill information*: May be regulated by federal law if the drug is a controlled substance; the physician must write on the script the number of times a refill is allowed
- *Physician's signature*: Must include the physician's manual signature, as well as his or her Drug Enforcement Agency (DEA) registration number when indicated

TABLE 33-3 Common Prescription Abbreviations

ABBREVIATION	MEANING	ABBREVIATION	MEANING	ABBREVIATION	MEANING
aa	of each	ID	intradermal	pt	patient
ac	before meals	IM	intramuscular	pt	pint
ad lib	as desired	IV	intravenous	pulv	powder
agit	shake, stir	K	potassium	qh	every hour
am	morning	kg	kilogram	q2h	every 2 hours
amp	ampule	KVO	keep vein open	q3h	every 3 hours
AD	right ear	L	liter	q4h	every 4 hours
AS	left ear	lb	pound	qid	four times a day
ASA	aspirin	LR	lactated Ringer's solution	qm	every morning
AU	both ears	ℳ	minim	qn	every night
aq	water	mcg	microgram	qod	every other day
bid	twice a day	med	medicine	qs	quantity sufficient
C	cup, Celsius	meq	milliequivalent	qt	quart
c̄	with	mg	milligram	R	rectal
cap	capsule	mL	milliliter	Rx	take, treatment
CC	chief complaint	MLD	minimum lethal dose	r/o	rule out
cc	cubic centimeter	mn	midnight	S, Sig	give the following directions
cm	centimeter	MO	mineral oil	s̄ or w/o	without
c/o	complaining of	MOM	milk of magnesia	SC, SQ, subQ	subcutaneous
D/C	discharge	MS	morphine sulfate	SOB	shortness of breath
Dx	diagnosis	MTD	maximum tolerated dose	s̄s̄	one-half
dil	dilute	NKA	no known allergies	stat	immediately
disp	dispense	noct	at night	sub-q	subcutaneous
dr	dram	NPO	nothing by mouth	T, tbs	tablespoon
EENT	eye, ear, nose, throat	NS	normal saline	t, tsp	teaspoon
ext	extract	N/V	nausea/vomiting	TAB	tablet
F	Fahrenheit	O$_2$	oxygen	tid	three times a day
FDA	Food and Drug Administration	OD	overdose	tinct	tincture
FE	iron	OD	right eye	TO	telephone order
fl	fluid	OS	left eye	tus	cough
fx	fracture	OU	both eyes	ung	ointment
gal	gallon	OTC	over-the-counter (drugs)	vag	vagina
gm, g	gram	oz	ounce	ves	bladder
gr	grain	pc	after meals	VO	verbal order
gtt	drops	PL	placebo	VS	vital signs
h	hour	pm	afternoon	W/O	water in oil
hs	at bedtime	PMI	patient medication instruction	WNL	within normal limits
HTN	hypertension	po	by mouth	x	times
Hx	history	pr	per rectum	y/o	years old
inj	injection	prn	as needed		

TABLE 33-4 The Joint Commission's "Do Not Use" List and Possible Future Inclusions

DO NOT USE	POTENTIAL PROBLEM	USE INSTEAD
U (for unit)	Mistaken as zero, four, or cc.	Write "unit"
IU (for international unit)	Mistaken as IV (intravenous) or 10 (ten)	Write "international unit"
Q.D., qd, Q.O.D., qod	Mistaken for each other. The period after the Q can be mistaken for an "I" and the "O" can be mistaken for "I"	Write "daily" and "every other day"
Trailing zero (X.0 mg), Lack of leading zero (.X mg)	Decimal point is missed	Never write a zero by itself after a decimal point (X mg), and always use a zero before a decimal point (0.X mg)
MS	Confused for one another	Write "morphine sulfate" or "magnesium sulfate"
MSO_4	Can mean morphine sulfate or magnesium sulfate	
$MgSO_4$		
Possible Future Inclusions		
> (greater than) or < (less than)	Misinterpreted as the number "7" or the letter "L"	Write "greater than" or "less than"
Abbreviations for drug names	Multiple drugs have similar abbreviations	Write drug names in full
Apothecary units	Unfamiliar to many practitioners; confused with metric units	Use metric units
@	Mistaken for the numeral "2"	Write "at"
c.c. or cc (for cubic centimeter)	Mistaken for U (units) when poorly written	Write "mL" or milliliters
μg (for microgram)	Mistaken for mg (milligrams), resulting in one thousand-fold dosing overdose	Write "mcg" or micrograms

From the Joint Commission. Accessed October 10, 2011, at www.jointcommission.org/PatientSafety/DoNotUseList/

TABLE 33-5 Top 50 Prescribed Drugs by Retail Sales in 2010

BRAND NAME	GENERIC NAME	CLASSIFICATION BY USE
Nexium	Esomeprazole	Antacid; inhibits gastric acid secretion
Lipitor	Atorvastatin calcium	Lowers cholesterol
Plavix	Clopidogrel bisulfate	Antiplatelet agent
Advair Diskus	Salmeterol xinafoate	Steroidal inhalant with bronchodilator
OxyContin	Oxycodone	Narcotic analgesic; extended release
Abilify	Aripiprazole	Antipsychotic
Singulair	Montelukast sodium	Anti-inflammatory; leukotriene inhibitor
Seroquel	Quetiapine	Antipsychotic
Crestor	Rosuvastatin	Lowers cholesterol
Cymbalta	Duloxetine	Antidepressant
Actos	Pioglitazone	Oral hypoglycemic
Lexapro	Escitalopram; Simvastatin	Antidepressant
Zyprexa	Olanzapine	Antipsychotic
Spiriva	Tiotropium inhalation	Anticholinergic agent; prevents bronchospasm
Lantus	Insulin glargine	Diabetes mellitus
Aricept	Donepezil	Alzheimer's disease
Lyrica	Pregabalin	Anticonvulsant; peripheral neuropathy

TABLE 33-5   Top 50 Prescribed Drugs by Retail Sales in 2010—cont'd

BRAND NAME	GENERIC NAME	CLASSIFICATION BY USE
Diovan	Valsartan hydrochlorothiazide	Antihypertensive
Concerta	Methylphenidate	Central nervous system stimulant
Levaquin	Levofloxacin	Antibiotic
Celebrex	Celecoxib	Antiarthritic
Diovan HCT	Valsartan	Antihypertensive
Januvia	Sitagliptin	Oral hypoglycemic
Suboxone	Buprenorphine and naloxone	Opiate analgesic
NovoLog	Insulin aspart	Diabetes mellitus
Viagra	Sildenafil	Erectile dysfunction
Atripla	Efavirenz, emtricitabine, and tenofovir	Antiviral; HIV medication
Tricor	Fenofibrate	Cholesterol lowering
Provigil	Modafinil	Stimulant; treat sleep apnea or narcolepsy
Zetia	Ezetimibe	Lowers cholesterol
Geodon oral	Ziprasidone	Antipsychotic
Vytorin	Ezetimibe	Lowers cholesterol
Ambien CR	Zolpidem tartrate	Hypnotic; sleep agent; controlled release
Lunesta	Eszopiclone	Hypnotic; sleep agent
Lidoderm	Lidocaine topical	Topical anesthetic
Lantus SoloStar	Insulin glargine	Long-acting form of insulin; diabetes mellitus
Vyvanse	Lisdexamfetamine	Central nervous system stimulant; treat attention deficit/hyperactivity disorder (ADHD)
Aciphex	Rabeprazole	Antacid; gastroesophageal reflux disease (GERD)
Nasonex	Mometasone	Steroidal decongestant
Lovenox	Enoxaparin	Anticoagulant
Adderall XR	Amphetamine and dextroamphetamine	Central nervous system stimulant; treat ADHD
ProAir HFA	Albuterol	Bronchodilator
Truvada	Emtricitabine and tenofovir	Antiviral; combination therapy for HIV
Niaspan	Nicotinic acid	B vitamin; lowers cholesterol
Humalog	Lispro insulin	Diabetes mellitus; fast-acting insulin
Cialis	Tadalafi	Erectile dysfunction
Namenda	Memantine	Alzheimer's disease
Symbicort	Budesonide and formoterol	Bronchodilator
Flovent HFA	Fluticasone HFA	Corticosteroid inhaler; anti-inflammatory

CRITICAL THINKING APPLICATION   33-3

Dr. Simon asks Kathy to prepare the following prescription for his signature: "Take one 20-mg tablet of Lipitor daily at bedtime. Dispense 4 weeks' worth, and the prescription may be refilled two times." How would Kathy write the prescription using the correct format, medical terminology, and abbreviations?

ELECTRONIC PRESCRIPTIONS

Electronic health records (EHRs) can be used to create, print paper copies, and/or send directly to a pharmacy the prescriptions for a patient. EHR programs are designed to automatically check a prescribed drug against the patient's allergies, identify possible drug-drug interactions, access current databases for the patient's medication history, review the patient's insurance drug **formulary** for coverage, and either print the prescription out for the patient to take to the pharmacy or electronically send the script to the patient's pharmacy to be filled. The Department of Health and Human Services (HHS) recognizes the importance of e-prescriptions in quality patient care because they reduce the possibility of misinterpreting physician handwriting and promote speed in filling prescriptions through the instant transfer of the script from the physician's office to the patient's pharmacy. It is possible to send controlled substance prescriptions to a pharmacy as long as the physician office and the pharmacy e-prescribing software package follow DEA regulations. HHS recommends that an individual—perhaps a medical assistant (MA) employee—be designated as the practice expert for e-prescribing, so the process runs smoothly and follows all regulations regarding the delivery of prescriptions electronically. More details on Medicare incentive programs to encourage physicians to adopt e-prescribing programs can be found at http://cms.gov/Medicare/E-Health/Eprescribing/index.html?redirect=/Eprescribing.

DRUG INTERACTIONS WITH THE BODY

Pharmacology is the study of drugs, their desired effects, and what happens to a drug while it is in the body. Different patients may react to the same dose of a drug in very different ways, and the same patient may react to the same dose of a drug differently at various times. Therefore, the management of medication therapy is concerned primarily with the effectiveness of a drug's action and the drug's potential side effects. *Pharmacokinetics* is the study of the movement of drugs throughout the body. Four basic actions occur when a drug is taken: absorption, distribution, metabolism, and excretion. By knowing what happens to the drug in the body, we can know the *onset* of a drug's activity (when the drug action starts), when the effects of the drug are likely to peak, the minimum amount of the drug needed to bring about the desired effect (therapeutic dose), and the *duration* of a particular drug's activity. All these factors help the physician determine the appropriate form, amount, route, and frequency of administration of a medication for a particular patient.

Drug Absorption

The rate at which drugs are absorbed from the site of administration into the bloodstream depends on many factors, including the drug's ability to be dissolved, the characteristics of the medication, the concentration of the dose, and the route of administration. Liquid oral medications are dissolved more rapidly than solid forms because they do not have to be dissolved by gastrointestinal (GI) fluids before they are absorbed. In addition, drugs that are soluble in fat pass more readily through the cell membrane, because cell membranes have a fatty acid layer. More acidic drugs are absorbed well in the stomach, whereas others cannot be absorbed until they reach the small intestine. For some medications, such as antibiotics, the physician may order an initial *loading dose* of the drug, usually twice the typical amount, so that the patient's blood levels reach the **therapeutic range** more quickly.

An important point to remember is that regardless of the route of administration, a drug can have one of two actions on the body:

local (restricted to one spot or part; not general) or *systemic* (affecting the body as a whole). Most drugs are used for their systemic effects. Even when drugs are used for local purposes, we know that no drug remains completely localized in the body. Any chemical that comes into contact with even the most superficial surface, such as the skin, has the potential to be absorbed into the bloodstream and to circulate to other tissues and organs.

Oral Route

Oral medications are convenient, safe, and relatively inexpensive. However, drugs that can be destroyed in any way by the digestive tract must be given by injection. Insulin and heparin are examples of drugs that are destroyed by the digestive process and therefore cannot be administered orally. Injection of medications leads to rapid absorption into the bloodstream, but this increases the danger of overdose or infection. Most oral medications are absorbed by the small intestine, but a few are absorbed more rapidly in the stomach. After absorption into the bloodstream from the small intestine, drugs are carried to the liver. Much of the drug's potency is inactivated in this organ before the drug circulates to the tissues. This inactivation by the liver often makes it necessary to administer higher doses orally than those given by injection.

Food slows the absorption of drugs; therefore, many medications are absorbed best when taken either 1 hour before or 2 hours after ingestion of food. Food also may bind with a medication or in some other way inactivate it. For example, tetracycline is destroyed by milk products and antacids containing calcium salts. Therefore, patients taking tetracycline should be advised not to eat dairy products or ingest liquid or solid forms of antacids. Stomach acid that naturally occurs during digestion may destroy certain drugs. Because some drugs are destroyed by the components of the digestive tract or irritate the empty lining of the stomach, oral drugs may be **enteric-coated** to keep them intact for passage into the small intestine or to prevent gastric irritation or vomiting.

Some drugs are not affected by digestive processes, but they cannot be absorbed through the intestinal walls into the bloodstream. For example, neomycin has no therapeutic effect when taken orally (unless it is used to sterilize the bowel before bowel surgery). Other drugs may be unable to cross the bowel mucosa because of their poor solubility in lipids (fats), or because they are inactivated by the pH of the GI tract.

It is important to remember these absorption factors when administering medication by the oral route. If a patient has previously responded to a drug but is no longer responding, it may be important to question the patient's food-medication cycle. It could be that the patient is no longer taking the medication on an empty stomach as directed.

Parenteral Route

Parenteral refers to the administration of drugs by injection. The parenteral route results in the fastest action, because the medication is administered directly into the bloodstream or into tissues with a rich blood supply. However, several factors determine the effectiveness and rate of absorption of injected medications.

A drug in an aqueous (water) solution is absorbed more quickly in an area with more blood vessels. Therefore, drugs deposited in the muscle are absorbed faster than drugs given subcutaneously. The *intramuscular* (IM) route is chosen in an emergency for fast action, or when larger amounts of the medication must be absorbed. The *subcutaneous* (SC) route is chosen when a slower, prolonged effect is desired.

Drug absorption also may be controlled physically. Absorption may be quickened by hand massage after injection, and it may be slowed by pharmaceutical preparation of the drug in a physical form that slows absorption. These methods include suspending the drug in a solution that prolongs absorption, such as **colloidal** substances, fatty substances (oil), or insoluble salts or esters. Drugs suspended in these substances slowly dissolve in the tissues over a long time, and the patient can be spared costly, frequent, and sometimes painful injections. Penicillin G is suspended with procaine (hydrochloride) salts for this purpose. Local anesthetics sometimes are mixed with epinephrine to keep the medication and its effects in an area longer, because epinephrine (adrenalin) constricts blood vessels at the site, reducing circulation and the rate of absorption.

The third parenteral route is the *intravenous* (IV) route, in which the medication is injected directly into the vein. Because of the dangers of IV administration, only members of the medical team who are licensed to do so may inject medication intravenously.

SAFETY ALERT

A medical assistant is not licensed to perform IV administration of medications to patients. Because IV administration is so dangerous, medications given intravenously usually are administered in small doses through an IV infusion (IV drip) so that the effects in the body can be monitored.

Other forms of parenteral routes include *intradermal* injection, which is injection of the drug within the dermal layer of the skin and superficial to the subcutaneous tissues. This route is used mostly for allergy testing and skin testing, such as testing for tuberculosis. *Intrathecal*, or *intraspinal*, injections are used for spinal anesthesia and for administering certain medications into the spinal column. *Intra-articular* injections are used for administering corticosteroids into joints, and *intralesional* medications are injected directly into a lesion, or an anticancer drug is administered into a cancerous tumor.

Mucous Membrane Absorption

Drugs may be absorbed by the mucous membranes of the mouth, throat, nose, eyes, rectum, vagina, and respiratory tracts. Some applications, such as nasal sprays, eye drops, and rectal suppositories for constipation, have a local effect. Others have a systemic effect, such as a rectal suppository given to control vomiting, or a nitroglycerin tablet dissolved under the tongue (sublingual) to dilate coronary arteries and relieve the pain of **angina pectoris**. *Inhalation* is used to concentrate drugs locally in the lower respiratory passages or to produce systemic effects, such as general anesthesia. For example, a **bronchodilator**, such as metaproterenol sulfate (Alupent), is inhaled during an asthma attack to relieve bronchospasms.

Topical Absorption

Topical routes include the application of medications to the skin, eyes, and ears. Drugs in ointments, creams, lotions, and aerosols can be applied for the treatment of skin itching, inflammation, or other discomforts, and for the treatment of skin infections with antibiotics. Nitroglycerin (for angina) can be absorbed through the skin from a dermal patch, which releases it systemically. Hormones such as testosterone and estrogen also can be administered via a dermal patch for systemic purposes.

TERMS RELATED TO DRUG INTERACTIONS

antagonism	The action of one drug diminishes the effect or shortens the duration of action of another drug.
synergism	A drug enhances the intensity or prolongs the action of another drug. This can have a positive effect, as when two different antibiotics are used to treat an infection, or a negative effect, as when two drugs lower blood pressure to dangerous levels.
potentiation	A form of synergism in which the effect of one drug is enhanced by the presence of another drug. In this case, the two drugs have different actions, but one increases the effect of the other.

Drug Distribution

Once a drug has been absorbed, it must be transported by the circulatory system to the area where it will have its effect. In the bloodstream, drugs can attach to plasma proteins and then are freed to pass from the blood into the site of action. Drugs are carried through the fluids into the cells of the tissues and organs. The blood supply to a part affects the speed with which drugs reach certain tissues.

The blood-brain barrier is a functional cellular barrier between the brain cells and the capillaries circulating blood through the brain. The barrier is poorly permeable to water-soluble materials, which makes it difficult for dissolved substances in the blood to pass through. For substances that do cross through, the barrier regulates the degree and rate of their absorption into the brain tissue. The general anesthetic thiopental (Pentothal) is able to cross the blood-brain barrier immediately and produces sleep within seconds, whereas other sleep-producing drugs, such as the barbiturates, cross slowly and may take as long as 30 minutes to 1 hour to produce the same effect. The blood-brain barrier is a mixed blessing. It provides a physical barrier that protects the brain from potentially dangerous chemicals, but it also makes it very difficult to treat central nervous system (CNS) disorders. In contrast, the placenta has no method for blocking substances, so whatever the mother consumes is readily passed through the placenta to the developing fetus. This means that childbearing women must be extremely careful of all chemicals they consume or inhale, because they are quickly transferred to the baby's bloodstream.

Drug Action

Multiple theories explain the actions of drugs. Drugs are believed to combine with body chemicals on the cell surface or within the cell itself. Pharmaceutical developers create compounds that have an affinity for a specific target cell. The target cell recipient is called a *receptor*, and the drug that has the affinity for it and produces a functional change in the cell is called an *agonist*. Not all drugs that bind to specific cells cause a functional change in the cell. These drugs act as an *antagonist* to the natural process and work by blocking a sequence of biochemical events.

Some drugs are believed to act by affecting the enzyme functions of the body. Drugs attach to enzyme substances and rob the enzymes from cells. As a result, the enzyme products needed for normal cellular function are not supplied, and the cell fails to function properly.

Certain anti-infective drugs have a selected toxicity for pathogens or parasites that have invaded the body. Penicillin and sulfonamides work because they poison or interfere with the life processes of bacteria without affecting the life processes of normal human cells. Research scientists continue to look for differences between cancer cells and normal cells so that they can apply the principle of selected toxicity in cancer treatment. Only recently have anticancer drugs been produced that are selective and therefore nontoxic to human cells.

Both drugs that have a selective affinity for cells and those that bind with enzymes may be counteracted by administering large amounts of natural substances with which the drugs compete. This process is known as administering an *antidote* to a drug that may be acting as a poison. For example, an antidote such as naloxone hydrochloride (Narcan) can be administered if a patient receives too much anesthesia or has taken a drug overdose.

Some drugs alter the function of a cell by affecting the physical properties of the cell membrane rather than altering biochemical processes within the cell. This is especially true of drugs that affect nerve cells, such as anesthetics and alcohol. A change in the cell membrane alters the permeability of the membrane, which in turn changes the flow of ions into and out of the cells. This change in ion flow alters the *polarity* (opposite effects at two extremities, the two extremities being inside and outside the cell membrane) on which nerve pulses are conducted, resulting in general sleep or stupor.

Drug Metabolism

After the drug has been absorbed and distributed, it is metabolized for excretion. During metabolism, the drug is converted into harmless byproducts, which are more easily eliminated by the kidneys. Most drugs are broken down by the enzyme activity of the liver. For oral medications that are absorbed in the small intestine, this process begins in the liver before distribution.

The ability to break down the chemical components of a drug varies among individuals. Factors that determine this ability include age, the presence of other drugs, and liver disease. Infants and aging individuals have more difficulty effectively metabolizing medications. Patients taking multiple medications also may be at increased risk for liver-related problems with metabolism because of the sheer number of chemicals the liver is exposed to on a daily basis. Individuals with chronic liver disease, such as **cirrhosis**, may not be able to metabolize even normal doses of medications. A cumulative effect, meaning the total amount of the drug present in the body after multiple doses, may result in a toxic condition if the drug is absorbed faster than it is metabolized. Because of these factors, drug therapy must be monitored closely in very young and aging patients, those taking multiple medications, and patients with chronic liver disease. In contrast, patients receiving long-term drug therapy may develop overstimulation of the enzyme activity of the liver. This results in rapid destruction of the drug, and the patient has to take larger and larger doses for the drug to be effective. This situation is called *tolerance.*

Drug Excretion

After the drug has been metabolized, its byproducts must be excreted from the body. The kidneys are the most important route for the elimination of drugs. Most drugs are filtered out of the blood, circulate through the kidneys, and are excreted in the urine. Because the kidneys are so important in the elimination of chemicals from the body, drug therapy must be carefully monitored in patients with kidney disease or malfunction. Drugs are also eliminated through the sweat glands, saliva, and feces. Exhalation, another mechanism for drug elimination, serves as the basis for measuring alcohol concentrations in the blood by the breathalyzer test. Drugs may be eliminated through the milk glands of a lactating mother, which means that a breastfeeding woman must be extremely careful about taking medications.

The combination of metabolism and excretion reduces the amount of drug in the body at any given time. The therapeutic dose of a medication depends on many factors, including the drug's half-life. The half-life is the amount of time it takes for half a dose of medication to be metabolized and excreted from the body. Some drugs have extremely short half-lives (only minutes), whereas others can take days to leave the body. The amount of drug lost during one half-life depends on how much drug is present. Physicians use the half-life of a drug to determine the timing of medication administration, or the dose intervals. The shorter the half-life of the drug, the closer are the times when it should be administered. If the next dose of the drug is not given within the half-life, blood levels drop and the patient does not receive adequate therapeutic effects from the treatment.

FACTORS THAT AFFECT DRUG ACTION

As was stated earlier, different people react to the same dose of medication in different ways, and the same patient can react to the same dose of the same drug differently on various occasions. A number of factors are important in determining the correct medication for a patient.

Body Weight

The effect of a medication is directly related to the person's weight. Basically, the same dose has a lesser effect on a patient who weighs more and a greater effect on a person who weighs less. Manufacturers of adult medications calculate dosages based on a normal adult weight (approximately 150 pounds). Sometimes the physician adjusts the dose to better suit the patient's body size. Pediatric medications are designed for the body weight or body surface area of children. If adult medications are used for children, the correct dose must be calculated and adjusted for the child's body weight (see Chapter 34).

Age

The most significant effect of age on the body's response to a drug occurs in newborns and elderly individuals. This usually is related to

TABLE 33-6 Effects of Medications on Geriatric Patients

PHYSIOLOGIC CHANGES ASSOCIATED WITH AGING	EFFECTS
Stomach takes longer to empty, and gastric acidity is reduced.	Increases the risk of stomach irritation and ulceration.
Increased percentage of adipose (fat) tissue in the body.	Increases likelihood of drug storage in fat; may lead to drug toxicity.
Fewer protein-binding sites available in bloodstream.	Reduces drug passage through cell membranes; increases blood level of drug; may lead to toxicity.
Liver function declines.	Slows rate of drug metabolism; increases risk of toxicity.
Kidney function declines.	Slows rate of elimination of drug byproducts; increases risk of toxicity and complications.
Peripheral vascular disease present; venous tone diminished.	Reduces distribution of drug to the periphery; may cause orthostatic hypotension.
Fat-soluble medications pass through blood-brain barrier more easily.	May affect central nervous system; increases risk of vertigo and confusion.

immature or deteriorating body systems. In addition, both patient groups are particularly sensitive to drugs that affect the CNS and are at risk of developing toxic drug levels. Consequently, dosage amounts for these two groups must be carefully calculated. The physician may opt to start therapy with very small doses and increase the dose over time based on the presence or absence of side effects. Table 33-6 summarizes the altered effects of medications on aging individuals. (Chapter 48 discusses in greater detail the effects of aging on body systems.)

Gender

Drugs may affect men and women differently. As has been mentioned, a pregnant woman must be extremely cautious when taking medications to prevent possible damage to the developing fetus. In addition, the side effects of some drugs can stimulate uterine contractions, causing premature labor and delivery. Intramuscular medications are absorbed faster by men because they generally have higher levels of muscle mass, which is rich in blood vessels. Because women typically have a higher body fat content and less muscle (therefore fewer blood vessels in peripheral tissues compared with men), intramuscular drugs remain in their tissues longer. In the past, most clinical trials were conducted only on men; therefore, until newer trial results are released that include women, the effect of gender on the action and safety of medications is impossible to predict accurately.

Time of Day

Diurnal refers to during the day or time of light. Diurnal body rhythms play an important part in the effects of some drugs.

Sedatives given in the morning are not as effective as those administered before bedtime, because the CNS is more alert in the morning, causing increased resistance to the effects of the drug. Corticosteroid administration is preferred in the morning, because this best mimics the body's natural pattern of corticosteroid production and elimination.

Pathologic Factors

Patients may adversely respond to drugs if they have liver or kidney disease, because the body is unable to detoxify and excrete chemicals properly. Drugs may also produce pathologic conditions of the liver or kidneys, and patients may need monitoring for potentially serious drug complications. For example, patients taking statin medications (e.g., atorvastatin calcium [Lipitor]) for **hypercholesterolemia** should have liver function studies done routinely, because these drugs are very hard on liver cells.

Patients with liver or kidney disease have an increased risk of drug toxicity, which may result in unconsciousness or death. Reactions in patients with other diseases or disorders may be quite different from the expected response. Therefore, a thorough medical history of the patient must always be taken before medications are prescribed and administered.

Immune Responses

The presence of a drug can stimulate a patient's immune response, causing the patient to develop antibodies to a particular chemical. If the same drug is administered again, the patient will have an allergic reaction to the drug, ranging from a mild reaction to anaphylaxis, a serious respiratory and circulatory emergency. Antibiotics are the group of drugs that most commonly cause allergic responses. A typical low-level allergic response to an antibiotic is urticaria, or the formation of hives.

Psychological Factors

People may respond differently to a medication because of the way they feel about the drug. If a patient believes in the therapy, even a placebo (a sugar pill or sterile water thought to be a drug) may help or bring about relief. In addition, a patient's personality can affect whether he or she will be cooperative in following the directions for a particular drug, and a patient's negative mindset, or mental attitude, can reduce an expected response to a drug.

Tolerance

Tolerance is the phenomenon of reduced responsiveness to a drug. Acquired tolerance occurs after a particular drug has been taken for a period of time. Cross-tolerance occurs when a patient acquires a tolerance to one drug and becomes resistant to other, similar drugs. Physical dependence, such as occurs with narcotic addictions, often accompanies tolerance. The body becomes so adapted to the presence of the drug that it cannot function properly without it. To withdraw the drug is to throw the body out of its equilibrium, causing withdrawal symptoms.

Accumulation

When a drug is taken too frequently to allow for proper elimination, it accumulates in the tissues. The result is a more intense effect and a longer duration. Accumulation can cause overdose and/or toxic effects. An example of a toxic accumulation of medication is ototoxicity (a toxic condition affecting the ears), which results in nausea, vomiting, **tinnitus**, and vertigo. Proper dosage and timing of administration are the best methods of preventing drug accumulation.

Idiosyncrasy

Occasionally a person reacts to a drug in a manner that is unexpected and peculiar to that individual only. An idiosyncratic response may manifest in many different ways, such as a hypnotic drug keeping a person awake, acting as a stimulant to this person rather than as a depressant. Usually these reactions cannot be explained.

Drug-Drug Interactions

Special care must be taken with patients who take more than one drug on a regular basis. One medication may increase or decrease the effects of another or may cause unexpected side effects. To safeguard patients from potentially negative drug interactions, it is important at each visit to record a complete list of all drugs the patient is taking, including OTC medications and herbal products. However, because many patients do not know or get confused about the names and dosages of their medications, the best way to maintain an accurate record is to ask that patients bring their medication containers with them to each office visit. This way, you can list information about their medications in the medical record and at the same time ask whether they have any questions about their treatment. It is also a good idea to advise patients to fill prescriptions at the same pharmacy, because the pharmacist can monitor medications for potential drug interactions. One of the positive aspects of EHR implementation is that the computer program will review possible drug-drug interactions if a correct list of all patient medications is included in the patient's electronic record.

An example of a drug interaction is the effect of some antibiotics on oral contraceptives. Certain antibiotics can interact with birth control pills, making the birth control pills less effective and pregnancy more likely. Patients should be told that spotting (midcycle bleeding) may be the first sign that an antibiotic is interfering with the effectiveness of birth control pills. Examples of antibiotics that interact with birth control pills include penicillin (Veetids), amoxicillin (Amoxil), ampicillin (Omnipen), sulfamethoxazole plus trimethoprim (Septra or Bactrim), tetracycline (Sumycin), minocycline (Minocin), metronidazole (Flagyl), and nitrofurantoin (Macrobid or Macrodantin). If a woman wants to prevent pregnancy while taking an antibiotic, the physician may recommend that she use a condom or **spermicide** as a backup birth control method while taking the medication and for at least 1 week after the completion of treatment.

CRITICAL THINKING APPLICATION   33-4

Sylvia Kramer, a 72-year-old patient of Dr. Simon, calls today and asks Kathy how she should be taking her heart medicine, diltiazem HCl (Cardizem). Mrs. Kramer has diabetes, hypertension, and a history of heart disease. She is overweight, has the potential for kidney disease, and takes a number of other prescriptions. What factors may have an impact on the potential effect of Mrs. Kramer's medication?

CLASSIFICATIONS OF DRUG ACTIONS

Clinical pharmacology is a complex subject. To make the subject easier, drugs are classified into groups according to their actions in the body (e.g., diuretics, emetics), the symptoms they relieve (e.g., antihistamine), or the body system they affect (e.g., drugs that act on the cardiovascular system). Following is a glossary of terms that describe some basic drug actions. As you read some of the examples, remember that a drug classified as one type of agent may have other uses and actions in other body systems. For example, a drug classified as a diuretic may also be an antihypertensive drug, and a vasodilator may also be a respiratory antispasmodic. It takes time to understand not only the basic classification of a particular drug, but also the many secondary uses and effects the drug has on the human body.

These are just a few examples of the different classifications of medications. Remember to research and review all medications before administering them.

PHARMACOKINETIC TERMS

absorption	The movement of a drug into the bloodstream. The rate of absorption depends on many factors, including the route of administration.
distribution	The transport of a drug from the site of administration to the location in the body where it is meant to act (i.e., the *target tissue*).
metabolism	The inactivation of a drug, including the time required for a drug to be detoxified and broken down into byproducts. The liver typically metabolizes medications.
excretion	The elimination of a drug from the body, including the route of elimination and the time required for this process. The kidneys typically excrete drug metabolites.

Examples of Drug Classifications

Adrenergics

Actions: Vasoconstriction (i.e., narrow the **lumen** of a blood vessel); dilate pupils and bronchioles; relax muscles of the GI and urinary tracts.

Examples: Those used to treat hypotension: isoproterenol (Isuprel); metaraminol (Aramine); norepinephrine (Levophed). Those used for nasal and ophthalmic decongestion: naphazoline (Privine or Naphcon); phenylephrine (Neo-Synephrine); pseudoephedrine (Sudafed); tetrahydrozoline (Visine).

Primary uses: Stop superficial bleeding; raise and sustain blood pressure; relieve nasal congestion and relieve redness, burning, irritation, and dryness of the eyes.

General side effects: Chest pain, tachycardia, headache, increased blood glucose levels, nervousness, tremors.

Adrenergic Blockers

Actions: Vasodilation; reduce blood pressure; increase muscle tone of GI walls.

Examples: propranolol (Inderal); atenolol (Tenormin); carvedilol (Coreg); tamsulosin (Flomax); metoprolol (Lopressor).

Primary uses: Control hypertension and peripheral vascular disease; treat prostatic hyperplasia.

General side effects: Confusion, lowering of blood pressure, lowering of blood glucose levels, fatigue, reduced heart rate.

Analgesics

Actions: Lessen the sensory function of the brain; block pain receptors.

Examples: *Nonnarcotic OTCs:* aspirin; acetaminophen (Tylenol); ibuprofen (Advil, Motrin). *Narcotic:* hydrocodone w/APAP (Tylenol with codeine); oxycodone (OxyContin); propoxyphene N/APAP (Darvocet); meperidine (Demerol); hydrocodone (Vicodin); propoxyphene (Darvon).

Primary use: Relieve pain.

General side effects: *Nonnarcotic:* GI disorders, liver and kidney disorders, tinnitus. *Narcotic:* suppression of vital signs, agitation, blurred vision, confusion, constipation, oversedation, restlessness.

Anesthetics

Actions: Produce insensibility to pain or the sensation of pain; block nerve impulses to the brain, resulting in unconsciousness; dilate pupils; lower blood pressure; reduce respiratory and pulse rates.

Examples: *Local:* benzocaine (Dermoplast, Solarcaine); lidocaine (Xylocaine); bupivacaine (Marcaine); lidocaine topical (Lidoderm); procaine (Novacaine). *General:* thiopental (Pentothal); midazolam (Versed).

Primary uses: Produce local anesthesia (absence of sensation without loss of consciousness) or general anesthesia (loss of consciousness).

General side effects: Hypotension, cardiopulmonary depression, sedation, nausea, vomiting, headaches.

Antacids

Action: Reduce acidity in the stomach.

Examples: omeprazole (Prilosec); esomeprazole (Nexium); rabeprazole (Aciphex); lansoprazole (Prevacid); pantoprazole (Protonix). *OTCs:* magaldrate (Riopan); calcium carbonate (Maalox).

Primary use: Treat gastric hyperacidity.

General side effects: Constipation, diarrhea, electrolyte imbalance, flatulence, kidney stones, osteoporosis.

Antianxiety Agents

Action: Reduce anxiety and tension.

Examples: chlordiazepoxide (Librium); clonazepam (Klonopin); chlorazepate (Tranxene); diazepam (Valium); alprazolam (Xanax); temazepam (Restoril); triazolam (Halcion).

Primary uses: Produce calmness and release muscle tension; sedation.

General side effects: Agitation, amnesia, bizarre behaviors, confusion, reduced white blood cell (WBC) count, depression, drowsiness, lethargy, oversedation, tremors, photosensitivity.

Antibiotics

Action: Kill or inhibit growth of microorganisms.

Examples: azithromycin (Zithromax); levofloxacin (Levaquin); cefaclor (Ceclor); tetracycline (Sumycin); amoxicillin (Amoxil); amoxicillin/clavulanic acid (Augmentin); cefadroxil (Duricef); ciprofloxacin (Cipro); cephalexin (Keflex); doxycycline (Vibramycin).

Primary uses: Treat bacterial invasions and infections.

General side effects: Hypersensitivity reaction, nausea, diarrhea, GI distress, light sensitivity, urticaria.

Anticholinergics

Actions: Parasympathetic blocking agents; reduce spasms in smooth muscles.

Examples: scopolamine or atropine sulfate; tiotropium inhalation (Spiriva); dicyclomine (Bentyl); ipratropium (Atrovent).

Primary uses: Dry secretions before surgery; prevent bronchospasm.

General side effects: Blurred vision, confusion, reduced GI and genitourinary motility, dilation of pupils, fever, flushing, headache, increased heart rate.

Anticoagulants

Action: Delay or block clotting of blood.

Examples: heparin; enoxaparin sodium (Lovanox); warfarin sodium (Coumadin); tinzaparin (Imnohep).

Primary uses: Treat blood clots, thrombophlebitis; prevent clot formation.

General side effects: Increased bleeding; blood irregularities; GI, liver, and kidney disease.

Anticonvulsants

Actions: Prevent seizures; reduce excessive stimulation of the brain.

Examples: clonazepam (Klonopin); gabapentin (Neurontin or Lyrica); phenytoin (Dilantin); phenobarbital; carbamazepine (Tegretol); lamotrigine (Lamictal); pregabalin (Lyrica); topiramate (Topamax); valproic acid (Depakane).

Primary uses: Treat epilepsy and other neurologic disorders (e.g., peripheral neuropathy).

General side effects: Sedation, vertigo, visual disturbances, GI disturbances, liver complications.

Antidepressants

Action: Treat depression.

Examples: venlafaxine hydrochloride (Effexor); sertraline (Zoloft); escitalopram (Lexapro); duloxetine (Cymbalta); bupropion (Wellbutrin); trazodone HCl (Desyrel); fluoxetine (Prozac); imipramine pamoate (Tofranil); amitriptyline (Elavil); citalopram (Celexa).

Primary uses: Elevate mood; treat other neurologic disorders (e.g., migraines).

General side effects: Anorexia, anxiety, sexual dysfunction, fatigue, drowsiness, vertigo, weight gain, confusion, blurred vision.

Antiemetics

Action: Act on hypothalamic center in the brain.

Examples: prochlorperazine (Compazine); trimethobenzamide (Tigan); metoclopramide (Reglan); granisetron (Kytril); ondansetron (Zofran); promethazine (Phenergan).

Primary uses: Prevent and relieve nausea and vomiting; manage motion sickness.

General side effects: Dry mouth, sedation, drowsiness, diarrhea, blurred vision.

Antifungals

Action: Slow or retard multiplication of fungi.
Examples: miconazole (Monistat); nystatin (Mycostatin); fluconazole (Diflucan); ketoconazole (Nizoral); nystatin (Mycostatin); terbinafine (Lamisil).
Primary use: Treat systemic or local fungal infections.
General side effects: Anemia, chills, hypotension, vertigo, fever, kidney and liver damage, malaise, photophobia, muscle and joint pain.

Antihistamines

Actions: Counteract the effects of histamine by blocking action in tissues; may be used to inhibit gastric secretions.
Examples: cetirizine (Zyrtec); fexofenadine (Allegra); loratadine (Claritin, Alavert); chlorpheniramine (Chlor-Trimeton); diphenhydramine (Benadryl); promethazine (Phenergan); cimetidine (Tagamet); ranitidine (Zantac).
Primary uses: Relieve allergies; prevent gastric ulcers.
General side effects: CNS depression, muscle weakness, epigastric distress, dry mouth.

Antihypertensive Agents

Actions: Block nerve impulses that cause arteries to constrict; slow the heart rate, reducing its contractility; restrict the hormone aldosterone in the blood.
Examples: amlodipine (Norvasc); atenolol (Tenormin); doxazosin mesylate (Cardura); metoprolol (Lopressor or Toprol); methyldopa (Aldomet); valsartan (Diovan); amlodipine plus benazepril (Lotrel); propranolol (Inderal); diltiazem (Cardizem); nifedipine (Procardia); benazepril (Lotensin); lisinopril (Prinivil, Zestril); losartan (Cozaar).
Primary use: Reduce and control blood pressure.
General side effects: Headache, vertigo, GI disturbances, rash, hypotension, nonproductive cough.

Anti-inflammatory Agents

Action: Reduce inflammation.
Examples: *Nonsteroidal anti-inflammatory drugs (NSAIDs):* ibuprofen (Advil, Motrin); naproxen (Naprosyn); celecoxib (Celebrex); indomethacin (Indocin). *Steroidal anti-inflammatory drugs (SAIDs):* dexamethasone (Decadron); prednisone (Cortisone); methylprednisolone (Medrol, Depo-Medrol); montelukast sodium (Singulair); fluticasone propionate (Flonase); mometasone (Nasonex). *Inhalers:* flunisolide (Aerobid); triamcinolone (Azmacort).
Primary use: Treat arthritis and other inflammatory disorders, including asthma and allergic rhinitis.
General side effects: GI upset, GI bleeding, hepatitis, drowsiness, tinnitus, irregular heart rate, kidney disorders.

Antimigraine Agents

Action: Alter circulation to the brain.
Examples: topiramate (Topamax); sumatriptan (Imitrex); zolmitriptan (Zomig).

Primary use: Treatment or prevention of migraine headaches.
General side effects: Confusion, psychomotor slowing, difficulty concentrating, memory problems, rare but serious cardiac events.

Antineoplastics

Action: Inhibit development of and destroy cancerous cells.
Examples: interferon alfa-2a (Roferon-A); hydroxyurea (Hydrea); cyclophosphamide (Cytoxan); fluorouracil (Adrucil); chlorambucil (Leukeran); cytarabine (Cytosar-U); raloxifene (Evista).
Primary use: Cancer chemotherapy and/or prevention.
General side effects: Nausea, vomiting, bone marrow depression, aplastic anemia, hair loss, GI ulcers.

Antipsychotics

Action: Alter chemical actions in the brain.
Examples: quetiapine (Seroquel); risperidone (Risperdal); aripiprazole (Abilify); olanzapine (Zyprexa); chlorpromazine (Thorazine); haloperidol (Haldol).
Primary use: Treat the symptoms of schizophrenia and bipolar disorder.
General side effects: GI distress, hypotension, electrocardiographic (ECG) changes, vertigo, sedation, headache, photosensitivity.

Antipruritics

Action: Relieve itching.
Examples: calamine lotion; hydrocortisone ointment; Benadryl.
Primary use: Treat allergies or topical exposures that cause itching.
General side effects: Topical agents have no side effects; Benadryl can cause vertigo, sedation, and nervousness.

Antipyretics

Action: Lower body temperature.
Examples: aspirin; acetaminophen; ibuprofen.
Primary use: Reduce fever.
General side effects: GI disturbance, liver disease; with aspirin, possibility of Reyes' syndrome if given during or after a viral disease.

Antispasmodics

Actions: Relieve or prevent spasms from musculoskeletal injury or inflammation.
Examples: methocarbamol (Robaxin); carisoprodol (Soma); cyclobenzaprine (Flexeril).
Primary use: Treat sports injuries.
General side effects: CNS suppression, drowsiness, vertigo.

Antitussives

Action: Inhibit the cough center.
Examples: *Narcotic:* codeine sulfate. *Nonnarcotic:* dextromethorphan (Romilar, Robitussin DM).
Primary uses: Temporarily suppress a nonproductive cough; reduce the thickness of secretions.
General side effects: Codeine cough suppressants cause CNS depression and constipation.

Antiviral Agents

Action: Inhibit the growth or reduce the spread of viral cells.

Examples: acyclovir (Zovirax); interferon; valacyclovir (Valtrex); oseltamivir (Tamiflu); famciclovir (Famvir); includes the human immunodeficiency virus (HIV) medications efavirenz (Sustiva), abacavir (Ziagen), and ritonavir (Norvir); Atripla; Truvada.

Primary use: Treat viral infections, including oral and genital herpes, influenza, and HIV.

General side effects: Confusion, diarrhea, headache, kidney disease, urticaria, vomiting.

Bronchodilators

Action: Relax the smooth muscle of the bronchi.

Examples: aminophylline (Aminophyllin); theophylline (Theo-Dur); epinephrine (Adrenalin, Sus-Phrine); albuterol (Ventolin, Proventil, ProAir HFA); budesonide and formoterol (Symbicort); isoproterenol (Isuprel).

Primary uses: Treat asthma, bronchospasm; promote bronchodilation.

General side effects: CNS stimulation, tremors, tachycardia, increased blood glucose level, elevated blood pressure.

Cathartics (Laxative)

Action: Increase peristaltic activity of the large intestine.

Examples: magnesium hydroxide (Milk of Magnesia); bisacodyl (Dulcolax); casanthranol (Peri-Colace).

Primary uses: Increase and hasten bowel evacuation (defecation).

General side effects: Nausea, bloating, flatulence, cramping.

Central Nervous System Stimulants

Action: Affect chemicals in the brain that contribute to hyperactivity and impulse control.

Examples: methylphenidate (Concerta, Ritalin); modafinil (Provigil); lisdexamfetamine (Vyvanse).

Primary use: Treat attention deficit disorder (ADD) and attention deficit hyperactivity disorder (ADHD).

General Side Effects: Irregular heartbeat, rash, sore throat, aggression, hypertension, numbness, fainting.

Contraceptives

Action: Inhibit conception.

Examples: medroxyprogesterone acetate (Depo-Provera); norgestrel (Ovrette); ethinyl estradiol and ethynodiol diacetate (Demulen 1/35); Ortho Evra; etonogestrel/ethinyl estradiol (NuvaRing); ethinyl estradiol (Yasmin).

Primary use: Prevent pregnancy.

General side effects: Breast enlargement and tenderness; cardiovascular risk; GI upset; headache; irregular menstrual bleeding; deep vein thrombosis; pulmonary embolus (PE).

Decongestants

Action: Relieve local congestion in the tissues.

Examples: ephedrine or phenylephrine (Neo-Synephrine); pseudoephedrine (Sudafed); oxymetazoline (Afrin); mometasone (Nasonex).

Primary use: Relieve nasal and sinus congestion caused by common cold, hay fever, or upper respiratory tract disorders.

General side effects: Arrhythmias, hypertension, headache, nausea, dry mouth.

Diuretics

Actions: Inhibit reabsorption of sodium and chloride in the kidneys; promote excretion of excess fluid in the body.

Examples: hydrochlorothiazide (Dyazide, Esidrix, HydroDiuril); furosemide (Lasix); triamterene (Dyrenium).

Primary uses: Increase urinary output; lower blood pressure.

General side effects: Dehydration, muscle weakness, fatigue, gout, hyperglycemia.

Expectorants

Action: Liquefy secretions in the bronchial tubes so that they can be coughed out.

Examples: dextromethorphan (Benylin); guaifenesin guaiacolate (Fenesin, Robitussin).

Primary use: Relieve upper respiratory tract congestion.

General side effects: Vomiting, diarrhea, abdominal pain.

Hematopoietic Agents

Action: Promote red blood cell production.

Examples: epoetin alfa (Epogen, Procrit).

Primary use: Treat anemia in patients undergoing chemotherapy.

General side effects: Headache, arthralgia, nausea, hypertension, diarrhea.

Hemostatic Agents

Actions: Control bleeding; act as a blood coagulant.

Examples: phytonadione, vitamin K (Konakion); absorbable hemostatic agents (e.g., Gelfoam, Surgicel) are applied directly to a wound.

Primary uses: Control acute or chronic blood-clotting disorder; promote formation of absorbable, artificial clot.

General side effects: Hypersensitivity reactions, transient flushing, dizziness; newborn hyperbilirubinemia.

Hormone Replacement Agents

Actions: Replace hormones or compensate for hormone deficiency.

Examples: insulin (Humulin, NovoLog, Lantus, Humalog); levothyroxine sodium (Synthroid or Levoxyl); estrogen (Premarin); vasopressin (Pitressin).

Primary use: Maintain adequate hormone levels.

General side effects: *Estrogen replacement therapy:* hot flashes, decreased sex drive, nausea, vomiting.

Hypnotics (Sedatives)

Actions: Induce sleep; lessen the activity of the brain.

Examples: zolpidem tartrate (Ambien); eszopiclone (Lunesta); secobarbital (Seconal); flurazepam (Dalmane); temazepam (Restoril); barbiturates.

Primary uses: Treat insomnia; obtain sedation (lower doses).

General side effects: Daytime sedation, confusion, dry mouth, vertigo.

Lipid-Lowering Agents

Actions: Reduce blood cholesterol levels and/or increase high-density lipoprotein (HDL) level.

Examples: atorvastatin calcium (Lipitor); simvastatin (Zocor); ezetimibe (Vytorin or Zetia); rosuvastatin (Crestor); fenofibrate (Tricor).

Primary use: Manage high blood cholesterol.

General side effects: GI discomfort, muscle pain and weakness, liver complications.

Miotics

Action: Cause the pupil to contract.

Examples: carbachol (Isopto Carbachol); isoflurophate (Floropryl); pilocarpine (Isopto Carpine).

Primary use: Counteract pupil dilation.

General side effects: Corneal edema, clouding, stinging, tearing, headache.

Mydriatic Agents (Anticholinergic)

Action: Dilate the pupil.

Examples: atropine sulfate (Isopto Atropine).

Primary use: Ophthalmologic examinations.

General side effects: Stinging, burning, photosensitivity.

Narcotics

Action: Depress the CNS, causing insensibility or stupor.

Examples: *Natural narcotics:* opium group (codeine phosphate, morphine sulfate); buprenorphine and naloxone (Suboxone); oxycodone (OxyContin). *Synthetic narcotics:* meperidine (Demerol), methadone (Dolophine), propoxyphene HCl (Darvon).

Primary use: Relieve pain.

General side effects: Suppression of vital signs, agitation, blurred vision, confusion, constipation, oversedation, restlessness.

Oral Hypoglycemic Agents

Action: Reduce blood glucose level by increasing insulin production and/or reducing target cell resistance to insulin, or by delaying glucose absorption.

Examples: pioglitazone (Actos); rosiglitazone (Avandia); sitagliptin (Januvia); metformin HCl (Glucophage); acarbose (Precose); chlorpropamide (Diabinese); glimepiride (Amaryl); glipizide (Glucotrol); glyburide (Micronase).

Primary use: Manage diabetes mellitus type 2.

General side effects: GI irritation, fatigue, hypoglycemia, vertigo; possible hypersensitivity reactions.

Osteoporosis Agents

Actions: Inhibit bone reabsorption and/or promote use of calcium.

Examples: alendronate (Fosamax); risedronate (Actonel); calcitonin (Miacalcin nasal spray and Calcimar); ibandronate (Boniva); zoledronic acid (Reclast, Zometa).

Primary use: Promote bone mineral density and reverse progression of osteoporosis.

General side effects: GI disorders, esophageal irritation.

HERBAL AND ALTERNATIVE THERAPIES

The use of alternative therapies, often called *complementary* or *holistic medicine,* has become very popular in the United States. According to estimates, more than 42% of adult patients use some form of alternative therapy, such as herbal medicine, acupuncture, massage therapy, chiropractic care, or mind-body therapies. Even though only limited scientific studies prove the effectiveness of herbs, their use to relieve the symptoms of common patient complaints is definitely on the rise. It is estimated that 15 million adults take prescription drugs along with herbal and vitamin supplements. Patients typically are hesitant to discuss their use of herbal products with their physician, which makes it difficult for physicians to assess potential drug-herb interactions. Therefore, it is important that medical assistants become familiar with common alternative therapies and that they include questions about the use of these therapies when gathering information about the patient's medication history.

Herbal Products

Regulation of Herbal Products

Herbal medicine uses plant-based products to promote health and treat the symptoms of a wide range of diseases. These remedies typically are marketed by manufacturers and are regulated by the federal government as dietary supplements. The FDA is responsible for regulating dietary supplements under the Dietary Supplement Health and Education Act of 1994 (DSHEA). Under DSHEA, manufacturers are responsible for performing tests and ensuring the safety of dietary supplements before they are sold. However, these products are not registered with the FDA and do not have to go through the rigorous process of FDA approval that new drugs face before they are produced and sold. In addition, there is no federal control over the standardization of herbal dietary supplements. Pharmaceutical companies must prove that each batch of a drug is standardized or consistent with previous batches. Because this is not the case with dietary supplements, there are no guarantees that the amounts of active ingredients in an herbal supplement remain the same over time or are similar to the amounts found in the same supplement produced by a different company.

This lack of government oversight recently was addressed by Congress, and new regulations implemented in June 2010 give the FDA the authority to oversee the manufacture of domestically made and foreign-made supplements. Supplement manufacturers must provide evidence that their products actually contain what the labels claim, and that the products are free of contaminants.

According to FDA regulations, dietary supplement labels must list the following:

- Product name with the word "supplement" on the label
- Name and location of the manufacturer or distributor
- Structure/function claim: Claims of specific benefits may be made, but the following statement must be included: *This statement has not been evaluated by the Food and Drug Administration. This product is not intended to diagnose, treat, cure, or prevent any disease.*
- Directions for use
- For plant-based herbal preparations, name of the plant or the part of the plant used

- For blended products created by the manufacturer, components and the weight of each ingredient
- All nondietary ingredients (e.g., fillers, artificial colors, sweeteners, flavors) listed in descending order of weight
- The label may include warnings about use, but the lack of cautionary statements does not mean that no adverse effects are associated with the supplement.

Commonly Used Herbal Products

Table 33-7 summarizes the most commonly used herbal products. Information about herbal remedies is constantly changing, but the federal government has several Web sites that can be used as references. These include the National Center for Complementary and Alternative Medicine (http://nccam.nih.gov/) and the National Institutes of Health Office of Dietary Supplements (http://ods.od.nih.gov/index.aspx).

Alternative Therapies

Acupuncture

Acupuncture treatments are part of traditional Chinese medicine, which is based on the concept that disease is caused by a disruption in the flow of life force and an imbalance between yin and yang. Acupuncture treatments use thin metal needles inserted through the skin to stimulate specific points in the body to restore and maintain health. Studies indicate that acupuncture may help reduce pain and relieve the nausea associated with chemotherapy treatments. Therapy involves a series of treatments with the placement of as many as 12 needles in various locations on the body.

During the procedure, the patient is placed supine, prone, or in Sims' position, depending on the needle insertion site. Although the procedure is not painful, the patient may notice a sharp sensation when the needles initially are placed. After the needles have been in place for a time, they may be rotated gently, heated, or electrically stimulated to achieve the benefit sought by the treatment. The needles usually are left in place for 5 to 20 minutes, and after they have been removed, the practitioner typically discusses the results of treatment with the patient.

Chiropractic Care

Chiropractic practitioners apply techniques that focus on the body's physical structure (usually the spine) and perform manipulations or anatomic adjustments to correct alignment problems and help the

TABLE 33-7 Commonly Used Herbal Products

NAME	USE	SIDE EFFECTS AND CAUTIONS
Acai	Weight loss and anti-aging; antioxidant	Little scientific information about the safety of acai; no scientific evidence to support use for any health-related purpose
Black cohosh	Relieve symptoms of menopause; treat menstrual irregularities and premenstrual syndrome; induce labor	Headaches, gastric complaints, heaviness in the legs, weight problems; safety unknown for pregnant women or those with breast cancer.
Echinacea	Treat or prevent colds, flu, and other infections; believed to stimulate the immune system	Most studies indicate it does not appear to prevent colds or other infections; some people experience allergic reactions, including rashes, increased asthma, and anaphylaxis; gastrointestinal side (GI) effects.
Flaxseed	Laxative; treat hot flashes and breast pain; flaxseed oil used to treat arthritis; both flaxseed and flaxseed oil used to treat high cholesterol levels and prevent cancer	Few reported side effects; contains soluble fiber, like that found in oat bran, and is an effective laxative; should be taken with plenty of water; may diminish body's ability to absorb medications taken by mouth; should not be taken at same time as oral medications.
Garlic	Treat high cholesterol, heart disease, hypertension; prevent certain types of cancer, including stomach and colon cancer	Some evidence indicates garlic can slightly lower blood cholesterol levels and may slow development of atherosclerosis. Side effects include breath and body odor, heartburn, GI upset, and allergic reactions. Acts as a mild anticoagulant (similar to aspirin); may be a problem during or after surgery; avoid dietary and supplemental garlic for at least 1 week before surgery. Interferes with effectiveness of saquinavir, a drug used to treat infections with the human immunodeficiency virus (HIV).
Ginger	Treat stomach aches, nausea, diarrhea; ginger extract a component of many cold and flu dietary supplements; used to alleviate nausea associated with postoperative state, motion sickness, chemotherapy, and pregnancy; used for rheumatoid arthritis, osteoarthritis, and joint and muscle pain	Short-term use can safely relieve pregnancy-related nausea and vomiting. Side effects most often reported are gas, bloating, heartburn, and nausea.

Continued

TABLE 33-7   Commonly Used Herbal Products—cont'd

NAME	USE	SIDE EFFECTS AND CAUTIONS
Asian ginseng	Support overall health and boost immune system; improve mental and physical performance; treat erectile dysfunction, hepatitis C, and menopause symptoms; lower blood glucose and control blood pressure	Some studies show it may lower blood glucose and possibly boost immune function. When taken by mouth, ginseng usually is well tolerated; most common side effects are headaches; sleep disorders; GI problems; possible allergic reactions. Patients with diabetes using medications for treatment should use ginseng with caution.
Gingko biloba	Treat a variety of conditions including asthma, bronchitis, fatigue, and tinnitus (ringing or roaring sounds in the ears); typically used to improve memory; treat or help prevent Alzheimer's disease and other types of dementia; decrease intermittent claudication (leg pain caused by narrowing arteries); treat sexual dysfunction and multiple sclerosis	Some studies show helps in Alzheimer's disease, dementia, and intermittent claudication. Side effects may include headache, nausea, GI upset, diarrhea, dizziness, or allergic skin reactions; severe allergic reactions occasionally are reported; can increase bleeding risk, so people who take anticoagulant drugs, have bleeding disorders, or have scheduled surgery or dental procedures should use caution. Uncooked ginkgo seeds contain a toxic chemical that can cause seizures.
Glucosamine plus chondroitin sulfate	Natural substances found in and around the cells of cartilage; used to treat arthritis/joint pain	Recent study shows participants with moderate to severe pain had significant relief with the combined supplement. Most common side effect is GI upset.
Melatonin	Treatment of sleep disorders	May help individuals with normal sleep patterns but has limited or no effect on those with sleep disorders. Most common side effects are nausea and drowsiness.
Milk thistle (silymarin)	Promote liver health, treat cirrhosis, chronic hepatitis, and gallbladder disorders; lower cholesterol; reduce insulin resistance	Studies suggest it may benefit the liver; associated with fewer and milder symptoms of liver disease in patients with hepatitis C; may lower blood glucose levels; can cause allergic reaction.
Saw palmetto	Primarily used to treat urinary symptoms associated with an enlarged prostate gland; also used for chronic pelvic pain, bladder disorders, reduced sex drive, hair loss, and hormone imbalance	Studies suggest it may be effective for treating prostate symptoms, but no evidence indicates that it reduces the size of an enlarged prostate; does not appear to affect readings of prostate-specific antigen (PSA) level, which is used as screening tool for cancer of the prostate. May cause mild GI upset and tender breasts and decline in sexual desire in male patients.
St. John's wort	Traditionally used to treat mental disorders and nerve pain; may be used as a sedative; treatment for malaria; balm for wounds, burns, and insect bites; currently used for depression, anxiety, and/or sleep disorders	Some scientific evidence shows it helps treat mild to moderate depression; not effective in treating major depression. Side effects include photophobia (increased sensitivity to sunlight), anxiety, dry mouth, dizziness, GI symptoms, fatigue, headache, or sexual dysfunction. Affects way the body processes or breaks down many drugs; may speed or slow a drug's metabolism. When combined with certain antidepressants, it may increase side effects such as nausea, anxiety, headache, and confusion. Drugs that can be affected include: Antidepressants Birth control pills Cyclosporine (prevents rejection of transplants) Digoxin (strengthens myocardial contractions) Indinavir and possibly other drugs used for HIV Irinotecan and possibly other drugs used to treat cancer Warfarin and related anticoagulants St. John's wort is not a proven therapy for depression. If depression is not adequately treated, it can become severe.

Modified from the National Center for Complementary and Alternative Medicine. Accessed October 12, 2011, at http://nccam.nih.gov/

body heal itself. Many patients combine chiropractic therapy with conventional medical treatment to obtain relief of chronic pain in the lower back and neck and to relieve persistent headaches. Chiropractors must earn a Doctor of Chiropractic degree at an accredited college and pass a state licensing examination before they can practice. Besides spinal adjustments, patient treatment plans may include a combination of hot and cold therapies; electrical stimulation; rest and rehabilitation exercises; dietary and lifestyle counseling; and the use of dietary supplements.

Mind-Body Therapy

Mind-body therapy uses biofeedback to teach patients to use their thoughts to control certain body reactions. It is based on the scientific principle that our thoughts can influence the body's involuntary functions. For example, a child experiencing the sudden onset of an asthma attack may become extremely anxious because he or she is having serious difficulty breathing. Panic and anxiety increase the urgency to breathe. If the child can be taught to relax and keep breathing at a normal rate, the asthma attack will not be influenced by the child's anxiety, and medications taken to relieve bronchospasm will be more effective.

Biofeedback specialists use special monitoring equipment to demonstrate the body's reaction to certain stimuli and to help teach patients how to control physical responses to stress. During a biofeedback session, the practitioner applies electrical sensors to various locations on the body. These sensors monitor and provide feedback about the body's physiologic responses to stress. For example, if a patient is experiencing chronic tension headaches, the sensors demonstrate that the headache is just part of overall muscular tension. Tension that is registering throughout the body may cause a beeping sound or lights flashing from the equipment as a cue for the patient to associate muscular tension with development of the headache. The goal is to help patients recognize that one body action results in another. Once this goal has been achieved, patients are taught relaxation techniques designed to prevent the stressful response. Biofeedback methods are effective in managing multiple stress-related conditions, including muscle tension, headaches, chronic low back pain, altered heart rates, and hypertension.

Homeopathic Medicine

Homeopathy, or homeopathic medicine, is a medical approach that was developed in Germany over 200 years ago. The primary principle of homeopathic medicine is to administer very dilute substances that are designed to stimulate the body's ability to heal itself. Homeopaths work individually with clients to administer the lowest dose of medication possible, believing that the lower the dose, the more effective the treatment. Remedies are created from plants, minerals, or animals, and include red onion, arnica (mountain herb), and stinging nettle plant.

Homeopaths assess clients holistically and gather details on individual and family health histories, body type, and current physical, emotional, and mental symptoms. Treatments are specifically designed for each client; therefore, it is not unusual for people with the same condition to have different treatment protocols. People seek homeopathic assistance for a wide range of health problems, including allergies, asthma, chronic fatigue syndrome, depression, digestive disorders, ear infections, headaches, and skin rashes.

Homeopathic remedies are regulated in the same manner as OTC drugs. They do not have to comply with the strict testing guidelines required for prescription drugs. However, the FDA does require that homeopathic remedies meet strength, purity, and packaging standards. Labels must identify at least one health condition that the remedy can treat, provide an ingredient list, indicate the dilution of the ingredients, and delineate safety instructions.

Homeopathic remedies are not known to interfere with prescription and OTC medications; however, it is important to gather information from patients regarding homeopathic use and to document the details in the patient record for physician review.

CLOSING COMMENTS

Patient Education

It is important for the patient to be aware of the effects a drug may have and should have on his or her system. The medical assistant plays an important role in helping patients understand their medications, promoting compliance with treatment, and preventing complications. The following should be considered when interviewing a patient and documenting in the patient's chart:

- Make a comprehensive list of all medications, including OTC agents and alternative therapies that the patient takes regularly.
- Ask the patient whether she is pregnant or breastfeeding.
- Pre-assess the patient for any adverse effects, such as drug allergies and drug-drug or drug-food interactions.
- Observe the patient for any adverse effects for a minimum of 20 minutes after administration of a medication in the office; also, inform the patient of possible adverse reactions to the medication that may occur at home.
- Discuss with the patient how and when the prescribed drug is to be taken, and whether any special storage precautions are required.
- Reassess that the patient is taking the medication properly.
- Provide comfort, encouragement, and guidance to patients to ensure their understanding, safety, and cooperation while taking drug therapy.
- Answer any questions asked. Remember: If you are not sure of the answer, consult the prescribing physician.

Therapeutic Communication With Patients From Diverse Cultures

Health beliefs can affect compliance with medication therapy. Patients from various cultures may be using home remedies or herbal treatments that could interfere with the effectiveness and safety of medications prescribed by the physician. Guidelines that the medical assistant may find helpful include the following:

- Investigate the healing practices of the primary cultures in your area, so that you are better equipped to discuss these practices with your patients.
- Encourage cultural sensitivity in your co-workers.
- Provide patients with educational materials in their native language.
- Ask patients if they are using home remedies or are consulting a healer from their culture. If so, get as much detail as possible so that you can share this information with the physician.

Legal and Ethical Issues

The medical assistant plays a key role in the management of controlled substances in the ambulatory care setting. It is important that all rules for record keeping, inventory, prescribing, dispensing, and documentation of scheduled drugs be followed according to state and federal regulations. The medical assistant may be responsible for requesting the physician's initial DEA registration and for continuing certification renewal. The area DEA office can provide instructions on this. Each DEA number is specific to a site, so multiple practice locations require a DEA number for each facility.

Accurate, complete documentation is essential for correct management of patient medications. Each time the patient is prescribed or administered a medication, complete details must be included in the patient's chart using approved medical terminology and abbreviations. Failure to do this may result in a serious error that could harm the patient and result in litigation.

HIPAA Applications

According to the Health Insurance Portability and Accountability Act (HIPAA), patients have the right to request restrictions on the disclosure of protected health information (PHI) for treatment, payment, and healthcare operations (TPO). For example, if a patient has a history of substance abuse and this information is not pertinent to current TPO circumstances, the patient can request that this information not be disclosed. The facility does not have to agree to the patient's request; however, a process must be established within the practice to review the demand and explain the physician's decision to the patient. If the physician agrees not to release this information, the specific restriction must be documented in the patient's chart, and staff members must review and comply with the restrictions each time material is sent out of the facility for TPO purposes.

SUMMARY OF SCENARIO

Kathy has a great deal of responsibility in managing medications in the ambulatory care setting. She must be familiar with and follow DEA regulations governing the management of controlled substances. In addition, she must be able to use drug reference materials; identify the general clinical uses of prescribed drugs and OTC products; understand the parts of a prescription and use accepted medical terms and abbreviations; recognize the significance of patient education in the safe use of OTC drugs; and understand the factors that affect drug action.

SUMMARY OF LEARNING OBJECTIVES

1. **Define, spell, and pronounce the terms listed in the vocabulary.**
   Spelling and pronouncing medical terms correctly bolsters the medical assistant's credibility. Knowing the definitions of these terms promotes confidence in communication with patients and co-workers.

2. **Apply critical thinking skills in performing the patient assessment and care.**
   Completing the Critical Thinking Application exercises throughout the chapter can help the student medical assistant become more adept at critical analysis of real-life situations.

3. **Distinguish among the government agencies that regulate drugs in the United States.**
   Several federal agencies combine forces to regulate drugs in the United States. The FDA regulates the development and sale of all prescription and OTC drugs; the DEA enforces laws designed to prevent drug abuse and educates the public about drug abuse prevention; and the FTC regulates OTC advertisement.

4. **Cite the areas covered in the regulations established by the Drug Enforcement Administration (DEA) for the management of controlled or regulated substances.**
   DEA regulations for the management of controlled substances include specific record-keeping guidelines and information on physician registration and the inventory, storage, and disposal of controlled substances.

5. **List the DEA regulations for prescription drugs for each of the five schedules of the Controlled Substance Act.**
   Prescriptions written for controlled substances must comply with both state and federal regulations. The prescription must include details about the patient; information about the physician, including the DEA number; and the amount of the drug, written out ("ten" not "10"). The prescription must be manually signed by the physician. Orders for Schedule II drugs cannot be phoned in except in an absolute emergency, and these prescriptions cannot be refilled. Schedule III, IV, and V drugs may be prescribed by phone and refilled up to five times in a 6-month period. In some states, Schedule V drugs can be dispensed by the pharmacist without a physician's prescription.

6. **Explain the medical assistant's role in preventing drug abuse.**
   The medical assistant should keep track of patients who repeatedly call for prescription refills of controlled substances and should request their medical records from other physicians when necessary to track the substance abuse history; keep prescription pads in a safe place and not use them for any other purpose; maintain a small supply of controlled substances in the office and accurately record their administration.

7. **Differentiate among a drug's chemical, generic, and trade names.**
   The chemical name is the drug's formula. The generic, or official, name is assigned to the drug and may reflect the chemical name. The trade,

or brand, name is given to the compound by the pharmaceutical company that developed it and is protected by law for 17 years.

8. **Describe the use of drug reference materials.**

The use of drug reference materials is crucial for the safe administration of medications. Most drug reference books include actions, indications, contraindications, precautions, adverse reactions, dosage, administration guidelines, and method of packaging. The most frequently used drug reference guide is the *Physicians' Desk Reference* (PDR), but package inserts also can be used.

9. **Explain the five pregnancy risk categories for drugs.**

Refer to Table 33-2.

10. **Define the five medical terms used to describe the clinical use of drugs.**

Clinically, drugs are used as therapeutic, or curative, medications; palliative medications, to relieve symptoms; prophylactic medications, to prevent the occurrence of a condition; diagnostic medications, to help determine the cause of a disease; and replacement medications, to provide substances that normally occur in the body.

11. **Cite safety measures for the use of OTC drugs.**

OTC drugs may interfere or interact with prescription drugs. Some safety measures for the use of OTC drugs include carefully reading directions, taking only the recommended dose, discarding the drug when it expires, informing the physician of OTC drug use, and being aware of contraindications to OTC drug use in certain conditions.

12. **Diagram the parts of a prescription.**

A prescription consists of the following parts: superscription, inscription, subscription, signature, refill information, and physician's signature. A prescription also must provide the patient's name and address and the date the drug is prescribed.

13. **Demonstrate the ability to transcribe a prescription accurately.**

Procedure 33-1 outlines the method for transcribing a prescription for the physician's signature. It is important that the medical assistant follow a written order; look up information about the medication in a drug reference text; ask the patient about drug allergies and record the patient's personal information on the prescription note; and correctly write the name of the drug, form, dosage, strength, route of administration, amount of the drug to be given to the patient, specifics about time of administration if appropriate, and the number of refills. The prescription should be reviewed and signed by the physician before it is given to the patient.

14. **Relate the principles of pharmacokinetics to drug use.**

Pharmacokinetics comprises the actions of absorption, which depends on the route of administration (oral, parenteral, mucous membrane, or topical); distribution through the bloodstream; metabolism in the liver; and excretion, primarily by the kidneys.

15. **Describe factors that affect the action of a drug.**

Multiple factors affect drug action, including weight, age, gender, diurnal rhythms, pathologic factors, immune responses, psychological factors, tolerance, accumulation, idiosyncrasy, and drug-drug interactions.

16. **Compare the therapeutic classifications of medications.**

Drugs are classified into groups according to their actions in the body, by the symptoms they relieve, or according to the body system that they affect. Drugs may have multiple actions and therefore multiple classifications.

17. **Differentiate among commonly used herbal remedies and alternative therapies.**

Table 33-7 summarizes common herbal remedies, their uses, and possible side effects. Acupuncture treatments use thin metal needles inserted through the skin to stimulate specific points in the body to restore and maintain health. Chiropractic practitioners perform manipulations or anatomic adjustments to correct alignment problems and help the body heal itself. Mind-body therapy uses biofeedback to teach the patient to use his or her thoughts to control certain body reactions. The primary principle of homeopathic medicine is to administer very dilute substances that are designed to stimulate the body's ability to heal itself.

18. **Examine the role of the medical assistant in drug therapy education.**

The medical assistant plays an important role in helping patients understand their medications, promoting compliance with treatment, and preventing complications. Conducting comprehensive interviews that ask detailed questions about patient use of drugs and documenting this information on the chart provides vital information for the physician. Culturally sensitive interviews with patients help the medical assistant gather details about home remedies and patient belief systems that may affect compliance with drug therapy.

19. **Identify the medical assistant's legal responsibilities in medication management in an ambulatory care setting.**

The medical assistant's legal responsibilities in medication management include documenting compliance with DEA regulations for controlled substances; maintaining complete and accurate documentation on all medications administered and prescribed for each patient; and following HIPAA regulations on the release of confidential information.

CONNECTIONS

Study Guide Connection: Go to the Chapter 33 Study Guide. Read and complete the activities.

Evolve Connection: Go to the Chapter 33 link at *evolve.elsevier.com/kinn* to complete the Chapter Review and Chapter Quiz. Peruse other resources listed for this chapter to increase your knowledge of Principles of Pharmacology.

34

PHARMACOLOGY MATH

SCENARIO

Heather Izacco, a recent graduate of a medical assistant program in the area, has just been hired by a local cardiologist, Dr. Angio. One of her responsibilities will be to administer medications under Dr. Angio's supervision. Heather is confident of her ability to administer medications but is unsure of her accuracy in pharmacology math. Heather never did well in math at school and had a difficult time calculating accurate doses and converting between math systems during her medical assisting training. Her supervisor, Mrs. Allison, suggests that Heather review the math section of her textbook at home and be prepared to work out some sample problems next week.

While studying this chapter, think about the following questions:

- How can Heather be sure that she has calculated the correct dosages?
- What are the parts of a drug label and why are they important?
- Is it important that Heather be able to convert dosages from one system to another?
- What is the standard formula for determining the correct dose of a drug?
- Are there any differences between calculating an adult dose and calculating a pediatric dose?
- How would Heather go about reconstituting an injectable powder?

LEARNING OBJECTIVES

1. Define, spell, and pronounce the terms listed in the vocabulary.
2. Apply critical thinking skills in performing patient assessment and patient care.
3. Summarize the important parts of a drug label.
4. Differentiate among the terms used in dosage preparation.
5. Perform basic math skills.
6. Demonstrate methods of verifying the accuracy of calculations.
7. Describe and perform conversions among the various systems of measurement.
8. Calculate the correct dose of a drug using the standard formula.
9. Determine accurate pediatric doses of medication.
10. Diagram how to reconstitute powdered injectable medications.
11. Specify the legal responsibilities of a medical assistant in calculating drug dosages.

dispense To prepare a drug for administration.
nomogram Graph on which variables are plotted so that a particular value can be read on the appropriate line.
stat Immediately.

surface area The total area of the body exposed to the outside environment.
unit dose Method used by the pharmacy to prepare individual doses of medication.

Medical assistants are responsible for being absolutely certain that the medication they prepare and administer to a patient is exactly what the physician ordered. Although drugs often are delivered by the pharmacy or supplied by pharmaceutical representatives in **unit dose** packs, the dosage ordered may differ from the dosage on hand. In this case, the medical assistant must be prepared to calculate the correct dose accurately before dispensing and administering the medication. There is never a margin of error in drug calculations, because even a minor mistake may result in serious complications for the patient. The medical assistant, therefore, must take meticulous care in calculating all drug dosages.

DRUG LABELS

The first step in safely calculating a drug dosage is to accurately read the label of the drug on hand to determine whether the physician's order and the packaged drug are in the same system of measurement. Starting at the top, the label shows the drug's name with the brand name capitalized and typically in bold print. The brand name is copyright protected; therefore, it is followed by either a registered trademark (®) or trademark (™) symbol. The generic name is printed in lowercase letters under the brand name in smaller print. If a medication has been on the market for a long time, the generic name may be the only one listed (e.g., meperidine instead of Demerol, diazepam rather than Valium). If the medication is ordered from the pharmacy and stocked as a generic drug, only the generic name is printed on the label. In the label examples in Figure 34-1, Cardizem is the brand name of the generic drug diltiazem HCl; on the second label, cephalexin is the generic name for Keflex, and because copyright protection has ended, only the generic name is listed on the label.

Under the name of the drug, the dosage strength of the medication is given. Whether listed in milligrams (mg), milliliters (mL), or another unit of measure, the label states how much of the drug is contained in each of the identified units. This is what you must compare with the physician's order to determine whether you must calculate the amount to administer to match the ordered dose of the drug. For example, the physician orders 250 mg of cephalexin, and the label states that the dosage strength is 250 mg per 5 mL; no calculation is needed—you simply administer 5 mL of the medication. However, if the physician orders 500 mg of the medication for a *loading dose* of the antibiotic, you must make sure you administer the correct amount of the medication to match the order. Sometimes the label helps by providing different but equivalent units of measurement for the dosage strength. For example, if the physician orders 250 mg of cephalexin and asks you to make sure the mother understands how much of the medication she should administer to her sick child, the label may state that 5 mL is equivalent to 1 teaspoon (according to the label, 250 mg of the drug is present in 5 mL of solution); therefore, you can confirm with the parent that the child should receive 1 teaspoon without having to do any calculation.

The label identifies the *route,* or method of administration, for the drug. If the medication is packaged as a tablet or a capsule, you can assume it should be given orally; liquid medication is labeled if it is for oral or parenteral use. If it is a powdered drug *(solute)* and it must be mixed with liquid *(solvent)* before administration, the label provides instructions on how to prepare the medication. Special storage precautions, such as light or heat sensitivity, are identified as well. At the bottom of the label is the total amount of the drug contained in the package. For example, a multidose bottle of cephalexin may contain as much as 200 mL of solution when mixed (e.g., 250 mg of cephalexin in each 5 mL of solution), and a single-dose bottle would contain one dose of the medication (250 mg in 5 mL of solution).

The name of the drug's manufacturer appears on the label, as does an expiration date that must be checked each time the medication is dispensed. Dispose of all medications that have reached the label's expiration date. The label also has a lot number stamped on the package so that it can be identified as belonging to a batch of drugs manufactured at the same time. This number becomes important if problems are noted with a particular batch and the medication is recalled. Depending on your employer's preferences, you may need to include the lot number in the documentation of the medication on the patient's chart. Finally, federal law requires that all labels have a national drug code (NDC) that identifies that particular drug.

Some of the basic information provided on drug labels includes the following:

- *Strength:* The potency of the drug stated as a percentage of drug in the solution (2% epinephrine), as a solid weight (grams, milligrams, pounds, grains), or as a milliequivalent or unit
- *Dose:* The size or amount of the drug available in the drug package. This could be expressed in milliliters, teaspoons, or number of tablets. For example, the label may read "Imitrex, 6 mg/0.5 mL," which means that there is 6 mg of the drug in each 0.5 mL.
- *Solute:* The pure drug that is dissolved in a liquid to form a solution
- *Solvent* or *diluent:* The liquid (usually sterile water or sterile saline) that dissolves the solute

MATH BASICS

You may need to review some basics of arithmetic before you tackle drug calculations. You must thoroughly understand the addition,

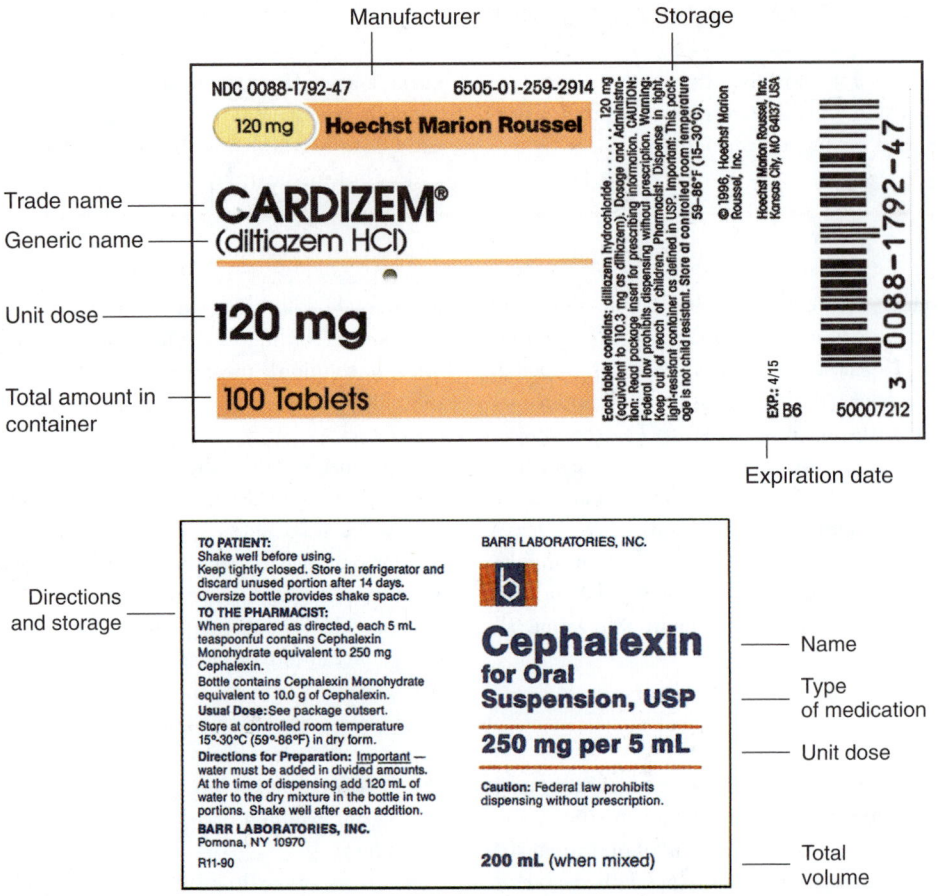

FIGURE 34-1 Drug labels. (From Brown M, Mulholland JM: *Drug calculations: process and problems for clinical practice*, ed 7, St Louis, 2004, Mosby.)

subtraction, multiplication, and division of fractions and decimals; the relationship of decimals and fractions; and how they are converted from one to the other.

Fractions

A fraction is a part of a whole, that is, fractions are a way of dividing a whole unit into parts. For example, think of dividing a small cherry pie into equal parts for friends after dinner. Four people want dessert, so you can divide the pie into four equal parts; each person receives ¼ of the pie. If only three people want dessert, you can divide the pie into three equal parts; each person receives ⅓ of the pie.

The top number in a fraction is the *numerator*, and the bottom number is the *denominator*. In a *proper fraction*, the numerator is smaller than the denominator. If we go back to the pie example, ¼ and ⅓ of the pie are proper fractions.

In *improper fractions*, the numerator is equal to or greater than the denominator. Another way of looking at improper fractions is that the numerator is so large that it is equal to or greater than 1. For example, the improper fraction ⁵⁄₄ is greater than 1. It is equal to ⁴⁄₄ (the entire pie that was cut into 4 pieces, or 1 whole pie) plus ¼ of another pie. Therefore, if you wanted everyone to have ¼ of a pie for dessert, you would need two pies: one whole pie for four guests (⁴⁄₄) and ¼ of another pie for yourself (1¼ pies). To convert improper fractions into whole numbers, divide the numerator by the denominator. In this case, you need ⁵⁄₄ of pie: 5 + 4 = 1¼ pies.

Review the following examples. Identify the proper and improper fractions. If the fraction is improper, perform the math to get the whole number equivalent.

½ ——————   ⅜ ——————
⅔ ——————   ⁶⁄₄ ——————
⁹⁄₁₀ ——————   ¹⁴⁄₁₂ ——————

Fractions typically are written in their lowest terms. For example, can you reduce the fraction ⁵⁄₁₅ to its lowest term? To reduce a fraction, you must divide the numerator and the denominator by the largest number that goes into each equally. In the case of ⁵⁄₁₅, 5 divides into 15 three times, which means that ⁵⁄₁₅ can be reduced to ⅓. Other examples include the following:

$$\frac{25}{100} \div \frac{25}{25} = \frac{1}{4} \qquad \frac{9}{45} \div \frac{9}{9} = \frac{1}{5}$$

$$\frac{30}{100} \div \frac{10}{10} = \frac{3}{10} \qquad \frac{6}{8} \div \frac{2}{2} = \frac{3}{4}$$

In some cases, you may have to multiply fractions. For example, let's say you want to multiply ⅓ of the contents of one bottle times ¾ of the contents of another. All you have to do in this case is multiply the numerators and denominators of each fraction and reduce the answer to its lowest terms. For example:

$$\frac{1}{3} \times \frac{3}{4} = \frac{3}{12} = \frac{1}{4}$$

To divide fractions, you must invert the divisor (the second fraction) before you multiply the numerators and denominators. For example:

$$\frac{1}{3} \div \frac{3}{4}$$

$$\frac{1}{3} \times \frac{4}{3} = \frac{4}{9}$$

Decimals

A decimal is similar to a fraction, but it is expressed in units of tenths (0.1), hundredths (0.01), and thousandths (0.001). To perform drug calculations, fractions first must be converted into decimals. To convert a fraction into a decimal, simply divide the numerator by the denominator. For example, rather than ordering ¾ of a dose for a patient, the physician orders the decimal equivalent. To perform this math, you may need to add zeroes after the decimal point at the end of the numerator.

$$\frac{3}{4} = 0.75$$

If the answer is less than a whole number, it is crucial to place a zero before the decimal point to prevent a medication error. For example, if you are to administer .5 mL of a medication and the zero is not placed before the decimal point, you may miss the decimal point and think that the correct dose is 5 mL. Also, a zero should never be placed after the decimal point of a whole number. Mathematically, a whole number such as 1 mL is actually 1.0 mL. However, if the decimal point and a zero follow the whole number, the dose may be misinterpreted as 10 mL.

Percent

A percent is a number expressed as part of 100. Decimal numbers can be converted to percentages by dividing the number by 100 *or* by simply moving the decimal point two spaces to the right. For example:

$$0.25 = \frac{25}{100} = 25\% \quad 0.48 = \frac{48}{100} = 48\%$$

$$0.03 = \frac{3}{100} = 3\% \quad 0.005 = \frac{5}{1,000} = 0.5\%$$

Ratio and Proportion

A ratio is one way of expressing a fraction or a division problem; it shows the relationship of the numerator to the denominator. The comparison of two ratios is called a *proportion*. A proportion is written as follows:

$$\frac{4}{16} = \frac{1}{4} \quad or \quad 4:16 = 1:4$$

This is read as 4 divided by 16 equals 1 divided by 4, or 4 is to 16 as 1 is to 4. The physician's order for a medication may be a ratio different from that of the medication in stock. To determine the correct proportion for administration, the ordered ratio must be compared with the available ratio (what is in stock).

The preceding proportion example has all the answers in it; there is nothing to solve. In calculating dosages, mathematical proportions are used, but with one element unknown. We must solve for that unknown, or *x*. For example:

$$\frac{4}{16} = \frac{1}{x}$$

Always in a proportion, the problem is solved by *cross-multiplication*. Do not confuse this with plain multiplication. An equals sign (=) between two fractions indicates that this is an equation to be cross-multiplied.

$$4 \times x = 16 \times 1$$

therefore, $4x = 16$.

We know what $4x$ equals, but next we must find what $1x$, or x, equals. To find the value of x, we must find a way to leave x (or $1x$) alone on the left side of the equation. We can change $4x$ to $1x$ by dividing the number 4 by itself:

$$4x \div 4 = 1x$$

However, what we do on one side of an equation, we must do on the other side, or the equation will not be equal anymore. Therefore, we also divide 16 by 4:

$$16 \div 4 = 4$$

therefore, $x = 4$ and $\frac{4}{16} = \frac{1}{4}$.

Another way to make sure your proportion answer is correct is to check your answer by multiplying the *means* (the middle numbers of the equation) and the *extremes* (the outer numbers of the equation). If your answer is correct, multiplication of the means and extremes produces answers that are equal. For example:

$$3:5 = 6:x$$

If the problem is solved by cross-multiplication, the equation looks like this:

$$\frac{3}{5} = \frac{6}{x}$$

After cross-multiplying, we have:

$$3x = 30 \text{ (divide each side by 3 to find } x)$$
$$x = 10$$

therefore, our equation is $3:5 = 6:10$.

To check the accuracy of your equation, multiply the means (5 × 6 = 30) and the extremes (3 × 10 = 30). Because the answers are equal, you know you have the correct proportion. Table 34-1 provides some examples of the relationships between percents, decimals, fractions, and ratios.

Determine the following equivalents:

0.20	= _____ (percent)	= _____ (fraction)	= _____ (ratio)
37%	= _____ (decimal)	= _____ (fraction)	= _____ (ratio)
⅔	= _____ (ratio)	= _____ (percent)	= _____ (decimal)
3:4	= _____ (fraction)	= _____ (decimal)	= _____ (percent)

Rounding Calculations

What should you do if the dose of the supplied drug does not exactly match your calculation? For example, what if you calculate a tablet dose as 1.75 tabs, but you have only whole tablets available? First,

TABLE 34-1 Mathematic Equivalents

PERCENTAGE	DECIMAL	FRACTION	RATIO
25	0.25	¼	1:4
50	0.5	½	1:2
60	0.6	⅗ (⁶⁄₁₀)	3:5
0.5	0.005	¹⁄₂₀₀	1:200
0.1	0.001	¹⁄₁₀₀₀	1:1,000
85	0.85	¹⁷⁄₂₀	17:20
1	0.01	¹⁄₁₀₀	1:100

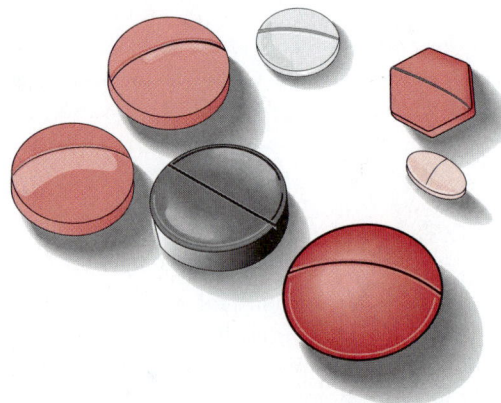

FIGURE 34-2 Examples of scored tablets. (From Fulcher EM, Fulcher RM, Soto CD: *Pharmacology: principles and applications,* ed 2, St Louis, 2007, Saunders.)

check your calculation for accuracy, then check the stocked supply of the drug to make sure no other dosages are available. If the calculation is correct and no other dosages of the drug are available, you will have to round your answer to the nearest amount that matches the dose available. *If the calculation is 0.5 or greater, round up to the next whole number.* For 1.75 tablets, 0.75 would be rounded up to 1, and the patient should be given two tabs of the medication. However, make sure you check with the physician before administering a rounded dose of medication.

Determine the correct doses for the following examples:

1.2 tabs = _____ tablet(s)	1.55 tabs = _____ tablet(s)
1.37 tabs = _____ tablet(s)	0.56 tab = _____ tablet
1.64 tabs = _____ tablet(s)	0.81 tab = _____ tablet

Some tablets are *scored,* which means that the medication was manufactured with an impression or groove down the center of the tablet. This type of tablet can be accurately divided into two equal parts; therefore, calculations can be rounded to the closest half-tab (Figure 34-2). For example, 0.4 tab would be rounded up to one-half of a scored tab, and 1.7 tabs would be 2 tabs. *Never* give a partial dose of a tablet unless the tablet has been scored, and then the dose can be given rounded to the nearest ½.

If a liquid medication is to be administered, it usually is acceptable to round the dose to the *nearest tenth.* For example, if the correct calculation for an injection of an antibiotic is 1.46 mL, administer

1.5 mL of the drug (the calculation is greater than 0.05). The *exceptions* to this rule are (1) pediatrics, because accurate doses for children may be much smaller than adult doses; and (2) if the dose is less than 1 mL and the syringe you are using is calibrated in hundredths, the medication is rounded to the nearest hundredth. What are the correct doses of the following medications, rounded to the nearest tenth?

1.47 cc = _____ cc	1.33 mL = _____ mL
2.62 mL = _____ mL	2.15 cc = _____ cc
1.08 mL = _____ mL	1.15 mL = _____ mL

SYSTEMS OF MEASUREMENT

If the dosage ordered by the physician is different from the dosage on hand, the medical assistant must follow three basic steps to calculate the prescribed dose accurately:

1. Compare the system printed on the drug label with the physician's order to determine whether the order is in the same mathematical system of measurement. If the systems are different (e.g., the order is in teaspoons but the label states that the medication is prepared in milliliters), accurately convert the order so that it matches the system used on the label.
2. Perform the calculation in equation form using the appropriate formula.
3. Check your answer for accuracy and ask someone you trust to confirm your calculations.

All three steps must be completed before the medication is dispensed and administered. Confirm your calculations with the physician if you have any doubt of their accuracy.

Sometimes the physician orders a medication in a strength completely different from the one on the drug label. For example, the physician may order 1 gr (grain) of a drug, but the available dosage form is in milligrams. Before the medical assistant can use the ratio and proportion formulas to arrive at the amount to administer, he or she first must convert to one system or the other. The medical assistant must convert the ordered dose to the measurement system on the drug label (i.e., what is available), because that system must be used to **dispense** the drug.

Three different systems of measurement are used for medications: the metric system, the apothecary system, and the household system. Table 34-2 presents abbreviations and symbols used in the apothecary and metric systems.

Metric System

The metric system of weights and measures is used throughout the world as the primary system for weight (mass), capacity (volume), and length (area). In the United States, the metric system is used for scientific work, including most tasks involving pharmaceuticals. However, some medication forms still use the older apothecary system; therefore, the medical assistant must learn the two systems and the relationships (conversions) between them.

The metric system of weights and measures is a decimal system based on the number 10, and all calculations are completed by moving decimal points to the right or to the left. Each higher measure is 10 times the measure at hand; each lower measure is 0.1 (¹⁄₁₀) the measure. The basic units are multiplied or divided by units of 10. The fraction is always written as a decimal, and the number

TABLE 34-2   Abbreviations and Symbols for Selected Weights and Measures

APOTHECARY SYSTEM			METRIC SYSTEM	
℞	Min (M)	minim	g	gram
ʒ	dr	dram	L	liter
fl ʒ	f dr	fluid dram	cc	cubic centimeter
ʒ	oz	ounce	mL	milliliter
fl	fl oz	fluid ounce		
O	Pt	pint		
C	gal	gallon		
	Gr	grain		

1 dg = 0.1 g or $\frac{1}{10}$ of a gram
1 dL = 0.1 L or $\frac{1}{10}$ of a liter
1 cg = 0.01 g or $\frac{1}{100}$ of a gram
1 cL = 0.01 L or $\frac{1}{100}$ of a liter
1 mg = 0.001 g or $\frac{1}{1,000}$ of a gram
1 mL = 0.001 L or $\frac{1}{1,000}$ of a liter

RULES FOR METRIC SYSTEM CONVERSIONS

1. To convert from a smaller unit of measurement to a larger unit of measurement, move the decimal point three places to the left. Your answer will always be a smaller number. Example: 62.4 mg = 0.0624 g

2. To convert from a larger unit of measurement to a smaller unit of measurement, move the decimal point three places to the right. Your answer will always be a larger number. Example: 1.7 g = 1,700 mg.

3. To prevent dosage errors, use a zero before a decimal point to clarify its presence; however, never leave a zero after a decimal point, because it may not be noticed, and too much medication may be administered.

precedes the letters designating the actual measure. Thus 1½ liters would be written 1.5 L. The cubic centimeter (cc) and the milliliter (mL) are interchangeable; however, the Joint Commission (formerly the Joint Commission on Accreditation of Healthcare Organizations [JCAHO]) advises against the use of the *cc* abbreviation in documenting medications in the patient's record.

In the metric system, 1 cc is a measurement of area, and an area this size holds exactly 1 mL, or 0.001 ($\frac{1}{1,000}$) of a liter of fluid. The milliliter measures the *amount* of liquid medication, or the volume, that is to be given orally or by injection. The gram (g) measures the weight, or *strength,* of a solid medication, such as a tablet, powder, or topical preparation. The meter is the measurement for *length* in the metric system. A meter is equal to 39.37 inches, which is slightly longer than a yard, or 3.28 feet. One inch is equal to 2½ centimeters (cm). The medical assistant may use centimeter measurements when measuring the depth and borders of a wound.

The units of measurement in the metric system are based on their prefixes: *kilo-* means 1,000, and *milli-* means 0.001. The prefixes mean the same whether used to measure volume or weight. For example, a kilogram (kg) is 1,000 grams (g), and a kiloliter (kL) is 1,000 liters (L); a milligram (mg) is 0.001 ($\frac{1}{1,000}$) of a gram, and a milliliter (mL) is 0.001 ($\frac{1}{1,000}$) of a liter.

Conversions within the metric system may be necessary if the physician orders a unit that is different from the one on the drug label. Units in the metric system are converted by moving the decimal point in multiples of 10. When *larger units of measurement are converted to smaller ones* (e.g., grams to milligrams), the answer is a larger number, so the *decimal point is moved three places to the right* (0.35 g = 350 mg). When *smaller units of measurement are converted to larger ones,* the answer is a smaller number, so the *decimal point is moved three places to the left* (e.g., 150 mL = 0.15 L). The following equivalents can be used to make conversions within the metric system.

1 kg = 1,000 g
1 kL = 1,000 L
1 g = 1,000 mg
1 L = 1,000 mL
1 mg = 1,000 micrograms (mcg)
1 mL = 1,000 microliters (mcL)

CRITICAL THINKING APPLICATION   34-1

The first problems Heather reviewed were conversions within the metric system. Yesterday, Dr. Angio ordered 0.45 L of a drug, but the label gave the contents in milliliters. How many milliliters should Heather have given? Review the examples below. If your answer is *less than* a whole number, make sure you place a zero before the decimal point so that the number is not mistaken for a whole number.

Examples:

6 g	=	6,000 mg	3,200 mL =	3.2 L		
0.6 g	=	600 mg	320 mL	=	0.32 L	
0.06 g	=	60 mg	32 mL	=	0.032 L	

Convert the following measurements:

2.5 g	=	_____ mg	42 g	=	_____ mg
0.21 g	=	_____ mg	150 mcg	=	_____ mg
1.7 g	=	_____ mg	55 mg	=	_____ g
3 mg	=	_____ mcg	74 L	=	_____ mL
0.28 L	=	_____ mL	950 mL	=	_____ L

Apothecary System

In the apothecary system, the basic unit of weight for a solid medication is the *grain,* and the basic unit of volume for a liquid medication is the *minim.* As in the metric system, these two units are related: The grain is based on the weight of a single grain of wheat, and the minim is the volume of water that weighs 1 grain (gr). Roman or Arabic numerals may be used, but they should not be used together in the same prescription. Symbols or abbreviations are used; for example, 1½ drams might be written ʒ or dr 1½. The number follows the symbol or abbreviation. Table 34-3 compares units of weight and volume in the metric and apothecary systems. Fluid ounces (oz) are used to differentiate liquids from solid weight.

TABLE 34-3 Approximate Equivalents for Some Commonly Used Measures

GRAINS	GRAMS	MILLIGRAMS	APOTHECARY		METRIC (mL [cc])	
			LIQUID MEASURE			
15	1.0	1,000	1	quart	1,000	mL (cc)
10	0.6	600	1	pint	500	mL
7½	0.5	500	8	fl oz	250	mL
5	0.3	300	7	fl oz	200	mL
4½	0.25	250	3.5	fl oz	100	mL
3	0.2	200	1	fl oz	30	mL
2	0.12	120	4	fl dr	15	mL
1½	0.1	100	2.5	fl dr	10	mL
1	0.06	60	2	fl dr	8	mL
¾	0.050	50	1	fl dr	4	mL
½	0.030	30	45	M	3	mL
⅜	0.025	25	30	M	2	mL
¼	0.015	15	15	M	1	mL
⅙	0.010	10	12	M	0.75	mL
⅛	0.008	8	10	M	0.6	mL
¹⁄₁₀	0.006	6	8	M	0.5	mL
¹⁄₁₂	0.005	5	5	M	0.3	mL
¹⁄₂₀	0.003	3	4	M	0.25	mL
¹⁄₃₀	0.002	2	3	M	0.2	mL
¹⁄₆₀	0.001	1	1.5	M	0.1	mL
¹⁄₁₀₀	0.0006	0.6	1	M	0.06	mL
¹⁄₁₂₀	0.0005	0.5	0.75	M	0.05	mL
¹⁄₁₅₀	0.0004	0.4	0.5	M	0.03	mL
¹⁄₂₀₀	0.0003	0.3				
¹⁄₂₅₀	0.00025	0.25				
¹⁄₃₀₀	0.0002	0.2				
¹⁄₄₀₀	0.00015	0.15				
¹⁄₅₀₀	0.00012	0.12				
¹⁄₆₀₀	0.0001	0.1				

Weight conversions: 1 lb = 0.45 kg; 1 kg = 2.2 lb; 10 lb = 4.5 kg; 10 kg = 22 lb; 30.0 g = 1 oz; 15.0 g = 4 dr; 7.5 g = 2 dr; 4 g = 1 dr; 4 g = 60 gr.
Domestic equivalents: 1 tsp = 5 mL (cc) = 1 fl dr; 1 Tbsp = 15 mL = 0.5 fl oz; 1 measuring cup = 250 mL = 8 fl oz; 4 measuring cups = 1,000 mL = 1 quart.

Household Measurements

The household system is used in most American homes. This system of measurement is important for a patient at home who has no knowledge of the metric or apothecary system; however, household measurements are not precise, so they should never be used in the medical setting. Nevertheless, a medical assistant must understand the conversions between medical and household measurements, so the patient can be instructed in how to measure the medication most accurately at home.

The basic measure of weight in the household system is the pound (lb); the basic measure of volume is the drop (gtt). The household drop is equal to an apothecary minim, so these two systems sometimes can be easily interchanged. Both household and apothecary systems use the term *ounce* as a unit of measurement, so the medical assistant must always be sure which system is being used.

TABLE 34-4 Common Household Measures

60	drops*	1 teaspoon
1	dash	Less than ⅛ teaspoon
3	teaspoons	1 tablespoon
2	tablespoons	1 ounce
4	ounces	1 juice glass
6	ounces	1 teacup
8	ounces	1 glass or cup
16	tablespoons or 8 ounces	1 measuring cup
2	cups	1 pint
2	pints	1 quart
4	quarts	1 gallon

*Drop (gtt) is an approximate liquid measure, depending on the kind of liquid measured and the size of the opening from which it is dropped.

TABLE 34-5 Household Equivalents

60	gtt	=	1 t or tsp			
3	t or tsp	=	1 T			
180	gtt	=	1 T	=	½ oz	
2	T	=	1 oz	=	6 t or tsp	
360	gtt	=	2 T			
1	oz	=	30 cc or 30 mL			
6	oz	=	1 tsp			
8	oz	=	1 C or 1 glass			
2	C	=	1 pt	=	16 oz	
2	pt	=	1 qt	=	32 oz	
4	C	=	1 qt	=	32 oz	
4	qt	=	1 gal	=	128 oz	

Medications are not measured in household weights, but many prescriptions contain directions using the household measurements of volume. Liquid oral medications are taken by the drop, teaspoon, or tablespoon and are supplied in bottles labeled in ounces or pints. Pediatric medications frequently are packaged as liquids, and the label gives instructions for the medication to be given in household measurements (e.g., teaspoon [tsp], tablespoon [Tbsp]). The medical assistant should know that 60 gtt = 1 tsp = 5 mL, and 180 gtt = 3 tsp = 1 Tbsp = 15 mL. Tables 34-4 and 34-5 show the household system of measurement. Based on these equivalents, convert the following orders:

2 tsp = _____ mL	120 gtt = _____ tsp
10 mL = _____ tsp	20 mL = _____ Tbsp
3 mL = _____ tsp	4 Tbsp = _____ mL

Conversions Among Systems of Measurement

Medication orders may have to be converted from one system to another if the order is written in one system and the drug label is in another. Using the conversions in Table 34-3, many measurements can be directly converted, or an equivalent can be chosen and the order mathematically converted to the system on the drug label. The conversion is calculated by multiplication or by division. For example, if the physician orders 30 grains of a drug but the label states that each tablet is equivalent to 2 grams, you must convert the order in grains to grams to know how many tablets to give the patient. To convert grains to grams, Table 34-3 tells us that 15 grains equals 1 gram. Therefore, you know that 15 grains equals 1 gram, and the physician has ordered 30 grains; to calculate the amount of the dose in tablets, you must divide the order by the conversion factor.

$$30 \text{ gr} \div 15 \text{ gr} = 2 \text{ g}$$

The label shows that each tablet contains 2 grams of the medication; therefore, the patient would be given 1 tablet.

Conversions between units of measurement also can be done by placing the numbers in an algebraic formula. We know that 15 grains equals 1 gram, and we are looking for the number of grams that is equivalent to 30 grains. If the amount ordered is placed on the left side of the equation and the conversion factor on the right side, similar units can be cancelled when cross-multiplied, and we can determine the dose.

$$30 \text{ gr} \times \frac{1 \text{ g}}{15 \text{ gr}}$$

Cross-multiply and the grain unit cancels out:

$$30 \times \frac{1 \text{ g}}{15} = \frac{30 \text{ g}}{15} = 2 \text{ g}$$

How would you convert a metric order for a medication into a household unit of measurement that a parent could administer to a sick child? For example, the physician orders 30 mL of an oral antibiotic. What is the equivalent household unit of measurement? As has been stated previously, 1 tablespoon equals 15 mL. Thus you can determine the answer in two ways. Either divide the order by the conversion factor:

$$30 \text{ mL} \div 15 \text{ mL} = 2 \text{ Tbsp}$$

or set the problem up as an equation with the ordered amount on the left side of the equation and the conversion factor on the right side:

$$30 \text{ mL} \times \frac{1 \text{ Tbsp}}{15 \text{ mL}}$$

Cross-multiply and the mL units cancel out; therefore, you have:

$$30 \times \frac{1 \text{ Tbsp}}{15} = \frac{30 \text{ Tbsp}}{15} = 2 \text{ Tbsp}$$

The following formula is another method of converting drug orders from one unit of measurement to the label unit:

$$\text{Drug have} \times \frac{\text{Wanted}}{\text{Have}} = \text{Unit wanted in new system}$$

The elements of this formula are:
- **Drug have**—unit of measurement on the drug label
- **Wanted**—amount or strength ordered by the physician
- **Have**—conversion (15 gr = 1 g)

Example:

Physician's order: Administer 30 gr of Lasix

Label: 1 g Lasix/tab

You must convert the ordered unit of measurement to match the unit of measurement on the drug label.

$$1 \text{ g (unit of measurement on label)}$$
$$\times \frac{30 \text{ gr (strength ordered by physician)}}{15 \text{ gr (conversion factor)}} = 2 \text{ g} = 2 \text{ tabs}$$

Complete the following conversion problems:

1. A patient with risk factors for heart disease is told to take a baby aspirin equivalent to gr 5 every morning. How many milligrams is the patient taking?
2. A patient scheduled for urinary tract diagnostic tests needs to drink a minimum of 2 L of water over the next 12 hours. How many ounces should the patient drink?
3. A pediatric patient is prescribed 8 mL of amoxicillin qid for 10 days. What is the equivalent dose in household measurements?

CALCULATING DRUG DOSAGES FOR ADMINISTRATION

The correct dosage of a medication may depend on the patient's age, weight, and state of health, or on what other drugs the patient is taking. Frequently the physician orders a medication in a dosage that is different from the dosage of the drug in stock. The difference may be in the system of measurement, the strength, or the form. Formulas and mathematical tables of conversion are available for calculating the correct dosage of medication to be administered. It is helpful to look at how the correct calculation is performed, one step at a time.

Calculating Dosages

A standard set of formulas is used for calculating dosages (Procedures 34-1 and 34-2). These formulas use the *strength* (potency) and *dose unit* (amount) of the drug. If the drug label reads "5 gr/tab," the strength is 5 grains, and the dose unit is 1 tablet. For liquids, the drug strength is an amount of *solute*, which is dissolved in a liquid called the *solvent*. Therefore, if a vial of injectable drug reads "500 mg/mL," 500 mg (strength) of the drug is present in every milliliter (amount) of liquid.

We can use these two examples and the proportion formula previously reviewed to work out two problems: (1) preparing an injectable medication and (2) determining an oral dose.

Problem 1: Preparing an Injectable Dose.

Order: Administer 250 mg of cephalexin IM

Available: A vial marked 500 mg/mL

Standard formula:

$$\frac{\text{Available strength}}{\text{Ordered strength}} = \frac{\text{Available amount}}{\text{Amount to give}}$$

When the standard formula is used, the *Available strength* is the strength of the drug that is written on the medication label. In this case, the cephalexin vial states on the label, "500 mg/mL," meaning there is 500 mg of cephalexin in each milliliter of the medication. The *Ordered strength* is the dose ordered by the physician (i.e., 250 mg). The *Available amount* is the amount of the drug that must be used to deliver the strength identified on the label. Because the label states, "500 mg/mL," we know that the available amount for 500 mg is 1 mL.

Problem: Given the strength of the drug needed (the physician's order of 250 mg), the amount of fluid to be withdrawn must be determined.

PROCEDURE 34-1

Prepare Proper Dosages of Medication for Administration: Apply Mathematic Computations to Solve Equations

GOAL: *To calculate the correct dose amount and choose the correct equipment when the physician orders 2.4 million IU of penicillin G benzathine (Bicillin).*

EQUIPMENT and SUPPLIES

- Premixed syringes of Bicillin, available as:
- 0.6 million IU/syringe
- 1.2 million IU/syringe

PROCEDURAL STEPS

Read the order in quiet surroundings to make sure that you fully understand it.

1. Write out the order.
2. Examine the drug labels to see what strengths and amounts are available.

3. Write down the standard formula.

$$\frac{\text{Available strength}}{\text{Ordered strength}} = \frac{\text{Available amount}}{\text{Amount to give}}$$

PURPOSE: To eliminate the chance of error, orders should never be carried out unless the calculations are completed in writing.

4. Rewrite the formula, replacing the unknown values with the known quantities. The unknown *x* will be the amount of the drug to give.
5. Work the proportion problem by cross-multiplying to solve for *x*.
6. State your answer by filling in the following blanks:
   To administer 2.4 million IU of Bicillin, I would select _____ of the premixed syringe labeled _____.

PROCEDURE 34-2

Prepare Proper Dosages of Medication for Administration: Convert Among Measurement Systems

GOAL: *To choose the correct system of measurement and calculate the correct dose amount when the physician orders 120 mg of a drug to be administered to a patient. (The label reads 1 gr/tab.)*

EQUIPMENT and SUPPLIES

- Tablets labeled 1 gr (grain) each
- Standard mathematical formula:

$$\frac{\text{Available strength}}{\text{Ordered strength}} = \frac{\text{Available amount}}{\text{Amount to give}}$$

- Conversion equivalent: 1 gr = 60 mg

Procedural Steps

1. Read the order in quiet surroundings to make sure you fully understand it.
2. Write out the order.
3. Examine the drug labels to see what strengths and amounts are available.
4. Convert the ordered system of measurement to the system of measurement on the label.
5. Place the amount ordered on the left side of the equation and the conversion factor on the right side so that similar units (in this problem, mg) can be cancelled.

$$120\,\text{mg} \times \frac{1\,\text{gr}}{60\,\text{mg}} = 120\,\text{gr} \div 60 = 2\,\text{gr}$$

6. Write down the standard formula:

$$\frac{\text{Available strength}}{\text{Ordered strength}} = \frac{\text{Available amount}}{\text{Amount to give}}$$

   <u>PURPOSE:</u> To eliminate the chance of error, orders should never be carried out unless the calculations are completed in writing.

7. Rewrite the formula, replacing the unknown values with the known quantities and using the system of measurement on the label. The unknown *x* will be the amount of the drug to give (amount to give).

$$\frac{1\,\text{gr}}{2\,\text{gr}} \times \frac{1\,\text{tab}}{x\,\text{tab}}$$

8. Work the proportion problem by cross-multiplying to solve for *x*.
9. State your answer by filling in the blank:
   To administer 120 mg of a drug from tablets labeled "1 gr/tab," give _____ tablet(s).

Set up a proportion with the three known quantities: (1) the strength of the drug in the vial, (2) the unit of fluid in which that strength is contained, and (3) the strength of the drug the physician has ordered for administration.

Apply the standard formula to the problem. If you get confused about where to place the numbers in the equation, remember that like units of measurement (in this case, mg) must be placed on the same side of the equation.

$$\frac{\text{Available strength}}{\text{Ordered strength}} = \frac{\text{Available amount}}{\text{Amount to give}} \quad \frac{500\,\text{mg}}{250\,\text{mg}} = \frac{1\,\text{mL}}{x\,\text{mL}}$$

The mg units in the numerator and denominator on the left side of the equation cancel each other out. Cross-multiply the equation.

$$500 \times x = 250 \times 1$$
$$500x = 250\,\text{mL}$$

To find *x* (the amount to be administered), you must divide each side of the equation by 500.

$$\frac{500x}{500} = \frac{250\,\text{mL}}{500}$$

$$x = \frac{1}{2}\,\text{mL} = 0.5\,\text{mL}$$

Solution: Administer 0.5 mL of cephalexin.

Problem 2: Determining an Oral Dose.

Order: Give 10 gr (grains) of a drug
Available: A bottle with tablets labeled 5 gr each
Standard formula:

$$\frac{\text{Available strength}}{\text{Ordered strength}} = \frac{\text{Available amount}}{\text{Amount to give}}$$

Problem: Given the strength of the drug needed, the number of tablets to be administered must be determined.

Set up a proportion with the three known quantities: (1) the strength of the drug in each tablet, (2) the unit amount in 1 tablet, and (3) the strength of the drug the physician has ordered for administration.

Apply the standard formula to the problem:

$$\frac{\text{Available strength}}{\text{Ordered strength}} = \frac{\text{Available amount}}{\text{Amount to give}}$$

$$\frac{5\,\text{gr}}{10\,\text{gr}} = \frac{1\,\text{tablet}}{x\,\text{(number of tablets)}}$$

The grain units in the numerator and denominator on the left side of the equation cancel each other out. Cross-multiply the equation.

$$5 \times x = 10 \times 1$$
$$5x = 10$$

To find x (i.e., the amount to be administered), you must divide each side of the equation by 5.

$$\frac{5x}{5} = \frac{10}{5}$$
$$x = 2 \text{ tablets}$$

Solution: Administer 2 tablets.

The standard formula can be used for any type of calculation. You may be using strengths that are measured in international units (IU), as with penicillin, as well as grams, milligrams, grains, or percentages. The forms in which drugs may be prepared include cubic centimeters (cc) or milliliters (mL), minims, drops, drams, ounces, pints, gallons (for making up diluted stock solutions from concentrated solutions, as with alcohol and hydrogen peroxide), and spoonfuls.

Follow the steps previously shown and, above all, discipline yourself to write down each step with complete calculations. This is the only way to ensure maximum accuracy and the safety of your patients. If you have difficulty with the calculation or the answer does not seem quite right, ask the physician to check your calculation. A double check is always preferred.

An alternative formula for calculating drug dosages may be used by your co-workers. Regardless of the formula used, the answer will be the same: $D/H \times Q$.

- **D**—desired dose (the physician's order)
- **H**—what is on hand (the dosage strength listed on the medication label)
- **Q**—quantity in the unit (identified on the label as 1 tablet, 5 mL, and so one)

More Sample Problems

Problem 1. Dr. Angio orders 500 mg of an antibiotic **stat**. The label states that the dosage strength is 250 mg/2 mL. How much should the patient receive?

$$\frac{D}{H} \times Q = \frac{500 \text{ mg (physician's order)}}{250 \text{ mg (dosage strength on hand)}} \times 2 \text{ mL (label quantity)}$$

The mg quantities cancel out:

$$\frac{500}{250} \times 2 \text{ mL} = 2 \times 2 \text{ mL}$$
$$= 4 \text{ mL of the medication should be administered}$$

Problem 2. Dr. Angio orders 50 mg of Imitrex to be given stat for a patient with a severe migraine. The label states, "25 mg/tab."

$$\frac{\text{Dose ordered}}{\text{Dose on hand}} \times \text{Quantity} = \text{Amount to give}$$

or $\quad \dfrac{D}{H} \times Q = \text{Amount to give}$

$$\frac{50 \text{ mg}}{25 \text{ mg}} \times 1 \text{ tab} = 2 \text{ tabs}$$

Calculate the following doses.

1. Administer 0.25 mg of Lanoxin. The label reads "0.125 mg/tab." How many tablets should you give?
2. The patient is prescribed 15 mEq of KCl, and the label reads "5 mEq/5 mL." How many milliliters should the patient receive?
3. The phenobarbital label states "15 mg/5 mL." The patient is prescribed 45 mg of the drug. How many milliliters should be administered?
4. The physician orders 25 mg of Compazine IM. The label reads "10 mg/mL." How much medicine should be injected?

CRITICAL THINKING APPLICATION   **34-2**

At work the next day, Dr. Angio orders Heather to administer Acetaminophen Elixir 70 mg stat to a 6-year-old patient with a fever of 102.6° F. Heather checks the label of the Acetaminophen Elixir in the drug cabinet and discovers that the bottle contains 120 mg per 5 mL in a 100-mL bottle. Using the standard formula presented earlier, how many milliliters should the child receive? If Heather is concerned about her calculation, what should she do?

PEDIATRIC DOSAGES

Calculating the Dose

Pediatric doses are calculated differently from those for other age groups because of multiple factors, including differences in absorption and drug metabolism. Although formulas have been used in the past that based the dose calculation on age, pediatric doses are much more accurate when based on weight, because children of any age can vary greatly in size and body weight. Therefore, the factor used to calculate pediatric doses is the child's body **surface area** (BSA) or weight. You must be especially careful in calculating dosages for children, because even a minor miscalculation can be dangerous.

Clark's Rule

Clark's rule is based on the weight of the child. It uses 150 pounds (68 kg) as the average adult weight and assumes that the child's dose is proportionately less. The formula is as follows:

$$\text{Pediatric dose} = \frac{\text{Child's weight (in lb)}}{150 \text{ lb}} \times \text{Adult dose}$$

For example, a child who weighs 32 lb is prescribed Tylenol. The normal adult dose of the drug is 240 mg. How much Tylenol should the child be given?

$$\text{Dose} = \frac{32 \text{ lb}}{150 \text{ lb}} \times 240 \text{ mg} \left(\begin{array}{l} \text{The pounds cancel out. First divide 32 by} \\ \text{150, then multiply that figure by 240 mg.} \end{array} \right)$$
$$= 0.2 \text{ (rounded from 0.213)} \times 240 \text{ mg}$$
$$= 48 \text{ mg}$$

West's Nomogram

West's **nomogram** uses a calculation of the BSA of infants and young children to determine the pediatric dose. Many physicians use the

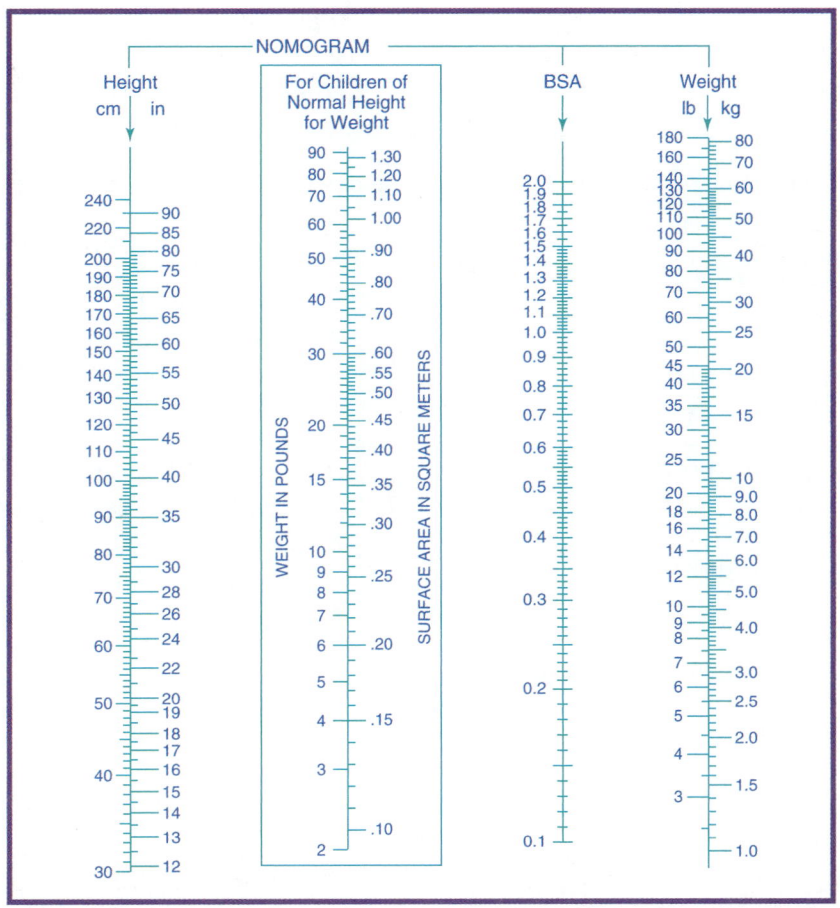

FIGURE 34-3 West's nomogram for estimating body surface area. (From Fulcher EM, Fulcher RM, Soto CD: *Pharmacology: principles and applications*, ed 3, St Louis, 2012, Saunders.)

nomogram as a quick reference for pediatric doses (Figure 34-3). The formula is based on the estimated adult BSA of 1.7 m². If the child is of normal height and weight, the BSA in square meters is the point at which the child's weight in pounds intersects with the surface area in the box on the left. Therefore, if the child weighs 15 lb (and that is normal for his or her age and height), the BSA is 0.36 m². If the child is underweight or overweight according to standard growth charts (see Chapter 42), the BSA is determined by intersecting the point on the nomogram between the child's height (in either centimeters or inches) in the left column and the child's weight (in pounds or kilograms) in the right column. For example, if a child is overweight at 45 lb and 40 inches in height, the BSA is 0.78 m².

After the child's BSA has been determined from the nomogram, it should be divided by 1.7 m² and that calculation multiplied by the adult dose to determine the amount of medication for the child (Procedure 34-3).

$$\text{Pediatric dose} = \frac{\text{BSA of child (in m}^2)}{1.7 \text{ m}^2 \text{ (average adult BSA)}} \times \text{Adult dose}$$

Sample problem: A child who weighs 10 lb and is 30 inches in height (underweight for height) is prescribed erythromycin. The normal adult dose of the drug is 400 mg. How much of the antibiotic should the child receive in a single dose?

1. According to the nomogram, the child's BSA is 0.31 m².

2. $\text{Dose} = \dfrac{32 \text{ lb}}{150 \text{ lb}} \times 240 \text{ mg}$ $\left(\begin{array}{l}\text{The pounds cancel out. First divide 32 by} \\ \text{150, then multiply that figure by 240 mg.}\end{array}\right)$

   $= 0.2 \left(\text{rounded from } 0.213\right) \times 240 \text{ mg}$

   $= 48 \text{ mg}$

   $= 0.18.$ (Because this is a pediatric dose, round to the nearest hundredth for greater accuracy.)

3. $0.18 \times 400 \text{ mg} = 72 \text{ mg}$

Dosages Based on Body Weight

Although Clark's rule and West's nomogram provide quick methods of determining pediatric doses, the most frequently used calculation method relies on the child's accurate weight in kilograms. Kilogram measurements are necessary because most pediatric medication dosages are based on the metric system, with a designated number of milligrams to be administered per kilogram of body weight (mg/kg). Several steps are involved in this type of calculation, but if you follow them closely, you will determine the most accurate amount of medication to administer to a child (Procedure 34-4).

1. Before you begin the dose calculation, carefully weigh the child to make sure you have an accurate weight. If the scale provides a reading in pounds, convert the child's weight to kilograms by dividing the number of pounds by 2.2 (1 kg = 2.2 lb). For

PROCEDURE 34-3

Apply Mathematic Computations to Solve Equations: Calculate the Correct Pediatric Dosage Using the Body Surface Area

GOAL: *To calculate the correct dose amount using the body surface area (BSA) method for a 90-lb child who is 48 inches tall when the adult dose is 250 mg/mL.*

EQUIPMENT and SUPPLIES

- Accurate scale with length measurement
- West's nomogram
- Adult dose 250 mg/mL

$$\text{Pediatric dose} = \frac{\text{BSA of child}\,(m^2)}{1.7\ m^2\ (\text{average adult BSA})} \times \text{Adult dose}$$

PROCEDURAL STEPS

1. Read the order in quiet surroundings to make sure you fully understand it.
2. Write out the order.
3. Examine the drug labels to see what strengths and amounts are available.

4. Write down the BSA formula.
   <u>PURPOSE:</u> To eliminate the chance of error, orders should never be carried out unless the calculations are completed in writing.
5. Using the BSA method, determine the BSA in m^2 by intersecting the child's height in the left column with the weight in the right column (child is overweight).
6. Divide the child's BSA by 1.7 m^2 (the average adult BSA).
7. Multiply this calculation by the adult dose (250 mg).
8. State your answer by filling in the blank:
   To administer an adult medication labeled 250 mg/mL to a 90-lb child, give _____ mg.

PROCEDURE 34-4

Apply Mathematic Computations to Solve Equations: Calculate the Correct Pediatric Dosage Using Body Weight

ORDER: *Zithromax suspension 5 mg/kg bid 5 days for a patient who has a diagnosis of otitis media. The patient weighs 22 lb. The suspension is labeled 100 mg/5 mL. Weight conversion: 2.2 lb = 1 kg.*

GOAL: *To calculate the correct pediatric dosage by using the body weight method.*

EQUIPMENT and SUPPLIES

- Suspension labeled 100 mg/5 mL
- Balance scale
- Formula for conversion of pounds to kilograms
- Standard math formula:

$$\frac{\text{Available strength}}{\text{Ordered strength}} = \frac{\text{Available amount}}{\text{Amount to give}}$$

- Paper and pencil

PROCEDURAL STEPS

1. Read the order in quiet surroundings to make sure you fully understand it.
2. Write out the order.
3. Examine the drug label to check the strength and amount.
4. Convert the patient's weight from pounds to kilograms.
   22 lb ÷ 2.2 lb/kg = 10 kg

5. Calculate the total daily amount of medication by multiplying the weight in kilograms by the mg/kg factor.
   5 mg × 10 kg = 50 mg of Zithromax daily for 5 days
6. Calculate the individual dose of Zithromax; divide the daily dose by 2 (bid is twice a day).
   50 mg ÷ 2 = 25 mg/dose
7. Compare the ordered daily dose with the dose information on the medication label. The suspension is labeled 100 mg/5 mL. (100 mg = 5 mL)
8. Write down the standard formula.
   <u>PURPOSE:</u> To eliminate the chances of error.
9. Rewrite the formula, replacing the unknown values with the known quantities. The unknown *x* will be the amount of the drug to give.
10. Work the problem by cross-multiplying to solve for *x*.
11. State your answer by filling in the blank:
    To administer 5 mg of Zithromax per kilogram of body weight from a suspension labeled 100 mg/5 mL, I would give _____ mL.

example, 36 lb is equal to 16.4 kg (36 × 2.2 = 16.36 = 16.4 kg [rounded up]). If the child's weight is in pounds and ounces, you must convert the ounces to pounds as a decimal and add it to the pounds. For example, if an infant weighs 9 lb 7 oz, first convert 7 oz to the nearest tenth of pounds (1 lb = 16 oz; 7 oz × 16 = 0.4 lb) and then add it to 9 lb; thus the baby weighs 9.4 lb. Then convert pounds to kilograms by dividing 9.4 by 2.2 (9.4 ÷ 2.2 = 4.3 kg).

2. Calculate the total daily dose of the medication by multiplying the child's weight in grams by the amount of drug stated on the label that should be administered per kg per day. For example, if the label states that the child should receive 4 mg per kg per day, multiply the child's weight in kg by 4 to determine the daily dose of the drug.

3. Calculate a single dose of the drug based on how frequently the medication is to be given throughout the day. For example, if the drug is ordered *qid*, divide the total daily dose by 4; if the medication is ordered for every 8 hours, divide the total daily dose by 3, because there are three 8-hour periods in a 24-hour day.

4. After calculating the amount of a single dose, compare the ordered amount with the drug label. If necessary, apply the standard formula to calculate the amount of medication that should be administered.

Example. An infant who weighs 12 lb 6 oz is prescribed erythromycin q6h. The label states that there is 200 mg of the drug in 5 cc of suspension. The recommended dose of the medication for infants is 30 mg/kg/day. How much should the child receive per dose?

1. Convert 12 lb 6 oz to kg.

$$6 \text{ oz} \div 16 \text{ oz} = 0.375 \text{ (converted to the nearest tenth} = 0.4)$$
$$0.4 \text{ lb} + 12 = 12.4 \text{ lb}$$
$$12.4 \div 2.2 = 5.6 \text{ kg}$$

2. The total daily dose of the medication is 30 mg times the weight in kilograms.

$$30 \times 5.6 = 168 \text{ mg/day}$$

3. A single dose of the drug is the total daily dose divided by 4 (there are four 6-hour periods in a 24-hour day).

$$168 \text{ mg} \div 4 = 42 \text{ mg/dose}$$

4. The amount of the medication that should be administered in a single dose is determined by the drug label, which states that there are 200 mg in every 5 cc of the suspension. The standard formula can be used as follows to find the answer:

$$\frac{\text{Available strength}}{\text{Ordered strength}} = \frac{\text{Available amount}}{\text{Amount to give}}$$
$$\frac{200 \text{ mg}}{42 \text{ mg}} = \frac{5 \text{ cc}}{x \text{ (number of cc)}}$$
$$200x = 210$$
$$x = 210 \div 200$$
$$x = 1.05 \text{ or } 1.1 \text{ cc}$$

RECONSTITUTING POWDERED INJECTABLE MEDICATIONS

Some medications are packaged in a vial as crystals or powder (solute) that must be mixed with sterile isotonic saline or sterile distilled water (solvent) to form a solution before it can be injected. In such cases, it is essential to *read the label directions carefully* to determine how much sterile solvent must be added to the solute to create the ordered dosage strength (see Procedure 35-6 for directions on administering the medication).

Example. The physician orders 500 mg of a drug. The label reads, "Add 5.5 mL of sterile water to make 250 mg/mL; total volume of available solution will be 6 mL."

1. Inject 5.5 mL of sterile water into the vial of medication. Rotate the vial between your hands to mix the solutes and the solvent. The total volume in the vial is now 6 mL.

2. According to the label, every milliliter in the vial contains 250 mg of the drug.

3. On the vial, write the date and time of reconstitution, because the guidelines on the drug label state that once the medication has been mixed, it must be discarded within a short time.

4. Using the standard formula, calculate the number of milliliters to withdraw from the vial to fulfill the physician's order for 500 mg of the drug.

$$\frac{\text{Available strength}}{\text{Ordered strength}} = \frac{\text{Available amount}}{\text{Amount to give}}$$
$$\frac{250 \text{ mg}}{500 \text{ mg}} = \frac{1 \text{ mL}}{x}$$
$$250x = 500$$
$$x = 500 \div 250 = 2 \text{ mL}$$

Answer: To administer 500 mg from a vial labeled 250 mg/mL, give 2 mL of medication.

CLOSING COMMENTS

Legal and Ethical Issues

A medical assistant who is responsible for administering medications must have completely mastered the calculation of dosages, whether the prescribed dose is for a child or for an adult. If the medical assistant is ever in doubt about the accuracy of a calculation, he or she should always have a trusted colleague or the physician check the calculations.

A medical assistant who prepares and administers medications is ethically and legally responsible for his or her own actions. Laws vary from state to state; therefore, it is essential that medical assistants become familiar with the laws in the states where they are employed before they administer medications. In some states, legislation gives physicians broad authority to delegate responsibility for giving medications. In such a case, the medical assistant acts as the "agent" of the physician. However, the assistant is responsible and accountable for the acts performed and may be subject to penalties.

Regardless of the differences in state authorization laws, the courts do not allow the carelessness of healthcare workers to go unpunished, especially when such actions result in harm or death for the patient.

SUMMARY OF SCENARIO

Heather recognizes how important it is to be able to calculate drug dosages correctly. To do so, she must understand the terms involved in dosage preparation, must be able to read a drug label correctly, and must follow the various steps in calculating a correct dose. The drug label contains a great deal of information, including brand and generic names; dosage strength; route of administration; instructions on mixing solvents if appropriate; storage guidelines; total amount of drug in the container; name of the drug manufacturer; expiration date; and both the lot number and the NDC identification number.

Heather also must be able to make conversions within and between measuring systems; use the standard formula to determine drug doses; accurately calculate pediatric doses based on the child's weight; and reconstitute powdered drugs for administration by following the label directions regarding the amount of solvent that should be added to the solute. She continues to ask Mrs. Allison or Dr. Angio to check her calculations for accuracy before dispensing and administering any drug order that differs from the medication label.

SUMMARY OF LEARNING OBJECTIVES

1. **Define, spell, and pronounce the terms listed in the vocabulary.**
   Spelling and pronouncing medical terms correctly bolsters the medical assistant's credibility. Knowing the definitions of these terms promotes confidence in communication with patients and co-workers.

2. **Apply critical thinking skills in performing the patient assessment and patient care.**
   Completing the Critical Thinking Application exercises throughout the chapter can help the student medical assistant become more adept at critical analysis of real-life situations.

3. **Summarize the important parts of a drug label.**
   The drug label contains a great deal of information, including brand and generic names; dosage strength; route of administration; instructions on mixing solvents if appropriate; storage guidelines; total amount of the drug in the container; name of the drug manufacturer; expiration date; and both the lot number and the NDC identification number.

4. **Differentiate among the terms used in dosage preparation.**
   Drug label terms must be understood to implement pharmacology math formulas. The strength of the drug is its potency; the dosage is the amount available in the drug package; the solute is the crystal or powdered form of the drug; the solvent is the sterile liquid that is combined in the vial with the solute to create the drug solution.

5. **Perform basic math skills.**
   The medical assistant must thoroughly understand the addition, subtraction, multiplication, and division of fractions and decimals; the relationships of decimals and fractions; and how they are converted from one to the other.

6. **Demonstrate methods of verifying the accuracy of calculations.**
   It is essential to verify the accuracy of calculations before dispensing and administering all medications. First, the medical assistant must check the drug label against the physician's order to verify the systems of measurement. If the physician's order is in a different unit of measurement, the ordered dose must be converted to match the system on the label. Next, the calculation is completed using the appropriate formula. Finally, the calculation is checked for accuracy.

7. **Describe and perform conversions among the various systems of measurement.**
   Three systems of measurement are used for drugs. The metric system is based on units of 10. The liter is a measure of the liquid volume of a drug, and the gram is a measure of the weight or strength. Units are converted within the metric system by moving the decimal point to the right or to the left. The apothecary system measures liquid volume in minims and weight in grains. Household measurements are based on pounds and drops. Table 34-3 can be used to convert from one system of measurement to another, or drug measurements can be converted by using the conversion formula.

8. **Calculate the correct dose of a drug using the standard formula.**
   The correct dose of an ordered drug can be calculated by using basic arithmetic involving fractions, ratios, and proportions. The standard formula for calculating drug dosage uses information about the drug's strength and amount (found on the label) and the strength of the drug ordered, with the unknown (x) being the answer sought. The only way to gain confidence in using the standard formula is to practice dose calculations frequently until you become comfortable with the math.

9. **Determine accurate pediatric doses of medication.**
   The medical assistant must be especially vigilant in calculating pediatric doses, because even a minor error may be dangerous to a child. West's nomogram can be used to determine the pediatric dose if the child's height and weight and the adult dose of the drug are known. However, the most accurate method for determining a pediatric dose is based on the child's weight. Procedure 34-4 describes how to calculate a pediatric dose based on the child's weight.

10. **Diagram how to reconstitute powdered injectable medications.**
    In reconstituting powdered injectable medications, the medical assistant must add a particular amount of solvent (as recommended on the drug label) to a vial of powdered or crystalloid medication. Once the solute and the solvent have been combined and mixed in the vial, a solution of medication is formed; the strength is based on equivalents printed on the drug label. After the medication has been mixed, it is important for the medical assistant to read the label carefully to determine how much of the drug must be withdrawn to fulfill the physician's order. This process

frequently requires use of the standard conversion formula to determine the accurate dose for administration.

11. **Specify the legal responsibilities of a medical assistant in calculating drug dosages.**

A medical assistant who prepares, dispenses, and administers medications is ethically and legally responsible for his or her own actions. If any doubt exists about the accuracy of calculations, it is essential that the medical assistant have the physician or another trusted employee review the math before the medication is dispensed and administered. Medical assistants must be aware of state laws that monitor medication administration by allied health workers.

CONNECTIONS

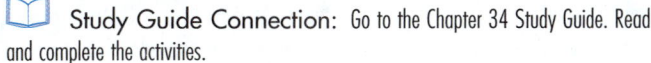 **Study Guide Connection:** Go to the Chapter 34 Study Guide. Read and complete the activities.

Evolve Connection: Go to the Chapter 34 link at *evolve.elsevier.com/kinn* to complete the Chapter Review and Chapter Quiz. Peruse other resources listed for this chapter to increase your knowledge of Pharmacology Math.

35

ADMINISTERING MEDICATIONS

Dr. Anna Thau just opened a new primary care office in the community. She is in the process of hiring office staff, and Dorothy Gaston, CMA (AAMA), is being interviewed for a clinical assisting position. One of Dr. Thau's chief requirements is that the medical assistants working in the clinical area be familiar with medications and competent in their administration. Her primary concern is the safety of her patients, so she requires that employees perform appropriate safety measures when dispensing and administering oral, topical, and parenteral drugs.

While studying this chapter, think about the following questions:

- What safety guidelines should Dorothy incorporate into her practice each time she receives a drug order from Dr. Thau?
- What information must be included in comprehensive documentation of the administration of medication?
- Are there patient assessment factors that might affect medication administration?
- Why does Dorothy have to understand the details of various drug forms and their administration guidelines?

- What practices mandated by the Occupational Safety and Health Administration (OSHA) must be followed in preparing and administering medications?
- Are there intravenous (IV) principles that Dorothy should understand?
- Does Dorothy need to be aware of the legal implications of drug administration?

LEARNING OBJECTIVES

1. Define, spell, and pronounce the terms listed in the vocabulary.
2. Apply critical thinking skills in performing the patient assessment and patient care.
3. Follow safety precautions in the management of medication administration in the ambulatory healthcare setting.
4. Analyze safety guidelines for specific patient populations.
5. Document the administration of a medication.
6. Summarize patient assessment factors that can affect medication administration.
7. Identify various drug forms and their administration guidelines.
8. Administer oral medications.

9. Specify parenteral administration equipment, including details about needles and syringes.
10. Follow OSHA guidelines in the management of parenteral administration.
11. Describe and demonstrate the types and locations of parenteral administrations.
12. Outline the principles of IV therapy.
13. Recognize the medical assistant's role in patient education about the administration of drugs.
14. Assess legal and ethical issues in drug administration in the ambulatory care setting.

VOCABULARY

aqueous (ak´-wee-uhs) A waterlike substance; a medication prepared with water.

asymptomatic Without symptoms of a disease process.

bevel (bev´-uhl) The angled tip of a needle.

bronchoconstriction Narrowing of the bronchiole tubes.

edema (i-dee´-muh) An abnormal accumulation of fluid in the interstitial spaces of tissues.

hermetically (hur-met´-ik-lee) **sealed** Sealed so that no air can enter.

immunosuppressant Substance that suppresses or prevents an immune system response.

immunotherapy Administration of repeated injections of diluted extracts of a substance that causes an allergy; also called *desensitization.*

induration (in-doo-rey´-shuhn) An abnormally hard, inflamed area.

loading dose Large dose administered as the first dose of a medication; it usually is used in antibiotic therapy to quickly achieve therapeutic blood levels of the drug.

meniscus (meh-nis´-kus) The curved surface of liquids in a container.

phlebitis (fluh-bi´-tis) Inflammation of a vein, with the possible complication of clot formation at the site (thrombophlebitis).

polyuria (pah-le-yur´-e-uh) Excretion of an unusually large amount of urine.

scored Slashed (e.g., a tablet manufactured with an indentation for division through the center).

vasodilation An increase in the diameter of a blood vessel.

viscosity (vis-kos´-uh-te) The quality of being thick and of lacking the capability of easy movement.

volatile (vol´-uh-tl) Capable of vaporizing at a low temperature, such as an explosive substance.

wheal (weel) A localized area of edema or a raised lesion.

Previous medication chapters in this text explained general pharmacologic principles and pharmacology math. In this chapter, you will learn about safety factors in drug administration, documentation guidelines, the forms of medications, and how they are administered. It is important to remember that medications can cause serious harm to a patient. Therefore, the process of dispensing and administering medications must always be treated with great care. Each member of the healthcare team involved in medication administration must be constantly vigilant to prevent errors and to deliver high-quality patient care.

No matter the type of medication administered, the order first must come from the physician. If the physician delegates drug administration to the medical assistant, this must be allowable under state law. Each state has a medical practice act that defines whether a medical assistant can administer drugs under the supervision of a physician. Some states allow medical assistants to administer only certain types of medications; some prohibit medical assistants from giving injections. You should obtain from your local government or medical society information about the scope of practice for medical assistants in your particular state. You should know what the law states and how your duties fit into that law.

SAFETY IN DRUG ADMINISTRATION

To ensure patient safety in drug administration, the medical assistant must perform certain procedures every time a medication is ordered. First, it is essential that the medical assistant understand the physician's order. Safety starts with a clearly written order that can be easily read and understood. Ask the physician for clarification if you have any questions about the medication, dose, strength, or route of administration. Once the order has been clarified, the medical assistant is responsible for looking up the drug in a pharmacology

reference, such as the *Physicians' Desk Reference* (PDR) (see Chapter 33). A medication should never be given until its purpose, possible side effects, precautions, and recommended dose are known.

After the medical assistant learns about the drug ordered, the medication is dispensed and administered. To safeguard the patient during this process, the medical assistant uses the "seven rights" of proper drug administration. Remember, however, that the patient always has the right to refuse to take a medication. If this occurs, make sure you inform the physician immediately, because he or she may want to follow up with the patient about the importance of the prescribed medication. If a patient refuses to take an ordered medication, be sure to document this refusal in the patient record. The seven rights of drug administration are as follows:

1. *The right patient.* The easiest way to make sure the medication is being given to the correct individual is to ask the patient his or her name or to address the patient by name before administering the drug.

2. *The right drug.* This begins with clarification of the physician's order if needed. *Every* time a drug is dispensed, the label must be checked *three times* to confirm the right drug, dose, and strength. You must be competent in reading and understanding the information on the drug label. The drug's name and strength on the label must exactly match the physician's written order. Compare the physician's written order with the medication label when you:
   - Take the medication from the storage area
   - Dispense the medication from the container
   - Replace the container to storage or before discarding the used container

3. *The right dose.* If the dose ordered does not match the dose available according to the drug label, perform appropriate pharmacology math procedures to determine the accurate dose. *Remember*

to have your calculations checked if you have any doubt about the accuracy of the dose.

4. *The right route.* Check the physician's order to clarify the route of administration, whether it is oral, via mucous membrane, or parenteral. Patient assessment includes determining whether this is an appropriate route for that particular patient.

5. *The right time.* In the ambulatory care setting, most medications are ordered *stat*. However, it is important to check the physician's order to clarify the time of administration and to refer to this information when looking up the drug to clarify any questions the patient may have about home administration of the drug.

6. *The right technique.* A medical assistant must be familiar with the proper techniques for all routes of administration. If you have any doubts about your ability to administer a particular drug, always ask for help.

7. *The right documentation.* Immediately after administering the drug, document the date and time of administration; the drug's name, strength, dose, and route of administration; any reactions the patient has to the medication; and the details of patient education about the drug. For parenteral medications, inspect the site of injection before administration for scarring, altered pigmentation, or any other indication of a possible problem with medication absorption. The exact site of administration must be charted. If the patient calls in for a prescription refill, document all pertinent information on the patient's chart as well. Procedures 35-1 and 35-2 present the safety measures to be followed in preparing and administering a medication and documenting it properly.

ADDITIONAL SAFETY STEPS FOR MEDICATION ADMINISTRATION

- Prepare medications in a quiet, well-lit area.
- Pay close attention to all the steps involved in dispensing drugs.
- Never substitute a drug or drug strength. Consult the physician for any discrepancy between the medication ordered and the medication available.
- Store medications as ordered on the package, and return containers to the proper storage area immediately after dispensing the dose.
- The person who administers the medication is responsible for any drug errors. Never administer a medication that you have not personally prepared.
- If ordered to prepare a medication for the physician to administer, place the container with the dispensed drug so that the physician can verify the seven rights.
- The physician should write every medication order before the medication is dispensed.
- Routinely check expiration dates when verifying the seven rights. Properly discard expired drugs.
- Discard medications with damaged labels to avoid errors caused by inaccurate reading of label information.
- If a medication is not administered after it is dispensed, discard it rather than returning it to the container.

- Before administering any medication, ask the patient about drug allergies. These can change over time.
- Patients should be observed for untoward effects for 20 to 30 minutes after a medication is administered. Any reactions must be reported to the physician and documented on the patient's chart.
- Always provide and document patient education about the medication, time of administration, side effects, and so on, when administering a drug.

CRITICAL THINKING APPLICATION   35-1

Dr. Thau asks Dorothy what safety precautions she would routinely follow when administering a dose of Plavix. Based on the information you have learned about safe drug administration, what steps should Dorothy follow in dispensing and administering the ordered medication?

Patient Assessment Factors

Although medications are given only under the direct order and supervision of the physician, the medical assistant is part of the assessment and problem-solving process. In medicine, assessment never ends, and it is never the responsibility of just one person. A physician gives the order to administer medication to a patient based on a medical assessment, but you must continue to assess the patient and the patient's environment as you follow through with that order. The physician depends on the medical assistant to be alert to patient changes or to new information that could mean that the use of a particular drug should be reconsidered. For example, perhaps the patient denied having any allergies to medications, but right before you administer an injection of penicillin, the patient mentions that she developed a rash after the last penicillin shot. You should stop right then and go back to the physician with this new information. It is vital to continuing patient safety that you assess the patient, the drug, and the environment before giving any medication.

Drug therapy should be based on a holistic approach to patient treatment. The patient is more than a particular disease. Many factors may have an impact on the patient's compliance with drug treatment, as well as the safety and effectiveness of medication therapy. The first step in holistic medication treatment is collecting a complete and accurate history. This includes gathering details about the patient's health history, current and past use of both prescription and over-the-counter (OTC) drugs, and any negative responses to medications, especially drug allergies. Every time a patient is seen in the office, he or she should be asked about drug allergies. Most medical practices have a specific place on the patient's chart to document drug allergies (e.g., in red ink in the upper right corner of each documentation sheet), as well as a special label on the front of the patient's chart that alerts the physician and staff to medication allergies. Electronic health records (EHRs) have a specific area on the chart for updating allergies. It is crucial that the physician have current and accurate information about drug allergies to prevent serious complications and possibly death.

Patient assessment does not end with the administration of the drug. Observe patients carefully for drug reactions after the administration of all medications, especially those that are injected. Patients

PROCEDURE 35-1

Administer Medications and Document Patient Care: Safety Measures in Preparing, Administering, and Documenting Medications

GOAL: To safely prepare, administer, and document completion of a medication order.

SCENARIO: Dr. Thau writes the following order: Administer Recombivax 10 mcg IM to Chris MacCarthy.

EQUIPMENT and SUPPLIES

- Written physician's order, including the drug name, strength, dose, and route of administration
- PDR
- Container of ordered medication
- Correct equipment for dispensing the drug
- Patient's medical record

PROCEDURAL STEPS

1. Read the order and clarify any questions with the physician.
2. If you are unfamiliar with the drug, refer to the PDR or the package insert to determine the purpose of the drug, common side effects, typical dose, and any pertinent precautions or contraindications. Recombivax is a hepatitis B immunization. Use the seven rights to prevent errors.
3. Take the written order with you to the medication room and compare the Recombivax label with the physician's order. Based on the information printed on the medication label, perform calculations needed to match the physician's order. Confirm the answer with the physician if you have any questions.
4. Dispense the medication in a well-lit, quiet area.
   PURPOSE: To prevent distractions and possible errors.
5. Sanitize your hands.
6. Compare the written order with the label on the multidose vial when you remove it from storage. Check the expiration date on the container and, if it was used previously, the date of first use; dispose of the medication if indicated.
   PURPOSE: To check the medication the first of three times.
7. Compare the order with the label on the multidose vial just before drawing up the medication into the appropriate syringe unit. Make sure the strength on the label matches the order or that you dispense the correctly calculated dose.
   PURPOSE: To check the medication the second of three times.

8. Compare the label and the physician's order before returning the vial to storage.
   PURPOSE: To check the medication the third of three times.
9. Greet and identify Chris by name and inform him you are going to administer a hepatitis B immunization.
   PURPOSE: To make sure you have the right patient.
10. Mention the name of the drug and why it is being given and ask the patient whether he is allergic to the medication.
    PURPOSE: To educate the patient about drug treatment and to verify that the patient is not allergic to the prescribed medication.
11. If necessary, help the patient into a sitting position.
12. Administer the medication into the left deltoid muscle using correct administration techniques and following OSHA precautions.
13. Conduct patient education on the purpose of the drug, typical side effects, and dosage and storage recommendations if appropriate. Consult the physician to clarify information if needed.
    PURPOSE: To ensure compliance with home drug therapy and to monitor for side effects.
14. The patient must remain in the office for 20 to 30 minutes after drug administration as a precaution against untoward effects.
15. If the patient experiences any discomfort after taking a medication, the physician should be notified immediately and the incident documented completely and accurately.
16. Sanitize your hands.
17. Document the administration of the drug, including the date and time; the drug name, dose, strength, and route of administration; any patient side effects; and patient education provided about the drug.

1/12/XX 11:22 AM Administered 10 mcg Recombivax to ① deltoid. Pt informed this is the first of 3 doses. No side effects noted. Appointment scheduled for patient to return in 1 mo for second dose. ———————————— D. Gaston, CMA (AAMA) _____

---

receiving penicillin (a drug with a high incidence of allergic response) or **immunotherapy** must remain in the office for 20 to 30 minutes after administration in case of an acute anaphylactic reaction. An acute anaphylactic reaction can result in respiratory failure and circulatory collapse within minutes if not reversed with epinephrine. Lesser allergic reactions that may occur include hives, swelling, and itching. The physician may order an antihistamine, such as diphenhydramine (Benadryl), if these reactions occur.

Because patient factors such as age, weight, and height may be used to determine the correct therapeutic dose, accurate recordings

of this information should be documented on the chart. As discussed in Chapter 33, chronic conditions, especially liver and kidney disease, may affect the body's ability to metabolize and excrete medications. Therefore, a complete and accurate medical history is crucial to patient safety.

Besides the patient's physical state, other holistic factors play a role in successful drug therapy. The patient must understand the drug regimen, may require family support to follow treatment guidelines, and must be able to afford the prescribed medication. Unless these criteria can be met, the patient may be unable to follow

Document Patient Care and Patient Education: Maintain Medication Records

GOAL: *To document completion of medication orders.*

SCENARIO: *Dr. Thau writes the following orders to control Mrs. Lange's hypertension:*

> *Lasix 20 mg PO qd*
> *Potassium chloride 20 mEq PO qd to Alice Lange*
> *You review the orders for clarification, complete the three label checks, confirm the identity of the patient, ask the patient about drug allergies, administer the medications as ordered, and answer the patient's questions about continuation of drug therapy at home. Now, you must document this process in the patient's medical record.*

EQUIPMENT and SUPPLIES

- Written physician's order, including the name, strength, dose, and route of administration of the medication ordered
- PDR
- Patient's medical record

PROCEDURAL STEPS

1. Greet and identify Mrs. Lange by name and inform her that you are going to administer a diuretic and a potassium supplement.
   <u>PURPOSE:</u> To make sure you have the right patient.
2. Mention the names of the drugs and why they are being given, and ask Mrs. Lange if she is allergic to the medication.
   <u>PURPOSE:</u> To educate the patient about drug treatment and to verify that the patient is not allergic to the prescribed medication. Follow office policy to update the patient's medical record about any newly reported medication allergies.
3. Sanitize your hands.
4. Administer the medications orally as ordered, making sure Mrs. Lange swallows the pills without difficulty.
5. Conduct patient education about the purpose of the drugs, typical side effects, and dosage and storage recommendations. Consult the physician to clarify information if needed.
   <u>PURPOSE:</u> To ensure compliance with home drug therapy and to monitor for side effects.
6. The patient must remain in the office for 20 to 30 minutes after drug administration as a precaution against untoward effects.
7. If the patient experiences any discomfort after taking a medication, the physician should be notified immediately and the incident documented completely and accurately.
8. Sanitize your hands.

9. Document the administration of the medications, including the date and time; the drug names, dose, strength, and route of administration; any patient side effects; and patient education provided about the drug.

Practice documenting the following orders:

1. Tylenol elixir 120 mg PO to Anthony Baker, 8 years old, for a fever

   _____

2. Gantrisin Pediatric 500 mg PO to Samantha Carpassi, 3 years old, for a urinary tract infection

   _____

3. Dilaudid cough syrup 2 mg PO to Roberto Alphonse, 43 years old, for bronchitis

   _____

4. Diflucan 400 mg PO loading dose to Anastasia Smith, 19 years old, for a vaginal yeast infection

   _____

   _____

4/02/XX 9:30 AM Administered Lasix 20 mg and potassium chloride 20 mEq PO without difficulty. Pt informed of importance of taking medications as prescribed for treatment of hypertension; warned she will have to urinate more frequently. No side effects noted. Appointment scheduled for patient to return in 1 mo for f/u. D. Gaston, CMA (AAMA) _____

---

through with the treatment protocol. It is important that the medical assistant investigate these issues and offer appropriate community support, if available, to help the patient maintain proper drug therapy.

Approaches to Special Patient Populations

Pregnant and breastfeeding women must be especially careful when taking OTC and prescription drugs, because medications are known to cross the placenta and may affect the developing fetus. A pregnant woman should not take any medication without the knowledge and

approval of her physician. As discussed in Chapter 33, the Food and Drug Administration (FDA) identifies five pregnancy risk categories of drugs. The medical assistant should be familiar with the specific drug category before administering any medication to a pregnant woman. Besides passing through the placenta, medications also are transmitted through breast milk. Therefore, similar precautions must be taken when the physician prescribes medications for a lactating mother.

As discussed in Chapter 34, special precautions must be followed in determining the correct dose of medication for children. Pediatric doses are determined primarily by the child's weight; therefore, it is important to measure and record the child's weight accurately at each office visit. A child's body manages drug absorption, distribution, metabolism, and excretion differently from an adult's body, and the physician considers these factors when prescribing pediatric doses.

Aging people also are more sensitive to the effects of medications, so certain factors must be considered when prescribing and administering drugs to this patient population. The metabolic rate typically slows with the aging process, resulting in increased susceptibility to a buildup of chemicals in the body that may lead to toxic conditions. Part of the normal aging process is loss of subcutaneous fat, which may affect the route of administration of some medications, especially parenteral sites. In addition, many elderly people have accompanying chronic diseases, such as circulatory, liver, or kidney disease, that may affect the distribution, metabolism, and excretion of medications. Geriatric patients frequently take multiple medications prescribed by more than one practitioner, which increases the risk of drug contraindications and interactions.

A holistic approach to aging patients should include a nutritional evaluation, because a poor diet or restricted fluid intake affects drug actions.

Another very real concern for aging patients is the cost of drug therapy. Many patients on fixed incomes may not be able to afford the ordered drug but hesitate to inform the physician of this problem. It may be up to the medical assistant to ask the patient about his or her ability to pay for the ordered medication and to offer available assistance for prescription drugs. This includes offering stocked drug samples with physician approval and/or investigating drug coverage offered by pharmaceutical companies.

SUGGESTIONS FOR SUCCESSFUL MEDICATION ADMINISTRATION TO CHILDREN

- Explain why the medication is needed and how it will make the child feel.
- Attempt to gain cooperation by getting down on the child's level and using a soft but firm voice.
- When possible, offer choices of care, such as, "Would you like your medicine in your right or left leg?"
- Divert the child to relieve stressful moments.
- If the child refuses to cooperate, get help as needed to restrain the child so the medication can be given safely.
- Encourage parents to participate as much as possible, and make sure that both parents and the child (if of an appropriate age) understand the prescribed drug therapy.
- Offer a "treat," such as a sticker, at the end of the visit.

GUIDELINES FOR ADMINISTRATION OF MEDICATION TO GERIATRIC PATIENTS

- Educate the patient and family about the purpose of the drug; the time, dose, and route of administration; and common side effects. Instructions should be written clearly for home reference.
- If the patient has difficulty swallowing the medication, crush (if allowed) the medication or mix it into applesauce or pudding.

- Encourage the patient to drink plenty of fluids (at least eight glasses of water per day) while taking the medication.
- Reinforce that the patient should take the medication as prescribed and should not skip or double doses.
- Request that patients bring to every physician visit all of the medications they are currently taking in their labeled containers, including OTCs, so a current medication record can be accurately maintained in the patient record.
- If patients are taking multiple medications, suggest the use of daily or weekly medication dispensers. These can be purchased in drugstores and restocked by family members on a weekly basis. It is safest if all prescriptions are filled at the same pharmacy so the pharmacist can keep track of possible drug interactions or contraindications.
- Encourage patients not to share or "save" medications. All leftover medications should be discarded to avoid use beyond the expiration date.

CRITICAL THINKING APPLICATION 35-2

Dr. Thau serves both pediatric and geriatric patients. Summarize key items that Dorothy should consider when administering medications to these specialty patient population groups.

Assessment of the Patient's Environment

The patient's surroundings affect the success of medication therapy. The patient may be uncooperative when you attempt to administer a medication (imagine a young child due for immunization updates), or the patient's family may protest the use of the drug. Administration of certain medications requires the presence of the physician. For example, because of the risk of anaphylactic shock, allergy injections should not be given unless a physician is in the facility. In addition, the environment must be safe for drug administration. Make sure the patient is comfortable and protected from accidental injury. If a patient is to receive an injection, take care to place the patient in a position that best exposes the site and protects the patient from injury in case he or she faints or has a drug reaction. If the patient is to take an oral medication with water, make sure he or she is seated in a position that prevents choking. Because any medication is potentially dangerous to a patient, emergency drugs must be readily available to counteract any adverse effects that might occur immediately after the administration of a medication. Emergency drugs should be in injectable form for rapid effect. Emergency carts typically include adrenergics (e.g., epinephrine), anticholinergics (e.g., atropine), bronchodilators, and histamine blockers. (The pharmaceutical management of emergencies is discussed in Chapter 36.)

The following section presents suggested questions that can be asked to obtain as much information as possible from the patient about medication therapy. Any information gathered should be included in your documentation.

Suggested Questions for Gathering Medication Information

- *What physician-prescribed drugs are you currently taking?* Record the names, doses, strengths, and routes of administration.

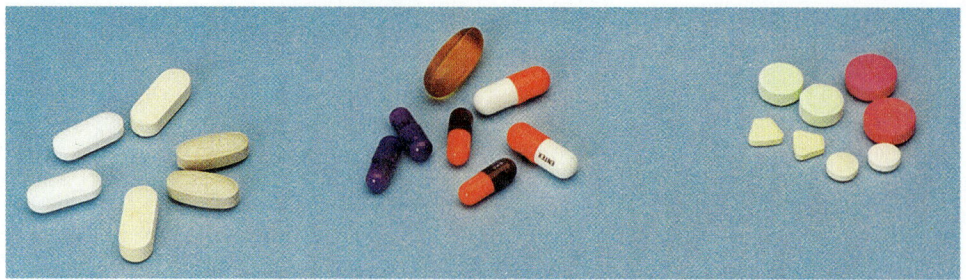

FIGURE 35-1 *Left to right,* Caplets, capsules, and tablets.

- *Do you take any OTC drugs on a regular basis?* Record the purpose, amount, and frequency of use. If appropriate, ask when the last dose was taken. For example, if a mother reports that her child has a fever but the temperature is normal at the time of the visit, perhaps she gave the child a dose of Tylenol before the visit.
- *What medications, including OTC drugs, have you taken over the past 6 months to 1 year, and why?* Ask this question to gather a history of medication use and perhaps to discover health problems that have not been recorded previously.
- *Do you regularly use any alternative or herbal products? What are they? How much do you use and how frequently are they used? For what purpose are they used?* Herbal products or alternative methods of treatment may interfere with prescribed medications.
- It is important that patients take their medications as prescribed, so focus a few questions on how currently prescribed drugs are taken. *What time of day do you take your medicine? How do you remember to take it? Are you having any problems or do you notice side effects from the medication? Can you afford to take the medication as prescribed? Are you having the desired response to the medication (e.g., pain relief, breathing better, lowered blood pressure)?*
- *Where do you store your medications at home?* Review any special storage precautions for prescribed drugs. Most medications should be stored away from any heat source and sunlight.
- *Have you checked the expiration dates on your containers?* Patients often neglect to dispose of unused medication and may take it after the expiration date if not informed of this precaution.
- *Can you tell me why you are taking the prescribed medication?* You should periodically check on the need for patient education about drug therapy. Patients are more likely to be compliant with treatment protocols if they understand the importance of taking the medication as prescribed.
- *Do you use the same pharmacy to fill all of your prescriptions?* Patients may see more than one physician. An excellent method of keeping track of all prescribed drugs, their contraindications, and possible drug-drug interactions is to strongly suggest that the patient use only one pharmacy. The pharmacist then can monitor overall medication safety.

DRUG FORMS AND ADMINISTRATION

As discussed in Chapter 33, the chosen route of drug administration determines the rate and intensity of the drug's effect. A drug prepared for one route but administered by another route may not have any effect at all and is potentially dangerous. Each route requires different dosage forms.

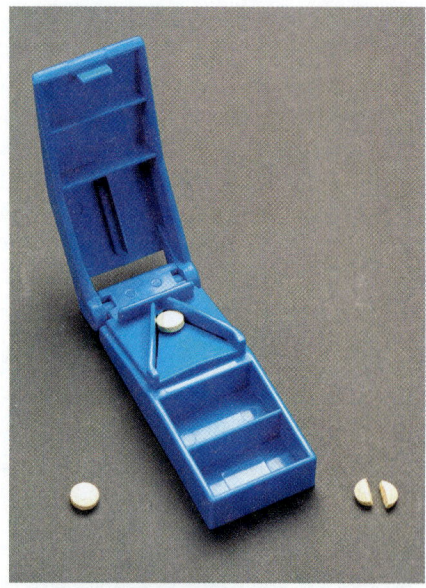

FIGURE 35-2 Pill cutter.

Solid Oral Dosage Forms

The basic forms for solid oral dosage are tablets, capsules, and lozenges (troches). Figure 35-1 depicts typical caplets, capsules, and tablets. Tablets are compressed powders or granules that, when wet, break apart in the stomach—or in the mouth if they are not swallowed quickly. Tablets may be sugar-coated to taste better, or enteric-coated (e.g., Ecotrin) to protect the stomach mucosa. Buffered tablets are also designed to prevent stomach irritation by combining the drug with a buffering agent that reduces the amount of acidity in the compound. Buffered or enteric-coated tablets should never be crushed or dissolved. Only **scored** tablets can be cut in half. This is accomplished with a pill cutter (Figure 35-2).

Some tablets are coated with a **volatile** liquid that helps the medication quickly dissolve in the mouth, such as certain antacid tablets and Claritin RediTabs, which are designed to dissolve on the tongue rather than to be swallowed. Caplets are tablets without a coating; they are solid and oblong, similar in shape to capsules.

Capsules are gelatin-coated and dissolve in the stomach, or they may be enteric-coated to protect them from stomach acids. Timed- or sustained-release (SR) capsules or spansules are designed to dissolve at different rates over a period of time to reduce the number of times a patient has to take a medication. These drugs should never be crushed or dissolved, because this negates their timed-release action. Another form of oral medication, the lozenge (or troche), is a flattened disk that is dissolved in the mouth to coat the throat, such as a lozenge for a sore throat.

Liquid Oral Dosage Forms

Many liquid forms of medication are available. They differ mainly in the type of substance used to dissolve the drug: water, oils, or alcohol.

A solution is a mixture of a liquid (usually water) and a powdered drug product (e.g., Amoxicillin solutions for pediatric patients). A solution separates if left standing, so you must shake the container before administering the medication. Liquid forms include the following:

- *Syrups:* A syrup is a solution of sugar and water, usually containing flavoring and medicinal substances. Cough syrups, such as Robitussin, are the most common.
- *Suspensions:* Suspensions are insoluble drug substances contained in a liquid. Examples include the following:
  - *Emulsions:* An emulsion is a mixture of oil and water that improves the taste of otherwise distasteful products (e.g., cod liver oil).
  - *Gels* and *magmas:* Gels and magmas consist of minerals suspended in water. Minerals settle; therefore, products containing minerals must be shaken before use. Milk of magnesia is an example.

A drug substance can be mixed with alcohol to enhance the drug's properties. Examples include the following:

- *Fluid extracts:* Fluid extracts are combinations of alcohol and vegetable products that are more potent than tinctures. For example, belladonna fluid extract has a higher percentage of the powdered belladonna leaf than tincture of belladonna.
- *Tinctures:* A tincture is an alcoholic preparation of a soluble drug or chemical substance, usually from plant sources. Examples include tincture of benzoin and tincture of iodine, which are applied externally.
- *Extracts:* Extracts are very concentrated combinations of vegetable products and alcohol or ether that are evaporated until a syrupy liquid, a solid mass, or powder is formed. Extracts are many times stronger than the crude drug.
- *Elixirs:* An elixir is an aromatic, alcoholic, sweetened preparation. Elixir of phenobarbital is one example; others include the alcoholic cough medicines terpin hydrate with codeine and plain elixir of codeine. Elixirs differ from tinctures in that they are sweetened. They should be used with caution in patients with diabetes or a history of alcohol abuse. Some pediatric medications retain the name *elixir,* although they no longer contain alcohol.

CRITICAL THINKING APPLICATION   35-3

Dorothy is ordered to administer a loading dose of cephalexin to a 17-year-old patient with acute bronchitis. The physician's order reads, "Administer cephalexin 500 mg cap PO stat." The patient is sent home with a prescription for Keflex, 250 mg cap q6h times 7 days. Document the details that should be included in Dorothy's note.

_____

_____

_____

Oral Administration

If the drug is not intended to coat the oral cavity or throat, oral medications should be taken with enough water to transport the drug to the stomach. Make sure the patient is able to swallow the medication. It may be helpful to place the medication on the back part of the tongue. Liquid medications are ideal for children. Solid drugs should not be administered to children until they reach the age at which they can safely swallow a solid drug form without the danger that they will aspirate the drug. Oral syringes are the best way to give liquid medications to children because there is less likelihood the medication will be spilled (Figure 35-3). Liquid medications, especially those that stain the teeth, can be taken through a straw. If the patient has been vomiting or is nauseated, an alternative route of administration may be necessary. Always remain with the patient until all of the medication has been swallowed. Procedure 35-3 outlines how to dispense and administer oral medications.

Mucous Membrane Forms

Some mucous membranes are selected for their ability to absorb medication for a systemic effect. The most commonly used areas are the gums, the cheeks (buccal), under the tongue (sublingual), the rectum, and the respiratory mucosa (inhalation). Nasal, ophthalmic, rectal, and vaginal preparations may also be applied to these mucous membranes for their localized effects. Inhalation drugs are discussed in Chapter 46.

Rectal Administration

The rectal mucosa allows rapid absorption of a drug, even though the surface of the rectum is small. Drugs are absorbed directly into the bloodstream without being altered, as they would be by the digestive processes, and without irritating the patient's gastric mucosa. Rectal medications are useful if the patient is nauseated, vomiting, or unconscious. For example, Tylenol or Compazine suppositories may be prescribed for a child who has fever, nausea, and vomiting. Manufacturers supply rectal medications in the form of

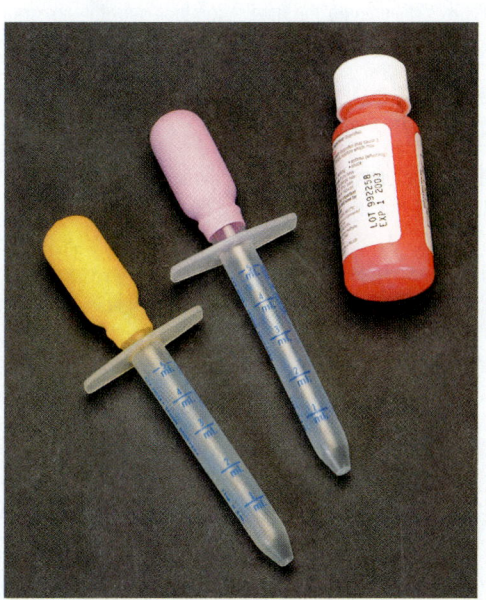

FIGURE 35-3 Sample oral syringes.

PROCEDURE 35-3

Administer Oral Medications

ORDER: *Administer hydrochlorothiazide (HydroDiuril) 100 mg PO tab stat for hypertension.*
GOAL: *To safely dispense, administer to a patient, and document the administration of an oral medication.*

EQUIPMENT and SUPPLIES

- Container of ordered medication
- Calibrated medication cup
- Written physician's order, including the drug name, strength, dose, and route
- Water if appropriate
- Patient's medical record

PROCEDURAL STEPS

1. Read the order and clarify any questions with the physician.
2. If you are unfamiliar with HydroDiuril, refer to the PDR or the package insert to determine the purpose of the drug, common side effects, typical dose, and any pertinent precautions or contraindications. Be prepared to answer any questions the patient may have about the medication. Use the seven rights to prevent errors.
3. Perform calculations needed to match the physician's order. Confirm the answer with the physician if you have any questions.
4. Dispense the medication in a well-lit, quiet area.
   PURPOSE: To prevent distractions and possible errors.
5. Sanitize your hands.
6. Compare the order with the label on the container of medicine when you remove it from storage. Check the expiration date on the container and dispose of the medication if it has expired.
   PURPOSE: To compare the medication label and the physician's order the first of three times.
7. Compare the order with the label on the container of medicine just before dispensing the ordered dose. Make sure the strength on the label matches the order or that you dispense the correctly calculated dose.
   PURPOSE: To compare the medication label and the physician's order the second of three times.

DISPENSING SOLID ORAL MEDICATIONS (HYDRODIURIL TABLET)

8. Gently tap the prescribed dose into the lid of the medication container. Do not touch the inside of the lid or the medication (Figure 1).

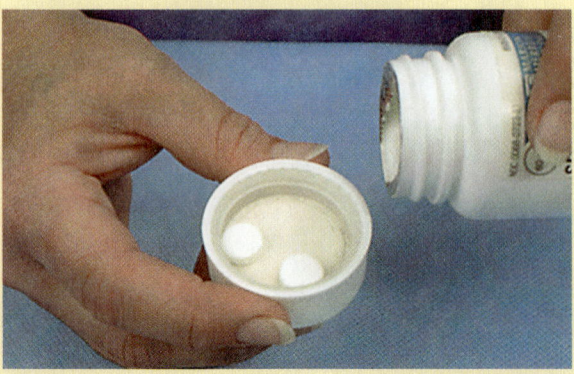

PURPOSE: Touching the medication or the inside of the container contaminates the drug.

9. Empty the medication in the container lid into a medicine cup.

DISPENSING LIQUID ORAL PREPARATIONS (HYDRODIURIL SOLUTION)

10. Mix medication well if required.
11. When liquid medications are poured, the label should be held in the palm of the hand.
    PURPOSE: To protect the label from medication spills. The medication must be discarded if staff members are unable to read the drug label clearly.
12. Place the medicine cup on a flat surface and, at eye level, pour the medication to the prescribed dose mark on the medicine cup (Figure 2).

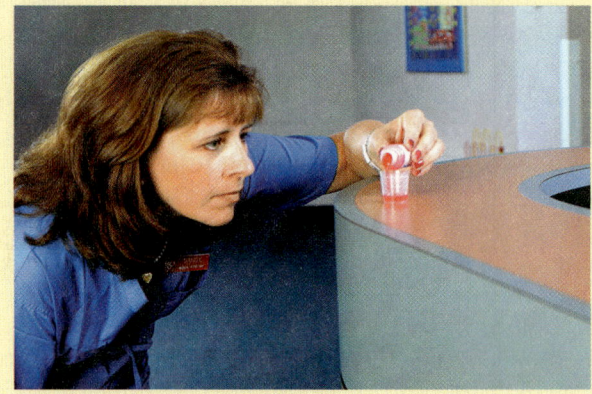

PURPOSE: At eye level, the base of the meniscus is where the prescribed dose should be measured.

FOR BOTH SOLID AND LIQUID ORAL MEDICATIONS

13. Recap the container and compare the label with the physician's order before replacing the container in storage.
    PURPOSE: To compare the medication label and the physician's order the third of three times.
14. Transport the medication to the patient.
15. Greet and identify the patient by name.
    PURPOSE: To make sure you have the right patient.
16. Mention the name of the drug and why it is being given and ask the patient whether she or he has any allergies to the medication.
    PURPOSE: To educate the patient about drug treatment and to verify that the patient is not allergic to the prescribed medication.
17. If necessary, help the patient into a sitting position.
18. Administer tablets, capsules, or caplets with water. If the patient is receiving liquid medication, offer water after the medication has been taken if appropriate. Make sure the patient swallows the entire dose.

19. Provide patient education about the purpose of the drug, typical side effects, and dosage and storage recommendations. Consult the physician to clarify information if needed.
    <u>PURPOSE:</u> To ensure compliance with home drug therapy and to monitor for side effects.
20. The patient must remain in the office for 20 to 30 minutes after drug administration as a precaution against untoward effects.
21. If the patient experiences any discomfort after taking a medication, the physician should be notified immediately and the incident documented completely and accurately.

22. Sanitize your hands.
23. Document the administration of the drug, including the date and time; the drug name, dose, strength, and route of administration; any patient side effects; and patient education provided about the drug.

6/8/XX 9:45 AM HydroDiuril 100 mg tab administered PO per physician order. Pt ed conducted; pt had no questions. Dorothy Gaston, CMA (AAMA) _____

---

gelatin- or cocoa butter–based suppositories, which melt in the warmth of the rectum and release the medication (Figure 35-4). Suppositories may also be used to soften the stool or to stimulate evacuation of the bowel; enemas are used to cleanse and evacuate the bowel.

The best time to administer a rectal drug intended for a systemic effect is after a bowel movement or enema. The patient should be cautioned to remain lying down for 20 to 30 minutes to prevent accidental evacuation of the drug. Of course, suppositories intended to treat constipation are administered to bring about bowel evacuation. The patient should be instructed to remove the outer wrapping and insert the suppository approximately 2 inches above the rectal sphincter muscles; a little mineral oil or vegetable oil may be used as a lubricant. If suppositories are individually wrapped in foil, make sure the patient knows that the foil is the wrapper and is not part of the treatment. Suppositories are typically stored in the refrigerator to keep them firm.

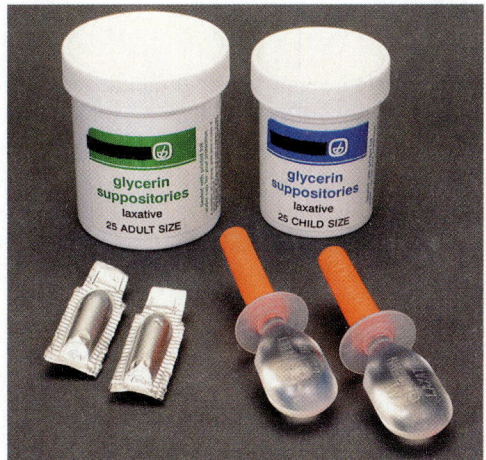

FIGURE 35-4 Sample rectal suppositories.

Vaginal Administration

Vaginal suppositories, tablets, creams, and fluid solutions are used to treat local infections. Irrigating solutions (douches) may be used as anti-infective treatments. Creams and foams are available as local contraceptives. Vaginal instillation is most effective if the patient remains lying down after administration to prevent leakage; many preparations, therefore, are intended to be used at bedtime. The patient may need to wear a pad to absorb drainage. Solid suppositories and tablets may be lubricated or moistened with water and inserted by hand or with an applicator. Creams are instilled with applicators. Prepackaged, disposable irrigation kits are available for douching.

When instructing patients, confirm that the patient can differentiate the urinary meatus from the vaginal orifice and the rectum. Mistakes could result in vaginal infections or in damage to or infection of the urinary tract. A simple drawing and explanation may be required.

Oral Administration

Mouth and throat agents come in the form of sprays, swabs, sublingual tablets, and buccal tablets. The mouth and throat membranes may be treated locally with antiseptics for oral hygiene and local infection, with anesthetics for pain relief, and with astringents that form a protective film over the mucous membranes. The patient may have to gargle, or the area may be painted or sprayed. To paint or spray the throat, first look for the area of inflammation to be treated. Otherwise, the part needing treatment may be missed entirely. Avoid touching the posterior pharynx (back of the throat); this causes gagging and possibly vomiting.

Sublingual (SL) tablets are placed under the tongue, where they are rapidly absorbed into the bloodstream by the rich supply of capillaries. Sublingual absorption is systemic and bypasses the acids in the stomach. Nitroglycerin, used for treating the chest pains of angina pectoris, may be administered sublingually. Patients should not chew or swallow sublingual medications. The patient should be instructed not to smoke, eat, or drink immediately before administration of these drugs. Buccal tablets are placed between the cheek and the upper molars and are quickly absorbed by the oral capillaries.

Nasal Administration

Nose drops and nasal sprays may be used for localized effect, but, like the inhalation drugs, they can spill over into the bloodstream. Some nasal preparations, such as decongestants, can cause an increased heart rate, elevated blood pressure, or central nervous system stimulation. Nasal medications are commonly used for blocked nasal passages (decongestants) and nosebleeds (hemostatics). Instillation of nasal medications is covered in Chapter 37. Nasal decongestant sprays are often misused by patients. Be sure to teach the patient not to exceed the amount or frequency ordered by the physician. If too much is used, these drugs can dry the mucosa and make congestion worse. Nasal inhalants can also be used for their systemic effect, such as the corticosteroid Flonase, which may be prescribed as part of asthmatic treatment.

Topical Forms

Topical drugs are prescribed for both local and systemic effects. Skin medication forms include lotions, liniments, ointments, and transdermal patches. The medical assistant should wear gloves when applying any topical treatment, to prevent self-administration of the drug.

Lotions

Often used to control itching, lotions are applied by dabbing with a soft cloth, a cotton ball, or a tongue blade. Calamine is an example. Some lotions are used to relieve inflammation and pain in muscles and joints. After the lotion has been applied, the area may be covered with a thick cloth to retain heat. However, the therapeutic value of these preparations is controversial. The effects of musculoskeletal lotions are limited to the skin surface where the medication is applied.

Liniments

Liniments (emulsions) have a higher portion of oil than lotions, and volatile active ingredients may be added. Liniments are often used to protect dried, cracked, or fissured skin.

Ointments

Ointments, such as bacitracin, are semisolid medications containing bases such as petrolatum and lanolin. An ointment should be removed from a jar or tube with a tongue blade to prevent contamination of the remaining medication.

Transdermal Patches

Certain medications can be absorbed slowly through the skin to create a constant, time-released systemic effect (Figure 35-5). The nitroglycerin patch is particularly useful for patients with frequent attacks of angina. Hormone patches, such as estrogen and testosterone, also can be absorbed slowly through the skin. With dermal patches, drugs can be administered in a time-released manner for as long as 7 days. The date and time the patch was applied should be written on the patch and documented in the patient's record.

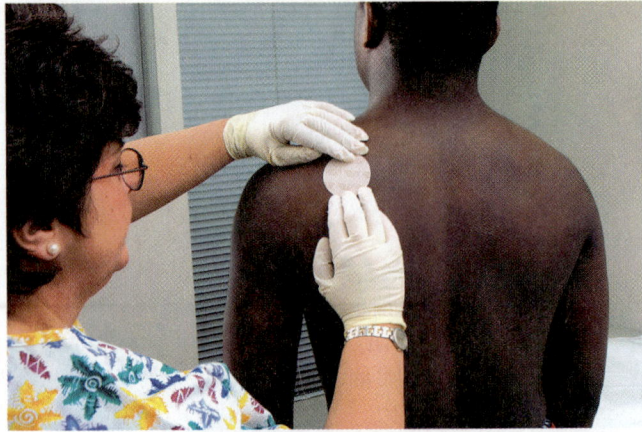

FIGURE 35-5 Transdermal patch.

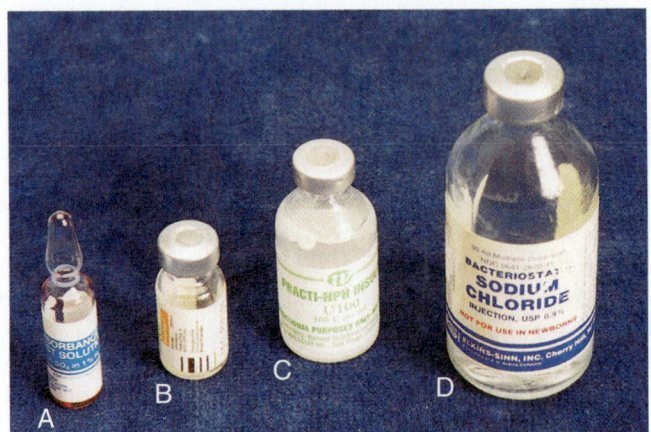

FIGURE 35-6 A, Ampule. B, Single-dose vial. C and D, Multidose vials.

- If the patch is to remain on for 24 hours for an extended number of days, apply a new patch at the same time every day and keep the old patch on for 30 minutes after applying the new patch to maintain therapeutic blood levels of the medication.
- Dispose of used patches appropriately, out of the reach of children or pets, because the old patch may still contain medication.

Parenteral Medication Forms

Injectable medications must be sterile and in liquid form. These medications may be supplied in an ampule, a single-dose vial, or a multidose vial (Figure 35-6). The drug usually is in a solution that is minimally irritating to human tissues (e.g., physiologic saline solution, sterile water) and may contain a preservative or a small amount of antibiotic to prevent bacterial growth in the vial. All injectable medications are dated. Before use, check the expiration date and examine the solution for possible deterioration. If the medication is discolored or if any sediment has formed at the bottom of the vial, the vial should be discarded. A parenteral medication is administered with a sterile syringe and needle. Occupational Safety and Health Administration (OSHA) guidelines must be followed when any sharp is used, including all types of needles, because every needle used on a patient is contaminated with blood and body fluids. The

PATIENT TEACHING RECOMMENDATIONS FOR TRANSDERMAL PATCHES

- The patient may shower with the patch in place.
- Rotate sites to prevent skin irritation. Follow package insert directions on where to apply the patch, avoiding scars and areas with a great deal of body hair.

medical assistant must wear disposable gloves when administering parenteral injections, must immediately dispose of the needle and syringe unit into a sharps container after use, and must never recap used needles.

Ampule

An *ampule* is a small, **hermetically sealed** glass flask that contains a single dose of medication. Its neck has a scored weak point where the ampule is broken just before use (Figure 35-6, *A*). Procedure 35-4 explains the special technique required for opening an ampule of medication and withdrawing medication for administration.

Single-Dose Vial

A single-dose vial is a small bottle with a rubber stopper through which a sterile needle is inserted to withdraw the single dose of medication inside. Before a sterile syringe and needle unit can be introduced into the solution, the rubber stopper must be wiped in a circular motion with alcohol or another suitable disinfectant (Procedure 35-5).

Multidose Vial

A multidose vial is a bottle with a rubber stopper that contains enough medication for multiple injections. The medical assistant should write on the bottle the date the first dose from a multidose

vial is used and should follow the manufacturer's guidelines or the facility's policy on how long the vial can remain on the shelf. Because multidose vials are used more than once, extreme caution must be taken every time a needle is inserted into the medication, to protect the medication from contamination, which could cause very serious infection in subsequent patients. If at any time you feel that an error has been made, or you suspect possible contamination, discard the vial. Never return unused medication to the vial. Learn to withdraw fluids to the correct mark. If you have more medication than you need in the syringe, eject the excess after you remove the unit from the vial.

Vials are vacuum sealed. Each time you withdraw medication from a vial, you first must replace the portion of withdrawn medication with the same portion of air. Not enough replaced air makes it difficult to withdraw medication, and too much replaced air increases pressure within the vial, forcing medication into the syringe. Procedure 35-5 describes how to safely and accurately withdraw medication from a vial.

Prefilled Syringe

A prefilled syringe is a sterile, disposable syringe and needle unit packaged by the manufacturer with a single dose of medication that is ready to administer. Some prefilled syringe units are designed to fit into a reusable cartridge injection system (Figure 35-7). Tubex

---

PROCEDURE 35-4

Administer Parenteral (Excluding IV) Medications: Fill a Syringe From an Ampule

GOAL: *To correctly and safely remove medication for administration from a glass ampule.*

EQUIPMENT and SUPPLIES

- Syringe and needle unit
- Medication ampule
- Filter needle
- Physician's order
- Sterile gauze squares
- Alcohol squares
- Sharps container
- Disposable gloves
- Biohazard waste container
- Patient's medical record

PROCEDURAL STEPS

1. Review the physician's medication order for clarity. If unfamiliar with the drug, look it up in a reference book.
   <u>PURPOSE:</u> The medical assistant should never dispense or administer a drug without making sure the physician's order is legible and the details of the drug are known.
2. Sanitize your hands and assemble the equipment.
3. Perform medication label and physician's order check when removing the ampule from storage. Check the expiration date on the ampule.
   <u>PURPOSE:</u> To complete the first check of the order. Dispose of any medication with an expiration date that has passed.

4. Gently tap the top of the ampule with your fingers to settle all the medication to the bottom portion of the flask (Figure 1).

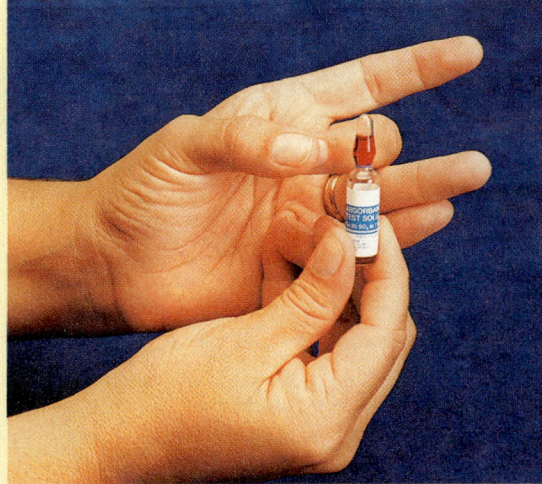

5. Thoroughly disinfect the neck of the ampule with alcohol squares. Check the label against the order a second time.
   <u>PURPOSE:</u> Disinfection prevents possible contamination of the medication.

6. Wrap the top of the ampule with a gauze square or alcohol swab to protect yourself from the glass. Hold the covered ampule between your thumb and finger, in front of you and above waist level (Figure 2).

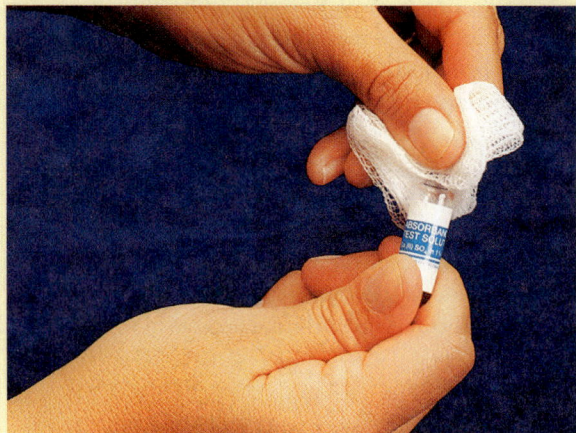

PURPOSE: To protect your fingers and maintain eye contact with the medication ampule at all times.

7. Push the top of the ampule away from your body to break the neck. You will hear a pop, because the ampule is vacuum sealed. The glass is designed not to shatter, and the medication will not spill out. Dispose of the gauze square and the glass top in the sharps container.

8. Open the sterile syringe and needle unit. Touching the needle covers only, unscrew the needle from the syringe, place it on the counter, and attach the sterile filter needle.
PURPOSE: To maintain the sterility of the unit, only the needle covers are touched. The filter needle is needed to withdraw the medication

from the ampule to prevent accidental aspiration of glass fragments into the injection unit.

9. Without touching the sides of the opened ampule, insert the syringe unit with the filter needle attached into the ampule and withdraw the ordered dose. Then recover the needle.
PURPOSE: Touching the needle with anything except the sterile interior of the ampule contaminates the needle. If this happens, start over again with a new filter needle.

10. Before discarding the ampule in the sharps container, check the physician's order against the label one more time to complete the three label checks. If you are drawing the medication up for the physician to administer, take the ampule and the syringe unit to the physician for the final safety check.

11. Change the filter needle, safeguarding the sterility of the injection unit, for a needle of the appropriate length and gauge based on the physician's ordered route of administration and patient characteristics. Discard the used filter needle into the sharps container.
PURPOSE: A new needle is used to prevent the possible injection of glass particles on or inside the filter needle.

12. Dispose of used alcohol and gauze squares.

13. Transport the ordered medication in the injection unit to the patient. Identify the patient. Put on gloves and administer the medication as ordered. Discard the used syringe unit into a sharps container in the patient room. Remove the gloves, discard them in a biohazard waste container, and sanitize your hands.

14. Answer any questions the patient has and document the procedure in the medical record.

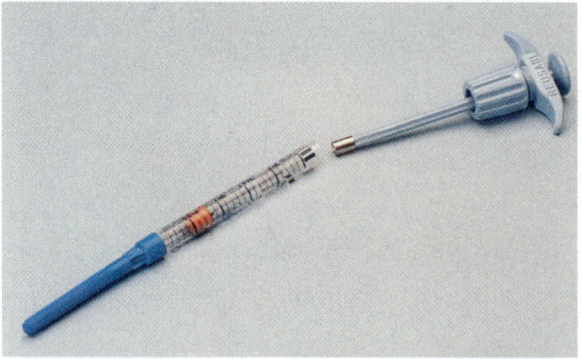

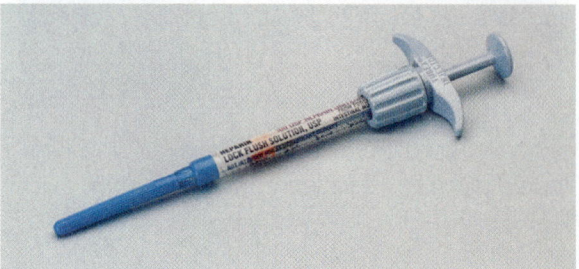

FIGURE 35-7 The Tubex injector system with disposable sterile medication cartridge.

and Carpuject are two examples of cartridge systems. Most prefilled syringe units are overfilled with medication or may contain more medication than was ordered by the physician. Before administration, carefully check the unit and expel any excess medication or air to make sure the patient receives an accurate dose.

Parenteral Medication Equipment

Syringes and needles are manufactured in countless varieties for specific purposes and sometimes for specific medications. For example, a special syringe unit used for insulin is calibrated in units of measurement and packaged with a micro-needle. Hypodermic needles are manufactured in many lengths and gauges, depending on the depth of the injection, the **viscosity** of the medication to be injected, the ordered route of administration, and patient characteristics. Needles may be purchased separately or as part of a needle-syringe unit. Figure 35-8 shows the parts of a needle and the three common types of **bevel** points. Needles are measured for length from the place where the cannula or shaft joins the hub to the tip of the point.

Needle Gauge

The diameter, or lumen size, of a needle is called its *gauge*. Needle gauges range in size from 14 (the largest) to 31 (the smallest). *The*

PROCEDURE 35-5

Administer Parenteral (Excluding IV) Medications: Fill a Syringe From a Vial

GOAL: *To fill a syringe from a multidose vial using sterile technique.*

EQUIPMENT and SUPPLIES

- Multidose vial containing the medication ordered
- Alcohol wipes
- Sterile needle and syringe unit
- Written physician's order, including the drug name, strength, and route of administration

PROCEDURAL STEPS

1. Sanitize your hands.
2. Read the order and choose the correct vial of medication.
   <u>PURPOSE:</u> To compare the medication label and physician's order the first of three times.
3. Choose the correct syringe and needle size, depending on the site, patient characteristics, and the amount of medication to be injected (Figure 1).

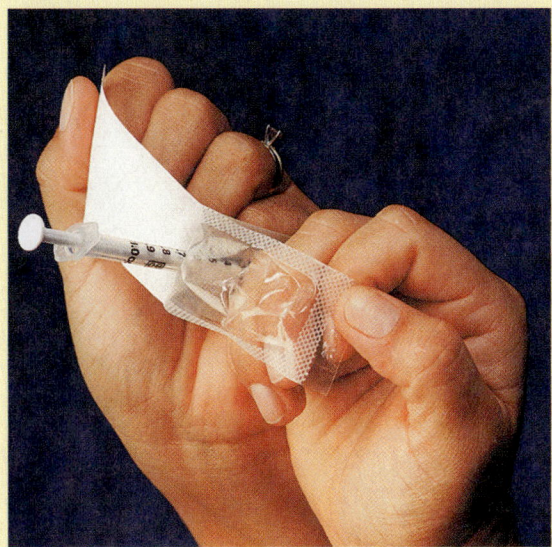

4. Compare the order with both the name of the drug on the vial of medication and the amount to be withdrawn in the syringe.
   <u>PURPOSE:</u> To compare the medication label and the physician's order the second of three times.

5. Gently agitate the medication by rolling the vial between your palms (Figure 2).

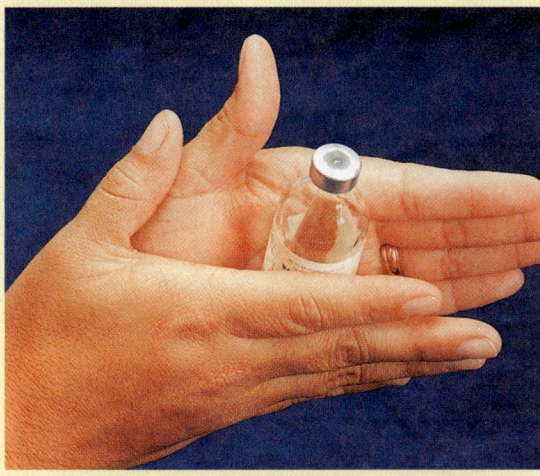

   <u>PURPOSE:</u> To mix any medication that may have settled.
6. Check the quality of the medication and the expiration date.
   <u>PURPOSE:</u> Dispose of the medication if it appears contaminated, contains sediment, or is outdated.
7. Clean the rubber stopper of the vial with the alcohol wipe using a circular motion (Figure 3). Place the vial on a secure, flat surface, leaving the alcohol swab over the rubber stopper.

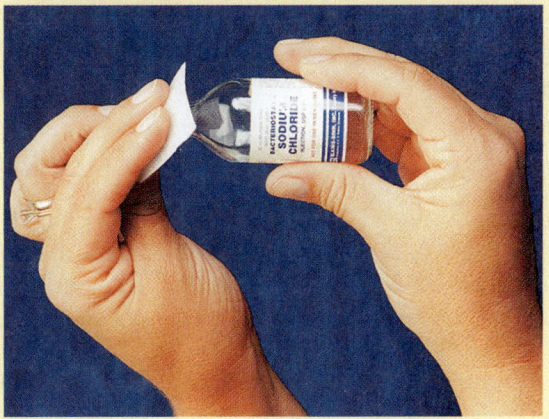

8. With the needle cover in place, grasp the syringe plunger and draw up an amount of air equal to the amount of medication ordered.
   <u>PURPOSE:</u> Not enough replaced air makes it difficult to withdraw the medication; too much replaced air increases the pressure in the vial so that medication is forced into the syringe without the plunger being pulled to withdraw it.

9. Remove the needle cover and insert the needle into the center of the rubber stopper. Hold the vial firmly against a flat surface and watch carefully that the needle touches only the cleaned rubber area.
   <u>PURPOSE:</u> To maintain the sterility of the needle.
10. Inject the aspirated air in the syringe into the vial.
11. Keeping the syringe unit in the vial, pick up and invert them (Figure 4). Slowly pull back on the plunger with the unit at eye level until the proper amount of medication has been withdrawn.

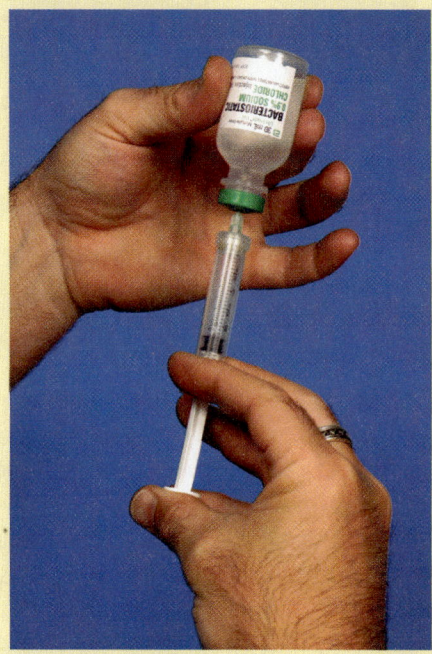

<u>PURPOSE:</u> Withdrawing medication rapidly causes air bubbles to form in the syringe.

12. While the needle is still in the vial, check that no air bubbles are in the syringe.
    <u>PURPOSE:</u> Air bubbles displace medication, and the patient will not receive the proper amount of medication.
13. If air bubbles are present, slip the fingers holding the vial down to grasp the vial and syringe as a single unit.
    <u>PURPOSE:</u> This frees your dominant hand.
14. With your free hand, tap the syringe until the air bubbles dislodge and float into the tip of the syringe.
15. Gently expel these tiny air bubbles through the needle, then continue withdrawing until the accurate amount of medication has been withdrawn.
16. Withdraw the needle from the vial and carefully replace the needle cover without letting the needle touch the outside of the cover.
17. Return the medication to the shelf or the refrigerator, checking that you have the correct drug and dosage.
    <u>PURPOSE:</u> This is the third of the three drug label and order checks.

larger the gauge number, the smaller is the diameter of the needle. Gauges 27 and 28 are used for intradermal (ID) injections, as is screening for tuberculosis (TB), when a very small opening is desired. These fine needle widths leave a small amount of medication just below the surface of the skin with a minimum amount of injury. Gauges 25 and 26 are commonly used for subcutaneous (SC) injections. Insulin needles may be as small as 31 gauge.

Medications in an **aqueous** solution and with low viscosity are easily injected through a small opening. In addition, these two gauges cause minimal tissue damage, and the patient experiences less pain. Larger needles (gauges 20 to 23) usually are necessary for intramuscular (IM) injection when the medication is thick (e.g., penicillin), or when the needle length requires the extra support of a thicker gauge. A patient cannot feel the difference between a 20- and a 22-gauge needle. In fact, the medication is not forced as strongly into the tissues with the larger 20-gauge needle as with the 22-gauge needle, and the patient actually experiences less pain. Needles larger than 20-gauge are not used for drug therapy. They are used mostly for venipuncture, blood donations, and blood transfusions.

Needle Length

Needle lengths range from ⅜ inch to 4 inches, depending on the area of the body to be injected, the patient's size, and the route (depth) used. ID injections require only the short ⅜-inch needle. Needles that are ½ or ⅝ inch long are used for SC injections. Longer needles are needed to deposit drugs intramuscularly. The choice of a 1-inch, 1½-inch, 2-inch, 2½-inch, or 3-inch length depends on both the muscle used and the patient's size.

Syringes

Parts of a syringe include the barrel, a calibrated scale (or scales), the flange, the plunger, and the tip (Figure 35-9). The typical syringe holds up to 3 mL and may be calibrated with two scales: milliliters (cubic centimeters), with each calibrated line marked at 0.1 mL, and minims. Larger syringes are calibrated in milliliters only. The

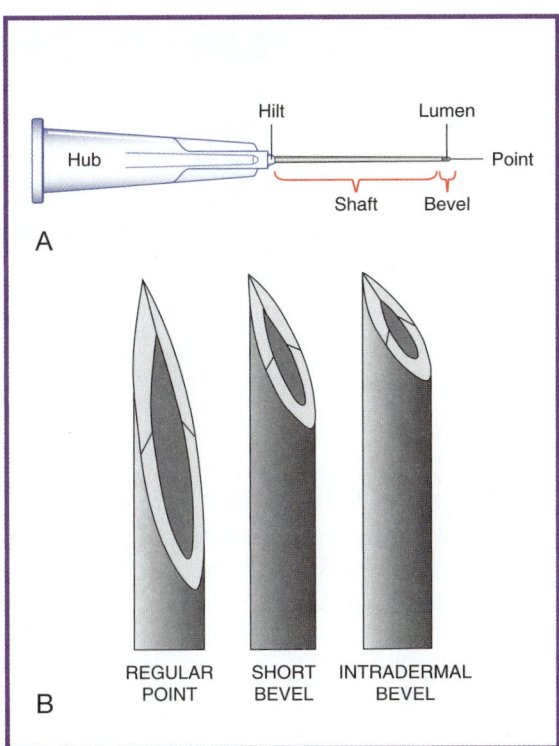

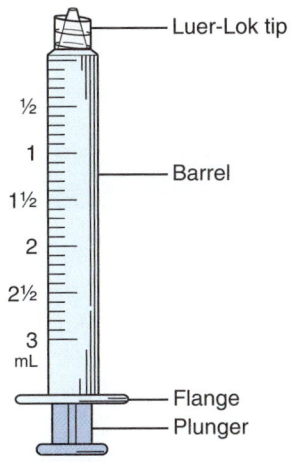

FIGURE 35-9 Parts of a syringe.

FIGURE 35-8 **A**, The construction of a hypodermic needle. **B**, Needle points. (**A** from Bonewit-West K: *Clinical procedures for medical assistants*, ed 6, Philadelphia, 2004, Saunders.)

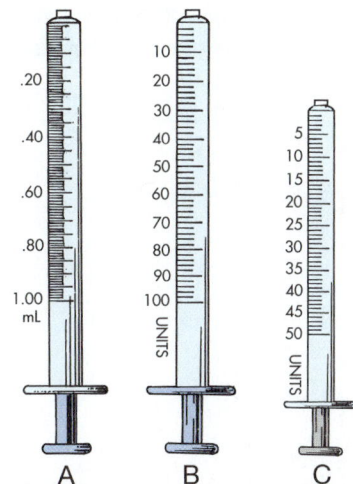

FIGURE 35-10 Types of syringes. **A**, 1-mL syringe. **B**, 100-unit insulin syringe. **C**, 50-unit insulin syringe. (From Perry AG, Potter PA: *Clinical nursing skills and techniques*, ed 6, St Louis, 2006, Mosby.)

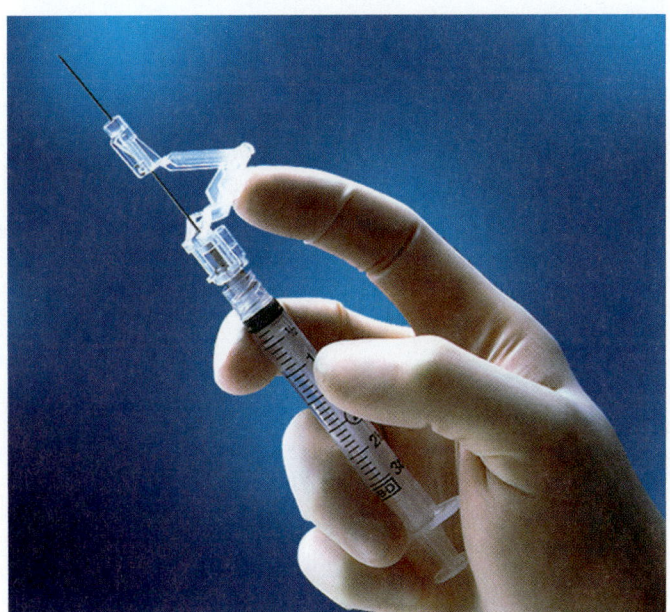

FIGURE 35-11 Disposable syringe with retractable needle cover.

tuberculin syringe, which is used for small amounts of drug, holds up to 1 mL of injectable material, and each calibrated line is marked at 0.01 mL (Figure 35-10, *A*).

The insulin syringe is calibrated in units specifically for the use of patients with diabetes. Insulin syringes are calibrated to hold 30 U, 50 U, or 100 U of insulin (Figures 35-10, *B* and *C*). The type of calibration chosen depends on the total amount of insulin to be injected in one dose. When less than 30 units is to be drawn up, the 30-U syringe should be used; for 30 to 50 units, the 50-U syringe is used; and for more than 50 units, the 100-U syringe is used.

Establishment of Standard Precautions and recognition of the danger of needlesticks prompted the development of syringes with retractable needle covers (Figures 35-11 and 35-12); these must

be made available to employees as an OSHA safeguard against accidental needlesticks.

Disposable syringe and needle units are packaged in sealed, rigid plastic containers or in peel-apart paper wrappers. Both individual needles and syringe-needle units are color-coded for easy identification. Table 35-1 summarizes the needle and syringe sizes used for injections.

TABLE 35-1 Needle and Syringe Sizes for Injection

ROUTE	GAUGE	LENGTH (IN)	SYRINGE
Intradermal	27-28	3/8	1 mL; tuberculin
Subcutaneous	25-26	1/2, 5/8	2 mL; insulin
Intramuscular	20-23	1-3	2-5 mL

EXAMPLE DEVICES WITH SAFETY FEATURES

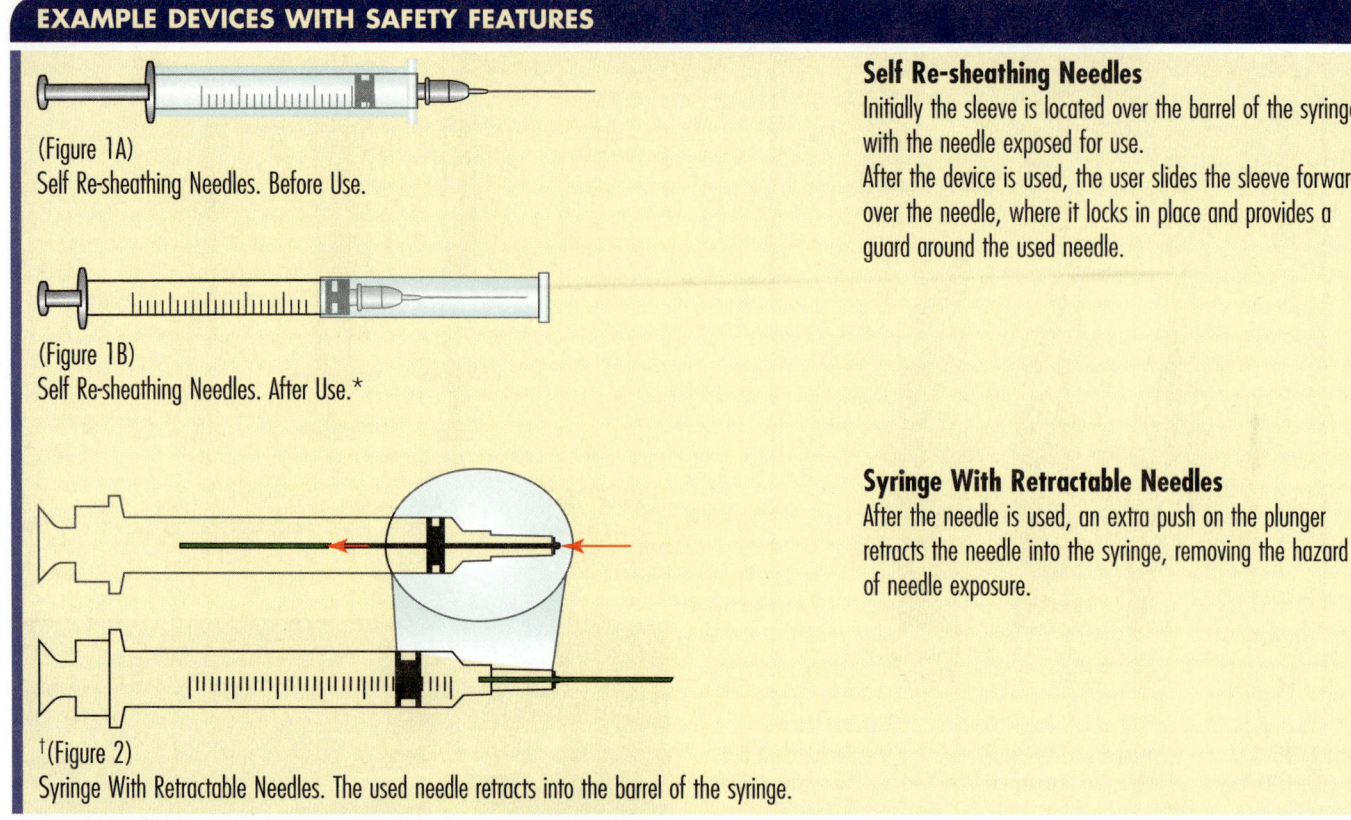

(Figure 1A)
Self Re-sheathing Needles. Before Use.

(Figure 1B)
Self Re-sheathing Needles. After Use.*

†(Figure 2)
Syringe With Retractable Needles. The used needle retracts into the barrel of the syringe.

Self Re-sheathing Needles
Initially the sleeve is located over the barrel of the syringe with the needle exposed for use.
After the device is used, the user slides the sleeve forward over the needle, where it locks in place and provides a guard around the used needle.

Syringe With Retractable Needles
After the needle is used, an extra push on the plunger retracts the needle into the syringe, removing the hazard of needle exposure.

From Occupational Safety and Health Administration, http://www.osha.gov/SLTC/etools/hospital/hazards/sharps/sharps.html#safer
*Please note that these safety devices lock in place and do not reset in actual use situations.
†Please note that these safety devices lock in place and do not reset in actual use situations.

FIGURE 35-12 Examples of safety needles.

Specialty Syringe Units

Because of concern about needlesticks, proper disposal of needles, and cross-contamination of individuals through needle misuse, devices now are available that do not require needle disposal; these can be used by patients who must give themselves injections away from home. An example of such a device is the injector pen. Different types are available, depending on the amount of medication to be dispensed per injection and the type of medication used. Administering insulin away from home has become easier with the development of the insulin pen (Figure 35-13), which contains a predetermined type and amount of insulin that can be injected with minimal preparation. (Different types of insulin are discussed in Chapter 45.)

The EpiPen is an automatic injector system that contains a dose of epinephrine (Figure 35-14). It must be prescribed by a physician and comes packaged with the correct dose for an adult (0.3 mg of epinephrine) or for a child (0.15 mg of epinephrine). The EpiPen is carried as a safety precaution by individuals who have anaphylactic reactions to such allergens as bee stings or certain types of foods. Anaphylactic reactions can be fatal if not treated immediately, so patients and their family members should be educated on the signs and symptoms of anaphylaxis and how to manage the EpiPen injection. The steps for EpiPen injection are quite simple:

1. Pull back the gray end of the autoinjector. This sets the device for use.

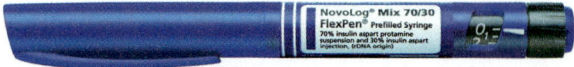

FIGURE 35-13 NovoPen.

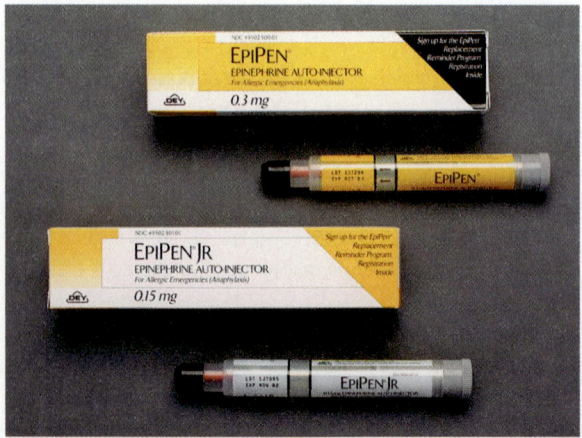

FIGURE 35-14 EpiPen prepackaged autoinjector.

2. The injector can go through clothing. Firmly press the black tip on the outer aspect of the thigh and hold in place for 10 seconds. The injector automatically administers the prepackaged dose.

3. Remove the EpiPen and massage the injection area for a few minutes to promote absorption of the epinephrine.

4. The patient still should call a physician or go to the emergency department of a nearby hospital for follow-up care.

It is important that patients or family members periodically check the expiration date of the autoinjector. If the device is near its expiration date, another prescription should be filled and the old, unused device discarded. To be of service in an emergency, the EpiPen must be readily available at all times.

SIGNS AND SYMPTOMS OF AN ANAPHYLACTIC REACTION

- Hypotension resulting from systemic vasodilation
- Hives, or *urticaria*
- Difficulty breathing *(dyspnea)*, resulting from bronchoconstriction
- Difficulty swallowing, as a result of edema
- Vomiting and diarrhea

Parenteral Administration

With practice, giving medications by injection becomes easy and even automatic. However, the medical assistant must always follow the physician's orders, perform the order and label checks while dispensing the medication, and strictly adhere to the seven rights throughout the procedure.

Practice developing techniques that provide maximum safety and comfort for the patient. Injections are least painful when the needle is inserted swiftly, the medication is injected slowly, and the needle is removed quickly, with counterpressure when needed. Remember that the same aseptic conditions necessary for minor surgery are necessary whenever you penetrate the protective skin barrier with an injection.

Never give an injection near bones or blood vessels. Avoid areas that have scar tissue; a change in skin pigmentation or texture; or excess tissue growth (e.g., a mole, a wart). The point of injection should be as far as possible from any major nerve, and the site selected should be capable of holding the amount of medication to be injected. Large doses of medication are given in muscle, because muscles have a larger tissue mass than SC tissue and a more extensive blood supply; these factors allow for faster absorption and systemic distribution.

Make sure all materials are ready for use. Many offices have a central room where medications are prepared. The medication then is taken to the waiting patient in another room. Handling medication administration in this way has many advantages, but care must be taken that the syringe and the needle unit are transported with sterile technique. After filling a syringe, replace the cap for transport to the patient, taking care to keep the needle sterile. Never transport more than one injection at a time unless two or more are for the same patient, or unless you have a special medication tray that has a named position for each syringe. Never combine two medications in a single syringe unless specifically ordered to do so

by the physician, and unless you have checked in the PDR or the medication package insert for contraindications on mixing different types of medications. If you are preparing a medication for the physician to give, place the vial or empty ampule beside the filled syringe. This shows what medication is in the syringe and offers a double-check for safety (see Procedure 35-5).

Some medications for injection are packaged in vials as sterile powders or crystals that must be mixed with sterile water or saline before they can be administered (see Chapter 34); the amount of solvent to be added to the dry form of the drug (solute) depends on the physician's order and the label directions. After calculating the correct amount of liquid that must be added to the dry form of the drug to create the dose ordered by the physician, follow the guidelines in Procedure 35-6 to prepare the drug and administer it to the patient.

GUIDELINES FOR PARENTERAL ADMINISTRATION OF MEDICATIONS

1. Use a professional approach and explain what you are going to do.
2. Small talk can keep the patient's mind off the procedure.
3. Never tell a patient that it will not hurt; you may destroy your credibility.
4. Make the patient as comfortable as possible, and allow for privacy.
5. Never allow the patient to stand during the procedure.
6. Keep the syringe unit out of the patient's sight as much as possible.
7. Always wear disposable gloves.
8. Immediately after the injection, cover the contaminated needle with the syringe unit safety device, and dispose of it in a sharps container.
9. *Never* recap a contaminated needle.
10. Sanitize your hands before and after the procedure.
11. Provide patient education as needed.
12. Document complete details about the procedure in the patient record.

Intradermal Injections

Intradermal injections are given within the skin layers (Figure 35-15 and Procedure 35-7). The ID site is used for allergy testing and tuberculin screening. The tine test is no longer used to screen for tuberculosis (TB), because it was found to be unreliable in diagnosing exposures to the TB bacillus. The Mantoux (purified protein derivative [PPD]) ID test now is used routinely to screen for TB exposure. It is the only widely used test for detecting **asymptomatic** TB infection, currently termed *latent tuberculosis infection* (LTBI). With the Mantoux test, a 0.1-mL solution of PPD is injected into the intradermal layers. If the person being tested was infected with the TB bacillus in the past, his or her immune system developed antibodies that recognize and fight the bacteria. When a PPD skin test is performed, these antibodies move to the injection site to try to stop the infection. This immune reaction causes swelling and **induration** in the area approximately 48 hours after administration of the skin test. An induration of 5 mm in diameter or larger is considered positive in patients at increased risk of being infected and in individuals who are most likely to develop active disease if infected

PROCEDURE 35-6

Administer Parenteral (Excluding IV) Medications: Reconstitute a Powdered Drug for Administration

GOAL: *To reconstitute a powdered drug for intramuscular injection as ordered by the physician.*

EQUIPMENT and SUPPLIES

- Vial containing the ordered powdered medication
- Diluent: sterile saline
- Alcohol wipes
- Cotton ball
- Two sterile needle and syringe units
- Disposable gloves
- Sharps container
- Written order, including the patient's name, when to give the drug, the route of administration, and the name and strength of the drug

PROCEDURAL STEPS

1. Sanitize your hands. Follow Standard Precautions.
2. Select the correct vial of powdered medication from the shelf and the recommended diluent for reconstitution. Perform the three drug label and physician's order checks during preparation and verify the seven rights throughout the procedure.
3. Read the label to determine the correct amount of diluent to add to create the dose ordered by the physician (see Chapter 34 for help with calculations). Calculate the correct dose, if necessary, and continue with the three label checks.
4. Remove the tops from each vial and clean each with an alcohol wipe. Leave the wipes in place on top of each vial.
5. Using one of the syringe units with the needle cover in place, grasp the syringe plunger and draw up the amount of air equal to the amount of diluent needed to reconstitute the drug.

PURPOSE: Not enough replaced air makes it difficult to withdraw the diluent; too much replaced air forces the diluent into the syringe without the plunger being pulled to withdraw it.

6. Remove the needle cover and insert the needle into the center of the rubber stopper of the diluent. Hold the vial firmly against a flat surface and watch carefully that the needle touches only the cleaned rubber area.
7. Inject the aspirated air in the syringe into the diluent vial.
8. Invert the diluent vial and aspirate the calculated or recommended amount of diluent.
9. Remove the needle from the diluent vial and inject the diluent into the center of the rubber stopper of the drug vial. Remove the needle from the vial and discard the syringe unit into the sharps container.

PURPOSE: An unused syringe unit should be used to administer the medication to the patient, because the needle on the used unit may not be as sharp as that on a new syringe unit.

10. Roll the vial with the drug and diluent mixture between the palms of your hands to mix it thoroughly. Do not shake the vial unless directed to do so on the drug label. When the medication is completely mixed, no residue or crystals are seen on the bottom of the vial.
11. Aspirate air into the second syringe unit that is equal to the calculated amount of medication to be administered.
12. Inject the air into the mixed drug vial, invert the vial, and withdraw the ordered amount of medication.
13. Proceed as outlined in steps 6 to 22 in Procedure 35-10 to administer the medication.

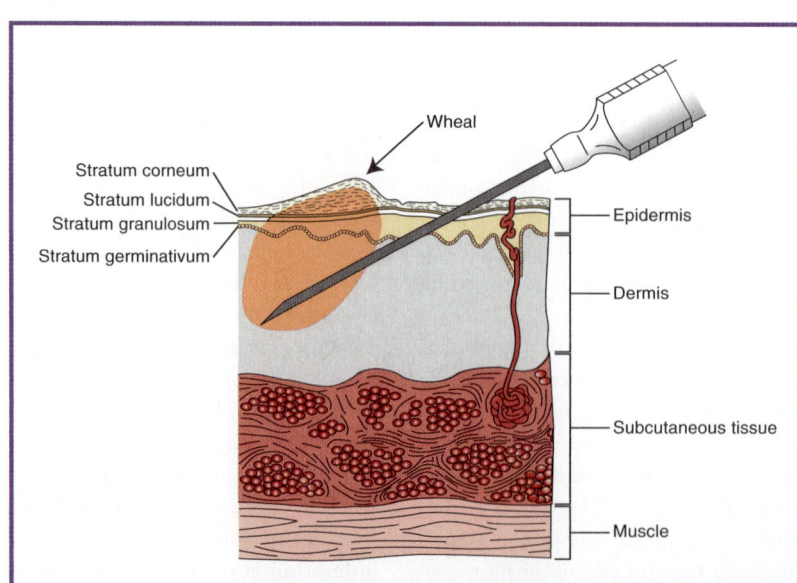

FIGURE 35-15 The intradermal injection is administered just under the epidermis. The drug is dispersed in an area where many nerves are present; therefore, it causes momentary burning or stinging. Minute amounts of medication are injected. This method is used to test for allergies, drug sensitivities, and susceptibility to some diseases.

PROCEDURE 35-7

Administer Parenteral (Excluding IV) Medications: Give an Intradermal Injection

ORDER: *Administer 0.1 mL PPD ID for a Mantoux test for TB screening.*
GOAL: *To inject 0.1 mL of purified protein derivative (PPD) ID to perform a Mantoux test as ordered by the physician.*

EQUIPMENT and SUPPLIES

- Vial of tuberculin PPD
- Alcohol wipes
- 27-gauge, ⅜-inch sterile needle and 1-mL syringe unit with safety needle cover device
- Physician's order, including the patient's name, when to give the drug, the route of administration, and the name and strength of the drug
- Disposable gloves
- Gauze squares
- Sharps container
- Patient's medical record
- Written patient instructions for follow-up

ORDER: *Administer 0.1 mL PPD ID for a Mantoux test for TB screening.*

PROCEDURAL STEPS

1. Sanitize your hands. Follow Standard Precautions.
2. Select the correct medication from the shelf or the refrigerator.
   PURPOSE: Some medications must be refrigerated.
3. Read the label to make sure you have the right drug (PPD) and the right strength. Perform the three label and order checks as the medication is dispensed.
   PURPOSE: Confirm that the medication label matches the physician's order. One medication may be manufactured and prepackaged in different strengths; for instance, an allergen may be available in 1:1,000, 1:100, and 1:10 dilutions.
4. Warm refrigerated medications by gently rolling the container between your palms.
5. Prepare the syringe as described in Procedure 35-5 and withdraw the correct dose of 0.1 mL.
6. Transport the medication to the patient.
7. Greet and identify the patient by name.
   PURPOSE: To make sure you have the right patient.
8. Ask the patient whether he or she has ever had a positive reaction to a PPD injection (TB test). If yes, report this information to the physician before administering the medication. An individual with a history of a positive PPD test result always has a positive result because of antibody action.
9. Put on gloves and position the patient comfortably.
   PURPOSE: To create a wheal successfully, it is easier if the patient is sitting and the medical assistant is lower than the patient (e.g., on a stool) with the anterior surface of the patient's arm extended straight out and angled downward.

10. Locate the antecubital space, then find a site several fingerwidths down the midanterior aspect of the forearm. Avoid any scarred, discolored, or pigmented areas.
11. Loosen the needle cover so that the needle can be picked up with one hand after the site is cleansed.
    PURPOSE: Once the site is grasped and cleaned, you must keep your hand in place on the patient's arm to avoid injecting the PPD solution into an area that was not cleansed with alcohol.
12. Wrap the thumb and the first two fingers of your nondominant hand around the patient's forearm, pulling downward and apart to stretch the skin of the forearm taut at the location of the injection.
    PURPOSE: Stretching the skin tightens the surface and facilitates insertion of the needle with minimum discomfort to the patient. The skin is not stretched tightly enough if it begins to wrinkle as you start to insert the needle.
13. Cleanse the patient's skin with an alcohol wipe using a circular motion, moving from the center outward (Figure 1).

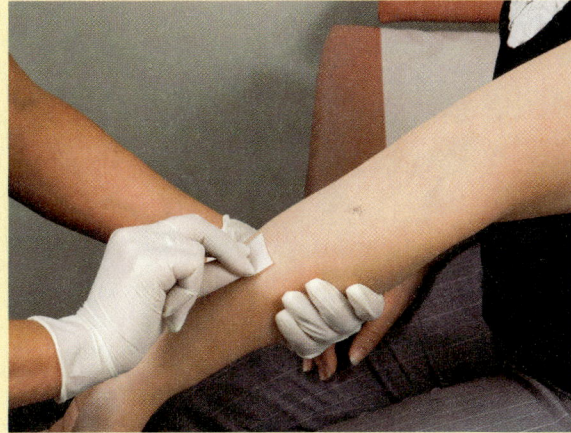

14. Allow the antiseptic to dry.
15. Pick up the syringe unit, shaking off the already loosened needle cover.
16. Wrap the thumb and first two fingers of your nondominant hand around the patient's forearm, pulling downward and apart to stretch the skin of the forearm taut at the location of the injection.
    PURPOSE: Stretching the skin tightens the surface and facilitates insertion of the needle with minimum discomfort to the patient. The skin is not stretched tightly enough if it begins to wrinkle as you start to insert the needle.
17. Grasp the syringe between the thumb and first two fingers of your dominant hand, palm down, with the needle bevel upward. Hold the syringe close to the plunger end.

18. At a 15-degree angle (Figure 2, *A*), with the syringe unit parallel to the surface of the skin, carefully insert the needle just until the bevel point is under the skin surface (Figure 2, *B*).

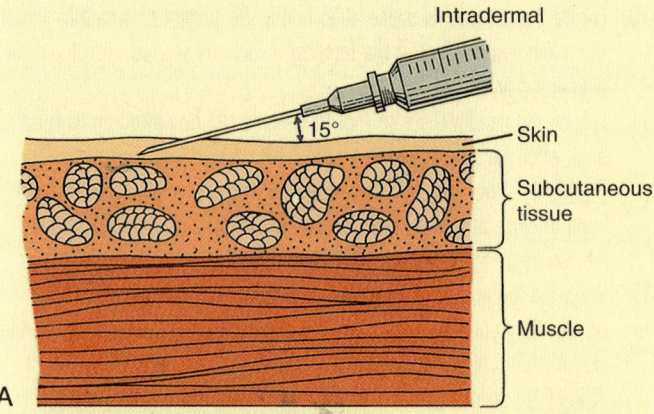

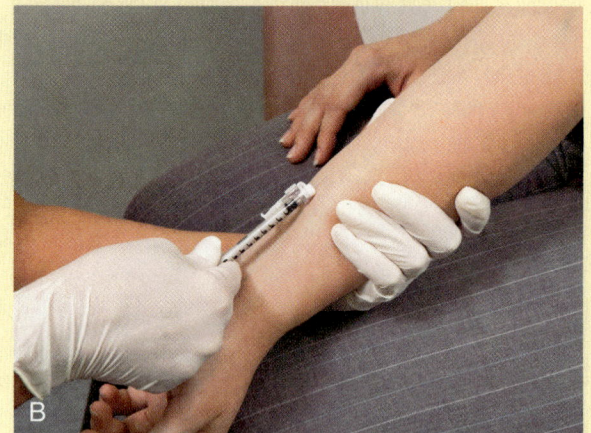

19. Slowly and steadily inject the medication by depressing the plunger with your ring or little finger. Do not aspirate. A wheal should appear.
    <u>PURPOSE:</u> A rapid injection may force the substance through to the surface.
20. After administering all of the medication (0.1 mL), withdraw the needle.
21. Immediately cover the contaminated needle with the syringe unit safety device and discard the unit in the sharps container.
22. Do not massage, but you may blot the area with a cotton ball or a gauze square. Do not cover the site with a bandage.
    <u>PURPOSE:</u> Massaging disturbs the wheal and interferes with the intended results.
23. Make sure your patient is comfortable and safe.
24. Observe the patient for any adverse reaction.
25. Dispose of the gloves in the biohazard container and sanitize your hands.
26. Record in the patient's medical record the procedure and any reactions that occurred at the site of the injection. Include the exact site of the injection.
    <u>PURPOSE:</u> A procedure is not considered done until it is recorded. The exact site must be known to monitor for reactions to the PPD in 48 to 72 hours.
27. Tell the patient when to return to the office for any reaction to be read.
    <u>PURPOSE:</u> Patient education must be provided to obtain intended results.

READING THE MANTOUX TEST RESULTS

28. Put on latex gloves; using good lighting and with the patient's arm slightly flexed, measure the induration at the site of the injection. Measure only the raised area; do not include any areas of inflammation (Figure 3).

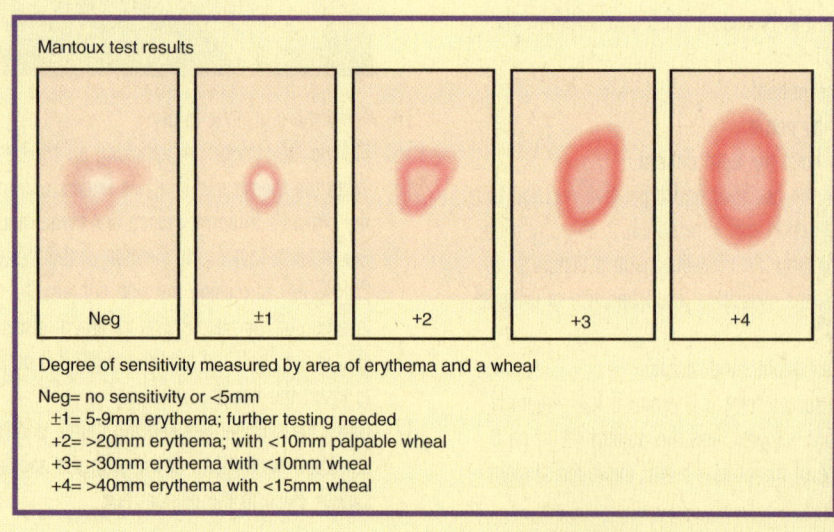

Mantoux test results

Neg   ±1   +2   +3   +4

Degree of sensitivity measured by area of erythema and a wheal

Neg= no sensitivity or <5mm
±1= 5-9mm erythema; further testing needed
+2= >20mm erythema; with <10mm palpable wheal
+3= >30mm erythema with <10mm wheal
+4= >40mm erythema with <15mm wheal

PROCEDURE 35-7—cont'd

PURPOSE: A positive Mantoux reaction occurs if the induration is inflamed, raised, and 15 mm or larger; an induration of 5 mm or larger is considered positive in patients with human immunodeficiency virus (HIV) infection, those in recent contact with a person who has TB, patients with a positive chest x-ray, those who have received organ transplants, and anyone who is immunosuppressed. An induration of 10 mm or larger is considered positive in recent immigrants, IV drug users, and children younger than 4 years of age. Further diagnostic tests are ordered to rule out or to confirm the diagnosis of tuberculosis (see Chapter 46).

29. Discard the gloves in the biohazard waste container and sanitize your hands.

30. Document in the patient's medical record the results of the Mantoux test, including a complete description of the size of the induration, if any, and the appearance of the test site. Notify the physician.

8/22/XX 9:10 AM Administered Mantoux TB test as ordered, 0.1 mL ID, lot #MF4780D, exp date 2/XX, to ® anterior forearm. Pt tolerated procedure well. No questions. Appointment made to return 8/24 for reading. Dorothy Gaston, CMA (AAMA) _____

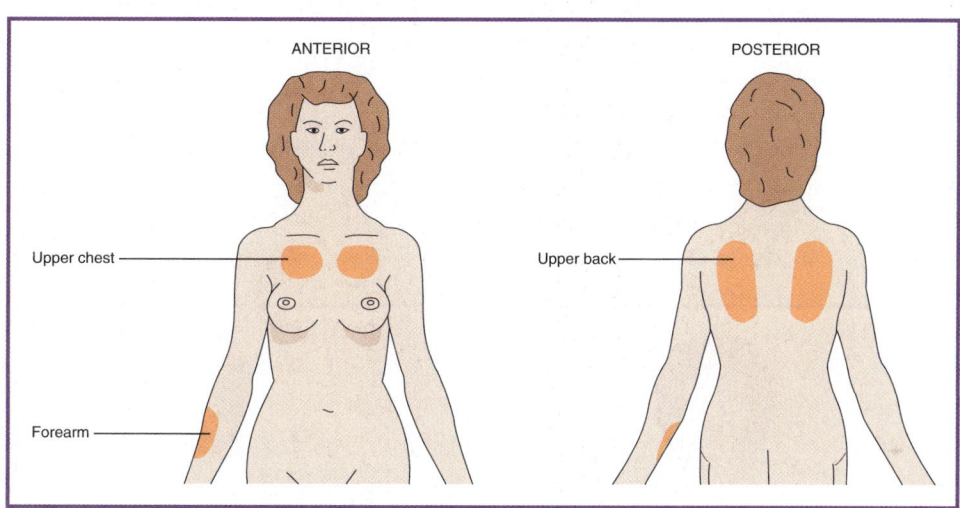

FIGURE 35-16 Sites recommended for intradermal injections.

with TB bacteria. This would include those infected with the human immunodeficiency virus (HIV); anyone in close contact with a newly diagnosed patient (e.g., family members); and patients who have undergone recent organ transplantation or are taking **immunosuppressant** medications. A 10-mm or greater induration is read as positive if the person has a moderate likelihood of TB exposure and infection, including recent immigrants from countries in which TB is prevalent; IV drug users; residents and employees of correctional institutions, homeless shelters, and healthcare facilities (including medical personnel); and children younger than 4 years of age. Regardless of risk factors, anyone with an induration of 15 mm or greater is considered positive. Patients must return to the office after the specified period for the staff to read the results (see Procedure 35-7, Figure 3). Many healthcare facilities now require employees to have a two-step tuberculin skin test (TST) to more accurately diagnose individuals who have been previously exposed to TB. The employee is tested as explained and then 48 to 72 hours later is retested. The first TST may be negative because the immune system did not immediately identify the TB bacillus. However, the second dose helps trigger the immune response and identifies individuals

who have been previously exposed to TB. (TB is discussed further in Chapter 46.)

When an ID injection is administered correctly, a small **wheal** is raised on the skin. A ⅜-inch, 27- or 28-gauge needle is used for ID injections. The angle of insertion is 15 degrees, almost parallel to the skin surface. The best site for injection is the center of the anterior forearm, but the upper chest and back are frequently used for allergy testing (Figure 35-16). (Allergy testing is discussed in Chapter 38.)

CRITICAL THINKING APPLICATION   35-4

Dorothy is ordered to give her first Mantoux test since being hired by Dr. Thau. Document the details that Dorothy should include in the patient's medical record. She administered 0.1 mL of PPD by ID injection into the patient's right midforearm and instructed the patient on when to return to the office to have the test read.

_____

_____

_____

Subcutaneous Injections

Subcutaneous injections are given between the epidermis and the muscle, into the fatty areolar layer called *adipose tissue* (Figure 35-17 and Procedure 35-8). Smaller doses of less irritating drugs (i.e., no more than 2 mL) are given by this method. A ½- to ⅝-inch, 25- or 26-gauge needle is used for SC injections. Insulin micro-needles are 31-gauge. The angle of insertion is 45 degrees; however, heparin and insulin may be administered at a 90-degree angle when a micro-needle is used or if the patient is obese. The posterior upper arm is the typical injection site, but the abdomen, the anterior aspect of the thighs, and the upper back may be used as well (Figure 35-18).

When multiple or frequent injections are ordered, as with routine insulin administration that requires the patient to receive up to four injections a day, the sites must be rotated to prevent tissue damage and problems with absorption of the medication. It is best to keep a rotation record (Figure 35-19). It might be helpful for patients to mark the site of the last injection with a spot bandage or a piece of tape. The easiest way to rotate sites is to give subsequent injections in a circular pattern around the site of the first injection in a particular location, such as the right anterior thigh. The goal is to avoid using the same location again for another month. Patients with diabetes typically have to administer two different types of insulin at one time. Procedure 35-9 explains how to perform this technique.

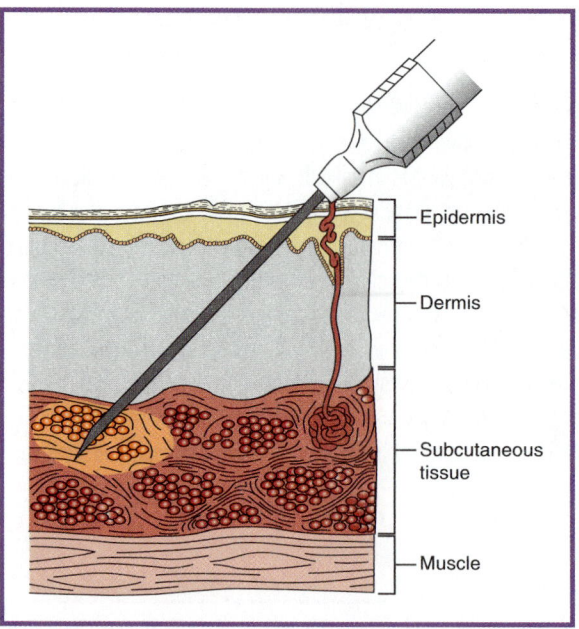

FIGURE 35-17 The subcutaneous injection is administered with a 25- or 26-gauge, ½- or ⅝-inch needle. The method is used for small amounts of nonirritating medications in aqueous solution. It is injected at a 45-degree angle (at a 90-degree angle for insulin and heparin). The most common site is the posterior upper arm.

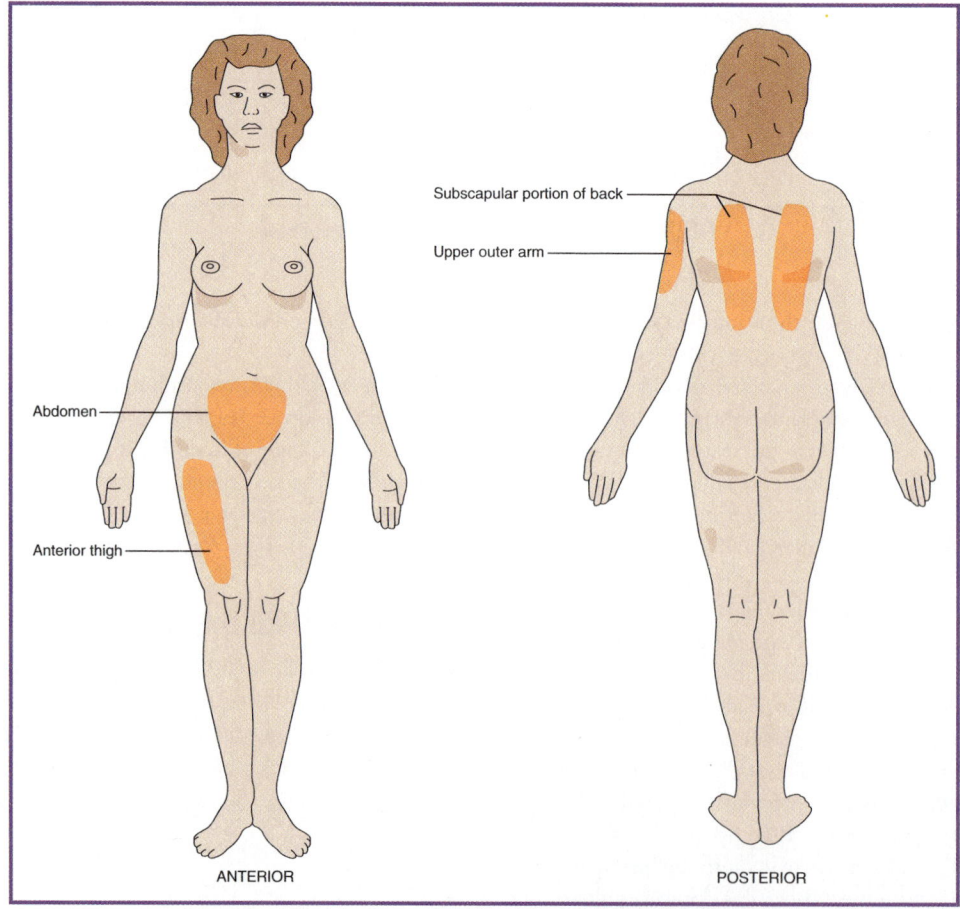

FIGURE 35-18 Areas of the body commonly used for subcutaneous injections.

Select the Proper Sites for Administering a Parenteral Medication: Give a Subcutaneous Injection

ORDER: *Administer 0.5 mL varicella vaccine SC stat to Mandy Leno, age 11.*
GOAL: *To inject 0.5 mL of medication into the subcutaneous tissue using a 25-gauge, ⅝-inch needle and syringe of correct size and type as directed by the physician.*

EQUIPMENT and SUPPLIES

- Vial of ordered medication
- Alcohol wipes
- Gauze squares or cotton balls
- A sterile needle and syringe unit with safety cover device
- Disposable gloves
- Sharps container
- A written order, including the patient's name, when to give the drug, the route of administration, and the name and strength of the drug
- Patient's medical record

PROCEDURAL STEPS

1. Sanitize your hands. Follow Standard Precautions.
2. Select the correct medication from the shelf or the refrigerator.
   PURPOSE: Some medications must be refrigerated or stored under special conditions.
3. Read the label to make sure you have the right drug and the right strength. Perform the three label and order checks while dispensing the medication and verify the seven rights. Perform any necessary dose calculations.
   PURPOSE: To promote safety and accuracy in drug therapy. One medication may be manufactured and prepackaged in different strengths. For instance, a particular drug may be available in vials of 250 mg/mL and 500 mg/mL.
4. Warm refrigerated medications by gently rolling the container between your palms.
5. Prepare the syringe and withdraw the correct dose.
6. Document the vaccine dose on the vaccination log. Each physician's office has a policy for vaccination documentation.
   PURPOSE: The immunization record or vaccination log must be completed each time a vaccine is administered. Information includes the manufacturer; batch and lot numbers, which are stamped on the container; expiration date; dose administered; route of administration; and whether a patient reaction occurred. (More details about immunization records are presented in Chapter 42.)
7. Transport the medication to the patient.
8. Greet and identify the patient by name. Explain the purpose of the immunization.
   PURPOSE: To make sure you have the right patient and to gain cooperation.
9. Ask the patient to sit upright and to help position her comfortably if necessary.
10. Expose the upper posterior arm.

11. Put on gloves, and with the thumb and fingers of your nondominant hand, grasp the tissue of the posterior upper arm. Cleanse the patient's skin with the antiseptic sponge, using a circular motion and moving outward from the center (Figure 1).

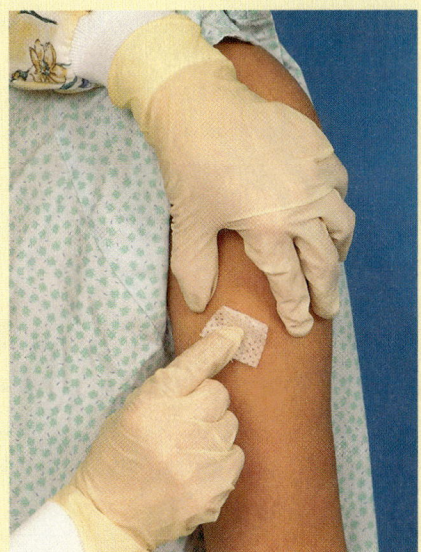

12. Remove the cap from the needle.
13. Hold the syringe between the thumb and the first two fingers of your dominant hand, and with one swift movement, insert the entire needle up to the hub at a 45-degree angle.
    PURPOSE: The depth of the injection is determined by the choice of needle length, not by how far you insert the needle. Once the needle is at the tissue layer, do not move the needle while injecting the medication.
14. Aspirate (except when administering heparin or insulin) by withdrawing the plunger slightly to be sure that no blood enters the syringe.
    PURPOSE: Blood in the syringe means that the needle is in a blood vessel and is not in the subcutaneous tissue.
15. If blood appears, immediately withdraw the unit without injecting the medication and dispose of it in the sharps container. Compress the injection site with an alcohol swab or gauze bandage.
    PURPOSE: To minimize bleeding and bruising.
16. Begin again with Step 1.
17. If no blood appears in the syringe, push in the plunger slowly and steadily until all medication has been administered.
    PURPOSE: A rapid injection may damage the tissues and may be uncomfortable for the patient.

PROCEDURE 35-8—cont'd

18. Place the gauze square next to the needle and withdraw it at the same angle of insertion. Immediately cover the contaminated needle with the syringe unit safety device and discard the unit in the sharps container.
19. Gently massage the site with the gauze square (do not massage insulin or heparin injections).
    PURPOSE: Massage helps increase absorption and reduce pain.
20. Make sure your patient is comfortable and safe.
21. Dispose of the gloves in the biohazard waste container and sanitize your hands.
22. Observe the patient for any adverse reaction. You may need to keep the patient under observation for 20 to 30 minutes.
23. Record the drug administration in the patient's medical record, including the exact injection site, and on the immunization record.

PURPOSE: A procedure is not considered done until it is recorded. It is important to keep an accurate record of vaccines administered. Include in the documentation the name of the vaccine, dose, route of administration and location, lot number, and any observed patient reactions. The caregiver must be given a Vaccine Information Sheet (VIS), and it must be documented that the VIS was received.

6/14/XX 11:35 AM 0.5 mL varicella virus vaccine administered SQ to ® posterior upper arm, lot #V5829K, exp date 9/xx. VIS form given to mother. She had no questions. Pt tolerated procedure well. ———————— Dorothy Gaston, CMA (AAM) _____

PROCEDURE 35-9

Administer Parenteral (Excluding IV) Medications: Mix Two Different Types of Insulin in One Syringe

ORDER: *Administer 5 U of Lispro and 15 U NPH insulin to Gregor Thomas stat.*
GOAL: *To mix two different types of insulin from two different multidose vials in one injection unit for administration.*

EQUIPMENT and SUPPLIES

- Multidose vial of Lispro insulin
- Multidose vial of NPH insulin
- Alcohol wipes
- Gauze squares or cotton balls
- Sterile needle and insulin syringe unit with safety cover device (because the total amount of insulin ordered is 20 U, use a 30-U insulin syringe)
- Disposable gloves
- Sharps container
- A written order, including the patient's name, when to give the drug, the route of administration, and the name and strength of the drug
- Patient's medical record

PROCEDURAL STEPS

1. Sanitize your hands. Follow Standard Precautions.
2. Select the correct multidose vials of insulin from the refrigerator.
   PURPOSE: Insulin is always stored in the refrigerator.
3. Read the label to make sure you have the right types of insulin. Perform the three label and order checks for each vial while dispensing the medication and verify the seven rights.
   PURPOSE: To promote safety and accuracy in drug therapy.

4. Inspect the appearance of the medication in each vial. Lispro and Regular insulin are clear and colorless. NPH is opaque or cloudy and colorless.
   PURPOSE: To make sure the Lispro vial is not contaminated with NPH. If the Lispro vial is cloudy, or if either vial has sediment in the mixture, dispose of the contaminated vial or vials.
5. Mix the insulin vials by gently rolling the containers between your palms.
   PURPOSE: Mixing ensures an equal concentration of medication throughout the vial. Shaking insulin vials can turn the medication frothy, making it difficult to measure the dose accurately.
6. Check to make sure the total amount of insulin ordered is less than the insulin syringe chosen.
   PURPOSE: Insulin syringes are available in 30-U, 50-U, and 100-U calibrations. The total amount of insulin ordered in this case is 20 units, so the 30-U syringe is the most appropriate.
7. Clean the tops of each vial with individual alcohol wipes, leaving the wipe on the top of each vial.
   PURPOSE: To disinfect the top of each vial before drawing up the ordered dose.

PROCEDURE 35-9—cont'd

8. Remove the alcohol swab and inject 15 units of air into the NPH vial, being careful not to touch the insulin in the vial with the needle, and withdraw the needle (Figure 1).

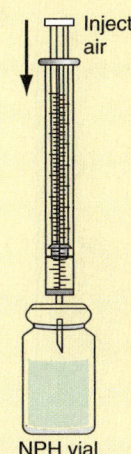

Inject air

NPH vial

PURPOSE: The NPH dose is drawn up last to avoid adding NPH insulin to the Lispro vial. Inject air into the vial before drawing up the Lispro order so that it is ready for dispensing. Touching the NPH insulin with the needle contaminates the Lispro vial.

9. Remove the alcohol swab and inject 5 units of air into the Lispro vial, keeping the needle in the vial (Figure 2). Invert the vial and withdraw the ordered dose of 5 U (Figure 3).

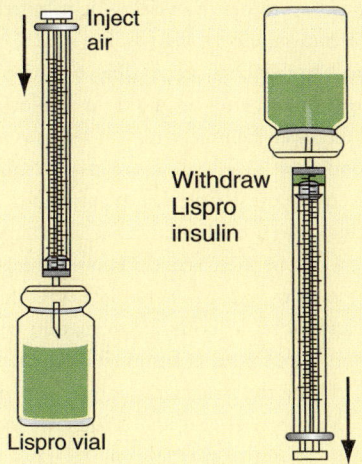

Inject air

Withdraw Lispro insulin

Lispro vial

10. Reinsert the needle into the NPH vial and carefully withdraw the ordered 15-U dose (Figure 4).

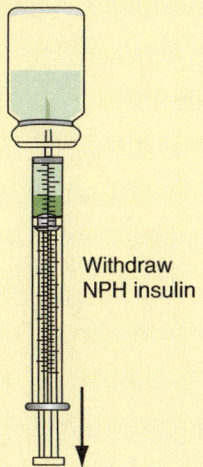

Withdraw NPH insulin

11. Complete the final label check and return the two insulin vials to the refrigerator.
12. Transport the syringe unit to the patient.
13. Administer the medication according to the steps explained in Procedure 35-8, Steps 8 through 13. If a micro-needle is used, insulin can be administered at a 90-degree angle.
14. Do not aspirate when administering insulin.
15. Immediately cover the contaminated needle with the syringe unit safety device and discard the unit in the sharps container.
16. Do not massage the site after administration.
    PURPOSE: Massage promotes blood flow to the site, which increases the rate of absorption. Different types of insulin are designed to be distributed at a varied rate to maintain coverage for the patient throughout the day.
17. Make sure the patient is comfortable and safe.
18. Dispose of the gloves in the biohazard waste container and sanitize your hands.
19. Observe the patient for any adverse reaction. You may need to keep the patient under observation for 20 to 30 minutes.
20. Record the drug administration in the patient's medical record, including the exact injection site.
    PURPOSE: A procedure is not considered done until it is recorded. It is important to keep an accurate record of all medications administered.

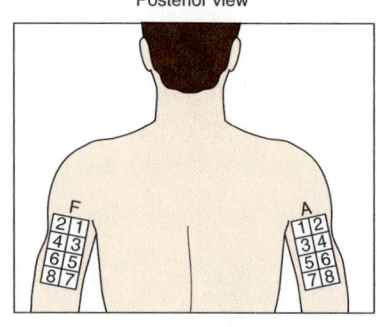

Posterior view

Anterior view

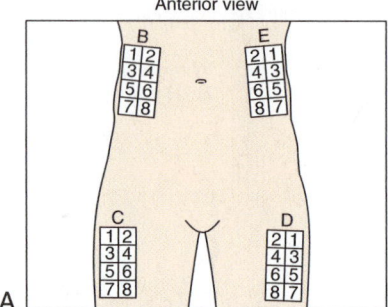

INJECTION LOG

SITE		1	2	3	4	5	6	7	8
Right arm	A								
Right abdomen	B								
Right thigh	C								
Left thigh	D								
Left abdomen	E								
Left arm	F								

B

FIGURE 35-19 **A**, Rotation sites for insulin injections. **B**, Rotation log.

INSULIN ADMINISTRATION GUIDELINES

- Typically more than one type of insulin is ordered for immediate administration. Check labels carefully, and follow office policy when mixing insulins in the same syringe. Not all insulin products can be mixed.
- Diabetes mellitus is discussed in detail in Chapter 45. Refer to Procedure 35-9 for details on how to mix two different types of insulin in one syringe.
- Insulin is always ordered in unit amounts. Use the appropriate insulin syringe—30 U, 50 U, or 100 U—depending on the total amount of insulin ordered.
- Insulin should be stored in the refrigerator and gently rotated between hands to warm before dispensing.
- Do not massage the site after injection.

Intramuscular Injections

Injections are given into muscle if the drug would irritate the SC tissues, if more rapid absorption is desired, or if a large volume of medication is to be injected. The angle of insertion is 90 degrees (Figure 35-20), and the preferred sites in an adult are the vastus lateralis, deltoid, ventrogluteal, and gluteus medius muscles (Figure

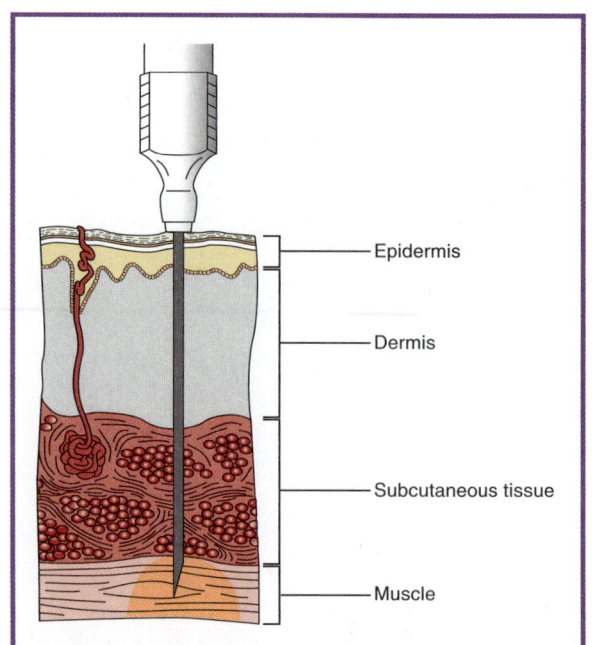

FIGURE 35-20 Anatomic illustration of the intramuscular injection. Note that the needle is inserted at a 90-degree angle, which deposits the medication into the large central part of the muscle.

35-21); in an infant or child, the preferred site is the vastus lateralis. It is important to select a needle that is long enough, especially for obese patients, to ensure that the medication is injected into the muscle and is not deposited in the upper adipose tissue. Fatty tissue does not absorb medication well, and the medication may remain at the site of the injection rather than being distributed systemically as intended. The recommended gauge is 20 to 23, and the needle length should be 1 to 3 inches, depending on the patient's size.

In adults, the deltoid region can hold up to 2 mL of medication, and the vastus lateralis and gluteal sites can hold up to 5 mL. Infants and children should be given no more than 2 mL in the vastus lateralis or the ventrogluteal site. The most important criterion in choosing an IM site is to use one that is not near large nerves, bones, or blood vessels. If any of these structures are damaged by the injection, the patient may experience nerve injury with lingering pain, or may develop an abscess or bone inflammation with infection.

When locating a site for an IM injection, expose the site so that you can see and palpate the landmarks correctly. If the patient must receive repeated IM injections, the sites should be rotated to prevent damage to the muscle and to surrounding tissues.

Deltoid Site. The deltoid muscle, the muscular cap of the shoulder, is located at the top of the upper arm. The muscle mass is somewhat limited, so it can hold only 1 to 2 mL of medication. This triangular muscle is located between the acromion and the deltoid tuberosities, and the injection site is approximately 2 fingerbreadths below the acromial process (Figure 35-22). The major nerves and blood vessels, especially the radial nerve and artery, must be avoided. Aqueous medications, such as vitamin B_{12}, are most appropriate here; hepatitis B and flu vaccines are also given in the deltoid.

If frequent injections are ordered, rotate the site and alternate the right and left arms. The deltoid site is acceptable for adults and older children, but it should not be used when the muscle is small or underdeveloped. For a small arm, you may need only a 25-gauge, ⅝-inch needle; the 23-gauge, 1-inch needle most often is used for

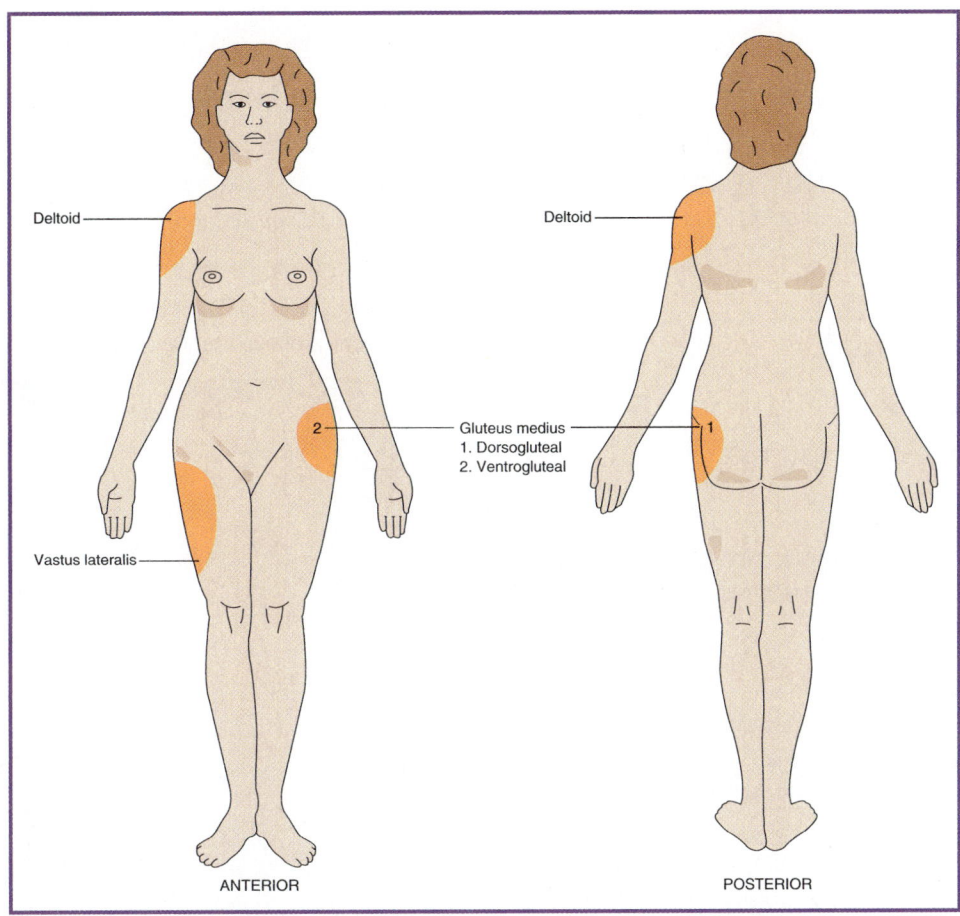

FIGURE 35-21 The muscles commonly used for intramuscular injection.

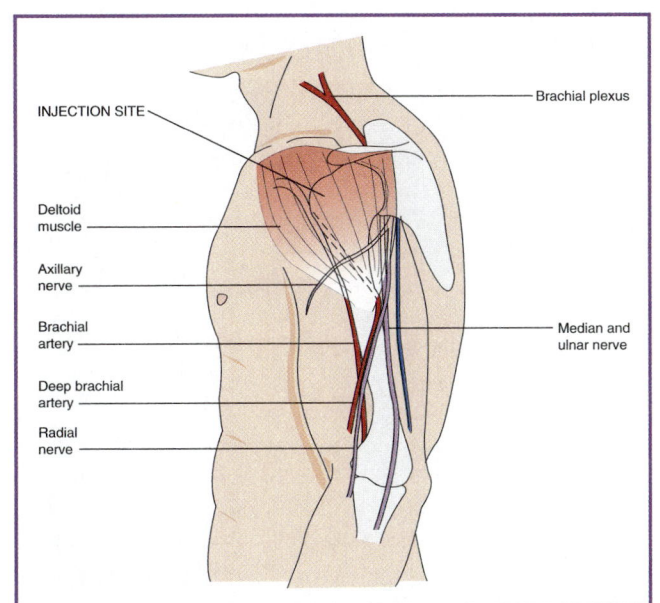

FIGURE 35-22 The deltoid muscle intramuscular site. This site is not recommended for infants, because the muscle is not well developed until later in childhood.

an arm of average size. The patient may be seated or lying down. When injecting, expose the entire shoulder rather than rolling up the sleeve. Rest the palm of your hand across the shoulder, and grasp the muscle before injecting the medication at a 90-degree angle (Procedure 35-10).

Vastus Lateralis (Thigh) Site. The vastus lateralis muscle is part of the quadriceps group of the thigh. It is one of the body's largest muscles, and because it is developed at birth, it is considered the safest IM injection site for infants. Many experts believe that as a site for adult IM injections, the vastus lateralis is better than the deltoid or the dorsogluteal sites, because fewer major nerves and blood vessels are in the vastus lateralis. The vastus lateralis muscle fills the midportion of the upper, outer thigh. In an adult, it can be located from 1 handwidth below the proximal end of the greater trochanter to 1 handwidth above the top of the patella (knee cap), or the middle third of the upper outer leg.

Administering injections to infants and small children requires some special considerations. The choice of a site is based on muscular development and the absence of major nerves and blood vessels. As has been mentioned, the most popular site for IM injections in children and infants is the vastus lateralis muscle. Other sites are avoided for the following reasons:

- Infants do not have well-developed deltoid muscles.
- The sciatic nerve, located near the dorsogluteal site, is proportionately larger in the infant.
- The gluteus medius is not well developed until the child is walking.

If you have any doubts, the best policy is to ask the physician to show you exactly where to inject the medication or vaccine. Any site selected for infants and children involves greater risk of error, because the muscles are smaller than the muscles of adults.

Infants should be restrained by a co-worker or a parent to prevent injury. If the child is old enough to understand, be honest and

Administer Parenteral (Excluding IV) Medications: Give an Intramuscular Injection Into the Deltoid

ORDER: *Administer 300,000 U penicillin G IM stat to Liz Anderson, age 23.*
GOAL: *To inject ordered medication into the muscle using a 22-gauge, 1½-inch needle and a 3-mL syringe as directed by the physician.*

EQUIPMENT and SUPPLIES

- Vial containing ordered medication
- Alcohol wipes
- Cotton ball
- Sterile needle and syringe unit with safety needle cover
- Disposable gloves
- Sharps container
- Written order, including the patient's name, when to give the drug, the route of administration, and the name and strength of the drug
- Patient's medical record

Procedural Steps

1. Sanitize your hands. Follow Standard Precautions.
2. Select the correct medication from storage.
3. Read the label to make sure you have the right drug and the right strength.
   PURPOSE: To perform the first of three drug label and order checks. One medication may be manufactured and prepackaged in different strengths; for instance, penicillin G is packaged in vials of 300,000 U/ mL and 600,000 U/mL.
4. Warm refrigerated medications by gently rolling the vial between your palms.
5. Calculate the correct dose, if necessary, and continue with the three label checks while drawing the medication into the syringe.
6. Transport the medication to the patient.
7. Greet and identify the patient by name.
   PURPOSE: To make sure you have the right patient.
8. Ask the patient whether she is allergic to penicillin or any other antibiotics.
   PURPOSE: Antibiotics, especially the penicillin family, are the most likely group of drugs to cause allergies. The patient's response can change over time, so it is important to request allergy information before each administration of an antibiotic.
9. Help the patient into an upright sitting position.
10. Put on gloves and expose the deltoid site. The mid-deltoid site is located approximately 2 to 3 fingerwidths below the acromial process.

11. Clean the patient's skin with the alcohol wipe using a circular motion and moving outward from the center (Figure 1).

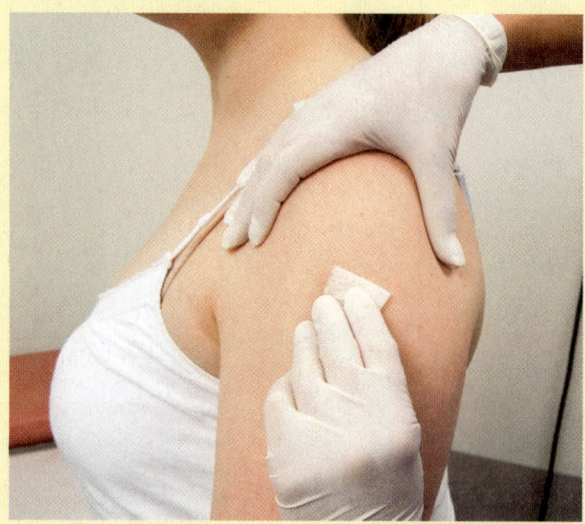

12. Remove the needle cover. Place your nondominant hand on the patient's shoulder, and with the thumb and first two fingers, spread the skin tightly and grasp the muscle deeply on each side (Figure 2).
    PURPOSE: To compress fat and stabilize the muscle.

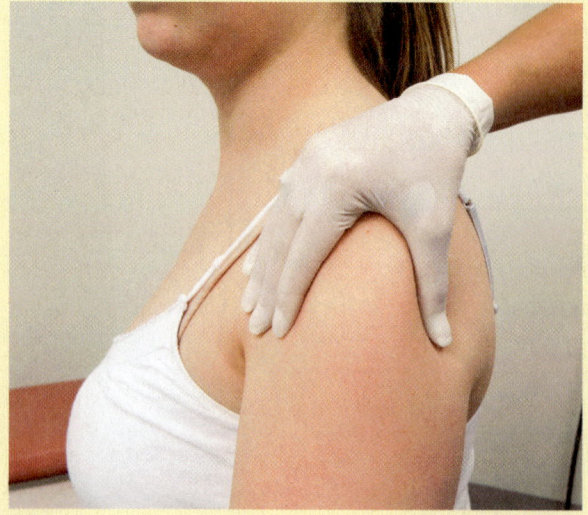

13. Grasp the syringe as you would a dart and with one swift movement, insert the entire needle up to the hub, at a 90-degree angle, into the muscle.
    PURPOSE: The depth of the injection is determined by the choice of needle length, not by how far you insert the needle. Once the needle is at the tissue layer, stabilize the syringe unit with the nondominant hand so that the needle does not move during aspiration and injection of the medication.

14. Aspirate; withdraw the plunger slightly to make sure no blood enters the syringe.
    PURPOSE: Blood in the syringe means that the needle is in a blood vessel and is not in the muscle tissue. You may not administer an intramuscular medication by the IV route.

15. If blood appears, immediately withdraw the syringe, discard it in the sharps container, and compress the injection site with the cotton ball.

16. Begin again with Step 1.

17. If no blood appears in the syringe, push in the plunger slowly and steadily until all medication has been administered.
    PURPOSE: A rapid injection is uncomfortable for the patient.

18. Place the cotton ball next to the needle and apply counterpressure to the area while you withdraw the needle at the same angle used for insertion. Immediately cover the contaminated needle with the syringe unit safety device and discard the syringe unit in the sharps container.

19. Gently massage the site with the cotton ball.
    PURPOSE: Massage helps promote absorption and reduce pain.

20. Make sure your patient is comfortable and safe.

21. Observe the patient for any adverse reaction. You may need to keep the patient under observation for 20 to 30 minutes.

22. Dispose of the gloves in the biohazard waste container and sanitize your hands.

23. Record the drug administration in the patient's medical record and in the required Drug Enforcement Agency (DEA) record if the medication is a controlled substance.
    PURPOSE: A procedure is not considered done until it is recorded.

9/8/XX 8:35 AM 300,000 U penicillin G administered IM to ® deltoid without complication. Pt observed for allergic reaction and none noted. Pt had no questions. Instructed to call office if she experiences any problems from injection. D. Gaston, CMA (AAMA)

---

explain that the injection may sting for a minute, but that it is important to hold very still. Always get help if giving an injection to an uncooperative child.

The recommended site for vastus lateralis injections in infants and children is below the greater trochanter of the femur but within the upper lateral quadrant of the thigh (Figure 35-23, *A*). When the vastus lateralis site is used in an adult, the needle should be inserted at a 90-degree angle; however, with infants and children, the needle should be inserted at a 45-degree angle, with the needle point directed toward the feet (Figure 35-23, *B*). Needle gauges for adults range from 20 to 23, and lengths range from 1 to 1½ inches; the muscle can hold as much as 5 mL of medication. In pediatric patients, the needle gauge should be 22 to 25, and the length should be ⅝ inch; the muscle can hold 0.5 mL in infants and 0.5 to 2 mL in children (Procedure 35-11). An adult patient may sit or lie supine, but the vastus lateralis is easier to locate in pediatric patients with the child lying down.

CRITICAL THINKING APPLICATION   35-5

Dr. Thau wants to make certain that Dorothy is comfortable with the procedure for administering IM injections to infants. She orders Dorothy to give the first dose of diphtheria, tetanus, pertussis (DTaP) vaccine IM to a 2-month-old infant in the office today for a well-baby checkup. Dorothy administers the injection in the right vastus lateralis. Document the information Dorothy should include on the child's record.

_____

_____

_____

Dorsogluteal (Gluteus Medius) Site. The dorsogluteal region is the traditional site for deep IM injections. However, complications from sciatic nerve injury are common enough that experts have suggested that use of this site be discontinued, and that the vastus lateralis and ventrogluteal sites be used instead. Regardless, the dorsogluteal site continues to be popular and is still acceptable for adults if care is taken to locate the exact site. This site should not be used for pediatric patients.

The patient should lie in Sims' position with the bottom leg straight and the top leg slightly bent. To locate the site, put the palm of your nondominant hand on the greater trochanter of the femur and point your fingers toward the posterior iliac spine. Palpate these bony prominences to make sure you are at the correct site, and draw an imaginary line between these two anatomic markings. The injection is made into the gluteus medius muscle above the imaginary line (Figure 35-24). Needle gauges 20 to 23 and a needle length of 1 to 3 inches should be used; the site can hold as much as 5 mL of medication. Procedure 35-12 can help you practice finding the dorsogluteal site.

Ventrogluteal (Gluteus Medius) Site. Although considered safe, the ventrogluteal region is not used as frequently as the others previously discussed. This technique uses a larger mass of the gluteus medius muscle than is used for the dorsogluteal site. The area is free of major nerves and blood vessels, and it is considered safe for both infants and adults (Figure 35-25). All types of IM medications can be injected here, including thick, oily preparations. Needle gauges 20 to 23 and needle lengths 1 to 3 inches should be used; the site can hold as much as 5 mL of medication.

To locate the site, place the patient in Sims' position and put the palm of your hand on the greater trochanter of the femur, pointing

Select the Proper Sites for Administering a Parenteral Medication: Administer a Pediatric Intramuscular Vastus Lateralis Injection

ORDER: *Administer 0.5 mL of Haemophilus influenzae type B (Hib) vaccine IM to Lizzy Dearborne, age 4 months, stat.*
GOAL: *To inject 0.5 mL of vaccine into the vastus lateralis muscle using a 22-gauge, ⅝-inch needle.*

EQUIPMENT and SUPPLIES

- Vial containing Hib vaccine
- Alcohol wipes
- Cotton ball or 2 × 2-inch gauze square
- Sterile needle and syringe unit with safety device
- Disposable gloves
- Sharps container
- Written order, including the patient's name, when to give the drug, the route of administration, and the name and strength of the drug
- Patient's medical record

PROCEDURAL STEPS

1. Check the patient's medical record for a previous allergic reaction to Hib vaccine; check the baby's temperature and ask the caregiver about recent illnesses, because patients with a moderate to severe illness should not be vaccinated.
2. Sanitize your hands. Follow Standard Precautions.
3. Select the correct medication from storage.
4. Read the label to make sure you have the right drug and the right strength; check the expiration date.
   <u>PURPOSE:</u> To perform the first of three drug label and order checks.
5. Warm refrigerated medications by gently rolling the vial between your palms.
6. Calculate the correct dose, if necessary, and continue with the three label checks while drawing the medication into the syringe. Follow the steps explained in Procedure 35-5 to correctly draw up the vaccine.
7. Complete the vaccination log according to office procedure.
   <u>PURPOSE:</u> The immunization record or vaccination log must be completed each time a vaccine is administered. Information includes the manufacturer; batch and lot numbers, which are stamped on the Hib container; expiration date; dose administered; route of administration; and whether there was a patient reaction. (More details about immunization records are presented in Chapter 42.)
8. Transport the medication to the patient.
9. Greet and identify the patient's caregiver and the child by name.
   <u>PURPOSE:</u> To make sure you have the right patient.
10. Explain the procedure to the child's caregiver.
    <u>PURPOSE:</u> To promote cooperation; also, this is a form of implied consent to the procedure.
11. Position the infant on her back. Ask the caregiver to remove any clothing necessary to expose the infant's thighs. Choose the right or the left thigh for the injection.
    <u>PURPOSE:</u> It is important to expose the entire vastus lateralis muscle to prevent injury to the child. The pediatric vastus lateralis site is located below the greater trochanter of the femur but within the upper lateral quadrant (fourth) of the thigh.
12. Put on gloves and clean the patient's skin with the alcohol wipe, using a circular motion and moving outward from the center.

13. Ask for the caregiver's assistance in holding the child still if necessary.
14. Remove the needle cover, and with the thumb and first two fingers of the nondominant hand, spread the skin at the site tightly.
15. Grasp the syringe as you would a dart, and with one swift movement, insert the needle at a 45-degree angle into the muscle, with the needle pointing toward the feet.
    <u>PURPOSE:</u> Once the needle is at the tissue layer, do not move it while injecting the medication.
16. Aspirate; withdraw the plunger slightly to make sure no blood enters the syringe.
    <u>PURPOSE:</u> Blood in the syringe means that the needle is in a blood vessel and is not in the muscle tissue. You may not administer an intramuscular medication by the IV route.
17. If blood appears, immediately withdraw the syringe, discard it in the sharps container, and compress the injection site with the cotton ball. Begin again with Step 2.
18. If no blood appears in the syringe, push in the plunger slowly and steadily until all medication has been administered.
    <u>PURPOSE:</u> A rapid injection is uncomfortable for the patient.
19. Place the cotton ball next to the needle and apply counterpressure to the area while you withdraw the needle at the same angle used for insertion. Immediately cover the contaminated needle with the syringe unit safety device and discard the syringe unit in the sharps container.
20. Gently massage the site with the cotton ball.
    <u>PURPOSE:</u> Massage helps promote absorption and reduce pain.
21. Make sure the infant is safely held by the caregiver.
22. Dispose of the gloves in the biohazard waste container and sanitize your hands.
23. Record the drug administration in the patient's medical record and in the vaccination log according to office procedure.
    <u>PURPOSE:</u> A procedure is not considered done until it is recorded. It is important to keep an accurate record of vaccinations performed so that the next dose is timed properly. Include in the documentation the name of the vaccine, dose, route of administration and location, lot number, and any observed patient reactions. The caregiver must be given a Vaccine Information Sheet (VIS), and it must be documented that the VIS was received.
24. Observe the patient for 20 to 30 minutes for any adverse reaction.

3/27/XX 1:30 PM Hib lot #98525, exp date 10/XX, administered IM to Ⓛ vastus lateralis. Caregiver given HIB VIS, answered questions regarding follow-up care. No adverse effects noted. Appointment made for next immunizations in 1 month. D. Gaston, CMA (AAMA) _____

PROCEDURE 35-12

Administer Parenteral (Excluding IV) Medications: Give a Z-Track Intramuscular Injection into the Dorsogluteal Site

ORDER: *Administer 1 mL of INFeD Z-track into the dorsogluteal site to Carlos Langa, age 63, stat.*
GOAL: *Inject 1 mL of medication into the gluteus medius muscle via the Z-track injection using a 23-gauge, 2-inch needle.*

EQUIPMENT and SUPPLIES

- Vial containing the ordered medication
- Alcohol wipes
- Cotton ball
- Disposable gloves
- Sharps container
- Sterile needle and syringe unit with safety needle cover
- Additional sterile needle
- Written order, including the patient's name, when to give the drug, the route of administration, and the name and strength of the drug
- Patient's medical record

PROCEDURAL STEPS

1. Sanitize your hands. Follow Standard Precautions.
2. Select the correct medication from the shelf or the refrigerator.
3. Perform the three order and label checks and verify the seven rights.
4. Warm refrigerated medications by gently rolling the container between your palms.
5. Draw up the ordered amount of medication into the syringe unit.
6. Replace the needle cover and give a slight turn to loosen the needle. Secure a new needle, still in its sheath, to the tip of the syringe, being careful to not contaminate the needle or hub of the syringe. Discard the contaminated needle.
   PURPOSE: The needle that was used to withdraw the medication is covered with the drug, which might be irritating to the skin and subcutaneous tissues.
7. Transport the medication to the patient.
8. Greet and identify the patient by name.
   PURPOSE: To make sure you have the right patient.
9. Position the patient comfortably in Sims' position.
10. Expose the site and put on gloves.
11. The dorsogluteal site is found by placing the palm of the nondominant hand on the greater trochanter of the femur, while pointing your fingers toward the posterior iliac spine and index finger toward the anterior iliac spine. The injection site is in the upper outer area of the gluteus medius. Visualize the area for the Z-track injection.
12. Clean the patient's skin with the alcohol wipe, using a circular motion and moving outward from the center. Make sure to clean the actual area of injection.
13. Remove the needle cover.
14. Push the skin to one side and hold it firmly in place. If the skin is slippery, use a dry gauze sponge to hold the skin in place.
    PURPOSE: Displacing the skin prevents medication from leaking back to the surface. This method is used for medications that irritate or stain surface tissues.

15. Grasp the syringe as you would a dart and with one swift movement, insert the entire needle up to the hub at a 90-degree angle into the upper outer area of the gluteus medius muscle.
    PURPOSE: The depth of the injection is determined by the choice of needle length, not by how far you insert the needle. Once the needle is at the tissue layer, do not move it while injecting the medication. Inserting the needle as far as the hub helps keep the needle in place.
16. Aspirate; withdraw the plunger slightly to make sure no blood enters the syringe.
    PURPOSE: Blood in the syringe means that the needle is in a blood vessel and not in the muscle tissue. You may not administer an intramuscular medication by the IV route.
17. If blood appears, immediately withdraw the syringe, dispose of the syringe unit in the sharps container, and compress the injection site with a gauze square or cotton ball.
    PURPOSE: To minimize bleeding and bruising.
18. Begin again with Step 1.
    PURPOSE: Blood is now mixed with the medication, and the medication is considered contaminated. Blood may interact with the drug and may be irritating to the intramuscular tissues.
19. If no blood appears in the syringe, push in the plunger slowly and steadily until all medication has been administered.
20. Wait 10 seconds for the medication to be dispersed, then withdraw the needle at the same angle used for insertion. As the needle is withdrawn, release the displaced skin to prevent the tracking of medication to the surface.
21. Immediately cover the contaminated needle with the syringe unit safety device and dispose of the needle and syringe unit in a sharps container.
22. If the manufacturer recommends it, gently massage the site with the gauze square or cotton ball. Many medications requiring Z-track administration should not be massaged.
23. Make sure your patient is comfortable and safe.
24. Dispose of the gloves in the biohazard waste container and sanitize your hands.
25. Observe the patient for any adverse reaction. You may need to keep the patient under observation for 20 to 30 minutes.
26. Record the drug administration in the patient's medical record, including the exact site of injection.

7/13/XX 1:25 PM 1 mL INFeD administered Z-track in ® dorsogluteal site. Injection site not massaged after administration. No evidence of skin discoloration after administration. Dorothy Gaston, CMA (AAMA) _____

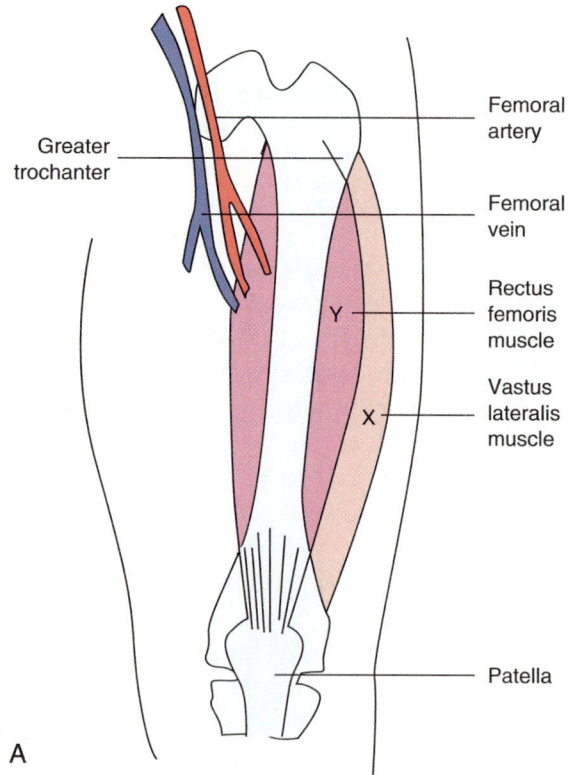

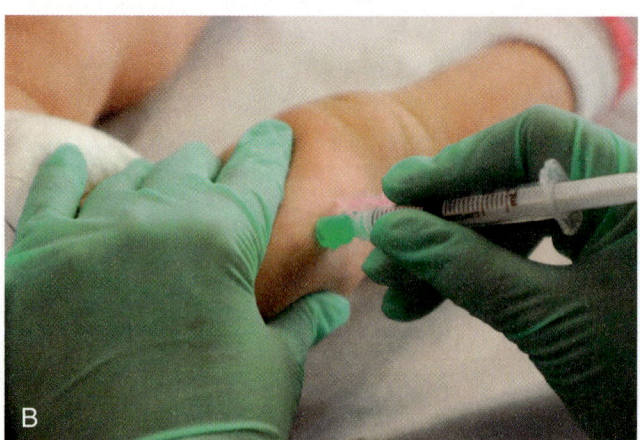

FIGURE 35-23 A, The vastus lateralis intramuscular site. B, The recommended site for vastus lateralis injections in infants and children. (From Bonewit-West K: *Clinical procedures for medical assistants*, ed 8, St. Louis, 2012, Saunders.)

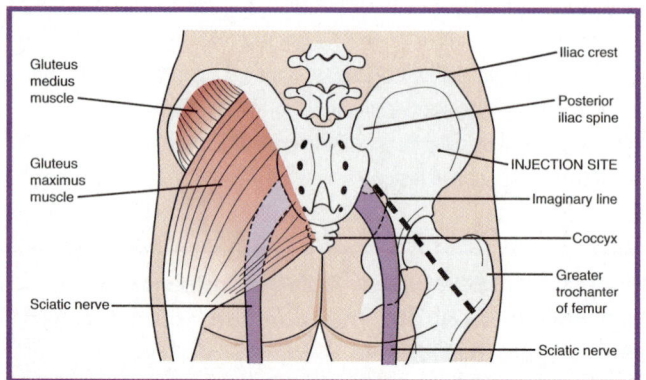

FIGURE 35-24 The dorsogluteal (gluteus medius) site is still preferred by many physicians.

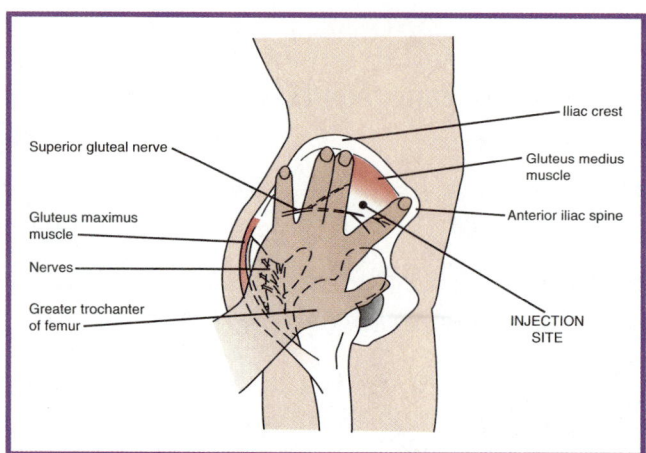

FIGURE 35-25 The ventrogluteal site can be used for most intramuscular injections.

your index finger toward the anterior iliac spine. Spread your middle finger back as far as possible from your index finger to form a triangular injection area. For a child you will need a 1-inch needle, whereas for an obese adult patient, you may need a 2½- to 3-inch needle, to reach the depth of the muscle. Table 35-2 summarizes the details of parenteral administration of medication.

Z-Track Intramuscular Injection

Some IM medications are irritating to the skin and SC tissues; others, such as iron replacement products, leak to the surface and stain surrounding tissues. These medications should be injected in such a way as to prevent any leakage from the deep muscle back into the upper SC layers. The Z-track method displaces the upper tissue laterally before the needle is inserted.

Prepare the medication according to safety guidelines and then put on gloves. Palpate the site using anatomically correct markings, and localize the injection site visually. Push the skin to one side, and clean it as described for IM injections. Insert the needle into the anatomically correct location, and slowly release the medication into the deep muscular tissue (see Procedure 35-12). After withdrawing the needle, release the tissue so that the needle track is to the side of the point where the medication was deposited in the muscle. This process prevents a direct pathway to the surface for the medication, which protects SC and surface tissues from the irritating and/or staining properties of the drug.

The medications for which Z-track injection is appropriate require a large muscle mass, so they should be injected only into the dorsogluteal site. Because the medication is so irritating to tissues, the needle should be changed after the medication has been drawn up from the vial and before the injection is given. Some facilities require personnel to use the Z-track method when administering abdominal heparin injections, because leakage of the drug at the site may cause localized bleeding. Although heparin is administered by SC injection, the technique of pushing the surface tissue to the side before injection is the same.

Medications that require the Z-track method of administration (e.g., heparin) should not be massaged after injection, because massaging encourages spread of the medication. Use alternate sides for multiple or frequent injections, to prevent tissue damage.

TABLE 35-2 Parenteral Administration of Medications

ROUTE OF ADMINISTRATION	SITE	NEEDLE GAUGE	NEEDLE LENGTH (IN)	SYRINGE	DRUG AMOUNT	EXAMPLE DRUGS
Intradermal	Midanterior forearm	27-28	⅜	1 mL: tuberculin	0.1 mL: allergy tests	Tuberculosis skin test (Mantoux)
Subcutaneous	Posterior upper arm, thigh, abdomen	25-26	½, ⅝	2-3 mL: insulin	Adult: 0.1-2 mL Child: 0.5 mL	Insulin, heparin, vaccines
Intramuscular	Adult deltoid	20-23	1-3	2-5 mL	1-2 mL	Epinephrine, vitamin B₁₂, antibiotics (e.g., penicillin), meperidine, morphine, vaccines
	Child deltoid	20-23	⅝-1	1-3 mL	0.5-2 mL	
	Adult vastus lateralis, dorsogluteal, ventrogluteal	20-23	1-1½ 1-3 1-3	3-5 mL	2-5 mL	
	Infant or child vastus lateralis	22-26	⅝	1-3 mL	0.5-2 mL	

PRINCIPLES OF INTRAVENOUS THERAPY

Administration of IV fluids or medication bypasses the absorption phase of pharmacokinetics, because the fluid and/or medication is administered directly into the bloodstream. IV therapy often is the route of choice if the physician wants to speed up the action of a drug. After administration into a vein, the medication is quickly distributed to the target tissue by the circulatory system and, depending on the medication and its purpose, may start acting within seconds to minutes. This very quality makes IV drug administration the most dangerous route of administration; one minor mistake could be life threatening to a patient. For this reason, state medical practice acts and the policies of individual healthcare facilities strictly define the types of professionals qualified to perform IV-related procedures and to administer IV medications. The medical assistant must be familiar with both legal restrictions and employer policies before having anything to do with IV therapy. However, regardless of whether you are responsible for IV therapy, you may work in a facility where patients have IV lines; therefore, it is important that you understand some basic principles of IV administration.

Intravenous Terminology and Practices

The administration of IV fluid is closely monitored by the physician to maintain homeostasis. Three basic types of fluids are used for IV therapy (Figure 35-26):

- *Isotonic solutions,* such as 0.9% sodium chloride (NaCl, also called *normal saline),* contain the same salt level as normal body fluids. Isotonic fluids are used for patients who need replacement of lost body fluids, such as those with gastrointestinal disease or burns. If the patient needs glucose for nutrients, dextrose can be added in either (D₅W) or saline (D₅NS) to meet the patient's caloric needs. Another type of isotonic IV solution is Ringer's lactate, which contains no dextrose (or calories) but provides electrolytes, including sodium, potassium, calcium, and chloride ions.
- *Hypertonic solutions* contain higher concentrations of NaCl than those found in normal body fluids; this higher level causes extracellular fluid to shift from the cells into the bloodstream. For example, 3% or 5% NaCl solution may be used in a patient with extensive peripheral edema. The concentrated solution in the

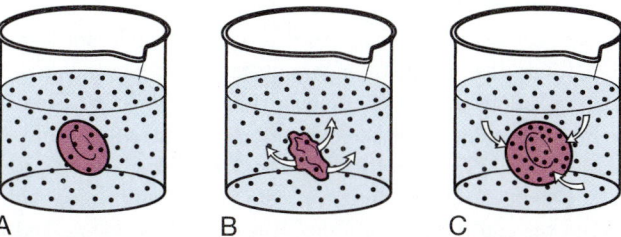

FIGURE 35-26 Basic types of fluids for IV therapy. **A,** Isotonic. **B,** Hypertonic. **C,** Hypotonic. (From Applegate E: *The anatomy and physiology learning system,* ed 3, Philadelphia, 2006, Saunders.)

blood vessels attracts excess intracellular and interstitial fluid into the bloodstream to dilute the highly concentrated plasma. These solutions are helpful in reducing edema, but they may lead to increased pressure in the blood vessels from the increased volume of fluid, ultimately causing hypertension.

- *Hypotonic solutions,* including 10% dextrose in water (D₁₀W) and 5% dextrose in 0.3% sodium chloride, contain less salt (NaCl) than body fluids. Hypotonic IV fluids promote cellular hydration by shifting fluid from blood vessels into the interstitial spaces surrounding cells; they are administered to maintain fluid intake when the patient does not require electrolyte replacement.

The physician carefully prescribes the type of IV solution based on the patient's systemic needs. It is crucial that anyone responsible for hanging, changing, or replacing IV fluids carefully follow the physician's orders to prevent serious complications for the patient.

Dangers of Intravenous Treatment

Poor aseptic technique may result in infection or inflammation at the IV site and/or systemic infection. Healthcare workers must be extremely careful in dealing with IV equipment and fluids, because material is being injected directly into the bloodstream.

Localized phlebitis may lead to clot formation at the site (thrombophlebitis). Local inflammation of the vein typically occurs because of poor aseptic technique when the IV is started or use of a contaminated bandage over the injection site. A vein may also become inflamed because of irritation from medication administered through the IV, the IV solution itself, or patient movement of the site. Signs of **phlebitis** must be reported to the physician immediately, because phlebitis can lead to serious complications, including thrombus formation and/or systemic infection. Indicators of phlebitis include inflammation, edema, warmth, and tenderness at the site; the vein feels hard and ropelike.

Infiltration can also occur if the IV needle or catheter becomes dislodged from the vein. The IV fluid escapes into surrounding tissues, causing edema and discomfort. If you notice this, close the roller clamp on the IV tubing and notify the physician immediately.

Fluid overload may be caused by too rapid infusion of the solution. This may cause serious complications in patients with hypertension, heart disease, or congestive heart failure.

Medication errors can occur. IV fluids and/or medication circulates throughout the entire body within 1 minute after administration. It is not possible to take back an error in IV therapy.

Intravenous Equipment

The medical assistant may be asked to gather supplies for starting the IV infusion, so it is important that you become familiar with the various pieces of equipment needed. Whoever is starting the IV infusion must follow strict sterile technique. All IV infusion equipment is individually packaged and disposable. This equipment includes skin-cleansing solution; needle or catheter; tubing with a spike at the end to insert into the IV bag; sterile dressings; and IV fluids. Typically, everything you need except for the ordered IV fluid is packaged in a sterile IV infusion kit. Check the package for the desired needle and catheter gauge, infusion rate of administration, expiration date, and package integrity (if the package is moist or torn, it is no longer considered sterile and must be discarded) (Figure 35-27). Additional supplies include a tourniquet, disposable gloves, a biohazard waste container, and an IV pole. Most ambulatory care facilities do not use infusion pumps, but one may be needed, depending on your facility's practice.

Most infusion sets in ambulatory care settings contain butterfly infusion needles that have winged extensions for grasping during placement of the needle into the vein (Figure 35-28).

These are available in a variety of gauges and lengths (25 to 17 gauge, length of 0.5 to 1 inch) and are used for short-term IV administration, as with a single dose of IV medication. The short, hard needle is relatively easy to dislodge from the vein when the patient moves, which may lead to infiltration of IV fluids. The physician prescribes a certain number of drips per minute of the IV solution, depending on the patient's condition and the reason for fluid administration. The macrodrip size, which delivers 8 to 20 drops/mL, is used for adult fluid replacement, whereas the microdrip unit (50 to 60 drops/mL) is used for children and/or for slow administration of medications to patients of any age. The length of the IV tubing that connects the fluid bag to the venous catheter varies according to the patient's need for mobility and freedom.

To prepare the solution for administration, insert the spike at the end of the IV tubing into the ordered fluid bag. Just below the spike is a drip chamber; this is an enlarged, flexible plastic container in the tubing that is squeezed so that it partially fills with fluid. The drop orifice leading into the drip chamber determines the size of the fluid drops. The rate at which the drops fall into the chamber and from there through the filled tubing into the patient is regulated by compressing the roller clamp on the tubing until the number of drops per minute prescribed by the physician is falling into the drip chamber (Figure 35-29). The distal end of the tubing is connected to the needle or catheter after the needle is in place, and after the tube has been filled with IV fluid so that all air bubbles are expressed. This step prevents the injection of air into the vein. If the patient is

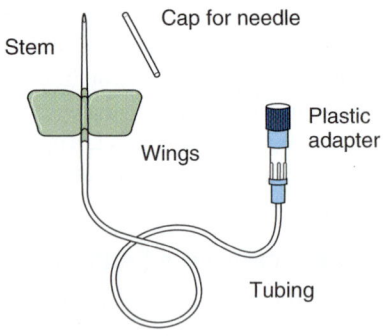

Steel needle ("butterfly") set

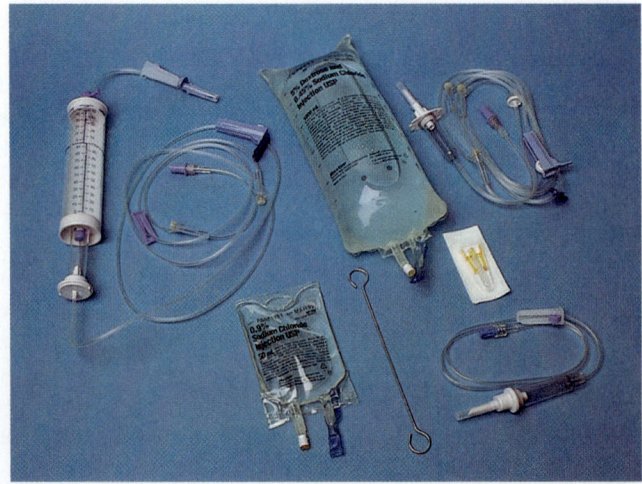

FIGURE 35-27 Intravenous administration set. (From deWit S: *Fundamental concepts and skills for nursing,* ed 3, St Louis, 2009, Saunders.)

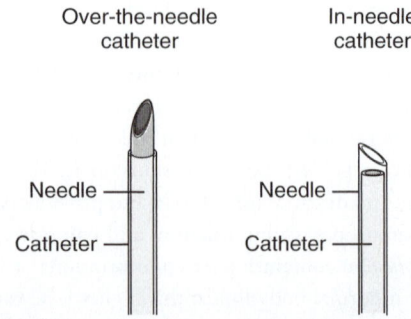

FIGURE 35-28 Intravenous cannulas: steel needle ("butterfly"), over-the-needle catheter, and in-needle catheter. (From Klieger DM: *Saunders textbook of medical assisting,* St Louis, 2005, Saunders.)

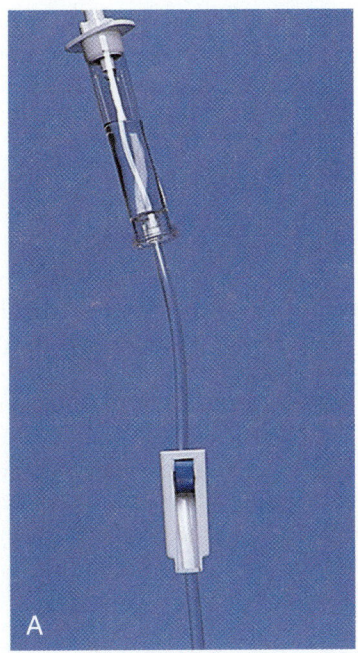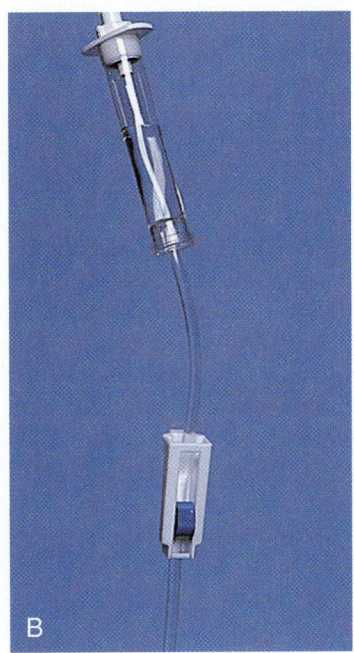

FIGURE 35-29 A, Roller clamp in the open position. **B,** Roller clamp in the closed position. (From Perry AG, Potter PA: *Clinical nursing skills and techniques,* ed 6, St Louis, 2006, Mosby.)

receiving medication, the IV tubing will have an injection port, which is a rubber extension to which another IV bag of medication can be connected, or through which the caregiver can inject medication by inserting a needle into the port.

When the desired fluid or medication infusion is complete, the IV system must be disconnected. To do this, put on gloves before clamping the IV tubing, carefully remove the dressing, and gently slide the needle and catheter out of the vein. Apply pressure to the site with a sterile gauze square to prevent the formation of a hematoma. Discard the contaminated materials in a biohazard waste container (the needle or catheter in a sharps container), and chart the completion of IV therapy.

Role of the Medical Assistant in Assisting With Intravenous Therapy

- Follow state practice acts. The medical assistant should not perform any task, even when it is legal, unless he or she understands the principles behind the procedure and has the technical skill to perform it safely.
- Gather a comprehensive health history to determine the indications for IV therapy.
- Weigh the patient before and monitor vital signs during the infusion so that the physician can be alerted if possible complications arise; do not take the blood pressure reading in the arm with the IV line.
- Be alert for signs of infiltration and phlebitis.
- Monitor the equipment for problems.
- Watch for too rapid infusion of fluids, which might lead to circulatory overload.
- Document all pertinent information in the patient's record.

CLOSING COMMENTS

Patient Education

It is extremely important to teach the patient how to take a prescribed drug, and to make sure he or she understands the purpose of the medication. Ideally, the physician informs the patient, but the medical assistant should be prepared to reinforce the physician's information or to explain parts of the information the patient did not understand. When a patient does not understand the need for the medication or the directions for taking it, the risk is greater that the medication will be taken incorrectly. As a result, the physician's orders will not be carried out, and the desired therapeutic effect will not be achieved. The patient should fully understand the type of medication, its route of administration, its desired effect, and the side effects that need to be reported if they occur.

If the patient receives medication in the physician's office, he or she should understand the expected results or possible side effects. For example, if a patient is given a diuretic in the office, he or she needs to know what the immediate effect is going to be. This prepares the patient for the urinary urgency and **polyuria** that will occur within a relatively brief period. When a pain medication is given, the patient should have full knowledge so that the possibility of personal injury can be prevented. Any medication given in the ambulatory care setting that affects the patient's ability to walk or drive must be used with caution. The patient must be able to get home safely, and if that is not possible, the medication should not be given.

The medical assistant should instruct the patient to take all of the medication prescribed. Often if a prescription is not completed, the treatment objectives may not be achieved. Patients should also be instructed to take their medication in the time sequence prescribed. This keeps the optimum level of the drug circulating in the bloodstream.

When sample medications are dispensed to the patient in the office, the package contains inserts that can be helpful in education efforts. If the patient should reread certain parts of the inserts, highlight this information for quick reference. If the physician has specific written instructions for the patient to follow, read over the material with the patient before discharge so that any areas of confusion can be cleared up before the patient leaves the office. Always remember that the more the patient knows and understands about how to take the medication and why it has been prescribed, the greater is the likelihood that the patient will comply with medication therapy, and the more likely it is that the drug treatment will be successful.

This also would be a good time to suggest that the patient check the status of medications at home. The National Association of Retail Druggists recommends that the medicine cabinet be checked once a month to determine the age and quality of medications. At that time, the patient should discard any medications that fall into the following categories:

- Medicines for past illnesses
- Any expired medicines, unidentified medications, or medications that are more than 2 years old
- Hydrogen peroxide that no longer bubbles or has changed color; ointments or salves that have separated or are crumbly; vinegary smelling aspirin; antiseptic solutions that are cloudy or have a solid residue on the bottom; and any medicine of uncertain quality

The Association also suggests the following:

- Keep medicines stored away from light, heat, air, and moisture.
- Use medicine from the original container until it is completely used or expired.

- Do not combine medicines from several containers.
- Keep medicine locked away from children.
- Make sure childproof medicine caps are used properly.

Legal and Ethical Issues

A medical assistant must be extremely knowledgeable when administering medications in the physician's office. Follow all of the physician's orders exactly as written. If you have a question about the order, ask for clarification before you proceed. It is advisable to give a medication only after the order has been written in the patient's chart. This helps eliminate errors and possible omissions in medication therapy.

Legal responsibilities in medication practice include preventing error by carefully following safe practice procedures in pouring and administering drugs. Always implement the seven rights and perform the three drug order and label checks when dispensing and administering medications. Anyone administering a drug must know the possible serious complications related to the drug and must be alert for side effects. The medical assistant must demonstrate compliance with individual state laws regulating medications and their administration. Precise charting of the administration of medications, as well as of the management of prescriptions, cannot be overemphasized.

The administration of drugs involves ethical principles. The patient always comes first. With that foremost in mind, never risk giving an incorrect medication. There is no such thing as a small error, because any mistake may result in serious harm or possible death. If an error is made, it must be reported immediately to the physician, so that measures can be taken to help the patient. It is difficult to admit that a mistake has been made, but it is absolutely necessary. For this reason, be sure to double-check your calculations with a co-worker or the physician before dispensing the drug. If a mistake is made, it must be documented completely, including the details of the error, to whom the error was reported, any action taken, and subsequent observations of the patient.

SUMMARY OF SCENARIO

Dorothy understands the importance of careful management of medications. Because of her concern for patient safety, she asks Dr. Thau to check all of her calculations and refers to the physician if she has any questions about medication orders or patient education. Because Dr. Thau is a primary care physician, it is important for Dorothy to understand the factors that affect the administration of medication to all age groups of patients. She routinely employs the standard three label checks when dispensing medications and implements the seven rights throughout medication administration procedures.

Dorothy recognizes the importance of complete and accurate documentation of medications, whether they are administered in the physician's office or given

to the patient as a prescription order. In addition, she consistently applies the rules of standard precautions when preparing and administering parenteral medications. Although as a medical assistant Dorothy cannot administer IV medication, she understands the principles of IV therapy just in case there is a patient in the facility who is receiving IV fluids or medications. All those administering a drug must know the possible serious complications related to the drug and must be alert for side effects. The medical assistant must demonstrate compliance with individual state laws governing medications and their administration. Precise charting of the administration of medications as well as the management of prescriptions cannot be overemphasized.

SUMMARY OF LEARNING OBJECTIVES

1. **Define, spell, and pronounce the terms listed in the vocabulary.**
   Spelling and pronouncing medical terms correctly bolsters the medical assistant's credibility. Knowing the definition of these terms promotes confidence in communication with patients and co-workers.

2. **Apply critical thinking skills in performing the patient assessment and patient care.**
   Completing the Critical Thinking Application exercises throughout the chapter can help the student medical assistant become more adept at critical analysis of real-life situations.

3. **Follow safety precautions in the management of medication administration in the ambulatory healthcare setting.**
   The three label checks and seven rights must always be performed. Medications are prepared in a quiet, well-lit area. A substitute is never used for the ordered drug or drug strength. Medications are stored as ordered on the package. Medical assistants must never administer a medication they have not prepared personally. If preparing a medication for the physician to administer, the medical assistant places the container with the dispensed drug. Only written physician's orders are followed. The medical assistant must check expiration dates and discard expired drugs. Medications with damaged labels are discarded. Dispensed medication that is not given is discarded. Patients must be consistently asked about drug allergies. Patients are observed for at least 20 minutes after administration of a drug. Drug reactions are reported and documented. Patient education about drug therapy is provided and documented.

4. **Analyze safety guidelines for specific patient populations.**
   Safety precautions in the management of medication administration should be applied consistently. Safe drug administration includes understanding the physician's order, looking up the drug if the medical assistant is unfamiliar with it, and using the three label checks and the seven rights every time a drug order is completed.

5. **Document the administration of a medication.**
   Immediately after administering a drug, the medical assistant should document the date and time of administration; the drug's name, strength, dose, and route of administration; any reactions the patient has to the drug; and patient education about the medication. For parenteral medications, the exact site of administration must be charted.

6. **Summarize patient assessment factors that can affect medication administration.**
   Such factors include continual evaluation of the patient's physical condition, as well as holistic factors, such as the patient's history, an accurate list of drug allergies, the patient's ability to understand the drug regimen and to afford the treatment, and special factors based on age, weight, and condition.

7. **Identify various drug forms and their administration guidelines.**
   Drugs are packaged in a variety of forms with a variety of administration guidelines. Oral medications include both solid and liquid preparations; mucous membrane medications are absorbed rectally, vaginally, orally, nasally, or topically through the skin. Each form of medication has specific guidelines for administration, but all require consistent use of the three label checks and the seven rights.

8. **Administer oral medications.**
   See Procedure 35-3.

9. **Specify parenteral administration equipment, including details about needles and syringes.**
   Parenteral medications are manufactured in ampules and in single-dose or multidose vials. The ordered route of administration, the drug's characteristics, and individual patient factors determine the correct gauge and needle length used for administration. The appropriate syringe is determined by the type of medication ordered and the amount of drug to be administered. Specialty syringe units, such as the insulin pen and the EpiPen, are designed for quick administration of certain medications. Tables 35-1 and 35-2 provide further details.

10. **Follow OSHA guidelines in the management of parenteral administration.**
    OSHA guidelines include using syringe units with safety needle covers; wearing disposable, nonsterile gloves and other appropriate protective gear when administering any medication that involves coming into contact with blood or body fluids; never recapping a contaminated needle and immediately discarding it into a sharps container; disposing of contaminated nonsharp materials in biohazard containers; disinfecting contaminated work areas; and washing hands before and after procedures.

11. **Describe and demonstrate the types and locations of parenteral administrations.**
    Parenteral routes of administration include intradermal (ID), subcutaneous (SC), and a variety of intramuscular (IM) sites. The type of medication, the physician's order, and the unique characteristics of individual patients determine the route and site of administration. Each requires specific administration practices, which are described in Procedures 35-4 through 35-12.

12. **Outline the principles of IV therapy.**
    IV therapy bypasses the absorption phase of pharmacokinetics, because the fluid and/or medication is placed directly into the bloodstream. After instillation into a vein, the medication is quickly distributed to the target tissue by the circulatory system; depending on the medication and its purpose, the drug may start acting within seconds to minutes. State medical practice acts and individual healthcare facility policies strictly define the individuals qualified to perform IV-related procedures. IV fluids are isotonic, hypotonic, or hypertonic.

13. **Recognize the medical assistant's role in patient education about the administration of drugs.**
    Patient education is crucial if patients are to administer medications correctly at home. The patient should understand the purpose of the drug; the time, frequency, and amount of the dose; any special storage requirements; and the typical side effects. The more the patient knows and understands about how to take the medication and why it has been prescribed, the greater is the chance that drug treatment will be successful.

14. **Assess legal and ethical issues in drug administration in the ambulatory care setting.**

The medical assistant must be extremely knowledgeable when preparing and administering medications in the physician's office. If any questions arise about the order, the medical assistant must ask for clarification before proceeding. Legal responsibilities include preventing error by carefully following safe practice procedures in dispensing and administering drugs. The medical assistant must comply with individual state laws regulating medications and their administration. Precise charting of the administration of medications and the management of prescriptions cannot be overemphasized.

CONNECTIONS

Study Guide Connection: Go to the Chapter 35 Study Guide. Read and complete the activities.

Evolve Connection: Go to the Chapter 35 link at *evolve.elsevier.com/kinn* to complete the Chapter Review and Chapter Quiz. Peruse other resources listed for this chapter to increase your knowledge of Administering Medications.

EMERGENCY PREPAREDNESS AND ASSISTING WITH MEDICAL EMERGENCIES

36

SCENARIO

Cheryl Skurka, CMA (AAMA), has been working for Dr. Peter Bendt for approximately 6 months. During that time, a number of patient emergencies have occurred in the office, and even more potentially serious problems have been managed by the telephone screening staff. Cheryl is concerned that she is not prepared to assist with emergencies in the ambulatory care setting. She decides to ask Dr. Bendt for assistance, and he suggests that she work with the experienced screening staff to learn how to manage phone calls from patients calling for assistance.

Dr. Bendt is participating in a community-wide preparedness effort focused on both natural and human-made disasters, and he expects his practice and employees to be ready to respond if needed. This includes both creating plans to maintain the safety of patients and employees in the facility and providing assistance as needed in a community emergency.

While studying this chapter, think about the following questions:

- What should Cheryl learn about the medical assistant's responsibilities in an emergency situation?
- What are some of the general rules for managing a medical emergency in an ambulatory care setting?
- What types of questions does the telephone screening staff ask if a patient calls with a medical emergency?
- What information from these phone calls should be documented?
- Is it important for Cheryl to be able to recognize life-threatening emergencies and to be prepared to respond to them?
- What are some of the typical patient emergencies that occur in a healthcare facility?

- How should Cheryl instruct a patient to control bleeding from a hemorrhaging wound?
- What safety practices should be followed in the healthcare facility to protect patients and employees from potential harm?
- What is the medical office's responsibility in preparing for community emergencies?
- Are there common health emergency topics for patient education that Cheryl should be prepared to present?
- What legal factors should Cheryl keep in mind when handling ambulatory care emergencies?

LEARNING OBJECTIVES

1. Define, spell, and pronounce the terms listed in the vocabulary.
2. Apply critical thinking skills in performing the patient assessment and patient care.
3. Describe patient safety factors in the medical office environment.
4. Evaluate the work environment to identify safe and unsafe working conditions.
5. Identify environmental safety issues in the healthcare setting.
6. Develop environmental, patient, and employee safety plans.
7. Discuss fire safety issues in a healthcare environment.
8. Demonstrate the proper use of a fire extinguisher.
9. Describe the fundamental principles for evacuation of a healthcare facility.
10. Role-play a mock environmental exposure event and evacuation of a physician's office.
11. Discuss the requirements for proper disposal of hazardous materials.
12. Define the important features of emergency preparedness in the ambulatory care setting.
13. Maintain an up-to-date list of community resources for emergency preparedness.

14. Describe the medical assistant's role in emergency response.
15. Summarize the typical emergency supplies and equipment.
16. Demonstrate the use of an automated external defibrillator.
17. Summarize the general rules for managing emergencies.
18. Demonstrate telephone screening techniques and documentation guidelines for ambulatory care emergencies.
19. Recognize and respond to life-threatening emergencies in the ambulatory care setting.
20. Perform professional-level cardiopulmonary resuscitation (CPR).
21. Administer oxygen through a nasal cannula to a patient in respiratory distress.
22. Identify and assist a patient with an obstructed airway.
23. Determine the appropriate action and documentation procedures for common ambulatory care emergencies.
24. Assist and monitor a patient who has fainted.
25. Control a hemorrhagic wound.
26. Apply patient education concepts to medical emergencies.
27. Discuss the legal and ethical concerns arising from medical emergencies.

VOCABULARY

arrhythmia (uh-rith′-mee-uh) An abnormality or irregularity in the heart rhythm.

asystole (ay-sis′-toh-le) The absence of a heartbeat.

cyanosis (si-an-oh′-sis) A blue coloration of the mucous membranes and body extremities caused by lack of oxygen.

diaphoresis (di-uh-fuh-re′-sis) The profuse excretion of sweat.

ecchymosis (e-ki-moh′-sis) A hemorrhagic skin discoloration commonly called *bruising*.

emetic (eh-met′-ik) A substance that causes vomiting.

fibrillation Rapid, random, ineffective contractions of the heart.

hematuria (hi-ma-tuhr′-e-uh) Blood in the urine.

idiopathic Pertaining to a condition or a disease that has no known cause.

mediastinum (meh-de-ast′-uhn-um) The space in the center of the chest under the sternum.

myocardium (my-oh-kar′-de-um) The muscular lining of the heart.

necrosis (neh-kroh′-sis) The death of cells or tissues.

photophobia An abnormal sensitivity to light.

polydipsia Excessive thirst.

thrombolytics Agents that dissolve blood clots.

transient ischemic attack (TIA) Temporary neurological symptoms caused by gradual or partial occlusion of a cerebral blood vessel.

The medical assistant typically is responsible for making the healthcare facility as accident-proof as possible. This requires attention to a number of factors. For example, cupboard doors and drawers must be kept closed; spills must be wiped up immediately; and dropped objects must be picked up. The medical assistant also should make sure that all medications are kept out of sight and away from busy patient areas. If children are in the office, all sharp objects and potentially toxic substances must be kept out of reach. In addition, the medical assistant should never leave a seriously ill patient or a restless, depressed, or unconscious patient unattended.

SAFETY IN THE HEALTHCARE FACILITY

Patient Safety

Patient safety is a critical component of the quality of care provided in a healthcare facility. The U.S. Department of Health and Human Services (DHHS) has conducted extensive research on the features of safe patient environments in physicians' offices. The DHHS has found the following factors to be crucial to patient safety:

- Open lines of communication must be established among all employees about possible safety issues, and employees must work together to solve these problems before a patient is injured.
- If an injury occurs (e.g., a medication is administered to the wrong patient), policies and procedures must be in place so that all employees recognize the potential for an error and protocols are established for preventing a similar problem in the future.
- Procedures must be standardized in the facility's policy and procedures manual so that all employees can refer to specific guidelines on how procedures should be performed. For example, in the case of a blood spill, the policy and procedures manual must outline a specific, step-by-step procedure for cleaning up the spill that safeguards both patients and staff members.
- The facility must provide ongoing staff training in patient safety factors.
- Staff members must work as a team to maintain a safe environment for patients. For example, all staff members must follow Standard Precautions to prevent the spread of disease in the facility.

Throughout this text, you have learned about situations that could result in serious harm to your patients. You must constantly be on guard to protect patients from possible injury. For example, studies have shown that healthcare workers frequently confuse drug names, which results in administration of the wrong medication; they also fail to identify a patient correctly before performing a procedure and neglect to perform hand sanitization consistently, thus promoting the spread of infectious diseases. The medical assistant is an important link in the delivery of quality and *safe* care. Can you think of anything you have learned thus far in your studies that could help keep patients safe in the physician's office? Procedure 36-1 presents a scenario about patient safety. Follow the step-by-step procedure to learn what you can do to protect your patients from possible harm.

Employee Safety

The healthcare facility should safeguard patients as well as staff members from the possibility of accidental injury. Data compiled by the Occupational Safety and Health Administration (OSHA) reveal that the leading causes of accidents in an office setting are slips, trips, and falls. You must think and work safely to prevent accidents. Following are some suggestions from OSHA for vigilant accident prevention methods (Procedure 36-2):

1. Use proper body mechanics in all situations (see Chapter 32). For example, bend your knees and bring a heavy item close to you before lifting rather than bending from your back; push heavy items rather than pulling them; and ask for assistance when transferring patients.
2. Constantly check the floors and hallways for obstructions and possible tripping hazards, such as telephone and computer cables or boxes.
3. Store supplies inside cabinets rather than on top, where they can fall off and injure someone; store heavier items on lower shelves so they do not have to be lifted any higher than necessary.
4. Clean up spills immediately; slippery floors are a danger to everyone.

PROCEDURE 36-1

Develop a Patient Safety Plan: Order the Correct Medication From the Pharmacy

GOAL: *To telephone the correct medication prescription into the pharmacy.*

SCENARIO: *The physician writes an order to be phoned into the pharmacy for a new patient diagnosed with depression. You think the order reads, Avinza, 30 mg po bid. The pharmacist asks you for the physician's DEA number, because Avinza is a narcotic analgesic. You ask the physician for clarification and are told the order was for Avanza, an antidepressant. Look up both medications in a drug reference. What could have happened if a powerful narcotic had been ordered for the patient instead of the antidepressant the physician intended?*

EQUIPMENT and SUPPLIES

- Notepad and pen
- Patient's record
- PDR or other drug reference

PROCEDURAL STEPS

1. Review the physician's written order for a prescription or repeat the order back to the physician if it is a verbal order. If it is a verbal order, write the order down and have the physician review it to make sure you have the correct medication before calling the pharmacy.
   PURPOSE: To make sure you can clearly read the order and/or have adequately verified a verbal order.

2. If you are unfamiliar with the medication, look it up in a drug reference.
   PURPOSE: To prevent possible errors, you should be familiar with all medications ordered.

3. After you have become familiar with the medication, if the order does not match the patient's diagnosis, ask the physician for clarification.
   PURPOSE: If you are not absolutely sure what the physician's handwriting means, do not hesitate to ask for clarification.

4. Refer to the office's policies and procedures manual to review the procedure for calling in a prescription order to the pharmacy.

5. Clarify any questions with the office manager to prevent any future errors.

PROCEDURE 36-2

Evaluate the Work Environment to Identify Safe and Unsafe Working Conditions: Develop an Environmental Safety Plan

GOAL: *To assess the healthcare facility for possible safety issues and develop a safety plan.*

SCENARIO: *Work with a partner to evaluate environmental safety in the laboratory at your school. Record your results and discuss them with the class. After all members of the class have shared their observations, develop a safety plan for your laboratory.*

EQUIPMENT and SUPPLIES

- Pen and paper
- Policies and procedures for environmental safety issues in the facility

PROCEDURAL STEPS

1. Check the floors and hallways for obstructions and possible tripping hazards, including torn carpets, possible spills, protruding electrical cords, and so on.
   PURPOSE: To prevent accidental falls.

2. Check storage areas to make sure the tops of cabinets are clear, and that heavier items have been stored closer to the floor.
   PURPOSE: To prevent injuries from items falling off shelves and to limit the lifting of heavy items.

3. Assess the location and security of handrails placed around the facility. They should be placed at all stairs, in restrooms, and in any other areas where staff members or patients may need assistance.
   PURPOSE: Handrails help safeguard staff members and patients and provide assistance where needed.

4. Examine all electrical plugs and outlets to prevent electrical overload.
   PURPOSE: Overloading electrical outlets could cause a fire.

5. Check all equipment to make sure it is in safe working condition.

6. Make sure all lights are working (both inside and outside the facility), that lighting is adequate, and that light fixtures are in good condition.
   PURPOSE: Adequate lighting both inside and outside the facility helps prevent accidents, and faulty fixtures can be a fire hazard.

7. Check the working condition of smoke alarms and examine all fire extinguishers.
   PURPOSE: To monitor the function of smoke detectors and make sure fire extinguishers are charged.

8. Make sure evacuation routes are posted throughout the facility, along with floor plans with clearly marked exit routes.
   PURPOSE: Every room in the facility must have a map with exit routes marked on it to make sure even those who are unfamiliar with the facility's floor plan can safely reach an exit in case of an emergency.

9. Record your observations and share them with the class.
   PURPOSE: To compile a comprehensive list of problem areas.

10. Based on group discussion, develop a plan of action for improving the safety of the laboratory.
    PURPOSE: The student-generated safety plan can be incorporated into the laboratory's policies and procedures manual.

5. Use a step stool to reach for things, not a chair or a box that could collapse or move.

6. Have handrails available as needed in the facility; use them and encourage patients to use them.

7. Do not overload electrical outlets.

8. Perform a safety check of the facility routinely; look for unsafe or defective equipment, torn carpeting that could catch heels, adequate lighting both inside and outside the facility, and so on.

A primary concern for personnel and patient safety is infection control. Chapter 27 discussed Standard Precautions in detail and the responsibility of employers to provide appropriate and adequate personal protective equipment (PPE). The goal is to protect staff members from occupational exposure to blood-borne pathogens while at the same time safeguarding patients in the facility. OSHA's guidelines include managing sharps and providing current safety-engineered sharps devices; providing hepatitis B immunization free of charge to all employees at risk of exposure to blood and body fluids; using latex-free supplies as much as possible to prevent allergic reactions in both staff members and patients; identifying all chemicals in the facility with Material Safety Data Sheets (MSDS; see Chapter 51) and adequately storing potentially dangerous substances; and performing proper hand hygiene consistently throughout the workday.

Another serious concern that faces all of us today is the prevention of workplace violence. Unfortunately, rarely does a week go by without reports of violence in a public place. Employees in a healthcare facility are no exception. We started the text with information about and exercises in communication techniques in the workplace—problem solving, therapeutic communication, and assertive behavior. All of these are helpful in dealing with a difficult patient. Employers should provide training on how to identify potentially violent patients and should discuss safe methods for managing difficult patients. Many employers offer training on how to manage assaultive behaviors.

In addition to these concerns, staff members should constantly be on the alert for possible safety hazards in and around the building, such as improper lighting, unlimited access to the facility, and inadequate use of security systems. Procedure 36-3 presents a scenario that deals with employee safety. Follow the steps of this procedure to learn how to handle such a situation.

Environmental Safety

Personal safety guidelines were discussed in Chapter 12. These include numerous work safety practices, such as office security, management of smoke detectors and fire extinguishers, posting of designated fire exit routes, and securing certain items (e.g., narcotics, dangerous chemicals) in locked storage areas in the facility.

The medical assistant must be prepared to use a fire extinguisher to prevent injury to patients and to protect the medical facility (Procedure 36-4). An ABC fire extinguisher is effective against the most common causes of fire, including cloth, paper, plastics, rubber, flammable liquids, and electrical fires. Most small extinguishers empty within 15 seconds, so it is important to call 911 immediately if the facility fire is not small and confined. If the fire is small, no heavy smoke is present, and you have easy access to an exit route, use the closest fire extinguisher. However, do not hesitate to evacuate the facility if you believe any danger exists to yourself or to others.

METHODS OF FIRE PREVENTION AND RESPONSE

- Properly store potentially flammable chemicals and supplies according to manufacturers' guidelines.
- Properly maintain electrical equipment, cords, and outlets throughout the facility.
- If a fire is suspected, immediately disconnect oxygen supplies or turn off oxygen tanks to prevent an explosion.
- Smoke alarms should be located throughout the facility, checked periodically, and replaced as needed.
- Make sure that fire safety equipment is available and current; fire extinguishers should be inspected at least annually; if an extinguisher is discharged, it must be replaced immediately.
- Fire extinguishers should be located in multiple sites throughout the facility and mounted on the wall for easy access.
- If you smell smoke or suspect a fire, immediately notify the fire department (or call 911) and evacuate the facility. Do not use elevators if a fire is suspected.

CRITICAL THINKING APPLICATION   36-1

Cheryl is in the middle of a busy day; patients are in all of the examination rooms, and the waiting room is full. She walks past the patient bathroom and smells smoke. She opens the door and sees smoke and flames coming from the waste basket. What should she do? Write down your response to this scenario and share it with your classmates.

Each facility should have a policy and procedure in place for evacuating the building. According to OSHA, the facility's plan first should identify the situations that might require evacuation, such as a natural disaster or a fire. The following provisions should be included in the facility's evacuation plan:

- An emergency action coordinator must be designated, and all employees must know who this individual is. This person is in charge if an emergency occurs.
- The coordinator is responsible for managing the emergency at the facility and for notifying and working with community emergency services.
- Evacuation routes with clearly marked exits must be posted in multiple locations throughout the facility. Maps of floor diagrams with arrows pointing to the closest exits are an easy means of finding the closest door out, even for individuals unfamiliar with the facility.
- Exit doors must be clearly marked, well lit, and wide enough for everyone to evacuate.
- Identify hazardous areas in the facility that should be avoided during an emergency evacuation.
- Designate a meeting place outside the facility for all those evacuating to make sure everyone got out of the facility safely.
- Employees should be trained to assist any co-worker or patient with special needs.
- A designated individual must check the entire facility, including restrooms, before exiting. He or she must make sure to close all

PROCEDURE 36-3

Develop an Employee Safety Plan: Manage a Difficult Patient

GOAL: *To communicate with an angry patient in a safe, therapeutic manner. The following procedure is part of an overall employee safety plan.*

SCENARIO: *You are working at the admissions desk when an extremely angry patient comes storming into the office, screaming about a mistake on his bill. Although the facility uses an outside billing center, you recognize that you should attempt to help the patient and try to diffuse the situation. Remember: Call 911 immediately and alert any available security if you or one of your co-workers is being threatened with violence.*

EQUIPMENT and SUPPLIES

- Telephone
- Patient record
- Policies and procedures manual

PROCEDURAL STEPS

1. Although it is important to safeguard patient privacy, do not ask an angry patient into an isolated room; do not close the door.
   PURPOSE: To protect yourself, remain in an open area. If you are in a room with an angry patient, keep the door open and stand close to the door so that you can leave the room quickly if necessary.
2. Alert other staff members to the situation, if possible.
   PURPOSE: To have assistance nearby; call 911 immediately if you feel physically threatened.
3. If you do not feel physically threatened, allow the patient to blow off steam.
   PURPOSE: Attempting to interrupt the patient to give a logical reason for the problem will only make him angrier. Allowing him to continue to yell helps him release the anger so that you can work on a reasonable solution to the problem. Call 911 if at any time you feel threatened.
4. When the patient begins to slow down, offer supportive statements, such as, "I understand it is frustrating to receive a bill you think is unfair." Continue to make supportive statements until the patient is calmer (think of it as the patient screaming his way up a mountain; sooner or later, he is going to run out of steam; when he begins to slow down, you can then start offering supportive statements).

PURPOSE: Providing verbal support helps diffuse the situation and gives the patient the opportunity to become calmer and reach a rational level where you can discuss the problem.

5. Once you can discuss the situation, ask the patient for the details of the problem. Gather as much information as possible so you can work together on a possible solution.
6. After determining the problem, suggest a possible solution to the patient. For example, tell him that you will contact the billing office with the information and will make sure they get back to the patient as soon as possible.
   PURPOSE: Use therapeutic techniques, including restatement, reflection, and clarification, to gather details and work on a possible solution with the patient. Make sure you follow up with the action to prevent future outbursts.
7. Report the incident to your supervisor and document the patient's problem and the agreed-upon action in the patient's medical record, taking care not to use judgmental statements.
   PURPOSE: Documenting the patient's problem and the agreed-upon solution allows for continuity of care if follow-up is needed. The patient's medical record is a legal document, and all judgmental statements must be avoided.
8. Discuss your approach to managing the difficult patient at the next staff meeting. With your supervisor's permission, summarize your approach and include it as part of the facility's Employee Safety Plan.
   PURPOSE: The safety plan should be reviewed frequently, and revisions should be made as needed.

PROCEDURE 36-4

Demonstrate the Proper Use of a Fire Extinguisher

GOAL: *To role-play the safe and proper use of a fire extinguisher.*

EQUIPMENT and SUPPLIES

- Portable, office-size ABC fire extinguisher that has been discharged

PROCEDURAL STEPS

Role-play the following with a discharged ABC fire extinguisher.
1. Pull the pin from the handle of the extinguisher.

2. Aim the discharge from the extinguisher toward the bottom of the flames.
   PURPOSE: Aiming the fire extinguisher directly onto the fire may spread the flames.
3. Squeeze the handle of the extinguisher so that it begins to discharge.
4. Sweep the extinguisher from side to side toward the base of the fire until it is out or until fire officials arrive.
5. Check on the safety of all patients and other personnel.

PROCEDURE 36-5

Participate in a Mock Environmental Exposure Event: Evacuate a Physician's Office

GOAL: *To role-play an environmental disaster and implement an evacuation plan.*

SCENARIO: *Role-play the following scenario with your lab group: The building next door to the physician's office where you work is on fire. One member of the group is the designated emergency action coordinator, two individuals are responsible for helping patients with special needs out of the facility, and one person is designated to be the last to leave after the building is clear. In a community emergency situation, certain staff members may be designated to provide immediate assistance to survivors. Two medical assistants are sent to help with fire victims. How could medical assistants help in this situation? After the evacuation is complete, meet in a designated spot to discuss the process and see whether any aspects of the evacuation plan could be improved. Document the steps taken throughout the mock environmental event.*

EQUIPMENT and SUPPLIES

- Pen and paper
- Policies and procedures for evacuation of the facility and response to an environmental disaster

PROCEDURAL STEPS

1. In an actual emergency, an emergency action coordinator is in charge.
   <u>PURPOSE:</u> All employees must know who this individual is (usually it is the office manager) and must follow his or her lead in safely responding to the emergency situation.

2. The coordinator is responsible for managing the emergency at the facility and for notifying and working with community emergency services.
   <u>PURPOSE:</u> The coordinator or someone designated by the coordinator must notify community emergency services of the fire; the coordinator works with emergency services to provide care at the scene.

3. Fire victims are being cared for across the street, where a triage and treatment center has been set up by the police, fire, and emergency responder units in the city. Two medical assistant staff members are sent to assist with the victims, as follows:
   - Use therapeutic communication techniques to calm and care for victims
   - Implement appropriate Standard Precautions
   - Monitor and record vital signs
   - Gather pertinent health histories
   - Observe victims for possible complications, such as breathing problems, shock, angina, and so on.
   - Immediately report to emergency responders any life-threatening changes in a patient's status
   - Use first aid skills as needed

4. The coordinator designates an employee to shut down any combustibles (e.g., oxygen tanks) immediately.
   <u>PURPOSE:</u> To prevent an explosion if the fire spreads.

5. Using the posted evacuation routes, staff members follow floor plan diagrams to the closest safe exit. Any hazardous areas in the facility that should be avoided during the emergency evacuation are identified.
   <u>PURPOSE:</u> Evacuation routes must be posted throughout the facility, and exit doors must be clearly marked, well lit, and wide enough for everyone to evacuate. The doors facing the building on fire should not be used, because this could be a hazard.

6. Assistance is provided for employees and patients with special needs who may require extra help during the evacuation.

7. One staff member is delegated to check that everyone has left the facility and that fire doors have been closed before he or she leaves the building.
   <u>PURPOSE:</u> To make sure the building is clear and that any fire is contained. This person should leave immediately if there is danger.

8. All evacuated personnel and patients should meet in a designated area to count heads and make sure everyone exited the facility safely.
   <u>PURPOSE:</u> To make sure everyone safely evacuated the facility.

9. After everyone has been accounted for and the office patients are secure, staff members who are not needed should report to the triage area to provide assistance to rescue workers and victims.

10. Discuss with the class the evacuation exercise and response to a community disaster.

11. Document your role in the exercise. What were the strengths and weaknesses of the group's response to an environmental emergency?
    <u>PURPOSE:</u> To reflect on the learning activity.

---

doors when leaving to try to contain the fire or other disaster (Procedure 36-5).

DISPOSAL OF HAZARDOUS WASTE

Chapter 27 explained the management of biohazardous waste; the use of PPE when the potential exists for exposure to blood and body fluids; the importance of flushing the eyes with an eye wash unit if they are exposed to potentially infectious material; and the consistent use of sharps containers. Regardless of individual responsibilities in the facility, all employees must be aware of potentially dangerous situations and must comply with all safety measures to protect themselves and their patients.

OSHA defines regulated waste as any contaminated item that might release blood or other potentially infectious material; contaminated supplies that are caked with dried blood or other potentially infectious material; contaminated sharps; and waste products that contain blood or other potentially infectious material.

Healthcare facilities must make special arrangements for the disposal of regulated waste, which often costs as much as 10 times more than regular garbage disposal. It therefore is important to put only supplies contaminated with blood or body fluids into red bag collection systems and sharps containers. Steps for the proper disposal of hazardous materials in the physician's office include the following:

- Place signs on or near the biohazard container to identify its purpose and the materials that should be deposited there. All biohazardous waste containers should display a biohazard label.
- Make sure all biohazardous waste containers are covered and have a foot pedal for opening and closing the container. This prevents the spread of infectious material and reduces the likelihood that noninfectious material will be tossed inside. Biohazard containers should be kept only in treatment areas where contaminated materials are likely to be produced.
- Place a regular garbage container next to a biohazard container to encourage staff to use the biohazard bags only as needed.
- Place only sharps in sharps containers; gauze, bandages, and so on belong in a contaminated waste container. Noninfectious packaging material and other items belong in the regular trash.

EMERGENCY PREPAREDNESS

Ambulatory care centers and hospitals may be the first to recognize and initiate a response to a community emergency. If an infectious outbreak is suspected, Standard Precautions should be implemented immediately to control the spread of infection. If the problem has the potential to affect a large number of individuals in the community (e.g., suspected food contamination), a communication network should be established to notify local and state health departments and perhaps federal officials. Your employer may participate in an annual community disaster preparedness drill designed to help facilities improve their response to natural disasters and other emergencies.

Local governments are responsible for creating a Local Emergency Management Authority (LEMA) that coordinates police, fire, emergency medical services, public health, and area healthcare response to community-wide emergencies. These agencies are responsible for developing an all-hazards response plan that would be appropriate for any community emergency. Local officials turn to state, regional, or federal officials for assistance as needed.

Every healthcare facility should have a policy that includes specific procedures for the management of emergencies on site. When a new employee starts on the job, part of the orientation process is to review the site's policies and procedures manual. As a new employee, be sure to get answers to any questions you have about emergency management in that particular facility.

Staff members should discuss emergencies that may occur and should have an emergency action plan for rapid, systematic intervention. For instance, local industries may present unique problems that call for very specialized care. Plan for these, and ask the physician's advice on the procedures to follow and the supplies to have on hand. If the facility has several employees, each should be assigned specific duties in the event of an emergency. Organization and planning make the difference between systematic care for patients and complete chaos.

EMERGENCY PLAN FOR A NATURAL DISASTER OR OTHER EMERGENCY IN AN AMBULATORY CARE FACILITY

- Evacuate the facility as needed.
- Include procedures for the protection of patients' medical records. If the facility uses electronic health records (EHRs), make sure this information is backed up on other systems or on flash drives.
- In the case of a community emergency, provide care to the extent possible within the facility.
- Coordinate services between the ambulatory facility and other local healthcare systems, including hospitals and public health departments.
- Provide staff and supplies as needed to help in a community emergency.
- Maintain up-to-date phone trees to notify staff members of an emergency.
- Educate patients on emergency preparedness.

CRITICAL THINKING APPLICATION   36-2

A chemical plant is located about 3 blocks from Dr. Bendt's office. The office staff is brainstorming ideas about what should be done if an accident occurs at the plant. Based on what you have learned so far about emergency preparedness, what do you think should be included in the office's emergency plan?

Community Resources for Emergency Preparedness

Most communities have an emergency medical services (EMS) system. This system includes an efficient communications network (e.g., the emergency telephone number 911), well-trained rescue personnel, properly equipped ambulances, an emergency facility that is open 24 hours a day to provide advanced life support, and a hospital intensive care unit for victims.

More than 100 poison control centers in the United States are ready to provide emergency information for the treatment of victims of poisoning. Every healthcare facility is required to post a list of local emergency numbers. This list should be kept in plain sight and should be known to all office personnel. A good place to post this vital information is next to all the phones in the facility. Include on the list the numbers for the local EMS system, poison control center, ambulance and rescue squad, fire department, and police department (Procedure 36-6).

TELEPHONE NOTIFICATION NUMBERS FOR EMERGENCY PREPAREDNESS

- Local hospital numbers, including emergency department, infection control officer, administration contacts, and public affairs office
- Local and state Health Department numbers
- Centers for Disease Control and Prevention (CDC) Emergency Response Office: 770-448-7100

PROCEDURE 36-6

Maintain an Up-to-Date List of Community Resources for Emergency Preparedness

GOAL: *To develop and maintain a list of community agencies that would respond to a natural disaster or other emergency.*

SCENARIO: *Your employer asks you to develop a list of groups in your community that are part of the community-wide emergency preparedness plan that has been mandated by the state and federal governments. Using multiple resources, develop a comprehensive list of emergency services for your area.*

EQUIPMENT and SUPPLIES

- Telephone
- Internet access
- Pen and paper
- Electronic record

PROCEDURAL STEPS

1. Start with an online search for the area Local Emergency Management Authority (LEMA) office, sponsored by the Department of Homeland Security. If available, investigate the Web site for information about the emergency preparedness plan in your community. You can begin the search at www.ready.gov/america
   PURPOSE: To develop emergency preparedness plans by starting with the federal and state governments.

2. Gather contact information for local police, fire, and emergency medical services (EMS); post this information next to all telephones in the facility.
   PURPOSE: To ensure that emergency services contact information is immediately available in case of an emergency in the facility.

3. Investigate services provided by your local Public Health office and the American Red Cross.
   PURPOSE: To coordinate services available to potential victims in the community.

4. Organize the information gathered about community resources for emergency preparedness. With your supervisor's approval, post a copy of this information in all appropriate locations in the facility. Prepare a database in the computer that can be updated as the information changes.

The Centers for Disease Control and Prevention (CDC) recommends that all healthcare facilities be aware of possible agents of bioterrorism, including anthrax, botulism, plague, and smallpox. The physician is responsible for diagnosing and reporting any suspected cases, but the medical assistant may be involved in patient care and certainly will participate in preventing the spread of infection in the facility. As with any suspected infectious disease, Standard Precautions (see Chapter 27) should be used to control disease transmission. These precautions should be implemented with all patients, regardless of their diagnosis or possible infection status.

Infection control procedures for bioterrorism threats include the following:

- Sanitize hands routinely.
- Wear disposable gloves when the potential exists for contamination with blood and body fluids.
- Use masks/eye protection or face shields if the potential exists for being splashed by secretions or blood and body fluids.
- Wear gowns to protect skin and clothes as needed; remove them promptly and wash the hands to prevent transmission of infectious material.
- Sanitize, disinfect, and sterilize equipment, supplies, and environmental surfaces.
- Dispose of contaminated waste in appropriate biohazard containers.

Community emergency preparedness plans are required by the federal government so that a coordinated response is in place if a natural disaster occurs, such as Hurricane Katrina, which devastated New Orleans. The federal government requires all healthcare facilities, including private physicians' offices, to be prepared to provide medical services and to contribute medical supplies if a natural disaster or other emergency occurs in the area.

Emergency preparedness plans are designed to coordinate the care provided by all healthcare facilities and agencies in the community, including local emergency management agencies, EMS, fire departments, law enforcement agencies, the American Red Cross, and the National Guard. Each of these groups can provide crucial services during any community emergency.

Medical assistants also can contribute to rescue and emergency efforts. Services that might be performed by trained medical assistants include providing emergency first aid at the site of a disaster; conducting patient interviews in an empathetic manner while using therapeutic communication to help calm victims and gather important health-related information; helping with mass vaccination efforts or antibiotic distribution; performing documentation and electronic health record management; ensuring compliance with the procedures required by Standard Precautions; assisting with patient education efforts; and performing phlebotomy and laboratory procedures according to their skill level.

PSYCHOLOGICAL ASPECTS OF AN EMERGENCY SITUATION

Everyone involved in an emergency situation experiences a certain amount of anxiety and stress. The Centers for Disease Control and Prevention (CDC) recommends that a facility's emergency preparedness plan consider the following steps to minimize these negative psychological effects on both healthcare workers and patients:

- Provide fact sheets for employees and patients to help them understand the dangers of certain emergencies, and encourage employee participation in disaster drills.

- Plan in advance for effective communication and action in response to an emergency; the plan should include methods for coordinating a response with local and state agencies and media sources.
- Put into place a method for clearly explaining emergency situations to patients and healthcare workers; offer immediate evaluation and treatment of an infectious outbreak.
- Treat acute anxiety with reassurance and explanation; provide follow-up counseling for employees as needed.

Further information on emergency preparedness can be found at the following CDC sites:

- Emergency preparedness planning: www.bt.cdc.gov/planning
- Coordinating Office for Terrorism Preparedness and Emergency Response (COTPER): www.bt.cdc.gov

ASSISTING WITH MEDICAL EMERGENCIES

First aid is defined as the immediate care given to a person who has been injured or has suddenly taken ill. Knowledge of first aid and related skills often can mean the difference between life and death, temporary and permanent disability, or rapid recovery and long-term hospitalization. The medical assistant may be responsible for initiating first aid in the office and continuing to administer first aid until the physician or the trained medical team arrives. Every medical assistant should successfully complete a course for the professional in cardiopulmonary resuscitation (CPR) and should continue to hold a current CPR card as long as he or she is employed.

Basic knowledge of CPR and life support skills needs to be updated regularly, because procedures change as new techniques are developed. For example, both the American Red Cross and the American Heart Association (AHA) now recommend the inclusion of training on automated external defibrillators for all healthcare workers.

Medical assistants need up-to-date training in current emergency practices. They should encourage their local professional chapters to offer workshops on management of emergencies in the ambulatory care setting, as well as community-wide emergency preparedness. Being prepared for both types of emergencies is important. The facility's employees must be ready to respond both to emergencies on site and to natural disasters or other emergencies that affect the community.

Medical assistants are not responsible for diagnosing emergencies, especially over the telephone, but they are expected to make decisions about emergency situations on the basis of their medical knowledge and training. If any doubt exists about how to manage a particular situation or emergency phone call, the medical assistant should not hesitate to consult the physician, the office manager, or some other more experienced member of the healthcare team.

THE MEDICAL ASSISTANT'S ROLE IN PERFORMING EMERGENCY PROCEDURES

- Perform only the emergency procedures for which you have been trained.
- If an emergency occurs in the facility, notify the physician.
- If a physician cannot be located, immediately contact the local emergency medical services (EMS) team.

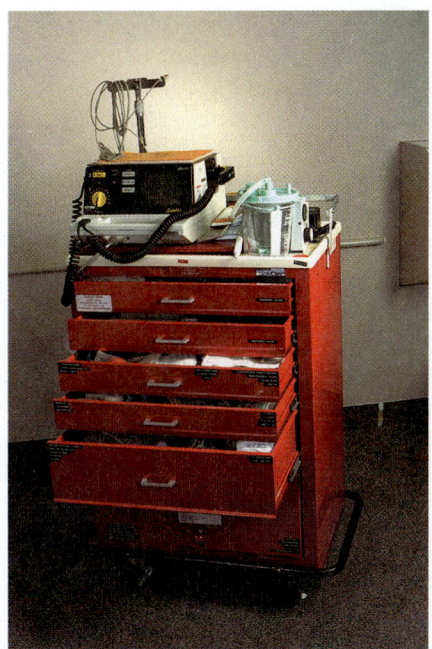

FIGURE 36-1 Office emergency cart with defibrillator. Drawers are marked for easy retrieval of emergency supplies.

Emergency Supplies

Emergency supplies consist of a properly equipped "crash cart" or box of items needed for a variety of emergencies (Figure 36-1). The contents vary to some degree, depending on the types of emergencies the particular office might expect to encounter. Emergency supplies should be kept in an easily accessible place that is known to all personnel in the office, and the supplies should be inventoried regularly. Expiration dates of medications and sterile supplies must be checked weekly or monthly, along with the status of available oxygen tanks and related supplies, and the cart should be replenished with fresh supplies after every use.

Emergency pharmaceutical supplies should include certain basic drugs, such as epinephrine, which has multiple uses in emergency situations. As a vasoconstrictor, it controls hemorrhage, relaxes the bronchioles to relieve acute asthma attacks, is administered for an acute anaphylactic reaction, and is an emergency heart stimulant used to treat shock. Epinephrine should be available in a ready-to-use cartridge syringe and needle unit. These units are supplied in 1-mL cartridges.

Other drugs used include atropine, digoxin (Lanoxin), nitroglycerin (Nitrostat), and lidocaine (Xylocaine). Atropine reduces secretions, increases respiratory rate and heart rate, and is a smooth muscle relaxant. It is administered in a cardiac emergency for **asystole**, or it can be used to treat bradycardia. Digoxin is a cardiac drug used to treat **arrhythmia** and congestive heart failure (CHF); it is good for emergency use because it has a relatively rapid action. Nitroglycerin is a vasodilator that is given to relieve angina; it acts by dilating the coronary arteries so that an increased volume of oxygenated blood can reach the **myocardium**. Lidocaine is used intravenously to treat a cardiac arrhythmia and locally as an anesthetic, and sodium bicarbonate corrects metabolic acidosis, which typically occurs after cardiac arrest.

Emergency medical supplies also should include an **emetic**, such as syrup of ipecac, which causes vomiting soon after the syrup is swallowed, and activated charcoal, an antidote that is swallowed to absorb ingested poisons. Narcan, an antidote administered intravenously for narcotic drug overdoses, acts to raise blood pressure and increase respiratory rate. Antihistamines for the treatment of allergic reactions and for anaphylaxis need to be available to treat any allergic responses to medications administered in the facility. Such antihistamines include Benadryl for minor reactions and Solu-Medrol, a corticosteroid, for severe anaphylactic reactions.

Other medications also may be found on a crash cart. These include isoproterenol (e.g., Isuprel, Medihaler-Iso, Norisodrine), an antispasmodic used to treat bronchospasms (such as those experienced during an asthma attack) that also is effective as a cardiac stimulant; metaraminol (Aramine) (50%, in a prefilled syringe) for severe shock; phenobarbital, amobarbital sodium (Amytal), and diazepam (Valium) for convulsions and/or sedative effects; furosemide (Lasix) for CHF; and glucagon, which is used primarily to counteract severe hypoglycemic reactions (low blood glucose) in diabetic patients taking insulin.

BASIC EMERGENCY SUPPLIES

Equipment
- Adhesive tape in 1- and 2-inch widths
- Airways—variety of types and sizes
- Alcohol wipes
- Ambu bag with assorted sizes of facial masks
- Antimicrobial skin ointment
- Bandage scissors
- Cotton balls and cotton swabs
- Cardiopulmonary resuscitation (CPR) masks—both adult and pediatric
- Defibrillator
- Elastic bandages in 2- and 3-inch widths
- Filter needles
- Flashlight with batteries
- Gauze pads, 2 × 2- and 4 × 4-inch widths, and roller bandage—both sterile and nonsterile
- Gloves, sterile and nonsterile, in multiple sizes
- Hot and cold packs (instant type)
- Intravenous catheters, tubing, solutions (variety of types, including D_5W and Ringer's lactate), and tourniquet
- Laryngoscope with blades
- Lubricant
- Personal protective equipment (PPE), including impervious gowns, splash guards or goggles, and booties
- Portable oxygen tank with regulator, mask, and nasal cannula
- Roller gauze (Ace bandages and gauze dressing) in various sizes
- Sharps container
- Sphygmomanometer—both pediatric and adult regular and large sizes
- Splints—various sizes
- Sterile dressings—miscellaneous sizes, including two abdominal pads
- Steri-Strips or suturing material
- Suction machine and catheters
- Syringes and needles in assorted sizes and gauges
- Tongue blades
- Tubex cartridge system
- Venipuncture supplies and butterfly units

Medications
- Activated charcoal, bottle of 30 to 50 g
- Amobarbital (Amytal)
- Antihistamine, injectable and oral
- Atropine
- Dextrose
- Diazepam (Valium)
- Digoxin (Lanoxin), injectable
- Diphenhydramine (Benadryl)
- Epinephrine (Adrenalin), injectable
- Furosemide (Lasix)
- Glucagon and/or glucose tablets
- Ipecac syrup
- Isoproterenol (Isuprel), aerosol inhaler and injectable
- Lidocaine (Xylocaine), injectable and spray
- Metaraminol (Aramine)
- Narcan
- Nitroglycerin tablets
- Phenobarbital, injectable
- Sodium bicarbonate, injectable
- Solu-Medrol
- Sterile water and saline for injection

Defibrillators

The medical assistant may be required to assist the healthcare team with defibrillation of emergency patients. Defibrillation is indicated when a patient is in ventricular **fibrillation** (VF). VF is a severe cardiac arrhythmia that is caused by uncoordinated, rapid firing of the electrical system of the heart, which makes it impossible for the ventricles to empty. In the absence of ventricular emptying, the patient has no pulse, blood pressure drops to zero, and the patient could die within 4 minutes unless help is given immediately.

Defibrillators are devices that send an electrical current through the myocardium by means of handheld paddles (in a healthcare facility) or self-adhesive pads applied to the chest. This electrical shock causes momentary asystole, giving the heart's natural pacemaker an opportunity to resume the heart rate at a normal rhythm.

An automated external defibrillator (AED) has a computerized system that analyzes a cardiac rhythm and delivers voice-prompt instructions on how to operate the device (Figure 36-2 and Procedure 36-7). AEDs uses self-adhesive pads that record and monitor the cardiac rhythm, and the device instructs the rescuer when to deliver the electrical charge. The apex-anterior position is the most commonly used paddle position, with the anterior (sternum) pad placed to the right of the upper sternum, and the apex pad placed under the patient's left nipple at the left middle axillary line (Figure 36-3). To defibrillate a female patient, the apex pad is placed next to or underneath the left breast.

Precautions for Automated External Defibrillators

- Neither the patient nor the caregiver should be in contact with any metal during defibrillation. Do not place the AED pad over jewelry, and remove the patient's glasses to prevent injuries.
- When available, a pediatric-dose AED system should be used for children 1 to 8 years of age (it should not be used on infants younger than 1 year old). These systems deliver a reduced shock dose for victims up to about 8 years old or weighing 55 pounds.

- All clothing (including bras) must be removed; pads must be applied directly to the skin. If the individual has a great deal of hair on the chest, try to push the hair aside before applying the pads; or, apply the pads and quickly remove them to remove hair form the area, then reapply new pads. The machine will prompt you by stating "Check electrode" if the connection is poor.
- To prevent burns, make sure the patient is lying on a dry surface and the chest is dry before applying the pads.
- If the patient has an implanted defibrillator or pacemaker, it will be obvious from the bulged area under the surface of the skin on

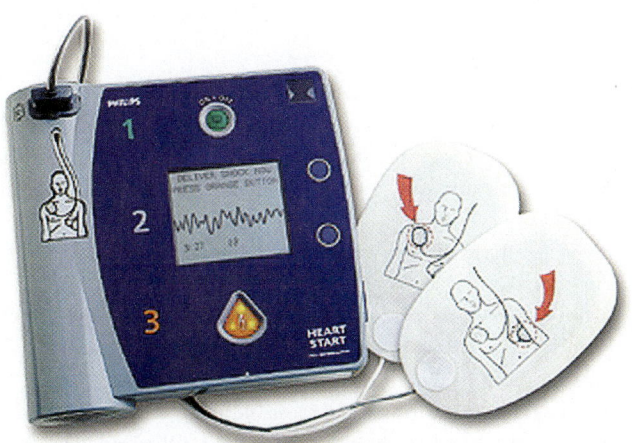

FIGURE 36-2 Fully automated external defibrillator. (From Aehlert B: *Mosby's comprehensive pediatric emergency care*, St Louis, 2005, Mosby.)

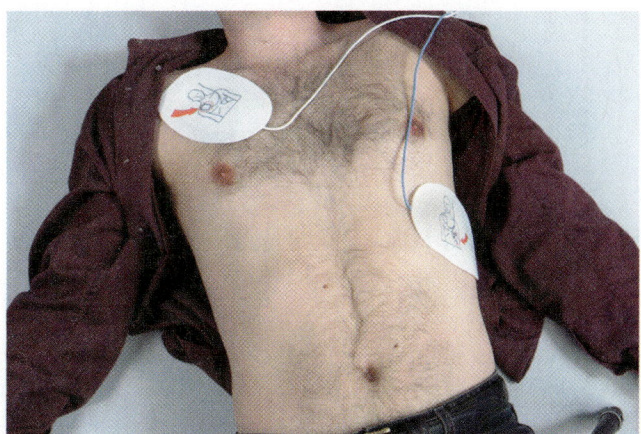

FIGURE 36-3 Connect the adhesive pads to the automated external defibrillator (AED) cables; apply the pads to the patient's chest at the upper right sternal border and at the lower left ribs over the cardiac apex. (From Chapleau W: *Emergency medical technician: making the difference*, St Louis, 2007, Mosby.)

PROCEDURE 36-7

Maintain Provider/Professional-Level CPR Certification: Use an Automated External Defibrillator

GOAL: *To defibrillate adult victims with cardiac arrest. Most adult victims in sudden cardiac arrest are in ventricular fibrillation. The survival rate for victims with ventricular fibrillation is as high as 90% when defibrillation occurs within the first minute of collapse; however, the survival rate declines 7% to 10% with every minute defibrillation does not occur.*

EQUIPMENT and SUPPLIES

- Practice automated external defibrillator (AED)
- Approved mannequin

PROCEDURAL STEPS

These steps are to be performed only on an approved mannequin.

If the healthcare worker witnesses a cardiac arrest, an AED should be used as soon as possible. If cardiopulmonary resuscitation (CPR) has already been started, continue performing CPR until the AED machine is turned on, pads are applied, and the machine is ready.

1. Place the AED near the victim's left ear. Turn on the AED.
2. Attach electrode pads to the victim's bare dry chest as pictured on the AED. Place the electrodes at the sternum and apex of the heart. Make sure the pads are in complete contact with the victim's chest and that they do not overlap (see Figure 36-3).

3. All rescuers must clear away from the victim. Press the ANALYZE button. The AED analyzes the victim's coronary status, announces whether the victim is going to be shocked, and automatically charges the electrodes (Figure 1).

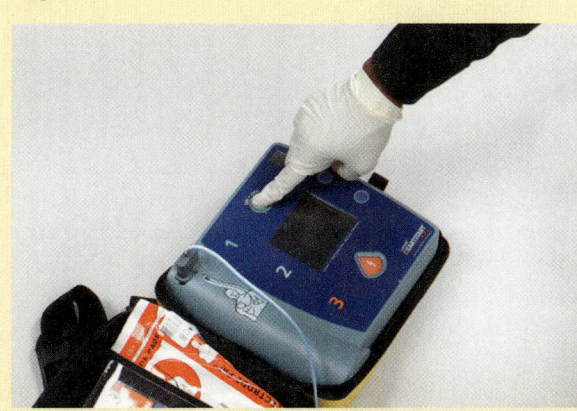

(From Chapleau W: *Emergency medical technician: making the difference*, St Louis, 2007, Mosby.)

PROCEDURE 36-7—cont'd

4. All rescuers must clear away from the victim. Press the SHOCK button if the machine is not automated. You may repeat 3 analyze-shock cycles.

5. Deliver 1 shock, leaving the AED attached, and immediately perform CPR, starting with chest compressions.

6. After 5 cycles (about 2 minutes) of CPR, repeat the AED analysis and deliver another shock, if indicated. If a nonshockable rhythm is detected, the AED should instruct the rescuer to resume CPR immediately, beginning with chest compressions.

7. If the machine gives the "No Shock Indicated" signal, assess the victim. Check the carotid pulse and breathing status and keep the AED attached until EMS arrives.
   <u>PURPOSE:</u> Continue to monitor breathing and circulation, because these can stop at any time. Keep the AED pads in place to diagnose ventricular fibrillation quickly if it occurs.

---

the chest. Apply the AED pads at least 1 inch away from implants to prevent interference.

GENERAL RULES FOR EMERGENCIES

A medical assistant will face two types of emergencies in the ambulatory care setting: office emergencies and home emergencies. Common office emergencies and their management are discussed later in this chapter. Besides dealing with actual emergency situations on site, a medical assistant frequently is the first person to interact with patients facing potential emergencies at home. It is estimated that one-third of the telephone calls received in a physician's office involve some type of problem that requires attention. An immediate decision must be made on how to manage that problem: by giving home care advice, scheduling an appointment, or, in life-threatening cases, notifying EMS. Many facilities, under the direction and approval of the physician, create a reference list of appropriate questions for specific patient complaints.

Regardless of how emergency phone calls are managed in the facility where you work, consider the following general rules when faced with an emergency:

- It is most important to stay calm. Reassure the patient and make him or her as comfortable as possible.
- Assess the situation to determine the nature of the emergency. Decide whether the need is immediate. This decision requires calm judgment and medical knowledge.
- Obtain as much information as possible to determine the appropriate action.
- Immediately refer any concerns to the office supervisor or physician.

Telephone Screening

Each time the phone rings in a healthcare facility, a person with a possible life-or-death situation may be on the other end of the line. One of the most important tasks performed by medical assistants every day is answering the phones and managing patients' needs efficiently and appropriately. Emergency action principles serve as a guide for managing emergency phone calls in an ambulatory care setting:

- If the patient's situation is life-threatening, activate EMS/911.
  - *Never put a caller with a life-threatening emergency on hold, and always be the last to hang up.*

- Remain on the line until help arrives and you have talked to EMS personnel.
- Immediately record the names of the caller and the patient, the location, and the phone number in case the connection is lost.
- If you are unsure how to manage the emergency situation, contact the physician.
- If the patient is referred to an emergency department (ED), call the ED to notify the staff of the patient's arrival, and make a follow-up call to determine the patient's condition.
- Gather as much information as possible about what is wrong with the patient and when the problem started. Obtain details about the patient's condition, including:
  - What is the patient's level of consciousness? Alert, responsive, lethargic, or confused? Did the patient lose consciousness at any time? If so, for how long?
  - What is the character of the patient's respirations (and pulse if the caller is able to determine this): normal, rapid, shallow, or difficult?
  - Is there bleeding? If so, how much and from where?
  - Is there a suspected head or neck injury? If so, has the patient been moved? Is there a suspected fracture? Where?
  - Does the patient have a history of this problem?
  - Any there other symptoms, such as fever, vomiting, diarrhea, or pain?
- Details about what has been done for the patient:
  - Medication: What, when? Dose, effectiveness? Current allergies?
- Thoroughly document the information gathered and any actions taken, including notification of EMS, whether the patient was sent to the ED or an appointment was scheduled, all home care recommendations, and whether the physician was notified and when.

Based on the outcome of the telephone interaction, a decision is made about when the practitioner will see the patient (Procedure 36-8). Emergency calls require activation of EMS or immediate attention as soon as the patient arrives. Urgent calls require a same-day appointment if the patient has an acute condition or is in severe discomfort. This would include a young child with a high fever or a patient who complains of moderate to severe abdominal pain. The new patient will have to be worked into the day's schedule, which may cause a delay in currently scheduled appointments. Patients

PROCEDURE 36-8

Perform Patient Screening Using Established Protocols: Telephone Screening and Appropriate Documentation

GOAL: To assess the direction of emergency care and to document information appropriately in the patient's record.

SCENARIO: Cheryl is working with the telephone screening staff when they receive a call from the mother of a 5-year-old patient. The mother reports that her son fell and cut his arm. What type of information should Cheryl gather about the injury? What action should be taken? How should the incident be documented?

EQUIPMENT and SUPPLIES

- Notepad and pen or pencil
- Patient's medical record
- Facility's emergency procedures manual
- Appointment book or computer program
- Area emergency numbers

PROCEDURAL STEPS

1. Stay calm and reassure the caller.
   PURPOSE: To enable you to gather accurate details about the patient's condition.
2. Verify the identity of the caller and the injured patient.
3. Immediately record the name of the caller and the patient, the location, and the phone number.
   PURPOSE: To be able to contact the caller if the connection is lost.
4. Determine whether the patient's condition is life threatening. Quantify the amount of blood loss, whether the patient is alert and responsive, and whether breathing is normal. Notify emergency medical services (EMS) if necessary.
   PURPOSE: Notify emergency services immediately if the patient is in danger.
5. If EMS is notified, stay on the line with the caller until EMS personnel arrive at the scene.
   PURPOSE: Never break a phone connection in the case of a life-threatening emergency.
6. If emergency services are not needed, gather details about the injury to determine whether the patient can be seen in the office or should be referred to an emergency department (ED). Consider the following questions:

- Is there a suspected head or neck injury? Has the patient been moved?
- Is there a possible fracture? If so, where?
- Are there any other symptoms?
- Is there anything pertinent in the patient's health history that would complicate the situation?
- Has the caller administered any first aid? If so, what was done?

7. Based on the information gathered, determine when the patient should be seen in the office if he or she has not been referred to an ED.
   PURPOSE: Most emergencies are scheduled for an immediate office visit. This may require altering the current appointment schedule.
8. At any point in this process, do not hesitate to consult the physician or experienced staff or refer to the facility's emergency procedures manual to determine how to manage the patient's problem.
9. Always allow the caller to hang up first, just in case more information or assistance is needed.
10. Document the information gathered, the actions taken or recommended, any home care recommendations, and whether the physician was notified.
    PURPOSE: To have a legal record of the management of the emergency and a comprehensive description of the patient's condition and recommended management.

7/13/XX 1:25 PM Patient's mother reports child fell against a window and lacerated his arm. Bleeding is moderate but controlled. No reported signs of dyspnea or altered consciousness. Mother will bring child to office immediately for physician assessment. Cheryl Skurka, CMA (AAMA)

---

with other, less urgent problems can be scheduled for appointments within the next 3 to 4 days.

Management of On-Site Emergencies

An emergency can occur at any time to anyone. Always follow Standard Precautions when at risk for coming into contact with blood or body fluids. When an emergency occurs, it is impossible to determine the level of infection. All body fluids must be considered infectious, and appropriate precautions must be taken to prevent cross-contamination. If the situation is life-threatening, notify EMS and stay with the patient until you are relieved by the EMS provider or the physician. It is important to document all details of the incident in the patient's medical record.

DOCUMENTATION OF AN ON-SITE EMERGENCY

1. Patient's name, address, age, and health insurance information
2. Allergies, current medications, and pertinent health history
3. Name and relationship of any person with the patient
4. Vital signs and chief complaint
5. Sequence of events, beginning with how the problem occurred, any changes in the patient's overall condition, and any observations made regarding the patient's condition
6. Details regarding procedures or treatments performed on the patient

CRITICAL THINKING APPLICATION   36-3

Cheryl is working the front desk when a patient comes into the office limping. She tells Cheryl that she fell in the parking lot and hurt her ankle. Cheryl helps the patient into an exam room and begins to interview her. Role-play the situation with a classmate and make a list of at least 10 questions Cheryl should ask the patient.

Life-Threatening Emergencies

If a patient in the facility shows any signs of unresponsiveness, the clinician must be brought to the patient immediately. If no clinician is available in the facility, EMS must be activated. Even when a physician is present, the physician may order you to call 911 for immediate emergency care. Put on gloves before you begin to assess the patient, because any emergency situation may involve exposure to blood or body fluids.

Unresponsive Patient

If a patient is able to talk to you, he or she has an open airway. If the patient does not respond to a simple question (e.g., "Are you OK?"), gently shake the person's shoulder to check responsiveness. If the patient does not respond, you must assume that the patient is unconscious. Immediately call for help and activate EMS if that is office policy.

To care for an unresponsive patient, first assess the patient's respirations to determine whether the person is breathing. When the patient collapsed, the tongue may have gone limp and occluded the trachea. Just by changing the individual's position and opening the airway, you may provide all the assistance the patient needs to breathe independently.

If the patient is face down, roll the victim onto his or her back while supporting the head, neck, and back. Apply the head tilt–chin lift movement to open the airway. The tongue is attached to the lower jaw, so moving the jaw forward automatically opens the patient's airway. If a head or neck injury is suspected, the neck should be manipulated as little as possible; therefore, the airway should be open with the jaw-thrust maneuver. Both of these actions relieve possible obstruction of the trachea by the tongue.

Check for breathing no longer than 10 seconds by looking for a rise in the chest and by listening or feeling for air exchange (Figure 36-4). Breathing may stop suddenly for a variety of reasons, including shock, disease, and trauma. If no breaths are detected, artificial ventilation must be started immediately, because death can occur within 4 to 6 minutes. Barrier devices should be kept on hand for artificial respiration (Figure 36-5), and these should be used if rescue breaths are required (Procedure 36-9).

After giving the patient 2 slow breaths, check for signs of normal breathing or movement. If no signs of responsiveness are evident, check for cardiac circulation at the carotid pulse (in an adult or a child) or at the brachial pulse (in an infant) (Figure 36-6). Gently feel for the pulse while continuing to assess the patient for possible signs of recovery for 5 to 10 seconds. If a pulse is present, continue ventilating the lungs with slow breaths every 4 to 5 seconds (adult) or every 3 seconds (child or infant). If the pulse is absent, begin cycles of 30 chest compressions at a rate of about 100 per minute followed by 2 slow breaths.

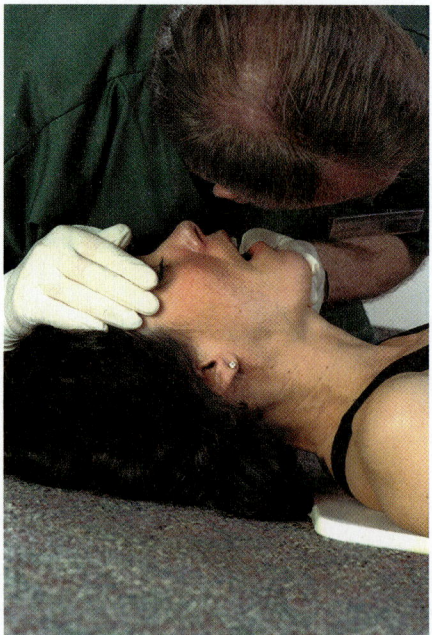

FIGURE 36-4 Checking for breathing in an unconscious patient.

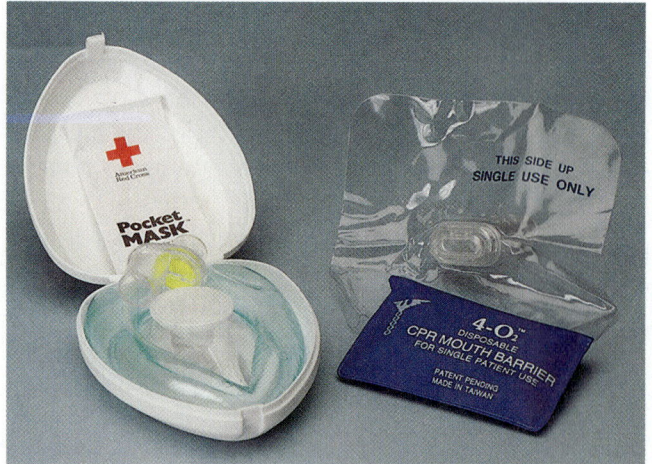

FIGURE 36-5 Cardiopulmonary resuscitation (CPR) mouth barriers.

When both breathing and pulse stop, the victim has suffered sudden death. Sudden death has many causes, including heart disease, choking, drowning, poisoning, suffocation, electrocution, and smoke inhalation. CPR must be started immediately to attempt to revive the patient and to prevent permanent damage to body organs, especially the brain. Continue CPR until the victim begins to move, an AED is available and ready to use, professional help arrives, or you are too exhausted to continue. If the patient has a pulse but is not breathing, continue rescue breathing and occasionally monitor the pulse until help arrives.

Refer to the *Standard First Aid Manual* of the American Red Cross or the *American Heart Association CPR Manual*, or the organizations' Web sites, for specific procedures and precautions in the management of respiratory and cardiac emergencies. As stated earlier, all healthcare workers should have a current Certification for the Professional in CPR.

PROCEDURE 36-9

Maintain Provider/Professional-Level CPR Certification: Perform Adult Rescue Breathing and One-Rescuer CPR; Perform Pediatric and Infant CPR

GOAL: *To restore breathing and blood circulation when respiration or pulse (or both) has stopped.*

EQUIPMENT and SUPPLIES

- Disposable gloves
- Cardiopulmonary resuscitation (CPR) ventilator masks for adults, children, and infants
- Approved mannequins

PROCEDURAL STEPS

These steps are to be performed only on approved mannequins.

TO PERFORM CPR ON AN ADULT VICTIM

1. Establish unresponsiveness. Tap the victim and ask, "Are you OK?" Wait for the victim to respond.
   <u>PURPOSE:</u> To determine whether the victim is conscious.
2. Activate the emergency response system. Put on gloves and get a ventilator mask.
   <u>PURPOSE:</u> As soon as it is determined that an adult victim requires emergency care, activate emergency medical services (EMS). Most adults with sudden, nontraumatic cardiac arrest are in ventricular fibrillation. The time from collapse to defibrillation is the single most important predictor of survival.
3. Tilt the victim's head by placing one hand on the forehead and applying enough pressure to push the head back; with the fingers of the other hand under the chin, lift up and pull the jaw forward. Look, listen, and feel for signs of breathing. Place your ear over the mouth and listen for breathing. Watch the rising and falling of the chest for evidence of breathing (Figure 1). If breathing is absent or inadequate, open the airway and place the ventilator mask over the victim's mouth and nose.
   <u>PURPOSE:</u> To open the airway and determine whether the victim is breathing.

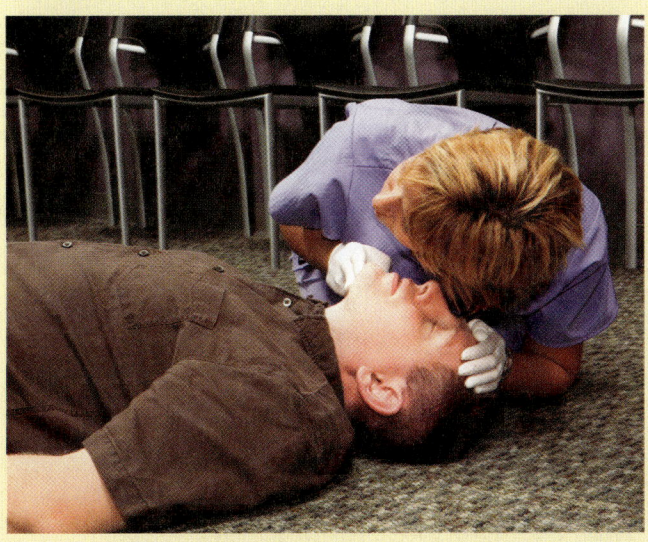

4. Give 2 slow breaths (1½ to 2 seconds per breath for an adult; 1 to 2 seconds per breath for an infant or child), holding the ventilator mask tightly against the face while tilting the victim's chin up to keep the airway open (Figure 2). Remove your mouth from the mouthpiece between breaths to allow time for the patient to exhale between breaths.

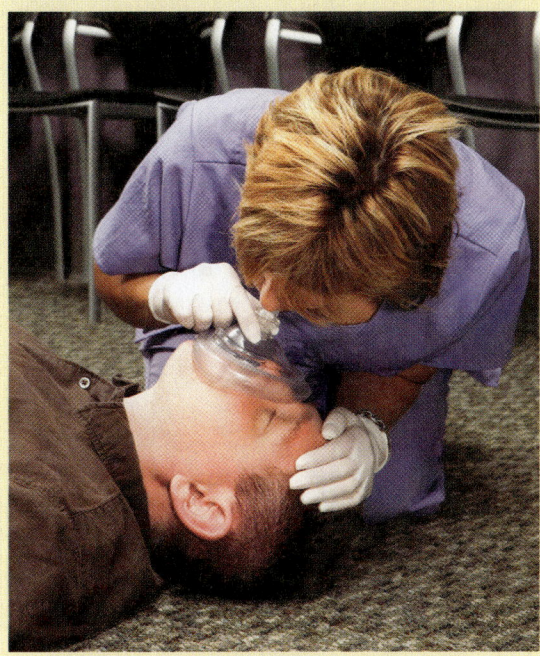

5. Check the patient's pulse (at the carotid artery for an adult or older child; at the brachial artery for an infant). If a pulse is present, continue rescue breathing (1 breath every 4 to 5 seconds—about 10 to 12 breaths per minute for an adult; 1 breath every 3 seconds—about 12 to 20 breaths per minute for an infant or child). If no signs of circulation are present, begin cycles of 30 chest compressions (at a rate of about 100 compressions per minute for an adult) followed by 2 slow breaths.
6. To deliver chest compressions, kneel at the victim's side a couple of inches away from the chest. Hand placement is over the sternum, between the nipples but above the xiphoid process.
7. Place the heel of your hand on the chest over the lower part of the sternum.
8. Place your other hand on top of the first and interlace or lift your fingers upward off the chest (Figure 3).
   <u>PURPOSE:</u> This position gives you the most control, allowing you to avoid injuring the victim's ribs as you compress the chest.

PROCEDURE 36-9—cont'd

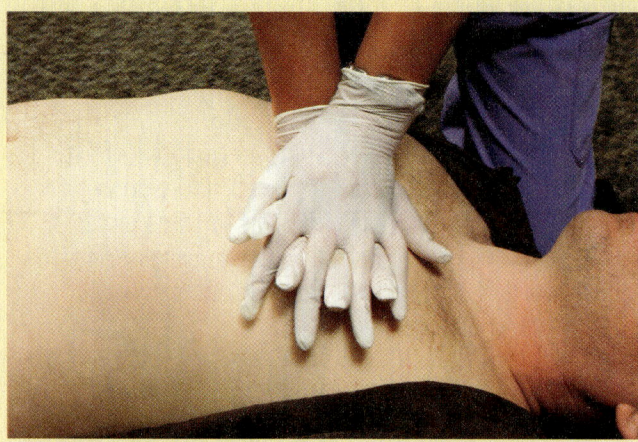

9. Bring your shoulders directly over the victim's sternum as you compress downward, keeping your elbows locked (Figure 4).

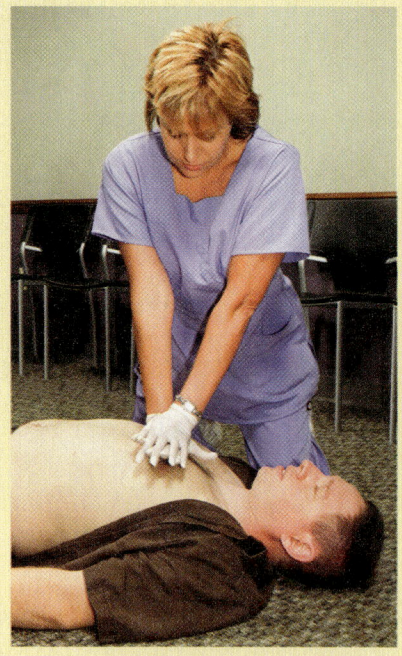

10. Depress the sternum at least 2 inches in an adult victim. Relax the pressure on the sternum after each compression but do not remove your hands from the sternum.
    PURPOSE: The depth of compression is needed to circulate blood through the heart. Movement of the hands may cause injury to the victim.

11. After performing 30 compressions (at a rate of about 100 compressions per minute), perform the head tilt–chin lift maneuver to open the airway, and give 2 slow rescue breaths.

12. After 5 cycles of compressions and breaths (30:2 ratio, about 2 minutes) recheck the breathing and carotid pulse (Figure 5). If a pulse is present but breathing is not, continue rescue breathing (1 breath every 5 seconds, about 10 to 12 breaths per minute) and re-evaluate the victim's breathing and pulse every few minutes. If no signs of circulation are present, continue 30:2 cycles of compressions and ventilations, starting with chest compressions. Continue giving CPR

until an automated external defibrillator (AED) is available or EMS relieves you.

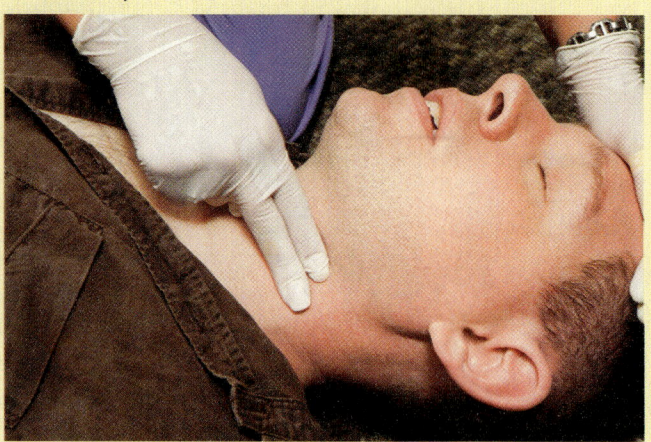

TO PERFORM CPR ON A CHILD

The procedure for giving CPR to a child ages 1 through 8 is essentially the same as that for an adult. The differences are as follows:

- Perform 5 cycles of compressions and breaths on the child (30:2 ratio, about 2 minutes) before calling 911 or the local emergency number or using an AED. If another person is available, have that person activate EMS while you care for the child.
  PURPOSE: It is important to provide immediate circulation of oxygenated blood to a child to prevent brain damage. Most pediatric cardiac arrests occur because of a secondary problem, such as airway occlusion, rather than a cardiac problem. If you know there is an airway obstruction, clear the obstruction and then proceed with CPR.
- Use only one hand to perform chest compressions (Figure 6).
  PURPOSE: The pediatric sternum requires less force to achieve the needed depression.

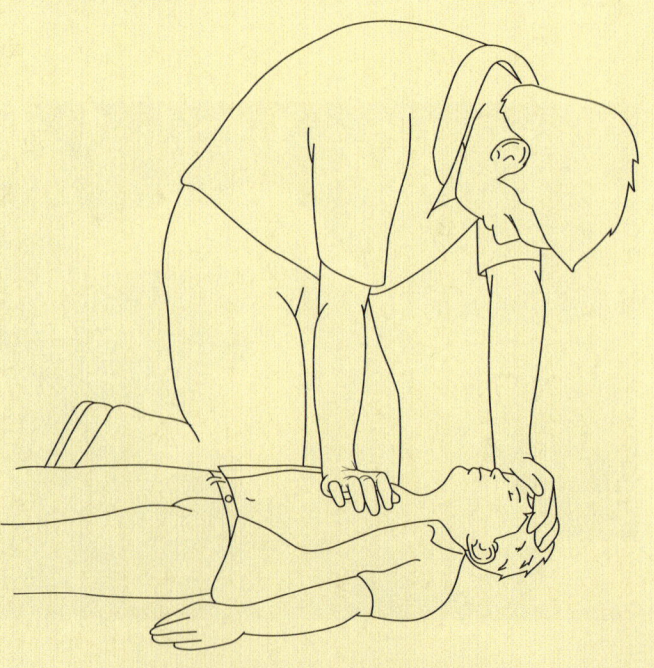

PROCEDURE 36-9—cont'd

- Breathe more gently.
- Use the same compression-to-breath ratio as used for adults, 30 compressions followed by 2 breaths per cycle; after 2 breaths, immediately begin the next cycle of compressions and breaths.
- After 5 cycles (about 2 minutes) of CPR without response, use a pediatric AED if available.
- Continue until the child responds or help arrives.

INFANT CPR

Infant cardiac arrest typically is caused by lack of oxygen from drowning or choking. If you know the infant has an airway obstruction, clear the obstruction; if you do not know why the infant is unresponsive, perform CPR for 2 minutes (about 5 cycles) before calling 911 or the local emergency number. If another person is available, have that person call for help immediately while you attend to the baby.

RESCUE BREATHING FOR AN INFANT

Use an infant ventilator mask or cover the baby's mouth and nose with your mouth.

- Give 2 rescue breaths by gently puffing out the cheeks and slowly breathing into the infant's mouth, taking about 1 second for each breath (Figure 7).

TO PERFORM CPR ON AN INFANT

- Draw an imaginary line between the infant's nipples. Place two fingers on the sternum just below this intermammary line.
- Gently compress the chest.
- Compression rate should be 100 to 120 per minute.
- Administer 2 breaths after every 30 compressions.
- After about five 30:2 cycles, activate EMS.
- Continue CPR until the child responds or help arrives.
13. Remove your gloves and the ventilator mask valve, and discard them in the biohazard container. Disinfect the ventilator mask per the manufacturer's recommendations. Sanitize your hands.
14. Document the procedure and the patient's condition.

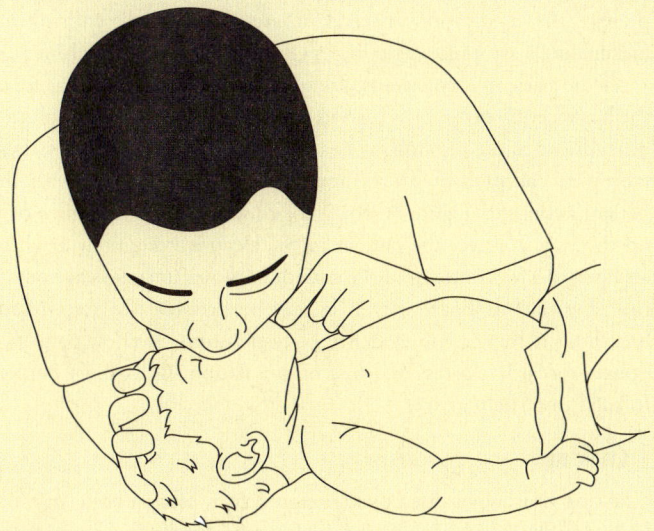

Cardiac Emergencies

Chest pain or angina can be associated with heart and lung disease, as well as a few other conditions. It can be quite serious; a patient with chest pain is treated as a cardiac emergency until a physician has ruled this out. A heart attack, or *myocardial infarction*, usually is caused by blockage of the coronary arteries, which reduces the amount of blood delivered to the myocardium. The most common signal of a heart attack is an uncomfortable pressure, squeezing, fullness, or pain in the center of the chest. This may spread to the shoulder, neck, jaw, or arms. The pain may not be severe. The lips and fingernails may be blue, which is a sign of **cyanosis** (Figure 36-7), or the patient may have a gray, ashen appearance. Frequently, the patient clutches the chest in pain. This pain may radiate from the **mediastinum** down the left arm and up the left side of the neck. The pulse may be rapid and weak, and the patient often complains of nausea. Other symptoms include sweating *(diaphoresis)*; indigestion; shortness of breath (SOB); cold, clammy skin; and a feeling of weakness *(general malaise)*. Unfortunately, most people deny that the problem is serious until they require immediate medical attention.

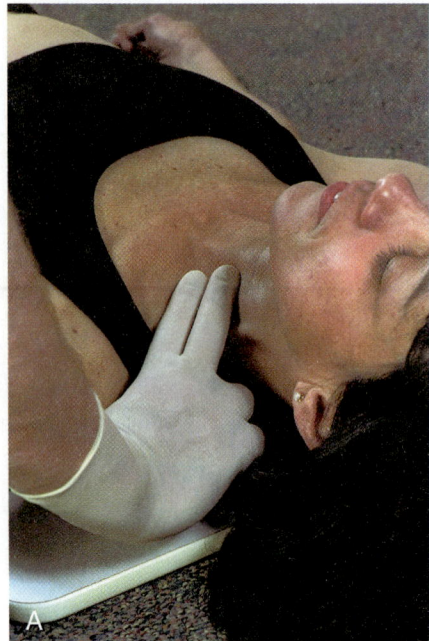

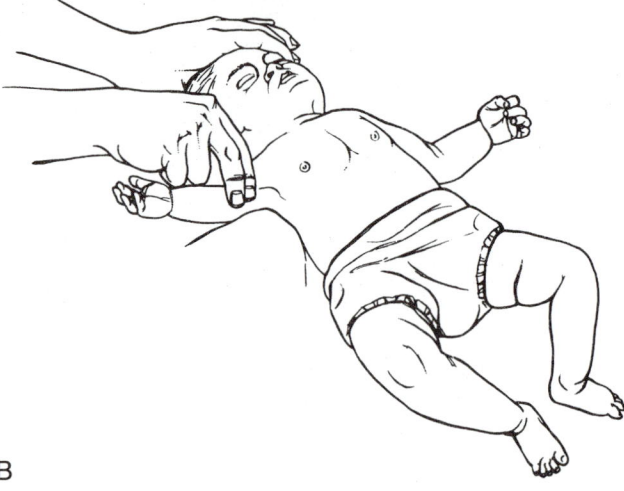

FIGURE 36-6 A, In an adult, check for a carotid pulse. **B,** In an infant, check for a brachial pulse.

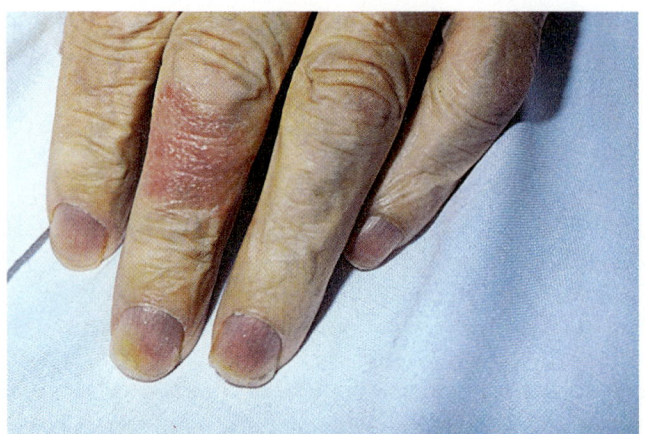

FIGURE 36-7 Cyanosis of the nail beds. (From Henry MC, Stapleton ER: *EMT prehospital care*, ed 3, Philadelphia, 2004, Saunders.)

SIGNS AND SYMPTOMS OF MYOCARDIAL INFARCTION IN WOMEN

Women may experience symptoms that are different from those traditionally associated with a heart attack. These include a combination of the following:

- Back pain or aching and throbbing in the biceps or forearms
- Shortness of breath (SOB)
- Clammy perspiration
- Dizziness (vertigo)—unexplained light-headedness or syncopal episodes
- Edema, especially of the ankles and/or lower legs
- Fluttering heartbeat or tachycardia
- Gastric upset
- Feeling of heaviness or fullness in the mediastinum

Immediately report any of these signs or symptoms to the physician. If the physician is not available, activate EMS. Use a wheelchair to move the patient to an examination room. Breathing will be easier if the patient's head is slightly elevated, or if the patient is in Fowler's position. Keep the patient quiet and warm. Loosen all tight clothing. Take vital signs, including both apical and radial pulses. The physician may order oxygen started on the patient to relieve dyspnea (Procedure 36-10). Bring the emergency cart into the room and open the medication drawer so that the physician can quickly prepare the medications needed. These may include epinephrine (adrenaline), atropine, digitalis, calcium chloride, or morphine.

If the patient is conscious, ask about any medication that he or she has recently taken or is carrying. If the patient has an established heart disorder, the person may be carrying nitroglycerin tablets; these tablets are administered sublingually and may be given with the patient's consent (Figure 36-8). If the physician is in the office or is on the way, connect the patient to the electrocardiograph machine and record a few tracings. If the patient becomes unresponsive before the physician or EMS arrives, it may be necessary to start rescue breathing if there is no evidence of respirations. If chest pain progresses to cardiac arrest and loss of circulation, CPR must be performed until help arrives.

Choking

Choking is usually caused by a foreign object, often a bolus of food, lodged in the upper airway. The victim may clutch the neck between the thumb and the index finger (Figure 36-9); this universal distress signal should be viewed as a sign the victim needs help. If the victim has good air exchange or only partial airway obstruction and can speak, cough, or breathe, do not interfere, but encourage the patient to continue coughing until the object is expelled. Monitor the patient for signs of respiratory distress, such as pallor and cyanosis. If the patient has a pronounced wheeze or a very weak cough, he or she has a partial airway obstruction with poor air exchange and may need help. If the patient is unable to speak, breathe, or cough, a complete airway obstruction exists, and quick action must be taken to clear the airway. With complete obstruction, the patient eventually loses consciousness from lack of oxygen to the brain. This condition may lead to respiratory and cardiac arrest. If the object is not

PROCEDURE 36-10

Perform First Aid Procedures: Administer Oxygen

GOAL: *To provide oxygen for a patient in respiratory distress.*

EQUIPMENT and SUPPLIES

- Portable oxygen tank
- Pressure regulator
- Flow meter
- Nasal cannula with connecting tubing
- Physician's order
- Patient's medical record

PROCEDURAL STEPS

1. Gather equipment and sanitize your hands.
2. Greet and identify the patient, introduce yourself, and explain the procedure.
   <u>PURPOSE:</u> A nasal cannula is applied with a nasal prong in each nostril and the tab resting above the upper lip. Patients who will be using oxygen at home need to be taught how to open an oxygen tank or to use an oxygen compressor. It is vital that patients and their families understand the dangers of oxygen use in the home. They must avoid open flames and not smoke when oxygen is in use, because it is combustible. The physician typically writes an order for the number of liters of oxygen to be delivered and for home healthcare services to set up the equipment in the patient's home.
3. Check the pressure gauge on the tank to determine the amount of oxygen in the tank.
4. If necessary, open the cylinder on the tank one full counterclockwise turn, then attach the cannula tubing to the flow meter.
5. Adjust the administration of the oxygen according to the physician's order. Usually the flow meter is set at 12 to 15 liters per minute (LPM). Check to make sure oxygen is flowing through the cannula.

6. Insert the tips of the cannula into the nostrils and adjust the tubing around the back of the patient's ears (Figure 1).

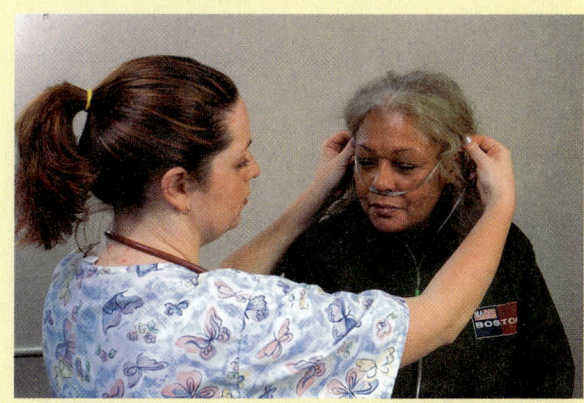

7. Make sure the patient is comfortable, and answer any questions he or she may have.
8. Sanitize your hands.
9. Document the procedure, including the number of liters of oxygen being administered and the patient's condition. Continue to monitor the patient throughout the procedure and document any changes in condition.

7/24/XX 3:05 PM R — 28 and labored. Oxygen initiated at 4 L/min via nasal cannula per physician order. Pt observed for signs of dyspnea and tachypnea. Cheryl Skurka, CMA (AAMA)

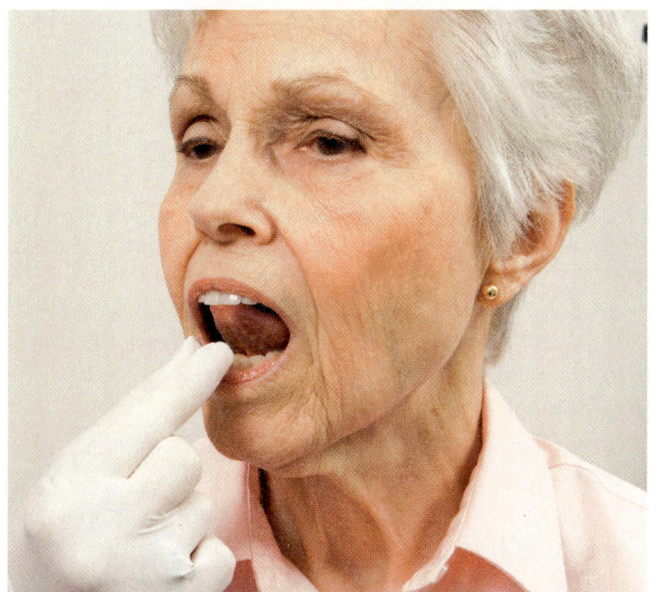

FIGURE 36-8 Nitroglycerin is administered beneath the patient's tongue.

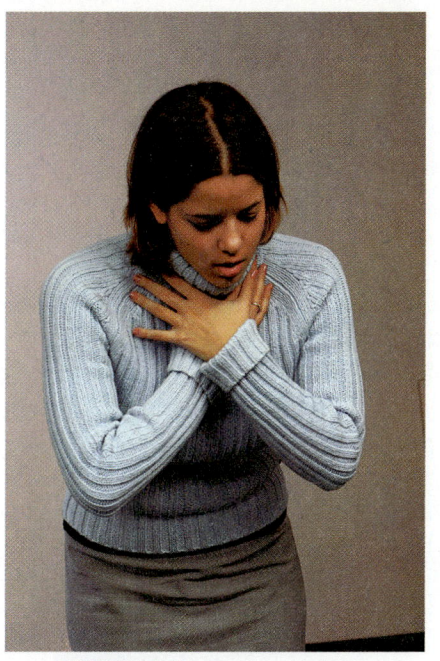

FIGURE 36-9 Universal sign of choking.

removed, the victim may die within 4 to 6 minutes. Procedure 36-11 presents the steps involved in clearing an obstructed airway in an adult. The procedure for removal of a foreign airway obstruction is exactly the same for a child older than 1 year of age.

To dislodge a foreign object from the airway of an infant up to 1 year of age, place the baby face down over your forearm and across your thigh. The head should be lower than the trunk, and you should support the baby's head and neck with one hand. Using the heel of your other hand, deliver 5 blows to the back, between the infant's shoulder blades (Figure 36-10, *A*). Holding the baby between your arms, turn the infant face up, keeping the head lower than the trunk. Using two fingers, deliver 5 thrusts to the midsternal area at the infant's nipple line (Figure 36-10, *B*). Examine the infant's mouth, and if the object is visible, pluck it out with your fingertips. *Never perform a finger sweep on an infant.* A baby's oral cavity is too small for a finger sweep, and such an action may only push the obstruction farther into the airway. If the obstruction is not visible, administer 2 rescue breaths by covering the baby's nose and mouth with your

mouth, or use a pediatric ventilator mask if available. Repeat the sequence until the foreign body is expelled or help arrives.

If a choking victim is in the late stages of pregnancy, chest compressions should be delivered to prevent possible trauma to the infant. If the patient is obese and you are unable to wrap your arms around the abdomen, perform chest compressions as you would for a pregnant woman.

The abdominal thrust maneuver also can be performed on yourself if you are choking and no one is nearby to help you. Press your fist into your upper abdomen with quick, upward thrusts, or lean forward and press the abdomen quickly against a firm object, such as the back of a chair.

Cerebrovascular Accident (Stroke)

A cerebrovascular accident (CVA), or stroke, is a disorder of the cerebral blood vessels that results in impairment of the blood supply to part of the brain. This interruption in normal circulation of blood through the brain leads to some degree of neurological damage,

---

PROCEDURE 36-11

Perform First Aid Procedures: Respond to an Airway Obstruction in an Adult

GOAL: *To remove an airway obstruction and restore ventilation.*

EQUIPMENT and SUPPLIES

- Disposable gloves
- Ventilation mask (for unconscious victim)
- Approved mannequin to practice unconscious foreign body airway obstruction (FBAO) removal

PROCEDURAL STEPS

The technique for an unresponsive victim is to be performed only on an approved mannequin.

1. Ask, "Are you choking?" If the victim indicates yes, ask, "Can you speak?" If the victim is unable to speak, tell the victim you are going to help.
   PURPOSE: If the victim is unable to speak, is coughing weakly, and/or is wheezing, he or she has an obstructed airway with poor air exchange, and the obstruction must be removed before respiratory arrest occurs.
2. Stand behind the victim with your feet slightly apart.
   PURPOSE: With an obstructed airway, the victim may lose consciousness at any time. The rescuer must be prepared to lower the unconscious victim to the floor safely.
3. Reach around the victim's abdomen and place an index finger into the victim's navel or at the level of the belt buckle. Make a fist of the opposite hand (do not tuck the thumb into the fist) and place the thumb side of the fist against the victim's abdomen above the navel. If the victim is pregnant, place the fist above the enlarged uterus. If the victim is obese, it may be necessary to place the fist higher in the abdomen. It may be necessary to perform chest thrusts on a victim who is pregnant or obese.
   PURPOSE: The fist should be placed in the soft tissue of the abdomen to avoid injury to the sternum or rib cage.

4. Place the opposite hand over the fist and give abdominal thrusts in a quick inward and upward movement (Figure 1).
   PURPOSE: Abdominal contents pushing against the diaphragm force trapped air out of the lungs, and with it the obstruction.

(From Chapleau W: *Emergency medical technician: making the difference,* St Louis, 2007, Mosby.)

5. Repeat the abdominal thrusts until the object is expelled or the victim becomes unresponsive.

Unresponsive Adult Victim

1. Carefully lower the patient to the ground, activate the emergency response system, and put on disposable gloves.
2. Immediately begin cardiopulmonary resuscitation (CPR) with 30 compressions and 2 breath cycles using the ventilator mask.
   PURPOSE: Higher airway pressures are maintained with chest compressions than with abdominal thrusts.

PROCEDURE 36-11—cont'd

3. Each time the airway is opened to deliver a rescue breath during CPR, look for an object in the victim's mouth and remove it if visible. If no object is found, immediately return to the cycle of 30 chest compressions.

4. A finger sweep should be used only if the rescuer can see the obstruction.

5. Continue cycles of 30 compressions to 2 rescue breaths until the obstruction is removed or emergency medical services (EMS) arrives.

6. If the obstruction is removed, assess the victim for breathing and circulation. If a pulse is present but the patient is not breathing, begin rescue breathing.

7. Once the patient has been stabilized or EMS has taken over care, remove your gloves and the ventilator mask valve and discard them in the biohazard container. Disinfect the ventilator mask per the manufacturer's recommendations. Sanitize your hands.

8. Document the procedure and the patient's condition.

7/22/XX 8:35 AM Pt in waiting room clutching throat and coughing weakly. After confirming pt choking, abdominal thrusts performed until foreign body expelled. Pt breathing without difficulty; R – 18 and regular. Incident reported to physician. Cheryl Skurka, CMA (AAMA) _____

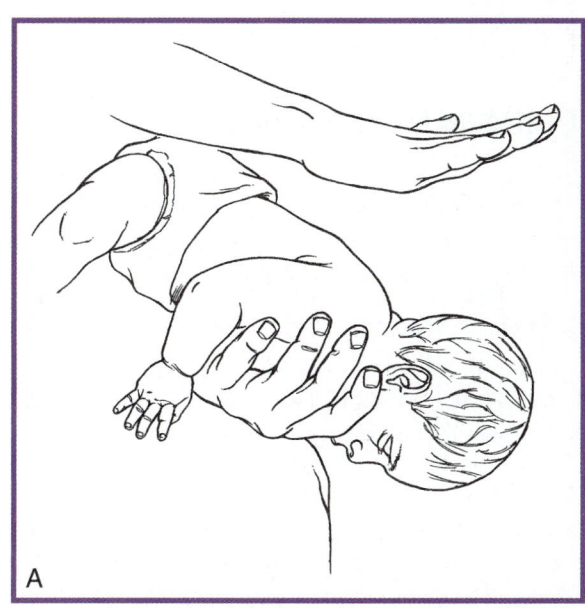 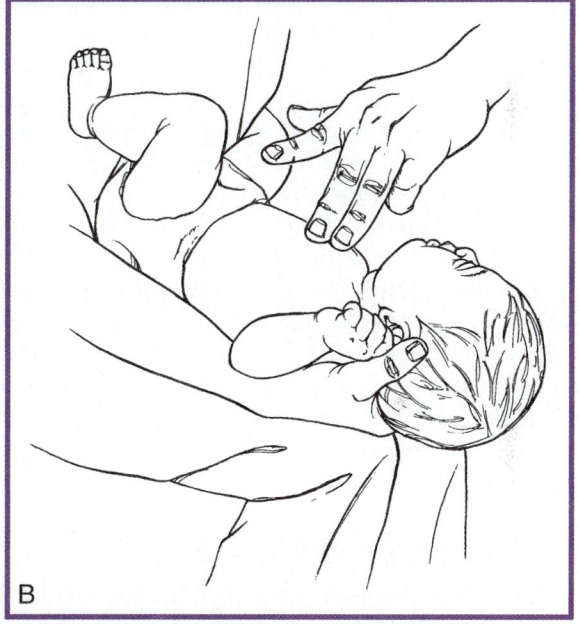

FIGURE 36-10 A, Back blows are administered to an infant supported on the arm and thigh. **B,** Chest thrusts are administered in the same position as for cardiac compressions. (From Henry MC, Stapleton ER: *EMT prehospital care,* ed 3, Philadelphia, 2004, Saunders.)

temporary or permanent, depending on the severity of oxygen deprivation to the brain cells.

A minor stroke, or **transient ischemic attack (TIA)**, usually does not cause unconsciousness, and symptoms depend on the location of the circulatory problem in the brain, as well as the amount of brain damage. TIA symptoms are temporary and may include headache, confusion, vertigo, ringing in the ears *(tinnitus)*, temporary paralysis or weakness of one side of the body, transient limb weakness, slurred speech, and vision problems. TIA episodes indicate that the patient is at risk for a major stroke.

Symptoms of a major stroke include unconsciousness, paralysis on one side of the body, difficulty breathing and swallowing, loss of bladder and bowel control, unequal pupil size, and slurring of speech.

Home recommendations for a patient who has suffered a major stroke should begin with notifying the physician and/or activating EMS. Keep the patient lying down and lightly covered. Maintain an open airway. To prevent choking, position the head so that any secretions drain from the side of the mouth. If the patient is lying on the floor, did not fall, and shows no indications of a head or neck injury, he or she can be placed in the recovery position as follows (Figure 36-11):

1. Place the patient's arm that is farthest from you alongside and above the head; place the other arm across the chest.

2. Bend the leg that is closest to you, and after placing one arm under the patient's head and shoulder and the other hand on the flexed knee, roll the patient away from you while you stabilize

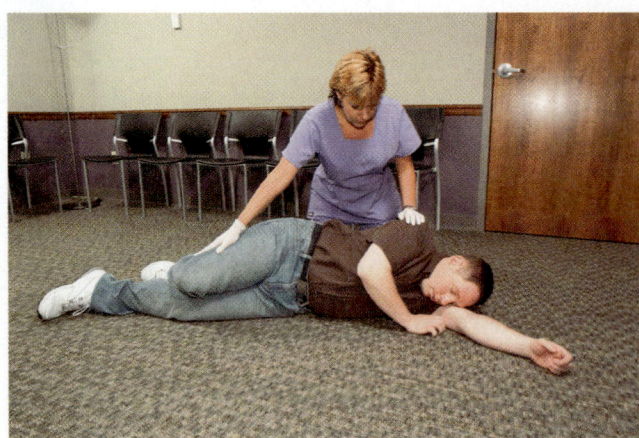

FIGURE 36-11 Recovery position.

the head and neck. The patient's head should be resting on the extended arm.

The recovery position uses gravity to drain fluids from the mouth and keep the trachea clear. Keep the patient in this position until the person is alert or help arrives. Do not give the patient anything to eat or drink. Vital signs should be measured at regular intervals and recorded for the physician.

Advances in early treatment of strokes show great promise in preventing long-term neurological deficits. However, to prevent permanent brain damage, **thrombolytics** must be administered intravenously within 3 hours of the onset of symptoms. If a patient does not know when the symptoms began (e.g., the person woke up with the symptoms) or cannot accurately tell the physician when the symptoms started, the time allotted for administration begins from the point at which the patient last was known to be asymptomatic. Intracranial hemorrhage must be ruled out before treatment begins. The earlier the treatment starts, the better are the neurological outcomes. The best possible outcomes are seen in patients who received thrombolytic therapy within 90 minutes of the onset of symptoms.

> **CRITICAL THINKING** APPLICATION   36-4
>
> Thomas Antonio, a 67-year-old patient, calls to report that when he woke up this morning, the left side of his face was drooping and he had difficulty seeing out of his left eye. The symptoms went away in about 2 hours, and he is feeling fine now. The schedule does not show any openings for 2 days. When should Cheryl make an appointment for Mr. Antonio? What questions should Cheryl ask him?

Shock

Shock is a state of collapse caused by failure of the circulatory system to deliver enough oxygenated blood to the body's vital organs. Injury, hemorrhage, infection, anesthesia, drug overdose, burns, pain, fear, or emotional stress can cause this physiologic reaction. Shock can be immediate or delayed, and it is potentially fatal. Many different types of shock can occur, but the signs and symptoms are universal. The most common indicators are a pale, gray, or cyanotic appearance; moist but cool skin; dilated pupils; a weak, rapid pulse; marked hypotension; shallow, rapid respirations; lethargy or restlessness; nausea and vomiting; and extreme thirst.

If a patient shows signs of shock, maintain an open airway and check for breathing and circulation. Place the patient supine with the legs elevated approximately 1 foot to return the blood from the legs to vital organs. Loosen all tight clothing and cover the patient with a blanket for warmth. Do not move the patient unnecessarily. Fluids may be given by mouth if the patient is alert. Because shock can evolve into a life-threatening situation, only basic first aid should be administered, and the patient should be transported to the hospital as soon as possible.

TYPES AND CAUSES OF SHOCK

- Anaphylactic—a severe allergic reaction
- Insulin—severe hypoglycemia caused by an overdose of insulin
- Psychogenic or mental—excessive fear, joy, anger, or emotional stress
- Hypovolemic or hemorrhagic—excessive loss of blood
- Cardiogenic—myocardial infarction, pulmonary embolism, or severe congestive heart failure
- Neurogenic—dilation of blood vessels as a result of brain or spinal cord injury
- Septic—systemic infection

COMMON OFFICE EMERGENCIES

The remainder of this chapter highlights typical emergencies seen in the ambulatory care setting or in telephone triage situations. Table 36-1 summarizes common emergencies, the questions that should be asked, and possible actions for home care.

Fainting (Syncope)

Fainting, or *syncope*, is a common emergency. It usually is caused by a transient loss of blood flow to the brain (e.g., a sudden drop in blood pressure), which results in a temporary loss of consciousness. It can occur without warning, or the patient may appear pale; may feel cold, weak, dizzy, or nauseated; and may have numbness of the extremities before the incident. The greatest danger to the patient is an injury from falling during the attack. Therefore, if a patient has syncopal symptoms, immediately place the individual in a supine position. Loosen all tight clothing and maintain an open airway. Apply a cold washcloth to the forehead. Measure and record the patient's pulse, respiratory rate, and blood pressure, and report the findings to the physician. Keep the patient in a supine position for at least 10 minutes after the person regains consciousness. A complete patient history can help determine the possible causes of the attack (e.g., a history of heart disease or diabetes). Document the details of the episode and how long it took the patient to recover completely (Procedure 36-12).

If the patient does not recover quickly, the physician may activate EMS for transport to the hospital. Syncope might be a brief episode in the development of a serious underlying illness, such as an abnormal heart rhythm, that could lead to sudden cardiac death.

Poisoning

Poisonings are considered medical emergencies and are the sixth leading cause of accidental pediatric death in the United States. Poisoning can occur by oral intake, absorption, inhalation, or

TABLE 36-1 Telephone Screening of Possible Emergency Situations

EMERGENCY SITUATION	SCREENING QUESTIONS	HOME CARE ADVICE
Syncope	• Was the patient injured? • Does the patient have a history of heart disease, seizures, or diabetes?	• Does not necessarily indicate a serious disease. If injured by a fall, the patient may need to be evaluated and treated. • The patient should get up very slowly to prevent a recurrence, take it easy, and drink plenty of fluids. • If the patient is to be seen, someone should accompany him or her to the physician's office.
Animal bites	• What kind of animal (pet or wild)? • How severe is the injury? • Where are the bites? • When did the bites occur?	• The health department or police should be notified. Every effort must be made to locate the animal and monitor its health. • If the skin is not broken, wash well and observe for signs of infection.
Insect bites and stings	• Does the patient have a history of anaphylactic reaction to insect stings? • Does the patient have difficulty breathing, have a widespread rash, or have trouble swallowing?	• If the patient has a history of anaphylaxis and an EpiPen, the EpiPen should be used immediately and emergency medical services (EMS) notified. • Activate EMS if the patient is having systemic symptoms. • An antihistamine (Benadryl) relieves local pruritus.
Asthma	• Does the patient show signs of cyanosis? • Has the patient used prescribed inhalers?	• If a patient with asthma is unable to speak in sentences, has poor color, and is struggling to breathe even after using an inhaler, he or she should be seen immediately, or EMS should be activated.
Burns	• Where are the burns located, and what caused them? • Are signs of shock present: moist, clammy skin, altered consciousness, rapid breathing and pulse? • Are signs of infection present (foul odor, cloudy drainage) in a burn more than 2 days old?	• Activate EMS for burns on the face, hands, feet, or perineum; those caused by electricity or a chemical; and burns associated with inhalation. Activate EMS if signs of shock are present. • The patient must receive a tetanus shot if he or she has not had one in more than 10 years. • Schedule an urgent appointment if signs of infection are reported.
Wounds	• Is the bleeding steady or pulsating? • How and when did the injury occur? • Does the patient have any bleeding disorders or is the patient taking anticoagulant drugs? • Is the wound open and deep?	• Pulsating bleeding usually indicates arterial damage; activate EMS. • If the injury was caused by a powerful force, other injuries also may have resulted. • For patients taking anticoagulants or with diabetes or anemia, schedule an urgent appointment. • A gaping, deep wound requires sutures.
Head injury	• Did the patient pass out or have a seizure? Is the patient confused or vomiting? Is a clear fluid draining from the nose or ears?	• If the answer is "yes" to any of these questions, EMS should be activated.

injection. Over-the-counter (OTC) medications (e.g., acetaminophen); detergents and bleach; plants; cough and cold medicines; and vitamins cause most cases of poisoning seen in young children. Other typical household poisons include drain cleaner, turpentine, kerosene, furniture polish, and paint (Figure 36-12). Signs and symptoms of poisoning, which vary greatly, include burns on the hands and mouth, stains on the victim's clothing, open bottles of medicines or chemicals, changes in skin color, nausea or stomach cramps, shallow breathing, convulsions, heavy perspiration, dizziness or drowsiness, and unconsciousness.

If you receive a phone call about a suspected poisoning, tell the caller not to hang up and not to leave the victim unattended. Call the local poison control center and forward all directions to the caller. Syrup of ipecac, which causes vomiting within 15 to 20 minutes, should be used only if ordered by the physician or the poison control center, because some chemicals can cause serious

Perform First Aid Procedures: Care for a Patient Who Has Fainted

GOAL: *To provide emergency care for and assessment of a patient who has fainted.*

EQUIPMENT and SUPPLIES

- Patient's record
- Sphygmomanometer
- Stethoscope
- Watch with second hand
- Blanket
- Footstool or box
- Pillows
- Oxygen equipment, if ordered by physician:
  - Portable oxygen tank
  - Pressure regulator
  - Flow meter
  - Nasal cannula with connecting tubing

PROCEDURAL STEPS

1. If warning is given that the patient feels faint, have the patient lower the head to the knees to increase the blood supply to the brain (Figure 1). If this does not stop the episode, have the patient lie down on the examination table or lower the patient to the floor. If the patient collapses to the floor when fainting, treat with caution because of possible head or neck injuries.

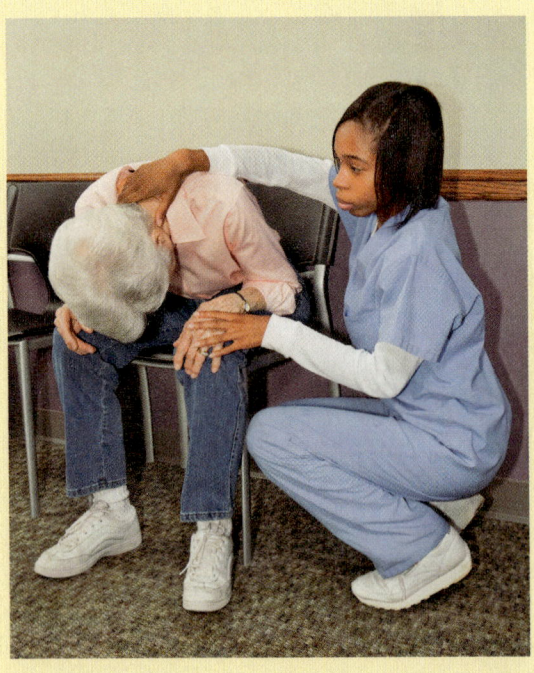

2. Immediately notify the physician of the patient's condition and assess the patient for life-threatening emergencies, such as respiratory or cardiac arrest. If the patient is breathing and has a pulse, monitor the patient's vital signs.

3. Loosen any tight clothing and keep the patient warm, applying a blanket if needed.

4. If a head or neck injury is not a factor, elevate the patient's legs above the level of the heart using the footstool with pillow support if available (Figure 2).
   PURPOSE: Elevating the legs assists with venous blood return to the heart. This may relieve symptoms of fainting by elevating the blood pressure and increasing blood flow to vital organs.

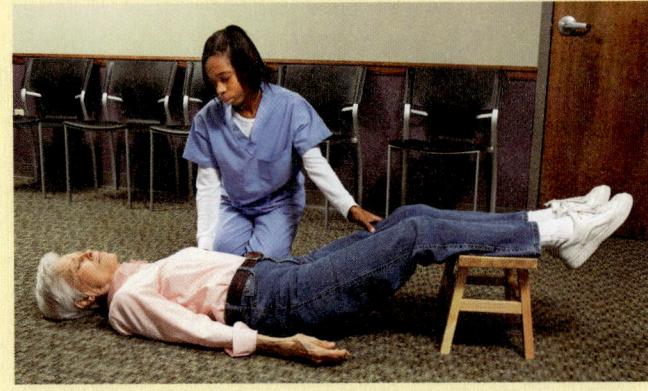

5. Continue to monitor vital signs and apply oxygen by nasal cannula if ordered by the physician.

6. If vital signs are unstable or the patient does not respond quickly, activate emergency medical services (EMS).
   PURPOSE: Fainting may be a sign of a life-threatening problem.

7. If the patient vomits, roll the patient onto his or her side to prevent aspiration of vomitus into the lungs.

8. Once the patient has completely recovered, assist the patient into a sitting position. Do not leave the patient unattended on the examination table.

9. Document the incident, including a description of the episode, the patient's symptoms and vital signs, the duration of the episode, and any complaints. If oxygen was administered, document the number of liters and how long oxygen was administered.

7/29/XX 4:18 PM Pt in waiting room states she feels faint. Pt lowered to floor, clothing loosened, legs elevated. Physician notified. P 88 and regular, R 22, BP 112/60. Syncopal episode persisted for 90 sec, feeling of vertigo lasted 10 min post syncope. Pt transferred to exam room via wheelchair after recovery. Cheryl Skurka, CMA (AAMA) _____

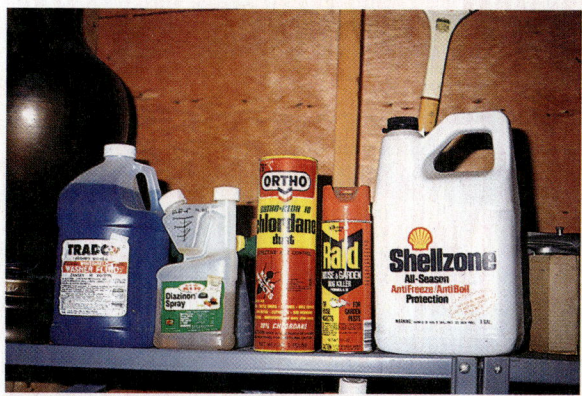

FIGURE 36-12 Hazardous household materials. (From Henry MC, Stapleton ER: *EMT prehospital care,* ed 3, Philadelphia, 2004, Saunders.)

irritation to the tissues if vomited. Do not induce vomiting if the victim is semiconscious or is experiencing convulsions, because of the risk of aspiration of stomach contents into the lungs. If syrup of ipecac is recommended, give 2 teaspoons to infants 9 to 12 months old after the child drinks about 4 ounces of warm water. For a child 1 to 4 years old, administer 1 tablespoon after the child drinks 4 to 8 ounces of warm water. If the patient is to be seen by the physician or sent to the hospital, tell the caller to bring the container of poison or a sample of the vomitus with him, so that the chemical contents of the substance can be verified.

WHAT TO ASK WHEN A POISONING IS REPORTED

- Victim's name, weight, and age
- Name of the poison taken and any information on the label
- How much was taken
- How long ago the poison was ingested
- Whether vomiting has occurred
- Any pertinent symptoms, such as difficulty breathing or an altered state of consciousness
- Any first aid that has been given

CRITICAL THINKING APPLICATION   36-5

A young mother calls in a panic to report that her 18-month-old daughter swallowed at least half a bottle of cough syrup. The child is fussy and very sleepy, and the mother wants to give her ipecac immediately. What should Cheryl do?

Animal Bites

Potential complications from animal bites include rabies, tetanus, and local skin infection. Any animal bite that is extensive or deep should be seen by a physician. Human infection with rabies is rare; however, if the bite is made by a domestic animal, the animal should be kept quarantined and under observation for 10 days for monitoring for signs of the disease. The animal should not be killed, because a positive finding of rabies is almost impossible to make if the animal has been dead for an extended time. If the bite is that of a bat,

raccoon, or any other wild animal, the animal is assumed to be rabid, and the patient must undergo a series of rabies vaccine injections. Local skin infection can be prevented by immediately cleansing the area with antimicrobial soap and water. If the bite breaks the skin (including human bites), the patient's tetanus immunization status must be checked and, if needed, a booster or the entire four-dose tetanus series must be administered as indicated.

Insect Bites and Stings

The bite or sting of an insect can be irritating and painful because of the chemical toxin injected by the insect, but it usually is not serious. Typical symptoms—inflammation, itching *(pruritus)*, and edema—are local and are confined to the area of the bite. In rare cases, a severe allergic reaction may occur; this is a potentially dangerous situation that can lead to anaphylaxis. Signs and symptoms of a systemic allergic reaction include a dry cough, a feeling of tightening in the throat or chest, swelling or itching around the eyes, widespread hives *(urticaria)*, wheezing, dyspnea, and hypotension. Difficulty talking is a sign of urticaria or edema in the throat and may indicate the onset of complete airway obstruction. This is a sign of a true emergency. Epinephrine and oxygen should be ready for immediate administration on the physician's orders. Antihistamines and corticosteroids may be used, but these agents act considerably slower than epinephrine. If acute anaphylactic shock develops, death may occur within 1 hour without medical intervention.

If the stinger is still lodged in the skin, scrape it off with a dull knife, a credit card, or a fingernail. Be careful not to squeeze the stinger, because this injects more venom into the skin. Apply an ice bag to the site to relieve pain and slow absorption of venom. Calamine lotion or hydrocortisone cream may be applied to relieve itching. If the patient has a history of allergies, especially to insect venom, he or she should have access to an EpiPen injection system; this should be used immediately after the sting. The patient should be transported to the nearest hospital for immediate care.

REMOVAL OF A TICK

Ticks can cause a number of diseases, including Rocky Mountain spotted fever and Lyme disease. The tick embeds its head into the skin to obtain blood, and it should be removed intact by the following method:

1. Do not handle ticks with uncovered fingers; use tweezers to prevent personal contamination.
2. Place the tips of the tweezers as close as possible to the area where the tick has entered the skin.
3. With a slow, steady motion, pull the tick away from the skin. Try not to squeeze or crush the tick. If the tick's entire body is not removed, make an appointment with a physician to have the site evaluated.
4. After removal, place the tick directly into a sealable container. Disinfect the area around the bite site using standard procedures.
5. If the tick is removed at home, the physician may suggest that it be brought to the office to be tested for disease.

Asthma Attacks

Asthma is characterized by expiratory wheezing, coughing, a feeling of tightness in the chest, and shortness of breath (SOB). During an asthma attack, two different physiologic responses occur. The lining of the respiratory tract becomes inflamed and edematous and produces mucus, which results in narrowing of the air passages. At the same time, bronchospasms occur, which also constrict the airways. The quality and severity of attacks vary greatly among patients, and treatment must be individualized to minimize or eliminate chronic symptoms (see Chapter 46). If the patient is prescribed a bronchodilator inhaler, it should be used at the first indication of symptoms. Depending on the severity of the attack, give the patient an appointment for the same day as the call, or consult the physician. The physician may recommend that the patient go directly to the ED for emergency respiratory care.

Seizures

Seizures may be **idiopathic**, or they may result from trauma, injury, or metabolic alterations, such as hypoglycemia or hypocalcemia. A *febrile* seizure is transient and occurs with a rapid rise in body temperature over 101.8° F (38.8° C). Febrile seizures typically occur in children between 6 months and 5 years of age. Many different types of seizures occur, but all are caused by a disruption in the electrical activity of the brain. (The different types of seizures are discussed in Chapter 44.)

If a patient suffers a grand mal seizure, which involves uncontrolled muscular contractions, the most important point is to protect the patient from possible injury. Clear everything away from the patient that could cause accidental injury, and observe him or her until the seizure ends. Do not place anything into the person's mouth, because it may damage the teeth or tongue and force the tongue back over the trachea. Do not hold the patient down, because this may result in muscle injuries or fractures. If unconsciousness persists after the seizure has subsided, place the patient in the recovery position to maintain an open airway and allow drainage of excess saliva. After the seizure is over, let the patient rest or sleep, but never leave the person alone. If the physician is not in the office, check the office policies and procedures manual to determine how to manage the situation.

Call 911 for emergency assistance in any of the following situations:

- The patient does not regain consciousness within 10 to 15 minutes.
- The seizure does not stop within a few minutes.
- The patient begins a second seizure immediately after the first one.
- The patient is pregnant.
- Signs of head trauma are present.
- The patient is known to have diabetes.
- The seizure was triggered by a high fever in a child.

Abdominal Pain

Abdominal pain is a symptom caused by many different problems, which can range from acute discomfort to life-threatening complications. The clinician should see every patient who reports abdominal pain; the question is how soon the patient should be seen. A patient with acute onset of severe, persistent abdominal pain, especially when this is accompanied by fever, should receive medical attention as soon as possible. Abdominal pain has a variety of causes, including intestinal infection, appendicitis, ectopic pregnancy, inflammation, hemorrhage, obstruction, and tumor.

Treatment in the ambulatory care setting depends on the cause of the pain; however, the medical assistant should observe the following general guidelines:

- Keep the patient warm and quiet.
- Have an emesis basin available.
- Administer nothing by mouth (NPO).
- Do not apply heat to the abdomen unless so instructed by the physician.
- Administer analgesics as ordered.
- Check and record the patient's vital signs and follow the physician's orders.

SCREENING GUIDELINES FOR ASSESSING ABDOMINAL PAIN

- Assess for shock-related signs and symptoms: **diaphoresis**; cold, clammy skin; cyanosis or gray pallor; rapid respirations; altered state of consciousness
- Is the pain severe and constant or does it come in waves?
- Has the patient had any bloody or tarry stools?
- Is the patient's temperature higher than 101° F?
- Could the patient be pregnant or has she missed a menstrual period?
- Has the patient experienced continuous vomiting or severe constipation?
- Are any urinary symptoms present, such as frequency, hematuria, or flank pain?
- Does the patient have chest pain, shortness of breath, or a continuous cough?
- Does the patient have a history of serious illness, such as diabetes, heart disease, or cancer?

Sprains and Strains

Sprains are tears of the ligaments that support a joint; *strains* are injuries to a muscle and its tendons. Both types of injury may damage surrounding soft tissues and blood vessels, as well as nearby nerves. With a sprain, the victim develops edema and **ecchymosis** around the injury, and any movement of the joint, especially a twisting one, produces pain. Usually no swelling or discoloration is seen with a strain, and only mild tenderness is noted unless the injured muscle or tendon is used.

Tendon strains and ligament sprains take several weeks to heal, whereas muscle tears usually heal in 1 to 2 weeks, because muscle has such a rich blood supply. (The details of orthopedic injuries are discussed in Chapter 43.) These injuries are treated by elevating the affected area and applying mild compression and ice. Swelling is reduced if ice is applied within 20 to 30 minutes of the injury. After 24 to 36 hours, alternating applications of mild heat and ice usually are indicated. The patient may be advised to immobilize the part.

Fractures

A fracture is a break or crack in a bone, which can result from trauma or disease. Fractures are very painful and affect the patient's ability to freely move the injured part. When a patient with a fracture is brought into the office, the medical assistant should make the patient as comfortable as possible. Place the patient in a position that supports the affected area at the joints above and below the suspected fracture and does not place strain on the injury. Notify the physician immediately and proceed according to the orders given. Emergency treatment for fractures includes preventing movement of the injured part through splinting, elevation of the affected extremity, application of ice, and control of any bleeding. If a patient with an open fracture is seen in an ambulatory care setting, he or she should be transported to the ED. (Fractures are discussed in greater detail in Chapter 43.)

Burns

Burns are among the most common causes of injury in the United States. Burn injuries can result from flame, heat, scalds, electricity, chemicals, or radiation. The skin surface may be reddened, blistered, or charred. The depth and extent of a burn are the major determinants in classifying its severity. The extent of the pain is directly proportional to the extent of the surface area burned, as well as the depth and nature of the burn.

To screen a burn injury, the medical assistant must know what caused the burn, its location and approximate size, the depth of the burn, and whether any additional injuries occurred. If the patient reports a chemical burn, it is important to have the person immediately remove all clothing that may have come into contact with the chemical and flood the affected area with running water to flush the irritant off the skin. If the chemical is not quickly flushed away or remains in the patient's clothing, the agent will continue to burn the skin and may do very serious damage.

The percentage of the body surface area burned can be estimated using the Rule of Nines (Figure 36-13). This is an assessment tool that helps caregivers quickly calculate the amount of burned tissue. With the Rule of Nines, the body is divided into areas approximately equal to 9% of the total body surface area. When a burn

victim is assessed, the affected regions are combined to yield an estimate of the total percentage of burned tissue. Partial-thickness burns over 15% of the total body surface and full-thickness burns of less than 2% can be treated in the ambulatory care setting if the patient can be seen immediately. Patients with larger body surface area involvement or other complications should be transported immediately to a hospital, preferably one with a burn unit. (A complete description of burns and their management is given in Chapter 38.)

Tissue Injuries

Patients may report any of several different types of wounds. A *contusion* is a closed wound with no evidence of injury to the skin; it typically is caused by blunt trauma, appears swollen and discolored, and is painful. A contusion results in a painful bruise, but the skin remains intact. A scrape on the surface of the skin (e.g., a skinned knee, rug burn) is called an *abrasion*. A deeper, more jagged wound is called a *laceration*. Additional tissue damage may occur around a laceration, and, depending on its depth, the wound may need to be repaired surgically. A *puncture* wound occurs when an object is forced into the body (e.g., stepping on a nail). If an object is lodged in body tissues, the best course is to leave it there, stabilize it as much as possible with rolled-up material, and transport the individual to a clinic or ED. The puncture may have severed blood vessels, and if the object is removed, considerable bleeding may occur. An injury in which tissue is torn away (e.g., complete or partial removal of a finger) is known as an *avulsion*.

Lacerations are common presentations in a primary care physician's office. A lacerated wound shows jagged or irregular tearing of the tissues. The severity depends on the cause of the laceration, the site and extent of the injury, and whether the area is contaminated. The injury that caused the laceration also may have damaged blood vessels, nerves, bones, joints, and organs in the body cavities.

When the patient arrives at the facility, put on gloves and notify the physician immediately. Have the patient lie down, and cover the injured area with a sterile dressing; use a dressing that is thick enough to absorb the bleeding (Procedure 36-13). Reassure the patient and explain your actions as much as possible. Ask the patient when he or she last received a tetanus inoculation, and record the date in the patient's record. If it has been longer than 10 years, the physician probably will want a booster injection given.

Wounds that are not bleeding severely and that do not involve deep tissue damage should be cleaned with antimicrobial soap and water to remove bacteria and other foreign matter. If the laceration is extremely dirty, the physician may want the area irrigated with sterile normal saline solution.

A butterfly closure strip may be used over small lacerations to hold the edges together. If the wound is superficial and has straight edges, it may be closed with a microporous tape (e.g., Steri-Strips) (Figure 36-14), which eliminates the discomfort of suturing and suture removal. Another wound closure option is a tissue adhesive product such as Dermabond fluid or Liquiband, which forms a strong, flexible closure similar in strength to nylon suture material. Tissue adhesive products are very useful for closing simple lacerations in children while providing an antimicrobial and waterproof coating to the wound site that lasts several days, even with repeated washing.

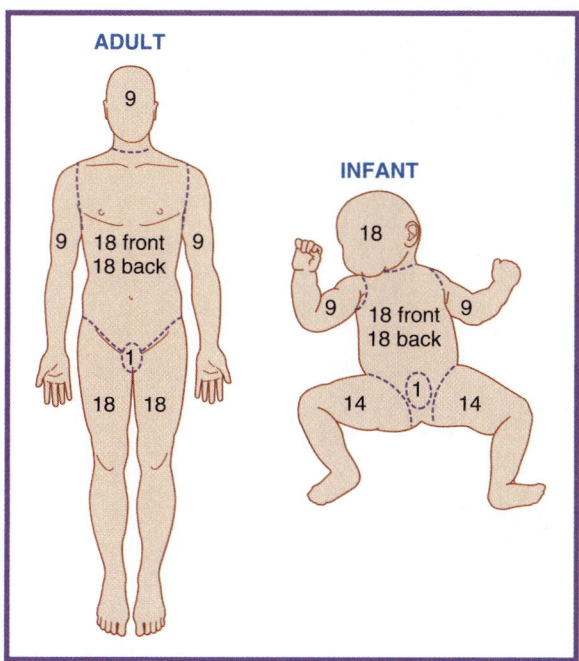

FIGURE 36-13 Rule of Nines classification of burns.

PROCEDURE 36-13

Perform First Aid Procedures: Control Bleeding

GOAL: *To stop the hemorrhaging from an open wound.*

EQUIPMENT and SUPPLIES

- Gloves, sterile if available
- Appropriate personal protective equipment (PPE) according to Occupational Safety and Health Administration (OSHA) guidelines, including:
  - Impermeable gown
  - Goggles or face shield
  - Impermeable mask
  - Impermeable foot covers if indicated
- Sterile dressings
- Bandaging material
- Biohazard waste container
- Patient record

PROCEDURAL STEPS

1. Sanitize your hands and put on appropriate PPE.
   PURPOSE: To follow Standard Precautions.
2. Assemble equipment and supplies.
3. Apply several layers of sterile dressing material directly to the wound and exert pressure.
   PURPOSE: Direct pressure to a wound slows or stops the bleeding. Sterile supplies are needed to prevent wound infection.
4. Wrap the wound with bandage material. Add more dressing and bandaging material if the bleeding continues.
5. If bleeding persists and the wound is on an extremity, elevate the extremity above the level of the heart. Notify the physician immediately if the bleeding cannot be controlled.
6. If the bleeding still continues, maintain direct pressure and elevation; also apply pressure to the appropriate artery. If the bleeding is in the arm, apply pressure to the brachial artery by squeezing the inner aspect of the middle upper arm. If the bleeding is in the leg, apply pressure to the femoral artery on the affected side by pushing with the heel of the hand into the femoral crease at the groin. If the bleeding cannot be controlled, emergency medical services (EMS) may need to be activated.
7. Once the bleeding has been brought under control and the patient has been stabilized, discard contaminated materials in an appropriate biohazard waste container.
8. Disinfect the area, then remove your gloves and discard them in a biohazard waste container.
9. Sanitize your hands.
10. Document the incident, including details of the wound, when and how it occurred, the patient's symptoms and vital signs, treatment provided by the physician, and the patient's current condition.

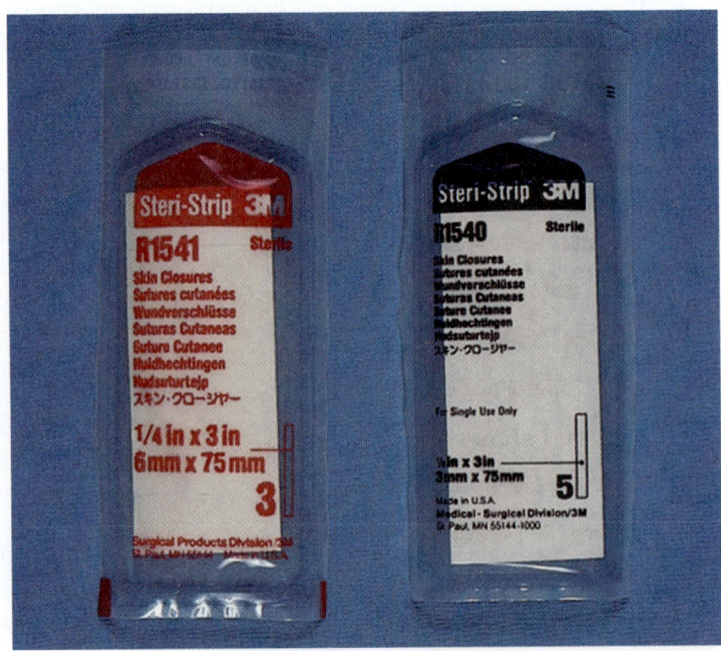

FIGURE 36-14 Steri-Strips.

After the clinician closes the wound, the medical assistant typically applies a sterile dressing to the site. The size and thickness of the dressing depend on the type of wound. (Various wound dressings and techniques for their application are discussed in Chapter 57.)

Nosebleeds (Epistaxis)

A nosebleed, or *epistaxis*, is a hemorrhage that usually results from the rupture of small vessels in the nose. Nosebleeds can be caused by injury, disease, hypertension, strenuous activity, high altitudes, exposure to cold, overuse of anticoagulant medications (e.g., aspirin), and nasal recreational drug use. Bleeding from the anterior nostril area usually is venous, whereas bleeding from the posterior region usually is arterial and is more difficult to stop. Treatment of epistaxis varies according to the amount of bleeding and the presence of other conditions, as well as the use of anticoagulant medications.

If the bleeding is mild to moderate and from one side of the nose, the patient should sit up, lean slightly forward, and apply direct pressure to the affected nostril by pinching the nose. Continue constant pressure for 10 to 15 minutes to allow clotting to take place. Repeat if the bleeding cannot be controlled, insert a clean gauze pad into the nostril, and notify the physician. If the physician is not available, proceed with standard EMS protocols. Bleeding should be considered a medical emergency if it is bilateral and continuous, or if it occurs in a patient who has a bleeding disorder or is undergoing anticoagulant therapy.

Head Injuries

The severity of head injuries can vary greatly. The history of the injury (i.e., details about what it is and how it happened) is crucial for determining appropriate management. With a head injury, the patient may appear normal; may experience dizziness, severe headache, mental confusion, or memory loss; or may even be unconscious. Loss of consciousness may be brief or prolonged; it may appear immediately or may be delayed. The victim may experience vomiting; loss of bladder and bowel control; and bleeding from the nose, mouth, or ears. The pupils of the eyes may be unequal and nonreactive to light.

All head injuries must be considered serious. Notify the physician or contact EMS immediately. If evidence of a neck injury is seen, stabilize the neck and do not attempt to move the victim. Do not administer anything by mouth. Keep the patient warm and quiet. Watch the pupils of the eyes and record any changes. Measure vital signs and record the extent and duration of any unconsciousness. If the patient is at home or is sent home after the physician's assessment, he or she should be watched closely for 24 hours after the injury for any change in mental status.

Foreign Bodies in the Eye

The eye is a delicate organ with a unique structure that demands special handling. This kind of emergency is most uncomfortable, and it often is extremely difficult to keep the patient from rubbing the eye. Tell the patient not to touch the eye in any way. The physician may order ophthalmic topical anesthetic drops to relieve pain. The patient should be placed in a darkened room to wait for the physician because **photophobia** is common with eye irritations. If a contusion and swelling are present, cold, wet compresses can help.

Ask the patient to close both eyes and cover them with eye pads until the physician arrives. The physician may order an eye irrigation to remove the object. Unless the foreign object is clearly visible, do not attempt to search for it or to remove it. (Eye care is presented in greater detail in Chapter 37.)

Heat and Cold Injuries

Exposure to extremes in temperature can cause minor to severe injuries. Heat injuries occur most often on hot, humid days and result in cramps, heat exhaustion, or heatstroke. Heat-related muscle cramps may be the first sign of *heat exhaustion*, which is a serious heat-related condition. Patients with heat exhaustion appear flushed and report headaches, nausea, vertigo, and weakness. *Heatstroke,* the most dangerous form of heat-related injury, results in a shutdown of body systems. Patients with heatstroke have red, hot, dry skin; altered levels of consciousness; tachycardia; and rapid, shallow breathing. This is a true medical emergency. If heat-related problems are recognized in the early stages and are adequately treated, the patient does not usually develop heatstroke. Management of heat-related conditions includes getting the person out of the heat; loosening clothing or removing perspiration-soaked clothing; and giving the person cool drinks if he or she is alert. An effective way to lower the victim's temperature is to apply cool, wet cloths and then fan the moist skin, so that heat is released from the body by evaporation.

The two types of cold-related injuries are frostbite and hypothermia. *Frostbite*, which is the actual freezing of tissue, occurs when skin temperature falls to a range of 14°F to 25°F (−10°C to −3.9°C). Prolonged exposure of the skin to cold causes damage similar to a burn. The tissue may appear gray or white, may be swollen, and may have clear blisters, or, in full-thickness frostbite, may show signs of tissue **necrosis**, including blackened areas and severe deformity. The more advanced the frostbite, the more serious is the tissue damage and the more likely the body part will be lost. Frozen tissue has no feeling, but as thawing occurs, the patient reports itching, tingling, and burning pain. Mild frostbite can be managed by applying constant warmth to the affected areas by immersing the area in warm water (no warmer than 105°F [40.6°C]) or by wrapping it in warm, dry clothing. Friction should never be used, because this would increase tissue damage. If blisters have formed, or if evidence of full-thickness frostbite is seen, the patient should be transported to the nearest ED.

Hypothermia is a medical emergency that may result in death unless the patient receives immediate assistance. Systemic hypothermia occurs when the core body temperature drops below 95°F (35°C). Signs and symptoms of hypothermia include shivering, numbness, apathy, and loss of consciousness. If hypothermia is suspected, activate EMS and care for any life-threatening conditions until help arrives. Remove the victim's wet clothing and wrap the victim in blankets while moving him or her to a warm place. If the victim is alert, give warm liquids and apply heating pads (using a barrier to prevent burns) to help slowly raise the core body temperature.

Dehydration

A person dehydrates when more water is excreted than is taken in. Dehydration can be a very serious health emergency, leading to convulsions, coma, and even death. Infants, young children, and older adult patients are at greatest risk of developing serious complications from dehydration. Severe dehydration may be caused by excessive heat loss, vomiting, diarrhea, or lack of fluid intake. Symptoms include vertigo; dark yellow urine or no urine output for 8 to 10 hours; extreme thirst; lethargy or confusion; and abdominal or muscle cramps. If the patient shows any of these symptoms and is unable to retain fluids, schedule an urgent appointment or recommend that the patient be taken to the ED. Replacement of lost fluids is vital, so the patient should be encouraged to drink water, tea, sports drinks, fruit juice, or Pedialyte.

Diabetic Emergencies

Diabetes mellitus is caused by a malfunction in the production of insulin in the pancreas or by an inability of the cells to use insulin. Insulin is required on the cellular level so that glucose can be used for energy. Two different diabetic emergencies are caused by *hyperglycemia* (high blood glucose levels) or by *hypoglycemia* (low blood glucose levels).

Insulin shock is caused by severe hypoglycemia, because the patient with diabetes has taken too much insulin, has not eaten enough food, or has exercised an unusual amount. Signs and symptoms, which have a rapid onset, include tachycardia, profuse sweating (diaphoresis), headache, irritability, vertigo, fatigue, hunger, seizures, and coma. It is important to provide glucose immediately, preferably in the form of glucose tablets, because they have a known concentrated quantity of glucose.

Diabetic coma results from severe hyperglycemia, which develops because the body is not producing enough insulin; the patient ate too much food or is very stressed; or the patient has an infection. Symptoms of impending diabetic coma develop more slowly than those of insulin shock; these include general malaise, dry mouth, polyuria, **polydipsia**, nausea, vomiting, SOB, and breath with an acetone (or "fruity") smell. If the patient or caregiver calling for an appointment reports these symptoms, notify the physician immediately, because the patient typically would be admitted to the hospital.

In an emergency situation, if a patient diagnosed with diabetes mellitus shows signs and symptoms of a diabetic emergency, the patient should be given glucose. If the problem is caused by insulin shock (hypoglycemia), the patient will improve quickly after receiving glucose; if it is caused by diabetic coma (hyperglycemia), a small amount of added glucose will not affect the patient's condition, and he or she must be transported to the hospital regardless. (Diabetes mellitus is covered in detail in Chapter 45.)

CLOSING COMMENTS

Patient Education

Emergencies can occur anywhere. Patients need to learn how to handle emergency situations both by the example of healthcare workers and through instruction. The medical assistant must remain calm, screen the situation, call for help, and be prepared to administer appropriate first aid. Brochures on home safety can be used to help teach patients methods for preventing accidents in the home.

All patients, even children, should understand how to contact EMS. This is especially important for families with members who have chronic diseases that are potentially life threatening, such as heart conditions, severe allergic reactions, diabetes, and asthma. Patients should be encouraged to post next to the telephone emergency numbers such as those for the local EMS and poison control center, and for the primary care physician. Families with young children need to "child-proof" their homes, being especially careful to keep potentially poisonous substances stored where children cannot get into them. Placing "Mr. Yuk" stickers on containers of poisonous substances can be an excellent educational tool for young children.

Medical assistants must remember to keep their American Red Cross or American Heart Association certifications current, and they should take advantage of community workshops to maintain and extend their skills. Post a list of community safety workshops in an area where it can be seen by patients, and encourage them to attend. Your participation in emergency care workshops, as well as encouraging others to participate, may help to save lives.

Legal and Ethical Issues

The medical assistant works in the healthcare environment as the physician's agent. Although you are responsible for your own actions, the physician is legally responsible for the care you administer to patients while working in the healthcare facility. You are responsible for knowing the limitations placed on medical assistants in your state and for adhering strictly to your employer's emergency care policies and procedures. Medical assistants are not qualified to diagnose a patient problem but are responsible for acting appropriately in a medical emergency. In addition to legal responsibilities, you have an ethical responsibility to your patients to provide the highest standard of care. Always act in the best interest of the patient, and never hesitate to ask the physician and/or the office manager for immediate assistance when faced with a medical emergency.

Most states have enacted Good Samaritan laws to encourage healthcare professionals to provide medical assistance at the scene of an accident without fear of being sued for negligence. These statutes vary greatly, but all have the intent of protecting the caregiver. A physician or other healthcare professional is not legally obligated to provide emergency care at the site of an accident, regardless of the ethical and moral considerations. Legal liability is limited to gross neglect of the victim or willfully causing further injury to the victim. As a caregiver, you are required to act as a reasonable person and cannot be held liable for personal injury resulting from an act of omission. Good Samaritan statutes provide for evaluation of the caregiver's judgment but are in effect only at the site of an emergency, not at your place of employment.

If you have not been trained in CPR, you cannot be expected to perform the procedure at the emergency site. However, in many states, a healthcare provider with CPR training and skills who is present at the scene can be declared negligent if cardiac arrest occurs and he or she does not administer CPR to the victim.

If the victim is conscious, or if a member of his or her immediate family is present, obtain verbal consent to perform emergency care. Consent is implied if the patient is unconscious and no family member is present.

Many types of emergencies can be handled in the physician's office. In an emergency situation, decisions that must be made quickly can determine whether the patient lives. A medical assistant must be prepared to act calmly and efficiently in all emergency situations.

Medical assistants also can play a key role in community response to natural or human-made disasters. The medical assistant is cross-trained to perform multiple administrative and clinical duties that would prove very useful in an emergency. These include management of medical records, interacting professionally with patients, performing diagnostic tests, performing phlebotomy and administering medications, assisting with procedures, and administering first aid and CPR as needed. Because of this wide range of skills, medical assistants serve as useful volunteers on local emergency response teams. Investigate agencies and organizations that are committed to emergency preparedness in your community, and see how a medical assistant could help these organizations if an emergency arises.

SUMMARY OF SCENARIO

Cheryl has learned through her work with the telephone screening team and involvement with emergencies in the office how important it is to gather complete information about emergency situations and to act calmly and knowledgeably when managing patient problems. She knows she needs to maintain her certification in CPR for the Professional and to continue to participate in workshops on emergency care to be prepared for the wide variety of patient problems seen in the ambulatory care setting. Working with the screening staff has reinforced the importance of documenting all interactions on the telephone and information gathered during patient visits.

Cheryl recognizes that medical assistants in the office must follow the facility's policies and procedures manual for handling emergencies. They must plan ahead and complete their designated duties if an emergency occurs; use community emergency services as needed; and keep emergency supplies and equipment well stocked and ready for any potential emergency situation. She recognizes that understanding first aid practices for common patient emergencies allows her to assist patients by providing instruction on the phone or by performing specific skills when emergencies occur in the facility.

Cheryl has investigated her legal standing as a medical assistant in her home state and recognizes her responsibilities when a patient calls or shows up at the office with a medical emergency. She will continue to refer to the more experienced screening staff or to Dr. Bendt when she has questions, but she now feels more confident in managing emergency situations at work. She also recognizes her role as part of the healthcare team if an emergency situation arises in her community.

SUMMARY OF LEARNING OBJECTIVES

1. **Define, spell, and pronounce the terms listed in the vocabulary.**
   Spelling and pronouncing medical terms correctly bolsters the medical assistant's credibility. Knowing the definitions of these terms promotes confidence in communication with patients and co-workers.

2. **Apply critical thinking skills in performing the patient assessment and patient care.**
   Completing the Critical Thinking Application exercises throughout the chapter can help the student medical assistant become more adept at critical analysis of real-life situations.

3. **Describe patient safety factors in the medical office environment.**
   The medical assistant must be constantly on guard to protect patients from possible injury. Methods for achieving this goal include communicating openly about patient safety issues; following standard procedures when delivering patient care; and working as part of a team to secure patients' safety (see Procedure 36-1).

4. **Evaluate the work environment to identify safe and unsafe working conditions.**
   See Procedure 36-2.

5. **Identify environmental safety issues in the healthcare setting.**
   Medical assistants must be constantly on the alert for potentially unsafe conditions; must consistently follow the guidelines established by OSHA for infection control; and must follow safety procedures to prevent workplace violence.

6. **Develop environmental, patient, and employee safety plans.**
   See Procedures 36-1 to 36-3.

7. **Discuss fire safety issues in a healthcare environment.**
   Combustibles should be stored properly; electrical equipment must be monitored for safety; smoke detectors and fire extinguishers should be checked routinely; and the facility should be evacuated if a fire breaks out.

8. **Demonstrate the proper use of a fire extinguisher.**
   See Procedure 36-4.

9. **Describe the fundamental principles for evacuation of a healthcare facility.**
   An emergency action coordinator should be designated. This person is in charge of delegating duties to staff members. Exit maps should be posted in multiple areas around the facility. Patients and staff members should be evacuated safely and should meet in a designated spot to make sure all staff members and patients have escaped.

10. **Role-play a mock environmental exposure event and evacuation of a physician's office.**
    See Procedure 36-5.

11. **Discuss the requirements for proper disposal of hazardous materials.**
    OSHA has established specific rules about biohazard waste disposal including the use of sharps containers and red bag collection systems. These must be used properly to avoid disease transmission.

12. **Define the important features of emergency preparedness in the ambulatory care setting.**

    Ambulatory care centers may be the first to recognize and initiate a response to a community emergency. Standard Precautions should be implemented immediately to control the spread of an infection. A communication network should be established to notify local and state health departments and perhaps federal officials. Every healthcare facility should have a standard policy with specific procedures for the management of emergencies on site. The CDC recommends that a facility's safety plan consider multiple steps to minimize the negative psychological effects of an emergency situation.

13. **Maintain an up-to-date list of community resources for emergency preparedness.**

    See Procedure 36-6.

14. **Describe the medical assistant's role in emergency response.**

    Medical assistants can be of considerable help in a community emergency. They can provide therapeutic communication to gather patient data; monitor injured victims; perform first aid and monitor vital signs; and help with any medically related service.

15. **Summarize the typical emergency supplies and equipment.**

    A physician's office must have a centrally located crash cart or emergency bag stocked with all emergency supplies, equipment, and medication. This material must be inventoried consistently and maintained. This chapter provides a detailed list of materials that should be readily available for an on-site emergency, including a defibrillator if indicated by the physician's practice.

16. **Demonstrate the use of an automated external defibrillator.**

    See Procedure 36-7.

17. **Summarize the general rules for managing emergencies.**

    Management of emergencies requires a calm, efficient approach. The medical assistant should assess the nature of the emergency and determine whether EMS should be activated, or whether the patient requires an immediate or urgent appointment. As many details about the situation as possible should be gathered, and the physician should be consulted when the medical assistant is in doubt.

18. **Demonstrate telephone screening techniques and documentation guidelines for ambulatory care emergencies.**

    Telephone screening is one of the medical assistant's most important tasks. Emergency action principles should be used to determine the level of a patient's emergency. These include determining whether the situation is life threatening and obtaining the patient's contact information, as well as all pertinent information about the injury and the patient's signs and symptoms. This information must be shared with the physician, and all details must be documented in the patient's chart (see Procedure 36-8).

19. **Recognize and respond to life-threatening emergencies in the ambulatory care setting.**

    Life-threatening emergencies require immediate assessment, referral to the physician, and, if the physician is not present, activation of EMS.

While waiting for assistance, the medical assistant should check for breathing and circulation. Rescue breaths or CPR is administered if indicated. Depending on the patient's signs and symptoms, the patient should be monitored for signs of a heart attack; the Heimlich maneuver is performed for an airway obstruction; the patient is evaluated for signs of a CVA and is assessed for shock. The medical assistant should ask for help when indicated and should perform appropriate procedures based on the patient's presenting condition.

20. **Perform professional-level CPR.**

    See Procedure 36-9 for instruction on performing adult, pediatric, and infant rescue breathing and CPR.

21. **Administer oxygen through a nasal cannula to a patient in respiratory distress.**

    See Procedure 36-10.

22. **Identify and assist a patient with an obstructed airway.**

    Procedure 36-11 presents instructions for assisting an adult with an obstructed airway. Infants with an obstructed airway should receive alternating back blows and chest thrusts with attempted rescue breaths until the item is dislodged or help arrives.

23. **Determine the appropriate action and documentation procedures for common ambulatory care emergencies.**

    The medical assistant should always follow Standard Precautions when caring for a patient with a medical emergency. Documentation of emergency treatment should include information about the patient; vital signs; allergies, current medications, and pertinent health history; the patient's chief complaint; the sequence of events, including any changes in the patient's condition since the incident; and any physician's orders and procedures performed.

24. **Assist and monitor a patient who has fainted.**

    See Procedure 36-12.

25. **Control a hemorrhagic wound.**

    See Procedure 36-13.

26. **Apply patient education concepts to medical emergencies.**

    Patients should know how to contact emergency personnel, and families with young children should have telephone numbers for poison control posted. Educating patients about how to care for minor emergencies at home is an important part of telephone triage in the ambulatory care setting. Encouraging patients to participate in community safety workshops and to become certified in CPR may help prevent emergencies and save lives.

27. **Discuss the legal and ethical concerns arising from medical emergencies.**

    Good Samaritan laws, which vary from state to state, are designed to protect any individual from liability, whether a healthcare professional or a layperson, if he or she provides assistance at the site of an emergency. The law does not require a medically trained person to act, but if emergency care is given in a reasonable and responsible manner, the healthcare worker is protected from being sued for negligence. This protection, however, does not extend to the workplace.

CONNECTIONS

Study Guide Connection: Go to the Chapter 36 Study Guide. Read and complete the activities.

Evolve Connection: Go to the Chapter 36 link at *evolve.elsevier.com/kinn* to complete the Chapter Review and Chapter Quiz. Peruse other resources listed for this chapter to increase your knowledge of Emergency Preparedness and Assisting With Medical Emergencies.

37

ASSISTING IN OPHTHALMOLOGY AND OTOLARYNGOLOGY

Kim Tau, CMA (AAMA), works in an out-patient clinic that specializes in the diagnosis and treatment of eye and ear disorders. Kim has been asked by her supervisor to help orient Amy Ling to the practice. Amy recently graduated from a medical assistant program and is familiar with basic eye and ear procedures, but she has many questions about her responsibilities at the clinic. Amy will be responsible for performing initial Snellen and Ishihara screening examinations on new patients, and for assisting the ophthalmologist and the optician in the practice with eye treatments. She also will have to be comfortable performing audiometry hearing screening on pediatric patients, performing ear irrigations, and administering otic medications. Kim recognizes that it is important that Amy be able to perform these skills with accuracy and confidence, but she also must be sensitive to the communication and patient education needs of patients with eye and ear disorders.

While studying this chapter, think about the following questions:

- What is the basic anatomy and physiology of the eye and of the ear?
- What are the major types of refractive errors?
- With what disorders of the eye and ear does Amy need to be familiar?
- How is a Snellen test performed?
- What are the important steps Amy should follow in performing eye and ear irrigations and medication applications?
- How is an examination with an audiometer conducted?
- How should Amy perform a throat culture?
- How should Kim prepare Amy to care for patients with sensory loss?

LEARNING OBJECTIVES

1. Define, spell, and pronounce the terms listed in the vocabulary.
2. Apply critical thinking skills in performing patient assessment and patient care.
3. Explain the differences among an ophthalmologist, an optometrist, and an optician.
4. Identify the anatomic structures of the eye.
5. Describe the process of vision.
6. Differentiate among the major types of refractive errors.
7. Summarize typical disorders of the eye.
8. Define the various diagnostic procedures for the eye.
9. Conduct a vision acuity test using the Snellen chart.
10. Assess color acuity using the Ishihara test.
11. Explain the purpose of eye irrigations and instillation of medications.
12. Properly irrigate a patient's eyes.
13. Accurately instill eye medication.
14. Identify the structures and explain the functions of the external, middle, and inner ear.
15. Describe the conditions that can lead to hearing loss, including conductive and sensorineural impairments.
16. Define the major disorders of the ear, including otitis, impacted cerumen, and Ménière's disease.
17. Explain diagnostic procedures for the ear.
18. Use an audiometer to accurately measure the hearing acuity of a patient.
19. Identify the purpose of ear irrigations and instillation of ear medications.
20. Demonstrate the procedure for performing ear irrigations.
21. Accurately instill medicated ear drops.
22. Summarize the nose and throat examination.
23. Perform a throat culture.
24. Describe the effect of sensory loss on patient education.
25. Discuss legal and ethical issues that might arise when caring for a patient with a vision or hearing deficit.

accommodation Adjustment of the eye that allows a person to see various sizes of objects at different distances.

amblyopia (am-ble-o′-pe-uh) Reduction or dimness of vision with no apparent organic cause; often referred to as *lazy eye syndrome.*

audiologist (au-de-ah′-lah-jist) Allied healthcare professional who specializes in evaluation of hearing function, detection of hearing impairment, and determination of the anatomic site of impairment.

cones Structures in the retina that make the perception of color possible.

fovea centralis (fo′-ve-uhl/sen-trah′-luhs) Small pit in the center of the retina that is considered the center of clearest vision.

gonioscopy (goh-nee-os′-kuh-pee) Procedure in which a mirrored optical instrument is used to visualize the filtration angle of the anterior chamber of the eye; the procedure is used to diagnose glaucoma.

hertz Unit of measurement used in hearing examinations; a wave frequency equal to 1 cycle per second.

miotic (mi-ah′-tik) Any substance or medication that causes constriction of the pupil.

mydriatic (mid-ree-at′-ik) Topical ophthalmic medication that dilates the pupil; it is used in diagnostic procedures of the eye and as treatment for glaucoma.

optic disk Region at the back of the eye where the optic nerve meets the retina; it is considered the blind spot of the eye, because it contains only nerve fibers and no rods or cones, and thus is insensitive to light.

optic nerve The second cranial nerve, which carries impulses for the sense of sight.

otosclerosis (o-tuh-skluh-ro′-suhs) The formation of spongy bone in the labyrinth of the ear, which often causes the auditory ossicles to become fixed and unable to vibrate when sound enters the ears.

ototoxic (o-tuh-tahk′-sik) Medicine or substance capable of damaging the eighth cranial nerve or the organs of hearing and balance.

psoriasis (suh-ri′-uh-suhs) A usually chronic, recurrent skin disease marked by bright red patches covered with silvery scales.

rods Structures in the retina of the eye that form the light-sensitive elements.

seborrhea (se-buh-re′-uh) An excessive discharge of sebum from the sebaceous glands, forming greasy scales or cheesy plugs on the body.

tonometer (toh-nom′-i-ter) An instrument used to measure intraocular pressure.

A medical assistant is responsible for performing a wide variety of procedures in an ophthalmologic or otorhinolaryngologic practice. First, the medical assistant must be familiar with the normal anatomy and physiology of the eyes, ears, nose, and throat. With an understanding of how these specialty sensory organs function, the medical assistant can master the skills needed to become a valuable asset to the physician who specializes in the treatment of eye and ear disorders.

This chapter covers the conditions most frequently seen in the ambulatory care setting. Many subspecialty areas are available to medical assistants in the eye, ear, nose, and throat (ENT) medical practice. Learning the fundamental procedures now will provide you with a base on which to build the advanced techniques you will need if you choose to concentrate your expertise in these areas.

EXAMINATION OF THE EYE

Ophthalmology is the science of the eye and its disorders and diseases. A physician who specializes in the diagnosis and treatment of disorders and diseases of the eye is an *ophthalmologist.* An ophthalmologist is a licensed medical physician who can diagnose eye disorders, prescribe medication, conduct eye screenings, prescribe glasses or contact lenses, and perform optic surgery. An *optometrist* is not a medical doctor but is licensed and has earned a degree as a Doctor of Optometry (OD). An optometrist can perform eye examinations, diagnose vision problems and eye diseases, and treat visual defects through corrective lenses and eye exercises. *Opticians* are trained to fill prescriptions written by ophthalmologists and optometrists for corrective lenses by grinding the lenses and dispensing eyewear.

Anatomy and Physiology of the Eye

The eyes are the smallest, yet the most detailed and complex, organs of the body. Each is located within a bony cavity (or *orbit*) in the skull. The bony orbit protects and supports the eye. Only approximately one-sixth of the eye lies outside the orbit. The eyelid helps protect the eye from trauma. The eyebrows help keep irritants out of the eyes. The eyelashes line the margins of the eyelids and help trap foreign particles.

The conjunctiva is a thin mucous membrane that lines the eyelid and covers the outside of the eyeball except for the most central portion, which is covered by the cornea. The mucus secreted from the conjunctiva helps keep the eye moist. The eye blinks every 2 to 3 seconds, causing the lacrimal gland, located in the superior outer portion of the upper eyelid, to secrete tears. Tears move across the eyes, cleansing and moistening the surface, and drain into the lacrimal canals in the medial corner of the eye. The tears then drain into the nasal cavity through the nasolacrimal duct. Consequently, when a person cries, the excess tears ultimately empty into the nose, producing a watery nasal discharge.

The Eyeball

The eyeball consists of three layers. The outermost layer is made up of the white, opaque sclera and the transparent cornea. The sclera is a tough, fibrous lining that protects the entire eyeball lying within the orbit, whereas the transparent cornea covers the exposed one-sixth of the eyeball. The cornea acts as a clear window that allows light to enter the eye. The cornea also *refracts,* or changes, the direction of light rays after they enter the eye. The cornea was one of the first tissues to be transplanted, and corneal transplants now are common. Long-term success after corneal implant surgery is excellent.

The choroid is the posterior portion of the middle layer of the eye. It is the eye's vascular layer, and it contains many blood vessels that supply nutrients to the outer layers of the retina. The choroid also has a brown pigment that absorbs excess light rays that could interfere with vision. In the anterior part of this layer, the choroid creates the iris and the ciliary body. The iris is the colored portion of the eye. It is doughnut shaped, with the opening of the pupil in the center. The iris contains muscles that regulate the size of the pupil according to the intensity of the light; it becomes smaller in bright light and opens wider in dim light. The ciliary body contains both the ciliary muscle, which regulates the shape of the lens, and the ciliary processes, which secrete aqueous humor.

The inner layer of the eye includes the retina in the posterior portion and the lens in the anterior portion. The **rods** and **cones, optic nerve, optic disc**, and **fovea centralis** are located in the retina. The delicate tissue of the retina is composed of light-sensitive neurons that convert light into neurological impulses. These impulses travel by means of the optic nerve to the brain, where they are converted into a visual form. Any damage to the retina has the potential to cause partial or complete blindness, because the neurological center of vision is located in the retina.

The lens is a transparent, biconvex body that helps focus light after it passes through the cornea. The lens and the ciliary body divide the eye into two cavities. The posterior cavity, which is between the lens and the retina, contains the transparent, gel-like vitreous humor. Vitreous humor maintains the shape of the posterior eyeball. The anterior cavity, between the cornea and the lens, is filled with aqueous humor, which is continuously produced by the ciliary processes. Aqueous humor helps maintain normal pressure within the eye and provides nutrients to the lens and the cornea (Figure 37-1).

Vision

Vision requires light and depends on the proper functioning of all parts of the eye (Table 37-1). A visual impulse begins with the passage of light through the cornea, where the light is refracted; it then passes through the aqueous humor and the pupil into the lens. The ciliary muscle adjusts the curvature of the lens to again refract the light rays so that they pass into the retina, triggering the photo-receptor cells of the rods and cones. At this point, the light energy is converted into an electrical impulse, which is sent through the optic nerve to the visual cortex of the occipital lobe of the brain; there, the light impulse is interpreted and a picture is created.

Disorders of the Eye

Refractive Errors

Four major types of refractive errors result when the eye is unable to focus light effectively on the retina. *Refraction* is the ability of the lens of the eye to bend parallel light rays coming into the eye so that

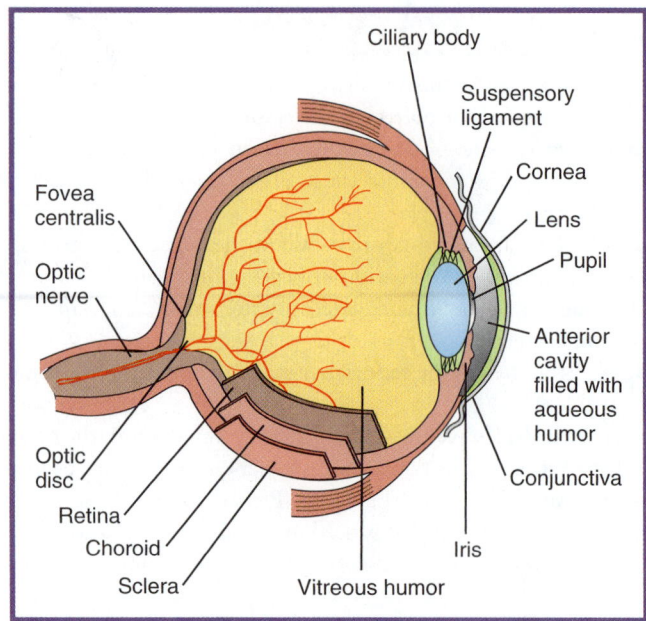

FIGURE 37-1 Anatomy of the eye.

TABLE 37-1 Functions of the Major Parts of the Eye

STRUCTURE	FUNCTION
Sclera	External protection
Cornea	Light refraction
Choroid	Blood supply
Iris	Light absorption and regulation of pupil width
Ciliary body	Secretion of vitreous fluid; changes the shape of the lens
Lens	Light refraction
Retinal layer	Light receptor that transforms optic signals into nerve impulses
Rods	Distinguish light from dark and perceive shape and movement
Cones	Color vision
Central fovea	Area of sharpest vision
Macula lutea	Center of the retina; contains the fovea centralis, the area of most highly acute vision
External ocular muscles	Move the eyeball
Optic nerve	One of a pair of nerves that transmit visual stimuli to (cranial nerve II) the brain
Lacrimal glands	Produce tears
Eyelid	Protects eye

Modified from Damjanov I: *Pathology for the health-related professions,* Philadelphia, 1996, Saunders.

the rays are focused simultaneously on the retina. An *error of refraction* means that the light rays are not refracted or bent properly and consequently do not focus correctly on the retina. Defects in the shape of the eyeball can cause a refractive error. Most refractive errors can be corrected with corrective lenses (Figure 37-2).

Hyperopia (Farsightedness). When light enters the eye and focuses behind the retina, a person has *hyperopia.* This disorder occurs when the eyeball is too short from the anterior to the posterior wall. An individual with hyperopia has difficulty seeing objects that are close, at reading or working level. A convex corrective lens helps the eye's internal lens place objects directly on the retina and creates a sharp, detailed image, or refractive surgery may be done to correct the shape of the lens.

Myopia (Nearsightedness). Myopia occurs when light rays entering the eye focus in front of the retina, causing objects at a distance to appear blurry and dull. Objects viewed at reading or working level are seen clearly. In this disorder, the eyeball is elongated from the anterior to the posterior wall, and the image cannot be sharpened by the internal lens of the eye. A concave corrective lens is used to focus the light rays on the retina, or surgery can be done to change the shape of the lens. However, the surgery is performed only on adults who have had a stable eye prescription for at least 1 year.

Presbyopia. As people age, the lens of the eye becomes less flexible, and the ciliary muscles weaken; consequently, changing the point of focus from distance to near becomes difficult; this is called *presbyopia.* The condition results in difficulty seeing at reading level. A combination corrective lens, known as a *bifocal lens* or a *progressive lens correction,* is used to focus both distal and proximal objects directly on the retina. Presbyopia actually starts at approximately age 10, but most people do not report an alteration in vision until their early forties. Conductive keratoplasty is the new laser procedure used to treat presbyopia.

Astigmatism. *Astigmatism* occurs when light rays entering the eye are focused irregularly. This usually occurs because the cornea or the lens is not a smooth sphere, but rather has an irregular shape. Ophthalmologists describe the lens as being shaped like a football rather than a sphere, such as a basketball. This causes light rays to be unevenly or diffusely focused on the retina, resulting in blurred vision. It is like attempting to focus on objects seen through a wavy piece of window glass. Astigmatism can be corrected with glasses, contacts, or surgery. Surgical correction attempts to reshape the cornea into a more spherical or uniformly curved surface.

Signs and Symptoms of Refractive Errors

Refractive errors in vision can lead to squinting, frequent rubbing of the eyes, and headaches. The individual notices blurred vision or fading of words at reading level, or both. Some refractive errors are familial in nature.

Treatment of Refractive Errors

Eyeglasses and contact lenses are the traditional treatments for visual acuity problems caused by refractive errors. However, problems with the shape of the lens can be corrected surgically. Surgery is performed on an outpatient basis and requires only a short stay in the facility. Medical assistants employed in an outpatient eye surgery facility must be trained to fulfill this specialized role.

> **CRITICAL THINKING** APPLICATION   **37-1**
>
> Amy is assisting Dr. Hanser with visual acuity examinations. He asks her whether she understands the cause of refractive errors. Amy doesn't really know, so later she asks Kim over lunch what the different refractive disorders are and why they occur. What information should Kim include in her answer?

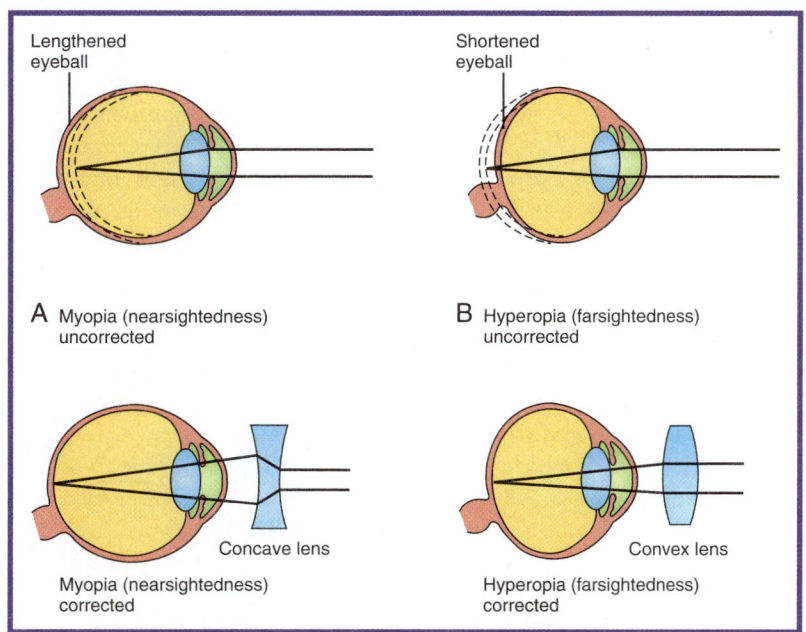

FIGURE 37-2 Errors in refraction. **A,** Myopia. **B,** Hyperopia.

SURGICAL CORRECTION OF REFRACTIVE ERRORS

Most types of health insurance do not cover surgery for refractive corrections. On average, each eye costs $1,500 to $3,000.

- Photorefractive keratectomy (PRK): PRK was the first surgical procedure developed to treat refractive errors. The epithelium layer of the cornea is removed, and a computer-controlled laser reshapes the central cornea into a flatter surface (for people who are myopic) or a more curved surface (for people who are hyperopic). Patients experience discomfort for 24 to 48 hours after the procedure while the epithelium regenerates, and they typically wear bandages for a few days to help control pain. This procedure has been replaced by the more advanced LASIK procedure.
- Laser-assisted in situ keratomileusis (LASIK): LASIK is a more advanced procedure in which an excimer laser is used to reshape the central cornea to treat myopia, hyperopia, and astigmatism. A thin, hinged flap of cornea is created, the flap is lifted, and the exposed surface of the cornea is reshaped. After the corneal curvature has been corrected, the flap is replaced, and the area heals without stitches.
- Laser-assisted epithelium keratomileusis (LASEK): LASEK is the most recent laser surgery development. The surface epithelial cells of the eye are softened with an alcohol solution, allowing the epithelial layer to be rolled back and the cornea to be exposed. A laser then is used to reshape the cornea and treat myopia, hyperopia, and astigmatism. The epithelial flap is returned to its original position, and a contact lens is placed on the cornea as a bandage for several days to aid healing and reduce pain.
- Conductive keratoplasty (CK): CK uses heat created by a laser to reshape the cornea. Heat is applied to the cornea's outer edge to tighten and steepen the cornea. CK is used in patients older than 40 years of age who need correction for hyperopia, presbyopia, and myopia. The procedure causes little or no discomfort and improves vision almost instantly. The corneal changes are not permanent, and retreatment may be required.

Strabismus

Strabismus is failure of the eyes to track together, which means that both eyes do not look in the same direction at the same time. Adults can develop strabismus because of a condition or disease elsewhere in the body, such as diabetes mellitus, muscular dystrophy, or hypertension, or as the result of a head injury. In children, strabismus is caused by weakness in the muscles that control eye movement. If the condition appears in infancy or childhood, it is most commonly associated with **amblyopia**. Amblyopia often is correctable until approximately age 7 or until the retina is fully developed. Treatment involves having the child wear a patch over the unaffected eye so that the muscles of the "lazy" eye are strengthened. The main symptom in all age groups is *diplopia* (double vision).

Nystagmus

A constant, involuntary movement of one or both eyes is called *nystagmus*. The eye can move in any direction and the movement is accompanied by blurred vision. A child may be born with the problem (congenital nystagmus), or the condition may be acquired as a result of a brain tumor, an inner ear lesion, multiple sclerosis, or substance abuse. Nystagmus is caused by an abnormal function in the part of the brain that controls eye movements. Congenital nystagmus is more common than acquired nystagmus, is usually milder, does not worsen over time, and is not associated with any other disorder. A patient with signs and symptoms of nystagmus first should undergo neurological evaluation to determine the cause of the disorder, with treatment based on those findings. However, congenital nystagmus has no cure. Affected individuals typically are not aware of the eye movements, but they may have a decrease in visual acuity that can be corrected with surgery or corrective lenses.

Infections of the Eye

Many acute disorders of the eye are seen in the ophthalmologist's office. These include the following:

- *Hordeolum* (stye): A localized, purulent infection of a sebaceous gland of the eyelid. The area is inflamed, swollen, and painful. The infection usually is caused by staphylococci, and it is treated with warm compresses and topical or systemic antibiotics.
- *Chalazion:* A small cyst that results from blockage of a meibomian gland (sebaceous gland) that lubricates the posterior margin of each eyelid. The cyst can become infected, inflamed, swollen, and painful. It may disappear spontaneously or may need to be removed surgically.
- *Keratitis*: Inflammation of the cornea that results in superficial ulcerations. It can be caused by the herpes simplex virus, bacteria, or fungi, or it may develop as a result of corneal trauma (e.g., intense light). Symptoms include inflammation, tearing, pain, and photophobia. The condition is treated with ophthalmic ointments, eye drops, and use of an eye patch.
- *Conjunctivitis*: Inflammation of the conjunctiva caused by irritation, allergy, or bacterial infection. Bacterial conjunctivitis (pinkeye) is highly contagious and produces a purulent discharge. Symptoms include inflammation, swelling and itching of the sclera, photophobia, and tearing. Bacterial infections are treated with antibiotic ophthalmic preparations.
- *Blepharitis:* Inflammation of the glands and lash follicles along the margins of the eyelids that may be caused by staphylococcal infection, allergies, or irritation. Symptoms include itching and inflammation along the eyelash margins, and the condition is treated with antibiotic ophthalmic ointment.

Disorders of the Eyeball

Corneal Abrasion

The cornea, the transparent outer covering of the eye, is prone to abrasion because of its location. Symptoms of corneal abrasion include pain, inflammation, tearing, and photophobia. The abrasion usually is caused by a foreign body in the eye or by direct trauma, such as from poorly fitting or dirty contact lenses. A corneal ulcer may form and become infected.

Diagnosis is based on the patient's signs and symptoms, but it can be confirmed with the instillation of fluorescein stain (Figure 37-3). After instillation of the stain, the physician uses a cobalt blue filtered light to visualize the abrasions, which appear green

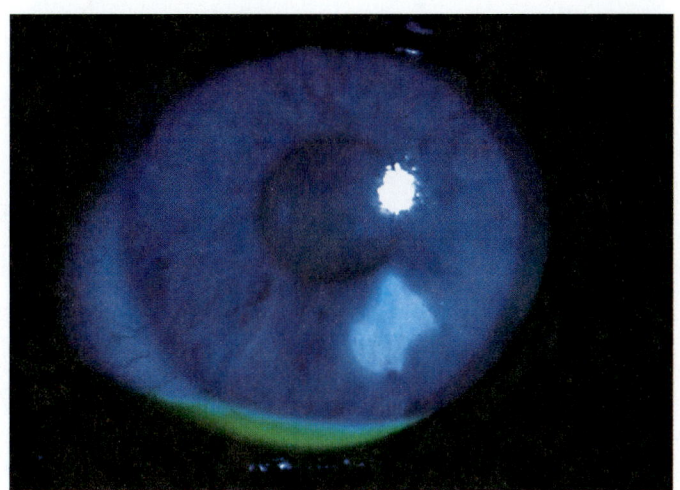

FIGURE 37-3 Corneal abrasion stained with fluorescein.

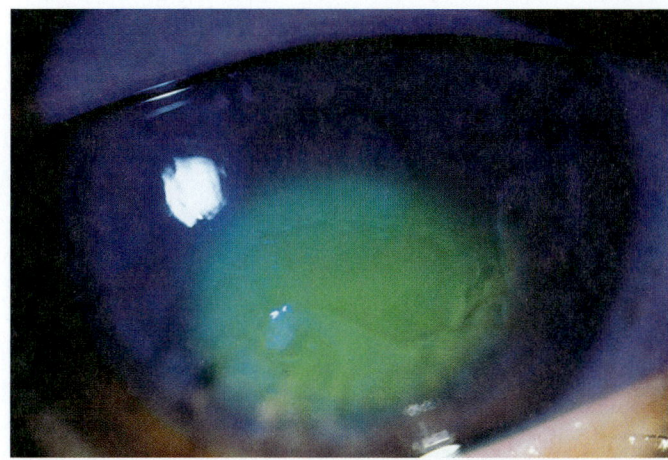

FIGURE 37-4 Corneal abrasion stained with fluorescein and highlighted by cobalt blue light.

(Figure 37-4). If the abrasions are caused by a foreign body, it must be removed first; the eye then can be treated with antibiotic ophthalmic ointment to prevent infection. Although patching the affected eye has been recommended in the past, studies now show that patching does not reduce the patient's pain and may actually prolong healing time. Corneal abrasions are quite painful, so the patient may be prescribed topical nonsteroidal antiinflammatory ophthalmic ointments (ung), such as diclofenac (Voltaren) and ketorolac (Acular), as well as oral analgesics. Most corneal abrasions heal in 24 to 72 hours, but the patient should be aware that symptoms can worsen if the affected eye is exposed to bright light, if excessive blinking occurs, or if the patient rubs the injured surface of the cornea against the inside of the eyelid. Because the patient may develop a secondary infection from the corneal injury, topical antibiotics, including bacitracin, erythromycin, or gentamicin ointments, may be prescribed. Patients with contact lenses may be prescribed oral antibiotics and should not wear their contacts until the abrasion has healed and the course of antibiotics has been completed.

Cataract

A cataract is a cloudy or opaque area in the normally clear lens of the eye that blocks the passage of light into the retina, causing impaired vision. This condition may result from injury to the eye, exposure to extreme heat or radiation, or inherited factors. However, most cataracts develop slowly and progressively as a result of the natural aging deterioration of the lens of the eye and typically occur after age 60. With advanced cataracts, the pupil of the eye appears white or gray.

Blurred and dimmed vision is the initial symptom of a cataract. The patient may need a brighter reading light or must hold objects closer to the eyes for better viewing. Continued clouding of the lens may cause diplopia. The patient also needs frequent changes of eyeglass prescriptions. Patients with cataracts report difficulty with night vision (nyctalopia), seeing halo images around lights, and increased sensitivity to glare. If left untreated, cataracts ultimately can lead to blindness.

When the patient's vision becomes distorted or appears to be deteriorating, the ophthalmologist performs a *slit lamp* procedure,

in which he or she examines the structures at the front of the eye using a combination of a low-power microscope and a high-intensity light that shines into the eye as a slit beam.

The only known effective treatment for a cataract is surgical removal of the lens. This is performed as an outpatient procedure in a clinic or hospital. After the eye has been anesthetized, the inner portions of the lens—the nucleus and the cortex—are removed. The physician may use an extracapsular extraction, in which the cataract is removed in one piece, or phacoemulsification, in which an ultrasonic probe is used to break up the cataract and the pieces are aspirated, before an artificial intraocular lens (IOL) is implanted. The incision may be closed with fine sutures, or it may be sutureless and self-sealing. The procedure usually takes 15 minutes, and the patient typically can leave the facility after 1 hour. Patients should be aware that they will not be able to drive until cleared by the ophthalmologist, and that they may need help at home until their vision is clear.

The patient is seen in the office the day after surgery and as frequently as needed for the next month. Vision gradually improves until it stabilizes, usually within 2 to 6 weeks; the patient then is fitted with new corrective lenses to match the improved vision.

Glaucoma

One of the most common and serious ocular disorders is a group of diseases known as *glaucoma*. Glaucoma is characterized by increased intraocular pressure (IOP), which damages the optic nerve and causes blindness if left untreated. It rarely occurs in people younger than age 40 and usually is seen in individuals older than age 60. The cause is unknown, but a hereditary tendency toward development of the most common forms has been noted. Glaucoma is responsible for approximately 12% of all cases of blindness. It is the leading cause of blindness among African-Americans, and it strikes approximately 2% of all individuals older than age 40 and 8% of those older than age 70 in the United States.

The ciliary body constantly produces aqueous humor, which should circulate freely between the anterior and posterior chambers of the eye and eventually empty into the general circulation. A healthy eye is filled with fluid in an amount carefully regulated to maintain the shape of the eyeball. In chronic open-angle glaucoma, the channels that drain the fluid malfunction, and over time aqueous humor builds up, resulting in increased pressure, which affects the blood supply to the retina and the optic nerve. With acute closed-angle glaucoma, the opening of the drainage system narrows or closes completely, causing a sudden increase in IOP (Figure 37-5).

Patients can have chronic open-angle glaucoma for a long time before symptoms occur. Early detection through regular ophthalmic examinations that include IOP measurements is crucial to prevent permanent vision loss. The need to change eyeglass prescriptions frequently, loss of peripheral vision, mild headaches, and impaired adaptation to the dark are some of the signs and symptoms that may be seen with chronic glaucoma.

Acute closed-angle glaucoma has more obvious symptoms; the patient complains of severe pain, headaches, inflammation, photophobia, and seeing halos around lights. If left untreated, acute glaucoma can cause permanent blindness in a matter of days. Screening for glaucoma is conducted during a complete eye examination. The ophthalmologist first uses a **tonometer** with a slit lamp to measure IOP. The air puff tonometer records the degree of indentation of the cornea from a puff of pressurized air without touching the eye. An applanation tonometer records the pressure needed to indent the cornea when the instrument is applied to the front surface of the eye. Electronic tonometry is the most recently developed technique. The ophthalmologist gently places the rounded tip of a tool that looks like a pen directly on the cornea, with results evident on a small computer panel. **Gonioscopy** also can be used to examine the aqueous fluid drainage system and to determine whether the glaucoma is the open- or closed-angle type. In addition, an ophthalmoscopic examination can identify cupping of the optic disk, which indicates atrophy of the optic nerve.

Open-angle glaucoma can be relieved with **miotic** and beta-blocker eye drops. The combinations of drugs used to treat glaucoma can vary considerably. Miotic medications increase the outflow of aqueous humor, and beta blockers reduce the production of aqueous humor (Table 37-2). It is imperative that the patient use prescribed eye drops and take oral medications daily to prevent further damage to the optic nerve. Laser surgery may be performed to create an opening or to build a new channel for drainage of the aqueous humor. The goal of treatment in any type of glaucoma is to diagnose the disease early and to effectively treat its progression, because any loss of sight that has occurred as the result of increased IOP cannot be regained. In closed-angle glaucoma, medications to lower IOP are prescribed so that surgery can be performed to create a channel in which aqueous fluid can circulate. This is a medical emergency, because the pressure must be relieved within a few hours or permanent vision damage occurs.

Macular Degeneration

The macula lutea, the part of the retina near the optic nerve, defines the center of the field of vision. Macular degeneration is progressive deterioration of the macula lutea, which causes loss of central vision; the patient can see only the edges of the visual field. It affects more than 10 million Americans and is the leading cause of blindness in those older than 55.

Two types of macular degeneration can occur. The dry form accounts for 90% of cases; it is painless and develops slowly, affecting sharp vision over time, so that reading and other activities that require fine detailed vision become impossible. Wet macular degeneration causes 90% of all severe vision losses from the disease and has a very acute onset and rapid progression. Dry macular degeneration is caused by the breakdown of light-sensitive cells in the region of the macula; the wet form is seen when new blood vessels behind the retina form and leak blood and fluid into the macula. The condition is age related, but additional risk factors include cigarette smoking, obesity, family history, cardiovascular disease, elevated blood cholesterol levels, light eye color, and excessive sun exposure. The disease has no known cure, but recent research indicates that antioxidants, including beta-carotene and vitamins C and E with zinc and copper, may prevent the condition or may slow its progress.

TABLE 37-2 **Ophthalmic Medications**	
DRUG NAME	**CLASS AND USE**
Neosporin ung	Antiinfective and steroid combination
Chloroptic, Ciloxan, erythromycin, and Garamycin ung	Topical antibiotic ointments
Viroptic	Antiinfective, antiviral
Pred-G, TobraDex	Antiinflammatory agents, corticosteroids
Ocufen, Acular, Voltaren	Topical antiinflammatory agents, nonsteroidal antiinflammatory drugs, analgesics
Isopto Atropine	Mydriatic eye drops; eye examinations
Betagan, Ocupress	Beta-blocker eye drops; glaucoma treatment
Alphagan	Alpha-adrenergic agonist eye drops; glaucoma treatment
Xalatan, Travatan, Lumigan	Prostaglandin analog eye drops; glaucoma treatment
Isopto Carpine, Pilocar	Miotic eye drops; glaucoma treatment

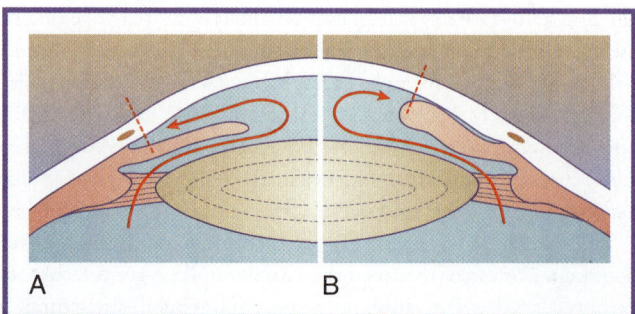

FIGURE 37-5 A, Open-angle glaucoma. **B,** Closed-angle glaucoma. (From Damjanov I: *Pathology for the health-related professions,* ed 3, Philadelphia, 2006, Saunders.)

ung, Unguent or ointment.

Diagnostic Procedures

A complete examination of the eye is technical and requires expensive equipment and the expertise of an ophthalmologist. However, a primary care physician performs some basic examinations and treatments of the eye. The ophthalmoscope is used to examine the interior of the eye. It projects a bright, narrow beam of light through the lens and illuminates the interior parts of the eye and retina. It is helpful for detecting disorders of the eyes and certain systemic disorders, such as diabetes mellitus.

The eyelids are examined for edema, which may be the result of nephrosis, heart failure, allergy, or thyroid deficiency. *Blepharoptosis,* also called *ptosis,* is drooping of the upper eyelid that can be caused by a disorder of the third cranial nerve, muscular weakness as seen in muscular dystrophy, or myasthenia gravis.

The pupils of the eyes are normally round and equal. Normal pupils constrict rapidly in response to light. This is demonstrated by shining a bright, pinpoint light into one eye from the side of the patient's head. The pupil of an illuminated eye constricts, and the pupil of the other eye constricts equally. This test is called *light and* **accommodation** (L&A). An older patient's eyes do not accommodate as well as those of a younger person. Each eye is checked this way. The patient then is asked to look at the physician's finger as it is moved directly toward the patient's nose to check for eye coordination. If the pupils are equal and round, respond normally to light, and adjust and focus on objects at different distances in a reasonable length of time, the physician charts the acronym PERRLA.

PERRLA

P — Pupils
E — Equal
R — Round
R — Reactive to
L — Light and
A — Accommodation

Special techniques used in the ophthalmologist's office include examinations performed with a slit lamp biomicroscope (Figure 37-6). This device is used to view fine details in the anterior segments of the eye. It may be used to view a foreign body, because it gives a well-illuminated and highly magnified view of the area. For this examination, the physician first orders administration of a **mydriatic** eye drop to dilate the pupil and enhance visualization of eye structures.

A patient with *exophthalmia* (abnormal protrusion of the eye, possibly resulting from an overactive thyroid or a tumor behind the eyeball) is checked with an exophthalmometer. This instrument measures how far the eye protrudes beyond the edge of the eye socket and helps determine the level of tissue swelling and enlargement behind the eye.

Distance Visual Acuity

Distance visual acuity frequently is part of a complete physical examination (Procedure 37-1). It is widely used in schools and industry and is the best single test available for vision screening. Many cases of myopia, astigmatism, and hyperopia have been detected with this routine test. The chart most commonly used is the Snellen alphabetical chart (Figure 37-7, *B*). This chart displays various letters of the alphabet, which the patient must identify in ever smaller font sizes. Patients with limited knowledge of the English alphabet can be tested with the E chart. In addition, a chart that uses pictures as symbols is available. This chart is used for young children or individuals who do not know the alphabet. The symbol on the top line of the chart can be read at 200 feet by persons with normal vision. In each of the succeeding rows, from the top down, the size of the symbols is reduced so that a person with normal vision can see them at distances of 100, 70, 50, 40, 30, and 20 feet, consecutively.

The patient must not be allowed to study the chart before taking the test. The room or hall should be long enough that the 20-foot distance can be marked off accurately and without interruptions from patient and staff traffic. The chart should be hung at the patient's eye level and illuminated with maximum light, without glare on the chart. Most adults do not need the standard Snellen chart explained, but if the E chart is used, an explanation must be given as to how the E's are to be read. The patient may point up or down or right or left toward the part of the letter that is open. If the E chart is to be used for a child, practice with an index card that has a large E drawn on it before the child is tested. Turn the card in different directions to simulate the position of the "fingers" of the E on the chart, and give the child the opportunity to demonstrate the direction of the E fingers by pointing his or her own fingers in the same direction (Figure 37-8).

Because this is a gross screening of distance visual acuity, the eyes typically are tested with corrective lenses; the patient therefore should not remove glasses or contact lenses unless the physician requests it. Indicate in the patient's medical record whether the assessment was done with or without corrective lenses. Record the results of each eye separately and as fractions. The numerator (top number) is the distance of the patient from the chart (always 20 feet), and the denominator (bottom number) is the lowest line read satisfactorily by the patient. For example, if the patient reads the 20 line at 20 feet, the fraction 20/20 is recorded for that eye. The last line the patient can read without squinting or straining and with no more than two mistakes is the line recorded in the patient's chart for that eye. The medical assistant should document the outcomes of the test with appropriate abbreviations, using OD (right eye), OS (left eye), and OU (both eyes).

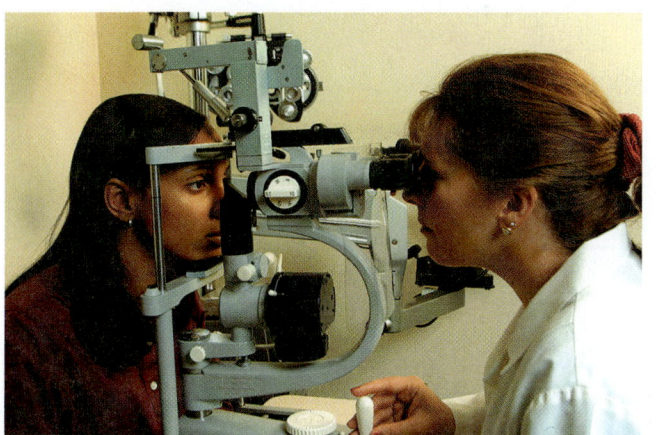

FIGURE 37-6 Slit lamp.

PROCEDURE 37-1

Perform Patient Screening Using Established Protocols: Measure Distance Visual Acuity With the Snellen Chart

GOAL: *To determine the patient's degree of visual clarity at a measured distance of 20 feet using the Snellen chart.*

EQUIPMENT and SUPPLIES

- Snellen eye chart
- Eye occluder
- Pen or pencil and paper
- Patient's record

PROCEDURAL STEPS

1. Sanitize your hands.
   PURPOSE: To ensure infection control.
2. Prepare the examination room. Make sure the room is well lit, and that a distance marker is 20 feet from the chart.
3. Identify the patient and explain the procedure. Instruct the patient not to squint during the test, because this temporarily improves vision. The patient should not have an opportunity to study the chart before the test is given. If the patient wears corrective lenses, they should be worn during the test.
   PURPOSE: Explanations help gain patient cooperation and alleviate apprehension.
4. Position the patient in a standing or sitting position at the 20-foot marker.
   PURPOSE: Twenty feet is the standard testing distance.
5. Check that the Snellen chart is positioned at the patient's eye level.
6. Instruct the patient to cover the left eye with the occluder and to keep both eyes open throughout the test to prevent squinting (Figure 1).
   PURPOSE: Traditionally, the right eye is tested first.

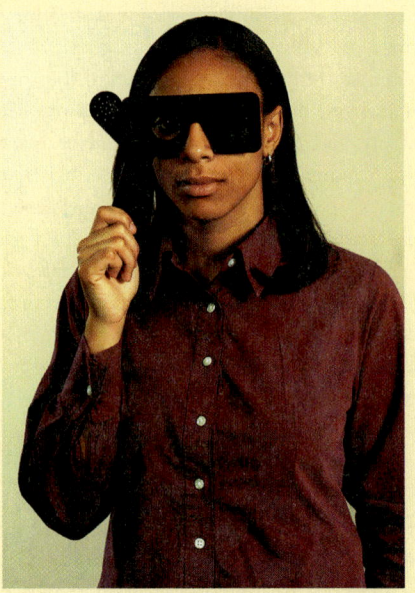

7. Stand beside the chart and point to each row as the patient reads aloud down the chart, starting with the 20/70 row (Figure 2).

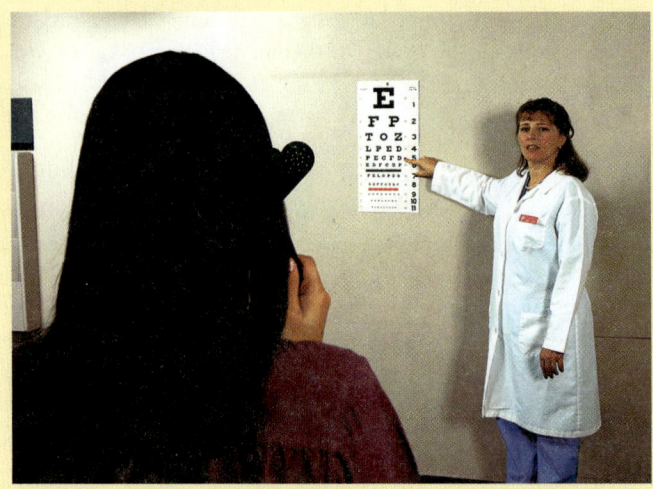

PURPOSE: Starting with larger letters gives the patient confidence and allows for accommodation of vision.

8. Proceed down the rows of the chart until the smallest row the patient can read with a maximum of two errors is reached. If one or two letters are missed, the outcome is recorded with a minus sign and the number of errors (e.g., 20/40–2). If more than two errors are made, the previous line should be documented.
9. Record any of the patient's reactions while reading the chart.
   PURPOSE: Reactions such as squinting, leaning, tearing, or blinking may indicate that the patient is having difficulty with the test.
10. Repeat the procedure with the left eye.
11. Repeat the procedure with both eyes.
12. Document the procedure in the patient's record, including the date and time, visual acuity results, and any reactions by the patient. Also record whether corrective lenses were worn.
    PURPOSE: Procedures that are not recorded are considered not done.

DOCUMENTATION EXERCISE

The medical assistant conducted a Snellen exam on Carlene Anderson, who wears contacts. The results were: right eye 20/60; left eye 20/30, but she missed one letter at the 20/30 line; both eyes 20/40. Carlene did not squint or strain during the exam.

8/01/XX 2:20 PM Visual acuity completed c̄ Snellen chart. OD 20/60, OS 20/30–1, OU 20/40 c̄ corrective lenses. No squinting noted. Kim Tau, CMA (AAMA)

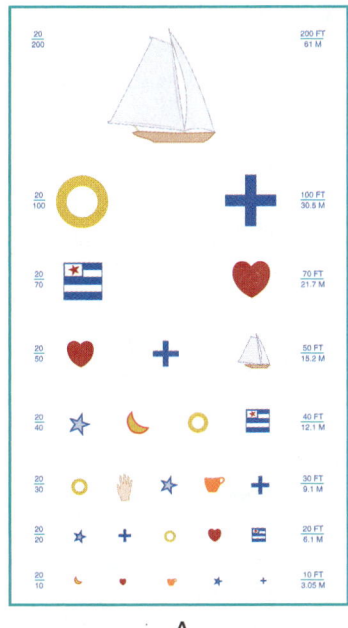

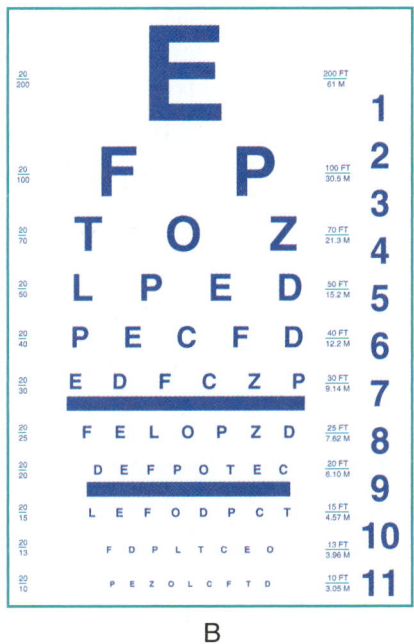

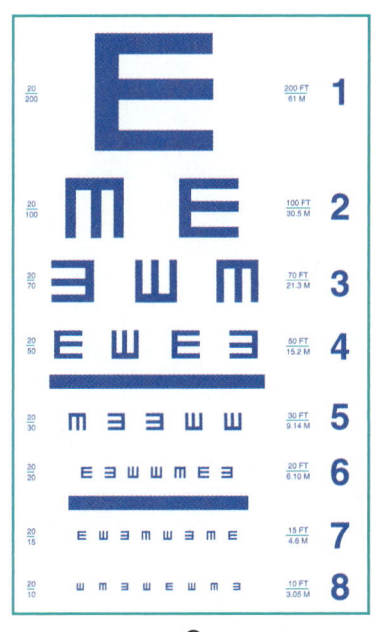

A   B   C

FIGURE 37-7 Different types of Snellen charts.

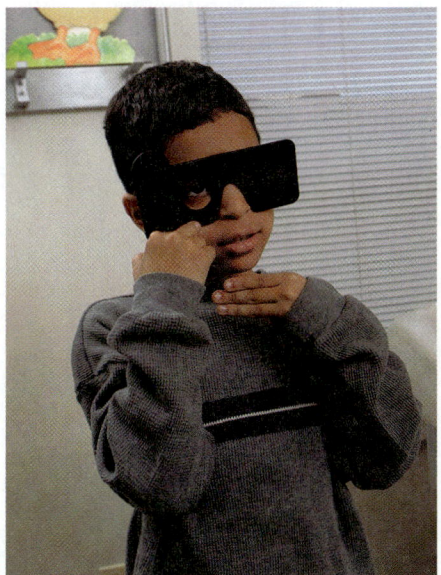

FIGURE 37-8 Visual acuity test with the E chart.

INTERPRETING SNELLEN OUTCOMES

- The patient always stands 20 feet from the chart.
- Each outcome is a record of how well the patient can see compared with normal vision.
- Example: A patient with a 20/40 reading can see that line correctly standing at 20 feet, but an individual with normal vision can see the same line correctly at 40 feet.
- Example: A patient with a 20/15 reading can see that line accurately standing at 20 feet, but a person with normal vision must stand at 15 feet to have the same vision.

CRITICAL THINKING APPLICATION   **37-2**

Susie Anthony, a 19-year-old patient, is seen today for a general eye examination. The physician orders a routine Snellen test, and Kim administers it. Susie wears contacts. With her right eye, she reads without errors to the 20/25 line; however, she squints and makes three errors at the 20/20 line. With her left eye, Susie makes two mistakes at the 20/30 line. How should Kim document this procedure?

Near Visual Acuity

Near visual acuity can be tested with the near vision acuity chart (Figure 37-9). This test frequently is given to patients initially to screen for presbyopia or hyperopia. If the patient wears corrective lenses, they should be worn during the test. The size of the type on the card varies from newspaper headlines to print similar to that found in telephone books. The test should be given in a well-lit room, with the patient holding the card approximately 14 to 16 inches away. As with the Snellen examination, the near visual acuity test is given for each eye, starting with the right eye. The eye not being tested should be covered but left open. The patient should be monitored for indications of difficulty, such as squinting or tearing. The patient reads the card, starting at the top, until reaching the smallest print that can be read. The medical assistant should document the number at which the patient stopped reading for each eye, whether corrective lenses were worn, and any signs of eye strain.

Ishihara Color Vision Test

Defects in color vision are classified as congenital or acquired. Congenital defects are caused by an inherited color vision defect and are found most often in males. Acquired defects are caused by eye injury or disease. The Ishihara test is a simple, convenient, and accurate procedure that detects total color-blindness as well as the red-green

60

Nothing can take the place of "the only pair of eyes you will ever have." That is why you are exercising such good judgment in taking care of them as you are now doing.

50

For this reason, you will welcome the suggestion about lenses which are designed and made to give you "greater comfort and better appearance." In man's earliest days he had little use for glasses. He used his eyes chiefly for long distance.

40

He worked by daylight and at tasks with little detail. But now, you use your eyes for much close work—reading, writing, sewing and many other uses which the eyes of primitive man did not know. Now your eyes meet all sorts of lighting conditions, artificial and natural.

30

Many of these conditions produce "overbrightness" or glare. Sometimes it is the direct or reflected glare of sunlight; often it is direct or reflected from artificial light. And very often this glare is uncomfortable—impairs your efficiency. But special lenses, developed by America's leading optical scientists, combat this glare.

25

These lenses give you more comfortable vision and blend harmoniously with your complexion. These lenses are less conspicuous. We are glad to recommend them because they will give you greater comfort and better appearance. Thousands of satisfied wearers testify to their real benefits.

20

You are wise in taking good care of "the only pair of eyes you will ever have." You know how valuable they are, that you can never have another pair. For this reason, you will welcome the suggestion about lenses which are designed and made to give you "greater comfort and better appearance." In man's earliest days he had little use for glasses.

The above letters subtend the visual angle of 5' at the designated distance in inches.

FIGURE 37-9 Near vision acuity chart.

blindness that is prevalent in congenital blindness (Procedure 37-2). The test assesses the perception of primary colors as well as shades of colors.

The test booklet contains polychromatic plates made up of colored dots in numeric patterns. The numbers are one color, and the background dots are a different color. Patients with average visual acuity can read the numbers within the dot matrix without difficulty. Patients with color vision defects are unable to read the number, or they see a totally different number. A section of plates is included that contains colored line trails through a background of dots. These plates are designed to be used with children and adults who are unable to read numbers. In this situation, the patient uses a finger to follow the dotted trail through the picture.

The test should be administered in a quiet room that is well illuminated by sunlight, not by artificial lighting. If this is not possible, create the best situation possible. If a quiet outside patio area is available, use it or try to set the electrical lights to create an artificial sunlight effect. The test uses 14 color plates. The basic test consists of plates 1 through 11. Plates 12 through 14 are used if the patient appears to be having difficulty with red-green differentiations. The medical assistant records the number of plates read correctly. If the score is 10 or higher, the patient is within the average

range. If the score is 7 or lower, the patient is suspected of having a color deficiency, and the ophthalmologist performs additional assessment tests using more precise color vision testing equipment.

Treatment Procedures

Eye Irrigation

The eye is irrigated to relieve inflammation, remove drainage, dilute chemicals, or wash away foreign bodies. Sterile technique and equipment must be used to prevent contamination (Procedure 37-3). Follow the procedure as prescribed, making sure the patient is comfortable. Record the treatment in the patient's medical record immediately after it has been determined. Remember, if it is not recorded, it has not been done.

Foreign bodies in the eye are very irritating and may cause considerable pain. Most foreign bodies are superficial and can be removed easily. Occasionally, a foreign particle may be deeply embedded, requiring eye surgery. Notify the physician immediately if a patient comes into the office with something in his or her eye.

The first objective of the physician's examination is inspection. The patient is asked to look to either side and up and down so that the anterior surface of the eye can be inspected. For the physician to fully inspect under the upper lid, the patient must cooperate by looking downward while the physician everts the upper lid using a cotton-tipped applicator. While the lid is maintained in an everted position, any foreign materials may be rinsed away with sterile water or saline solution. If the physician's order is for you to remove the foreign body, do so with irrigation only. If this technique is unsuccessful, cover both of the patient's eyes with a gauze dressing and notify your supervisor immediately.

SAFETY ALERT
Never attempt to remove a foreign body from the cornea using an applicator. Scratches to the cornea may result, causing scar formation and impaired vision.

CRITICAL THINKING APPLICATION   37-3
The physician tells Kim to irrigate the left eye of a 22-year-old patient to remove a foreign body. She is to irrigate the eye with sterile normal saline solution until clear. How should Kim document this procedure?

Instillation of Eye Medication

Medication may be instilled into the eye to treat an infection, soothe an eye irritation, anesthetize the eye, or dilate the pupils before examination or treatment (Procedure 37-4). Ophthalmic medications are available in several forms. Liquid drops usually are supplied in small squeeze bottles with tips that allow one drop at a time to be dispensed; or, the bottle may contain a dropper with a small rubber attachment used to dispense the medication by drops. Eye ointments are dispensed in small metal or plastic tubes with an ophthalmic tip that allows them to be dispensed in a small ribbon of ointment directly into the bottom eyelid (see Table 37-2).

PROCEDURE 37-2

Perform Patient Screening Using Established Protocols: Assess Color Acuity Using the Ishihara Test

GOAL: *To assess a patient's color acuity correctly and record the results.*

EQUIPMENT and SUPPLIES

- Room area with natural light
- Ishihara color plate book
- Pen, pencil, and paper
- Watch with a second hand
- Patient's record

PROCEDURAL STEPS

1. Assemble the equipment and prepare the room for testing. The room should be quiet and illuminated with natural light.
   <u>PURPOSE:</u> Natural light is needed to test colors correctly.
2. Greet the patient by name and explain the procedure. Use a practice card during the explanation and make sure the patient understands that he or she has 3 seconds to identify each plate.
   <u>PURPOSE:</u> To make sure you have the right patient. Also, an informed patient is a cooperative patient. The first plate is a practice plate and is designed to be read correctly.
3. Hold up the first plate at a right angle to the patient's line of vision and 30 inches from the patient. Be sure both of the patient's eyes are kept open during the test (Figure 1).

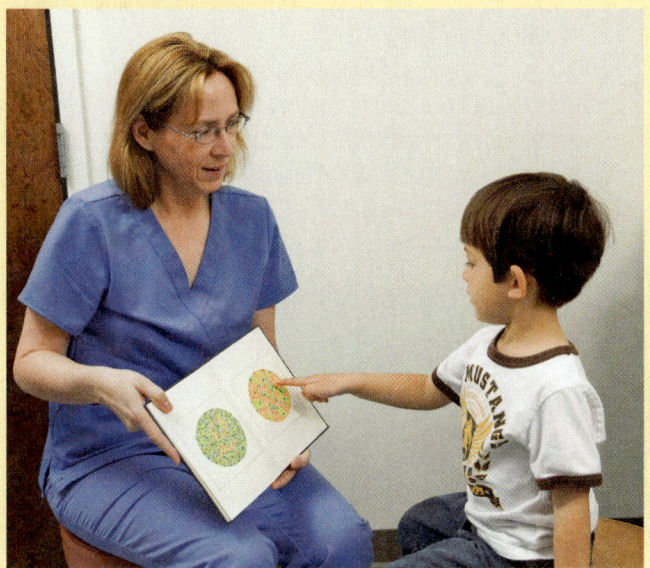

4. Ask the patient to tell you the number on the plate. Record the plate number and the patient's answer (Figure 2).

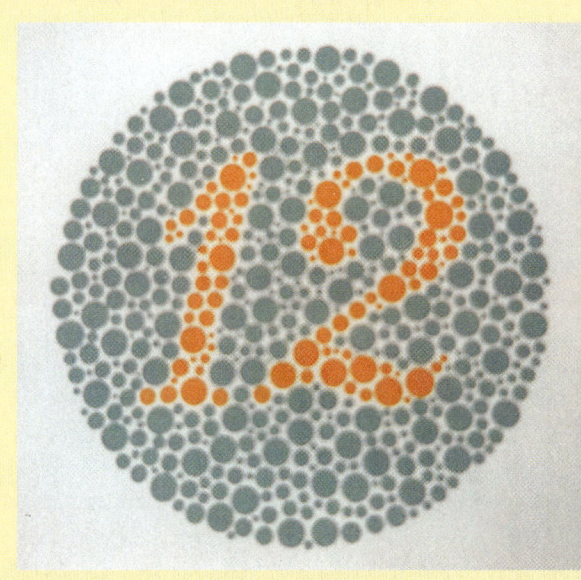

5. Continue this sequence until all 11 plates have been read. If the patient cannot identify the number on the plate, place an X in the record for that plate number. Your record should look like this:
   Plate 1 = pass, Plate 2 = pass, Plate 3 = X, Plate 4 = pass, and so on.
6. Include any unusual symptoms in your record, such as eye rubbing, squinting, or excessive blinking.
7. Place the book back in its cardboard sleeve and return it to its storage space.
   <u>PURPOSE:</u> The Ishihara color plates need to be stored in a closed position away from external light to protect the colors.
8. Record the procedure in the patient's record, including the date and time, the testing results, and any patient symptoms shown during the test.
   <u>PURPOSE:</u> Procedures that are not recorded are considered not done.

SAFETY ALERT

Whatever the medication, the dispenser should never touch the eye while the prescribed amount of medication is administered. This can traumatize the eye and can contaminate the medication applicator.

CRITICAL THINKING APPLICATION 37-4

Amy is ordered to administer Humorsol 0.25%, 1 drop to the left eye, to a 75-year-old patient recently diagnosed with glaucoma. How should Amy document this procedure?

PROCEDURE 37-3

Assist the Physician With Patient Care: Irrigate a Patient's Eyes

GOAL: *To cleanse one or both eyes as ordered by the physician.*

EQUIPMENT and SUPPLIES

- Prescribed sterile irrigation solution
- Sterile irrigating bulb syringe and sterile basin or prepackaged solution with dispenser
- Basin for drainage
- Sterile gauze squares
- Disposable drape
- Towel
- Nonsterile disposable gloves
- Biohazard waste container
- Patient's record

PROCEDURAL STEPS

1. Sanitize your hands.
   PURPOSE: To ensure infection control.
2. Check the physician's orders to determine which eye requires irrigation (or whether both eyes require it) and the type of solution to be used.
   PURPOSE: To check the abbreviations: OD (right eye), OS (left eye), OU (both eyes).
3. Assemble the materials needed.
4. Check the expiration date of the solution; read the label three times.
   PURPOSE: To follow the rules for administering medications.
5. Greet the patient by name and explain the procedure.
   PURPOSE: To make sure you have the right patient. Also, explanations help gain the patient's cooperation and ease apprehension.
6. Assist the patient into a sitting or supine position, making sure that the head is turned toward the side of the affected eye. Place the disposable drape over the patient's neck and shoulder.
   PURPOSE: This position causes the solution to flow away from the unaffected eye, reducing the chance of cross-contamination of the healthy eye.
7. Put on gloves and rinse your gloved hands under warm water to remove all powder from the gloves, or wear powder-free gloves.
   PURPOSE: Gloves help hold the eye open, but powder may irritate the eyes.
8. Place or have the patient hold a drainage basin next to the affected eye to receive the solution from the eye. Place a polylined drape under the basin to prevent the solution from getting on the patient.
9. Moisten a gauze square with solution and cleanse the eyelid and lashes. Start at the inner canthus (near the nose) and move to the outer canthus (farthest from the nose). Dispose of the gauze square in the biohazard container after each wipe (Figure 1).

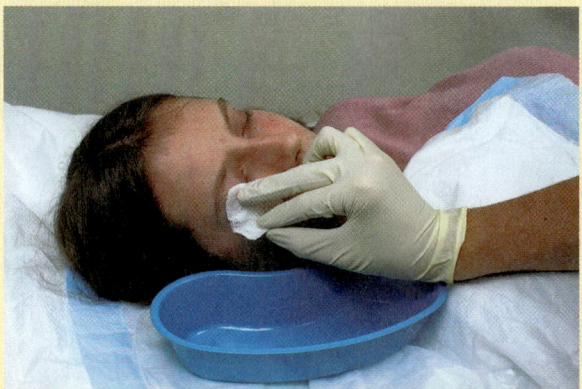

PURPOSE: Debris on the lids or lashes must be cleaned away before the conjunctiva is exposed.

10. If using a bulb syringe, pour the required volume of room temperature irrigating solution into the basin and draw the solution into the bulb syringe. If an irrigating solution in a prepackaged dispenser is used, remove the lid.
    PURPOSE: Cold solution causes the patient pain and discomfort.
11. Separate and hold the eyelids with the index finger and thumb of one hand. With the other hand, place the syringe or dispenser on the bridge of the nose parallel to the eye.
    PURPOSE: To support and steady the dispenser.
12. Squeeze the bulb or dispenser, directing the solution toward the lower conjunctiva of the inner canthus; allow the solution to flow steadily and slowly from the inner to the outer canthus. Do not touch the eye or eyelids with the applicator (Figure 2).
    PURPOSE: To prevent possible injury to the eye.

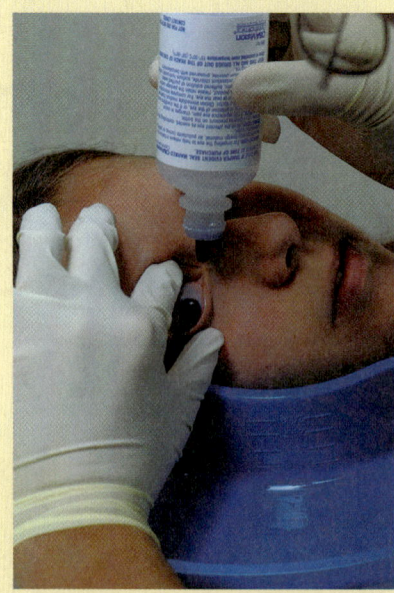

PROCEDURE 37-3—cont'd

13. Refill the syringe or continue to gently squeeze the prepackaged bottle and continue the procedure until the amount of solution ordered by the physician has been administered, or until drainage from the eye is clear.
14. Dry the eyelid with sterile gauze, moving from the inner canthus to the outer canthus. Do not use cotton balls, because fibers might remain in the eye.
15. Dispose of the irrigation results and clean the work area.
16. Remove your gloves and sanitize your hands.
    PURPOSE: To ensure infection control.
17. Document the procedure in the patient's record using appropriate abbreviations; include the date and time, the type and amount of solution used, which eye was irrigated, any significant reactions by the patient, and the results.
    PURPOSE: Procedures that are not recorded are considered not done.

DOCUMENTATION EXERCISE

Toby Kramer is ordered eye irrigations until clear because of sand in both eyes. You use 50 mL of irrigation solution in the right eye and 125 mL in the left eye. After the procedure is complete, the sclera appears red and Toby complains of irritation in both eyes.

8/06/XX 9:00 AM OD irrigated c̄ 50 mL normal saline sol and OS c̄ 125 mL. Postprocedure sclera appears inflamed and pt c/o bilateral irritation. Kim Tau, CMA (AAMA)

PROCEDURE 37-4

Assist the Physician With Patient Care: Instill an Eye Medication

GOAL: *To apply medication to one or both eyes as ordered by the physician.*

EQUIPMENT and SUPPLIES

- Sterile medication with sterile eye dropper or ophthalmic ointment
- Disposable drape
- Sterile gauze squares
- Disposable nonsterile gloves
- Patient's record

PROCEDURAL STEPS

1. Sanitize your hands.
   PURPOSE: To ensure infection control.
2. Check the physician's order to determine which eye requires medication (or whether medication is ordered for both eyes) and the name and strength of the medication to be used.
   PURPOSE: To prevent a medication error.
3. Assemble the equipment and supplies.
4. Read the label of the medication three times.
   PURPOSE: To follow the rules for administering medications.
5. Greet the patient by name and explain the procedure.
   PURPOSE: To make sure you have the right patient. Also, explanations help gain the patient's cooperation and ease apprehension.
6. Put on nonsterile gloves and rinse your gloved hands under warm water to remove all powder from the gloves, or wear powder-free gloves.
   PURPOSE: Gloves help hold the eye open, but powder may irritate the eyes.
7. Assist the patient into a sitting or supine position. Ask the patient to tilt the head backward and look up.

PURPOSE: Looking up helps prevent the applicator's tip from touching the cornea. It also helps keep the patient from blinking as the medication is instilled. For eye drops, draw the medication into the dropper. For an eye ointment, remove the cap.

8. Pull the lower conjunctival sac downward (Figure 1).
   PURPOSE: To create a pocket for the medication.

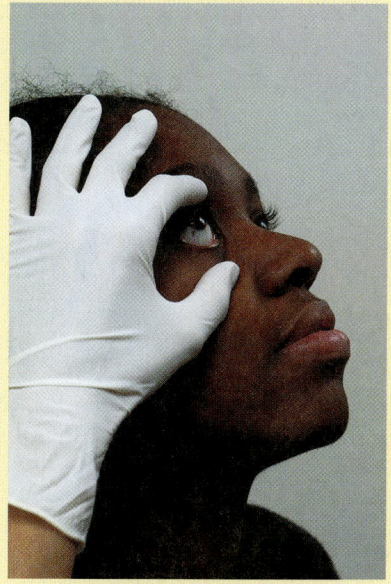

9. Administer the prescribed number of drops or amount of ointment into the eye. For eye drops, place the drops in the center of the lower conjunctival sac, with the tip of the dropper held parallel to the eye and ½ inch above the eye sac. For eye ointment (ung), squeeze a thin ribbon along the lower conjunctival sac from the inner canthus to the outer canthus, making sure not to touch the eye with the applicator.
PURPOSE: Placing the medication in the conjunctival sac rather than on the eyeball prevents injury to the cornea. Touching the eye with the applicator could injure the eye and contaminates the applicator (Figure 2).

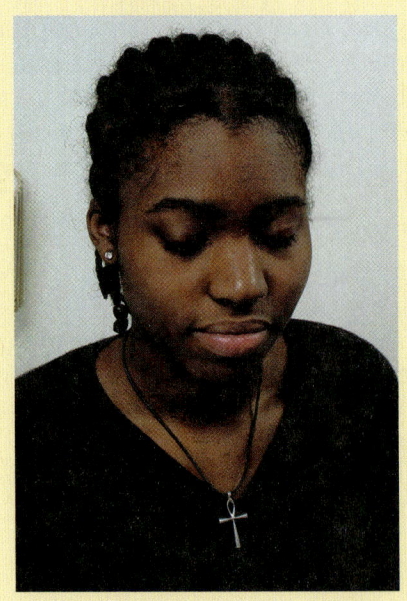

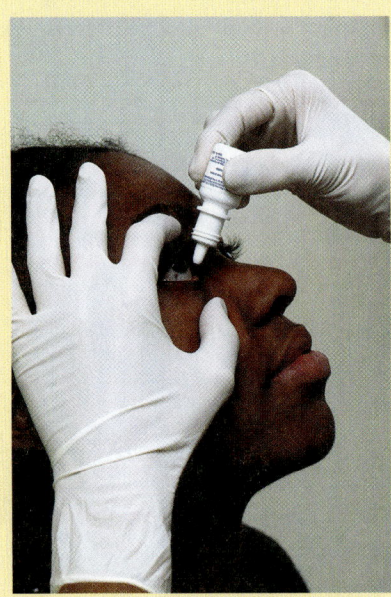

10. Instruct the patient to close the eye gently and rotate the eyeball.
PURPOSE: Gently closing the eye prevents the medication from being dispelled, and rotating the eyeball distributes the medication evenly (Figure 3).

11. Dry any excess drainage from the inner canthus to the outer canthus and explain that the medication may temporarily blur vision.
12. Discard the unused medication and clean the procedure area.
13. Remove your gloves and sanitize your hands.
PURPOSE: To ensure infection control.
14. Record the procedure in the patient's medical record, including date and time, name and strength of the medication, dose administered, eye treated, teaching instructions given (if treatment is to continue at home), and any observations.
PURPOSE: Procedures that are not recorded are considered not done.

8/8/XX 1:45 PM Thin ribbon of Neosporin ophthalmic ung applied in lower conjunctival sac of OS. No pt complaints. Pt instructed on home care application of med, including washing hands before and after procedure and taking care not to touch eye c̄ applicator. Kim Tau, CMA (AAMA)

Aseptic Procedures in Ophthalmology

A major concern in ophthalmologic procedures is the contamination of eye medication applicators. Because of the concern of cross-contamination, use of stock ophthalmic medications is discouraged. The sterility of all eye medications is critical for good patient care. Newly opened sterile solutions should be used for each patient and should be discarded after instillation or given to the patient for home use. All instruments used to remove a foreign body should be sterile.

EXAMINATION OF THE EAR

Otorhinolaryngology is the medical specialty that deals with the ear, nose, and throat. It frequently is referred to as *otolaryngology* or even as a single specialty of otology or laryngology. Usually, the specialty otorhinolaryngology is referred to simply as *ear, nose, and throat* (ENT).

Anatomy and Physiology of the Ear

The ears are only a small part of the actual organ of hearing. Most of this structure lies hidden in the temporal bone. Anatomically, the organ of hearing is divided into three sections: the outer ear, the middle ear, and the inner ear (Figure 37-10).

Outer or External Ear

The outer ear consists of the auricle, or pinna, the fleshy part of the ear that can be seen on the side of the head, and the external auditory canal, the tube that extends from the auricle to the tympanic membrane (eardrum).

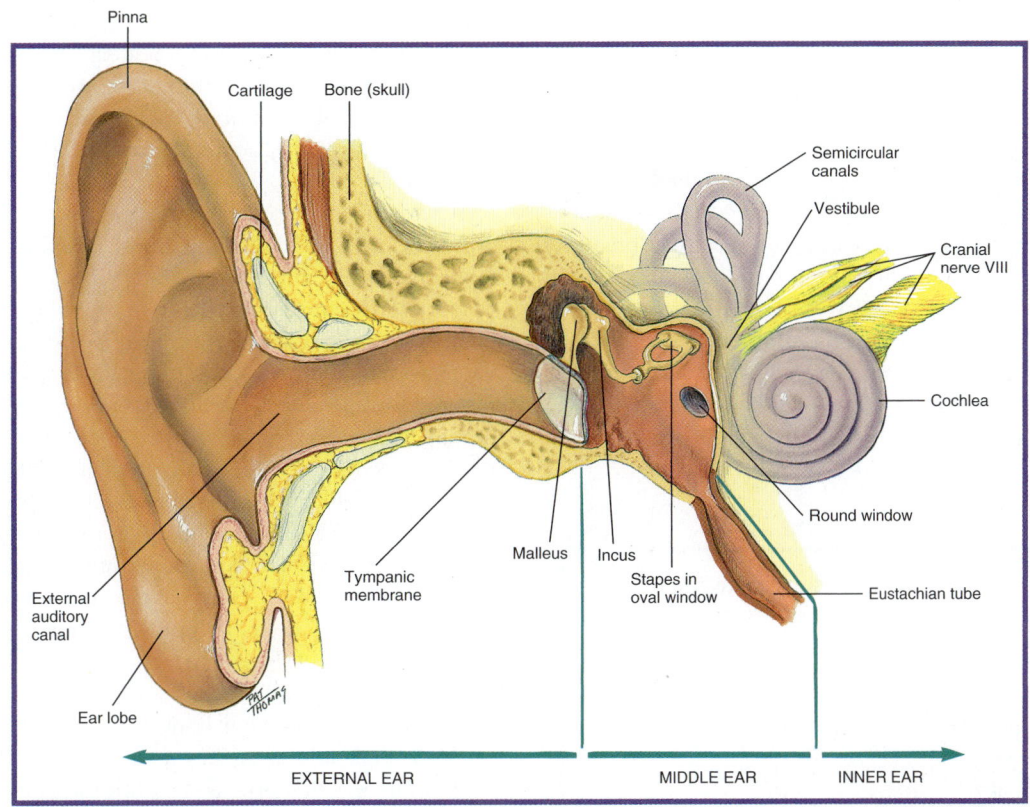

FIGURE 37-10 Anatomy of the ear. (Modified from Jarvis C: *Physical examination and health assessment,* ed 4, Philadelphia, 2004, Saunders.)

The auricle collects sound waves and sends them down the auditory canal. The skin that lines the auditory canal contains numerous hair follicles and many nerve endings, as well as ceruminous glands that secrete cerumen (commonly called *ear wax),* which lubricates the canal. Both the hair and the waxy cerumen help prevent foreign objects from reaching the eardrum. The canal has a slight S shape and is approximately 1 inch (2.5 cm) long.

Middle Ear

The middle ear, sometimes called the *tympanic cavity,* is an air-filled chamber that begins with the tympanic membrane and terminates at the oval window. The middle ear contains the auditory ossicles or bones: malleus, incus, and stapes. These three tiny bones are linked by minute ligaments to form a bridge across the space of the tympanic cavity. The malleus is next to the tympanic membrane, and the stapes is against the oval window. The eustachian tube opens into the middle ear cavity and connects to the nasopharynx. It is designed to equalize pressure in the middle ear with that in the external auditory canal. This equalized pressure makes hearing possible. Throat infection may spread to the middle ear through the eustachian tube; this is a very common occurrence in young children.

The tympanic membrane is a thin, disk-shaped tissue that totally seals off the outer ear from the middle ear. Sound waves conducted through the external auditory canal hit this membrane and cause it to vibrate. These vibrations are picked up by the three ossicles and are changed from air-conducted sound waves to bone-conducted sound waves. The ossicles transmit the bone-conducted sound waves through the middle ear to the oval window, which is the membrane that connects the middle ear and the inner ear. At the oval window, the sound waves move into the fluids of the inner ear. This fluid motion excites the receptors, changing the bone-conducted sound into sensorineural impulses.

Inner Ear

The inner ear, called the *labyrinth,* is divided into the cochlea and the semicircular canals, which are joined by the vestibule. The semicircular canals function to maintain equilibrium, and the cochlea is responsible for the sense of hearing.

The organ of Corti, which contains the receptors for sound, is located within the cochlea. It is made up of hairlike sensory cells surrounded by sensory nerve fibers that form the cochlear branch of the eighth cranial nerve. Sound impulses cause the hairs to bend and rub against the nerve fibers, which initiate stimuli to travel through the cochlear nerve into the brain for sound interpretation.

The eighth cranial nerve transmits auditory impulses to the medulla oblongata. These impulses then travel to the thalamus and on to the auditory cortex of the temporal lobe of the brain, where they are interpreted into audible sound and speech patterns.

The semicircular canals are responsible for evaluating the position of the head in relation to the pull of gravity. The three canals are positioned at right angles to one another, on different planes (Figure 37-11). When the head turns rapidly, these fluid-filled canals must rapidly adjust and send the stimulated change into the central nervous system, which interprets the information and initiates the desired response to maintain balance. With repetitive or excessive stimulation to the equilibrium receptors, some people become nauseated and may vomit. This condition is known as *motion sensitivity* or *motion sickness*.

Disorders of the Ear

Hearing Loss

Two problems result in hearing loss: a conduction problem and a sensorineural impairment. Some individuals have both conditions.

Conductive hearing loss is caused by a problem that originates in the external or middle ear, which prevents sound vibrations from passing through the external auditory canal, limits the vibration of the tympanic membrane, or interferes with the passage of bone-conducted sound in the middle ear. Some common causative factors in conductive hearing loss include impacted cerumen; trauma to the tympanic membrane, especially with scar formation; hemorrhage or fluid in the middle ear; **otosclerosis**; and recurrent chronic ear infections. Patients with conductive hearing loss receive the greatest benefit from a hearing aid. If the hearing loss is caused by a malfunction or congenital abnormality of the ossicles, a surgical procedure can be performed to replace the damaged ossicles with manufactured models.

A sensorineural hearing loss results from an abnormality of the organ of Corti or of the auditory nerve. Viral infection (e.g., rubella, influenza, herpes) can result in hearing loss, as can head trauma or certain **ototoxic** medications. The first sign of ototoxic drug complications usually is tinnitus, a ringing in the ears. This sometimes occurs with high doses of aspirin, certain antibiotics (erythromycin and vancomycin), and chemotherapeutic agents. A sensorineural hearing loss also can occur because of prolonged exposure to loud noise, such as repetitive noise in the workplace, or loud music, which damages the delicate cilia lining the organ of Corti. *Presbycusis,* the hearing loss that affects aging people, is caused by a reduction in the number of receptor cells in the organ of Corti and also is classified as a sensorineural loss. Children can be born with a congenital hearing deficit or deafness because of intrauterine infection or trauma (Figure 37-12).

If the sensorineural hearing loss cannot be improved by hearing aids, an option is surgical implantation of an artificial cochlea. Cochlear implants are complex devices that use electrical impulses to stimulate the auditory nerve, which then carries the current to the brain to be interpreted as sound. These implants do not create normal hearing but provide increased sound for a person with profound or complete hearing loss.

Mixed hearing loss is a combination of conductive and sensory deafness. This type of loss can result from tumors, toxic levels of certain medications, hereditary factors, and stroke.

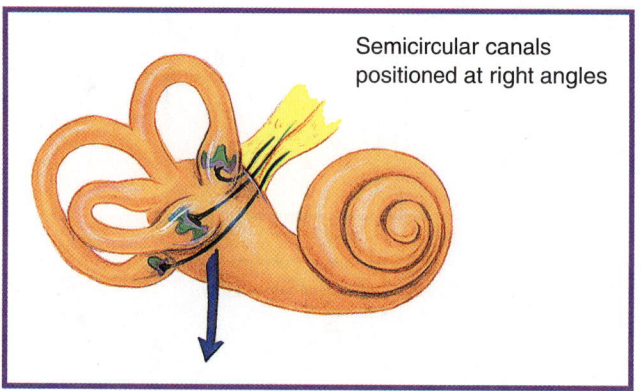

Semicircular canals positioned at right angles

FIGURE 37-11 Semicircular canals. (From Applegate EJ: *The anatomy and physiology learning system,* ed 3, Philadelphia, 2006, Saunders.)

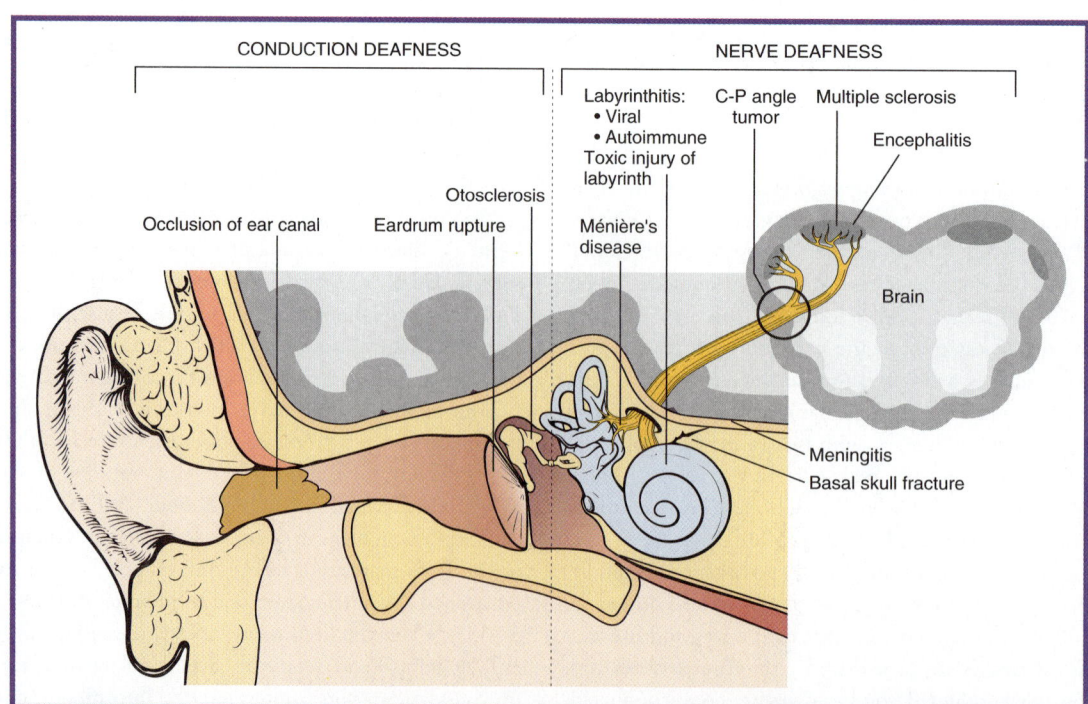

FIGURE 37-12 Causes of deafness. (From Damjanov I: *Pathology for the health-related professions,* ed 3, Philadelphia, 2006, Saunders.)

Otitis

Two common types of otitis are seen in patients in an otology or family practice. The first affects the external ear canal and is called *otitis externa,* or swimmer's ear. Otitis externa may be caused by dermatologic conditions, such as **seborrhea** or **psoriasis**, trauma to the canal, or continuous use of earplugs or earphones. Swimmers frequently have otitis externa because water collects in the ears and mixes with cerumen to form an ideal culture medium for bacteria and fungus. Patients with otitis externa complain of severe pain and have inflammation and swelling of the external auditory canal, hearing loss, and possibly *purulent* (containing pus) or serous drainage. The inflammation is treated with antibiotic or steroid ear drops, and the canal must be kept clean and dry, or the condition can become chronic.

Otitis media is an inflammation of the normally air-filled middle ear that results in a collection of fluid behind the tympanic membrane. Otitis media can be serous or suppurative. Serous otitis media occurs because of a buildup of clear fluid in the middle ear; patients complain of a full feeling and some hearing loss. In suppurative otitis media, purulent fluid is present in the middle ear, and the patient has fever, pain, and hearing loss. Otitis media often is associated with an upper respiratory tract infection caused by a virus or an allergic reaction that results in swelling and inflammation of the sinuses and eustachian tubes. A child's eustachian tube is shorter and narrower than that of an adult. The small size increases the chance that inflammation will block the tube and cause fluid to collect in the middle ear, which not only is uncomfortable but also interferes with the conduction hearing process (Figure 37-13).

RISK FACTORS FOR OTITIS MEDIA

Factors That Cannot Be Controlled
- Gender (male)
- Age (infants and younger children [6 to 18 months])
- Premature birth
- Family history
- Siblings
- Underlying disease (cleft palate, Down syndrome, asthma, allergies)
- Ethnicity (American Indian and Alaskan Inuit because of the shape of the eustachian tubes)
- Cochlear implants

Factors That Can Be Controlled
- Limit exposure to large-group child care settings.
- Do not expose the child to second-hand smoke.
- Hold the child upright during bottle feeding.
- Do not use a pacifier.
- Wash the hands frequently to prevent colds and flu.
- Have the child immunized with pneumococcal conjugate vaccine (Prevnar).

An otoscopic examination reveals that the normally pearly gray tympanic membrane is inflamed and bulging. Areas of fluid or pus may be visible through the membrane. A *tympanogram* may be done to determine the air pressure of the middle ear and the

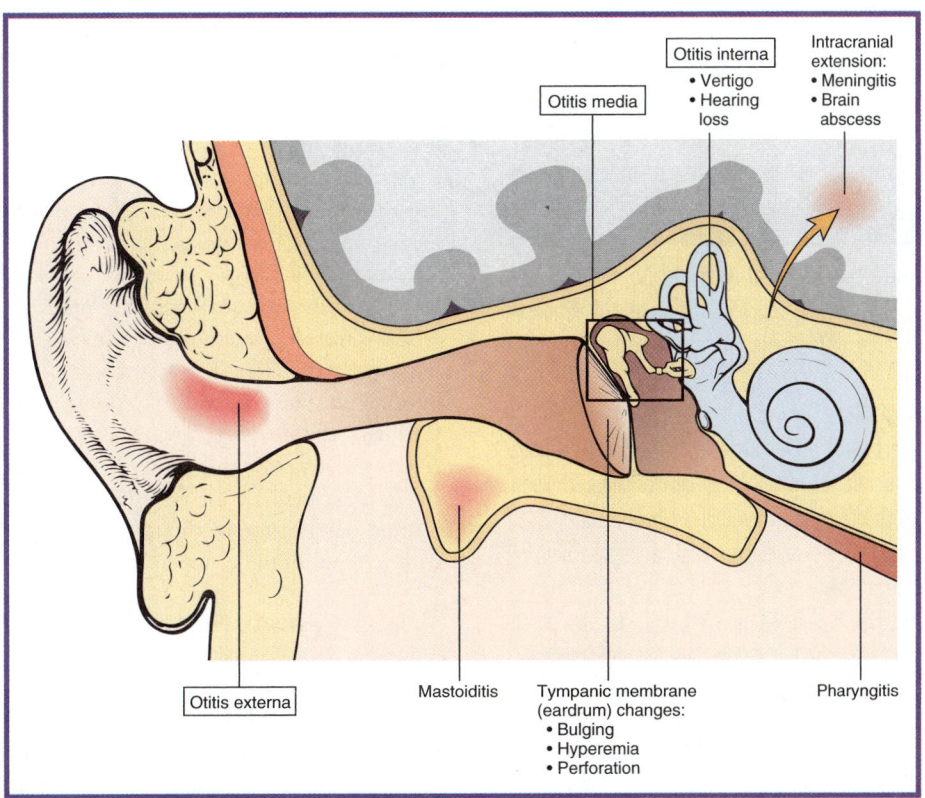

FIGURE 37-13 Inflammation and infection of the ear and surrounding tissues. (From Damjanov I: *Pathology for the health-related professions,* ed 3, Philadelphia, 2006, Saunders.)

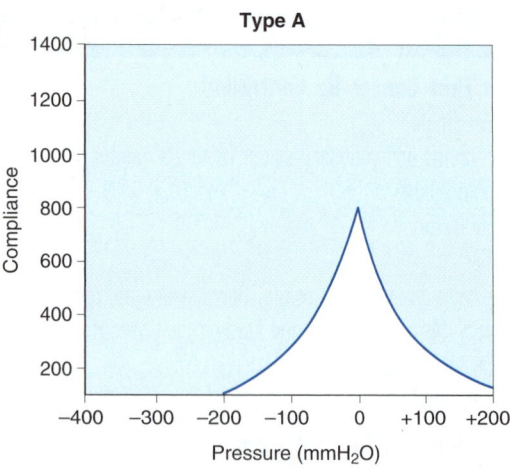

FIGURE 37-14 A normal tympanogram shows a peak at normal pressure (0). An ear with fluid produces a flat tympanogram.

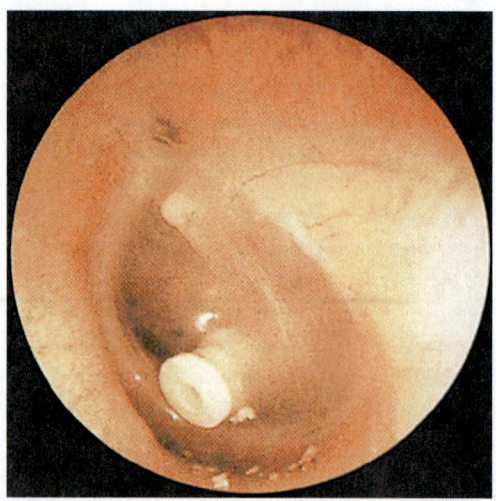

FIGURE 37-15 Tympanic membrane with a tympanostomy tube. (From Frazier MS, Drzymkowski JW: *Essentials of Human Diseases and Conditions*, ed 5, St Louis, 2013, Saunders.)

mobility of the tympanic membrane. During a tympanogram test, a small earphone is placed into the ear canal and the air pressure is gently changed. This test is helpful for showing whether an ear infection or fluid is present in the middle ear (Figure 37-14). If fluid is present in the canal, it can be cultured to determine the causative pathogen. The individual may be given antibiotics, analgesics, and often a decongestant to promote drainage. If this condition becomes chronic, the physician may recommend a *myringotomy*, which is the creation of a surgical incision in the tympanic membrane to drain the fluid, followed by insertion of a tympanostomy tube to continually drain the middle ear of fluid. This may be necessary to prevent permanent hearing loss caused by damage to the ossicles (Figure 37-15).

RECOMMENDATIONS FOR TREATING OTITIS MEDIA

The development of drug-resistant strains of bacteria as a result of over-prescription of antibiotics is a growing concern. Therefore, the American Academy of Pediatrics recommends the following for the treatment of otitis media:

- Delay treatment with antibiotics, giving the child's immune system a chance to fight the infection by itself: this delay should last 24 hours in children 6 to 24 months old and 72 hours for older children. Approximately 61% of children improve within 24 hours regardless of whether they are treated. If the child's condition does not improve, prescribe an appropriate antibiotic.
- The child typically improves within 48 to 72 hours, but the parent should understand how important it is to complete the antibiotic medication as ordered to prevent the infection from recurring.
- The physician may decide to treat otitis media with a short course of antibiotics (i.e., 5 days) but at a higher dose. The drugs of choice include amoxicillin (Amoxil), azithromycin (Zithromax), and cefuroxime (Rocephin).

- Antibiotics will not help if otitis is caused by a virus. The child should be observed for possible complications, and analgesics should be administered for pain control. Viral otitis media typically resolves within 7 to 14 days.

The medical assistant plays a key role in helping parents understand why antibiotic therapy may not be recommended and in educating parents about the importance of administering a prescribed antibiotic at the time ordered using the correct dose and completing the entire prescription.

Impacted Cerumen

Cerumen normally is a soft, yellowish, waxy substance that lubricates the external auditory canal. Excessive secretion of cerumen can gradually cause hearing loss, tinnitus, a feeling of fullness, and *otalgia* (ear pain). Impacted cerumen that has been pushed up tightly against the eardrum is a common cause of conductive hearing loss, because sound vibrations cannot pass through the cerumen to initiate movement of the tympanic membrane. Individuals with psoriasis, abnormally narrow ear canals, or an excessive amount of hair growing in the ear canals are more prone to this condition.

An otoscopic examination quickly reveals this problem. If impacted cerumen is found, it must be removed. This can be done by softening the wax with oily drops, such as carbamide peroxide (Debrox), and then irrigating the ear with warm water until the plug is removed. Because this condition can recur, the patient may need to schedule periodic examinations. If the patient is experiencing hearing loss because of the impaction, it is immediately remedied with removal of the cerumen.

Ménière's Disease

The semicircular canals of the inner ear, in coordination with the eighth cranial nerve, control balance and give a sense of how the body is positioned. The canals contain fluid (the endolymph), the filtration and excretion of which are controlled by the part of the canal called the *endolymphatic sac*. Ménière's disease causes swelling and edema in this part of the semicircular canals, along with an overproduction or collection of excess endolymph. When this occurs, the patient shows signs. Although the cause of this problem is unknown, Ménière's disease is a chronic, progressive condition that triggers episodes of recurring attacks of vertigo, tinnitus, a sensation of pressure in the affected ear, and advancing hearing loss. During an acute attack, patients experience nausea, vomiting, and problems with balance. These attacks can last a few hours to several days, and they increase in severity over time.

During active periods of the disease, the patient is treated symptomatically with medications for nausea and vomiting. A salt-restricted diet, diuretics, and antihistamines may be prescribed to control edema in the labyrinth. Surgical destruction of the affected labyrinth is an option. Although this relieves symptoms, it may also result in permanent deafness if the cochlea is damaged.

USEFUL QUESTIONS FOR GATHERING A HISTORY OF EAR PROBLEMS

- Are you experiencing nausea, vomiting, dizziness, ear pain, fever, headache, upper respiratory infection, ringing of the ears, drainage, loss of balance, or hearing loss?
- What are the onset, duration, and frequency of symptoms?
- Have you taken any medication for the symptoms? What? Has it been helpful?
- Do you have the problem in both ears?
- Are you experiencing pain? On a scale of 1 to 10, with 10 being the worst pain, how would you rate the pain? Is it localized or radiating, in one ear or both?
- Has anything you have tried relieved the symptoms?

Diagnostic Procedures

An ear examination involves viewing the external auditory canal with an otoscope covered by an ear speculum (Figure 37-16). Disposable plastic speculum covers should be used each time to prevent disease transmission. A normal otoscopic examination reveals an external auditory canal with a small amount of cerumen and a pearly gray and concave tympanic membrane. In addition to performing the otoscopic examination, the physician palpates the area around the pinna for abnormalities or sensations. A number of tests are used to

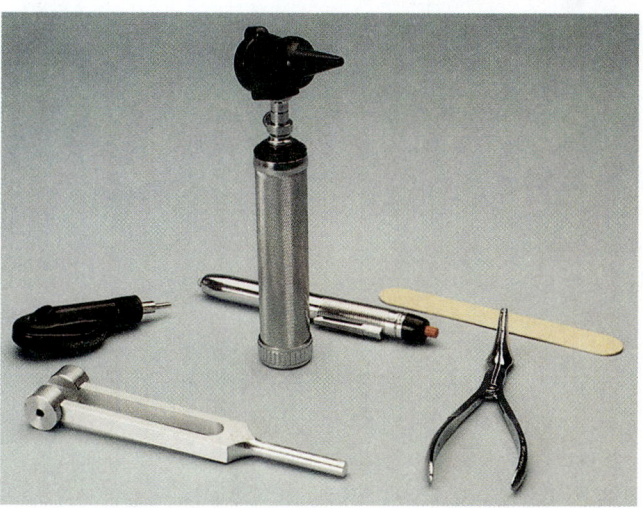

FIGURE 37-16 Instruments used in an otoscopic examination.

assess hearing acuity, ranging from simple tuning fork tests to quantitative and qualitative audiometric testing. If a hearing loss is suspected, the next test usually is performed with a tuning fork.

Tuning Fork Testing

As is mentioned in Chapter 32, tuning fork tests measure hearing by air conduction and bone conduction. Remember that in bone conduction, the sound vibrates through the cranial bones to the inner ear. Tuning forks are available in different sizes, each with a different frequency. The most commonly used tuning fork is the 512 Hz (**hertz**), which means that it vibrates 512 cycles per second—the level of normal speech patterns. To activate the fork, the physician holds it by the stem and strikes the tines softly on the palm of the hand. Striking the tines too forcefully creates a tone that is too loud for diagnostic use. The two tests used to evaluate hearing are the Weber and Rinne tests. Both of these procedures are commonly used to evaluate conductive and sensory losses.

The Weber test is used if the patient reports that hearing is better in one ear than in the other. The vibrating fork is placed in the center of the top of the head, and the patient is asked in which ear the tone is louder, or if the tone is the same in both ears. Because the patient is hearing the tone by bone conduction through the head, a normal result is hearing the sound equally in both ears.

The Rinne test is designed to compare air conduction sound with bone conduction sound. In this test, the stem of the vibrating fork is placed on the patient's mastoid process, and the patient is instructed to raise a hand when the sound disappears. The fork is quickly inverted so that the vibrating tines are approximately 1 inch in front of the external ear canal. If hearing is normal, the patient should still hear a sound. In normal hearing, the sound is heard twice as long by air conduction as by bone conduction.

Audiometric Testing

An audiometric test may be done in an otology or family practice and is performed by medical assistants who have received additional training. Audiometry measures the lowest intensity of sound an individual can hear (Figure 37-17, *A*). The patient, frequently a child, is assisted in placing headphones over the ears (Figure 37-17, *B*). Each ear is tested by delivering a single frequency at a specific intensity, starting with low-frequency tones and going up to very high frequencies. The patient is asked to signal when he or she hears the sound. The results are printed on a graph, called an *audiogram,* or the medical assistant charts the results on a graph sheet (Procedure 37-5). An adult with normal hearing can hear tone frequencies below 25 decibels, and children with normal hearing can hear those below 15 decibels.

If initial screening indicates a hearing deficit, the physician may recommend an appointment with an **audiologist** for audiometric evaluation. The evaluation consists of a battery of tests that assesses the level of hearing impairment and provides valuable information as to how the patient may be helped. The first test evaluates speech comprehension and assesses the patient's ability to follow verbal instructions. Once this evaluation is complete, the patient is placed in a soundproof booth with earphones over the ears. From this point on, the audiologist speaks to the patient and conducts all testing through the earphones. The assessment includes testing the frequency, intensity, and audibility of sound. This process takes approximately 1 hour.

Aseptic Procedures in Otology

Routine examination instruments should be disinfected or sterilized after each use according to office policy and stored in a clean area. Surgical asepsis must be practiced when dressings are changed and minor surgery is performed. Medications, such as ear drops and nose drops, must be handled carefully to prevent contamination.

Treatment Procedures

Ear Irrigation

Irrigation of the ear is done to remove excessive or impacted cerumen, to remove a foreign body, or to treat the inflamed ear with an antiseptic solution (Procedure 37-6). When an ear irrigation is ordered by the physician, the medical assistant may perform the procedure if he or she has had the proper training and is competent in the technique. To prevent discomfort for the patient, it is important to administer the irrigating solution with the applicator tilted up, toward the top of the external canal, so that the solution is not directed at the tympanic membrane. Some discomforts the patient may experience during ear irrigation include vertigo, ear discomfort, coughing, or a tickle in the back of the throat. Perform the procedure as prescribed, making sure the patient is comfortable. Always chart the treatment and its results immediately after completion.

> ### CRITICAL THINKING APPLICATION   37-5
>
> Kim is instructed to perform bilateral ear irrigation on a 68-year-old patient with impacted cerumen. Before the procedure, she uses an otoscope to check the auditory canal and sees a large amount of dark brown cerumen in the right ear, completely covering the tympanic membrane. The left ear has a moderate amount of golden brown cerumen covering the bottom half of the tympanic membrane. After the procedure, both membranes are visible, and the patient tolerated the procedure without complaints. How should Kim document the procedure?

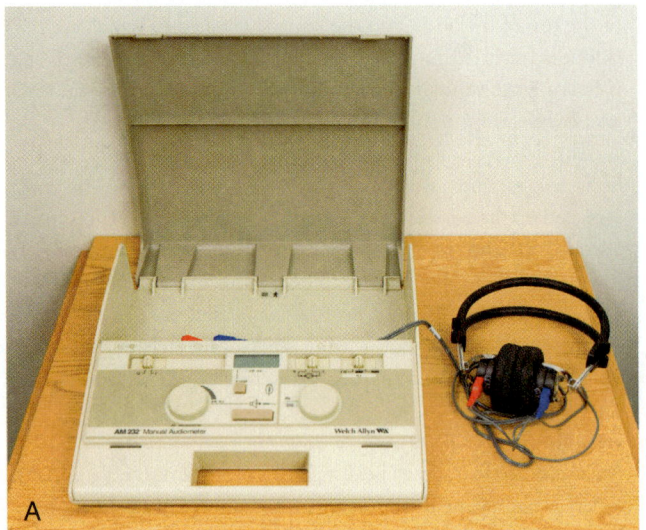 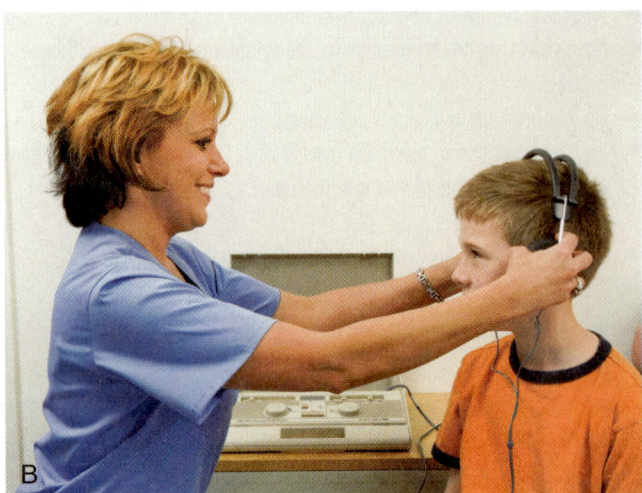

FIGURE 37-17 A, An audiometer. **B,** Placing the headphones.

PROCEDURE 37-5

Perform Patient Screening Using Established Protocols: Measure Hearing Acuity With an Audiometer

GOAL: *To perform audiometric testing of hearing acuity.*

EQUIPMENT and SUPPLIES

- Audiometer with adjustable headphones and graph paper
- Quiet area
- Patient's record

PROCEDURAL STEPS

1. Sanitize your hands, assemble the equipment, and bring the patient into a quiet area (see Figure 37-17, *A*).
   <u>PURPOSE:</u> The testing room should be free of distractions and noise so the patient can concentrate completely on the hearing evaluation.
2. Explain that the audiometer measures whether the patient can hear various sound wave frequencies through the headphones. Each ear is tested separately. When the patient hears a frequency, he or she should raise a hand to signal the medical assistant.
   <u>PURPOSE:</u> Patient education is needed for compliance with the examination.
3. Place the headphones over the patient's ears, making sure they are adjusted for comfort (see Figure 37-17, *B*).
4. The audiometer tests each ear separately, starting at a low frequency. If the results are not automatically recorded by the machine, the medical assistant documents the patient's response to the frequencies on a graph or audiogram. Results for the left ear are marked with an X, and those for the right ear are marked with an O (Figure 1). The medical assistant must have specialized training to conduct this test.

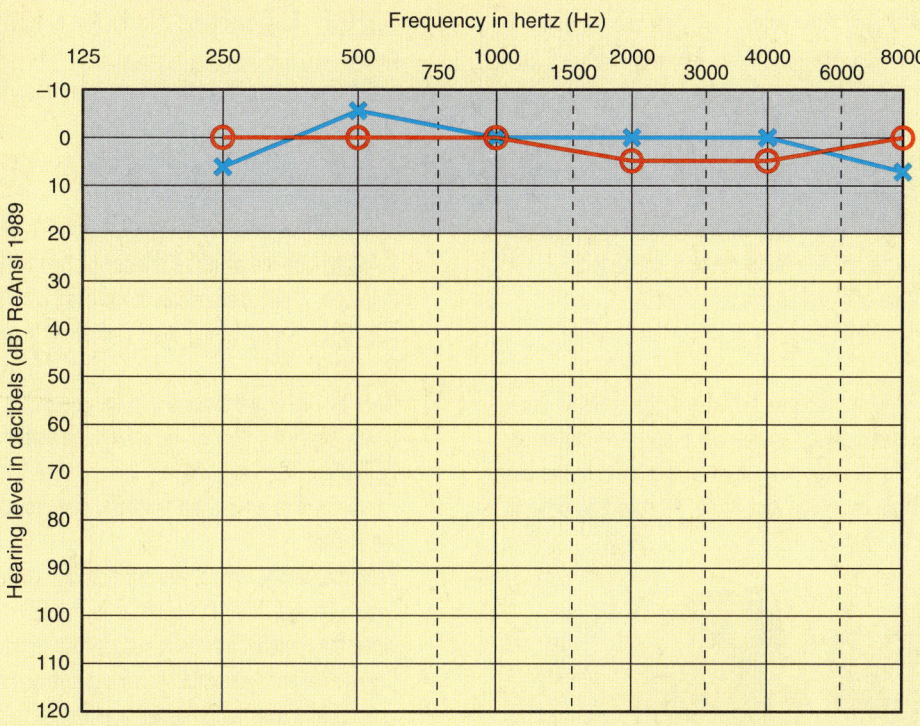

5. Frequencies are increased gradually to test the patient's ability to hear. Each response by the patient is documented.
6. After one ear has been tested, the other ear is then tested, and the results are documented using the appropriate abbreviations: AU (both ears), AD (right ear), AS (left ear).
7. The results are given to the physician for interpretation.
8. The equipment is disinfected according to the manufacturer's guidelines.
9. Sanitize your hands.

PROCEDURE 37-6

Assist the Physician With Patient Care: Irrigate a Patient's Ear

GOAL: *To remove excessive or impacted cerumen from one or both of the patient's ears.*

EQUIPMENT and SUPPLIES

- Irrigating solution
- Basin for irrigating solution
- Bulb syringe or an approved otic irrigation device
- Gauze squares
- Otoscope
- Drainage basin
- Disposable drape with polylined barrier
- Cotton-tipped applicators
- Disposable gloves
- Patient's record

PROCEDURAL STEPS

1. Sanitize your hands.
   PURPOSE: To ensure infection control.

2. Check the physician's order and assemble the materials needed (Figure 1).

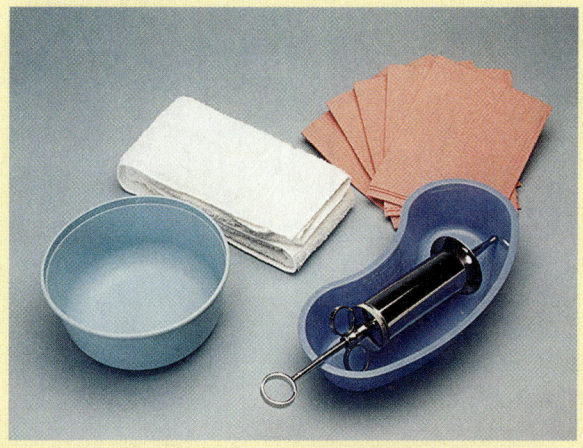

3. Check the label of the solution three times: (1) when you remove it from the shelf; (2) when you pour it; and (3) when you return it to the shelf.
   PURPOSE: To prevent a medication error.
4. Prepare the solution as ordered. The solution should be kept at body temperature to help loosen the cerumen.
   PURPOSE: Solutions at 100° F are most comfortable for the patient. Ask the patient whether the solution temperature is comfortable.
5. Greet the patient by name and explain the procedure.
6. Inspect the affected ear with an otoscope to locate the cerumen impaction.
7. Place the patient in a sitting position with the head tilted toward the affected ear. Place a water-absorbent towel over a polylined barrier on the patient's shoulder, and the collecting basin on the towel at the base of the ear. The patient can assist you by holding the collecting basin in place (Figure 2).

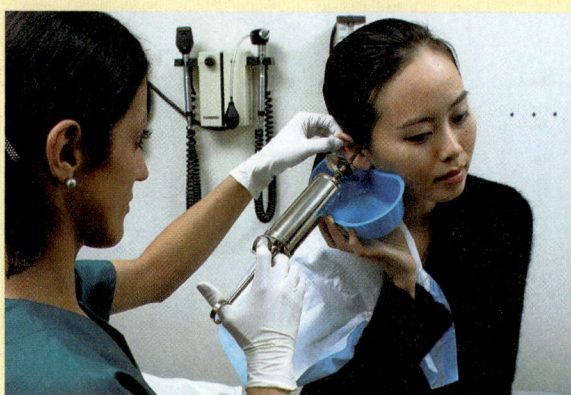

PURPOSE: To minimize the risk of getting the patient's clothing wet and to direct the flow of water into the collecting basin.

8. Put on gloves and wipe any particles from the outside of the ear with gauze squares.

PURPOSE: To prevent the introduction of foreign material into the ear canal.

9. Test to make sure the solution is warm; then fill the syringe and expel air.
   PURPOSE: Trapped air in the syringe increases the pressure of the irrigation, causing discomfort.
10. Straighten the external ear canal. For adults and children older than age 3, gently pull the pinna of the ear up and back; for children younger than age 3, pull the earlobe down and back (Figure 3).
    PURPOSE: Straightening the canal allows the irrigating fluid to circulate through it.
11. Place the tip of the syringe into the meatus of the ear.
12. Gently direct the flow of the solution toward the roof of the canal.
    PURPOSE: This helps prevent injury to the tympanic membrane, aids in the removal of embedded material, and provides the most comfort for the patient.
13. Refill the syringe with warm solution and continue until the material has been removed. Note the particles in the collecting basin to be evaluated when the material has been successfully removed.
14. Dry the patient's external ear with gauze squares and the visible ear canal gently with cotton-tipped applicators.
    PURPOSE: Inserting the applicator into the canal may cause serious trauma.
15. Inspect the ear with an otoscope to determine the results (Figure 4).

16. Place a clean, absorbent towel on the examination table and allow the patient to rest quietly with the head turned to the irrigated side while you wait for the physician to return to check the affected ear.
17. Clean the work area and return all equipment after it has been properly disinfected. Sanitize your hands.
    PURPOSE: To ensure infection control.
18. Document the procedure in the patient's record, including the date and time; the ear irrigated, using the appropriate abbreviations: AU (both

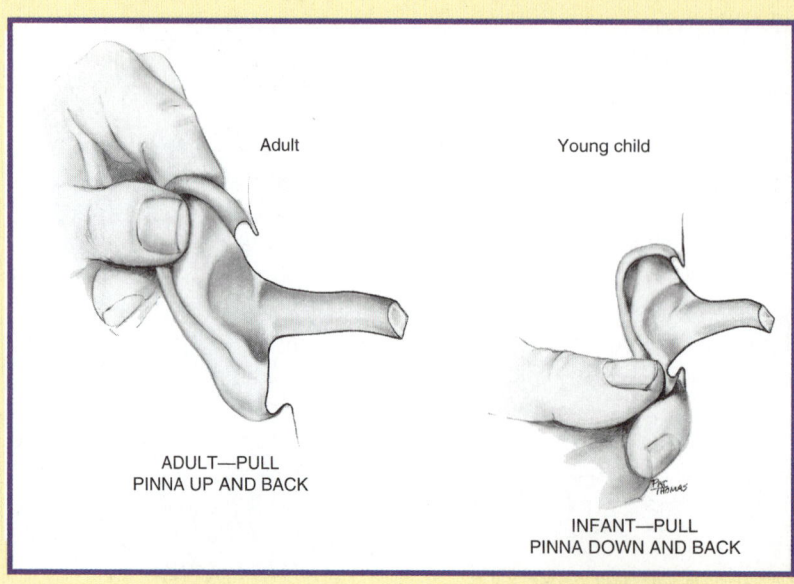

Adult

Young child

ADULT—PULL
PINNA UP AND BACK

INFANT—PULL
PINNA DOWN AND BACK

PROCEDURE 37-6—cont'd

ears), AD (right ear), AS (left ear); the type and amount of irrigating solution used; the characteristics of the material returned from the irrigation; the visibility of the tympanic membrane after irrigation; and any reactions by the patient.

<u>PURPOSE:</u> Procedures that are not recorded are considered not done.

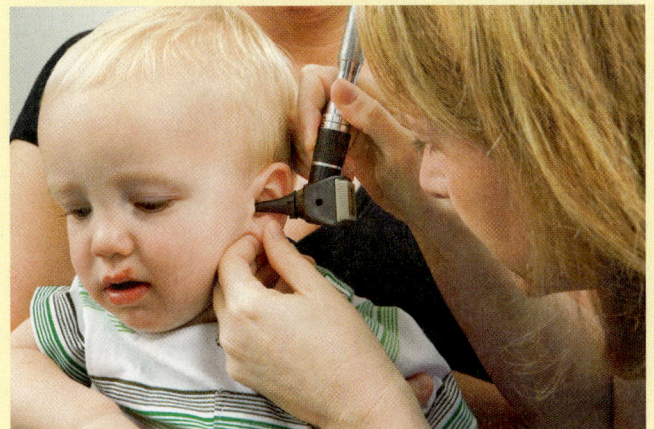

DOCUMENTATION EXERCISE

You are ordered to perform an irrigation of both ears on Mrs. Ophelia Black because of impacted cerumen. Otoscopic examination before the irrigation revealed a large amount of dark brown ear wax in both ears. After irrigation, both tympanic membranes were visible, and Mrs. Black had no complaints of discomfort.

8/12/XX 10:15 AM AD and AS irrigated c̄ 500 mL saline sol bilaterally. Lrg amt dark brown cerumen expelled; post irrigation both TMs visible and pearly gray. No c/o discomfort. Kim Tau, CMA (AAMA)

Instilling Otic Medications

Medication ordered for ear instillation is given to soften impacted cerumen, to relieve pain, or as an antibiotic drop for an infectious pathogen (Procedure 37-7). Patients with ear conditions may be in considerable pain and may have difficulty hearing, which makes health teaching a challenge. Wait until after the procedure has been completed and the patient is more comfortable to reinforce health behaviors.

EXAMINATION OF THE NOSE AND THROAT

If you are working in an ENT specialty office, you also will assist in the examination of the nasal cavity and the throat. The nasal cavity is examined to inspect the mucous membrane of the nostrils. The common cold and allergies are the main causes of changes in the mucosa. The physician may use a nasal speculum to visualize the nostrils and examines the nasal sinuses by palpation and transillumination.

The throat is the area that includes the larynx and pharynx; it can be viewed with the aid of a mirror and either a tongue depressor or a gauze square for grasping the tongue. In the nasopharynx, the physician looks for enlarged adenoids (pharyngeal tonsils) and for the orifices of the eustachian tubes. The physician may spray the patient's throat with a topical anesthetic before the examination to prevent the gag reflex.

Throat specimens frequently are collected in the physician's office to assist in the diagnosis of strep throat infections. Strep throat is caused by the group A beta-hemolytic streptococcal bacteria; if left untreated, it can cause serious complications. Throat cultures are collected by gently swabbing the back of the throat and the surfaces of the tonsils with a sterile swab. The mouth and tongue should be avoided to prevent contamination of the swab with the normal flora of the mouth (Procedure 37-8).

CLOSING COMMENTS

Patient Education

Patients with vision or hearing impairment face serious challenges. For these patients, the medical assistant must use good listening skills, appropriate nonverbal methods, and touch to communicate empathy and understanding. Teaching may have to be adapted to meet the special needs of these patients. A person with a vision loss benefits from large-print forms and handouts, increased levels of lighting, and verbal rather than written instructions to reinforce learning. For an individual with a hearing deficit, printed instructions, demonstrations of how to manage treatments, or even sign language interpretation should be available to ensure accurate communication. Including family members in the patient's treatment plan and offering referrals to appropriate community or professional resources may be very beneficial to a patient with sensory loss. Each patient must be assessed individually to determine the type of adaptation that he or she needs.

An important part of patient education for those receiving eye medications at home is stressing the need to maintain the sterility of the medication. Patients and/or family members must be taught how to apply the medication while preventing trauma to the eye and contamination of the applicator. Patients receiving ear treatments also must understand how to instill the medication.

PROCEDURE 37-7

Assist the Physician With Patient Care: Instill Medicated Ear Drops

GOAL: *To instill the correct medication in the accurate dose directly into the external auditory canal.*

EQUIPMENT and SUPPLIES

- Prescribed otic drops in dispenser bottle
- Cotton balls
- Disposable gloves
- Patient's record

PROCEDURAL STEPS

1. Sanitize your hands and gather the equipment and supplies.
   <u>PURPOSE:</u> To control infection and to reduce procedure time.
2. Check the medication label three times: (1) when you remove it from the shelf; (2) when you prepare it; and (3) when you return it to the shelf.
   <u>PURPOSE:</u> To prevent a medication error.
3. Greet the patient by name and explain the procedure.
4. Have the patient sit up and tilt head away from the affected ear or lie down on the side with the affected ear upward.
   <u>PURPOSE:</u> To expose the ear for treatment, allow gravity to help the medication flow into the canal, and ensure the patient's comfort.
5. Check the temperature of the medication bottle. If it feels cold, gently roll the bottle back and forth between your hands to warm the drops.
   <u>PURPOSE:</u> Cold medication may increase the pain level or cause symptoms of nausea and vertigo.
6. Hold the dropper firmly in your dominant hand. With the other hand, gently pull the pinna up and back if the patient is older than age 3 or the earlobe down and back if the patient is younger than age 3.
   <u>PURPOSE:</u> To straighten the ear canal and make it easier for the medication to reach the target tissue.
7. Place the tip of the dropper in the ear canal meatus and instill the medication drops along the side of the canal (Figure 1).

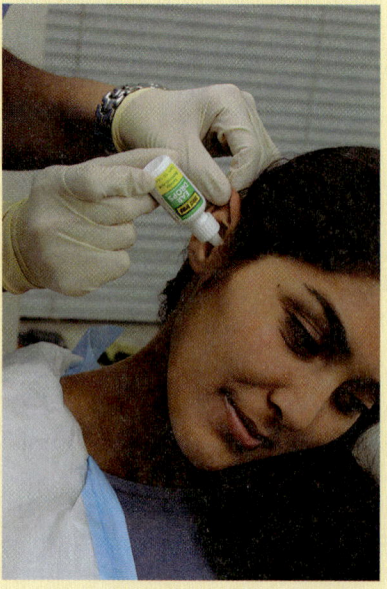

8. Instruct the patient to rest on the side opposite the affected ear and to remain in this position for approximately 3 minutes.
   <u>PURPOSE:</u> To help the medication reach the base of the canal and prevent it from immediately running out of the ear (Figure 2).

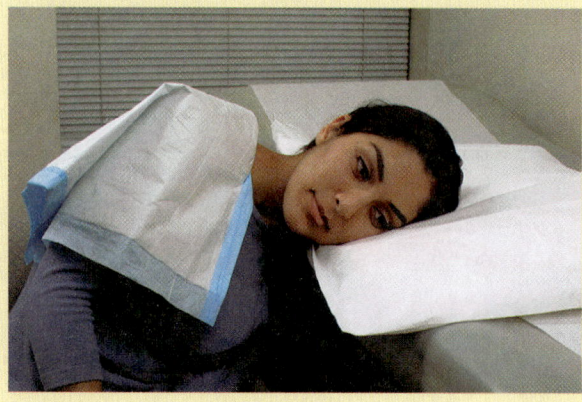

9. If instructed by the physician, place a moistened cotton ball into the ear canal.
   <u>PURPOSE:</u> To protect the ear canal and prevent medication from leaking out of the ear.
10. Clean the work area and sanitize your hands.
    <u>PURPOSE:</u> To ensure infection control.
11. Record the procedure in the patient's record using the appropriate abbreviations; include the date and time; name, dose, and strength of the medication; the ear treated; and any reactions by the patient.
    <u>PURPOSE:</u> Procedures that are not recorded are considered not done.

8/12/XX 3:22 PM ii gtts Auralgan otic sol administered to AD. No c/o discomfort. Pt instructed on home use. Kim Tau, CMA (AAMA)

Perform Patient Screening Using Established Protocols: Collect a Specimen for a Throat Culture

GOAL: To collect a throat culture using sterile technique for immediate testing or for transportation to the laboratory.

EQUIPMENT and SUPPLIES

- Nonsterile gloves
- Face protection barrier (if the patient is coughing or if there is danger of splattering body fluids)
- Sterile swab
- Sterile tongue depressor
- Transport medium
- Biohazard waste container
- Laboratory requisition if sample is being sent out for examination
- Patient's record

PROCEDURAL STEPS

1. Sanitize your hands.
   PURPOSE: To ensure infection control.
2. Gather the materials needed.
3. Put on gloves and face protection if needed.
   PURPOSE: To follow Standard Precautions.
4. Position the patient so that the light shines into the mouth.
   PURPOSE: To illuminate the area to be swabbed.
5. Remove the sterile swab from the sterile wrap with your dominant hand and grasp the sterile tongue depressor with your nondominant hand.
   PURPOSE: To achieve better control of the swabbing process.
6. Instruct the patient to open the mouth and say "Ah." Depress the tongue with the depressor.
   PURPOSE: Saying "Ah" helps elevate the uvula and reduces the tendency to gag. The tongue is depressed so that you can see the back of the throat and prevent contamination of the sterile swab.
7. Swab the back of the throat between the tonsillar pillars, especially any reddened, patchy areas of the throat, white pus pockets, purulent areas, and the tonsils; take care not to touch any other areas in the mouth (Figure 1).

PURPOSE: Pathogenic organisms are found in the back of the throat and on the tonsils.

8. Place the swab in the transport medium, label it, and send it to the laboratory (Figure 2). If direct slide testing is requested, return the labeled swab to the laboratory. (The rapid strep test procedure is described in Chapter 55.)

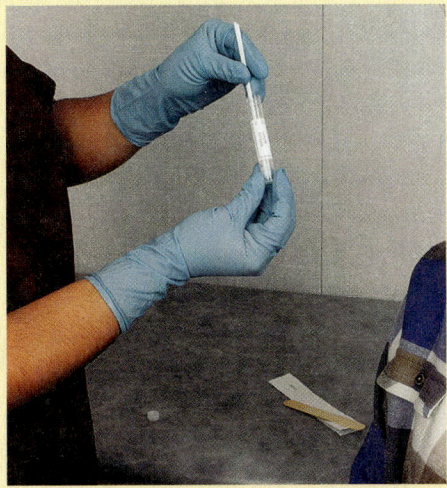

PURPOSE: Transport medium prevents the swab from drying. Labeling immediately after collection prevents specimens from becoming mixed up.

9. Dispose of contaminated supplies in the biohazard waste container.
   PURPOSE: To prevent the spread of infection.
10. Disinfect the work area.
11. Remove your gloves and discard them in a biohazard waste container.
12. Sanitize your hands.
    PURPOSE: To ensure infection control.
13. Record the procedure in the patient's record.
    PURPOSE: Procedures that are not recorded are considered not done.

Uvula

Palatine tonsil

Swab
held together

Tongue blade

8/14/XX 8:35 AM Throat specimen collected via swab from tonsillar area. Sent to University Laboratories for strep testing. Kim Tau, CMA (AAMA)

Legal and Ethical Issues

Diminished sight or hearing may render a patient seriously impaired. To prevent accidents and office injuries, always ask a sight- or hearing-impaired patient whether he or she requires assistance. When you escort the patient to an examination room, offer your arm and tell the patient the approximate distance you will be walking. If the patient is to have an examination that involves local anesthesia or eye drops that dilate the pupil, be sure the patient has recovered and someone is available to take the patient home before allowing him or her to leave the office. Never assume that the patient is capable of leaving alone. If the patient insists on leaving before the designated recovery time, inform the physician and record the time and circumstances surrounding the event in the patient's medical record. This information should be signed and witnessed. The physician may want a refusal of care form signed by the patient and placed in the medical record.

HIPAA Applications

Regardless of the patient's disability, the ambulatory care center must follow the guidelines for Notice of Privacy Practices (NPP) established by the Health Insurance Portability and Accountability Act (HIPAA). The NPP is a form developed by the facility that outlines the patient's rights and the facility's legal responsibilities to safeguard the patient's protected health information. The facility must give the NPP to each new patient at the first office visit. To comply with HIPAA guidelines, the document must be in a language the patient easily understands. The staff is responsible for obtaining the patient's signature on the form, which indicates the patient's agreement with the stipulations of the facility's privacy practice. An individual with a vision deficit may require a large-print form, or a staff member may need to read the document to the person and answer any questions. The staff must make sure that patients with hearing deficits understand the form before signing.

Americans With Disabilities Applications

The Americans With Disabilities Act (ADA) was first passed in 1990, and amendments were made in 2009. The ADA prohibits discrimination based on disability. An individual with a disability is defined by the ADA as a person who has a physical or mental impairment that substantially limits one or more major life activities, a person who has a history or record of such an impairment, or a person who is perceived by others as having such an impairment. The ADA does not specifically name all of the impairments that are covered under the law. Public facilities—including physicians' offices and other healthcare buildings—must comply with ADA requirements for physical accommodations. If appropriate, assistive devices must be provided for individuals with vision or hearing impairment. Refer to the ADA home page at http://www.ada.gov/ for additional details.

CRITICAL THINKING APPLICATION   37-6

Mr. Samuel Langton is a 77-year-old patient with profound hearing loss and severe glaucoma. How would you suggest that Amy communicate therapeutically with this patient? Role-play this interaction with one of your classmates.

SUMMARY OF SCENARIO

After observing Kim and asking many questions, Amy is beginning to understand her special responsibilities in the ophthalmology and otorhinolaryngology clinic. She recognizes the need to be familiar with the anatomy and physiology of both the eye and the ear, as well as the importance of being able to perform specialty-related skills, such as irrigations, medication instillations, and diagnostic procedures. Amy has become quite proficient at performing Snellen and Ishihara screening examinations and accurately documenting the results of each. Kim has taught her to use the audiometer and assisted her with the first few screenings, so she is now ready to do hearing tests on her own.

Although she learned about eye and ear medications in her medical assistant program, Amy found that instilling these medications in an actual patient is different from working on mannequins and classmates. Kim has reinforced the skills she learned in her program, continually emphasizing infection control procedures and reinforcing patient education information. Amy realizes that she needs to understand the pathologic conditions that can occur in the sensory organs so she will be able to assist the physician as needed and answer patients' questions.

After working with patients who have vision and hearing deficits, Amy understands the importance of adapting communication techniques to meet the needs of each patient. She has decided to take advantage of educational opportunities at the hospital and through her professional organization to continue to learn about this special area of practice.

SUMMARY OF LEARNING OBJECTIVES

1. **Define, spell, and pronounce the terms listed in the vocabulary.**
   Spelling and pronouncing medical terms correctly bolsters the medical assistant's credibility. Knowing the definition of these terms promotes confidence in communication with patients and co-workers.

2. **Apply critical thinking skills in performing the patient assessment and patient care.**
   Completing the Critical Thinking Application exercises throughout the chapter can help the student medical assistant become more adept at critical analysis of real-life situations.

3. **Explain the differences among an ophthalmologist, an optometrist, and an optician.**

   An *ophthalmologist* is a medical doctor who specializes in the diagnosis and treatment of the eye; an *optometrist* can examine and treat visual defects; and an *optician* fills prescriptions for corrective lenses.

4. **Identify the anatomic structures of the eye.**

   The anatomy of the eye begins with the outer covering, the conjunctiva, and three layers of tissue: sclera, choroid, and retina. The retina is where light rays are converted into nervous energy for interpretation by the brain.

5. **Describe the process of vision.**

   Vision begins with the passage of light through the cornea, where it is refracted. The light rays then pass through the aqueous humor and pupil into the lens. The ciliary muscle adjusts the curvature of the lens to again refract the light rays so that they pass into the retina, triggering the photoreceptor cells of the rods and cones. Light energy is converted into an electrical impulse that is sent through the optic nerve to the brain, where interpretation occurs.

6. **Differentiate among the major types of refractive errors.**

   Refractive errors include hyperopia, myopia, presbyopia, and astigmatism. All are caused by a problem with bending light so that it can be accurately focused on the retina. These conditions usually are caused by defects in the shape of the eyeball and can be corrected with glasses, contacts, or surgery.

7. **Summarize typical disorders of the eye.**

   Eye disorders can range from problems with eye movement, as in strabismus and nystagmus, to infections of the eye, including hordeolum, chalazions, keratitis, conjunctivitis, and blepharitis. Disorders of the eyeball include corneal abrasions, cataracts, glaucoma, and macular degeneration.

8. **Define the various diagnostic procedures for the eye.**

   Diagnostic procedures for the eye begin with a visual examination of the eye with an ophthalmoscope. Next, the eyelids are examined for abnormalities, and the pupils are tested for PERRLA. More advanced techniques include the use of a slit lamp to view the fine details of the eye and an exophthalmometer to measure the distance of the eyeball from the orbit. Distance visual acuity typically is assessed with a Snellen chart; near visual acuity is tested with a near vision acuity chart. A patient can be tested for a color vision defect with the Ishihara test.

9. **Perform a visual acuity test using the Snellen chart.**

   Procedure 37-1 explains the Snellen evaluation.

10. **Assess color acuity using the Ishihara test.**

    Procedure 37-2 outlines the color acuity examination.

11. **Explain the purpose of eye irrigations and the instillation of medications.**

    Eye irrigations relieve inflammation, remove drainage, dilute chemicals, or wash away foreign bodies. Sterile technique and equipment must be used to prevent contamination. Medication may be instilled into the eye to treat an infection, soothe an eye irritation, anesthetize the eye, or dilate the pupils before examination or treatment.

12. **Properly irrigate a patient's eyes.**

    Procedure 37-3 describes the method for eye irrigation.

13. **Accurately instill eye medication.**

    Procedure 37-4 explains how to administer eye medications.

14. **Identify the structures and explain the functions of the external, middle, and inner ear.**

    The external ear consists of the auricle, or pinna, and the external auditory canal, which transmits sound waves to the tympanic membrane. The middle ear is an air-filled cavity that contains the ossicles. The sound vibration passes through the tympanic membrane, causing the ossicles to vibrate. This bone-conducted vibration passes through the oval window into the inner ear. The organ of Corti in the cochlea of the inner ear converts sound waves into nervous energy, which is sent to the brain for interpretation. The semicircular canals in the inner ear maintain equilibrium.

15. **Describe the conditions that can lead to hearing loss, including conductive and sensorineural impairments.**

    Conductive hearing loss is caused by a problem that originates in the external or middle ear and prevents sound vibrations from passing through the external auditory canal, limiting tympanic membrane vibrations or interfering with the passage of bone-conducted sound in the middle ear. A sensorineural hearing loss results from damage to the organ of Corti or the auditory nerve and prevents vibrations from being converted into nervous stimuli.

16. **Define the major disorders of the ear, including otitis, impacted cerumen, and Ménière's disease.**

    Otitis externa is an inflammation of the auditory canal, and otitis media is an inflammation of the normally air-filled middle ear, resulting in the collection of serous or suppurative fluid behind the tympanic membrane. Impacted cerumen is a common cause of conductive hearing loss. Ménière's disease is a chronic, progressive condition that affects the labyrinth and causes recurring attacks of vertigo, as well as tinnitus, a sensation of pressure in the affected ear, and advancing hearing loss.

17. **Explain diagnostic procedures for the ear.**

    The ear examination begins with an otoscopic examination. It can include various tuning fork tests to detect conductive or sensorineural hearing deficits, as well as more advanced audiometric testing.

18. **Use an audiometer to measure a patient's hearing acuity accurately.**

    Procedure 37-5 explains the audiometry examination.

19. **Identify the purpose of ear irrigations and instillation of ear medications.**

    Irrigation of the ear is performed to remove excessive or impacted cerumen, to remove a foreign body, or to treat the inflamed ear with an antiseptic solution. Medication is instilled into the ear to soften impacted cerumen, relieve pain, or treat an infectious pathogen.

20. **Demonstrate the procedure for performing ear irrigations.**

    Procedure 37-6 describes how to perform an ear irrigation.

21. **Accurately instill medicated ear drops.**

    Procedure 37-7 explains how to administer otic drugs.

22. **Summarize the nose and throat examination.**

    Examination of the nose and throat begins with inspection of the nasal cavity; this is followed by visual examination of the throat and the nasopharynx. Throat cultures may be done to determine whether a streptococcal infection is present. The anterior and posterior neck regions are palpated for abnormalities.

23. **Perform a throat culture.**
    Procedure 37-8 explains how to perform a throat culture.

24. **Describe the effect of sensory loss on patient education.**
    Patients with vision and hearing impairments face serious challenges and require individualized attention to meet their health education needs. Patients with vision loss may need large-print forms and handouts, increased levels of lighting, or verbal instructions rather than written ones. Individuals with hearing deficits may benefit from printed instructions, demonstrations on how to manage treatments, or even sign language interpretation. Family members should be included in the patient's treatment plan, and referrals to appropriate community or professional resources may be very beneficial.

25. **Discuss legal and ethical issues that might arise when caring for a patient with a vision or hearing deficit.**
    Diminished sight or hearing may render a patient seriously impaired. To prevent accidents and office injuries, always ask a sight- or hearing-impaired patient whether he or she requires assistance. Regardless of the patient's disability, the ambulatory care center must follow the guidelines for Notice of Privacy Practices (NPP) established by the Health Insurance Portability and Accountability Act (HIPAA). Public facilities must comply with ADA requirements for physical accommodations. If appropriate, assistive devices must be provided for individuals with vision or hearing impairments.

CONNECTIONS

📖 **Study Guide Connection:** Go to the Chapter 37 Study Guide. Read and complete the activities.

ⓔ **Evolve Connection:** Go to the Chapter 37 link at *evolve.elsevier.com/kinn* to complete the Chapter Review and Chapter Quiz. Peruse other resources listed for this chapter to increase your knowledge of Assisting in Ophthalmology and Otolaryngology.

38

ASSISTING IN DERMATOLOGY

SCENARIO

Dr. Sam Lee is a dermatologist who employs several medical assistants in his busy private practice. Melissa Bauman, CMA (AAMA), has worked for Dr. Lee since graduating from a medical assisting program last year. Melissa works as a clinical specialist, whose primary responsibilities are to perform telephone screening, prepare patients for procedures, and assist Dr. Lee as needed. To fulfill her responsibilities in the dermatology practice, Melissa must be familiar with common diseases and disorders that affect the skin, must assist with dermatologic procedures, and must be prepared to reinforce patient education about the treatment and prevention of dermatologic conditions.

While studying this chapter, think about the following questions:

- What is the basic anatomy and physiology of the integumentary system?
- What are common diseases and disorders that affect the integumentary system?
- How can Melissa determine the difference between the levels of burn injuries?
- Why is it important that Melissa understand the concepts of staging and grading of malignant tumors?
- What are the primary malignancies of the skin?
- What dermatologic procedures should Melissa be prepared to perform?

LEARNING OBJECTIVES

1. Define, spell, and pronounce the terms listed in the vocabulary.
2. Apply critical thinking skills in performing the patient assessment and patient care.
3. Explain the major functions of the skin.
4. Describe the anatomic structures of the skin.
5. Compare various skin lesions and give examples of each.
6. Describe typical integumentary system infections.
7. Differentiate among various inflammatory and autoimmune integumentary disorders.
8. Recognize thermal injuries to the skin.
9. Compare the characteristics of benign and malignant neoplasms.
10. Explain the grading and staging of malignant tumors.
11. Conduct patient education on the warning signs of cancer.
12. Describe skin malignancies and their treatment.
13. Define the ABCDE rule for identifying a malignant melanoma.
14. Summarize allergy testing procedures.
15. Explain dermatologic procedures performed in the ambulatory care setting.
16. Describe the diagnosis and treatment of allergies.
17. Correctly obtain an exudate sample from a wound for laboratory analysis.
18. Discuss the medical assistant's role in patient education regarding the integumentary system.

VOCABULARY

alopecia (al-o-pe′-se-uh) Partial or complete lack of hair.

anaplastic Relating to an alteration in cells to a more primitive form; a term that describes cancer-producing cells.

bilirubin (bih-luh-roo′-bin) An orange pigment in bile; its accumulation leads to jaundice.

cryosurgery The technique of exposing tissue to extreme cold to produce a well-defined area of cell destruction.

debridement The removal of foreign material and dead, damaged tissue from a wound.

electrodesiccation The destruction of cells and tissue by means of short high-frequency electrical sparks.

eschar Devitalized skin that forms a scab or a dry crust over a burn area.

exacerbation An increase in the seriousness of a disease, marked by greater intensity of the signs and symptoms.

excoriated Skin that has been injured by scratching; abraded.

glomerulonephritis (glo-mer′-yoo-loh-nih-fri′-tuhs) Inflammation of the glomerulus of the kidney.

hyperplasia An increase in the number of normal cells.

jaundice A yellow discoloration of the skin and mucous membranes caused by deposits of bile pigments; these deposits occur because of excess bilirubin in the blood.

keloid A raised, firm scar formation caused by overgrowth of collagen at the site of a skin injury.

keratin A very hard, tough protein found in the hair, nails, and epidermal tissue.

keratinocytes The skin cells that synthesize keratin.

leukoderma Lack of skin pigmentation, especially in patches.

opaque Not translucent or transparent; murky.

petechiae (peh-te′-ke-uh) Small, purplish hemorrhagic spots on the skin.

postherpetic neuralgia Pain that lasts longer than a month after a shingles infection and is caused by damage to the nerve; the pain may last for months or years.

Raynaud's phenomenon Intermittent attacks of ischemia of the extremities, resulting in cyanosis, numbness, tingling, and pain.

teratogen (te-rah′-tuh-jen) Any substance that interferes with normal prenatal development, resulting in a developmental abnormality.

The skin is the largest organ of the human body. In an average-size adult, it covers a total area of about 20 square feet. Forming the outer boundary of the body, the skin performs several essential functions: it acts as a barrier to protect vital internal organs from infection and injury; it helps dissipate heat and regulate body temperature; and it synthesizes vitamin D when exposed to ultraviolet (UV) light. In addition, various sensory receptors present throughout the skin enable it to respond to such sensations as heat, cold, pain, and pressure.

The specialty of dermatology deals with the skin and its accessory structures—hair, nails, and sweat glands, and the subcutaneous tissue that lies beneath the skin. A physician who specializes in dermatology is called a *dermatologist.*

ANATOMY AND PHYSIOLOGY

The integumentary system is composed of the skin and its accessory organs. Each square inch of the skin contains millions of cells, numerous specialized nerve endings, hair follicles, muscles, sweat glands to cool the body, and sebaceous glands, which release sebum, an oily substance that lubricates the skin. These diverse structures and glands are nourished by a permeating, elaborate network of blood vessels. The thickness of human skin varies markedly at different parts of the body, ranging from fairly thin over protected areas, such as the eyelids, to very thick over areas subject to abrasion, such as the palms of the hands and the soles of the feet.

Skin is composed of three layers: the epidermis—the thin, uppermost layer; the dermis—the thicker layer beneath that makes up about 90% of the skin mass and often is referred to as the *true skin;* and the subcutaneous layer—the layer composed primarily of fatty, or adipose, tissue (Figure 38-1).

Epidermis

New skin cells, called **keratinocytes,** are found in the basal cell layer of the epidermis and migrate upward over about 4 weeks. As the cells move toward the surface, they grow flatter and scalier, eventually losing their nuclei and changing into dead skin cells that contain an inert protein called **keratin.** Keratin makes up the outermost layer of the epidermis and forms a protective barrier across the surface of the skin that helps control water loss from the body. Ultimately, the outermost keratin layer sloughs off as a result of washing and friction. Hair and nails, which are also composed of keratin, are products of the epidermis.

About 95% of the cells in the epidermis are keratinocytes. The other 5% of epidermal cells are pigmented cells, or melanocytes. Melanin is a protein manufactured in the body that gives coloring to the skin and protects the body from UV radiation. Skin coloring is determined not by the total number of melanocytes, which is relatively constant for all races, but rather by the rate at which these cells produce melanin. The amount of melanin produced depends on genetics and exposure to UV light. Individuals with albinism, an inherited recessive trait, are unable to produce melanin, so they have white hair and skin and lack pigment in the iris. Because they have no protection from UV light, they must stay out of the sun.

Dermis

The underlying dermis is a thick layer of connective tissue that contains collagen and elastin fibers, as well as water and jellylike materials that make the skin compressible. Collagen fibers help prevent tearing of the skin, and elastin is a flexible fiber that makes the skin resilient. Distributed throughout the dermis are blood vessels, lymph vessels, muscle cells, hair follicles, and sebaceous and

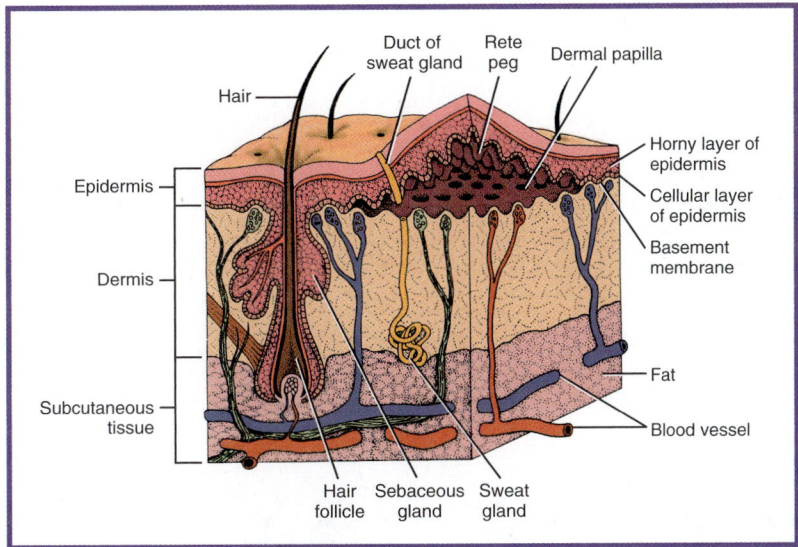

FIGURE 38-1 The three layers of the skin.

Labels in figure: Hair · Duct of sweat gland · Rete peg · Dermal papilla · Horny layer of epidermis · Cellular layer of epidermis · Basement membrane · Epidermis · Dermis · Subcutaneous tissue · Fat · Blood vessel · Hair follicle · Sebaceous gland · Sweat gland

sweat glands. The two types of sweat glands are *exocrine glands,* which excrete sweat through skin pores to release heat or create sweat in response to stress, and *apocrine glands,* which open into hair follicles and are located in specific areas, including the axilla, scalp, face, and genitalia. Sweat is odorless when excreted; bacterial action results in odor.

A variety of microorganisms, called *normal* or *resident flora,* are found on the skin and may increase the risk of integumentary system infection. Healthcare workers are encouraged to sanitize their hands before and after each procedure to prevent transient microbes picked up throughout the day from becoming resident flora. If transient microorganisms are not destroyed and/or removed by good hand sanitization techniques, they eventually become part of the individual's resident flora. Sensory receptors for the nervous system that detect pain, temperature, pressure, or texture also are located in the dermis.

Subcutaneous Layer

The subcutaneous layer contains fat cells, which provide insulation and serve as a depository for reserve calories. It also contains blood vessels, nerves, and the base of the appendages of the skin. Subcutaneous tissue is distributed unevenly, and as the human body ages, it thins considerably, which can make administering injections or drawing blood more difficult in aging patients. This loss of subcutaneous tissue is one reason elderly people are unable to compensate for changes in temperature, so they are colder when temperatures drop and hotter when temperatures rise. Aging skin is very fragile; it is easily traumatized and damaged by items such as the tourniquets used for drawing blood and bandage adhesives. The medical assistant must be very careful to avoid injuring the skin of an elderly person.

DISEASES AND DISORDERS

Skin is continuously exposed to the environment and may be affected by a wide range of disorders, including infections, inflammatory processes, allergic reactions, and tumors. Many skin problems resolve spontaneously, others can be managed with drug therapy, and still others, such as tumors, large cysts, or moles, may require surgical intervention.

Skin Lesions

Skin lesions can be caused by a systemic problem, such as an allergic reaction to medication, or they may develop from a localized infection. When communicating with the physician, documenting in the patient's chart, or doing telephone screening, always use correct medical terminology to describe skin lesions, such as, "The patient reports a widespread maculopapular rash across the anterior trunk" rather than, "The patient has a red raised rash on his stomach."

When you gather details from the patient about the characteristics of lesions, some questions you should consider include the following:

- Describe the color, elevation, and texture of the lesion.
- Is there any pain or pruritus (itching)? If pruritus is present, is the area **excoriated** or inflamed?
- Is there any drainage? If so, what are its characteristics?
- What is the exact anatomic location of the lesion? Have there been changes over time?

Primary lesions are those that appear immediately. Macules, papules, plaques, nodules, cysts, wheals, and pustules all are primary lesions. *Secondary lesions* are the result of alterations in a primary lesion. Examples of secondary lesions include scales, crusts, fissures, erosions, ulcerations, and scars (Figure 38-2). For instance, vesicles from a partial-thickness burn are primary lesions, but if the blisters break and ulcerations form, healing ends in a scar. Ulcerations and scars are secondary lesions.

Infections

Bacterial Infections

Impetigo. Impetigo is a common, superficial infection caused by streptococci or *Staphylococcus aureus* that usually affects children. Initially, impetigo looks like small vesicles on the face, especially around the nose and mouth, which quickly enlarge and rupture, excreting a honey-colored exudate. The exudate forms crusty lesions, and beneath the crust, the area is inflamed and moist (Figure 38-3).

PRIMARY LESIONS

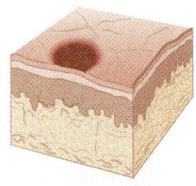

MACULE
Flat area of color change (no elevation or depression)

Example: Freckles

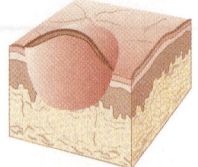

PAPULE
Solid elevation less than 0.5 cm in diameter

Example: Allergic eczema

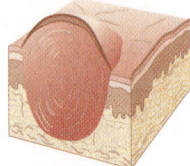

NODULE
Solid elevation 0.5 to 1 cm in diameter. Extends deeper into dermis than papule

Example: Mole

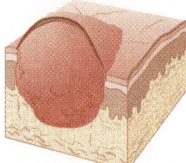

TUMOR
Solid mass—larger than 1 cm

Example: Squamous cell carcinoma

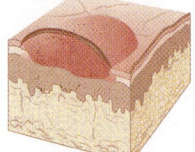

PLAQUE
Flat elevated surface found on skin or mucous membrane

Example: Thrush

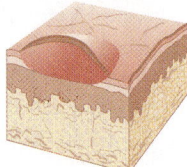

WHEAL
Type of plaque. Result is transient edema in dermis

Example: Intradermal skin test

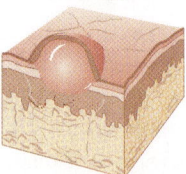

VESICLE
Small blister—fluid within or under epidermis

Example: Herpesvirus infection

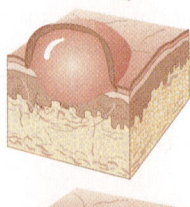

BULLA
Large blister (greater than 0.5 cm)

Example: Burn

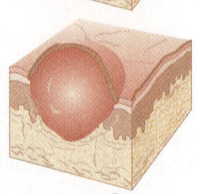

PUSTULE
Vesicle filled with pus

Example: Acne

SECONDARY LESIONS

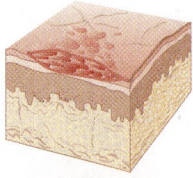

SCALES
Flakes of cornified skin layer

Example: Psoriasis

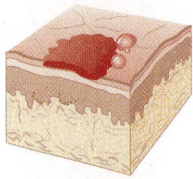

CRUST
Dried exudate on skin

Example: Impetigo

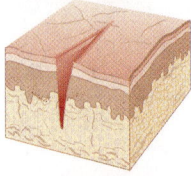

FISSURE
Cracks in skin

Example: Athlete's foot

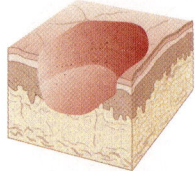

ULCER
Area of destruction of entire epidermis

Example: Decubitus (pressure sore)

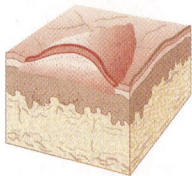

SCAR
Excess collagen production after injury

Example: Surgical healing

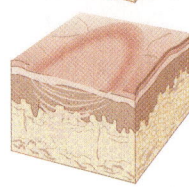

ATROPHY
Loss of some portion of the skin

Example: Paralysis

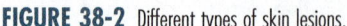

FIGURE 38-2 Different types of skin lesions.

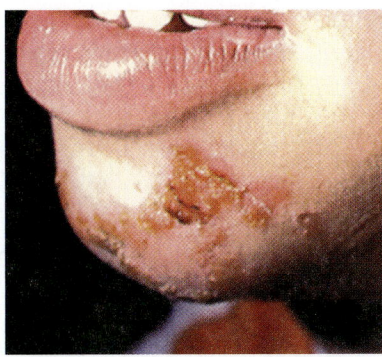

FIGURE 38-3 Impetigo. (From Marks J, Miller J: *Lookingbill's principles of dermatology,* ed 4, Philadelphia, 2006, Saunders.)

Pruritus accompanies the infection, and scratching helps spread the lesions at the site. Impetigo is contagious, and bacteria are transmitted by direct contact with the drainage, whether at other sites or with other children through the sharing of toys and touching. Consistent hand washing is required to help break the chain of infection. It also is important to keep personal items that may be contaminated, such as washcloths, linens, and drinking glasses, away from other members of the family. If the areas of infection are limited, topical treatment with an antibiotic ointment may be effective. However, impetigo caused by streptococci may result in **glomerulonephritis;** more involved infections may require treatment with oral antibiotics.

CRITICAL THINKING APPLICATION   **38-1**

Mrs. Allio calls the office because she is concerned that her children have been exposed to a child in the neighborhood who was diagnosed with impetigo. She tells Melissa that her 3-year-old woke up this morning with blisters around his mouth. Dr. Lee prescribes polymixin-bacitracin-neomycin (Neosporin) ointment to be applied three times daily to the affected areas. What should Melissa tell Mrs. Allio about preventing the spread of infection to her other children?

Acne. *Acne vulgaris* typically begins at puberty and is caused by a number of factors, including inherited predisposition, hormonal fluctuations, exposure to heat and humidity, and the use of oily creams (Figure 38-4). Acne is a disorder of the hair follicle and sebaceous gland unit. It develops when sebum, which reaches the skin surface through the hair follicles, stimulates the follicle walls, causing more rapid shedding of skin cells. Cells and sebum stick together and form a plug that promotes the growth of staphylococcal organisms in the follicles. The result is the formation of comedones (blackheads), pimples, pustules, or larger abscesses at the site.

Acne treatment begins with twice-daily face washes with benzoyl peroxide or salicylic acid. Medications include topical antibiotic cream such as erythromycin or application of a retinoid such as Retin-A (tretinoin) or adapalene (Differin). Oral antibiotics, such as tetracycline and doxycycline, at a maintenance dose of 250 mg once or twice daily, can be prescribed to control comedones and pustules. Severe cystic acne can be treated with isotretinoin (Accutane or

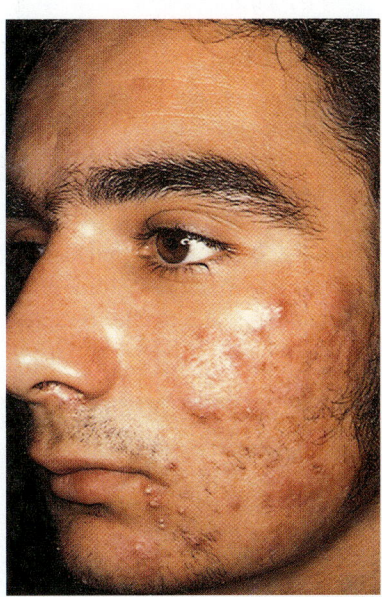

FIGURE 38-4 Acne. (From Paller A, Mancini A: *Hurwitz clinical pediatric dermatology: a textbook of skin disorders in childhood and adolescence,* ed 3, Philadelphia, 2006, Saunders.)

Sotret), but this drug is a strong **teratogen** and should never be prescribed for pregnant women or women who are not using contraceptives. The use of oral contraceptives, such as Ortho Tri-Cyclen, and Yaz, may reduce acne outbreaks as well. Laser resurfacing can be performed to smooth out shallow acne scars that form as the result of extreme cases of acne vulgaris.

Acne conglobata is a severe form of acne that typically occurs later in life and results in lesions across the back, buttocks, thighs, face, and chest. Abscesses or cysts may form between affected sites, and healing frequently results in **keloid** formation. This type of acne requires more aggressive treatment with systemic corticosteroids (e.g., prednisone), oral antibiotics, oral retinols (Accutane), and laser resurfacing or **debridement** to treat excessive scarring.

Rosacea. Rosacea is a chronic disease seen most frequently in women between the ages of 30 and 60. It causes inflammation and pustule formation and begins as frequent flushing across the nose, forehead, cheeks, and chin. As the condition progresses, capillaries of the face dilate and are visible across affected areas as small, red, edematous lines; these are accompanied by eye inflammation and photosensitivity. Over time, the face appears red, eye inflammation is more apparent, and painful nodules and pustules form. Men with rosacea may develop rhinophyma, a large, inflamed, bulbous nose caused by **hyperplasia** of sebaceous nasal tissue (Figure 38-5). Individuals with rosacea eventually may develop an obvious thickening of the skin across the forehead, nose, cheeks, and chin. The condition is treated with topical antibiotics and, as symptoms progress, with oral antibiotics, such as tetracycline, erythromycin, or doxycycline. Antibiotics help treat the pustule formation but do not affect the redness and flushing, which may cause the patient greatest concern.

Furuncles and Carbuncles. A *furuncle,* or boil, is a localized staphylococcal infection that begins as an inflammation of a hair follicle (*folliculitis*) or a skin gland. The affected area is raised, inflamed, and painful and eventually may produce purulent drainage. A *carbuncle* is a collection of furuncles that have joined to form a large infected area that may drain through multiple sites or form an abscess. Both infections are treated with oral antibiotics, frequent cleansing of the area, application of an antibiotic ointment, and, in some cases, surgical incision and drainage of the purulent material.

Cellulitis. Cellulitis, also called *erysipelas,* is an acute infection of the skin and subcutaneous tissue caused by staphylococci or streptococci. It begins from a small cut or as a result of a skin injury, or it develops at the site of a furuncle or ulcer. The area surrounding the site becomes inflamed, edematous, and painful with red streaks along the lymph vessels that lead from the infection. The condition is treated with oral antibiotics. Warm compresses applied locally aid healing, and analgesics may be needed to relieve discomfort. Cellulitis must be treated with caution, because a systemic infection can develop if the lymph glands become involved.

Fungal Infections (Dermatophytoses)

Fungal, or mycotic, infections such as *tinea pedis* (athlete's foot) (Figure 38-6, *A*), *tinea cruris* (jock itch) (Figure 38-6, *B*), and *tinea corporis* (ringworm) (Figure 38-6, *C*) are extremely common. These pathogens, which tend to live off dead tissue in the keratin layer of the epidermis, the hair, or the nails, cause almost no inflammation in the underlying skin. The fungus invades the skin, where it has been damaged or is consistently moist. All of these lesions are pruritic and are characterized by a distinct border with scaling areas that have a clear center. Secondary bacterial infections may occur with excoriation.

The physician typically diagnoses a fungal infection by noting the way the skin looks and the patient's complaints of pruritus. The skin may be scraped to obtain cells for examination under a microscope, and sometimes the physician may order a skin culture, for which a suspicious area is swabbed or scraped using sterile technique and the sample is sent to the laboratory for analysis. Treatment consists of topical antifungal agents, such as clotrimazole (Lotrimin), ketoconazole (Nizoral), econazole (Spectazole), or nystatin (Mycostatin). Antibiotics may be necessary if a secondary infection occurs. Because mycotic infections thrive in dark, moist areas, the patient should be advised to keep the site clean and dry and to wear loose clothing if possible. All types of dermatophytoses can become chronic infections if not managed carefully.

Tinea unguium, or *onychomycosis,* is a fungal infection of the toenails and fingernails. Unlike athlete's foot, which occurs on the skin's surface, nail fungus lives in the nail bed and the nail plate.

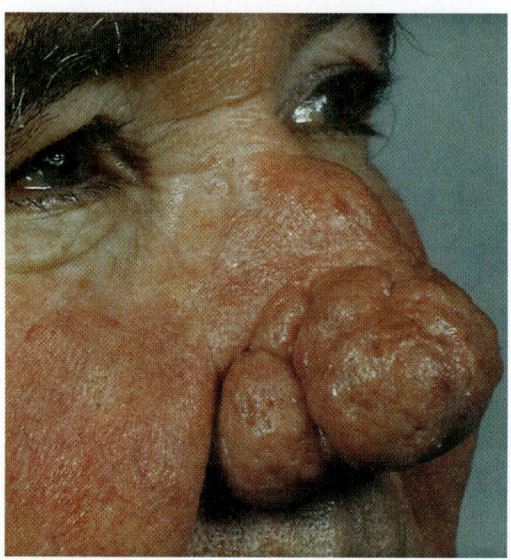

FIGURE 38-5 Rhinophyma. (From du Vivier A: *Atlas of clinical dermatology,* ed 2, London, 1993, Gower Medical Publishing.)

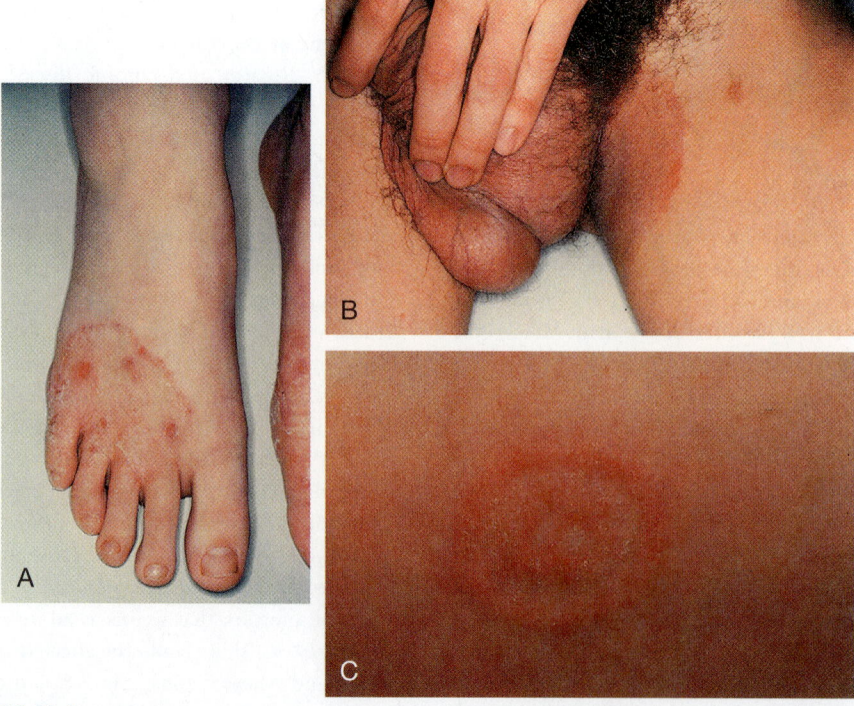

FIGURE 38-6 Fungal infections. **A,** Tinea pedis. **B,** Tinea cruris. **C,** Tinea corporis. (From Callen J, Greer K, Hood A et al: *Color atlas of dermatology,* ed 2, Philadelphia, 2000, Saunders.)

The nail provides the fungus with an extremely well-protected place to live, which is why nail fungus may be especially difficult to treat. The primary sign of nail fungus is the appearance of the nail, which turns yellow, white, or **opaque** (Figure 38-7). The texture also changes, and the nail becomes thick and brittle. If the fungus has been present for a long time, the nail can become twisted or distorted. The most effective treatment for nail fungus is oral terbinafine hydrochloride (Lamisil), which inhibits the production of fungal cells. However, the drug must be taken for 6 weeks to treat fungal infection of a fingernail and for 12 weeks for infection of a toenail; treatment carries the risk of liver complications.

Viral Infections

Warts. Warts, or verrucae, are caused by the human papilloma virus (HPV). Infection with HPV results in hyperplasia of the epidermis and a raised, cauliflower-like appearance. Verrucae can develop anywhere, but the most common sites are the fingers and the soles of the feet (plantar warts). (Genital warts are addressed in Chapter 40.) Most warts resolve over time, but they can be treated with topical chemicals, excised surgically, vaporized with lasers, or removed with **cryosurgery.**

Herpes Simplex (Cold Sores). Cold sores or fever blisters are caused by the herpes simplex virus type 1 (HSV-1). The initial infection may be asymptomatic or may cause painful ulcers along the gumlines of the mouth or on the lips. After the primary infection, the virus remains dormant in the trigeminal nerve and can be reactivated by exposure to the sun or to cold; by the presence of another infection, such as an upper respiratory infection; or when the patient is under stress. The patient reports a feeling of burning, tingling, or numbness before the eruption of vesicles. The blisters heal in 2 to 3 weeks, but the process may be speeded up by the use of topical antiviral drugs, such as acyclovir (Zovirax) or penciclovir cream (Denavir), or with oral antivirals, including Zovirax or valacyclovir (Valtrex). If applied at the first indications of a cold sore, the topical antiviral creams can limit the duration and severity of the outbreak.

Herpes Zoster (Shingles). Herpes zoster is an acute inflammatory disorder characterized by highly painful vesicular eruptions on the trunk of the body and occasionally on the face (Figure 38-8). The lesions develop on one side of the body and follow the course of the peripheral nerve, or dermatome, which has been infected by the varicella virus, the same virus that causes chickenpox. If the virus is not completely destroyed by the immune system, it lies dormant in dorsal root ganglia and is reactivated in later years. The cause of this reactivation is unclear, although it appears to be related to stress, immune system problems, and aging.

The onset of the disorder usually is marked by pain along the nerve pathway, and lesions appear in approximately 3 days. Inflammation lasts 10 days to 5 weeks. The patient is diagnosed by the characteristic pattern of painful lesions, and the diagnosis may be confirmed by isolating the virus in cell cultures. The condition also can be detected by the presence of varicella zoster antibodies in the blood.

Treatment focuses on promoting patient comfort with analgesic and antipruritic medications. Corticosteroid medications (prednisone) and antiviral drugs, including topical or oral acyclovir (Zovirax) and oral famciclovir (Famvir) or valacyclovir (Valtrex), also can be prescribed. One of the most serious complications of herpes zoster is postherpetic neuralgia, which causes chronic pain after resolution of the initial outbreak and may require treatment with a combination of medications, including topical calamine (Caladryl) lotion, capsaicin cream (Zostrix), topical lidocaine (Xylocaine), narcotics, a tricyclic antidepressant (e.g., Elavil, Tofranil), and anticonvulsants (including Dilantin, Tegretol, and Neurontin).

Two vaccines are available that may help prevent shingles. The chickenpox (varicella virus) vaccine (Varivax) is given to babies 12 to 18 months old and to older children and adults who have not had the chickenpox; this vaccine reduces the risk and severity of both chickenpox and shingles. A new varicella-zoster vaccine (Zostavax) is recommended for all adults over age 60, regardless of whether they have had shingles. This vaccine does not guarantee protection against shingles, but it can reduce the duration and severity of the outbreak, and it helps prevent **postherpetic neuralgia**.

Other Infections

Scabies and Pediculosis. The itch mite (which causes scabies) and lice (which cause pediculosis) are the two most common parasites

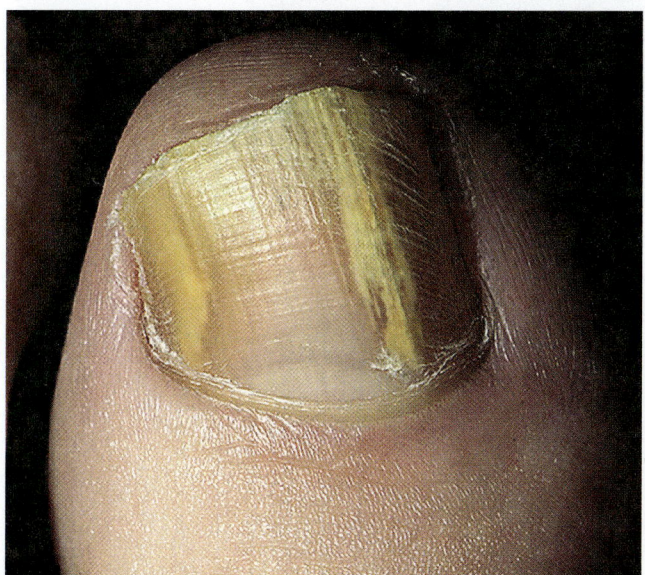

FIGURE 38-7 Tinea unguium. (From Habif TP: *Clinical dermatology,* ed 5, St Louis, 2010, Mosby.)

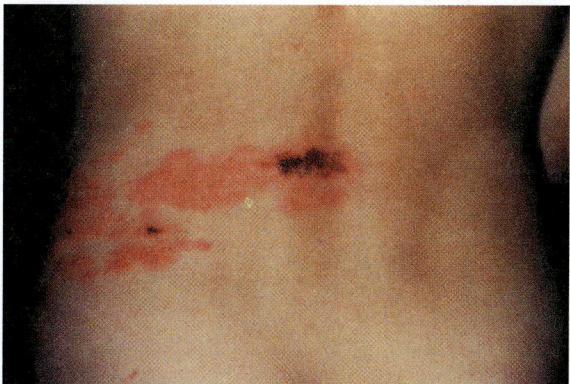

FIGURE 38-8 Herpes zoster (shingles). (From Callen J, Greer K, Hood A, et al: *Color atlas of dermatology,* ed 2, Philadelphia, 2000, Saunders.)

that infest human beings. Scabies mites are tiny organisms, barely visible to the eye, that burrow into the epidermis (Figure 38-9). Pediculosis can be caused by three different types of lice: head lice (*Pediculus humanus capitis;* Figure 38-10, *A*), body lice (*Pediculus humanus corporis*), and pubic lice (*Pthirus pubis;* Figure 38-10, *B*). Both scabies and lice infestations are highly contagious. The diagnosis of scabies may require scraping the skin at an inflamed area and examining the mites under a low-power microscope. Lice can be seen on the hair shafts. Patients describe symptoms of intense itching, possibly a body rash, and a sensation of something crawling on the skin. Treatment consists of ridding the body of the parasite, controlling the pruritus, and disinfecting the home environment to prevent reinfestation.

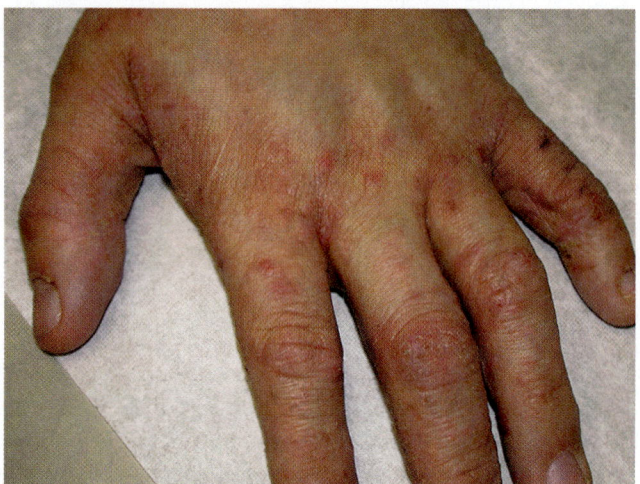

FIGURE 38-9 Scabies rash of the hand. (From Zaoutis LB, Chiang VW, editors: *Comprehensive pediatric hospital medicine,* Philadelphia, 2007, Mosby.)

CDC RECOMMENDATIONS FOR THE TREATMENT OF LICE

The Centers for Disease Control and Prevention (CDC) has established the following recommendations for treating lice:

1. Apply a lice medication (e.g., Nix, Rid, Ovide, Lindane). Do not use cream rinse or a conditioner before applying the medication. Do not rewash the hair for 1 to 2 days after treatment.
2. After treatment, check the hair and use a nit comb to remove nits and lice every 2 to 3 days. Continue to check for 2 to 3 weeks to make sure all lice and nits are gone. Head lice survive less than 1 to 2 days, and nits die within 1 week if they are not on a person.
3. Retreatment is recommended after 9 to 10 days to kill any surviving hatched lice before eggs are produced.
4. The following measures should be taken to prevent reinfestation:
   - Machine wash in hot water and dry on high heat: all clothing, bed linens, and other items worn or used for 2 days before treatment; and dry-clean items that cannot be washed; or seal all exposed items in a plastic bag for 2 weeks.
   - Soak combs and brushes in hot water for 5 to 10 minutes.
   - Vacuum floors and furniture.

Scabies is treated with a single application of 5% permethrin cream (Elimite) or crotamiton (Eurax) all over the body, from the neck down. Because the medication should be left on for a minimum of 8 hours, it typically is applied before bedtime. Treatment must be repeated in 7 to 10 days to destroy the nits (eggs). If a secondary infection occurs, antibiotics may also be prescribed. All family members and other individuals who have had direct personal contact

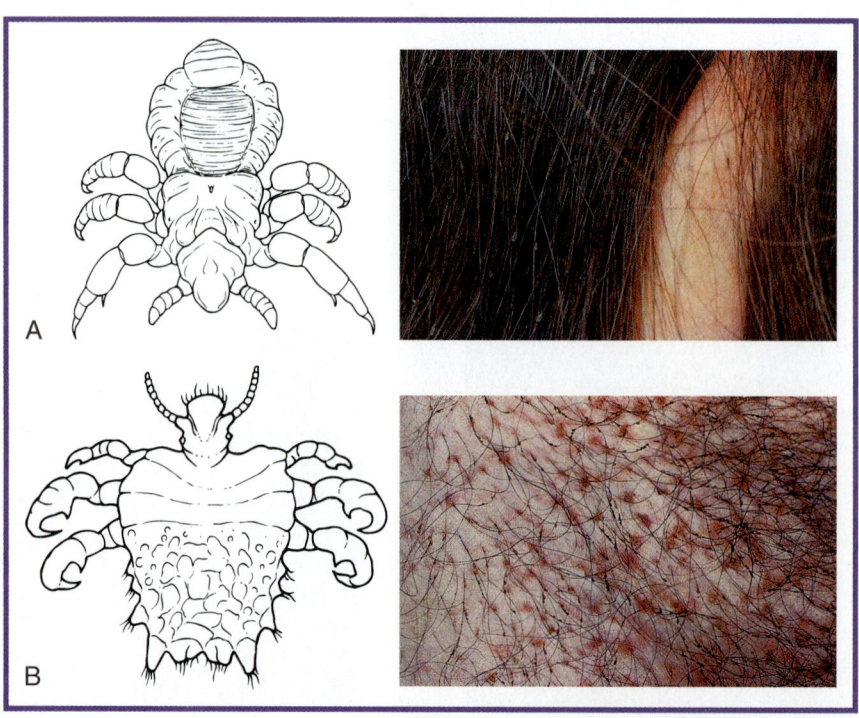

FIGURE 38-10 Pediculosis. **A,** *Pediculus humanus capitis* (head louse) and lice in the hair. **B,** *Phthirus pubis* (pubic or crab louse) and pubic lice rash. (From Callen J, Greer K, Hood A et al: *Color atlas of dermatology,* ed 2, Philadelphia, 2000, Saunders.)

with the infested person must be treated. Lindane lotion (Kwell) should be used only if permethrin treatment has failed, because it carries the risk of neurotoxicity, including seizures in children.

Inflammatory and Autoimmune Disorders

Seborrheic Dermatitis

Seborrheic dermatitis is one of the most common chronic inflammatory conditions of the sebaceous glands. It alters the amount and quality of the sebum, resulting in dry or moist, greasy-appearing scales and yellowish crusts on the scalp, eyebrows, eyelids, and sides of the nose, behind the ears, and in the middle of the chest. The condition has many different forms, including cradle cap in infants and dandruff in adults. Seborrheic dermatitis of the scalp can be treated with tar- or sulfur-based shampoos; inflammations of the skin usually are treated with topical corticosteroids, such as triamcinolone diacetate (Aristocort), betamethasone valerate (Valisone), or fluocinolone acetonide (Synalar). Seborrheic keratosis (age spots) is characterized by benign, slightly raised, tan to black lesions that occur with aging.

Contact Dermatitis

Contact dermatitis is an acute inflammatory response to a skin irritant or to exposure to a substance that causes an allergic reaction. An individual who is allergic to latex gloves or who has been exposed to poison ivy shows the signs and symptoms of contact dermatitis. The patient complains of redness (erythema), edema, pruritus, and vesicles. The patient should be encouraged to wash the affected area immediately after exposure to remove the irritant if possible. Medical treatment includes application of a corticosteroid cream or the use of oral corticosteroid medications (e.g., prednisone, methylprednisolone [Medrol]) if the symptoms are severe.

Eczema (Atopic Dermatitis)

Eczema is an idiopathic inflammatory skin disease that tends to occur in patients with a family history of allergies. In young children, it may be caused by food allergies, and in older children, stress or temperature extremes can trigger flare-ups. The condition usually improves and may disappear as the child ages. Eczema is characterized by a vesicular rash on the face, neck, and elbows and behind the knees and ears. It causes pronounced pruritus that, if left untreated, results in excoriation of the affected area from constant scratching.

Eczema is diagnosed with a comprehensive family history and examination of the skin. The patient may be asked to investigate possible allergens by making a list of all items that might be responsible for the outbreak, or the physician may recommend allergy testing. The goal of treatment is to reduce the frequency and number of eruptions and to relieve the pruritus so that affected areas do not become excoriated. The primary inflammation usually is treated with topical corticosteroids and oral antihistamines (e.g., diphenhydramine [Benadryl], cetirizine [Zyrtec], fexofenadine [Allegra]) to control itching. The physician may recommend controlled exposure to sunlight or UV rays to prevent and treat outbreaks. Inflamed plaques indicate a secondary staphylococcal infection, which should be treated with an oral antibiotic.

Psoriasis

Psoriasis is a chronic skin disease that produces discrete pink or red lesions covered with silvery scales (Figure 38-11). The disease may begin at any age, although most patients develop the problem before age 40. The lesions are not infectious, and the disease is characterized by periodic flare-ups throughout life. Psoriasis is caused by an autoimmune reaction that speeds up the maturation rate of skin cells. Normal skin cells mature, die, and are shed every 28 to 30 days, but in patients with psoriasis, cells mature in 3 to 6 days, and instead of sloughing off the surface of the skin, they build up and form the classic psoriasis silvery patch. The affected skin is dry, cracked, and encrusted. Lesions may appear on the scalp, chest, buttocks, and extremities.

Outbreaks of psoriatic plaques are associated with triggers that the patient may be able to identify and therefore avoid, such as infection (e.g., strep throat); an injury to the skin or bug bite; stress; cold weather; smoking and heavy alcohol consumption; and certain medications, such as lithium for mood disorders or beta blockers for hypertension. Psoriasis is diagnosed by observation of the skin, a careful patient history (a familial link has been established), and/ or a skin biopsy. Treatment is palliative, because the disease has no cure. Exposure to UV light may slow cell production, and coal tar preparations help relieve irritation when applied to affected areas. The physician also may order a combination of therapies, including methotrexate; a retinoid, such as acitretin (Soriatane); the immunosuppressant cyclosporine (Neoral); low-dose antihistamines; and oatmeal baths to promote patient comfort. Newer drugs called biologics may be prescribed if other treatments do not work. Biologics target the body's immune system and include adalimumab (Humira), etanercept (Enbrel), and infliximab (Remicade). Excimer

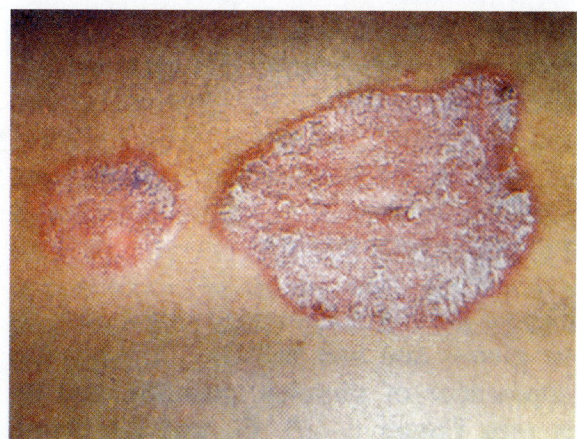

FIGURE 38-11 Psoriasis. (From Callen J, Greer K, Hood A et al: *Color atlas of dermatology,* ed 2, Philadelphia, 2000, Saunders.)

laser treatments that localize high-intensity wavelengths of UV light to targeted plaques, reducing both cell production and inflammation, may also be effective.

Systemic Lupus Erythematosus

Systemic lupus erythematosus (SLE) is a chronic autoimmune inflammatory disease of the connective tissue. The cause is unknown, although women are nine times more likely to develop the disease than men. It can affect any connective tissue in the body but typically causes inflammatory changes in the skin, joints, muscles, and kidneys. SLE usually involves more than one organ, and the patient experiences periods of **exacerbation** and remission. A diagnostic characteristic of the disease is a butterfly-shaped rash that stretches from one cheek across the nose to the other cheek (Figure 38-12). Other integumentary system symptoms include erythematous patches and plaques, **alopecia,** and photosensitivity.

The prognosis for SLE depends on organ involvement; patients who develop renal, cardiovascular, or neurological complications have a poor prognosis. Treatment includes the use of nonsteroidal antiinflammatory drugs (NSAIDs), including ibuprofen (Advil), diclofenac (Voltaren), and etodolac (Lodine), or controlled low doses of corticosteroids (prednisone) when needed. Serious cases are treated with cytotoxic drugs (cyclophosphamide [Cytoxan]) and antimalarial drugs, such as hydroxychloroquine (Plaquenil) or chloroquine hydrochloride (Aralen), and oral corticosteroids (prednisone) as needed to control inflammatory reactions.

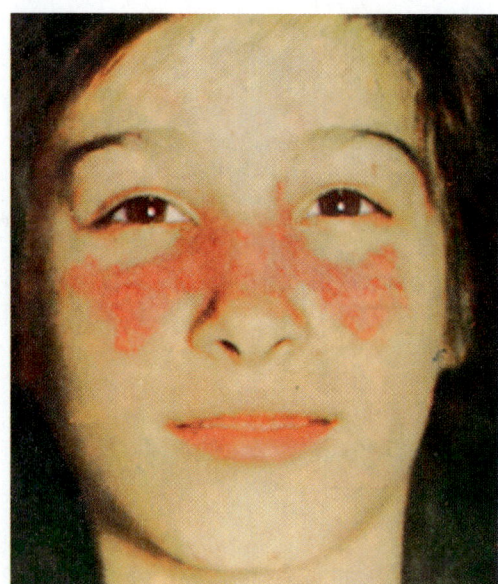

FIGURE 38-12 Butterfly rash of systemic lupus erythematosus (SLE). (Modified from Kliegman RM et al: *Nelson textbook of pediatrics,* ed 18, Philadelphia, 2007, Saunders.)

SLE DIAGNOSIS

The American Rheumatism Association has developed 11 criteria for the diagnosis of systemic lupus erythematosus (SLE):

- Malar or "butterfly" rash
- Discoid skin rash—patchy redness with hyperpigmentation and hypopigmentation
- Photosensitivity—skin rash in reaction to sunlight
- Mucous membrane ulcers of the lining of the mouth, nose, or throat
- Arthritis
- Pleuritis or pericarditis—inflammation of the tissue that lines the heart or lungs
- Kidney abnormalities
- Brain irritation—seizures and/or psychosis
- Low blood cell counts
- Abnormal immune studies
- Positive antinuclear antibodies (ANAs) in the blood

Scleroderma

Collagen is a fibrous protein that forms the body's connective tissues, including the skin. Scleroderma is caused by overproduction and accumulation of collagen in the body's tissues. It is a chronic, progressive, autoimmune disease that causes generalized inflammation of blood vessels throughout the body, leading to narrowing and destruction of smaller arteries and ultimately fibrotic circulatory changes. Scleroderma also causes destruction of the connective tissue lining and formation of scar tissue in all major organs, including the

gastrointestinal system, heart, lungs, and kidneys. Integumentary system symptoms include fibrous changes in the skin that result in sclerosis (hardening) of the skin, edema, pallor, pigmentation, and fixation to subcutaneous tissues. These same sclerotic changes can occur in any organ in the body. **Raynaud's phenomenon** may be the first symptom of the disease. The cause of scleroderma is unknown, but it usually occurs in middle-aged women.

The disease has no cure and no specific treatment. Drugs are used to treat inflammation and circulatory symptoms of the disease, and analgesics are prescribed for pain. Physical therapy helps maintain muscle strength, but the prognosis is poor. Patients with scleroderma usually die as a result of cardiac, pulmonary, or renal involvement.

Thermal Injuries

Skin can be damaged and injured by exposure to moderately high or low temperatures over an extended period. It also can be injured in a relatively short time when exposed to very high or low temperatures. The most common thermal injuries are burns, which are classified as superficial thickness (first degree), partial thickness (second degree), or full thickness (third degree), depending on the depth of the wound (Figure 38-13). With severe burns, all three types commonly are seen in the same location: superficial burns along the edges, partial-thickness burns with vesicles closer to the center, and full-thickness burns at the center of the area.

Superficial-Thickness (First-Degree) Burn

A superficial-thickness burn affects only the epidermis, is erythemic (red), blanches with pressure, and is painful but does not have blisters at the site. A mild sunburn and a steam burn without vesicle formation are examples of superficial burns.

Partial-Thickness (Second-Degree) Burn

A partial-thickness burn destroys the entire epidermal layer and varying depths of the dermis and causes blister formation and

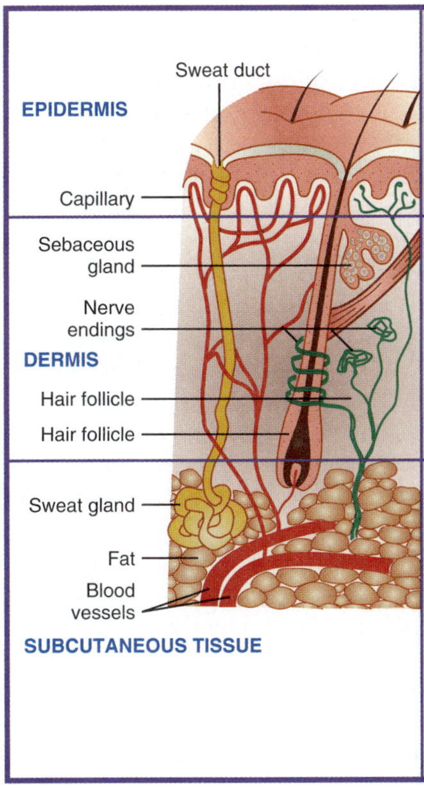

	APPEARANCE	SENSATION	COURSE
SUPERFICIAL BURN	Mild to severe erythema; skin blanches with pressure Skin dry Small, thin-walled blisters	Painful Hyperesthetic Tingling Pain eased by cooling	Discomfort lasts about 48 hours Desquamation in 3–7 days
PARTIAL-THICKNESS BURN	Large thick-walled blisters covering extensive area (vesiculation) Edema; mottled red base; broken epidermis; wet, shiny, weeping surface	Painful Hyperesthetic Sensitive to cold air	Superficial partial-thickness burn heals in 10–14 days Deep partial-thickness burn requires 21–28 days for healing Healing rate varies with burn depth and presence or absence of infection
FULL-THICKNESS BURN	Variable, e.g., deep red, black, white, brown Dry surface Edema Tissue disrupted	Little pain Anesthetic	Full-thickness dead skin suppurates and liquefies after 2–3 weeks Spontaneous healing impossible Requires removal of **eschar** and skin grafting Scarring deformities and function loss Beneath eschar capillary tufts and fibroblasts organize into granulating tissue

FIGURE 38-13 Classification of burns.

subcutaneous edema and pain. The danger of infection in the blistered area also is a concern. If a burn is deep enough, some destruction of the hair follicles and the sebaceous glands may occur.

Treatment of Minor Burns

Because burns damage the natural protection of the skin, preventing infection at the site is a primary concern. Superficial-thickness burns typically heal on their own within a week, as long as they are kept clean and infection does not occur. Medical treatment of partial-thickness burns includes gentle cleansing of the site with a bactericidal solution and debridement of broken blisters or dead skin. Intact blisters should be left alone. Partial-thickness burns may be treated with a thin layer of silver sulfadiazine cream and application of a nonadherent, multilayered dressing for several days to 1 week. The patient's tetanus immunization status should be reviewed, and a tetanus injection should be given if needed. The physician also may order analgesics to relieve pain. Patients with partial-thickness burns (those reporting blisters at the site of the burn) should be seen by the physician for treatment.

CRITICAL THINKING APPLICATION 38-3

Thomas Rangoso, a 66-year-old patient, calls the office to report a burn on his right hand and forearm. He fell while passing the stove and burned himself on the hot surface. Mr. Rangoso tells Melissa that the area is very red and painful and has blisters in the center. He wants to break the blisters and put butter on the burn. Should Mr. Rangoso be seen by Dr. Lee? What should Melissa tell him about how to care for the burn?

PATIENT EDUCATION FOR BURN CARE

- Warning signs of infection include fever, malaise, inflammation, swelling, increased pain, odor, and drainage from the burn area. Any of these should be reported to the physician immediately.
- Review wound care with the patient, including gentle cleansing with bactericidal solution (e.g., povidone-iodine solution [Betadine]) and covering the wound with an antibiotic ointment (silver sulfadiazine) so that the dressing does not stick to the burn.
- The patient should eat a high-calorie, high-protein diet to maintain weight and promote healing.
- For partial-thickness burns, the development of new skin takes 6 weeks, and complete healing occurs in 6 to 12 months, depending on the extent of the burn.

Full-Thickness (Third-Degree) Burn

A full-thickness burn destroys all layers of the skin and may involve underlying fat, muscle, nerves, blood supply, and bone. The area appears charred or white and has a firm, leathery texture. The patient feels no pain, because nerve endings have been destroyed. Full-thickness burns have the potential to cause major complications, including dehydration, circulatory collapse, respiratory distress, and septic shock. Treatment of major burns includes maintaining the patient's airway, replacing fluids, preventing infection, and administering oxygen. Debridement of affected tissue, including areas of **eschar,** and skin grafts are required for wound healing. Depending on the extent of the burns, the patient may be hospitalized in an intensive care unit or a specialty burn unit.

Burns are classified according to the percentage of body surface involved, based on the Rule of Nines (see Chapter 36).

Cold Injuries

Cold injuries usually are less severe than burns, but prolonged exposure to cold temperatures can result in infection, gangrene, amputation, and, in severe situations, death. Frostbite is caused by exposure to subfreezing temperatures. Damage occurs at the level of the capillaries, which become permanently dilated and unable to regulate local blood flow. Signs and symptoms of superficial frostbite include burning, tingling, numbness, and a white or grayish color of the skin. With deep frostbite, blisters form and the area is hard, mottled, edematous, and blue or gray after thawing.

The extent of injury is determined by visual examination and the history of the exposure. Treatment consists of warming the area with immersion in warm water (100°F to 106°F [38°C to 41°C]). The affected site should never be rubbed, because this increases cellular destruction. Vital signs should be monitored and the physician's orders followed explicitly.

Benign and Malignant Neoplasms

A neoplasm is an abnormal growth or tumor that may be benign or malignant. Table 38-1 outlines the differences between benign and malignant tumors. Invasion and metastasis are the principal criteria used to distinguish between cancerous and noncancerous tumors. Benign masses are encapsulated, and although they may increase in size, they remain confined within a shell; malignant tumors, on the other hand, invade and take over surrounding tissues. Local invasion of surrounding tissue occurs when malignant cells break through the basement membrane that separates epithelial cells from connective tissue. Here the cancerous cells can invade blood and lymph vessels, which carry the malignant cells to organs throughout the body.

Patients diagnosed with carcinoma in situ have a malignant tumor that is confined to the original site of growth without invasion of the basement membrane. Patients with regional spread have evidence of malignant cells in surrounding tissues but no evidence of lymph node involvement. Patients with distant spread, or metastasis, show positive lymph node involvement locally and the development of secondary tumors in other organs, including lungs, liver, brain, or bones.

Malignant tumors are classified according to their grade and stage. A biopsy sample of the tumor is obtained and is sent to a pathologist. The pathologist examines the cells under a microscope and grades the sample according to its histologic, or cellular, classification of differentiation. Differentiation is the process that normal cells go through to mature. Immature, or primitive, cells never mature and are classified as **anaplastic,** or cancerous. Therefore, the more poorly differentiated the cells (i.e., the less they look like normal cells), the more likely it is that the tissue is cancerous. If the physician receives a grading report that indicates anaplastic cancerous cells, the next step is to determine whether the cancerous cells have spread from the original site; this is called *staging* the tumor. With staging, a physical examination and diagnostic tests (e.g., bone, liver, or positron emission tomography [PET] scans) are done to determine the degree of tumor spread to a secondary location. The size and depth of the primary tumor, the degree of lymph node involvement, and the presence of metastatic spread determine whether the patient has carcinoma in situ (i.e., a tumor localized to the organ of origin), direct spread beyond the primary organ, lymph node metastasis, or confirmed secondary tumor growth in a distant metastatic site. Grading and staging determine the extent of malignant involvement, which allows the physician to plan appropriate treatment.

Three methods are used to obtain a small piece of tissue for examination under a microscope. In an excision biopsy, such as removal of a mole, the entire lesion may be removed for analysis. A punch biopsy involves removal of a small section from a designated location in the lesion; the center usually is the optimum site. This is done with a scalpel-like circular punch instrument if the lesion is on the surface of the skin, as with a mole (Figure 38-14), or a large-gauge needle and syringe unit is used to aspirate cells and fluid from a suspicious area, as in a breast biopsy. A shave biopsy is performed with a scalpel by cutting or shaving off the growth or lesion just above the skin line. This method is used to biopsy a possible squamous cell carcinoma lesion. The medical assistant may help the physician perform these procedures.

The protocol for the treatment of cancer depends on staging, grading, and type of carcinoma. Possible treatments include surgical removal of the tumor, radiation therapy, chemotherapy, hormone therapy, and immune system boosters. These approaches may be used singly or in combination and usually are determined by an oncologist, who is a specialist in the study and treatment of cancer.

TABLE 38-1 Differences Between Benign and Malignant Tumors		
CHARACTERISTIC	BENIGN TUMOR	MALIGNANT TUMOR
Cellular structure	Same as surrounding tissue	Anaplastic changes and poor cellular differentiation
Type of growth	Encapsulated mass that expands over time	Infiltrates and metastasizes; distant spread through the bloodstream or lymph system to other body tissues and organs can occur
Rate of growth	Usually slow; rarely fatal	May be slow, rapid, or very rapid; almost always fatal if left untreated
Destruction of localized tissue	None	Common; ulceration and necrosis of surrounding tissue

ASSISTING WITH A TISSUE BIOPSY

1. Assemble the necessary supplies for the procedure.
2. Prepare the patient with proper gowning, draping, and positioning and make sure the patient understands the procedure.

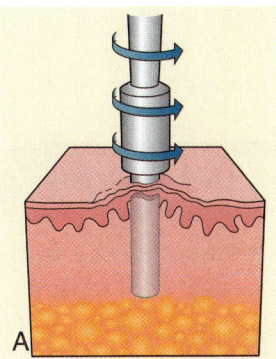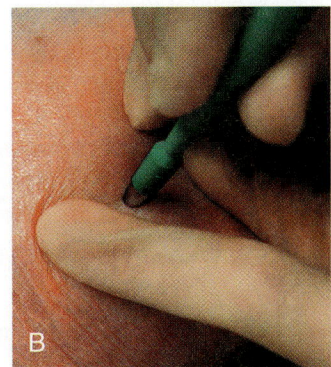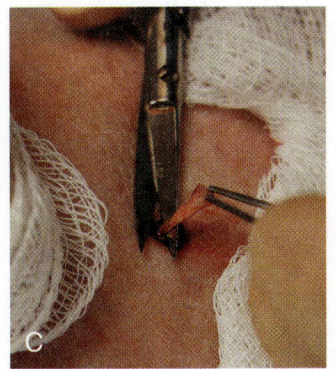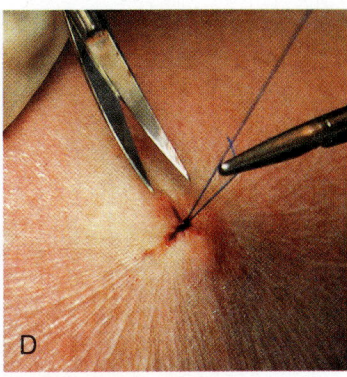

FIGURE 38-14 **A,** Punch biopsy diagram. **B,** Punch biopsy instrument rotated into the skin. **C,** Cutting the base of the specimen. **D,** Closure of the biopsy wound with a simple epidermal stitch. (Modified from Bolognia J: *Dermatology*, ed 2, Edinburgh, 2008, Mosby.)

3. Confirm that the physician has obtained the patient's informed consent.
4. Prepare the site of the biopsy according to office protocol.
5. Assist the physician as needed, using appropriate personal protective equipment according to Standard Precautions.
6. Label the sample container and prepare it for transport to the testing laboratory. Remember to include laboratory request forms.
7. Clean the procedure area, properly dispose of all waste materials, and disinfect and sterilize equipment used in the procedure.
8. Sanitize your hands and document the procedure, including the patient education provided on biopsy site care.

PATIENT EDUCATION: CANCER'S SEVEN WARNING SIGNS

The initial letters of the warning signs spell out the word CAUTION. Any of these warning signs should be reported to the physician immediately. Early detection and self-examination are crucial to cancer survival.

- Change in bowel or bladder habits
- A sore that does not heal
- Unusual bleeding or discharge
- Thickening or a lump in the breast or elsewhere
- Indigestion or difficulty in swallowing
- Obvious change in a wart or mole
- Nagging cough or hoarseness

Neoplasms of the Skin

Neoplasms of the skin may be benign or malignant. Examples of benign tumors include birthmarks and moles *(nevi)*. However, a tumor may be benign but have a predisposition to be cancerous, which means that it can change from a benign state to a malignant one. Whenever a neoplasm is discovered, the physician usually performs a biopsy of the lesion to establish the type of cells involved.

Three cancerous lesions of the skin can occur: basal cell carcinoma, squamous cell carcinoma, and malignant melanoma. Basal cells line the deepest layer of the epidermis. Basal cell carcinoma is very slow growing and is the most frequently seen form of skin cancer. The most common sites are areas of the body exposed to the sun, such as the face and forearms. The typical basal cell carcinoma appears as a small, pearly, dome-shaped nodule with small, visible

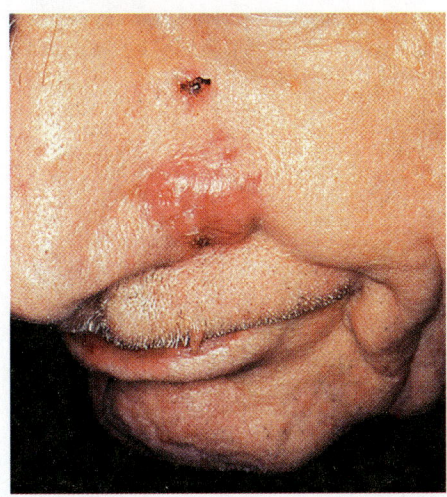

FIGURE 38-15 Basal cell carcinoma. (Modified from Damjanov I: *Pathology for the health-related professions,* ed 3, Philadelphia, 2006, Saunders.)

blood vessels called *telangiectasis*. However, it also can appear as a persistent sore that does not heal and that has a reddish, irritated appearance (Figure 38-15).

Squamous cell carcinoma grows rapidly and is more serious because it has a tendency to metastasize. It appears as a firm, red nodule with visible scales, and it may ulcerate and form a crust (Figure 38-16). Patients typically report both basal and squamous cell skin cancers as sores that persist and never heal.

Malignant melanoma develops from a change in a mole. Sunburns increase the risk of melanoma, and individuals with more moles than average (more than 100) are at greater risk. Individuals with congenital nevi (moles present at birth) are more likely to develop a melanoma. Additional risk factors include an inability to tan, light or red hair, fair skin, family history, and a large number of childhood sunburns. Many forms of melanoma occur, but all are pigmented lesions (usually brown, tan, blue, red, black, or white) that are asymmetric (i.e., have irregular borders) and usually are larger than 6 mm (Figure 38-17). Staging of the disease depends on the depth of the mass, not on the surface size of the mole. If cancerous cells have invaded the basement membrane, risk of metastasis via the blood and lymph vessels located in the dermis is greater. The incidence of malignant melanoma has doubled in the past 10 years, and the disease causes more deaths than all other skin diseases. Melanomas often recur or metastasize within 5 years of diagnosis.

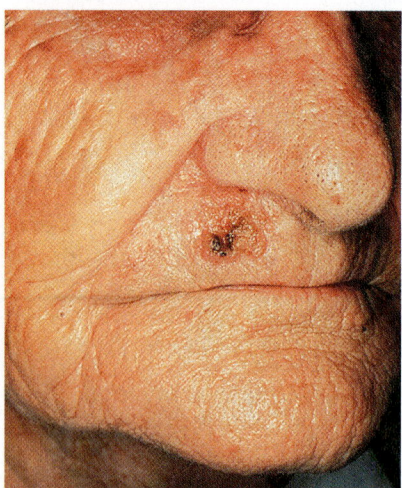

FIGURE 38-16 Squamous cell carcinoma. (Modified from Damjanov I: *Pathology for the health-related professions*, ed 3, Philadelphia, 2006, Saunders.)

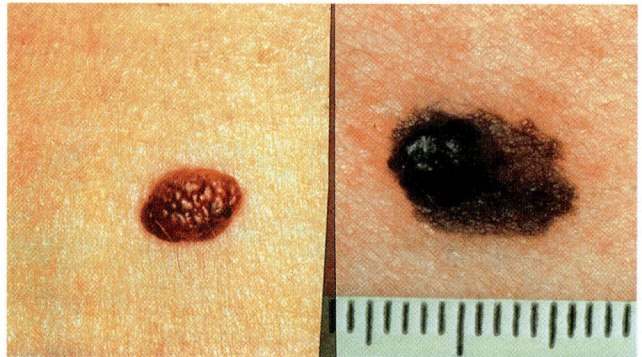

FIGURE 38-17 Pigmented skin lesions. *Left,* Benign pigmented nevus (mole). *Right,* Malignant melanoma. (Courtesy National Cancer Institute, Bethesda, Md.)

The patient should be routinely examined for at least 10 years after removal of a melanoma.

All skin cancers are diagnosed by the appearance of the lesions, with confirmation through biopsy. Treatment depends on the type, the level of invasion, and the location of the mass. The physician may choose to remove the tumor surgically or eradicate it with cryosurgery, **electrodesiccation,** or application of chemotherapeutic agents. A relatively new procedure, Mohs micrographic surgery, is an effective, precise method for treating and removing basal and squamous cell carcinomas. The Mohs technique is performed by specially trained dermatologists, who use a microscope during the surgical procedure to systematically trace the cancerous lesion down to its roots and remove the tumor layer by layer; this minimizes the chance of regrowth and reduces scar formation.

The National Cancer Institute has stated that the best way to prevent skin cancer is to protect the skin from the sun, starting at an early age. People of all ages should do the following:

- Stay out of the midday sun (10 AM to 4 PM).
- Use protection against UV rays reflected off water and snow.
- Use protection against UV rays even on cloudy days, on which exposure can still occur.
- Wear protective clothing and a wide-brimmed hat when in the sun and protect the eyes with sunglasses.

- Use a sunscreen that filters both UVB and UVA rays with a sun protection factor (SPF) of at least 15.
- Avoid using artificial sun lamps and tanning beds.

EARLY WARNING SIGNS OF MALIGNANT MELANOMA: ABCDE RULE

If a mole displays any of the following characteristics, a dermatologist should examine it immediately.

A	Asymmetry	One-half of the mole does not match the other half.
B	Border	The edges of the mole are blurred or irregular.
C	Color	The mole is not the same color throughout and has shades of tan, brown, black, red, white, or blue.
D	Diameter	The mole is larger than 6 mm, about the size of a pencil eraser.
E	Elevation	A mole that once was flat against the skin now is raised and elevated.

DERMATOLOGIC PROCEDURES

The integumentary system can reflect both internal and external reactions and disease processes. The skin holds information about the body's circulation and nutritional status, and signs of systemic diseases. It also acts as a mirror, reflecting aging changes that occur in all organs of the body. For many people, self-esteem is linked to a youthful appearance, and dermatologic conditions may be very threatening to feelings of self-worth. As you prepare patients for a dermatologic examination, allow them to express their anxieties. The impairments that most frequently bring a patient to the dermatologist's office are cosmetic disfigurements caused by a skin disease, pain and pruritus, and interference with sensations or movements.

Assisting With a Dermatologic Examination

During a dermatologic examination, the physician inspects the entire body, beginning with the scalp and continuing to the soles of the feet, including the genital area. Inspection of the skin is followed by detailed examination of suspicious areas through palpation, diascopy, and special tests. A diascope is a glass plate held firmly against the skin to permit observation of changes produced in underlying areas when pressure is applied. Inspection may include the use of a magnifying lens and a bright light to closely examine a suspicious lesion or growth. The dermatologist frequently asks the medical assistant to take photographs of moles and/or to chart specific measurements and locations of suspicious lesions. These are placed in the medical record for comparison when the patient returns for follow-up visits.

In the physical examination, concerns about the integumentary system include abnormal coloring, such as cyanosis, pallor, erythema, **leukoderma,** or excessive brown patches. **Jaundice** may indicate an increase in the level of **bilirubin** in the blood. Decreased pigmentation is found in vitiligo, an acquired loss of melanin characterized by blotchy white patches on the skin. Lesions, ulcers, and bruises may be the result of pathologic conditions. Localized red or purple changes may be the result of vascular neoplasms, birthmarks, or subcutaneous hemorrhages (**petechiae** and ecchymoses). Palpation helps confirm findings of the inspection. Therefore, inspection and palpation are interrelated in confirming the diagnosis of an integumentary system disorder. Palpated findings may include the skin's texture or elasticity or the presence of edema or a neoplasm.

Gowning and draping of a patient for a skin examination depend on the area to be examined. Remember to expose the area adequately but also to protect the patient's privacy. Try to make the patient as comfortable as possible and offer support when it is needed.

Skin Testing for Allergies

Skin testing to detect allergies requires percutaneous application or intradermal injection of a small amount of antigen (or groups of antigens) and later examination of the test sites for a visible reaction. The larger the localized skin reaction, the more profound is the patient's allergic response to the tested allergen.

Percutaneous Test. A percutaneous, or scratch, test may be performed on the forearm, upper arm, or back. The back is favored in young children because of the large area of skin available. It also is easier to immobilize the child in this position. The skin surface is labeled or numbered in rows 1½ to 2 inches apart, and a small amount of allergen is placed on the skin, which is then scratched or pricked to place the allergen just under the skin surface. Many allergists use a plastic device that is dipped into the designated allergens and lightly pressed into the skin so that the prick and allergen deposition occur at the same time. Seventy or more tests may be done at one time. It is essential to follow a pattern so that the site of each allergen can be easily identified. This type of allergy testing is used for allergic rhinitis, asthma, and detection of food allergies.

A reaction usually occurs within 10 to 30 minutes of exposure to the allergen. If the reaction is positive, a wheal (hive) forms at the site of the scratch (Figure 38-18). Interpretation of the test result should always be based on a comparison of this reaction with that of the control, which is a scratch with a plain base fluid free of any allergy-producing extract.

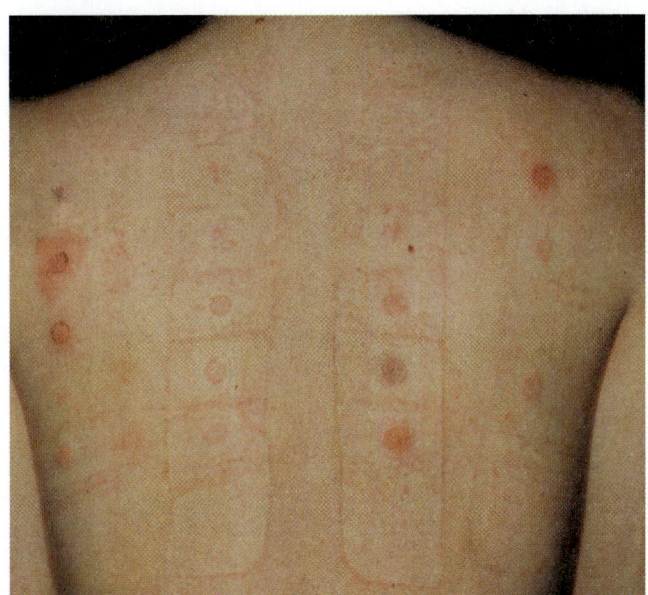

FIGURE 38-18 Results of allergy testing. (From Habif TP: *Clinical dermatology*, ed 5, St Louis, 2010, Mosby.)

The interpretation, or reading, of the skin tests is performed by the physician or a trained technician. Reactions commonly are graded from 2 to 4. No precise definition of a reaction can be given, and the intensity of the response may vary among individuals. However, as a general rule, a 2 reaction implies a wheal that is definitely larger than that of the control. A larger wheal is interpreted as a 3, whereas the presence of pseudopods (fingerlike extensions around the periphery of the wheal) may be read as a 4. If a strong reaction occurs, the allergen extract should be carefully wiped off to prevent any further exposure. Erythema around the wheal usually is disregarded in the interpretations. Frequently, large or significant reactions are accompanied by local itching. Patients should remain in the office for at least 30 minutes after completion of the test in case a delayed systemic allergic response occurs.

Patch Test. This test uses an allergen that is applied to a patch that is placed on the skin. Patch testing helps detect delayed allergic reactions such as a substance that causes contact dermatitis. The patches are placed on the arms or back and must remain in place for 48 hours. The patient needs to avoid bathing and activities that cause heavy sweating. The patches are removed at a subsequent office visit. Skin irritation at the patch site indicates an allergy to that particular substance.

GUIDELINES FOR ALLERGEN SKIN TESTING

- The patient should stop taking all antihistamines or allergy medications 3 to 10 days before testing to prevent false-negative results.
- Recommended sites for injection or application of the allergen are the anterior forearm, the upper arm, and the back.
- Allergen sites must be specifically labeled and spaced approximately 1½ to 2 inches apart.
- If the patient shows signs of anaphylaxis, notify the physician immediately and prepare emergency supplies. Allergy testing should be performed only when the physician is on site.
- Skin testing may cause a mild systemic allergic response, resulting in rhinitis, wheezing, and sneezing. The patient should contact the physician if a more severe reaction occurs.

Intradermal (Intracutaneous) Test. The intradermal test is more sensitive than the percutaneous test and usually is used to diagnose allergies to penicillin and insect venom, such as in bee stings. Extracts are injected into the intradermal layer of the skin in doses of 0.1 to 0.2 mL. This method also is used for the tuberculin (purified protein derivative [PPD]) test and the Valley Fever coccidioidomycosis test. When intradermal injections are used for allergy testing, 10 to 15 allergens may be tested at one time on each arm. The reaction time is identical to that of the scratch test; however, the antigen is more dilute.

Radioallergosorbent Test. The radioallergosorbent test (RAST) measures the level of antibodies created when a sample of the patient's blood is mixed with allergens in the laboratory. The RAST is easier to perform than skin testing, because it requires a single venipuncture. Although skin testing remains the preferred method of diagnosing hypersensitivity, the RAST may be indicated when the patient cannot stop antihistamine medications, when a skin disorder makes accurate interpretation of skin test results difficult, or when skin test results are negative but the patient's signs and symptoms support further investigation. RAST blood tests are primarily used to identify food allergies.

Treatment of Allergies

The classic treatment of allergies is to encourage the patient to avoid known or suspected allergens. Unfortunately, this is not always possible, so the physician may prescribe antihistamine medications, such as Xyzal (levocetirizine) or Clarinex (desloratadine) for relief of allergy symptoms. Over-the-counter antihistamines include Allegra, Zyrtec, and Claritin. Another option is the use of immunotherapy, a series of injections in which minute doses of known allergens are administered subcutaneously over time to desensitize the patient's immune system and ultimately develop a resistance to the immune response. This usually requires weekly or bimonthly injections over several years. Some patients are cured, whereas others have only a minor reduction in allergic symptoms. Immunotherapy is controversial, because it is an expensive, invasive, and potentially dangerous treatment with unpredictable results. It is recommended only for patients with severe allergic symptoms that are not relieved by antihistamine medications.

If you are responsible for administering allergen injections, you must take great care to dispense the correct dose of each allergen; administer each subcutaneous injection in a separate site; accurately document the procedure and the exact location of each injection; record any local or systemic reactions; and observe the patient for at least 20 to 30 minutes after the injections to detect possible systemic allergic responses, including urticaria, wheezing, or hypotension. If the patient shows any localized or systemic reactions, the physician should be notified.

Obtaining a Wound Specimen for Culture

A wound culture specimen is obtained so that a microscopic analysis of the organisms at the site of a lesion can be performed to determine the causative infectious agent. The physician may order a culture if the wound is inflamed or has purulent drainage, or if the patient has a fever. Aerobic cultures are performed to detect organisms that grow in the presence of oxygen and are usually found on superficial surfaces of the wound. Anaerobic cultures check for the presence of organisms that require little or no oxygen and appear in deeper wound sites or in areas that have a poor blood supply, such as ulcers or compound fractures (Procedure 38-1). Wound culture results help the physician prescribe the most effective antibiotic for the infection.

Appearance Modification Procedures

Chemical Peel (Chemexfoliation). Topical agents are used in chemical peels to minimize or remove minor skin features, such as acne scars, hyperpigmentation, and fine wrinkles. Agents used for chemical peels include tretinoin cream 0.05% to 0.1% concentration (Retin-A), alpha hydroxy acid, trichloroacetic acid, and phenol (carbolic acid). During application, care must be taken to prevent the solution from entering the eyes. The use of chemical exfoliating agents may cause the skin to appear inflamed and dry with crusting and edema. The patient may complain of stinging and burning at the beginning of the treatment regimen. The patient should avoid sun exposure for the length of treatment and should use a sunscreen with a minimum SPF of 15, because photophobia (light sensitivity) is a typical side effect of treatment.

Dermabrasion. A dermabrader is a handheld device that mechanically evens the layers of dermal tissue. It is effective in the treatment of scars from acne vulgaris. Topical anesthetics (e.g., ethyl chloride) or locally injected anesthetics are used for the procedure. Besides the dermabrader, the dermatologist may use a variety of wire brushes, abrasive disks, or other devices to smooth scar tissue. Standard Precautions must be followed, including the use of face and eye guards, to prevent aerosol or splatter contamination from the site. The patient should be educated about wound care, signs of infection, and the presence of photophobia for 6 to 12 months after the procedure.

Laser Resurfacing (Photothermolysis). Laser therapy may be used for fine lines and wrinkles, pigmented areas, shallow scars, and tattoo removal. Typically, the patient is instructed to prepare the site 3 to 6 weeks before the procedure with tretinoin (Retin-A), alpha hydroxy solutions, or bleaches. Laser procedures are performed with the patient under local, regional, or general anesthesia. During the procedure, it is extremely important that the patient and all personnel wear the type of eye protection recommended by the laser manufacturer. After the procedure, cool packs are applied to help reduce swelling, and topical antibiotic ointment is used to prevent infection. The treated area appears inflamed and edematous and can take up to 2 weeks to heal; it can take as long as 6 months for the inflammation to fade.

Botox Injections. Botox is a strong neurotoxin (a substance toxic to nerves) produced by *Clostridium botulinum,* a bacterium that causes food poisoning. Two strains of the botulism bacterium are used in dermatologic procedures for appearance modification. Botox treatments involve injection of the substance around the eyes, mouth, and forehead. The toxin interferes with nervous stimulation, which temporarily paralyzes the muscles of the face that cause wrinkles to form. It also smoothes out the skin and makes it look younger and fresher. The effects are short term, so treatments must be repeated every 3 to 4 months, and some patients complain of an inability to show facial expression because of muscle paralysis.

CLOSING COMMENTS

Patient Education

The field of dermatology offers medical assistants many opportunities and topics for patient education. Skin care products are advertised in the newspaper, on billboards, in magazines, and on television. Consult the dermatologist for whom you work and get approval of skin care products the office can recommend to patients. Sometimes companies that manufacture skin care products will provide samples if contacted and informed that the office recommends a certain

PROCEDURE 38-1

Obtain Specimens for Microbiologic Testing: Collect a Wound Specimen for Testing and/or Culture

GOAL: *To obtain an adequate sample for culture without contaminating the specimen.*

EQUIPMENT and SUPPLIES

- Sterile culture kit containing tube, swabs, and transport medium (for swabbing)
- Sterile culture kit containing syringe and transport medium (for aspirating)
- Laboratory requisition
- Sterile gauze squares
- Recommended wound-cleansing solution
- Sterile dressing
- Gloves
- Biohazard container
- Face guard
- Patient's record

PROCEDURAL STEPS

1. Sanitize your hands, gather supplies (Figure 1), and put on gloves and face protection.

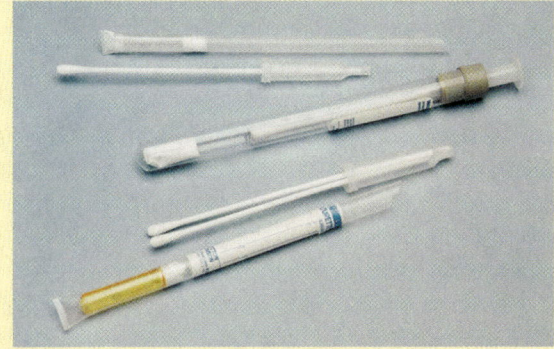

   PURPOSE: To follow Standard Precautions.
2. Remove the dressing from the wound and dispose of it in a biohazard waste container.
   PURPOSE: To ensure infection control.
3. Observe the wound and make note of the color, odor, and amount of exudate present.
   PURPOSE: To note this information in the patient's record.

4. *Aspirating.* Remove the syringe from the kit, insert the tip into the wound exudate, and draw back the plunger, drawing the exudate up into the syringe. Remove the needle and dispose of it in a sharps container. Place the labeled syringe in a biohazard bag for transport to the clinical laboratory with the appropriate physician order.
5. *Swabbing.* Remove the swab from the culture kit, insert it into the wound, and saturate it with the exudate. If necessary, use more than one swab, properly labeling each container, to obtain exudates from the entire wound. If preparing an anaerobic culture, place the specimen in the culture tube as quickly as possible to prevent oxygen exposure and possible destruction of microbes.
6. Place the swab into the culture tube and crush the transport medium ampule, which is in the transport tube, by squeezing the walls of the transport tube slightly, or place the exudate-filled syringe directly into the transport tube (Figure 2).

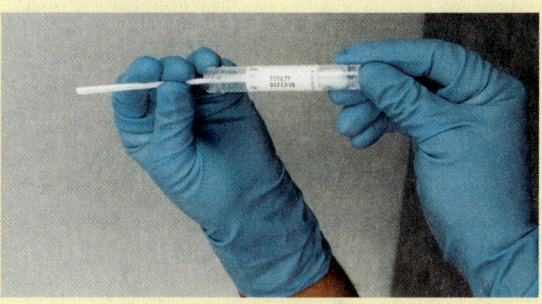

7. Label the culture tube accurately. Include on the laboratory slip the patient's recent antibiotic therapy and the wound site.
8. Clean the wound as ordered by the physician and apply a sterile dressing to the area (see Chapter 57 for the sterile dressing procedure).
9. Clean the area and dispose of all waste materials in a biohazard waste container. Remove your gloves and sanitize your hands.
   PURPOSE: To ensure infection control.
10. Place the culture tube in the laboratory collection area. Document the procedure and all wound data in the patient's record.
    PURPOSE: A procedure is not done until it is recorded.

---

product to patients. Patients enjoy receiving samples and encouragement to try a new skin care technique.

Another area of patient education involves the potentially dangerous effects of sunlight and tanning beds. Obtain literature showing how UV rays cause premature aging and may cause cancerous lesions later in life. You can explain the meaning of the sun protective factor in sun-tanning lotions. Tanning beds should be avoided, especially by individuals with a skin disorder and by those taking medications that cause photophobia. Providing patients with information about the warning signs of cancer also is a vital part of patient education in a dermatology practice.

▌ Legal and Ethical Issues

While working in a dermatology practice, you will hear many patients express concern about skin disorders. Allowing patients to express their concerns and using therapeutic listening techniques are always helpful; however, be careful when offering encouragement about the course and outcome of treatment. No treatment can restore youth. The improvement achieved may be slow and gradual. Keep encouragement on a positive level. Compliment the patient on small improvements, but remember that it is the physician's role to explain potential treatment outcomes.

SUMMARY OF SCENARIO

Melissa enjoys her work with Dr. Lee, and she recognizes that she needs to keep up with new developments in the field of dermatology. She has learned the importance of giving patients accurate information while conducting telephone screening and always refers questions or concerns to Dr. Lee. Melissa especially enjoys the patient education aspects of working for a dermatologist, including teaching patients the importance of using sunscreen, controlling sun exposure, and checking for the warning signs of cancer. Melissa also has learned how to assist Dr. Lee with dermatologic procedures, including performing allergy skin testing, obtaining wound cultures, and assisting with biopsies, chemical peels, dermabrasions, and laser resurfacing.

SUMMARY OF LEARNING OBJECTIVES

1. **Define, spell, and pronounce the terms listed in the vocabulary.**
   Spelling and pronouncing medical terms correctly bolsters the medical assistant's credibility. Knowing the definition of these terms promotes confidence in communication with patients and co-workers.

2. **Apply critical thinking skills in performing the patient assessment and patient care.**
   Completing the Critical Thinking Application exercises throughout the chapter can help the student medical assistant become more adept at critical analysis of real-life situations.

3. **Explain the major functions of the skin.**
   The skin acts as a barrier to protect vital internal organs from infection and injury. It also helps dissipate heat and regulate body temperature, and it synthesizes vitamin D when exposed to UV light. In addition, various sensory receptors all over the skin enable the body to respond to heat, cold, pain, and pressure.

4. **Describe the anatomic structures of the skin.**
   The skin is made up of three layers: the epidermis, which is the thin, uppermost layer; the dermis, which is the thicker layer beneath, which makes up approximately 90% of the skin mass; and the subcutaneous layer, which consists of primarily fatty or adipose tissue.

5. **Compare various skin lesions and give examples of each.**
   Figure 38-2 shows different types of skin lesions. The diagnosis of skin lesions is based on the color, level of elevation, and texture of the lesion; whether pruritus, excoriation, pain, or drainage is present; and whether the lesion is a primary or secondary growth.

6. **Describe typical integumentary system infections.**
   Integumentary system infections include bacterial infections, such as impetigo, acne vulgaris, furuncles, carbuncles, and cellulitis; fungal infections, including a variety of tinea growths; viral infections, which cause warts, herpes simplex, and herpes zoster outbreaks; and scabies or pediculosis infestations.

7. **Differentiate among various inflammatory and autoimmune integumentary disorders.**
   Inflammatory and vascular integumentary system disorders include a variety of seborrheic dermatitis inflammations; contact dermatitis; eczema; and autoimmune disorders.

8. **Recognize thermal injuries to the skin.**
   The most common thermal injuries are burns, which are classified as superficial, partial-thickness, or full-thickness burns, depending on the depth of the wound. The most important concern in the treatment of burns is the prevention of infection. Cold injuries usually are less severe than burns, but prolonged exposure can result in infection, gangrene, amputation, and death.

9. **Compare the characteristics of benign and malignant neoplasms.**
   Benign masses are encapsulated, whereas malignant tumors invade and take over surrounding tissues. Local invasion of surrounding tissue occurs when malignant cells break through the basement membrane that separates epithelial cells from connective tissue. This allows the cancerous cells to invade blood and lymph vessels, and blood and lymph then can carry the malignant cells to organs throughout the body.

10. **Explain the grading and staging of malignant tumors.**
    Grading is the histologic, cellular classification of a tumor. The more poorly differentiated the cells, the closer the biopsy sample is to an anaplastic cancerous mass. Staging involves using physical examination and diagnostic tests (such as bone or liver scans) to determine the presence of tumor spread.

11. **Conduct patient education on the warning signs of cancer.**
    The warning signs of cancer include any change in bowel or bladder habits; a sore that does not heal; unusual bleeding or discharge; a thickening or a lump in the breast or elsewhere; indigestion or difficulty swallowing; an obvious change in a wart or mole; or a nagging cough or hoarseness. Any of these warning signs should be reported to the physician immediately. Early detection and self-examination are crucial to cancer survival.

12. **Describe skin malignancies and their treatment.**
    Three cancerous lesions of the skin can occur: basal cell carcinoma, which is very slow growing and the most frequently seen form of skin cancer; squamous cell carcinoma, which grows rapidly and is more serious because it has a tendency to metastasize; and melanomas, which are pigmented lesions that are asymmetric, have irregular borders, and usually are larger than 6 mm. Treatment depends on the type of lesion, the level of invasion, and the location. The physician may surgically remove the tumor or may destroy it with cryosurgery, electrodesiccation, laser treatment, or the application of chemotherapeutic agents.

13. **Define the ABCDE rule for identifying a malignant melanoma.**
    The ABCDE rule includes examination of the site for any of the following: *a*symmetry, irregular *b*order, change in *c*olor, increase in *d*iameter, and

elevation. If a mole displays any of these characteristics, a dermatologist should check it immediately.

14. **Summarize allergy testing procedures.**

Allergy testing is done by exposing the patient to suspected allergens through a scratch on the skin or an intradermal injection, and then observing the exposure site to see whether a localized allergic reaction develops. The patient must be off antihistamine drugs for several days before testing. Sites for allergen exposure include upper arms, anterior forearms, and back. A physician must be present in the facility while allergy testing is being done because of the potential for local or systemic allergic reactions in sensitized individuals.

15. **Explain dermatologic procedures performed in the ambulatory care setting.**

Dermatologic procedures include allergy skin testing that can be done with scratch, patch, or intradermal tests; drawing blood for a RAST test; treating allergies with immunotherapy; performing a wound culture; and appearance modification procedures, including chemical peels, dermabrasion, and laser resurfacing.

16. **Describe the diagnosis and treatment of allergies.**

Skin testing to detect allergies requires percutaneous application or intradermal injection of a small amount of antigen and later examination of the test sites for a visible reaction. The larger the localized skin reaction, the more profound is the patient's allergic response to the tested allergen. The classic treatment of allergies consists of avoiding known or suspected allergens and prescribing antihistamine medications or immunotherapy.

17. **Correctly obtain an exudate sample from a wound for laboratory analysis.**

Procedure 38-1 summarizes the steps for collecting a wound sample for culture.

18. **Discuss the medical assistant's role in patient education regarding the integumentary system.**

Areas for possible patient education include dermatologist recommendations for skin care products, the dangers of UV exposure, and information about the warning signs of skin cancer.

CONNECTIONS

Study Guide Connection: Go to the Chapter 38 Study Guide. Read and complete the activities.

Evolve Connection: Go to the Chapter 38 link at *evolve.elsevier.com/ kinn* to complete the Chapter Review and Chapter Quiz. Peruse other resources listed for this chapter to increase your knowledge of Assisting in Dermatology.

39

ASSISTING IN GASTROENTEROLOGY

SCENARIO

Joan Rothman, CMA (AAMA), was recently hired by United Community Hospital to work for a group of internists. Joan works primarily with Dr. Raj Sahani, a physician who specializes in gastroenterology. Although Joan did very well in school, she has had to learn more advanced information about disorders of the gastrointestinal (GI) tract so that she can answer patients' questions and understand the diagnostic procedures ordered by Dr. Sahani.

Dr. Sahani has asked Joan to research and develop educational packets for common gastrointestinal studies and to work with other staff members on understanding procedures related to the GI system. Part of the role of the medical assistant working in a gastroenterology practice is to conduct routine patient education so that patients are properly prepared for diagnostic procedures. Joan also is expected to help in the orientation of new staff members.

While studying this chapter, think about the following questions:

- What does Joan need to include in the educational packets so that patients are prepared for GI examinations?
- What are some of the GI disorders Joan can expect to see in this specialty practice?
- What information should be included in a pamphlet on infectious viral hepatitis?
- What should a new medical assistant know about the GI examination, including instructions for patients on how to collect fecal specimens?

LEARNING OBJECTIVES

1. Define, spell, and pronounce the terms listed in the vocabulary.
2. Apply critical thinking skills in performing the patient assessment and patient care.
3. Describe the primary functions of the GI system.
4. Identify the anatomic structures that make up the GI system and describe the physiology of each.
5. Differentiate among the abdominal quadrants and regions.
6. Summarize the typical symptoms and characteristics of GI complaints.
7. Perform telephone screening for patients with GI complaints.
8. Distinguish among cancers of the GI tract.
9. Describe common esophageal and gastric disorders, the signs and symptoms, diagnostic tests, and treatments.
10. Describe intestinal disorders, the signs and symptoms, diagnostic tests, and treatments.
11. Classify disorders of the liver and gallbladder and list the signs and symptoms, diagnostic tests, and treatments.
12. Describe the similarities and differences among the various forms of infectious viral hepatitis.
13. Summarize the medical assistant's role in the GI examination.
14. Explain the common diagnostic procedures for the GI system.
15. Demonstrate the procedure for assisting with an endoscopic colon examination.
16. Perform the procedural steps for assisting with the collection of a fecal specimen.
17. Describe the medical assistant's role in the proctologic examination.

VOCABULARY

adhesions (ad-he'-zhuns) Bands of scar tissue that bind together two anatomic surfaces that normally are separate.

anastomosis (uh-nas-tuh-mo'-suhs) The surgical joining of two normally distinct organs.

anorexia (a-nuh-rek'-se-uh) A lack or loss of appetite for food.

ascites (uh-si'-tez) An abnormal collection of fluid containing high levels of protein and electrolytes in the peritoneal cavity.

carcinogens (kar-si'-nuh-juhns) Substances or agents that cause the development or increase the incidence of cancer.

endemic (en-de'-mik) Term describing a disease or microorganism that is specific to a particular geographic area.

esophageal varices (i-sah-fuh-je'-uhl var'-uh-sez) Varicose veins of the esophagus that occur as a result of portal hypertension; these vessels can easily hemorrhage.

fecalith (fe'-kuh-lith) A hard, impacted mass of feces in the colon.

fissures Narrow slits or clefts in the abdominal wall.

fistula (fis'-chuh-luh) An abnormal, tubelike passage between internal organs or from an internal organ to the body's surface.

flatus Gas expelled through the anus.

gangrene The death of body tissue as a result of loss of nutritive supply, followed by bacterial invasion and putrefaction.

hematemesis (hi-mat-uh-me'-sis) Vomiting of bright red blood, indicating rapid upper gastrointestinal (GI) bleeding; associated with esophageal varices or peptic ulcer.

hematocrit The percentage by volume of packed red blood cells in a given sample of blood after centrifugation.

hemoglobin (he'-muh-glo-buhn) A protein found in erythrocytes that transports molecular oxygen in the blood.

hepatomegaly (he-puh-to-me'-guh-le) Abnormal enlargement of the liver.

ileostomy The surgical formation of an opening of the ileum onto the surface of the abdomen, through which fecal material is emptied.

jaundice Yellowing of the skin and mucous membranes caused by the deposition of bile pigment; jaundice is not a disease but rather is a sign of a number of diseases, especially liver disorders.

lithotripsy (li'-thuh-trip-se) A procedure for eliminating a kidney stone or gallstone by crushing or dissolving it in situ through the use of high-intensity sound waves.

lymphadenopathy (lim-fa-duh-nah'-puh-the) Any disorder of the lymph nodes or lymph vessels.

peristalsis The rhythmic, involuntary serial contraction of the smooth muscles lining the GI tract.

polyps (pah'-lips) Tumors or outgrowths found in the mucosal lining of the colon; they are considered precancerous.

portal circulation The pathway of blood flow through the portal vein from the GI system to the liver.

portal hypertension Increased venous pressure in the portal circulation caused by cirrhosis or compression of the hepatic vascular system.

pyloric sphincter A muscular ring at the distal end of the stomach that separates the stomach from the duodenum of the small intestine.

sclerotherapy (skluh-rah-ther'-ah-pe) The treatment of hemorrhoids, varicose veins, or esophageal varices by means of injection of sclerosing solutions.

Valsalva's maneuver Occurs when a person strains to defecate or urinate, uses the arms and upper trunk muscles to move up in bed, or strains during laughing, coughing, or vomiting; causes trapping of blood in the great veins, preventing it from entering the chest and right atrium, and may cause heart attack and death.

Internal medicine is a nonsurgical specialty consisting of several subspecialties. Gastroenterology, one of these subspecialties, covers an extremely wide area known as the *gastrointestinal (GI) system*, or the *alimentary canal.* Gastroenterologists are concerned with diseases and disorders of the stomach, small intestine, large intestine (colon), appendix, and accessory organs of the liver, gallbladder, and pancreas. Proctology, a subspecialty of gastroenterology, is concerned with disorders of the rectum and anus. The major purpose of the GI system is to prepare, digest, and absorb the necessary nutrients to maintain homeostasis and excrete waste products through the feces.

ANATOMY AND PHYSIOLOGY

The GI system is basically a long, hollow tube with the same structural organization from its beginning to its termination (Figure 39-1). The muscles lining the GI tract are closely regulated by the autonomic nervous system, which gives the entire system its unique ability to move slowly in some locations and to have increased movement in other sections.

The GI system is divided into two parts: the upper digestive system, which includes the mouth, esophagus, and stomach, and the lower digestive system, which consists of the small and large intestines. The GI tract is rich in lymphatic tissue, which is very important for the absorption of nutrients from ingested food. Unfortunately, the lymphatic vessels also are the main route for the spread of cancer.

As mentioned, the GI organs have three primary functions: digestion, absorption, and elimination. When food is taken in through the mouth, it is chewed, or masticated, and moistened with saliva. Salivary amylase, an enzyme released by the salivary glands, mixes with the food and begins carbohydrate digestion. This mass, now called a *bolus,* is swallowed, and the food enters the esophagus. Contractions of the smooth muscles are activated, and the bolus is moved by **peristalsis** down the esophagus and into the stomach.

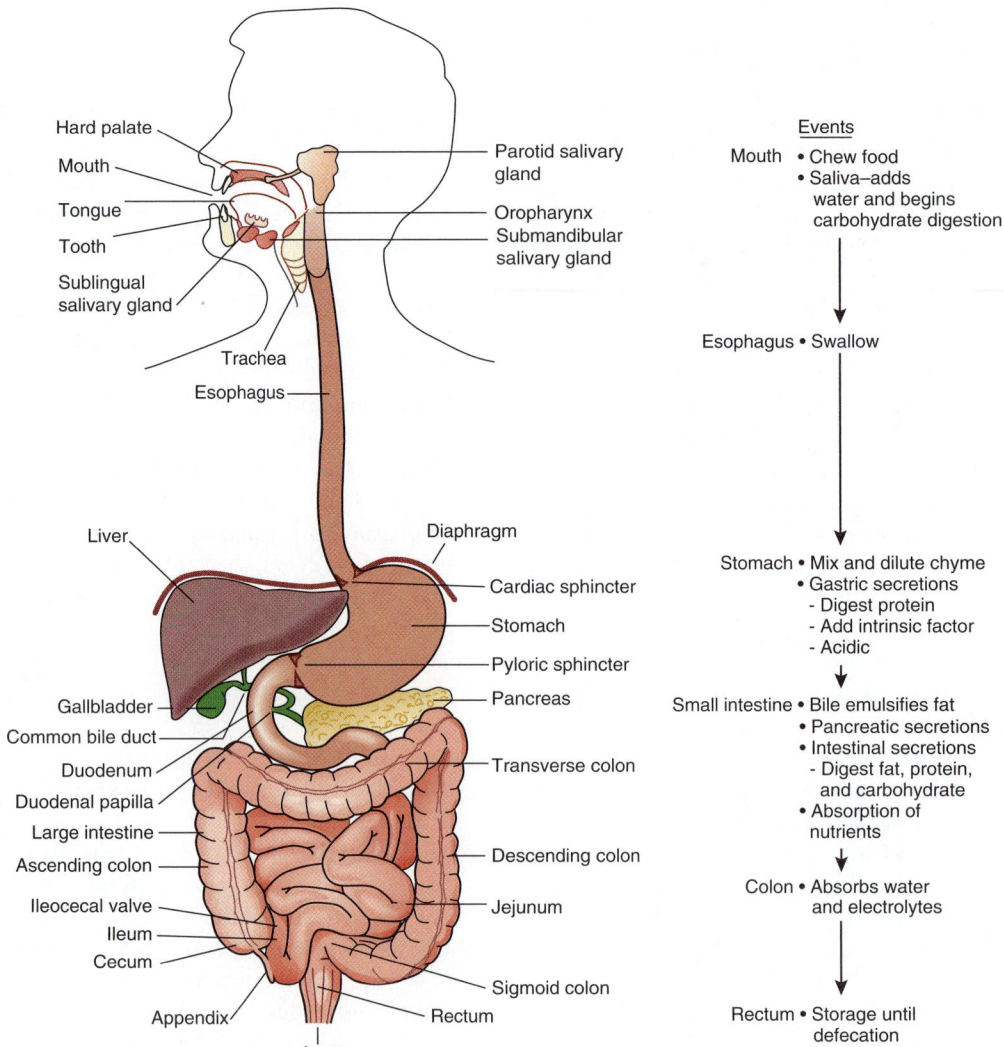

FIGURE 39-1 Anatomy of the digestive system, with associated events. (From Gould B: *Pathophysiology for the health professions,* ed 3, Philadelphia, 2006, Saunders.)

At the distal end of the esophagus is the gastroesophageal or cardiac sphincter, which relaxes as the bolus is swallowed so that it can pass into the stomach. The muscular walls of the stomach overlap in folds, or rugae, which permit the stomach to expand and to hold as much as 1 to 1.5 L of food and liquid. The gastric glands in the stomach mucosa secrete hydrochloric acid, pepsinogen (which begins the digestion of protein), and intrinsic factor, which is needed for the absorption of vitamin B_{12}. The gastric contents, called *chyme,* are slowly emptied through the **pyloric sphincter** into the small intestine. The small intestine is made up of the duodenum at the proximal end, the jejunum, and the ileum at the distal end.

The common bile duct delivers bile, which is produced in the liver and stored in the gallbladder, to the duodenum. Bile acids emulsify fat, that is, they break down large fat molecules into smaller molecules that can be chemically digested by fat enzymes. The pancreatic duct delivers digestive enzymes to the duodenum, including amylase for carbohydrate digestion, trypsin for protein breakdown, and lipase for fats. This mixture of bile and pancreatic enzymes in the duodenum completes the digestion of nutrients, converting

carbohydrates into glucose, protein into amino acids, and fats into fatty acids and glycerol.

Once digestion has been completed in the duodenum, the second function of the GI tract, absorption of nutrients, begins. The small intestine is lined with transverse folds of tissue called *villi.* Approximately 25,000 of these overlapping projections greatly increase the surface area available in the small intestine for nutrient absorption. Each villus is rich with blood vessels that absorb digested nutrients into the **portal circulation** system and carry them directly to the liver for processing. Lymph vessels along the villi absorb fat and deposit it into the systemic circulation. By the time the chyme reaches the terminal end of the small intestine, every nutrient the body needs should have been absorbed. This mass enters the colon, or large intestine, which is made up of the cecum (extending from it is the vermiform appendix), ascending colon, transverse colon, descending colon, sigmoid colon, rectum, and anus. The colon absorbs large amounts of fluids and electrolytes to prevent dehydration of body tissues. Once fluid has been reabsorbed, the remaining solid waste materials, called *feces,* are moved into the sigmoid colon and rectum, and elimination occurs through the anus. This final function is called *defecation*.

DISEASES OF THE GASTROINTESTINAL SYSTEM

GI disorders probably are the most common problems seen in a medical office. Most conditions of the GI system are managed by a primary care physician. About 5% to 10% of patients with GI problems are referred to a gastroenterologist for diagnosis and treatment. It is assumed that problems that stem from dental disorders are treated by dental professionals. This chapter concentrates on the GI problems most frequently seen, diagnosed, and treated in an ambulatory care center.

CHARACTERISTICS OF THE GI SYSTEM

- The abdominal cavity can be divided into four quadrants or nine regions (see Figure 39-2).
- The *peritoneum* is a membrane that lines the abdominal wall and covers the organs of the abdominal cavity.
- The *mesentery* is a dorsal peritoneal fold that attaches the jejunum and ileum to the posterior abdominal wall.
- The *omentum* is a fold of fatty peritoneal tissue with multiple lymph nodes. It hangs from the stomach like an apron, covering the anterior transverse colon and the small intestine. Inflammation of the omentum results in the formation of scar tissue and adhesions.
- The GI system digests and absorbs nutrients for the entire body; if it becomes diseased, all other systems are affected.

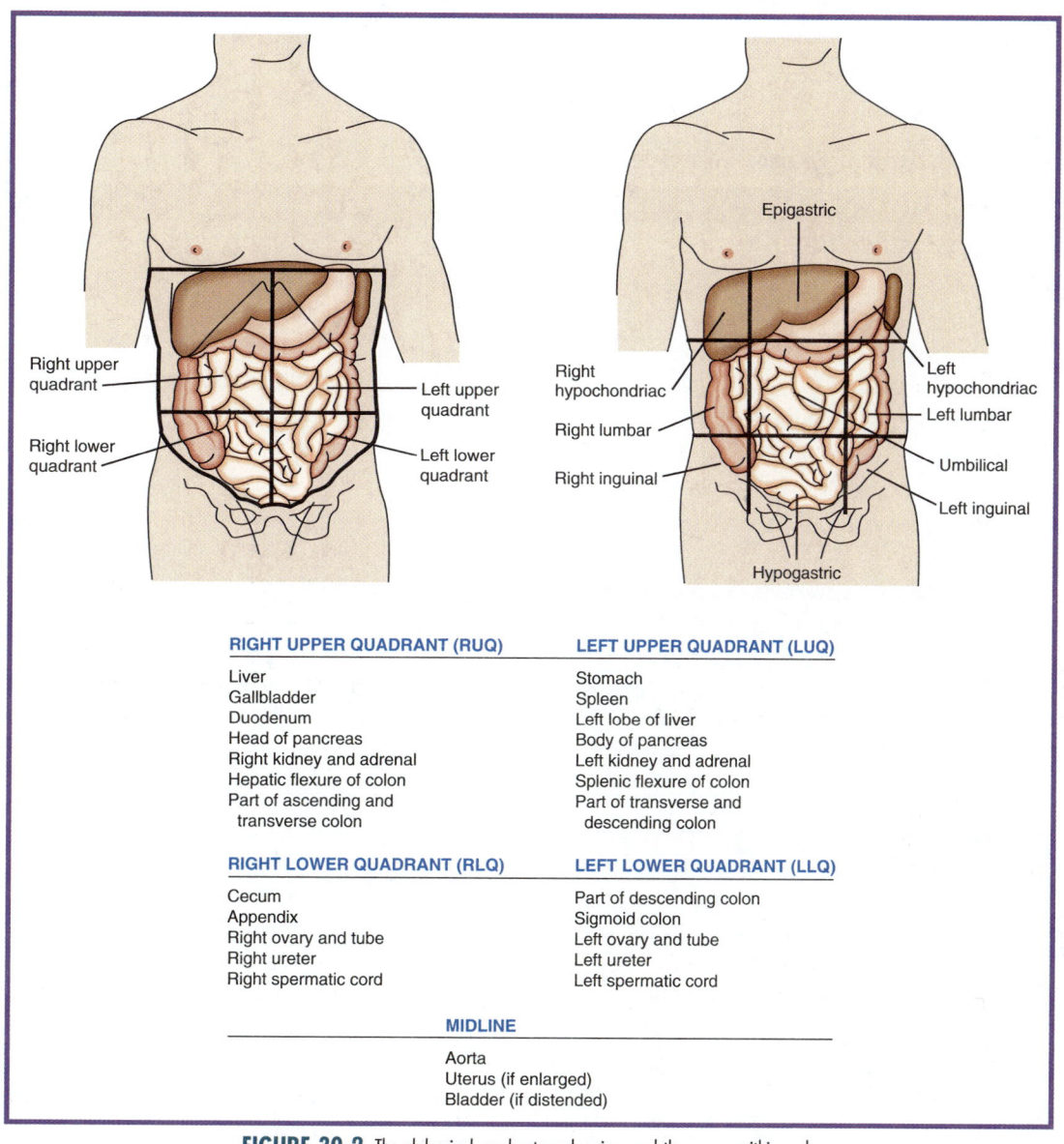

FIGURE 39-2 The abdominal quadrants and regions and the organs within each.

COMMON SIGNS AND SYMPTOMS

A patient with a GI problem may complain of multiple discomforts, including nausea, vomiting, **anorexia**, diarrhea, constipation, and abdominal pain. The medical assistant may find it difficult to identify the exact location and quality of the patient's discomfort. When discussing abdominal pain with the patient, ask the patient to point to or touch the area where the pain is located. This is one way of making sure the correct quadrant or region is identified and the patient is properly prepared for the physician's examination. If possible, document the location of the patient's complaint using the abdominal regions (Figure 39-2), because this is most accurate. For example, if the patient complains of heartburn after eating, this can be charted as: Pt c/o epigastric discomfort after meals; 6 on a pain scale of 10.

CRITICAL THINKING APPLICATION   39-2

Two days a week, Joan works in the telephone screening area of the practice, where she is responsible for the initial management of calls from Dr. Sahani's patients. The following problems from patients are typical of a call day. What are some questions Joan should ask and subsequently document in each patient's chart?
- The mother of a 7-year-old patient is concerned because her son has been vomiting since yesterday.
- The father of an 18-month-old infant reports that the child has had diarrhea for 2 days.
- A 72-year-old patient is concerned about constipation that has not been relieved with laxatives.

Table 39-1 outlines the typical signs, symptoms, and characteristics seen in patients with GI complaints. Using Procedure 39-1, outline how you would respond to the scenarios in Critical Thinking Application 39-2.

Cancers of the Gastrointestinal Tract

Any organ of the digestive tract can develop cancer. The features of malignant tumors and their treatments are described in Chapter 38. These characteristics, including the ability to invade surrounding tissues and metastasize through the blood or lymph system, are true of all cancerous tumors.

TABLE 39-1 Characteristics of Common Gastrointestinal Complaints

COMPLAINT	CHARACTERISTICS	COMPLAINT	CHARACTERISTICS
Nausea	Pallor, diaphoresis, tachycardia	Constipation	*Caused by:*
Vomiting (emesis)	*Caused by:*		Lack of dietary fiber
	GI irritation		Inadequate intake of fluids
	Pain or stress		Lack of exercise
	Inner ear disturbance		Neurologic disorders, including spinal cord injury and multiple sclerosis
	Increased intracranial pressure (ICP)		Side effect of medications (e.g., codeine, iron, antacids)
	Important characteristics to report and record:		Bowel obstruction or tumor
	Onset, frequency, duration of the problem		*Important characteristics to report and record:*
	Yellow or greenish color (indicates bile from the duodenum)		Onset, frequency, duration of the problem
	Pyloric stenosis (causes vomiting of undigested food)		Treatment and effectiveness of over-the-counter medications
	Projectile vomiting (may indicate pyloric stenosis or increased ICP		Diet and fluid intake
	Hematemesis (vomitus that looks like coffee grounds)		Presence of watery diarrhea (may indicate fecal impaction)
Diarrhea	*Caused by:*	Abdominal pain	*Caused by:*
	Infection or inflammation		Ulcerative disease
	Food allergies		Tumor
	Malabsorption syndromes		Appendicitis
	Important characteristics to report and record:		Bowel obstruction
	Onset, frequency, duration of the problem		Food poisoning
	Dehydration (may occur if diarrhea is persistent; occurs more often in infants and older adults)		Infection or inflammatory process
	Presence of blood, mucus, or pus in the stool		*Important characteristics to report and record:*
	Steatorrhea (large, foul-smelling, greasy stools)		Onset, frequency, duration
	Melena (tarry stools from bleeding higher in the digestive tract)		Exact location (using quadrants or abdominal regions)
			Quality of the pain (e.g., burning, cramping, sharp, dull)
			Degree of pain (on a scale of 1 to 10)

Perform Patient Screening Using Established Protocols: Telephone Screening of a Patient with a Gastrointestinal Complaint

GOAL: *To answer the telephone professionally and to manage patients' phone calls according to the physician's guidelines.*
SCENARIO: *A 22-year-old woman reports acute abdominal pain.*

EQUIPMENT and SUPPLIES

- Telephone
- Message pad
- Pen
- Access to the appointments schedule
- Access to the patient's record
- Physician's policy manual for managing patients' phone calls

PROCEDURAL STEPS

1. Answer the telephone by the third ring, speaking directly into the mouthpiece.
   PURPOSE: Answering promptly conveys interest in the caller. Proper positioning of the mouthpiece allows for an audible tone.
2. Speak distinctly, using a pleasant tone and expression, at a moderate rate, and with sufficient volume.
3. Greet the caller, identify the office and/or the physician as well as yourself, and offer to help the caller.
   PURPOSE: So the patient knows she has reached the correct number, as well as the staff member to whom she is speaking.
4. Verify the identity of the caller and access the patient's record.
   PURPOSE: To have the patient's medical record ready for reference regarding the health history and recent care.
5. Determine the caller's needs using therapeutic communication skills.
   PURPOSE: To gather comprehensive information about the caller's complaint and to communicate empathetically regarding the caller's needs.
6. Upon learning the patient's complaint, formulate questions designed to gather the information required to make a decision about when the patient should be seen and the physician notified. On the basis of the patient's gender, age, and complaint of acute abdominal pain, consider the following questions:
   - What are the onset, frequency, and duration of the abdominal pain?
   - What is the exact anatomic location of the discomfort?
   - What is the quality of the pain (e.g., sharp, dull, stabbing)?
   - On a scale of 1 to 10, with 10 being the worst pain, how does she rate the pain?
   - Does the patient have a history of this occurrence? Does she have a history of gynecologic or pelvic disorders?
   - Has she taken any medication for the discomfort and has it been effective?
7. Refer to the physician's policies for patients' phone calls as needed.
   PURPOSE: The medical assistant is not qualified to diagnose the patient. The policies and procedures manual developed by the facility should be used to guide appropriate management of individual patient problems.
8. Depending on the patient's answers to your questions and the physician's policies for the management of abdominal discomfort, refer to the appointment schedule and make an appointment or take a message for the physician to return the patient's call.
9. Document the details of the interaction and the results in the patient's medical record.
   PURPOSE: All communications with a patient, including phone calls, are part of the record of care. Students should document based on role-play answers to questions in Step 6.

Documentation Practice

_____

_____

Table 39-2 describes some of the common malignant tumors found in the GI system. The exact cause of a malignancy may not be known, but exposure to **carcinogens** increases the risk of developing a cancerous tumor. Examples of carcinogens include tobacco and alcohol, as well as exposure to chemicals and radiation. The family history and lifestyle factors, such as consuming a diet high in fat and low in fiber, also can increase a person's risk of developing certain types of cancer.

Disorders of the Esophagus and Stomach

Hiatal Hernia

A hernia is the abnormal protrusion of part of an organ or tissue through the structures that normally contain it. These protrusions can develop in various parts of the body but most frequently are seen in the abdominal region. Causes of herniation include congenital weakness of the structures, trauma, relaxation of ligaments and skeletal muscles, and increased upward pressure from the abdomen. Herniation most often is found in middle-aged or older individuals.

The location of the hernia determines the term by which the protrusion is identified. In patients with a *hiatal hernia*, the upper part of the stomach protrudes through the esophageal opening, the hiatal sphincter of the diaphragm (Figure 39-3). With a *sliding hiatal hernia*, part of the stomach moves above the diaphragm when the individual is supine and slides back down into the abdominal cavity when the person stands. Part of the fundus of the stomach moves through the weakened hiatus in a *paraesophageal hiatal hernia*. Food may lodge in the herniated part of the stomach, causing reflux of

TABLE 39-2   Cancers of the Gastrointestinal Tract

TUMOR	CHARACTERISTICS	CAUSE OR CONTRIBUTING FACTORS
Oral tumor	White mass in or on the mouth that bleeds easily; ulcer or fissure that does not heal; the mass usually is not painful	Cancer of the lip (pipe smoking), cancer of the tongue or gums (chewing tobacco)
Esophageal cancer	Typically found in the distal esophagus; initial sign is dysphagia (difficulty swallowing)	Associated with chronic irritation resulting from chronic esophagitis, alcohol abuse, or smoking
Gastric cancer	Asymptomatic in early stages; usually not diagnosed until well advanced; poor prognosis; marked by anorexia, indigestion, weight loss, fatigue; tests positive for occult blood in the stool	Food preservatives, long-term use of nitrates, smoked foods; genetic association; chronic gastritis
Liver cancer	Primary malignant tumors rare, usually a metastasized secondary tumor; initial symptoms mild; anorexia, vomiting, weight loss, fatigue, hepatomegaly, splenomegaly, portal hypertension; usually advanced when diagnosed	Primary tumor caused by cirrhosis from hepatitis or chemical exposure
Pancreatic cancer	Weight loss, jaundice; usually advanced when diagnosed; metastasis occurs early; no effective treatment	Cigarette smoking
Colorectal cancer	Usually develops from polyps in the colon; metastasis to the liver common; initial signs depend on location of tumor, may include changes in the character of stool, iron-deficiency anemia, fatigue, weight loss, frank bleeding, or melena	Genetic or familial link; diet high in fat, sugar, and red meat and low in fiber; usually occurs in patients over age 55

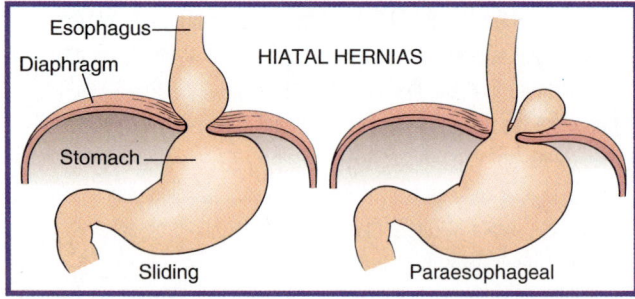

FIGURE 39-3 Hiatal hernias. (From Damjanov I: *Pathology for the health professions*, ed 3, St Louis, 2006, Saunders.)

highly acidic stomach contents into the esophagus, dysphagia, and chronic esophagitis, which may cause fibrosis and stricture. Patients complain of heartburn, frequent belching, and increased discomfort when they cough, bend over, or lie down after eating. Patients with hiatal hernias are treated medically with Prilosec, Nexium, Pepcid, Tagamet, or Zantac. Treatment may include dietary modifications, such as avoiding caffeine, cigarettes, and alcohol; eating six small meals a day; losing weight; avoiding lying down after meals; and raising the head of the bed 6 to 8 inches.

Gastroesophageal Reflux Disease

Gastroesophageal reflux disease (GERD) occurs when the gastro-esophageal sphincter (cardiac sphincter) at the distal end of the esophagus does not close properly, allowing acidic stomach contents to leak back, or reflux, into the esophagus. The regurgitated acidic contents of the stomach irritate the esophageal lining, causing heartburn symptoms. Occasional heartburn is not a problem, but a patient who experiences heartburn more than twice a week is

diagnosed with GERD. All age groups can be diagnosed with GERD; however, it is seen most frequently in adults and is associated with alcohol use, pregnancy, and smoking; it is very common in overweight patients. Besides persistent heartburn, patients may report chest pain, hoarseness in the morning, difficulty swallowing, a feeling of tightness in the throat or a choking sensation, dry cough, and bad breath from the reflux of partly digested food. GERD frequently is seen in patients with hiatal hernias, and treatment protocols are similar in the two conditions.

Laparoscopic repair of the gastroesophageal sphincter may be recommended if lifestyle changes and medication are not effective in curing the problem. The U.S. Food and Drug Administration (FDA) has approved an Enteryx implant, which is placed next to the sphincter with an endoscope. The Enteryx device releases a solution that helps strengthen the muscle. The most important concern with chronic GERD is the potential for developing Barrett's esophagus, a precancerous condition caused by long-term exposure of esophageal cells to gastric contents. Patients diagnosed with GERD are followed regularly by a gastroenterologist so that these abnormal cells can be detected early and removed before cancerous changes occur.

Gastric and Duodenal Ulcers

Peptic ulcers occur most frequently in the proximal duodenum (duodenal ulcer) but may also be found in the stomach (gastric ulcer). Both types are characterized by an area of breakdown of the mucosal membrane, which leads to ulceration of the epithelial lining of the duodenum or stomach (Figure 39-4).

The first sign of a peptic ulcer may be iron-deficiency anemia or a positive stool test for occult blood, which results from erosion of blood vessels in the organ wall. Patients typically complain of gnawing or burning pain in the epigastric area between meals.

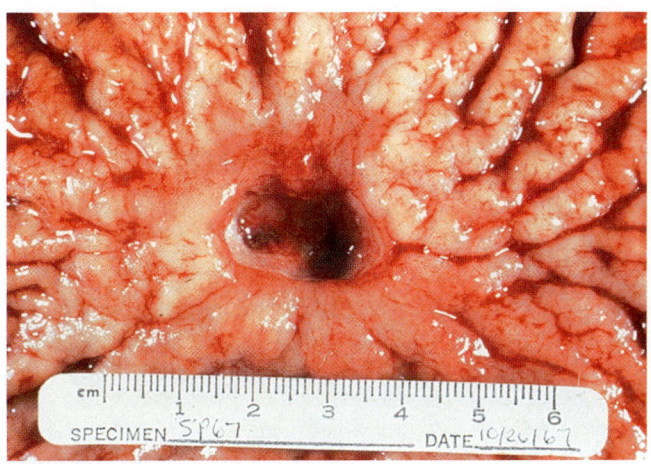

FIGURE 39-4 Peptic ulcer. (From Leonard P: *Building a medical vocabulary: with Spanish translations,* ed 7, St Louis, 2009, Saunders.)

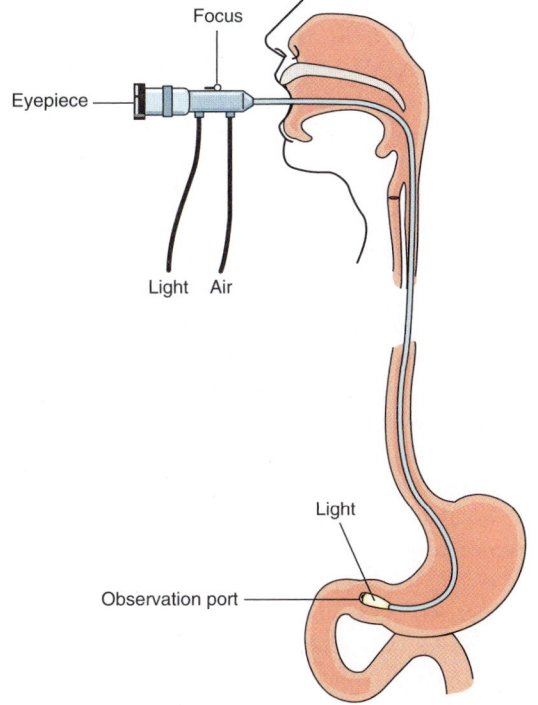

FIGURE 39-5 Fiberoptic endoscopy of the stomach. (From Phipps WJ, Sands JK, Marek JF, editors: *Medical-surgical nursing: health and illness perspectives,* ed 7, Philadelphia, 2003, Saunders.)

occult (hidden) blood. Blood tests also are ordered to establish the **hemoglobin** and **hematocrit** levels.

Peptic ulcers can appear under a variety of predisposing circumstances, including use of alcohol, smoking, use of nonsteroidal anti-inflammatory drugs (NSAIDs) or corticosteroids (e.g., prednisone), and genetic predisposition. However, research indicates that 80% of gastric ulcers and 90% of duodenal ulcers are caused by the *Helicobacter pylori* bacterium. *H. pylori* can be diagnosed either by a blood test that measures the presence of antibodies to the bacteria or by a breath test that is done after the patient swallows a drink containing urea and carbon. Expired air is examined to detect the bacteria. The diagnosis is confirmed with biopsy samples of the gastric and duodenal mucosa obtained during an endoscopic examination.

Peptic ulcers caused by *H. pylori* are treated with a combination of medications, including antibiotics to kill the bacteria and drugs to reduce the production of hydrochloric acid and protect the stomach lining. The most effective treatment is a triple therapy method that lasts 2 weeks and includes two antibiotics (e.g., amoxicillin, Flagyl, Biaxin) and either a histamine blocker (e.g., Tagamet, Zantac) or a proton pump inhibitor (e.g., Prilosec, Prevacid). Surgery may be indicated in severe cases, such as with perforation of the gastric wall. Any ulcer that does not heal is re-evaluated periodically through gastroscopy to rule out cancer.

GI SYSTEM MEDICATIONS

- Histamine stimulates acid-secreting cells to release hydrochloric acid; histamine (H_2)-blockers reduce the amount of hydrochloric acid released into the stomach. Prescription and over-the-counter (OTC) H_2-blockers include ranitidine (Zantac), famotidine (Pepcid), cimetidine (Tagamet), and nizatidine (Axid).
- OTC antacids neutralize existing stomach acid and provide rapid pain relief.
- Proton pump inhibitors reduce acid by blocking the action of "pumps" within acid-secreting cells; these drugs include omeprazole (Prilosec), lansoprazole (Prevacid), rabeprazole (Aciphex), esomeprazole (Nexium), and pantoprazole (Protonix).
- Cytoprotective agents help protect tissues lining the stomach and small intestine; they include Pepto-Bismol and the prescription medications sucralfate (Carafate) and misoprostol (Cytotec).

Gastric ulcers may cause weight loss, whereas duodenal lesions often cause nausea and vomiting. If the ulcerative area is bleeding internally, the patient may have **hematemesis** (blood in the vomitus) or melena (coffee ground–like vomitus and/or tarry black stools).

The description of the patient's pain gives the physician a suspicion of the disorder. Examination often shows that the patient is guarding the painful area, characterized by clutching the upper abdominal area and drawing the knees up toward the chest. A definitive diagnosis is based on an upper GI series (x-ray evaluation) or endoscopy (visualization) of the upper GI tract (Figure 39-5). A biopsy sample of the affected area may be taken during the endoscopy to rule out cancer. A stool test may be ordered to check for

Pyloric Stenosis

Pyloric stenosis, which is narrowing and hardening of the pyloric sphincter at the distal end of the stomach, can be caused by scar tissue produced by chronic conditions but typically is seen as a congenital defect in infants. The difficulty becomes apparent in newborns within 2 to 6 weeks of birth, because the infant has projectile vomiting immediately after feeding, as a result of the stomach's inability to empty effectively. Consequently, the baby displays symptoms of failure to thrive, becomes dehydrated, has small and infrequent stools, and is very irritable. Congenital pyloric stenosis typically occurs in first-born males and can be corrected by surgery.

TABLE 39-3 Food-Related Gastrointestinal Disorders

MICROORGANISM	CAUSE	INCUBATION PERIOD	SIGNS AND SYMPTOMS
Staphylococcus aureus	Improper hand washing by food handlers; insufficient refrigeration of salads or improper cooking of meats	4-6 hours	Low body temperature; hypotension; acute, severe nausea, vomiting, cramps
Escherichia coli	Fecal contamination of food or water; improper cooking of meat or washing of fruits and vegetables	24-72 hours	Vomiting; abdominal cramps; diarrhea, may contain blood or mucus
Salmonella sp.	Fecal contamination of food; contaminated work areas; undercooked or raw poultry, eggs, or shellfish	8-48 hours	Acute diarrhea; sometimes vomiting; abdominal cramping and pain; fever
Campylobacter jejuni	Consumption of contaminated food or water; often raw poultry, fresh produce, or unpasteurized milk	2-4 days	Cramping abdominal pain; watery diarrhea; fever
Clostridium botulinum	Bacterial spores in improperly canned or prepared food	12-36 hours	Vomiting or diarrhea possible; neurologic complications (e.g., vision problems, paralysis, respiratory failure)

Intestinal Disorders

Food Poisoning

Food poisoning occurs when food that contains bacteria or toxic material is eaten. This includes poisoning from eating mushrooms, foods that contain poisonous insecticides, and foods that have been contaminated with bacteria or have partially decomposed. The condition usually is self-limiting and subsides within 48 hours. Occasionally, it can be much more severe and even life threatening. The more severe cases usually are seen in young children and in individuals in a weakened state of health. Food poisoning causes generalized gastroenteritis with sudden, intense symptoms (Table 39-3).

A complete patient history is crucial in determining the diagnosis. Stool and blood cultures may be performed to verify the causative pathogen. If the patient has a remaining portion of the suspected ingested food, it should be sent to the laboratory for analysis. In severe cases, the physician may order an endoscopic examination of the GI system to determine the extent of the damage or the condition of the mucosal lining of the system.

The patient is stabilized and symptoms are treated so that dehydration is minimized and electrolyte balance is maintained. Antiemetics, such as prochlorperazine (Compazine) and trimethobenzamide (Tigan) rectal suppositories, may be prescribed to control vomiting. Other medications, such as furazolidone (Furoxone), loperamide (Imodium), or diphenoxylate with atropine (Lomotil), may be used to control diarrhea. If vomiting and diarrhea cannot be corrected within a reasonable time (as determined by age, body size, and health condition), the patient may be hospitalized so that intravenous (IV) fluid replacement can be administered.

Dumping Syndrome

A postsurgical complication of weight loss surgery is rapid gastric emptying, or dumping syndrome. This occurs when the jejunum fills too quickly with undigested food, resulting in intestinal distention and increased intestinal motility. Signs and symptoms include nausea, abdominal cramps, diarrhea, vertigo, tachycardia, and **diaphoresis.** The condition typically occurs after the individual eats sweets or high-fat foods. Patients undergoing weight loss surgery should be instructed to eat frequent small meals that are high in protein and low in simple sugars and to drink fluids between meals rather than with meals. These dietary modifications usually can prevent dumping syndrome.

Irritable Bowel Syndrome

Irritable bowel syndrome (IBS) is a recurrent functional bowel disorder; this means that the bowel does not work as it should, but diagnostic studies fail to show an organic cause for the symptoms. The diagnosis of IBS is made if the patient complains of recurrent abdominal discomfort of at least 3 months; abdominal pain that is relieved by defecation; feeling bloated; a change in bowel habits with constipation, diarrhea, and mucous discharge; and increased flatulence. The most common site of abdominal pain is the left lower quadrant. Diagnostic studies, such as a complete blood count, stool testing for occult blood, urinalysis, barium enema, and colonoscopy, are performed to rule out other GI diseases that have an organic cause.

IBS is more common in women. Symptoms usually appear in late adolescence or early adulthood. The condition seems to have a familial pattern, and IBS may account for up to 50% of referrals to gastroenterologists because of concern about possible organic disease. IBS is quite common; an estimated 9% to 20% of the adult population is affected. The syndrome is associated with food intolerances, menstruation, and stress levels.

Treatment is primarily pharmaceutical, with bulk-forming agents (Metamucil) given for constipation; loperamide (Imodium) or diphenoxylate and atropine (Lomotil) for diarrhea episodes; Lactaid if the patient is lactose intolerant; antispasmodic agents (dicyclomine [Bentyl]) for cramping; and anticholinergic agents (hyoscyamine [Levsin]) and simethicone (Mylicon) for bloating and flatulence. Lubiprostone (Amitiza) may be indicated for women who have IBS with constipation. It increases fluid secretion in the small intestine to help relieve constipation.

Alternative therapies for IBS include acupuncture to relieve cramping and improve bowel function; the herb peppermint to relax intestinal smooth muscles; and probiotic foods, such as yogurt, to provide bacteria that make up the natural flora of the intestinal tract to help relieve symptoms. The patient should be encouraged to keep a food diary in an effort to identify foods that exacerbate the symptoms; to increase fluid and fiber intake; and to avoid spicy and fatty foods and caffeine. Routine exercise also can be very helpful in relieving symptoms.

Patients with IBS can become very frustrated and need confirmation that this is a real problem, even though no organic or anatomic changes are apparent. Patients should be encouraged to follow lifestyle recommendations, including actively working to reduce stress. The medical assistant plays an important role in providing understanding and support to the patient with IBS.

WEIGHT LOSS SURGERY

Bariatric, or weight loss, surgery creates a smaller stomach pouch (about the size of an egg) and bypasses the duodenum, where most of digestion is completed. After the surgery, patients can eat only small amounts of food at one time, which reduces the number of calories consumed. Because the duodenum is bypassed, fewer nutrients are absorbed. The most common gastric bypass surgery is the Roux-en-Y procedure, in which surgical staples or a plastic band is used to create a small pouch at the top of the stomach. The smaller stomach then is anastomosed to the jejunum. This surgery can be done either as an open procedure or with a laparoscope, although the laparoscopic procedure is preferred because it is associated with fewer surgical risks and complications.

Bariatric surgery is an option for patients with a body mass index (BMI) of 40 or higher or those with a BMI of 35 or higher who have a serious medical condition, such as diabetes, hypertension, or sleep apnea. Patients interested in the procedure must undergo a battery of examinations, including a psychological evaluation, and must show that they have been unable to lose weight with other methods.

Recent studies indicate that weight loss after stomach-reduction surgery can drastically improve diabetes mellitus; the greater the weight lost, the more likely the patient is to improve.

Patients begin to lose weight shortly after the procedure and continue to lose for approximately 12 to 24 months. Most individuals lose 60% to 80% of their excess body weight, and most experience resolution of weight-related health issues as the weight comes off, including relief of heartburn, reduced musculoskeletal discomfort, improved breathing, reduced sleep apnea, and lower blood pressure. Because of malabsorption problems, patients may be prone to vitamin B_{12} deficiency, which may necessitate vitamin B_{12} injections on a regular basis; iron deficiency anemia; lack of calcium absorption, which may contribute to osteoporosis; and other vitamin and mineral deficiencies. Patients should take daily vitamin and mineral supplements to reduce the effects of these malabsorption problems.

The FDA recently approved a weight loss procedure, the adjustable gastric band (or AGB), for patients with BMI of 30 or greater who also have at least one condition linked to obesity, such as heart disease or diabetes. With the AGB, the amount of food that can be consumed at one time is reduced by placing a small braceletlike band around the top of the stomach. A circular balloon inside the band can be inflated or deflated with saline solution, allowing the surgeon to control the size of the opening into the stomach.

CRITICAL THINKING APPLICATION 39-3

Dr. Sahani frequently sees patients with IBS. He asks Joan to prepare a handout for patients describing the disorder, making sure to include possible treatments. What should Joan include?

Acute Appendicitis

The vermiform appendix is a narrow pouch approximately 3½ inches long that extends off the cecum of the large intestine. It has no known function but can become inflamed and ultimately infected because of obstruction by a **fecalith** or by foreign material. As bacteria multiply, the appendix becomes inflamed and swollen, causing ischemia and necrosis of the appendix wall. If the infectious material leaks out or bursts from the appendix, a localized infection forms that may become regional if the abdominal peritoneum becomes involved, resulting in peritonitis. Peritonitis is a serious infection that may become life threatening.

Classic signs of appendicitis include right lower quadrant pain; nausea and vomiting; tenderness at McBurney's point, which is located between the umbilicus and the right anterior superior iliac spine; low-grade fever; and leukocytosis (an increase in the white blood cell count). Other conditions that might cause similar symptoms include ectopic pregnancy or ovarian cyst, a kidney stone lodged in a ureter, and Crohn's disease. Appendicitis is confirmed with computed tomography (CT) or ultrasound. The infected appendix is removed surgically (appendectomy), typically in a laparoscopic procedure, in which a pencil-thin tube with its own lighting system and a miniature video camera is inserted through a small incision in the abdomen to visualize the area. The surgeon removes the appendix with tiny instruments that are inserted through one or two other small abdominal incisions. However, if the appendix has ruptured, a larger incision is needed to clean the abdominal cavity. After surgery, the patient is treated with broad-spectrum antibiotics to prevent or treat infection at the site.

Crohn's Disease

Crohn's disease, also called *regional ileitis* or *regional enteritis*, is an inflammation that may be located anywhere in the alimentary tract but most commonly is found in the ileum. The inflammation begins with a localized area of ulcer development, with healthy tissue interspersed with areas of affected tissue. Inflammation results in the formation of ulcers that eventually invade deeper into the walls of the intestine, creating scar tissue and partial or complete obstruction at the affected site. If this occurs in the small intestine, the damaged wall reduces the intestine's ability to digest and absorb nutrients; if it occurs in the colon, increased motility prevents reabsorption of fluids. Scar tissue from the localized ulceration ultimately can lead to a bowel obstruction, or the ulcer may completely invade the intestinal wall, resulting in perforation and leakage of intestinal contents into the abdominal cavity. **Adhesions** may develop from chronic inflammation, or **fistulas** may form between two loops of the intestine or between the intestine and adjacent organs.

Signs and symptoms of Crohn's disease include loose, semiformed stool; melena if the ulcers break through blood vessels; pain or tenderness in the right lower quadrant; anorexia; weight loss; anemia; and fatigue. Most patients cycle through periods of remission and relapse. The cause of the disease is unknown, although some theories associate the disease with either a viral or bacterial immune response or a genetic predisposition. Risk factors include age (most cases are diagnosed between 15 and 35 years of age), smoking, Jewish or European descent, a family history of the disorder, and residence in a developed country or urban area. The diagnosis is made from a barium enema, a small bowel series, abdominal CT scan, and colonoscopy and is confirmed with a biopsy.

The goals of treatment are to reduce inflammation, manage symptoms, and provide nutritional support. Antiinflammatory drug therapy includes sulfasalazine (Azulfidine), mesalamine (Asacol), and corticosteroids (e.g., prednisone, budesonide [Entocort]), which are used during the acute phases. Immune system suppressors, including azathioprine (Imuran) and infliximab (Remicade), also are recommended to control the immune system's reaction to the inflammatory process. Metronidazole (Flagyl) and ciprofloxacin (Cipro) are antibiotics prescribed for fistulas, and antidiarrheal agents (e.g., Imodium, Lomotil) may provide symptomatic relief. Surgical intervention that involves resection of the diseased bowel and **anastomosis** may be necessary if an intestinal obstruction occurs, a fistula is present, or abscess formation is seen. Unfortunately, the disease usually recurs at the site of the anastomosis. The patient may require dietary supplements with a high-protein, high-calorie diet to maintain a normal weight and vitamin B_{12} shots if ulcerations occur in the distal ileum, where the vitamin is absorbed.

Ulcerative Colitis

Ulcerative colitis causes inflammation that usually starts in the rectum and moves proximally through the colon, affecting the lining of the colon in a continuous pattern. The disease causes the formation of ulcers that invade the mucosal and submucosal layers but do not advance through the entire wall of the colon (Figure 39-6). Ulcerative colitis can affect people of any age; although a familial tendency exists, the cause is unknown. The patient complains of abdominal pain, mucoid stools, and intermittent episodes of bloody

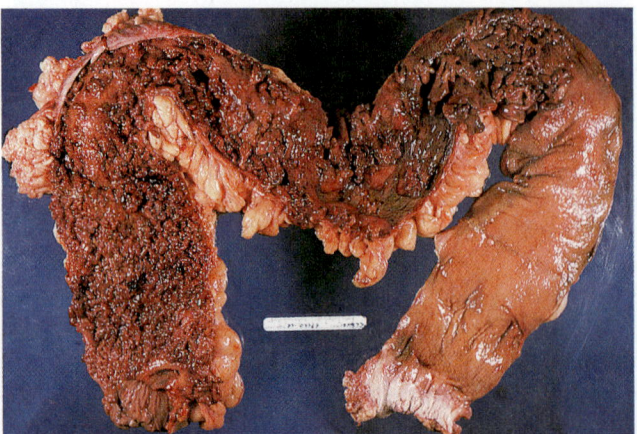

FIGURE 39-6 Ulcerative colitis. (From Damjanov I: *Pathology for the health professions,* ed 3, St Louis, 2006, Saunders.)

diarrhea. As the disease progresses, the patient may experience as many as 10 to 20 stools a day, along with weight loss, fever, and general malaise.

Drug therapy is similar to that for Crohn's disease, but surgical removal of the colon with an **ileostomy** is considered curative for ulcerative colitis. A new surgical procedure, the ileoanal pouch anastomosis, has been developed. In this procedure, a pouch is formed out of the ileum and then is connected directly to the anus. This results in multiple watery bowel movements a day, because the colon is not there to absorb fluid; however, the patient has a continuous GI tract and does not need to wear a collection bag on the abdomen. Patients with ulcerative colitis must be screened annually with a colonoscopy because they have an increased risk of colon cancer.

Celiac Disease

Celiac disease, also known as *celiac sprue,* is a malabsorption syndrome caused by a genetic defect in the intestinal enzyme that metabolizes gluten. Celiac disease can occur at any age once gluten is present in the diet, or it may develop after some form of traumatic event, such as infection, injury, pregnancy, severe stress, or surgery. Gluten is found in all grains, including any products made from wheat, barley, rye, and possibly oats. If the affected individual eats a product that contains gluten, even a small amount, an antigen-antibody reaction occurs that causes destruction of the villi in the small intestine. The intestine is unable to absorb nutrients, and the result is malnutrition. The patient has steatorrhea, abdominal pain, and weight loss. Celiac disease can be treated with strict adherence to a gluten-free diet; rice, soy, corn, and potato flours can be substituted for gluten products. Although oats may not be harmful, oat products frequently are contaminated with wheat, so these should be avoided as well. Gluten-free products, identified by food label claims, are becoming more widely available.

Diverticular Disease

Diverticula are outpouchings or herniations of the muscular lining of the colon, usually the sigmoid colon. Diverticula develop because of chronic constipation and muscular hypertrophy in the colon and become more common as people age. *Diverticulosis* is an asymptomatic diverticular disease in which multiple diverticula are present in the colon but the patient has no complaints other than mild discomfort, diarrhea, constipation, or flatulence. However, if the herniations become blocked with feces and inflammation develops, *diverticulitis* occurs. Signs and symptoms include lower left quadrant cramping, tenderness, or pain; nausea and vomiting; low-grade fever; and leukocytosis. A barium enema or colonoscopy may be done to confirm the presence of diverticula.

Patients with diverticulosis are encouraged to eat a diet high in roughage, to drink plenty of fluids, and to avoid foods with kernels or seeds such as nuts, popcorn, and sunflower, pumpkin, and sesame seeds. Keeping a food diary may help the patient identify problem foods. The goals of dietary management are to prevent the collection of waste in the herniations and to encourage regular, soft bowel movements. The physician may recommend that the patient take a daily fiber product (e.g., Citrucel, Metamucil) to increase the amount of fiber regularly consumed. If diverticula become inflamed,

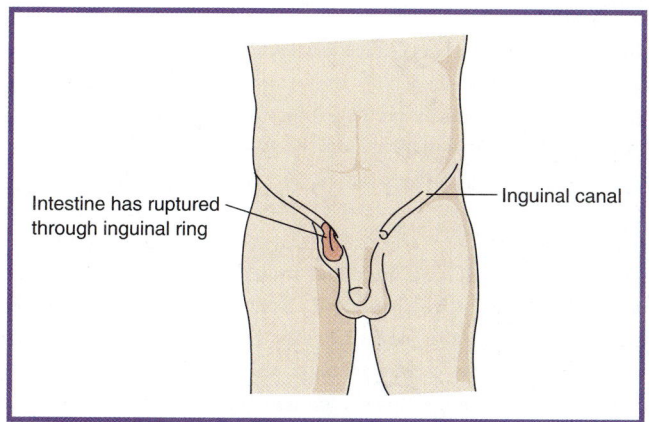

FIGURE 39-7 Herniated inguinal canal.

Intestine has ruptured through inguinal ring

Inguinal canal

antibiotics are prescribed to treat the infection. An acute attack with severe pain and infection may require hospitalization, IV antibiotic therapy, and pain management. Surgery may be necessary if the colon perforates.

Hernias of the Abdomen

Hernias can develop in various parts of the body but most frequently are seen in the abdomen when an organ or part of an organ protrudes through a weakened area in the abdominal muscle wall. The causes of herniation include congenital weakness of the structures, trauma, relaxation of ligaments and skeletal muscles, and increased upward pressure from the abdomen. They most often are found in middle-aged or older individuals. The location of the hernia establishes the term by which the protrusion is identified. Types of hernias include umbilical hernias; incisional hernias at the site of a previous surgery; and inguinal hernias, in which a loop of the bowel protrudes into the inguinal canal (Figure 39-7).

The usual sign of an abdominal hernia is an abnormal lump or bulge that the patient finds while bathing. This bulge is tender, but the pain is mild. The patient also may discover that the bulge can be pushed back into the abdomen, where it remains until some type of moving activity is performed and it reappears. If severe pain is present, the hernia may be trapped or strangulated if blood flow has been compromised. If immediate surgical intervention is not performed, the tissue may die, and **gangrene** will set in.

The physician uses palpation to assess an abdominal or inguinal hernia for size and inspects the area with the patient standing and lying down. An inguinal hernia can be detected in a male by having him perform **Valsalva's maneuver.** The most common treatment is surgical repair in the form of a herniorrhaphy or a hernioplasty.

Hemorrhoids

Hemorrhoids are varicose veins of the anus and rectum. They affect approximately 5% of all adults. The disorder has a familial, hereditary predisposition, and it is common in people with varicose veins of the lower extremities and inguinal hernias. Hemorrhoid formation is related to increased pressure in the rectum, often caused by

constipation. If the swollen veins are within the rectal wall, they are considered internal hemorrhoids, which usually do not cause uncomfortable symptoms; if they are firm and protruding and can be felt and/or seen, they are external hemorrhoids, which usually prompt complaints of pain and itching.

Some patients experience no pain, and other patients experience rectal irritation and discomfort. Frequently, the patient reports that anal itching and burning occur immediately after a bowel movement. If the patient must strain to defecate, bleeding and a protrusion of the swollen mass can occur. Patients often state that the anal area must be bathed or even soaked in warm water after every bowel movement to relieve the itching and pain.

A proctologic examination and inspection of the anal area reveals external hemorrhoids. Proctoscopy is performed to detect internal hemorrhoids of the rectum. A hemoglobin level and red blood cell count may be ordered to determine whether any significant blood loss has occurred. Hemorrhoids are treated with stool softeners (e.g., docusate sodium [Colace]); fiber supplements (e.g., Metamucil, Citrucel); a high-fiber diet; increased fluid intake; and an analgesic ointment applied locally or by suppository to relieve swelling. If these measures do not correct the problem, the next step may be **sclerotherapy** with a chemical injection, cryosurgery, infrared coagulation to burn hemorrhoidal tissue, ligation, or hemorrhoidectomy.

DISEASES OF THE LIVER AND GALLBLADDER

Cirrhosis

The liver is located in the right upper quadrant of the abdomen. Its primary functions are to metabolize nutrients and detoxify drugs or other harmful substances. The liver also excretes proteins that aid in blood clotting and produces bile for fat metabolism. Cirrhosis is a chronic liver disease in which the lobes of the liver become fibrous and hard, and liver cells degenerate, causing deterioration of liver function. Cirrhosis is the twelfth leading cause of death by disease and the fourth most common cause of death in men 40 to 60 years of age. The primary causes of the disease in the United States are chronic alcoholism and hepatitis C. Cirrhosis also can be caused by chronic hepatitis B; nonalcoholic steatohepatitis (NASH), which is characterized by a buildup of fat in the liver, which eventually causes scar formation and loss of function; blocked bile ducts; and severe reactions to prescription drugs or exposure to environmental toxins.

The patient is asymptomatic in the early stages of cirrhosis, but as scar tissue replaces normal hepatocytes, the liver begins to fail and the patient has fatigue, anorexia, weight loss, and abdominal pain. Complications associated with advanced cases of liver failure include dependent edema (fluid retention in the legs); **ascites** (Figure 39-8); bleeding abnormalities; **jaundice**; pruritus from deposits of bile salts on the skin; sensitivity to medication, because the liver is unable to metabolize drugs; **portal hypertension**; **esophageal varices**; insulin resistance, with the development of diabetes mellitus type 2; and cancer of the liver. Treatment is based on the cause of the problem, but avoiding alcohol and eating a nutritious diet are key factors. With advanced cases, the only cure is a liver transplant.

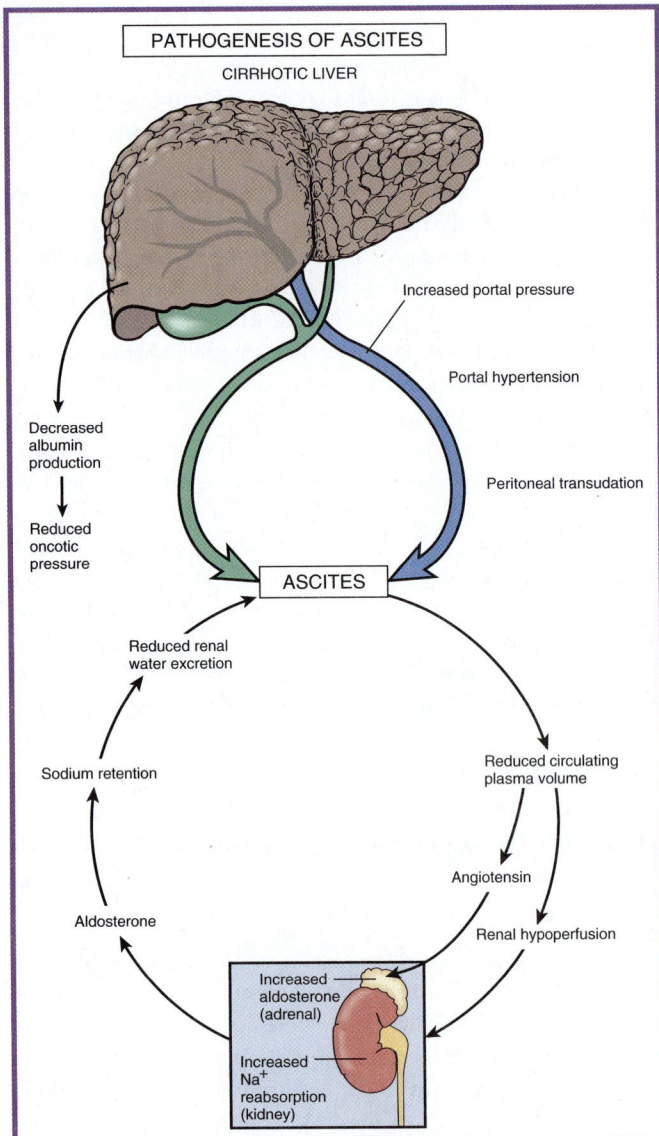

PATHOGENESIS OF ASCITES

CIRRHOTIC LIVER

Increased portal pressure

Portal hypertension

Peritoneal transudation

Decreased albumin production

Reduced oncotic pressure

ASCITES

Reduced renal water excretion

Sodium retention

Aldosterone

Increased aldosterone (adrenal)

Increased Na⁺ reabsorption (kidney)

Reduced circulating plasma volume

Angiotensin

Renal hypoperfusion

FIGURE 39-8 Pathology of ascites. (From Damjanov I: *Pathology for the health professions,* ed 3, St Louis, 2006, Saunders.)

NONALCOHOLIC FATTY LIVER DISEASE

- Accumulation of fat in the liver causes inflammation, which may lead to scar formation, cirrhosis, and liver cancer.
- The condition affects all age groups, including children, but is seen most often in middle-aged people who are overweight or obese and may be diabetic.
- Symptoms are rare in the early stages; the disease often is detected because of abnormal liver blood test results.
- Treatment includes weight loss, exercise, improved diabetes control, and anticholesterol medications.
- The disease can be life threatening; approximately 25% of patients develop serious liver disease that requires a transplant.

Hepatitis

Inflammation of the liver, called *hepatitis,* may be caused by a localized infection (viral hepatitis), a systemic infection, chemical exposure, or a complication of drug metabolism. Mild inflammation temporarily impairs function, but severe inflammation may lead to necrosis and serious complications.

Viral Hepatitis

Acute viral hepatitis is an infection of the liver that causes a sudden onset of hepatocyte inflammation. Several forms of the hepatitis virus are categorized as hepatitides A, B, C, D, E, and G (Table 39-4). Hepatic cells can regenerate; therefore, depending on the degree of liver involvement, the patient may recover completely or could develop widespread necrosis, cirrhosis, and liver failure. Chronic inflammation, defined as the presence of the disease for longer than 6 months, can occur with hepatitis B, C, or D. This usually results in permanent liver damage and an associated increased risk of liver cancer. Individuals infected with hepatitis B, C, or D may become lifelong carriers of the disease. Hepatitis carriers are asymptomatic but can transmit the virus to others.

The hepatitis A virus (HAV) is transmitted through contaminated water or shellfish. Some parts of the world are **endemic** for the disease, and a vaccine is available. The hepatitis B virus (HBV) has a relatively long incubation period, which makes tracking the source of the infection difficult. Because the virus is found in all blood and body fluids, it can be transmitted in many ways, including needlesticks, human bites from individuals infected with the virus, sexual contact, and fetal transmission. Immunization of individuals at increased risk is highly recommended. All healthcare personnel are included in this group, because they are at increased risk for infection through exposure to blood or blood products and body fluids. HBV immunization is included as part of the pediatric immunizations (see Chapter 42).

As a healthcare professional, the medical assistant cares for sick people on a daily basis who may be carriers of the hepatitis virus. Changing dressings, collecting specimens, holding a patient's hand that was just used to cover the mouth, and discarding a wet baby diaper all are possible ways that exposure can occur. The first line of defense, regardless of whether the medical assistant has been immunized, is frequent sanitization of the hands and wearing gloves when exposure to blood or body fluids is possible.

Diagnosis and Treatment

Hepatitides A, B, and C are diagnosed through identification of the virus or antibodies to the virus in the blood. Another useful diagnostic test is a liver biopsy. Once the infection has been diagnosed, liver function tests are done periodically throughout the course of the disease to determine the degree of liver damage. Patients with hepatitis B, C, or D must be monitored for possible chronic hepatitis and the development of a carrier state. Prescription medications include interferon, which stimulates the immune response, and antiviral drugs (e.g., telbivudine [Tyzeka], entecavir [Baraclude]) to prevent viral cell replication. Otherwise, the treatment for all forms of hepatitis generally consists of bed rest and a high-protein diet.

The best form of treatment for hepatitis B is prevention through vaccination against the disease. The vaccine is given intramuscularly in three doses. The first two are given 30 days apart, and the third

TABLE 39-4   Characteristics of the Types of Viral Hepatitis

HEPATITIS TYPE	MODE OF TRANSMISSION	INCUBATION PERIOD	SYMPTOMS
A	Fecal-oral (food or water contaminated by feces from infected person); contaminated raw shellfish; infected household members or sexual partners	2-7 weeks	Fatigue, weakness, anorexia; some patients have joint pain, hepatomegaly, lymphadenopathy, jaundice
B (serum hepatitis)	Blood and body fluids; placental transfer	1-6 months	General malaise, joint swelling, pruritic rash, hepatomegaly, anorexia, nausea, vomiting, dark yellowish-brown urine, jaundice; may become chronic
C (non-A non-B)	Blood and body fluids; most frequent type of posttransfusion hepatitis	2 weeks-6 months	Acute onset of fever, chills malaise, nausea, vomiting; frequently becomes chronic
D (delta virus)	Blood and body fluids	Seen only in patients with hepatitis B	Similar to those of hepatitis B; increases the severity of hepatitis B
E	Fecal-oral	2-9 weeks	Similar to those in hepatitis A; seen in India, Asia, Africa, and Central America; mild form but can cause death in pregnant women
G	Blood and blood products	Not known	Similar to those of hepatitis C; may become chronic but does not appear to be an important cause of clinical liver disease

is given 6 months after the first. As discussed in Chapter 27, the Occupational Safety and Health Administration (OSHA) requires healthcare employers to make the vaccine available to employees free of charge. Medical assistant programs encourage students to be vaccinated, because they also are at risk for acquiring the disease.

GROUPS AT RISK FOR HEPATITIS A, B, AND C

- **Hepatitis A:** day care workers and clients, institutionalized residents, individuals traveling to infected areas
- **Hepatitis B:** IV drug users, homosexual men, hemodialysis patients, hemophiliac individuals, healthcare workers, individuals with a history of frequent sexual partners
- **Hepatitis C:** patients receiving frequent blood transfusions, homosexual men, IV drug users, healthcare workers

CRITICAL THINKING APPLICATION   39-4

As a healthcare worker who may be exposed to blood and body fluids, Joan is quite concerned about contracting viral hepatitis. For what types of hepatitis is she at risk in Dr. Sahani's office? What can she do to reduce her risk and protect herself from contracting these diseases?

Cholelithiasis (Gallstones)

The gallbladder is an accessory organ of the GI system that stores the bile excreted by the liver. Cholelithiasis, or gallstones, form in the gallbladder from insoluble cholesterol and bile salt. These stones vary in size and number. The reasons for formation are not always clear, although gallstones are more common with a

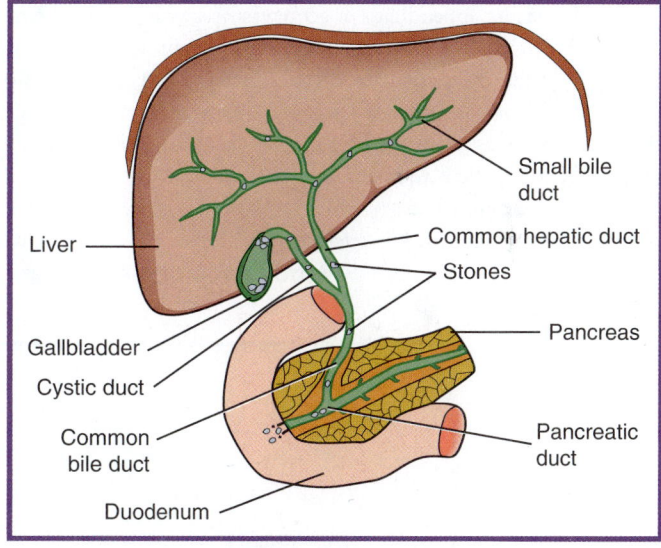

FIGURE 39-9 Gallstones.

high-calorie, high-cholesterol diet and are associated with obesity (Figure 39-9). About 20% of people older than age 65 develop cholelithiasis, and the risk is three times higher for women than for men.

Signs and Symptoms

Most gallstones are asymptomatic and are discovered incidentally during a routine x-ray. Pain usually occurs when the stones move and obstruct the cystic or common bile ducts. The pain is felt in the epigastric region and the right upper quadrant, often radiating into the right upper back area, and is worse after a high-fat meal. Nausea and vomiting may accompany the pain. The pain hits in a wavelike pattern and is called *colicky pain* or *biliary colic*. If the obstruction is not corrected, jaundice may develop.

Diagnosis and Treatment

The physician bases the preliminary diagnosis on the patient's symptoms and on the signs noted on palpation of the upper right quadrant. To confirm the diagnosis, blood tests may be done to detect signs of infection, obstruction, pancreatitis, or jaundice, and an abdominal sonogram is performed to visualize the stones. CT scan may show gallstones, and magnetic resonance (MR) cholangiography may be ordered to diagnose blocked bile ducts. In addition, cholescintigraphy (a hepatobiliary iminodiacetic acid [HIDA] scan) can be ordered to diagnose biliary tract obstruction. The patient is given an IV injection of radioactive material (HIDA), which is taken up by the liver and is excreted into the biliary tract. A nuclear scanner then takes pictures of the biliary tract over a 2-hour period.

Treatment is surgical removal of the gallbladder (cholecystectomy), which usually is done laparoscopically. Gallstones may be fragmented by **lithotripsy** procedures.

THE MEDICAL ASSISTANT'S ROLE IN THE GASTROINTESTINAL EXAMINATION

Emotional factors play an important part in many GI problems, often making the separation of functional and organic disorders difficult. Some forms of GI disease may demand immediate attention, such as acute appendicitis or acute gastritis with possible hemorrhage. Both may require surgical therapy. Careful questioning is needed to guide the patient to a more precise description of the symptoms. In the role of liaison between the patient and the physician, the medical assistant can help the physician make the diagnosis and can get the patient the treatment needed.

General abdominal discomfort (colic) is common, because abdominal pain frequently is referred pain (Figure 39-10), that is, the pain felt in the abdomen actually is generated from an organ elsewhere. The pain may not be located directly over the involved organ or the point of the disorder. The patient's pain is referred to the site of the organ during fetal development. Even though the organ moves during fetal development, its nerves persist in referring sensations to its primitive location.

Assisting with the Examination

When a patient describes and points to the location of the pain, the medical assistant must know the underlying organs that may be involved. Record the quadrant or region in which the pain is located so that the physician can immediately assess this area when the examination begins. The physician's inspection of the abdomen begins with noting any change in skin color, such as jaundice. Striae (silver stretch marks), petechiae (small, purple hemorrhagic spots), scars, and visible masses may be seen. The contour of the abdomen may be flat, rounded, or bulging in localized areas.

The physician uses palpation and percussion to evaluate the entire abdominal area. As this is done, the medical assistant should remove the drape from the area to be examined and should redrape the patient once the physician has completed this segment of the examination. In addition, the physician may want findings noted as the examination progresses. If the physician wants to examine the anal area, have the patient turn onto his or her left side, and then assist the patient into Sims' position. As this is done, make sure the patient remains draped. After the patient is in Sims' position, adjust the drape on an angle so that it can be easily lifted for the final part of the examination.

> ### CRITICAL THINKING APPLICATION   39-5
>
> Joan is responsible for initially questioning patients about complaints and clearly documenting this information in the patient's chart. What information should Joan include that details each patient's problem and would be helpful for the physician in determining the patient's diagnosis?

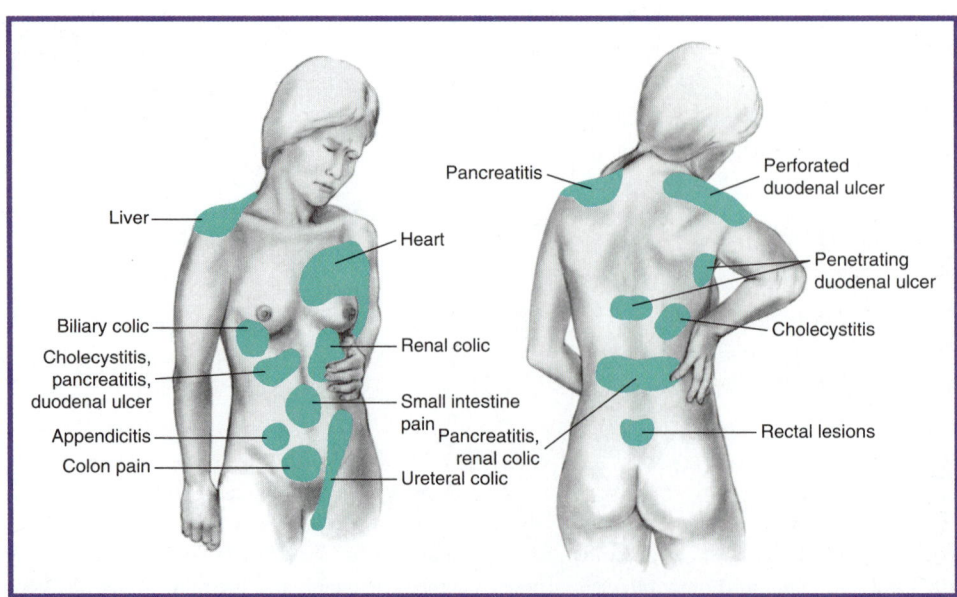

FIGURE 39-10 Common site of referred abdominal pain. (From Jarvis C: *Physical examination and health assessment*, ed 4, Philadelphia, 2004, Saunders.)

Diagnostic Procedures

Typical diagnostic procedures for the GI system are summarized in Table 39-5. Although most of these procedures are not performed in the ambulatory care setting, the medical assistant must understand the procedure and the recommended patient preparation so that adequate patient education can be provided. If the patient does not prepare adequately for these procedures, the results will be inconclusive, and an expensive, time-consuming, uncomfortable test may have to be rescheduled. It is very important that patients completely understand what is required; the patient should be given a handout to review at home that repeats the verbal instructions given in the office. Physicians may vary in their preferences for patient preparation for GI diagnostic tests. It is important that the medical assistant refer to the office procedures manual or ask the physician his or her preference before providing patient education.

The most conclusive diagnostic procedure of the GI system is an endoscopic analysis. In this procedure, the upper GI system is examined by passing a soft, flexible tube down the esophagus into the stomach. The colon is examined through an ascending technique, with entrance through the anus. Fiberoptic technology allows the examiner to view the tissues, take images, and collect laboratory samples (e.g., biopsied tissue, gastric fluid, pathogens, bile crystals, cytology samples) during the procedure with only minor discomfort to the patient.

Endoscopic procedures are performed to allow the clinician to observe the function of the gallbladder, biliary ducts, and pancreatic ducts. A dye is injected directly into the ducts of the gallbladder and the pancreas, and examination confirms ductal patency and functioning of the organs.

Sigmoidoscopy and Colonoscopy Examinations

Sigmoidoscopy is used to diagnose hemorrhoids, polyps, and diverticular disorders. Examination with a flexible sigmoidoscope can be performed in the physician's office, because the patient does not undergo anesthesia for the procedure. The patient is positioned in left-lying Sims' position and is draped appropriately. The physician

---

TABLE 39-5 Common Diagnostic Procedures for the Gastrointestinal System

TEST	DESCRIPTION AND PURPOSE	PATIENT PREPARATION
Barium swallow	X-ray or fluoroscopic examination of the pharynx and esophagus after the patient swallows barium sulfate; to diagnose hiatal hernia, esophageal varices, strictures, and tumors; takes 15-20 minutes.	NPO after midnight; remove all metal objects; do not take medication for GERD. Cathartics given after examination to help with excretion of barium.
Upper gastrointestinal (UGI) and small bowel series; air-contrast UGI	X-ray and fluoroscopic examination of esophagus, stomach, and small intestine after patient swallows barium sulfate; to diagnose ulcers, tumors, regional enteritis, and malabsorption syndrome; takes approximately 30 minutes.	Low-fiber diet 2-3 days before, NPO after midnight, no smoking before test. No medications after midnight unless approved by physician. Remove all metal objects. Stool will be chalky and light colored 24-72 hours after the test. Cathartics given after examination to help with excretion of barium. Explain to patient that he or she will swallow a carbonated powder that creates carbon dioxide in the stomach, which helps in visualizing the stomach mucosa.
Barium enema; air-contrast barium enema (ACBE)	X-ray evaluation of large intestine after rectal instillation of barium sulfate; to diagnose colorectal cancer, inflammatory disease of the colon; to detect polyps, diverticula, or obstructions; takes approximately 45 minutes.	No dairy products and liquid diet 24 hours before the test. Take bowel preparation as supplied by radiology department; enemas until clear in the morning. No breakfast; mild laxative or enema after procedure to remove barium. Light-colored stool for 24-72 hours after test. Explain to patient that air is insufflated into the colon after instillation of the barium to aid visualization of the colonic mucosa.
Cholescintigraphy (HIDA scan)	Nuclear scan following IV injection of radioactive material. Pictures of biliary tract are taken over a 2-hour period to determine whether an obstruction caused by cholelithiasis exists. Best tool for diagnosing acute cholecystitis in patients with acute RUQ pain. Gallbladder visualized 60 minutes after injection of radionuclide; takes 4 hours to get all images. IV morphine during nuclear scanning speeds up bile movement to reduce scanning time to 1 hour.	NPO 2 hours before the test; ensures that patient exposure to radioactivity during the procedure is minute. Patient may be given a fatty meal during scanning to determine gallbladder ejection fraction (measures percentage of isotope ejected when gallbladder empties).

Continued

TABLE 39-5 Common Diagnostic Procedures for the Gastrointestinal System—cont'd

TEST	DESCRIPTION AND PURPOSE	PATIENT PREPARATION
Ultrasonography of the liver, gallbladder, biliary system, pancreas	High-frequency sound waves from a transducer penetrate the organ, bounce back to the transducer, and are electronically converted into an image that is recorded on film. Used to diagnose neoplasm of the liver; cholelithiasis in the gallbladder or ducts; pancreatic tumor, abscess, or inflammation.	Does not use contrast or radiation; useful in patients who are allergic to contrast media or are pregnant. Must be performed before barium contrast studies because barium and gas distort sound waves and alter test results. Patient must fast before gallbladder and biliary ultrasound tests.
Sigmoidoscopy	Endoscopic examination of distal sigmoid colon, rectum, and anal canal. Used to diagnose inflammatory, infectious, and ulcerative bowel disease and tumors; and to detect hemorrhoids, polyps, fissures, fistulas, and abscesses in the rectum and anal canal. Air insufflated to distend and visualize the lower intestinal tract. Biopsy specimens may be collected and polyps removed; takes 15-20 minutes.	Light breakfast the morning of the examination; oral cathartic and 2 Fleet enemas. Usually done without sedation in the physician's office or outpatient clinic. Patient may experience gas pains after procedure from air instillation. May have slight rectal bleeding if specimen is collected.
Colonoscopy	Endoscopic examination of the large intestine to detect or monitor inflammatory or ulcerative disease; to locate the site of GI bleeding; and to diagnose tumors or strictures. Air insufflated for better visualization. Biopsy samples collected and polyps removed. Recommended for patients with positive Hemoccult test result and for those at high risk for colon cancer; takes 30-60 minutes.	Clear liquid diet for 48 hours before the test; laxatives; enemas until clear or 1 gallon of Colyte the day before. Large intestine must be completely cleansed. Monitor vital signs before and during procedure. Done with IV sedation in a hospital or outpatient clinic. May have pre-sedation injection of Demerol and Versed. Must drink large amount of fluid to prevent dehydration from test preparation. Patients with valvular heart disease should have prophylactic antibiotics.
Endoscopy	Fiberoptic view of the esophagus and upper GI tract to diagnose or monitor cancer, Barrett's esophagus, peptic ulcers, polyps. Biopsy samples collected and polyps removed; takes 45-60 minutes.	No food or fluids for 8 hours before test; back of throat sprayed with local anesthesia to reduce gag reflex as tube is passed.

GERD, Gastroesophageal reflux disease; *GI,* gastrointestinal; *HIDA,* hepatobiliary iminodiacetic acid; *IV,* intravenous; *NPO,* nothing by mouth; *RUQ,* right upper quadrant.

inserts a short, flexible, lighted tube into the rectum and slowly guides it into the sigmoid colon. The scope transmits an image of the inside of the rectum and colon, allowing the physician to examine the lining of these organs carefully. The scope also blows air into the colon to inflate the organ and improve visualization. The physician may remove polyps or biopsy tissue samples during the procedure. The procedure takes 10 to 20 minutes, during which the patient may complain of pressure and slight cramping in the lower abdomen (Procedure 39-2).

A colonoscope is used to examine the entire length of the large intestine (Figure 39-11). The American Cancer Society recommends that all patients over age 50 have a colonoscopy to screen for colorectal cancer. This procedure usually is performed in a hospital outpatient area, because it requires the use of an IV sedative.

Laboratory Tests

Many of the diagnostic tests for GI disorders are noninvasive. The physician may order a variety of radiographs taken of the digestive system (see Table 39-5). Urine is tested for bilirubin and urinary

amylase levels. The stool is tested for occult blood, intestinal ova and parasites, fat excretion, and color.

Occult Blood Screening

Fecal examination is one means of evaluating patients with GI bleeding, obstruction, parasites, dysentery, colitis, or increased fat excretion. The test for ova and parasites is described in Chapter 55. The American Cancer Society recommends that all patients over age 50 be screened for occult blood in the stool. This test may be performed on younger patients if a family history indicates a need. Blood is not found in the stool of healthy individuals. If the person is experiencing bleeding of the intestinal wall, the blood is likely to be *occult,* or hidden, which means that it cannot be seen with the naked eye. A Hemoccult test is done to screen for microscopic bleeding that might occur because of precancerous or cancerous changes in the bowel.

The physician may collect a random stool sample during a routine examination. However, if GI bleeding is suspected, the recommendation is to test three different samples for occult blood. Seven days before the test, the patient should stop taking aspirin and NSAIDs,

PROCEDURE 39-2

Prepare a Patient for Procedures and/or Treatments: Assist with an Endoscopic Examination of the Colon

GOAL: *To assist the physician with the examination, to prepare collected specimens as requested, and to ensure the patient's comfort and safety.*

EQUIPMENT and SUPPLIES

- Nonsterile gloves (for the medical assistant and the physician)
- Appropriate instrument: sigmoidoscope or proctoscope
- Water-soluble lubricant
- Drape and patient gown
- Long cotton-tipped swabs
- Suction source
- Sterile biopsy forceps
- Rectal speculum
- Specimen containers with appropriate preservative added
- Laboratory requisition forms
- Tissue wipes
- Biohazard container
- Patient's record

PROCEDURAL STEPS

1. Sanitize your hands and assemble all required equipment and supplies.
   PURPOSE: To ensure infection control.
2. Identify the patient and explain the procedure. Make sure the patient has completed the proper preparation procedures.
3. Ask the patient to empty the bladder.
   PURPOSE: To aid patient comfort during the examination.
4. Give the patient an examination gown and instruct him or her to remove all clothing below the waist and to put on the gown with the opening to the back. Provide a drape for additional privacy.
5. Obtain and record the patient's vital signs.
   PURPOSE: Baseline vital signs allow detection of variations that might occur during the examination.
6. Assist the patient onto the table. When the physician is ready, place the patient in Sims' position.
7. Drape the patient so that only the anus is exposed. A fenestrated drape (a drape with a circular opening placed over the anus) may be used in place of the rectangular drape.

8. Put on gloves and assist the physician as requested during the examination, including:
   - Lubricating the physician's gloved index finger for the digital examination
   - Lubricating the obturator tip of the instrument before insertion
   - Plugging in the scope's light source when the physician is ready
   - Handing supplies to the physician
   - Collecting specimens by holding the container to accept the sample
   - Labeling specimens immediately, because several specimens may be taken from different areas
   - Disposing of contaminated supplies as you are given them by the physician
9. Throughout the examination, observe the patient for any undue reactions. Encourage the patient to breathe slowly through pursed lips to facilitate relaxation.
10. On completion of the examination, provide the patient with tissues to cleanse the anal area. Remove your gloves, sanitize your hands, and assist the patient into a resting position. Allow the patient time to recover from the procedure. Monitor the patient's blood pressure if indicated.
    PURPOSE: A drop in blood pressure, which often occurs after an invasive procedure, may cause fainting.
11. Once the patient's condition has stabilized, assist the patient off the table and instruct him or her to get dressed. Show the patient where the sink, towels, and tissues are, and provide assistance if needed.
12. Complete all laboratory request forms and specimen container labels, and place specimens in the appropriate location for laboratory pickup.
13. Put on gloves and clean the work area and all equipment used. The endoscope first is sanitized and then is sterilized according to the manufacturer's recommendations. Dispose of gloves in a biohazard waste container and sanitize your hands.
    PURPOSE: To ensure infection control.
14. Record the procedure and any pertinent information in the patient's record.
    PURPOSE: Procedures that are not recorded are considered not done.

---

such as ibuprofen and naproxen (Naprosyn). Starting 72 hours before the stool collections, the patient should not take any more than 250 mg of vitamin C a day; should not eat red meat, including processed meats and cold cuts; and should not eat raw fruits and vegetables, especially melons, radishes, turnips, and horseradish. These restrictions should continue throughout the time the patient is collecting the ordered fecal samples (Procedure 39-3). Failure to follow dietary guidelines or instructions on the use of identified medications can cause false-positive test results.

CRITICAL THINKING APPLICATION   39-6

Dr. Sahani wants to update patient handouts on the preparations necessary for common GI tract diagnostic procedures. He asks Joan to do the initial research and gather pertinent information that should be included. What should Joan include regarding patient preparation for these examinations?

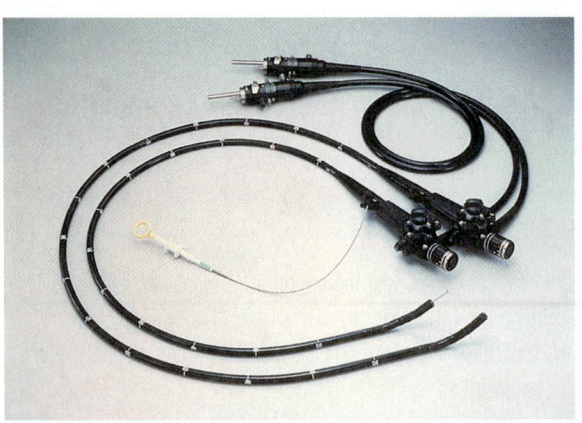

FIGURE 39-11 Flexible colon fiberscopes. (From Phipps WJ, Sands JK, Marek JF, editors: *Medical-surgical nursing: health and illness perspectives*, ed 7, Philadelphia, 2003, Saunders.)

Proctologic Examination

Proctology is the branch of internal medicine that is concerned with diseases and disorders of the colon, rectum, and anus. The anal area is examined with a proctoscope, which allows detection of hemorrhoids, **polyps**, **fissures**, fistulas, and abscesses. The rectum and the sigmoid colon are examined with a flexible sigmoidoscope, and the descending, transverse, and ascending colon sections (or the entire colon) are examined with a colonoscope.

Many people are apprehensive about colorectal examinations. To alleviate this anxiety, instruct the patient in exactly what to do before the examination, and provide support during the procedure. Let the patient know that some discomfort, such as cramping, may be experienced. Furthermore, the sensation of expelling **flatus** or of an impending bowel movement may be felt. These sensations are caused by the instrument and the procedure.

PROCEDURE 39-3

Instruct Patients According to Their Needs to Promote Health Maintenance and Disease Prevention: Instruct Patients in the Collection of a Fecal Specimen

GOAL: *To assist the physician with the collection of a fecal sample, to process the sample for hemoccult screening, and to instruct the patient in hemoccult screening at home.*

EQUIPMENT and SUPPLIES

- Hemoccult slides
- Hemoccult developer
- Applicator sticks
- Disposable examination gloves
- Biohazard waste container
- Patient's record

PROCEDURAL STEPS

1. Sanitize your hands and assemble all required equipment and supplies.
   <u>PURPOSE:</u> To ensure infection control.
2. Identify the patient and explain the procedure.
3. Give the patient an examination gown; instruct him or her to remove all clothing below the waist and to put on the gown with the opening to the back. Provide a drape for additional privacy.
4. Assist the patient onto the table. When the physician is ready, place the patient in the appropriate position for the type of examination ordered.
5. Drape the patient so that only the anus is exposed. A fenestrated drape (drape with a circular opening placed over the anus) may be used in place of the rectangular drape.
6. Put on gloves and assist the physician as requested during the examination, including:
   - Handing the physician supplies
   - Collecting specimens by holding the Hemoccult card to accept the sample
   - Placing a thin smear of fecal material inside Box A
   - Applying a second sample from a different part of the stool inside Box B

- Closing the cover and disposing of contaminated supplies as you are given them by the physician
7. On completion of the examination, remove your gloves, sanitize your hands, and assist the patient into a sitting position.
8. Wait 3 to 5 minutes before developing the sample.
9. Put on gloves and open the flap in the back of the card. Apply 2 drops of Hemoccult developer directly over the smear.
10. Interpret the results in 60 seconds.
11. The Hemoccult test is negative if no trace of color is detectable on or at the edge of the smear; it is positive if any trace of blue is seen on or at the edge of the smear (Figure 1).

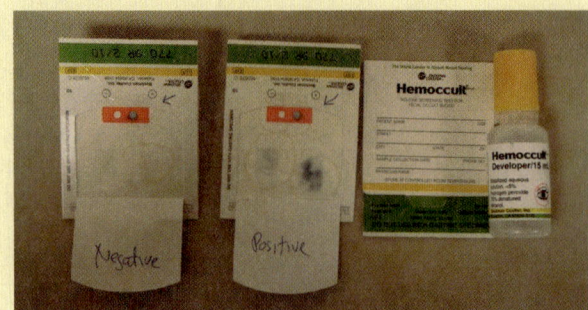

(From Roberts J, Hedges J: *Clinical procedures in emergency medicine*, ed 5, Philadelphia, 2010, Saunders.)

12. Put on gloves and clean the work area and all equipment used. Dispose of the gloves in a biohazard waste container and sanitize your hands.
    <u>PURPOSE:</u> To ensure infection control.
13. Record the procedure and any pertinent information in the patient's record.
    <u>PURPOSE:</u> Procedures that are not recorded are considered not done.

PROCEDURE 39-3—cont'd

PATIENT INSTRUCTIONS FOR HOME COLLECTION OF HEMOCCULT SAMPLES

1. Give the patient a kit for collecting stool samples as ordered by the physician. Typically, the physician orders a sample from three different bowel movements. The patient must follow the recommended medication restrictions and dietary guidelines throughout the testing period, because false-positive results can occur if the recommended medication and dietary restrictions are not followed. These include:
   - No aspirin or nonsteroidal antiinflammatory drugs (NSAIDs) for 7 days before the test
   - No more than 250 mg of vitamin C per day; avoid eating red meats, including processed meats or cold cuts; and avoid raw fruits and vegetables, especially melons, radishes, turnips, and horseradish, for 72 hours before the stool collections

   The patient then is instructed as follows:
2. Store the kit in the bathroom at home or carry it with you while you are away from home until the three different stool samples have been collected.
3. Write your name and other required information on the front of the collection cards.
4. Flush the toilet twice before your bowel movement or cover the toilet with plastic wrap to collect the stool specimen.
5. Use one of the applicator sticks to collect a small fecal sample. Place a smear of stool on the designated area in the first card.
6. Close the card and store it away from heat, light, and strong chemicals such as bleach. Do not place it in a plastic bag.
   PURPOSE: Strong chemicals will affect the slide. The stool sample must air dry to be processed properly.
7. Repeat this procedure for 2 more days or two more bowel movements, as ordered by the physician, using a different card for each sample.
   PURPOSE: To test multiple stool samples for minute amounts of bleeding.
8. After collecting all samples as ordered, seal the test envelope and return the kit to the physician's office. Do not send stool samples in the mail unless you have a special envelope from the physician.
   PURPOSE: To prevent contamination of the mail.

The patient must be given specific instructions on how to prepare the colon for any endoscopic examination (see Table 39-5). You should refer to your employer's procedures manual to determine the preferred method of patient preparation for each test, because physicians' orders may vary.

CLOSING COMMENTS

Patient Education

The GI system is responsible for the nourishment of the entire body. When disease interferes with this process, the individual may become ill and develop serious pathologic disorders. Listen for patients' concerns that may indicate a problem within the system and its accessory organs. Report these concerns to the physician or note them on the patient's medical record for the physician to read. If the office has information that may assist the patient in dealing with a particular problem, lay out the information for the physician to give to the patient; or with the physician's authorization, talk to the patient and offer suggestions that might help the person deal with a particular concern. Learning to perform and assist with diagnostic procedures allows the medical assistant to aid the physician in the diagnostic sequence and to assist the patient in maintaining a healthy GI system.

Legal and Ethical Issues

Legally and ethically, the medical assistant's responsibility is to assist the physician and act as the patient's advocate. All information discussed between the patient and the physician, as well as all testing procedures ordered and done, must remain confidential. Confidentiality and trust are very closely linked, and these two issues form the basis of a sound patient-physician relationship. The medical assistant is an important part of that relationship and can strengthen it through ethical professional conduct.

SUMMARY OF SCENARIO

Joan enjoys working with Dr. Sahani and his GI patients but is constantly challenged to maintain and update information about diseases and disorders of the GI system, as well as their diagnosis and medical management. Joan must consistently work at applying correct medical terminology when documenting patient complaints and must use her knowledge of GI disorders to ask pertinent, detailed questions when gathering patient information.

Joan has also had to update her knowledge of patient preparation for diagnostic procedures so that patients are adequately educated and prepared for scheduled examinations. She participates in workshops offered by her local professional organization to stay up-to-date on medications and treatments for GI diseases, especially current research on infectious hepatitis. Joan is looking forward to active involvement in patient care as she continues to prepare patient education materials and to assist Dr. Sahani as needed in providing high-quality patient care.

SUMMARY OF LEARNING OBJECTIVES

1. **Define, spell, and pronounce the terms listed in the vocabulary.**
   Spelling and pronouncing medical terms correctly bolsters the medical assistant's credibility. Knowing the definitions of these terms promotes confidence in communication with patients and co-workers.

2. **Apply critical thinking skills in performing patient assessment and patient care.**
   Completing the Critical Thinking Application exercises throughout the chapter can help the student medical assistant become more adept at critical analysis of real-life situations.

3. **Describe the primary functions of the GI system.**
   The GI system is responsible for the digestion of food, the absorption of nutrients, and the excretion of waste materials.

4. **Identify the anatomic structures that make up the GI system and describe the physiology of each.**
   The GI system begins at the mouth and ends at the anal canal. The digestive process starts in the mouth with mastication and enzyme action; the bolus of food is swallowed and passes from the esophagus into the stomach, where digestion continues with the addition of hydrochloric acid and further enzyme action. Digestion ends in the duodenum, with pancreatic juices and emulsification of fat by bile, which is excreted by the liver and stored in the gallbladder. Absorption of nutrients takes place in the ileum and jejunum, and fluids are absorbed in the large intestine. Ultimately, waste materials are excreted through the anus.

5. **Differentiate among the abdominal quadrants and regions.**
   The abdominal cavity can be divided into four sections, or quadrants: the right and left upper quadrants and the right and left lower quadrants. More specifically, the abdominal cavity can be divided into nine regions: the right hypochondriac, epigastric, and left hypochondriac; the right lumbar, umbilical, and left lumbar; and the right inguinal, hypogastric, and left inguinal. These anatomic markers are important for clearly identifying the location of a GI problem.

6. **Summarize the typical symptoms and characteristics of GI complaints.**
   Patients with GI disorders may complain of nausea with pallor, diaphoresis, and tachycardia; vomiting because of pain, stress, GI upset, or an inner ear or intracranial pressure disturbance; diarrhea caused by an infection, an allergy, or a malabsorption problem; constipation that occurs because of a low-fiber diet or inadequate fluids, as a side effect of medication, or because of a bowel obstruction or tumor; and abdominal pain that varies in intensity and quality. It is important for the medical assistant to identify the location of the patient's discomfort, using either the abdominal quadrants or the abdominal regions, and to note the onset, duration, and frequency of all symptoms.

7. **Perform telephone screening for patients with GI complaints.**
   Telephone screening for GI complaints involves following the physician's policy manual for management of disorders; gathering detailed information about the onset, duration, and frequency of the problem and the pertinent patient history; recording the interaction in the patient's chart, including use of medications for relief, a pain scale, if

appropriate, and the course of action based on the physician's recommendations.

8. **Distinguish among cancers of the GI tract.**
   Cancers of the GI tract can occur in any of the primary or accessory organs of the system. These can include oral tumors, which manifest as a white mass or as an ulcer; esophageal tumors, which cause dysphagia; gastric tumors, which cause anorexia and weight loss but are difficult to diagnose in the early stages; liver tumors, which usually occur secondary to metastasis from another cancerous site, accompanied by hepatomegaly and portal hypertension; pancreatic cancer, which usually is advanced when diagnosed; and colorectal cancer, which causes changes in bowel function and anemia.

9. **Describe common esophageal and gastric disorders, the signs and symptoms, diagnostic tests, and treatments.**
   Esophageal and gastric disorders include hiatal hernias, in which part of the stomach pushes through the hiatal sphincter of the diaphragm, causing GERD; peptic ulcers, associated with *H. pylori* infections, which are treated with a combination of antibiotics and proton pump inhibitors; and pyloric stenosis, seen most frequently in firstborn male infants, which causes projectile vomiting and must be corrected by surgery. These disorders usually are diagnosed symptomatically and with the use of a barium swallow or an upper GI series of x-ray films. Medical treatment includes the use of omeprazole (Prilosec), esomeprazole (Nexium), famotidine (Pepcid), cimetidine (Tagamet), or ranitidine (Zantac). Surgery may be indicated for repair of a hiatal hernia or gastric ulcers if perforation occurs.

10. **Describe intestinal disorders, the signs and symptoms, diagnostic tests, and treatments.**
    Intestinal disorders include a variety of conditions. Food poisoning causes mild to severe gastroenteritis, and the symptoms are controlled with antiemetics and antidiarrheal medications. Dumping syndrome, which may occur as a postsurgical complication of weight loss surgery, results in widespread GI complaints. IBS is a recurrent functional bowel disorder that causes alternating bouts of diarrhea, flatulence, and constipation; it is treated pharmaceutically with bulk-forming agents, antidiarrheals, antispasmodics, and anticholinergics. Acute appendicitis is diagnosed through a positive McBurney's sign and ultrasonography or CT scan and is treated surgically. Regional enteritis, or Crohn's disease, causes localized areas of ulceration in the intestinal tract and is treated medically to reduce inflammation, manage symptoms, and maintain nutritional status. Ulcerative colitis causes inflammatory ulcers from the anus that move proximally through the colon; it is treated as is Crohn's disease, but surgical removal of the colon is curative. Celiac disease is a malabsorption disorder caused by a genetic defect in the ability to metabolize gluten. Diverticular disease consists of small herniations of the muscular lining of the colon and is managed with dietary changes and surgery if diverticulitis is advanced. The abdominal musculature can become weakened and hernias that require surgical repair can develop. Hemorrhoids, which are varicose veins of the anus, are treated with stool softeners, a high-fiber diet, or surgical repair.

11. **Classify disorders of the liver and gallbladder and list the signs and symptoms, diagnostic tests, and treatments.**

    Disorders of the liver include hepatitis from either viral infection or a chemical reaction, such as alcohol abuse, or as a complication of drug metabolism. Mild inflammation temporarily impairs liver function, but severe inflammation may lead to necrosis and serious complications, including jaundice, cirrhosis, and portal hypertension. The gallbladder stores bile that is excreted by the liver to aid in fat metabolism. If cholelithiasis or cholecystitis develops, the gallbladder may have to be removed surgically to relieve symptoms.

12. **Describe the similarities and differences among the various forms of infectious viral hepatitis.**

    Viral hepatitis is an infection of the liver that causes acute inflammation of hepatocytes. Six forms of this virus exist: A, B, C, D, E, and G. Hepatic cells can regenerate; therefore, depending on the degree of liver involvement, the patient may recover or develop widespread necrosis, cirrhosis, and liver failure. Chronic inflammation can occur with hepatitis B, C, or D. This usually results in permanent liver damage and an associated increased risk of liver cancer. Vaccinations are available for hepatitis A and B.

13. **Summarize the medical assistant's role in the GI examination.**

    The medical assistant provides patient support and education, gathers and records specific details about the patient's complaints, and assists the physician with the examination and diagnostic procedures performed in the ambulatory care setting.

14. **Explain the common diagnostic procedures for the GI system.**

    Diagnostic procedures for the GI system include laboratory studies, such as liver panels and urinary tests for bilirubin and amylase, and stool tests for occult blood, intestinal parasites, and fat excretion. Radiologic and endoscopic tests include barium swallow, upper GI series, barium enema, cholescintigraphy, sigmoidoscopy, and colonoscopy.

15. **Demonstrate the procedure for assisting with an endoscopic colon examination.**

    The endoscopic colon examination is described in Procedure 39-2. The medical assistant prepares the room, equipment, and patient for the procedure; assists the physician throughout the procedure by positioning the patient, monitoring vital signs as indicated, helping with equipment, and labeling specimens for transport to the laboratory; assists the patient after the examination; cleans the equipment and the room; and documents the procedure in the patient's medical record.

16. **Perform the procedural steps for assisting with the collection of a fecal specimen.**

    Procedure 39-3 presents the steps in the procedure. Patient education includes information on proper dietary and drug restrictions and collecting three different stool specimens for analysis for hidden blood in the stool.

17. **Describe the medical assistant's role in the proctologic examination.**

    The medical assistant supports and prepares the patient; positions and drapes the patient for the procedure; monitors vital signs before and during the procedure; and assists the physician with the procedure.

CONNECTIONS

Study Guide Connection: Go to the Chapter 39 Study Guide. Read and complete the activities.

Evolve Connection: Go to the Chapter 39 link at *evolve.elsevier.com/ kinn* to complete the Chapter Review and Chapter Quiz. Peruse other resources listed for this chapter to increase your knowledge of Assisting in Gastroenterology.

Sara Ricci, a CMA (AAMA) with 10 years' experience, works for Dr. Samuel Fineman, a urologist who also manages male reproductive disorders. Dr. Fineman relies on Sara to handle telephone calls from patients, to have a clear understanding of the anatomy and physiology of the renal system, and to assist him in the clinical area of the practice. Although Sara has worked for Dr. Fineman for almost 2 years, occasionally problems still arise that she is not sure how to manage. Sara attends workshops and conferences to earn continuing education units to maintain her CMA credential and tries to choose topics that focus on urologic issues. In addition, she keeps up to date on new diagnostic procedures and treatments for sexually transmitted infections (STIs), including human immunodeficiency virus (HIV) infection and acquired immunodeficiency syndrome (AIDS). Sara helps train other medical assistants in the practice and makes sure adequate patient education supplies are available for self-testicular examination.

While studying this chapter, think about the following questions:

- What is the basic anatomy and physiology of the renal and male reproductive systems?
- What should Sara know about common adult and pediatric urologic disorders so that she is able both to assist the physician in the practice and to answer patients' questions?
- What are some of the genital pathologic conditions seen in men?
- What are the typical signs, symptoms, and treatments for sexually transmitted infections in men?
- How can Sara provide patient education and support for individuals with renal and male reproductive system disorders?

LEARNING OBJECTIVES

1. Define, spell, and pronounce the terms listed in the vocabulary.
2. Apply critical thinking skills in performing the patient assessment and patient care.
3. Describe the anatomy and physiology of the urinary system.
4. Explain the susceptibility of the urinary system to diseases and disorders.
5. Identify the primary signs and symptoms of urinary problems.
6. Detail common diagnostic procedures of the urinary system.
7. Compare and contrast infections and inflammations of the urinary system.
8. Describe urinary tract disorders and cancers.
9. Distinguish between the two methods of treating renal failure.
10. Summarize the typical pediatric urologic disorders.
11. Identify the male organs of reproduction.
12. Determine the causes and effects of prostate disorders.
13. Outline common types of genital pathologic conditions in men.
14. Perform patient education for the testicular self-examination.
15. Analyze the effects of sexually transmitted infections in men.
16. Summarize the characteristics of HIV infection and the diagnostic criteria and treatment protocols.
17. Describe the medical assistant's role in urologic and male reproductive examinations.
18. Discuss HIPAA applications in the urology practice.

VOCABULARY

albuminuria (al-byu-muh-nur-e'-uh) The abnormal presence of albumin protein in the urine.

azotemia (a-zo-te'-me-uh) The retention of excessive quantities of nitrogenous wastes in the blood.

casts Fibrous or protein material molded to the shape of the part in which it has accumulated and thrown off into the urine in kidney disease.

copulation Sexual intercourse.

creatinine (kre'-a-tuhn-en) Nitrogenous waste from muscle metabolism that is excreted in urine.

dysuria Painful or difficulty urination.

erythropoietin (i-rith-ruh-poi-e'-tuhn) A substance released by the kidneys and liver that promotes red blood cell formation.

Kaposi's sarcoma A malignant tumor of endothelial cells that begins as brown or purple papules on the feet and slowly spreads in the skin.

renin An enzyme produced and stored in the glomerulus; it is released by a homeostatic response to raise the blood pressure when needed.

urgency A sudden, compelling desire to urinate and the inability to control the release of urine.

wasting syndrome Physical deterioration resulting in profound weight loss, fatigue, anorexia, and mental confusion.

Urology is the study of the urinary tract in both male and female patients. A physician who specializes in the diseases and disorders of the urinary system is a urologist. Urologists also specialize in conditions associated with the male reproductive system.

ANATOMY AND PHYSIOLOGY OF THE URINARY SYSTEM

The urinary tract consists of bilateral kidneys and ureters, the urinary bladder, and the urethra (Figure 40-1). The main function of the urinary system is to remove waste products from the body. Waste materials are byproducts of the body's metabolic processes, and if left to accumulate in the bloodstream, they can become toxic. The urinary system removes salts and nitrogenous wastes (nitrogen is the product of protein metabolism) from the blood, forming urea, which is excreted. Besides excreting waste material, the urinary system performs other functions, such as:

- Helping to maintain homeostasis by regulating water, electrolyte, and acid-base levels
- Activating vitamin D, which is needed for calcium absorption
- Producing **erythropoietin**, which helps control the rate of red blood cell formation
- Helping to maintain blood pressure by secreting the enzyme **renin**

The kidneys are red-brown, bean-shaped glandular organs. They are located posterior to the peritoneum (retroperitoneal) and against the muscles of the back, roughly between the T12 and L3 vertebrae. The left kidney is situated about 1 inch (2 cm) higher than the right because of the location of the liver.

The kidneys remove unwanted substances from the blood and form urine for excretion. For this crucial function, a great deal of blood circulates through the kidneys—approximately 15% to 30% of the total cardiac output. The blood is delivered to the two kidneys by the renal artery and is distributed through the kidneys by a highway of smaller arteries. The blood then is returned through a

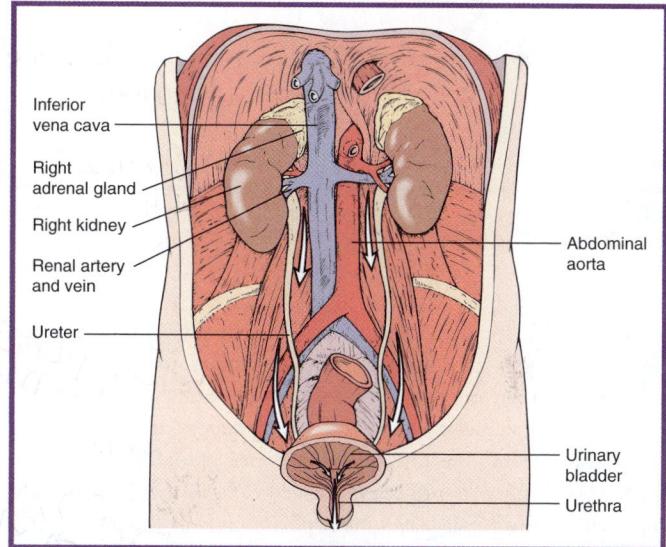

FIGURE 40-1 The urinary system. (From Frazier MS, Drzymkowski JA: *Essentials of human diseases and conditions*, ed 5, St Louis, 2013, Saunders.)

pathway of veins, including the renal vein, which flows into the inferior vena cava in the abdominal cavity.

The outer layer of the kidney, the cortex, contains the functional unit of the kidney, the nephron, where urine is formed as fluid and dissolved substances move between its vascular and tubular structures. Three processes are involved in urine formation: filtration, reabsorption, and excretion. The nephron consists of the glomerulus, a cluster of capillaries extending from the distal renal artery that is partly surrounded by Bowman's capsule. Fluid and dissolved substances are filtered from the glomerulus to Bowman's capsule and then into the proximal convoluted tubules, where most of the fluid is reabsorbed by venules and arterioles surrounding the tubules and sent back into the general circulation. Based on the homeostatic needs of the body, the kidneys determine the type and quantity of

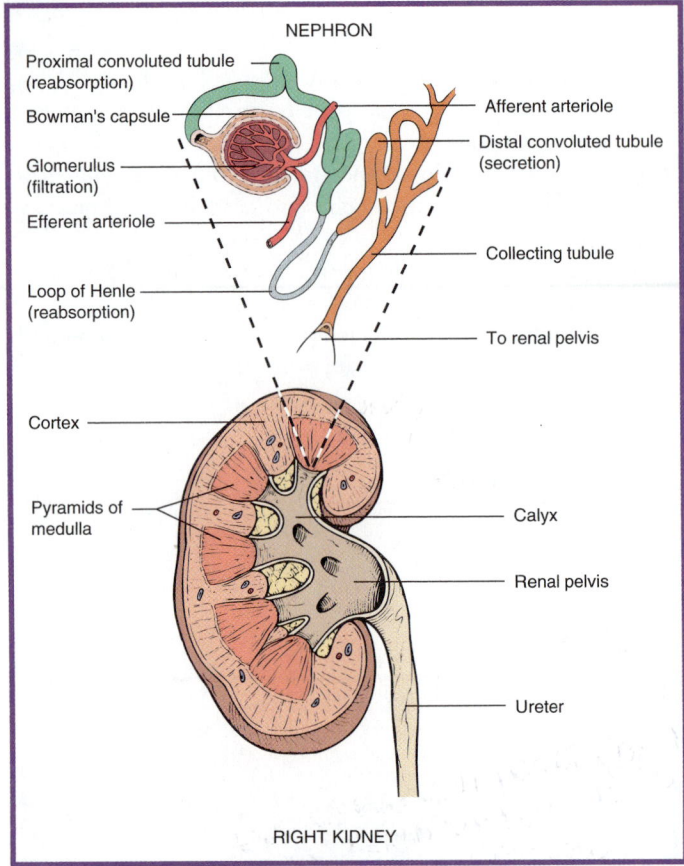

FIGURE 40-2 The kidney. (From Frazier MS, Drzymkowski JA: *Essentials of human diseases and conditions,* ed 5, St Louis, 2013, Saunders.)

substances that are reabsorbed. Finally, the remaining substances are excreted through the distal convoluted tubules to the collecting tubules and then on to the medulla of the kidney. The medulla contains the renal pelvis, where the urine is deposited before passing down the ureters. The distal collection area of the renal pelvis is made up of fingerlike projections, called the *calyces,* where urine is first deposited when it leaves the nephron units of the renal cortex (Figure 40-2).

The bilateral ureters are tubular organs approximately 10 inches (25 cm) long; with the aid of peristaltic waves generated by the ureter's muscle layer, the bilateral ureters move the urine from the kidneys to the urinary bladder. The urinary bladder is a hollow organ lined with smooth muscle that overlaps in rugae formation, which enables the bladder to expand as it fills. When the bladder is full, sphincters open and urine flows into the urethra. The urethra is lined with a mucous membrane, and in males it functions both as the urinary canal and as a passageway for cells and secretions from various reproductive organs. The male urethra is about 8 inches (20 cm) long and is divided into three sections: the prostatic urethra (which passes through the prostate gland at the base of the bladder), the membranous urethra, and the penile urethra. In a female, the urethra is about 1 to 1½ inches (3 to 4 cm) long. Its proximity to the vagina and anus exposes the renal system to microorganisms that can cause infection. The urethra passes the urine from the bladder to the urinary meatus and outside the body. The process of urination is known as *voiding* or *micturition.*

CRITICAL THINKING APPLICATION   **40-1**

Dr. Fineman wants Sara to review a number of pamphlets on the anatomy and physiology of the urinary system for patient education purposes. Sara has researched the available pamphlets and must decide which is best suited to the practice. What material should be included in a comprehensive pamphlet? Are diagrams important for patient understanding?

DISORDERS OF THE URINARY SYSTEM

The urinary tract is made up of a continuous mucosal lining that gives organisms entering the urethra a direct pathway through the system. Of the wide range of symptoms that occur in patients with disorders of the renal system, the most common involve changes in the frequency of urination. **Dysuria**, **urgency**, retention, and incontinence all are common symptoms. Abnormal functions of any part of the urinary tract often can be determined through urinalysis, blood urea nitrogen (BUN) levels, and analysis of **creatinine** clearance. (Urinalysis is discussed in Chapter 52.) Radiologic and endoscopic studies also are important in detecting urinary tract diseases. Table 40-1 summarizes common diagnostic tests of the urinary system.

Urinary Incontinence

Urinary incontinence, which is a temporary or chronic loss of urinary control, can be the result of many conditions, including urinary tract infections, brain disorders, and tissue damage. This disorder also can be caused by straining or coughing in postsurgical patients and in patients with weak pelvic musculature; in such situations, the condition is called *stress incontinence.*

The treatment of incontinence depends on the causative factor. Behavioral approaches include bladder or habit training that teaches the patient to urinate according to an established schedule rather than when he or she has the urge to void. This is helpful for patients who are incontinent as a result of strokes, Parkinson's disease, Alzheimer's disease, central nervous system lesions, or cystitis. Pelvic muscle exercises (Kegel exercises) that strengthen the muscles of the pelvic floor are helpful for patients with stress incontinence. Patients are trained to simulate stopping the flow of urine and holding that contraction for 10 seconds, in sets of 20, three times a day.

Patients with neurogenic bladder, who have lost control of urination because of central nervous system trauma or disease, may have to be catheterized to remove urine from the bladder. Intermittent catheterization to empty the bladder is preferable to indwelling catheters, which often lead to infection. External (condom) catheters can be used for male patients, but they are associated with an increased incidence of urinary tract infections (UTIs). If possible, the patient should be taught to perform routine catheterization throughout the day, or a family member may be involved in care.

Chronic incontinence can be treated pharmacologically with antispasmodic preparations, including tolterodine (Detrol), oxybutynin chloride (Ditropan), solifenacin (Vesicare), or darifenacin (Enablex). When all other treatments have failed, surgical intervention may be the answer. Several different suburethral sling

TABLE 40-1 Common Diagnostic Tests of the Urinary System

TEST	DESCRIPTION	PATIENT PREPARATION
Kidney-ureter-bladder (KUB) x-ray	Flat plate films of the abdomen; show the size, shape, location, and any malformations of the kidneys and bladder; used to visualize calculi.	No specific patient preparation; contraindicated in pregnancy.
Renal scanning	Nuclear scans to determine the size, shape, and function of the kidney or to diagnose obstruction or hypertension; radioisotope is administered intravenously, and images are taken to show distribution.	Patient should void before the procedure; no sedation or fasting required; patient drinks two or three glasses of water before scanning; contraindicated in pregnancy.
Cystography and voiding	X-ray evaluation with contrast dye to study bladder structure or function.	Clear liquids for breakfast; Foley catheter cystourethrogram inserted; may take x-ray films while patient is voiding (voiding cystourethrogram); after procedure, patient forces fluids to eliminate dye and prevent infection.
Intravenous pyelography (IVP); may be called *intravenous urography* (IUG)	Intravenous injection of dye, then x-ray films taken at intervals to show passage through kidneys and ureters into bladder; used to diagnose tumors, calculi, obstructions, and congenital renal problems.	Contraindicated in pregnancy and with iodine allergies; laxative evening before; liquid diet 8 hours before; adequate fluids after; may have enema morning of the study.
Arteriography (angiography)	Injection of dye into the renal artery. Computerized fluoroscopy permits visualization of the blood flow of the kidneys, and serial x-ray films are taken. Used to diagnose stenosis of the renal artery and highly vascular renal cancers.	Nothing by mouth (NPO) 2 to 8 hours before procedure; administer preprocedural medications as ordered; void before the study; warm flush may occur when dye is injected; check for allergies to iodine and shellfish.
Renal computed tomography (CT)	Can be done with or without contrast dye; transverse views of the kidney are taken by CT to detect tumors, abscesses, cysts, and hydronephrosis.	If contrast medium is used, fast 4 hours before procedure; scanner may make loud clicking sounds as it rotates; dye may cause flushing, metallic taste, and headache; check for allergies to iodine and shellfish; remove all metal objects.
Renal ultrasonography	High-frequency sound waves are transmitted through the kidneys to detect abnormalities; used to determine kidney size and to diagnose hydronephrosis, polycystic kidneys, and obstructions of ureters and bladder.	No food or fluid restrictions; noninvasive and painless.
Cystoscopy	Endoscopic view of urethra and bladder for biopsy; used to measure bladder capacity, to find or remove calculi, for dilation of urethra and ureters, and for placement of ureteral stents.	Enemas to clear bowel; force fluids before procedure if local anesthesia is used; for general anesthesia, NPO after midnight; preprocedural sedative to reduce bladder spasms; aftercare: monitor urinary output for 24 hours.
Retrograde pyelography	Injection of dye into the bladder, ureters, and kidneys through a cystoscope to detect stones and other obstructions; can replace an IVP for patients with renal failure, obstructions, or allergies to IV dye.	Same as cystoscopy; check for iodine and shellfish allergies.

procedures have proved successful in treating female incontinence. The surgeon uses a piece of abdominal tissue or a strip of synthetic material to compress the urethra so that urine does not leak during a stressful event, such as jumping or coughing. An artificial urinary sphincter is helpful for men with incontinence. A device shaped like a doughnut is implanted around the neck of the bladder; it keeps the urinary sphincter closed until the patient presses a valve implanted under the skin. This deflates the ring and releases urine from the bladder.

CRITICAL THINKING APPLICATION   40-2

Sara is responsible for scheduling and providing patient preparation instructions for diagnostic radiologic and endoscopic procedures. With Dr. Fineman's approval, she has prepared patient handouts that summarize the correct procedures to follow when scheduled for specific urologic tests. Today she has a patient who needs to be scheduled for both a cystogram and an intravenous pyelogram (IVP). How should the patient prepare for both of these examinations?

Urinary Tract Infections and Inflammations

UTIs occur frequently because the urinary system has a direct opening to the outside, and urine is an excellent medium for bacterial growth. Most UTIs are ascending, that is, they start with pathogen exposure in the perineal area, infecting the continuous mucosa of the urinary system, which in turn allows the pathogen to travel up through the urethra, bladder, and ureters to the kidneys. Infection and inflammation of the urethra is called *urethritis* and that of the bladder is *cystitis*. The resident flora of the colon, *Escherichia coli,* is the usual causative agent.

Women are more susceptible than men to UTIs because of the female anatomy (i.e., a short urethra and the proximity of the anus) and as a result of irritation caused by tampon use, the ingredients of bubble bath formulas, and sexual activity. Older men with prostatic hyperplasia and resultant urinary retention also are at risk for frequent urinary tract infections.

GENERAL SIGNS AND SYMPTOMS OF URINARY TRACT INFECTION

- Overwhelming urge to urinate (urgency)
- Burning on urination (dysuria)
- Urgency with frequent, small amounts of urine
- Blood in the urine (hematuria) or cloudy, dark, foul-smelling urine
- Frequent urination at night (nocturia)

Urethritis

Urethritis, or inflammation of the urethra, is more common in men. It typically is caused by chlamydia or gonorrhea bacteria. Symptoms include the discharge of pus, an itching sensation at the opening of the urethra, and burning on urination. Infectious urethritis can cause cystitis in women, so sexual partners also should be treated. Urinalysis may show hematuria as well as pyuria (pus in the urine).

Cystitis

Cystitis, an infection of the urinary bladder, causes inflammation of the bladder wall and urinary urgency. Symptoms include very mild to acute discomfort in the lower abdomen, urinary frequency, and painful urination (dysuria). The patient may have signs of a systemic infection, including fever, general malaise, and leukocytosis. A positive diagnostic urinalysis shows more than 100,000 bacteria per milliliter of urine, pyuria, and hematuria. An infection of the urinary bladder is especially difficult to eliminate because of the bladder's overlapping rugae walls. It is very important that patients understand that, to prevent a recurrence of the infection, they must complete the entire antibiotic prescription to destroy all the bacteria in the folds of tissue.

Pyelonephritis

Pyelonephritis, an inflammation of the renal pelvis and kidney, is the most common type of renal disease. It is caused by bacteria that ascend from the lower urinary tract and is associated with conditions such as urinary retention or obstruction that promotes urinary stasis and the growth of bacteria. It frequently is preceded by urethritis and cystitis. With pyelonephritis, pus collects in the renal pelvis, and abscesses form. Symptoms include fever, chills, nausea, vomiting, and flank (lateral lumbar) pain. The patient reports foul-smelling, dark urine with frequency and urgency.

Diagnostic studies include urinalysis of a clean-catch urine sample. It reveals hematuria, pyuria, increased white and red blood cells, **albuminuria**, **casts**, and bacteria. Urine cultures usually are done to determine the causative agent.

Treatment of Urinary Tract Infections

UTIs are treated with antibiotics, such as ciprofloxacin (Cipro), nitrofurantoin (Macrodantin, Furadantin), sulfamethoxazole (Bactrim, Septra), and levofloxacin (Levaquin). Patients may also be prescribed a urinary tract analgesic, such as phenazopyridine hydrochloride (Pyridium), which is rapidly excreted in the urine and has a topical analgesic effect that helps relieve pain, burning, urgency, and frequency. However, Pyridium gives the urine an orange to red color, which initially may be misinterpreted as hematuria. Patients diagnosed with UTIs are encouraged to force fluids to dilute the urine and flush the urinary tract. A follow-up urinalysis should be run to confirm the effectiveness of antibiotic therapy in curing the infection. UTIs tend to recur unless the cause of the infection is removed.

The medical assistant should instruct the patient to finish the entire antibiotic prescription as ordered, to maintain proper hygiene, to empty the bladder completely when the urge to void arises, and, for female patients, to wipe the bottom from front to back to discourage the spread of *E. coli* from the anal area toward the urethral region. Cranberry juice may be recommended as a prophylactic measure, because it contains substances that discourage *E. coli* growth and help maintain the acidity of urine.

CRITICAL THINKING APPLICATION   40-3

Tabitha Allison, a 22-year-old patient of Dr. Fineman, was diagnosed today with her third UTI in as many months. Patient education on prevention and treatment of UTIs is needed. What should Sara tell her?

Glomerulonephritis

Acute glomerulonephritis, or degenerative inflammation of the glomeruli, usually develops in children and adolescents about 2 weeks after a streptococcal infection, such as strep throat or scarlet fever. Symptoms include low-grade fever, anorexia, general malaise, and flank pain. Hypertension and edema may occur because of reduced renal function. Urinalysis shows hematuria and proteinuria. Diuretics, such as triamterene and hydrochlorothiazide (Dyazide) or furosemide (Lasix), may be given to control hypertension and reduce edema. The prognosis usually is good; most patients recover spontaneously, but in some patients, the condition progresses to a chronic state.

Chronic glomerulonephritis may also be called *nephritis* or *nephrotic syndrome.* It typically develops over many years and may be associated with chronic diseases that affect the blood vessels, such as systemic lupus erythematosus (SLE) and diabetes mellitus. Chronic glomerulonephritis causes progressive, irreversible nephron damage that frequently results in renal failure. At first the patient is asymptomatic, but as the disease progresses and more glomerular damage occurs, the patient develops anorexia, fatigue, hypertension, hematuria, proteinuria, oliguria (scanty urination), and edema. The cause of chronic glomerulonephritis is unknown, but it may be associated with an antigen-antibody reaction in the glomerular capsule that ultimately destroys the nephron unit. Treatment is supportive and involves an attempt to control symptoms by administering antihypertensives and diuretics, as well as prescription of a diet low in protein with limited sodium and potassium to slow the progression of the disease. Glomerulonephritis is a leading cause of kidney failure; ultimately, many patients require kidney dialysis. The only cure for the disease is a kidney transplant.

Urinary Tract Disorders and Cancers

Renal Calculi

Renal calculi, or kidney stones, are created when crystals in the urine (e.g., calcium, oxalate, uric acid) collect in the kidney, or when fluid intake is low, creating a highly concentrated filtrate. The tendency to develop kidney stones runs in families, and patients with a history of renal calculi are at increased risk for developing more stones in the future. Small stones usually do not cause any difficulty until they grow large enough to lodge in the ureters or renal pelvis. If a stone blocks the flow of urine, infection can develop from the resultant stasis. This blockage also can result in hydronephrosis, a backup of urine that causes dilation of the ureters and calyces and increases pressure on the nephron units. Other signs and symptoms include hematuria; cloudy, foul-smelling urine; nausea and vomiting; a persistent urge to urinate; and fever and chills if an infection is present.

If stones are located in the kidney or bladder, the patient often is asymptomatic, and frequent infections are the only presenting problem. If the calculi begin to move or are lodged in the ureters, the patient experiences renal colic, which is severe pain in the flank region that fluctuates in intensity over periods of 5 to 15 minutes. As the calculi progress down the ureter, the pain radiates to the lower abdomen, groin, and genital areas on the affected side. If the stone stops moving, the pain stops until it starts to move again. This pattern continues until the stone is passed or it is treated medically. The patient may be able to pass small stones by drinking large amounts of fluid (2 to 3 quarts of water a day). However, larger

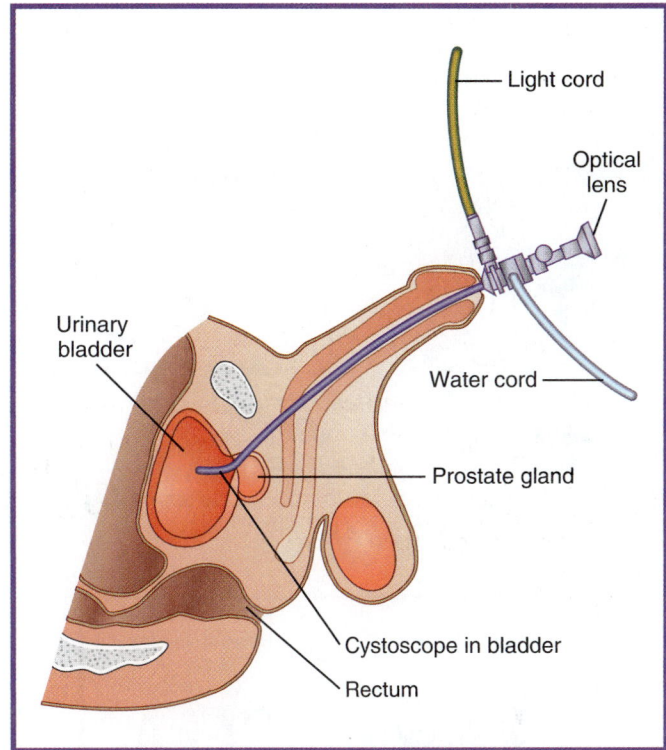

FIGURE 40-3 Cystoscopy.

stones or calculi that cause bleeding, kidney damage, or persistent infection require medical intervention.

The physician may perform a cystoscopic examination to visualize the urethra and bladder and to remove any stones found (Figure 40-3). The most common procedure for treating calculi is extracorporeal shock wave lithotripsy (ESWL), which uses vibrations of powerful sound waves to break the stones into fragmented pieces that can be passed through the renal system. Diagnostic studies are performed to identify the exact location of the calculi, and x-rays or ultrasound is used during the procedure to keep track of the calculi and to monitor treatment progress. The patient may be immersed in water during the procedure or may lie on a water-filled cushion as high-energy sound waves are passed through the body toward the exact location of the calculi (Figure 40-4). The procedure causes moderate pain, so the patient usually is pre-sedated or is given a light anesthetic. The patient wears earphones during the treatment because of the loud noise created each time a shock wave is generated. Side effects of the treatment include flank tenderness, hematoma formation across the treatment site, and hematuria. Measures for preventing recurrence include drinking 3 to 4 quarts of fluid a day, preferably water, and following a diet that is low in sodium and animal protein.

Hydronephrosis

Hydronephrosis, or swelling of the kidney caused by inability of urine to drain from the renal pelvis, usually results from blockage caused by renal calculi, but it may also be caused by an enlarged prostate or a tumor. Hydronephrosis can occur bilaterally or unilaterally. The condition frequently is asymptomatic, or patients may complain of mild flank pain as the renal capsule is distended. Urine testing detects hematuria and, if infection develops from stagnant

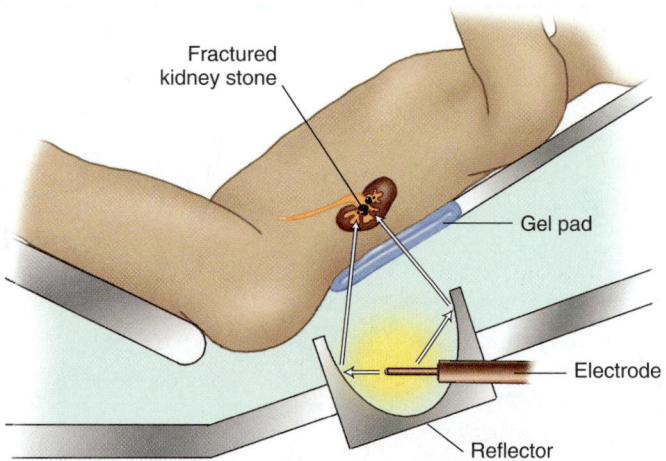

FIGURE 40-4 Extracorporeal shock wave lithotripsy. (From Leonard P: *Building a medical vocabulary: with Spanish translations,* ed 7, St Louis, 2009, Saunders.)

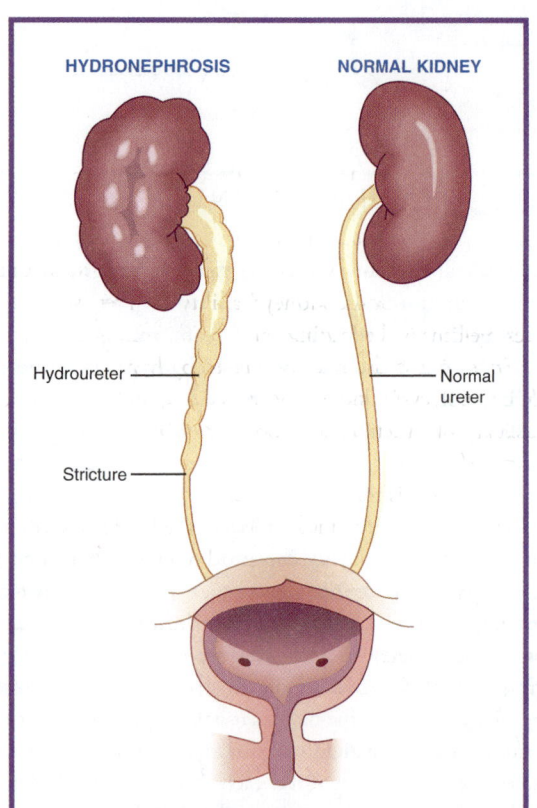

FIGURE 40-5 Hydronephrosis.

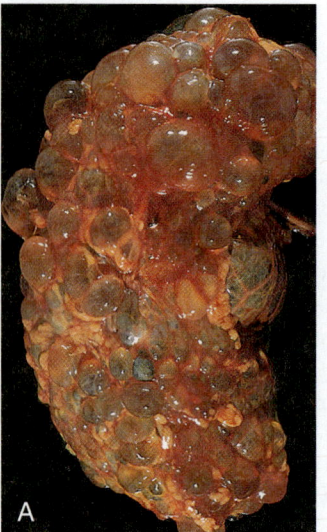
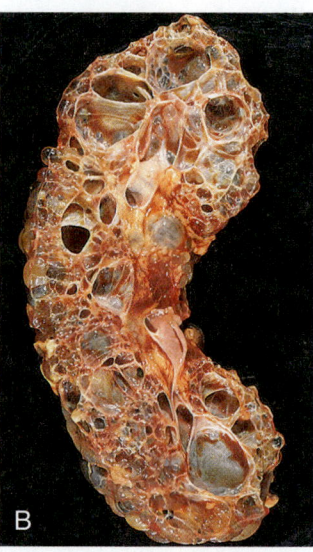

FIGURE 40-6 Polycystic kidney (adult autosomal dominant). **A,** Cysts on the external surface of the enlarged kidney. **B,** Bisected kidney showing large interior cysts. (From Cotran RS, Kumar V, Collins T: *Robbin's pathologic basis of disease,* ed 6, Philadelphia, 1999, Saunders.)

nephrons and collecting tubules become dilated, fused, and infected. As the cysts enlarge, they compress the surrounding tissue, causing necrosis, uremia, and renal failure. Symptoms do not usually become apparent until the individual reaches adolescence or adulthood. Patients with polycystic disease have a family history of kidney disease or renal failure, flank pain, hematuria, and hypertension. They also are more likely to develop UTIs and renal calculi. Because cyst formation is progressive, these patients eventually require renal dialysis or kidney transplantation.

Bladder Cancer

The most common cancer of the urinary tract affects the bladder (Figure 40-7) and is two to three times more common in men than in women. Bladder cancer is characterized by one or more tumors that can metastasize through the blood or surrounding pelvic lymph nodes. Because 50% to 90% of patients experience a recurrence of bladder tumors, follow-up testing that can identify recurrence is extremely important. NMP22 is a urine test that screens for recurrence of the disease. It identifies a protein in bladder cells that are either precancerous or cancerous. Ninety percent of bladder cancers are attributed to these particular cells, which are called *transitional cells* because they are cubelike when the bladder is empty and flat when it is full. The test can be performed in the physician's office, and the results are available in 1 hour. If the NMP22 test result is positive, cystoscopy is performed to confirm the presence of abnormal cells.

Smoking is the greatest single risk factor for the development of bladder cancer. The carcinogens from tobacco become concentrated in the bladder and eventually cause cellular changes in the walls of the organ. Other risk factors include occupational exposure to chemical carcinogens (e.g., oil, rubber, dyes), drinking pesticide-contaminated water, treatment with certain anticancer drugs, and recurrent parasitic infections of the bladder. If the cancerous cells are confined to the inner lining of the bladder, a transurethral resection of the bladder tumor (TURBT) is performed. The physician passes

urine, pyuria. It is important to treat hydronephrosis aggressively, because continued pressure from blocked urine flow can cause tissue necrosis and ultimately can lead to irreversible kidney damage. Removing the blockage corrects the condition (Figure 40-5).

Polycystic Kidneys

Polycystic kidney disease typically is an autosomal dominant genetic disorder, which means that one parent has the disease and each child has a 50% chance of inheriting it. No indications of the disease occur in children, but as time goes on, normal renal tissue in both kidneys is replaced by multiple, benign, fluid-filled cysts (Figure 40-6). The

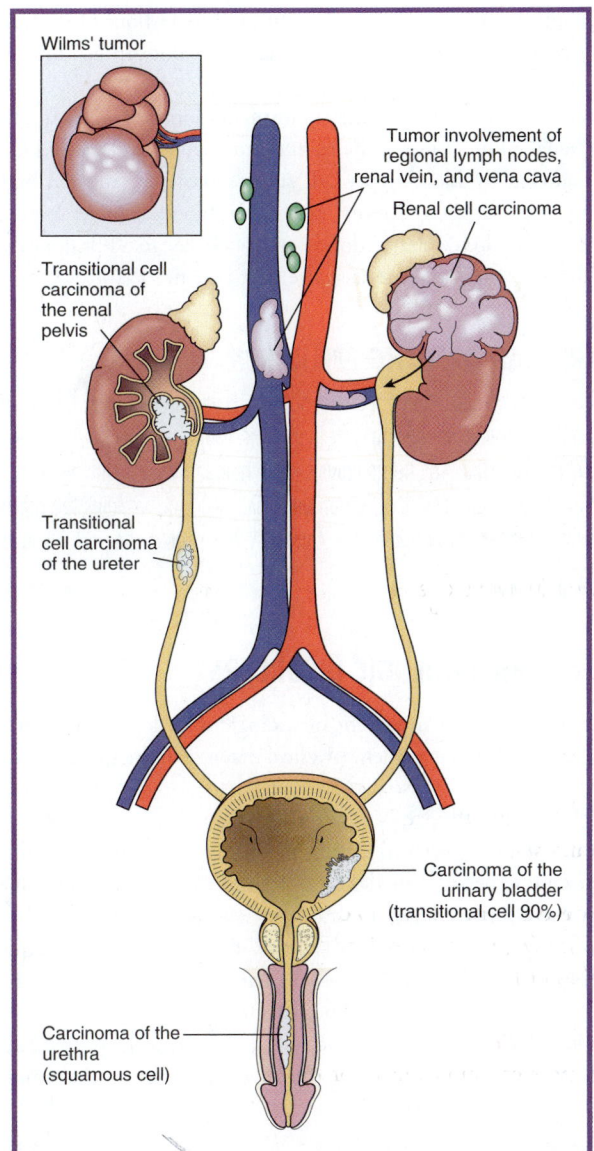

Wilms' tumor

Tumor involvement of regional lymph nodes, renal vein, and vena cava

Renal cell carcinoma

Transitional cell carcinoma of the renal pelvis

Transitional cell carcinoma of the ureter

Carcinoma of the urinary bladder (transitional cell 90%)

Carcinoma of the urethra (squamous cell)

FIGURE 40-7 Neoplasms of the urinary tract. (From Damjanov I: *Pathology for the health-related professions,* ed 4, St Louis, 2010, Saunders.)

of the disease include flank pain, anorexia, anemia, hematuria, and an increased white blood cell count. Surgical nephrectomy is the treatment of choice. Although the prognosis for patients with the tumor has improved, the 5-year survival rate is still only approximately 40%.

Wilms' Tumor

Wilms' tumor, or nephroblastoma, is cancer of the kidney in children. Although the condition appears to be caused by a genetic defect, very few of the children diagnosed with Wilms' tumor have a family history of the disease. It usually occurs unilaterally, is diagnosed most frequently at age 3, and rarely occurs after age 8. The tumor may be noticed by parents as a mass in the child's abdomen or by a physician during a routine physical examination. The preferred treatment is a partial or complete nephrectomy combined with chemotherapy. The survival rate for children diagnosed and treated for Wilms' tumor is greater than 90%.

Renal Failure

Acute renal failure has a sudden, severe onset caused by exposure to toxic chemicals; circulatory collapse from serious burns or heart disease; acute bilateral kidney infection or inflammation; occlusion of the renal arteries; or complications from surgery. Blood tests show high BUN and creatinine levels, and the patient experiences acute onset of oliguria. The primary problem must be resolved as quickly as possible to prevent necrosis and permanent kidney failure.

Chronic renal failure is a slowly progressive process caused by gradual destruction of the kidneys' ability to filter waste materials. Diabetes mellitus is the leading cause of chronic renal failure in the United States, but it also may be caused by hypertension, glomerulonephritis, polycystic kidneys, long-term hydronephrosis resulting from urinary obstruction, lead poisoning, or renal artery stenosis. Symptoms of the condition may not be evident until as much as 75% of the kidney is no longer functioning.

Patients with chronic renal failure pass through several stages, starting with an early stage of decreased reserve in which no clinical signs are apparent but serum creatinine levels are consistently higher than average. The middle stage of renal insufficiency is marked by hypertension, elevated BUN and creatinine levels, and a low urine specific gravity. End-stage renal failure (uremia) is marked by oliguria that progresses to anuria (no urine output), edema, hypertension, acidosis, and **azotemia**. The end result is that the kidneys can no longer remove waste products from the blood, and toxicity develops. To survive, the patient must be placed on dialysis or receive a kidney transplant.

Treatment

Dialysis, or cleansing of the blood, is used to treat acute renal failure until the problem is reversed, or, for patients in end-stage renal disease, until they receive a transplant. The two forms of dialysis are hemodialysis and peritoneal dialysis. Hemodialysis usually is done in an outpatient clinic or hospital. The process uses a machine known as an *artificial kidney,* or *dialyzer,* to filter waste products from the blood and return the cleansed blood to the body (Figure 40-8). A surgically placed cannula or shunt creates an internal fistula between an artery and a vein. During the procedure, approximately 1 cup of blood at a time passes from the shunt through a tube to

a small wire loop through the urethra and uses an electrical current or a laser to burn away the cancer cells. The procedure may cause dysuria or hematuria for a few days. If the tumor has invaded the walls of the bladder, treatment may require a partial or complete cystectomy (removal of the bladder), chemotherapy, and the use of interferon to boost the patient's immune system. The current treatment of choice is implantation of radioactive seeds in the bladder to destroy the affected tissue.

Renal Carcinoma

Adenocarcinoma of the kidney, or renal cell cancer, is a primary tumor that can be cured if it is diagnosed and treated in the early stages. However, affected patients frequently are asymptomatic, which gives the tumor the opportunity to metastasize to the lungs, liver, male urogenital system, bone, or brain before it is diagnosed. Renal cell carcinoma typically occurs in patients over age 50 and is seen more often in men and in smokers. Signs and symptoms

the semipermeable membrane of the dialysis machine. The membrane filters the waste out of the blood, which then is returned to the patient's vein. Patients on hemodialysis require anticoagulant therapy to prevent clots from forming during the blood transfer process. Hemodialysis usually is needed three times a week; the procedure takes approximately 3 to 4 hours each time.

Peritoneal dialysis uses the capillaries in the peritoneal cavity to filter the blood by infusing the patient's abdomen with a dialyzing fluid through a surgically implanted catheter. The highly concentrated dialyzing fluid attracts and absorbs waste products from the blood vessels and then is drained from the abdominal cavity by gravity into a container (Figure 40-9). This procedure can be done at home in two different ways. With continuous ambulatory peritoneal dialysis (CAPD), the patient exchanges the dialysis solution in the abdomen four times a day, 7 days a week. Continuous cycling peritoneal dialysis (CCPD) uses a cycler machine at night to automatically infuse the dialysis solution into and out of the peritoneal cavity. This process takes 10 to 12 hours but can be done while the patient is sleeping.

Although successful kidney transplantation is curative for end-stage renal failure, finding the right donor can be a problem. Donors are matched by blood type, cell surface proteins, and antibodies. Siblings are the best donors, but other blood relatives may also match. If no blood relative donors are available, an adult donor who matches the patient's criteria is the next best fit.

> ### CRITICAL THINKING APPLICATION   40-4
>
> Aloysius Gonzales, a 59-year-old patient, is in chronic renal failure. His family is trying to decide whether their father should be brought to the dialysis clinic for hemodialysis, or whether they should try to keep him at home and assist with peritoneal dialysis. Sara explains the mechanism of each procedure to the family. What should she include in her description?

PEDIATRIC UROLOGIC DISORDERS

Early detection and treatment of urologic disorders in children can drastically reduce permanent physical damage to the urinary system.

Nocturnal Enuresis

One of the most common reasons parents bring a child to a pediatric urologist is enuresis, or bed-wetting. Enuresis is the lack of voluntary control of urination at night or during the day by a child considered to be beyond the age when control should have been acquired (usually after age 6). This problem has a familial tendency and is more common in boys than in girls. The urologist first determines whether the problem is physical or psychological. With primary enuresis, bladder control was never established in the child. It

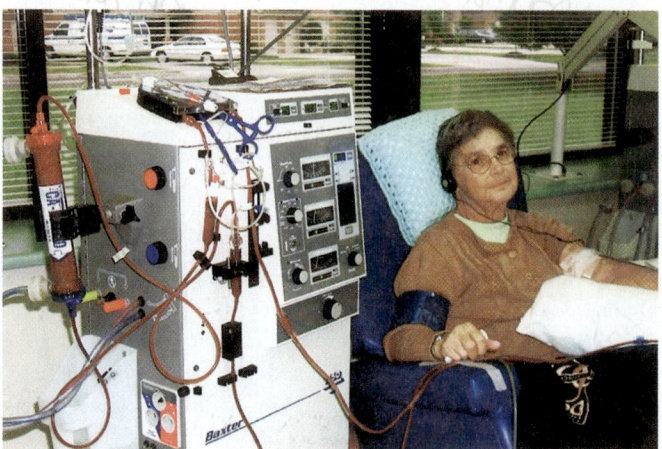

FIGURE 40-8 Dialysis. (From Ignatavicius D: *Medical-surgical nursing: patient-centered collaborative care, single volume,* ed 6, St Louis, Saunders.)

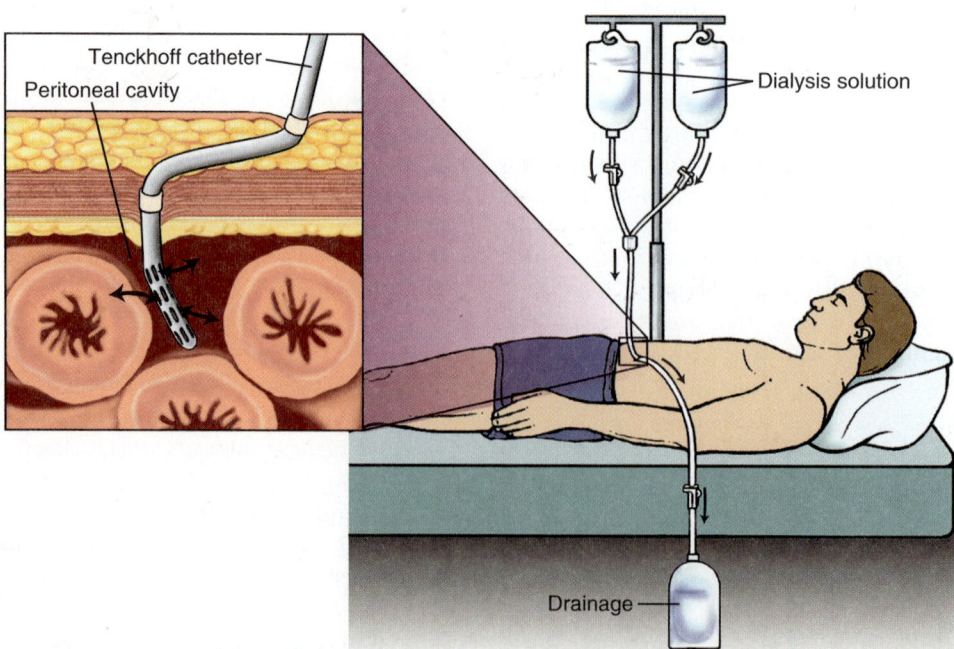

FIGURE 40-9 Peritoneal dialysis. (From Linton AD: *Introduction to medical-surgical nursing,* ed 5, St Louis, 2012, Saunders.)

may be caused by a physiologic problem with bladder control, such as an immature bladder with small capacity, a neurologic deficit, diabetes mellitus or insipidus, a UTI, or sleep apnea, or it may be a result of stressful events. Secondary enuresis, in which loss of bladder control occurs in a child who has been consistently dry for at least 6 months, can develop because of stressful events, UTIs, diabetes, or sexual abuse.

A physical and neurologic examination and urinalysis with a urine culture help determine whether any physical abnormality or disease process is causing the problem. If a psychological problem is suspected, help from a pediatric mental health professional may be needed. If no known causative factors are present, medications that relax the bladder muscles or that reduce urine production at night may be useful. Unfortunately, these may have side effects, so parents may refuse drug therapy. Parents should positively reinforce dryness and should not punish or embarrass the child. A moisture alarm can be used to help train the child to get up at night to go to the bathroom. This is a small, battery-operated device that connects to a moisture-sensitive pad placed in the pajamas or on the bed that beeps when the pad becomes wet. The goal is to wake the child just as he or she starts to urinate so that the child can stop urinating and get to a toilet. The success rate is high (80%), but the device must be used for at least 2 weeks before any change occurs and for up to 12 weeks to stop accidents.

Urinary Reflux Disorder

Urinary reflux disorder may be another reason for pediatric urology referrals. Reflux nephropathy occurs if the kidneys are damaged by a backward flow of urine. Each ureter has a one-way valve where it enters the bladder that is designed to prevent urine from flowing backward. Reflux may be caused by faulty formation of or damage to the valves, or it may be associated with cystitis, neurogenic bladder, or bladder overfilling because of an obstruction. It may be detected with ultrasonography, computed tomography (CT) scan of the kidneys, or a voiding cystourethrogram (VCUG) (Figure 40-10). A VCUG is performed by placing a urinary catheter in the bladder and injecting a contrast medium that helps visualization of the bladder and the flow of urine. X-ray films are taken in several positions, the catheter is removed, and the child is asked to void. X-ray films are taken while the bladder empties to determine whether urinary reflux is present. Although a VCUG is an uncomfortable procedure, the benefit of early detection and reduced damage to the kidneys makes the screening worthwhile. Untreated reflux nephropathy can lead to renal failure.

The treatment for urinary reflux usually is determined by grading its severity on a scale of 1 to 5, with 5 being the most severe. Prophylactic antibiotics may be given daily in low doses to prevent damaging kidney infections, which can cause low-grade reflux. However, with higher grade reflux that persists after 4 or 5 years of age, or for patients who have breakthrough infections despite the antibiotics, surgical repair of the valves of the ureters is necessary. Parents and physicians also may opt for surgery because the procedure has a 95% success rate and poses little risk.

Cryptorchidism

Cryptorchidism, or undescended testicles, is fairly common in premature infants and occurs in about 4% of full-term infants

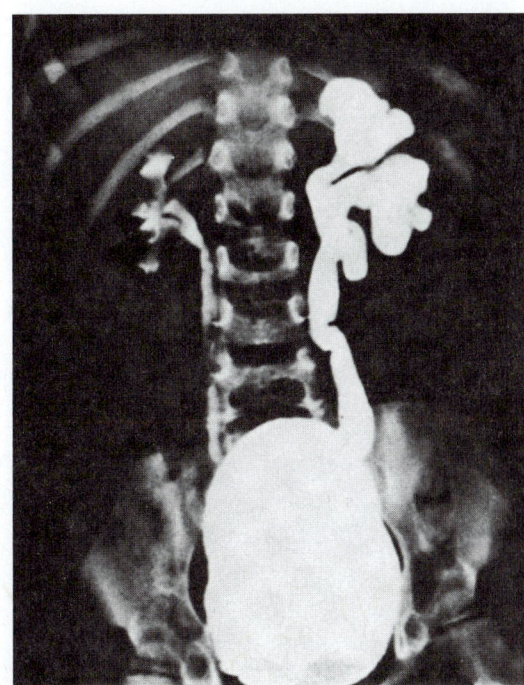

FIGURE 40-10 Voiding cystourethrogram. (From James AE Jr, Squire LF: *Nuclear radiology*, Philadelphia, 1973, Saunders.)

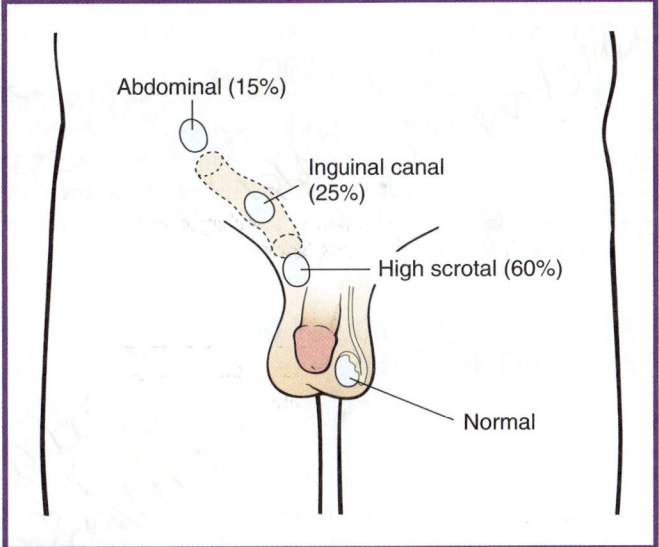

FIGURE 40-11 Cryptorchidism. (From Damjanov I: *Pathology for the health-related professions*, ed 4, St Louis, 2010, Saunders.)

(Figure 40-11). The testes develop in the abdominal cavity of the fetus and descend into the scrotum near the end of the pregnancy. If an infant is born with an undescended testicle, the testicle usually drops without treatment by 9 months of age. However, persistent cryptorchidism should be treated, because infertility may result from exposure of the sperm to the slightly warmer temperature in the abdominal cavity. In addition, it increases the risk of testicular cancer in adolescence. The current recommendation is that surgical attachment of the testicle should be done by 1 year of age to reduce the chance of permanent testicular damage. Parents need to recognize

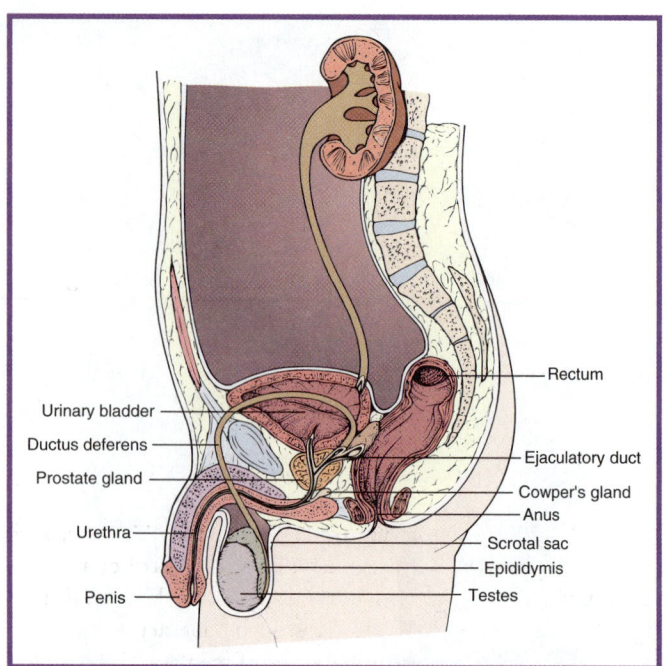

FIGURE 40-12 Male reproductive anatomy. (From Frazier MS, Drzymkowski JA: *Essentials of human diseases and conditions,* ed 5, St Louis, 2013, Saunders.)

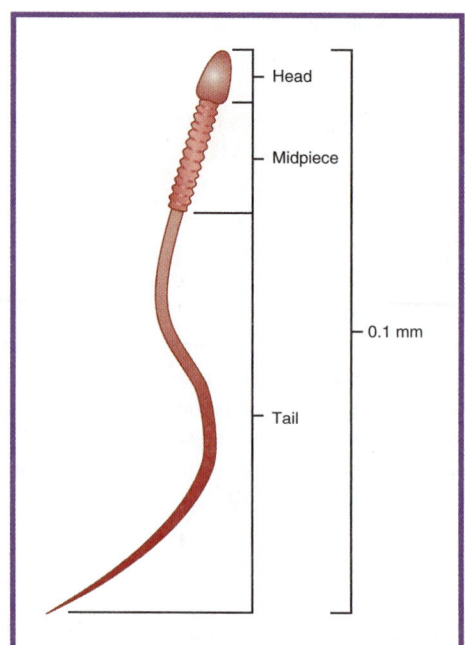

FIGURE 40-13 Sperm.

that this child is considered at increased risk for testicular carcinoma even after treatment and should be taught testicular examination procedures.

The outpatient surgical procedure known as *orchiopexy* involves suturing the undescended testicle in the scrotum. If the testicle is impalpable (cannot be felt), laparoscopic surgery is necessary to locate it. The laparoscope is inserted into the abdomen through a small incision near the navel, and the testicle is moved into proper position or is removed.

ANATOMY AND PHYSIOLOGY OF THE MALE REPRODUCTIVE SYSTEM

The male reproductive system plays an important role in the continuation of the human species (Figure 40-12). Although not necessary for individual survival, the production, sustenance, and transport of male sex cells are vital to the creation of life.

The primary reproductive organs in the male are a pair of testes. The testis is an oval structure about 1⅗ to 2 inches (4 to 5 cm) long and 1 to 1⅕ inches (2.5 to 3 cm) in diameter. Each testis is surrounded by a white, fibrous capsule, and they are contained together in the retractable, saclike scrotum. Lobules in the testes hold the seminiferous tubule, where spermatozoa, the male sex cells, are produced. These cells have 23 chromosomes, or half of the deoxyribonucleic acid (DNA) chain needed to form a complete cell. Sperm cells are tadpolelike structures less than 0.1 mm long that are carried to the epididymis for maturation (Figure 40-13).

The epididymis is a coiled tube almost 20 feet (6 m) long that rests on the top and lateral side of each testis. Peristaltic waves in the epididymis help the sperm move into the vas deferens, where the spermatozoa, which are now capable of movement, are stored until ejaculation. Each vas deferens is a muscular tunnel about 18 inches

(45 cm) long that connects to the epididymis at the base of that structure and passes along the side of the testes. The vas deferens becomes the spermatic cord that passes through the pelvic cavity and ends behind the urinary bladder. Uniting there with the seminal vesicle just outside the prostate gland, it passes through the prostate and into an ejaculatory duct that empties its contents into the urethra. The male urethra is an organ of two body systems—the urinary and reproductive systems.

The adult prostate gland is roughly 1⅗ inches (4 cm) wide and 1⅕ inches (3 cm) thick. It surrounds the urethra at the base of the bladder. The prostate gland is about the size of a pea at birth but grows rapidly at puberty to its full size, about the size of a walnut, by age 20. The central part of the gland may start to grow again after age 45. The primary function of the prostate gland is to secrete a thin fluid with an alkaline pH that neutralizes vaginal secretions to provide the optimum pH for fertilization. Secretions from the prostate gland, vas deferens, seminal vesicles, and bulbourethral glands combine with sperm cells to form semen. The volume of semen in one ejaculate ranges from 2 to 6 mL and averages roughly 100 million to 200 million sperm cells.

Penis

The organ of male **copulation** is the penis. It is a cylindrical organ consisting of an elongated body with a slightly enlarged end, called the *glans penis.* Around the glans penis is a fold of skin that begins just behind the glans and extends forward to cover it like a sheath. This is called the *prepuce,* or foreskin, which sometimes is removed in a surgical procedure known as *circumcision.* The penis carries both urine and semen through the urethra and outside the body. When transmitting semen to the female tract, the penis must enlarge and stiffen for insertion. This occurs when three columns of erectile tissue in the penis become stimulated. The arteries in the penis dilate, and the veins compress; this compression reduces blood flow away from the penis, causing it to swell. Motor impulses are stimulated by swelling of the urethra as a result of semen collection, and contraction of the urethra causes ejaculation of the semen through the penis.

Hormone Production

Hormone production is also an important aspect of the male reproductive system. As a group, the male sex hormones are called *androgens.* Testosterone is the primary male hormone. During pubescence, when the male becomes reproductively functional, the anterior pituitary gland produces gonadotropic hormones that stimulate the testes to produce testosterone. Testosterone stimulates enlargement of the testes, growth of body hair, thickening of the skin and bones, increased muscle growth, and maturation of sperm cells.

DISORDERS OF THE MALE REPRODUCTIVE TRACT

Many diseases and disorders of the male reproductive tract are known. The most common of these involve enlargement or inflammation of certain organs and malignant tumors. The prostate is the most widely affected organ.

Diseases of the Prostate

Prostatitis

The cause of inflammation of the prostate is not always known, but it usually develops in the presence of infection. Bacterial causes may be *E. coli* or, in patients with gonorrhea, gonococci. Infection or inflammation of the prostate gland puts pressure on the urethra, causing dysuria, tenderness, and secretion of pus from the tip of the penis. The condition usually is treated with an antibiotic, such as penicillin. Chronic prostatitis may develop as a result of repeated UTIs, urethral obstruction, or urinary retention.

Benign Prostatic Hyperplasia

As men age, the cells of the prostate gland that surround the urethra can start to reproduce more rapidly, causing the organ to enlarge (hyperplasia). This nonmalignant process, also known as *benign prostatic hyperplasia* (BPH), is seen in about half of men in their 60s and in more than 90% of men in their 70s and 80s. Enlargement of the prostate gland partly blocks the flow of urine, creating a medium for bacterial infection that can lead to cystitis. Signs and symptoms include urinary urgency and frequency; difficulty starting urination; hematuria; and repeated UTIs. The diagnosis is made from the patient's complaints and a digital rectal examination (DRE), during which the physician can palpate the enlarged gland (Figure 40-14).

Treatment includes the use of alpha-adrenergic blockers, such as doxazosin mesylate (Cardura), tamsulosin (Flomax), or alfuzosin (Uroxatral), which relax the smooth muscles of the bladder, making it easier to urinate. Finasteride (Proscar) or dutasteride (Avodart) may also be prescribed to reduce the size of the prostate, increasing urine flow and providing symptomatic relief. Nonsurgical therapies include laser treatment or placement of a prostatic stent to keep the urethra open. Because enlargement of the gland can be a sign of prostate cancer, it is important that the prostrate be biopsied to rule out possible cancerous cells. If drug therapy and alternative treatments are not successful in relieving the patient's prostate enlargement, surgery is recommended. Transurethral resection of the prostate (TURP), the most common surgical treatment, involves threading a small instrument (a resectoscope) through the urethra to the prostate and scraping away the excess tissue.

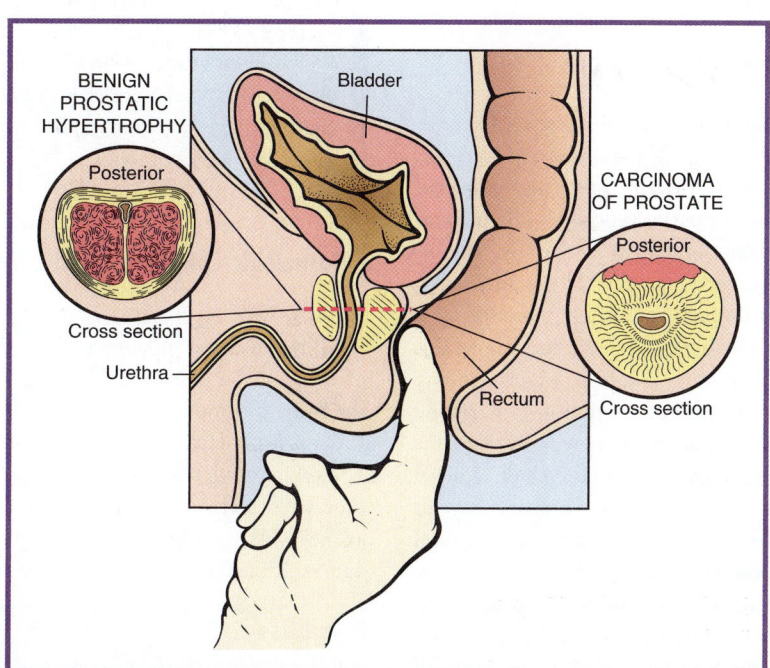

FIGURE 40-14 Digital rectal examination to diagnose benign prostatic hyperplasia and carcinoma of the prostate. (From Damjanov I: *Pathology for the health-related professions,* ed 4, St Louis, 2010, Saunders.)

Prostate Cancer

Cancer of the prostate is common in men over age 50 and ranks as the second highest cause of cancer deaths in men, behind lung cancer. The patient is asymptomatic in the early stages and may not become symptomatic until the cancer has spread outside the prostate gland. Once symptoms develop, they include urinary obstruction with difficulty urinating, frequent UTIs and nocturia (the need to void at night), hematuria, and generalized pain in the pelvic region. Prostate cancer spreads locally to the bladder, rectum, and lymph nodes of the pelvis, causing metastasis to the bones, lungs, and brain. The prognosis is poor unless the tumor is discovered in its early stages of development, when it is still confined to the prostate gland.

The first indication of a problem may come with a routine DRE, when the physician notices a firm or irregular area in the prostate. The primary screening tool for cancer of the prostate is the prostate-specific antigen (PSA) blood test. Blood levels of PSA, a protein produced by the prostate, are elevated with prostatitis, BPH, and cancer of the prostate. The higher the PSA level, the more likely it is that the patient has prostate cancer. However, because the PSA level can be elevated with other disorders, one abnormal screening value is not enough to diagnose cancer. The test should be repeated over time, and if levels continue to rise, further diagnostic studies should be done. If tests indicate cancer, the physician may order a transrectal ultrasound, which involves inserting a small transducer into the rectum to bounce sound waves off the prostate, creating a picture. The ultrasound pictures are used to help pinpoint areas of concern during a tissue biopsy. If the transrectal ultrasound does not indicate any suspicious areas, the physician takes multiple biopsies (usually eight) from different sections of the prostate gland. Tissue samples are sent to the pathologist for analysis and diagnosis.

The American Cancer Society recommends that the PSA test be used in conjunction with a DRE annually for all men over age 50. In addition, PSA screenings should be performed yearly in men over age 40 who have a family history of the disease and in African-American men over age 45, because they are at increased risk for developing the disease.

The treatment for prostate cancer depends on its stage of spread. Radiation may be delivered directly to the cancer cells through external beam radiation therapy (EBRT), which uses high-powered x-rays to kill the cancer cells. An alternative procedure is implantation of radioactive seeds, a variant of radiation therapy. In this procedure, 40 to 100 rice-sized radioactive seeds are implanted directly into the prostate gland through a precisely placed hollow needle. The radiation is quite strong but has a very short range; this allows it to destroy the tumor but minimizes damage to surrounding tissue. Testosterone can stimulate growth of the tumor, so hormone therapy frequently is prescribed to block the action of testosterone or to stop its production. Surgical treatment options include removal of the prostate gland by transurethral resection; orchiectomy, in which the testosterone-producing testicles are removed; and radical prostatectomy, in which the prostate and local lymph nodes are removed. These are debilitating surgical procedures that have serious side effects, including urinary incontinence and erectile dysfunction; therefore, they typically are used as a last measure. As with all cancers, chemotherapy may be prescribed for advanced cases or for recurrence.

IMPORTANT INFORMATION ABOUT PROSTATE-SPECIFIC ANTIGEN (PSA) STUDIES

- Most men have a PSA level below 4; a level between 4 and 10 indicates a 25% chance of prostate cancer; a level higher than 10 increases the chance to 50%.
- Because an elevated PSA level can have many possible causes, if no other indicators of cancer are present, the physician may recommend that the digital rectal examination (DRE) and the PSA test be repeated to determine whether the level increases over time.
- If the PSA level increases with repeated testing, or if the DRE reveals an abnormal prostate, additional diagnostic studies should be done.
- If cancer is suspected, biopsies (typically needle aspiration) are performed.
- Part of the controversy with PSA testing is that it may diagnose a slow-growing tumor that is not life threatening, which can result in aggressive and life-changing surgery.
- The PSA test has a significant false-positive outcome (patients who do not have cancer are told that they do). False-positive results lead to further diagnostic testing that is both expensive and stressful for the patient and his family. Only 25% to 30% of biopsies done because of elevated PSA levels actually reveal cancer.
- At this point, it is not clear whether PSA screening saves lives, or if the benefits of screening outweigh the risks of follow-up diagnostic studies and cancer treatment for potentially slow-growing tumors that are not life threatening.
- The most common complications of prostate surgery are erectile dysfunction and urinary incontinence.

CRITICAL THINKING APPLICATION   40-5

Dr. Fineman frequently sees patients for prostate-related conditions. Sara decides to review the information on disorders that affect the prostate gland so that she is better able to assist the physician and answer patients' questions. What are the important details of prostate disease that Sara should remember?

Pathologic Conditions of the Genital Organs

Epididymitis

Epididymitis is an inflammation of the tubular epididymis. It most often is attributed to a UTI in men over age 40; in younger men, the most common cause is a sexually transmitted infection (STI). Patients experience severe low abdominal and testicular pain, as well as swelling and tenderness of the scrotum. If abscesses form and produce scar tissue, sterility can occur. Antibiotics, including ceftriaxone (Ceftin), ciprofloxacin (Cipro), doxycycline (Vibramycin), and azithromycin (Zithromax), are prescribed for treatment.

Balanitis

Inflammation of the glans penis and the mucous membrane beneath it is known as *balanitis*. It occurs most often in uncircumcised patients with narrow foreskins that do not retract easily and in men

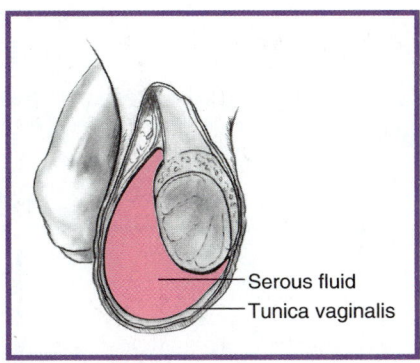

FIGURE 40-15 Hydrocele. (From Jarvis C: *Physical examination and health assessment,* ed 4, Philadelphia, 2004, Saunders.)

with diabetes. It has many causes, including an allergic reaction to certain chemicals (e.g., contraceptive foam), poor personal hygiene that results in a buildup of skin secretions (smegma) around the glans penis, and urinary tract and yeast infections. Treatment depends on the cause of the problem: Antibiotics are used for infections, and cleansing is used for smegma buildup; avoiding chemicals that cause reactions can help prevent the problem.

Hydrocele

During the descent of the testes, a small canal develops for them to pass through. If the canal does not close after birth, fluid from the peritoneal cavity may pass through and collect in the scrotum. This is called a congenital *hydrocele,* which must be corrected surgically (Figure 40-15). Acquired hydroceles usually occur after middle age because of a scrotal injury or tumor and can form in men who sit for extended periods (e.g., aging men in long-term care facilities), causing painful scrotal swelling.

Testicular Cancer

Testicular carcinoma is the most common cancer in Caucasian men 15 to 34 years of age. The cause is unknown, but the primary predisposing factor is cryptorchidism. The patient complains of a mass in either testicle; a heavy sensation in the scrotum accompanied by a sudden collection of fluid; pain in a testicle or in the scrotum, abdomen, or groin; and unexplained fatigue. Testicular cancer can be treated successfully if diagnosed early; the survival rate for stage I testicular cancer is approximately 95%. Unfortunately, because young men may hesitate to go to the physician to report a mass in the testicle, the cancer may have reached an advanced stage before it is diagnosed. In advanced stages, treatment usually involves a combination of orchiectomy, radiation therapy, and chemotherapy. Testicular cancer can be detected early with monthly self-examination. Men should be taught to do this 3-minute examination beginning in puberty or by age 15 (Procedure 40-1).

The physician may provide pamphlets or a shower card showing the steps of testicular self-examination (Figure 40-16). The medical assistant can approach this teaching intervention in two ways. One way is to take the information to the patient and tell him to follow the pictures, and if he has any questions, he should call for clarification. Will he call? Would you? The second way is to go over the instructions with the patient. Demonstrate the procedure on a model, if one is available, or a male medical assistant could observe

the patient doing the examination for the first time and provide feedback to answer any questions.

Erectile Dysfunction

The inability to achieve and maintain an erection sufficient for sexual intercourse is a condition known as *erectile dysfunction* (ED). It has many causes, both psychological and physiologic. Stress, anxiety, fear of unsatisfactory performance, and physical diseases that affect the vascular system, including arteriosclerosis, alcoholism, and diabetes mellitus, all can lead to ED. Changes in erectile function are normal as men age. Also, impotency is a side effect of certain medications, such as some hypertensive drugs. ED can be treated pharmaceutically with sildenafil (Viagra), tadalafil (Cialis), or vardenafil (Levitra). However, these medications are contraindicated in patients with a history of uncontrolled hypertension, myocardial infarction (heart attack), a cerebrovascular accident (stroke), or a life-threatening arrhythmia. In addition, they cannot be taken if the patient is prescribed nitrate drugs, such as nitroglycerin, because the combination of these medications can cause heart complications. If the patient is taking an alpha blocker (e.g., Flomax, Cardura) for treatment of an enlarged prostate, ED drugs must be used with caution, because the combination of these medications can cause dangerous hypotension.

Infertility

Fertility peaks in men at age 25. Infertility can be caused by a problem in the man, a problem in the woman, or a combination of the two. About 10% to 20% of male infertility cases have no known cause. For the remaining cases, many causative factors may be involved. Cryptorchidism, stricture, and varicoceles (dilated spermatic cord veins); a low sperm count and poor motility; obstruction of the vas deferens; and hormonal imbalances all are factors in infertility.

Examination of semen specimens is helpful in making a diagnosis of infertility. These tests determine the presence of sperm, the number of sperm in an ejaculation, and the health and motility of the sperm. Ultrasonography also is helpful for detecting blockage of the vas deferens.

Sexually Transmitted Infections

Diseases of the male reproductive system can be acquired during sexual intercourse (Table 40-2). No one is immune to these diseases, and an individual can be infected with more than one at a time. No cure is available for viral STIs, such as human immunodeficiency virus (HIV) infection, herpes, and venereal warts. Bacterial infections are increasingly becoming resistant to antibiotic therapy. STIs frequently are asymptomatic in men, although they can cause serious health problems and are infectious regardless of whether symptoms are present (see Chapter 41 for pathologic conditions of the female reproductive tract).

Bacterial Sexually Transmitted Infections

STIs caused by bacterial infections include chlamydia, gonorrhea, and syphilis. Gonorrhea and chlamydia organisms tend to coexist, so a patient who has tested positive for one of the organisms typically is treated for both. Symptoms are similar to those for urethritis and epididymitis, such as painful and frequent urination, discharge from

PROCEDURE 40-1

Instruct Patients According to Their Needs to Promote Health Maintenance and Disease Prevention: Teach Testicular Self-Examination

GOAL: *To instruct the patient in the steps of testicular self-examination.*

EQUIPMENT and SUPPLIES

- Self-examination pamphlet and shower card
- Demonstration model
- Nonsterile gloves
- Patient's record

PROCEDURAL STEPS

1. Sanitize your hands and collect the required supplies.
   <u>PURPOSE:</u> To ensure infection control.
2. Explain to the patient what you are going to do.
   <u>PURPOSE:</u> Understanding helps with cooperation.
3. Begin by explaining to the patient that testicular cancer may cause no symptoms in the early stages, so it is important to examine the testes once a month for abnormal changes and early detection of the disease. This should begin at puberty, or approximately 15 years of age. It is best to do the examination in the shower or in a warm bath. The total examination takes about 3 minutes.
   <u>PURPOSE:</u> Heat causes the scrotal skin to relax, making the examination easier.
4. *Examination of the testis:* Using the demonstration model, start by holding the scrotum in the palms of the hands. Then feel one testicle. Apply a small amount of pressure. Slowly roll it between the thumb and fingers and feel for any hard, painless lumps (Figure 1).

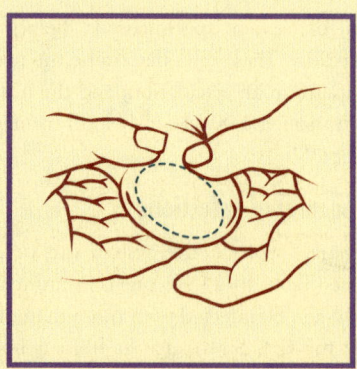

5. *Examination of the epididymis:* This comma-shaped cord is found on top of and behind the testis. Its job is to store and transport sperm. Tender when touched, it is the location of most noncancerous problems. Check for hard spots and lumps (Figure 2).

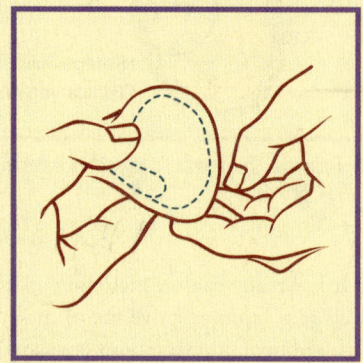

6. *Examination of the vas deferens:* Continue by examining the sperm-carrying tube that runs up the epididymis. Normally the vas feels like a firm, movable, smooth tube (Figure 3).

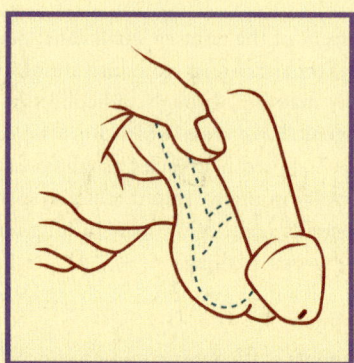

7. Now repeat the entire examination on the other testis.
8. After completing the examination on the model, ask the patient to do a return examination using the model. A male assistant can have the patient do a self-testicular examination.
9. Give the pamphlet to the patient, along with the shower card, with instructions to hang it in the shower as a monthly reminder and guide.
10. Record the instructional interaction in the patient's medical record.
    <u>PURPOSE:</u> If it is not recorded, it was not done.

8/19/XX 11:12 AM Pt shown and successfully demonstrated testicular self-exam on model; no questions. Pt given pamphlet and shower card for home use. Dorothy Gaston, CMA (AAMA)

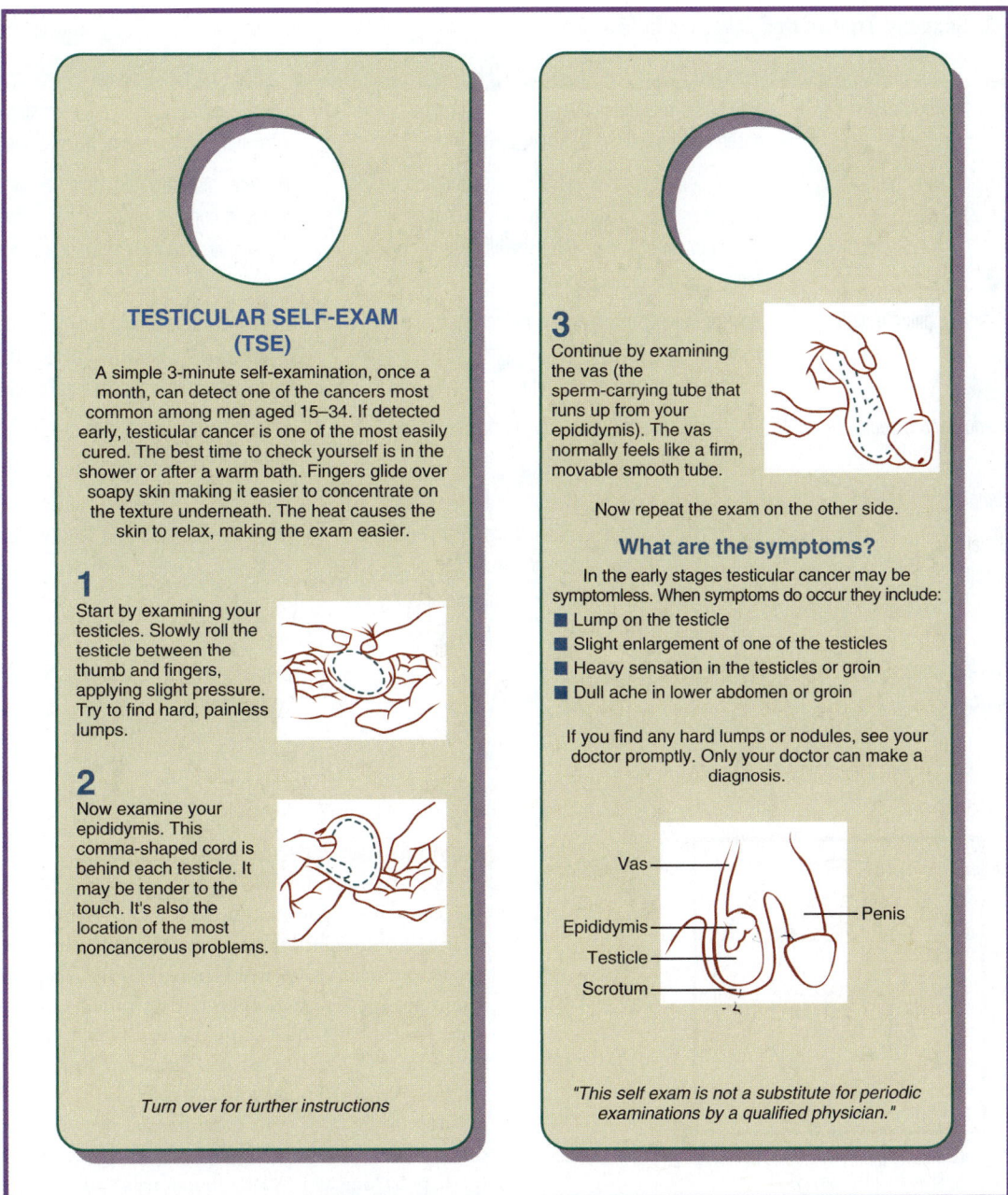

FIGURE 40-16 Testicular self-examination shower card.

the penis, and lower abdominal pain. Chlamydia is resistant to penicillin; therefore, a regimen of antibiotics other than penicillin (e.g., Zithromax, doxycycline, erythromycin) is prescribed if the patient has both conditions. Sexual partners must also be treated, or the infection will continue to be transmitted back and forth.

A syphilitic lesion, called a *chancre,* develops on the male genitalia, usually the penis, a few days to a few weeks after exposure (Figure 40-17). Syphilis initially is diagnosed through the Venereal Disease Research Laboratory (VDRL) or the rapid plasma reagin (RPR) antibody blood test. If the results of these are positive, the diagnosis is confirmed with a fluorescent *Treponema* absorption (FTA) test, which is specific for antibodies to the *Treponema* microorganism. Syphilis can be treated successfully with penicillin but may go unnoticed or unreported. Without treatment, it advances to a secondary

phase, which is marked by low-grade fever, headache, and sore throat, as well as a rash that does not itch but that can affect any part of the body. In the secondary phase, the disease is highly contagious but still can be treated with penicillin. The more advanced stages of the disease can remain undetected or dormant for years. Symptoms that appear years after the primary infection show multisystem involvement, including neurologic and cardiovascular complications. Syphilis is not curable in advanced stages.

Viral Sexually Transmitted Infections

Viral STIs include hepatitis B, C, and D (see Chapter 39), genital herpes, genital warts (caused by the human papilloma virus [HPV]), and HIV infection. With genital herpes, the herpes simplex virus (HSV) enters the body through small breaks in the skin or mucous

TABLE 40-2 Sexually Transmitted Diseases in Men

DISEASE (CAUSATIVE ORGANISM)	SIGNS AND SYMPTOMS	TREATMENT
Chlamydia (*Chlamydia trachomatis*) — bacteria	May be asymptomatic; dysuria; itching and white discharge from penis; testicular pain.	Curable with antibiotic therapy: single dose of Zithromax or 1 week of doxycycline (Vibramycin).
Genital herpes simplex virus (herpes simplex virus type 2)	Painful genital vesicles and ulcers; erythema and pruritus; tingling or shooting pain 1 to 2 days before cycle through episodes. Viral shedding may occur during asymptomatic periods.	No cure, but antiviral therapy during episodes shortens duration of lesions: acyclovir (Zovirax), famciclovir (Famvir), or valacyclovir (Valtrex).
Genital warts (human papilloma virus [HPV])	Most prevalent sexually transmitted disease; period of communicability is unknown; pinhead lesions may or may not be visible; warts tend to recur.	Goal of treatment is to remove symptomatic warts; cryotherapy for lesions; podofilox (Condylox) solution or imiquimod (Aldara) cream for lesions.
Gonorrhea (*Neisseria gonorrhoeae*) — bacteria	Dysuria and urinary frequency; thick, cloudy, or bloody discharge from penis.	Curable with antibiotic therapy: cefixime (Suprax), azithromycin, doxycycline.
Syphilis (*Treponema pallidum*) — spirochete bacteria	Six stages that can affect multiple body systems; 10- to 90-day incubation; initial sign is a painless lesion, or *chancre*, at the exposure site (penis); serous discharge from chancre; lymphadenopathy; if left untreated, advances to later stages.	Penicillin G (Wycillin); if patient is allergic to penicillin, doxycycline or tetracycline.
Trichomoniasis (*Trichomonas vaginalis*) — protozoa	Asymptomatic in men.	Single oral dose of metronidazole (Flagyl).

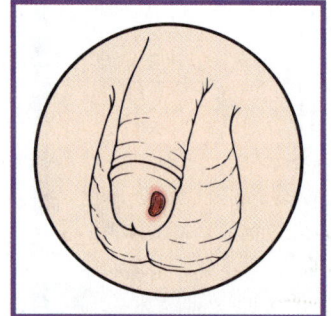

FIGURE 40-17 Syphilitic chancre. (From Frazier MS, Drzymkowski JA: *Essentials of human diseases and conditions,* ed 5, St Louis, 2013, Saunders.)

membranes. Most individuals with HSV are asymptomatic, or signs and symptoms are so mild that they go unnoticed. If symptoms are experienced, the first episode typically is the worst, with the formation of a blistered, inflamed, painful rash on the penis, scrotum, and urethra. After several days, the vesicles rupture, resulting in painful, ulcerated areas. The lesions heal in 3 to 4 weeks, but the herpes virus then migrates to a nerve dermatome. Many factors can reactivate the disease at any time (e.g., stress, upper respiratory infection), making the individual infectious again. However, HSV can be spread even when sores are not present.

Genital warts often are asymptomatic in men and require preliminary treatment with acetic acid to be seen. The incubation period for HPV infection may be as long as 6 months. In women, these infections greatly increase the risk of cervical cancer (see Chapter 41).

Acquired Immunodeficiency Syndrome

AIDS is the most deadly STI. It is caused by the human immunodeficiency virus. The virus invades CD4 T lymphocytes, destroying their ability to fight infection on the cellular level. Individuals may be asymptomatic when first exposed to HIV. Those who do develop symptoms may complain of a fever, arthralgia (joint pain), myalgia (muscle pain), lymphadenopathy, rash, night sweats, and malaise approximately 2 to 6 weeks after exposure to the virus.

The goal of treatment of HIV infection is to reduce the amount of virus in the body with antiretroviral drugs, thereby slowing the destruction of the immune system. It is unclear how many years (perhaps as long as 17 years) individuals with an early diagnosis and consistent, appropriate medical treatment with advanced drug therapy can remain HIV positive before developing AIDS. AIDS is diagnosed when evidence appears of a wide range of opportunistic infections that develop because of depressed T-cell counts. These include *Pneumocystis carinii* pneumonia (PCP), candidiasis (yeast infection), **Kaposi's sarcoma**, dementia, and **wasting syndrome**. A patient is considered to be HIV positive when antibodies to the virus are detected; however, the diagnosis of AIDS is not made until the CD4 T-cell count drops below 200 mm^3 (the normal count is 600 to 1,000 mm^3) and/or opportunistic infections have been diagnosed. Current HIV management includes monitoring of CD4 T-cell counts at diagnosis and every 3 to 6 months thereafter.

HIV is transmitted when infected blood or blood products, semen, or vaginal secretions come in contact with the mucous membranes or the broken skin of an uninfected person. It also can be passed in utero from an infected mother to her fetus, during delivery, or by breast-feeding. Intravenous drug users who share needles and anyone who has unprotected sex of any kind are at increased risk for contracting HIV. Healthcare workers are also at risk for accidental exposure in the workplace and should consistently follow Standard Precautions to protect themselves and their patients from this deadly disease. HIV is a fragile virus; it cannot survive outside the body, and it is easily destroyed by chemical disinfectants such as household bleach.

All HIV tests screen for antibodies to the virus, and any positive result, regardless of the type of test used, is followed up with the more definitive Western Blot test before a positive diagnosis is made. The most widely used screening test for HIV infection is the enzyme immunoassay (EIA; also called the *enzyme-linked immunosorbent assay* [ELISA]), which typically is performed on a venous blood sample. EIA tests also can be done on other body fluids, including oral fluid and urine, although urine screening is not as accurate or as sensitive to antibody levels. The physician may also order a viral load test that reflects the amount of HIV in the blood. Generally, the higher the viral load, the more aggressive the HIV infection.

Newer developments in rapid HIV screening use either blood or oral fluid (not the same as saliva) and can produce results within 20 to 60 minutes with accuracy rates similar to those of traditional EIA screening tests. The U.S. Food and Drug Administration (FDA) has approved the OraQuick Advance HIV1/2 Antibody Test for use on both oral fluid and plasma specimens. To perform the oral test, a single gentle swab is done around both upper and lower outer gums, the swabbing device is inserted into a vial containing a developer solution, and the result is positive if two reddish purple lines appear in a small window after 20 minutes. This test is not designed for home screening, because it is restricted to use by trained individuals, such as medical assistants. However, an FDA-approved home test called the *Home Access HIV-1 Test System* is available at most drug stores. The kit provides the materials for collection of a specimen at home rather than in a healthcare facility. To perform the test, the individual pricks a finger, places a blood drop on a specially treated card, and then mails the card to a licensed laboratory for testing. The individual uses an identification number provided with the kit to call the laboratory for results. As with all other HIV screening tools, a positive result must be followed by a Western blot test to confirm the diagnosis.

HIV infection can be treated with medications, but it cannot be cured. However, recent research indicates that HIV positive individuals taking antiretroviral medications are less contagious than those not being treated. Once patients begin antiretroviral treatment, they must continue to take these drugs for the rest of their lives. The medications must be taken at the time and frequency prescribed to be effective in controlling the spread of the virus and to prevent drug-resistant strains from developing. The FDA currently has approved more than 30 medications for the treatment of HIV infection in adults and adolescents. Six classes of FDA-approved antiretroviral medications are designed to prevent HIV replication or to block entry of the virus into the body's T cells. Examples of these drugs include delavirdine (Rescriptor, DLV), zidovudine (Retrovir, AZT, ZDV), amprenavir (Agenerase, APV), enfuvirtide (Fuzeon, T-20), and raltegravir (Isentress). Current FDA guidelines recommend a combination of three or more antiretroviral drugs in a regimen called *highly active antiretroviral therapy* (HAART). Examples of combination drugs include Combivir (Zidovudine and Lamivudine), Trizivir (Zidovudine, Lamivudine, and Abacavir), Epzicom (Abacavir and Lamivudine), and Truvada (Tenofovir and Lamivudine). Unfortunately, HIV medications can cause multiple side effects, including fever, nausea, fatigue, liver abnormalities, diabetes mellitus, hypercholesterolemia, decreased bone density, skin rash, pancreatitis, and neurologic disorders. Patients must be educated on the importance of strictly following their prescribed treatment regimen and of immediately reporting any side effects to the physician.

The psychosocial needs of a patient diagnosed with HIV infection are far reaching. Treatment is designed to control duplication of the virus in the body, but the patient will always be infectious. Transmission of the disease is prevented by sexual abstinence or consistent use of condoms and precautions with blood spills; these options must be discussed and consistently reinforced with the patient. Community organizations can serve as a source of counseling and support for patients who test HIV positive and for their families. As mandated by federal law, the medical assistant must remember that all information regarding a patient's HIV status must be kept in strict confidence, and no documentation in the medical record can indicate the patient's HIV or AIDS status.

TRENDS IN REPORTABLE SEXUALLY TRANSMITTED INFECTIONS

- The Centers for Disease Control and Prevention (CDC) estimates that there are 19 million new STIs every year, costing the healthcare system an estimated $17 billion.
- Chlamydia is the most frequently reported infectious disease in the United States, with 1.3 million cases reported in 2010; it is estimated that twice that number are infected but are not diagnosed or treated; improved testing and treatment among men could help reduce transmission to women. The infection can be diagnosed with a urine test, and complications among men are rare.
- Gonorrhea is the second most commonly reported infectious disease in the United States, with more than 300,000 cases reported in 2010. The CDC estimates that twice as many new infections occur each year. The number of reported cases is 19 times higher in African-Americans than in Caucasians. Antibiotic resistance (especially to such drugs as ciprofloxacin [Cipro] and Levaquin) is a serious concern; if the disease goes untreated, epididymitis and possibly infertility can result. Studies indicate that the presence of gonorrhea increases the likelihood of HIV transmission.
- Syphilis is highly infectious in the early stages but is easily curable; left untreated, it can lead to serious long-term complications, including nerve, cardiovascular, and organ damage and even death. The incidence of syphilis is increasing among young black men and homosexual individuals.
- Males typically are asymptomatic or have minimal signs or symptoms of herpes infection. With symptoms, the initial outbreak consists of one or more blisters on or around the genitals that break, leaving tender ulcers that last 2 to 4 weeks. The outbreaks may lessen in severity over time. The virus is present in the body indefinitely, but the

frequency of outbreaks declines over time. The virus can be transmitted by an infected partner who does not have a visible sore, and who may not know that he or she is infected.

- Herpes simplex virus type 1 (HSV-1) can cause genital herpes, but it more commonly causes oral herpes or cold sores. HSV-1 infection of the genitals can be caused by oral-to-genital contact with a person who has an HSV-1 infection. Condoms do not completely prevent the transmission of genital herpes.

- Most human papilloma virus (HPV) infections are asymptomatic in males; the man may be unaware of the infection but can transmit it to a sex partner. Genital warts may disappear without treatment. Because no diagnostic test for HPV is available for men, the diagnosis is based on evidence of wart development. Condoms do not completely prevent transmission of HPV. New research indicates that the rising rate of oral and throat cancers can be linked to the oral transmission of one of the cancer-causing types of HPV.

- The human immunodeficiency virus (HIV) cannot reproduce outside a living host, and no record exists of infection from environmental contact. Also, no evidence indicates that the virus can be transmitted by insects. Latex or polyurethane condoms used consistently and correctly provide a highly effective mechanical barrier to HIV. According to 2009 data, HIV is most prevalent in gay and bisexual men, as seen in 61% of new cases; African-Americans represent approximately 14% of the U.S. population but accounted for 44% of new HIV infections; Hispanic/Latinos accounted for 20% of all new infections, and 27% of new cases were reported in heterosexuals. Individuals with an STI are at two to five times greater risk of contracting HIV if exposed; if an HIV-infected individual has another STI, HIV transmission is more likely. Treating STIs in HIV-infected individuals decreases the amount of HIV in genital secretions.

Summary from STD Trends in the US. http://www.cdc.gov/std/stats10/trends.htm. Accessed March 1, 2013.

CRITICAL THINKING APPLICATION   40-6

The number of patients seen weekly in Dr. Fineman's practice who have STIs continues to rise. Sara is responsible for telephone screening and for clinical medical assisting practices. She is constantly being asked questions about the signs and symptoms of STIs and their treatment. What should Sara know about bacterial and viral STIs and their treatment?

THE MEDICAL ASSISTANT'S ROLE IN UROLOGIC AND MALE REPRODUCTIVE EXAMINATIONS

Much of the diagnosis of urinary dysfunction depends on the patient's history, which may include frequency or urgency of urination, dysuria, or incontinence. A major part of the urologic examination is urinalysis, and the medical assistant must be able to instruct the patient in how to obtain a clean-catch urine specimen (see Chapter 52). It is best to have the patient collect the specimen during an office visit so that it can be examined immediately. The urologist may need to examine a catheterized specimen, which is collected using sterile technique. This procedure requires advanced training.

Assisting with a Urologic Examination

No special instrument setup is required for a routine urologic examination unless a special procedure is ordered, such as obtaining a catheterized urine specimen or a specimen for culture. Most offices use prepackaged, disposable packs for catheterization and bladder irrigation.

Both male and female patients disrobe and are given a gown. A woman is placed in the dorsal recumbent position, and a man is seated on the examining table. The physician explains what is required to the patient. With female patients and male physicians, a female medical assistant must remain in the room while the patient's genital area is exposed and examined. The primary responsibility during the examination process is to assist the physician with any supplies and equipment needed and to maintain proper draping of the patient.

Assisting with a Male Reproductive Examination

The medical assistant needs to understand the male reproductive system and to provide patient support throughout the examination. The patient should empty his bladder and disrobe before the physician begins the examination. A drape sheet is placed around the patient's waist, covering the lower extremities. A female medical assistant is present only if requested by the physician. The physician inspects the foreskin (if the patient has not been circumcised) and the glans penis. The penis and scrotum are palpated for possible masses and tenderness. The patient also is examined for possible inguinal hernias. A DRE completes the physical assessment.

A male medical assistant may assist the physician with the examination and help with patient draping and positioning. The medical assistant should watch the patient for signs of discomfort or anxiety, answer the patient's questions, and reinforce the physician's orders as needed.

Vasectomy

A vasectomy is a surgical procedure for sterilizing a male patient (Figure 40-18). It is performed by surgically removing a section of each vas deferens to stop sperm from reaching the prostate and mixing with semen. Sexual function is not affected by the procedure.

The procedure can be performed in a physician's office using a local anesthetic agent, such as lidocaine (Xylocaine). In the standard procedure, which takes approximately 30 minutes, the physician makes a small incision on both sides of the scrotum with a scalpel, clips both vasa deferens, and closes the site by cauterization or with sutures.

The no-scalpel vasectomy is a newer technique that takes approximately 10 minutes. The physician palpates and clamps the vas deferens under the scrotal sac, makes a tiny puncture through the skin, pulls the vas deferens out and cuts it, replaces the tube, and seals the site. The procedure is repeated on the other side. Patients must be informed that sterility is not achieved immediately, because sperm may be present in the ducts; it may take as long as 1 month for the semen to be sperm free. Patients should use a backup method of birth control until two sperm counts 4 to 6 weeks apart show no evidence of sperm.

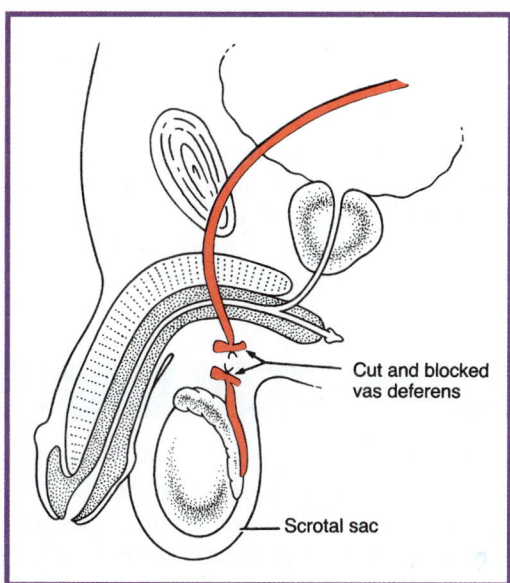

FIGURE 40-18 Vasectomy. (From Chabner DE: *The language of medicine*, ed 7, Philadelphia, 2004, Saunders.)

Labels in figure: Cut and blocked vas deferens; Scrotal sac

CRITICAL THINKING APPLICATION   40-7

Sara routinely assists Dr. Fineman with urologic and male reproductive examinations. She is also responsible for orienting new employees and helping them learn the procedures that typically occur in the office. Summarize the role of a medical assistant in helping with these examinations.

CLOSING COMMENTS

Patient Education

Most men younger than 50 years of age have not seen a physician in years. Medical studies reveal that attitude, not biology, has a lot to do with the difference between men's and women's life spans. Men just do not go to the doctor as often as women and tend to ignore symptoms of disease. The solution to maintaining good health is preventive care, and the first step is establishing a good rapport with a physician of choice. As a general rule, a man in good health should have three checkups in his twenties, three to four checkups in his thirties, and a checkup every other year in his forties. After the age of 50, a yearly checkup is recommended. In addition to testing for conditions such as cancer, heart disease, and diabetes, patient education can help male patients make responsible healthcare decisions.

The American Cancer Society recommends that men age 50 or older have an annual fecal occult stool test and a flexible sigmoidoscopy every 5 years; a double-contrast barium enema every 5 years; and a colonoscopy every 10 years to screen for colorectal cancer. Prostate screening (DRE and PSA blood test) is recommended for all men over age 50, but it also should be done at age 45 in African-Americans and in men with a family history of prostate cancer.

The urinary system is a very private, personal part of the patient's body. Patients often feel embarrassed to ask questions about how to obtain the requested urine or semen sample. The medical assistant can provide this information in a sincere, confidential manner to relieve the patient's anxiety and worry. Diagrams, models, and handouts help the patient understand disease process and the treatments and also encourages patient compliance.

Legal and Ethical Issues

When working in a urology office, the medical assistant must be very careful to ensure that patients have provided informed consent for ordered procedures. If the patient refuses a procedure, the assistant must have the patient sign the appropriate informed refusal forms, which are then included in the medical record. All patient education should be done after the physician has completed the explanation and has given the assistant instructions to do so. Never diagnose, prescribe, or offer comment about a patient's condition. Medical assistants who overstep their professional boundaries may place the physician and themselves in legal jeopardy. Remember that the patient who is legally informed and satisfied with the care received is less likely to take legal action.

A urology practice manages many sensitive patient issues that require strict adherence to confidentiality guidelines. This is especially true for a patient who has a functional disorder with the reproductive system or who has been diagnosed with an STI. In addition, special legal guidelines regarding patients diagnosed with HIV must be strictly followed to prevent litigation. The medical assistant caring for patients with HIV naturally is concerned about possible exposure. Discuss your concerns with your physician employer and remember that Standard Precautions have been developed to prevent the accidental spread of communicable diseases. If you strictly follow the standards established by the Centers for Disease Control and Prevention (CDC), you need not fear contamination.

HIPAA Applications

Staying up-to-date on confidentiality restrictions regarding a patient's HIV status is a major challenge. The Health Insurance Portability and Accountability Act (HIPAA) provides minimum requirements for protecting personal health information, but state laws can override HIPAA regulations if the state law is considered more stringent. In addition, individual healthcare institutions (hospitals, universities, physicians' practices) may have their own policies and procedures for managing confidential information about HIV and AIDS. For example, if a physician believes that a person who tests HIV positive will not disclose his or her HIV status to significant others, most states permit the physician to act. First, the physician must attempt to notify the patient that the information is going to be disclosed. Then the physician can inform the patient's spouse, sexual partner or partners, child, or needle-sharing partner or partners at risk of being infected with HIV about their risk of exposure. However, the state may limit this disclosure by not permitting the physician to identify the name of the individual who is HIV positive.

- Confidential HIV information includes any records that could reasonably identify the individual as a person who has had an HIV test, is HIV positive, has opportunistic diseases related to HIV, or has AIDS.

- HIPAA protects the patient's confidential *information,* not just the paper or electronic records of that information. This means that verbal disclosure of the individual's HIV and AIDS status is limited to only the personnel who have the right to that information according to individual state laws. For example, if you learn about your neighbor's HIV status at work and you go home and discuss it with your family, your employer is responsible for your disclosure of this information, and both you and your employer may be fined by the state or sued by the patient.

- Disclosure of HIV and AIDS status for treatment, payment, or healthcare operations can be made only with the specific written consent of the patient.
- Depending on state laws, written consent may not be needed to release HIV information if a court order for the information is issued; if the case is being reported to state or local vital statistics or public health agencies; or if the information is to be provided to certain employees of correctional institutions or residential treatment facilities, funeral directors, or emergency personnel.

SUMMARY OF SCENARIO

Sara enjoys working with Dr. Fineman and the patients seen in his urology practice. She recognizes the need to stay current with information about disorders of the urologic system and their treatment. Sara continues to learn on the job and through workshops about the urinary system and current therapies. Her expertise is constantly growing, and she uses this knowledge to help with patient education, manage telephone screening, and assist Dr. Fineman with procedures in the office. She also is working on building a database with local resources, support groups, and Internet sites that could be helpful for patients confronted with urologic or male reproductive system problems.

SUMMARY OF LEARNING OBJECTIVES

1. **Define, spell, and pronounce the terms listed in the vocabulary.**
   Spelling and pronouncing medical terms correctly bolsters the medical assistant's credibility. Knowing the definitions of these terms promotes confidence in communication with patients and co-workers.

2. **Apply critical thinking skills in performing the patient assessment and patient care.**
   Completing the Critical Thinking Application exercises throughout the chapter can help the student medical assistant become more adept at critical analysis of real-life situations.

3. **Describe the anatomy and physiology of the urinary system.**
   The urinary system is made up of two kidneys, the ureters, the urinary bladder, and the urethra. The functions of the urinary system include removing waste products; regulating water, electrolyte, and acid-base levels; activating vitamin D; and secreting erythropoietin and renin. The three processes involved in urine formation are filtration, reabsorption, and excretion. The cortex contains the nephron unit where urine is formed, and the medulla is the collection site for urine.

4. **Explain the susceptibility of the urinary system to diseases and disorders.**
   The urinary tract is made up of a continuous mucosal lining, which gives organisms that enter the urethra a direct pathway through the system.

5. **Identify the primary signs and symptoms of urinary problems.**
   The most common signs and symptoms of urinary problems include changes in the frequency of urination, dysuria, urgency, retention, and incontinence. Abnormal function of any part of the urinary tract can be determined with urinalysis, BUN levels, and creatinine clearance.

6. **Detail common diagnostic procedures of the urinary system.**
   Diagnostic procedures are summarized in Table 40-1.

7. **Compare and contrast infections and inflammations of the urinary system.**
   Most UTIs are ascending; they start with pathogens in the perineal area and infect the continuous mucosa, up through the urethra, bladder, and ureters to the kidneys. Infections and inflammations include urethritis, cystitis, pyelonephritis, and acute or chronic glomerulonephritis.

8. **Describe urinary tract disorders and cancers.**
   Renal calculi are created when salts in the urine collect in the kidney, or when fluid intake is low. They can block the flow of urine, causing hydronephrosis. Polycystic kidney disease, a slowly progressive and irreversible genetic disorder, causes the formation of multiple grapelike cysts in the kidney. Bladder cancer is invasive and can metastasize through the blood or surrounding pelvic lymph nodes. Adenocarcinoma of the kidney initially is asymptomatic and therefore frequently has metastasized before it is diagnosed. Wilms' tumor is cancer of the kidney in children.

9. **Distinguish between the two methods of treating renal failure.**
   Acute renal failure has a sudden, severe onset caused by exposure to toxic chemicals, severe or prolonged circulatory or cardiogenic shock, or acute bilateral kidney infection. Chronic renal failure is a slowly progressive process caused by gradual destruction of the kidneys' ability to filter waste materials. Dialysis is used to treat acute renal failure until the problem is reversed or, for those patients in end-stage renal disease, until transplantation can be performed. The two forms of dialysis are hemodialysis and peritoneal dialysis.

10. **Summarize the typical pediatric urologic disorders.**
    Pediatric urologic disorders include enuresis, urine reflux disorder, and cryptorchidism.

11. **Identify the male organs of reproduction.**

The male reproductive system is made up of a pair of testes that contain the seminiferous tubule, where spermatozoa are produced and carried to the epididymis for maturation and into the vas deferens for storage. The prostate gland secretes seminal fluid, which is ejaculated with sperm by the penis. Testosterone stimulates the development of secondary male characteristics and matures sperm.

12. **Determine the causes and effects of prostate disorders.**

Inflammation of the prostate usually develops because of an infection, such as an STI. Common symptoms are dysuria, tenderness, and secretion of pus from the tip of the penis. Benign prostatic hyperplasia partially blocks the flow of urine and is diagnosed from patient complaints and with a DRE. Treatment includes the use of medication or surgery. Cancer of the prostate is common in men older than age 50 and is the second highest cause of male cancer deaths; complaints include urinary obstruction, UTIs, and nocturia. Prostate cancer is diagnosed by a DRE, elevated PSA level, and biopsy; treatment includes radioactive seed implantation, hormone therapy, or prostatectomy.

13. **Outline common types of genital pathologic conditions in men.**

Male genital pathologic conditions include epididymitis, balanitis, prostatitis, and STIs. Testicular tumors usually occur in young men and generally are malignant. Erectile dysfunction (ED) typically is treated with medication. Male infertility may be caused by cryptorchidism, stricture, varicoceles, low sperm count and motility, and hormonal imbalances.

14. **Perform patient education for the testicular self-examination.**

Patient education for testicular self-examination is summarized in Procedure 40-1.

15. **Analyze the effects of sexually transmitted infections in men.**

Table 40-2 summarizes the signs, symptoms, and treatment of STIs in men. There is no cure for viral STIs, and bacterial causes of infection are becoming increasingly resistant to antibiotic therapy. STIs in male patients frequently are asymptomatic. Bacterial STIs include gonorrhea, chlamydia, and syphilis. Viral infections include hepatitis B, C, and D; genital herpes; genital warts; and HIV. Trichomoniasis is a protozoal infection that is asymptomatic.

16. **Summarize the characteristics of HIV infection and the diagnostic criteria and treatment protocols.**

HIV invades the CD4 T lymphocytes, destroying their ability to fight infection on the cellular level. Initial exposure may cause flulike symptoms, but after this it could be many years before clinical symptoms of AIDS occur. A patient is considered to be HIV positive when antibodies are detected and to have full-blown AIDS when T-cell counts are below 200 mm^3 and/or opportunistic infections are diagnosed. HIV is transmitted when infected blood or blood products, semen, or vaginal secretions come in contact with the mucous membranes or broken skin of an uninfected person; it also is transmitted from an infected mother to her fetus in utero, during delivery, or by breast-feeding. Many methods of HIV testing are available, but all must be confirmed with the Western blot test. A combination of antiviral drugs is used to control the virus, but the disease has no cure.

17. **Describe the medical assistant's role in urologic and male reproductive examinations.**

In a urology practice, the medical assistant is responsible for taking a complete patient history that details urinary symptoms, providing patient instruction for diagnostic tests, assisting with a urologic or male reproductive examination, and answering patients' questions.

18. **Discuss HIPAA applications in the urology practice.**

Staying up-to-date on confidentiality restrictions regarding a patient's HIV status varies from state to state. It is the medical assistant's responsibility to manage HIV/AIDS patient confidentiality according to the laws in the state of practice.

CONNECTIONS

Study Guide Connection: Go to the Chapter 40 Study Guide. Read and complete the activities.

Evolve Connection: Go to the Chapter 40 link at *evolve.elsevier.com/kinn* to complete the Chapter Review and Chapter Quiz. Peruse other resources listed for this chapter to increase your knowledge of Assisting in Urology and Male Reproduction.

41

ASSISTING IN OBSTETRICS AND GYNECOLOGY

SCENARIO

Betsy Davis, CMA (AAMA), recently was hired by the University Women's Hospital to work for Dr. Erin Beck, an obstetrician/gynecologist for a busy family-centered healthcare facility in her community. Betsy has worked for a family practice physician for 3 years, but this is her first position in a specialty practice. Betsy is excited about the opportunity to focus on women's health issues and is especially interested in helping in the obstetric area of the practice. Betsy's responsibilities will include understanding current methods of contraception and the patient education factors that are important for each. She also needs to develop expertise in gynecologic diseases and conditions, including diagnostic and treatment protocols for cancers of the female system. Medical assistants in the practice are expected to be able to teach breast self-examination and to answer the questions of pregnant patients concerning a healthy pregnancy, labor, and delivery.

While studying this chapter, think about the following questions:

- What is the basic anatomy and physiology of the female system?
- What does Betsy need to learn about contraceptives to be able to answer patients' questions?
- Betsy needs to become familiar with which gynecologic disorders?
- What are the primary malignancies of the female system?
- How should Betsy assist Dr. Beck with a Pap smear?

- How can Betsy teach patients to perform a breast self-examination?
- What are the stages of pregnancy and birth?
- How can Betsy help patients understand issues that can arise with menopause?
- What are the typical diagnostic procedures used in obstetrics and gynecology?

LEARNING OBJECTIVES

1. Define, spell, and pronounce the terms listed in the vocabulary.
2. Apply critical thinking skills in performing the patient assessment and patient care.
3. Explain the anatomy and physiology of the female reproductive system.
4. Trace the ovum through the three phases of menstruation.
5. Compare current contraceptive methods.
6. Summarize menstrual disorders and conditions.
7. Distinguish among different types of gynecologic infections.
8. Differentiate between benign and malignant neoplasms of the female reproductive system.
9. Prepare for and assist with the female examination, including obtaining a Papanicolaou (Pap) smear.
10. Demonstrate patient preparation for a cryosurgery procedure.

11. Teach the patient the technique for a breast self-examination.
12. Compare the positional disorders of the pelvic region.
13. Summarize the process of pregnancy and parturition.
14. Describe the common complications of pregnancy.
15. Specify the signs, symptoms, and treatments of conditions related to menopause.
16. Outline the medical assistant's role in gynecologic and reproductive examinations.
17. Demonstrate how to assist with a prenatal examination.
18. Distinguish among diagnostic tests that may be done to evaluate the female reproductive system.
19. Summarize patient education guidelines for obstetric patients.
20. Discuss the legal and ethical implications in a gynecology practice.

VOCABULARY

adnexal (add-neks-uhl) Pertaining to adjacent or accessory parts.

Bartholin's cyst A fluid-filled cyst in one of the vestibular glands that are located on either side of the vaginal orifice.

clitoris (kli'-tuh-ris) A small, elongated erectile body above the urinary meatus at the superior point of the labia minora.

coitus Sexual union between male and female; also called *intercourse*.

colostrum (koh-lahs'-trum) A thin, yellow, milky fluid secreted by the mammary glands a few days before and after delivery.

dilation The opening of the cervix through the process of labor, measured as 0 to 10 cm dilated.

dilation and curettage (D&C) The widening of the cervix and scraping of the endometrial wall of the uterus.

dysplasia An alteration in cell growth, causing differences in size, shape, and appearance.

effacement The thinning of the cervix during labor, measured in percentages from 0% to 100% effaced.

endocervical curettage The scraping of cells from the wall of the uterus.

fundus The curved, top portion of the uterus; the fundal height can be used as a measurement of fetal growth and estimated gestation.

human chorionic gonadotropin (HCG) A hormone secreted by the placenta that is found in the urine of pregnant females.

lymphedema (limf-uh-de'-muh) Swelling caused by the accumulation of lymph fluid in soft tissues.

mons pubis The fat pad that covers the symphysis pubis.

multiparous Pertaining to women who have had two or more pregnancies.

myelomeningocele A herniation of a portion of the spinal cord and its meninges that protrudes through a congenital opening in the vertebral column.

neural tube defects Congenital malformations of the skull and spinal column caused by failure of the neural tube to close during embryonic development; the neural tube is the origin of the brain, spinal cord, and other central nervous system tissue.

nonstress tests (NSTs) Fetal monitoring used in combination with maternal reports of fetal movement to evaluate the fetal heart rate response.

parturition (par-too-rih'-shun) The act or process of giving birth to a child.

stereotactic Pertaining to an x-ray procedure used to guide the insertion of a needle into a specific area of the breast.

vulva The external female genitalia, which begins at the mons pubis and terminates at the anus.

The branch of medicine that deals with pregnancy, labor, and the postnatal period is known as *obstetrics,* and the branch of medicine that deals with diseases of the genital tract in women is called *gynecology.* Frequently, a physician practices both specialties and is known as an *OB/GYN physician.* Assessment of the female reproductive system is an important part of healthcare. Patients often are hesitant and uncomfortable about talking about sexual matters, so they wait until symptoms are intolerable or disease is advanced before seeking medical care. In addition to the signs and symptoms of disease, the medical assistant must be aware of the patient's emotional state and must give support when needed.

ANATOMY AND PHYSIOLOGY

Female Reproductive System

The female reproductive system includes both internal and external organs. The internal organs are located in the pelvis and cannot be seen without special instruments, such as a vaginal speculum or a laparoscope. The external organs can be seen during the physical examination.

The primary parts of the female reproductive system are the **vulva**, vagina, uterus, fallopian tubes, and ovaries (Figure 41-1). The vulva includes the **clitoris**, the urethral meatus, and the vaginal orifice. These structures are covered by two sets of lips of tissue. The

inner set, the *labia minora,* is a thin layer of skin that extends from the top of the clitoris to the base of the vaginal opening. The external set, the *labia majora,* and the **mons pubis** are covered with hair in the adult.

The vagina connects the internal and external organs. This tube-like structure is constructed to receive the penis during **coitus**. It is lubricated by a mucous membrane lining, and its walls are made up of overlapping tissue in the form of rugae, which allows the vagina to expand during the birth of an infant. At the distal end of the vagina is the cervix, often called the *neck of the uterus,* which is approximately 1 to 1½ inches long. The uterus is an upside-down, pear-shaped muscular organ, and its sole purpose is to house and nourish the fetus from implantation shortly after conception until **parturition**. The uterine walls have three layers. The inner layer, the endometrium, is rich in blood and changes in consistency during the menstrual cycle. The middle layer, the myometrium, is the powerful muscular layer that contracts to make the birth of a baby possible. The outer layer, the perimetrium, protects the structure and attaches to ligaments that support and hold the uterus in place (Figure 41-2).

On both sides of the **fundus** of the uterus are the fallopian tubes, also called the *oviducts.* These tubes extend from the uterus to the ovaries but do not attach to the ovaries. The distal end of the tube opens freely into the abdominopelvic cavity and acts as a passageway for the ovum to the uterus and for the sperm as they search for the ovum. At the distal end of the fallopian tubes are fingerlike

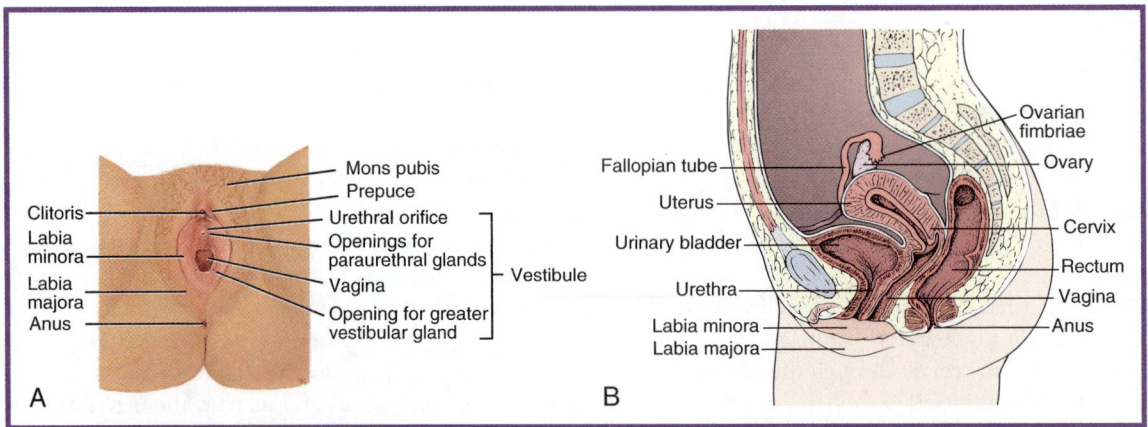

FIGURE 41-1 A, Female external genitalia. **B**, Normal female reproductive system. (**A**, from Applegate EJ: *The anatomy and physiology learning system,* ed 3, Philadelphia, 2006, Saunders; **B**, from Frazier MS, Drzymkowski JA: *Essentials of human diseases and conditions,* ed 5, St Louis, 2013, Saunders.)

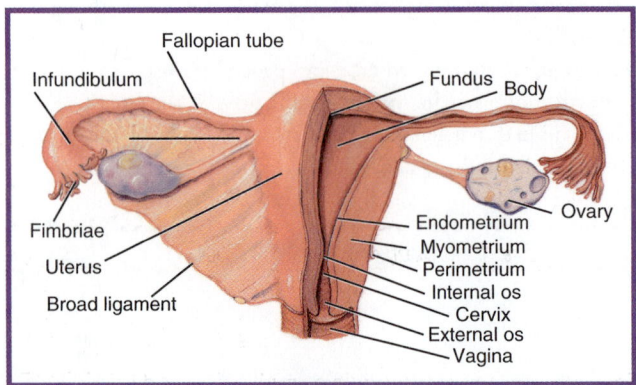

FIGURE 41-2 Uterus and fallopian tubes. (Modified from Applegate EJ: *The anatomy and physiology learning system,* ed 3, Philadelphia, 2006, Saunders.)

projections, called *fimbriae,* which move in a wavelike pattern to draw the released ovum into the fallopian tube.

The ovaries are almond-shaped organs that produce and release the egg (ovum) and excrete the hormones necessary for the development of secondary sexual characteristics and the maintenance of a pregnancy. The ovaries secrete the hormones progesterone and estrogen, which regulate reproductive function. For pregnancy to occur, the vagina must receive the sperm from the male; the sperm move up through the opening in the cervix (the cervical os), through the uterus, and into the fallopian tubes. As many as 200 million to 600 million sperm can be deposited, and about 100,000 survive the acidic environment of the vagina to swim toward the egg.

Fertilization occurs when one sperm cell penetrates and fertilizes an egg. Fertilization usually takes place in the distal third of the fallopian tube. The tiny fertilized ovum, now called a *zygote,* moves by peristalsis and the massaging motion of the cilia that line the fallopian tube into the uterus and implants itself into the uterine wall. After implantation, the placenta forms; this structure supplies the new life with all the nourishment needed for development. Once pregnancy begins, the serum levels of **human chorionic gonadotropin (HCG)** rise, and the hormone spills into the woman's urine, where it can be detected with a pregnancy test.

Breast Tissue

Mammary tissue develops from the increased estrogen secretion that occurs during puberty. In the center of each breast is a nipple surrounded by a pigmented region called the *areola.* Inside the breast are 15 to 20 lobes and their subunits—the lobules of glandular tissue that are separated by connective support tissue and surrounded by adipose tissue. The amount and distribution of adipose tissue determine the size and shape of the breast (Figure 41-3). Breast tissue also contains mammary glands, modified sweat glands that become the organs of milk production, and a system of ducts for delivery of milk to the nipple. Mammary ducts respond to elevated levels of estrogen and progesterone produced during the menstrual cycle by increasing in size, resulting in premenstrual fullness and tenderness of the breasts.

Four hormones control the mammary glands: *Estrogen* is responsible for the increase in size; *progesterone* stimulates the development of the duct system; *prolactin* stimulates the production of milk; and *oxytocin* causes the ejection of milk from the glands.

Menstruation

When a girl enters puberty, one of the many changes that occur is *menarche,* or the beginning of the menstrual cycle. Menstruation is a normal body process that occurs in every female. It is the physiologic means by which the body rids itself of the thickened endometrial wall that develops during the average 28-day cycle. The menstrual cycle involves a series of events controlled by hormones from the pituitary gland and the ovaries. The cycle is divided into three phases: the follicular phase, the luteal phase, and the menstrual phase.

Follicular Phase (Proliferative Phase)

The hypothalamus begins the follicular phase by secreting gonadotropin-releasing hormone (GnRH), stimulating the anterior pituitary to release follicle-stimulating hormone (FSH) and luteinizing hormone (LH). These hormones mature a graafian follicle in an ovary that contains an ovum. The ovarian follicle secretes estrogen, which stimulates the growth of the endometrium. It takes approximately 9 days (to day 14 of the menstrual cycle) for the

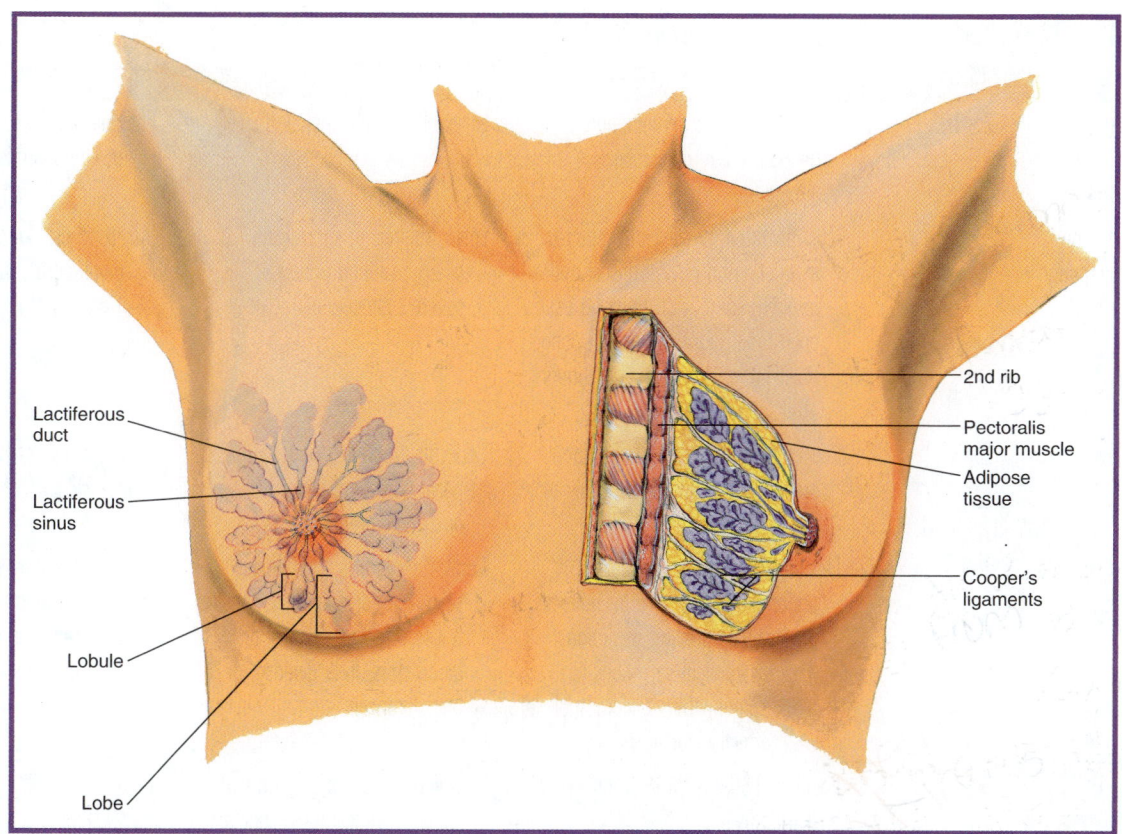

FIGURE 41-3 Normal female breast. (From Jarvis C: *Physical examination and health assessment,* ed 4, Philadelphia, 2004, Saunders.)

graafian follicle to ripen and bulge out from the ovarian wall. The ovarian wall becomes thinner as the follicle enlarges until it bursts, allowing the ovum to be liberated into the abdominal cavity. Expulsion of the egg ends the follicular phase. The fallopian fimbriae begin their wavelike motion to fan the ovum into the fallopian tube. The rupture spot on the ovary, now called the *corpus luteum,* begins to secrete progesterone. Ovulation causes a rise in body temperature, and some women experience cramping and tenderness in the lower abdominal area at this time as a result of the rupture of the graafian follicle.

Luteal Phase (Secretory Phase)

Once ovulation is complete, the luteal phase begins (day 15). During this phase, progesterone secreted by the corpus luteum causes extensive growth of the endometrium as it prepares for a possible pregnancy. If conception occurs, the corpus luteum continues to secrete progesterone until the placenta is well established and can secrete progesterone and HCG to maintain the pregnancy. If conception does not occur, HCG is not secreted, and the corpus luteum atrophies. Without increased levels of progesterone and HCG, the endometrium breaks down, and menstruation begins.

Menstrual Phase

Menstruation begins on day 28. This discharge is made up of necrotic endometrial tissue, mucus, and the blood from the endometrial engorgement. As the uterus contracts to shed the excess tissue, a woman may experience cramping pain and irritability. This phase usually lasts approximately 5 days, and then the follicular phase begins again.

CONTRACEPTION

A woman's choice of a contraceptive method is based on many factors. To make an informed choice, a patient should know the risks, benefits, side effects, costs, failure rates, and convenience of each available method. In addition, although condoms are only moderately successful at preventing pregnancy, they should be used consistently to prevent transmission of sexually transmitted infections (STIs). The medical assistant may help provide patient education on contraceptive methods. Table 41-1 summarizes the characteristics of various contraceptive methods.

Barrier Methods

Barrier methods of contraception either kill sperm through the use of a chemical spermicide or prevent them from entering the cervical os. These methods, which are relatively inexpensive, include the condom, diaphragm, and cervical cap or sponge. Each method must be used every time the person has intercourse, which means the patient must be motivated to follow through on using it. Patient education on the use of a diaphragm includes the following instructions:

- Examine the diaphragm before each use by holding it up to a bright light to check for holes or cracks.

TABLE 41-1 Characteristics of Various Contraceptive Methods

TYPE	FAILURE RATE	CHARACTERISTICS	CONTRAINDICATIONS	SIDE EFFECTS
Condom (barrier method)	2%-10%	No prescription or examination needed; easily available; inexpensive	Latex allergy in either partner	Possible allergic response to latex or spermicide
Diaphragm, cervical cap, cervical sponge (barrier method)	2%-19%	Must be fitted by clinician; requires instruction on how to insert and remove; spermicide must be used each time; diaphragm and sponge must be left in place for 6 hours after intercourse	Latex, rubber, or spermicide allergy; uterine prolapse; severe cystocele or rectocele	Increased risk for UTI (diaphragm); increased risk of abnormal Pap test result (cap)
Intrauterine device (IUD)	2%-6%	Causes endometrial inflammation, preventing implantation of a fertilized egg	Cervicitis, vaginitis, endometriosis, pelvic infection, history of STI or ectopic pregnancy	Increased risk of PID; spotting in 10%-15% of users
Implanon	1%	Flexible plastic implant inserted under skin of upper arm; releases progestin to prevent ovulation, thickens cervical secretions to block semen, thins endometrial wall; effective for up to 3 years	Certain antibiotics, HIV drugs, seizure medications may make it less effective; history of blood clots, liver disease, or breast cancer	Irregular bleeding in first 6-12 months; nausea, headache, sore breasts, scarring at implantation site
Depo-Provera (DMPA)	0.5%	Requires 150-mg IM injection every 3 months	Intention of becoming pregnant within 1 year; breast cancer; liver disease	Return of fertility may be delayed 10-18 months; headache, weight gain, possibly depression
Oral contraceptives (OCPs) Hormonal patch Vaginal ring	1%	Suppress ovulation; atrophy of the endometrium	Thrombolytic, liver, or coronary artery disease; breast, liver, reproductive tract cancer; smoker over age 35; diabetes; sickle cell disease	Nausea, breakthrough bleeding, breast tenderness, fluid retention; hypertension, elevated lipid levels, blood clots, strokes

HIV, Human immunodeficiency virus; *IM*, intramuscular; *PID*, pelvic inflammatory disease; *STI*, sexually transmitted infection; *UTI*, urinary tract infection.

- Place 1 to 2 tablespoons of spermicidal jelly or cream into the diaphragm dome before insertion.
- Leave the diaphragm in place for 6 hours after intercourse; do not douche until after you have removed it.
- Before repeated intercourse, add spermicide to the outside of the diaphragm with an applicator. Do not remove the diaphragm until 6 hours after the last intercourse.
- After removal, wash the diaphragm with soap and water, allow it to air dry, and inspect it for breaks or holes before storing.
- Have the diaphragm refitted if (1) you gain or lose more than 10 to 15 pounds; (2) you have a miscarriage, give birth, or undergo any type of pelvic surgery; or (3) you have difficulty voiding or moving your bowels with the diaphragm in place.

The cervical cap is a thimble-sized, domed barrier device that fits over the end of the cervix. It also is used with spermicidal jelly. It is 92% to 96% effective if used properly. An advantage of this barrier method is that the cap can be inserted up to 12 hours before intercourse and can stay in place up to 72 hours without affecting effectiveness or safety. The cervical sponge contains spermicide and also can be inserted hours before intercourse and is effective for 24 hours. The sponge is 80% to 91% effective if always used as directed.

Hormonal Contraceptives

Hormonal contraceptives are a highly effective and reversible form of contraception. They work by inhibiting ovulation, changing the cervical mucosa, affecting sperm mobility, and preventing thickening of the endometrial wall. Hormonal contraceptives include the birth control pill or patch, the vaginal ring, Depo-Provera injections, and the Implanon implant.

Besides being a highly effective method of birth control, oral contraceptives can be used to treat a wide range of gynecologic conditions, including menstrual irregularities, premenstrual syndrome (PMS) symptoms, and anovulation; they also can be used to prevent ovarian cysts and may be prescribed to increase bone density. However, to be effective, the pills must be taken daily. Failure rates are associated with noncompliance and can range from less than 1% in highly compliant women to greater than 15% in those who do not take the pills as prescribed. Oral contraceptive pills (OCPs) can have serious side effects, so patients should be informed of conditions that require immediate medical attention. These can be remembered with the mnemonic ACHES: **a**bdominal pain (new and severe), **c**hest pain (new and severe), **h**eadaches (new or more frequent), **e**ye problems (blurred vision or vision loss), and **s**evere leg pain. These symptoms may indicate the formation of a blood clot in the abdomen, chest, or leg, or they may be signs of a stroke; blood clot formation and stroke are the most serious complications of OCPs.

A type of oral contraception, Seasonale, limits the number of menstrual periods to four a year, although patients are more likely to have spotting and breakthrough bleeding with this hormone therapy than with the traditional 28-day birth control pill. Seasonale is designed to be taken once a day for 84 days, and then an inactive dose is taken for a week, during which the woman would menstruate. A recently released OCP, Yaz, may be prescribed for women suffering from a severe form of PMS called premenstrual dysphoric disorder (PMDD) and also is useful for treating acne in female patients at least 14 years of age who have started menstruating.

As mentioned, hormonal contraception also can be delivered via a transdermal patch, the Ortho Evra patch. The patch is a 1¾-inch square that slowly releases estrogen and progestin through the skin and into the bloodstream. It is considered as effective as oral contraceptives in women who weigh less than 198 pounds. Women who choose the patch as a birth control method are exposed to 60% more estrogen than those who take OCPs. For this reason, patch users may be at greater risk of side effects. The side effects of the patch are similar to those of birth control pills, but the risks for heart attack, stroke, and blood clots may be slightly greater. Cigarette smoking increases the risk of serious cardiovascular side effects, especially if the patient is over age 35. Patients should be told not to apply any creams or oils at the application site, to change the patch weekly for 3 consecutive weeks, and to go patch free the fourth week, allowing menstruation to occur. The patch can be applied to the buttocks, lower abdomen, and upper body but not to the breasts. The woman can bathe, shower, and swim while wearing the patch, but if it comes off, it should be replaced immediately.

The vaginal ring (NuvaRing) contraceptive device is made of flexible plastic and is inserted into the vagina. The ring slowly releases estrogen and progestin to prevent pregnancy and provide effective contraceptive action for 1 month after insertion. The device is 2 inches in diameter and can be inserted anywhere in the vagina; however, the deeper it is placed, the less likely it is to be felt after insertion. Side effects of the NuvaRing are similar to those of other hormonal contraceptives, and it may increase the risks of heart attack, stroke, and blood clots. When the patient first starts using the ring, an additional method of birth control must be used for the first week. If the ring falls out, it should be rinsed with warm water and reinserted within 3 hours. If it is out for longer than 3 hours, contraception is not certain and the patient should use another birth control method for 1 week.

Depo-Provera is an injectable contraceptive that contains high doses of progestin. Each dose prevents pregnancy for up to 3 months, but women must be compliant in returning to the healthcare facility for follow-up and repeat doses every 9 to 13 weeks. The first injection should be administered within the first 5 days of the menstrual period for birth control coverage. This is a highly effective method of contraception and is ideal for women who either do not comply with a birth control regimen or do not want to take a pill every day. However, using Depo-Provera for 2 years or longer may increase the risk of bone loss and the eventual development of osteoporosis. Almost all patients using the injections experience some menstrual irregularities, but these usually subside after two doses. Women using this form of hormonal contraception are not at risk for the side effects of estrogen exposure, such as increased risk of blood clots and cardiovascular disease.

The Implanon implant is a single rod about the size of a match that is inserted under the skin of the upper arm. Implanon releases a low, steady dose of progestin, which suppresses ovulation, thickens cervical mucus to block the passage of sperm, and thins the endometrial wall to prevent implantation. It is currently the only contraceptive implant that is approved by the FDA and is designed to prevent pregnancy for up to 3 years after insertion. The Implanon implant has similar risks and contraindications as other hormonal types of contraception.

Intrauterine Devices

The intrauterine device (IUD) (Figure 41-4) is a T-shaped plastic frame with threads attached that is inserted by the physician into the uterus to prevent pregnancy. Two types of IUDs currently are available: the copper type (ParaGard) and the hormonal type (Mirena). Both products inhibit fertilization by blocking the sperm's journey to the fallopian tubes, and if fertilization does occur, they prevent the embryo from implanting in the uterine wall. In addition, ParaGard releases copper, which acts to slow sperm in the cervix, and Mirena releases progestin, which reduces sperm mobility and prevents thickening of the endometrial wall during the menstrual cycle. Both types of IUDs are extremely effective at preventing pregnancy (over 99%); the copper type can remain in place as long as 10 years, whereas hormonal IUDs must be replaced every 5 years. The copper IUD may increase vaginal bleeding and menstrual pain, and the hormonal IUD results in both decreased menstrual flow and cramping. Shortly after placement of an IUD, the risk of infection is greater, so the physician may prescribe antibiotics before insertion to reduce this risk. To remove an IUD, the physician gently

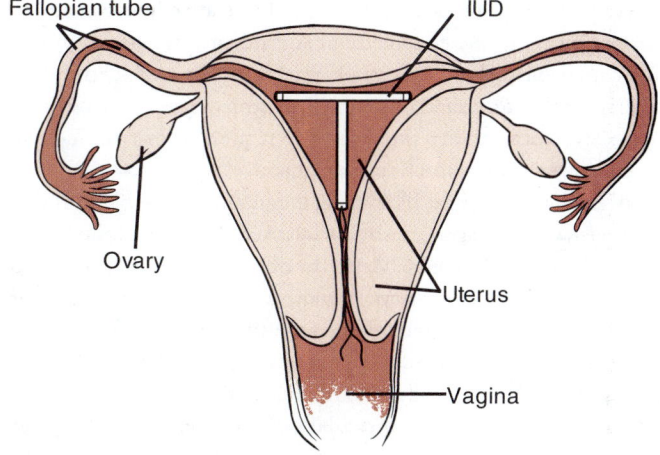

FIGURE 41-4 Intrauterine device (IUD). (From Goodman C, Snyder T: *Differential diagnosis for physical therapists: screening for referral,* ed 4, St Louis, 2007, Saunders.)

withdraws it by pulling on the IUD string. In rare instances, it must be removed surgically.

Permanent Methods

Both male and female patients can undergo surgical procedures that are considered permanent contraceptive methods. Vasectomies in the male were addressed in Chapter 40. For the female, a bilateral tubal ligation can be performed in which a portion of both fallopian tubes is excised or ligated. The cost and rate of complications are higher for tubal ligations than for vasectomies. In addition, tubal ligations must be done on an outpatient basis with general anesthesia, so the woman has that additional risk. Both procedures can be reversed, but not always successfully.

CRITICAL THINKING APPLICATION   41-1

Dr. Beck's patients often ask questions about birth control methods, including the pros and cons of each. Although Betsy's former employer also prescribed contraceptives, Betsy was not involved in patient education. Dr. Beck expects Betsy to be aware of all birth control options, their characteristics and side effects, and any patient education details that might be requested or appropriate. Betsy has decided to create a reference sheet for herself that includes all these details. What should she include?

GYNECOLOGIC DISEASES AND DISORDERS

Menstrual Disorders and Conditions

Amenorrhea is the absence of menstruation for a minimum of 6 months; in oligomenorrhea, the woman has not experienced a period for 35 days to 6 months. The absence of menstruation outside pregnancy could be the result of a number of factors, including hormonal imbalance, thyroid disease, ovarian failure, or structural defects in the female sex organs. If a patient has established menstruation that stops, this usually is the result of a problem with the hypothalamus or the pituitary. Suppression of the hypothalamus can occur as the result of an eating disorder, stress, or extreme exercise that results in low body fat content.

Women who do not ovulate and therefore do not go through a monthly shedding of the endometrial wall of the uterus are at greater risk for cancer of the endometrium and the breast. Patients usually are started on oral contraceptives that artificially provide the hormones needed to create a monthly menstrual cycle. These women may experience fertility problems and require further testing and medical intervention to become pregnant.

Abnormal menstrual bleeding is a common cause of OB/GYN visits. Menorrhagia is excessive menstrual blood loss, such as a menses lasting longer than 7 days. The physician may ask the patient to count the number of tampons and pads used for several cycles to establish a method of determining an estimate of blood loss. Iron-deficiency anemia is a sign that a woman is losing excessive amounts of blood. Metrorrhagia is spotting or bleeding between menstrual cycles. The physician may prescribe oral contraceptives to atrophy the endometrium and lessen the bleeding. Surgical options for excessive menstrual flow include **dilation and curettage (D&C)** or, in extreme cases, hysterectomy.

Endometriosis

Endometriosis is characterized by the presence of functional endometrial tissue outside the uterus. It commonly is found attached to the ovaries, urinary bladder, fallopian tubes, uterosacral ligaments, intestines, and peritoneum. Many hypotheses have been offered to explain this migration of endometrial tissue, but the most widely accepted is a retrograde flow during menstruation that causes menstrual fluid and stray endometrial cells to migrate out of the fallopian tubes and implant in the pelvic region. The use of tampons has been suggested as a possible cause. A familial tendency also has been noted; a woman with a first-degree relative (a mother or sister) who has the condition has a 10 times greater risk of developing the disorder.

The ectopic endometrial tissue responds to routine hormonal changes; it proliferates, degenerates, and bleeds just as does the endometrium of the uterus throughout the menstrual cycle. This causes inflammation at the site of the implantation that recurs with each cycle, ultimately leading to adhesions and obstruction of the affected tissue. The primary symptom of endometriosis is dysmenorrhea (painful menstruation). More than one third of affected patients also report dyspareunia (painful intercourse), and others complain of contact pain in the lower abdomen, pelvis, and back beginning 7 days before menses and lasting 3 days after onset. Other symptoms can include profuse menses, hematuria, rectal bleeding, nausea, vomiting, and abdominal cramps. Infertility is a serious problem for approximately 70% of women afflicted with endometriosis because of the buildup of scar tissue and adhesions in and around the fallopian tubes.

Conservative treatment through the use of hormones is recommended when the woman wants to have children. Treatment may consist of a laparoscopy to remove the ectopic endometrial tissue. Pharmaceutical treatment includes continuous use of oral contraceptives to prevent menstruation or Depo-Provera injections. Leuprolide acetate (Lupron) injections may be prescribed intramuscularly every month for 6 months; however, Lupron puts the patient into a state of artificial menopause and can cause menopausal symptoms, including hot flashes, vaginal dryness, and bone density loss. Another medication that causes induced menopause is oral danazol. Danazol lowers estrogen levels and increases androgen levels, which stops ovulation and shrinks endometrial growths; however, it can cause the development of male physical traits, an elevated cholesterol level, and liver disease. In severe cases, a total hysterectomy may be indicated. No cure for endometriosis is known, but pregnancy, breastfeeding, or natural menopause frequently causes remission (Figure 41-5).

CRITICAL THINKING APPLICATION   41-2

Melissa Steiner, a 19-year-old patient of Dr. Beck's, was diagnosed with endometriosis when she was 17. She has had two laparotomy procedures and continues to complain of moderate to severe pain before and during menstruation. What can Betsy tell her about the disease to help her understand why she has the pain? Melissa also wants to know about long-term complications, including the impact of the disease on fertility. She asks Betsy to help her understand Dr. Beck's explanation of the disease.

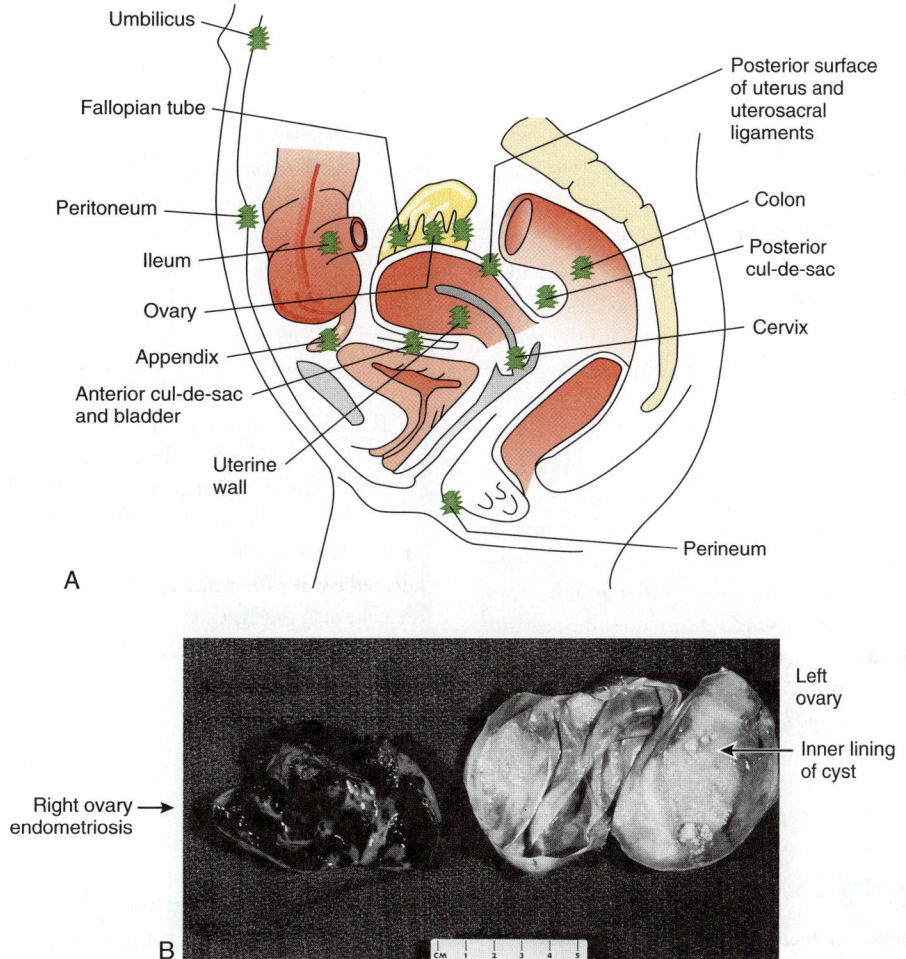

Umbilicus

Fallopian tube

Peritoneum

Ileum

Ovary

Appendix

Anterior cul-de-sac
and bladder

Uterine
wall

Posterior surface
of uterus and
uterosacral
ligaments

Colon

Posterior
cul-de-sac

Cervix

Perineum

A

Left
ovary

Inner lining
of cyst

Right ovary
endometriosis

B

FIGURE 41-5 Endometriosis. **A,** Possible ectopic sites. **B,** Endometriosis involving the right ovary (chocolate cyst) and the left ovary, showing the inner lining of a large cyst with excrescences. (**A,** From Gould BE: *Pathophysiology for the health professions,* ed 3, Philadelphia, 2006, Saunders; **B,** courtesy RW Shaw, MD, North York General Hospital, Toronto, Ontario, Canada.)

Infections

Candidiasis

Candida albicans is the yeastlike fungus responsible for this candidiasis. *Candida* organisms are commonly part of the normal flora of the mouth, skin, intestinal tract, and vagina. Overgrowth of the organism can be caused by antibiotic use, high estrogen levels, oral contraceptive use, diabetes mellitus, and immunosuppressive disorders, including acquired immunodeficiency syndrome (AIDS). Candidiasis also can be spread through sexual contact. Symptoms include vulvovaginal itching; dry, bright red vaginal tissue; and an odorless, white, "cottage cheese" vaginal discharge. This infection can be treated with prescription antifungal medications, such as oral Diflucan or miconazole or terconazole vaginal suppositories, as well as with over-the-counter (OTC) creams or suppositories, such as Gyne-Lotrimin or Monistat. Women prescribed an antibiotic for a different infection may develop vaginal candidiasis as a side effect. To help prevent the development of a fungal infection during antibiotic therapy, the patient can eat active-culture yogurt and drink acidophilus milk.

Bacterial Vaginosis

Bacterial vaginosis (BV) occurs when the normal level of bacteria in the vagina is disrupted and secondary bacteria begin to grow and infect the tissue lining. Signs and symptoms include vaginal discharge, odor, pain, pruritus, or burning. Although BV is the most common vaginal infection in women of childbearing age in the United States, it does not usually cause complications. However, an infection of the vagina appears to make women more susceptible to STIs, including infection with the human immunodeficiency virus (HIV); it may lead to pelvic inflammatory disease (PID) if the infection spreads; and in pregnant women, it is associated with a premature or low-birth-weight infant. For these reasons, antibiotic therapy is especially important for pregnant women. The antibiotic of choice is either metronidazole (Flagyl) or clindamycin (Cleocin).

Cervicitis

Cervicitis is an inflammation of the cervix caused by an invading organism. The main sign is a thick, purulent, whitish discharge with an acrid odor. Dysuria may also be noted. Cervicitis can occur after vaginal delivery as a result of an infected cervical laceration, but most cases are caused by an STI. Treatment consists primarily of antibiotics, although cauterization may be indicated when cervical erosion exists.

Pelvic Inflammatory Disease

PID is any acute or chronic infection of the reproductive system that ascends from the vagina (vaginitis), cervix (cervicitis), uterus (endometritis), fallopian tubes (salpingitis), and ovaries (oophoritis). These infections may cause the fallopian tubes to fill with pus, and chronic episodes can result in scarring of the fallopian tubes and the formation of adhesions. PID is caused by advanced, untreated vaginosis, gonorrhea, or chlamydial infection; or it can develop from infection after pelvic surgery, tubal examination, or abortion. PID is responsible for a large percentage of cases of infertility in women, primarily resulting from adhesions that form in the fallopian tubes, preventing the ovum from migrating through the tube. The patient may be asymptomatic or may complain of purulent vaginal discharge, fever, malaise, dysuria, lower abdominal pain, bleeding, nausea, and vomiting. Cultures of cervical discharge typically are done to determine the pathogenic organism. Treatment should include broad-spectrum antibiotic therapy, such as ofloxacin (Floxin) with Flagyl or ceftriaxone (Rocephin) with doxycycline (Vibramycin). If cultures are positive for an STI, treatment of the patient's sexual partner is necessary to prevent reinfection.

TRENDS IN REPORTABLE SEXUALLY TRANSMITTED INFECTIONS

- Inflammatory STIs can facilitate the transmission of infection with the human immunodeficiency virus (HIV).
- Chlamydia is known as the "silent" STI because 75% of infected women and 50% of infected men are asymptomatic. An estimated 40% of women with untreated chlamydia infections develop pelvic inflammatory disease (PID), with resultant infertility in 20% of those. The condition is diagnosed in African-American women almost eight times more frequently than in Caucasian women. The highest rates are seen in 15- to 19-year-olds. The Centers for Disease Control and Prevention (CDC) recommends yearly chlamydia screening for sexually active women younger than 26 years of age and for those older with risk factors, including new or multiple sex partners. Women infected with chlamydia are up to five times more likely to become infected with HIV if exposed. If chlamydia is diagnosed, the patient and partner should abstain from sexual intercourse until treatment has been completed to prevent reinfection.
- Gonorrhea is a major cause of PID. Most affected women are asymptomatic. Transmission can occur during vaginal birth, causing fetal blindness, joint infection, or a life-threatening blood infection. Pregnant women should be treated as soon as gonorrhea is diagnosed to reduce these risks.
- Congenital syphilis can cause stillbirth, neonatal death, physical deformities, and neurologic complications.
- Approximately one in five women 14 to 49 years of age have a genital herpes simplex virus (HSV) infection, which can cause potentially fatal infections in babies. Initial exposure during pregnancy carries a greater risk of fetal transmission. Transmission from an infected male to his female partner is more likely than from female to male. Studies show that individuals with HSV are more susceptible to HIV infection; an HIV-positive person with HSV is more infectious.
- At least 50% of sexually active men and women acquire genital human papilloma virus (HPV) infection at some point. By age 50, at least 80% of women will have acquired a genital HPV infection. Each year, about 12,000 women are diagnosed with cervical cancer; almost all of these are caused by HPV.
- Trichomoniasis is the most common curable STI in young, sexually active women. Symptoms usually appear in women within 5 to 28 days of exposure. Pregnant women with trichomoniasis may have premature or low-birth-weight (less than 5 pounds) infants.
- HIV can cross the placenta during pregnancy, can infect the baby during birth, and is found in breast milk. An elective cesarean birth at 38 weeks may be recommended to reduce the risk of transmission during the birth process.
- Women who test negative for hepatitis B may receive the hepatitis B vaccine during pregnancy.

Summarized from the CDC Sexually Transmitted Diseases (STD) Fact Sheets at http://www.cdc.gov/std/default.htm. Accessed March 1, 2013.

Sexually Transmitted Infections

The list of infectious diseases spread by sexual contact continues to grow. These diseases are considered the most common contagious diseases in the United States. All STIs are transmitted from one person to another through body fluids such as blood, semen, or vaginal secretions during vaginal, anal, or oral sex (Figure 41-6). A summary of STIs was included in Chapter 40. This chapter focuses on the impact of STIs on women.

The human papilloma virus (HPV), which causes genital warts, is a matter of special concern in women. The infection may be asymptomatic up to 2 years after exposure; however, regardless of whether the virus causes symptomatic wart development, the infection can lead to serious complications in women. HPV infection typically is first diagnosed by abnormal Pap test results, because all 40 HPV types that are sexually transmitted can cause Pap test abnormalities. A positive Pap test result is followed up with an HPV DNA test to diagnose the specific strain of HPV that caused the infection. Although most women have a healthy immune system that can successfully clear the virus without the development of future health problems, approximately 15 high-risk HPV types are linked to the development of cervical carcinoma. Women diagnosed with one of these carcinogenic strains must have regular Pap testing, usually every 3 to 6 months, for early detection and treatment of precancerous and cancerous cells on the cervix.

The vaccine Gardasil is available to protect women from the four HPV types that cause 90% of genital warts, as well as cancers of the cervix, anus, vagina, vulva, and throat. Gardasil is routinely recommended for 11- and 12-year-old girls, as well as for those females between the ages of 13 and 26 who have not completed the vaccination series. The goal is to vaccinate young girls before they are

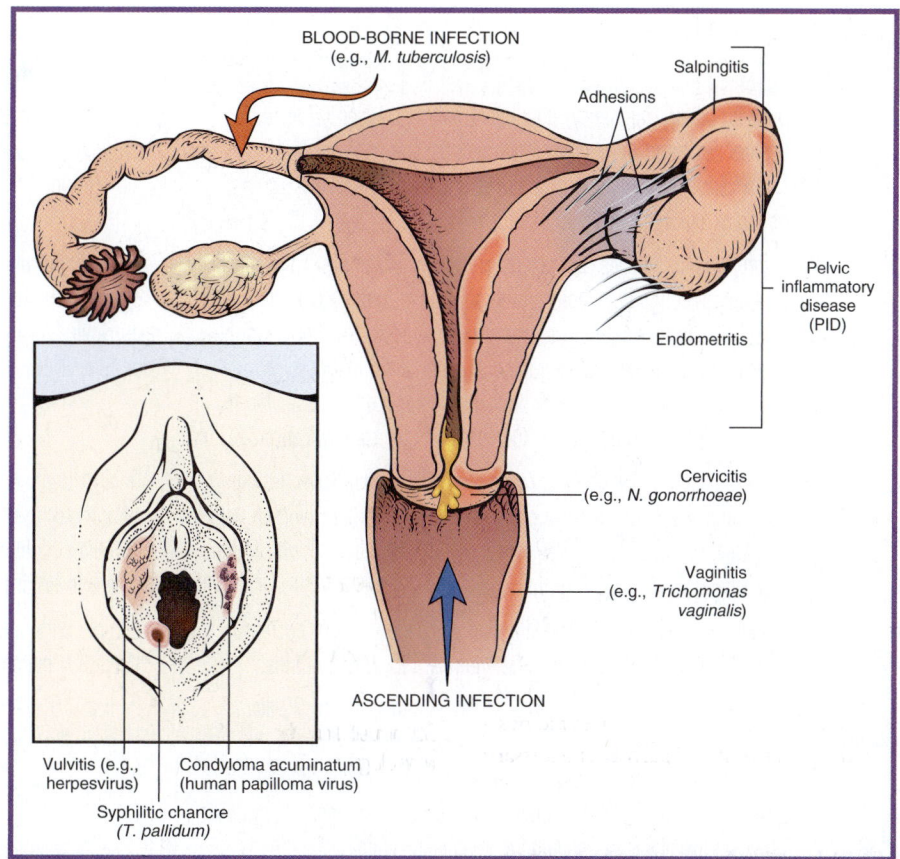

FIGURE 41-6 Ascending infections of the female genital organs are usually caused by sexual contact, pregnancy, or instrumentation. Descending infections usually begin in the blood or lymph nodes. (From Damjanov I: *Pathology for the health-related professions*, ed 3, Philadelphia, 2006, Saunders.)

sexually active. Even if a patient has been infected with one or more HPV types, she should still be vaccinated because this will give her protection from the HPV types not yet acquired. The Advisory Committee on Immunization Practice of the Centers for Disease Control and Prevention (CDC) recently made recommendations that males 9 through 26 years of age should also receive the Gardasil vaccine. The goal is to prevent the transmission of HPV to partners and to affect the rapid increase in the incidence of HPV-related throat and anal cancers. The vaccine is administered in three separate injections over a 6-month period, and total costs can range from $320 to $500.

Table 41-2 summarizes the effects of STIs on women. Individuals 35 to 44 years of age have the highest reported incidence of HIV infection and AIDS. The percentage of women and girls infected with HIV is declining, largely because of educational emphasis on the use of condoms; however, women account for 27% of HIV cases diagnosed each year. Because HIV can be transmitted through the placenta to the developing fetus, it is crucial that women be diagnosed either before pregnancy or as early in the pregnancy as possible. Treatment of HIV-positive pregnant women with a three-part ZDV regimen (zidovudine, AZT, or Retrovir) can cut the risk of transmission to below 2%. Even where resources are limited, a single dose of medicine given to mother and baby can reduce the risk of HIV infection in the infant by 50%. According to this treatment protocol, the pregnant woman should start taking ZDV at 14 to 34

weeks; it should be administered intravenously during labor and delivery; and it should be given to the infant every 6 hours for 6 weeks after birth. Because some AIDS drugs are very dangerous for developing infants, the medication regimen of a woman currently receiving treatment may be changed during pregnancy. Women who are HIV positive should never breastfeed, because the virus is present in breast milk.

> ### CRITICAL THINKING APPLICATION 41-3
> A 28-year-old patient recently was diagnosed with an acute gonorrheal and chlamydial infection. She first tested positive for HPV when she was 22. Dr. Beck asks Betsy to give the patient education materials, including the potential long-term complications of HPV, and to confirm that she understands the signs and symptoms of STIs in herself and her partner. What should Betsy include in the information?

Benign Tumors

Fibroid Tumors

Uterine fibroid tumors, also called *fibromyomas*, *leiomyomas*, or *myomas*, are idiopathic benign tumors composed mainly of smooth muscle and some fibrous connective tissue. These tumors appear to have a genetic link, because they tend to run in families. Fibroids vary in number, size, and location in the uterus and are quite

TABLE 41-2   Sexually Transmitted Infections in Women

INFECTION (CAUSATIVE ORGANISM)	SIGNS AND SYMPTOMS	TREATMENT
Chlamydia (*Chlamydia trachomatis*)	Dysuria; urinary frequency; abdominal pain; increased or decreased vaginal discharge. May cause endometritis, PID, and urethritis. Transmission to newborn can occur during vaginal delivery; causes neonatal eye infections and pneumonia.	Curable with antibiotic therapy; azithromycin (Zithromax), tetracycline, or Vibramycin
Genital herpes simplex virus (HSV-2) infection	Painful genital vesicles and ulcers; erythema and pruritus; tingling or shooting pain 1-2 days before outbreak; cycle through episodes. Viral shedding may occur during asymptomatic periods. Newborns can be infected by active lesions in vagina at birth. Brain damage, blindness, or death of the newborn may occur. Cesarean section if active lesions at time of birth. Increases risk for cervical cancer.	No cure, but antiviral therapy during episodes shortens duration of lesions; acyclovir (Zovirax), famciclovir (Famvir), or valacyclovir (Valtrex)
Genital warts (HPV)	Most prevalent STI; period of communicability is unknown; lesions seen more frequently in women; tend to recur; 25% of women with HPV develop invasive cervical cancer, should be followed with routine Pap smears (every 3-6 months).	Goal of treatment is to remove symptomatic warts; cryotherapy to lesions; podofilox solution or imiquimod cream to lesions
Gonorrhea (*Neisseria gonorrhoeae*) — bacteria	Dysuria; urinary frequency; abdominal pain; increased or decreased vaginal discharge. May cause endometritis, PID, and urethritis.	Curable with antibiotic therapy; cefixime (Suprax), azithromycin, doxycycline
Syphilis (*Treponema pallidum*) — spirochete bacteria	Six stages that can affect multiple body systems; 10- to 90-day incubation; initial sign is a painless lesion, or chancre, at the exposure site (vulva or vagina); serous discharge from chancre; lymphadenopathy. If not treated, advances to later stages. Can infect fetus via the placenta, resulting in congenital syphilis.	Penicillin G (Wycillin); if patient is allergic to penicillin, doxycycline or tetracycline
Trichomoniasis (*Trichomonas vaginalis*) — protozoa	May be asymptomatic; urinary frequency, urgency, and dysuria; frothy yellow-green vaginal discharge; pruritus.	Metronidazole (Flagyl); partner must be treated

HPV, Human papillomavirus; *PID*, pelvic inflammatory disease; *STI*, sexually transmitted infection.

common. Menorrhagia is the primary symptom, although the patient may experience bladder or rectal pressure, pelvic pressure, pain, abdominal distortion, and infertility. Fibroid tumors affect premenopausal women, because they consist of estrogen-sensitive cells. Fibroid tumors do not recur and do not undergo malignant transformation; therefore, patients with fibroid tumors have an excellent prognosis. Treatment depends on the severity of the symptoms and the patient's age, because fibroid tumors tend to become smaller and to calcify after menopause. The masses can be removed surgically, or a hysterectomy may be indicated if bleeding is a serious problem (Figure 41-7).

Ovarian Cysts

Ovarian cysts are sacs of fluid or semisolid material that form on or near the ovaries. They can occur in the follicle or the corpus luteum at any time between puberty and menopause. Most cysts are benign, and small, asymptomatic cysts do not require treatment. Large or multiple cysts may cause discomfort, low back pain, nausea, vomiting, and abnormal uterine bleeding. These can be treated with birth control pills over a period of several months to reduce the size of the cysts or to prevent the development of new cysts. If pharmaceutical therapy is not sufficient, laparoscopic procedures can be done to drain or remove large cysts. Surgery may be indicated if a cyst

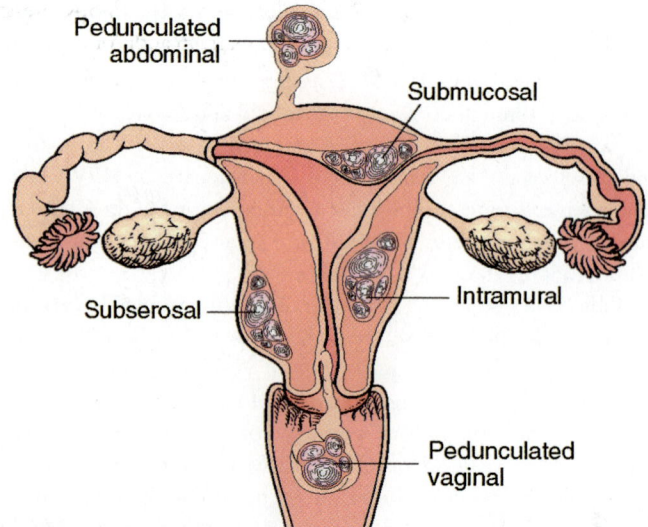

FIGURE 41-7 Uterine fibroid tumors are composed of hormone-sensitive cells and are designated subserosal, intramural, submucosal, or pedunculated, depending on their location. (From Salvo SG: *Mosby's pathology for massage therapists*, ed 2, St Louis, 2009, Mosby.)

ruptures, or in cases of torsion of the ovary, in which twisting cuts off the blood supply to the ovary.

Polycystic ovary syndrome is a hormonal problem that may cause cysts to develop over enlarged ovaries. The diagnosis depends on the presence of two or more indicators, including irregular or no menstruation, high testosterone levels, hirsutism (excessive body hair in a masculine pattern), acne, and male pattern baldness (alopecia). Women affected by this disorder have unusually high levels of testosterone, estrogen, and LH and decreased amounts of FSH. They initially may be diagnosed because of fertility problems. The combination of hormone irregularities causes the symptoms associated with the disorder; however, some women are diagnosed by menstrual irregularity alone. These women are at greater risk of uterine cancer, because the endometrium does not slough off monthly. Also, there appears to be a link with insulin and cholesterol metabolism, so women with this disorder are at greater risk of developing diabetes mellitus type 2 and heart disease. The condition is treated with OCPs to stimulate menses artificially, to lower androgen levels, and to reduce masculine-type symptoms if present.

Fibrocystic Breast Disease

Fibrocystic breast disease is characterized by the presence of multiple, palpable nodules in the breasts; these nodules usually are associated with pain and tenderness and fluctuate with the menstrual cycle (Figure 41-8). Over time, the cysts enlarge, and the connective tissue of the breast is replaced with dense, firm fibrous tissue. The masses may be fibrous tumors that have degenerated or sacs filled with fluid. The cysts feel firm and movable, and the degree of tenderness and the size depend on the point in the menstrual cycle, with tenderness peaking just before and during the secretory phase. Several different cellular types of cysts can form, but fibrocystic changes in the breast are not considered precancerous.

Although the risk of breast cancer is not increased with fibrocystic breast disease, the diagnosis of cancerous breast masses becomes more complicated. Because the breasts consistently feel lumpy, breast examinations may not isolate a suspicious mass. In addition, accurate

mammography screening is complicated by the dense nature of the cysts, making visualization of a cancerous area more difficult. Because caffeine and high-fat diets aggravate the symptoms of fibrocystic breast disease, diet therapy often is recommended. Patients should be encouraged to perform monthly breast self-examination (BSE) and to report any changes in the breast immediately.

Malignant Tumors

Most problems encountered with the female reproductive organs are related to abnormal cell growth. Early screening and preventive intervention are essential. Most malignant tumors require surgical removal. Radiation, chemotherapy, and hormone therapy are alternative treatment choices.

Cervical Cancer

Almost all cervical carcinomas are caused by HPV. The first stage of cervical cancer is asymptomatic, but early diagnosis of cervical cellular changes is possible with a Papanicolaou (Pap) smear (Procedure 41-1). During the invasive stage, the patient reports abnormal vaginal bleeding and persistent discharge, as well as bleeding and pain during intercourse. The average age of diagnosis for carcinoma in situ (cancerous cells restricted to the original site) currently is 35; however, it continues to drop, because the number of cases in young women is increasing. Women with HPV infection may be tested every 3 to 6 months, depending on previous Pap results.

> ### THE AMERICAN COLLEGE OF OBSTETRICIANS AND GYNECOLOGISTS (ACOG) NEW PAP SMEAR GUIDELINES
>
> - The first screening Pap smear should be performed at age 21 unless there is a history of an abnormal Pap smear.
> - Pap smears should be performed every 2 years (assuming prior Pap smears have been normal) for women in their 20s.
> - Women age 30 and older with three consecutive normal Pap smears should have a Pap smear every 3 years.
> - Women who have had a hysterectomy for noncancerous reasons do not need a Pap smear unless they have a cervix.
> - Follow these guidelines whether the patient has received the human papilloma virus (HPV) vaccine or not.
> - Women should have a yearly physical examination, including breast exam, pelvic exam (with or without a Pap smear), and sexually transmitted infection (STI) screening if indicated.
> - Patients must have an annual exam to receive birth control.
> - Patients with a history of an abnormal Pap smear should consult with their physician regarding how often to schedule Pap smears.

From http://www.niu.edu/healthservices/forms/pdfs/PapSmearHandout.pdf. Accessed May 8, 2012.

The patient should be informed of factors that can interfere with Pap test results, including menstruation and the use of vaginal creams, spermicidal foams, and douching 2 to 3 days before the examination. Also, the patient should refrain from vaginal intercourse for 24 hours before the examination because it may cause inflammation. The medical assistant should include in the patient

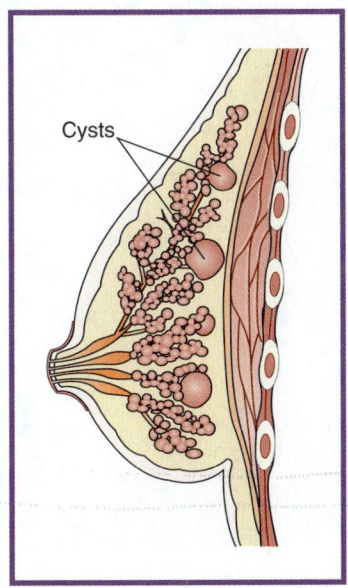

Cysts

FIGURE 41-8 Fibrocystic breast disease.

Prepare a Patient for Procedures and/or Treatments: Assist with the Examination of a Female Patient and Obtain a Pap Smear

GOAL: *To assist the physician in the examination of a female patient and in obtaining a diagnostic Pap smear.*

EQUIPMENT and SUPPLIES

- Patient gown
- Lubricant
- 4 × 4-inch gauze squares
- Laboratory requisition slips
- Drape sheet
- Examination light
- Cervical spatula and Cytobrush
- ThinPrep container
- Vaginal speculum
- Uterine sponge forceps
- Disposable examination gloves
- Urine specimen container, if needed
- Stool for occult blood test, if needed
- Biohazard waste container
- Appropriate patient education materials
- Patient's record

PROCEDURAL STEPS

1. Assemble the materials needed and prepare the room. Prepare the equipment and supplies needed for the Pap smear (Figure 1).

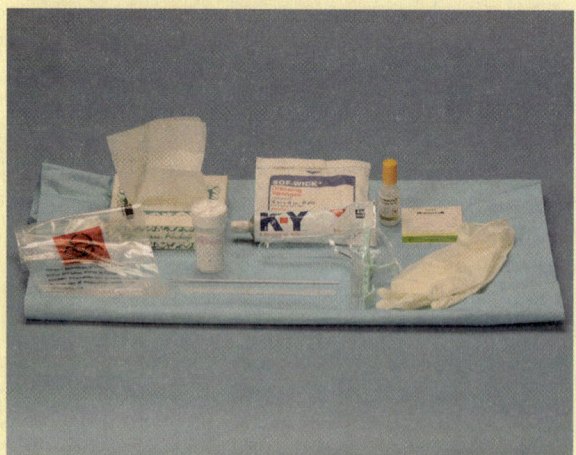

(From Bonewit-West K: *Clinical procedures for medical assistants*, ed 7, St Louis, 2008, Saunders.)

2. Sanitize your hands and follow Standard Precautions.
   PURPOSE: To ensure infection control.
3. Identify the patient and briefly explain the procedure.
   PURPOSE: Explanations gain the patient's cooperation and alleviate apprehension.
4. Instruct the patient to empty the bladder and collect a urine specimen if needed.
   PURPOSE: The physician's bimanual examination (see Figure 41-15) is performed on an empty bladder.

5. Instruct the patient to disrobe completely and to put on a gown with the opening in the front.
6. Assist the physician with the breast examination. To start, have the patient sit at the end of the examination table. Drape the patient and assist the physician with the examination. Reassure the patient as needed.
7. When the physician is ready to examine the breasts and the abdomen with the patient in the supine position, assist the patient into the supine position and drape as needed.
   PURPOSE: To prevent unnecessary exposure of the patient.
8. When the physician is ready to begin the vaginal examination, assist the patient into the lithotomy position. Have the patient slide down to the end of the table; then adjust the stirrups as needed so that the knees are relaxed and rotated outward. Remember always to position the patient while she is underneath the drape.
9. Direct the light source onto the perineum.
   PURPOSE: To facilitate better viewing of the cervix.
10. Put on gloves. Warm the stainless steel vaginal speculum in warm water (the physician may prefer a disposable plastic speculum). Pass the proper instruments to the physician in the proper sequence. The physician will need the Cytobrush for cervical cells and the spatula for the cervical sample.
    PURPOSE: Teamwork enhances efficiency.
11. Assist the physician with ThinPrep preparation by swirling the cervical specimen in the preservative solution at least 10 times to ensure that the specimen has been mixed with the preservative solution (Figure 2).

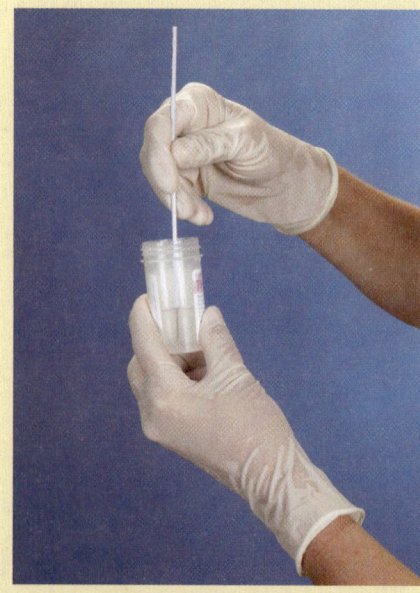

(From Bonewit-West K: *Clinical procedures for medical assistants*, ed 7, St Louis, 2008, Saunders.)

PROCEDURE 41-1—cont'd

12. Label the specimen container and place it in a biohazard bag.
13. Apply water-soluble lubricant to the physician's fingers.
    <u>PURPOSE:</u> To facilitate the bimanual examination.
14. The physician may prepare a stool sample for occult blood testing after the rectal examination. Have the materials ready.
15. Instruct the patient to breathe deeply through the mouth with the hands crossed over the chest.
    <u>PURPOSE:</u> To help relax the muscles.
16. Place the soiled instruments in a basin.
    <u>PURPOSE:</u> To help create better aesthetic surroundings.
17. Assist the patient off the table and with dressing if needed.
18. While the patient is in the dressing room, clean the examination room, removing used equipment.
19. Sanitize and sterilize stainless steel equipment. Remove your gloves and sanitize your hands.
    <u>PURPOSE:</u> To ensure infection control.

20. Prepare the Pap smear and other samples for transportation to the laboratory. Complete the requisitions, including the date of the patient's last menstrual period (LMP) and whether she is on hormone therapy.
21. Record all procedures in the patient's medical record.
    <u>PURPOSE:</u> A procedure is not done until it is entered into the patient's record.

8/23/XX 2:00 PM Pap smear and pelvic examination completed by physician. ThinPrep specimen placed for pickup by University Laboratory for cytology. Pt tolerated procedure well. Betsy Davis, CMA (AAMA) _____

---

history the use of certain medications, such as tetracycline, which may interfere with results; whether the patient has a latex allergy; the date of the last menstrual period (LMP); whether the patient has a history of a bleeding disorder or is taking anticoagulant medications; and whether the patient is pregnant or may be pregnant.

The physician obtains the cervical smear with a Cytobrush or a small wooden spatula that is inserted and rotated in the cervical canal to obtain endocervical cells for cytology. The ThinPrep Pap Test has replaced the traditional slide preparation method for analyzing these cells, because it is more accurate in diagnosing precancerous and cancerous lesions and rarely has to be repeated because of an inadequate cellular sample. The physician uses the same technique to collect the cellular sample, but instead of fixing it onto a glass slide, the collection device is rinsed into a vial containing a preservative solution. In the laboratory, a processor filters the sample and creates a slide with a thin layer of cervical cells that is more uniform and better preserved than is possible with the traditional method.

The pathologist examines the slide to determine whether cellular abnormalities are present. The results are classified into one of five categories: negative or normal, atypical squamous cells, abnormal with low-grade squamous lesions, abnormal with high-grade lesions (precancerous), or carcinoma cells. Inflammation or an STI infection can cause abnormal changes in cervical cells, so the physician decides how to manage abnormal results on the basis of other diagnostic studies.

If the Pap test indicates abnormal cells, the pathologist can grade cervical changes using a cervical intraepithelial neoplasia (CIN) system of I to III, depending on the degree of cellular **dysplasia** (Figure 41-9). CIN I indicates mild to moderate dysplasia; CIN II, moderate and moderate to severe dysplasia; and CIN III, carcinoma in situ. Patients whose Pap smears indicate dysplasia of any severity should have a colposcopy with biopsy if indicated and possibly an **endocervical curettage**. If adequately diagnosed and treated, carcinoma in situ of the cervix has a 100% survival rate at 5 years.

Carcinoma of the cervix is classified into the following stages:
- Stage 0: Carcinoma in situ
- Stage I: Carcinoma of the cervix with no **adnexal** involvement
- Stage II: Carcinoma of the cervix that has not spread into the pelvic wall or vagina
- Stage III: Carcinoma of the cervix that has spread into the lower part of the vagina; may be blocking the ureters
- Stage IV: Carcinoma of the cervix that has spread to nearby organs, such as the bladder or rectum, with involvement of structures outside the pelvic area

Colposcopy is the visual examination of the vagina and cervical surfaces through the use of a colposcope (Figure 41-10). The colposcope is a microscope with a light source and a magnifying lens that can be used during a vaginal examination to locate and evaluate abnormal cells and to detect cancer of the cervix in the early stages, to examine tissue from which an abnormal Pap smear has been obtained, and to monitor areas of the cervix where malignant lesions have been removed. Colposcopy also can be used to monitor women at risk of developing cervical cancer because their mothers were given diethylstilbestrol (DES) during their pregnancy. A cervical biopsy may be performed in conjunction with a colposcopy. A major advantage of obtaining a biopsy during colposcopy is that the instrument permits visualization of the suspicious area so that the biopsy can be taken from the most atypical site.

Colposcopy is a relatively safe, painless procedure performed in the physician's office. Discomfort may occur when the speculum is inserted into the vagina to improve visualization of the tissue. Discomfort and bleeding can occur when tissue is taken for biopsy. Depending on the results of a previous biopsy, the patient may need a more extensive procedure or conization, in which a cone-shaped wedge of cervical tissue is removed for treatment or further analysis. More often, a less invasive loop electrosurgical excision procedure (LEEP) is performed with injection of a local anesthetic to the cervix

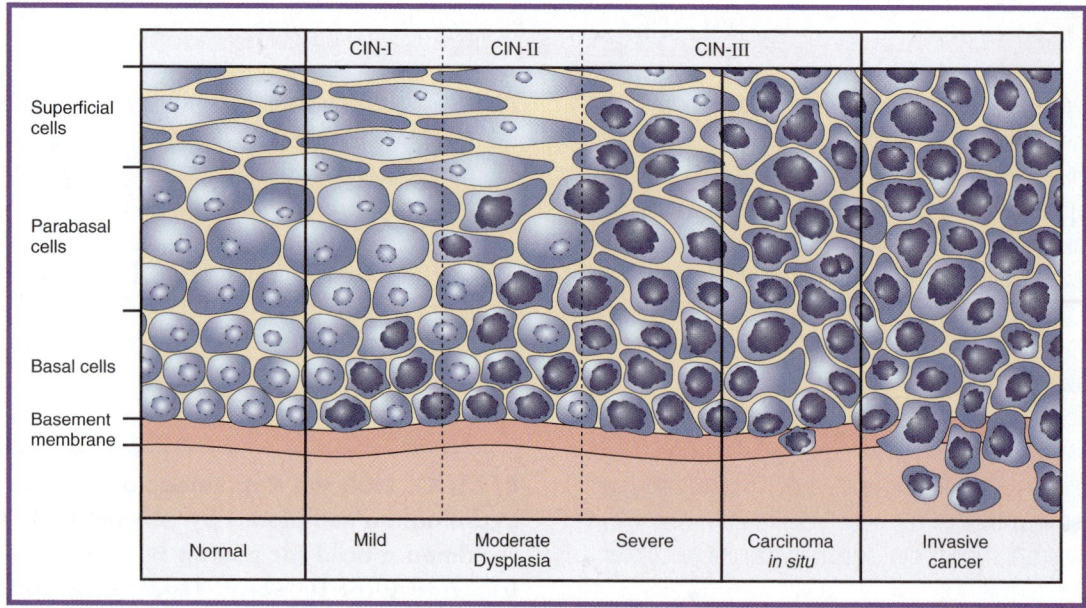

	CIN-I	CIN-II	CIN-III	

FIGURE 41-9 Cervical dysplasia and carcinoma. (From Damjanov I: *Pathology for the health-related professions,* ed 3, Philadelphia, 2006, Saunders.)

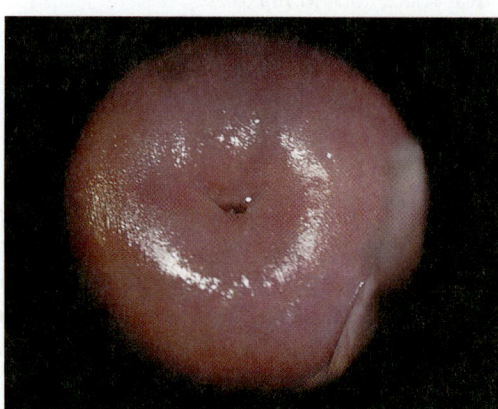

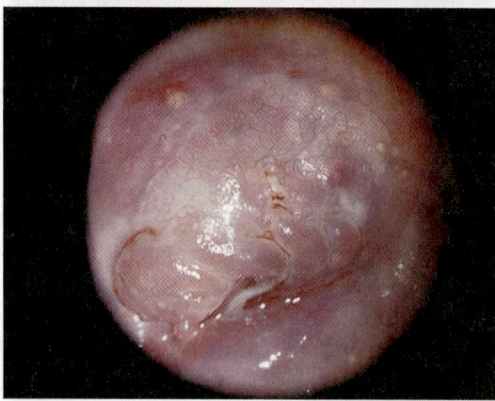

FIGURE 41-10 Colposcopic appearance of normal cervix *(top)* and abnormal cervix *(bottom).* (From Damjanov I: *Pathology for the health-related professions,* ed 3, St Louis, 2006, Saunders.)

and insertion of a wire loop into the vagina. A high-frequency electrical current running through the wire is used to remove abnormal tissue from both the cervix and the endocervical canal. Like conization, LEEP can be used as a diagnostic tool to collect biopsy samples and as a treatment to remove abnormal tissue.

Depending on the condition of the cervix, cryosurgery, or the application of freezing temperatures, may be used to treat chronic cervicitis and cervical erosion. Freezing causes cellular necrosis, and in approximately 1 month, the dead cells are replaced with healthy cells. The procedure involves placing a probe against the problem area on the cervix and applying liquid nitrogen to the area for approximately 3 to 4 minutes or until the site is frozen (Procedure 41-2). The patient may experience some pain for 30 minutes or so after the procedure and a slight watery discharge for up to a week. If any signs of infection, foul discharge, or pain develop, the patient should call the physician's office. She is advised not to engage in sexual intercourse for 1 month and to expect a heavier than usual menstrual flow for the first cycle after the procedure.

Endometrial Cancer

The inner lining of the uterus, the endometrium, is at increased risk for dysplasia in postmenopausal women who have never had children and in those who experienced early menarche and late menopause. Endometrial cancer also is seen more frequently in obese women and in those with a history of irregular ovulation. This slow-growing cancer begins with hyperplasia of the endometrial wall, followed by dysplasia. Early signs are irregular vaginal bleeding and leukorrhea (white or yellow) vaginal discharge. The diagnosis usually is made with an endometrial biopsy. Treatment involves a complete hysterectomy with radiation therapy and chemotherapy. Because most of these tumors develop after menopause, vaginal bleeding is unusual, and the woman is more likely to seek medical attention. Because of this, early diagnosis and treatment lead to a survival rate of almost 90%.

Ovarian Cancer

Ovarian neoplasms are the most important pathologic disorder of the ovaries. Ovarian cancer is the second most common gynecologic cancer but is ranked first in gynecologic cancer deaths. In fact, it

PROCEDURE 41-2

Prepare a Patient for Procedures and/or Treatments: Prepare the Patient for Cryosurgery

GOAL: *To prepare the patient and assist the physician in cryosurgery.*

EQUIPMENT and SUPPLIES

- Cryosurgery machine equipped with liquid nitrogen canister
- Cryoprobe
- Cervical tenaculum
- Cervical ring forceps or disposable cervical swabs
- Vaginal speculum
- 4 × 4-inch gauze squares
- Disposable examination gloves
- Gowns and face protection, appropriate personal protective equipment (PPE)
- Specimen containers
- Biohazard waste container
- Cytology request forms
- Patient's record

PROCEDURAL STEPS

1. Assemble the necessary equipment.
   PURPOSE: To expedite the procedure.
2. Sanitize your hands.
   PURPOSE: To ensure infection control.
3. Take the patient's temperature and blood pressure and record them in the patient's record.
   PURPOSE: To establish a baseline for vital signs.
4. Drape the patient and assist her into the lithotomy position. Put on gloves.
5. Assist the physician with the procedure by handing equipment as needed.

6. Encourage the patient to take deep breaths to promote relaxation of the pelvic muscles during the procedure. Observe the patient for any signs of distress.
   PURPOSE: To ensure patient safety.
7. When the procedure is complete, place the patient in a supine position and allow her to rest while you tidy the room and remove the used supplies. Retake her temperature and blood pressure.
   PURPOSE: To ensure that vital signs and blood pressure return to baseline levels.
8. Help the patient sit up and assist her in dressing if needed.
   PURPOSE: To ensure patient safety.
9. Remove your gloves and sanitize your hands.
   PURPOSE: To ensure infection control.
10. Disinfect and sterilize equipment per the manufacturer's directions and return the equipment to the proper storage area.
11. Provide instructions on follow-up care as ordered by the physician.
12. Record the procedure and the final vital sign measurements in the patient's record.
    PURPOSE: A procedure is not done until it is recorded.

7/22/XX 10:25 AM Cervical cryosurgery procedure completed by physician without incident. Pt stable, T 98.6°, BP 118/72. No c/o discomfort. Pt to call office if any problems noted. Betsy Davis, CMA (AAMA) _____

---

causes more deaths than all other tumors of the reproductive system combined. Metastasis has occurred in 71% of cases before the tumor is diagnosed. Symptoms do not appear until the tumor has enlarged enough to exert pressure on nearby structures; patients complain of vague abdominal discomfort, bloating, urinary urgency, weight loss, and general malaise.

Researchers are working to perfect a blood test that can be used to screen for ovarian cancer so the disease can be diagnosed in earlier, more treatable stages. Currently, ovarian cancer is diagnosed by a combination of a pelvic examination that indicates a mass in an ovary; a cancer antigen CA125 blood test, which identifies a protein found in abnormally high levels in women with ovarian cancer (although the test can produce false-positive and false-negative results); and a pelvic or transvaginal ultrasound to evaluate the size and shape of the ovaries. The ultimate diagnosis is based on a biopsy to confirm the presence of cancerous cells.

Little is known about how or why ovarian cancer occurs, but pregnancy, breastfeeding, and oral contraceptive use may reduce the risk. Treatment includes a complete hysterectomy (removal of the

uterus, fallopian tubes, and ovaries), radiation therapy, and chemotherapy. Ovarian tumors are classified on the basis of their biologic features. About 20% of all ovarian tumors are cancerous, and the recovery rate is linked to the location, the stage of tumor development, and the patient's age.

Breast Cancer

Breast cancer is the second leading cause of cancer deaths in women. According to the American Cancer Society, 1 in 8 women has a lifetime risk of developing breast cancer and a 1 in 28 risk of dying from the disease. Predisposing factors include a family history of breast cancer (especially in the mother or a sister), early menarche and late menopause, first pregnancy after age 30 or no pregnancy, prolonged use of estrogen replacement therapy, excess alcohol intake, smoking, and obesity.

Because recent research has failed to link reduced death rates from breast cancer with monthly breast self-examinations (BSE), the American Cancer Society now recommends that women have their physician perform a clinical breast examination (CBE) rather than rely on monthly BSEs for early detection. However, although a monthly BSE is now considered optional, women still should be aware of the normal appearance and texture of the breasts and should immediately report to the physician any changes or new breast symptoms. The medical assistant should be prepared to teach the BSE technique (Procedure 41-3). CBEs should be done every 3 years from age 20 to 39 and annually at 40 years of age and over. A mammogram should be done annually starting at age 40 and each year after that. If a woman has an increased risk of breast cancer (e.g., family history), the physician may recommend annual mammography screening before age 40 or other diagnostic procedures, such as ultrasound or magnetic resonance imaging (MRI). An MRI scan can

reveal tumors too small to detect with a breast examination that may not show up clearly on a mammogram. The American Cancer Society recommends MRI screening for women at high risk for developing breast cancer.

Indications of breast cancer include a palpable breast mass that is firm and immovable, breast pain, tissue thickening, nipple retraction or dimpling, nipple discharge, and axillary lymphadenopathy. If a breast mass is palpated, a mammogram or ultrasound of the area is ordered and, if indicated, a biopsy is performed. The physician may perform a needle biopsy to remove cells and/or tissue from a palpated mass for evaluation by the pathologist. If a nonpalpable mass is found on a mammogram, a **stereotactically** guided needle

PROCEDURE 41-3

Instruct Patients According to Their Needs to Promote Health Maintenance and Disease Prevention: Teach the Patient Breast Self-Examination

GOAL: *To teach the patient how to palpate her breasts to check for possible abnormalities.*

EQUIPMENT and SUPPLIES

- Instruction pamphlet/shower card
- Teaching model (to demonstrate the technique before a return demonstration by the patient)
- Patient's record

PROCEDURAL STEPS

1. Assemble the necessary equipment.
2. Instruct the patient to examine her breasts while bathing or showering in warm water, because the fingers glide more easily over wet tissue. The best time to perform this examination is immediately after the end of the menstrual period, when breast engorgement is minimal. Nonmenstruating women should examine their breasts the first of each month.
3. Instruct the patient to raise one arm, using the right hand to examine the left breast and the left hand for the right breast. Using the finger pads of the three middle fingers, move in a small circular pattern up and down the breast. Starting at the axillary region, work down the area and back up again from the axillary to the ribs below the breast, back up to the clavicle, and repeatedly across to the sternum bilaterally (Figure 1).

4. After finishing her bath or shower, the patient should continue the examination in front of a mirror with the arms at the sides. Then, with her arms raised above her head, she should look carefully for changes in the size, shape, and contour of each breast. She should look for puckering, dimpling, or changes in skin texture (Figure 2).

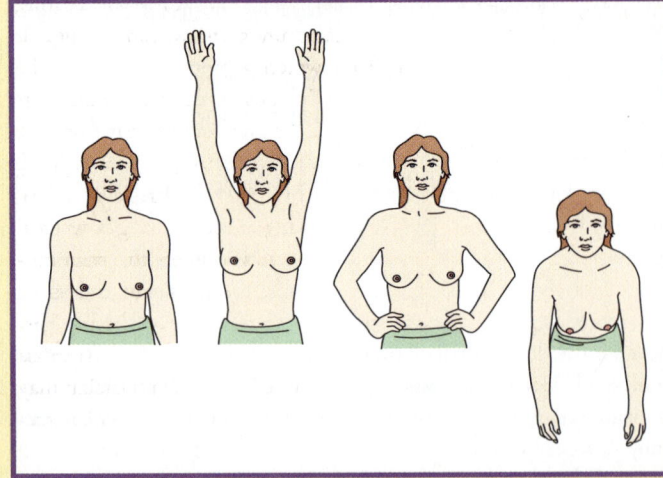

5. Instruct the patient to squeeze both nipples gently and to look for discharge (Figure 3).

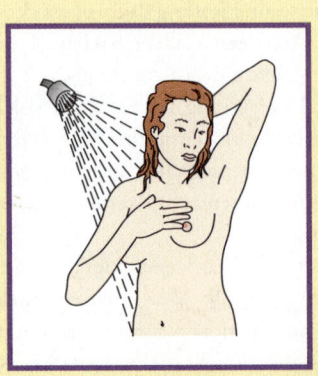

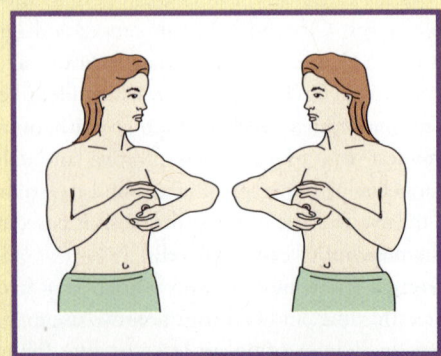

6. Before dressing, the patient should lie on a bed. A towel or pillow is placed under the right shoulder, and the right hand is placed behind the head. The right breast is examined with the left hand. Instruct the patient to press gently in small circles, starting at the top outermost edge, including the axillary region, and spiraling in toward the nipple. This is repeated with the left breast (Figure 4).

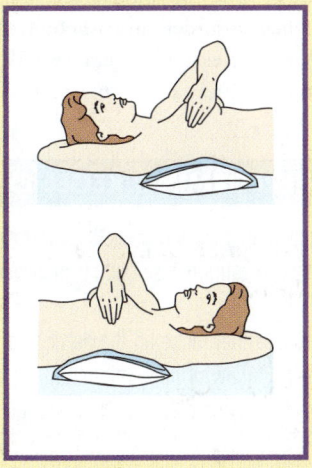

7. The patient should return the demonstration using the teaching model to confirm her understanding.
8. Give the patient an instruction pamphlet to use at home. If you have given her a shower card to follow, show her how it will hang inside the shower on a faucet or the shower nozzle and serve as a quick reference guide.
9. Record the patient education intervention in the patient's medical record.
   PURPOSE: Patient education interventions should always be documented; a procedure is not done until it is entered into the patient's record.

---

aspiration is done, and surgical biopsy is a possible follow-up. During this procedure, the physician uses a mammogram to guide the needle toward the suspicious mass, from which a biopsy sample can be taken. If a tissue sample cannot be obtained through a needle, wire localization may be done to pinpoint the areas of concern from the mammogram. During this diagnostic procedure, a thin wire is passed through the breast to the point of concern (based on mammogram visualization). This wire marking is used during a surgical procedure to pinpoint tissue that was suspicious on the mammogram. If a biopsy shows malignant cells, the physician orders an estrogen and progesterone receptor test to determine whether hormones affect the way the cancer grows. If the cancer cells increase growth patterns when exposed to hormone levels, the physician may recommend treatment with a drug such as tamoxifen, which prevents estrogen from binding to these sites.

Treatment of breast cancer depends on the type of carcinoma and its staging. Treatment almost always begins with surgery, but the type of surgery and the extent of the tissue removed depend on several factors. Breast-saving surgeries include lumpectomy, in which only the suspicious mass plus a surrounding area of normal tissue is removed, and radiation therapy is used as a follow-up to destroy any remaining cancerous cells. A partial mastectomy may be done for more advanced cases; this procedure involves removal of the tumor and tissue surrounding it, part of the chest muscle beneath the mass, and some of the lymph nodes in the axillary region. A complete mastectomy, which involves removal of the entire breast, chest muscle, and axillary lymph nodes, may still be indicated if the mass has spread. However, removal of multiple axillary lymph nodes greatly increases the risk that subsequent **lymphedema** and recurrent infections will develop in the arm on the affected side. New

techniques recommend the removal of the sentinel lymph node, the first lymph node to which the cancer is likely to spread from the tumor. The sentinel node is found by injecting a blue dye near the tumor; the lymph vessels absorb the dye and carry it toward the lymph nodes, and the first node to receive the dye and turn blue is the one that is removed for pathologic testing. If the sentinel node is cancer free, there is very little chance that the breast tumor has metastasized, and no other nodes need to be removed. If cancer cells are evident, further diagnostic procedures are indicated to determine possible locations of metastatic tumors.

Many patients now opt for breast reconstruction after a partial or complete mastectomy. This procedure typically is performed by a plastic surgeon and can be done using a variety of methods, including implantation of a silicone or gel material or the use of fat and other tissue from another part of the body, such as the abdomen, to reconstruct breast tissue. After the breast has been re-formed, the physician uses tattoo techniques to create the areola and nipple. The patient must discuss these options with her surgeon before the mastectomy is performed; therefore, the medical assistant may be involved in the referral process.

INFLAMMATORY BREAST CANCER

- Inflammatory breast cancer is a rare, aggressive cancer that causes the sudden onset of discoloration and warmth in the affected breast, along with edema, dimpling of the skin, enlarged axillary lymph nodes, and pain.
- The condition is easily confused with a breast infection, so patients should contact their physician as soon as symptoms appear.

- Cancer cells spread rapidly and block lymph vessels in the skin, which results in the classic symptoms.
- The condition is diagnosed by an excisional biopsy to confirm the presence of clumped cancer cells in the area lymph vessels.
- Inflammatory breast cancer typically is diagnosed as stage II, which means that the cancer has spread to local lymph nodes. However, one third of patients are diagnosed with stage IV carcinoma, in which metastasis already has occurred.

Positional Disorders of the Pelvic Region

The correct anatomic position for the uterus is tipped slightly anteriorly (anteverted) and bent over the bladder, with the cervix down and back. However, the uterus may be positioned at various angles because of a congenital anomaly, aging, or the effects of childbirth. With the aging process and/or multiple pregnancies, the muscles and ligaments that support the uterus, bladder, and rectum can stretch or weaken. This weakening of the supportive structures of the pelvic floor can result in multiple structural disorders.

A cystocele is a protrusion of the bladder into the anterior wall of the vagina. The bladder becomes angled, and urinary retention is common, along with frequent cystitis. The diagnosis can be made by having the patient bear down as the vaginal opening is examined; this allows the physician to feel the bladder protrusion. A cystocele can result from injury during childbirth, obesity, heavy lifting, chronic coughing, and poor musculature that comes with aging (Figure 41-11).

A rectocele is a protrusion of the rectum into the posterior wall of the vagina. The patient complains of difficulty with bowel movements and pressure in the pelvic region. The diagnosis can be made by having the patient bear down as the vaginal opening is examined so that the physician can palpate the posterior wall. Rectoceles are most often seen in postmenopausal women. A rectocele may result

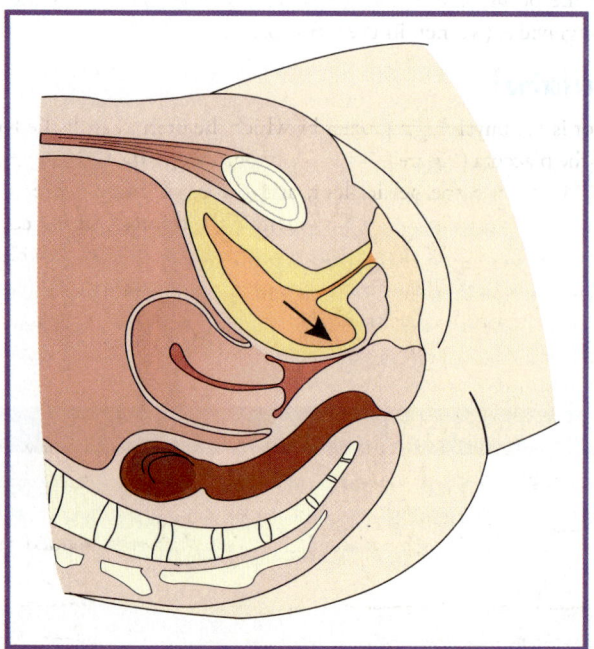

FIGURE 41-11 Cystocele.

from pregnancy, difficult delivery, prolonged labor, obesity, chronic coughing, and lifting of heavy objects.

The uterus also may lose supportive structure and drop into the vagina. This structural disorder is called *uterine prolapse*. The prolapse may involve only descent of the cervix into the vaginal area, or it may progress to protrusion of both the uterus and the cervix from the vaginal opening.

The first step in the treatment of pelvic positional disorders is to teach the patient how to perform pelvic floor muscle exercises, or Kegel exercises. The patient may be referred to a physical therapist who specializes in female disorders and uses biofeedback to help train the patient to perform the exercises accurately. If severe, all three of these structural abnormalities can be corrected with surgery.

STEPS FOR PERFORMING KEGEL EXERCISES

Kegel exercises help strengthen the pelvic floor muscles and are done to prevent or treat pelvic organ prolapse and incontinence. The steps are as follows:

1. Contract the muscles that make up the pelvic floor by visualizing that you are stopping the flow of urine midstream.
2. Hold the contraction to the count of three and then slowly relax for a count of three.
3. Repeat the exercise until you are performing 10 to 15 contractions in a set, with up to three sets throughout the day.

PREGNANCY

Anatomy and Physiology

Fertilization usually takes place in the distal third of the fallopian tube when one sperm cell penetrates and fertilizes an egg, which is then called a *zygote*. The zygote, which is made up of 23 chromosomes from the ovum and 23 chromosomes from the sperm, forms the first complete cell. This cell begins to grow and multiply immediately. The zygote travels down the fallopian tube and reaches the uterus in 5 to 6 days, implanting in the uterine endometrium. Enzymes are secreted by the zygote to aid the implantation process.

After implantation, the placenta forms within the uterine wall. It is derived from maternal endometrial tissue and from the chorion, the outermost membrane that surrounds the developing zygote. The amnion, the innermost layer of the membranes, holds the fetus suspended in an amniotic cavity surrounded by a fluid called *amniotic fluid*. The amnion and the fluid sometimes are called the "bag of water." In about 25% of pregnancies, breaking of the amniotic sac signals the onset of labor.

Within 2 weeks of fertilization, the zygote has undergone mitosis and is well established in the uterus. The next stage of development is the embryonic period, which includes the third to twelfth weeks of pregnancy (the first trimester). The embryonic period is a crucial time for the developing fetus, because this is when all tissues and organs develop. During the second and third trimesters, the embryo becomes a fetus; this is when cells develop and begin their primary functions, organs mature, and the fetus gains weight and grows in length.

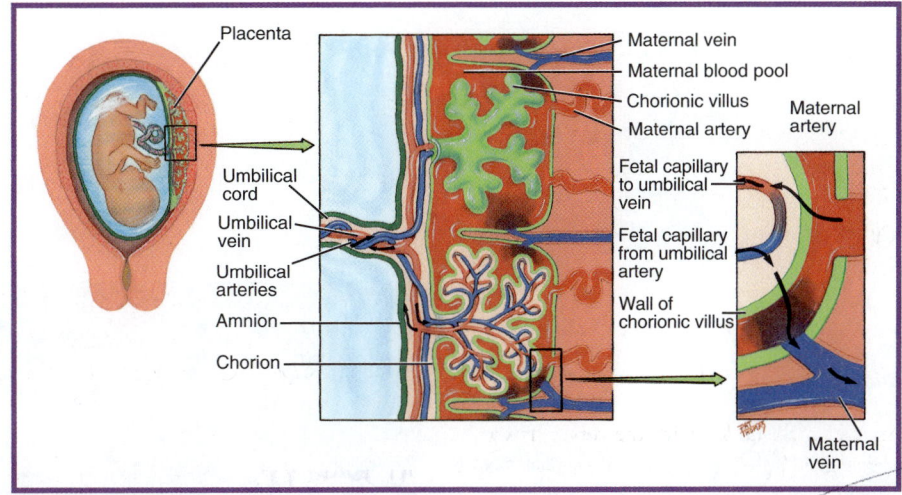

FIGURE 41-12 Structural features of the placenta and exchange of nutrients and wastes between maternal and fetal blood. (From Applegate EJ: *The anatomy and physiology learning system,* ed 3, Philadelphia, 2006, Saunders.)

Throughout the pregnancy, maternal and fetal blood never mix. Nutrients and oxygen diffuse from the mother's blood across the placental membrane into the blood vessels of the fetus's umbilical cord. Carbon dioxide and waste materials pass from the umbilical cord, through the placenta, and into the mother's circulatory system for excretion (Figure 41-12).

The placenta also acts as a gland by producing HCG and progesterone to maintain the pregnancy. Low levels of progesterone can lead to spontaneous abortion in pregnant women and menstrual irregularities in nonpregnant women. The average gestation is calculated at 9 calendar months, 10 lunar months, or 266 to 280 days. As previously mentioned, it is divided into three trimesters.

First Trimester

The first trimester is the period from the beginning of the LMP through the fourteenth week. It is a time of multiple physical and psychological changes for the woman and a crucial time for fetal organ development. It is essential that the pregnant woman understand the importance of a nutritious diet and of avoiding potential teratogens. The woman may complain of breast tenderness, constipation, headaches, urinary frequency, and nausea and vomiting. Rest, relaxation exercises, plenty of fluids, regular exercise, and small, frequent meals help relieve these discomforts. During this time, the obstetrician obtains a complete health history of the patient, including family, medical, menstrual, and obstetric histories. The obstetric history includes the number of times the patient has been pregnant (gravida) and the number of times she has given birth to a live infant (para).

Second Trimester

The second trimester extends from the fifteenth through the twenty-eighth week after the LMP. The uterus has enlarged to above the umbilicus, and the patient feels the first fetal movements, called *quickening*. In addition to the basic health history and physical examination, assessment is performed by abdominal palpation and fetal heart monitoring. The height of the fundus may be measured in centimeters from the symphysis pubis to the fundus. At each office visit, a urine sample is screened with a dipstick to detect protein or glucose, and the woman's blood pressure is monitored for signs of hypertension. The mother may complain of backache, dizziness, leukorrhea, and leg cramps from the increasing size of the uterus.

Third Trimester

The third trimester begins at the twenty-eighth week and lasts until delivery. This period is marked by rapid fetal growth, with the baby gaining close to 1 pound per week. The patient continues to be closely monitored. Childbirth preparation classes usually begin during this time. The patient experiences noticeable breast enlargement and may have an occasional discharge from the nipples of the clear, sticky fluid **colostrum**. The pregnant woman may complain of uterine cramping (Braxton-Hicks contractions), heartburn, edema, and frequent urination. Lightening, the dropping of the fetus into the pelvis, may occur a few weeks before birth, especially in primigravidas (women in their first pregnancy).

Parturition

Labor is the physiologic process by which the uterus expels the fetus and the placenta (Figure 41-13). To be born vaginally, the baby must drop down into the pelvic floor, and the cervix must efface (thin out) and dilate (open up). **Effacement** is the thinning of the cervix from its prelabor length of 1 to 1½ inches to a completely thin tissue (Figure 41-13, *A*). This occurs when uterine contractions pull cervical tissue upward as labor progresses so that the bottom uterine segment (the cervix) becomes thinner and the top uterine segment (the fundus) becomes thicker. Effacement is measured as a percentage; the cervix is said to be 0% to 100% effaced. **Dilation** (sometimes called *dilatation*) is the opening of the cervix, which allows the infant to pass out of the uterus and into the vaginal birth canal. Dilation is measured in centimeters, which are estimated during vaginal examinations by manual palpation. Labor is divided into three stages:

- Stage I—from the onset of labor through complete dilation and effacement of the cervix (Figure 41-13, *B*). During this time, uterine contractions become longer, stronger, and closer together

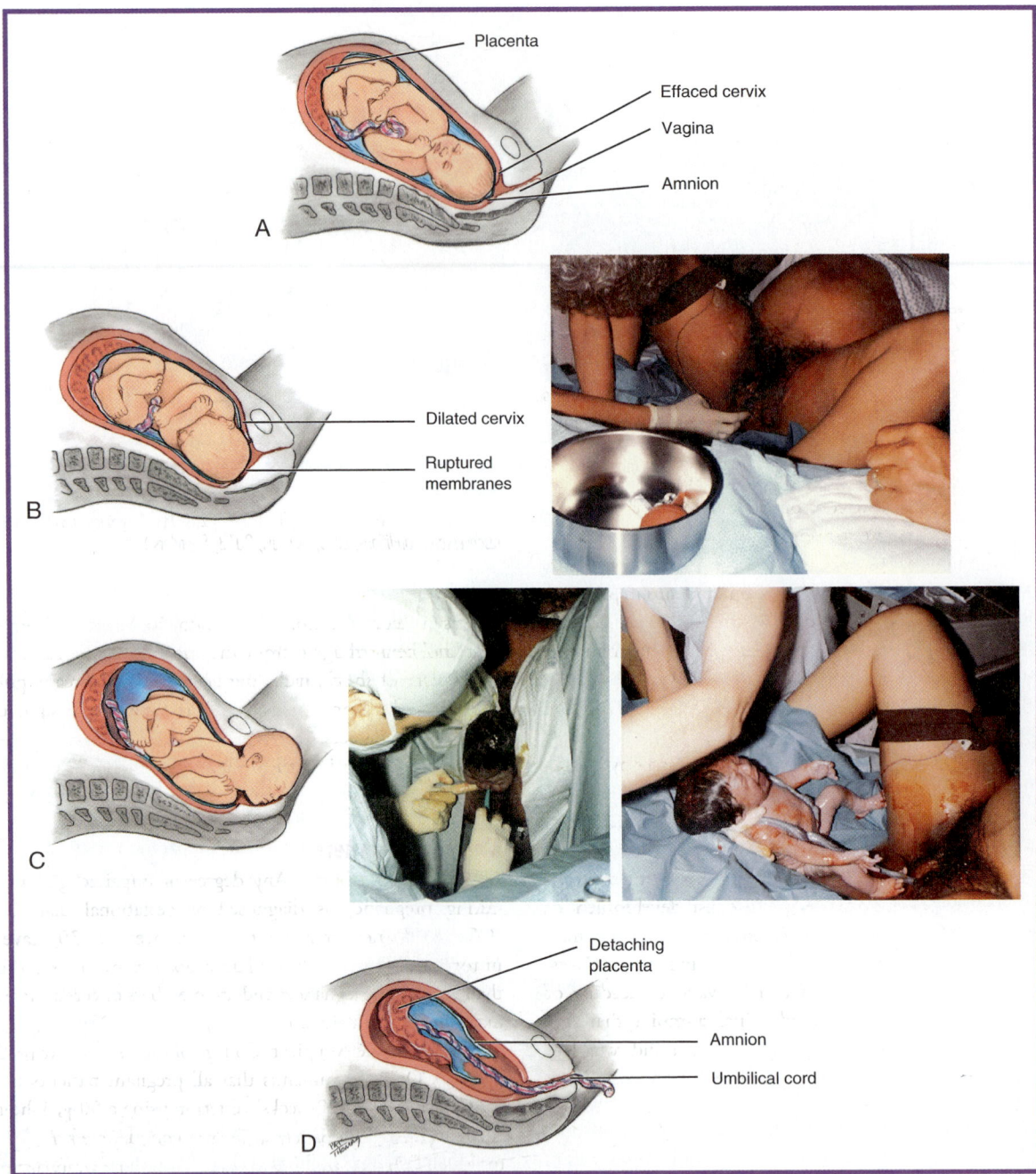

FIGURE 41-13 **A**, Effaced cervix. **B**, Dilation stage. **C**, Expulsion stage. **D**, Placental stage. (From Applegate EJ: *The anatomy and physiology learning system*, ed 3, Philadelphia, 2006, Saunders.)

until complete dilation and effacement occur and pushing begins. Stage I is divided into early active (up to 3 cm dilation and 80% to 100% effaced), active (4 to 7 cm dilation and completion of effacement), and transition (8 to 10 cm dilation). The average length of time for primigravidas in stage I is 9 to 11 hours.

- Stage II—from complete dilation and effacement of the cervix through the birth of the fetus (Figure 41-13, *C*). This is the pushing stage, which lasts approximately 1 hour for primigravidas.
- Stage III—from the birth of the fetus through expulsion of the placenta (Figure 41-13, *D*). This occurs approximately 20 minutes after the birth of the baby.

Pregnancy Complications

Infertility and Abortions

Fertility problems in women can occur for many different reasons, including a history of STIs that have caused scarring or adhesions of the fallopian tubes, failure to ovulate or irregular ovulation, congenital anomalies of the reproductive organs, endometriosis, medications that reduce fertility, and advancing age.

Problems in becoming pregnant can occur at several points in time, the first being abnormal fertilization. Some couples are unable to have a child because of the inability of the sperm and the ovum to unite. Ovarian factors are not totally understood; however, it is known that as women age, the ova become less viable. If the couple is able to fertilize an egg, another problem that can occur is improper implantation.

An ectopic pregnancy is one that occurs outside the uterus. Although an ectopic pregnancy can develop on or near the ovary or in the abdominal cavity, most occur in the fallopian tube. As the zygote develops, the cells that form the placenta begin to erode the muscle layer of the tube, bleeding and destruction of the muscular layer occur, and the tube ruptures. Rupture of the fallopian tube containing an ectopic pregnancy is a serious event that requires immediate surgical intervention to prevent fatal hemorrhage.

Once a woman becomes pregnant, problems can occur with carrying the infant to term. Interruption of a pregnancy before the term of fetal viability is called an *abortion,* which is identified in lay terms as a miscarriage. There are several different categories of naturally occurring abortions, including the following:

- Spontaneous—Abortions do not have an identifiable cause.
- Complete—Complete expulsion of both fetus and placenta occurs with no medical intervention.
- Incomplete—Expulsion of only parts of the fetus and placenta occurs. A D&C must be done to remove the remaining pieces or the mother will continue to bleed.
- Missed—The fetus dies in utero and must be removed surgically.
- Threatened—Cervical bleeding occurs, but dilation does not, and the pregnancy continues uninterrupted.

It is estimated that one in three pregnancies terminates by a naturally occurring abortion, and in most cases, the causes are not clear. Chromosomal anomalies frequently are detected in an aborted fetus or placenta and may be the primary reason for the abortion. Spontaneous abortion is the loss of a pregnancy before the twentieth week of fetal development. Common causes are defective development of the embryo, abnormalities of the placenta, endocrine disorders, malnutrition, infection, drug reaction, blood group incompatibilities, severe trauma, and shock. Symptoms include vaginal bleeding of varying degrees of severity and lower abdominal cramping that progresses to cervical dilation with rupture of membranes and complete expulsion of the products of conception. Induced abortions involve evacuation of the uterus at the request of the mother.

Placental Abnormalities

Pregnancy complications can occur because of the site of placental implantation. In placenta previa, the placenta implants in the lower uterine segment. If the condition is diagnosed early in the pregnancy from routine sonograms, the placenta may migrate with uterine wall enlargement. However, if the previa persists throughout the pregnancy and the placenta is implanted on or near the cervix when the mother goes into labor, dilation and effacement of the cervix can cause the placenta to tear loose (Figure 41-14). Complete dilation and effacement cannot progress without serious oxygen deprivation in the fetus and hemorrhaging in the mother. The signs of placenta previa include painless, bright red vaginal bleeding during or near the last trimester. The diagnosis is confirmed with a sonogram. A cesarean section is done as close to term as possible to prevent complications in both mother and fetus.

Another placental problem, abruptio placentae, occurs when the placenta detaches from the uterine wall. The pregnant woman

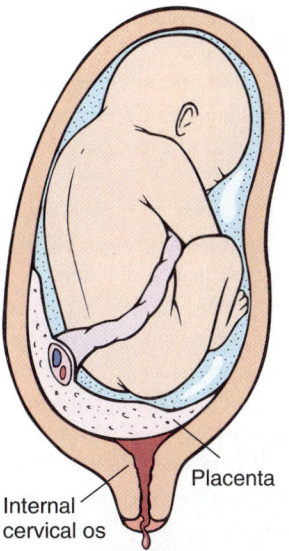

FIGURE 41-14 Placenta previa. (From Frazier MS, Drzymkowski JW: *Essentials of human diseases and conditions,* ed 5, St Louis, 2013, Saunders.)

reports an acute onset of severe abdominal pain; firmness on palpation and hemorrhaging from the vagina also are factors. She also shows signs of shock, including tachycardia, a thready pulse, hypotension, and clammy, cool skin. The fetus shows signs of distress from lack of oxygen, including a decreased fetal heart rate and lack of movement. This is a true obstetric emergency and requires immediate cesarean delivery to save the infant and the mother.

Maternal Disorders

Gestational Diabetes. Any degree of impaired glucose tolerance during pregnancy is diagnosed as gestational diabetes mellitus (GDM). Women at greatest risk are over age 30; have a family history of diabetes mellitus; had a body mass index (BMI) greater than 25 before pregnancy; and are members of certain racial groups, including African-Americans, Hispanics, and Native Americans.

Currently, the American College of Obstetricians and Gynecologists (ACOG) recommends that all pregnant patients be screened for GDM at 24 to 28 weeks' gestation using a 50-g, 1-hour glucose challenge test. The patient is given a concentrated drink equivalent to 50 g of glucose, and blood is drawn 1 hour afterward to measure blood glucose levels. A level greater than 140 mg/dL is indicative of GDM, but these patients are retested with a 3-hour glucose challenge. Blood is checked every hour for 3 hours after the patient drinks a concentrated glucose solution, and elevation in two of these blood draws is considered positive for GDM.

It is very important that women diagnosed with GDM carefully monitor their blood glucose levels regularly using a glucometer. This requires the patient to place a drop of blood on a machine that analyzes it and reports the current blood glucose level. Patients may be able to achieve normal glucose levels with diet therapy and exercise, although some patients require medication. Studies indicate that the best medical treatment for GDM is insulin therapy. The mother's problem with glucose metabolism typically goes away after the birth of the infant, but these women are at greater risk of developing diabetes mellitus type 2 later in life. Patient education on healthy lifestyles, including the importance of a nutritious diet, weight management, and exercise, is needed to help prevent adult-onset diabetes mellitus type 2.

The medical assistant's responsibilities include performing blood tests as ordered, completing routine urinary dipstick tests at each visit, and providing referral to a dietician for help with diet therapy management.

Hypertension. Most women who develop hypertension during pregnancy have normal blood pressure before becoming pregnant and also during early pregnancy but develop hypertension in the second half of the pregnancy. Gestational hypertension (pregnancy-induced hypertension) can be mild to severe and occurs in approximately 10% to 15% of pregnancies.

If hypertension is accompanied by proteinuria after 20 weeks of pregnancy, the patient is diagnosed with pre-eclampsia or toxemia, which occurs in approximately 2% to 3% of pregnancies. Pre-eclampsia usually shows up unexpectedly during a routine prenatal visit. The patient has an elevated blood pressure with protein or albumin in the urine and may also have uremia, altered liver function, and a reduced platelet count. The birth of the baby cures pre-eclampsia, with blood pressure returning to normal within a few days of delivery. However, if indicators of pre-eclampsia occur early in the pregnancy, the physician attempts to balance the need to prevent premature birth of the infant with what is best for the mother. The baby is monitored with routine **nonstress tests (NSTs)**, sonograms, and maternal reports of fetal movement. If pre-eclampsia persists, the patient is at risk of severe headaches, vision disturbances, oliguria, and convulsions either before or during labor, and an emergency cesarean section may be required to prevent serious maternal complications.

The medical assistant is responsible for monitoring the pregnant woman's vital signs at each visit, including any report of a sudden weight gain that may indicate edema, and for performing routine urine dipstick tests. Complete and accurate documentation of findings helps alert the physician to possible problems with hypertension.

MENOPAUSE

Menopause is the permanent ending of menstruation as a result of cessation of ovarian function. It usually occurs between 45 and 55 years of age but can occur as early as the 30s and as late as the 60s. Menses may stop suddenly, flow may decrease over time, or the time between menses may lengthen until complete cessation occurs. Menopause can be diagnosed only retrospectively. Only after 12 months of amenorrhea is a woman said to be in menopause, and the years after this are called *postmenopause.*

Perimenopause begins when hormone-related changes start to appear, and it lasts until the final menses; this can be as long as 10 years before menopause. During this time, women are still ovulating, but the uneven rise and fall of estrogen and progesterone may cause symptoms. Some women experience few or no symptoms, whereas others have hot flashes, concentration problems, mood swings, irritability, migraines, vaginal dryness, urinary incontinence, dry skin, and sleep disorders. Treatment focuses on relieving these signs and symptoms. The physician may prescribe low-dose oral contraceptives (Alesse) to balance estrogen and progesterone levels or short-term hormone replacement therapy (HRT) (e.g., Premarin, Prempro) to

treat symptoms. The physician also may recommend that the patient consume soy products or take soy supplements for a plant source of estrogen. Vitamin E may help alleviate hot flashes, and vitamin B_6 helps create natural serotonin, a neurotransmitter that affects mood. Other methods that help alleviate symptoms include avoiding caffeine and spicy foods to reduce hot flashes, using relaxation techniques to aid with sleep disorders, consuming a low-fat diet high in calcium, and performing regular weight-bearing exercise to help prevent osteoporosis and heart disease.

Medical treatment of menopause focuses on managing uncomfortable symptoms and preventing conditions associated with a drop in blood levels of estrogen, such as osteoporosis and coronary artery disease. Physicians traditionally treated perimenopause and menopause with long-term HRT for most women; however, studies indicate that although HRT does protect the menopausal woman from osteoporosis, hip fracture, and colon cancer, at the same time it increases the risk of heart attack, stroke, breast cancer, and blood clotting. It is now recommended that physicians prescribe HRT to meet individual patient needs over a short term (i.e., no longer than 5 years) rather than as routine treatment for all menopausal women. Studies show that the risk for heart disease and other complications increases after 5 years of HRT. The medical assistant must be aware of the physician's recommendations regarding HRT.

Other medications that may be prescribed include antidepressants, such as venlafaxine (Effexor) or fluoxetine (Prozac, Sarafem), to prevent hot flashes. Gabapentin (Neurontin) and clonidine (Catapres) also may be prescribed to reduce the frequency of hot flashes. Because the development of osteoporosis is a concern in perimenopausal and postmenopausal women, the physician may prescribe alendronate (Fosamax), risedronate (Actonel), or ibandronate (Boniva) to reduce bone loss and the risk of fracture. Another drug that may be used to improve postmenopausal bone density is raloxifene (Evista); however, hot flashes are a common side effect of this medication. Vaginal dryness can be treated with estrogen administered locally by vaginal tablet, ring, or cream, or the patient can use K-Y Jelly or some other vaginal moisturizer as a lubricant.

> ### CRITICAL THINKING APPLICATION   41-4
>
> Rose Conrad, a 53-year-old patient of Dr. Beck's, calls because she read recently that the hormone replacement therapy she has been taking for 3 years may be dangerous. Dr. Beck has reviewed her case and agrees that if she is concerned, she can stop taking the medication; however, she recommends that Mrs. Conrad try some alternative therapies. What suggestions might Dr. Beck make for nonpharmaceutical treatment of perimenopausal symptoms?

THE MEDICAL ASSISTANT'S ROLE IN GYNECOLOGIC AND OBSTETRIC PROCEDURES

As the female progresses from menarche through the childbearing years and then into menopause, her medical concerns change, and the focal point of the physical examination may change as well. The overall goal of the medical office is to keep her physically and mentally healthy. Being able to assist the physician in identifying possible problems before the problem becomes a threat to the patient's health is a major priority of care. This is best accomplished by listening to the patient. Remember, to the patient, there is no such thing as a routine examination.

Examination Preparation

An annual or semiannual examination of the female reproductive system is done to ensure normality of the reproductive organs or to diagnose and treat abnormalities of these organs. Before the physician begins the examination, the medical assistant should obtain a complete gynecologic history. After documenting the patient's history and chief complaint, the medical assistant should prepare the room and the patient for the examination (see Procedure 41-1).

The following should be included in the gynecologic history:

- Age at menarche
- Details about the regularity of the menstrual cycle; the amount and duration of menstrual flow; and a history of menstrual disturbances and their treatment
- Any current indicators of infection, including vaginal discharge, pelvic pain, urinary difficulties, and so on
- Feedback on any breast abnormalities and the date of the patient's last mammogram
- Date of the last Pap test
- Sexual history; STI history
- Number of pregnancies and live births
- Date of LMP
- Lifestyle factors, including diet, exercise, smoking, alcohol use, and so on

The physical examination during a first prenatal visit includes an overall assessment of the woman's health status, including vital signs, weight, and urinalysis. The medical assistant must prepare the patient and also the supplies and equipment necessary to obtain pelvic measurements, perform serologic tests, and prepare for laboratory tests (Procedure 41-4). The physician assesses heart, lung, and thyroid function and performs a physical examination to rule out any other abnormality. Next, the practitioner performs an obstetric examination that includes palpation of the mother's abdomen, measurement of the height of the uterus, and an internal or pelvic examination.

A series of blood tests also is performed during the initial prenatal visit. In follow-up prenatal visits, the medical assistant should collect a urine specimen for urinalysis, weigh the patient, measure the blood pressure, and answer questions about diet and health habits. The mother should gain approximately 10 to 12 pounds in the first half of pregnancy and another 15 to 17 pounds during the second half. Experts believe that a healthy weight gain is somewhere between 25 and 35 pounds. The baby's heart tones can be picked up through a specialized method, called *Doppler ultrasound*, somewhere between 9 and 12 weeks of pregnancy. Once recorded, the fetal heart rate is assessed at each subsequent visit.

Prenatal blood and laboratory tests include the following:

- Hematocrit and hemoglobin levels to check for anemia
- Blood type and Rh with antibody screening for possible Rh incompatibility
- Rubella titer to determine whether the mother is immune to German measles; rubella infection during pregnancy can cause multiple birth defects, including deafness, vision disorders, and mental retardation

- Syphilis screening; if the result is positive, antibiotic treatment is initiated to protect the fetus from congenital syphilis
- Hepatitis B screening, because this virus can be passed to the fetus in utero
- HIV screening is suggested; if the result is positive, treatment of the mother greatly reduces the risk of transmission to the fetus
- Pap smear to check for abnormal cervical cells
- Gonorrhea and chlamydia cultures to prevent infection of the baby at birth
- Urinalysis to detect protein, white blood cells, or glucose
- Group B streptococcus culture of the lower vagina for strep B infection, performed between the thirty-second and thirty-sixth weeks; if the result is positive, the mother is treated with antibiotics to prevent fetal exposure during vaginal birth
- NST to evaluate the fetal heart rate; the mother is attached to a fetal monitor, with the goal of seeing accelerations in the fetal heart rate with movement
- Stress test or oxytocin challenge test (OCT) if the NST is abnormal; a small amount of oxytocin (which causes the uterus to contract) is administered intravenously while the mother is attached to a fetal monitor to see how the fetus will respond to the normal stresses of labor

Any concerns the patient has should be noted and reported to the physician. The medical assistant should be prepared to suggest community resources that can provide assistance to new parents, such as childbirth and parenting classes; infant cardiopulmonary resuscitation (CPR) courses; nutritional counseling if needed; and contact information for the Special Supplemental Nutrition Program for Women, Infants, and Children (WIC), which helps lower income expectant mothers get nutritious food.

The examination room must be adequately equipped and the surroundings pleasant. A dressing area with an adjacent toilet should be provided. The dressing area should ensure privacy and should be equipped with tissues and sanitary protection items, as well as disposable examination gowns and drapes. The medical assistant should restock supplies as needed throughout the day.

Assisting with the Examination

The female reproductive system examination is probably the most emotionally charged medical experience the average woman undergoes. Even women with relatively sophisticated attitudes toward their bodies and sexuality may be embarrassed by the casual, impersonal approach of the medical team during this procedure. Many women fear the physician's findings. Anxieties and fears are best handled through explanations and by showing a genuine interest in the patient's concerns.

If the physician is male, a female medical assistant should be present during the examination. The only exception to this rule is when the patient requests that the medical assistant leave the room; if this is done, the request is noted on the patient's medical record. A male medical assistant is not usually in the room during the examination except when he must assist with a procedure. The physician makes the decision regarding the male assistant's role in the female reproductive system examination. The medical assistant is responsible for supporting the patient and assisting the physician during the procedure. The procedure should be fully explained to

PROCEDURE 41-4

Prepare a Patient for Procedures and/or Treatments: Assist with a Prenatal Examination

GOAL: *To promote a healthy pregnancy for the mother and fetus and to screen for potential problems.*

EQUIPMENT and SUPPLIES

- Scale with height measure
- Sphygmomanometer
- Stethoscope
- Tape measure
- Doppler fetoscope
- Ultrasound gel
- Urine specimen container
- Disposable examination gloves, vaginal speculum, and lubricant if vaginal examination is to be performed
- Sexually transmitted infection (STI) test setups
- Laboratory requisition slips
- Biohazard waste container
- Biohazard bags for specimen transport
- Patient education materials
- Patient's medical record

PROCEDURAL STEPS

1. Sanitize your hands, assemble equipment, and identify the patient.
2. Weigh the patient and record the weight.
   PURPOSE: An expectant mother's weight reflects both maternal nutritional status and fetal growth; an unusual weight gain may indicate fluid retention.
3. Collect a urine specimen and perform a urinalysis to detect protein, glucose, or ketones in the urine; record the urinalysis results.
   PURPOSE: Protein, glucose, or ketones in the urine may indicate problems with the pregnancy.
4. Measure and record the mother's blood pressure.
5. Instruct the patient to disrobe from the waist down and to put on a gown open to the front so that the uterine fundal height can be measured.

PURPOSE: The physician will palpate the abdomen and may use a tape measure to assess the fundal height as a determinant of fetal growth.

6. Assist the patient onto the examination table if needed and provide a drape for privacy.
7. Assist the physician as needed throughout the examination. If a Doppler fetoscope is to be used to listen to the fetal heart tones, apply a liberal amount of ultrasound gel to the patient's abdomen and hand the fetoscope to the physician. After the procedure, clean the Doppler head with a paper towel and offer the patient tissues to wipe the gel off of her abdomen.
8. After the examination is complete, assist the patient off the examination table; make sure to observe for signs of dizziness or problems with balance.
   PURPOSE: Lying supine or in the lithotomy position puts pressure on the aorta, which may result in momentary vertigo when the patient sits or stands.
9. Answer the patient's questions and provide patient education materials as needed.
   PURPOSE: To take advantage of "teaching moments" to provide information on diet, health habits, and community resources.
10. Collect and package all specimens for transport. Complete labels as needed.
11. Discard supplies and disinfect the equipment according to the manufacturer's guidelines. Wear disposable examination gloves and follow Occupational Safety and Health Administration (OSHA) guidelines if handling any contaminated items.
12. Sanitize your hands.
13. Document the pertinent information in the patient's medical record.
    PURPOSE: A procedure is not done until it is recorded.

---

the patient to prevent unnecessary embarrassment and discomfort. During the explanation, the assistant has the opportunity to conduct patient teaching.

In preparation for the examination, the patient should empty her bladder, completely disrobe, and put on an examination gown that opens in the front. The patient should have been advised at the time the appointment was made not to douche or have sexual intercourse for 24 hours before the examination so that vaginal discharges can be evaluated properly and to ensure accurate results of cytologic studies.

Breast Examination

Begin the examination by assisting the patient into a sitting position and by adjusting the gown so that the breast tissue can be easily exposed. The physician will instruct the patient to place her arms above her head, and the assistant should be present to assist the patient if she has difficulty following these instructions. The physician may prefer to examine the breasts with the patient in the supine position. When the patient is instructed to assume a supine position, help the patient, adjust the gown, and drape as needed to assist the physician and to protect the patient's privacy. A small pillow may be placed under the patient's head for comfort. When the examination is complete, the gown is readjusted to cover the breasts. The physician may choose to discuss breast self-examination with the patient at this time or may inform the patient that you will be explaining the technique at the end of the examination (see Procedure 41-3).

Abdominal Examination

After the breasts have been examined, cover them and position the drape to allow the physician to palpate the abdomen; this is done to confirm normal symmetry and to detect any masses. In the case of pregnancy, the level of the fundus is measured to determine fetal growth. For this examination, the patient's arms should be placed at her sides to achieve better relaxation of the abdominal muscles.

Pelvic Examination

The medical assistant should remain in the examination room to provide reassurance to the patient and as legal protection for a male physician while the patient's vaginal and perineal areas are examined. Furthermore, the lithotomy position is awkward to assume without assistance and may be embarrassing to the patient. Never place the patient in the lithotomy position until the physician is ready to begin the examination. When you assist the patient into the lithotomy position, always keep her totally covered.

You should stand at the patient's side so that you can observe the patient, yet still be able to move quickly if needed by the physician. First, the physician inspects the external genitalia and palpates the perineal body. The patient may be asked to bear down to show any muscular weaknesses that may be the result of lacerations of the perineal body during childbirth. A third-degree laceration may have involved the rectal sphincter and may cause rectal incontinence.

Next, the vaginal speculum, without lubrication, is inserted for examination of the cervix and the vaginal canal and for obtaining the Pap specimen. The speculum should be prewarmed with warm water. Have the patient take some deep breaths to help relax the abdominal muscles. The normal cervix points posteriorly and has smooth, pink, squamous epithelium. Abnormalities most frequently seen are ulcerations (erosions), **Bartholin's cysts**, and cervical polyps. Because erosions cannot be palpated, inspection is the only method of detecting them. Healed lacerations from childbirth are common in a **multiparous** patient. Pregnancy increases the size of the cervix, and hormone deficiency causes it to atrophy. The vaginal wall is reddish pink and has a corrugated appearance from the overlapping tissue (rugae) lining. Vaginal infections change the appearance of the vaginal mucosa. After the Pap specimen has been obtained, you may be responsible for labeling the specimen and preparing it for transport to the cytology laboratory. Be sure to follow laboratory instructions during the preparation to avoid having to repeat the examination.

After removal of the vaginal speculum, the physician does a bimanual examination; that is, two gloved fingers are lubricated with a water-soluble jelly (lubricant) and inserted into the vaginal canal, and the other hand palpates the abdomen over the pelvic organs and the mons pubis (Figure 41-15). The uterus is examined for shape, size, and consistency, and its position is noted. A normal uterus is freely movable with limited discomfort. A laterally displaced uterus usually is the result of pelvic adhesions or displacement caused by a pelvic tumor. The fallopian tubes and ovaries are evaluated. Normal tubes and ovaries are difficult to palpate, which is why the physician may have to press firmly in the pelvic area, causing minor discomfort for the patient. The physician completes the examination by performing a rectovaginal abdominal examination. A stool test for occult blood may be done at this time.

Postexamination Duties

When the examination is finished, help the patient into a sitting position and into the dressing room if needed. Following the

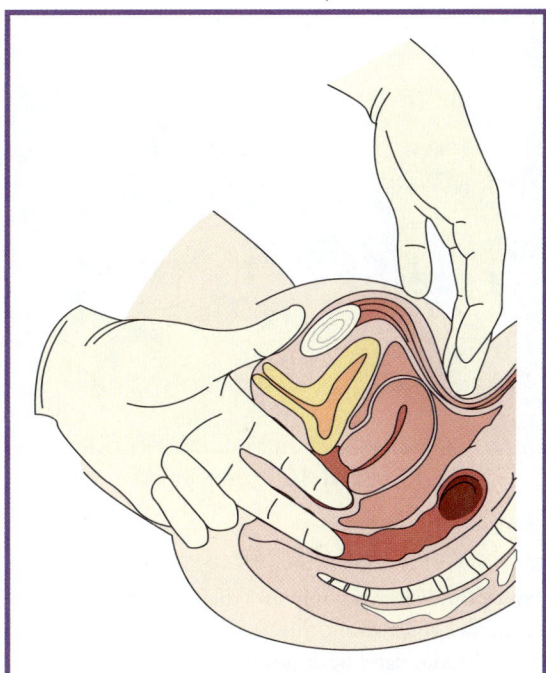

FIGURE 41-15 Bimanual examination.

Standard Precautions established by the Occupational Safety and Health Administration (OSHA), remove the examination equipment and supplies while the patient is dressing so that when the physician returns to talk to the patient, the room is neat and clean. Once the patient has left, the room should be cleaned and restocked as necessary and made ready for the next patient.

SAFETY ALERT

Instruments that come in contact with a patient, including vaginal speculums, should be sanitized, disinfected, and sterilized before they are used for another patient. If the instrument does not penetrate tissue, it can be stored under clean or medically aseptic conditions. Some physicians prefer to use disposable speculums for routine pelvic examinations. Instruments that penetrate tissue (e.g., uterine biopsy punch, uterine tenaculum, cervical dilators and sounds) must be sterilized and stored and handled under sterile conditions.

DIAGNOSTIC TESTING

Sonography

Sonography is a technique in which high-frequency sound waves are used to produce images of the body's soft tissues. It can be used to distinguish between cysts and tumors, and it is used during pregnancy to determine the number of fetuses and their age and gender; fetal abnormalities; and the position of the placenta. The skin over the area to be studied is coated with conductive gel or lotion, and the transducer is pressed lightly against the area. Sound waves emitted by the transducer bounce off the structure being studied and

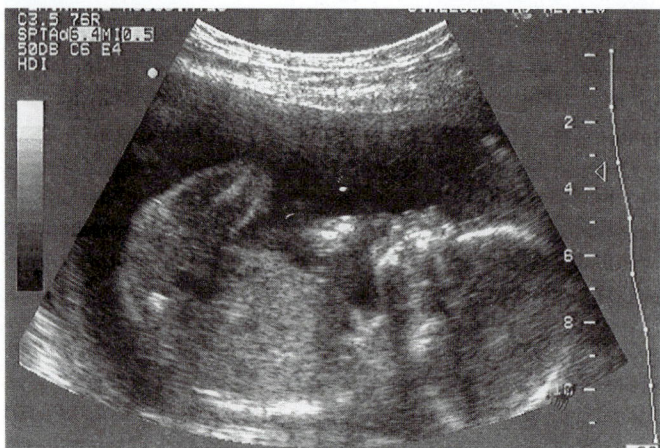

FIGURE 41-16 Sonogram of a fetus.

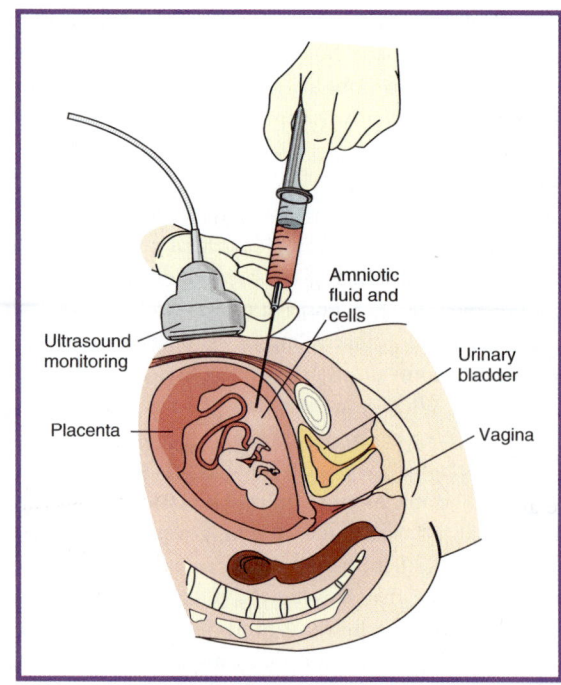

FIGURE 41-17 Amniocentesis.

are converted into electrical impulses that create a picture for analysis. The mother must drink three to four glasses of water 1 hour before the procedure and must not void so that the full bladder can be used as a reference point.

Sonograph technology is divided into two methods. The grayscale image converts sound wave echoes into graphs or dots that form pictures of organs and blood vessels (Figure 41-16). The Doppler method converts the ultrasound into audible sounds that are heard as pulsations and is used in the obstetrician's office to monitor the heartbeat of the fetus. Color-coded Doppler signals, three-dimensional imaging, and contrast medium enhancement of ultrasound images provide more accurate images and data on organ structure and function.

FETAL DIAGNOSTIC TESTS

- *Chorionic villus sampling:* Chorionic villi are tiny placental projections, the cells of which have the same genetic material that is found in fetal cells. Cellular screening at 8 to 12 weeks' gestation provides early detection of genetic or chromosomal disorders. Potential complications include accidental abortion, infection, bleeding, and fetal limb deformities. Results are available within several days.
- *Amniocentesis:* This procedure involves needle aspiration of approximately 2 tablespoons of amniotic fluid after week 14 of pregnancy to detect genetic and chromosomal abnormalities or inherited metabolic disorders (Figure 41-17). Potential complications include miscarriage, fetal injury, infection, premature labor, and maternal hemorrhage. Results usually are not available for 2 weeks.
- *Alpha-fetoprotein (AFP):* Maternal blood sample is analyzed between 16 and 18 weeks; elevated level indicates a neural tube defect such as a myelomeningocele. Levels also increase with multiple pregnancies (twins) or fetal congenital anomalies. The test is controversial because it has a high rate of false-positive results.
- *Percutaneous umbilical cord blood sampling (PUBS):* Under ultrasound guidance, a sample of fetal blood is removed from the umbilical cord to detect blood diseases not diagnosed by amniocentesis.

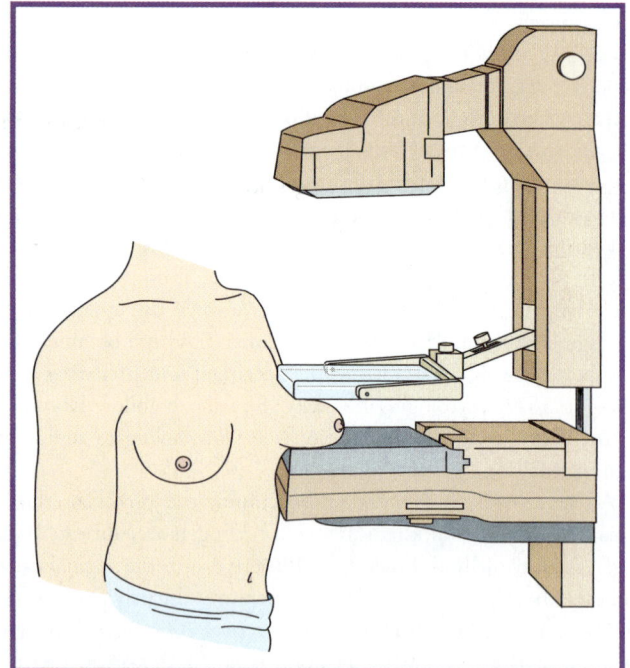

FIGURE 41-18 Proper position of the breast for a mammogram.

Mammography

Mammography is a specialized x-ray technique that provides images of breast tissue and is performed to identify abnormal masses that would go undetected in a breast palpation examination (Figure 41-18). Special x-ray equipment is used that compresses the breast firmly during each exposure. Compression is essential to provide the high degree of detail needed to visualize the significant but often subtle signs of a tumor. This process is not usually painful, but some patients, especially those with fibrocystic breast disease, may find it uncomfortable. If pain persists after the examination, aspirin or ibuprofen is recommended for relief. Women with fibrocystic breast disease may find it helpful to avoid caffeine 24 to 72 hours before the procedure.

Patients with breast implants should follow routine guidelines for mammography; however, implants may make diagnosing breast cancer more difficult, because they tend to obscure the breast image. It is recommended that women with implants have mammograms done at a facility where the radiologist is experienced at interpreting these particular studies. In addition, women with silicone implants should have an MRI examination every 2 years to check for rupture of the implants.

In preparation for mammography, patients are instructed not to use underarm deodorant and not to apply powder or lotion on the breasts or axillary areas. These products may contain ingredients that produce artifacts on mammographic images. This is especially true of antiperspirants that contain aluminum salts. When previous mammograms are available, every effort must be made to obtain them, because comparative evaluation often is significant in the radiologic diagnosis.

Pregnancy Testing

Pregnancy tests are designed to detect HCG, which is secreted after the ovum has been fertilized. It appears in the blood and urine of pregnant women as early as 10 days after conception. Once pregnancy has been confirmed, the patient undergoes a complete medical and obstetric examination, which includes a number of laboratory tests. The estimated day of delivery (EDD) is calculated at the first office visit (the EDD frequently is called the *expected due date*). The EDD typically is determined with a gestational wheel (Figure 41-19). However, most obstetricians rely on fetal sonograms to determine the expected due date.

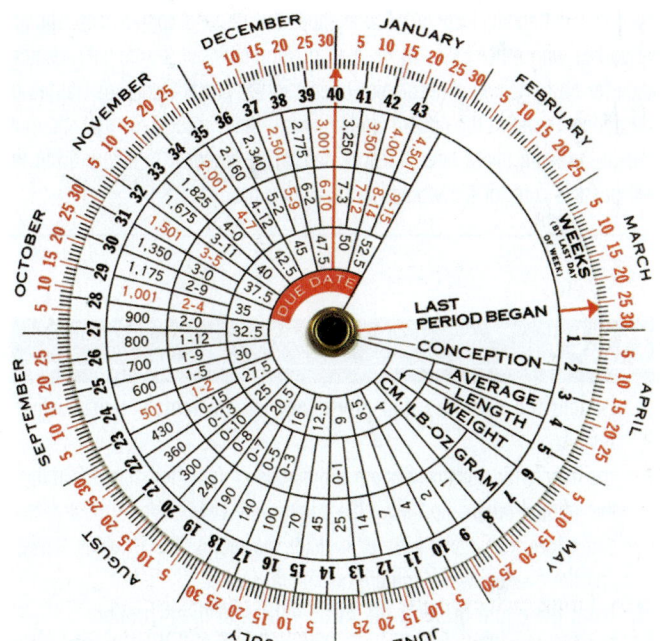

FIGURE 41-19 Gestational wheel. (From Jarvis C: *Physical examination and health assessment*, ed 5, St Louis, 2007, Saunders.)

CLOSING COMMENTS

Patient Education

The medical assistant can assist the physician by providing the patient with information that promotes sexual health and prevents gynecologic and obstetric disorders throughout the patient's life.

A woman who is planning a pregnancy or who has just found out that she is pregnant may benefit from some simple guidelines for healthy living.

- *Nutrition:* Before pregnancy, emphasize the need for folic acid to prevent **neural tube defects**. The woman can take a supplement or can eat dark green, leafy vegetables. Many women have iron-deficiency anemia, and eating foods high in iron (red meat, spinach, or enriched cereal) is helpful. A pregnant woman must meet the calcium needs of both herself and her fetus; therefore, she needs about 1,000 mg of calcium a day. Most pregnant women should consume about 2,500 calories a day. Women of average weight should gain 25 to 35 pounds, but underweight women should gain 28 to 40 pounds for a healthy infant.
- *Alcohol:* Alcohol passes through the placenta to the fetus and can cause serious problems. No one knows how much is safe, so it is a good idea for pregnant women to avoid alcohol completely.
- *Smoking:* Smoking can cause premature birth and low-birth-weight full-term infants. Smoking is linked to increased risk of otitis media, heart problems, and upper respiratory infection in infants, as well as sudden infant death syndrome (SIDS). Pregnant women should not smoke and should not be exposed to secondhand smoke.
- *Medicine:* All chemicals pass through the placenta; therefore, a pregnant woman should never take any medicine (even over-the-counter drugs) without the knowledge and approval of her obstetrician. If the medical assistant is managing telephone screening, having a list of physician-approved medications next to the phone helps in answering patients' questions.
- *STI screening:* STI screening should be done before a woman becomes pregnant. Many STIs are asymptomatic in women but treatable. Infants are at risk for serious health problems if exposed to certain STIs in utero or during the birth process.

ADVANTAGES OF BREASTFEEDING

For the Infant
- Completely digestible nutrition source for the infant
- Protects against gastrointestinal infection
- Protects against food allergies
- Provides newborn with mother's antibodies to infectious disease
- Associated with higher infant IQ
- Promotes muscular eye and facial development
- Promotes maternal-infant bonding

For the Mother
- Simple, safe, and economical
- Promotes uterine involution, which reduces postpartum bleeding
- Reduces the incidence of breast cancer
- Promotes maternal-infant bonding

Pregnant women usually are searching for information about pregnancy and wellness both during and after the birth. Use the waiting room as an education center with videos, books, and pamphlets on health issues and parenting. Keeping an up-to-date list of community education and support programs also is helpful. The obstetric patient who is interested in breastfeeding may need education and support to be successful. The American College of Pediatricians recommends breast milk as the optimum food for newborns. Referral to a breastfeeding support group or a lactation consultant can help a new mother solve her breastfeeding problems and find answers to her questions.

Legal and Ethical Issues

Many ethical and legal issues arise as a result of missed communication. Listen to what every patient reports, and write down any information that will assist the physician in treating the patient. The issue may appear to be an insignificant problem, but to the patient, it may be a major concern. Let the physician be the judge of whether the problem is relevant. As the patient's advocate and the physician's assistant, the medical assistant plays an important role in establishing good communication as a vital link in patient care.

Confidentiality is crucial in dealing with obstetric and gynecologic disorders. Only healthcare professionals directly involved in the patient's care should know the purpose of the patient's visit, diagnosis, or treatment. Maintaining patient confidentiality is not just an ethical responsibility; in the case of HIV status, it is a legal requirement.

The medical assistant may be in the position to recognize and provide assistance to women who are being mistreated. Battered women seldom come forward and tell healthcare workers they are being abused. If the patient reports such problems to the medical assistant, or if an abusive situation is suspected, the medical assistant should not hesitate to report this information to the physician. The American Medical Association (AMA) has developed guidelines to help caregivers recognize victims of abuse.

- *Know what to look for:* Suspicious findings include multiple injuries at different sites, especially areas that normally are covered by clothing. Also, the patient may be frightened, anxious, and passive and may have a history of "accidents."

- *Know what to ask when obtaining a patient history:* Even patients who show no signs of abuse should be asked whether they have ever been in an abusive relationship; if verbal arguments ever become physical; if their partner acts differently when drinking or using drugs; and if their partner is overprotective and jealous.

- *Know what to say and do:* A battered woman suffers both physical and emotional abuse. She may begin to believe that she deserves to be mistreated, and she needs unconditional and nonjudgmental emotional support from the healthcare worker. She needs to be treated with warmth and respect and encouraged to develop a plan of action to deal with the next violent episode. Suggestions include having immediate access to important documents, keys, money, transportation, the address of a safe house, and phone numbers for the police and local domestic violence hotline if available. The National Domestic Violence Hotline can be reached at 1-800-799-SAFE (7233). It provides 24-hour help for victims seeking local shelters.

SUMMARY OF SCENARIO

Having worked with obstetric and gynecologic patients, Betsy has learned that a wide range of disorders and conditions can affect a woman's health and pregnancy. She also has learned how to assist with a number of different diagnostic procedures performed in the ambulatory care setting. An integral role of the medical assistant in the OB/GYN practice is reinforcing the physician's patient education efforts. Betsy enjoys this part of the practice but realizes that it involves extensive reading and discussion with Dr. Beck to determine her preferred method of practice. Betsy stays up-to-date on current contraceptive practices by attending local AAMA workshops and regional conferences. She has networked with other CMAs to develop a comprehensive community resource guide for obstetric and gynecologic patients in the practice and has created an educational center in the patient waiting room. Betsy recognizes that she must continue to learn about new practices and recent research to help provide the best possible care for the women in Dr. Beck's practice.

SUMMARY OF LEARNING OBJECTIVES

1. **Define, spell, and pronounce, the terms listed in the vocabulary.**
   Spelling and pronouncing medical terms correctly bolsters the medical assistant's credibility. Knowing the definitions of these terms promotes confidence in communication with patients and co-workers.

2. **Apply critical thinking skills in performing the patient assessment and patient care.**
   Completing the Critical Thinking Application exercises throughout the chapter can help the student medical assistant become more adept at critical analysis of real-life situations.

3. **Explain the anatomy and physiology of the female reproductive system.**
   The female reproductive system is made up of the external genitalia and the internal organs, including the vagina; the cervix, which must dilate and efface for vaginal birth of a child; the uterus; the fallopian tubes; and the ovaries, which mature and produce ova.

4. **Trace the ovum through the three phases of menstruation.**
   The follicular phase matures a graafian follicle so that an ovum can be released at the same time the endometrial wall is thickening; the luteal

phase causes extensive growth of the endometrium; if conception does not occur, the menstrual cycle begins with the breakdown of the endometrium and menstrual flow.

5. **Compare current contraceptive methods.**

   Barrier contraceptive methods include the use of condoms, diaphragm, cervical cap, or cervical sponge; all of these are relatively inexpensive and reversible, but they must be used with each instance of intercourse. Hormonal contraceptives include Depo-Provera injections, the Implanon implant, oral and patch contraceptives, and the vaginal ring, all of which are very effective but have side effects and contraindications. Contraceptive methods are summarized in Table 41-1.

6. **Summarize menstrual disorders and conditions.**

   Menstrual disorders include amenorrhea and oligomenorrhea; abnormal menstrual bleeding includes menorrhagia and metrorrhagia; endometriosis is characterized by the presence of functional endometrial tissue outside the uterus.

7. **Distinguish among different types of gynecologic infections.**

   Gynecologic infections include candidiasis; BV; cervicitis; and PID, which is any acute or chronic infection of the reproductive system that ascends from the vagina (vaginitis), cervix (cervicitis), uterus (endometritis), fallopian tubes (salpingitis), or ovaries (oophoritis). STIs are summarized in Table 41-2.

8. **Differentiate between benign and malignant neoplasms of the female reproductive system.**

   Benign tumors of the reproductive system include uterine fibroids; ovarian cysts; the hormonal disease of polycystic ovary syndrome; and fibrocystic breast disease, the presence of multiple palpable nodules in the breasts. Malignant tumors include cervical, endometrial, and ovarian cancers that vary in their diagnostic features and symptoms. Breast cancer can have multiple origins. Treatment of all forms of reproductive cancer depends on staging and grading of the tumors.

9. **Prepare for and assist with the female examination, including obtaining a Papanicolaou (Pap) smear.**

   Procedure 41-1 explains the steps for assisting with examination of a female patient.

10. **Demonstrate patient preparation for a cryosurgery procedure.**

    Procedure 41-2 describes how to prepare a patient for cryosurgery.

11. **Teach the patient the technique for a breast self-examination.**

    Procedure 41-3 explains how to teach breast self-examination.

12. **Compare the positional disorders of the pelvic region.**

    Positional disorders of the pelvic region include cystocele or rectocele, which causes protrusion of the bladder or the rectum into the vaginal wall, and uterine prolapse, in which the cervix or uterus drops into the vaginal area. Kegel exercises van help improve these problems, but if they are severe, all three structural abnormalities can be corrected with surgery.

13. **Summarize the process of pregnancy and parturition.**

    Pregnancy occurs when the ovum and the sperm meet in the fallopian tube and a zygote is formed. The zygote implants in the uterine wall, and the placenta begins to form, which provides hormonal support for the pregnancy. The fetus is surrounded by an amniotic sac and floats in amniotic fluid. Oxygen and nutrients for the fetus pass through the placenta to the umbilical cord. The embryonic period ends at 12 weeks; by then, all tissues and organs have developed. During the remainder of the pregnancy, the organs mature and begin to function, and the fetus grows. Pregnancy is divided into three trimesters. The first trimester is a crucial time for fetal organ development; the second trimester brings quickening and many physiologic changes in the mother; during the third trimester, the fetal organ systems mature. The three stages of labor are dilation and effacement of the cervix, birth, and expulsion of the placenta.

14. **Describe the common complications of pregnancy.**

    Complications of pregnancy include potential loss of the pregnancy as a result of different types of abortions (miscarriages). Placental abnormalities include placenta previa, in which the placenta covers the cervical os, and abruptio placentae, in which the placenta breaks away from the uterine wall. Both cause maternal hemorrhage, threaten the fetal oxygen supply, and require a cesarean birth to protect the fetus and mother. Maternal disorders include GDM, which requires dietary changes and possible insulin therapy, and hypertension, which may progress to toxemia, a life-threatening rise in blood pressure accompanied by edema, uremia, and possibly seizure activity.

15. **Specify the signs, symptoms, and treatments of conditions related to menopause.**

    Menopause is the permanent ending of menstruation caused by the cessation of ovarian function. Perimenopause begins when hormone-related changes start to appear and lasts until the final menses. Some women experience few or no symptoms, whereas others have hot flashes, concentration problems, mood swings, irritability, migraines, vaginal dryness, urinary incontinence, dry skin, and sleep disorders. The physician may prescribe low-dose oral contraceptives or HRT, weight-bearing exercise, soy products or vitamin supplements, dietary changes, and medication to manage hot flashes, mood swings, and vaginal dryness and to prevent osteoporosis.

16. **Outline the medical assistant's role in gynecologic and reproductive examinations.**

    The medical assistant prepares the patient for the examination, equips the room, makes sure supplies are available and properly prepared, positions and drapes the patient as needed, assists with the Pap smear or any other procedures, and provides support and understanding for the patient.

17. **Demonstrate how to assist with a prenatal examination.**

    Procedure 41-4 explains how to assist with a prenatal examination.

18. **Distinguish among diagnostic tests that may be done to evaluate the female reproductive system.**

    Diagnostic tests for the female reproductive system include sonography during pregnancy to determine the number of fetuses, fetal age and gender, fetal abnormalities, and the position of the placenta; chorionic villus sampling, amniocentesis, or umbilical blood sampling to perform genetic testing; AFP blood tests to diagnose neural tube defects; mammography, which provides an x-ray image of the breast tissue to identify cancerous tumors; colposcopy procedures that permit visualization of abnormal cervical tissue for evaluation or biopsy; and a variety of tests done during pregnancy.

19. **Summarize patient education guidelines for obstetric patients.**
    A woman who is planning a pregnancy or who has just found out she is pregnant may benefit from some simple guidelines about nutrition, alcohol consumption during pregnancy, medications that might affect the developing fetus, STI screenings, and breastfeeding.

20. **Discuss the legal and ethical implications in a gynecology practice.**
    Confidentiality is crucial in dealing with obstetric and gynecologic disorders. Only healthcare professionals directly involved in the patient's care should know the purpose of the patient's visit, diagnosis, or treatment. The medical assistant may be in the position to recognize and provide assistance to women who are being mistreated. If the patient reports such problems to the medical assistant, or if an abusive situation is suspected, the medical assistant should not hesitate to report this information to the physician.

CONNECTIONS

📖 **Study Guide Connection:** Go to the Chapter 41 Study Guide. Read and complete the activities.

🅔 **Evolve Connection:** Go to the Chapter 41 link at *evolve.elsevier.com/kinn* to complete the Chapter Review and Chapter Quiz. Peruse other resources listed for this chapter to increase your knowledge of Assisting in Obstetrics and Gynecology.

ASSISTING IN PEDIATRICS

42

SCENARIO

Susie Kwong, CMA (AAMA), who has 2 years of experience, has accepted a new position with North Hills Pediatrics, a large multiphysician practice. Susie's primary responsibility will be to assist in the clinical area, but she also will have to rotate through the message screening center in the office. Office policy states that telephone screening employees should manage problems as much as possible, but if patient callbacks are needed, they are to be referred to the physician on call that day by noon for morning calls and no later than 5 PM for afternoon calls. Although the physicians in the practice have developed specific guidelines for managing patient problems, Susie is anxious about this responsibility, so she asks to work with the screening staff for several days before she starts answering incoming calls.

While studying this chapter, think about the following questions:

- What other clinical responsibilities should Susie be prepared to perform?
- Are patient and caregiver health education an important part of delivering high-quality care in a pediatric setting?
- Does Susie need to be clinically competent to perform immunizations and document their administration?
- How can Susie maintain her skill level and continue to learn about patient-centered pediatric care?

LEARNING OBJECTIVES

1. Define, spell, and pronounce the terms listed in the vocabulary.
2. Apply critical thinking skills in performing the patient assessment and patient care.
3. Describe childhood growth patterns.
4. Summarize the important features of the Denver II Developmental Screening Test.
5. Identify four different growth and development theories.
6. Explain common pediatric gastrointestinal disorders and their signs, symptoms, and treatment.
7. Classify disorders of the respiratory system in children.
8. Distinguish among pediatric infectious diseases.
9. Recognize the etiologic factors and signs and symptoms of the two primary pediatric inherited disorders.
10. Summarize the immunizations recommended for children by the Centers for Disease Control and Prevention (CDC).
11. Demonstrate how to document immunizations and maintain accurate immunization records.
12. Compare and contrast a well-child and a sick-child examination.
13. Outline the medical assistant's role in a pediatric examination.
14. Measure the circumference of an infant's head.
15. Obtain accurate length and weight measurements and plot pediatric growth patterns.
16. Accurately measure pediatric vital signs and perform vision screening.
17. Correctly apply a pediatric urine collection device.
18. Describe the characteristics and needs of the adolescent patient.
19. Specify child safety guidelines for injury prevention and management of suspected child abuse.
20. Summarize patient education guidelines for pediatric patients.
21. Discuss the legal and ethical implications in a pediatric practice.

VOCABULARY

anomaly A congenital malformation that occurs during fetal development.

attenuated (uh-ten-yuh-wat'-ed) Weakened or changed; refers to the virulence of a pathogenic microorganism.

fontanelles A space covered by thick membranes between the sutures of an infant's skull; called the baby's "soft spots"; there are both anterior and posterior fontanelles.

hydrocephaly (hi-dro-suh'-fuh-le) Enlargement of the cranium caused by abnormal accumulation of cerebrospinal fluid within the cerebral system.

laryngoscopy (lar-uhn-gahs'-kuh-pe) Visual examination of the voice box area through an endoscope equipped with a light and mirrors for illumination.

microcephaly Small size of the head in relation to the rest of the body.

serous A thin, watery, serumlike drainage.

stridor A shrill, harsh respiratory sound heard during inhalation when a laryngeal obstruction is present.

suppurative Characterized by the formation and/or discharge of pus.

Pediatrics is the medical specialty that deals with the development and care of children and with the treatment of childhood diseases. Pediatric patients range in age from newborn to puberty. Some practices continue to see the child until he or she graduates from high school. Subspecialties within pediatrics include surgery, cardiology, and psychiatry.

Approximately 50% of the patients in a pediatric office are there for well-baby or well-child visits. The roles of the pediatrician and the medical office staff are to supervise and help maintain the health of these patients. Parents must be involved in the care and development of their young children for treatment to be a success. The medical assistant can help by encouraging therapeutic communication among the patient, parents, and medical staff. The trust a child develops in the relationships and consideration received in the physician's office forms the basis of good medical care.

Pediatric care actually starts before the child is born, with promotion of good general health for mothers before conception and during pregnancy. The confidence and enthusiasm of parents can have a significant impact on an infant's physical and emotional well-being.

NORMAL GROWTH AND DEVELOPMENT

The terms *growth* and *development* often are used together. They refer to the combination of changes a child goes through as he or she matures. *Growth* refers to measurable changes, such as height and weight. The first determinant of these physical characteristics is the genetics inherited from the parents; however, a child's growth can be influenced by many factors, including nutritional status, environmental factors, and the presence of disease. *Development* considers qualitative maturation in motor, mental, social, and language skills. A child's development is determined by a combination of prenatal, environmental, and caregiver factors. Each child has his or her own pattern of growth and development. Pediatric assessments are individualized for each child according to age, developmental level, health condition, family characteristics, and past experiences with healthcare professionals. The pediatrician checks for indications of irregularities in growth and development by comparing a child's physical, intellectual, and social levels with published national standards. This comparison indicates whether the child is at the appropriate stage of growth and development for his or her chronologic age.

Growth Patterns

Physical growth is one of the most visible changes in childhood. The average birth weight is 7 to 7½ pounds, and in 6 months, the baby's birth weight doubles. Growth then slows slightly; by 1 year of age, the birth weight has tripled and length has increased by 50%. By age 2, the child has reached approximately 50% of his or her adult height. Between ages 1 and 2, the child gains approximately ½ pound per month. Between ages 2 and 3, weight gain averages 3 to 5 pounds and height increases 2 to 2½ inches. Most children slim down during this period, so that by the time the third birthday arrives, the potbellied toddler has become the characteristic preschooler.

THERAPEUTIC APPROACHES FOR INFANTS (NEWBORN TO 12 MONTHS)

- Crying is normal; use distraction, but do not overstimulate.
- It is important to keep the infant close to the caregiver; either have the parent hold the infant or keep the parent in the child's line of vision.
- Involve the parent as much as possible, depending on the task and the parent's level of comfort.
- Place a familiar object near the infant and keep frightening ones out of view.
- An infant's negative response to strangers usually develops at approximately 8 months; do not take the rejection personally.
- Do not restrain the infant any more than necessary, but be ready to use restraint at times (e.g., when giving an injection) to keep the infant safe.
- Encourage the caregiver to cuddle and hug the child after the procedure is complete.
- Unpleasant procedures are associated with other objects, so do not use play areas for treatment and do not use a favorite toy or object during the procedure; offer it afterward for comfort.

During the preschool period, ages 3 to 6 years, weight increases 3 to 5 pounds per year; height increases at a slower but steady rate of 1½ to 2½ inches per year. By age 4, the child usually has doubled the birth length. During this time, the legs are the fastest growing part; fatty connective tissue continues to increase slowly until approximately age 7. This same growth rate continues through the school-aged period, 6 to 12 years, and as this period of development ends, the child usually is into a growth spurt that indicates impending puberty.

is determined by the presence of sperm in the semen. The timing of sexual maturity in both genders varies greatly.

Skeletal growth is complete in girls between 15 and 16 years of age and in boys between ages 17 and 18. Skeletal growth is considered complete when the growth plates (epiphyseal plates) of the long bones of the extremities have fused completely.

THERAPEUTIC APPROACHES FOR TODDLERS AND PRESCHOOLERS (2 TO 6 YEARS)

- Toddlers and preschoolers often fear visits to the doctor; ignore temper tantrums and negative behavior.
- Praise the child as much as possible.
- Perform unpleasant procedures as quickly as possible; the fear of the procedure is worse than the actual discomfort.
- Allow the child to keep on as much clothing as possible for security and comfort.
- Use words familiar to the child and do not use words the child could misinterpret (e.g., "the test uses dye"—the child may think you mean "die"; "the doctor will put you to sleep so it doesn't hurt"—the family dog may have been put to sleep).
- Explain a procedure as the child would sense it; that is, what it will look like, how it will smell, how it will feel, and so on.
- Allow the child to handle equipment when possible.
- Do not use the child's favorite doll or stuffed animal to demonstrate; the child may believe the toy feels pain.
- Explain procedures to the parents away from the child when possible; the child may misinterpret the information.

THERAPEUTIC APPROACHES FOR SCHOOL-AGED CHILDREN (7 TO 10 YEARS)

- Allow choices when possible, such as which arm to use for an injection.
- A parent or caregiver should always be present during examinations.
- Remove only as much clothing as needed for the examination or procedure.
- Explain procedures in concrete terms; use pictures and diagrams when possible.
- Give the child time to ask questions.
- School-aged children often are curious, and they can be cooperative if they know what is expected of them.
- Address the conversation to the child; involve the child in decision making as much as possible.
- Provide privacy.

The growth spurt continues for approximately 2 years, and the child then reaches adolescence (ages 12 to 18 years). During this period, the adolescent gains almost half of his or her adult weight, and the skeleton and organs double in size. Weight increases in girls by 20 to 25 pounds and in boys by 15 to 20 pounds. Girls grow 5 to 6 inches, and boys grow 4 to 5 inches. As the growth spurt is completed, the teenager reaches sexual maturity. In girls, sexual maturity is signaled by the onset of the menstrual cycle; in boys, it

THERAPEUTIC APPROACHES FOR ADOLESCENTS (12 TO 18 YEARS)

- Adolescents are self-conscious and strongly influenced by peers.
- Privacy is very important to them.
- Address how a procedure might affect the adolescent's appearance.
- Do not be judgmental; listen without condemning.
- Encourage the adolescent to verbalize his or her concerns and fears.
- The adolescent may regress to more childish behaviors when sick.
- Teenagers want to be treated as adults; they want to know what is being done and why.
- Encourage the teenager to see the physician without the parent present.

CRITICAL THINKING APPLICATION   42-1

Based on what you have learned about therapeutic approaches for the pediatric patient, what would be the best way to deal with the following patient situations?
1. A crying 3-month-old being seen for a well-child visit
2. A 10-month-old with otitis media
3. A 2-year-old who needs the dressing changed on an infected wound
4. A 5-year-old scheduled for vision and hearing screening
5. An 8-year-old who needs a throat culture to rule out a strep infection
6. A 12-year-old who needs a penicillin injection in the dorsogluteal site
7. A 15-year-old girl who complains of abdominal pain and is accompanied by her mother

Growth charts that can be used to compare the child's individual growth pattern with national standards have been used since 1977, but in 2000 the Centers for Disease Control and Prevention (CDC) revised the charts to reflect cultural and racial diversity (samples are available at *www.cdc.gov/growthcharts*). The CDC charts take into account whether an infant was formula fed or breast-fed, because breast-fed infants may grow differently during the first year of life.

In addition, the CDC growth charts include information on the average body mass index (BMI) for infants and young adults 2 to 20 years of age, giving pediatricians another weapon in the fight against childhood obesity. As was discussed in Chapter 30, the BMI is a means of assessing the relationship between height and weight. BMI conversion charts typically are available, but the BMI can be calculated by dividing the child's weight in kilograms by the height in meters squared, or

$$BMI = \frac{Weight\ (kg)}{Height\ (m)^2}$$

Denver II Developmental Screening Test

Each child develops individually and attains developmental plateaus differently. The Denver II Developmental Screening Test is a standardized tool used to screen for developmental delays, to investigate concerns about an infant's development, or to monitor high-risk children for potential problems (Figures 42-1 and 42-2). The test should be given at ages 3 to 4 months, 10 months, and 3 years. Although it is not difficult to administer, only those trained in the procedure and interpretation of results should give it. The assessment focuses on four developmental areas:

- *Gross motor skills:* Evaluates the child's ability to control large muscle groups (e.g., standing, kicking, running, and balance).
- *Language:* Assesses the child's verbal comprehension (e.g., word comprehension, following simple commands, use of subjects, and counting).
- *Fine motor skills:* Tests the child's coordination of fine motor muscles (e.g., reaching, grasping, piling blocks, and drawing).
- *Personal skills:* Examines the child's self-confidence and socialization (e.g., playing games, using a fork and spoon, dressing, and brushing the teeth).

The results of the test are analyzed and determined to be normal or suspect, or the child is diagnosed as untestable. With an abnormal finding, the child should be rescreened in 1 to 2 weeks to rule out temporary developmental delays caused by fatigue or anxiety. If those results are abnormal, the child may be retested with other developmental tests, either by the pediatrician or by a professional pediatric testing agency.

Developmental Patterns

General patterns of child development occur rapidly during the first year of life as the infant progresses from reflex activities (e.g., grasping fingers and sucking) to learning to manipulate simple objects (e.g., pulling open drawers or throwing toys out of the crib). In addition to these motor skills, the child learns verbal patterns, progressing from cooing and crying for attention to speaking his or her first words.

By age 3, the child is showing increased autonomy. Now the child can walk, is toilet trained, sits at the table and eats with the family, can make simple sentences, understands the word "no," and even imitates the parent by using verbal gestures that he or she has seen used. The child's vocabulary consists of up to 900 words.

During the preschool stage the child becomes increasingly independent and initiates activities. Preschoolers have mastered many gross motor skills and are perfecting their fine motor development. Verbal communication has increased to full simple and even complex sentences but remains quite literal. For example, if you tell a preschool child that you are going to fly to visit Aunt Sue, the child thinks you are going to flap your arms and fly. Nonverbal communication skills are also being mastered. The vocabulary now includes more than 2,000 words. During this period, children need to develop social skills, such as sharing and taking part in peer group activities.

The school-aged child has perfected fine motor skills and can paint, draw, and play an instrument, enjoys team activities, and expands reading and writing skills. His or her intellectual skills are developing, and social skills are going through refinement as a sense of self-achievement and self-worth is developed. During this time the child learns and tests the rules for socializing outside the immediate family as an independent individual.

Adolescence, or the transition stage, is the time when the individual attempts to establish an adult identity. The teenager proceeds by trial and error, experimenting with adult roles and behavior patterns. Traditional values learned in childhood may be questioned, and peer relationships take on new importance. During this time teenagers must develop the emotional maturity and motivation to make reasonable decisions. The teen looks to family members for encouragement and guidance in making decisions that will help develop self-confidence and to become patient and less impulsive and self-centered.

> **CRITICAL THINKING** APPLICATION   **42-2**
>
> Susie receives a call from the mother of a 6-month-old child. She is concerned that her child may not be reaching his developmental milestones. What type of information about the child's growth and development should Susie gather? If Susie is unable to answer the mother's questions, what should she do?

Developmental Theories

Psychologists have been researching and developing theories about human behavior since the beginning of the twentieth century. The first of these theorists to gain influence was Sigmund Freud, who believed that the motivating stimulus for human behavior is the libido, which is defined as an individual's pleasure-seeking instincts. Freud's theory describes four major components of the mind: the *unconscious mind,* which cannot be accessed but affects our behavior; the *id,* which focuses on immediate self-gratification; the *ego,* which develops throughout life and balances the immediate desires of the id with the reality of the social world; and the *superego,* the individual's conscience, which helps the child incorporate social expectations and norms. Freud also was the first therapist to identify developmental stages that all individuals must achieve, including the oral, anal, phallic, latency, and genital stages.

The next developmental theory to gain general acceptance was the psychosocial approach of Erik Erikson. Erikson expanded Freud's work to recognize cultural and social influences on individual development. His theory is based on eight stages of development that the individual must pass through and master. Each stage focuses on a developmental crisis, starting in infancy and ending in old age. According to Erikson, the stages that children must master include:

- *Trust versus mistrust*—Infants learn to rely on caregivers; mistrust occurs if needs are not met.
- *Autonomy versus shame and doubt*—Toddlers learn language skills and gain independence; they may feel shame and doubt if they cannot meet parental expectations or are overprotected.
- *Initiative versus guilt*—Preschoolers actively seek out new experiences; children become hesitant if restrictions or reprimands make them feel guilty or afraid to try more challenging skills.

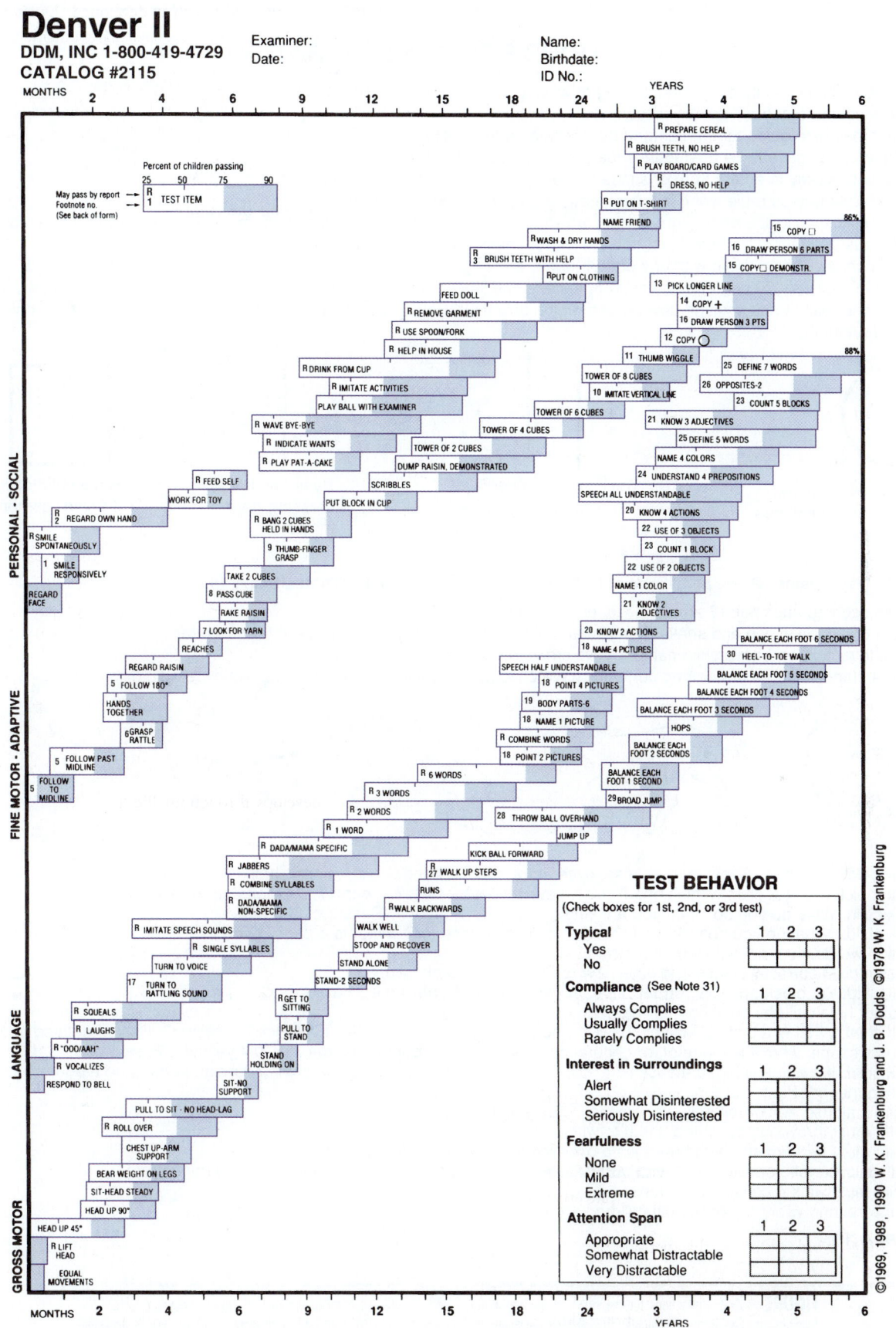

FIGURE 42-1 Denver II Developmental Screening Test (DDST). (Copyright 1969, 1989, 1990 WK Frankenburg and JB Dodds. Copyright 1978 WK Frankenburg. Copies can be obtained from Denver Developmental Materials, Inc, (800) 419-4729. Accessed April 17, 2010. Available at www.denverII.com.)

DIRECTIONS FOR ADMINISTRATION

1. Try to get child to smile by smiling, talking or waving. Do not touch him/her.
2. Child must stare at hand several seconds.
3. Parent may help guide toothbrush and put toothpaste on brush.
4. Child does not have to be able to tie shoes or button/zip in the back.
5. Move yarn slowly in an arc from one side to the other, about 8" above child's face.
6. Pass if child grasps rattle when it is touched to the backs or tips of fingers.
7. Pass if child tries to see where yarn went. Yarn should be dropped quickly from sight from tester's hand without arm movement.
8. Child must transfer cube from hand to hand without help of body, mouth, or table.
9. Pass if child picks up raisin with any part of thumb and finger.
10. Line can vary only 30 degrees or less from tester's line.
11. Make a fist with thumb pointing upward and wiggle only the thumb. Pass if child imitates and does not move any fingers other than the thumb.

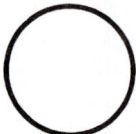
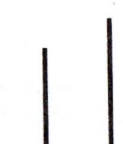
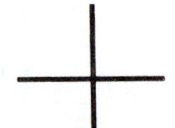

12. Pass any enclosed form. Fail continuous round motions.

13. Which line is longer? (Not bigger.) Turn paper upside down and repeat. (pass 3 of 3 or 5 of 6)

14. Pass any lines crossing near midpoint.

15. Have child copy first. If failed, demonstrate.

   When giving items 12, 14, and 15, do not name the forms. Do not demonstrate 12 and 14.

16. When scoring, each pair (2 arms, 2 legs, etc.) counts as one part.
17. Place one cube in cup and shake gently near child's ear, but out of sight. Repeat for other ear.
18. Point to picture and have child name it. (No credit is given for sounds only.)
    If less than 4 pictures are named correctly, have child point to picture as each is named by tester.

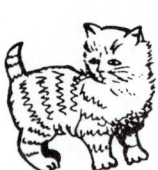
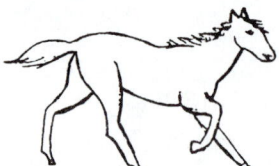
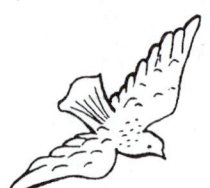
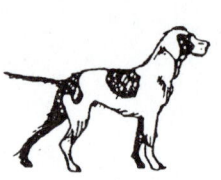
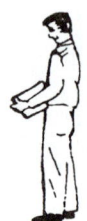

19. Using doll, tell child: Show me the nose, eyes, ears, mouth, hands, feet, tummy, hair. Pass 6 of 8.
20. Using pictures, ask child: Which one flies?... says meow?... talks?... barks?... gallops? Pass 2 of 5, 4 of 5.
21. Ask child: What do you do when you are cold?... tired?... hungry?   Pass 2 of 3, 3 of 3.
22. Ask child: What do you do with a cup? What is a chair used for? What is a pencil used for?
    Action words must be included in answers.
23. Pass if child correctly places <u>and</u> says how many blocks are on paper. (1, 5).
24. Tell child: Put block **on** table; **under** table; **in front of** me, **behind** me. Pass 4 of 4.
    (Do not help child by pointing, moving head or eyes.)
25. Ask child: What is a ball?... lake?... desk?... house?... banana?... curtain?... fence?... ceiling? Pass if defined in terms of use, shape, what it is made of, or general category (such as banana is fruit, not just yellow). Pass 5 of 8, 7 of 8.
26. Ask child: If a horse is big, a mouse is __? If fire is hot, ice is __? If the sun shines during the day, the moon shines during the __? Pass 2 of 3.
27. Child may use wall or rail only, not person. May not crawl.
28. Child must throw ball overhand 3 feet to within arm's reach of tester.
29. Child must perform standing broad jump over width of test sheet (8 1/2 inches).
30. Tell child to walk forward, ⚬⚬⚬⚬⚬⚬➡ heel within 1 inch of toe. Tester may demonstrate.
    Child must walk 4 consecutive steps.
31. In the second year, half of normal children are non-compliant.

OBSERVATIONS:

FIGURE 42-2 Instructions for the DDST. (Copyright 1969, 1989, 1990 WK Frankenburg and JB Dodds. Copyright 1978 WK Frankenburg. Copies can be obtained from Denver Developmental Materials, Inc, (800) 419-4729. Accessed April 17, 2010. Available at www.denverII.com.)

- *Industry versus inferiority*—School-aged children enjoy finishing projects and receiving recognition; they develop feelings of inferiority if not accepted by peers or if they cannot please their parents.
- *Identity versus role confusion*—Adolescents face many physical and hormonal changes in this stage. Teenagers work at figuring out who they are and where they fit; they are looking for a direction for their lives. If they are unable to establish an identity and sense of direction, they become role confused.

Jean Piaget's developmental theory focuses on intellectual growth, with four stages of cognitive development. From birth to 24 months, children progress through the *sensorimotor stage,* which starts with reflexive behavior and advances to learning by doing. The *preoperational stage* (2 to 7 years) is characterized by language development and using play to understand the world. In the *concrete operational stage* (7 to 11 years), children develop logical thinking and become less egocentric. Finally, the *formal operational stage* (11 years or older) brings abstract thinking and deductive reasoning to establish values and determine the meaning of life.

Lawrence Kohlberg's theory, which focuses on moral reasoning, involves levels similar to Piaget's cognitive development theory, yet recognizes the influence of culture and interpersonal relationships on the child's moral development. In *preconventional morality,* the child's behavior is based on the external control of authority figures. The child perceives the goodness or badness of a behavior based on parental reaction. In the *conventional level,* the child wants to follow the rules of the group or society and internalizes the values of others. As the child reaches adolescence, the *postconventional level,* he or she develops individual morality and values, and behavior is regulated internally rather than externally. Table 42-1 summarizes these growth and development theories.

POSTPARTUM DEPRESSION

- The incidence is not clear but it is believed that more than 1 in 10 new mothers experience significant postpartum depression, and fewer than half of them are diagnosed in routine office visits.
- Postpartum depression can be diagnosed a month to a year after childbirth.
- Risk factors include a history of depression, abuse, or mental illness; smoking or alcohol use; anxiety during pregnancy and fears over child care; lack of financial resources and secure relationships; a fussy or colicky infant; and lack of social support.
- As symptoms of postpartum depression, the mother may experience anorexia and insomnia; irritability and anger; overwhelming fatigue; loss of interest in sex and lack of a feeling of joy in life; feelings of shame, guilt, or inadequacy; severe mood swings; difficulty bonding with the baby; withdrawal from family and friends; and thoughts of harming herself or the baby.
- Postpartum depression must be detected as soon as possible so that treatment can begin; untreated postpartum depression may last for a year or longer. Treatment includes both counseling and antidepressant medication.

PEDIATRIC DISEASES AND DISORDERS

The disease process in pediatric patients poses special problems, because children are constantly changing both physically and functionally. As a child grows and develops, the immune system matures, and with the aid of routine prophylactic immunizations, the child acquires long-term protection against certain infectious diseases.

Gastrointestinal Disorders

Colic

Colic usually is seen in the newborn period or in early infancy. The problem is intermittent. The classic situation is an infant between 2 weeks and 4 months of age who has crying episodes that occur at least three times a week for longer than 3 hours a day and lasting 3 weeks. During an attack, the infant draws up the legs, clenches the fists, and cries inconsolably. The abdominal distress of colic usually occurs in the late afternoon and evening. Many theories have been suggested for why infants have colic, but none has been proven correct. If the baby is fed infant formula, pediatricians recommend switching formulas, perhaps to a non–cow's milk type, because this may help relieve the infant's discomfort. Treatment consists of determining the cause; however, the child frequently outgrows the condition before the causative agent can be identified. Drugs are not helpful and in some cases may be dangerous for the infant. Parents need reassurance that they are not responsible for the child's discomfort, and they may find counseling and assistance in developing coping techniques helpful.

Diarrhea

Diarrhea can be caused by a variety of microorganisms, including bacteria, viruses, and parasites. However, children sometimes can have diarrhea without having an infection, such as when diarrhea is caused by food allergies or by certain medications, such as antibiotics. Diarrhea is diagnosed when the child has two or more watery or apparently abnormal stools within 24 hours. The child may not show other signs of illness or may have nausea, vomiting, stomach aches, headache, or fever. If the diarrhea continues for longer than 2 days, medical intervention is needed, because prolonged diarrhea, in which fluid loss becomes excessive, can cause dehydration and electrolyte imbalance. In addition, a resultant diaper rash and excoriation can make defecating painful.

Pediatric diarrhea needs to be followed closely with observation and, in the case of bloody stools, laboratory analysis to determine the causative factors. Infants and small children should be followed up by telephone in 12 hours and then daily until the diarrhea has stopped. Parents should know the indications of dehydration, including lack of tears when crying, lethargy, fewer wet diapers or decreased urination, dry mouth and lips, and weight loss. The physician may recommend the use of oral rehydration therapy, such as Pedialyte or Infalyte; small amounts (approximately 2 tablespoons) are offered at a time (i.e., every 15 minutes) to prevent vomiting. Soft drinks, juices, sport drinks, and tea should be avoided, because they lack electrolytes and may lead to even more diarrhea. Parents should be informed that the child's diarrhea may not stop when the child is given oral rehydration therapy, but the fluids prevent the child from becoming dehydrated. It is important to continue to feed the child, because lack of food can cause damage to the villi in the

TABLE 42-1 Summary of Growth and Development Theories

AGE GROUP	FREUD (1856-1939) PSYCHOSEXUAL THEORY	PIAGET (1896-1980) COGNITIVE THEORY	ERIKSON (1902-1994) PSYCHOSOCIAL THEORY	KOHLBERG (1927-1987) MORAL REASONING
Infant	Oral stage; child operates with the pleasure principle, and the id develops.	Sensorimotor level; uses reflexive behavior; has to do things to learn.	Building basic trust versus mistrust; learning drive and hope.	Avoids punishment and obeys for obedience's sake.
Toddler	Passes through oral aggressive stage to anal stage; elimination is used to control and inhibit.	Coordinates more than one thought at a time; uses thought to create new solutions.	Autonomy versus shame and doubt; learning self-control and willpower.	Avoids punishment and the power of authority figures.
Preschool to early school years	From phallic stage, in which the ego (conscious reality) develops, to latent stage, in which superego (morality) develops.	Intuitive-preoperational; preschoolers are egocentric and have magical thinking. Early school-aged children begin to develop understanding of cause and effect. Child functions symbolically using language; develops understanding of life events and relationships.	Preschool processing initiative versus guilt and attempting to develop direction and purpose. Children mimic others and are more purposeful in establishing goals.	Develops preconventional morality; follows the standards of others to avoid punishment or to earn a reward; recognizes some things are self-satisfying and some are done to satisfy others.
School age	Latent stage continues; superego develops morality or a conscience; represses the sexual drive.	Concrete operations: uses mental reasoning to solve problems; attempts to reach logical solutions; tests beliefs to establish values.	Industry versus inferiority; establishing methods for solving problems and a feeling of competence; mastering tasks and using hands to create things.	Conventional morality; doing what is expected is important. Children need to be good in their own eyes as well as doing what they perceive others expect of them; they want to please others.
Adolescence	Genital stage	Formal operations developing; adolescents are determining values that will guide their lives and religious affiliations; they develop abstract ideas that can be based in reality.	Identity versus role confusion; developing self-identity that will determine devotion and fidelity in future relationships.	Postconventional morality; developing a respect for the laws of society; adolescents are learning to consider the greatest good for the greatest number; values are related to one's group. Behavior is controlled internally.

small intestine. If breast-fed, the baby should continue to nurse, and formula feeding also should be continued.

For older children, a diet of bananas, rice, applesauce, and toast (the BRAT diet) or foods high in carbohydrate are most helpful in enhancing fluid and sodium absorption in the child's irritated gastrointestinal tract. The child should not be given over-the-counter (OTC) antidiarrheal medications, such as Pepto-Bismol, Kaopectate, Imodium, or Lomotil, because these can cause serious side effects, including decreased motility of the bowel, respiratory depression, and drowsiness. The physician may prescribe antibiotics if stool cultures test positive for pathogens. Children with severe dehydration require hospitalization with intravenous (IV) hydration to replace electrolytes and fluids.

CRITICAL THINKING APPLICATION   42-3

Susie receives a call from the grandmother of a 3-year-old child who has had diarrhea since last night. What are some questions Susie should ask to determine the seriousness of the problem? Should the child be seen today, even though appointments are already overbooked?

Failure to Thrive

Failure to thrive is a symptom more than a disease. It is diagnosed in an infant or young child whose weight is consistently below the 3rd percentile on standardized growth charts or one who is 20% below the ideal body weight for length. Physical, mental, and social skills also are delayed in these children. Manifestations include failure to roll over, smile, coo, stand, or walk at age-appropriate developmental levels. Failure to thrive can be caused by a physiologic factor (e.g., malabsorption disease or cleft palate), or it may be related to a problem with the parent-child relationship. The physician needs an accurately recorded history of the child's birth weight and subsequent length, weight, and head circumference measurements. A comprehensive family history is important to rule out genetic growth abnormalities or a history of malabsorption problems, such as cystic fibrosis or celiac disease.

Children with failure to thrive need more calories than usual—approximately 150% of their normal calorie load—to catch up to their target weight. Both medical and social factors are evaluated in the treatment of children with this problem. Experts believe that infants may suffer from this problem if they are being neglected; however, low weight gains also are possible with extremely attentive and cautious parents. The family must be considered as a whole to treat nonorganic causes effectively. Treatment may include the use of support groups and parental counseling.

Obesity

Just as with adult weight patterns, children are assessed according to their BMI. A child's level of body fat varies as the child grows; for example, children normally slim down as they reach school age, and very often their weight increases as they mature from adolescence to adulthood. In addition, body fat levels vary between boys and girls as they reach puberty. Pediatricians therefore use growth charts that plot the child's BMI-for-age to determine whether the child's weight, in comparison with height, is within healthy limits. A child is considered overweight if the BMI-for-age is between the 85th and 94th percentiles; the child is identified as obese if the BMI is at or greater than the 95th percentile. It is estimated that more than 30% of school-aged children are overweight, and almost 16% are considered obese.

The reasons for childhood obesity vary; they include a family history of obesity, inactivity, high-calorie diets, and stress. In rare cases, childhood obesity may be caused by metabolic or endocrine disorders. Overweight and obese children are at greater risk of developing serious health conditions, including asthma, diabetes mellitus type 2, sleep apnea, and hypercholesterolemia, which increases the risk of cardiovascular disease and hypertension. The psychosocial impact of obesity can be overwhelming for many children, because isolation, loneliness, and lack of self-esteem are common. Studies have shown that 70% to 80% of overweight teenagers become overweight adults, with all the health risks and psychological issues that come with weight problems. The pediatrician can provide assistance by recommending a comprehensive diet and exercise program that emphasizes healthy living. The medical assistant can help by providing educational materials, encouragement for the child and parents, and referral to community education and support programs.

Respiratory Disorders

Common Cold

The common cold, or infectious rhinitis, has more than 100 causative pathogens and is highly contagious. It is spread through respiratory droplets from rhinitis, sneezing, or coughing, either from direct contact or from touching contaminated items. The signs include

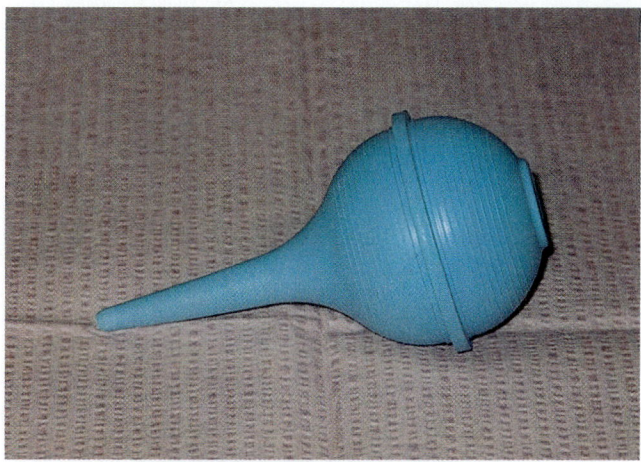

FIGURE 42-3 Nasal bulb syringe.

nasal congestion, low-grade fever, and general malaise. Most colds are self-limiting and run their course in about a week. In infants and young children, the primary concerns are nasal congestion and loss of appetite. The parent may need to be shown how to use a nasal bulb syringe to suction the nose of an infant (Figure 42-3). Secondary infections in the lower respiratory tract or in the middle ear can occur.

One of the secondary infections that can occur is strep throat, which is caused by group A *Streptococcus* bacteria. It is easily spread when an infected person coughs or sneezes contaminated droplets into the air and another person inhales them. A person also can become infected by touching such secretions and then touching the mouth or nose. Symptoms of strep throat infections may include severe sore throat, fever, headache, and lymphadenopathy; also, the throat appears bright red, and pustules may be present on the tonsils. If they are not treated with antibiotics, strep infections can lead to scarlet or rheumatic fever; infections of the skin, bloodstream, or ears; and pneumonia. Scarlet fever is characterized by a bright red, rough-textured rash that spreads over the child's body. Rheumatic fever is a serious disease that can damage the heart valves.

Otitis Media

Infection or inflammation of the middle ear usually is a side effect of a cold or other upper respiratory tract disorder, but it also can be caused by allergies. Otitis media usually occurs in children younger than 3 years of age. Signs include inflammation of the middle ear, with fluid building up behind the tympanic membrane. The child may cry persistently, tug at the ear, have a fever, be irritable, and have diminished hearing in the affected ear. These symptoms sometimes may be accompanied by diarrhea, nausea, and vomiting.

Otitis media is classified as either **serous** (Figure 42-4) or **suppurative** (Figure 42-5), depending on the composition of the accumulated fluid in the middle ear. Because the condition may be caused by bacteria or a virus, determining the most appropriate treatment can be difficult. Traditionally, children with indications of a middle ear infection were treated with antibiotics; however, if the infection is caused by a virus, antibiotics do not help. Because of concern over the growing problem of antibiotic-resistant strains of bacteria, current recommendations call for treatment with acetaminophen or ibuprofen if the child is in pain or has a fever, but the use

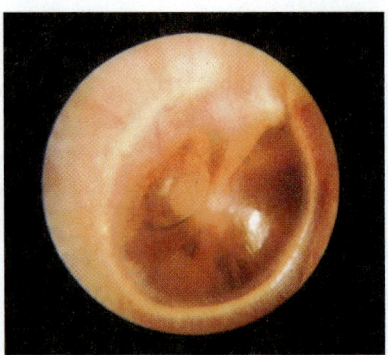

FIGURE 42-4 Serous otitis media. (From Swartz MH: *Textbook of physical diagnosis,* ed 5, Philadelphia, 2006, WB Saunders.)

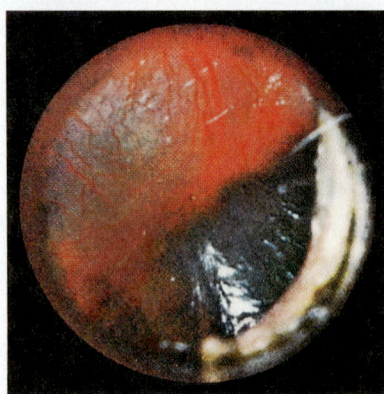

FIGURE 42-5 Suppurative otitis media. (Courtesy Dr. Richard A. Buckingham and Dr. George E. Shambaugh, Jr.)

of antibiotics is delayed for 48 to 72 hours to give the body a chance to fight the infection by itself. Children 6 to 24 months old who show no improvement in symptoms within 24 hours and children older than 24 months who do not improve within 72 hours should be prescribed antibiotics (typically amoxicillin or azithromycin [Zithromax]). The medication usually is ordered for a shorter course (i.e., 5 days rather than 10 to 14 days), because patients and their parents comply better with short-term treatment. Regardless of the length of treatment, it is very important that the complete prescription be administered to prevent a relapse.

If fluid in the middle ear persists for longer than 3 months and/or if the child experiences hearing loss, the physician may recommend a myringotomy; in this operation, a small incision is made in the tympanic membrane and a tube is inserted to drain the fluid and balance the pressure between the outer and middle ear. The tube typically stays in the eardrum for 6 to 12 months and falls out as the child grows. While tubes are in place, it is important to keep water out of the child's ears and to report any drainage to the physician.

CAUTIONS ON THE USE OF OVER-THE-COUNTER COUGH AND COLD MEDICINES IN CHILDREN

The U.S. Food and Drug Administration (FDA) strongly recommends that over-the-counter (OTC) cough and cold products not be given to children under 2 years of age. A number of serious complications may occur, including death, convulsions, rapid heart rate, and diminished levels of consciousness. These medications are given for symptomatic relief and have not been proven to be safe or effective for very young children. Manufacturers have responded to the FDA's recommendation by voluntarily removing the products from shelves.

The FDA also is concerned about the use of these products in children ages 2 to 11 years. Parents need to know that many OTC cough and cold products contain the same active ingredients. Giving a child more than one product that contains the same active ingredient can result in overdose, especially if the wrong dose is given or the product is administered too frequently. Parents of older children are encouraged to read the *Drug Facts* section on the label of each product to familiarize themselves with the active ingredients in the product and to follow dosing guidelines strictly to reduce the risk of complications.

CRITICAL THINKING APPLICATION   42-4

A young mother calls, extremely upset about her 4-year-old son. His symptoms started 3 days ago with a cold, but now the child complains of a sore throat and an earache. What questions should Susie ask to determine whether the child should be seen today?

Croup

Croup is a viral inflammation of the larynx and the trachea that causes edema and spasm of the vocal cords. This varying degree of obstruction of the cords produces hoarseness, a harsh barking cough, and **stridor** during inhalation. The episodes usually occur at night, and symptoms ease by morning. The infection usually is self-limiting, and the child typically recovers without treatment. Mild croup can be relieved by using a cool mist humidifier in the child's room, sitting with the child in a steamy bathroom, or even taking the child outside if the air is cool. Children with allergies may require medical treatment. If the problem becomes chronic or continues for a period of time, the child may need to be treated with corticosteroids (e.g., prednisone). The physician may recommend **laryngoscopy** to visualize the vocal cords or may order throat cultures to determine the underlying cause of the inflammation.

Bronchiolitis

Bronchiolitis is a viral infection of the small bronchi and bronchioles that usually affects children younger than 3 years of age. The infection varies in severity and is seen in children with a family history of asthma and children exposed to cigarette smoke. The child typically has a previous history of rhinitis and cough with an acute onset of wheezing and dyspnea. Symptoms occur because of inflammation, edema, increased secretions, and bronchospasm in the respiratory pathway. Treatment includes acetaminophen for discomfort and fever and a bronchodilator inhaler (albuterol sulfate [Proventil]) or nebulizer treatment for relief of wheezing. Most children fully recover in 2 weeks, but as many as 50% have recurrent wheezing and coughing.

Asthma

Asthma is the most common chronic health problem among children. It is the result of two specific reactions, bronchospasm and inflammation. During an asthma attack, the bronchial tubes begin to spasm, which reduces the amount of air that can pass through them. At the same time, the tissue lining the bronchioles becomes edematous and secretes mucus; therefore, in an asthma attack, the smaller airways are filling up with mucus and secretions. Air passing through these secretions causes the classic symptom of asthma—wheezing on expiration. Asthma has a strong hereditary link. Factors that can trigger an attack include:

- Respiratory infections, including infections caused by common cold viruses
- Exposure to cigarette smoke
- Stress
- Strenuous exercise
- Weather conditions, including cold, windy, or rainy days and extreme humidity
- Allergies to animals, dust, pollen, or mold
- Indoor air pollutants, such as paint, cleaning materials, chemicals, or perfumes
- Outdoor air pollutants, such as ozone

Children with asthma have a nonproductive cough accompanied by an expiratory wheeze and shortness of breath. Shallow breathing makes it difficult for the child to speak more than a few words at a time. The child complains of tightness or pressure in the chest, and the physician hears rhonchi on auscultation. An asthma attack can last minutes to days and may develop into a medical emergency. Each child and each attack must be evaluated independently.

The therapeutic plan is determined by the severity and frequency of attacks. Children with mild to moderately persistent disease (i.e., symptoms that occur less often than twice a week to daily symptoms) should be referred to a specialist. A child who experiences symptoms two or more times a week should take daily medication to prevent asthma attacks. Such medications may include inhaled corticosteroids that deliver an antiinflammatory directly to the bronchioles (e.g., fluticasone [Advair Diskus, Flovent]); long-acting bronchodilators, including salmeterol (Serevent); and oral medications such as montelukast (Singulair) or zafirlukast (Accolate). The child also is prescribed a quick-acting medication, or "rescue inhaler," such as albuterol (Proventil, Ventolin) for acute relief of bronchospasm or exercise-induced asthma; this inhaler should be readily available at all times. Further management of asthma is covered in Chapter 46.

Influenza

Influenza (the "flu") is an acute, highly contagious viral infection of the respiratory tract. The highest incidence is seen in school-aged children, but it is most severe in infants and toddlers. It is transmitted by direct contact with moist secretions. Children tend to have high fevers with influenza and are susceptible to pulmonary complications. Influenza can vary widely in severity, ranging from very mild to life-threatening. The virus can destroy the respiratory epithelium, which is one of the body's defense mechanisms against bacterial invasion. With the loss of this protective mechanism, bacteria can invade any part of the respiratory tract and cause pneumonia.

No medication cures influenza. Some drugs can shorten the duration of the disease, but they must be taken at the onset of symptoms to be effective. Examples of these are zanamivir (Relenza), which is inhaled every 12 hours, and oseltamivir (Tamiflu), which is available in pill form. However, Relenza cannot be prescribed for children under 5 years, and Tamiflu cannot be prescribed for children younger than 1 year. Antibiotics are prescribed only if a secondary bacterial infection develops, such as sinusitis. The usual treatment for influenza is bed rest, increased fluids, and a nonaspirin analgesic to reduce fever and relieve discomfort.

Flu vaccines are available but are beneficial only if the individual is vaccinated before the onset of the disease, and annual vaccines do not provide immunity from all strains of the flu virus. The CDC recommends annual flu vaccinations for all healthy children from age 6 months up to the nineteenth birthday and for their caregivers. The flu vaccine also is recommended for any child over 6 months of age who has a chronic health problem, such as children with chronic heart or lung diseases (including asthma); those undergoing long-term aspirin therapy; children with diabetes mellitus or sickle cell anemia; and those with kidney, blood, or suppressed immune system diseases. The first influenza immunization for children age 6 months to 9 years requires two doses given about 1 month apart. Influenza strains continually change, so the child must receive an updated version of the vaccine each year.

Infectious Diseases

Conjunctivitis

Pinkeye, also called *conjunctivitis,* was discussed in Chapter 37. It is a common infection in children and is highly contagious, especially in day care centers and schools. It can be caused by a bacterial or viral infection that produces white or yellowish pus that may cause the eyelids to stick shut in the morning. Health teaching for caregivers of infected children includes the following:

- Use good hand sanitization practices and hygiene, including proper use and disposal of tissues.
- Do not share towels or any other item that comes in contact with the child's face.
- Disinfect any articles that may have been contaminated.
- Children diagnosed with infectious conjunctivitis should be treated with an antibiotic for at least 24 hours before returning to day care or school.

Tonsillitis

Tonsillitis is caused by many infectious agents, but the most common is *Streptococcus A.* The onset is sudden, and the disorder can cause intense pain within a short time, in addition to fever and general malaise. The tonsils appear enlarged and inflamed and may be covered with pustules. A throat culture usually is performed to determine the causative organism. Treatment consists of bed rest, a liquid to soft diet, an analgesic throat spray, and oral antibiotics if the causative organism is a bacterium. The danger lies in the secondary problems that can occur, which include rheumatic heart disease and kidney disease if the streptococcal infection is not treated with antibiotics.

Fifth Disease

Fifth disease, also called *erythema infectiosum, parvovirus infection,* or *slapped cheek disease,* is an infection caused by parvovirus B19. Outbreaks are most common in the winter and spring. Symptoms begin with a mild fever and general malaise. After a few days, the cheeks take on a flushed appearance, making the face look as if it had been slapped. A lacy rash also may be seen on the trunk, arms, and legs, but not all those infected develop the rash.

Most children who get fifth disease are not very ill and recover without any serious consequences. However, children with sickle cell anemia, chronic anemia, or an impaired immune system may become seriously ill when infected and require medical care. If a pregnant woman becomes infected with parvovirus B19, she has an increased risk of miscarriage, and the fetus may suffer from severe anemia. The woman herself may have no symptoms or may have a mild illness with a rash and/or arthralgia (joint pain).

Fifth disease is spread through direct contact or by breathing in respiratory secretions from an infected person. Patients are most contagious before the onset of the rash; once the rash appears, they are no longer considered contagious.

Hand-Foot-and-Mouth Disease

Hand-foot-and-mouth disease is caused by the coxsackievirus, which is ingested and transmitted by direct contact with nose and throat drainage, saliva, or the stool of an infected individual. The disease is seen most often in day care settings, where children can easily come in contact with infected bodily secretions. Symptoms include a combination of fever; sore throat; painful red blisters on the tongue, mouth, palms, and soles; headache; anorexia, and irritability. Most cases of hand-foot-and-mouth disease are not serious.

The most common complication of the infection is dehydration. Young children may stop eating and drinking because sores in the mouth make swallowing painful. Because the infection is caused by a virus, antibiotic therapy is not helpful, and the disease must run its course. Supportive therapy is recommended, consisting of plenty of rest, fluids, and acetaminophen or ibuprofen for fever or discomfort. To prevent the spread of the disease, family members should be instructed to wash their hands thoroughly, especially after diaper changes, and disinfect shared items such as toys frequently. Individuals with the disease are highly contagious during the first week; however, the virus may be spread for weeks after symptoms have cleared. Children with hand-foot-and-mouth disease should be kept out of day care or school until the fever is gone and mouth sores have healed.

Varicella (Chickenpox)

Chickenpox is caused by a member of the herpes virus group and is transmitted by direct or indirect droplets from the respiratory tract of an infected person. The incubation period is 14 to 21 days. The child usually runs a slight fever for up to 3 days before the skin eruptions occur and is contagious at this time. Skin lesions continue to erupt for 3 to 4 days and cause intense itching. The infection lasts approximately 2 weeks and in most cases leaves the child with lifetime immunity. The disease is so contagious in its early stages that an exposed person who is not immune to the virus has a 70% to 80% chance of contracting the disease.

The varicella virus vaccine, Varivax, is available for protection against chickenpox. Varivax is very effective; 80% to 90% of those vaccinated are completely protected from chickenpox. If a child does get chickenpox after vaccination, it is usually a very mild case lasting only a few days with limited skin lesions, low-grade or no fever, and few other symptoms.

The CDC recommends that children receive two doses of the vaccine, the first between 12 and 15 months of age and the second between 4 and 6 years. Adolescents and adults who have never had chickenpox also should receive two doses of the vaccine. Varivax has proved to be safe and effective and can be administered at the same time as the measles, mumps, and rubella vaccine.

Chickenpox is not a serious disease for most children. However, newborns and individuals with an impaired immune system (e.g., those undergoing chemotherapy for cancer, those with acquired immunodeficiency syndrome [AIDS], and those who take steroid medications [e.g., prednisone]) may have a severe case or can even die. Chickenpox can be very dangerous for pregnant women, causing stillbirths or birth defects, and can be spread to their babies during childbirth. Occasionally chickenpox can cause serious, life-threatening illnesses, such as encephalitis or pneumonia, especially in adults. After infection, the virus migrates to a dermatome and may cause "shingles" or herpes zoster (see Chapter 38).

Meningitis

Meningitis is an inflammation of the membranes that cover the brain and spinal cord. It is caused by a bacterial, fungal, or viral infection. Viral meningitis usually is mild and clears up on its own within 10 to 14 days. Fungal meningitis can be quite serious and typically is seen in immunocompromised individuals, such as those with AIDS. Meningitis caused by a bacterial infection (sometimes called *spinal meningitis*) is one of the most serious types, sometimes leading to permanent brain damage or even death. Bacterial meningitis most often is caused by three different bacteria: *Neisseria meningitidis* (meningococcal meningitis), *Streptococcus pneumoniae,* and *Haemophilus influenzae* serotype b (*H. influenzae* meningitis). These bacteria are carried in the upper back part of the throat (nasopharynx) of an infected person and are spread either through the air (when the person coughs or sneezes) or by direct contact with secretions, such as through kissing or sharing eating or drinking utensils. However, transmission usually occurs only after very close contact with the infected person. Signs and symptoms of bacterial meningitis include a sudden onset of fever, headache, neck pain or stiffness, vomiting (often without abdominal complaints), and irritability. These signs and symptoms may quickly progress to a decreased level of consciousness (the person is difficult to rouse), convulsions, and death. For this reason, if any child displays symptoms of possible meningitis, he or she should receive medical care immediately. Bacterial meningitis is treated with immediate hospitalization and IV antibiotic therapy.

Meningitis caused by *H. influenzae* serotype b (Hib) can be prevented with the Hib vaccine, which is given as part of the routine childhood immunizations in three or four doses starting at 2 months of age. Some cases of meningococcal meningitis also can be prevented by vaccination. However, this vaccine is not used routinely; it usually is given only during outbreaks or to high-risk children. Many states require reporting of bacterial meningitis cases to the health department, which probably will recommend preventive antibiotics for potentially exposed persons.

Hepatitis B

Infection with the hepatitis B virus (HBV) can lead to a serious, chronic infection of the liver. The virus can be transmitted across

TABLE 42-2 Five Stages of Reye's Syndrome

STAGE	SIGNS AND SYMPTOMS
1	Restlessness, vomiting, liver malfunction
2	Elevated respiratory rate, hyperactive reflexes, increased liver dysfunction
3	Internal organ tissue changes, coma
4	Loss of brain function, deepening coma
5	Seizures, respiratory arrest, death

the placenta or during the birth process if the mother is infected. HBV also can be transmitted sexually, by blood transfusion, or by direct contact. A child can carry the virus for years and only later develop liver failure or liver cancer. Many states now include immunization for HBV in the recommended immunization schedule, which usually is begun in the newborn nursery.

Reye's Syndrome

The cause of Reye's syndrome is unknown, but the disorder has been linked to the use of aspirin during a viral illness. Reye's syndrome is an acute and sometimes fatal illness characterized by fatty invasion of the inner organs, especially the liver, and swelling of the brain. It most often is seen in children from infancy through puberty (age 16). The syndrome moves through five stages (Table 42-2).

Prevention is the best treatment, which means children should never be given aspirin. Parents should be advised to use nonsalicylate analgesics and antipyretics, such as ibuprofen and acetaminophen, for fevers or discomfort. Parents should also be warned to read the labels of OTC medications carefully, because cold and flu remedies may contain aspirin.

CRITICAL THINKING APPLICATION   **42-5**

The father of a 10-year-old girl calls this morning, concerned about his daughter's symptoms. She has a sore throat, fever, and bright red cheeks. He wants to give her aspirin for the fever. What advice should Susie give the father? What questions should she ask to determine the seriousness of the child's problem? Should she list this call on the physician's call back list?

AUTISM

- The American Academy of Pediatrics (AAP) recommends that all children be screened for developmental delays and disabilities during regular well-child doctor visits at 9, 18, and 24 to 30 months of age. By age 2, a diagnosis by an experienced professional is considered very reliable.
- An estimated 3 to 6 in 1,000 children are diagnosed with autism; it occurs four times more often in boys.
- The cause of this developmental disorder is unknown, but researchers believe it is due to a combination of genetic errors and environmental factors, perhaps a problem with fetal brain development. Although many parents are concerned about a connection with vaccines, extensive studies have failed to show a link between the two.
- Children with autism have impaired social interaction, do not respond to their name, avoid eye contact, and show limited interest in their surroundings. They rarely communicate with others and display repetitive movements or mannerisms such as rocking or twirling. They may also have self-abusive behaviors, such as biting and head banging. Many children with autism have a very high pain tolerance but are extremely sensitive to noise, touch, or other sensory stimulation.
- Treatment involves coordinated educational and behavioral interventions to help the child develop social and language skills. Medications may be prescribed to treat depression, anxiety, and obsessive-compulsive behaviors.

Inherited Disorders

Cystic Fibrosis

Cystic fibrosis (CF) is an autosomal recessive genetic disorder (i.e., both parents are carriers but do not have the disease) that prevents the normal movement of sodium chloride (salt) into and out of cells. The lungs and pancreas are primarily affected, causing a buildup of abnormally thick secretions in the lungs and blockage of the pancreatic ducts, which prevents the excretion of pancreatic digestive enzymes and results in malabsorption problems. The child is prone to developing an emphysema-like lung condition because of the obstruction of the air pathways with mucus. There is also an abnormality in the sweat glands, which produce sweat that is very high in sodium chloride.

Signs and symptoms of cystic fibrosis include a salty taste to the skin, which may be noticed when parents kiss the child, steatorrhea (large, greasy, foul-smelling stools), abdominal distention, failure to thrive, chronic cough, and frequent respiratory infections.

All states screen newborns for CF using either a genetic or blood test. The genetic test shows whether the newborn has the CF gene, whereas the blood test evaluates pancreatic function. If either of these tests suggests CF, the diagnosis is confirmed using a sweat test, which shows an elevated chlorine level. Treatment of the disease is complicated and requires a multispecialty approach, because so many systems are involved. The first line of treatment is prevention of bronchial obstruction through routine chest percussion therapy (CPT). Mechanical devices have been developed to assist with CPT. Two examples are an electric chest clapper, known as a *mechanical percussor*, and an inflatable therapy vest that uses high-frequency airwaves to force the mucus that is deep in the lungs toward the upper airways. Medical treatments include bronchodilators and antibiotics for signs of infection. More recent therapies have included medications such as aerosolized dornase alfa (Pulmozyme) to make mucus thinner and easier to cough up. The child also is given pancreatic enzymes to improve digestion and absorption of nutrients. Cystic fibrosis is a chronic, progressive disease that has no cure; the life expectancy is 35 to 40 years. Genetic testing can identify carriers, and its presence can be detected through prenatal genetic testing with either chorionic villi sampling or amniocentesis. Cystic fibrosis usually occurs without any warning (parents have no idea they are carriers), so families need support and

MODIFIED CHECKLIST FOR AUTISM IN TODDLERS (M-CHAT)

The M-CHAT is validated for screening toddlers between 16 and 30 months of age, to assess risk for autism spectrum disorders (ASD). The M-CHAT can be administered and scored as part of a well-child checkup and also can be used by specialists or other professionals to assess the risk for ASD. Children who fail three or more items total or two or more critical items (particularly if these scores remain elevated after the M-CHAT follow-up interview) should be referred for diagnostic evaluation by a specialist trained to evaluate ASD in very young children. If the behavior is rare (only seen once or twice), answer as if the child does *not* do it.

1. Does your child enjoy being swung, bounced on your knee, etc.? Yes No
2. Does your child take an interest in other children? Yes No
3. Does your child like climbing on things, such as up stairs? Yes No
4. Does your child enjoy playing peek-a-boo/hide-and-seek? Yes No
5. Does your child ever pretend, for example, to talk on the phone or take care of a doll or pretend other things? Yes No
6. Does your child ever use his/her index finger to point, to ask for something? Yes No
7. Does your child ever use his/her index finger to point, to indicate interest in something? Yes No
8. Can your child play properly with small toys (e.g. cars or blocks) without just mouthing, fiddling, or dropping them? Yes No
9. Does your child ever bring objects over to you (parent) to show you something? Yes No
10. Does your child look you in the eye for more than a second or two? Yes No
11. Does your child ever seem oversensitive to noise? (e.g., plugging ears) Yes No
12. Does your child smile in response to your face or your smile? Yes No
13. Does your child imitate you? (e.g., you make a face-will your child imitate it?) Yes No
14. Does your child respond to his/her name when you call? Yes No
15. If you point at a toy across the room, does your child look at it? Yes No
16. Does your child walk? Yes No
17. Does your child look at things you are looking at? Yes No
18. Does your child make unusual finger movements near his/her face? Yes No
19. Does your child try to attract your attention to his/her own activity? Yes No
20. Have you ever wondered if your child is deaf? Yes No
21. Does your child understand what people say? Yes No
22. Does your child sometimes stare at nothing or wander with no purpose? Yes No
23. Does your child look at your face to check your reaction when faced with something unfamiliar? Yes No

© 1999 Diana Robins, Deborah Fein, & Marianne Barton

understanding to cope with the demands of caring for a child with the disease.

Duchenne's Muscular Dystrophy

Muscular dystrophy is an X-linked genetic disease (passed from mothers to sons) that causes progressive muscle degeneration. The disease usually develops before age 5 and is marked by muscular weakness, frequent falls, a waddling gait, possible swallowing problems, and difficulty climbing stairs. The disorder is diagnosed with a blood test that shows an elevated creatine phosphokinase (CPK) level, electromyography, muscle biopsy, and genetic testing. As the disease progresses and the necrotic skeletal muscles are replaced with fat and fibrous connective tissue, muscle function is gradually lost. Respiratory insufficiency and infections are common because of involvement of the diaphragm and intercostal muscles required for breathing. The disease has no cure and no specific treatment except for supportive care. Family counseling is helpful so that family members can learn to cope with the disease. Death usually occurs in the early 20s as a result of respiratory or cardiac complications.

IMMUNIZATIONS

Over the years, immunization has helped dramatically reduce potentially lethal childhood infections. Figure 42-6 summarizes the 2011 immunization recommendations from the CDC for children 0 through 6 years of age, which can be found at the CDC's Web site (*www.cdc.gov/vaccines/recs/schedules/downloads/child/0-6yrs-schedule-pr.pdf*). Figure 42-7 identifies the 2011 immunization recommendations for children age 7 through 18, which also can be found at the CDC's Web site (*www.cdc.gov/vaccines/recs/schedules/downloads/child/7-18yrs-schedule-pr.pdf*).

The schedules are updated periodically as new vaccines become available and/or research indicates a better method for giving the vaccine. For example, it is now recommended that both male and female children be immunized against the human papilloma virus (HPV) at 11 to 12 years of age. The CDC recommends immunization against infectious diseases for all children, except those for whom a particular vaccination would pose a risk. However, each state develops its own immunization program and methods of enforcement.

The vaccines used in immunizations consist of a suspension of **attenuated** organisms or their toxins, which is administered to stimulate an active immune response in the child's body, resulting in the production of antibodies against the specific pathogens. Booster doses usually are equivalent to a single dose of the initial immunization; for some immunizations, such as tetanus, boosters are prescribed at designated intervals to ensure maintenance of immune levels.

Vaccine manufacturers have trade names for each product and have established protocols to ensure potency and stability. All vaccines are tested for safety and effectiveness. In every package of vaccine is an insert that fully describes the vaccine, its use, the route of administration, adverse reactions, and signs and symptoms that the parent might observe after immunization that would indicate a potential problem. Untoward responses include high fever, swelling at the site of the injection, urticaria, breathing difficulties, severe headache, and convulsions. Any of these should be reported to the

Vaccine ▼ Age ►	Birth	1 month	2 months	4 months	6 months	9 months	12 months	15 months	18 months	19–23 months	2–3 years	4–6 years	
Hepatitis B[1]	Hep B	HepB			HepB								Range of recommended ages for all children
Rotavirus[2]			RV	RV	RV[2]								
Diphtheria, tetanus, pertussis[3]			DTaP	DTaP	DTaP		see footnote[3]	DTaP				DTaP	Range of recommended ages for certain high-risk groups
Haemophilus influenzae type b[4]			Hib	Hib	Hib[4]		Hib						
Pneumococcal[5]			PCV	PCV	PCV		PCV				PPSV		
Inactivated poliovirus[6]			IPV	IPV	IPV							IPV	
Influenza[7]					Influenza (Yearly)								
Measles, mumps, rubella[8]							MMR		see footnote[8]			MMR	Range of recommended ages for all children and certain high-risk groups
Varicella[9]							Varicella		see footnote[9]			Varicella	
Hepatitis A[10]							Dose 1[10]				HepA Series		
Meningococcal[11]							MCV4 — see footnote[11]						

This schedule includes recommendations in effect as of December 23, 2011. Any dose not administered at the recommended age should be administered at a subsequent visit, when indicated and feasible. The use of a combination vaccine generally is preferred over separate injections of its equivalent component vaccines. Vaccination providers should consult the relevant Advisory Committee on Immunization Practices (ACIP) statement for detailed recommendations, available online at http://www.cdc.gov/vaccines/pubs/acip-list.htm. Clinically significant adverse events that follow vaccination should be reported to the Vaccine Adverse Event Reporting System (VAERS) online (http://www.vaers.hhs.gov) or by telephone (800-822-7967).

FIGURE 42-6 Recommended immunization schedule for children ages 0 to 6 years. (From U.S. Centers for Disease Control, 2009. Accessed May 1, 2010, at www.cdc.gov/vaccines/recs/schedules.)

Vaccine ▼ Age ►	7–10 years	11–12 years	13–18 years	
Tetanus, diphtheria, pertussis[1]	1 dose (if indicated)	1 dose	1 dose (if indicated)	Range of recommended ages for all children
Human papillomavirus[2]	see footnote[2]	3 doses	Complete 3-dose series	
Meningococcal[3]	See footnote[3]	Dose 1	Booster at 16 years old	Range of recommended ages for catch-up immunization
Influenza[4]	Influenza (yearly)			
Pneumococcal[5]	See footnote 5			
Hepatitis A[6]	Complete 2-dose series			Range of recommended ages for certain high-risk groups
Hepatitis B[7]	Complete 3-dose series			
Inactivated poliovirus[8]	Complete 3-dose series			
Measles, mumps, rubella[9]	Complete 2-dose series			
Varicella[10]	Complete 2-dose series			

This schedule includes recommendations in effect as of December 23, 2011. Any dose not administered at the recommended age should be administered at a subsequent visit, when indicated and feasible. The use of a combination vaccine generally is preferred over separate injections of its equivalent component vaccines. Vaccination providers should consult the relevant Advisory Committee on Immunization Practices (ACIP) statement for detailed recommendations, available online at http://www.cdc.gov/vaccines/pubs/acip-list.htm. Clinically significant adverse events that follow vaccination should be reported to the Vaccine Adverse Event Reporting System (VAERS) online (http://www.vaers.hhs.gov) or by telephone (800-822-7967).

FIGURE 42-7 Recommended immunization schedule for children ages 7 to 18 years. (From U.S. Centers for Disease Control, 2009. Accessed May 1, 2010, at www.cdc.gov/vaccines/recs/schedules.)

physician immediately. Vaccine storage should follow the manufacturer's guidelines (e.g., some vaccines must be refrigerated; others must not be exposed to sunlight).

Some vaccines are grown in birds' eggs or in a medium made of animal organs or are weakened with chemicals. Therefore, a child who is allergic to eggs cannot receive some of the vaccines, such as those for measles, mumps, and rubella (MMR) and the vaccine for varicella. The medical assistant must know the potential allergic problems, common symptoms, and adverse reactions to immunizations and must make sure the parent is informed. Table 42-3 details guidelines for childhood immunizations.

Before a child or adult receives a vaccine, the healthcare provider is required by the National Childhood Vaccine Injury Act (NCVIA) to provide a copy of a Vaccine Information Sheet (VIS) to either the adult patient or the child's parent or legal guardian. A VIS provides information about the risks and benefits of each vaccine. If providing the parent or guardian with the VIS is the medical assistant's responsibility, he or she should do the following (Procedure 42-1):

- Before administering the vaccine, give the parent the most current VIS available for that particular vaccine. Give the parent enough time to review the information and then answer any questions or refer the parent's concerns to the physician before administering the vaccine.
- Document in the child's medical record the date the VIS was given and the publication date of the VIS (which appears on the bottom of the form).
- To make sure the office has the most current VIS forms, either call the state health department or refer to the CDC Web site (www.cdc.gov/nip/publications/VIS/default.htm). Forms can be printed directly from the site.
- An informed consent form must be signed and attached to the child's health record before immunizations are given. Documentation of immunization administration must include the date the vaccine was administered, the manufacturer of the vaccine, the manufacturer's lot number, the type of vaccine, the exact site of administration if an injection was

TABLE 42-3 Guidelines for Childhood Immunization

VACCINE AND DISEASE	ROUTE OF ADMINISTRATION	CONTRAINDICATIONS*	SIDE EFFECTS
DtaP Diphtheria, tetanus, pertussis (whooping cough)	IM; Td (tetanus and diphtheria) boosters at 11-12 yr if at least 5 yr since last dose; subsequent booster every 10 yr	Moderate or severe acute illness; neurologic problem; complication after previous dose (e.g., fever, convulsion)	Mild fever, anorexia, irritability, drowsiness
HAV Hepatitis A (can use either Havrix or Vaqta brands)	IM; all children 1 yr; two doses 6 mo apart	Hypersensitivity to product, acute infection or fever	Localized injection site reaction, fever, headache
HBV Hepatitis B (can use either Energix B or Recombivax HB brands)	IM; may give with all other vaccines but at a separate site; requires three injections	Moderate or severe acute illness; yeast allergy; severe cardiovascular disease	Fever, pain at site, headache, malaise, vomiting
Hib *Haemophilus influenzae* serotype B meningitis	IM; may give with all other vaccines but at a separate site	Not routinely given to children 5 yr; moderate or severe acute illness	Minimal
HPV Human papilloma virus (Gardasil)	IM; second dose 2 mo after first, third dose 6 mo after first	Hypersensitivity to ingredients; pregnancy	Relatively few; mild headache and GI upset
Influenza Trivalent inactivated vaccine for 6 months; at 2 years, use live, attenuated vaccine	IM; annually each fall	Allergy to eggs; recent fever	Uncommon; fever, local irritation at injection site, general malaise
IPV Inactive poliovirus for polio	SC or IM; four doses; may give with all other vaccines but at a separate site	Moderate or severe acute illness; egg allergy	Uncommon
MMR Measles, mumps, rubella	SC; may give with all other vaccines but at a separate site	Moderate or severe acute illness; immunocompromised patients (may be given if HIV positive); pregnancy or possible pregnancy in 3 mo; egg allergy	Fever
Pneumococcal Pneumococcal pneumonia	IM or SC; all children 2-23 mo; administer every 6 yr for high-risk patients		
Rotavirus (Rota) RotaTeq for prevention of rotavirus gastroenteritis	Oral; three doses at 6-12 wk; subsequent doses at 4-10 wk intervals	Hypersensitivity	Gastrointestinal upset and blood disorders
Varicella Varicella (chickenpox)	SC; may give with all other vaccines but at a separate site; all susceptible children 12 mo	Confirmed history of chickenpox; pregnancy or possible pregnancy in 1 mo; moderate or severe acute illness; immunocompromised patients; egg allergy	No salicylates for 6 wk afterward to prevent risk of Reye's syndrome

HIV, Human immunodeficiency virus; *IM*, intramuscular; *SC*, subcutaneous.
*Mild illness is not a contraindication.

given, any reported or observed side effects, the name and title of the person who administered the vaccine, and the address of the medical office where the vaccine was administered.

- An official immunization booklet should be given to the parent and updated as needed to reflect the child's current immunization status. The medical assistant should not only document the required details in the patient's medical record but also complete the parent's immunization booklet each time the child receives another vaccination or booster. These parent records help schools and day care centers determine the child's immunization status. Some states are developing computerized immunization record systems.

- It is very important that vaccine vials be handled and stored properly to maintain the compound's ability to fight disease. The CDC's recommendations for vaccine management practices are listed on p. 887.

CRITICAL THINKING APPLICATION 42-6

Susie will be administering pediatric immunizations during the well-baby visits scheduled for today. To prepare for this responsibility, she looked up the primary vaccinations, their routes of administration, contraindications, and possible side effects. The first child is here for her 4-month checkup. What immunizations should the child receive and how should they be administered? The baby's father asks whether she will get sick from the vaccines. What should Susie tell him? What does Susie need to do to meet the requirements of the National Childhood Vaccine Injury Act?

THE PEDIATRIC PATIENT

An infant's first physical assessment comes at the time of delivery, when the pediatrician assesses the newborn's ability to thrive outside the uterus. The Apgar score is a system for evaluating the infant's physical condition at 1 and 5 minutes after birth (Table 42-4). Developed by pediatrician Virginia Apgar, the scoring system evaluates the following: *a*ppearance (color); *p*ulse (heart rate); *g*rimace (reflex; response to stimuli); *a*ctivity (muscle tone); and *r*espiration (breathing). These parameters are each rated 0, 1, or 2. The maximum total score is 10. Infants with low scores require immediate medical attention.

Well-Child Visits

The frequency of well-child visits varies with the physician and the community. It may follow this pattern: 2 weeks, 4 weeks, 8 weeks, 4 months, 6 months, 12 months, 18 months, 2 years, 5 years, 10 years, and 15 years. These visits focus on maintaining the child's health through basic system examinations, immunizations, and upgrading of the child's medical history record.

The decision on whether the child is to be seen alone or with the parent depends on the pediatrician and the child's age. Often the child looks to the parent for approval before answering or performing a skill; for this reason, the physician may want to assess the child alone. If this is the case, explain to the parent that the physician wants to evaluate the child's independent abilities and that as soon as testing is complete, the physician will explain the results of the tests.

The medical history is an essential guide to the pediatric examination. With an infant, the physician depends on the caregiver for the

---

PROCEDURE 42-1

Maintain Medication and Immunization Records: Document Immunizations

GOAL: To document accurately the administration of a pediatric immunization.

SCENARIO: Samantha Anderson, a 5-week-old infant, has just received her second dose of the hepatitis B (HBV) vaccine. Document the administration of the vaccine.

EQUIPMENT and SUPPLIES

- Vaccine immunization administration record (Figure 1)
- Parent's immunization booklet
- Vaccine Information Sheet (VIS) form for hepatitis B
- Patient's record

PROCEDURAL STEPS

1. Gather the necessary forms.
2. Make sure the physician obtained informed consent from the parent, that the hepatitis B VIS form was given, and that all the parent's questions were answered.
   PURPOSE: To follow risk management practices.
3. After dispensing the vaccine dose and before administration, complete the information required on the Vaccine Administration Record, including the name of the vaccine, the date given, the route of administration and site, the vaccine lot number and manufacturer, the date on the VIS form, the date it was given to the parent, and your signature or initials.
   PURPOSE: To meet the legal requirements of the National Childhood Vaccine Injury Act.
4. Administer the vaccine intramuscularly (see Chapter 35).

5. Record the date of administration, the name and address of the physician's practice, and the type of vaccine administered in the parent's immunization booklet.
   PURPOSE: To maintain an accurate and comprehensive parental record of childhood immunizations for school and/or day care purposes.
6. After administration of the hepatitis vaccine, record in the child's medical record the following details:
   - Date the vaccine was administered
   - Vaccine's manufacturer, batch and lot numbers, and expiration date
   - Type of vaccine administered and dose
   - Route of administration and exact site if an injection was given
   - Any reported or observed side effects
   - Publication date of the VIS form given to the parent (on the bottom of the form)
   - Parent education about possible side effects of the vaccine
   - Name and title of the person who administered the vaccine

---

4/2/XX 3:25 PM Mother given VIS form for Hep B. Had no questions. Administered second dose of Hep B to ① vastus lateralis as ordered. No problems noted after injection. S. Kwong CMA (AAMA)

Vaccine Administration Record for Children and Teens

Patient name: _____

Birthdate: _____

Chart number: _____

Before administering any vaccines, give the parent/guardian all appropriate copies of Vaccine Information Statements (VISs) and make sure they understand the risks and benefits of the vaccine(s). Update the patient's personal record card or provide a new one whenever you administer vaccine.

Vaccine	Type of Vaccine[1] (generic abbreviation)	Date given (mo/day/yr)	Route	Site given (RA, LA, RT, LT)	Vaccine		Vaccine Information Statement		Signature/ initials of vaccinator
					Lot #	Mfr.	Date on VIS[2]	Date given[2]	
Hepatitis B[3] e.g., HepB, Hib-HepB, DTaP-HepB-IPV			IM						
			IM						
			IM						
			IM						
Diphtheria, Tetanus, Pertussis[3] e.g., DTaP, DT, Tdap, DTaP-Hib, DTaP-HepB-IPV, Td			IM						
			IM						
			IM						
			IM						
			IM						
			IM						
			IM						
***Haemophilus influenzae* type b**[3] e.g., Hib, Hib-HepB, DTaP-Hib			IM						
			IM						
			IM						
			IM						
Polio[3] e.g., IPV, DTaP-HepB-IPV			IM•SC						
			IM•SC						
			IM•SC						
			IM•SC						
Pneumococcal PCV (conjugate) PPV (polysaccharide)			IM						
			IM						
			IM						
			IM						
Measles, Mumps, Rubella[3] e.g., MMR, MMRV			SC						
			SC						
Varicella[3] e.g., Var, MMRV			SC						
			SC						
Hepatitis A HepA			IM						
			IM						
Meningococcal[4] MCV4 (conjugate) MPSV4 (polysaccharide)									
Influenza[5] TIV (inactivated) LAIV (live, attenuated)									
Other									

1. Record the generic abbreviation for the type of vaccine given (e.g., DTaP-Hib, PCV), *not* the trade name.
2. Record the publication date of each VIS as well as the date it is given to the patient. According to federal law, VISs must be given to patients (or parent/guardian of a minor child) before administering each dose of DTaP, Td, Hib, polio, MMR, varicella, PCV, or HepB vaccine, or combinations thereof. Use of the VISs for hepatitis A, influenza, and meningococcal vaccines will become mandatory in later 2005.
3. For combination vaccines, fill in a row for each separate antigen in the combination.
4. Give MCV4 via the IM route and MPSV4 via the SC route.
5. Give TIV via the IM route and LAIV intranasally (IN).

www.immunize.org/catg.d/p2022b.pdf • Item #P2022 (10/05)

Immunization Action Coalition • 1573 Selby Ave. • St. Paul, MN 55104 • (651) 647-9009 • www.immunize.org • www.vaccineinformation.org

SAFE HANDLING AND STORAGE OF VACCINES

The Centers for Disease Control and Prevention (CDC) has devised a list of important rules and steps to ensure safekeeping of a practice's vaccine supply. This list can be used as a checklist in the office.

_____ 1. One person should be in charge of the handling and storage of vaccines at the facility, with a backup person to ensure proper management.

_____ 2. A vaccine inventory log should be maintained that includes the following: (1) vaccine name, (2) number of doses, and (3) date received; (4) condition of vaccine on arrival; (5) vaccine manufacturer, (6) lot number, and (7) expiration date

_____ 3. A full-size refrigerator that has a separate freezer compartment door should be used for vaccine storage, or the facility should have a refrigerator and a separate freezer.

_____ 4. The vaccine refrigerator and freezer should not be used for food or drinks.

_____ 5. Vaccines should be stored in the middle of the refrigerator or freezer, not on the door.

_____ 6. New supplies should be placed behind the vials with the closest expiration date; the vials with the nearest expiration date should be used first.

_____ 7. A sign should be posted on the refrigerator door identifying which vaccines should be stored in either the refrigerator or the freezer.

_____ 8. A thermometer should be kept in the refrigerator and one in the freezer; the refrigerator temperature is maintained at 35° to 46°F (2° to 8°C) and the freezer at +5°F (−15°C) or colder.

_____ 9. Containers of water should be kept in the refrigerator and ice packs in the freezer to help maintain cold temperatures.

_____ 10. A temperature log should be kept on the refrigerator door; the refrigerator and freezer temperatures should be recorded twice a day: first thing in the morning and at the end of the day.

_____ 11. A "Do Not Unplug" sign should be posted next to the refrigerator's electrical outlet.

_____ 12. If the refrigerator stops working, the following steps should be taken:
- Immediately place the vaccines in another refrigerator; mark them so that they can be separated from vaccines that were not affected.
- Record the temperature of the refrigerator or freezer and contact the vaccine manufacturer or state health department; follow their instructions regarding the use, alteration of expiration dates, or disposal of the vaccines.

_____ 13. The facility should have a copy of the health department's general and emergency vaccine management policies.

TABLE 42-4 Apgar Scoring System*

CLINICAL SIGN	0	1	2
		ASSIGNED SCORE	
Heart rate	Absent	100	100
Respiratory effort	Absent	Slow and irregular	Good and crying
Muscle tone	Limp	Some flexion of the arms and legs	Active movement
Reflex irritability	No response	Grimace	Coughing and sneezing
Color	Blue and pale	Body pink and extremities blue	Pink all over

*Readings are taken by the pediatrician at 1 minute and 5 minutes after birth. At *1 minute:* If the score is 7 or lower, some nervous system problems are suspected. If the score is below 4, resuscitation usually is necessary. At *5 minutes:* If the score is at least 8, the child probably is reacting normally.

history, but as the child gets older, some history may be obtained from the child and clarified or amplified by the parent. Close observation also gives the physician considerable information.

LEAD PAINT EXPOSURE

Children are especially vulnerable to lead levels in their environment. High blood lead levels can result in serious brain injury, including seizures, coma, and death; lower levels can cause learning problems, stunted growth, and behavior disorders. Lead-based paint in homes and on imported toys and chronic exposure to lead-contaminated dust are the most common causes of lead exposure. The Centers for Disease Control and Prevention (CDC) recommends a screening blood lead test for all children between 1 and 2 years of age. For children who show elevated levels, follow-up should include home and school environmental testing to determine the cause of lead exposure.

Sick-Child Visits

Sick-child visits occur whenever needed, usually on short notice. For this reason, most pediatric offices keep open appointments in the schedule to accommodate calls for sick-child visits. The length and frequency of this type of visit depends entirely on the child and the illness. The medical assistant frequently is the first point of contact for a sick child and his or her caregiver.

Determining whether the child should be seen immediately or the problem can wait for an opening in the schedule is crucial to pediatric care. The medical assistant should follow established office policies, but when in doubt about the seriousness of the problem, he or she should ask the office manager or physician for advice. Usually the physician prefers to see the child rather than delay seeing a patient with a potentially serious condition. When the medical assistant conducts telephone screening, if the child is young (under

2 years old) and the parent reports frequent cycles of crying, lethargy, vomiting that lasts longer than 24 hours, diarrhea (more than six stools in the past 12 hours), or fever of 103°F (39.4°C) or higher, the best course is to see the child right away. He or she cannot verbalize associated pain or problems.

Table 42-5 summarizes some important questions for telephone screening of an older child who can communicate his or her symptoms. It is important to focus on the *onset* (when symptoms first started), *frequency* (are symptoms constant, or do they cycle through recurrences), and *duration* (how long the episodes last) of the problem, in addition to attempted treatments and their effectiveness. As with any other patient, all telephone communication should be documented to record the reason for the call; the information gathered; the action taken, including whether the physician was consulted; any orders given; and whether and when an appointment was scheduled.

TABLE 42-5	Important Questions for Telephone Screening of Pediatric Problems
COMPLAINT	**SCREENING QUESTIONS**
Pain	• What are the onset, frequency, and duration of the pain? • On a scale of 1 to 10, how severe is the pain? • Where is the exact location? • Was any accident involved? (include details) • Has the pain gotten worse over time? • Has the pain interfered with sleep? • Is there associated fever, vomiting, diarrhea, or rash?
Gastrointestinal	• What are the onset, duration, and frequency of the symptoms? Has the child been vomiting longer than 24 hr without improvement? • Is the child receiving clear liquids only? • Is the child dehydrated (e.g., dry mouth, no urination in 8-10 hr, listless)? • If the child has diarrhea, have there been more than five or six watery stools in 12 hr? • Does the child have other symptoms (e.g., vomiting, fever of 103°F [39.4°C], rapid breathing)?
Respiratory	• What are the onset, duration, and frequency of the symptoms? • How would you describe the child's breathing? • Has the child been diagnosed with a breathing disorder? • Is a prescribed treatment being used? • Are any other signs or symptoms present (e.g., severe headache, stiff neck, fever, cough)? • If the child is coughing, what does it sound like? • Are there signs of a sore throat or earache?

THE MEDICAL ASSISTANT'S ROLE IN PEDIATRIC PROCEDURES

The medical assistant is responsible for assisting the pediatrician with examinations; upgrading patient histories; performing ordered screening tests, such as vision, hearing, urinalysis, and hemoglobin checks; administering immunizations; measuring and weighing children as needed; and providing patient and caregiver support. A medical assistant must develop a relationship with the pediatric patient that encourages cooperation and compliance with tests and treatment plans. If the child becomes upset, everything that needs to be done during that visit will be done under duress, and the chance for future mistrust intensifies.

Interacting with children requires special techniques, depending on the child's age. A calm, unhurried manner is essential to gaining cooperation. The tone of voice should be gentle but confident. Using a firm, direct approach about expected behavior is important in gaining the cooperation of older children. Offer reasonable choices when possible, such as, "Would you like your shot in your left or right leg?" not, "Are you ready for your shot now?" Offering sincere praise for the child during the examination or procedures helps ease anxiety and builds self-esteem. If the child is having an unusually difficult time, try to discover the reason. If he or she has had a bad medical experience in the past, the child may be afraid of what might happen. Each step should be explained in a language the child (and parent) can understand. Children younger than age 2 feel better when the parent holds them or remains very close (Figure 42-8). Preschool children enjoy playing, so making a game out of the situation is helpful (Figure 42-9). Whatever the child's age, the medical assistant should be sensitive to his or her individual needs and should adapt the examination and procedures as much as possible to meet those needs.

The sequence of the physician's examination varies and frequently is adapted based on the child's cooperation. The pediatrician probably will leave procedures and tests that are likely to cause the most objections until the end of the appointment. The physician is constantly evaluating the child's growth and development. A child's alertness and responses tell the physician a considerable amount.

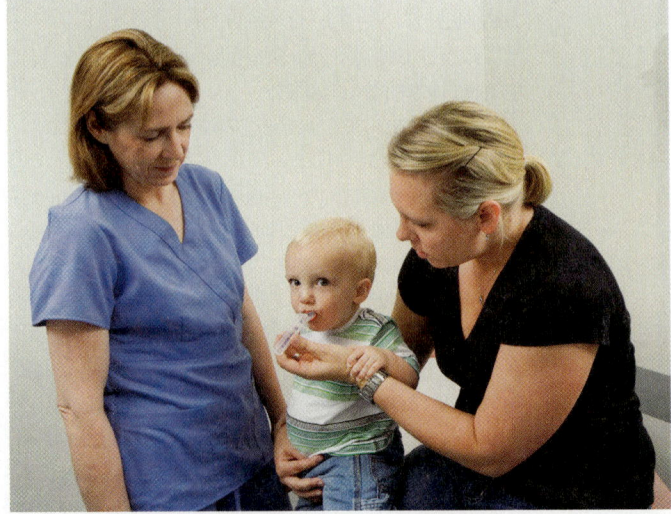

FIGURE 42-8 Sometimes a pediatric patient is more comfortable when held by a parent.

With infants and young children of preschool age, the parent is closely questioned about the child's eating, sleeping, and elimination habits. A school-aged child usually is a little more cooperative during an examination and can answer most questions without parental assistance. Adolescent patients should be given the option of not having parents present during an examination. This may permit teenagers to respond more honestly about lifestyle factors and also protects their privacy.

Measurement

Examination of the child during routine well-child care includes measurement of the circumference of the infant's head to determine normal growth and development (Procedure 42-2). The size of the child's head reflects the growth of the brain. Brain growth is 50% complete by 1 year of age, 75% by age 3, and 90% by age 6. Routine head measurement is recommended in children until 36 months of age and in older children whose head size is not within norms. If the circumference of the head deviates greatly from normal measurements, **hydrocephaly** or **microcephaly** may be suspected. It is important to discover any congenital problem as early as possible so that appropriate treatment can be started.

The medical assistant should record the child's length or height, weight, and head circumference on growth charts so that the physician can compare the child's measurement statistics with national standards (Procedure 42-3). Growth charts consist of a series of percentile curves that illustrate the distribution of selected body measurements.

The current version of the CDC's growth records consists of 16 charts (eight for boys and eight for girls) (Figures 42-10 and 41-11).

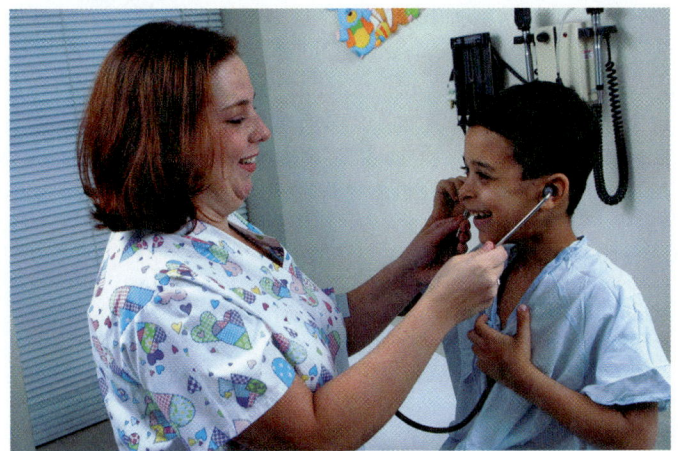

FIGURE 42-9 Making a game out of a procedure.

PROCEDURE 42-2

Maintain Growth Charts: Measure the Circumference of an Infant's Head

GOAL: To obtain an accurate measurement of the circumference of an infant's head and plot the result on the patient's growth chart.

EQUIPMENT and SUPPLIES

- Flexible disposable tape measure
- Age- and gender-specific growth chart
- Pen
- Patient's record with appropriate growth chart

PROCEDURAL STEPS

1. Sanitize your hands.
   PURPOSE: To ensure infection control.
2. Identify the patient. If he or she is old enough, gain the child's cooperation through conversation.
   PURPOSE: To alleviate anxiety and gain the child's trust.
3. Place an infant in the supine position, or the infant may be held by the parent. An older child may sit on the examination table.
4. Hold the tape measure with the zero mark against the infant's forehead, slightly above the eyebrows and the top of the ears. Ask the parent for assistance if necessary.
5. Bring the tape measure around the head, just above the ears, until it meets (Figure 1).
6. Read to the nearest 0.01 cm or ¼ inch.
7. Record the measurement on the growth chart and in the patient's medical record.
   PURPOSE: A procedure is not done until it is recorded.
8. Dispose of the tape measure.
9. Sanitize your hands.
   PURPOSE: To ensure infection control.

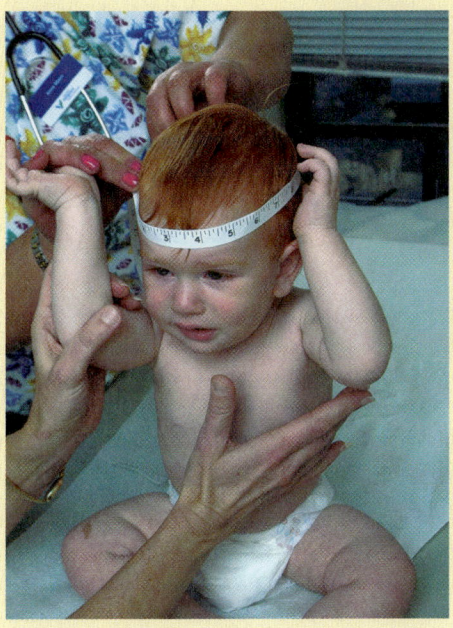

PROCEDURE 42-3

Maintaining Growth Charts: Measuring an Infant's Length and Weight

GOAL: *To measure an infant's length and weight accurately so that growth patterns can be monitored and recorded.*

EQUIPMENT and SUPPLIES

- Infant scale with paper cover
- Flexible measuring tape
- Examination table paper
- Pen
- Pediatric length board if available
- Gender-specific infant growth chart
- Biohazard waste container
- Patient's record

PROCEDURAL STEPS

Measuring an Infant's Length

1. Sanitize your hands, assemble the necessary equipment, and explain the procedure to the infant's caregiver.
2. Undress the infant. The diaper may be left on while the length is measured, but it must be removed before the infant is weighed.
3. Ask the caregiver to place the infant on his or her back on the examination table, which is covered with paper. If the table is a pediatric table with a headboard, ask the caregiver to hold the infant's head gently against the headboard while you straighten the infant's leg and note the location of the heel on the measurement area. If there is no headboard, ask the caregiver to gently hold the infant's head still while you draw a line on the paper at the back of the baby's head and at the heel after the leg is extended (Figure 1).

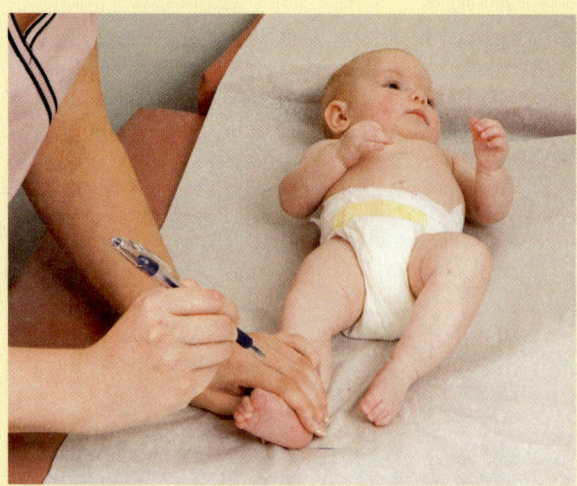

4. Measure the infant's length with the tape measure and record it.
5. Document the results in either inches or centimeters, depending on office policy, on the infant's growth chart, in the progress notes, and in the caregiver's record if requested. Complete the growth chart graph by connecting the dot from the last visit.

Weighing an Infant

1. Sanitize your hands, assemble the necessary equipment, and explain the procedure to the infant's caregiver.
2. Prepare the scale by sliding weights to the left; line the scale with disposable paper to reduce the risk of pathogen transmission.
3. Completely undress the infant, including removing the diaper.
4. Place the infant gently on the center of the scale, keeping your hand directly above the infant's trunk for safety (Figure 2).

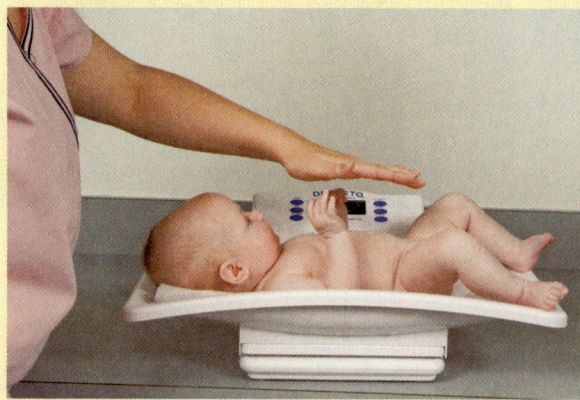

5. Slide the weights across the scale until balance is achieved. Attempt to read the infant's weight while he or she is still.
6. Return the weights to the far left of the scale and remove the baby. The caregiver can rediaper the baby while you discard the paper lining the scale. If the scale became contaminated during the procedure, follow Occupational Safety and Health Administration (OSHA) guidelines for use of gloves and disposal of contaminated waste. Disinfect the equipment according to the manufacturer's guidelines.
7. Sanitize your hands.
8. Document the results in either pounds or kilograms, depending on office policy, on the infant's growth chart, in the progress notes, and in the caregiver's record if requested. Complete the growth chart graph by connecting the dot from the last visit.

8/24/XX 10:20 AM Wt 17 lb 4 oz Length 27 in. S. Kwong, CMA (AAMA) _____

Birth to 36 months: Boys
Length-for-age and Weight-for-age percentiles

NAME ______________________

RECORD # ____________

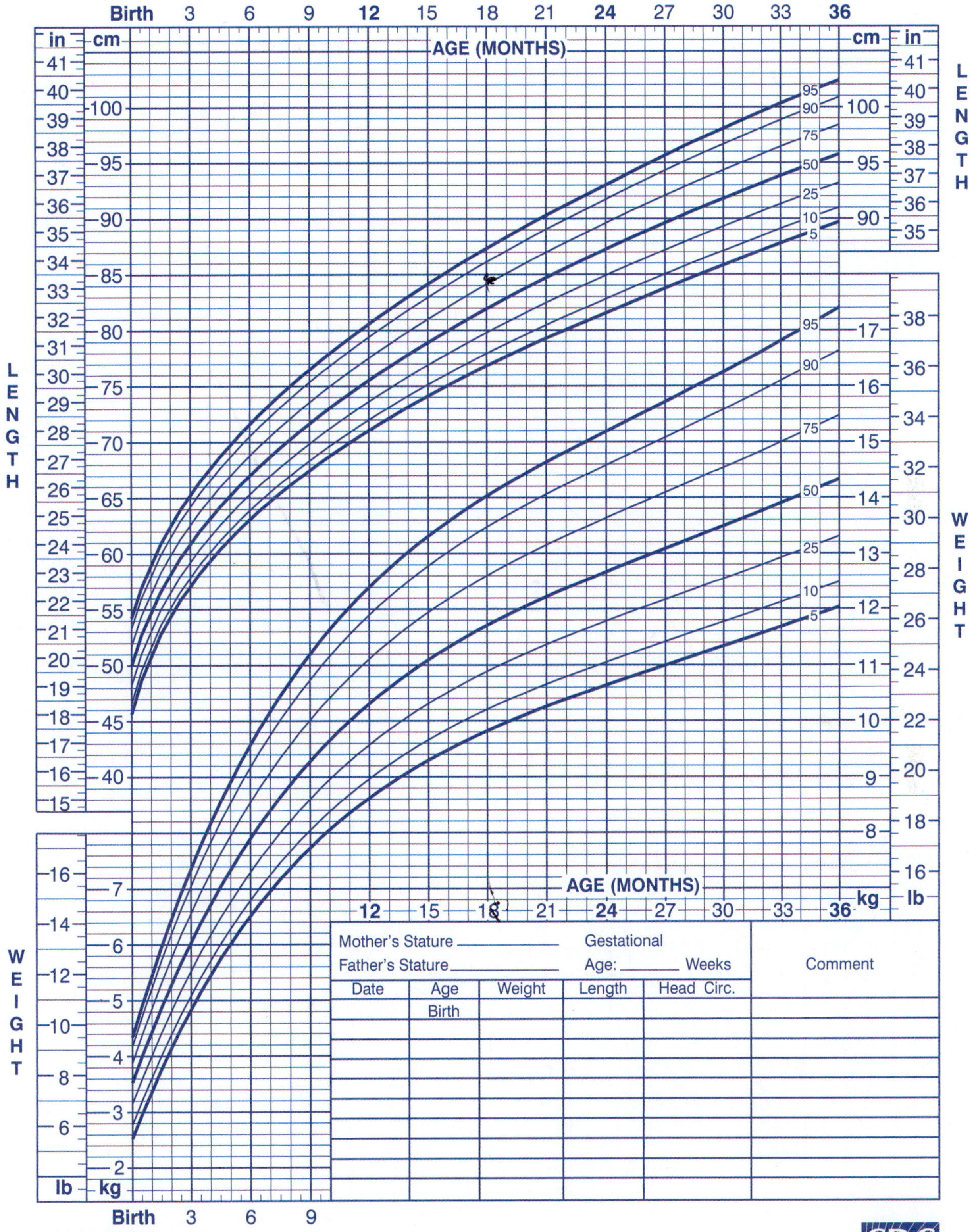

AGE (MONTHS)
Birth 3 6 9 12 15 18 21 24 27 30 33 36
in
cm
LENGTH
WEIGHT
95
90
75
50
25
10
5
kg
lb
Mother's Stature
Father's Stature
Gestational Age: Weeks
Date
Age
Weight
Length
Head Circ.
Birth
Comment

Published May 30, 2000 (modified 4/20/01).
SOURCE: Developed by the National Center for Health Statistics in collaboration with the National Center for Chronic Disease Prevention and Health Promotion (2000).
http://www.cdc.gov/growthcharts

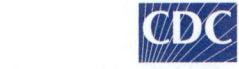

CDC
SAFER•HEALTHIER•PEOPLE™

FIGURE 42-10 Growth chart: males (birth to 36 months).

2 to 20 years: Girls
Stature-for-age and Weight-for-age percentiles

NAME _____

RECORD # _____

Mother's Stature _____ Father's Stature _____

Date	Age	Weight	Stature	BMI*

*To Calculate BMI: Weight (kg) ÷ Stature (cm) ÷ Stature (cm) x 10,000
or Weight (lb) ÷ Stature (in) ÷ Stature (in) x 703

AGE (YEARS)

STATURE

WEIGHT

Published May 30, 2000 (modified 11/21/00).
SOURCE: Developed by the National Center for Health Statistics in collaboration with
the National Center for Chronic Disease Prevention and Health Promotion (2000).
http://www.cdc.gov/growthcharts

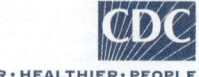

SAFER · HEALTHIER · PEOPLE™

FIGURE 42-11 Growth chart: females (2 to 20 years).

These charts represent revisions of the 14 previous charts and also the introduction of BMI-for-age charts for boys and for girls ages 2 to 20 years. As mentioned previously, the BMI is the recommended method of determining whether children or adults are overweight or obese. The BMI growth charts can be used beginning at 2 years of age, when height can be measured accurately.

Assisting with the Examination

The pediatrician will have a designated set of procedures that the medical assistant completes before the physician sees the child (Procedure 42-4). Vital signs are measured first (Table 42-6). Depending on the child's age and level of cooperation, the temperature may be obtained by the axillary, oral, rectal, tympanic, or temporal method. The rectal and temporal methods are considered most accurate in infants; however, the temporal method is easiest, quickest, and less invasive. It is important to remember that the younger the child, the more immature the ability to regulate body heat. Therefore the temperature of an infant may fluctuate easily and rapidly. The child's pulse rate is affected similar to that of an adult; it can increase as a result of activity, anxiety, illness, and environmental temperature. If the child is younger than age 2, the pulse is measured apically by placing the stethoscope on the left side of the chest medial to the nipple. Always count the beats for 1 full minute for accuracy.

An alternative method of obtaining the pulse of a very young child is to use the brachial artery in the upper arm. After age 2, the child's pulse may be taken at the radial pulse site. Anticipate a pulse rate higher than that of an adult; the younger the child, the faster the pulse. The respiratory rate is easily obtained in a child, because the chest can be readily observed. Expect the rate to be increased according to the child's age (the younger the child, the faster the normal respiratory rate) and health. The ratio of four pulse beats to one respiration should remain constant in a healthy child.

Blood pressure measurements are not included in most pediatric examinations. However, if the child has a heart or kidney **anomaly**, a blood pressure reading may be ordered. The cuff must be the appropriate width to obtain an accurate reading, and the bell of the stethoscope must be small enough to seal over the site. It is best to use a pediatric stethoscope with a pediatric bell when obtaining an infant's pressure. Blood pressure readings in a young child are lower than those in an adult.

To prevent a small child or infant from rolling the head from side to side during the physician's examination, stand at the head of the table and support the child's head between your hands, taking care not to press on the ears or on the anterior or posterior **fontanelles**. An infant need not be draped, but privacy is important to an older child. Sincere respect and friendly conversation at the child's level

---

PROCEDURE 42-4

Assisting the Physician with Patient Care: Obtain Pediatric Vital Signs and Perform Vision Screening

GOAL: *To accurately obtain vital signs and assess the vision of a pediatric patient.*

EQUIPMENT and SUPPLIES

- Digital, tympanic, or temporal thermometer
- Pediatric blood pressure cuff
- Wristwatch with sweep second hand
- Weight scale with height bar
- Stethoscope
- Snellen E eye chart and oculator
- Pen
- Patient's record

PROCEDURAL STEPS

1. Gather the necessary equipment.
2. Sanitize your hands.
   PURPOSE: To ensure infection control.
3. Explain the procedure to the parent, and if you want the parent to help by holding the child, explain how you want him or her to do that.
   PURPOSE: Explanations ahead of time save time and improve cooperation.
4. Help the child stand in the center of the scale, then weigh the child. Ask the child to turn around, then measure the child's height. Record your findings (see Chapter 31).
5. Obtain the tympanic, temporal, or axillary temperature using the procedure explained in Chapter 31 (Figure 1).

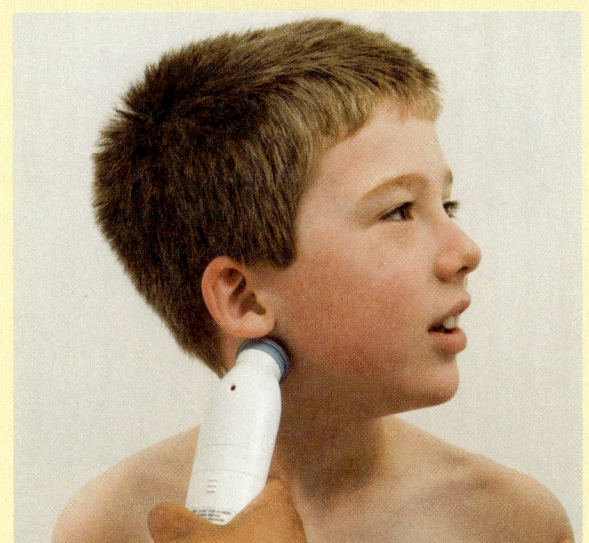

6. Record the temperature and indicate the method used.
   PURPOSE: A procedure is not done until it is recorded in the patient's record.
7. Place the stethoscope on the child's chest at the midpoint between the sternum and the left nipple. Listen for the apical beat (Figure 2).

PROCEDURE 42-4—cont'd

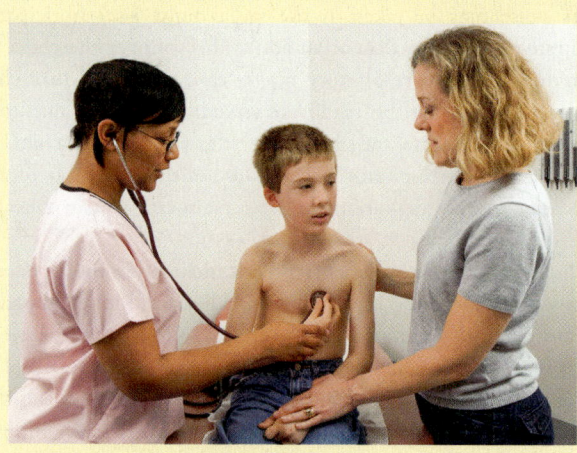

8. Count the apical beat for 1 full minute.
9. Record the apical pulse. Be sure to place "Ap" before the rate to indicate that this is an apical pulse reading.
   PURPOSE: A procedure is not done until it is recorded in the patient's record.
10. Observe the child's chest or place your palm on the child's chest and count the respirations for 1 full minute.
11. Record the respiratory rate.
    PURPOSE: A procedure is not done until it is recorded in the patient's record.
12. Check to make sure you have the correct-sized blood pressure cuff and then take the child's blood pressure (see the procedure in Chapter 31) (Figure 3).

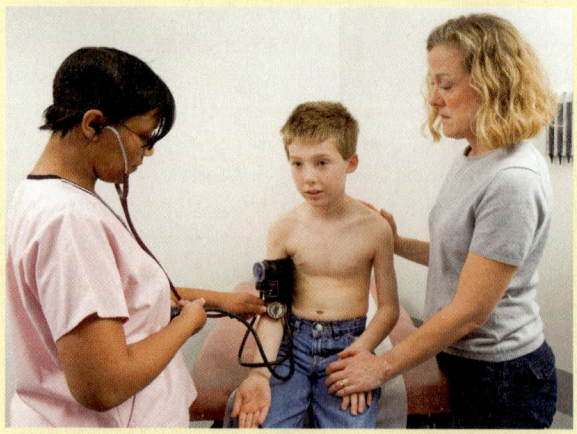

13. Record the blood pressure.
    PURPOSE: A procedure is not done until it is recorded in the patient's record.
14. If vision screening is to be done, familiarize the child with the E chart by asking him or her to make an E that points the same way your E is pointing. Then position the child in front of the pediatric Snellen E chart (Figure 4) and have the child match the E sign (using the fingers) with the E on the chart to which that you are pointing.

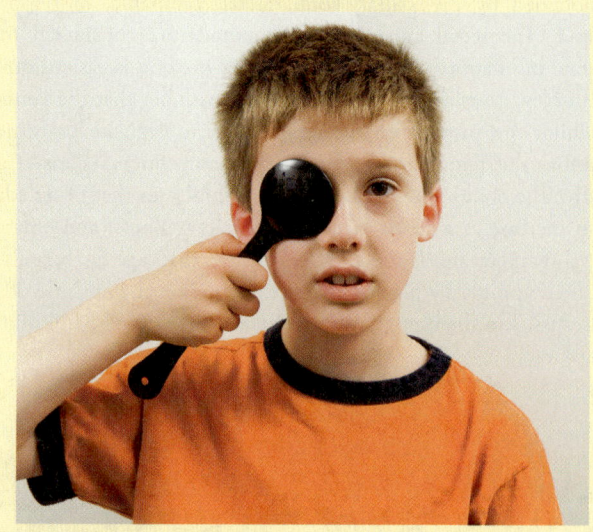

15. Record the vision results.
    PURPOSE: A procedure is not done until it is recorded in the patient's record.
16. Compliment the child on his or her performance, and if the parent is present, share the praise with the parent.
    PURPOSE: To build rapport and encourage self-confidence in the child.
17. Sanitize your hands.
    PURPOSE: To ensure infection control.
18. Perform appropriate disinfection and return all equipment to the proper storage area.

accomplishes a great deal. Always be patient with children. Make sure they understand what is expected. Always involve the parents or caregivers as much as possible.

Accurately judging the level of pain a young patient is experiencing can be difficult. If the child is able to communicate, the Wong-Baker Faces Pain Scale could be used, which shows simple drawings of faces that express varying levels of pain on a 0 to 10 scale (Figure 42-12).

Obtaining a Urine Sample

The easiest way to obtain a urine sample from a child older than age 2 who is toilet trained is to give the parent the container and

TABLE 42-6 Reference Ranges for Pediatric Vital Signs

VITAL SIGN	REFERENCE RANGE
Temperature	
Oral	98.6° F (37° C)
Aural	100.4° F (38° C)
Axillary	97.6° F (36.4° C)
Pulse	
Newborn	100-180 beats per minute
3 mo–2 yr	80-150 beats per minute
2-10 yr	65-130 beats per minute
Respirations	
Newborn	30-50 breaths per minute
1-3 yr	25-30 breaths per minute
4-6 yr	23-25 breaths per minute
7+ yr	16-20 breaths per minute
Blood Pressure	
Newborn	Systolic 90 mm Hg; diastolic 70 mm Hg
1-5 yr	Systolic 100 mm Hg; diastolic 70 mm Hg
6-12 yr	Systolic 120 mm Hg; diastolic 84 mm Hg
13+ yr	Systolic, 100 mm Hg + age; diastolic, 30-40 mm Hg less

instructions ahead of time. Then, when the child appears at the office for the examination, the sample is available to be tested. If the sample is needed while the child is at the office, consult with the parent for the best method to use. If the child is younger than age 2, a pediatric urine collection device can be put on him or her to collect the sample (Figure 42-13 and Procedure 42-5). This device is placed as soon as the child is checked in to increase the chance of obtaining the needed sample before the child leaves. Once the device is in place, the child can be diapered to help hold it properly. Make sure the adhesive sticks tightly so that the specimen collects in the device when the child urinates.

In some cases the child may need to be catheterized to obtain the specimen. Pediatric catheterization kits contain all the supplies needed for this procedure. When preparing the kit for the pediatrician's use, always remember that this is a sterile procedure. The pediatrician usually asks the parent to help with the infant while the medical assistant labels and prepares the specimen for the laboratory.

INJURY PREVENTION

Unintentional injuries are the leading cause of death and disability in children in the United States. Injuries cause more childhood deaths than all diseases combined. The primary causes of childhood injuries are motor vehicle accidents, drowning, burns, falls, poisoning, aspiration with airway obstruction, and firearm accidents. Childhood injuries are linked to the child's growth and development level and usually are preventable. Young children are totally dependent on caregivers to keep them safe, so constant supervision and a childproof environment are essential for this age group. Older children need to be aware of health hazards and should be encouraged to protect themselves from injury (e.g., use bike helmets, protective padding when skateboarding, seat belts, and so on). The highest incidence of accidental injuries is seen in children under age 9, but as children grow older, the percentage of deaths from injuries increases. Healthcare workers play a major role in injury prevention. The medical assistant is responsible for making sure the ambulatory care environment is safe and parents are educated about potential hazards.

CRITICAL THINKING APPLICATION 42-7

The office manager asks Susie to check the entire office for potential child safety problems. After inspecting the facility, Susie is concerned about some safety issues, so she decides to create a checklist for future use. What precautions or safety features should she include?

THE ADOLESCENT PATIENT

The adolescent patient may present the greatest challenge to health education and disease management. Adolescence begins with the onset of puberty, a time when the child's reproductive system matures, and is marked by rapid changes in the endocrine and musculoskeletal systems. The adolescent undergoes rapid growth spurts and the development of secondary sexual characteristics.

Health examinations for patients in this age group should include screening for height and weight; gathering details about diet and exercise routines; screening for sexually transmitted infections (STIs) and for sexually active female adolescents, a Pap test, especially to screen for infection with HPV; reviewing the vaccination history and administration of boosters as indicated; and assessing for high-risk behaviors, such as substance abuse and sexual behavior.

Some health problems most frequently seen in adolescent patients include eating disorders (anorexia nervosa and bulimia nervosa), obesity, and injury-related problems. Accidents are the leading cause of death and injury in adolescence, and suicide is the third leading cause of death. All healthcare personnel should be on the alert for indicators of suicide, including:

- Signs of depression, such as headaches, abdominal discomfort, anorexia, fatigue, aggressiveness, drug or alcohol abuse, and sexual promiscuity
- Verbal statements that hint at the adolescent's intention to commit suicide; talking about dying
- Actions such as giving away prized objects, withdrawing from social groups, sudden changes in normal behavior patterns, or writing a suicide note

CHILD ABUSE

The Child Abuse Prevention and Treatment Act states that all threats to a child's physical and/or mental welfare must be reported. This

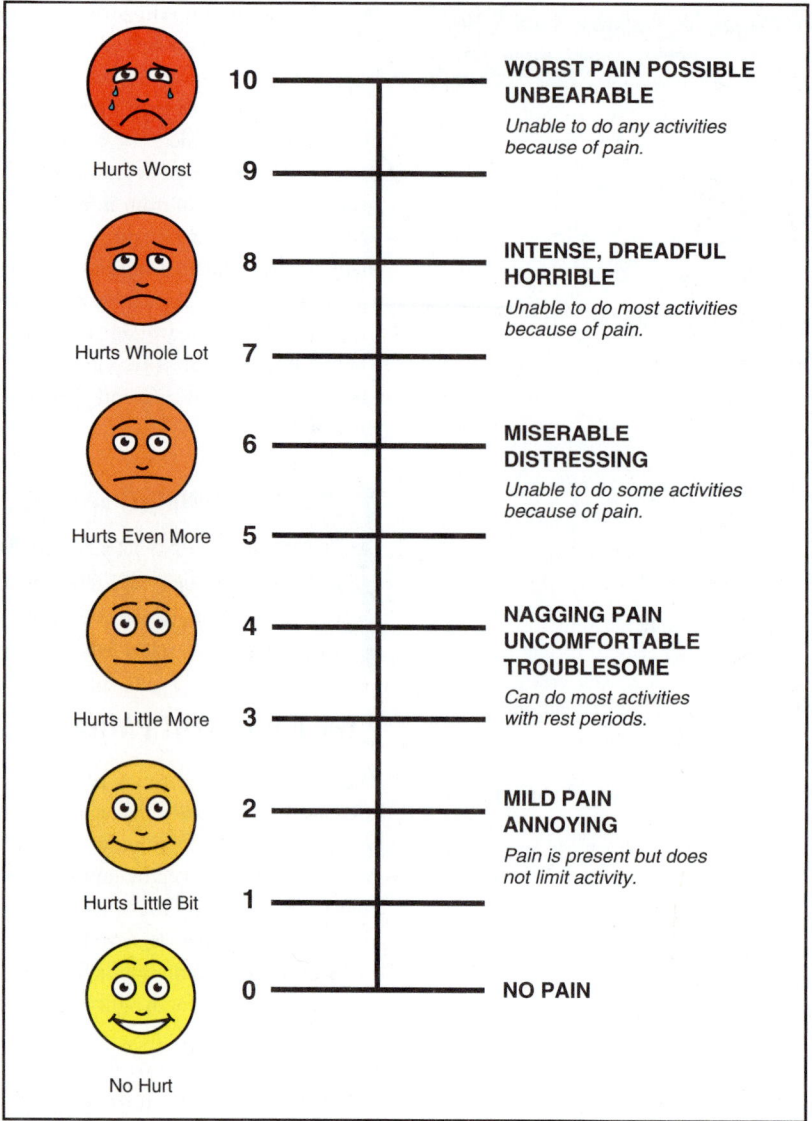

FIGURE 42-12 Wong-Baker Faces Pain Scale for children age 3 to 7 years. (From Hockenberry MJ, Wilson D: *Wong's essentials of pediatric nursing*, ed 8, St Louis, 2009, Mosby.)

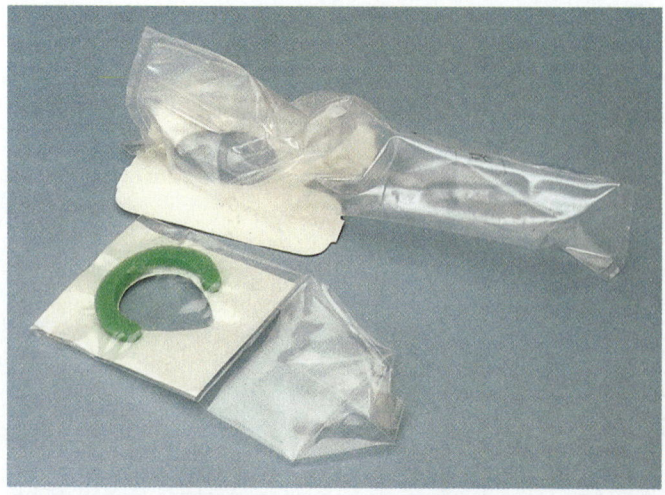

FIGURE 42-13 Urine collection devices.

means that every teacher, healthcare worker, and social worker—in fact, every citizen—who suspects that a child is being neglected or abused must report this to the proper authority. The agency must record the report, and after three similar reports, the agency must investigate.

When suspected abuse is reported, the individual must provide his or her name; however, this is considered confidential information and is not given to the child's parent or guardian, nor is it given to the investigating officer. The individual making the report also is protected under the law from any liability for reporting suspicions of child abuse.

If the medical assistant suspects that a child is a victim of abuse, he or she should consult with the pediatrician immediately. In most states, the medical assistant and the physician can make separate reports to the authorities. However, state laws vary, so state and local reporting protocols should be outlined in the office procedures manual.

<table>
<tr><td>

SIGNS OF CHILD ABUSE

Obvious Signs

- Previously filed reports of physical or sexual abuse of the child
- Documented abuse of other family members
- Different stories between parents and child on how an accident happened
- Stories of incidents and injuries that are suspicious
- Injuries blamed on other family members
- Repeated visits to the emergency department for injuries

Examination Findings

- Trauma to the nervous system
- Internal abdominal pain
- Discolorations/bruising on the buttocks, back, and abdomen
- Elbow, wrist, and shoulder dislocations

Changes in Behavior

- Too eager to please the parent
- Overly passive and too compliant
- Aggressive and demanding
- Parenting the parent (role reversal)
- Delays in the normal growth and development patterns
- Erratic school attendance

Physical Indicators

- Poor hygiene
- Malnutrition
- Obvious dental neglect
- Neglected well-baby procedures (e.g., immunizations)

</td></tr>
</table>

CLOSING COMMENTS

Patient Education

In a pediatric practice, the child usually is joined by one or both parents during visits to the physician. Parents need reinforcement, praise, and understanding in dealing with the health and welfare of their child. Provide parents with information to help them understand their children's behavior and improve their parenting skills. Understanding the normal behavioral characteristics of a particular developmental stage may increase the parents' confidence and reinforce expectations for the child.

The waiting room is an ideal place for parent education. Use the space and resources available to provide up-to-date information on child health issues and on local resources for support and assistance. If the pediatrician has pamphlets available, discuss them with the parents. Answer questions when possible, or alert the physician so that questions can be answered during the office visit. Every opportunity should be taken to teach parents about sound healthcare. Because so many ambulatory care visits involve infectious disorders, educating children and parents on the following infection control measures may help reduce the spread of disease:

- Children should cover their mouth with a disposable tissue when they cough and should blow the nose with disposable tissues.
- A tissue should be used only once and then immediately thrown away.
- Children should not be allowed to share toys they have put in their mouth.
- After a child has discarded a toy that was in the mouth, it should be placed in a bin for dirty toys that is out of reach of

---

PROCEDURE 42-5

Assisting the Physician with Patient Care: Applying a Urinary Collection Device

GOAL: *To apply a pediatric urinary collection device properly.*

EQUIPMENT and SUPPLIES

- Pediatric urine collection bag
- Labeled laboratory urinary container
- Laboratory test request form
- Antiseptic wipes
- Biohazard waste container
- Disposable examination gloves
- Patient's record

PROCEDURAL STEPS

1. Assemble all needed supplies.
   PURPOSE: To manage time efficiently.
2. Sanitize your hands and put on gloves.
   PURPOSE: To ensure infection control.
3. Ask the parent to remove the child's diaper or place the child in a supine position on the examination table and remove the diaper.

4. Cleanse the genitalia with antiseptic wipes.
   Male: Cleanse the urinary meatus in a circular motion, starting directly on the meatus and working in an outward pattern. Repeat with a clean wipe. If the child has not been circumcised, gently retract the foreskin to expose the meatus; when you have completed the cleansing, return the foreskin to its natural position. *Female:* Hold the labia open with your nondominant hand; with your dominant hand, cleanse the inner labia, from the clitoris to the vaginal meatus, in a superior to inferior pattern. Discard the first wipe and repeat with a clean wipe, cleaning both sides of the inner labia.
   PURPOSE: To prevent contamination of the urine specimen with surface pathogens.
5. Make sure the area is dry. Unfold the collection device, remove the paper from the upper portion, place this portion over the mons pubis, and press it securely into place. Continue by removing the lower portion of the paper and securing this portion against the perineum. Make sure

PROCEDURE 42-5—cont'd

the device is attached smoothly and that you have not taped it to part of the infant's thigh.

6. Rediaper the infant or, if the parent is helping, have the parent rediaper the infant at this time. The diaper will help hold the bag in place.

7. Suggest that the parent give the child liquids, if allowed; check the bag for urine at frequent intervals.
   PURPOSE: Increasing intake helps increase output.

8. When a noticeable amount of urine has collected in the bag, put on gloves, remove the device, cleanse the skin area where the device was attached, and rediaper the child.

9. Pour the urine carefully into the laboratory urine container and handle the sample in a routine manner.

10. Dispose of all used equipment in a biohazard waste container.

11. Remove your gloves, dispose of them in a biohazard container, and sanitize your hands.

12. Record the procedure in the patient's record.
    PURPOSE: A procedure is not done until it is recorded.

8/24/XX 10:45 AM Urine specimen collected for culture as ordered. Placed for pick up by North Hills Laboratory. S. Kwong, CMA (AAMA)

---

others. Wash and disinfect these toys before allowing children to play with them again.

- Make sure all children and adults follow good hand-washing practices.

Legal and Ethical Issues

In the United States, children are considered persons who are growing and developing physically, emotionally, and mentally. Our laws view children as a distinct group, and laws and customs have been established that deal with the protection of children's rights. Occasionally in the pediatric office, legal and ethical issues arise, and the entire office staff may be faced with an ethical situation. If this type of situation occurs, the first option is to talk it over with the pediatrician. It may be necessary to have an office staff meeting to identify the conflict, note pertinent laws and facts, consider possible options and the consequences of each, and decide on a course of action. Facing ethical issues confidently may reduce the risk of liability. If the pediatrician's feelings are different from yours, this might be a totally separate dilemma with which you will have to deal. Always remember that as your employer, the physician makes the final decision, and as long as you work in that office, you are required to do things according to that decision.

If something happens that you cannot ethically support, seek the help of your local medical assistant organization. You may find that others have been in similar situations and that they can suggest possible methods of solving the problem.

SUMMARY OF SCENARIO

After working with the telephone screening staff, Susie realizes the importance of becoming familiar with childhood diseases and disorders and the management policy of her physician-employers. Many times Susie has had to refer to the office disease manual to make sure she is asking the right questions and gathering all the information needed for the physician who will make the daily response calls. From working in the clinical area, Susie also has realized that a pediatric practice actually has two groups of patients: the child and the caregivers. She must be sensitive to the needs of both groups and develop communication skills that build trust with the child and his or her parents. Susie is working on developing a comprehensive education site in the office for interested parents and is creating a community resource guide for interested caregivers. She recognizes the need to stay up-to-date on the CDC's recommendations for childhood immunizations and routinely refers to the CDC Web site to make sure the office has the most recently published VIS forms. Susie regularly attends her local American Association of Medical Assistants (AAMA) chapter meetings to maintain her certification and to continue to learn about the pediatric practice specialty.

SUMMARY OF LEARNING OBJECTIVES

1. **Define, spell, and pronounce the terms listed in the vocabulary.**
   Spelling and pronouncing medical terms correctly bolster the medical assistant's credibility. Knowing the definitions of these terms promotes confidence in communication with patients and co-workers.

2. **Apply critical thinking skills in performing the patient assessment and patient care.**

Completing the Critical Thinking Application exercises throughout the chapter can help the student medical assistant become more adept at critical analysis of real-life situations.

3. **Describe childhood growth patterns.**
   By 6 months of age, the child's birth weight has doubled; at 1 year it has tripled, and the child's length has increased by 50%. By age 2 the

child has reached approximately 50% of adult height. This same growth rate continues through the school-aged period, 6 to 12 years, which leads into a growth spurt that indicates impending puberty. In adolescence, ages 12 to 18 years, the adolescent gains almost half of his or her adult weight and the skeleton and organs double in size.

4. **Summarize the important features of the Denver II Developmental Screening Test.**
   The Denver II Developmental Screening Test is a standardized tool used for children between 1 month and 6 years of age to screen healthy infants for developmental delays, to validate concerns about an infant's development, or to monitor high-risk children for potential problems.

5. **Identify four different growth and development theories.**
   Table 42-1 summarizes Freud's psychosexual, Piaget's cognitive, Erikson's psychosocial, and Kohlberg's moral reasoning theories.

6. **Explain common pediatric gastrointestinal disorders and their signs, symptoms, and treatment.**
   Pediatric gastrointestinal disorders include infant colic; diarrhea, which can be caused by a variety of different microorganisms and is treated medically when it continues for longer than 2 days; failure to thrive caused by a physiologic factor (e.g., malabsorption disease or cleft palate) or a nonorganic cause that is associated with the parent-child relationship; and obesity if the child's BMI is equal to or greater than the 95th percentile.

7. **Classify disorders of the respiratory system in children.**
   The common cold may lead to secondary bacterial infections, including strep throat or otitis media; croup is a viral disorder that affects the larynx; bronchiolitis is a viral infection of the bronchioles that causes acute onset of wheezing and dyspnea; asthma causes bronchospasms and inflammation of the bronchioles; and influenza is an acute, highly contagious viral infection of the respiratory tract.

8. **Distinguish among pediatric infectious diseases.**
   Pediatric infectious diseases include conjunctivitis, caused by a bacterial or viral infection; tonsillitis, typically caused by beta-hemolytic streptococci; fifth disease, also called *erythema infectiosum,* a mild infection caused by parvovirus B19; hand-foot-and-mouth disease, caused by the coxsackievirus, which causes multiple symptoms, including painful blisters on the tongue, mouth, palms of the hands, and soles of the feet; chickenpox, caused by a member of the herpes virus group; meningitis, an inflammation of the membranes that cover the brain and spinal cord, caused by bacteria or viruses (bacterial meningitis is the more dangerous); HBV, which can lead to serious and chronic infection of the liver and can be transmitted across the placenta; and Reye's syndrome, which is linked with the use of aspirin during a viral illness.

9. **Recognize the etiologic factors and signs and symptoms of the two primary pediatric inherited disorders.**
   Pediatric inherited disorders include cystic fibrosis, an autosomal recessive genetic disorder that causes exocrine glands to produce abnormally thick secretions and primarily affects the lungs and pancreas; and Duchenne's muscular dystrophy, an X-linked genetic disease that causes progressive muscle degeneration and subsequent replacement of muscle fibers with fat and fibrous connective tissue.

10. **Summarize the immunizations recommended for children by the Centers for Disease Control and Prevention (CDC).**
    The CDC's recommendations for childhood immunization are summarized in Table 42-3.

11. **Demonstrate how to document immunizations and maintain accurate immunization records.**
    Procedure 42-1 summarizes how to document immunizations in both the official vaccination record and the parent's immunization booklet. Documentation of immunization administration on the VIS form must include the date the vaccine was administered, the vaccine's manufacturer, the manufacturer's lot number, the type of vaccine, the route of administration and exact site if an injection is given, any reported or observed side effects, the name and title of the person administering the vaccine, the address of the medical office where the vaccine was administered, and the date.

12. **Compare and contrast a well-child and a sick-child examination.**
    Well-child visits are typically scheduled from age 2 weeks through 15 years to focus on maintaining the child's health with physical examinations, immunizations, and upgrading of the child's medical history record. Sick-child visits occur whenever the child needs to be seen because of illness or injury. Table 42-5 summarizes important questions for telephone screening of pediatric problems.

13. **Outline the medical assistant's role in a pediatric examination.**
    The medical assistant assists the pediatrician with examinations; maintains patient histories; performs ordered screening tests, such as vision, hearing, urinalysis, and hemoglobin checks; administers immunizations; measures and weighs children as needed; documents accurately; and provides support to patients and caregivers.

14. **Measure the circumference of an infant's head.**
    Procedure 42-2 outlines the steps for measuring an infant's head.

15. **Obtain accurate length and weight measurements and plot pediatric growth patterns.**
    Procedure 42-3 outlines the steps for measuring an infant's length and weight.

16. **Accurately measure pediatric vital signs and perform vision screening.**
    Procedure 42-4 summarizes the steps for obtaining accurate pediatric vital signs and performing vision screening on a child. Tympanic thermometers are the easiest and quickest method for measuring temperature; the apical pulse should be taken for a full minute, respirations observed and recorded, and blood pressures taken with the appropriate-sized cuff when indicated. After patient education, the Snellen E chart is used to perform vision screening and to record results accurately.

17. **Correctly apply a pediatric urine collection device.**
    Procedure 42-5 summarizes the steps for applying a urinary collection device.

18. **Describe the characteristics and needs of the adolescent patient.**
    Adolescents are going through extreme physical and emotional changes, and an extra measure of patience and understanding is required to establish therapeutic interactions. Ensuring their privacy, giving them the option of being seen without the parents, and providing pertinent

education materials all are important factors in patient-centered adolescent care.

19. **Specify child safety guidelines for injury prevention and management of suspected child abuse.**
The medical assistant should be involved in parent education regarding injury prevention for children. Childhood injuries are linked to the child's growth and development level and therefore are often predictable and many times preventable.

20. **Summarize patient education guidelines for pediatric patients.**
Parents need reinforcement, praise, and understanding in dealing with the health and welfare of their child. Provide parents with information to help them understand their children's behavior and improve their parenting skills.

21. **Discuss the legal and ethical implications in a pediatric practice.**
Occasionally in the pediatric office, legal and ethical issues arise, and the entire office staff may be faced with an ethical situation. If this type of situation occurs, the first option is to talk it over with the pediatrician. It may be necessary to have an office staff meeting to identify the conflict, note pertinent laws and facts, consider possible options and the consequences of each, and decide on a course of action.

CONNECTIONS

Study Guide Connection: Go to the Chapter 42 Study Guide. Read and complete the activities.

Evolve Connection: Go to the Chapter 42 link at *evolve.elsevier.com/ kinn* to complete the Chapter Review and Chapter Quiz. Check out the other resources listed for this chapter to make the most of what you have learned from Assisting in Pediatrics.

ASSISTING IN ORTHOPEDIC MEDICINE

43

SCENARIO

Kaiwan Tillman became interested in orthopedics before he even knew what the word meant. In the sixth grade, he broke his right femur in a bicycle accident. He spent 2 months in traction in the hospital on an orthopedic floor. On graduation from high school, he attended the local community college and enrolled in a medical assisting program that offered an associate's degree. Since earning his CMA (AAMA), Kaiwan has worked in a sports medicine clinic. The clinic staff at Sport Medicine Associates includes three orthopedic surgeons, two physical therapists, and two massage therapists. Kaiwan is very excited about working in the clinic, although he initially was somewhat intimidated. Dr. Steve Alexander is the team physician for a local professional baseball team, and Kaiwan's responsibilities include assisting Dr. Alexander with treating the team.

While studying this chapter, think about the following questions:

- What are the primary responsibilities of the medical assistant in an orthopedic practice?
- What clinical skills are required in this specialty practice?
- What are the common musculoskeletal injuries and disorders that the medical assistant should understand?
- What diagnostic and treatment procedures typically are used in an orthopedic practice?

LEARNING OBJECTIVES

1. Define, spell, and pronounce the terms listed in the vocabulary.
2. Apply critical thinking skills in performing patient assessment and patient care.
3. Describe the principal anatomic structures of the musculoskeletal system and their functions.
4. Differentiate among tendons, bursae, and ligaments.
5. Summarize the major muscular disorders.
6. Identify and describe the common types of fractures.
7. Explain the difference between osteomalacia and osteoporosis.
8. Classify typical spinal column disorders.
9. Differentiate among the various joint disorders.
10. Summarize the medical assistant's role in assisting with orthopedic procedures.
11. Explain the common diagnostic procedures used in orthopedics.
12. Compare and contrast therapeutic modalities used in orthopedic medicine.
13. Apply cold therapy to an injury.
14. Assist with hot moist heat application to an orthopedic injury.
15. Properly apply therapeutic ultrasound.
16. Explain the use of common ambulatory devices.
17. Properly fit a patient with crutches and explain the correct mechanics of crutch walking.
18. Prepare for and assist with the application of a cast.
19. Prepare for and assist with the removal of a cast.
20. Summarize patient education guidelines for orthopedic patients.
21. Discuss the legal and ethical implications in an orthopedic practice.

VOCABULARY

arthritis Inflammation of a joint.

articular (ar-ti′-kyuh-luhr) Pertaining to a joint.

bursae (bur′-suh) Fluid-filled, saclike membranes that provide cushioning and allow frictionless motion between two tissues.

cartilage A rubbery, smooth, somewhat elastic connective tissue that covers the ends of bones.

cervical (ser′-vi-kuhl) Pertaining to the neck region containing seven cervical vertebrae.

corticosteroids Antiinflammatory hormones, natural or synthetic.

crepitation (kre-puh-ta′-shun) A dry, crackling sound or sensation.

diaphysis (di-a′-fuh-suhs) The midportion of a long bone; it contains the medullary cavity.

epiphysis (i-pi′-fuh-suhs) The end of a long bone; it contains the growth (epiphyseal) plates.

goniometer An instrument for measuring the degrees of motion in a joint.

inflammation A tissue reaction to trauma or disease that includes redness, heat, swelling, and pain.

kyphotic (kahy-fot′-ik) Relating to the normal convex curvature of the thoracic spine.

ligaments Tough connective tissue bands that hold joints together by attaching to the bones on either side of the joint.

lordotic (lor-do′-tik) Relating to the normal concave curvature of the cervical and lumbar spines.

lumbar Relating to the lower back region that contains the five lumbar vertebrae.

luxation Dislocation of a bone from its normal anatomic location.

malaise (muh-laz′) An indefinite feeling of debility or lack of health, often indicative of or accompanying the onset of an illness.

medullary cavity The inner portion of the diaphysis; it contains the bone marrow.

periosteum The thin, highly innervated, membranous covering of a bone.

prosthesis (prahs-the′-suhs) An artificial replacement for a body part.

range of motion (ROM) The extent of movement possible in a joint; the degree of motion depends on the type of joint and whether a disease process is present; ROM exercises are applied actively (independently) or passively (with assistance) to prevent or treat joint problems.

reduction The return to correct anatomic position, as in reduction of a fracture.

scoliosis An abnormal lateral curvature of the spine.

striated Muscle that contains fibers divided by bands of cross stripes or striations because of overlapping myofilaments.

synovial fluid A clear fluid found in joint cavities that facilitates smooth movements and nourishes joint structures.

tendons Tough bands of connective tissue that connect muscle to bone.

A physician who specializes in orthopedics diagnoses and treats diseases and disorders of the musculoskeletal system and deals primarily with the bones. Rheumatologists are specialists in treating inflammatory joint disorders. Chiropractors are doctors of chiropractic (DC) but are not medical physicians; they use manual adjusting procedures to correct subluxations or misalignments of the spine to allow maximum nerve function, thus facilitating the body's ability to maintain homeostasis and prevent disease.

The musculoskeletal system includes all of the skeletal muscles, bones, joints, and supportive connective tissues (**cartilage**, **tendons**, and **ligaments**). The general functions of the musculoskeletal system are:

- Protection of internal organs
- Support for standing erect
- Movement
- Hemopoietic function (production of blood cells in the red bone marrow)
- Storage of the minerals calcium and phosphorus in the bones

ANATOMY AND PHYSIOLOGY OF THE MUSCULOSKELETAL SYSTEM

Muscles

More than 600 muscles attach to the human skeleton (Figure 43-1). These muscles account for approximately half of a person's weight, and they contribute to the body's distinct shape. This chapter discusses the skeletal muscles that attach to bones and allow movement. Skeletal muscle fibers are voluntary and **striated** (Figure 43-2, *A*). The body has two other types of muscle: smooth muscle (Figure 43-2, *B*), which lines organs and blood vessel walls and is nonstriated, and cardiac muscle (Figure 43-2, *C*), a striated muscle in the heart. Both of these types are involuntary muscles; that is, the individual cannot control their function. Skeletal muscles are voluntary and can be controlled when they contract or relax. Special fibers in skeletal muscles allow them to shorten (contract) and lengthen (relax), which creates movement (Table 43-1). These muscles are connected to bone with bands of tough, fibrous connective tissues called *tendons*.

Bones

The human skeleton is composed of more than 200 bones (Figure 43-3). Bones provide a framework that protects vital organs. In general, the size and shape of a bone is related either to how much it moves and how much body weight it must carry or to its protective function for the underlying organs.

Bones generally are categorized by shape: long, short, flat, rounded, or irregular. A long bone is made up of a **diaphysis** (shaft) with an expansion at each end called an **epiphysis** (Figure 43-4). The epiphysis is covered with **articular** cartilage and is attached by ligaments to the epiphysis of another bone, forming a joint. Articular cartilage reduces the stress of weight bearing and

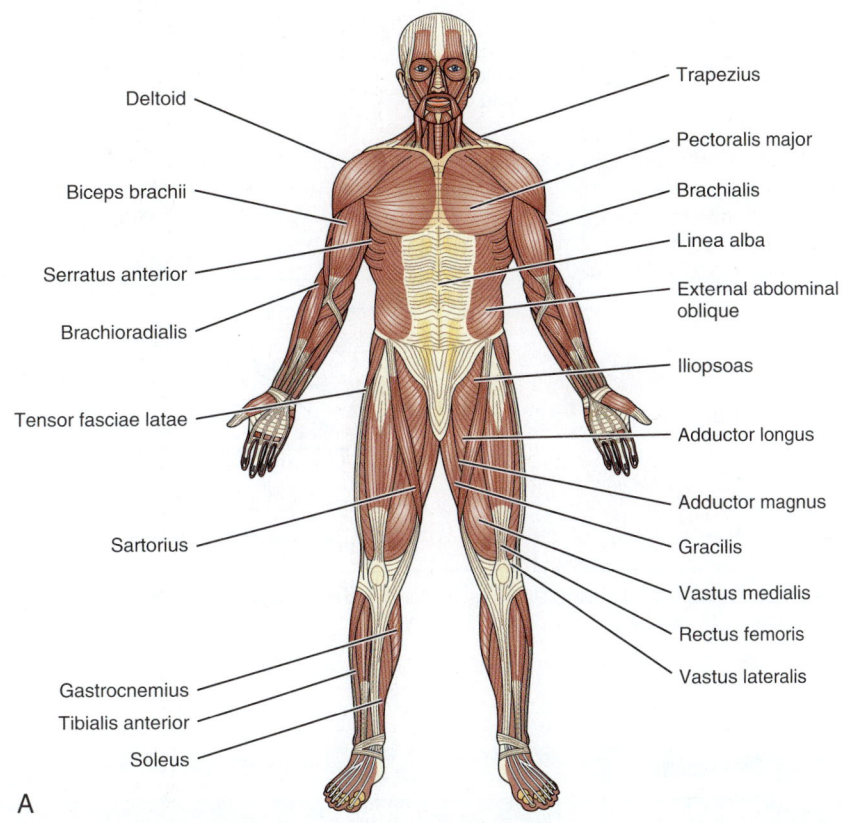

Deltoid

Biceps brachii

Serratus anterior

Brachioradialis

Tensor fasciae latae

Sartorius

Gastrocnemius
Tibialis anterior
Soleus

Trapezius

Pectoralis major

Brachialis

Linea alba

External abdominal oblique

Iliopsoas

Adductor longus

Adductor magnus

Gracilis

Vastus medialis

Rectus femoris

Vastus lateralis

A

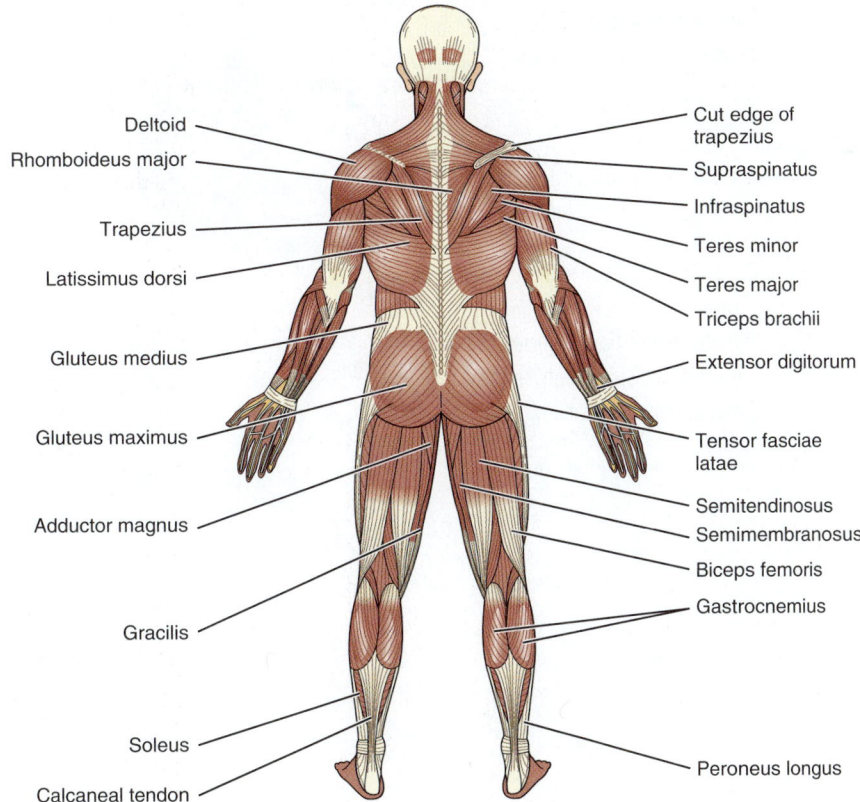

Deltoid

Rhomboideus major

Trapezius

Latissimus dorsi

Gluteus medius

Gluteus maximus

Adductor magnus

Gracilis

Soleus

Calcaneal tendon

Cut edge of trapezius

Supraspinatus

Infraspinatus

Teres minor

Teres major

Triceps brachii

Extensor digitorum

Tensor fasciae latae

Semitendinosus

Semimembranosus

Biceps femoris

Gastrocnemius

Peroneus longus

B

FIGURE 43-1 Muscles of the body. **A,** Anterior view. **B,** Posterior view. (From Chester GA: *Modern medical assisting,* Philadelphia, 1999, WB Saunders.)

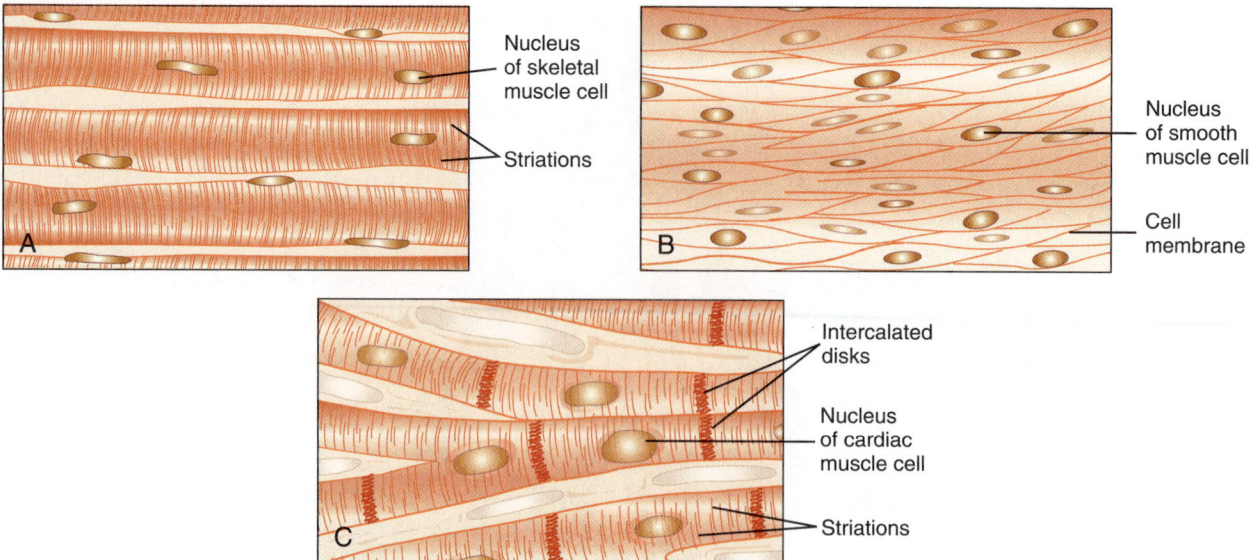

FIGURE 43-2 **A**, Skeletal muscle. **B**, Smooth muscle. **C**, Cardiac muscle. (From Applegate E: *The anatomy and physiology learning system*, ed 4, St Louis, 2011, Saunders.)

TABLE 43-1 **Types of Body Movement**

MOVEMENT	DEFINITION OR EXAMPLE	MOVEMENT	DEFINITION OR EXAMPLE
Flexion 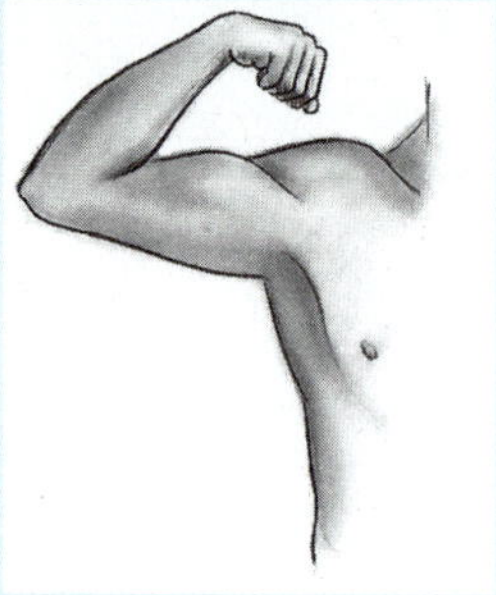	Reduces the angle of the joint and brings the two bones closer together.	Hyperextension 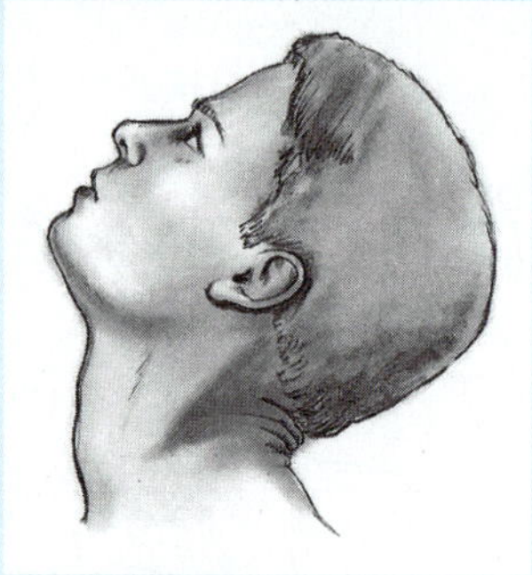	Extension 180 degrees (e.g., the neck is extended backward or the toes are pointed downward).
Extension 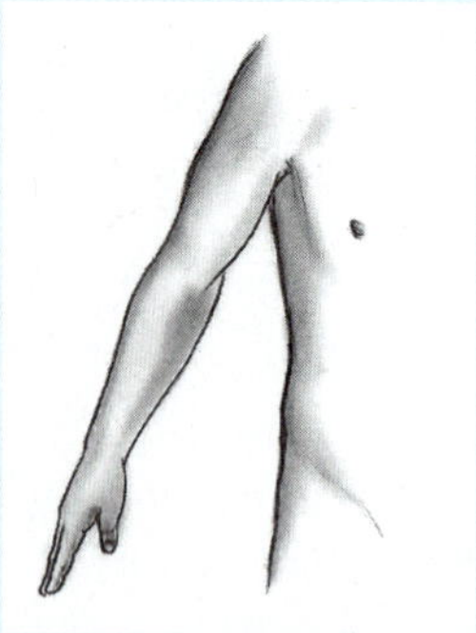	The opposite of flexion; increases the angle or distance between two bones or parts of the body.	Abduction 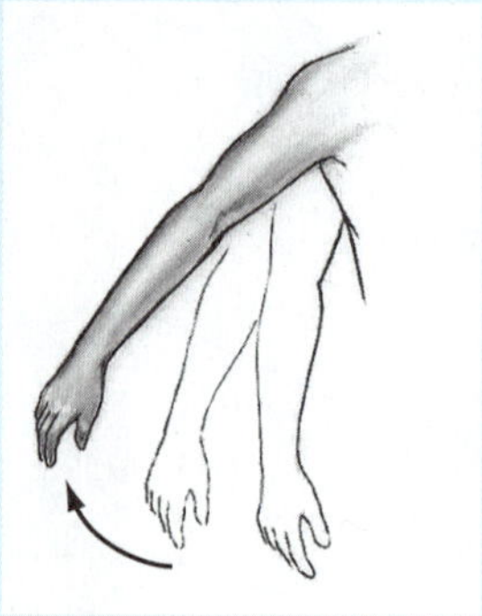	Moving the body part away from the midline or median plane of the body.

TABLE 43-1 Types of Body Movement—cont'd

MOVEMENT	DEFINITION OR EXAMPLE	MOVEMENT	DEFINITION OR EXAMPLE
Adduction	The opposite of abduction; moving the body part toward the midline of the body.	Plantar flexion	A toe-down movement of the foot at the ankle; increases the angle of the joint.
Rotation	Moving a bone around its central axis; common in ball-and-socket joints.	Eversion	Turning the sole of the foot laterally, or outward.
Circumduction	Circular movement of a limb; a combination of abduction, adduction, extension, and flexion.	Inversion	The opposite of eversion; turning the sole of the foot medially, or inward.
Dorsiflexion	Moving the instep of the foot up and dorsally, reducing the angle between the foot and the leg.	Pronation	Rotation of the forearm that turns the palm of the hand downward, or posteriorly.
		Supination	The opposite of pronation; rotation of the forearm that turns the palm of the hand upward, or anteriorly.

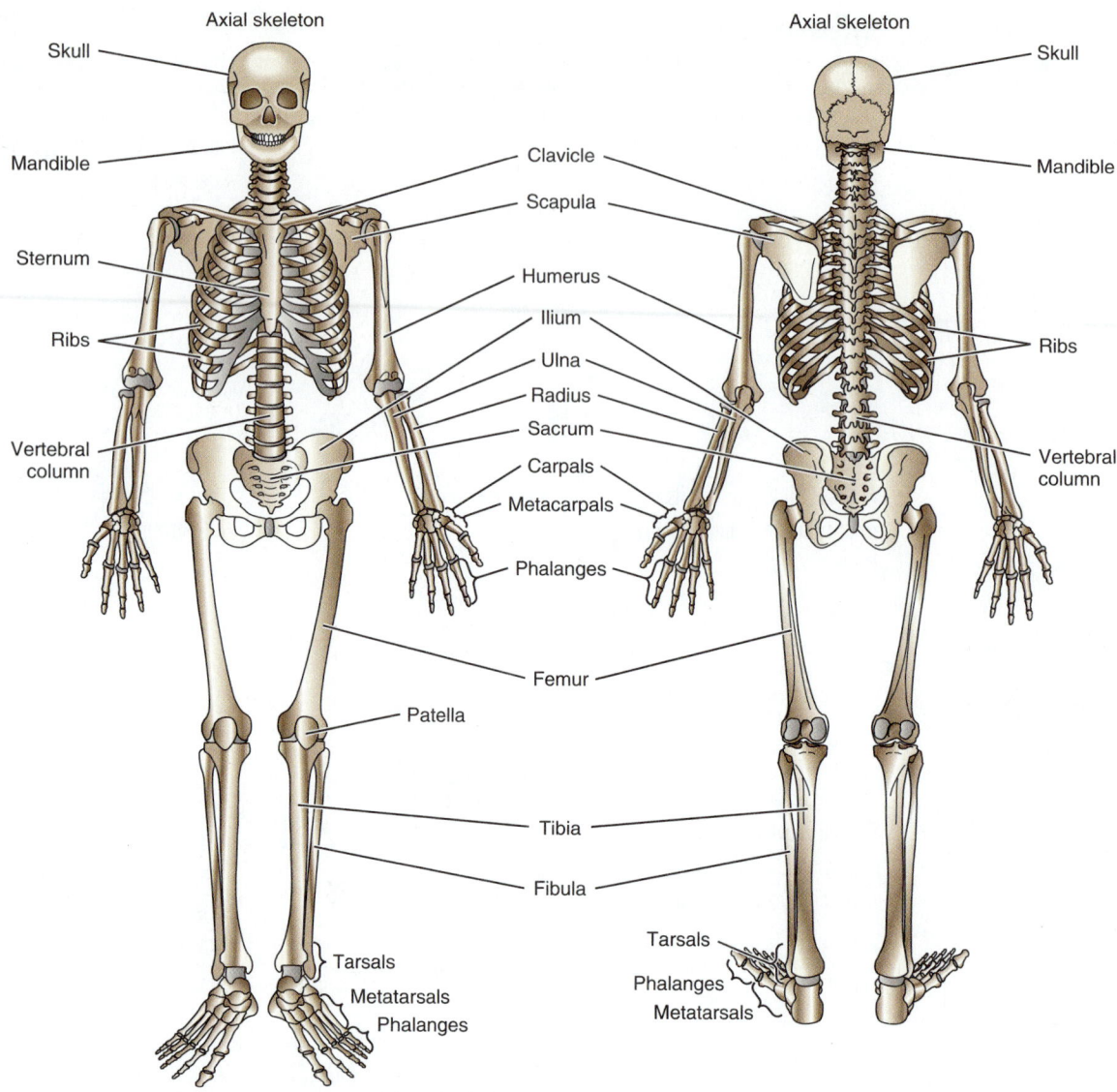

FIGURE 43-3 Axial skeletal bones *(outside columns)* and appendicular skeletal bones *(middle column)*. (From Chester GA: *Modern medical assisting,* Philadelphia, 1999, WB Saunders.)

the friction of movement. The thickness of the cartilage depends largely on the amount of stress placed on a particular joint. The **medullary cavity,** located within the diaphysis, contains yellow bone marrow.

Bone is living tissue that is constantly being remodeled in response to stress or injury. It also is a storage location for minerals, including calcium and phosphorus. Red bone marrow produces blood cells and is found in the spongy (cancellous) bone of the proximal epiphyses of the humerus and femur, sternum, ribs, and vertebrae of adults. Bones are covered with a thin, membranous tissue, the **periosteum,** which contains many sensory nerves.

CRITICAL THINKING APPLICATION   43-1

In what way does Kaiwan benefit by being familiar with the names and locations of the major bones of the extremities? How might this knowledge make his job at Sports Medicine Associates more interesting?

Joints

Bones are connected to each other at junctions known as *joints.* The two main kinds of joints are nonsynovial joints and synovial joints. In nonsynovial joints, the bones are joined with fibrous cartilage and are immovable (e.g., the sutures of the skull) or only slightly moveable (e.g., the vertebrae). Synovial joints are freely moveable, because the adjacent ends of two bones are covered with cartilage and are enclosed in a joint cavity that contains a viscous, slippery fluid called **synovial fluid,** which is an excellent lubricant. Synovial joints such as the elbow and the knee are hinge joints, which allow movement in only one plane (Figure 43-5). Other synovial joints, such as the hip and shoulder, allow movement in many planes, which permits a wider **range of motion (ROM)** than a hinge joint.

Types of Joints

Joints are classified by the way they are shaped or by their ability to move. The joints of the skull are known as *sutures.* Sutures permit

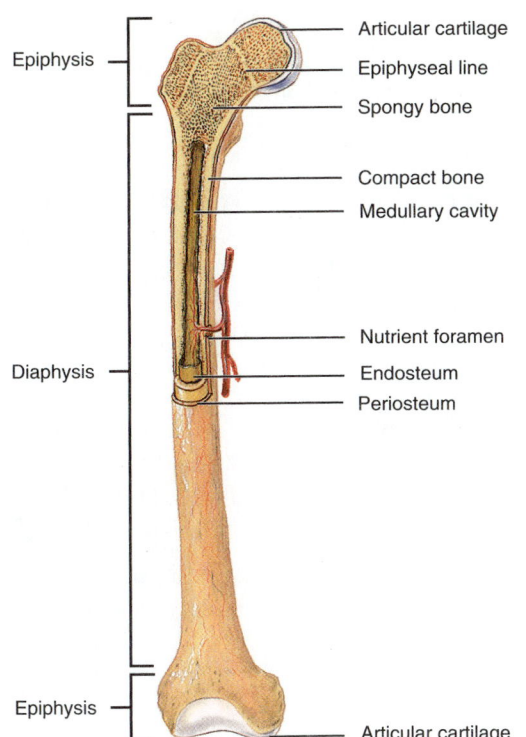

FIGURE 43-4 Long bone features. (From Applegate EJ: *The anatomy and physiology learning system,* ed 4, St Louis, 2011, Saunders.)

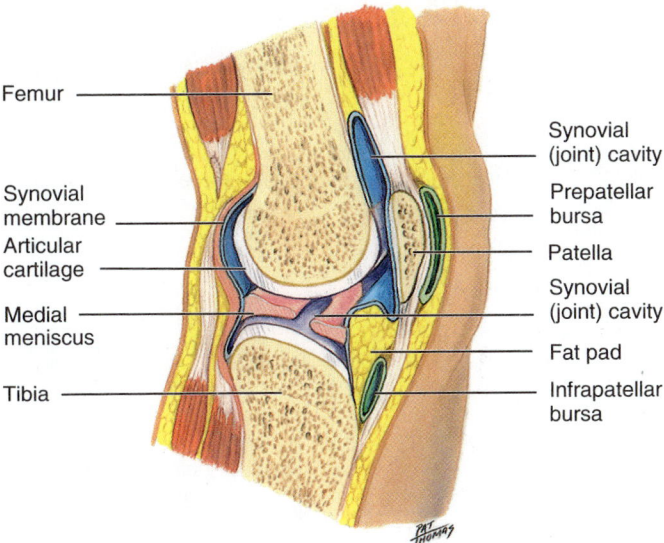

FIGURE 43-5 Sagittal section of the knee joint. (From Applegate EJ: *The anatomy and physiology learning system,* ed 3, St Louis, 2006, Saunders.)

the skull to grow with the child but have very limited flexibility. As mentioned, the hinge joints of the elbow and knee allow for movement in one plane, such as bending back and forth. A gliding joint, as in the wrist and foot, is made up of two flat-surfaced bones that slide over each other, allowing limited movement. Ball-and-socket joints, as in the shoulder and hip, allow for the greatest ROM by permitting the joint to rotate in a complete circle. Artificial joints have been successfully implanted to replace joints that have been damaged by disease or trauma, including the joints of the hip, knee, ankle, shoulder, elbow, wrist, and finger.

Ligaments, Tendons, and Bursae

Ligaments are powerful, strong, fibrous bands of connective tissue that connect bone to bone at the joint and encase the joint capsule. Ligaments allow purposeful joint movement and prevent excessive movement in any particular joint. Ligaments may be oblique or parallel to the joint, as in the knee, or may surround the joint, as in the hip.

A tendon is a strong bundle of connective tissue that attaches muscle to bone. Tendons can be flat or round and can pass between muscles, between bones, or through specialized openings between bones.

Bursae are fibrous sacs that lie between tendons and bones; they are lined with synovial membranes that secrete synovial fluid and act as cushions between a bone and a tendon or between a tendon and a ligament. Bursae reduce friction and help muscles and tendons glide smoothly over bone.

MUSCULOSKELETAL DISEASES AND DISORDERS

Musculoskeletal diseases and conditions can affect any of the muscles, bones, or joints. These problems are common and have a tremendous impact on an individual's quality of life. Brittle or deformed bones that are prone to fracture often mark bone disorders such as osteoporosis and osteomalacia. Joint disorders, such as osteoarthritis (OA), rheumatoid **arthritis** (RA), and gout, can lead to painful, swollen, or inflamed joints. Muscle problems, such as sprains and spasms, can bring on sudden pain or cause stiffness (Table 43-2).

Trauma to the musculoskeletal system can quickly lead to **inflammation** in the area of injury. This type of injury is one of the leading causes of time lost from work and for visits to primary care physicians and emergency departments. As soon as possible after injury, even before a patient is seen by a physician, treatment involving *r*est, *i*ce, *c*ompression, and *e*levation (RICE therapy) should be started. The combination of these measures can help reduce swelling and inflammation and enhance healing.

To maintain musculoskeletal health, a person must have a significant dietary intake of foods rich in calcium and vitamin D, avoid smoking, and include weight-bearing exercises (e.g., walking) in the daily routine. In addition to these lifestyle measures, medications sometimes are required for conditions that impair normal functioning of this system. The conditions discussed in the following sections are typically seen in an orthopedic practice.

USING FROZEN PEAS FOR AN ICE BAG

A bag of frozen peas (or corn) easily conforms to the shape of a body part and serves as an excellent means of immediately applying ice to a musculoskeletal injury. The vegetable ice bag should be wrapped in a towel to protect tissue from overexposure to the cold. It should be applied for 20 minutes, put back into the freezer for 30 to 60 minutes, and applied again.

TABLE 43-2 Common Musculoskeletal Conditions

DISEASE	SYMPTOMS AND SIGNS	DIAGNOSTIC PROCEDURES	LABORATORY TESTS	TREATMENT AND MEDICATIONS
Bursitis and tendonitis	Painful joint with reduced ROM	History, physical examination, x-ray studies to rule out fracture	CBC to rule out infectious arthritis	RICE, temporary immobilization, NSAIDs
Carpal tunnel syndrome	Hand and finger pain, numbness, tingling, difficulty grasping or holding objects, especially in the morning	History, physical examination, compression test	None	Rest, splint, forearm extensor strengthening exercises, surgical decompression in severe cases
Dislocation	Painful joint that is out of place and has severely reduced ROM	History of trauma, physical examination, x-ray studies	None	Reduce and temporarily immobilize joint
Fibromyalgia	Chronic, severe musculoskeletal pain, generalized weakness	History, physical examination to rule out other causes	As appropriate to rule out other conditions	NSAIDs, rest, reduce stress, muscle relaxants (Flexeril) and tricyclics (Elavil and Thorazine), SSRIs (Celexa, Paxil, Zoloft)
Fractures	Severe pain, swelling, reduced ROM	History, physical examination, x-ray studies	None	Reduction, immobilization, analgesics, NSAIDs
Gout	Painful joint inflammation, often affects great toe, very sensitive to touch and movement	History, physical examination, microscopic synovial fluid examination for uric acid crystals	Serum uric acid test	Analgesics, NSAIDs
Herniated disk	Depend on location and severity of herniation; back pain, extremity pain or weakness	History, physical examination, CT, MRI	None	Immobility, physical therapy, traction, muscle relaxants, surgical laminectomy in severe cases
Infectious arthritis	Severely inflamed joint	History, physical examination, microscopic synovial fluid examination for cell count and presence of bacteria	CBC, culture of joint fluid	NSAIDs, corticosteroids, appropriate antibiotic or antiviral agents
Lupus	Widely disparate presentations of symptoms with no known cause; very difficult to diagnose	Very careful history and physical examination to rule out possible causes of presenting symptoms; frequently a diagnosis of exclusion	Diagnostic tests as needed to rule out possible symptom causes	Symptomatic relief
Lyme disease	General malaise, fatigue, fever, headaches, myalgias, polyarthralgias	Careful history; physical examination to check for tick bite	CBC and perhaps other blood studies	Antibiotics and symptomatic relief
Myasthenia gravis	Profound muscular weakness, frequently starting with facial muscles; can involve any voluntary muscles	History, neurologic examination, EMG	Anti-AChR antibody test	Cholinesterase inhibitors, NSAIDs, steroids, immune inhibitors, thymectomy, plasmapheresis
Osteoarthritis	Gradually increasing joint pain, gradually decreasing ROM in affected joint	History, physical examination, x-ray studies, possibly CT	RA latex test to rule out rheumatoid arthritis, CBC to rule out infectious arthritis	NSAIDs, physical therapy, analgesics, ambulatory support
Osteomalacia	Fractures, muscle weakness, bone pain	History, physical examination, x-ray studies, bone scan	Serum vitamin D, serum calcium, serum alkaline phosphatase, PTH level, occasionally bone biopsy	Vitamin D and calcium supplementation

TABLE 43-2 Common Musculoskeletal Conditions—cont'd

DISEASE	SYMPTOMS AND SIGNS	DIAGNOSTIC PROCEDURES	LABORATORY TESTS	TREATMENT AND MEDICATIONS
Osteoporosis	Frequent fractures, exaggerated thoracic kyphosis, reduced height, back pain	History, physical examination, x-ray studies, bone density studies	DEXA scan, blood calcium level	Weight-bearing exercise, calcium supplementation, and pharmaceutical treatment with alendronate (Fosamax), etidronate (Didronel), calcitonin-salmon (Miacalcin), or raloxifene (Evista)
Rheumatoid arthritis	Severe joint pain and joint deformity	History, physical examination, x-ray studies	RA latex test	NSAIDs, analgesics, joint replacement in severe cases
Scoliosis	Lateral spinal deformity accompanied by back pain	Physical examination, radiographic studies	None	Braces, casts, surgery
Sprain, strain, spasm	Cardinal signs: inflammation, redness, heat, swelling, pain, reduced ROM	History, physical examination, including active and passive ROM, x-ray studies to rule out fracture	None	RICE and NSAIDs

AChR, Acetylcholine receptor; *CBC,* complete blood count; *CT,* computed tomography; *DEXA,* dual energy x-ray absorptiometry; *EMG,* electromyography; *MRI,* magnetic resonance imaging; *NSAIDs,* nonsteroidal antiinflammatory drugs; *PTH,* parathyroid hormone; *RA,* rheumatoid arthritis; *RICE,* rest, ice, compression, elevation; *ROM,* range of motion; *SSRIs,* selective serotonin reuptake inhibitors.

CRITICAL THINKING APPLICATION 43-2

Why is it important to obtain an accurate history from an injured patient who comes to the office for the first time? What is Kaiwan's responsibility in finding out the reason a new patient is being seen?

Muscular Disorders

Fibromyalgia

Fibromyalgia is a condition of widespread connective tissue and muscular pain and often includes severe fatigue of unknown origin. A patient with fibromyalgia usually complains of diffuse aches and pains all over the body. The disorder can affect people of all ages and is seen more frequently in women than in men. Chronic pain and fatigue are the cardinal signs in the absence of any other known cause. Associated conditions can include sleep disorders, irritable bowel syndrome, chronic headaches, temporomandibular joint (TMJ) problems, increased chemical sensitivity, and other musculoskeletal complaints.

Although the cause remains unknown, fibromyalgia can be triggered by an automobile accident or a bacterial or viral infection, or it can follow the diagnosis of other medical conditions, such as rheumatoid arthritis, lupus, or hypothyroidism. It is aggravated by changes in the weather or temperature, monthly hormonal variations, stress, anxiety, and depression. The diagnosis is made by eliminating any other cause for the symptoms and by finding 11 of 18 specific points to be extremely tender to palpation (Figure 43-6). Treatment goals include reducing pain, enhancing sleep, and reducing anxiety and stress. Pregabalin (Lyrica), an antiseizure medication, is the first drug that has been approved by the U.S. Food and Drug Administration (FDA) to treat fibromyalgia. Prescription sleeping pills, such as zolpidem (Ambien), are prescribed only for the short

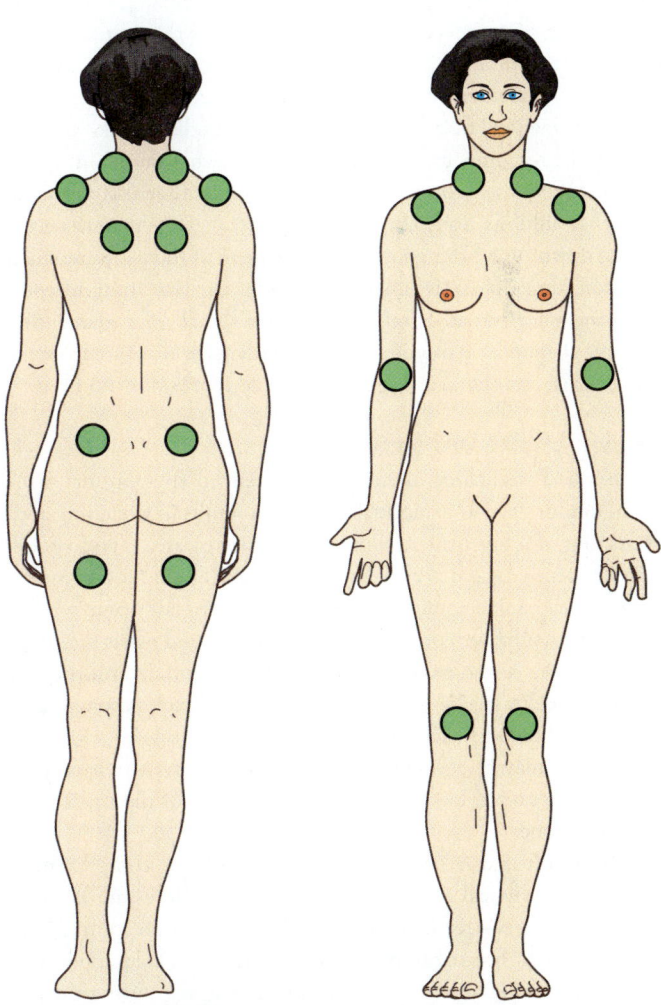

FIGURE 43-6 Tender points seen in fibromyalgia.

term, because the body eventually becomes tolerant to the medication, rendering it ineffective. Other medical treatments include over-the-counter analgesics and antiinflammatory agents, such as Tylenol or ibuprofen; tramadol (Ultram) for relief of pain; and antidepressants, such as duloxetine (Cymbalta) and milnacipran (Savella), to ease the pain and fatigue associated with fibromyalgia and fluoxetine (Prozac) to help promote sleep. Stress reduction and relaxation exercises help control symptoms. Fibromyalgia has no known cure.

Myasthenia Gravis

Myasthenia gravis is a chronic autoimmune neuromuscular disease of unknown origin that affects voluntary muscle contraction. It can occur at any age but most frequently affects young adult women (under age 40) and older men (over age 60). Often the patient experiences a sudden onset of weakness in the muscles that control eye and eyelid movement, facial expression, and swallowing. Symptoms vary in type and severity and may include drooping of one or both eyelids (ptosis); blurred or double vision (diplopia) as a result of weakness of the muscles that control eye movements; an unstable or waddling gait; weakness in the arms, hands, fingers, legs, and neck; altered facial expressions; difficulty swallowing; shortness of breath; and impaired speech (dysarthria).

Myasthenia gravis is caused by a defect in the transmission of nerve impulses to muscles. It occurs when a nervous stimulus is unable to stimulate a muscle at the neuromuscular junction, the place where nerve cells connect with the muscles they control. Normally, when impulses travel down the nerve, the nerve endings release acetylcholine (ACh), a neurotransmitter that activates muscular contraction. In myasthenia gravis, antibodies block, alter, or destroy the receptors for ACh at the neuromuscular junction, which prevents the muscle contraction. The primary treatment is a medication that inhibits acetylcholinesterase, the enzyme that normally breaks down ACh. This allows ACh to remain at the neuromuscular junction longer than usual so that more of the remaining receptor sites can be activated. Surgical removal of the thymus gland (thymectomy) reduces symptoms in most patients and may cure some individuals. Spontaneous improvement and remissions can occur.

Sprains, Strains, and Spasms

A *sprain* is a wrenching or twisting of a joint in an abnormal plane of motion or beyond its normal ROM that results in stretching and/or tearing of a ligament. Concurrent damage to area blood vessels, muscles, tendons, and nerves may occur. Probably the most common sprain is the ankle sprain (Figure 43-7), which can occur when a person steps off a curb or into a small depression and twists the ankle. Severe sprains are so painful the joint cannot be used, and they are accompanied by swelling and reddish to bluish discoloration because of ruptured blood vessels in the area.

A *strain* may be a simple overstretching of a muscle or tendon, or it can be caused by a partial or complete tear of the tissue away from the bone.

These soft tissue injuries are diagnosed by a comprehensive history and physical examination. Usually x-ray films are taken to rule out fractures. Treatment includes RICE: rest of the injured joint with no weight bearing to prevent further damage; cold application for 20 minutes at a time, four to eight times a day, during the first 24 to 48 hours to reduce pain and swelling; compression with an

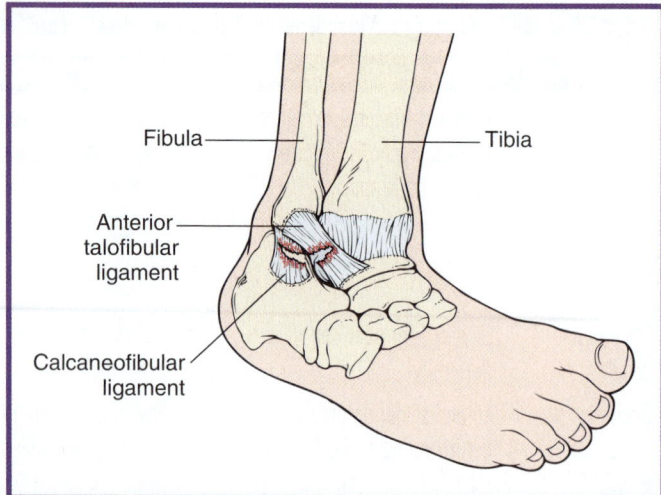

FIGURE 43-7 Ankle sprain. (From Frazier MS, Drzymkowski JW: *Essentials of human diseases and conditions*, ed 3, Philadelphia, 2004, Saunders.)

elastic wrap or air cast to reduce swelling; and elevation of the injured part. The physician also may recommend the use of over-the-counter (OTC) antiinflammatory drugs such as aspirin or ibuprofen to help reduce pain and inflammation at the site. If severe soft tissue injury occurs, immobilization by casting, surgical repair, or both may be required.

Treatment of a sprain or strain may also include rehabilitative exercises. The physician typically prescribes an exercise program designed to prevent stiffness, improve the joint's ROM, and restore normal flexibility and strength. Some patients may also be referred to physical therapy for complete return of function after the initial pain and swelling have subsided.

TELEPHONE SCREENING OF JOINT INJURIES

The following factors can help the medical assistant determine the need for an appointment when a patient calls to report a joint injury:

- Presence of severe pain and inability to put any weight on the injured joint
- Crooked appearance of injured area or unusual lumps and bumps
- Inability to move the injured joint
- Inability to walk more than four steps without significant pain
- Limb buckles or gives way if attempts are made to use the joint
- Numbness in any part of the injured area
- Inflammation that spreads out from the injured area
- History of injury to this particular joint
- Pain, swelling, or inflammation over a bony prominence

CRITICAL THINKING APPLICATION   43-3

A patient comes into the clinic hopping on one foot and holding the other in the air. She says she thinks she broke her ankle when she stepped off the curb wrong and fell. What is the first thing Kaiwan should do for this patient? What tests will Dr. Alexander most likely order? Why?

Muscle spasms occur spontaneously and may persist for hours. They typically are caused by heavy exercise and muscle fatigue, but they also can be caused by dehydration, hypothyroidism, lack of calcium or magnesium, kidney failure, and alcoholism. Muscle spasms can be quite painful. Treatment includes massage, direct pressure, ultrasound therapy, stress reduction, stretching exercises, and muscle relaxants in some cases.

RESTLESS LEG SYNDROME

A patient with restless leg syndrome (RLS) reports unpleasant sensations, such as tingling, aching, and twitching of the legs, during periods of inactivity, especially at night. The individual feels an overwhelming urge to move the affected leg (or legs) to relieve these abnormal feelings. Patients with nighttime leg twitching are diagnosed with periodic limb movements of sleep (PLMS), which causes involuntary flexion and extension of the legs during sleep. Most people with this disorder have difficulty getting to sleep or staying asleep.

Initial treatment plans include lifestyle changes, such as relaxation exercises, soaking in a warm bath, cutting back on caffeine, and moderate exercise. If these methods do not relieve the symptoms, patients may be prescribed medications, including ropinirole (Requip), anticonvulsants such as gabapentin (Neurontin), diazepam (Valium), or sleep agents like zolpidem (Ambien) or eszopiclone (Lunesta).

Skeletal Disorders

Fractures

A fracture is a break or crack in a bone that generally is the result of trauma or disease. Many different types of fractures occur, and each produces its own set of problems (Table 43-3). The common symptom of all fractures is pain. Other symptoms may include swelling, bleeding, inability to move, misalignment of the bone, and discoloration of the immediate area.

When a patient with a suspected fracture comes into the office, you should make the person as comfortable as possible. First aid includes RICE; positioning the patient to prevent stress on the injured area; elevating the injured extremity if possible; and controlling any bleeding but never applying pressure over a suspected fracture. Do not attempt to straighten the fracture or move it in any way. If the patient must be moved, either apply a splint or support the joints above and below the suspected fracture before and while moving the patient. The fracture must be confirmed by x-ray examination as soon as possible.

Treatment includes reduction, if necessary, and immobilization. **Reduction** places the fractured bone back into its correct anatomic alignment. Reduction may be closed or open. In a closed reduction, the physician manipulates the bone into its correct position. If this is not possible or if the fractured bones have pierced the skin, an open reduction is required, which is surgical realignment of the

TABLE 43-3 Types of Fractures

FRACTURE	DEFINITION	FRACTURE	DEFINITION
Closed, or simple	Broken bone is contained within intact skin.	Transverse	Break is caused by direct force applied perpendicular to a bone; fracture runs across the bone.
Open, or compound	Skin is broken above the fracture, which therefore is open to the external environment, creating the potential for infection.	Oblique	Break is caused by a twisting force with an upward thrust; fracture ends are short and run at an oblique angle across the bone.
Longitudinal	Fracture extends along the length of the bone.	Greenstick	Break is caused by compression or angulation forces in the long bones of children under age 10; because of its softness, the bone is cracked on one side and intact on the other side.

Continued

TABLE 43-3 Types of Fractures—cont'd

FRACTURE	DEFINITION	FRACTURE	DEFINITION
Comminuted	Break is caused by severe, direct force, which creates a fracture with multiple fragments.	Displaced	Bone ends are moved out of alignment.
Impacted	Break is caused by strong forces that drive bone fragments firmly together.	Spiral	Break is caused by a twisting or rotary force, which results in long, sharp, pointed bone ends; suspicious as a child abuse injury.
Pathologic	Break results from weakening of the bones by disease, as in osteoporosis or sarcomas.	Compression	Break is caused by transmitted forces that drive bones together.
Nondisplaced	Bone ends remain in alignment.	Avulsion	Break is caused by forceful contraction of a muscle against resistance, and a bone fragment tears at the site of muscle insertion.
		Depression	Bone fragments of the skull are driven inward.

From Chester GA: *Modern medical assisting*, Philadelphia, 1999, WB Saunders.

bone. During an open reduction, the orthopedic surgeon may have to install metal pins, plates, or screws to facilitate and maintain correct bone alignment. These metal implants may be temporary or permanent, depending on the extent of injury (Figure 43-8). After the fracture has been reduced, it must be immobilized by splinting, casting, taping, or wrapping the area to prevent movement of the fracture site and thereby facilitate healing.

Osteomalacia

The term *osteomalacia* literally means "softening of the bones." Osteomalacia is a metabolic disease in which inadequate calcium or phosphorus (or both) is available for building new bone during growth or remodeling. It is caused by either a lack of vitamin D or problems with its metabolism. The skeleton gradually loses calcium,

and the bones soften and become more flexible. Weight bearing gradually changes the shape of the softened bones. Symptoms can include reduced endurance, easy fatigability, **malaise,** and generalized bone tenderness and pain. Osteomalacia in children is called *rickets*.

Osteomalacia may be caused by a fat absorption problem in the gastrointestinal tract that prevents adequate absorption of dietary fats, resulting in steatorrhea and vitamin D deficiency. Vitamin D promotes the body's absorption of calcium, which is essential for normal development and maintenance of healthy teeth and bones. Vitamin D can be produced by the body with adequate sun exposure, and nearly all milk sold in the United States is fortified with vitamin D. Osteomalacia can occur in individuals who use very strong sunscreen, have limited exposure to sunlight, experience short

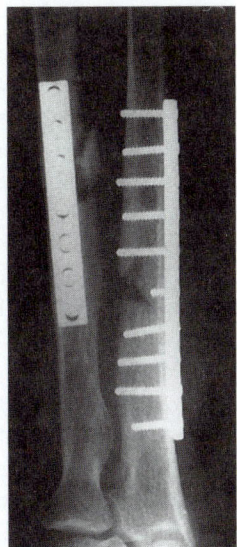

FIGURE 43-8 Orthopedic hardware from open reduction of fractures of the radius and ulna. (From Mettler MA: *Essentials of radiology,* ed 3, Philadelphia, 2004, Saunders.)

days of sunlight, live in a smoggy environment, or do not drink milk because of lactose intolerance. The condition is treated with vitamin D, calcium, and phosphorus supplements.

Osteoporosis

Osteoporosis is a disease in which calcium deposits in the bone gradually decline, and bones become increasingly weak and brittle so that even small stressors, such as bending over or coughing, can cause fractures. Bone strength depends on the size and density of the bone structure and the amount of calcium, phosphorus, and other materials deposited and maintained in the bone. Bones are constantly changing through a process called *remodeling,* or bone turnover. This process allows bones to grow and heal. As we age, remodeling breaks down bone more quickly than it forms new bone. Peak bone mass is reached by the middle 30s, so a person's risk of developing osteoporosis depends on the bone mass collected by age 25 to 35 and how rapidly bone tissue is lost after that. Lack of vitamin D and calcium in the diet results in a lower peak bone mass and a more rapid onset of bone loss later in life. People over age 50 are particularly at risk, and women are four times more likely to develop osteoporosis than men. Osteoporosis is a major public health threat in the United States, affecting more than 40 million individuals.

Osteoporosis often is called the "silent disease," because the progressive loss of bone density occurs without any symptoms. Osteopenia is mild bone loss that is not severe enough to be called osteoporosis but that increases the risk of osteoporosis. By the time fractures occur, the disease is quite advanced. Patients with osteoporosis complain of back pain because of a fractured or collapsed vertebra; loss of height over time, with stooped posture (kyphosis, or "dowager's hump"); and fractures typically of the vertebrae, wrists, and hips. Risk factors include being a postmenopausal woman over age 50; a slight build with a family history of osteoporosis; a history of amenorrhea; a low dietary calcium intake; an excessive intake of caffeinated soda; an inactive lifestyle; smoking; alcohol abuse; hyperthyroidism; a reduced lifetime exposure to estrogen; and long-term

treatment with certain medications, including antiseizure drugs, corticosteroids, and heparin. Men over age 50 with low testosterone levels also are at risk. Osteoporosis occurs in all races but is slightly more common in Caucasian and Asian individuals.

The diagnosis is made by a specialized form of x-ray evaluation that specifically measures bone density. This study allows the diagnosis of osteoporosis before a fracture occurs and thus intervention to prevent fractures. Readings are repeated annually to determine the rate of bone loss and to monitor the effectiveness of treatment. Intervention and treatment include increasing dietary intake of calcium and vitamin D; increasing weight-bearing exercise; and pharmaceutical treatment with bisphosphonates (alendronate [Fosamax], risedronate [Actonel]), zoledronic acid [Reclast] and ibandronate sodium [Boniva]); raloxifene (Evista), and calcitonin-salmon (Miacalcin). The best screening test is a dual energy x-ray absorptiometry (DEXA) scan, which measures the bone density of the spine, hip, and wrist. Other tests that can accurately measure bone density include ultrasound and quantitative computed tomography (CT) scanning.

The National Osteoporosis Foundation recommends that all women have a bone density test if they are not receiving estrogen replacement therapy and are in any of the following categories:

- Undergoing long-term treatment with medications that can cause osteoporosis, such as prednisone
- Have diabetes type 1, liver disease, kidney disease, or a family history of osteoporosis
- Experienced early menopause (in the early 40s)
- Are postmenopausal, over age 50, and have at least one risk factor for osteoporosis
- Are postmenopausal, over age 65, and have never had a bone density test

Spinal Column Disorders

Abnormal Spinal Curvatures

When the medical assistant looks at a patient's back, the spine should be vertically straight. Any abnormal deviation or curvature to the right or left is called **scoliosis.** Mild scoliosis generally causes no problems and usually is not even noticeable. When scoliosis is severe, it can cause significant back pain and possibly heart or lung problems because of the diminished space in the thoracic cavity on one side.

When the spine is viewed from a lateral position, four normal curves are seen (Figure 43-9). The **cervical** and **lumbar** regions should have curves toward the front of the body; these are called **lordotic** curves. The normal curves in the thoracic region of the spine and the sacrum are toward the back and are called **kyphotic** curves. Loss of cervical lordosis is called *military neck.* Excessive lumbar lordosis is called *swayback.* Excessive upper thoracic kyphosis is called *hunchback* (Figure 43-10).

These conditions are diagnosed by inspection and palpation and may be confirmed with x-ray studies. Treatment may include orthopedic devices, such as braces, shoe lifts, exercises, and electrical muscle stimulation. In severe cases, rigid casting with or without surgery may be necessary.

Herniated Disk

A herniated disk occurs when the soft nucleus of an intervertebral disk protrudes through a tear or weakened area in its tough outer cartilaginous covering (Figure 43-11). This condition occurs most often in the lumbar region, frequently in the cervical region, and rarely in the thoracic region of the spine. In children and young adults, disks have a high water content. As people age, this water content declines, and the structures begin to shrink and become less

flexible. This causes the spaces between the vertebrae to narrow. Factors that can weaken intervertebral disks include improper lifting; smoking; excessive body weight that places added stress on the disks of the lower back; sudden, possible slight pressure; and repetitive strenuous activities. Herniation may also occur gradually over time as a result of a progressive deterioration of the disks.

Symptoms depend on the location and extent of the protrusion of the nucleus beyond its normal location. If the herniation occurs in the lumbar region, it usually causes severe low back pain that can radiate down the leg and cause difficulty walking. If the herniated disk is in the cervical region, the person usually has a burning pain in the neck that can radiate down the arms to the fingers.

The diagnosis is made from a careful history, physical examination, either magnetic resonance imaging (MRI) or CT scans to confirm which disk is injured, or electromyography (EMG), which measures the nervous stimulation of affected muscles. Treatment depends on the severity of the herniation and the symptoms. Conservative treatments include chiropractic adjustments, physical therapy mobilization, and applications of cold until muscle spasms stop, then the use of heat. Traction of the affected area, especially of the neck, may help relieve pressure on affected nerves. Muscle relaxants, such as carisoprodol (Soma) and cyclobenzaprine (Flexeril), and/or analgesics may be given. If these measures are ineffective and the patient has recurring pain, numbness, and progressive weakness, surgery may be necessary.

Joint Disorders

Dislocation

Dislocation of a joint is also called a **luxation**, a condition in which two bones of a joint are no longer in approximation (Figure 43-12). A subluxation is an incomplete dislocation of a joint, meaning that the bones are only slightly out of proper alignment and location. It is possible to have a congenital dislocation, especially of the hip. Common dislocations occur in the finger, thumb, and shoulder and usually are caused by trauma, frequently while a person is playing sports. Symptoms include pain, swelling, loss of motion,

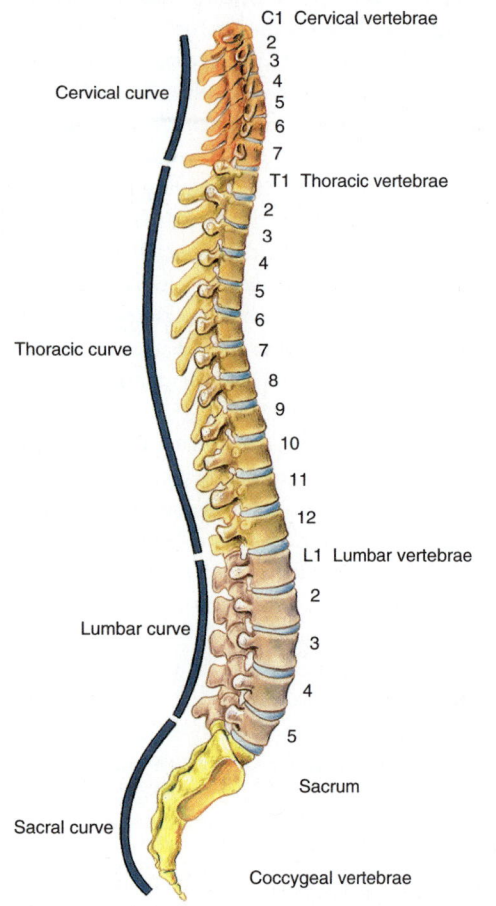

FIGURE 43-9 Normal curves of the spine. (From Applegate EJ: *The anatomy and physiology learning system*, ed 3, St Louis, 2006, Saunders.)

C1 Cervical vertebrae
2
3
4
Cervical curve
5
6
7
T1 Thoracic vertebrae
2
3
4
5
6
Thoracic curve
7
8
9
10
11
12
L1 Lumbar vertebrae
2
Lumbar curve
3
4
5
Sacrum
Sacral curve
Coccygeal vertebrae

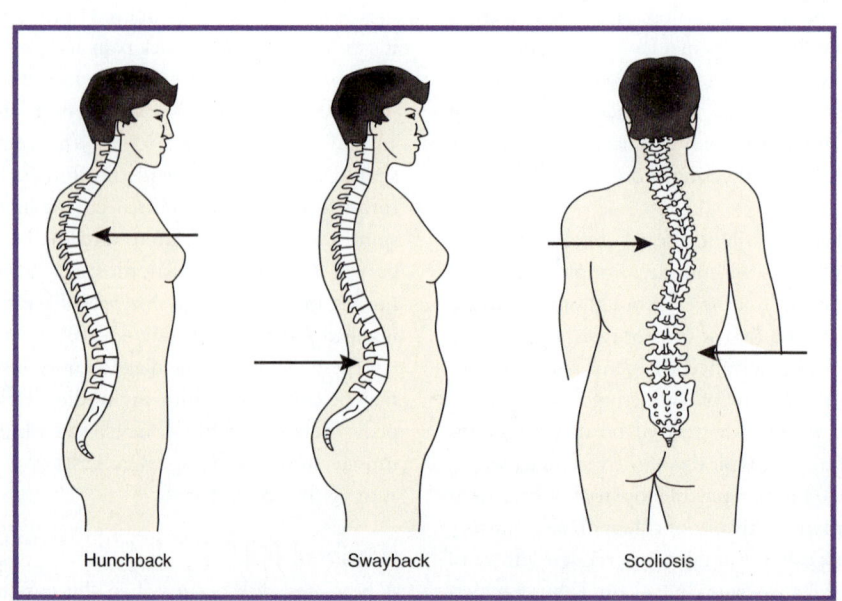

Hunchback   Swayback   Scoliosis

FIGURE 43-10 Spinal curve abnormalities.

and sometimes temporary paralysis of the affected part. A dislocation requires immediate reduction and immobilization to prevent permanent injury to nerves and major blood vessels near the joint. Occasionally, surgical reduction and repair may be necessary to stabilize the joint.

CRITICAL THINKING APPLICATION   43-4

A patient comes into the office after a softball game. After sliding into home plate, he immediately was unable to move his right arm, and he says that he has a lot of pain in his right shoulder. What steps should Kaiwan take to help this patient?

Gout

Gout, which may also be called *gouty arthritis*, is a metabolic disease involving overproduction or improper elimination of uric acid. Uric acid is a waste product formed from the breakdown of purines, which are found naturally in the body and in certain foods, including organ meats (liver, brains, and kidney), anchovies, herring, asparagus, mushrooms, cold cuts, sausage, and alcohol. Uric acid should dissolve in the blood so that it can be excreted as it passes through the kidneys. However, with gout, uric acid is not effectively excreted, and needlelike crystals of uric acid collect in the synovial fluid of the affected joint, causing extreme sensitivity to touch, pronounced inflammation, and severe pain. The most frequently affected area is the great toe (Figure 43-13). Risk factors include consumption of alcohol, obesity, untreated hypertension, diabetes, hypercholesterolemia, and a family history of the disease. Men are more likely to experience gout than women, but women become increasingly susceptible to gout after menopause.

In general, keeping uric acid levels within a normal range is the key to preventing future episodes of gout. Therefore, long-range treatment includes dietary modifications to eliminate foods containing purine. For treatment of an acute onset of inflammation, the patient may take nonsteroidal antiinflammatory drugs (NSAIDs), such as ibuprofen and naproxen (Aleve), for pain and joint inflammation. In severe cases the physician may prescribe prednisone. Pharmaceutical treatment to reduce the risk or lessen the severity of future episodes includes allopurinol (Zyloprim, Aloprim) and probenecid (Benemid). Taken daily, these drugs slow the rate of uric acid production and enhance its elimination from the body.

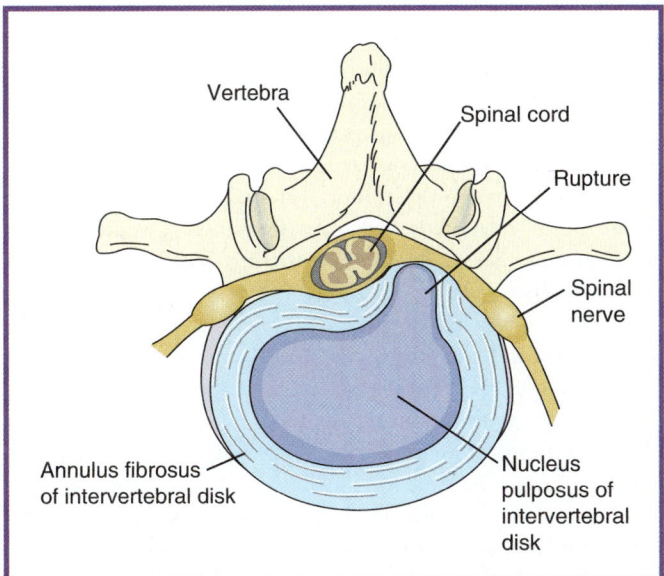

FIGURE 43-11 Herniation of a vertebral disk.

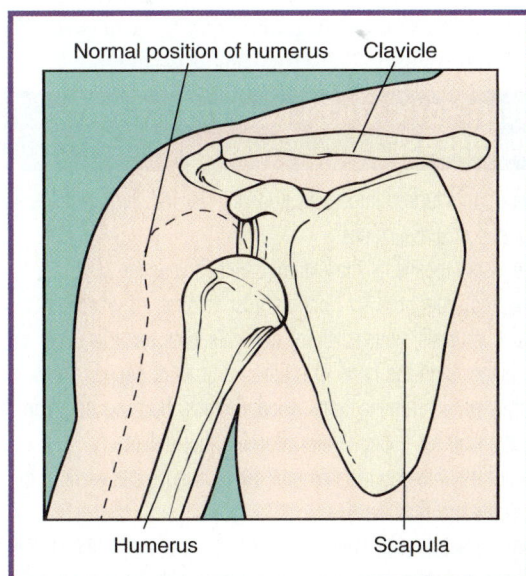

FIGURE 43-12 Luxation (dislocation) of the shoulder. (From Frazier MS, Drzymkowski JW: *Essentials of human diseases and conditions*, ed 3, Philadelphia, 2004, Saunders.)

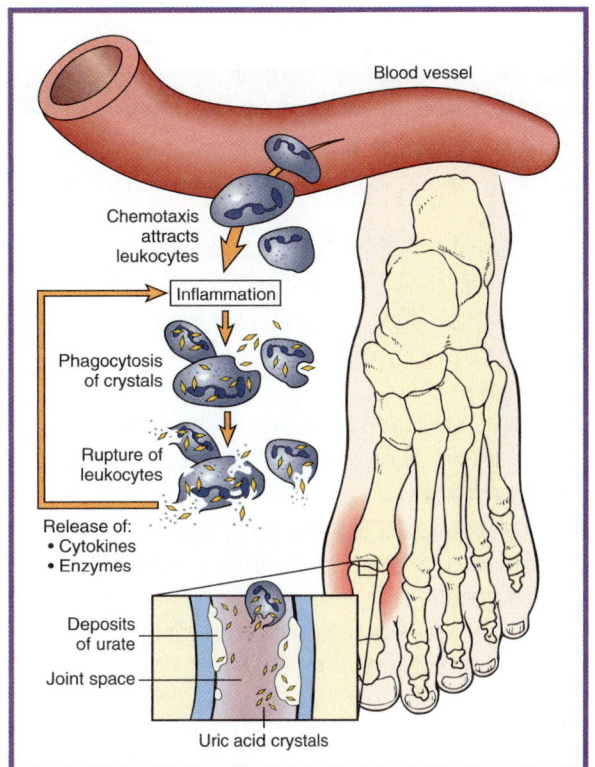

FIGURE 43-13 Gout is characterized by deposits of uric acid crystals in the connective tissue. The inflammation most often affects the joint of the big toe. (From Damjanov I: *Pathology for the health-related professions*, ed 3, St Louis, 2006, Saunders.)

Lupus

The three main types of lupus are systemic lupus erythematosus (SLE), discoid lupus erythematosus, and drug-induced lupus. Of these, SLE is the most common and serious form of the disease. SLE is an autoimmune disease of unknown cause. It occurs primarily in women 20 to 50 years of age, although it can occur in both younger and older individuals. Other risk factors include recurrent infections caused by the Epstein-Barr virus, a family history of the disease, and being an African-American.

SLE is difficult to diagnose and entirely unpredictable. The patient develops autoantibodies (antibodies to self) that can attack any tissue or organ in the body, which may result in severe inflammation with tissue changes and destruction. The progression and severity of the disease vary widely among patients. Furthermore, problems associated with SLE change over time and overlap with those of many other disorders. For these reasons, doctors may not initially consider lupus until the signs and symptoms become more obvious. At times the disease may become severe, and at other times it may subside completely. There is no known cure; the therapeutic goal is to maintain patient function as much as possible. The type of pharmaceutical treatment prescribed depends on which parts of the body are affected by the disease and the severity of the symptoms. Some medications used to treat SLE include NSAIDs, such as naproxen sodium and ibuprofen, to reduce joint pain and inflammation; antimalarials, such as hydroxychloroquine (Plaquenil), to treat skin and joint problems and the ulcers that some people develop in the mouth or nose; **corticosteroids** (prednisone) during acute inflammatory processes; and immunosuppressive medications, such as azathioprine (Imuran) and cyclophosphamide (Cytoxan), to suppress the immune system. The kidneys may fail even with treatment, which may necessitate either kidney dialysis or a kidney transplant.

DIAGNOSIS OF LUPUS

According to the American Rheumatism Association, the diagnosis and classification of lupus require four of the following 10 clinical and laboratory criteria:

- Malar rash (a butterfly-shaped rash that covers the bridge of the nose and spreads across the cheeks)
- Discoid rash (raised, scaly patches that may cause scarring)
- Marked sensitivity to sunlight
- Oral ulcers
- Arthritis that involves two or more peripheral joints
- Inflammation of the lining of the heart or lung (serositis)
- Renal disease
- Neurologic disorder (e.g., seizures or psychosis)
- Hematologic disorder (e.g., anemia, thrombocytopenia, or leukopenia)
- Elevated blood level of antinuclear antibodies (an indicator of an autoimmune disease)

Infectious Arthritis

Infectious arthritis usually occurs after some type of systemic or local infection in some other part of the body or after a joint has been violated by trauma or surgery. The infection can be caused by bacteria, fungi, or viruses. The joint usually shows signs of severe inflammation and significantly reduced ROM. To determine the diagnosis, the physician may order an x-ray evaluation and bone scan and may withdraw synovial fluid for microscopic examination and culture. The goals of treatment are to reduce inflammation, increase ROM, and treat the causative organism with the appropriate medication.

Lyme Disease

Lyme disease is an infection caused by the bacterium *Borrelia burgdorferi*. It is transmitted to humans by a bite from ticks of the *Ixodes* family. The disease is named after Lyme, Connecticut, where it was first identified in 1975 in a cluster of children who showed signs of what was thought to be rheumatoid arthritis. Eventually epidemiologists traced the cause of the problem to a bacterial infection. Signs and symptoms may include a "bull's-eye" lesion, called *erythema migrans*, surrounding the area of the tick bite; this lesion can appear within a few days or up to a month after exposure. The rash can last several days to several weeks and occurs in as many as 80% of people infected with Lyme disease. Additional indicators of the disease include flulike symptoms, such as fever, chills, fatigue, body aches, and headache. If the infection remains untreated, the patient complains of pain in multiple joints. Late-stage symptoms of Lyme disease include meningitis, Bell's palsy, numbness or weakness of the limbs, memory loss, difficulty concentrating, and changes in mood or sleep habits.

The diagnosis is made by taking a careful history, including the patient's level of outdoor exposure, locating the tick bite, and ruling out other causes for presenting symptoms. Laboratory tests to identify antibodies to the bacterium are used to help confirm the diagnosis. These tests are most reliable a few weeks after an infection, because it takes some time for antibodies to develop. The blood test most often used to screen for Lyme disease is the enzyme-linked immunosorbent assay (ELISA), which detects antibodies to *B. burgdorferi*. If the ELISA result is positive, the Western blot test is performed to confirm the diagnosis. Antibiotics, such as doxycycline (Doryx, Monodox) or amoxicillin (Amoxil, Trimox), are the standard treatment for Lyme disease in its early stages. If the disease has progressed to a later stage, the patient may be hospitalized for treatment with intravenous (IV) ceftriaxone (Rocephin).

PATIENT EDUCATION FOR PREVENTING LYME DISEASE

- Wear pants tucked into socks and long-sleeved shirts when walking in wooded or grassy areas.
- Use insect repellents that contain diethyltoluamide (DEET).
- Tick-proof your yard by clearing brush and leaves where ticks live.
- Check yourself, your children, and your pets for ticks; deer ticks are no bigger than the head of a pin or a grain of pepper; shower immediately after returning from wooded areas, because ticks can remain on the skin for hours before attaching themselves.
- Do not assume you are immune; Lyme disease can occur in the same person more than once.
- Remove a tick with tweezers by gently grasping it near the head or mouth; do not squeeze or crush the tick, but pull it out carefully and steadily. After removal, apply antiseptic to the bite area.

Osteoarthritis

OA, also called *degenerative joint disease* (DJD), is marked by significant thinning and degeneration of the articular cartilage of synovial joints. The symptoms range from mild to severe, depending on the amount of degeneration. As the articular cartilage disintegrates and wears away, the roughened surface of the bone is exposed, leaving bone rubbing against bone, with resultant pain and stiffness of the involved joint. Commonly involved joints include the fingers, the spine, and the weight-bearing joints of the hips, knees, and feet. Diagnosis frequently includes x-ray films, which show degenerative changes in the joint surfaces and asymmetric joint space narrowing.

Treatment goals include relieving pain, maintaining normal motion in the joint, and attempting to prevent crippling deformities. Medications may include analgesics, NSAIDs, and intra-articular steroid injections. Using a walker or cane may be helpful for maintaining mobility. Severe cases require surgery to remove the affected joint and replace it with a joint **prosthesis.**

Rheumatoid Arthritis

RA is an autoimmune inflammatory condition that involves an immune system response to the synovial membranes, causing synovitis. Proteins are released at the site of the joint inflammation, eventually resulting in thickening of the synovium and damage to the cartilage, bone, tendons, and ligaments of the affected joint. Gradually the joint loses its shape and alignment, causing deformity and pain. Researchers suspect RA is triggered by an infection in people with an inherited susceptibility to the disease.

Early symptoms include malaise, fever, weight loss, and morning stiffness of the affected joints. One or more joints may become painful and inflamed. Usually, bouts of arthritis increase in frequency and severity over time. As this occurs, the joints become damaged, and joint swelling and deformity occur. The patient ultimately loses the ability to move the affected joints, and a pronounced loss of strength occurs in the muscles attached to the inflamed joints. Small lumps, called *rheumatoid nodules,* may form at pressure points in the elbows, hands, feet, Achilles tendons, knees, and posterior scalp, and even in the lungs. Patients with RA may appear undernourished and chronically ill because of the formation of degenerative lesions in the collagen (connective tissues) in the lungs, heart, blood vessels, and pleura (Figure 43-14). Periods of increased disease activity, called *flare-ups,* alternate with periods of relative remission, during which the swelling, pain, difficulty sleeping, and weakness fade or disappear. X-ray findings show uniform joint space narrowing, which is different from the degenerative changes seen in OA.

Rest and exercise seem to be the key elements in treating RA. Therapeutic exercises are designed to prevent and correct deformities, control pain, strengthen weakened muscles, and improve joint function. The most frequently prescribed medications are NSAIDs, including aspirin (acetylsalicylic acid), indomethacin (Indocin), diclofenac (Voltaren), naproxen (Naprosyn), and ibuprofen (Motrin). Corticosteroids (prednisone and Medrol) may be prescribed for severe flare-ups. To limit the extent of joint damage early in the disease, the physician prescribes disease-modifying antirheumatic drugs (DMARDs), such as hydroxychloroquine (Plaquenil), etanercept (Enbrel), adalimumab (Humira), the gold compound auranofin

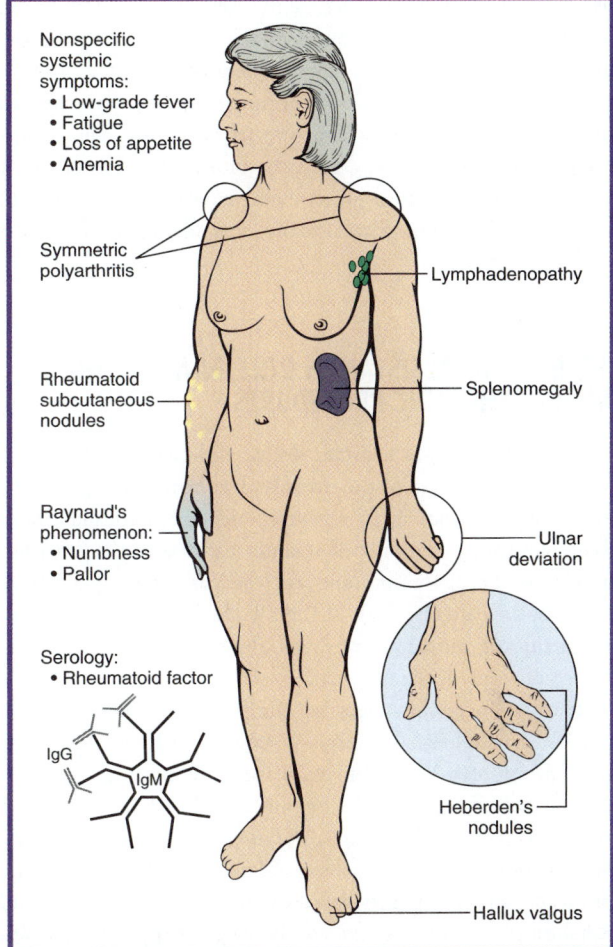

FIGURE 43-14 Signs and symptoms of rheumatoid arthritis. (From Damjanov I: *Pathology for the health-related professions,* ed 3, St Louis, 2006, Saunders.)

(Ridaura), and infliximab (Remicade). In severe cases, surgical joint replacement may be necessary.

CRITICAL THINKING APPLICATION   43-5

An 80-year-old male patient with arthritis comes into the office complaining of severe pain in his knees, hips, and lower back. The pain makes it impossible for him to get up onto the examination table. What should Kaiwan do? Is this patient required to get onto the examination table? Why or why not?

Tendonitis and Bursitis

Tendonitis is one of the most common causes of pain in the shoulder and elbow. Inflammation of tendons may be associated with calcium deposits in the bursae around the joint, causing concurrent bursitis. The diagnosis is made if the patient has increased severity of pain when abducting the arm beyond 50 degrees. Treatment includes pain relief and reducing the localized inflammation to make exercise possible and to prevent shoulder immobility, called *frozen shoulder.* Medications might include analgesics, NSAIDs, and injections of long-acting corticosteroids. Cold applications are helpful in relieving pain; heat applications are contraindicated because they tend to aggravate calcium tendonitis.

Bursitis is a painful inflammation of a joint bursa that most commonly follows a repetitive movement or prolonged pressure on a joint. The pain is increased with movement of the affected joint. It also can occur from staphylococcal or tubercular infections and with some joint diseases, including gout and arthritis. Treatment includes preventing the activity that caused the bursitis and protecting the affected site from excessive pressure and movement. NSAIDs may provide pain relief, but corticosteroid antiinflammatories may be needed in severe cases.

THE MEDICAL ASSISTANT'S ROLE IN ASSISTING WITH ORTHOPEDIC PROCEDURES

The role of the medical assistant begins with accurately recording the patient's description of the circumstances surrounding the onset of the problem, what measures were undertaken to alleviate the problem, and the patient's current concerns. Record the exact location of pain or discomfort and ask the patient to quantify the intensity of the pain on a scale of 1 to 10; also ask about medications taken, including the names of drugs, the dose and frequency, and the date and time of the last dose.

Offer assistance when escorting the patient to the examination room. Use a wheelchair if necessary. Assist the patient into a comfortable position in the examination room by offering a pillow or folded blanket to support the painful or injured body part. The patient may have limited mobility because of pain, so you may need to provide assistance with disrobing and getting into an examination gown. Make sure the patient is warm enough by offering an additional sheet or blanket. Explain clearly what is happening and what the patient can expect. Notify the physician as soon as the patient is ready for the examination.

Assisting with the Examination

The physician may use inspection, palpation, ROM testing, and muscle testing to examine the major skeletal muscles and joints. Much of the examination involves comparing muscles and joints on the affected side with those on the contralateral side for size, position, and strength. When the patient needs to assume a certain position, demonstrating the position or movement desired may be helpful. Watch the patient during the manipulative and palpatory portion of the examination for a facial grimace or physical jerk or jump, which may indicate pain.

As a general rule, the unaffected side is examined first, then the affected side, and the two are compared. You may be responsible for taking notes during the examination. Keep the patient properly draped and assist the physician by handing the equipment as needed. Most examinations require the use of a measuring tape, goniometer, blood pressure cuff, stethoscope, and felt-tipped washable marker. Be alert and ready to prevent the patient from falling during the examination, because some of the requested movements and positions may place the injured patient off balance.

The physician performs a gait analysis by watching the patient walk in a straight line with or without the patient knowing he or she is being observed. In addition to being associated with disorders of the musculoskeletal system, gait abnormalities may be caused by an associated neurologic condition.

SPECIALIZED DIAGNOSTIC PROCEDURES IN ORTHOPEDICS

Range-of-Motion Evaluation

Often orthopedic injuries severely affect the normal ROM of a joint. Measuring the ROM of specific joints is an objective measure of both the seriousness of an injury and the recovery progress. When the ROM of a particular joint is evaluated, usually both active and passive ROM results are measured and recorded.

The joint movement in a single plane is measured with a **goniometer**. A goniometer has two arms that are fixed together with a hinge joint at one end (Figure 43-15). Each of the arms is lined up with a bone on each side of the joint being tested. The degrees of motion are indicated on a scale on the hinged center of the instrument. To determine the active ROM of a joint, the patient is asked to move the joint as far as possible. For evaluation of passive ROM, the patient is asked to relax and the physician moves the joint as far as possible. All ROMs are measured in degrees. During these examinations, you may be asked to record the degrees of motion for active and/or passive ROM for specific joints and to note any pain, tenderness, or **crepitation** during the examination.

> ### CRITICAL THINKING APPLICATION   43-6
> How can Kaiwan best assist Dr. Alexander in testing upper extremity ROM in a new patient? What equipment should Kaiwan have ready? What patient position would best facilitate this examination? Why?

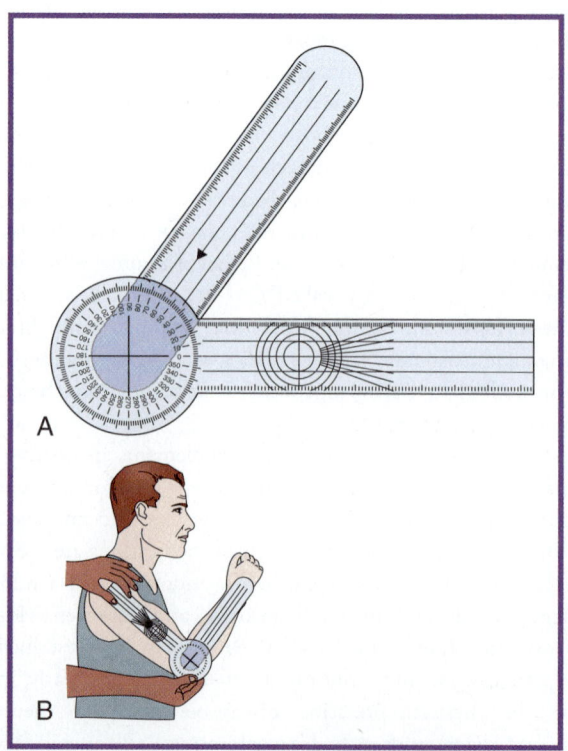

FIGURE 43-15 A, Goniometer. B, Correct position of the goniometer on the arm.

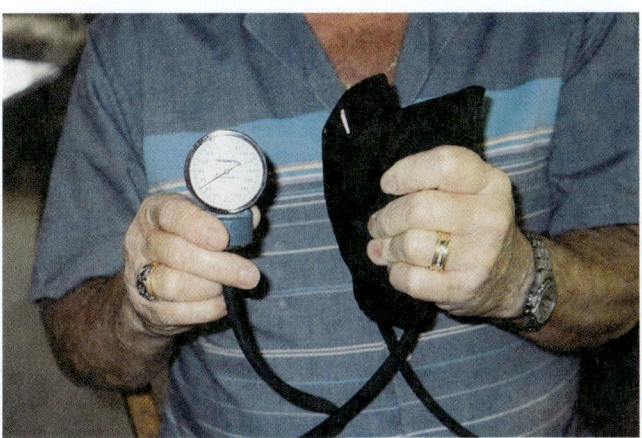

FIGURE 43-16 Assessing grip strength using a blood pressure cuff.

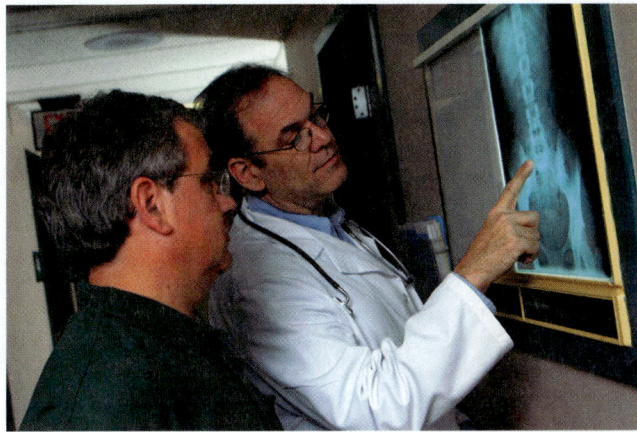

FIGURE 43-17 Reading a lumbar radiograph.

Muscle Strength Evaluation

During the ROM evaluation, the physician also assesses each muscle group for strength. Normal muscle strength allows for complete voluntary ROM despite resistance. This resistance can be gravity, as when rising from sitting to a standing position, or physical, as in pulling, pushing, or lifting an object. Muscle strength is bilaterally equal in normal conditions. The evaluation compares like muscles in each hemisphere of the body, such as using a blood pressure cuff to compare the grip of the right hand with the grip of the left hand (Figure 43-16).

ASSESSMENT OF GRIP STRENGTH USING A BLOOD PRESSURE CUFF

1. Roll up an aneroid blood pressure cuff and have the patient hold it in one hand.
2. Inflate the cuff to 20 mm Hg of pressure.
3. Ask the patient to squeeze the cuff as tightly as possible.
4. Note the increase in pressure on the dial (a normal grip registers above 150 mm Hg).
5. Record the hand tested and the results of the test.
6. Repeat on the other hand.

RADIOLOGY

Radiology and diagnostic imaging frequently are used to help diagnose orthopedic conditions (Figure 43-17). X-ray evaluation is necessary to diagnose fractures, dislocations, and bone and joint diseases accurately. X-ray films also can be used to track the healing of a fracture to determine when it has healed sufficiently to allow removal of a cast.

CRITICAL THINKING APPLICATION 43-7

A patient who has just undergone x-ray studies stops Kaiwan and wants to see his x-ray films. How should Kaiwan handle this situation? If a patient is in an examination room with her own x-ray film on the view box and she asks Kaiwan to show her where the break is, how should he respond to this request?

When one of these diagnostic tests is necessary, you should explain the procedure to the patient. Your explanation should include what will be done, how it is done, where it will take place, and approximately how long it will take. Patients always are concerned about whether the procedure will hurt. Tell the truth. If the procedure is painful, let the patient know so that he or she can prepare for it. Most painful procedures are performed only after the patient has been given a mild sedative. Discuss the procedure in a professional yet empathetic manner. If the patient wants to talk with the physician about the test, make sure this happens.

SPECIALIZED IMAGING TECHNIQUES USED IN ORTHOPEDICS

- Arthrograms—To visualize the joints.
- Bone scans—To evaluate areas of bone growth, bone tumors, and other bone disease patterns.
- Dual energy x-ray absorptiometry (DEXA) scan—To assess bone density used in the diagnosis and management of osteoporosis.
- Computed tomography (CT) scans—To visualize soft tissue such as tumors, lesions, or some spinal injuries.
- Electromyography (EMG) and nerve conduction velocity studies (NCS)—To evaluate muscle response to stimulus.
- Biopsies of bone and muscle—To identify cancerous tumors and other neoplasms and pathogens.

THERAPEUTIC MODALITIES

Physical treatment methods called *modalities* often are used in orthopedic, chiropractic, and physical therapy offices to treat orthopedic conditions. These can include the application of cold, heat, baths, electric currents, therapeutic ultrasonography, massage, and therapeutic exercises. Cold applications are recommended for the first 48 hours after an injury to help control pain and swelling. Heat application is used after this to help improve circulation, reduce pain, and maintain muscle and joint function (Table 43-4). *Diathermy* is a technique for creating deep tissue heat through the use of a high-frequency current, ultrasonic waves, or microwave radiation. As is surface heating, deep heat is used to reduce pain, relieve muscle spasms, resolve inflammation, and promote healing. Deep heat may be used to treat chronic arthritis, bursitis, fractures, and other musculoskeletal problems.

General Principles of Cold Application

Cold applications, such as ice packs and cold compresses, act as vasoconstrictors and also cause contraction of the involuntary muscles of the skin ("goose bumps"). These two actions reduce the blood supply to the area and exert a numbing effect on the sensory nerve endings. Cold applications can help control bleeding, prevent further swelling and inflammation, and reduce pain. Disposable, reusable, or homemade ice packs most commonly are used for cold application (Procedure 43-1).

Heat Modalities

Heat produces local vasodilation, which increases circulation. This accelerates the inflammatory process, promotes local drainage, reduces swelling, relaxes muscles, and repairs tissues and cells. The effects of external heat application depend on the type of heat used, the length of time it is applied, the frequency with which it is applied, the patient's general condition, and the size of the area treated. Heat application is an excellent therapeutic modality, but it must be used with caution to prevent overheating and burning of surface tissues. Special care must be taken in patients who have reduced sensation, because they may not sense a burn occurring. Therefore, heat application is contraindicated in the following circumstances:

- With acute inflammatory conditions, particularly during the first 48 hours
- In individuals with severe circulatory problems of any kind
- In those with diminished or abnormal sensation
- Over areas with encapsulated pus
- On blisters from previous burns
- Over scar tissue, because it does not have a normal blood supply and easily overheats
- In body areas with cancerous tumors

TABLE 43-4 Effects of Heat and Cold Application

APPLICATION	CAUSES	TISSUE RESPONSE	THERAPEUTIC EFFECT
Heat	Vasodilation Muscle relaxation Increased metabolism Local warmth	Increased blood flow More white blood cells to area Reduced muscle spasm Decreased pain	Increased nutrients to site Faster removal of wastes Phagocytosis Faster tissue repair
Cold	Vasoconstriction Numbness of nerve endings Reduced metabolism Increased blood viscosity	Reduced blood flow Local anesthesia Reduced oxygen need Faster blood clotting	Inhibition of swelling Reduced inflammation Reduced pain

PROCEDURE 43-1

Assist the Physician with Patient Care: Assist with Cold Application

GOAL: *To apply a cold compress to a body area to reduce pain, prevent further swelling, and/or reduce inflammation.*

EQUIPMENT and SUPPLIES

- Small ice cubes or ice chips
- Ice bag or closeable disposable plastic kitchen food bag
- Towel
- Patient's record

PROCEDURAL STEPS

1. Sanitize your hands.
2. Explain the procedure to the patient and answer any questions.
3. Check the bag for leaks.
4. Fill the bag with small cubes or chips of ice until it is about two thirds full.
   PURPOSE: Small chips conform more easily to the shape of the body.
5. Push down on the top of the bag to expel excess air and put on the cap or seal the plastic bag.
   PURPOSE: To remove as much air as possible from the bag, because air is a poor conductor of cold.

6. Dry the outside of the bag and cover it with one or two towel layers.
7. Help the patient position the ice bag on the injured area.
8. Advise the patient to leave the ice bag in place for about 20 to 30 minutes or until the area feels numb, whichever comes first.
   PURPOSE: Leaving the ice in place for longer than 20 to 30 minutes may cause tissue damage.
9. Check the skin for color, feeling, and pain.
   PURPOSE: If the treated area becomes very painful, remains numb, or is pale or cyanotic, the ice bag should be removed and the physician notified.
10. Record the procedure in the patient's medical record.
    PURPOSE: A procedure is not considered done until it is recorded.

8/27/XX 1:45 PM Ice pack applied to Ⓡ knee for 20 min. No c/o discomfort. Pt instructed to continue ice application at home q 3 hr while awake for 24 hr at 20-min intervals. Call physician if edema persists or pain increases. K. Tillman, CMA (AAMA)

- Over inflamed skin, because the initial erythema caused by a burn cannot be detected
- Over any metal jewelry or any area with metal implants

Body parts may safely be heated to 110°F (44°C) without any tissue damage. Redness appears, because the skin capillaries become congested at the skin's surface. Heat modalities may be either wet or dry and can have either superficial or deep effects. Dry heat therapies include heating pads, infrared radiation lamps, ultraviolet radiation, and hot water bottles. More penetrating methods of dry heat application include diathermy and ultrasound. Moist heat modalities include soaks, whirlpool treatments, hot moist compresses (Figure 43-18), and paraffin baths (Procedure 43-2).

Paraffin Bath

A paraffin bath is especially useful for treating chronic joint inflammation. A mixture of seven parts paraffin and one part mineral oil is melted and heated to approximately 125°F (52°C). The body part (usually a hand, an elbow, or a foot) is dipped into the warm paraffin mixture and removed immediately, leaving a thin coating on the skin. This dipping is repeated numerous times until a thick coating of paraffin remains on the body part (Figure 43-19). The part then is wrapped with plastic and a towel to allow the heat to penetrate the tissues. The paraffin is kept on for 30 minutes and then is peeled off. The process leaves the skin soft, warm, moisturized, and pliable, with slight erythema.

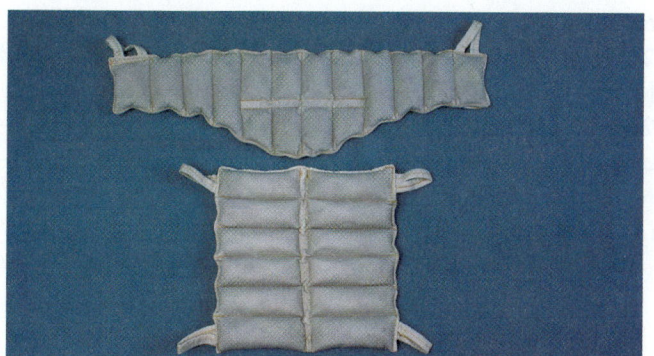

FIGURE 43-18 Commercial hot packs made of canvas that contain a silicone gel.

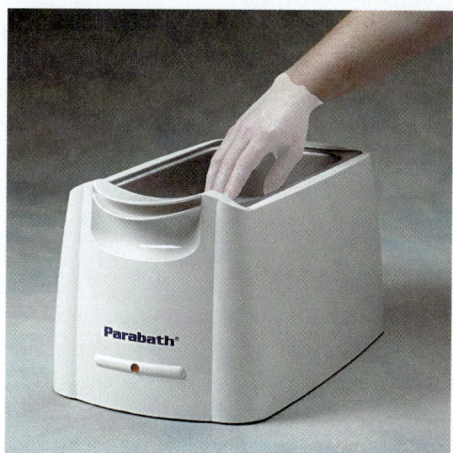

FIGURE 43-19 A paraffin bath is especially helpful for relieving pain in patients with arthritis. The hand is dipped in warm paraffin, which is left on for about 30 minutes and then peeled off.

CRITICAL THINKING APPLICATION   43-8

Kaiwan is helping a 56-year-old patient with RA who is receiving a paraffin bath treatment for both hands. He did not check the temperature before having the patient put her hands in the bath, and when she puts her hands in, she immediately pulls them out and complains that it is too hot. How should Kaiwan handle this situation? What should he say to the patient? What steps should he take to prevent this from occurring with another patient?

Hot Water Bottle

Hot water bottles often are used at home without any concern for correct technique. Patients should be cautioned to keep the water temperature below 125°F (52°C). The hot water bottle usually can be left in place until it becomes cold. If the patient is a child, the temperature should be kept below 115°F (46°C) to prevent burns. Generally a hot water bottle should not be applied to a child for longer than 15 minutes without a physician's instruction. A hot water bottle that is less than half full conforms better to the body surface and is more comfortable (Procedure 43-2).

SAFETY ALERT

To prevent burns, electric heating pads should be left in place no longer than 30 minutes.

Patient Instructions for Applying a Hot Compress at Home
1. Moisten a clean hand towel with warm water; it should be warm, not hot.
2. Wring it out and fold it to the appropriate size.
3. Place the folded warm moist compress directly on the skin.
4. Cover the towel with plastic to keep in the moist heat.
5. Cover the plastic with a dry towel to help maintain the heat.
6. Apply for as long and as often as the physician orders, usually 20 to 30 minutes at a time.

Therapeutic Ultrasonography

Ultrasound is the energy carried by very-high-frequency sound waves. Audible sounds are the result of sound waves vibrating from 100 to 12,000 hertz (Hz; cycles per second). Ultrasonic waves vibrate at a rate of up to 1 million Hz and cannot be heard by the human ear. The ultrasound transducer contains a quartz crystal that vibrates very rapidly when an electric current is passed through it. It is placed in contact with the body, and the vibrations are passed into the tissues. Because these waves do not travel through air, complete contact with the body must be maintained during treatment by using a coupling agent (a water-soluble gel) between the ultrasound transducer and the skin.

The ultrasound waves cause the tissue to vibrate, generating heat as they penetrate superficial tissues and speeding up circulation to the area. This increases the metabolism in the local area, which has a beneficial effect on the body's healing process. Because ultrasound waves travel best through water, they penetrate deeper into body

PROCEDURE 43-2

Assist the Physician with Patient Care: Assist with Moist Heat Application

GOAL: *To apply moist heat to a body area to increase circulation, increase metabolism, and relax muscles.*

EQUIPMENT and SUPPLIES

- Commercial hot moist heat packs
- Towel
- Patient's record

PROCEDURAL STEPS

1. Sanitize your hands.
2. Explain the procedure to the patient and answer any questions.
3. Ask the patient to remove all jewelry from the area to be treated.
   PURPOSE: To prevent trauma to the area and the collection of heat at the jewelry site.
4. Place one or two towel layers over the area to be treated.
   PURPOSE: To prevent trauma and a burn in the area.
5. Apply the commercial moist heat packs (Figure 1).

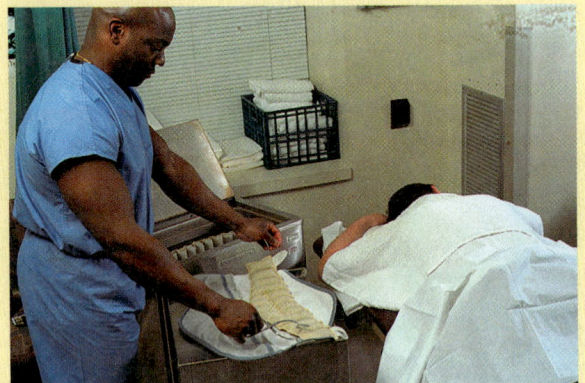

6. Cover with the remaining portion of the towel.
7. Advise the patient to leave the heat pack in place no longer than 20 to 30 minutes, off for the same amount of time, and then repeat if needed.
   CAUTION: Monitor the patient for complaints of discomfort or signs of a burn, including erythema and blister formation.
8. Record the procedure in the patient's medical record.
   PURPOSE: A procedure is not considered done until it is recorded.

9/2/XX 8:35 AM Commercial moist heat pack applied to cervical/thoracic region as ordered for 20 min. Pt states muscle cramps relieved. Instructed to continue moist heat packs at home q 2 hr for 20 min for relief of muscular pain. Cautioned pt about danger of accidental burn to the area. To return to office 9/6/XX for F/U. K. Tillman, CMA (AAMA) _____

---

tissues with a high water content, such as muscles. Ultrasonography may reduce pain and increase the rate of collagen synthesis, which promotes healing. Bone tissue contains almost no water, therefore ultrasonography must be used very carefully around bony areas, because the waves may concentrate and cause damage (Procedure 43-3).

Massage and Exercise

Massage is the systematic, therapeutic stroking or kneading of the body or a body part, which can effectively relieve or significantly reduce both localized and referred pain. Medical assistants are not usually asked to perform therapeutic massage on patients, but you should be familiar with the terminology.

A growing branch of healthcare uses exercise to aid muscle relaxation, promote healing, and provide relief from tension and pain caused by stress or a wide variety of physical disorders. Exercise also can be used to restore mobility, coordination, and strength. If the motion in a joint is restricted even for a short time, the joint tissues become dense, hard, and shortened. These changes can begin to

occur in as little as 4 days. This can be prevented or reduced by the use of active or passive exercises.

In active exercise, the patient initiates and controls movements of a particular part of the body. Special equipment may be used, such as stationary bicycles, treadmills, and/or weight machines. In passive exercise, the therapist moves the body part without the voluntary action of the patient. Both active and passive exercises can be performed to maintain normal ROM or to remedy diminished ROM after an injury.

Electrical Muscle Stimulation

An electrical stimulation unit is a low-voltage machine that creates a controlled electrical current, which is applied to the patient through disposable gel electrodes. This low-voltage current is useful for stimulating the motor and sensor nerves that supply muscles. Stimulation provides a passive means of exercising a muscle when a patient cannot activate the muscle voluntarily because of injury. Electrical muscle stimulation frequently is used to prevent atrophy of a normal muscle.

PROCEDURE 43-3

Assist the Physician with Patient Care: Assist with Therapeutic Ultrasonography

GOAL: *To apply ultra-high-frequency sound waves to deep tissues for therapy. (This is done only under the supervision of the physician or a physical therapist.)*

EQUIPMENT and SUPPLIES

- Ultrasound machine
- Ultrasound gel or lotion
- Paper towels
- Patient's record

PROCEDURAL STEPS

1. Prepare the equipment and sanitize your hands.
2. Confirm the patient's identity.
3. Explain the procedure and tell the patient to notify you of any discomfort during the procedure.
   <u>PURPOSE:</u> To ensure that the patient does not experience any pain or injury.
4. Ask the patient about the presence of any internal or external metal objects.
   <u>PURPOSE:</u> Metal objects must be avoided during the ultrasound procedure.
5. Position the patient comfortably, with the area to be treated exposed.
6. Apply a warmed ultrasound gel liberally over the area to be treated and to the applicator head.
   <u>PURPOSE:</u> To transmit the sound waves effectively through a water-based medium.
7. Begin the treatment with the intensity control at the lowest setting.
8. Set the timer on the machine to the ordered time.
   <u>PURPOSE:</u> The timer starts the machine.
9. Slowly increase the intensity control to the ordered amount.
10. Hold the applicator with the head firmly and completely against the patient's skin over the ultrasound gel in the treatment area (Figure 1).

11. Work the applicator over the area to be treated by moving it continuously in a circular fashion at a speed of 2 inches per second or as directed by the physician.
12. Keep the applicator head in contact with the patient's skin at all times while the machine is on and keep it moving continuously during the treatment time.
    <u>PURPOSE:</u> The applicator head becomes overheated when not in contact with the body and may burn the patient. Constant motion prevents hot spots from occurring as a result of the accumulation of excessive ultrasonic waves in one area.
13. When the timer sounds, the machine shuts off automatically. You then can safely lift the applicator head away from the patient.
14. Return the intensity control to zero.
15. Remove the ultrasound gel from the patient's skin and from the applicator head with a tissue or paper towel. Sanitize your hands.
16. Help the patient to dress if necessary.
17. Record the procedure in the patient's medical record, including the date, area treated, intensity setting, duration of treatment, and any unusual reactions that may have occurred during treatment. If none occurred, indicate that also.
    <u>PURPOSE:</u> A procedure is not considered done until it is recorded.

9/6/XX 4:33 PM Ultrasound Rx applied to ℞ shoulder @ 3 watts × 6 min. Pt denied discomfort during procedure. Pt states pain relieved, increased muscle relaxation. K. Tillman, CMA (AAMA)

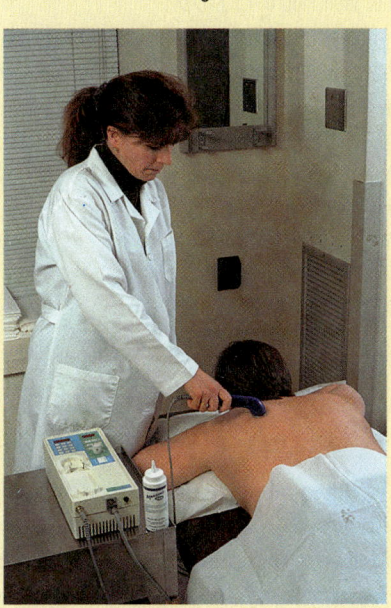

Another means of using electrical stimulation in orthopedics is called *transcutaneous electrical nerve stimulation* (TENS) (Figure 43-20). A TENS unit sends a controlled electrical current through electrodes attached to the skin to help relieve pain caused by arthritis, back injuries, and sports injuries. Because TENS units operate by electrical stimulation, they are not recommended for patients with heart disease and/or cardiac pacemakers.

AMBULATORY DEVICES

Crutches

Axillary crutches are made of wood or aluminum and must be measured to fit the patient as described in Procedure 43-4 and Figure 43-21. It is very important to fit the crutches properly and to make sure the patient understands the importance of not bearing weight

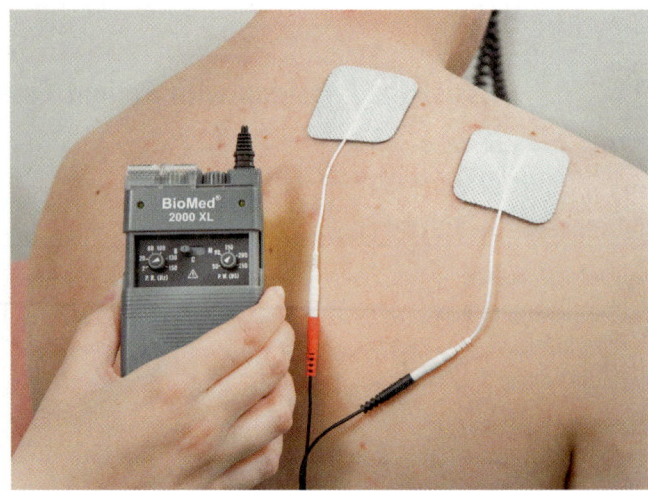

FIGURE 43-20 Transcutaneous electrical nerve stimulation (TENS) unit application.

PROCEDURE 43-4

Assist the Physician with Patient Care: Teach the Patient Crutch Walking and the Swing-Through Gait

GOAL: *To fit crutches accurately and to teach the patient to use the crutches properly in three-point walking.*

EQUIPMENT and SUPPLIES

- Crutches with arm pads and foam handgrips
- Patient's record

PROCEDURAL STEPS

1. Fit the crutches to the patient so that they are 1 to 1½ inches (2 fingerwidths) below the armpits when they are standing up straight. The handgrips should be even with the top of the hip line.
2. Make sure all wing nuts are tight.
3. Make sure the foam pads at the armpits and around the handgrips are comfortable.
4. Instruct the patient to keep the injured leg as relaxed as possible and slightly bent at the knee.
5. The patient's elbow should be bent approximately 30 degrees when holding the handgrip.
6. Place the crutch tips about 2 inches in front of each foot and approximately 6 inches to the side of each foot before beginning crutch walking.
7. Ask the patient to push down on the crutches and lift the body slightly, nearly straightening the arms. The patient should hold the top of the crutches tightly to the sides and use the hands to absorb the weight. Do not let the tops of the crutches press into the armpits.
   PURPOSE: To prevent injury to the muscles and nerves of the axillary region.
8. Have the patient swing the body forward about 12 inches (see Figure 43-21, C).
   PURPOSE: The swing-through gait is one of the fastest crutch gaits that can be used, but it requires a great deal of energy and upper body strength.
9. Instruct the patient to stand on the good leg, then move the crutches just ahead of the good foot, and repeat.

10. Additional crutch gait patterns can be taught as needed:
    - Two-point crutch gait: Move the left crutch and the right foot together, then the right crutch and the left foot together. Repeat. This gait is used if both legs are weak; it can be a challenge for the patient to learn the pattern (see Figure 43-21, A).
    - Three-point crutch gait: Move both crutches and the affected leg forward, then bear weight down through the crutches and move the unaffected leg forward. Repeat. This gait is used if the patient is unable to bear weight on one leg (see Figure 43-21, B).
    - Four-point crutch gait: Move the right crutch forward, then the left foot, followed by the left crutch and then the right foot. This gait provides the best stability but is slow; it can be helpful if both legs are weak (see Figure 43-21, D).
11. *Stairs:* Face the steps, hold the handrail with one hand, and tuck both crutches under the armpit on the other side. To go up the steps, start with the uninjured side, keeping the injured side raised behind. When going down, hold the injured foot up in front and hop down each stair on the good foot. If the stairway does not have handrails, use the crutches under both arms and hop up or down each step on the uninjured leg. If necessary, the patient can sit on the stairs and move up or down each step.
12. Document the patient education intervention in the patient's record.
    PURPOSE: A procedure is not considered done until it is recorded.

9/7/XX 3:17 PM Pt instructed in crutch walking using 3-point gait on steps and floor. Pt understands need to avoid weight bearing on ① leg. Pt demonstrated technique s̄ difficulty. K. Tillman, CMA (AAMA) _____

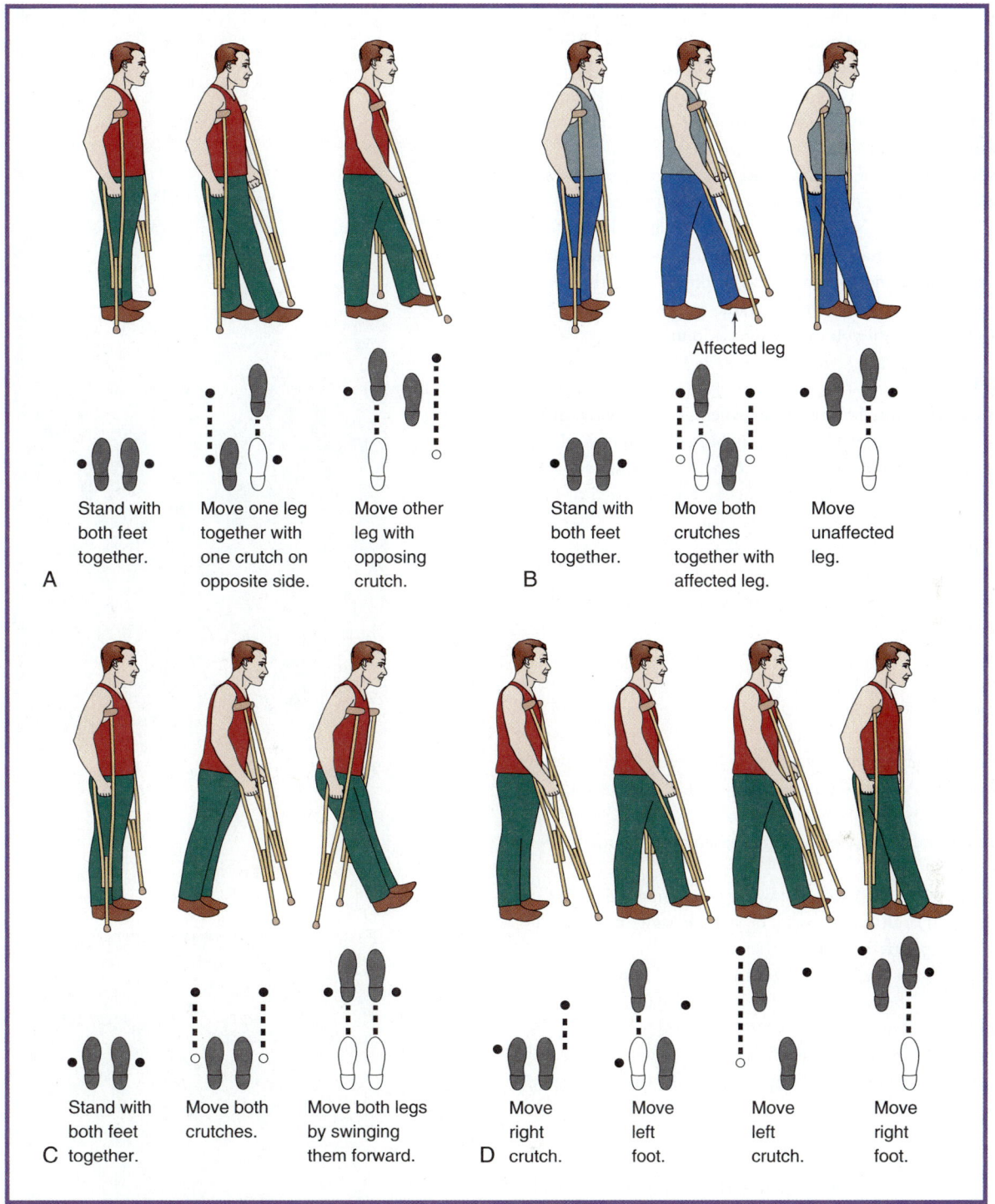

Affected leg

A
Stand with both feet together.

Move one leg together with one crutch on opposite side.

Move other leg with opposing crutch.

B
Stand with both feet together.

Move both crutches together with affected leg.

Move unaffected leg.

C
Stand with both feet together.

Move both crutches.

Move both legs by swinging them forward.

D
Move right crutch.

Move left foot.

Move left crutch.

Move right foot.

FIGURE 43-21 Crutch gaits. **A,** Two-point crutch gait. **B,** Three-point crutch gait. **C,** Swing-through gait. **D,** Four-point crutch gait.

in the axillary region. If the crutch is too long or the handgrips are too low or if the patient leans forward bearing weight on the armpit, serious injury can occur to the nerves in the brachial plexus. Patient guidelines for the correct use of crutches include the following:
- Wear flat shoes with nonskid soles to prevent accidents.
- Bear weight on your hands and the handgrips, not on your armpits.
- Report any numbness or tingling of the upper body or arms to the physician; this may indicate nerve damage from axillary weight bearing.

- Keep your elbows close to your body so that the crutches are against your side.
- Place the crutch tips about 2 inches to the side of each foot so that you do not trip over them.
- Keep your elbows slightly bent when doing crutch walking.
- Keep your head up; do not look at your feet when using your crutches.
- Make sure the crutch tips, handgrip pads, and axillary pads on your crutches are in good condition at all times.
- Remove all throw rugs to keep from tripping or sliding.

- To stand up from a chair: Place both crutches on the injured side, tilt forward and push off with the arm on your uninjured side while bearing weight on the uninjured leg.
- To sit down: Place both crutches on the uninjured side, ease yourself down onto the chair while bearing weight with the uninjured arm and leg.
- To get into and out of a car: Make sure the front seat is moved back as much as possible. Back up toward the seat until you feel its edge; hold both crutches on the side of the body closest to the car door; grab the seat's head rest, tilt your head forward so that you do not bump it, and sit down. Place the heel of your uninjured leg on the car frame and push yourself back into the seat until you can swing the injured leg into the car.

Walkers

Walkers are used primarily by geriatric patients to help with balance and support. A walker's wide base helps stabilize the gait of weakened patients and can support up to 50% of the patient's body weight. Walkers are made of aluminum and can easily be adjusted to fit an individual. They are lightweight, can fold flat for storage and traveling, and can be equipped with a front pack to carry personal items or supplies. They also can be fitted with a fold-down seat. The disadvantage of a walker is that it cannot be used in small, cramped quarters.

To adjust the height of a walker, have the patient stand by the examination table. The top of the walker should be just below the patient's waist at the same height as the top of the hip bone. If the walker has been correctly adjusted to the patient, the patient's elbows will bend about 30 degrees while he or she uses the walker (Figure 43-22). Patient guidelines for walker use include the following:

- Lift the walker and place it about an arm's length in front of you.
- Take your first step with the weaker leg, using the walker for support. If both legs are weak or you are using the walker for general support, start with either leg.
- Take smaller, slower steps than usual; if you step too close to the front of the walker, you can lose your balance.
- Hold your head up and look straight ahead.
- To sit down, back up with the walker until you feel the back of the chair against your legs; let go of the walker and reach back for the chair; slowly lower yourself into the chair.

Canes

Canes are available in a variety of designs (Figure 43-23). The single-tipped cane with a curved handgrip is indicated for individuals who need only minimal assistance with walking. Another type is the legged cane, which has a tripod or quad base. This base provides greater stability for the patient than does a single-tipped cane. It is heavier and is recommended for patients who need greater support.

To fit a cane properly, have the patient stand up straight and measure the distance from the wrist crease to the floor. If the patient is age 70 or older or finds that extra length would feel more comfortable, up to 2 inches can be added to the previous measurement. This is the total length of the cane fitted to the patient. The patient's elbow should be bent to approximately 20 to 30 degrees if the cane has been correctly adjusted.

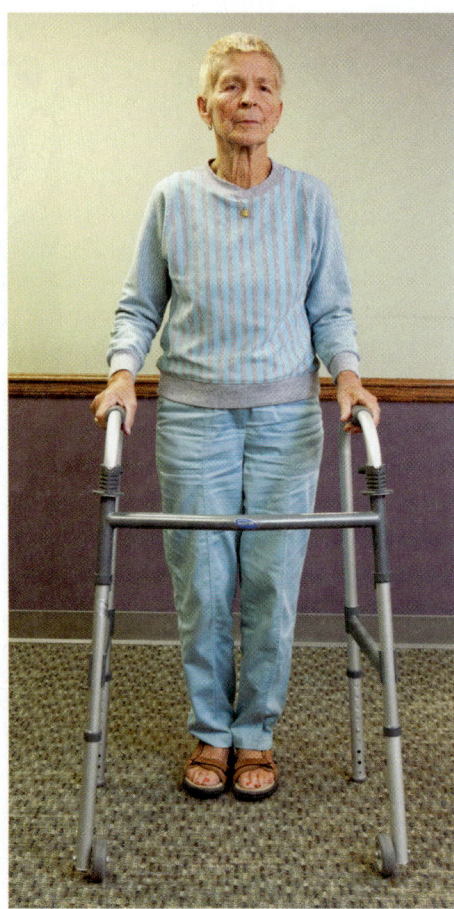

FIGURE 43-22 Properly fitted walker. Note the angle of the arms and the height of the walker.

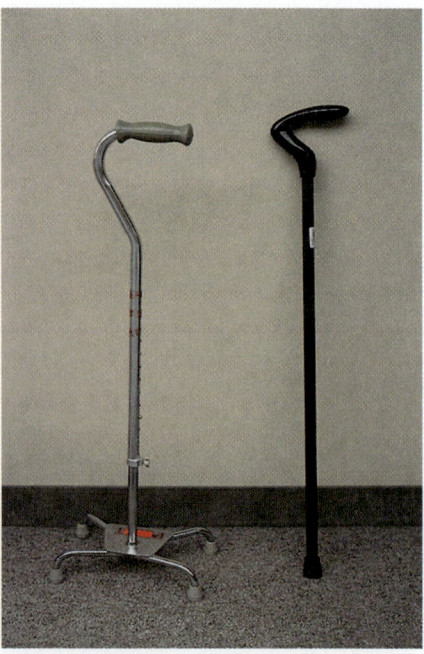

FIGURE 43-23 Types of standard canes. (From DeWit S: *Fundamental concepts and skills for nursing,* ed 3, St Louis, 2009, Saunders.)

Canes typically are used to help a patient with balance problems, to widen the base of support so that falls are less likely, and to reduce weight bearing on an affected leg. To walk safely with a cane, the patient needs to be taught the following steps:

- Always use the cane on the side opposite the affected leg so that it can provide additional support as you walk through the step.
- The cane and the injured or weak leg should be advanced at the same time so that the cane and the leg are hitting the ground at the same time.
- Start by positioning the cane one small stride ahead on the strong side and step off with the injured leg, finishing the step with the stronger leg.
- Bear weight with the arm holding the cane as needed.
- The unaffected leg should bear the weight through the step.

Wheelchairs

Wheelchairs provide mobility for patients who cannot walk or who are able to walk only short distances. With a manual wheelchair, the patient uses arm muscles for mobility. Wheelchairs also come with motors that can be controlled by the patient. The patient is referred to an orthopedic appliance store, where the appropriate wheelchair is fitted to the individual.

> **SAFETY ALERT**
> Always set the brakes on a wheelchair before transferring the patient into or out of the chair.

ASSISTING WITH CASTING

When a cast is to be used to immobilize a fracture or sprain, the medical assistant must know the type of cast to be applied (Procedures 43-5 and 43-6). Possibilities for casting material include plaster of paris, fiberglass or plastic, synthetic material, or air casts. Plaster of paris is the oldest casting material. It is formed by briefly soaking rolls of casting material that have been impregnated with calcium sulfate (i.e., plaster of paris) in warm water, then rolling them around the fracture site. This forms a wet bandage that easily conforms to the extremity; the surface is rubbed smooth and then allowed to dry and harden. Fiberglass casting material has fiber or resin impregnated in the roller gauze and is applied in a similar fashion. A fiberglass cast is stronger, weighs less, and is relatively waterproof.

Before any type of cast is applied, the area first is wrapped with cotton padding to protect the skin. To immobilize the injured area, the splint or cast must cover the joints above and below the fracture. If the site is edematous, a splint may be used until the swelling

---

PROCEDURE 43-5

Assist the Physician with Patient Care: Assist with Application of a Cast

GOAL: *To assist the physician in applying a fiberglass cast.*

EQUIPMENT and SUPPLIES

- Rolls of fiberglass
- Basin casting material
- Bandage
- Stockinette
- Gloves for physician and medical assistant
- Sheet wadding and/or spongy padding
- Stand to support foot (lower extremity)
- Tape
- Scissors
- Water
- Patient's record

Procedural Steps

1. Sanitize your hands.
2. Identify the patient.
3. Explain the procedure for applying a cast and answer any questions.
   PURPOSE: Knowing what to expect reassures the patient. Questions about the injury should be directed to the physician.
4. Assemble the necessary equipment.
5. Seat the patient comfortably, as directed by the physician. If the cast is being applied to the lower extremity, the toes must be supported by a stand.
   PURPOSE: The amount of flexion of the ankle can be controlled by supporting the toes so that the patient can more easily maintain the desired position without fatigue.
6. Clean the area that the cast will cover. Note any objective signs and ask about subjective symptoms (chart them at the end of the procedure).
   PURPOSE: The condition of the area under the cast must be noted before the cast is applied, so that it can be compared with the site when the cast is removed. Clean the area with a mild soap solution or as directed. Dry thoroughly.
7. Cut the stockinette to fit the area the cast will cover.

PROCEDURE 43-5—cont'd

8. Apply the stockinette smoothly to the area the cast will cover. Leave 1 or 2 inches of excess stockinette above and below the cast area to finish the cast (Figure 1).

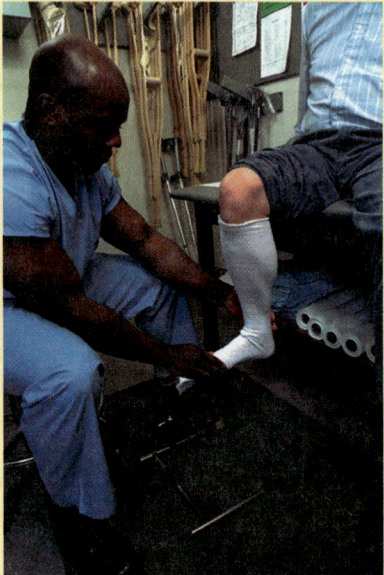

9. Excess stockinette may be cut away where wrinkles form, such as at the front of the ankle (Figure 2).

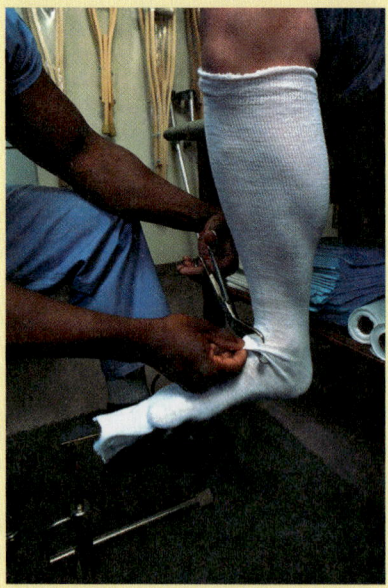

PURPOSE: Stockinette must lie smoothly and cannot be too bulky or wrinkled, because this may cause a pressure wound.

10. Apply sheet wadding along the length of the cast using a spiral bandage turn. Extra padding may be used over bony prominences, such as the bones of the elbow or ankle (Figure 3).

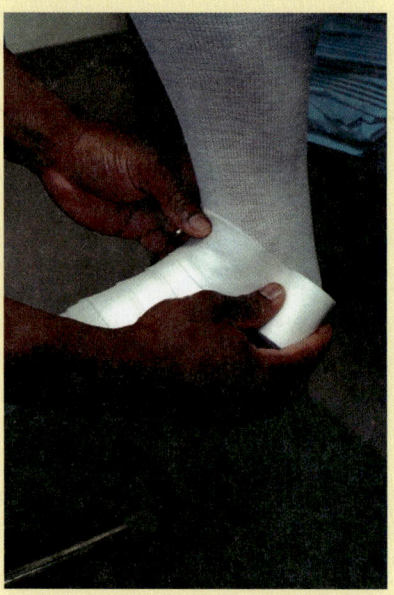

PURPOSE: Padding the cast helps reduce pressure against bony prominences, which could cause skin breakdown.

11. Put on gloves.
12. With lukewarm water in the basin, wet the fiberglass tape as directed by the physician (Figure 4).

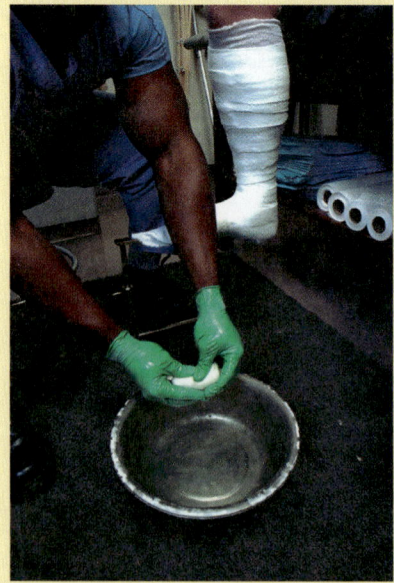

PURPOSE: Immersing the roll of fiberglass tape in water begins the chemical reaction that will cause the cast to harden. The cast can be shaped while wet and will harden in the shape that is formed.

13. Assist as directed as the physician applies the inner layer of fiberglass tape (shown in the photograph as beige). A length of 1 to 2 inches of stockinette is rolled over the inner layer of the cast to form a smooth edge when the outer layer is applied (Figure 5).

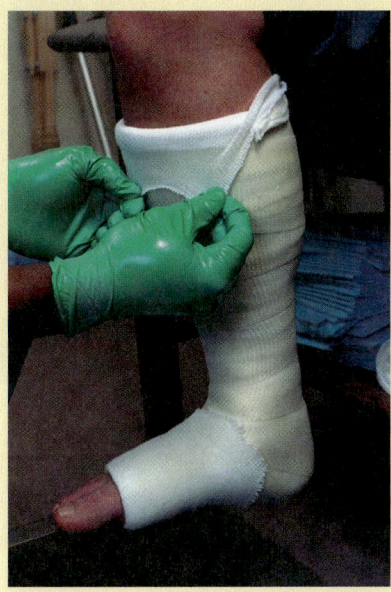

14. Assist as directed by the physician to open and apply an outer layer of fiberglass tape (shown in the photograph as blue) (Figure 6).

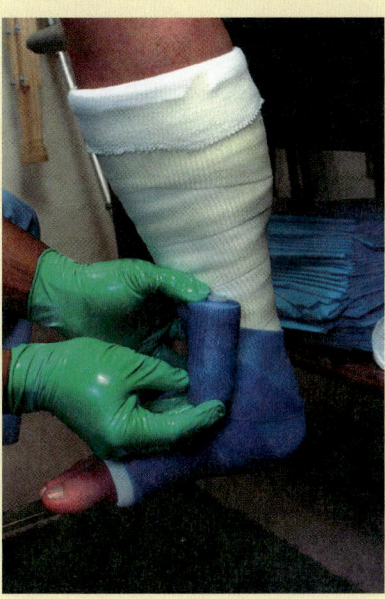

15. Help shape the cast as directed. All contours must be smooth (Figure 7).

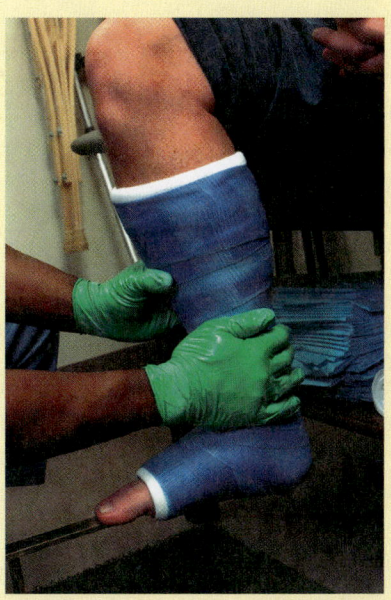

(Modified from Hunt SA: *Saunders fundamentals of medical assisting,* Philadelphia, 2001, WB Saunders.)

PURPOSE: If flat or dented areas develop on the cast, they may cause pressure on the skin below.

16. Discard the water and excess materials. Remove your gloves and wash your hands.

17. Reassure the patient, review cast care verbally, and provide written instructions.

18. Document observations and the procedure in the patient's record.

PURPOSE: A procedure is not considered done until it is recorded in the patient's medical record.

9/8/XX 1 PM Assisted with application of knee to toe cast to ℞ leg. Skin under cast dry and intact. Pt given written instructions on cast care. Material reviewed s̄ questions. Instructed to call physician if there is numbness, tingling, swelling of toes, blue discoloration. K. Tillman, CMA (AAMA)

PROCEDURE 43-6

Assist the Physician with Patient Care: Assist with Cast Removal

GOAL: *To remove a cast.*

EQUIPMENT and SUPPLIES

- Cast cutter
- Cast spreader
- Large bandage scissors
- Basin of warm water
- Mild soap
- Towel
- Skin lotion
- Patient's record

PROCEDURAL STEPS

1. Explain the procedure to the patient.
   <u>PURPOSE:</u> To allay the patient's anxiety and ensure cooperation.
2. Provide adequate support for the limb throughout the procedure.
   <u>PURPOSE:</u> To ensure the patient's comfort.
3. Make a cut on the medial and lateral sides of the long axis of the cast (Figure 1).

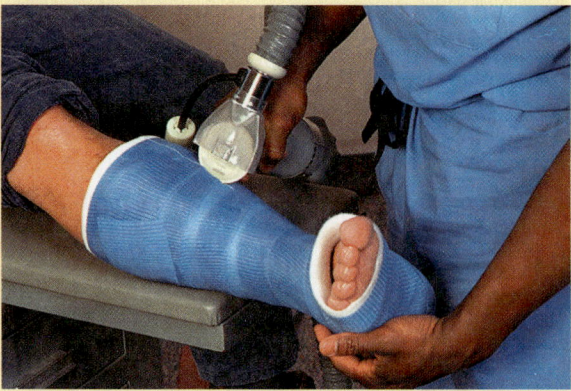

4. Pry the two halves apart using the cast spreader (Figure 2).

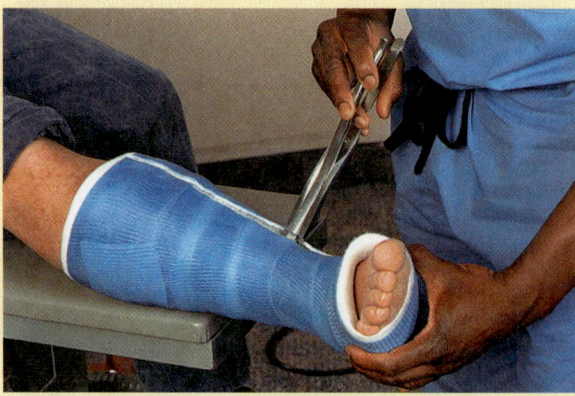

5. Carefully remove the two parts of the cast.
6. Use large bandage scissors to cut away the stockinette and padding remaining.
7. Gently wash the area that was covered by the cast with mild soap and warm water.
   <u>PURPOSE:</u> To ensure the patient's comfort.
8. Dry the area and apply a gentle skin lotion.
   <u>PURPOSE:</u> To ensure the patient's comfort.
9. Give the patient appropriate instructions about exercising and using the limb, as directed by the physician.
   <u>PURPOSE:</u> To enhance continued healing, restore lost strength, and prevent injury.
10. Record the procedure in the patient's medical record.
    <u>PURPOSE:</u> A procedure is not considered done until it is recorded.

---

subsides, at which time a full cast is applied. In some cases a cast may have to be replaced as the swelling diminishes if the patient reports that the cast is too big. As a fracture heals, the physician may decide to remove the cast and apply a splint until the fracture has mended completely. A patient may call the office complaining that the splint or cast feels tight. Swelling typically occurs in the first 48 to 72 hours after the injury. The patient should be told to elevate the injured part above the heart to help collected fluid drain from the site; to gently move the fingers or toes at the affected area to improve circulation; and to apply ice around the splint or cast in a plastic bag at the level of the injury to help reduce swelling.

If the patient needs to wear a cast only when using the limb, synthetic casts are available in the shape of a boot or sleeve with Velcro fasteners that fit like a sandwich over the fracture to immobilize the area. An air cast is a temporary cast that is inflated around the limb to immobilize it. The type of cast used depends on the location and severity of the injury, the patient's age and occupation, and the physician's preference.

WARNING SIGNS AFTER APPLICATION OF A SPLINT OR CAST

The patient should be told to contact the physician's office if any of the following occurs after the application of a splint or cast:

- Increased pain and/or a feeling that the splint or cast is too tight
- Numbness and tingling in the affected hand or foot, indicating pressure on the nerves
- Burning and stinging because of pressure on the skin
- Excessive swelling below the cast, which may mean the cast is slowing circulation
- Loss of active movement of toes or fingers (this requires an urgent evaluation by the physician)

CRITICAL THINKING APPLICATION 43-9

Kaiwan has just finished helping Dr. Alexander put a cast on the arm of a 6-year-old girl who fell out of her neighbor's tree house and fractured her radius. Her mother wants to take her home immediately. Should the patient be allowed to leave immediately? Why? What might happen?

- Do not stick objects (e.g., coat hangers) inside the splint or cast to scratch itching skin; if itching persists, contact your physician.
- Do not break off rough edges of the cast or trim the cast before asking your physician.
- Inspect the skin around the cast; if it is red or raw, contact your physician.
- Inspect the cast regularly; let your physician know if it becomes cracked or develops soft spots.

CLOSING COMMENTS

Patient Education

An informed patient is better prepared to continue with home care. Musculoskeletal conditions, particularly arthritis, can be so painful and debilitating that these patients may be easy prey for miracle drug promotions. It is important for you to recognize the need for patient education about the condition and to work diligently with the patient and family to encourage participation in effective care programs. When you work with the physician and the physical therapist in helping the patient, you become an important member of the healthcare team. This type of involvement leads to patient satisfaction and to personal satisfaction and achievement for the medical assistant.

PATIENT EDUCATION FOR THE CARE OF A SPLINT OR CAST

The American Academy of Orthopedic Surgeons has made the following recommendations for caring for a cast or splint:

- Keep the device dry; moisture weakens the plaster, and damp padding can irritate the skin. Use two layers of plastic or buy waterproof shields to keep the splint or cast dry while you shower or bathe. In special circumstances, the physician can apply a waterproof cast.
- Do not walk on a "walking cast" until it is completely dry and hard; it takes at least 1 hour for fiberglass and 2 to 3 days for plaster to become hard enough to walk on.
- Prevent dirt, sand, and powder from getting inside the splint or cast.
- Do not pull out the padding.

Legal and Ethical Issues

Working with orthopedic patients may involve assisting with assessments and performing procedures that directly involve the patient's recovery plan. Many of the procedures in this chapter are not the basic procedures you will be required to perform when you are first hired as a medical assistant. These techniques all involve additional on-the-job training and practice. Before performing any of the described procedures, you should check with your local and state medical assistant organizations about the laws in your state. Whenever you perform the procedures and techniques described in this chapter, you are responsible for them. The following steps are all required before you perform any procedure on a patient:

- You must have a written order before performing a procedure.
- You must follow the procedure precisely as it is ordered, without variation.
- Never advise the patient without permission.
- Make sure you know what instructions the physician gave the patient.
- Reinforce the instructions the physician gave the patient.
- If you have any concerns about a procedure, discuss them with the physician privately before proceeding.
- Do not perform a procedure if you are uncomfortable; get someone to help you.

Always remember: You are the assistant, and this is the physician's patient. The physician ultimately is responsible for every aspect of the patient's care. If you feel uncertain or unsure of any order the physician has written for a patient, you must get it clarified before you proceed. Always stay within the legal and ethical guidelines of the medical assisting profession in your state.

SUMMARY OF SCENARIO

Kaiwan is becoming more and more comfortable in his position as an orthopedic medical assistant at the sports medicine clinic. His enthusiasm is contagious. Patients consistently comment on his positive, upbeat manner. Kaiwan is motivated to learn new methods of better assisting the physicians with routine procedures. He always seeks answers to questions that occur with new patients. He has gained a great deal of confidence and now remembers always to check the temperature of the paraffin bath before starting a treatment. One of the most enjoyable aspects of his job continues to be assisting Dr. Alexander with treating the team members. Kaiwan has attended two continuing education seminars in sports medicine with Dr. Alexander. He now is thinking about continuing his education part time to become an athletic trainer while still working at the clinic. Kaiwan recognizes the importance of continuing education in maintaining orthopedic skills.

SUMMARY OF LEARNING OBJECTIVES

1. **Define, spell, and pronounce the terms listed in the vocabulary.**
   Spelling and pronouncing medical terms correctly bolster the medical assistant's credibility. Knowing the definitions of these terms promotes confidence in communication with patients and co-workers.

2. **Apply critical thinking skills in performing patient assessment and patient care.**
   Completing the Critical Thinking Application exercises throughout the chapter can help the student medical assistant become more adept at critical analysis of real-life situations.

3. **Describe the principal anatomic structures of the musculoskeletal system and their functions.**
   The main structures of the musculoskeletal system are the skeletal muscles, which provide movement; tendons, which connect muscles to bones; bones, which provide support, protection, mineral storage, and blood cell development; and ligaments, which connect bone to bone.

4. **Differentiate among tendons, bursae, and ligaments.**
   Tendons are the tough bands that connect muscles to bones; ligaments provide support by connecting bone to bone and preventing a joint from moving beyond its normal ROM. Bursae prevent friction between different tissues in the musculoskeletal system.

5. **Summarize the major muscular disorders.**
   Fibromyalgia is a condition of unknown origin that causes widespread connective tissue and muscular pain, along with sleep disorders and extreme fatigue. Myasthenia gravis is an autoimmune disorder that affects the use of ACh at the neuromuscular junction, resulting in muscular weakness, especially in the face and eyes. A sprain is the tearing of ligaments and a strain is the overstretching or tearing of a muscle or tendon.

6. **Identify and describe the common types of fractures.**
   The common types of fractures are explained in Table 43-3.

7. **Explain the difference between osteomalacia and osteoporosis.**
   Osteomalacia is softening of the bones, which occurs because of a problem with the metabolism or absorption of vitamin D, calcium, and phosphorus; in children the condition is called *rickets*. Osteoporosis is a reduction in bone density, which can be caused by many factors, including lack of dietary calcium early in life; it leads to brittle bones that fracture easily.

8. **Classify typical spinal column disorders.**
   Spinal column disorders are related to the shape of the spine: scoliosis is a lateral deviation; lordosis (swayback) is a pronounced curve of the lower back; and kyphosis is a pronounced cervical curve, or hunchback.

9. **Differentiate among the various joint disorders.**
   Joint disorders include dislocations, in which the two bones of the joint are no longer approximated; gout, which is a form of arthritis caused by the collection of uric acid crystals, most commonly in the synovial membrane of the great toe; SLE, which is a widespread autoimmune disorder that can affect any organ system in the body; Lyme disease, a form of infectious arthritis caused by bacteria transmitted via a tick bite, can cause extensive joint and neurologic problems if left untreated; OA,

caused by degeneration of the articular cartilage of synovial joints; RA, an autoimmune disorder that causes crippling pain and deformity of the joints; and tendonitis and bursitis, which are inflammatory reactions of supportive tissue typically caused overuse of a joint.

10. **Summarize the medical assistant's role in assisting with orthopedic procedures.**
    The medical assistant is responsible for gathering and recording a detailed history of the patient's presenting problem; providing the patient with assistance as needed; and assisting with the orthopedic examination.

11. **Explain the common diagnostic procedures used in orthopedics.**
    Common diagnostic procedures routinely performed in the orthopedic office include ROM evaluation, inspection, palpation, percussion, muscle strength evaluation, and x-ray studies. Other diagnostic tools include arthrograms, myelograms, bone scans, CT, MRI, electromyography, biopsies, and diagnostic ultrasonography.

12. **Compare and contrast therapeutic modalities used in orthopedic medicine.**
    Therapeutic modalities include the application of cold and heat; paraffin baths; hot water bottles and moist heat packs; therapeutic ultrasonography; massage and therapeutic exercise; and electric muscle stimulation.

13. **Apply cold therapy to an injury.**
    Cold should be used immediately after an injury to help reduce inflammation, inhibit additional swelling, and help relieve pain. The ice pack should remain in place for 20 minutes at a time, several times a day, and the area should be checked for feeling and color after each application (see Procedure 43-1).

14. **Assist with hot moist heat application to an orthopedic injury.**
    Procedure 43-2 lists the steps for the application of heat. Heat should be used on injuries after 48 hours to promote circulation and healing, reduce swelling, and promote soft tissue relaxation in the affected area. Care must be taken to prevent burns.

15. **Properly apply therapeutic ultrasound.**
    Therapeutic ultrasound applies deep tissue heat to an injured area (see Procedure 43-3). It is important to keep the applicator head constantly moving in a circular fashion over the injured site during the treatment.

16. **Explain the use of common ambulatory devices.**
    The most common ambulatory assistive devices are crutches, canes, walkers, and wheelchairs. The most important aspects of using these assistive devices in an orthopedic practice are to fit them properly to the patient and to instruct the patient adequately in how to use the device properly and safely.

17. **Properly fit a patient with crutches and explain the correct mechanics of crutch walking.**
    Procedure 43-4 presents the steps for properly fitting a patient with crutches and explaining the correct mechanics of crutch walking.

18. **Prepare for and assist with the application of a cast.**
    Preparing for and assisting with application of a cast are detailed in Procedure 43-5. The tissue beneath the cast must be safeguarded by

applying a stockinette and sheet wadding. The casting material then is immersed in water and carefully rolled around the limb.

19. **Prepare for and assist with the removal of a cast.**
    Procedure 43-6 presents the steps for preparing for and assisting with cast removal.

20. **Summarize patient education guidelines for orthopedic patients.**
    Musculoskeletal conditions are often painful and debilitating. The medical assistant should recognize the need for patient education and work with the patient, family and healthcare team to promote recovery.

21. **Discuss the legal and ethical implications in an orthopedic practice.**
    Before performing any orthopedic procedures, the medical assistant should check with local and state medical assistant organizations about applicable state laws. Procedures and techniques should be performed only under the direct supervision of the physician.

CONNECTIONS

📖 **Study Guide Connection:** Go to the Chapter 43 Study Guide. Read and complete the activities.

ⓔ **Evolve Connection:** Go to the Chapter 43 link at *evolve.elsevier.com/ kinn* to complete the Chapter Review and Chapter Quiz. Check out the other resources listed for this chapter to make the most of what you have learned from Assisting in Orthopedic Medicine.

44

ASSISTING IN NEUROLOGY AND MENTAL HEALTH

Mai Lee, CMA (AAMA), has been working in Dr. Kim Song's neurology practice for 2 years. Dr. Song has always been pleased with Mai's professional behavior toward all patients in the practice. She is conscientious about charting notes accurately for each of her patients. Dr. Song has just asked Mai to train a new medical assistant in the clinical procedures of the office. He is expanding his clinic hours and wants to have Mai more involved in assisting him with patients, particularly in patient education. She is excited to have additional responsibilities with Dr. Song's patients, and she is quite happy about the raise in salary that goes along with her new position.

While studying this chapter, think about the following questions:

- What is the basic anatomy and physiology of the neurologic system?
- Mai should familiarize herself with what neurologic disorders?
- What are the diagnostic and treatment procedures for typical nervous system disorders?
- What is the medical assistant's role in the neurologic examination?
- Is patient education a significant factor when working with patients diagnosed with either nervous system or mental health disorders?

LEARNING OBJECTIVES

1. Define, spell, and pronounce the terms listed in the vocabulary.
2. Apply critical thinking skills in performing the patient assessment and patient care.
3. Summarize the anatomy and physiology of the nervous system.
4. Differentiate between the central and peripheral nervous systems.
5. Identify the typical symptoms associated with neurologic disorders.
6. Distinguish among common nervous system diseases and conditions.
7. Describe the pathology of cerebrovascular diseases.
8. Identify the various types of epilepsy.
9. Compare and contrast encephalitis and meningitis.
10. Explain the dynamics of brain and spinal cord injuries.
11. Summarize the neurologic diseases that affect mobility.
12. Differentiate among common mental health disorders.
13. Analyze the medical assistant's role in the neurologic examination.
14. Explain the common diagnostic procedures for the nervous system.
15. Outline the steps needed to prepare a patient for an electroencephalogram (EEG).
16. Describe the steps for preparing a patient for and assisting with a lumbar puncture.
17. Discuss the implications of patient education in a neurologic and mental health practice.
18. Explain the legal issues and Health Insurance Portability and Accountability Act (HIPAA) applications associated with neurology and mental health.

VOCABULARY

anomalies (uh-noh'-muh-lez) Deformities or deviations from a normal condition, resulting from faulty development of a fetus.

ataxia (uh-taks'-e-uh) Failure or irregularity of muscle actions and coordination.

aura A peculiar sensation that precedes the appearance of a more definite disturbance.

benign Not cancerous and not recurring.

blood-brain barrier An anatomic-physiologic structure made up of astrocyte glial cells that prevents or slows the transfer of chemicals into the neurons of the central nervous system (CNS).

coma An unconscious state from which the patient cannot be aroused.

compression The state of being pressed together.

contralateral (kon-trah-la'-tehr-uhl) Pertaining to the opposite side of the body.

cryptogenic (krip-tuh-je'-nik) Pertaining to a disease with an unknown cause.

embolus A foreign material that blocks a blood vessel; frequently a blood clot that has traveled from some other part of the body.

ipsilateral (ips-uh-la'-tehr-uhl) Pertaining to the same side of the body.

malignant Cancerous.

myelin sheath A segmented, fatty tissue that wraps around the axon of the nerve cell and acts as an electrical insulator to speed the conduction of nerve impulses.

occlusion Complete obstruction of an opening.

papilledema Swelling of the optic disc from increased intracranial pressure.

paresthesia (par-uhs-thee'-zee-uh) An abnormal sensation of burning, prickling, or stinging.

paroxysmal (par-ehk-siz'-muhl) Pertaining to a sudden, recurrent spasm of symptoms.

plaque An abnormal accumulation of a fatty substance.

proprioception The sensation of awareness of body movements and posture; nerve impulses that provide the central nervous system with information about the position of body parts.

radiopaque A substance that can easily be visualized on an x-ray film.

thrombus A blood clot.

transection Cross-section; a division made by cutting across.

turbid Refers to a cloudy solution.

The human brain weighs about 3 pounds, requires about the same amount of energy needed to light a 20-watt bulb, stores more than 100 trillion bits of information, and works better than any computer. The matter that makes up the brain is approximately 85% water and therefore has a soft texture. Early scientists believed that the brain's function was to cool the blood. Today's scientists have shown us that even though the brain receives 20% of the body's blood supply, its function is much more complex than simply cooling blood.

Neurologists specialize in the diagnosis and treatment of medical disorders and conditions of the nervous system. A neurosurgeon provides surgical management and treatment for trauma and other conditions requiring surgery. A psychiatrist is a physician who treats behavioral disorders and neurologic conditions that affect behavior.

ANATOMY AND PHYSIOLOGY OF THE NERVOUS SYSTEM

The nervous system works with the endocrine system to integrate stimuli both from within the body and from the outside environment to regulate body systems so that homeostasis can be maintained. The nervous system is divided into two major parts: the *central nervous system* (CNS), which is made up of the brain and spinal cord, and the *peripheral nervous system* (PNS), which includes all the nervous tissue and neurologic responses found outside the CNS.

The brain is the "president" or "chief executive officer" of the body. It constantly receives information from the periphery, including all the organs and systems inside the body and on its surface. This information (i.e., stimuli) is carried to the brain by the peripheral nerves along the *afferent,* or ascending, tract. The brain monitors and interprets the stimuli received from the afferent nerves and sends appropriate responses back along *efferent* pathways to the organs or to the body's surface. These responses from the brain cause a specific reaction in the organ, in the glands, or in skeletal muscles. These reactions keep the body running smoothly and allow it to react instantly to both external and internal stimuli.

The functioning cell of the nervous system is the neuron (Figure 44-1). The brain contains billions of individual neurons. The nervous system begins very early in embryonic development, by week 3, as the neural tube, which eventually develops into the brain and spinal cord. Each neuron is made up of a main cell body that contains the nucleus and a relatively long extension of the cell, called the *axon,* which may be covered with a **myelin sheath**. Multiple filaments, called *dendrites,* extend from the neuron body. Dendrites receive the nervous impulse from a preceding neuron and carry it into the cell body. Impulses are carried away from the cell body through the axon to another neuron or to cells in another tissue. This transfer of stimuli begins as an electrical impulse that travels down an axon of one neuron and becomes a chemical impulse while moving across the synapse (the space between two neurons) to the dendrite of another neuron. The transfer of impulses from the end of one neuron to the dendrites of another is enhanced by chemical neurotransmitters, which bind to specific receptor sites on the dendrites of the next neuron. If the nerve impulse is traveling to a muscle or to any other organ or tissue instead of another neuron, the chemical neurotransmitters bind to special receptors in the target tissue. Messages move throughout the entire nervous system in this manner. Impulses in the neuron are electrical; the impulses become chemical as a specific

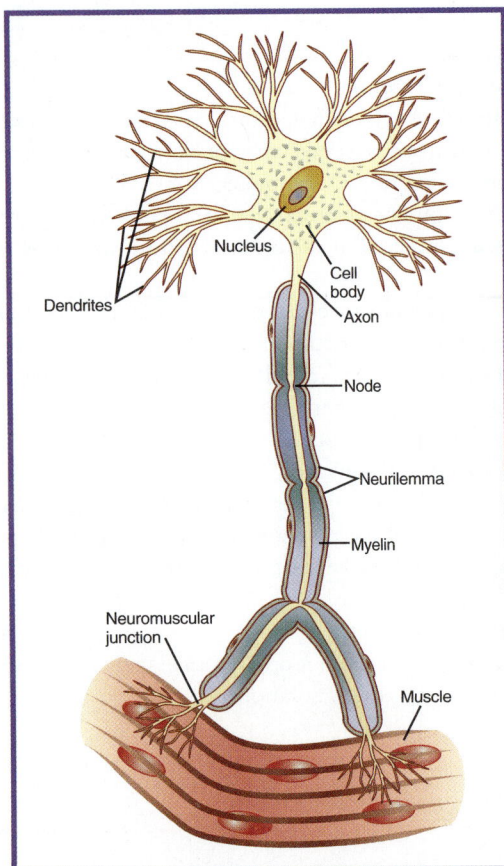

FIGURE 44-1 A neuron.

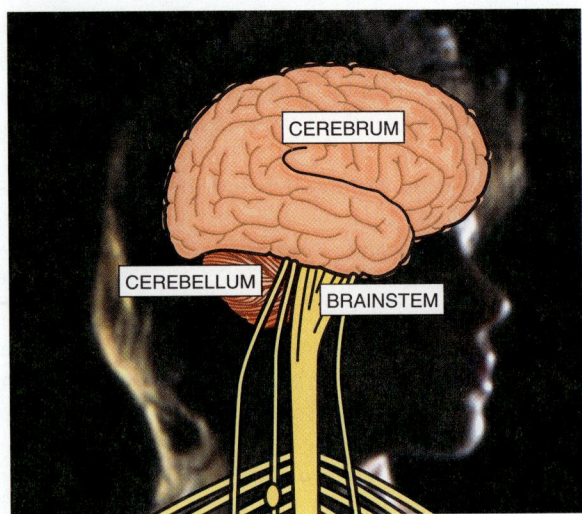

FIGURE 44-2 The brain. (Modified from Chester GA: *Modern medical assisting,* Philadelphia, 1999, WB Saunders.)

neurotransmitter is released at each synapse, and they become electrical again as they are picked up by the subsequent dendrites of another neuron or by the target tissue.

Supportive cells of the nervous system are called *glial* or *neuroglial* cells. These specialized cells perform specific functions in the nervous system; for example, Schwann cells form the myelin sheath, and astrocytes help form the **blood-brain barrier**. However, the glial cells do not carry on any of the functions of the nervous system. The blood-brain barrier closely regulates what substances enter the brain tissue. Oxygen, water, and glucose molecules easily pass into the brain, whereas many chemicals and drugs are prevented from moving into brain tissue. Brain inflammation can increase the ability of many drugs to cross the blood-brain barrier.

WHAT HAPPENS WHEN YOU ACCIDENTALLY TOUCH A HOT IRON

1. Impulses travel to the central nervous system (CNS) along an afferent (sensory neurons) nervous pathway, carrying the information "hot."
2. The CNS performs a hasty analysis and determines that a heat danger is present.
3. The CNS sends a quick, strong message back to skeletal muscles via the efferent (motor neurons) pathway to move the finger immediately.
4. You quickly pull your hand away from the hot iron, preventing a serious burn and maintaining homeostasis.

Central Nervous System

The brain and spinal cord together make up the CNS. The brain is encased within the skull in the cranial cavity. The spinal cord is a bundle of nervous tissue that extends inferiorly from the brainstem at the base of the brain and exits the skull at the foramen magnum. It descends for about 17 inches inside the spinal canal, which courses through the vertebrae of the backbone.

Brain

The brain accounts for only about 2% of a person's weight, but it consumes about 20% of the body's oxygen. The brain is divided into three main areas: the cerebrum, the cerebellum, and the brainstem (Figure 44-2). The cerebrum, the largest and uppermost section of the brain, has multiple convolutions along its surface, called *gyri,* which are formed by the folding in of the cerebral cortex. The gyri are separated by shallow grooves, called *sulci.* The gyri greatly increase the surface area of the cerebrum, which maximizes the potential of the CNS neurons in each area. The cerebrum is divided into lobes, which are named after the region of the skull under which they are located. The cerebrum is separated by a longitudinal fissure into left and right hemispheres. The right hemisphere usually controls artistic functions, such as drawing, rhythm, and picture memory. The left hemisphere controls verbal functions, such as reading, writing, speaking, and mathematic calculations. The diencephalon, located deep in the center of the cerebrum near the superior portion of the brainstem, is made up of the thalamus and the hypothalamus. The thalamus acts as a relay station between sensory neurons and the cerebral cortex. The functions of the hypothalamus include controlling the autonomic nervous system, regulating endocrine processes, and managing body temperature, sleep, and appetite to maintain homeostasis. Within the cerebrum are four spaces, called *ventricles,* which contain cerebrospinal fluid (CSF). CSF nourishes, lubricates, and provides some cushioning protection for the brain and the spinal cord.

The cerebellum is just inferior to the occipital lobe of the cerebrum and controls balance, equilibrium, posture, and muscle coordination. The brainstem controls reflexes and serves as a sensory relay station for input coming into the brain from the body. The brainstem plays a vital role in vision, hearing, respiration, heart rate, blood pressure, waking, and sleeping.

Spinal Cord

The spinal cord extends from the inferior portion of the brainstem to approximately the second lumbar vertebra. Thirty-one pairs of spinal nerves extend from the spinal cord through openings in the vertebrae. Starting just below the first cervical vertebra in the neck, a nerve extends from the spinal cord on each side; therefore, a pair of spinal nerves originates at each level. Each of these pairs of nerves innervates a specific organ or area of the body. The spinal cord carries messages between the spinal nerves and the brain.

Meninges

Because the brain and the spinal cord are critical to life, they are well protected. They both are encased in some of the thickest bones in the body; they also are surrounded by three membranes, called *meninges;* and they are cushioned by the CSF (Figure 44-3).

The outer layer of the meninges is called the *dura mater* ("hard mother"), because it is a tough membrane, similar to a very strong rubber band. The subdural space lies below the dura mater and contains small veins that have little support. Trauma to the head can cause bleeding of these tiny vessels, ultimately leading to the development of a subdural hematoma. Above the dura mater is the epidural space. The arterial supply to the meninges comes from blood

vessels that line the inner aspect of the skull. If the skull is fractured, these arteries can be damaged, resulting in a collection of blood between the skull and the dura mater called an *epidural hematoma.*

The middle meningeal layer is the arachnoid, which was given that name because of its fine spider web appearance. Beneath the arachnoid membrane in the subarachnoid space is the cerebrospinal fluid, a clear liquid that contains glucose, protein, and chloride produced by specialized cells in the ventricles (Table 44-1). CSF circulates continuously through the ventricles and around the brain and spinal cord, carrying nutrients and removing wastes.

The innermost layer, which covers the brain and spinal cord, is the delicate *pia mater* ("tender mother"); it is highly vascular and the thinnest of the three layers. The pia mater provides support for the blood vessels of the brain.

HYDROCEPHALUS

Hydrocephalus is the abnormal accumulation of cerebrospinal fluid (CSF) in the ventricles of the brain. It is the result either of overproduction of CSF or of failure of the fluid to drain properly. If left untreated, hydrocephalus causes gross enlargement of the skull and severe damage to brain tissue from increased intracranial pressure. The only treatment is surgery to place a shunt (tube) from a ventricle in the brain to the right atrium or to the abdominal cavity. The shunt allows the excess CSF to drain away from the brain.

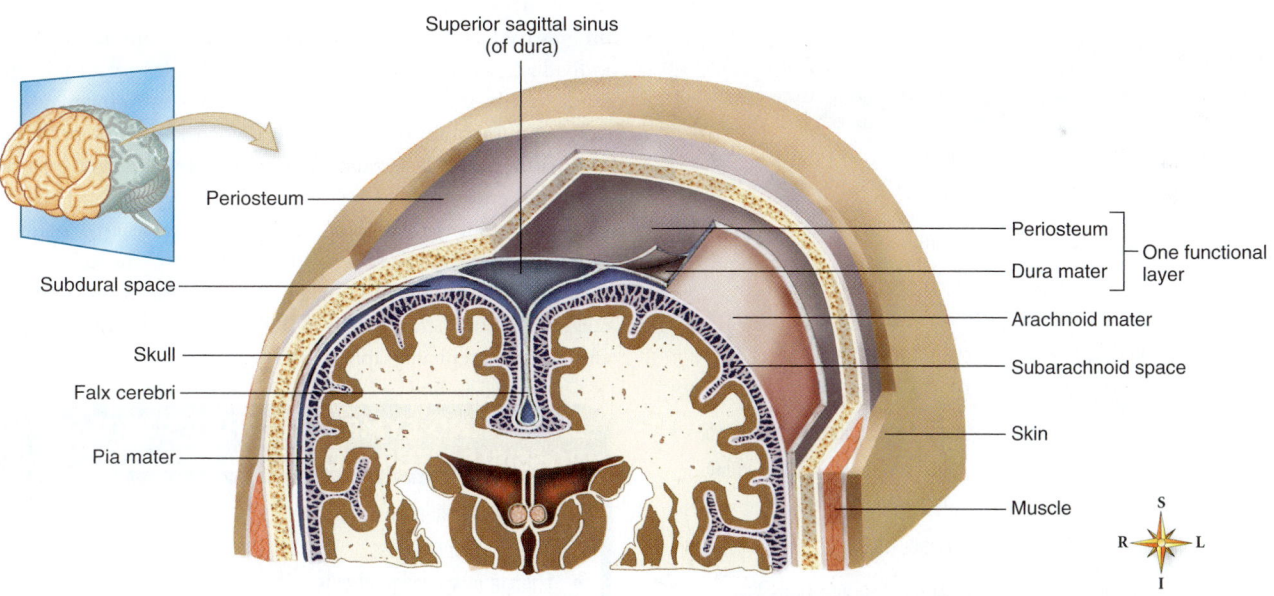

FIGURE 44-3 Protective coverings of the brain. (Modified from Patton K, Thibodeau G: *Anatomy and physiology,* ed 7, St Louis, 2010, Mosby.)

TABLE 44-1 Typical Laboratory Values for Cerebrospinal Fluid

CONDITION	PRESSURE (mm)	APPEARANCE	CELLS	PROTEIN (mg/dL)	GLUCOSE (mg/dL)
Normal	50-200	Clear, colorless	0-10 lymphocytes and monocytes	<45	50-80
Acute bacterial meningitis	200-500	Turbid	100-10,000 granulocytic neutrophils	50-500	Absent or low
Subarachnoid hemorrhage	200-500	Bloody	Red blood cells (RBCs)	50-1000	50-80

Peripheral Nervous System

The PNS is made up of the nerves that exit the brain or spinal cord. The peripheral nerves exiting the brain directly through the cranium are called *cranial nerves.* The spinal nerves from the spinal cord enter and exit the spinal canal through spaces between the vertebrae. Cranial nerves originate from the underside of the brain and relay information to and from the sensory organs and muscles of the face and neck (Table 44-2).

Spinal nerves carry information to and from the brain through the spinal cord. Sensory fibers in these nerves carry stimuli from the skin and internal organs to the CNS. Motor fibers carry messages from the CNS to skeletal muscles, causing them to contract.

The autonomic nervous system (ANS) is part of the PNS. Autonomic nerves control homeostasis, or keep the body running smoothly, much like a thermostat controls the temperature in a room. The ANS (Figure 44-4) is an automatic system that regulates body functions such as breathing, heart rate, sweating, circulation, and digestion. It also controls the actions of muscles in blood vessel walls, organs, and glands. Just as a thermostat can control both heating and cooling in a room to maintain a comfortable temperature, the autonomic system is made up of two divisions, called the *sympathetic system* and the *parasympathetic system.* The sympathetic system promotes responses geared toward protecting the individual ("fight or flight"), generally causing a stimulating effect: it speeds up the heart, raises blood glucose levels and blood pressure, reduces peristalsis, and widens the bronchioles, allowing more oxygen to enter the body quickly. The parasympathetic system generally promotes rest or a reducing effect: it slows the heart rate, constricts the bronchioles, and increases digestive system function.

> ### CRITICAL THINKING APPLICATION   44-1
> Dr. Song mentions a patient's nervous system function to Mai. The patient hears this conversation and asks Mai, "What does my nervous system do?" How should Mai answer this question? What resources could she use to help explain the nervous system to the patient?

DISEASES AND DISORDERS OF THE CENTRAL NERVOUS SYSTEM

Because the CNS and PNS are so complex, diseases and conditions that affect them can produce a wide range of signs and symptoms. Causes include trauma, infection, congenital **anomalies**, degeneration, tumors, and vascular disorders (Table 44-3). The medical assistant needs to listen carefully when a patient describes his or her neurologic symptoms. Many different types of symptoms can indicate a serious condition of the nervous system.

Cerebrovascular Disease

Cerebrovascular disease (CVD) is the third leading cause of death and the most frequent cause of crippling disease in the United States. Generally, CVD is related to arteriosclerosis or atherosclerosis of the cerebral arteries, but it also can be caused by untreated or uncontrolled hypertension, thrombi, or emboli. Arteriosclerosis causes progressive loss of elasticity of the arterial wall and is seen in elderly individuals with CVD. Atherosclerosis, the deposit of fatty **plaque** on the inside of the arterial wall, can involve any of the major arteries supplying the brain or any of their branches. Sudden narrowing, or **occlusion**, may occur when an artery becomes blocked by a **thrombus** or an **embolus**.

CVD usually is diagnosed through cerebral arterial angiography, in which a **radiopaque** dye is injected into the suspect vessel and a radiograph is immediately taken. Other confirming tests include magnetic resonance imaging (MRI), computed tomography (CT), and electroencephalography (EEG).

TABLE 44-2   Cranial Nerves and Their Functions

CRANIAL NERVE	NAME	FUNCTION
I	Olfactory	Smell
II	Optic	Vision
III	Oculomotor	Eye movement Pupil constriction and accommodation
IV	Trochlear	Eye movement
V	Trigeminal	Muscles of chewing General sensations from anterior half of head, including entire face and meninges
VI	Abducent	Eye movement
VII	Facial	Muscles of facial expression Tearing, salivation, and taste
VIII	Vestibulocochlear	Hearing and equilibrium
IX	Glossopharyngeal	Swallowing and taste
X	Vagus	Breathing, speech, sweating, regulating heartbeat, stimulating muscles of gastric region
XI	Spinal accessory	Shoulder and head movements
XII	Hypoglossal	Tongue movements

> ### SIGNS AND SYMPTOMS THAT SUGGEST POSSIBLE NEUROLOGIC PROBLEMS
>
> - Recurrent headache
> - Periodic memory loss
> - Change in sleeping patterns
> - Frequently dropping items
> - Difficulty with particular speech patterns
> - Numbness in a specific body area
> - Visual disturbances or abrupt changes in vision
> - Loss of consciousness
> - Confusion or disorientation as to date, time, and place

Transient Ischemic Attacks

Transient ischemic attacks (TIAs), also called *ministrokes,* occur when the blood supply to a particular part of the brain is inadequate

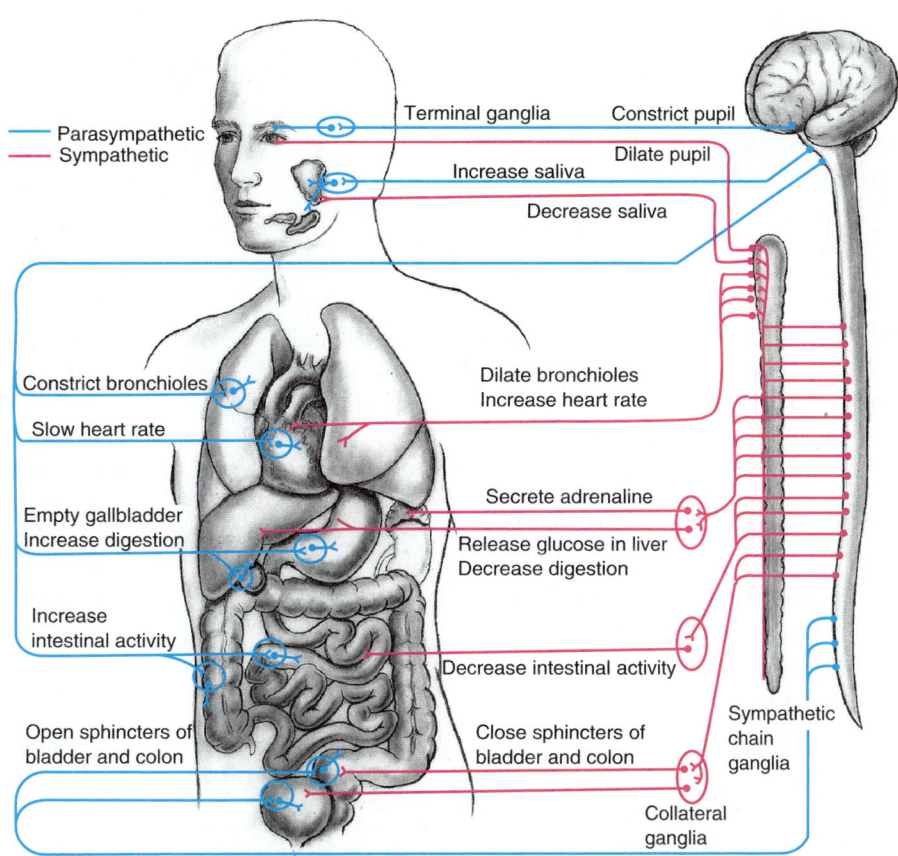

FIGURE 44-4 Structure and function of the autonomic nervous system. (From Applegate E: *The anatomy and physiology learning system,* ed 3, St Louis, 2006, WB Saunders.)

for a limited time, usually seconds to minutes. TIAs occur when brain tissue becomes ischemic for a short time, causing the same symptoms as a stroke. Because the cause of the ischemia is limited, the symptoms dissipate quickly. Symptoms can include numbness or weakness in the face, arm, or leg or on one side of the body; confusion or difficulty talking or understanding speech; vision abnormalities, including diplopia; difficulty walking; and vertigo or loss of balance and coordination.

These episodes may occur in the days, weeks, or months before a stroke. Patients and their families should understand that any strokelike symptom should be taken seriously. Individuals experiencing TIAs should be seen within an hour of the onset of symptoms so that they can be evaluated carefully and treated to prevent a possible stroke. Individuals with atrial fibrillation (an irregular rapid firing of electrical activity in the atria of the heart) may be prescribed anticoagulants (e.g., heparin or warfarin [Coumadin]), or they may be put on daily low-dose aspirin or clopidogrel (Plavix), because these individuals are at increased risk of emboli formation. TIAs are important warning signs that the patient is at serious risk of having a debilitating stroke. When TIAs occur, it is time for preventive treatment and patient education, including altering and/or treating such factors as hypertension, smoking, heart disease, diabetes, carotid artery disease (carotid artery occlusion with atherosclerotic plaques), and alcohol abuse.

Cerebrovascular Accident

A cerebrovascular accident (CVA) is the most important clinical manifestation of CVD. A CVA, commonly referred to as a *stroke,* occurs when a vessel in the brain either ruptures or occludes and the tissue on the other side of the damaged vessel becomes oxygen deprived. Cerebral artery ruptures are caused by uncontrolled hypertension or hemorrhaging of a weakened section of an artery in the brain. As a result of the rupture, the surrounding brain tissue fills with blood, damaging and possibly destroying the affected tissue. An occlusion occurs when an embolus or thrombus becomes wedged in an artery and obstructs the flow of blood to an area of the brain (Figure 44-5).

The patient's subsequent symptoms depend on the location of the arterial occlusion or rupture. Some of the more common symptoms include slurred speech; unexplained confusion; sudden, severe headache; difficulty swallowing; vertigo; diplopia; loss of consciousness; personality change; loss of bowel or bladder control; and paralysis on one side of the body.

Treatment of a stroke requires immediate emergency transport to the hospital. The initial emphasis is on minimizing the long-term disabilities often seen with strokes by providing immediate treatment to salvage as much brain tissue as possible. Thrombolytic drugs to dissolve the clot and anticoagulants may be given if the cause of the stroke was a thrombus or an embolus. However, thrombolytic

TABLE 44-3 Common Diseases and Conditions of the Nervous System

DISEASE	SIGNS AND SYMPTOMS	DIAGNOSTIC PROCEDURES	LABORATORY TESTS	TREATMENT AND MEDICATIONS
Alzheimer's disease	Short-term memory loss; progressive, irreversible confusion and disorientation	History	None specific; ordered to rule out other causes of dementia	Supportive care, tacrine (Cognex), donepezil (Aricept)
Brain tumor	Depend on location; generally caused by increased ICP	History, neurologic examination, imaging studies	None	Estrogen, surgery, radiation, chemotherapy
CVA	Depend on severity; speech difficulties, hemiplegia, confusion, loss of muscle coordination	History, neurologic examination, CT, MRI	Lumbar puncture	Thrombolytics, antiinflammatories, anticoagulants, hyperbaric oxygen, rehabilitation, supportive care
Encephalitis	Increased ICP, cerebral edema	History, neurologic examination, CT, MRI	Lumbar puncture	Antivirals, supportive care
Epilepsy	*Grand mal:* Tonic-clonic muscle contractions *Petit mal:* Momentary absence, stare, amnesia	History, neurologic examination, CT, MRI, EEG	Blood work	Anticonvulsants
Closed head injury caused by trauma	Depend on location and severity of injury; headache, increased ICP	History, neurologic examination, CT, MRI	Lumbar puncture	Diuretics; reduce ICP
Meningitis	Headache, nuchal rigidity	History, neurologic examination, Kernig's and Brudzinski's signs	Lumbar puncture	Antibiotics, anticonvulsants, antiinflammatories
Migraine	Unilateral throbbing sensation, nausea, vomiting, blurred vision	History, neurologic examination	Tests to rule out organic causes of headaches	Vasodilators, vasoconstrictors
Multiple sclerosis	Problems with vision, sensation, motor function	History, neurologic examination, MRI	None	Interferon, corticosteroids, antispasmodics, antidepressants
Parkinson's disease	Resting tremor, shuffling gait, masklike face	History, neurologic examination	None	Anticholinergics, dopamine agonists

CT, Computed tomography; *CVA,* cerebrovascular accident; *EEG,* electroencephalography; *ICP,* intracranial pressure; *MRI,* magnetic resonance imaging.

medication can effectively treat resulting ischemia only if it is given within the first 3 to 6 hours after the ischemia began. If cerebral edema is present, the patient is treated with corticosteroids and diuretics to reverse the swelling. Hyperbaric oxygen also can be used to increase oxygenation of the brain. An important part of the subsequent recovery is extensive treatment in a stroke rehabilitation program that includes physical, occupational, and speech therapies.

TYPES, CAUSES, AND RISKS OF CEREBROVASCULAR ACCIDENTS

Thrombotic stroke: A blood clot (thrombus) forms in a cerebral artery and blocks distal blood flow.
Embolic stroke: A blood clot from somewhere else in the body (e.g., the lower leg) or a piece of plaque (typically from the carotid arteries)

breaks away and flows through the bloodstream to the brain; the embolus eventually blocks a cerebral artery, causing distal ischemia.
Cerebral hemorrhage: An artery in the brain ruptures, possibly because of untreated or uncontrolled hypertension or a congenital aneurysm.

Any of the following factors can increase the risk of a stroke:
- Hypertension
- Diabetes (increases the risk by two to three times)
- Hypercholesterolemia
- Cigarette smoking (increases the risk by 50%)
- Obesity
- Family history of stroke
- Endocarditis (may promote thrombus formation)
- Arteriosclerosis and atherosclerosis

- Heart disease (e.g., atrial fibrillation, which increases the risk by five times)
- Sleep apnea
- Sickle cell anemia
- Cocaine abuse

Individuals with three or more of the following five health conditions are twice as likely to have a cerebrovascular accident: obesity, low high-density lipoprotein (HDL) cholesterol levels, high triglyceride levels, blood pressure of 130/85 mm Hg or higher, and diabetes and/or prediabetes (fasting blood sugar between 100 and 125 mg/dL).

CRITICAL THINKING APPLICATION   44-2

Mai answers the phone at the clinic. The caller is a patient, an anxious woman who is desperately trying to say something but appears unable to do so. Mai thinks the patient is trying to say something like "Help." Mai checks the number on the caller ID display, looks it up in the office computer, and finds that it belongs to a 50-year-old patient who came in 2 days earlier because of frequent, severe headaches. How should Mai handle this situation? Be sure to think about what she should do, why she should do it, and what might happen if she does nothing.

Migraine Headache

More than 28 million Americans suffer from migraine headaches, and the condition affects three times more women than men. Migraine headaches are **paroxysmal** attacks of headaches that can be completely incapacitating and frequently are associated with other symptoms, such as nausea, vomiting, visual disturbances, and throbbing pain on one side of the head. The manifestations of migraine headaches differ from one individual to another. The patient may experience a sensory warning sign (an **aura**) before the onset of the headache. An aura often consists of some form of visual disturbance, such as dark lines or spots within the visual field or a flash of light.

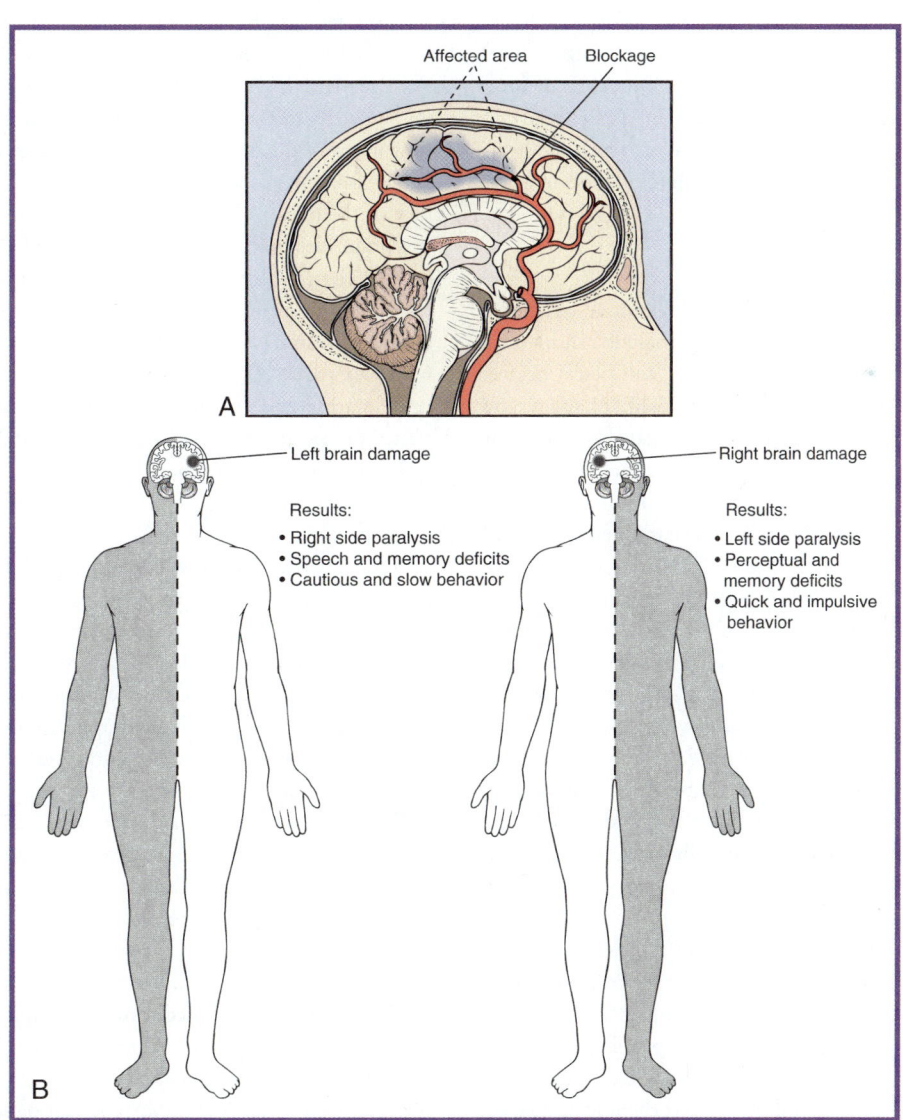

FIGURE 44-5 Cerebral artery occlusion **(A)** and hemiplegia **(B)**. (Modified from Frazier MS, Drzymkowski JW: *Essentials of human diseases and conditions*, ed 5, St Louis, 2013, Saunders.)

Medical science has not yet discovered the underlying cause of migraines. However, some researchers believe they may be caused by a combination of a problem with the trigeminal nerve and an imbalance of chemicals in the brain, especially the neurotransmitter serotonin; this causes cerebral blood vessels to become dilated and inflamed, resulting in the acute onset of a terrible headache. Individuals who suffer from migraine headaches report a number of different triggers, including changes in estrogen levels; certain foods, such as alcohol, chocolate, aspartame, caffeine, and monosodium glutamate (MSG); elevated stress levels; bright lights, sun glare, and certain smells; altered sleep patterns; and changes in the weather, especially with changing altitude levels and barometric pressures. The diagnosis usually is established from a complete medical history. EEG, a CT scan, or an MRI study can be performed as part of the diagnostic process to rule out other causes of the headaches.

Drugs used to treat migraines include nonsteroidal antiinflammatory drugs (NSAIDs) or triptans, such as sumatriptan (Imitrex), rizatriptan (Maxalt), or zolmitriptan (Zomig), which mimic the effects of serotonin, causing vascular constriction (these drugs must be taken at the onset of the headache to be effective). Other medications recommended for the prevention of migraines include beta blockers and antidepressants. Antiseizure medications, such as topiramate (Topamax) and gabapentin (Neurontin), may be effective in reducing the frequency and severity of the headaches. Other treatments include biofeedback techniques and elimination diets to avoid migraine triggers.

Dementia and Alzheimer's Disease

The term *dementia* describes a group of symptoms caused by altered brain function. Dementia symptoms may include short-term memory loss; disorientation about person, time, and place; neglect of personal hygiene, nutrition, and safety; personality changes; and inability to follow simple directions. Dementia can be caused by multiple conditions. Some can be reversed, such as nutrition disorders or disorientation caused by a minor head injury. Others are irreversible, such as multi-infarct (vascular) dementia and Alzheimer's disease.

Multi-infarct dementia is caused by a series of small strokes that interfere with the brain's blood supply, resulting in multiple areas of tissue necrosis. The location of the infarcts determines the degree of disability and the dementia symptoms that might occur. Symptoms of an acute onset of dementia typically are caused by this type of dementia. People with multi-infarct dementia are likely to show signs of improvement or remain stable for long periods and then quickly develop new symptoms if more strokes occur. Untreated or uncontrolled hypertension usually is the cause of this type of dementia.

Alzheimer's disease is the most common form of dementia among older people today. It is a devastating, chronic, progressive, and degenerative disease that begins in the parts of the brain that control thought, memory, and language. The patient exhibits slow, increasing loss of recent memory; loss of recognition of people, places, and events; confusion and disorientation; and physical deterioration that leads to death. The cause remains unknown, and there is no known cure. Treatment is supportive care only. (Alzheimer's disease is addressed in more detail in Chapter 48.)

CRITICAL THINKING APPLICATION   44-3

Mr. Jackson, a 75-year-old patient with Alzheimer's disease, is coming in for his first visit. He does not respond to verbal commands and is unable to answer direct questions. How can Mai get him into the examination room and into a patient gown while preserving his dignity?

Epilepsy and Seizure Disorders

Epilepsy is a chronic brain disorder associated with abnormal electrical impulses generated by some of the neurons in the brain. These errant impulses cause seizures (Figure 44-6). A seizure is characterized by abnormalities in levels of consciousness, sensory disturbances, and impaired motor function. A diagnosis of a seizure disorder is made if the individual has two or more seizures. Children may have a single seizure associated with a high fever (i.e., febrile seizure), but that alone does not mean that the child has a seizure disorder. However, most individuals with the disorder have an onset of seizures during childhood, although many children grow out of the problem as they get older. In many cases the cause is never identified; some known causes include brain tumors, CNS infections, anoxia, CVA, and traumatic head injury.

Seizures are classified as either partial or generalized, based on how much of the brain is involved in the abnormal electrical activity. Partial seizures result from abnormal electrical activity in just one part of the brain, whereas generalized seizures involve most or all of the brain. Seizure classifications are divided into more specific categories. Simple partial seizures originate in a small, localized area of the brain, do not cause loss of consciousness, and are identified by a routine action, such as shaking of an arm or a leg or altered speech. Complex partial seizures also begin in a small area of the brain but cause staring and repeated movements, such as hand rubbing, lip smacking, swallowing, and postseizure confusion or amnesia. Generalized seizures include petit mal seizures, which are brief episodes characterized by staring, subtle body movement, and brief lapses of awareness.

Probably the best-known seizure disorder is the generalized tonic-clonic form that causes grand mal seizures, with loss of consciousness, tonic (stiffening) muscle contractions, followed by clonic (twitching, jerking) muscle contractions of the limbs, clenched teeth, and/or loss of bowel or bladder control. After the shaking subsides, the individual may fall asleep or appear confused for a few minutes. The patient may experience an aura, usually a sensory warning such as a specific smell or taste, before a grand mal seizure occurs.

Diagnosis depends on an accurate seizure history, EEG, and CT or MRI scans. Seizures cannot be cured but usually can be controlled effectively by pharmaceutical treatment; however, finding the most effective medication at the right dose can be complex. Some individuals with epilepsy require more than one drug or have to try multiple medications until the most effective one is found. Antiseizure (anticonvulsant) medications include phenytoin (Dilantin), carbamazepine (Tegretol), valproic acid (Depakene), gabapentin (Neurontin), phenobarbital, clonazepam (Klonopin), and lamotrigine (Lamictal). It is very important that patients know never to stop taking their seizure medication without the physician's supervision, because this may trigger more frequent and severe seizure episodes.

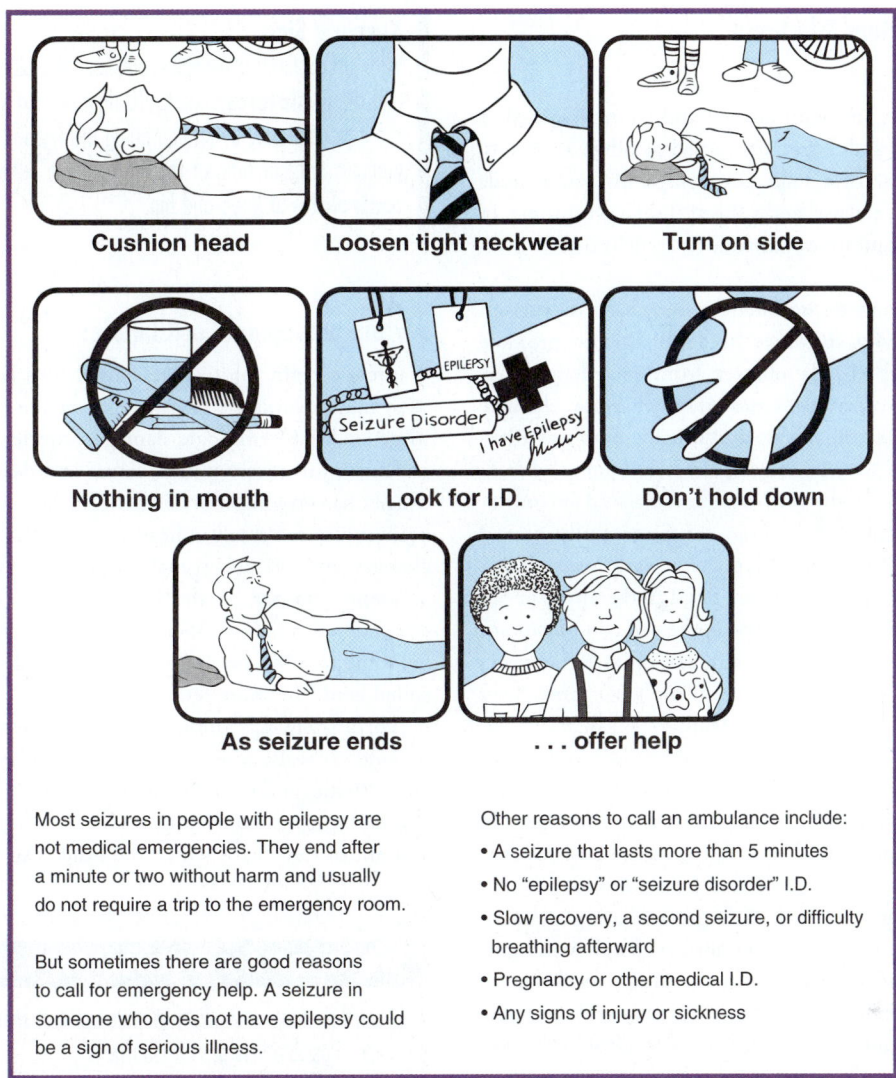

Cushion head   Loosen tight neckwear   Turn on side

Nothing in mouth   Look for I.D.   Don't hold down

As seizure ends   . . . offer help

Most seizures in people with epilepsy are not medical emergencies. They end after a minute or two without harm and usually do not require a trip to the emergency room.

But sometimes there are good reasons to call for emergency help. A seizure in someone who does not have epilepsy could be a sign of serious illness.

Other reasons to call an ambulance include:
• A seizure that lasts more than 5 minutes
• No "epilepsy" or "seizure disorder" I.D.
• Slow recovery, a second seizure, or difficulty breathing afterward
• Pregnancy or other medical I.D.
• Any signs of injury or sickness

FIGURE 44-6 First aid for seizures. (Modified from Epilepsy Foundation of America, Landover, Md.) www.epilepsyfoundation.org

WHAT IS ELECTROENCEPHALOGRAPHY?

Electroencephalography is used to record the brain wave activity of a patient suspected of having a seizure disorder or to determine the effectiveness of pharmaceutical treatment to control the brain's abnormal electrical activity. The particular pattern of brainwave activity helps diagnose the seizure disorder type. Electroencephalograms (EEGs) also are used to help localize the area of the brain that is causing a partial seizure disorder. During an EEG, 32 electrodes are placed on the patient's scalp with either paste or an elastic cap to record the electrical activity of the brain. The patient must remain very still during the examination, even sleep if possible, so that the electrodes can pick up the electrical impulses of the brain without interference. Sedation may be required for pediatric patients (Figure 44-7).

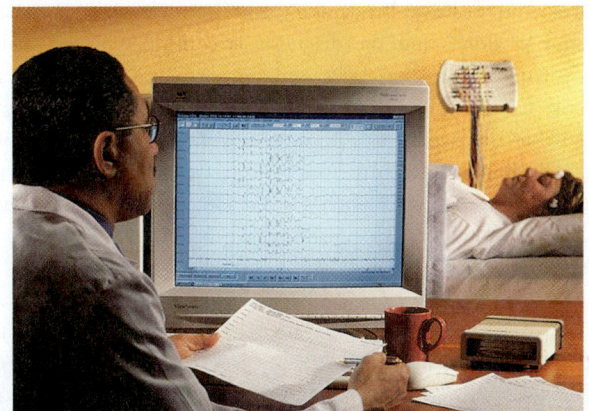

FIGURE 44-7 Patient undergoing electroencephalography. (From Linton A: *Introduction to medical-surgical nursing*, ed 4, St Louis, 2008, WB Saunders.)

Central Nervous System Infections

Encephalitis

Most cases of encephalitis are viral in origin and are transmitted to humans from mosquitoes and ticks or are caused by other infections, such as herpes infections. In a mild case symptoms can include headaches, muscle aches, malaise, and general flulike symptoms. In more severe cases, the symptoms can include fever, delirium, convulsions, **coma**, and even death.

A quiet, nonstimulating environment is necessary to prevent triggering of seizure activity, to relieve headache, and to promote rest. A patient with cerebral inflammation from encephalitis may suffer from confusion, disorientation, and other behavioral changes. These symptoms are part of the disease and usually disappear when the condition improves.

Patient management treats the symptoms and is aimed at controlling fever and seizure activity, as well as constant monitoring of respiratory and urinary functions. In patients with severe CNS damage, recovery usually is prolonged, and physical therapy is necessary to overcome the neurologic and musculoskeletal complications. If encephalitis is caused by the herpes simplex or varicella zoster virus, treatment includes the use of acyclovir (Zovirax) or ganciclovir (Cytovene).

Meningitis

Meningitis is an infection and inflammation of the meninges and CSF of the brain and spinal cord that can be caused by viruses, bacteria, or fungi. Meningitis is transmitted from an infected individual through coughing, sneezing, kissing, or sharing personal items, such as eating utensils or a toothbrush. Viral meningitis usually is mild and has flulike symptoms that typically resolve in 10 days or earlier. Fungal meningitis is seen in patients with immune deficiencies, such as acquired immunodeficiency syndrome (AIDS), and can be life-threatening. Acute bacterial meningitis can occur as a complication of an earlier infection of the ears, sinuses, or lungs, or it can be transmitted from an infected person.

Bacterial meningitis can be quite serious; symptoms can include a high fever, severe headache, stiff neck, photophobia, confusion, seizures, and positive Brudzinski's and Kernig's signs. A lumbar puncture is done, and the diagnosis is confirmed if the CSF is cloudy **(turbid)** and has large numbers of white blood cells and bacteria. Culturing the CSF usually identifies the causative organism so that the patient can be treated with the appropriate intravenous antibiotics. The patient also is treated with analgesics and medications to reduce cerebral edema. Despite treatment, meningitis can be fatal or can cause long-term neurologic damage in some patients.

TESTING FOR BRUDZINSKI'S AND KERNIG'S SIGNS

Brudzinski's Sign
The patient is placed in the supine position. The head is passively flexed toward the chest. Brudzinski's sign is seen if the patient spontaneously flexes the arm, hip, and knee in response to the neck flexion.

Kernig's Sign
With the patient in a supine position, the physician flexes both one hip and the **ipsilateral** knee to 90 degrees and then attempts to straighten the leg completely by straightening the knee. Kernig's sign is seen if pain prevents straightening of the leg or if the patient involuntarily flexes the **contralateral** knee and hip.

Brain and Spinal Cord Injuries

Traumatic brain injuries are caused by a blow or jolt to the head. They may be limited to a particular section of the brain or may result in generalized neurologic damage. Injuries can range from a mild concussion to severe injury, coma, and death. A minor concussion usually has no long-term side effects; however, a moderate to severe brain injury can result in headaches, amnesia, confusion, personality changes, and seizures. Spinal cord injuries usually result from severe, accidental trauma to the back or neck. These injuries are most common in the 16- to 30-year-old age group and are associated with automobile and sports accidents. The higher the damage to the spinal cord, the more serious the injury is.

Fortunately, CNS injuries can be prevented with the proper use of child car seats, adult safety belts, and helmets in childhood sports and activities and by reducing the frequency of drinking and driving. Several types of brain injuries can occur, depending on the type and amount of force with which the head is struck.

SIGNS OF A CONCUSSION

Signs that occur seconds to minutes after a head injury include:
- Possible loss of consciousness
- Difficulty focusing, with slowed responses
- Slurred speech
- Nausea and vomiting
- Headache
- Blurred vision
- Confusion and disorientation or amnesia

The patient should be seen immediately if he or she reports any of the following signs and symptoms days or weeks after a head injury:
- Persistent headache
- Vertigo (dizziness)
- Inability to concentrate
- Repeated problems with memory
- Nausea or vomiting (especially if vomiting is projectile)
- Unusual anger, irritability, anxiety, or depression
- Sleep disorders
- Seizures

Cerebral Concussion and Contusion

Concussion is the mildest and the most common type of brain injury. Trauma from an impact or a sudden change in motion can cause a concussion with loss of consciousness, which may last seconds to several minutes and may be followed by a period of disorientation that lasts up to 24 hours (Figure 44-8). A single concussion may disrupt the normal electrical activity in the brain, but the brain usually is not injured permanently. However, research has shown that the damage from multiple concussions may be cumulative, and neurologists recommend that children should be removed from all sporting activities if they have experienced three concussions.

A more serious injury to the brain can cause the formation of a contusion, or bruised area, usually because of a skull fracture. Symptoms can include headache, nausea, vomiting, vision disturbances, and sensitivity to light. Talking with the patient may reveal reduced levels of concentration, irritability, or periods of amnesia. The patient's initial assessment may include an evaluation of consciousness according to the parameters of the Glasgow Coma Scale (Table 44-4).

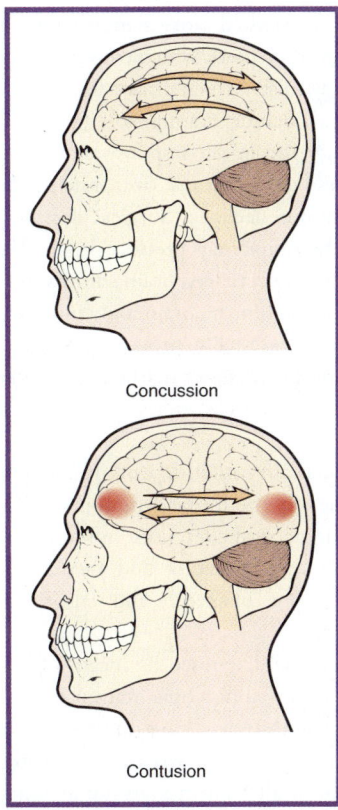

FIGURE 44-8 Brain concussion and contusion. (Modified from Frazier MS, Drzymkowski JW: *Essentials of human diseases and conditions*, ed 5, St Louis, 2013, WB Saunders.)

CRITICAL THINKING APPLICATION   **44-4**

■ Mai is putting together an information sheet on head injury for the family of a patient who recently suffered a minor concussion. The family should watch for what symptoms? When should the family seek additional medical care?

■ Dr. Song said he would approve the leaflet after Mai had completed it, but he was called away on an emergency before he saw it. A patient sees it behind the desk and asks to take one. Should Mai let him? Why or why not?

Open and Closed Head Injuries

In a closed head injury, a brain injury occurs but the skull is not fractured. A more serious brain injury can occur with an open head injury, because the skull is fractured or displaced. A serious head injury can cause life-threatening damage to the intracerebral structures. Subarachnoid hemorrhage may occur when the delicate meningeal blood vessels are ruptured, resulting in the collection of blood in the subarachnoid space. This causes a rapid increase in intracranial pressure, which may give rise to sudden, severe headache; nausea and severe projectile vomiting; motor disturbances; visual disturbances; and seizures. In addition to trauma, other predisposing factors that can cause subarachnoid hemorrhage include hypertension, a family history of the condition, and congenital malformations of cranial blood vessels. Treatment is designed to reduce the intracranial pressure, sometimes surgically.

A subdural hematoma develops when blood collects in the space between the dura mater and the arachnoid layers of the meninges, usually as a result of head trauma that has caused slow bleeding from ruptured blood vessels in the meningeal layers. Symptoms of increased intracranial pressure occur over a several days as the hematoma increases in size. Signs and symptoms build over time and include headache, motor disturbances, speech abnormalities, nausea and vomiting, seizures, and a decreased level of consciousness. Treatment requires surgery to stop the bleeding and reduce the pressure inside the skull. People age 75 or older are at greatest risk of developing a subdural hematoma after a minor fall or cranial impact.

Shaken Baby Syndrome

Shaken baby syndrome is the most common reason for serious head injury in infants. It is caused by violently shaking the infant back and forth, forcing the brain against opposite ends of the skull. Shaking is so dangerous for babies because of their small size in comparison to their relatively large head size, as well as their undeveloped neck

TABLE 44-4 Glasgow Coma Scale					
SCORE	1	2	3	4	5
Eye opening	No response	To pain	To voice	Spontaneously	
Best motor response (movement of arms and legs)	No response	Extension to pain	Flexion to pain	Localizes to pain	Follows commands
Best verbal response	No response	Incomprehensible sounds	Inappropriate words	Disoriented and converses	Oriented and converses

Scoring: 13 to 15, Mild head injury; 9 to 12, moderate head injury; 3 to 8, severe head injury.

muscles. The typical presentation is a child approximately 6 months old who is brought to the clinic or emergency department because of difficulty breathing or marked lethargy. Usually little or no external bruising or trauma is seen. Physical findings on examination or autopsy include a subdural hematoma and retinal hemorrhages. The history given by the caregiver usually indicates that the baby "fell" from the sofa, coffee table, or bed or was "dropped." Approximately one fourth of these infants die of their injuries.

Spinal Cord Injuries

If a traumatic accident completely transects the spinal cord, all CNS stimulation to nerves distal to the injury stops, resulting in paralysis of the areas below the injury. Paralysis because of cord **transection** is grouped into one of two categories (Figure 44-9). In *paraplegia,* transection occurs below the midpoint of the spinal cord, causing paralysis of both legs, loss of function below the level of injury, including loss of bladder and bowel control, and sexual dysfunction in males. In *quadriplegia,* transection occurs in the upper thoracic or cervical region of the spinal cord, causing paralysis of all four limbs, respiratory difficulty, and loss of function to all muscles below the injury points. *Hemiplegia* is unrelated to spinal cord injury and occurs when a CVA, a vascular injury such as a ruptured aneurysm, or a tumor occurs on one side of the brain, resulting in paralysis on the opposite side of the body.

No surgery or treatment can restore a transected cord, although much research currently is underway in this area. If the spinal cord is injured but not completely transected, the degree of paralysis depends on the degree of injury. Such patients usually respond well to physical therapy, and their ability to restore motor function is good, although they may always have some functional limitations.

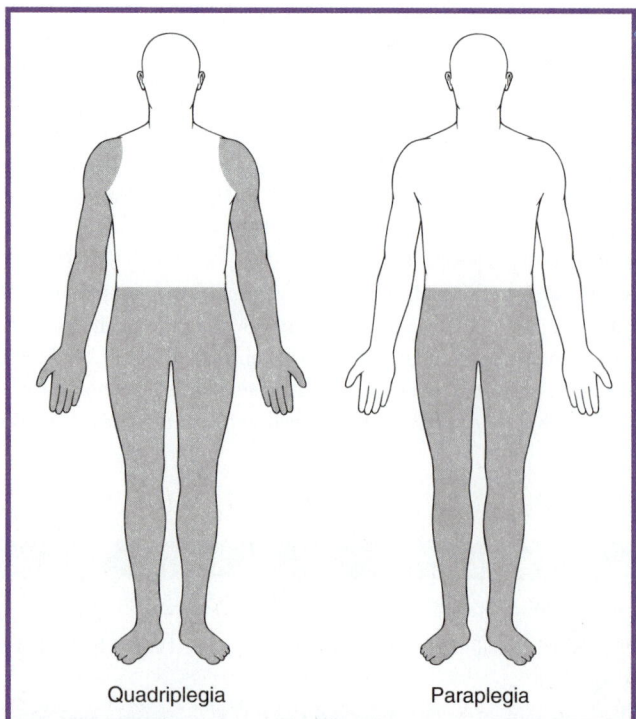

Quadriplegia   Paraplegia

FIGURE 44-9 Types of paralysis: quadriplegia and paraplegia. (Modified from Frazier MS, Drzymkowski JW: *Essentials of human diseases and conditions,* ed 5, St Louis, 2013, WB Saunders.)

Additional Central Nervous System Pathologies

Parkinson's Disease

Parkinson's disease (PD) is a chronic, progressive, debilitating disease that affects about 1 in 100 adults over age 60; more than 60,000 new cases occur annually in the United States. PD affects men more frequently than women. The four primary symptoms of PD are tremors of the hands, arms, legs, jaw, and face; rigidity of the limbs and trunk; bradykinesia, or slowness of movement; and postural instability with impaired balance and coordination. The typical presentation of PD includes a unilateral, pill-rolling tremor; a high-pitched, monotone voice; difficulty swallowing; a masklike facial expression; and bowed head and forward-bent posture. Tremors and rigidity increase in severity over time. Currently there are no laboratory tests specific for PD; therefore the diagnosis is based on a comprehensive medical history and neurologic examination.

Parkinson's disease is caused by a deficiency of the neurotransmitter dopamine in the brain. The disease has no cure, but various medications are prescribed for symptomatic relief, including carbidopa-levodopa (Sinemet), which converts into dopamine in the brain. Dopamine agonists, which mimic the effects of dopamine, are also prescribed and include pramipexole (Mirapex) and ropinirole (Requip). Although the initial response to medical treatment can show dramatic relief of symptoms, over time the body's response to Parkinson medications declines. Surgical destruction of the most affected area of the brain may produce some relief of symptoms. Another treatment option is deep brain stimulation (DBS), in which electrodes are implanted in the brain and connected to a small electrical device that is externally programmed to help control the tremors and gait problems associated with the disease.

Tumors

The symptoms of a brain tumor depend on the type and location of the mass, but generally the initial symptoms are headaches, vomiting, dizziness, diplopia, and alterations in muscle strength and coordination. Changes in personality and mental function, seizures, progressive paralysis, loss of speech, and sensory disorders appear as the tumor enlarges.

CNS tumors can be diagnosed by means of CT, MRI, EEG, or lumbar puncture. Ophthalmoscopic examination may reveal **papilledema**. Accurate diagnosis of a brain tumor includes determining its precise location in the brain and whether it is **benign** or **malignant**. Approximately half of all brain tumors are metastatic growths from other primary cancer sites in the body. Lung cancer, breast cancer, and melanoma frequently spread to the brain by metastasis. Regardless of whether the mass is benign or malignant, as brain tumors grow, they cause serious problems and complications for the patient because of the limited space inside the skull. Treatment of brain tumors can include surgery, chemotherapy, and radiation in any combination.

CRITICAL THINKING APPLICATION   44-5

A 34-year-old man has just found out that he has a brain tumor, and Mai is to schedule him for surgery next week. Before he leaves the office, he says he wants to talk to Mai privately. They go into an examination room, and he says, "Tell me the truth; this is cancer, and I'm going to die, right?" How should Mai respond to this frightened patient?

DISEASES OF THE PERIPHERAL NERVOUS SYSTEM

Multiple Sclerosis

The axon of a nerve cell in the PNS is covered with a myelin sheath to protect and insulate electrical stimulation as it is passed to the terminal end of the neuron. Multiple sclerosis (MS) is an autoimmune reaction that causes progressive inflammation and deterioration (demyelination) of the myelin sheath, leaving nerve fibers uncovered and resulting in a scattering of the nervous message as it passes down the axon. Early symptoms may include numbness, **paresthesia**, diplopia, **ataxia**, and bladder control problems. As the disease progresses, patients experience increased spasticity, vertigo, depression, gait problems, joint pain, fatigue, and varying degrees of paralysis. It most commonly begins in women in their early 30s. The cause remains unknown; however, it is more common in Northern climates, and it may be associated with a viral infection. MS frequently is diagnosed by the exacerbation and remission of neurologic symptoms characteristic of the condition. Patients cycle through remission and relapse, and an ever-increasing degree of dysfunction occurs after each episode. An MRI study may show plaques on nerve fibers where the myelin sheaths have been destroyed and areas of sclerosis from scar tissue at the inflammation sites.

MS has no cure; therefore, treatment focuses on alleviating symptoms and delaying the progression of the disease. Medications used to treat the disease include corticosteroids during periods of exacerbation, interferon (Betaseron, Avonex) to reduce the frequency and severity of relapses, and additional medications to treat fatigue, pain, spasticity, and bladder control problems. Some patients live an essentially normal life with only occasional attacks, whereas others experience rapidly progressive incapacitation.

Amyotrophic Lateral Sclerosis

Amyotrophic lateral sclerosis (ALS), or Lou Gehrig's disease, is a rapidly progressive, ultimately fatal neurologic disease that destroys the motor neurons responsible for voluntary muscle control. Without stimulation from motor neurons, muscles cannot function and gradually weaken and atrophy. ALS usually begins with small, local, involuntary muscle contractions in the forearms and hands. As the disease progresses, the patient has difficulty with speech, chewing, swallowing, and breathing. In most cases the disease does not affect a person's personality, intelligence, or memory, nor does it affect the ability to see, smell, taste, hear, or recognize touch. The first drug treatment for the disease, recently approved by the U.S. Food and Drug Administration (FDA), is riluzole (Rilutek), which reduces damage to motor neurons and prolongs survival, especially in patients with difficulty swallowing. Other treatments, which are palliative, include attempts to keep the individual as comfortable as possible and to help with pain, depression, sleep disturbances, and constipation. Death from failure of the respiratory muscles usually occurs within 3 to 5 years after the onset of symptoms. The cause is unknown, but the disease most commonly occurs in males over age 50.

Bell's Palsy

Bell's palsy is a temporary facial paralysis. It results from inflammation and edema of the seventh cranial nerve, which in turn are caused by a viral infection (e.g., herpes simplex or Epstein-Barr virus). The condition occurs suddenly, and symptoms reach their peak within 48 hours. The disorder usually subsides spontaneously over several weeks to months. Symptoms range in severity from mild weakness to complete paralysis on the affected side, depending on the degree of nervous involvement. The patient can experience facial twitching, eyelid drooping, excessive tearing of the affected eye, and drooping of the mouth with drooling of saliva. The patient is unable to close the eye on the affected side completely and may have taste disturbances. The antiviral drug acyclovir may be prescribed, in addition to prednisone to reduce the inflammation and control edema. The physician recommends an eye patch to protect the exposed eye, especially at night, to prevent corneal abrasions.

Peripheral Neuropathy

Peripheral neuropathy is not a disease in itself, but rather a condition of peripheral nerve dysfunction that can have more than 100 different known causes. It can be **cryptogenic**, or idiopathic, which means that the underlying cause cannot be identified. Conditions that can cause peripheral neuropathy include diabetes mellitus, human immunodeficiency virus (HIV) infection, nutritional deficiencies, and neurologic side effects of some medications. Symptoms usually affect the legs and arms and can include muscular weakness and pain or sensory disturbances such as burning, numbness, and tingling.

Symptoms can vary widely from person to person in both number and severity. Patients often feel extremely frustrated when they try to explain to the physician the abnormal sensations they are experiencing. Peripheral neuropathies can result from damage or injury to any portion of the neuron. Treatment of peripheral neuropathy is most effective when the causative condition is diagnosed and then treated successfully. Encouraging a healthy lifestyle, including weight control, exercise, a nutritious diet, and limiting or avoiding alcohol, helps control the physical and emotional effects of peripheral neuropathy.

Carpal Tunnel Syndrome

Carpal tunnel syndrome (CTS) results from **compression** of the median nerve as it passes through the carpal bones of the wrist. The carpal tunnel, which is about the size of the thumb, is an open area between the wrist bones that contains the flexor tendons of the forearm and the median nerve, which runs from the forearm to the hand. Compression of these structures within the carpal tunnel can occur spontaneously but more commonly is the result of repetitive movements. CTS is the most common repetitive strain injury (RSI). A frequently reported cause is daily use of the computer keyboard for prolonged periods. The symptoms of median nerve compression are pain, weakness, and numbness in the hand and wrist that radiates up the arm, and paresthesia of the radial-palmar region of the hand. As symptoms worsen, the individual may have reduced grip strength, which makes forming a fist, grasping small objects, or performing other fine motor tasks difficult.

Treatment includes taking breaks from repetitive hand or wrist activities, wearing a wrist support, taking NSAIDs, applying ice, and undergoing physical therapy. If these treatments do not resolve the problem, surgery may be required to relieve the pressure on the median nerve.

MENTAL HEALTH

Each year more than 44 million Americans are affected by a diagnosable mental condition that adversely affects their work, their relationships with family and friends, and their activities of daily living. Mental health disorders can be caused by a number of factors, alone or in combination, including changes in brain chemicals, hereditary makeup, psychological disposition, and life experiences. Emotional and physical symptoms can occur for no apparent reason and can be quite persistent. Emotional symptoms may include panic, apprehension, fear, anxiety, nightmares, withdrawal, flashbacks, and ritualized repetitive behaviors, such as constant hand washing. Possible physical symptoms include tachycardia, shortness of breath, sleep disturbances, gastrointestinal upset, muscular tension, and cold, clammy hands. Patients often do not associate these symptoms with a mental health disorder and therefore do not get the appropriate diagnosis and treatment.

Depressive Disorders

About 10% of adults in America experience depression each year. Almost twice as many women as men are affected by the disorder. Depression interferes with daily activities and causes pain and suffering not only to those who have the disorder, but also to those who care about them. Although multiple medications and psychosocial therapies are available to treat and manage depression, most individuals do not seek treatment. Depressive disorders affect the way a person thinks, feels, eats, and sleeps. People with depression cannot "snap out of it" and without treatment may experience symptoms that persist for weeks, months, or years.

Depressive disorders can be categorized as major depressive disorders, dysthymic disorders, and bipolar disorders. Individuals with major depression show a combination of symptoms that interfere with their ability to work, study, sleep, eat, and enjoy activities they once considered pleasurable. Dysthymic disorders are a less severe type of depression in which patients experience long-term, chronic symptoms that are not incapacitating but that affect their level of performance and daily emotions. Many people with dysthymia also experience major depression at some time in their lives. Individuals with bipolar disorders, also called *mood disorders* or *manic-depression*, cycle through a wide range of moods from extreme highs (mania) to extreme lows (depression). When in the depression cycle, they may show any or all of the symptoms of a depressive disorder. When cycling through mania, they may make decisions or act in a way that can be both embarrassing and dangerous. Manic individuals are extremely energetic and rarely sleep. If left untreated, the disorder can progress to a psychotic state.

Patients must understand that antidepressant medications take a minimum of 3 to 4 weeks for the full therapeutic effects of the drug to occur. Once they start to feel better, many individuals are tempted to stop taking the medication. *It is important to continue treatment for a minimum of 4 to 9 months to prevent a recurrence of the depression.* The patient should never stop taking antidepressant medication suddenly or without the direction of a physician. Individuals with bipolar disorders or chronic major depression may need maintenance therapy indefinitely.

Treatment for depression typically begins with a selective serotonin reuptake inhibitor (SSRI), because these medications have limited side effects. SSRIs include fluoxetine (Prozac) paroxetine (Paxil), sertraline (Zoloft), and citalopram (Celexa). If the patient does not experience relief of symptoms, the physician may order an older group of drugs called *tricyclic antidepressants* (TCAs), which inhibit the reabsorption of serotonin and norepinephrine.

Recently, concern has arisen about the association of suicidal thoughts with antidepressant medications in children and adults in the first few weeks of treatment and also when dosages are altered. The FDA has warned physicians to monitor patients closely when starting antidepressant therapy and to provide patient and family education on the importance of reporting to the physician any changes in symptoms.

SYMPTOMS OF DEPRESSION

According to the National Institute of Mental Health (NIMH), the severity of depressive symptoms varies among individuals and also with each episode. A discussion of the following symptoms can be found at te NIMH Web site (*www.nimh.nih.gov*).

- Persistent sad, anxious, or "empty" feeling
- Feelings of hopelessness and pessimism
- Feelings of guilt, worthlessness, and helplessness
- Loss of interest or pleasure in hobbies and activities that once were enjoyed, including sex
- Decreased energy and complaints of fatigue
- Difficulty concentrating, remembering, and making decisions
- Insomnia, early morning awakening, or oversleeping
- Either anorexia and weight loss or overeating and weight gain
- Thoughts of death or suicide, with possible suicide attempts
- Restlessness, irritability
- Persistent physical complaints that do not respond to treatment, such as headaches, gastrointestinal disturbances, or chronic pain

Anxiety Disorders

Anxiety disorders affect approximately 19 million American adults. The primary symptoms are an overwhelming, irrational feeling of anxiety and fear. Anxiety disorders include panic disorder, obsessive-compulsive disorder (OCD), post-traumatic stress disorder, and phobias. Individuals with panic disorder report feelings of terror that strike unexpectedly and are accompanied by nausea, chest pain, palpitations, diaphoresis, weakness, vertigo, syncope, and a fear of impending doom or loss of control. People with OCD experience anxious thoughts or images (obsessions) that they cannot control, so they resort to performing specific rituals (compulsions) to try to prevent or dispel the obsession. For example, an individual may be obsessed with germs or dirt, so he or she repeatedly washes the hands; or an individual may have to check repeatedly to make sure a door is locked because of fear that it will be left open. Performing the ritual does not bring pleasure, only temporary relief of the anxiety caused by the obsession, which will grow if the compulsion is not performed.

Post-traumatic stress disorder can occur after a patient is a part of or witnesses some terrifying, horrendous, or violent physical or emotional event, such as assault, battery, rape, war, natural disasters, acts of terrorism, and serious accidents during which many people are killed or injured. The person who survives the ordeal often has flashbacks; feelings of panic, fear, or guilt; constant replaying of the event in his or her mind; or deep feelings of emotional numbness. Severe depression and inability to function normally in daily activities also may be present.

A phobia is an intense, irrational fear of something that poses little or no actual danger. It may include such things as fear of heights, escalators, tunnels, and water. Although the individual may realize that the fear is unreasonable, just the thought of facing the feared object or situation causes a panic attack or severe anxiety. The two types of treatment for anxiety disorders are antianxiety medication, such as alprazolam (Xanax) or buspirone (BuSpar), and specific types of psychotherapy.

Schizophrenia

Schizophrenia is a chronic, severe, disabling brain disorder with symptoms that include hallucinations and delusions; difficulty speaking and expressing emotions; and cognitive deficits, such as problems with concentration and memory loss. Schizophrenia cannot be cured, but psychotic episodes can be reduced significantly by long-term, consistent pharmaceutical treatment. However, relapses are not unusual, because most individuals with schizophrenia stop taking their antipsychotic medication periodically because they feel better, they do not believe they need the medication, or they do not think that taking it regularly is important. In addition, the earliest antipsychotic medications, such as chlorpromazine (Thorazine) and haloperidol (Haldol), caused disturbing side effects, including rigidity, persistent muscle spasms, tremors, and restlessness. Newer drugs, which have limited side effects, include risperidone (Risperdal) and olanzapine (Zyprexa).

SUICIDE FACTS FROM THE NATIONAL INSTITUTE OF MENTAL HEALTH

- More than 90% of individuals who commit suicide have a diagnosable mental disorder, typically depression, or are substance abusers.
- The highest suicide rate in the United States is seen in Caucasian men over age 85.
- Suicide is the third leading cause of death in children ages 10 to 19 and in young adults ages 20 to 24.
- Although women attempt suicide two to three times more often than men, four times as many men are successful.
- Risk factors vary with age, gender, and ethnic group. They include serious depressive disorders; reduced levels of serotonin (a neurotransmitter); a prior suicide attempt; family violence, including physical or sexual abuse; and exposure to the suicidal behavior of others, including family members and peers.

www.nimh.nih.gov/health/publications/suicide

THE MEDICAL ASSISTANT'S ROLE IN THE NEUROLOGIC EXAMINATION

As with other physical examinations, a careful history provides the physician with valuable clues in diagnosing neurologic conditions. Such clues may include a record of seizures, syncope, diplopia, incontinence, or any of the previously mentioned subjective symptoms. The patient's general health often complicates a neurologic diagnosis.

The purposes of a neurologic examination are to determine whether a nervous system malfunction is present, to discover its location (or locations), and to identify the type and extent of the malfunction. During the examination, the physician may determine the effect of the symptoms on the patient's emotional status, intellectual performance, cognitive ability, and general behavior (Procedure 44-1). The patient's grooming and mannerisms are carefully observed, as is his or her ability to communicate effectively, including the appropriate use of speech, language, and writing skills. The medical assistant should listen carefully for difficulty putting words together, slurred speech, and whether conversation makes sense. If you notice inappropriate changes in the patient, note them on the patient's record for the physician's attention and evaluation.

The physical examination of the neurologic system includes evaluation of the cranial nerves. You can assist by helping the patient assume the proper position necessary for each test and by having the instruments the physician needs ready for use. For example, cranial nerve I (the olfactory nerve) is tested by determining the patient's ability to identify familiar odors such as coffee, tobacco, or cloves. Cranial nerve V (the trigeminal nerve) is checked by having the patient differentiate between warm and cold objects held against the right and left cheeks.

Peripheral nerve function is evaluated by examining the motor system, including muscular strength, gait, and movements. The diameters of the upper arms and the calves of the legs may be measured and compared to diagnose muscle atrophy. Motor functioning can be assessed through Romberg's test, in which the patient is asked to stand with the feet together, arms horizontal to the body, and eyes closed. The sensory system is examined by noting the patient's ability to perceive superficial sensations, such as a wisp of cotton brushed on the skin, a light pinprick, or hot and cold touching certain areas. Several deep tendon reflexes (DTRs), such as the patellar and Achilles reflexes, are tested (Figure 44-10). Babinski's reflex is tested by stroking the lateral aspect of the sole of the foot with a dull instrument (e.g., the handle of a reflex hammer or a tongue blade). In a positive Babinski's sign, the great toe dorsiflexes while the other toes fan out. This may indicate a possible stroke or brain lesion. Other diagnostic tests may include a skull radiograph, carotid arteriogram, EEG, and MRI and CT studies.

DIAGNOSTIC TESTING

Several diagnostic tests are used to help the physician accurately diagnose conditions and diseases of the neurologic system. The most common diagnostic procedures are the lumbar puncture and various radiographic studies (Table 44-5).

Electroencephalography

EEG is the recording of changes in electrical impulses in various areas of the brain by means of electrodes placed on the scalp. Every individual has a unique EEG pattern. In a healthy brain, most of the recorded waves are the occipital alpha waves coming from the back of the head. Irregular slow waves are called *delta waves,* which normally are found in people deeply asleep and in infants and young

PROCEDURE 44-1

Assist the Physician with Patient Care: Assist with the Neurologic Examination

GOAL: *To assist the physician in performing a neurologic examination of the patient.*

EQUIPMENT and SUPPLIES

- Patient gown
- Drape
- Otoscope
- Ophthalmoscope
- Percussion hammer
- Disposable pinwheel
- Penlight
- Tuning fork
- Cotton ball
- Tongue depressor
- Small vials of warm and cold liquids prepared according to the physician's instructions
- Small vials of sweet and salty liquids prepared according to the physician's instructions
- Small vials containing substances with distinct odors (e.g., instant coffee, cinnamon, vanilla) prepared according to the physician's instructions
- Patient's record

PROCEDURAL STEPS

1. Assemble and prepare the equipment and supplies needed for the neurologic examination and prepare the room.

2. Sanitize your hands and follow Standard Precautions.
   <u>PURPOSE:</u> To ensure infection control.
3. Identify the patient and briefly explain the procedure.
   <u>PURPOSE:</u> Explanations gain the patient's cooperation and ease apprehension.
4. Instruct the patient to disrobe as needed for the examination and to put on a gown with the opening in the back.
5. During the examination, be prepared to assist the patient in changing positions as necessary. Have the necessary examination instruments ready for the physician at the appropriate time during the examination. Record all results from the examination as indicated by the physician.
   <u>PURPOSE:</u> To facilitate a thorough, accurate neurologic examination.
6. A neurologic examination proceeds as follows but can be modified according to the physician's preference:
   - Mental status examination
   - **Proprioception** and cerebellar function
   - Cranial nerve assessment
   - Sensory nerve function
   - Reflexes
7. Record all procedures in the patient's medical record.
   <u>PURPOSE:</u> A procedure is not complete until it has been documented accurately in the patient's medical record.

---

children. A delta wave pattern is abnormal in an awake adult. Rhythmic slow waves, called *theta waves,* show a decrease in brain activity. Electrical silence (flatline EEG) indicates no evidence of brain activity and is one of the criteria used to determine brain death. EEG is valuable for diagnosing epilepsy, brain tumors, and other brain conditions (Procedure 44-2).

Lumbar Puncture

If the physician suspects that an infection or inflammation of the CNS is present, a lumbar puncture (spinal tap) is ordered to collect a CSF sample for culture, for analysis of glucose and protein, or to detect increased intracranial pressure or an area of intracranial bleeding. The patient is placed on the left side in the fetal position; using sterile technique, the physician injects the lumbar puncture site with a local anesthetic, and the puncture is performed by inserting a special needle into the subarachnoid space, usually between the L4 and L5 vertebrae (Figure 44-11). The pressure within the subarachnoid space is recorded, and a sample of CSF is collected for laboratory analysis.

After the procedure, the patient must remain flat in bed for approximately 8 hours to reduce the chances of developing a spinal headache. Medical practices usually have a specially equipped room where this procedure is performed. If you are working in such an office, you may be responsible both for assisting with the procedure and for monitoring the patient after the procedure until he or she

is sent home. Watch for side effects such as severe headaches, visual disturbances, and pain. You also will have particular office protocols to follow regarding the frequency of vital signs, liquid intake, urine output, and visitors. Lumbar punctures usually are performed in hospitals, outpatient clinics, or surgical centers (Procedure 44-3). On discharge, patients should be told to notify the physician immediately if they experience any numbness and tingling of the legs; drainage of blood or liquid from the injection site; inability to urinate; or a persistent headache.

CRITICAL THINKING APPLICATION   44-6

Dr. Song wants to perform a lumbar puncture on a 10-year-old girl who he suspects has bacterial meningitis. Her mother agreed to the procedure, but while Mai is preparing the girl, the mother changes her mind. She is afraid that inserting a needle into her daughter's spine will paralyze the girl. What should Mai do in this situation?

CLOSING COMMENTS

Patient Education

The nervous system is the major communication and control system in the human body. It influences and regulates all mental activity,

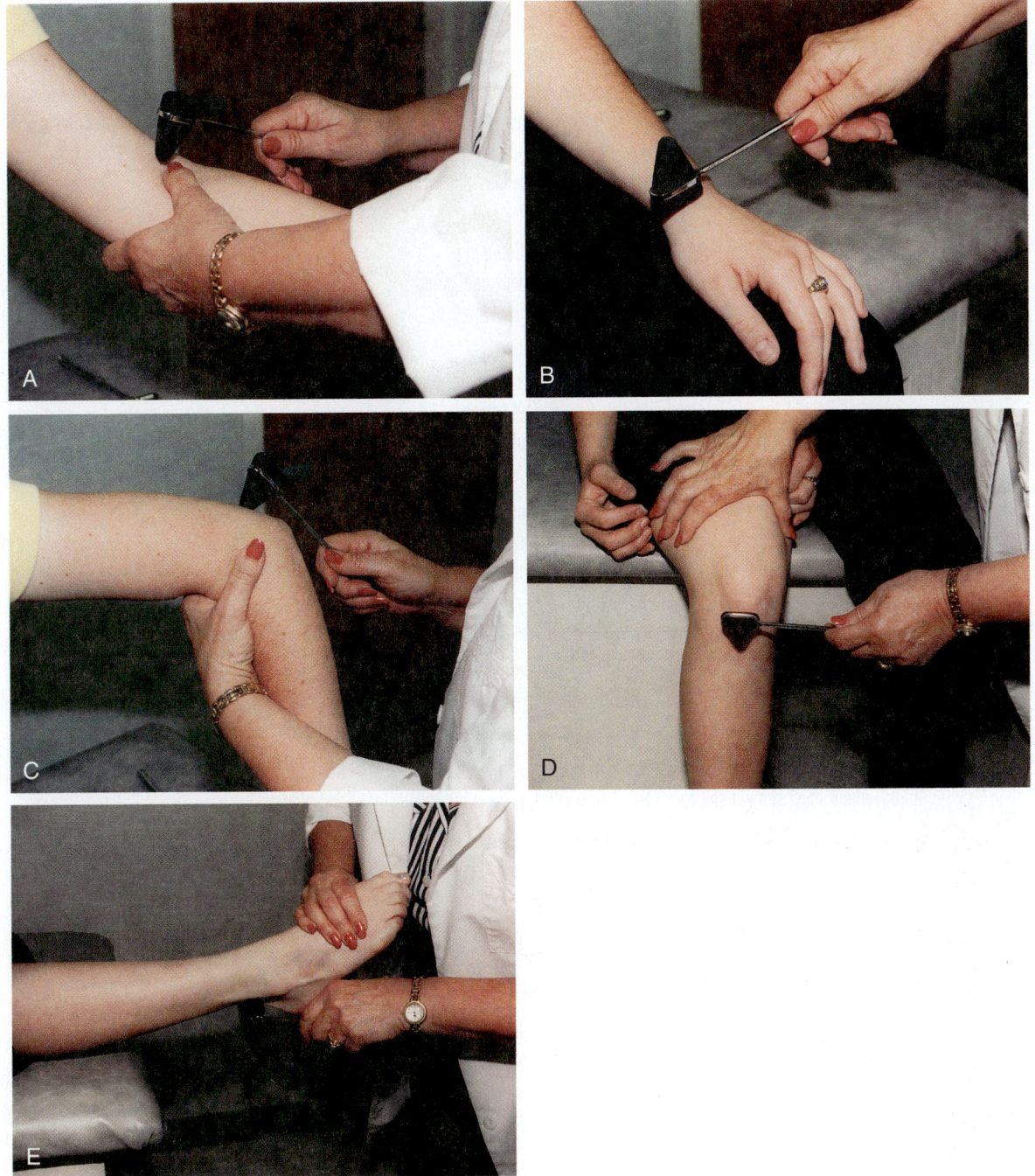

FIGURE 44-10 Testing deep tendon reflexes. **A,** Biceps reflex; results in flexion of the elbow. **B,** Brachioradialis reflex; results in flexion and supination of the forearm. **C,** Triceps reflex; results in extension of the arm. **D,** Patellar reflex; results in extension of the leg. **E,** Achilles reflex; results in plantar flexion of the foot.

TABLE 44-5 Diagnostic Tests for the Nervous System

TEST	PROCEDURE AND PATIENT PREPARATION	PURPOSE
Arteriography (angiography)	Patient usually is given a sedative. Then, after injection of a local anesthetic, a catheter is threaded into an artery toward the head. A contrast medium is injected, and videofluoroscopic studies are recorded. The patient must remain still during the procedure, which may last up to 1 hr.	To visualize the vertebral and carotid arteries, cerebral arterial circulation, leaking vessels, aneurysms, and occluded vessels
CT scan	Patient's head is strapped into a foam block to prevent movement, and patient lies on a moveable table. The table moves into the CT machine, which converts an x-ray study into a visual image of multiple transverse sections of the test structure. Procedure can last up to 1 hr, and the patient must remain still the entire time.	To visualize multiple, serial, radiographic sections of a structure, differentiating between bone and soft tissues
EEG	Patient relaxes comfortably on a recliner or bed. Electrodes are attached to the head. The examiner may ask the patient questions, give the patient various forms of visual or auditory stimulation, or have the patient sleep.	To record electrical activity of the brain to determine cerebral function or origin of seizure activity, diagnose sleep disorders, or determine lack of brain function
Lumbar puncture	With the patient in a side-lying fetal position, a local anesthetic is injected. A needle then is inserted into the subarachnoid space between the third and fourth lumbar vertebrae. Patient must remain very still during the procedure, which normally takes 5-20 min.	To determine CSF pressure, obtain CSF specimens for testing, reduce intracranial pressure, and inject contrast medium for radiographic studies
MRI	Patient should not have any metal in the body. Patient lies down on a moveable table, and the head is strapped into a foam block to prevent movement. The table moves into the MRI machine, which converts the cells' electromagnetic energy into a visual image. Patient must remain still during the procedure, which lasts up to 1 hr.	As with CT, to visualize multiple, serial, radiographic sections of a structure; shows images of the brain, spinal cord, and surrounding vascular and soft tissue
PET scan	Radioactive isotope is injected into the patient, and the brain is scanned to locate areas of isotope concentration. Patient must remain still during the procedure, which lasts up to 2 hr.	A radionuclide study that can identify areas of increased metabolic activity, vascular abnormalities, and space-occupying lesions
X-ray studies	Patient's head is placed in a specific position in front of the x-ray film; patient must remain still for about 1 min while x-ray is taken.	Bone studies to identify fractures and other bone pathologies

CT, Computed tomography; *EEG,* electroencephalography; *CSF,* cerebrospinal fluid; *MRI,* magnetic resonance imaging; *PET,* positron emission tomography.

PROCEDURE 44-2

Assist the Physician with Patient Care: Prepare the Patient for an Electroencephalogram

GOAL: *To prepare a patient physically and psychologically so that an accurate, useful EEG can be obtained.*

EQUIPMENT and SUPPLIES

- Patient's record

PROCEDURAL STEPS

1. Greet the patient and introduce yourself. Explain that you will go over what is going to happen step by step to ensure the best results.
2. Explain the purpose of the EEG, how the procedure is performed, and what is expected of the patient during the test.
3. Tell the patient that the electrodes pick up tiny electrical signals from the body and that there is no danger of electrical shock.
4. Explain that the test is painless, because the electrodes are attached to the scalp with paste.

5. If this is a sleep EEG, suggest that the patient stay up later than usual the night before the test so that it will be easier to fall asleep.
   PURPOSE: Sleep medications usually are not used, because they may alter the brain wave pattern.
6. Go over the physical preparation, including the diet to be followed for the 48 hours before the test. This usually includes no stimulants (e.g., coffee, chocolate, or sodas) and no skipping meals.
   PURPOSE: Meal skipping may cause hypoglycemia, which alters brain function.
7. Explain that a baseline EEG will be taken at the beginning of the test and during this time the patient will be asked to avoid all movement, even eye and tongue movement.

PROCEDURE 44-2—cont'd

PURPOSE: These activities can be very disruptive to the brain wave tracing.

8. If a stimulation examination is ordered, explain that the patient will be asked to view flickering lights to stimulate the brain. The EEG will measure the brain's response to this stimulation.

9. Ask the patient whether he or she has any questions. If so, answer the questions so that the patient understands the procedure clearly.

PURPOSE: Patients are more likely to cooperate if they understand the process so that they are not unduly apprehensive before and during the test.

10. Document the patient education intervention in the patient's record.
NOTE: Advanced training is required to perform an EEG.

PROCEDURE 44-3

Assist the Physician with Patient Care: Prepare the Patient for and Assist with a Lumbar Puncture

GOAL: *To prepare a patient physically and mentally for a lumbar puncture so that a specimen of CSF can be obtained for testing.*

EQUIPMENT and SUPPLIES

- Patient gown
- Drape
- Local anesthetic
- Sterile, disposable lumbar puncture kit
- Instrument stand
- Sterile gloves
- Permanent marker to label tubes
- Laboratory requisitions as needed
- Biohazard laboratory transport bag
- Patient's record

PROCEDURAL STEPS

1. Assemble the materials needed, and prepare the room. Prepare the equipment and supplies needed for the lumbar puncture.

2. Sanitize your hands and follow Standard Precautions.
PURPOSE: To ensure infection control.

3. Identify the patient and introduce yourself. Explain that you will go over what will happen step by step to ensure the best results.

4. Have the patient void just before the procedure.
PURPOSE: To improve the patient's comfort during the procedure.

5. Give the patient a hospital gown and have him or her put it on with the opening in the back.

6. Place the patient in a left side-lying fetal position for the lumbar puncture.
PURPOSE: To give the physician the easiest access to the lumbar region.

7. Support the patient's head with a pillow as necessary and provide a pillow for between the knees if needed.
PURPOSE: To make the patient as comfortable as possible for the procedure.

8. Perform a sterile skin preparation of the lumbar region in the usual manner.
PURPOSE: To prevent bacterial infection at the puncture site.

9. Place the sterile disposable lumbar puncture kit on an instrument stand and open it, establishing a sterile field. Drape a sterile fenestrated drape over the lumbar region so that only the L3-L4 region of the lower spine is exposed.
PURPOSE: To isolate the area of the procedure in a sterile field.

10. When the physician is ready to perform the lumbar puncture, hold the vial of local anesthetic for the physician.
PURPOSE: To maintain sterile technique and expedite the procedure.

11. Reassure the patient and help him or her hold still during injection of the local anesthetic and insertion of the spinal needle.
PURPOSE: To facilitate accurate insertion of the spinal needle.

12. Using the permanent marker, label the specimens #1, #2, and #3 in the order in which they are collected. This is a crucial step in the procedure.
PURPOSE: Different tests are done on different tubes. The accuracy of these tests depends on the tube on which they are performed.

13. Complete the laboratory requisition form and prepare the CSF specimens for transport to the laboratory.
PURPOSE: To ensure that all the necessary tests are ordered correctly.

14. Clean the area by disposing of sharps, biohazard materials, and regular waste in the normal manner.

15. Monitor the patient and give liquids as directed by the physician.

16. Document the procedure in the patient's medical record.
PURPOSE: A procedure is not complete until it has been documented accurately in the patient's medical record.

9/15/XX 8:32 AM Lumbar puncture performed by Dr. Song. 300 cc CSF labeled and placed for pick up by North Hills Laboratory. Pt stable, no c/o discomfort. Pt given instructions for home care before leaving office. M. Lee, CMA (AAMA)

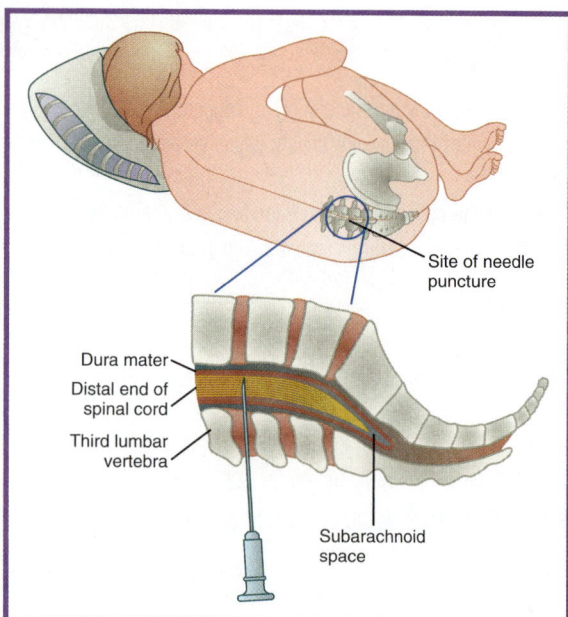

Site of needle
puncture

Dura mater
Distal end of
spinal cord
Third lumbar
vertebra

Subarachnoid
space

FIGURE 44-11 Lumbar puncture.

severe headache accompanied by vomiting may indicate a serious intracranial problem that requires immediate attention. The medical assistant in a neurology practice must remain alert to these types of situations at all times, because neurologic emergencies can develop quite rapidly.

Legal and Ethical Issues

In neurology you will be faced with a variety of behaviors and personality changes that frequently are a part of neurologic conditions. Often a patient is not aware of these changes and may appear as though nothing is wrong. You must treat this patient with the same dignity and respect as you would all other patients, despite how the patient may treat you. Some patients are concerned that loved ones have turned against them and are treating them in an abusive manner. A patient's family may be experiencing severe emotional stress in coping with the patient's behavior. You must remember the medical assistant's code of ethics and the need for total confidentiality. Whatever is discussed in the examination room cannot be repeated to other staff members in the office and can never be discussed outside the office. Confidentiality must be strictly maintained.

HIPAA Applications

Although patients typically have the right to obtain a copy of their confidential health information, under the HIPAA privacy regulations, access to psychotherapy notes is limited. HIPAA defines psychotherapy notes as the documentation completed by a mental health professional that describes and analyzes the conversations with a patient during counseling sessions. These notes are not supposed to be stored in the patient's general chart and should not be released to third-party payers. Disclosure of psychotherapy notes requires specific patient permission before any documentation can be released to an insurance provider. Under federal law, the therapist must decide whether to release the notes to the patient, and if the therapist decides not to release the information, the patient cannot appeal this decision. However, the final authority rests with individual state laws. If a state law is stricter than the federal mandate or gives the patient greater access to psychotherapy notes, state law takes precedence over federal law.

including thought, learning, and memory. It is responsible for maintaining homeostasis (constant internal environmental conditions that are compatible with life) among the body's systems. Through its many receptors, the nervous system constantly monitors what is going on inside the body and in the environment outside the body.

When the nervous system becomes damaged or diseased, signs and symptoms can appear in every other body system. Motor activity can become erratic, or activity level can decline to the point that the person becomes unable to communicate or function normally.

Your main responsibilities as a medical assistant in neurology are to observe, listen, and report any changes in patients. Even signs and symptoms that may seem rather slight can give the physician the one clue needed to put the puzzle together and arrive at a correct diagnosis before proceeding to the appropriate treatment. It is crucial that medical assistants working in a neurology practice recognize the importance and significance of a variety of symptoms. For example,

SUMMARY OF SCENARIO

Mai has excelled in her new position as clinical assistant and patient educator. With Dr. Song's approval, she has developed a series of patient information sheets that explain the functions of the nervous system, the symptoms to watch for after a head injury, the kinds and causes of headaches, and infections of the nervous system. Patients often ask for information sheets for other family members and for their friends and neighbors. She also developed a set of

information sheets to explain typical neurologic diagnostic tests and how best to prepare for them. Although the patient receives a copy of the information sheet, Mai still talks with each patient to make sure he or she understands exactly what will happen in the test and to answer all questions completely. Mai feels a great deal of personal satisfaction from working with patients and helping them understand their diagnosis and treatment protocols.

SUMMARY OF LEARNING OBJECTIVES

1. **Define, spell, and pronounce the terms listed in the vocabulary.**
   Spelling and pronouncing medical terms correctly bolster the medical assistant's credibility. Knowing the definitions of these terms promotes confidence in communication with patients and co-workers.

2. **Apply critical thinking skills in performing the patient assessment and patient care.**
   Completing the Critical Thinking Application exercises throughout the chapter can help the student medical assistant become more adept at critical analysis of real-life situations.

3. **Summarize the anatomy and physiology of the nervous system.**
   The main function of the nervous system is to control body functions so that homeostasis can be maintained. It does this by receiving messages in the CNS from the PNS, then sending a response to the appropriate location in the body, again via the PNS. The neuron is the functional cell of the nervous system, and neuroglial cells support and protect neurons throughout the system. The brain is made up of the cerebrum, cerebellum, and brainstem. The CNS is well protected, first by the skull and then by the dura mater, arachnoid mater, and pia mater meninges.

4. **Differentiate between the central and peripheral nervous systems.**
   The nervous system is made up of two parts: the CNS, which includes the brain and spinal cord, and the PNS, which includes all the nerves outside the CNS.

5. **Identify the typical symptoms associated with neurologic disorders.**
   Symptoms of potentially serious neurologic conditions include headache, nausea and vomiting, change in vision, altered level of consciousness, memory loss, sleep disorders, confusion or disorientation, and problems with mobility.

6. **Distinguish among common nervous system diseases and conditions.**
   Table 44-3 summarizes the most common diseases and conditions of the nervous system.

7. **Describe the pathology of cerebrovascular diseases.**
   CVD may be caused by atherosclerosis, hypertension, thrombi, emboli, or aneurysm. A TIA is a temporary limitation of function as a result of short-term ischemia. A CVA occurs when the blood supply to a particular part of the brain is cut off by an embolus, a thrombus, or an aneurysm that bursts. Migraine headaches are associated with a disturbance in the blood supply to the brain.

8. **Identify the various types of epilepsy.**
   Seizures are classified as either partial or generalized, based on how much of the brain is involved in the abnormal electrical activity. Partial seizures result from abnormal electrical activity in just one part of the brain, whereas generalized seizures involve most or all of the brain. Generalized seizures include petit mal seizures, which are brief episodes characterized by staring, subtle body movement, and brief lapses of awareness. Probably the best-known seizure disorder is the generalized tonic-clonic disorder that causes grand mal seizures.

9. **Compare and contrast encephalitis and meningitis.**
   Encephalitis is a viral infection of the brain that can cause serious CNS symptoms. Meningitis may be caused by viruses, bacteria, or fungi. Bacterial meningitis is most serious. Viral meningitis usually resolves without treatment or incident.

10. **Explain the dynamics of brain and spinal cord injuries.**
    Traumatic brain injuries can range from a mild concussion to severe injury, coma, and death. A minor concussion usually causes no long-term side effects; however, a moderate to severe brain injury can result in headaches, amnesia, confusion, personality changes, and seizures. The higher the damage to the spinal cord, the more serious the injury. Head injuries can be either open or closed, with possible serious intracerebral damage and potential complications within the meningeal layers. Shaken baby syndrome is caused by violently shaking an infant back and forth, forcing the brain against opposite ends of the skull.

11. **Summarize the neurologic diseases that affect mobility.**
    PD is a chronic, progressive, debilitating neurologic disease that is caused by lack of the neurotransmitter dopamine. MS causes progressive inflammation and demyelination of the axon, resulting in a scattering of the nervous message as it passes down the axon. ALS is a rapidly progressive, ultimately fatal neurologic disease that destroys the motor neurons responsible for voluntary muscle control. Bell's palsy causes temporary facial paralysis because of damage or trauma to cranial nerve VII. Peripheral neuropathies can result from damage or injury to any part of the neuron and typically are caused by other systemic diseases, such as diabetes. CTS results from compression of the median nerve as it passes through the carpal bones of the wrist.

12. **Differentiate among common mental health disorders.**
    Depressive disorders affect the way a person thinks, feels, eats, and sleeps. People with depression cannot "snap out of it" and without treatment may suffer from symptoms that last weeks, months, or years. Types of depressive disorders include major depression, dysthymia, and bipolar disorders. Anxiety disorders cause an overwhelming, irrational feeling of anxiety and fear; these include panic disorder, OCD, post-traumatic stress disorder, and phobias. Risk factors for suicide include serious depressive disorders; reduced serotonin levels; a prior suicide attempt; family violence; and exposure to the suicidal behavior of others. Schizophrenia is a chronic, severe, and disabling brain disorder with symptoms that include hallucinations and delusions; difficulty speaking and expressing emotions; and cognitive deficits.

13. **Analyze the medical assistant's role in the neurologic examination.**
    When assisting in neurology, the medical assistant must be particularly careful to recognize signs and symptoms, which frequently are quite subtle but yet can be extremely significant in helping to assess and diagnose the neurologic patient accurately (see Procedure 44-1).

14. **Explain the common diagnostic procedures for the nervous system.**
    Diagnostic tests for the neurologic system are summarized in Table 44-5. They include arteriograms, CT, MRI, and PET scans, EEG, lumbar puncture, and various x-ray studies.

15. **Outline the steps needed to prepare a patient for an electroencephalogram (EEG).**

    Procedure 44-2 outlines the steps for preparing a patient for an EEG.

16. **Describe the steps for preparing a patient for and assisting with a lumbar puncture.**

    Procedure 44-3 describes the procedural steps for preparing a patient for and assisting with a lumbar puncture.

17. **Discuss the implications of patient education in a neurologic and mental health practice.**

    When the nervous system becomes damaged or diseased, signs and symptoms can appear in every other body system. Motor activity can become erratic, or activity level can decline to the point that the person becomes unable to communicate or function normally. Your main responsibilities as a medical assistant in neurology are to observe, listen, and report any changes in patients.

18. **Explain the legal issues and HIPAA applications associated with neurology and mental health.**

    Whatever is discussed in the examination room cannot be repeated to other staff members in the office and can never be discussed outside the office. Confidentiality must be strictly maintained. Disclosure of psychotherapy notes requires specific patient permission. Under federal law, the therapist must decide whether to release the notes to the patient, and if the therapist decides not to release the information, the patient cannot appeal this decision. However, the final authority rests with individual state laws.

CONNECTIONS

Study Guide Connection: Go to the Chapter 44 Study Guide. Read and complete the activities.

Evolve Connection: Go to the Chapter 44 link at *evolve.elsevier.com/kinn* to complete the Chapter Review and Chapter Quiz. Check out the other resources listed for this chapter to make the most of what you have learned from Assisting in Neurology and Mental Health.

ASSISTING IN ENDOCRINOLOGY

45

SCENARIO

Miguel Vasco has been a certified medical assistant (CMA [AAMA]) for 10 years and has worked for the past 3 years with a multiphysician endocrinology and internal medicine practice. Although he has taken care of patients with many different disorders of the endocrine system, most of the practice's patients are individuals with diabetes mellitus type 2. One of Miguel's responsibilities is teaching patients newly diagnosed with diabetes how to monitor their blood glucose levels and maintain a healthy lifestyle.

While studying this chapter, think about the following questions:

- What are the primary responsibilities of a medical assistant in an internal medicine practice?
- What clinical skills are required in this specialty practice?
- What common diseases and disorders of the endocrine system should medical assistants working in this field be able to discuss and explain?
- What diagnostic and treatment procedures typically are used in an endocrinology practice?
- What information should the medical assistant know regarding the management of diabetes and the possible complications associated with the disease?

LEARNING OBJECTIVES

1. Define, spell, and pronounce the terms listed in the vocabulary.
2. Apply critical thinking skills in performing the patient assessment and patient care.
3. Summarize the anatomy and physiology of the endocrine system.
4. Explain the mechanism of hormone action.
5. Differentiate among the diseases and disorders of the endocrine system.
6. Describe the diagnostic criteria for diabetes mellitus.
7. Compare and contrast prediabetes, diabetes type 1, diabetes type 2, and gestational diabetes.
8. Outline the treatment plan and management of the different types of diabetes mellitus.
9. Perform blood glucose screening with a glucometer.
10. Identify the characteristics of hypoglycemia and hyperglycemia.
11. Describe the complications associated with diabetes mellitus.
12. Summarize patient education approaches to diabetes.
13. Discuss legal and ethical issues to consider when caring for patients with endocrine system disorders.

VOCABULARY

adrenocorticotropic hormone (ACTH) (uh-dren-o-cor-ti-ko-tro'-pik) A hormone that stimulates the production and secretion of glucocorticoids; it is released by the anterior pituitary gland.

follicle-stimulating hormone (FSH) A hormone secreted by the anterior pituitary; it stimulates oogenesis and spermatogenesis.

gluconeogenesis (glu-kuh-ne-uh-je'-nuh-suhs) The formation of glucose in the liver from proteins and fats.

glycogen The sugar (starch) formed from glucose; it is stored mainly in the liver.

glycosuria The abnormal presence of glucose in the urine.

growth hormone (GH) Also called *somatotropic hormone;* it stimulates tissue growth and restricts tissue glucose dependence when nutrients are not available.

luteinizing hormone (LH) (lu-te-uh-niz'-ing) A hormone produced by the anterior pituitary gland that promotes ovulation.

nocturia Excessive urination during the night.

polyphagia (pah-le-faj'-e-uh) Increased appetite.

prolactin (PRL) A hormone secreted by the anterior pituitary gland that stimulates the development of the mammary gland.

satiety The state of being satisfied or feeling full after eating.

specific gravity The density of urine compared with an equal volume of water.

thyroid-stimulating hormone (TSH) A hormone secreted by the anterior pituitary gland that stimulates the secretion of hormones produced by the thyroid gland.

Individuals with disorders of the endocrine system usually are seen first by the primary care physician (PCP), who may refer them to an internist or an endocrinologist for specialized care. Patients with certain endocrine disorders, such as diabetes mellitus (DM), also may be seen in a clinic for follow-up and treatment. A medical assistant employed in any of these ambulatory care settings assists with diagnostic procedures, specialized examinations, and patient education. It is important that medical assistants recognize the dynamics of endocrine system diseases so that they can help patients understand how to administer their medications and prevent long-term complications from the disease.

ANATOMY AND PHYSIOLOGY OF THE ENDOCRINE SYSTEM

Both the nervous system and the endocrine system control the body's physiologic responses to internal and external stimuli. The nervous system is electrical in nature and sends immediate messages along a nerve pathway to evoke a response; the endocrine system relies on the bloodstream to carry hormonal messages to a target cell for action. Through hormonal action, the endocrine system regulates all body functions. Endocrinology is the study of hormones, their receptor cells, and the results of hormone action.

The word part *endo-* means "in" or "within"; the suffix *-crine* means "secrete." The endocrine system consists of glands located throughout the body that produce and secrete chemicals known as *hormones.* Hormones are excreted directly into the bloodstream, which carries them to the target tissue. Hormones function as the body's chemical messengers, transferring information from one group of cells to another. Hormones control growth, mood, system functions, metabolism, sexual maturity, and reproduction. Hormone levels vary and can be affected by outside factors such as illness and stress.

Basic Anatomy

Glands are categorized as either exocrine or endocrine. *Exocrine glands,* such as sweat glands and salivary glands, secrete either

through a duct or directly onto the surface of the skin or in the mouth. *Endocrine glands* release hormones directly into the bloodstream, which transports the hormones to target cells for action.

The glands of the endocrine system are the hypothalamus, pituitary, pineal gland, thyroid, parathyroids, thymus, and adrenals and the reproductive glands (i.e., the ovaries and the testes) (Figure 45-1). Some nonendocrine organs, especially the pancreas, also can produce and release hormones. The hypothalamus, located in the inferior midportion of the brain, is the major connection between the nervous and endocrine systems. The hypothalamus controls the action of the pituitary, a pea-sized gland located below the hypothalamus. The pituitary often is called the "master gland" because it secretes hormones that regulate multiple endocrine glands.

The pituitary gland is separated into two parts, the anterior and posterior lobes. The anterior pituitary, or adenohypophysis, regulates the functions of the thyroid, adrenals, and reproductive glands. It produces **growth hormone (GH)**, **thyroid-stimulating hormone (TSH)**, **adrenocorticotropic hormone (ACTH)**, **prolactin (PRL)**, **follicle-stimulating hormone (FSH)**, and **luteinizing hormone (LH)**. The posterior lobe of the pituitary, or neurohypophysis, excretes oxytocin, which stimulates the contractions of the smooth muscle of the uterus that occur during labor and the flow of breast milk toward the nipple when an infant breastfeeds. The posterior pituitary also produces antidiuretic hormone (ADH), which helps control fluid balance by acting on the kidneys to reabsorb fluid as needed to maintain homeostasis (Figure 45-2).

The pineal gland, which is located deep within the brain, excretes the hormone melatonin. Melatonin helps regulate waking and sleeping patterns and also may affect seasonal reactions to alterations in the availability of sunlight.

When stimulated by TSH, the thyroid gland produces the thyroid hormones triiodothyronine (T_3) and thyroxine (T_4), which control the body's metabolic rate and are important factors in bone growth and nervous system development in children. On the dorsal aspect of the thyroid gland are several small parathyroid glands, which release hormones (parathyroid and calcitonin) that regulate the level of calcium in the blood. The parathyroid hormone (PTH) maintains

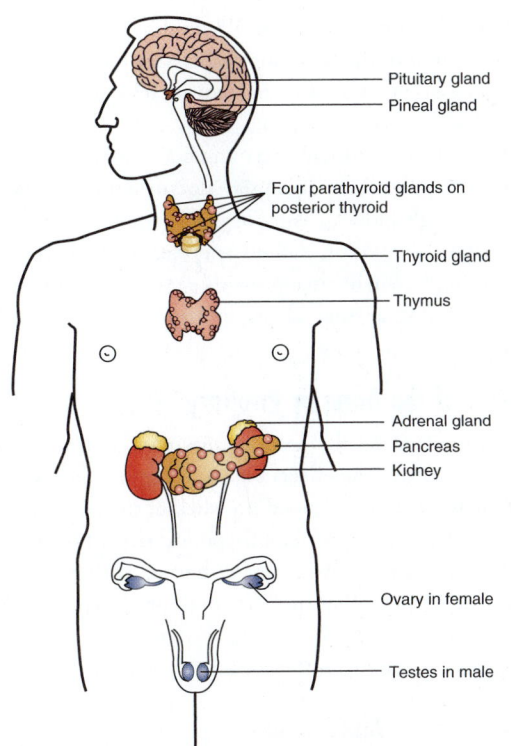

FIGURE 45-1 Location of the endocrine glands. (From Gould B: *Pathophysiology for the health professions,* ed 3, St Louis, 2006, WB Saunders.)

a constant concentration of calcium in the body by regulating the absorption of calcium from the gastrointestinal tract and stimulating the reabsorption of calcium stored in the bone as needed to maintain homeostasis. Calcitonin stimulates deposition of calcium into the bone when excess amounts of calcium are available.

The thymus gland, located behind the upper portion of the sternum, produces hormones that stimulate the production of specialized immune system cells called *T cells.* The thymus gland is present at birth, enlarges as the child ages, but begins to atrophy as the child reaches puberty. It once was thought that the thymus played no role in the physiology of adults, but we now know that its hormone action is crucial to T-cell maturation. (T cells are discussed in further detail in Chapter 54.)

On top of each kidney are the adrenal glands, which are triangular-shaped glands consisting of an outer layer, called the *adrenal cortex,* and an inner body, called the *adrenal medulla.* The adrenal cortex secretes corticosteroid hormones, including cortisol, aldosterone, and adrenal androgens, all of which influence a wide range of bodily functions. The adrenal medulla produces epinephrine, also called *adrenaline,* which activates the body's reaction to stress.

The gonads produce sex hormones. The male gonads are the testes; they secrete testosterone, which regulates the development of secondary sexual characteristics, such as voice changes and the growth of facial and pubic hair, and promotes the production of sperm. The female gonads, the ovaries, produce eggs or ova (oogenesis) and secrete estrogen and progesterone. The female hormones

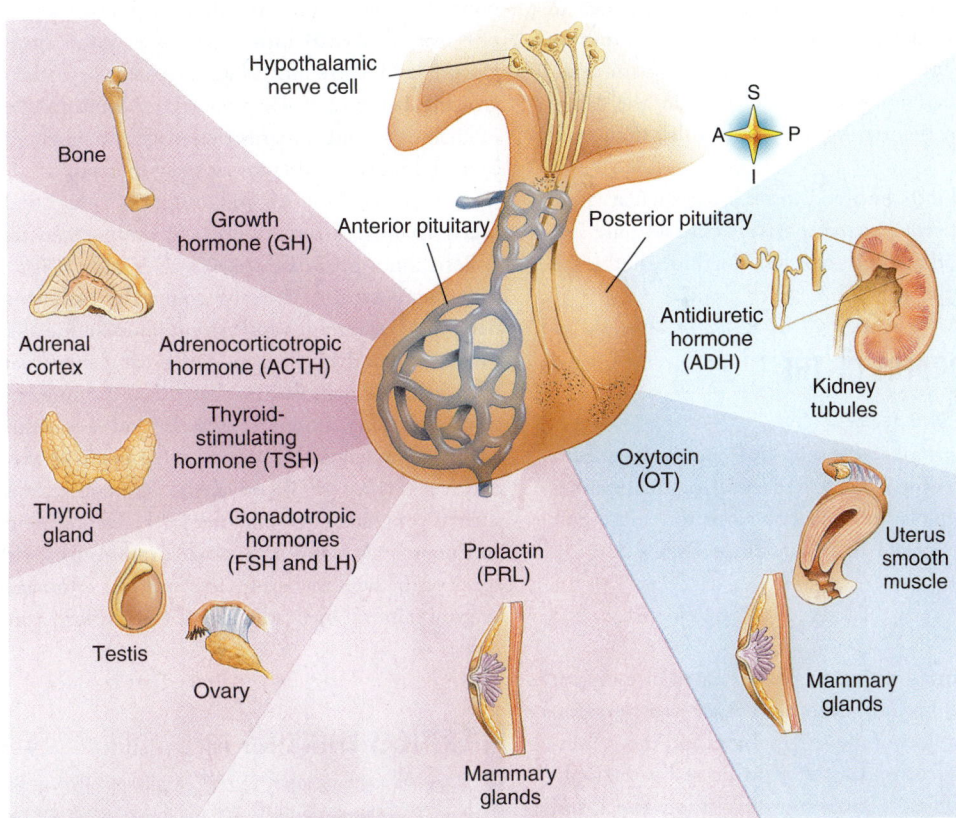

FIGURE 45-2 The principal anterior and posterior pituitary hormones and their target organs. (From Thibodeau GA, Patton KT: *The human body in health and disease,* ed 4, St Louis, 2005, Mosby.)

control the development of breast tissue and other secondary sexual characteristics, regulate menstruation, and play important roles during pregnancy.

The pancreas performs essential endocrine functions by producing insulin and glucagon, which work together to maintain normal blood glucose levels and store glucose for energy.

CRITICAL THINKING APPLICATION   **45-1**

Miguel is asked to order educational supplies for patients with endocrine system disorders. Because he thinks it is important for patients to understand their health problems, he wants to order a brochure that clearly depicts and describes the anatomy of the endocrine system. What glands and organs should be included in the handout?

Mechanisms of Hormone Action

The goal of hormone regulation is to maintain homeostasis. Hormone secretion is regulated by a number of mechanisms, including nervous stimulation, endocrine control (a hormone from one gland, such as the anterior pituitary, stimulates the release of a hormone from another gland), and feedback systems. An example of nervous system regulation of endocrine function is the release of adrenaline from the adrenal medulla in response to stimulation from the sympathetic nervous system during a stressful episode. In the most common feedback system, negative feedback, an endocrine gland is activated by an imbalance and acts to correct the imbalance by stopping the secretion process. For example, if calcium blood levels fall below normal, the parathyroid glands are stimulated to release PTH. PTH acts to increase blood calcium levels either by stimulating the absorption of calcium from the gut or by demineralizing bone to release stored calcium. This change in the blood calcium level is detected by the parathyroid gland, which then stops production of PTH.

Each hormone released into the bloodstream has particular target cells for action. The target cells have receptors that attract only specific hormones and permit the hormone to pass through the cell membrane and affect cellular action.

DISEASES AND DISORDERS OF THE ENDOCRINE SYSTEM

Faulty secretion of any hormone, whether too much or too little, can cause health problems for patients. The goal of treatment is either to control the hypersecretion of hormones or to replace hormones that are not being secreted at therapeutic levels.

Posterior Pituitary Gland Disorder

Diabetes Insipidus

When ADH (or vasopressin) is not produced or released in sufficient amounts, the patient develops a condition called *diabetes insipidus.* ADH increases the permeability of the renal tubules and the collecting tubules in the kidneys, permitting fluid to be reabsorbed and causing the urine to become more concentrated. Without the action of ADH, fluid is not reabsorbed from the renal tubules, which causes a large amount of fluid to be excreted in the urine, with the potential

onset of dehydration. A lack of ADH results from a tumor either in the hypothalamus or the posterior pituitary gland, or diabetes insipidus may develop because of an inadequate response to ADH in the renal tubules.

Diabetes insipidus usually has an acute onset, and the patient presents with polyuria, polydipsia, **nocturia**, low urine **specific gravity**, and high blood plasma osmolality (concentration). It can result in fatal dehydration if fluid and electrolyte levels cannot be controlled. Replacement therapy with a synthetic vasopressin (desmopressin) nasal spray, oral tablets, or injections can be used to treat the disorder.

Diseases of the Anterior Pituitary

Hormones secreted by the anterior pituitary control a number of glandular functions. The effects on the body of changes in anterior pituitary gland secretion depend on whether the hormones are produced at an abnormally low level (hypopituitarism) or at a very high level (hyperpituitarism). A patient diagnosed with panhypopituitarism has a deficiency of all the hormones produced by the anterior pituitary, and the symptoms reflect systemic inactivity of all the glands stimulated by the anterior pituitary hormones.

Growth Hormone Abnormalities

Hypopituitary dwarfism occurs when the pituitary gland fails to produce normal amounts of GH. The child's height is impaired, but he or she will have a normal-sized head and trunk. Hypersecretion of GH causes two different disorders, depending on the patient's developmental age. Oversecretion of GH in childhood, before closure of the epiphyseal plates in the long bones, causes the long bones to grow excessively. Affected individuals may reach a height of 8 feet or taller. Because GH has a secondary effect on the blood glucose level, these individuals may develop diabetes mellitus. Slow-growing, benign anterior pituitary adenomas frequently are the cause of gigantism, and treatment consists of removing the tumor if possible and radiation therapy or drug therapy.

If hypersecretion of GH occurs in adulthood, the disorder is called *acromegaly*. Because the epiphyseal plates are closed, the long bones cannot grow. Consequently, a wide range of manifestations can occur because of excessive connective tissue growth and overproduction of bone. Signs and symptoms include arthralgia, an enlarged tongue, overactive sebaceous and sweat glands, coarse skin, excessive body hair, and nerve damage caused by pressure on peripheral nerves from increasing amounts of bone and soft tissue. A gradual but noticeable enlargement occurs in the bones of the jaw, face, hands, and feet (Figure 45-3). Advanced acromegaly causes complications such as congestive heart failure, DM, cerebrovascular abnormalities, and neurologic symptoms as the tumor grows within the confined space of the hypothalamus. Treatment of acromegaly requires either surgical removal or irradiation of the pituitary tumor.

CRITICAL THINKING APPLICATION   **45-2**

Many different disorders can occur with problems with the anterior pituitary. Describe two such health problems using your knowledge of target organ action.

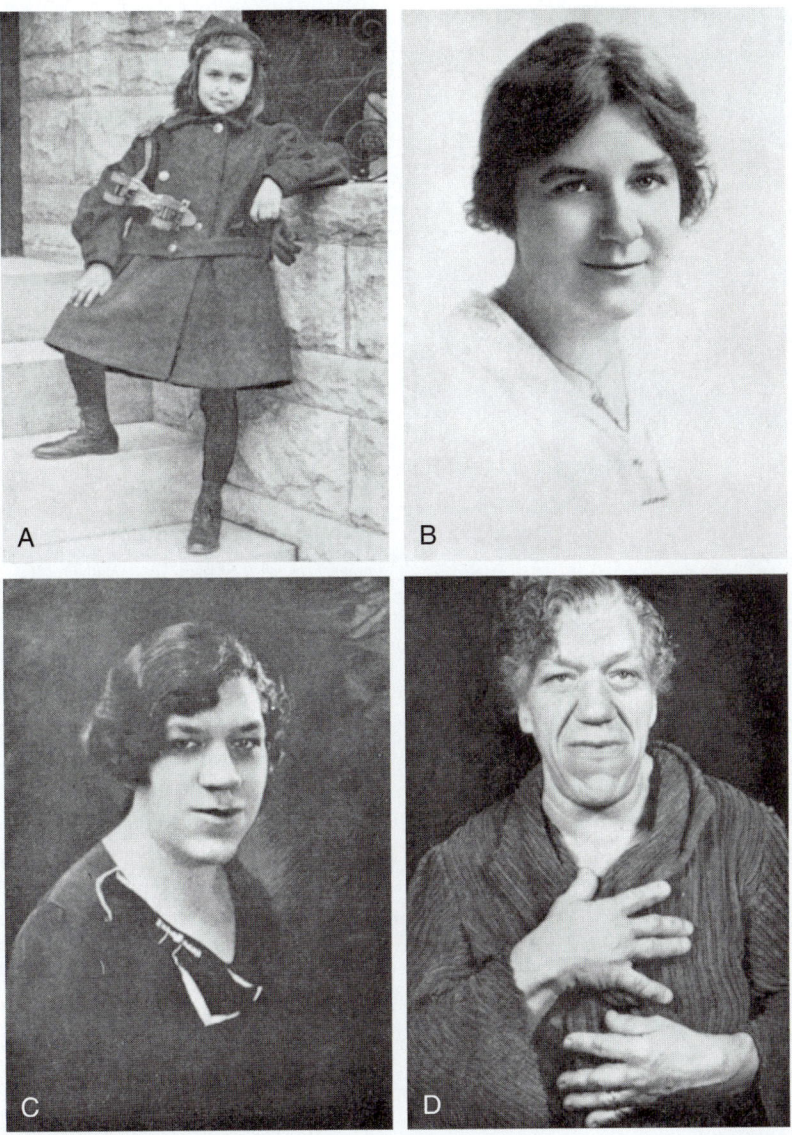

FIGURE 45-3 Progression of acromegaly. **A,** Patient at age 9. **B,** Patient at age 16, with possible early features of acromegaly. **C,** Patient at age 33, with well-established acromegaly. **D,** Patient at age 52, end-stage acromegaly. (From Clinical Pathological Conference, Am J Med 20:133, 1956.)

Disorders of the Thyroid

Hypothyroidism

Deficient secretion of the thyroid hormones may result from a number of factors. One cause of hypothyroidism is endemic iodine deficiency, a lack of iodine in the diet, resulting in the formation of a simple goiter. A *simple goiter* is any thyroid enlargement that has not been caused by an infection or neoplasm. Endemic goiters occur in certain geographic areas. If more than 10% of the children 6 to 12 years of age in a particular area have goiters, that geographic location is defined as endemic for goiters.

T$_3$ and T$_4$ are produced in the thyroid gland from iodine and are responsible for the regulation of metabolic activities in all body cells. When the thyroid gland is unable to obtain sufficient amounts of iodine from the circulating blood, it enlarges, or hypertrophies, in an attempt to produce the hormones needed by the body. A decreased amount of thyroid hormones results in a lower metabolic rate, heat loss, and poor mental and physical development. Iodine deficiency is rare in the United States because of the widespread use of iodized table salt and the distribution of foods from iodine-rich areas. The treatment for a simple goiter is to reduce its size by prescribing dietary supplements of iodine, thyroid hormone replacement, or surgery.

Improper development of the thyroid in an infant or young child usually is congenital. The absence of adequate levels of thyroid hormones results in a condition known as *cretinism*. Newborns have feeding problems, constipation, and a hoarse cry and sleep for extreme lengths of time. Symptoms include lethargy, bradycardia, stunted skeletal growth, and varying degrees of mental retardation, depending on the severity and the length of the hypothyroidism.

When severe or chronic hypothyroidism occurs in an adult or older child, the condition is called *myxedema*. The patient shows fatigue, weight gain, hair loss, a slower pulse rate, a lowered body temperature, muscle cramps, menorrhagia, and thick, dry, puffy

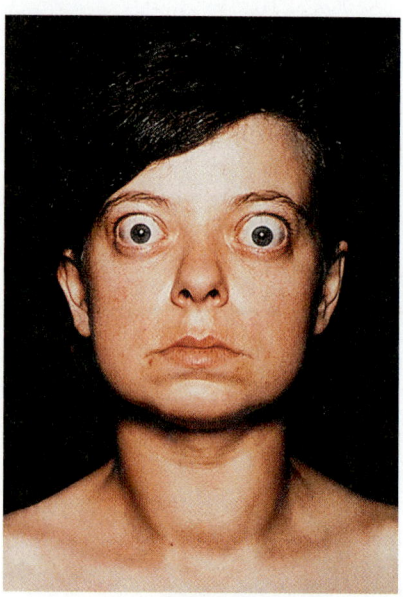

FIGURE 45-4 Exophthalmos in Graves' disease. (From Seidel HM et al: *Mosby's guide to physical examination*, ed 6, St Louis, 2006, Mosby.)

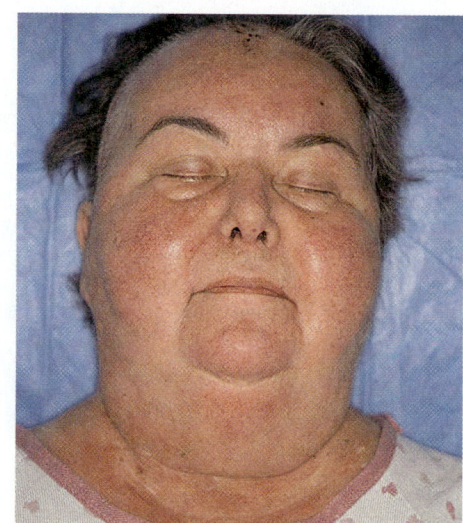

FIGURE 45-5 Cushing's syndrome. (From Seidel HM et al: *Mosby's guide to physical examination*, ed 6, St Louis, 2006, Mosby.)

skin. Routine tests to diagnose hypothyroidism include radioimmunoassay, a radiologic blood test, for T_3, T_4, and TSH. Adequate doses of thyroxine (Levothroid, Levoxyl, or Synthroid) restore normal function and appearance. Patients diagnosed with hypothyroidism must take hormone replacement therapy daily for the rest of their lives.

Hyperthyroidism

Thyrotoxicosis, a condition in which the serum levels of thyroid hormones are excessively high, can also be caused by a number of factors. Symptoms include weight loss, tachycardia, palpitations, hypertension, agitation, nervousness, depression, tremor, excessive sweating, goiter, and exophthalmia (protruding eyes) (Figure 45-4). Graves' disease, an autoimmune disorder that stimulates overactive thyroid hormone production, is the most common cause of thyrotoxicosis. The goal of treatment is to control excessive thyroid hormone production through drug therapy (methimazole and propylthiouracil); radioactive implants to destroy part of the gland; ingestion of radioactive iodine, which concentrates in the thyroid gland, causing it to shrink; or thyroidectomy, which is the surgical removal of a section of the gland. After irradiation or surgical removal of part of the thyroid gland, the patient's thyroid hormone levels are evaluated. The patient often must receive replacement hormone therapy (Levothroid, Levoxyl, or Synthroid) postoperatively to maintain normal thyroid hormone levels. Individuals who develop exophthalmia from hyperthyroidism may require orbital decompression surgery, in which the bone between the eye socket and sinuses is removed, giving the eyes room to return to their normal position.

> **CRITICAL THINKING APPLICATION   45-3**
> One of the internists, Dr. Misha, asks Miguel if he can describe the signs and symptoms of a patient with hypothyroidism or hyperthyroidism. Summarize Miguel's answer.

Disorders of the Adrenal Glands

Adrenal insufficiency is called *Addison's disease*. This condition is relatively rare and is caused by an autoimmune reaction that affects the adrenal cortex, which secretes corticosteroid hormones. Symptoms include hypoglycemia, increased pigmentation of the skin, muscle weakness, gastrointestinal disturbances, and fatigue. Cortisol and aldosterone deficiencies lead to retention of potassium and the excretion of water and sodium in the urine. Severe dehydration, low blood volume, low blood pressure, and circulatory shock can occur. Treatment includes replacement of cortisol with the long-term daily administration of glucocorticoids (e.g., prednisone) and replacement of aldosterone with fludrocortisone (Florinef) to control sodium and potassium levels while helping to maintain normal blood pressure levels. Patients should also be encouraged to eat a diet high in complex carbohydrates and protein and to maintain an adequate fluid intake. Patients with Addison's disease are at risk for addisonian crisis, a life-threatening drop in blood pressure, hypoglycemia, and high blood potassium levels. A crisis can be brought on by stressful situations, infections, minor illness, or surgery. Treatment requires immediate administration of an intravenous saline and dextrose solution with corticosteroids.

Hypersecretion of the adrenal cortex, causing increased levels of cortisol, is known as *Cushing's syndrome*. Usually a benign pituitary tumor causes the release of excessive amounts of ACTH. Symptoms associated with Cushing's syndrome may be seen in individuals taking corticosteroids for medical reasons, such as organ transplantation, severe asthma, or rheumatoid arthritis. Excessive levels of cortisol cause an accumulation of adipose tissue in the trunk, a round, or "moon," face, and fat pads in the cervical spine region, causing the formation of a "buffalo hump" (Figure 45-5). The patient also has glucose intolerance because of insulin resistance at the target cell level.

Additional symptoms include hyperpigmentation, muscle wasting, problems with wound healing, hypertension, kidney stones, and osteoporosis. Female patients have menstrual irregularity, and many patients with Cushing's syndrome experience mental disorders such as irritability, depression, or severe psychiatric disorders. Treatment depends on the cause of the disorder; it includes medication to control cortisol levels, radiation therapy to reduce the size of the tumor, and surgery to remove the tumor.

Endocrine Dysfunction of the Pancreas: Diabetes Mellitus

Diabetes mellitus is a common hormonal imbalance that has reached epidemic proportions in the United States. Approximately 24 million Americans, or close to 8% of the population, have DM, and the number is growing. Diabetes occurs in people of all ages and races but is more common in older adults (23% of individuals over age 60) and in African-Americans, Latinos, Native Americans, and Asian-Americans/Pacific Islanders. DM is characterized by chronic hyperglycemia and problems with carbohydrate metabolism. This problem with glucose management is caused by a lack of insulin production and/or resistance to insulin at the target cell level. The pancreas contains islets of Langerhans, which produce and secrete the hormones insulin and glucagon. When the blood glucose level is too high, beta islet cells secrete insulin, which is sent through the bloodstream to the target tissue site to conduct glucose into the cell. When blood glucose levels are low, glucagon is secreted by the alpha islet cells to stimulate the liver to convert **glycogen** (stored glucose) into circulating glucose.

If there is resistance to insulin at the target cell membrane or if not enough insulin is available to help transport glucose from the blood into the cells, the person experiences a variety of symptoms, including **glycosuria**, polyuria, polydipsia, **polyphagia**, rapid weight loss, drowsiness, fatigue, itching of the skin, visual disturbances, and skin infections. The American Diabetes Association has identified four major types of diabetes: prediabetes, DM type 1, DM type 2, and gestational diabetes. If left untreated or managed poorly, DM can have serious, life-threatening consequences, such as cardiovascular disease, stroke, hypertension, blindness, kidney disease, nervous system disorders, amputations, pregnancy complications, and diabetic coma. Patient education is crucial for compliance with treatment and prevention of life-threatening complications.

DIAGNOSTIC CRITERIA FOR DIABETES MELLITUS

- Plasma glucose level ≥ 200 mg/dL (norm is 80 to 120 mg/dL) with the classic symptoms of polyuria, polydipsia, and unexplained weight loss
- Fasting plasma glucose level ≥ 126 mg/dL (norm is 70 to 110 mg/dL) on more than one occasion
- Two-hour oral glucose tolerance test (OGTT) result ≥ 200 mg/dL
- Urinalysis positive for glucose and possibly ketones
- Glycosylated hemoglobin (HbA$_{1c}$) > 7% (normal is 4% to 6%)

Prediabetes

Prediabetes is a condition in which a person's blood glucose level is higher than normal but not high enough for a diagnosis of diabetes type 2. It is estimated that 54 million adults in the United States have prediabetes. Some of the long-term damage to vascular and cardiac systems may be occurring during prediabetes. Studies indicate that most individuals with prediabetes develop diabetes type 2

within 10 years. However, if patients lower their blood glucose levels, they can delay or prevent its onset. Experts recommend that patients with prediabetes lose 5% to 10% of their weight and perform moderate physical activity for 30 to 60 minutes daily. A loss of just 10 to 20 pounds can make a huge difference in blood glucose levels.

Two tests are used to diagnose prediabetes: the fasting plasma glucose (FPG) test and the oral glucose tolerance test (OGTT). A person with prediabetes has a fasting blood glucose level between 100 and 125 mg/dL; individuals with an FPG level of 126 mg/dL or higher are diagnosed as diabetic. A person with prediabetes has a 2-hour OGTT result of 140 to 199 mg/dL; diabetes is diagnosed if the OGTT is 200 mg/dL or higher.

Type 1 Diabetes

Diabetes type 1 most often develops in children and young adults. This disease previously was known as either *juvenile-onset diabetes* or *insulin-dependent diabetes*. In DM type 1 the pancreas is unable to produce insulin because of the destruction of the beta islet cells from autoimmune, genetic, or environmental factors. DM type 1 affects 5% to 10% of patients with diabetes, and it typically has an acute onset. Treatment of diabetes type 1 requires insulin administration. The goal for insulin therapy is to maintain blood glucose levels as close to normal as possible without causing hypoglycemia. Many types and brands of insulin are available, but to prevent allergic reactions, only genetically engineered human insulin should be used. At this time, the only method of insulin administration is injection, because gastrointestinal processes destroy insulin if it is given by mouth. However, multiple studies are underway on buccal, inhaled, and patch forms of the hormone. An inhaled form of insulin had been released but is no longer available because of concerns that the drug is associated with decreased pulmonary function. (Subcutaneous administration of insulin was presented in Chapter 35.)

The medical assistant usually is involved in teaching patients how to administer their insulin accurately. Table 45-1 summarizes the various types of insulin. Although insulin should be stored in the refrigerator, injecting the cold solution may be painful for the patient, and patients who must travel with insulin doses need to understand correct storage procedures. The physician may recommend that the patient store the bottle currently in use at room temperature. Depending on the type of insulin, it can be stored safely at room temperatures for 7 to 28 days. For example, Humalog and Regular insulins can be stored at room temperature for 28 days, whereas NPH and premixed solutions containing NPH can be stored this way only for 7 to 14 days. Extreme temperatures can damage the drug, so it should not be frozen, left in the sunlight, or carried in the glove compartment of a car. Temperatures below 59°F (15°C) or above 86°F (30°C) must be avoided.

Successful treatment of DM type 1 involves a complicated regimen in which various types of insulin are given in multiple injections (typically four) throughout the day. (See Procedure 35-9 for the steps for dispensing and mixing two different types of insulin in one syringe.) The insulin type and dosage are balanced by the patient's typical exercise regimen and diet (the diabetic diet is discussed in Chapter 30). The patient must monitor blood glucose levels with a glucometer periodically throughout the day to determine whether the levels are within the normal range. The physician typically prescribes glucometer testing in the morning before

TABLE 45-1 Types and Characteristics of Insulin

TYPE	ONSET OF ACTION	PEAK ACTION	EFFECTIVE DURATION	APPEARANCE	COMMENTS
Rapid Acting					
Humalog (Lispro), NovaLog (Aspart)	10-15 min	1-2 hr	2-5 hr	Clear	Take just before or just after eating
Short Acting					
Regular (Novolin R, Humulin R)	30-60 min	2-4 hr	3-5 hr	Clear	Take 30 min before meal
Intermediate Acting					
NPH (Novolin N, Humulin N)	2-4 hr	4-10 hr	10-16 hr	Cloudy	Take at bedtime to minimize nighttime hypoglycemia
Lente (Novolin, Humulin L)	3-4 hr	4-12 hr	12-18 hr	Clear	
Long Acting					
Ultralente	6-10 hr	Minimal peak	18-20 hr	Clear	
Glargine (Lantus)	4-6 hr	Peakless	24 hr	Clear	Do not mix with other insulins
Premixed					
Humulin, Novolin 70:30 (70% NPH, 30% Regular)	30-60 min	2-10 hr	10-16 hr	Cloudy	

breakfast, before dinner, and possibly before lunch and at bedtime if the patient is having difficulty keeping blood plasma levels stabilized. An important responsibility of the medical assistant is to teach the patient how to perform glucometer screening (Procedure 45-1).

ALTERNATIVE METHODS OF INSULIN ADMINISTRATION

- *Insulin pump:* An insulin pump is a computerized device that administers a constant dose of insulin using a small portable pump. The pump is programmed to deliver a measured dose of insulin by continuous subcutaneous infusion through a catheter, which is placed in the abdomen or buttocks areas. This method more closely resembles the body's normal surge of insulin and is designed to maintain blood glucose levels consistently within normal limits.
- *Injector pen:* Injector pens are preloaded with insulin cartridges for easy use (Figure 45-6). Insulin pens are disposable or refillable and easily portable and therefore can be used by patients with diabetes when they are away from home.

Glucometers are palm sized and use very small amounts of capillary blood from a site in the finger, forearm, upper arm, or abdomen (Figure 45-7). Many different types of glucometers are available, but all display test results within seconds, and the results are stored in the memory function of the machine for future reference. The medical assistant should stress that the accuracy of blood glucose results depends on following the instructions for the particular type of glucometer used by the patient. When teaching the patient about glucometer screening, the medical assistant must use the same machine the patient will use at home and must stress the importance of keeping a record of glucometer readings to determine long-term

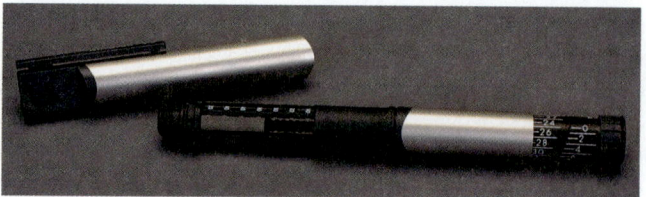

FIGURE 45-6 Nova Pen.

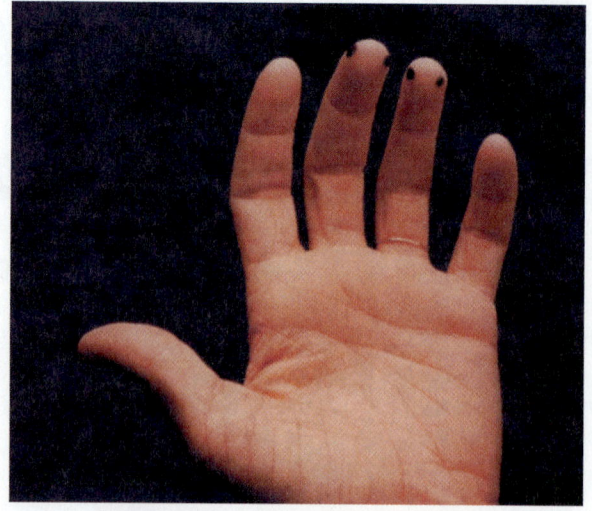

FIGURE 45-7 Capillary puncture sites on the fingers.

serum glucose control. Patients should be encouraged to bring their glucometers with them to each office visit so that the physician can review glucose levels.

The patient education for glucometer use should include not only the steps for successfully checking blood glucose levels but also quality-control mechanisms as suggested by the manufacturer of the

PROCEDURE 45-1

Assist the Physician with Patient Care: Perform a Blood Glucose Accu-Chek Test

GOAL: *To perform a blood test for diabetes mellitus accurately.*

EQUIPMENT and SUPPLIES

- Accu-Chek glucose monitor or similar glucose monitoring device
- Accu-Chek glucose testing strip
- Lancet and autoloading finger-puncturing device
- Alcohol preps
- Gauze squares
- Sharps container
- Disposable gloves
- Patient's record

PROCEDURAL STEPS

1. Check the physician's order and collect the necessary equipment and supplies. Perform quality control measures according to the manufacturer's guidelines and office policy.
2. Sanitize your hands and put on gloves.
   PURPOSE: To ensure infection control.
3. Ask the patient to wash his or her hands in warm soapy water and then rinse them in warm water and dry them completely.
   PURPOSE: To clean the area that will be punctured; also, warming the fingers may increase peripheral blood flow.
4. Check the patient's index and ring fingers and select the site for puncture.
   PURPOSE: To make sure the site of puncture is free of trauma.
5. Turn on the Accu-Chek monitor by pressing the ON button (Figure 1).

6. Make sure the code number on the LED display matches the code number on the container of test strips.
   PURPOSE: If the code numbers do not match, the device must be reprogrammed with the new code for the test results to be valid.
7. Remove a test strip from the vial and immediately replace the vial cover.
   PURPOSE: The vial must be kept closed to protect unused strips from possible contamination and decomposition from light exposure.
8. Check the strip for discoloration by comparing the color of the round window on the back of the test strip with the designated "unused" color chart provided on the label of the test strip vial.
   PURPOSE: To establish the validity of the testing procedure.
9. Do not touch the yellow test pad or round window on the back of the strip when handling the strip.
10. When the test strip symbol begins flashing in the lower right corner of the display screen, insert the test strip into the designated testing slot until it locks into place. If the test strip has been inserted correctly, the arrows on the test strip will face up and point toward the monitor (Figure 2).

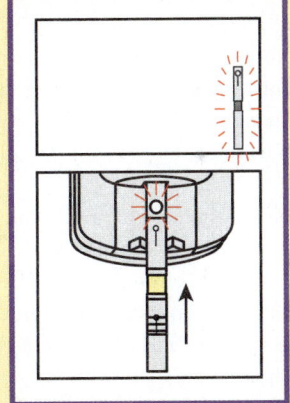

11. Cleanse the selected site on the patient's fingertip with the alcohol wipe and allow the finger to air dry.
12. Perform the finger puncture and wipe away the first drop of blood.
    PURPOSE: Tissue fluid may be present in the first drop of blood.
13. Apply a large, hanging drop of blood to the center of the yellow testing pad (Figure 3).

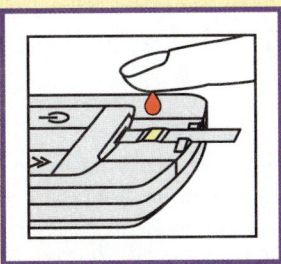

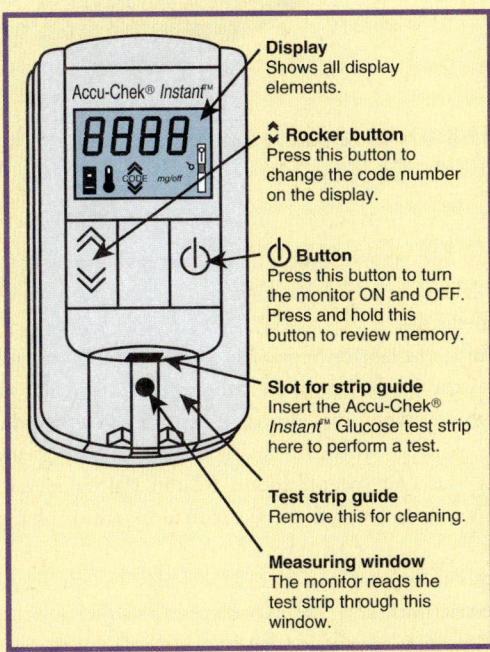

Display
Shows all display elements.

Rocker button
Press this button to change the code number on the display.

Button
Press this button to turn the monitor ON and OFF. Press and hold this button to review memory.

Slot for strip guide
Insert the Accu-Chek® *Instant*™ Glucose test strip here to perform a test.

Test strip guide
Remove this for cleaning.

Measuring window
The monitor reads the test strip through this window.

PROCEDURE 45-1—cont'd

- Do not touch the pad with the patient's finger.
- Do not apply a second drop of blood.
- Do not smear the blood with your finger.
- Make sure the yellow test pad is saturated with blood.

14. Give the patient a gauze square to hold securely over the puncture site.

15. The monitor automatically begins the measurement process as soon as it senses the drop of blood.

16. The test result will be shown in the display window in milligrams per deciliter (mg/dL).

17. Turn off the monitor by pressing the O button.

18. Discard all biohazardous waste in the proper waste containers.
   <u>PURPOSE:</u> To ensure infection control.

19. Clean the glucometer according to the manufacturer's guidelines, disinfect the work area, remove your gloves and dispose of them properly, and sanitize your hands.

20. Record the test results in the patient's medical record.
   <u>PURPOSE:</u> A procedure is considered not done until it is recorded.

8/16/XX 1:00 PM Glucometer screening completed as ordered. NFBS 144. Pt took routine dose of 10 U Humalog insulin at noon. Reinforced pt ed on using control methods. No questions. M. Vasco, CMA (AAMA) _____

From Stepp CA, Woods MA: *Laboratory procedures for medical office personnel,* Philadelphia, 1998, WB Saunders.

---

device (Figure 45-8). Some examples of quality controls include the following:

- Follow the manufacturer's instructions exactly.
- Perform the instrument maintenance specified by the manufacturer, including correct cleaning and storage of the instrument.
- Check the expiration dates on test strips and solutions and store these products correctly.
- Match and correctly enter the test strip code into the instrument before use.
- Contact the physician if test results do not match the person's symptoms.

Patients with diabetes also need to find the best method of disposing of their syringes and lancets. Local pharmacies or hospitals may offer assistance with disposal of used sharps. If the patient does not have access to a sharps return program, a puncture-resistant container with an opening that can be easily and tightly sealed before disposal is a good choice.

Regardless of the type of diabetes, for treatment to be successful, patients must play an active role in the management of their disease. The medical assistant should consistently encourage patients to be active participants in maintaining blood glucose levels within the normal range and constantly be on alert for possible complications from their disease. The ideal is to maintain blood plasma levels as close to the norm as possible to prevent complications. The American Diabetes Association recommends blood levels between 90 and 130 mg/dL before meals and below 180 mg/dL 2 hours after starting a meal, with a glycated (glycosylated) hemoglobin level (HbA_{1c}) below 7%.

Type 2 Diabetes

DM type 2, once called *adult-onset* or *non-insulin-dependent diabetes,* usually develops in adults but may be seen at any age. Factors that increase the risk of developing DM type 2 include a family history, a history of gestational diabetes, impaired glucose tolerance, physical inactivity, and obesity. In this type of DM, the pancreas produces

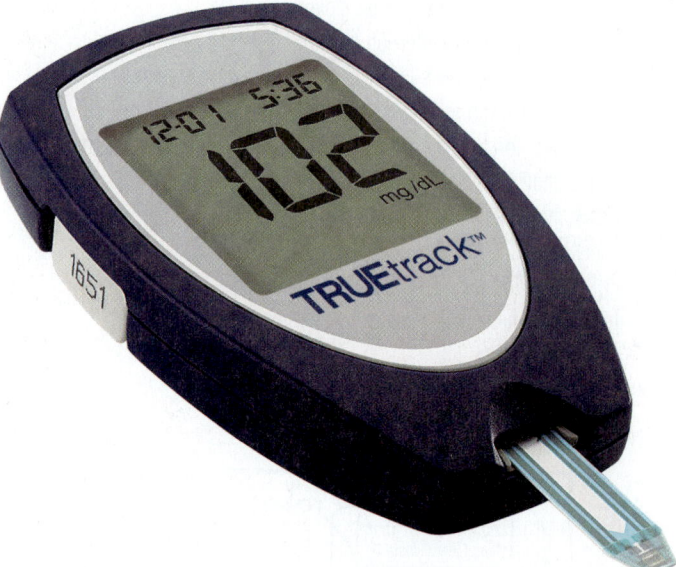

FIGURE 45-8 Blood glucose monitoring device (TrueTrack Smart System). (Courtesy Home Diagnostics, Fort Lauderdale, Fla.)

insulin, but not enough, and/or the target cells are resistant to insulin action. Diabetes type 2 is responsible for 90% to 95% of cases of diabetes mellitus.

This form of diabetes frequently goes undetected for many years because of the gradual onset of hyperglycemia and the absence of classic diabetic symptoms. However, because of this insidious onset over time, patients with diabetes type 2 are at even greater risk of developing vascular complications. Insulin resistance at the target cell level may improve with weight reduction and/or pharmacologic treatment.

Treatment for diabetes type 2 includes weight loss, exercise, dietary restrictions, and oral hypoglycemic medications that act to stimulate insulin production and/or improve tissue response to insulin (Table 45-2). Medications for diabetes type 2 have

TABLE 45-2 Oral Hypoglycemics Used in the Treatment of Diabetes Type 2

MEDICATION	CLASSIFICATION	ACTION	SIDE EFFECTS
Ornase, Tolinase, Diabanase	Sulfonylureas, first generation	Increase insulin production	Hypoglycemia, weight gain
Micronase, Glucotrol, Amaryl	Sulfonylureas, second generation	Increase insulin production	Hypoglycemia, weight gain
Prandin	Meglitinide	Increase insulin release from the pancreas	Hypoglycemia, weight gain
Metformin (Fortamet, Glucophage)	Biguanide	Reduce hepatic glucose production; slightly increase muscle glucose uptake	Nausea, diarrhea, metallic taste
Avandia	Thiazolidinediones	Reduce insulin resistance; increase glucose uptake; fat redistribution; reduce vascular inflammation; preserve beta cells in the pancreas	Minor weight increase; edema
Precose, Glyset	Alpha-glucosidase inhibitor	Slows absorption of complex carbohydrates	Gas and bloating, diarrhea
Glucovance (Micronase and Glucophage)	Sulfonylurea and biguanide	Reduce hepatic glucose production and increase insulin secretion	Hypoglycemia, weight gain
Avandamet (Avandia and Glucophage)	Thiazolidinedione and biguanide	Reduce hepatic glucose production; increase glucose uptake; reduce insulin resistance; preserve beta cells	Edema

Modified from the National Institutes of Health National Diabetes Education Program. Accessed May 1, 2010. Available at http://ndep.nih.gov/resources.

multiple functions, including stimulating insulin secretion from pancreatic islet cells in patients with some pancreatic function; reducing insulin resistance at the cellular level; improving sensitivity to insulin in muscle and adipose tissue; and inhibiting hepatic **gluconeogenesis**.

As with diabetes type 1, the goal of treatment is to maintain blood glucose levels within the normal range. For some patients, exercise, diet, and weight loss are sufficient to control blood glucose levels. Sometimes just the loss of 10 to 20 pounds is enough to bring blood glucose levels under control. Other patients may need medication to maintain normal blood glucose levels; however, levels must be monitored daily with a glucometer to determine the success of treatment. Over time, the individual with diabetes type 2 may require insulin to control hyperglycemia.

INJECTABLE DRUGS FOR THE MANAGEMENT OF DIABETES MELLITUS TYPES 1 AND 2

- *Pramlintide* (Symlin): A synthetic form of the hormone amylin that works with insulin and glucagon to maintain normal blood glucose levels. Injections administered before meals help improve A_{1c} levels by reducing the rate at which food moves through the stomach, thereby preventing a sharp increase in blood plasma levels after meals. The drug has been approved for people with diabetes type 1 who are not achieving the recommended A_{1c} levels and for those with diabetes type 2 who are using insulin but not achieving A_{1c} goals. The drug improves **satiety**, reduces caloric intake, and may assist with weight loss.
- *Exenatide* (Byetta): Lowers blood glucose levels by increasing insulin secretion. It is injected 60 minutes before breakfast and dinner. The drug helps patients achieve modest weight loss and improved glycemic control. It is not for use by patients with diabetes type 1.

CRITICAL THINKING APPLICATION   45-4

Carlos Vespa, a 47-year-old patient, recently was diagnosed with DM type 2. He has a BMI of 32; eats a high-fat, high-carbohydrate diet; and does not exercise. What health issues should Miguel include in his patient teaching intervention? Mr. Vespa tells Miguel he cannot afford the medication prescribed by the physician or the glucometer needed to monitor his blood glucose levels. Is there anything Miguel can do to help him with these issues?

Gestational Diabetes

A pregnant woman is diagnosed as having gestational diabetes if she meets either of two criteria:

- A fasting blood sugar (FBS) higher than 105 mg/dL
- During a 100-g OGGT: a 1-hour glucose level of 180 mg/dL or higher; a 2-hour glucose level of 155 mg/dL or higher; or a 3-hour glucose level of 140 mg/dL or higher.

Gestational diabetes affects about 4% of pregnant women in the United States each year, and it is considered a risk factor for the development of DM type 2 later in life. Factors that increase the risk of gestational diabetes are obesity; maternal age over 40; history of delivering infants who weigh more than 10 pounds at birth; a family history of diabetes; previous, unexplained stillbirth; previous birth with congenital anomalies; smoking; and belonging to certain ethnic groups, including Hispanics, Native Americans, Asian-Americans, and African-Americans. Some women are asymptomatic, whereas others show classic symptoms of diabetes. Because many pregnant women have gestational diabetes without obvious symptoms, all pregnant women are routinely screened between 24 and 28 weeks of pregnancy.

Gestational diabetes is precipitated by a buildup of insulin resistance at the cellular level, resulting in hyperglycemia. The elevated glucose in the mother's blood passes through the placenta into the baby, causing hyperglycemia with increased insulin production in the fetus. The extra carbohydrate energy is stored in the infant as fat and may result in a macrosomic, or "fat" baby who is at higher risk for breathing problems at birth, obesity, and diabetes type 2.

The treatment goal for gestational diabetes is to keep plasma glucose levels equal to those of pregnant women without the disorder. The treatment plan always includes diabetic diet counseling and regular physical activity. In obese women, a 30% calorie reduction reduces hyperglycemia. Some women may require insulin to maintain blood glucose levels within the therapeutic range and thereby reduce the possibility of fetal complications. Most women return to normal blood glucose levels after the baby is born; however, two out of three women experience gestational diabetes in future pregnancies. Because these women are at greater risk of developing diabetes type 2 later in life, patient education should stress the following:

- The patient should try to lose weight; if she is unable to reach a normal body mass index (BMI), losing 5% to 7% of her current body weight will make a big difference.
- The patient should exercise a minimum of 30 minutes a day.
- She should reduce her fat and calorie intake and increase her consumption of whole grains, complex carbohydrates, fruits, and vegetables.

Complications of Diabetes Mellitus

Acute Complications. Two acute complications can occur in patients with diabetes, depending on the level of glucose in the bloodstream. If an adult patient's blood glucose level is below 45 to 60 mg/dL, the symptoms seen are caused by hypoglycemia (Table 45-3). This reaction is related to insulin treatment and may also be called *insulin shock.* The goal is to prevent such episodes with adequate patient education and reinforcement of individualized medical management of diabetes, in addition to frequent blood glucose monitoring. The treatment for hypoglycemia is immediate glucose replacement. The recommended form of sugar supplement is glucose tablets, because each tablet contains a known amount of

glucose. The patient can use other sugar supplements, such as candy, orange juice with sugar, or nondiet soft drinks, but the amount of glucose in these items is unknown, and the patient actually may become hyperglycemic from ingestion of too much glucose. After the hypoglycemic crisis has ended, if the next meal is more than 1 hour away, the patient should have a mixed protein and carbohydrate snack (peanut butter crackers, cheese crackers) to maintain blood glucose levels until the next meal.

A second acute complication is diabetic ketoacidosis, or diabetic coma. In this case the person with diabetes is unable to use glucose for energy because insulin is absent or insufficient or there is resistance to insulin at the target cell site. Hyperglycemia results, with blood glucose levels rising to 300 to 750 mg/dL. Because cells cannot use carbohydrates for energy, the body begins to burn fat. Ketones are waste materials from fat metabolism that build up in the bloodstream and cause it to become more acidic. Although the development of ketoacidosis takes longer than insulin shock, it can become a medical emergency if the patient does not recognize the signs, monitor his or her blood glucose levels, and administer insulin as prescribed by the physician.

TREATING HYPOGLYCEMIA: THE RULE OF 15

1. Take 15 g of carbohydrate (CHO) if the glucometer reading is below 80 mg/dL.
2. Fifteen grams of CHO equals three glucose tablets, ½ cup of fruit juice, or five or six pieces of hard candy.
3. Wait 15 minutes and check the glucometer reading again; if the level is still low, repeat steps 1 and 2.
4. After the symptoms have been relieved, eat a regular meal as planned to maintain plasma glucose levels.
5. Treat hypoglycemia immediately, because it can cause fainting.
6. The physician may order injected glucagon to quickly raise blood plasma levels.

TABLE 45-3 Characteristics of Hypoglycemia and Hyperglycemia

DISEASE	CAUSES	ONSET	SIGNS AND SYMPTOMS	TREATMENT
Hypoglycemia (low serum glucose level)	Too much insulin; insufficient calories; excessive exercise; individual with diabetes type 2 using insulin-boosting medications	Slow	Shakiness, vertigo, palpitations, diaphoresis, headache, hunger, pallor, fatigue, confusion, irritability, poor judgment, visual disturbances, seizures, coma	Ingest sugar (glucose tablets recommended); monitor blood levels in 15 min. If still low and symptoms persist, take another glucose tablet. If patient passes out, physician may order injected glucagon; call for emergency services
Hyperglycemia (high serum glucose level)	Too little insulin; body not able to use insulin properly; excessive caloric intake; inadequate exercise; illness; stress	Rapid	Polyphagia, polyuria, glycosuria, ketonuria, weight loss, pruritus; possible ketoacidosis with shortness of breath, "fruity" breath, dry mouth, nausea and vomiting, lethargy	Exercise if blood glucose level <240 mg/dL. Reduce caloric intake. Physician may alter amount and timing of insulin

CRITICAL THINKING APPLICATION   45-5

Mr. Vespa returns to the office 1 week later and tells Dr. Misha that he has not been feeling well. Sometimes he feels very shaky, dizzy, and tired; he has been getting headaches and cannot think straight. Dr. Misha orders a glucometer reading, which shows Mr. Vespa's blood glucose level at 65. Dr. Misha's diagnosis is hypoglycemic episodes, and the physician asks Miguel to reinforce patient teaching about hypoglycemic and hyperglycemic signs and symptoms and treatment. What should Miguel include in the teaching intervention? How can he best reinforce the material so that Mr. Vespa will remember how to manage his disease?

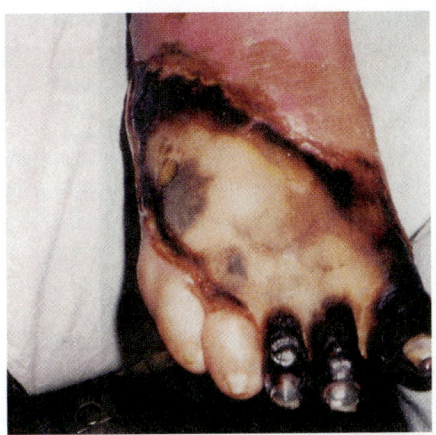

FIGURE 45-9 Patient with diabetes who has peripheral neuropathy and an insensate foot. Cold packs were applied to the patient's foot for treatment of a sprain. Frostbite developed, and the patient required a transmetatarsal amputation. (From Levin ME: Pathogenesis and general management of foot lesions in the diabetic patient. In Bowker JH, Pfeifer MA, editors: *Levin and O'Neal's the diabetic foot*, ed 6, St Louis, 2001, Mosby.)

Chronic Complications

Microvascular Disease. Arterial changes at the capillary level can occur within 1 to 2 years of the onset of DM. Hyperglycemic episodes combined with the duration of the disease cause degeneration of tissue arterioles, which results in multiple system disorders, including diabetic retinopathy. Diabetes is a leading cause of new blindness in people 20 to 74 years of age and is often a result of 8 to 10 years of diabetes. Ninety percent of patients with diabetes type 1 and 65% of patients with diabetes type 2 develop retinopathy.

Hyperglycemic episodes damage the blood vessels in the retina; therefore, close glucose control helps delay the onset of retinopathy and slows its progression. The vision disturbances occur as a result of vascular changes in the capillaries of the retina. These complications can lead to retinal detachment and blindness. In addition, people with diabetes are at much higher risk for developing glaucoma and cataracts and should have yearly eye screenings and frequent ophthalmologic examinations during routine office visits for early diagnosis of diabetic retinopathy.

Microvascular disease also can cause diabetic nephropathy. Kidney disease is present in 10% to 21% of individuals with diabetes and is the most common cause of kidney failure in the United States. Diabetic kidney disease is the greatest threat to life in adults with diabetes type 1. Diabetes damages the small blood vessels in the kidneys and impairs their ability to filter waste from the blood. Degenerative changes cause destruction of the glomerular unit and can lead to renal failure. High blood pressure and smoking often are associated with diabetic nephropathy. Because urinary protein usually is the first sign of kidney damage, frequent testing for albuminuria is suggested. Early treatment reduces the progression of kidney disease. Good glucose control often can reverse the early stages of diabetic nephropathy. With disease progression, renal failure may occur, resulting in the need for dialysis and possibly kidney transplantation.

Macrovascular Disease. Macrovascular disease, in the form of atherosclerosis, is a serious health issue for all patients with diabetes, especially those with DM type 2. People with diabetes are two to four times more likely to have atherosclerotic heart disease or strokes. Coronary artery disease (CAD) is the most common cause of death in those with diabetes type 2. The patients most affected are women at or before middle age. The longer the patient has had diabetes, the greater the risk of CAD. Cerebrovascular accidents (CVAs, or strokes) occur twice as often in patients with diabetes as in those without the disease. Hypertension is common in patients with diabetes and contributes to the rates of CAD and CVA.

Peripheral vascular disease (PVD), a disease process in blood vessels outside the heart, is associated with atherosclerotic changes in small arteries and arterioles and contributes to the incidence of gangrene and amputations in patients with diabetes. Patients with diabetes type 2 frequently have signs and symptoms of PVD when first diagnosed. Compromised circulation in the lower extremities causes the formation of ulcers, poor wound healing, and possible progression to gangrene. This progression of PVD may result in amputation of the toes, foot, or leg. Blockage of blood vessels can lead to impotence in men with diabetes. About 13% of men with diabetes type 1 and 8% of men with diabetes type 2 have impotence caused by diabetic vascular disease.

Diabetic Neuropathy. Diabetic neuropathy is the most common complication of diabetes; 60% to 70% of those with diabetes have some form of diabetic nerve damage. This type of nerve damage is caused both by vascular changes and by hyperglycemia. The chief areas that show pathologic changes are the nerves and blood vessels in the eyes, kidneys, legs, and feet. The first signs of diabetic neuropathy usually are numbness, pain, or tingling in the hands, feet, or legs. The loss of sensation in the extremities is important, because it affects the patient's ability to be aware of injuries, especially to the feet. Because of peripheral vascular compromise, foot injuries can develop into ulcers or lesions can become infected and ultimately lead to gangrene and amputation. Even a minor undetected injury, such as a foot blister, can lead to a serious problem for a patient with diabetes. Individuals with diabetes also may lose temperature sensation and thus are more susceptible to heat or cold injuries such as burns and frostbite (Figure 45-9). Patients with diabetes should have their feet inspected at every visit to the physician's office to ensure early detection and treatment of problems. Healthcare providers should provide verbal and written advice to help prevent or reduce these potentially serious injuries.

QUESTIONS TO ASK WHEN SCREENING FOR DIABETIC NEUROPATHY

- Can you feel your feet when walking?
- Have you noticed weakness in the muscles of your feet and legs?
- Do you have problems with balance when standing or walking?
- Do you have trouble feeling heat or cold in your feet or hands?
- Do you have open sores on your feet and legs that heal slowly?
- Have you noticed that your feet have changed shape?
- Do your feet tingle or feel like "pins and needles," or do you have burning or shooting pains in your feet? Do they hurt at night? Are they numb?
- Are your feet very sensitive to touch?
- Do your feet and hands get very cold or very hot?

American Diabetes Association. Accessed May 1, 2010. Available at www.diabetes.org/living-with-diabetes/complications/neuropathy.

Infection. All patients with diabetes are at increased risk for infection because of a number of different factors. Those with impaired vision and neuropathies have an increased risk of injury because they may not be able to see or feel potentially dangerous items to prevent injury. Once an injury occurs and the integrity of the skin has been compromised, damaged or atherosclerotic blood vessels are unable to deliver the blood needed for healing, and the thickened blood vessel walls impede the release of white blood cells (WBCs) to the area. The WBCs of patients with diabetes show reduced phagocytosis, so their ability to destroy pathogens is limited. In addition, some pathogens multiply rapidly in the glucose-rich environment of individuals with diabetes. Therefore, the best method of controlling infections in these patients is to prevent skin trauma or damage.

FOOT CARE FOR PATIENTS WITH DIABETES

Patients with diabetes need instruction in foot hygiene and also a foot inspection during each visit. Education guidelines should include the following:

- Wash your feet every day with warm (not hot) water and mild soap.
- Cut your nails straight across to prevent ingrown toenails and possible injuries.
- Apply lotion to the feet, especially the heels. If the skin is cracked or red, speak to your doctor.
- Check your feet every day, using a mirror if necessary. Call your doctor at the first sign of redness, swelling, or numbness.
- Speak with your doctor before treatment of corns, calluses, or bunions.
- Do not go barefoot or allow your feet to get too hot or cold.
- Check your shoes for foreign objects or rough areas before wearing them.
- Wear comfortable, well-fitting shoes.
- Stop smoking. Smoking causes vasoconstriction, which reduces circulation to the extremities.

CRITICAL THINKING APPLICATION   45-6

Mr. Vespa and his wife are scheduled for a long visit today so that Dr. Misha can review his treatment plan. Dr. Misha asks Miguel to reinforce the possible complications of DM and the elements of foot care. What should Miguel include in his teaching intervention? How can he make sure Mr. and Mrs. Vespa understand the disease, its management, and possible complications?

FOLLOW-UP FOR PATIENTS WITH DIABETES

Experts agree that the best method of preventing diabetic complications is to maintain blood glucose levels consistently at near-normal ranges. Several laboratory tests can be ordered to monitor a patient's blood glucose levels. The fasting blood sugar (FBS) test (or FPG, discussed earlier) measures the glucose levels in a blood specimen from a fasting individual. The test requires a 12-hour fast. The normal range for an FBS is 70 to 110 mg/dL. Even though the physician may order periodic FBS tests, patients with diabetes still need to check their blood glucose levels as ordered with a home glucometer.

A routine test for monitoring long-term diabetes therapy is the glycosylated hemoglobin (HbA_{1c}) test. This test has distinct advantages over routine FBS studies, because the FBS reflects glucose levels at a given point in time, whereas the glycosylated hemoglobin test reflects serum glucose control over several months. The test measures glucose levels that have been chemically bound to the hemoglobin molecule on the red blood cell (RBC) over a 120-day period (the lifespan of an RBC). The physician can assess average daily glucose levels over the preceding 2 to 3 months and evaluate treatment compliance and results. The patient does not need to restrict food or fluid intake for this test and should continue to take prescribed medication before the blood sample is drawn. The patient's total glycosylated hemoglobin level should be less than 7%. The higher the glycosylated hemoglobin result, the higher the risk the patient will develop diabetic complications.

CORRELATION BETWEEN A_{1c} LEVELS AND AVERAGE PLASMA GLUCOSE LEVELS

A_{1c} (%)	Average Plasma Glucose (mg/dL)
6	135
7	170
8	205
9	240
10	275

From American Diabetes Association. Accessed June 10, 2010. Available at www.diabetes.org/living-with-diabetes/treatment-and-care/blood-glucose-control.

Developing a Diabetic Patient Education Plan

The plan of care for individuals newly diagnosed with diabetes should be developed from a holistic point of view. Holistic care means that the diabetic team (including the medical assistant) considers all aspects of the patient's needs, including lifestyle factors,

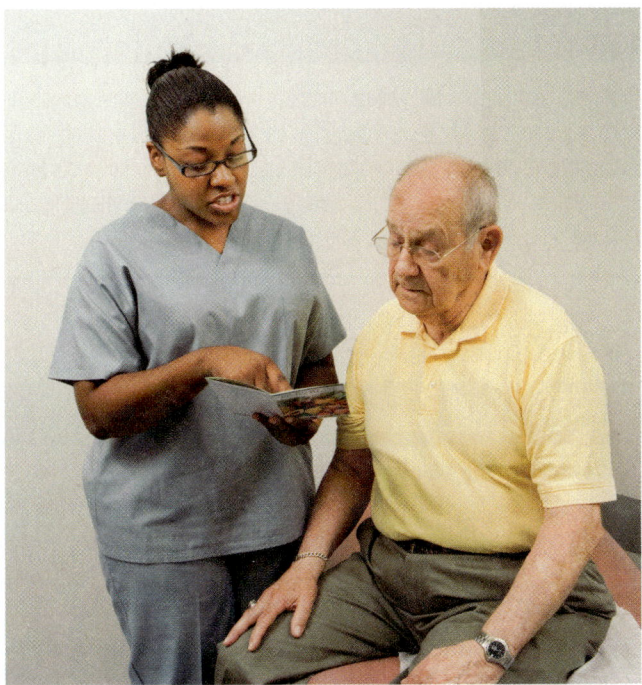

FIGURE 45-10 The medical assistant can use premade educational materials to discuss new lifestyle habits with a patient with diabetes.

such as diet and level of exercise; medications and the education needed to comply with their use; education that includes the details of the disease and its possible complications; demonstration and return demonstration as needed until the patient is proficient in glucometer testing and/or insulin administration; family involvement in the treatment process; and the use of community resources (e.g., a diabetic educator, support group, and dietitian) to assist with management of the disease (Figure 45-10). The equipment and supplies needed to treat diabetes effectively can be extremely expensive, so the medical assistant should investigate alternative methods of getting these materials if the patient is unable to afford them. The need for continuous daily glucose control must be emphasized at each patient visit. The medical assistant can research various Web sites and suggest that these be explored.

CLOSING COMMENTS

Patient Education

Because the management of endocrine disorders can be quite complicated, the medical assistant must make sure the patient understands the proper procedures for at-home treatment. By demonstrating a given procedure in the office, the medical assistant can address any inaccurate information or answer any questions the patient may have. Visual materials, such as brochures and procedure cards, also are helpful, because they can be taken from the office and used as a reminder. If the patient is taking medication, the medical assistant should review the dosage schedule with the individual, discuss the purpose of the treatment, and clear up any confusion over the physician's instructions. As always, if the medical assistant is uncertain of any procedures or information, he or she should ask the physician for assistance before explaining anything to the patient.

IMPORTANT POINTS IN PATIENT EDUCATION FOR PATIENTS WITH DIABETES

- Physical activity (too much or too little), stress, disease, medications, and diet all combine to affect blood glucose levels; following an effective dietary plan is the first step toward self-management.
- The medical assistant should weigh the patient and measure his or her height. The medical assistant also should reinforce the body mass index (BMI) recommended by the physician and provide information about the basic nutritional requirements needed to help the individual either to maintain his or her ideal body weight or to lose weight.
- The goal of a diet plan is to help maintain a homeostatic blood glucose level. If a healthy blood glucose level is maintained, the patient will avoid complications that can develop with hypoglycemia or hyperglycemia. Basic guidelines, according to the person's ethnic influences, age, gender, and physical activity, are used to establish a therapeutic meal plan (see Chapter 30). Family members should be involved in dietary health teaching, and appropriate community resources, such as a registered dietitian, should be used to help the patient understand and comply with the dietary guidelines.
- The medical management of diabetes can be quite complicated and overwhelming for many patients. People with diabetes type 2 who are prescribed oral hypoglycemics must understand the drugs' mechanism of action and accurate dosage. Patients with diabetes type 1 or type 2 who require daily insulin must be able to prepare and administer their medication accurately and must understand the connection between glucometer readings and insulin dosage. All patients with diabetes must be able to use a glucometer accurately and must be aware of the possible complications of the disease.

Legal and Ethical Issues

Pathophysiology of the endocrine system can have far-reaching effects on the body's ability to function. Patient education interventions should be documented completely to establish legal proof of the information shared with the patient. Never assume that the patient understands the disease process and treatment recommendations. The following suggestions can help ensure patient welfare and promote risk management:

- Advise patients that a Medic Alert bracelet with his or her diagnosis and medication information is an important safeguard.
- Patients must take medication as prescribed, following the directions for dosage, route of administration, and storage; they also must be alert for possible side effects.
- Patients newly diagnosed with diabetes should not drive until glycemic control has stabilized. These patients also should be warned about possible visual impairment from the disease.
- Remember that you are always representing your profession and employer and respond to each situation accordingly.
- Ask for assistance or further information if you feel unprepared to perform a procedure or to give accurate information.

SUMMARY OF SCENARIO

In his interactions with patients, Miguel has learned to pay attention to both verbal and nonverbal messages. He has used this technique consistently when interacting with Mr. Vespa. Miguel recognizes the complexity of endocrine system disorders and the importance of understanding the anatomy and physiology of the system and the most frequently seen endocrine disorders. As a concerned medical assistant, Miguel continues to read professional journals and attend workshops so that he is prepared to answer questions from patients. He is especially interested in DM, because the practice for which he works has so many patients with diabetes. Miguel never hesitates to ask the attending physicians questions about the disease and its management.

SUMMARY OF LEARNING OBJECTIVES

1. **Define, spell, and pronounce the terms listed in the vocabulary.**
   Spelling and pronouncing medical terms correctly bolster the medical assistant's credibility. Knowing the definitions of these terms promotes confidence in communication with patients and co-workers.

2. **Apply critical thinking skills in performing the patient assessment and patient care.**
   Completing the Critical Thinking Application exercises throughout the chapter can help the student medical assistant become more adept at critical analysis of real-life situations.

3. **Summarize the anatomy and physiology of the endocrine system.**
   The endocrine system consists of glands located throughout the body that produce and secrete chemicals known as *hormones.* The glands of the endocrine system are the hypothalamus, pituitary, pineal glands, thyroid, thymus, parathyroids, thymus, adrenals, and reproductive glands (i.e., the ovaries and the testes). Some nonendocrine organs, such as the pancreas, produce and release hormones. Through hormonal action, the endocrine system regulates all body functions.

4. **Explain the mechanism of hormone action.**
   Hormones are chemical transmitters produced by glands and transported to the target tissue by the bloodstream. Hormone secretion is regulated by a combination of nervous stimulation, endocrine control, and feedback systems. Each hormone released into the bloodstream has particular target cells on which it acts.

5. **Differentiate among the diseases and disorders of the endocrine system .**
   Hypersecretion or hyposecretion of hormones can cause endocrine disorders. When ADH is not produced or is not released in sufficient amounts, the patient develops diabetes insipidus. Gigantism and acromegaly are both diseases of the pituitary gland involving GH. When this condition affects children, gigantism is the result; in adults, acromegaly causes excessive growth of the facial area and extremities. Deficient secretion of thyroid hormone may be caused by an endemic iodine deficiency, resulting in a simple goiter. Improper development of the thyroid in an infant or young child causes cretinism; in an adult or older child, the condition is called *myxedema.* Hypersecretion of the thyroid gland causes thyrotoxicosis, or Graves' disease. Adrenal cortex insufficiency is called *Addison's disease.* Hypersecretion of the adrenal cortex, which results in elevated levels of cortisol, is known as *Cushing's syndrome.*

6. **Describe the diagnostic criteria for diabetes mellitus.**
   Diabetes is diagnosed if the patient has a plasma glucose level of 200 mg/dL or higher with polyuria, polydipsia, and unexplained weight loss; an FPG level of 126 mg/dL or higher on more than one occasion; a 2-hour OGTT of 200 mg/dL or higher; a positive urinalysis result for glucose and possibly ketones; or a glycosylated hemoglobin greater than 7%.

7. **Compare and contrast prediabetes, diabetes type 1, diabetes type 2, and gestational diabetes.**
   Prediabetes is a condition in which an individual has a higher than normal blood glucose level that is not high enough for a diagnosis of diabetes type 2. Diabetes type 1 is seen in children and young adults and is characterized by a complete absence of insulin production. Patients must receive daily injections of insulin to survive. Diabetes type 2 develops gradually because of an insufficient amount of insulin or resistance at the target cell site, or both. Weight management, diet therapy, exercise, and medications are used to control glucose levels. Gestational diabetes occurs in some pregnancies but typically resolves after the infant is born. Affected women may need insulin therapy for glucose metabolism.

8. **Outline the treatment plan and management of the different types of diabetes mellitus.**
   All patients with diabetes must monitor their blood glucose levels regularly to determine the effectiveness of treatment. The goal of treatment is to maintain plasma glucose levels as close to the normal range as possible, as much as possible. Management of DM is a complicated interaction involving exercise, a therapeutic diet, weight control, and medication. Patients with diabetes type 1 require daily injections of a combination of insulins. Patients with diabetes type 2 and gestational diabetes may be prescribed oral hypoglycemics or insulin if needed.

9. **Perform blood glucose screening with a glucometer.**
   Procedure 45-1 describes how to perform plasma glucose screening accurately with a glucometer. Many types of glucose meters are available, so it is important that the patient be taught how to perform testing using the type of device that will be used at home.

10. **Identify the characteristics of hypoglycemia and hyperglycemia.**
    With hyperglycemia, the patient experiences a sudden onset of polyphagia, polyuria, glycosuria, ketonuria, weight loss, pruritus, "fruity" breath, dry mouth, nausea and vomiting, and lethargy. This occurs as a result of an inadequate dosage of insulin, target cell resistance, overeating,

lack of exercise, illness, or stress. Hypoglycemia causes shakiness, vertigo, headache, hunger, pallor, fatigue, confusion, irritability, visual disturbances, seizures, and possibly coma.

11. **Describe the complications associated with diabetes mellitus.**
Complications of DM include hypoglycemia; hyperglycemia and diabetic coma; diabetic neuropathy; microvascular diseases, including diabetic retinopathy and nephropathy; macrovascular diseases, such as atherosclerosis, CAD, CVA, and PVD; and decreased resistance to infection.

12. **Summarize patient education approaches to diabetes.**
Patient education for patients with diabetes is an intricate mix of information on the dynamics of the disease; the importance of exercise, diet, and weight control in preventing complications and maintaining health; an understanding of the various types of insulin and when and how they should be administered; and for patients with diabetes type 2, a knowledge of oral medications, their side effects and dosage; home care management, including proper use of glucose meters and insulin administration; prevention of complications through effective control of blood glucose levels; proper foot care; and monitoring for and immediately contacting the physician about infections or other complications.

13. **Discuss legal and ethical issues to consider when caring for patients with endocrine system disorders.**
Pathophysiology of the endocrine system can have far-reaching effects on the body's ability to function. Patient education interventions should be documented completely to establish legal proof of the information shared with the patient. Never assume that the patient understands the disease process and treatment recommendations. Specific risk management procedures may be instituted depending on patient characteristics and diagnosis.

CONNECTIONS

📖 **Study Guide Connection:** Go to the Chapter 45 Study Guide. Read and complete the activities.

Ⓔ **Evolve Connection:** Go to the Chapter 45 link at *evolve.elsevier.com/kinn* to complete the Chapter Review and Chapter Quiz. Check out the other resources listed for this chapter to make the most of what you have learned from Assisting in Endocrinology.

46

ASSISTING IN PULMONARY MEDICINE

Michael McGuire, CMA (AAMA), works for a primary care physician, Dr. John Samuelson, in the small town in which he grew up. Dr. Samuelson's practice is open to all patients, but a large number of individuals with respiratory disease seek his help in managing their pulmonary problems. In the 6 months since he started with the practice, Michael has learned how to assist with pulmonary diagnostic tests and the special needs of patients with respiratory diseases. Michael has become familiar with the diagnosis and treatment of many common pulmonary problems and adept at accurately documenting respiratory system signs and symptoms. Many of Dr. Samuelson's patients smoke cigarettes, and the main employers in the community are coal mining and construction companies, so many patients are at risk for smoking and occupation-related respiratory problems.

While studying this chapter, think about the following questions:

- What are the common pathologic conditions of the pulmonary system? What medical terms must Michael know to identify and explain these patient disorders?
- What are the medical assistant's primary responsibilities in working with patients with pulmonary problems?
- What clinical skills are required in this specialty practice?
- What pulmonary complications are associated with smoking and occupational respiratory hazards?
- What diagnostic and treatment procedures typically are used in a pulmonary practice?

LEARNING OBJECTIVES

1. Define, spell, and pronounce the terms listed in the vocabulary.
2. Apply critical thinking skills in performing the patient assessment and patient care.
3. Describe the organs of the respiratory system and their functions.
4. Explain the process of ventilation.
5. Implement correct respiratory system terminology when documenting in the medical record.
6. Describe the major diseases of the respiratory system.
7. Explain the diagnosis and treatment of tuberculosis.
8. Summarize the disorders associated with chronic obstructive pulmonary disease and their treatments.
9. Teach a patient how to use a peak flow meter.
10. Administer a nebulizer treatment.
11. Detail patient teaching for the use of a metered-dose inhaler.
12. Describe the cancers associated with the pulmonary system.
13. Summarize the medical assistant's role in assisting with pulmonary procedures.
14. Distinguish among common diagnostic procedures for the respiratory system.
15. Perform a volume capacity spirometry test.
16. Correctly use a pulse oximeter.
17. Collect a sputum sample for culture.
18. Discuss legal and ethical issues associated with pulmonary medicine.

VOCABULARY

bifurcates Divides from one into two branches.

bronchiectasis (brong'-ke-ek-tuh-sis) Dilation of the bronchi and bronchioles associated with secondary infection or ciliary dysfunction.

chronic bronchitis Recurrent inflammation of the membranes lining the bronchial tubes.

cilia (sil'-e-uh) Hairlike projections capable of movement; in the lungs, cilia waves move unwanted substances (e.g., mucus, dust, and pus) upward; cilia are destroyed by smoking.

hypercapnia (hi-per-kap'-ne-uh) Excess levels of carbon dioxide in the blood.

pulmonary consolidation In pneumonia, the process by which the lungs become solidified as they fill with exudates.

rhinorrhea (ri-no-re'-uh) The discharge of nasal drainage.

tubercle (too'-buhr-kuhl) A nodule produced by the tuberculosis bacillus.

tracheostomy (tra-ke-os'-tuh-me) A surgical opening made through the neck into the trachea to allow breathing.

virulent (vir'-u-lent) Exceedingly pathogenic, noxious, or deadly.

The respiratory system has two primary functions. The first is to exchange oxygen from the atmosphere for carbon dioxide waste. The two types of respiration are *external respiration,* which brings oxygen into the lungs, where carbon dioxide exchange occurs in the blood vessels surrounding the alveoli, and *internal respiration,* in which oxygen is exchanged for carbon dioxide at the cellular level. Cells soon stop functioning and die if they are deprived of oxygen.

The second function of the respiratory system is to maintain the acid-base balance in the body. Failure of this function may result in respiratory acidosis or alkalosis. Respiratory acidosis occurs if the patient experiences hypoventilation and carbon dioxide levels increase in the body, causing **hypercapnia**. Respiratory alkalosis is related to an excess release of carbon dioxide caused by hyperventilation, which may be associated with anxiety or an acute asthma attack. Both conditions can be life-threatening if the underlying causes are not corrected. The respiratory and circulatory systems work together to supply body cells with oxygen and remove metabolic wastes. The ventilation process is controlled by the respiratory center in the central nervous system and assisted by the intercostal muscles and the diaphragm.

THE RESPIRATORY SYSTEM

The thoracic cage, sometimes called the *rib cage,* is a bony structure that is narrower at the top and wider at the base. It is held in place by the thoracic vertebrae of the spine in the center of the back and by the sternum in the center of the anterior aspect of the body. The first seven ribs attach directly to the sternum and are called the *true ribs.* Ribs 8, 9, and 10 fasten one to another, forming the false ribs, and ribs 11 and 12 are the "floating" ribs, or half ribs, because their only attachment is to the thoracic vertebrae. At the base or floor of the rib cage is the diaphragm, a musculotendinous membrane that separates the thoracic cavity and the abdominal cavity (Figure 46-1). The respiratory system is divided into two anatomic regions, the upper respiratory tract and the lower respiratory tract.

REQUIREMENTS FOR NORMAL RESPIRATION

- An open airway leading to the lungs
- Ability of the lungs to expand rhythmically
- Intact alveolar membranes
- Coordination of the intercostal muscles and the diaphragm
- Proper action of the central nervous system's respiratory control center

Upper Respiratory Tract

The upper respiratory tract, which transports air from the atmosphere to the lungs, includes the nose, pharynx (throat), and larynx (Figure 46-2). As air enters the nasal cavity, it is cleaned by the **cilia**, warmed by capillary blood vessels, and moistened by mucous membranes. The paranasal sinuses, hollow cavities that also are lined with mucous cells and cilia, open into the nasal cavity and help warm and moisten inhaled air. The filtered, warmed, and moistened air moves past the tonsils, which have an immunity function and help defend the body from potential pathogens, and through the pharynx. As the air continues toward the lungs, it passes through the larynx. The opening into the larynx is protected by a moveable piece of cartilage, the epiglottis. The larynx, or voice box, is made up of vocal cords, which vibrate when air is exhaled, creating the sound of the voice. Once the air passes through the larynx, it enters the lower respiratory tract.

Lower Respiratory Tract

The lower respiratory tract consists of the trachea, bronchial tubes, and lungs (see Figure 46-2). These structures are also lined with mucous tissue that is covered with cilia. The collection of dust and foreign particles in the cilia initiates the coughing reflex; this helps expectorate mucus, which may contain pathogens. Without these defense mechanisms, pathogens would remain in the lungs and may cause disease. Cigarette smoke and other air pollutants slow or paralyze the cleansing action of the cilia and damage the mucous membrane lining throughout the respiratory tract.

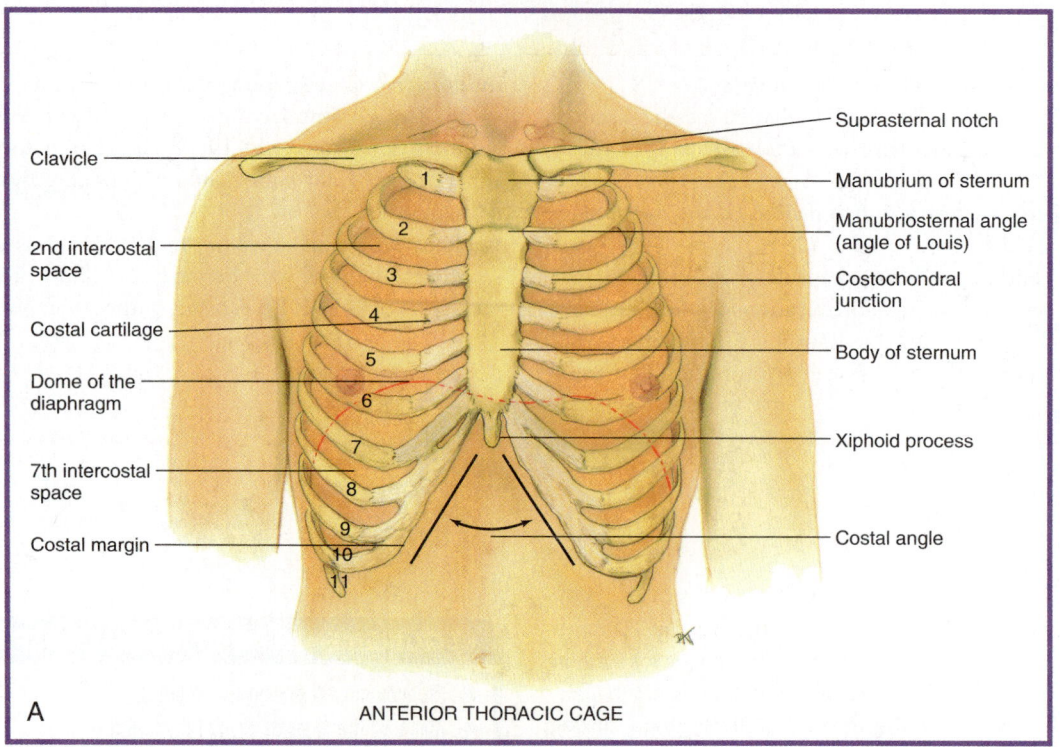

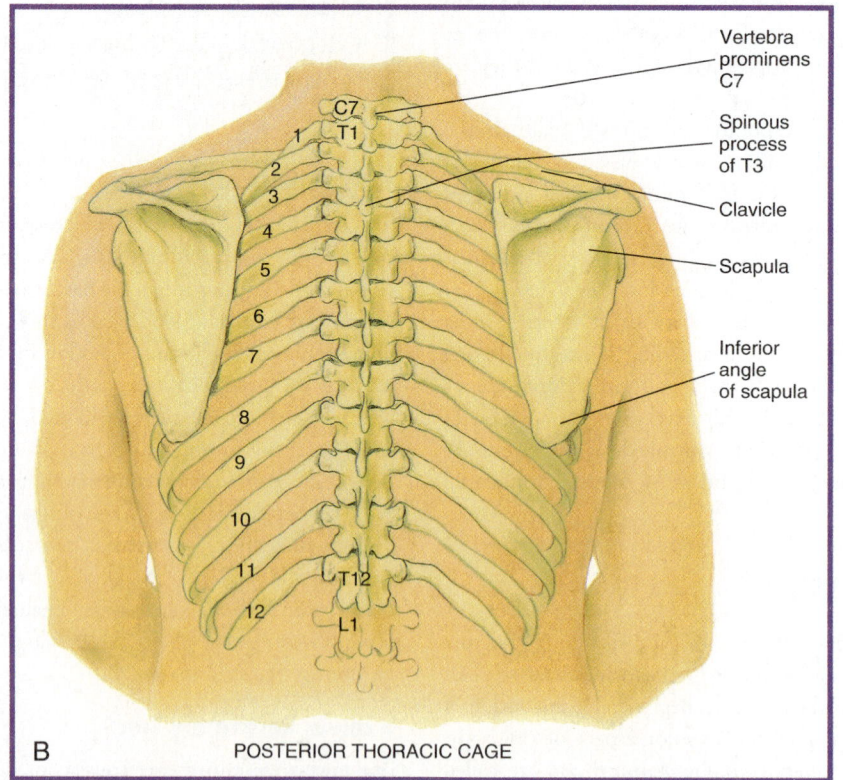

FIGURE 46-1 A, Anterior thoracic cage. **B,** Posterior thoracic cage. (From Jarvis C: *Physical examination and health assessment,* ed 5, St Louis, 2008, Saunders.)

The trachea (windpipe) is a tube that begins at the larynx and extends into the center of the chest, where it divides, or **bifurcates,** into the right and left bronchi. It is about 5 inches long and is surrounded by C-shaped cartilaginous rings. These rings hold the trachea open regardless of changes in air pressure.

It is often said that the bronchial tubes look like a tree hanging in the chest (Figure 46-3). The right bronchus is wider than the left to accommodate the right lung lobes, which also are larger. This means that foreign substances are more frequently seen in the right bronchus. Once the bronchi enter the lungs, they branch into

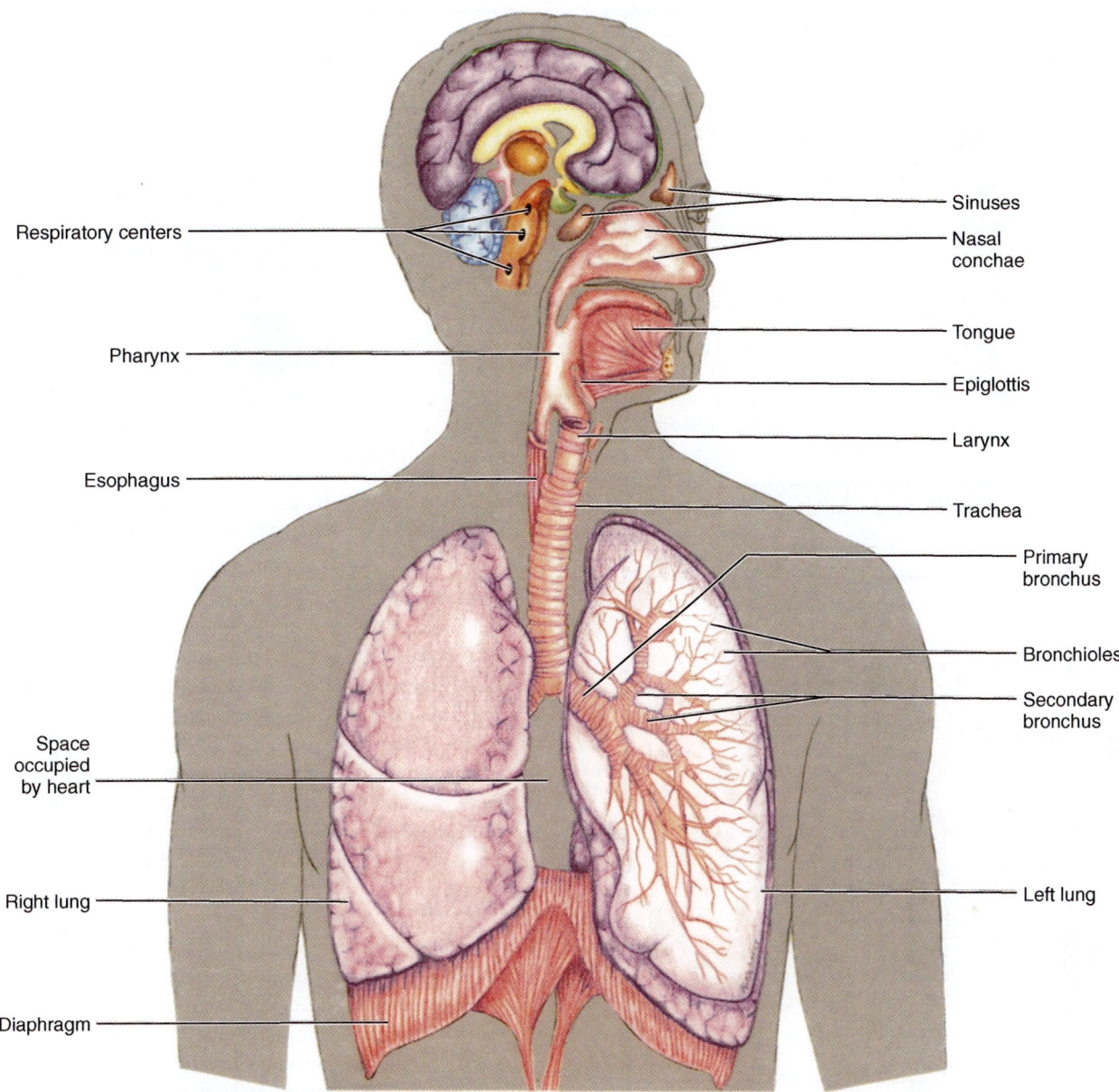

FIGURE 46-2 Anatomic structures of the respiratory system. (From Solomon EP: *Introduction to human anatomy and physiology,* ed 3, St Louis, 2009, Saunders.)

smaller and smaller passageways, much as blood vessels do in the circulatory system. This branching continues until it becomes microscopic. These very tiny bronchi are called *bronchioles.* Every bronchiole terminates in microscopic air sacs called *alveoli.* The alveoli are made of thin tissue, only one cell wall thick that allows for the exchange of oxygen and carbon dioxide through the cell membrane.

The bronchial tree and alveoli are the major structures housed within the right and left lungs. The lungs are soft and spongy because of the air sacs that make up most of their mass. They hang in the right and left sides of the chest, separated by the pericardial sac, which contains the heart. The right lung is divided into three lobes and has a greater volume capacity than the left lung. Because each lobe has its own bronchus and blood supply, the removal of one lobe (lobectomy) results in little or no damage to the rest of the lung.

The left lung is longer and narrower and has a distinct indentation in its center, known as the *cardiac notch,* where the left ventricle of the heart is located and an apical pulse is heard. The left lung has only two lobes, the upper and lower sections (Figure 46-4).

Each lung is encased in a double-layered sac called the *pleural membrane.* The membrane closest to the lung is called the *visceral pleura,* which doubles back to form the parietal pleural membrane. Small amounts of pleural fluid fill the space between the two membranes and provide lubrication for the movement of the lungs during inhalation and exhalation.

VENTILATION

In the very delicate lung tissue, the bronchioles deposit oxygenated air into the grapelike structures of the alveoli. Surrounding each

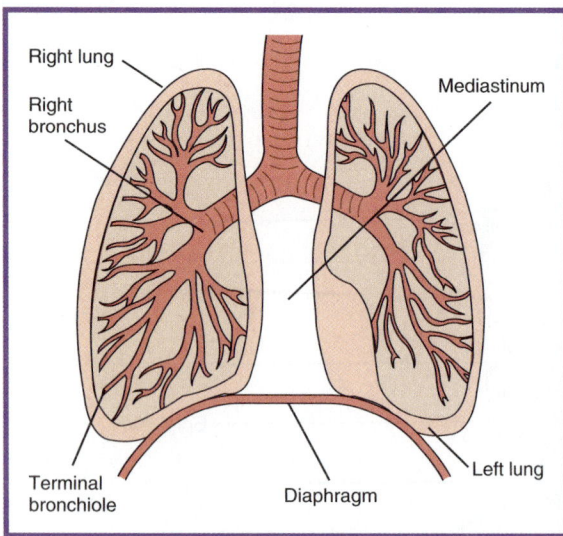

FIGURE 46-3 Bronchial tree.

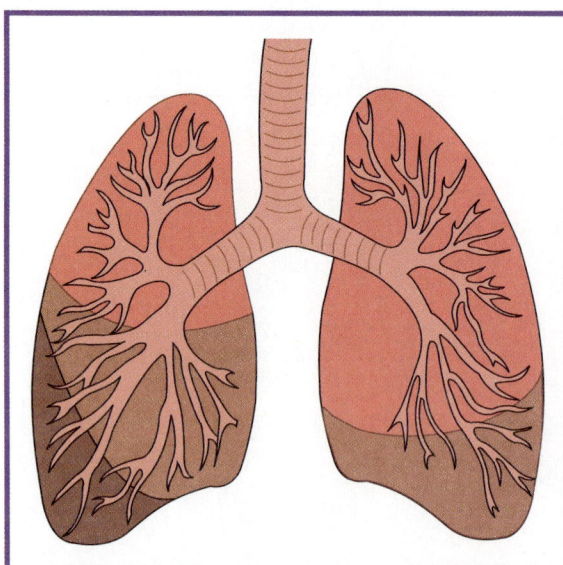

FIGURE 46-4 Lobes of the lungs.

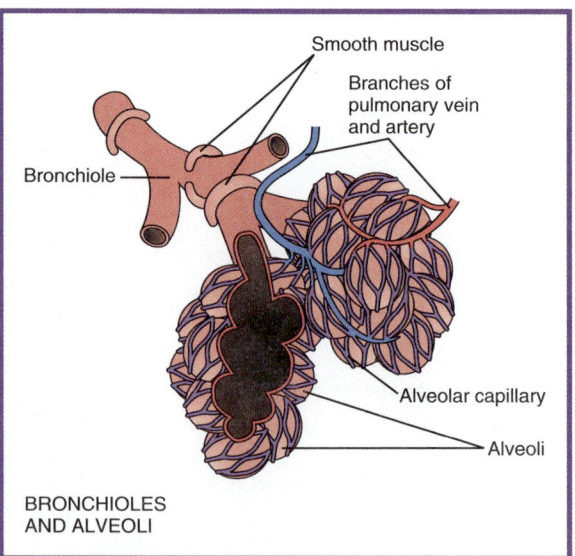

FIGURE 46-5 Alveoli with their capillary network.

alveolus is a network of pulmonary capillaries filled with waste air. The oxygenated air moves through the single-celled walls of the alveoli and into the single-celled walls of the pulmonary capillaries (Figure 46-5). As this is happening, the waste air is forced out of the capillaries, into the alveoli, and then into the bronchioles. This carbon dioxide–oxygen exchange provides oxygen-rich blood that is returned to the heart for distribution throughout the body; carbon dioxide wastes are excreted with exhalation. The process involved in this gaseous exchange is called *ventilation.* The movement of oxygen from the atmosphere into the alveoli is known as *inspiration,* and the movement of waste gases from the alveoli into the atmosphere is called *expiration.*

Inspiration

Inspiration begins with a signal from the medulla oblongata in the brainstem. The signal originates because of a decrease in blood oxygen levels or an increase in carbon dioxide levels. The stimulus

is carried by the phrenic nerve to the major muscle of inspiration, the diaphragm. When the diaphragm receives the signal, it flattens out and pulls downward. At the same moment, the intercostal muscles between the ribs contract, causing the ribs to move outward and the chest cavity to enlarge. This movement causes the lungs to expand and increase their volume. The more these muscles are contracted, the deeper the inhalation is and the greater the air volume becomes. Respiratory distress occurs when an individual is unable to move an adequate amount of air into the lungs, using the diaphragm and intercostal muscles, to meet the body's needs.

Expiration

The second half of ventilation is expiration. Once inspiration is complete, the diaphragm and intercostal muscles relax, causing the diaphragm to move upward into the thoracic cavity and the ribs to move inward, reducing lung capacity. This movement forces the waste air out of the lungs and back into the atmosphere. Expiration requires very little energy and takes place with minimal effort by the body. However, in certain respiratory conditions, such as asthma or emphysema, the person has difficulty getting air out of the lungs, and accessory muscles in the chest and abdomen are needed to assist the intercostal and diaphragm muscles for complete exhalation.

RESPIRATORY SYSTEM DEFENSES

Every part of the respiratory system has a defense mechanism. In the upper respiratory tract, the mucus-covered ciliated surface of the mucous membranes trap particles; through the continuous flow of the mucus back toward the nasopharynx, the particles are either sneezed outward or swallowed.

The lower respiratory tract is sterile, which is phenomenal considering that each day these airways are exposed to approximately 10,000 L of air containing an endless number of microorganisms and foreign material. The ever-changing airflow, inspiration to expiration, creates a turbulence that makes remaining in the bronchi very difficult for these invading substances. This, combined with

TABLE 46-1   Respiratory System Terms

MEDICAL TERM	DEFINITION
Apnea	Absence of breathing
Atelectasis	Collapsed lung
Dyspnea	Difficulty breathing
Empyema	Accumulation of pus in the pleural space
Hemoptysis	Expectoration of blood
Hemothorax	Accumulation of blood and fluid in the pleural cavity
Hypercapnia	Greater than normal amounts of carbon dioxide in the blood
Hyperpnea	Deep, rapid, labored respiration that may occur because of exercise or pain and fever
Hypoxemia	Low level of oxygen in the blood
Orthopnea	Person must sit or stand to breathe comfortably
Pleurisy	Inflammation of the parietal pleura, causing dyspnea and stabbing pain; friction rub may be auscultated
Pneumothorax	Collapse of the lung as a result of the collection of air or gas in the pleural space
Pyothorax	Collection of pus in the pleural cavity caused by infection
Rales	Bubbling or popping sound heard on auscultation; it is produced by the passage of air through bronchi that are constricted or contain secretions
Rhinoplasty	Plastic surgery to repair or alter the structure of the nose
Rhinorrhea	Excessive drainage from the nose
Rhonchi	Continuous rumbling sound heard on auscultation; it is caused by thick secretions or spasms
Tachypnea	Abnormally rapid rate of breathing
Thoracotomy	Surgical opening into the thoracic cavity

coughing, sneezing, and a functioning immune system, protects the respiratory tract and helps the body maintain homeostasis. Disease occurs when something disrupts the normal homeostatic chain of events.

MAJOR DISEASES OF THE RESPIRATORY SYSTEM

Many diseases affect the respiratory system. The major ones can be divided into infectious diseases, obstructive disorders, and tumors. Respiratory diseases cause common symptoms, including sneezing, a productive or nonproductive cough, sore throat or hoarseness, fever, general malaise, altered breath sounds, and changes in breathing patterns. The medical assistant must be familiar with common respiratory terms and use them in documenting a patient's signs and symptoms (Table 46-1).

CRITICAL THINKING APPLICATION   46-1

Michael is taking a patient history for a new patient, who reports the following problems: difficulty breathing; sometimes she has to sit up to breathe comfortably; occasionally she coughs up blood and has excessive nasal drainage. Six months ago, she experienced very rapid breathing and a blue color to her skin, so she was admitted to the hospital and diagnosed with blood and fluid around her right lung, which had become infected, causing her lung to collapse. Based on what Michael knows about respiratory system terminology, how should he document this information?

Infectious Diseases

Respiratory tract infections fall into two categories, depending on their location. Diseases of the nose and upper respiratory tract are more common than diseases of the lower respiratory tract (e.g., pneumonia). Respiratory tract infections account for approximately 75% of all clinically diagnosed infections. Only about 5% of these infections involve the lungs. Most lung infections are seen in hospitalized patients, the elderly, substance abusers, alcoholics, and patients with acquired immunodeficiency syndrome (AIDS). Pneumonia is the seventh leading cause of death in the United States and often is the cause of death for debilitated people.

Upper Respiratory Tract Infections

Common Cold. The common cold was discussed in Chapter 42 as an acute inflammatory process affecting the mucous membranes that line the nose, pharynx, larynx, and bronchus. Usually the term "cold" is used when only the membranes of the nose and pharynx are affected; however, the same virus can affect the larynx and lungs. The viral invasion can be followed by bacterial infections of the pharynx, sinuses, and middle ear. Common signs of an upper respiratory tract infection (URTI or URI) include nasal congestion and **rhinorrhea**, sneezing, watery eyes, pharyngitis (sore throat), laryngitis (hoarseness), and coughing. Nasal discharge usually is clear and watery in the early stage but can become greenish yellow as the virus becomes more **virulent** or when bacteria invade. The patient usually complains of headache, low-grade fever, chills, and anorexia.

Currently there is no cure for the common cold; the infection usually runs its course in 3 to 5 days. The best way to treat it is to get plenty of rest and drink fluids. An over-the-counter (OTC) cold remedy, cough syrup, and acetaminophen may lessen the discomfort of cold-related symptoms. Antibiotics are prescribed only if evidence of a secondary bacterial infection is present. As discussed in Chapter 33, although echinacea may be promoted as an effective preventive and/or treatment for the common cold, most studies show little or no evidence that it is effective.

Sinusitis. The paranasal sinuses are air-filled spaces in the skull located in the brow area over the eyes, inside each cheekbone, behind the bridge of the nose, and behind the eyes. Each sinus has an opening into the nose for the free exchange of air and is lined with a continuous mucous membrane. Healthy sinuses are sterile, but an infection or an allergic reaction can cause one or more of the sinuses to become inflamed or infected. Inflammation causes edema and the collection of mucus within the sinus cavity, creating a feeling of pressure, nasal congestion or rhinorrhea, and classic sinus headaches.

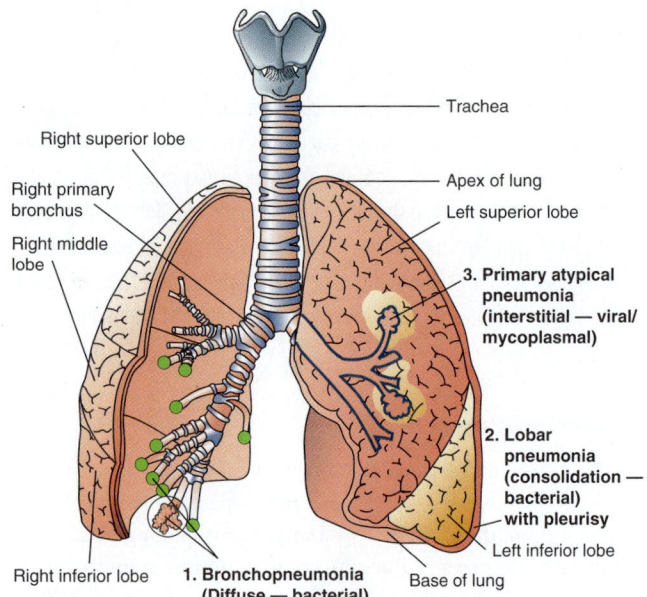

FIGURE 46-6 Types of pneumonia. (From Gould B: *Pathophysiology for the health professions,* ed 3, St Louis, 2006, Saunders.)

TABLE 46-2 Pathogens That Cause Pneumonia	
PATHOGEN	**TYPE OF INFECTION**
Bacteria	*Streptococcus pneumoniae*
	Haemophilus influenzae
	Staphylococcus aureus
	Mycobacteria
Virus	Influenza virus
Fungi	*Aspergillus fumigatus*
	Candida albicans
	Mycoplasma pneumoniae
Parasite	*Pneumocystis carinii* (opportunistic infection, seen in immunosuppressed, debilitated, or terminally ill patients)

The location of sinus pain depends on the sinus cavity involved but can be described as pain in the forehead (frontal sinuses), upper jaw and teeth discomfort (maxillary sinuses), pain between the eyes (ethmoid sinuses), and/or an earache and neck pain (sphenoid sinuses). The condition is treated with decongestants, antibiotics for bacterial infections, and analgesics. Sinusitis can be acute, lasting 2 to 8 weeks, or chronic, with symptoms lingering much longer.

Allergic Rhinitis (Hay Fever). Although not caused by a pathogenic organism, allergic rhinitis frequently is confused with infectious disease. This disorder affects millions of people every year. It is caused by a reaction of the nasal mucosa to an environmental allergen. The most common allergen is plant pollen; this is where the term "hay fever" originated. Signs and symptoms include sneezing, nasal congestion, nasal itching, and rhinorrhea. Symptoms can be controlled either with OTC treatments, such as Sudafed, Zyrtec, and fexofenadine hydrochloride (Allegra), or with prescription antihistamines, such as montelukast (Singulair), and fluticasone (Flonase) and cromolyn sodium (Nasalcrom) nasal sprays. The list of possible allergens is extensive. When this condition is seen in the respiratory practice, the patient usually is referred to an allergist for testing and possible immunotherapy.

Patients may have difficulty determining whether symptoms are caused by a cold or an allergy. The condition usually is an allergy if the eyes, ears, nose, throat, and roof of the mouth (palate) are itchy; the eyes are red and watery; a clear, thin nasal discharge is present; symptoms are seasonal and last for weeks or months; and the individual does not have a fever.

Lower Respiratory Tract Infections

Pneumonia. Pneumonia is both a specific disorder and a general term meaning inflammation of all or part of the lungs (Figure 46-6). Pneumonia can be caused by bacteria, viruses, or other pathogens (Table 46-2). It also can be caused by inhalation of irritants or poisonous gas and by aspiration of solids or fluids into the lungs. The most common causative organisms are staphylococci and streptococci.

Pneumonia can occur in any age group but most often affects preschoolers and the elderly (over age 65). It can range from a mild complication to a life-threatening illness. Risk factors include smoking, alcoholism, and immunosuppression caused by diseases or treatment. The patient usually comes to the office with symptoms of high fever, chills, and general malaise. Signs of the illness include dyspnea, tachypnea, chest pain during inspiration, and a relentless cough with possible hemoptysis. Auscultation of the chest reveals rales, rhonchi, and other signs of **pulmonary consolidation**. The infection may spread into the pleural cavity, causing empyema and pleurisy.

The diagnosis is confirmed with a chest x-ray evaluation; sputum culture and sensitivity testing to identify the invading organism and determine the appropriate antibiotic therapy; and a white blood cell (WBC) count, including a differential count to determine whether the pneumonia is viral or bacterial. If the pneumonia is viral, the number of WBCs does not increase; if it is bacterial, the greater the invasion, the higher the WBC count. With bacterial pneumonias, the differential count shows elevated neutrophil and monocyte levels. If the invading organism is bacterial, the treatment of choice is antibiotics and lung function therapy until the patient has recovered. If the organism is viral, the patient is given supportive care, such as antipyretics, fluids, and oxygen, until the immune system can control the spread of the virus.

Tuberculosis. According to the Centers for Disease Control and Prevention (CDC), approximately one third of the world's population is infected with tuberculosis (TB). TB causes more deaths than any other infectious agent in the world. For more than 50 years, the incidence of TB in the United States steadily declined; however, from the late 1980s through the 1990s, a resurgence in reported cases occurred. This increase was believed to be the result of increased travel and immigration; the number of individuals with AIDS, who have little resistance to disease; an increase in the number of homeless and malnourished people; and the overwhelming proliferation of drug-resistant TB bacilli. An international TB vaccine, bacille Calmette-Guérin (BCG), is available, but it is rarely used in the

United States. The vaccine does not always provide protection from the disease and those who are vaccinated may have a positive Mantoux test result.

TB is caused by the bacterium *Mycobacterium tuberculosis*. This organism is covered with a waxy substance that enables it to survive outside a living host for a long time. It is transmitted by droplets of sputum expectorated into the environment by an infected host that are inhaled by another person. In the warm, moist respiratory tract, these organisms again can become active if the individual is susceptible to the disease. TB also can be spread when an infected person coughs or sneezes, releasing airborne infected droplets, which are inhaled and cause an infection if the person is susceptible.

TB develops in two stages. The primary infection occurs when the person is first infected with the bacteria and the lungs become inflamed. Cell-mediated immunity ensues, isolating the bacteria and forming a **tubercle**. At this point a healthy individual can stop the spread of infection, causing the TB bacillus in the tubercle to become inactive. In this case, the person was exposed to the pathogen but never developed active disease and so is said to have a *latent* TB infection. Individuals with latent TB are asymptomatic and are not infectious. However, because an exposed person develops antibodies to the disease, he or she consistently tests positive on TB skin screening tests. Therefore, rather than the purified protein derivative (PPD), or Mantoux test, these patients should have chest x-ray studies to diagnose active TB.

At any time the bacilli in the tubercles can be reactivated, and secondary, or active, TB can develop. The patient now is actively infected with the disease, which can spread to the bones, brain, and kidneys (Figure 46-7). Some people develop active TB soon after becoming infected, before the immune systems can fight the TB bacteria; others develop it later in life, when the immune systems are weakened for other reasons.

TB is diagnosed most frequently in people living in crowded conditions with poor hygiene, those who are malnourished, and those who have other chronic conditions. It spreads most rapidly in large cities, in the elderly, alcoholics, and the homeless. Symptoms of an active infection include an intermittent fever that peaks in the afternoon, night sweats, weight loss, and general malaise. As the infection becomes virulent in the host, a productive cough develops, and thick, dark, frequently blood-tinged mucus is expectorated.

The primary diagnosis of TB is established through the patient's signs and symptoms. The infection is suspected with a positive chest x-ray film but is confirmed with a sputum culture. Traditional culture methods originally took 4 to 6 weeks, and this extended period allowed a potentially infectious individual to continue to spread the disease. New culture techniques identify the bacterium in as little as 36 to 48 hours. The physician also may order a blood test, the QuantiFERON-TB Gold test (QFT), to diagnose TB infection. The QFT measures the response to TB proteins when they are mixed with a small amount of blood. A two-step Mantoux test is recommended for individuals who are over age 45 and have never had a Mantoux test; those who have been vaccinated with BCG; and employees of hospitals and long-term care facilities. For this test, the initial intradermal skin test is administered and read in 48 to 72 hours. If the result is negative, a second Mantoux is performed on the opposite arm 1 to 3 weeks after the first test and again read in 48 to 72 hours.

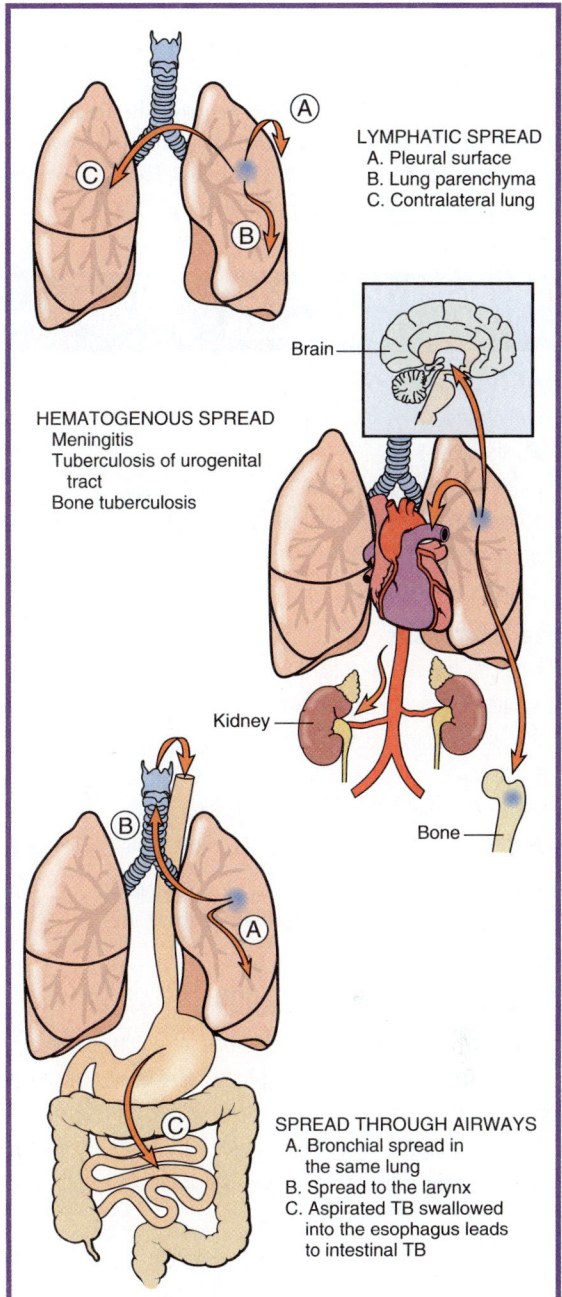

FIGURE 46-7 Spread of tuberculosis. (From Damjanov I: *Pathology for the health-related profession,* ed 4, St Louis, 2010, Saunders.)

Once a diagnosis of TB has been confirmed, the patient is prescribed long-term treatment with a combination of drugs to eradicate the bacilli. If the patient has tested positive for TB but does not have an active infection, the physician prescribes isoniazid (INH) and rifampin (RIF) for 6 months to treat any possible tubercle formations. If the patient has active pulmonary TB, the CDC recommends a four-drug regimen—INH, RIF, pyrazinamide, and ethambutol—daily for 2 months; this is then reduced to two drugs for an additional 4 to 7 months, depending on sputum culture outcomes. It is crucial that patients being treated with TB medications strictly comply with medication orders to prevent the creation of multidrug-resistant TB (MDR-TB). Resistant strains of TB develop because of skipped doses or failure to take the medication as long as prescribed. MDR-TB requires at least 2 years of drug therapy with medications that can cause serious side effects, especially liver damage. All tuberculin-negative healthcare workers should have a PPD annually; workers who show a positive reaction but are not actively infected with TB should have an annual chest x-ray evaluation to screen for the disease.

SIGNS AND SYMPTOMS OF LATENT AND ACTIVE TUBERCULOSIS

Latent Tuberculosis
- Asymptomatic
- Not infectious
- Positive purified protein derivative (PPD) test result
- Positive QuantiFERON-TB Gold blood test result
- Normal chest x-ray studies
- Negative sputum culture

Active Tuberculosis
- Symptoms include cough for 3 weeks or longer, chest pain, hemoptysis, fatigue, weight loss, anorexia, fever with chills, and night sweats
- Infectious (highest risk of infection is with close family members or associates)
- Positive PPD and QuantiFERON-TB Gold blood tests
- Abnormal chest x-ray studies and/or positive sputum culture

From the Centers for Disease Control and Prevention. Accessed August 10, 2012. Available at www.cdc.gov/tb/publications/factsheets/general/LTBIandActiveTB.htm.

CRITICAL THINKING APPLICATION   46-2

Dr. Samuelson is the primary care physician for a nursing home in the area. He is concerned, because one of the employees has had a positive result on a Mantoux test. What other tests will Dr. Samuelson order to confirm the diagnosis? If those tests come back positive, how will the patient be treated? What about the other employees and residents of the nursing home?

Chronic Obstructive Pulmonary Disease

Chronic obstructive pulmonary disease (COPD) is a group of diseases with the common characteristic of chronic airway obstruction. COPD is the fourth leading cause of death in America, and most of those deaths are related to smoking. Among the diseases in this group are **chronic bronchitis**, **bronchiectasis**, asthma, pneumoconiosis, and emphysema. Although the mechanism of the obstruction may vary, a patient with COPD is unable to ventilate the lungs freely, which results in an ineffective exchange of respiratory gases, dyspnea, and productive cough. Over time, eliminating carbon dioxide from the lungs during expiration becomes increasingly difficult.

Asthma

Pediatric asthma was addressed in Chapter 42. Asthma attacks occur in response to a number of triggers that cause inflammation and bronchospasm with resultant airflow obstruction. Asthma can develop into a chronic disease characterized by increased activity or sensitivity of the bronchial tubes to external factors, such as environmental irritants, poor air quality, and allergies, or to internal factors, such as stress, exercise, infection, and allergen inhalation. Asthma also has a strong hereditary factor.

Asthma attacks can be mild to severe and can last minutes to days. Bronchospasms trap air in the lungs while the inflammatory response creates edema and causes secretion of mucus into the constricted bronchioles. A patient with asthma complains of a nonproductive cough, dyspnea, expiratory wheezing, and chest tightness. Because the individual has difficulty breathing, tachycardia, pallor, and diaphoresis also may occur. The patient can speak only a few words at a time, stopping intermittently to regulate air intake. When the chest is auscultated, the physician hears diminished breath sounds with wheezes and rhonchi in the lungs. Spirometry can be used to measure the degree of airflow obstruction. Chest x-ray studies may show changes in the lungs from mucous obstructions. Blood tests include a complete blood cell count with a differential count to determine whether the attack is allergy related.

Regardless of their age, patients with asthma should be actively involved in the day-to-day management of their disease. The medical assistant may be responsible for teaching the patient how to perform peak flow measurements either daily or at the onset of an attack. Peak flow meters assess the individual's ability to move air into and out of the lungs. The physician may want the patient to keep a log of daily peak flow results or to use the instrument as an at-home monitoring device when chest tightness and wheezing occur. The meter measures the peak expiratory flow rate, which is the fastest speed at which the patient can blow air out of the lungs after taking in as big a breath as possible (Procedure 46-1). Peak flow readings provide an evaluation of bronchiole function that the patient can perform at home with limited assistance. Readings can help predict an asthma attack if levels are falling; can measure the degree of bronchospasm; and provide the physician with feedback regarding the effectiveness of asthma treatment.

The physician uses three zones of measurement to interpret peak flow rates. The green zone is considered normal: the reading is 80% to 100% of normal peak flow rates, indicating the patient's asthma is under control. The yellow zone signals caution: the patient's highest reading is 50% to 80% of normal. The physician makes treatment decisions and recommendations at this point, or the patient may already be instructed on how to manage medications if readings are within these levels. The red zone includes readings below 50% of the normal level, and immediate action must be taken to prevent severe bronchospasms.

If the patient is having an asthma attack, the bronchioles are constricting, becoming edematous, and filling up with mucus, so the patient is unable to exhale strongly enough to raise the peak flow indicator to a normal level. If readings are below normal, the physician prescribes a treatment plan that may include contacting the physician when peak flow levels are below a certain point or starting nebulizer treatments. The physician may recommend an increase in antiinflammatory medication if more than a 20% variation from normal is seen in the readings. The medication therapy chosen depends on the severity and frequency of acute attacks, but management is necessary to prevent permanent lung damage and emphysema-like changes in the lungs.

PROCEDURE 46-1

Instruct Patients According to Their Needs: Teach a Patient to Use a Peak Flow Meter

GOAL: *To instruct the patient in the proper method of performing a peak flow meter test.*

EQUIPMENT and SUPPLIES

- Peak flow meter
- Disposable mouthpiece
- Notebook with pen
- Biohazardous waste container
- Patient's record

PROCEDURAL STEPS

1. Sanitize your hands.
2. Place the mouthpiece on the peak flow meter and slide the marker to the bottom of the scale.
   PURPOSE: The indicator must be at the bottom of the scale for proper measurement of expiratory effort (Figure 1).

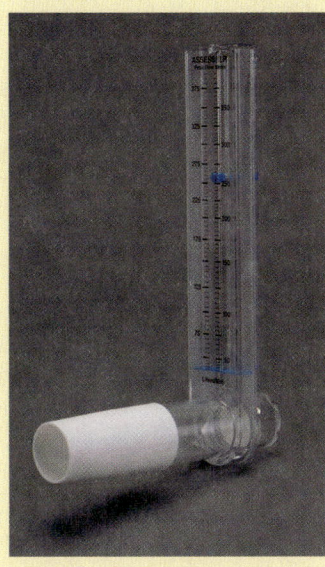

3. Introduce yourself and confirm the patient's identity.
4. Explain the purpose of the test.
   PURPOSE: To help reassure the patient.
5. Explain the actual maneuver of forced expiration.
   PURPOSE: The patient must understand the maneuver so that he or she can cooperate fully; this produces the best test results.
6. Make sure the patient is comfortable and in a proper position, either sitting upright or standing (standing is preferred).
   PURPOSE: Proper positioning ensures maximum lung expansion and accurate test results.
7. Loosen any tight clothing, such as a necktie, bra, or belt.
   PURPOSE: Tight clothing may restrict breathing capacity.
8. Hold the meter upright, taking care not to block the opening with the fingers (Figure 2).
   PURPOSE: To prevent obstruction of forced exhalation.

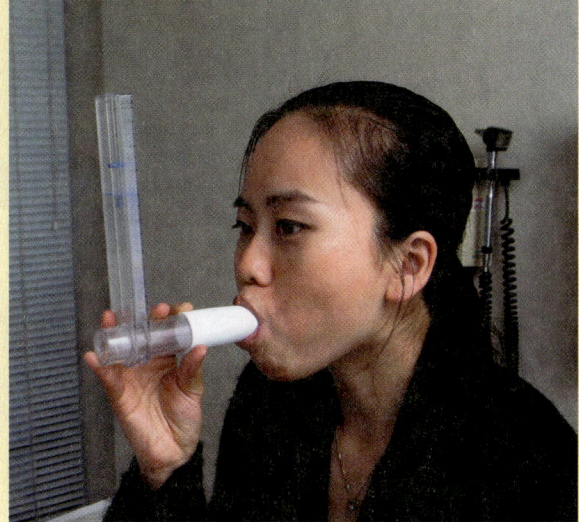

9. Instruct the patient to inhale as deeply as possible, to place the mouthpiece into the mouth beyond the teeth, and to form a tight seal with the lips. Caution the patient not to put the tongue in the mouthpiece when exhaling.
   PURPOSE: To prevent any leakage of air around the mouthpiece and any obstruction of airflow.
10. Instruct the patient to exhale as fast and as forcefully as possible into the peak flow meter.
11. The forced exhalation will move the marker up the scale and stop at the point of the peak expiratory flow. Record this number and return the marker to the bottom of the scale.
12. Repeat the procedure two more times, sliding the indicator to the bottom of the scale before each reading, and record each result.
13. Encourage the patient to inhale as deeply as possible and to exhale as fast and as forcefully as possible with each effort.
14. Place the test results on the patient's chart for the physician to review, noting the time and date of the highest reading.
15. Clean and disinfect the equipment, discarding waste in a biohazardous waste container, or give the patient the meter for continued use at home with instructions to follow the manufacturer's cleaning recommendations.
16. Sanitize your hands.
    PURPOSE: To ensure infection control.
17. Record the testing information in the patient's chart.
    PURPOSE: Procedures that are not recorded are considered not done.
    CAUTION: Peak flow readings may trigger bronchospasms or severe coughing in patients experiencing an asthma attack. If this occurs, instruct the patient to rest and try again. If the patient is unable to perform three readings because of bronchospasms and/or coughing, follow the physician's guidelines for managing this situation.

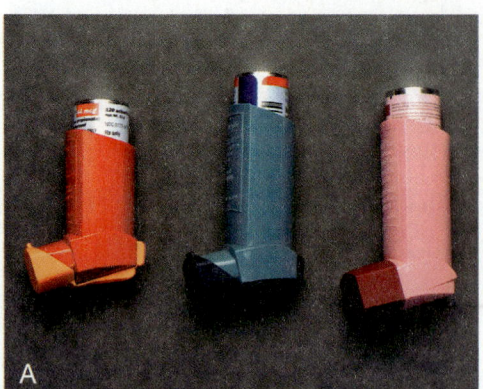
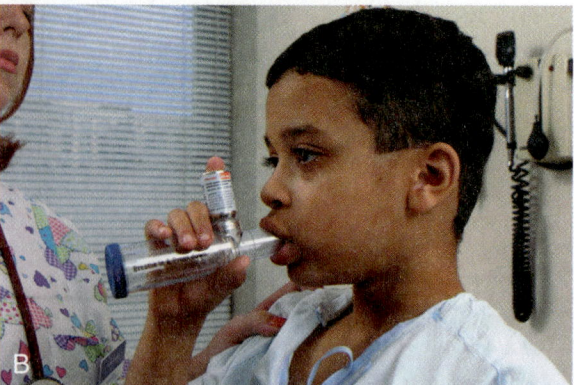

FIGURE 46-8 **A,** Inhalers. **B,** An inhaler with a spacer.

The treatment of asthma consists of a regimen of medications, including "rescue" inhalers (e.g., ipratropium bromide [Atrovent] or albuterol [Ventolin]), which are used to relieve bronchospasms or for exercise-induced asthma (Figure 46-8). Tissue inflammation can be treated with steroid inhalers (e.g., flunisolide [Aerobid], triamcinolone acetonide [Azmacort], or fluticasone [Flovent Diskus]) and/or an oral leukotriene-receptor antagonists such as zafirlukast (Accolate) or montelukast sodium (Singulair) taken daily. Another option is a combination inhaler, such as fluticasone and salmeterol (Advair Diskus), that contains both types of medications to prevent and treat bronchiole inflammation. A severe attack may require injections of epinephrine, oral corticosteroids (prednisone) and/or nebulizer treatments with a bronchodilator (Procedure 46-2). A nebulizer forces compressed air through a medication chamber that converts liquid medication (albuterol or budesonide [Pulmicort]) into an aerosol or mist form that can be inhaled though a mask or mouthpiece.

The physician prescribes an inhaler dose according to the number of "puffs" of a metered-dose inhaler (MDI) the patient should administer. MDIs consist of a pressurized canister containing medication and a mouthpiece. Most MDIs hold about 200 doses of medication combined with a pressurized gas propellant, which forces the drug out of the canister. When the canister is inverted and depressed, a metered dose (premeasured) is delivered through the mouthpiece in aerosol form. Patient teaching is very important to ensure that the patient operates the device correctly so that the medication can be administered as ordered. If both a steroid and a bronchodilator have been prescribed, the bronchodilator should be taken first, because this opens the airways so that the steroid is better distributed throughout the lungs.

3. Exhale normally. Then, while beginning to inhale slowly, depress the canister, releasing a metered dose of medication.
4. Continue to breathe in until your lungs are full; hold the breath to a count of 10, if possible, and then breathe out normally.
5. If a second dose has been prescribed, wait at least 1 minute between puffs.
6. Some inhalers come attached to spacers or can be adapted to meet the needs of children or older patients who have difficulty managing the technique. When the canister is depressed, the medication stays in the spacer, and the patient can take more time to inhale the particles (see Figure 46-8, *B*).

Pneumoconioses

Environmental causes of respiratory diseases include inhaled dusts, fumes, and various kinds of organic or inorganic matter. Most of these respiratory diseases are occupational; they are the consequence of long-term exposure to unsafe air in the workplace. Although the respiratory system is designed to filter and trap air contaminants, it can become overloaded after intense exposure. Subsequently, irritants enter the lungs, and the amount of damage to pulmonary tissue increases if the particles are very small and can enter the alveoli; if the individual is exposed to a large amount of contaminants over a long period; and when there is the added irritation of cigarette smoking.

Some occupations that can cause pneumoconiosis include coal mining (anthracosis); insulation manufacturing and shipbuilding (asbestosis); and stonecutting or sandblasting (silicosis). The tissue changes caused by inhalation of these substances into the lungs are irreversible. Patients develop dyspnea, cough, and emphysema-like changes and have an increased risk of lung cancer.

Emphysema

Emphysema is a progressive obstructive disease of the pulmonary system that is irreversible. Emphysema causes loss of elasticity in the walls of the alveoli, and eventually these walls stretch and break, creating air spaces that cannot conduct the oxygen–carbon dioxide exchange. The remaining alveoli become overinflated, and as time progresses, exhaling completely becomes very difficult. Cigarette smoking is the primary contributing factor, although patients who

---

PATIENT EDUCATION FOR A METERED-DOSE INHALER

Instruct the patient in the use of a metered-dose inhaler has follows:
1. Shake the canister vigorously and place it into the mouthpiece device.
2. Open your mouth and hold the inhaler approximately 1 inch away. (If the patient places the mouthpiece in the mouth, the gas propellant causes the drug to bounce off the back of the throat, and much of it will be lost around the mouth.)

Assist the Physician with Patient Care: Administer a Nebulizer Treatment

GOAL: *To perform a nebulizer treatment.*

EQUIPMENT and SUPPLIES

- Nebulizer machine
- Disposable connector tubing with medication dispenser
- Disposable mouthpiece or mask as ordered
- Medication as ordered
- Biohazardous waste container
- Patient's record and pen

PROCEDURAL STEPS

1. Plug the nebulizer into a properly grounded electrical outlet.
2. Introduce yourself and confirm the patient's identity.
3. Explain the purpose of the treatment.
   <u>PURPOSE:</u> To help reassure the patient.
4. Sanitize your hands.
5. Measure the prescribed dose of drug into the nebulizer medication cup (Figure 1).

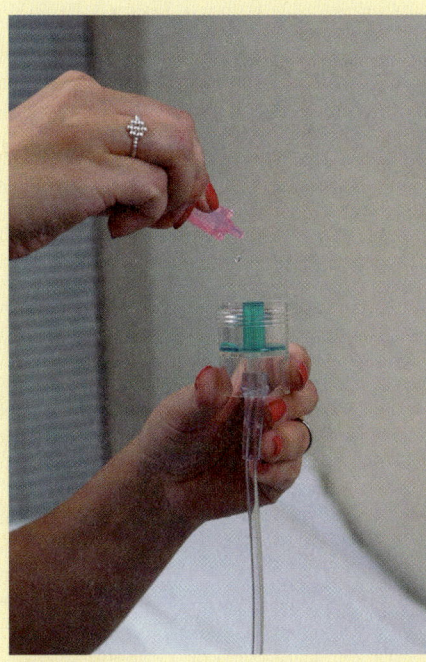

6. Replace the top of the medication cup and connect it to the mouthpiece or face mask.
7. Connect the disposable tubing to the nebulizer and the medication cup.
8. The patient should be sitting upright to allow for total lung expansion.
   <u>PURPOSE:</u> Proper positioning ensures adequate dispersal of the medication.
9. Turn on the nebulizer (a mist should be visible coming from the back of the tube opposite the mouthpiece or into the face mask).
   <u>PURPOSE:</u> The mist is the aerosolized medication.

10. If using a mask, position it comfortably but securely over the patient's mouth and nose.
11. If using a mouthpiece, instruct the patient to hold it between the teeth with the lips pursed around the mouthpiece (Figure 2).

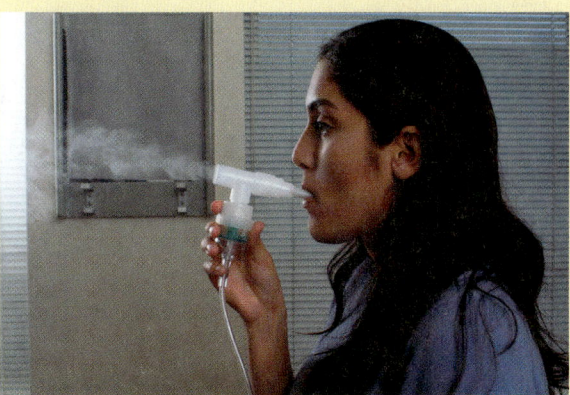

12. Encourage the patient to take slow, deep breaths through the mouth and to hold each breath 2 to 3 seconds to allow the medication to disperse through the lungs.
    <u>PURPOSE:</u> To ensure maximum distribution of the medication in the lung tissue.
13. Continue the treatment until aerosol is no longer produced (approximately 10 minutes).
    <u>CAUTION:</u> If the patient is receiving a bronchodilator (albuterol), he or she may experience dizziness, tremors, or tachycardia. Continue the treatment unless otherwise ordered by the physician.
14. Turn off the nebulizer.
15. Encourage the patient to take several deep breaths and to cough loosened secretions into disposable tissues.
16. Dispose of the mouthpiece or mask and tubing in a biohazard container and instruct the patient also to dispose of the contaminated tissues in the biohazard container.
    <u>PURPOSE:</u> To ensure infection control.
17. Sanitize your hands.
    <u>PURPOSE:</u> To ensure infection control.
18. Record the nebulizer treatment; the patient's response, including the amount of coughing and whether coughing was productive or nonproductive; and any side effects of the medication.
    <u>PURPOSE:</u> Procedures that are not recorded are considered not done.
19. If the patient is to continue home nebulizer treatments, provide patient education for both the patient and caregivers as appropriate. Make sure they demonstrate the treatment steps to confirm understanding.
    <u>PURPOSE:</u> Feedback through demonstration of technique ensures patient follow-through.

develop emphysema at an early age may have a genetic predisposition to the disease. Other contributors include exposure to pollutants (pneumoconioses) or chronic respiratory disorders (chronic bronchitis or asthma).

Symptoms may not be seen until irreversible damage has occurred. When signs and symptoms occur, they include dyspnea, shortness of breath (SOB), wheezing, production of thick mucus, restlessness, fatigue, anorexia, persistent cough (productive or nonproductive), and peripheral cyanosis with clubbing (Figure 46-9). The patient typically is diagnosed from presenting signs and symptoms and a chest x-ray examination, as well as a pulmonary function test (PFT)

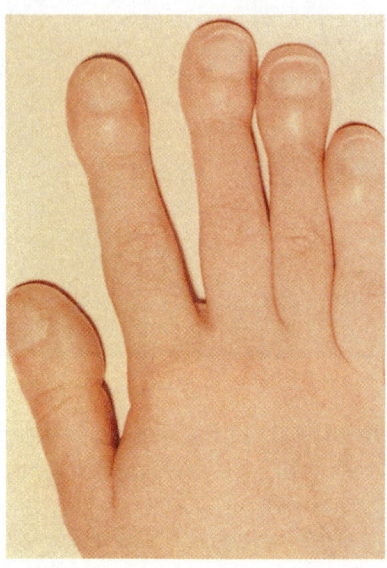

FIGURE 46-9 Clubbing. (From Zitelli B, Davis H: *Atlas of pediatric physical diagnosis,* ed 5, Philadelphia, 2007, Mosby.)

that shows increased residual volume and decreased forced expiratory volume (Table 46-3).

Patients with emphysema are encouraged to avoid respiratory irritants and individuals with respiratory infections and to stop smoking. Many of these patients require oxygen therapy and benefit from postural drainage and chest percussion to enable the patient to expectorate trapped mucus. Nebulizer treatments also may be prescribed.

Patients with emphysema expend a great deal of energy just to expel air from the lungs, so they should consume a high-calorie, high-fluid diet and perform certain exercises, such as pursed-lip breathing, to help them conserve energy. A patient with emphysema requires continuous care and support; therefore, encouraging family involvement in the treatment plan is important. Referral to a pulmonary rehabilitation program or support group can benefit both patient and family members.

Obstructive Sleep Apnea

Obstructive sleep apnea occurs when the muscles in the posterior pharynx that support the soft palate, uvula, tonsils, and tongue relax during sleep. This relaxation causes the trachea to narrow or close with inhalation, momentarily stopping breathing. Blood oxygen levels are lowered, and the brain senses hypoxemia so it stimulates the patient from sleep to reopen the trachea. The patient is awake so briefly he or she is not aware of the arousal, but this occurs repeatedly throughout the night, preventing the person from achieving a deeper, more restful level of sleep. Because of this interrupted sleep, the individual frequently complains of sleepiness during the day.

Individuals are at greater risk of developing obstructive sleep apnea if they are overweight, because a fat or thick neck may narrow the trachea; if they have enlarged adenoids or tonsils; if they are male, because men develop sleep apnea twice as frequently as women; if

TABLE 46-3 Pulmonary Function Tests

LUNG FUNCTION	DESCRIPTION	PATIENT INSTRUCTIONS
Tidal volume (TV)	Volume of air inspired and expired during a normal respiration	Patient breathes in and out normally with lips pursed around mouthpiece.
Vital capacity (VC)	Maximum amount of air that can be expired after maximum inspiration	Patient takes deep breath and exhales completely (not forcefully).
Inspiratory capacity (IC)	Maximum amount of air that can be inspired after a normal expiration	Patient breathes in and out normally, then forcibly inhales at the end of the TV.
Expiratory reserve volume (ERV)	Maximum volume of air that can be exhaled after a normal expiration	Patient breathes in and out normally, then exhales forcibly at the end of the TV.
Residual volume (RV)	Volume of air left in lungs after forced expiration	
Functional residual volume (FRV)	Amount of air left in the lungs after a normal expiration	FRV = ERV + RV
Forced vital capacity (FVC)	Amount of air that can be forcefully exhaled from a maximum inhalation	Patient inhales as deeply as possible, then forcibly exhales as much as possible.
Maximum volume ventilation (MVV)	Maximum volume the patient can breathe in and out in 1 minute	Patient breathes in and out as deeply and as frequently as possible for 15 seconds (total volume is multiplied by 4).

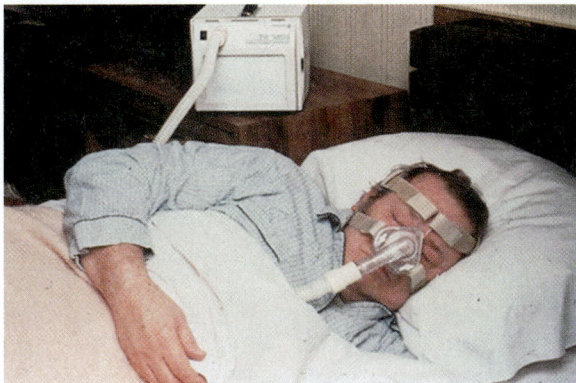

FIGURE 46-10 Patient with a CPAP machine. (Courtesy Respironics, Murrysville, Pa.)

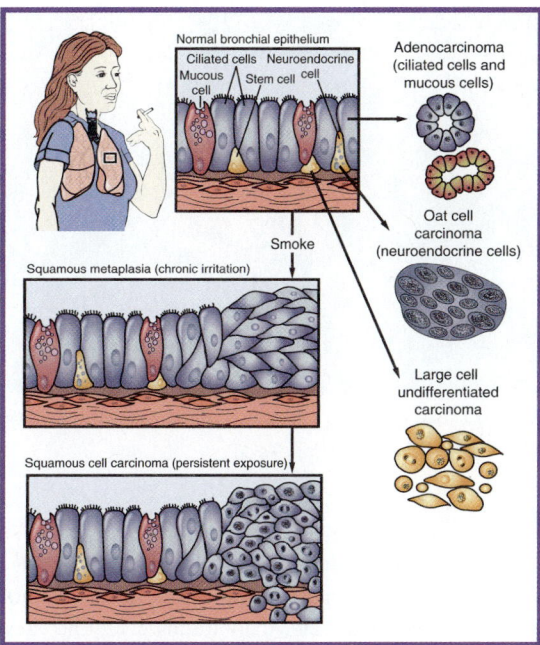

FIGURE 46-11 Classification of lung cancer. (From Damjanov IL: *Pathology for the health-related professions,* ed 4, St Louis, 2010, Saunders.)

they have a family history of sleep apnea; and if they drink alcohol or take sedatives, because these chemicals relax throat muscles.

Patients with suspected sleep apnea report chronic fatigue (from the constant startling out of a restful sleep) and pronounced snoring. Sleep apnea is diagnosed after the patient has been monitored during a sleep study, a process called *nocturnal polysomnography.* The patient is connected to equipment that monitors the pulse rate, brain activity, breathing patterns, blood oxygen levels, and limb movements during sleep.

Multiple complications in addition to chronic daytime fatigue can occur because of sleep apnea. Patients are more susceptible to hypertension and resultant heart disease because hypoxic episodes during sleep raise blood pressure and put a strain on the heart. Individuals with sleep apnea also tend to complain of memory problems, morning headaches, depression, and nocturia.

Sleep apnea typically is treated with a continuous positive airway pressure (CPAP) machine (Figure 46-10), which delivers air pressure through a mask placed over the mouth or through a cannula in the nose. The air pressure created by the machine is greater than that of the surrounding air, and it forces the upper airway passages open and prevents tracheal collapse. Although CPAP is the preferred method of treatment, it can be awkward and uncomfortable, making it difficult to sleep. Patients may have to experiment with different types of masks and need to be encouraged to follow through with the recommended treatment. Individuals with mild obstructive sleep apnea can try alternative treatment with a dental device that opens the throat by bringing the jaw forward. Surgery may also be an option to remove the uvula, tonsils, and adenoids, as well as excess tissue from the nose and back of the throat that vibrates during sleep, resulting in snoring.

COMMON SIGNS AND SYMPTOMS OF OBSTRUCTIVE SLEEP APNEA

- Excessive daytime sleepiness (hypersomnia)
- Persistently loud, disruptive snoring
- Snoring, choking, or gasping sounds while asleep
- Episodes of breathing cessation during sleep
- Dry mouth or sore throat on awakening
- Morning headache

CRITICAL THINKING APPLICATION 46-3

Dr. Samuelson has quite a few patients with either asthma or emphysema. Under Dr. Samuelson's direction, Michael is expected to reinforce patient education and answer patients' and family members' questions. Michael decides to make a file on pertinent health education information and review it with Dr. Samuelson before using it to help coordinate the care of these patients. What information should Michael include in the file? What community resources or groups should be included for patient support?

Cancer of the Pulmonary System

The most prevalent neoplasms of the respiratory system are lung cancer and carcinoma of the larynx.

Lung Cancer

Lung cancer is the leading cause of cancer-related deaths for both men and women in the United States. It is estimated that 90% of lung tumors are linked to cigarette smoking; other risk factors include chronic exposure to second-hand smoke, carcinogens (e.g., radon gas and asbestos), and a genetic predisposition. The risk of developing cancer is higher for patients who started to smoke at a young age and who have smoked more than a pack a day for a long period (Figure 46-11). Individuals who quit smoking can significantly lower their risk of lung cancer; after 10 years, the risk is reduced by one third. Female smokers are at greater risk of lung cancer than male smokers.

The lung is a common site of secondary tumors from metastasis in addition to primary carcinomas. Several different cellular types of tumors can develop in the lungs, but the one seen most frequently is bronchogenic carcinoma, which originates in the epithelial lining

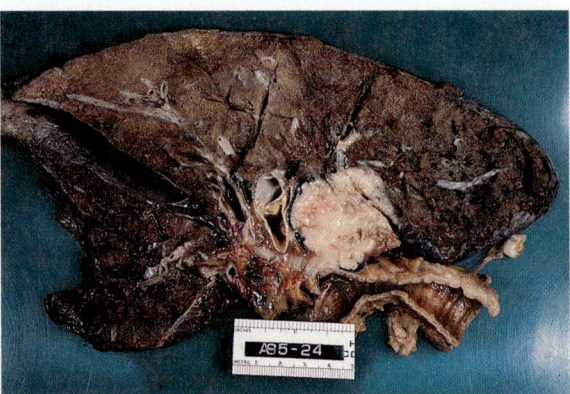

FIGURE 46-12 Lung cancer. (From Damjanov IL: *Pathology for the health-related professions*, ed 4, St Louis, 2010, Saunders.)

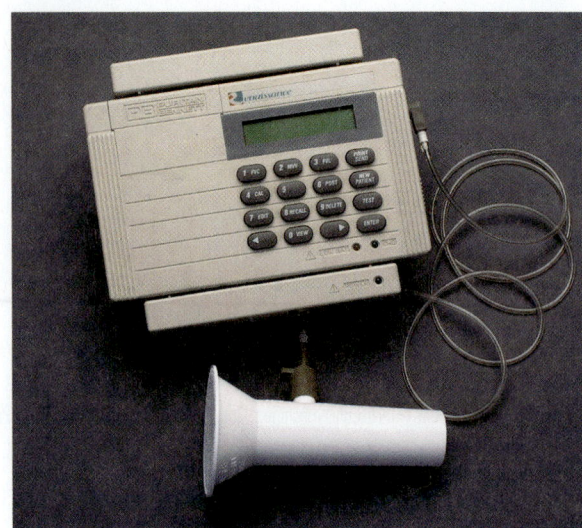

FIGURE 46-13 Spirometer.

of the bronchioles (Figure 46-12). The early symptoms of lung cancer (i.e., a chronic, productive cough; SOB; and chest tightness) are masked by symptoms regularly displayed by habitual smokers. A tumor may be discovered accidentally during a routine chest x-ray evaluation or may not be discovered until metastatic symptoms, such as anemia, weight loss, and fatigue, lead to the diagnosis of a primary lung tumor. Patients who show symptoms usually display local effects of a tumor in the chest, such as bronchial obstruction, atelectasis, hemoptysis, chest pain, and pleural membrane involvement. Unless the tumor is diagnosed very early, lung cancer has a poor prognosis. Treatment consists of surgery, radiation therapy, and chemotherapy.

Carcinoma of the Larynx

Carcinoma of the larynx is pathologically linked to smoking and chronic alcohol consumption. Ninety percent of cases of laryngeal cancer occur in men; most of those affected are 60 to 70 years of age. Patients show early signs of hoarseness, loss of voice, and dysphagia (difficulty swallowing), and occasionally, respiration becomes impaired. Because of these early symptoms, most laryngeal tumors are discovered in the early stages and can be removed, resulting in a very good prognosis. Surgical treatment consists of a partial or total laryngectomy. With a total laryngectomy, the voice is permanently lost, and a **tracheostomy** is performed. Patients undergoing such procedures need comprehensive preparation and benefit from meeting a laryngectomy survivor, in addition to participating in a support group to deal with postsurgical adjustments.

THE MEDICAL ASSISTANT'S ROLE IN PULMONARY PROCEDURES

Assisting with the Examination

Preparing a patient for a respiratory examination includes having the patient disrobe to the waist and put on a gown with the opening in the front or back, depending on the physician's preference. To assess the status of the respiratory system, the physician uses inspection, palpation, percussion, and auscultation on the anterior thorax, then repeats the process on the posterior and lateral thorax. The medical assistant is responsible for assisting the physician throughout the examination, providing privacy and support for the patient, and performing diagnostic tests as ordered.

Diagnostic Procedures

Tuberculosis

If the physician orders TB screening, the medical assistant administers the Mantoux test (see Chapter 35). An intradermal injection of PPD from a live tuberculin bacillus culture is given to test for the presence of tuberculin antibodies. A positive Mantoux reaction indicates the possibility of active or latent TB or exposure to the disease. Further testing by chest x-ray examination and sputum culture is required for a definitive diagnosis.

Spirometry

PFTs are performed to diagnose a pulmonary abnormality and/or to determine the extent of a pulmonary disease (see Table 46-3). In physicians' offices, lung function measurements are taken with a spirometer (Figure 46-13). Successful spirometry requires consistent methods of preparing the patient, explaining and performing the procedure, and determining the results. Patient preparation begins when the procedure is scheduled. The patient should be instructed not to smoke and to refrain from using bronchodilators and nebulizers for 6 hours before the test.

The medical assistant may be responsible for conducting this test in the ambulatory care setting (Procedure 46-3). Before the patient is scheduled for the procedure, the physician considers certain health problems that would contraindicate the test, such as a pneumothorax, a history of angina or recent myocardial infarction, or the presence of vascular aneurysms. When the patient arrives for testing, the medical assistant should explain the purpose of the test, obtain the patient's vital signs (including height and weight), and explain the maneuver. Spirometry should be described briefly, in simple terms. One statement that works well is, "I am going to have you blow into a machine to see how much air your lungs hold and how fast you can expel it. The test does not hurt, but it does require your cooperation and lots of effort." The patient should be in a comfortable upright position with the legs uncrossed and both feet on the floor. Dentures that fit poorly may be a nuisance and should be

PROCEDURE 46-3

Assist the Physician with Patient Care: Perform Volume Capacity Spirometry Testing

GOAL: *To perform volume capacity testing.*

EQUIPMENT and SUPPLIES

- Scale with height measuring device
- Sphygmomanometer and stethoscope
- Spirometer with recording paper in place
- External spirometric tubing
- Disposable mouthpiece
- Nasal clip if needed
- Biohazardous waste container
- Patient's record

PROCEDURAL STEPS

1. Sanitize your hands and assemble the spirometer.
2. Introduce yourself and confirm the patient's identity. Determine whether the patient needed any special preparation and if so, whether it was done.
   PURPOSE: If special procedures were not followed, the test may have to be rescheduled.
3. Explain the purpose of the test.
   PURPOSE: To help reassure the patient.
4. Measure and record the patient's vital signs, height, and weight.
5. Explain the actual maneuver.
   PURPOSE: The patient must understand the maneuver so that he or she can cooperate fully; this produces the best test results.
6. Make sure the patient is comfortable and either is standing or is sitting with the legs uncrossed and the feet on the floor.
   PURPOSE: Proper positioning ensures maximum lung expansion and accurate test results.
7. Loosen any tight clothing, such as a necktie, bra, or belt.
   PURPOSE: Tight clothing may restrict breathing capacity.
8. Show the patient the proper chin and neck position: the chin should be slightly elevated and the neck slightly extended.
9. Practice the maneuver with the patient before beginning the test.
   PURPOSE: To relieve apprehension and enhance understanding.
10. Place a soft nose clip on the patient's nose if this is part of the facility's procedure.
    PURPOSE: To prevent air from escaping through the nose during exhalation.

11. Instruct the patient to place the mouthpiece in the mouth and to seal the lips around it (Figure 1).

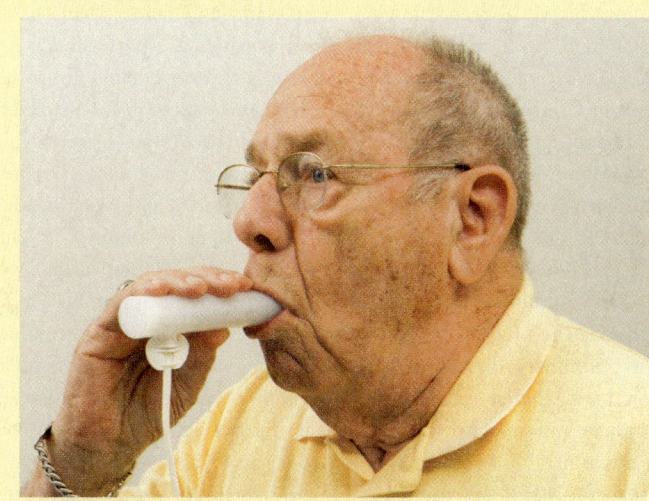

12. Tell the patient to inhale according to instructions.
13. Use active, forceful coaching during exhalation.
    PURPOSE: Coaching improves performance.
14. Provide the patient with feedback after he or she completes the maneuver.
    PURPOSE: Encouragement and explanations of mistakes in the maneuver can help improve the patient's compliance.
15. Carefully observe the patient for indications of vertigo or dyspnea or any other signs of difficulty. If complications occur, stop the test and inform the physician.
16. Continue testing until three acceptable maneuvers have been performed.
17. Place the test results in the patient's medical record for the physician to review.
18. Clean and disinfect the equipment. Discard waste in a biohazardous waste container.
19. Sanitize your hands.
    PURPOSE: To ensure infection control.
20. Record the testing information in the patient's medical record.
    PURPOSE: Procedures that are not recorded are considered not done.

removed if they might interfere. The chin should be slightly elevated and the neck slightly extended. This position should be maintained throughout the forced expiratory procedure.

Give specific instructions in simple, direct terms; for example, "I want you to take the deepest breath possible, put the mouthpiece in your mouth and seal your lips tightly around it, and then blow into the tube as hard and as fast as you can in one long, complete breath." An analogy that sometimes is helpful for further explaining the maneuver is, "It's like blowing out the candles on a birthday cake when they don't all go out; you need to keep blowing the same breath until they do."

Next, demonstrate the maneuver. Many patients forget some or all of the instructions they just received, so demonstration reinforces exactly what to do. Show the patient the proper chin and neck position, how to place the mouthpiece at the right time, and how to blow the air out and continue to blow.

When the demonstration is done, remind the patient of the following points:

- Take as deep a breath as possible.
- Blow air out hard.
- Do not stop blowing until you are told to stop.

Use active and forceful coaching while the patient is performing the maneuver. You may need to raise your voice with some urgency to improve the patient's performance, using such phrases as, "Blow, blow, blow!" "Keep blowing, keep blowing!" and "Don't stop blowing!" After the maneuver, give the patient some feedback on the quality of the test and describe what improvements could be made. Continue to repeat efforts until the patient has completed three acceptable maneuvers. The two best efforts are used to calculate pulmonary function. The physician calculates normal values for each patient based on the individual's age, height, weight, and gender; the test results are documented as a percentage. If the patient's best efforts are greater than 80% of pretest calculated values, pulmonary function is considered normal. Spirometry tests provide the physician information about the impact of obstruction or pulmonary disease on airflow. If the results are less than 60% of the predicted value, the patient may be given bronchodilators and be retested to determine the impact of the inhalant on function.

Test Results. Place the results of the maneuvers with the patient's medical record on the physician's desk when the tests are completed. Many physicians rely on the assistant to include comments pertinent to the testing, such as the patient's condition during the test and compliance with coaching. If any questions arise about the quality of the results, ask the patient to wait while the physician reviews the results. If the patient has delayed taking medication, check with the physician as to when the patient should resume taking it.

CRITICAL THINKING APPLICATION   46-4

Michael is teaching Cinda, a new employee, how to perform a spirometry test. He has summarized the steps of the procedure on a card, which is kept next to the machine for easy reference. Cinda knows nothing about the procedure. What would be the best way for Michael to teach her about the test? What information should he include?

Pulse Oximetry

Pulse oximetry is a noninvasive method of evaluating both the pulse rate and the oxygen saturation of hemoglobin in arterial blood. It identifies the percentage of hemoglobin that is oxygenated in comparison with the total amount of hemoglobin available. Many ambulatory settings use pulse oximeters to assess a patient's oxygenation status in such disorders as pneumonia, bronchitis, emphysema, or asthma (Figure 46-14, *A*).

To perform the procedure, the medical assistant clips a probe on the patient's earlobe or finger (Figure 46-14, *B*). Fingernail polish must be removed before the clip is applied. A beam of infrared light passes through the tissue, and the machine measures the amount of light absorbed by oxygenated hemoglobin, which is displayed on the digital screen as a percentage. At the same time the light measures the patient's pulse rate, which also is shown on the screen. A normal pulse oximetry reading is 95% or higher (meaning 95% of the total available hemoglobin attachments for oxygen are carrying oxygen).

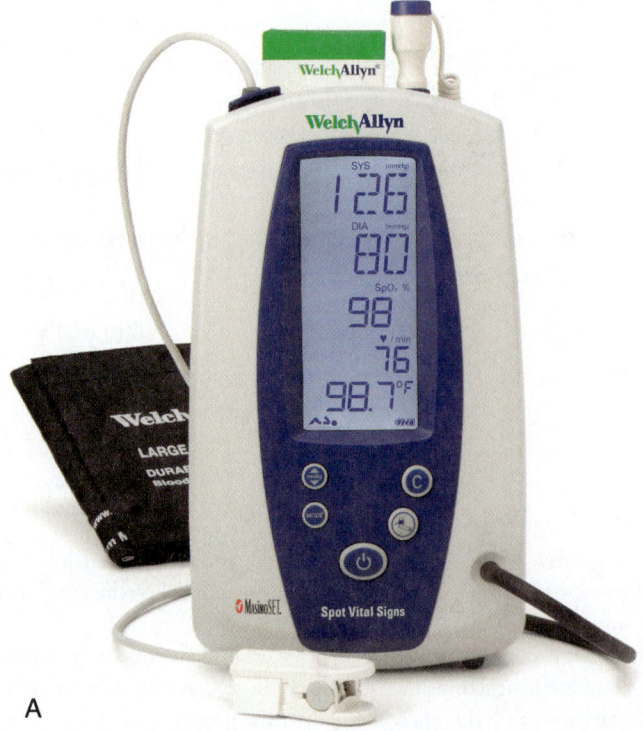

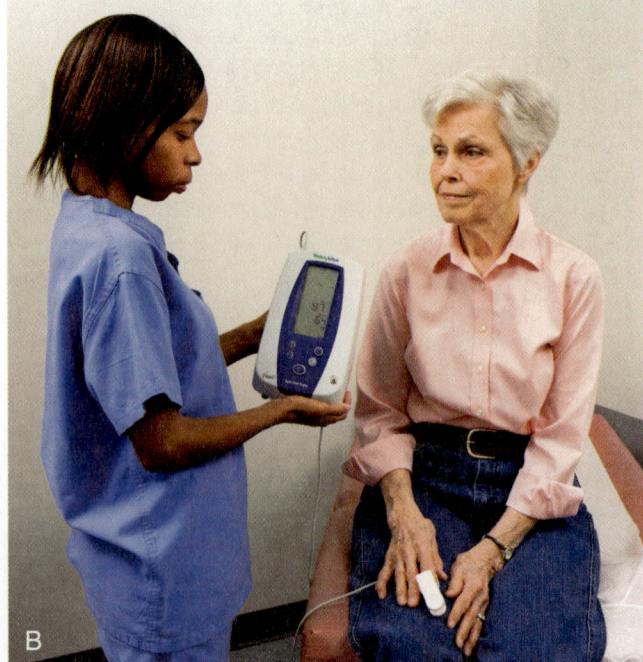

FIGURE 46-14 A, Spot Vital Signs with Masimo SET pulse oximeter. **B,** Pulse oximetry clip. (**A** courtesy Welch Allyn, Skaneateles Falls, N.Y.)

Treatment, such as oxygen or bronchodilator therapies, usually is started when readings are 90% to 92% or lower.

Obtaining Sputum for Culture

A sputum culture is requested when signs and symptoms are accompanied by physical evidence of pneumonia, TB, or other infectious diseases of the lower respiratory tract. The specimen is sent to a laboratory equipped to handle potentially infectious bacteriologic samples. The sample is cultured and incubated, and the pathogenic organism grown in the culture medium is identified. If possible, the physician refrains from starting antibiotic therapy until the sputum has been collected. The sample may also be sent to the laboratory for cytologic analysis, which may indicate a cancerous condition of the lungs or bronchi.

Methods of Collection. In the ambulatory care setting, the primary method of collecting a sputum sample is expectoration (Procedure 46-4). However, sputum also can be collected by tracheal suctioning and bronchoscopy. If the sample is to be collected by expectoration, most physicians have the patient perform the procedure at home with instruction. The medical assistant may be responsible for explaining the procedure to the patient or reinforcing the physician's instructions. The patient should understand that the best time for collecting a sputum specimen is in the morning when the patient first wakes up, before eating or drinking. The patient can rinse out the mouth with water before collecting the sample to reduce contamination from the oropharynx. The sample is collected from sputum coughed up from the lungs, not from saliva, so the patient should be encouraged to cough deeply and forcefully to collect a satisfactory sample. It may help to have the patient take several deep breaths and then cough. At least 1 teaspoon of sputum should be collected in a sterile specimen cup (the patient needs to know how to handle the specimen cup to maintain sterility), which must be returned to the office or laboratory as soon as possible after collection.

PROCEDURE 46-4

Obtain Specimens for Microbiologic Testing: Obtain a Sputum Sample for Culture

GOAL: *To collect a sputum sample while following Standard Precautions.*

EQUIPMENT and SUPPLIES

- Sterile laboratory specimen cup, accurately labeled
- Biohazard laboratory specimen bag with laboratory requisition
- Disposable examination gloves
- Face shield with goggles
- Impervious gown
- Biohazardous waste container
- Cup of water
- Ginger ale or juice
- Patient's record

PROCEDURAL STEPS

1. Assemble the equipment and label the specimen cup.
2. Identify the patient and explain the procedure.
   PURPOSE: An informed patient is more cooperative.
3. Sanitize your hands and put on gloves, a face shield with goggles, and an impervious gown.
   PURPOSE: Standard Precautions must be followed when potentially infectious materials are collected.
4. Have the patient rinse his or her mouth with water.
   PURPOSE: Any food particles in the mouth will contaminate the specimen.
5. Carefully remove the specimen cup lid, taking care not to touch the inside of the lid or the inside of the container, and place it upside down on a side table.
   PURPOSE: To maintain the sterile environment of the specimen cup.
6. Instruct the patient to take three deep breaths and then cough deeply to bring up secretions from the lower respiratory tract.
   PURPOSE: The organisms for culture must be from the lung fields in the lower respiratory tract.

7. Tell the patient to spit directly into the specimen container and to avoid getting any sputum on the exterior of the container. Do not touch the inside of the container during the procedure.
   PURPOSE: Sputum on the exterior of the container is considered hazardous. Prevent contamination of the inside of the container.
8. Place the lid securely on the container, taking care not to touch the inside of the lid, and then place the container in the plastic specimen bag.
   PURPOSE: To maintain the sterility of the container and to minimize the chance of spreading the potentially infectious organisms.
9. Offer the patient a glass of juice or ginger ale.
   PURPOSE: The patient may have a bad taste in the mouth after the test, and this may cause nausea.
10. If another sputum test is ordered for the next morning, instruct the patient when to come to the office or explain how to perform the procedure at home. Remind the person to follow the same instructions for preparation. Stress the importance of maintaining the sterility of the container and of collecting the specimen first thing in the morning.
11. Clean the work area and properly dispose of all supplies.
    PURPOSE: To follow Standard Precautions.
12. Sanitize your hands.
    PURPOSE: To ensure infection control.
13. Process the specimen immediately to ensure optimum test results or refrigerate the specimen until it is sent to the laboratory for analysis.
    PURPOSE: Microorganisms may propagate or die, which can result in a false-positive or false-negative result.
14. Record the procedure in the patient's record.
    PURPOSE: Procedures that are not recorded are considered not done.

If the patient is taking antibiotic medications at the time of the specimen collection, this information should be included on the laboratory slip. If the cough does not produce sputum, chest physiotherapy or nebulization may be ordered by the physician to induce it. In some cases the physician may order sputum collection for three consecutive mornings.

CRITICAL THINKING APPLICATION   46-5

Tomas Garcia, a 68-year-old patient, has a chronic cough, and Dr. Samuelson orders a sputum culture to rule out an infectious disease. Mr. Garcia is supposed to collect the specimens every morning for the next 3 days, but he is very hard of hearing and does not understand English very well. His daughter, who is bilingual, is with him at today's visit. How should Michael relay the information about how to collect the sputum sample? What important details should be reviewed with Mr. Garcia's daughter?

Bronchoscopy

Bronchoscopy typically is performed in an outpatient clinic or a hospital. However, the medical assistant should be familiar with the procedure, because he or she probably will schedule the test, instruct the patient on preparation, and help answer questions from the patient or family.

Bronchoscopy provides an endoscopic view of the larynx, trachea, and bronchi. A pulmonary specialist or a surgeon performs the procedure, using a flexible fiberoptic instrument through which the physician can visualize respiratory tissues and collect biopsy specimens or bronchial washings as needed for cytologic evaluation or culture. Laser therapy to treat endotracheal lesions also is possible through the flexible scope.

The patient should remain on nothing by mouth (NPO) status for 4 to 8 hours before the test to reduce the risk of aspiration. The patient should perform good mouth care before the procedure to reduce the number of bacteria present. Dentures should be removed. The patient receives medication before the procedure to aid relaxation and to dry up oral secretions. The patient should be reassured that the procedure does not interfere with breathing.

Before the instrument is inserted, the physician sprays a topical anesthetic (lidocaine) into the mouth and on the back of the throat to help suppress the gag reflex and reduce any discomfort from passage of the instrument. The tube can be inserted through the nose or mouth, and as it reaches the glottis, more lidocaine is sprayed to control the cough reflex. The physician continues to pass the tube through the bronchi and larger bronchioles, collecting biopsy specimens of any suspicious tissue and obtaining cellular washings if indicated. Because the patient is sedated, it is not an uncomfortable procedure, but the patient may complain of a sore throat and may experience hemoptysis for several hours after the procedure. Biopsy and culture reports usually are available in 2 to 7 days.

CLOSING COMMENTS

Patient Education

It is often said that the greatest fear a person has is the fear of the unknown. Patients frequently worry about tests the physician has ordered. The imagination can create all types of frightening scenarios with even more alarming outcomes. The medical assistant plays a vital role in allaying patients' fears by explaining diagnostic tests, making sure the patient understands how to prepare for the examination and what will be expected of him or her during the procedure. Make sure to give the patient brochures or handouts explaining the procedure that he or she can review at home. Answer all the patient's questions, and consult the physician about questions or concerns you cannot address before the patient leaves the office.

Legal and Ethical Issues

When the respiratory system is mentioned, people generally think of breathing; however, this is only one of the activities of the respiratory system. The cells of the body need a continuous supply of oxygen to maintain life. The respiratory system works with the circulatory system to supply this oxygen and to remove the waste products of metabolism. Too often people take breathing for granted and assume that nothing could possibly happen to their ability to breathe. Sadly, respiratory diseases are a leading cause of death, and that means that people we know and love will suffer from and die of some of the diseases discussed in this chapter.

If the pulmonary test ordered is an invasive test, such as bronchoscopy, make sure a written consent form is obtained from the patient and is in the patient's medical record. If the patient is to see another specialist, a consent form must be signed giving permission to copy and forward patient information to the consultant. If oxygen therapy is ordered, the physician must write a prescription that specifies the amount of oxygen to be given and the type of device to be used for delivery. The physician also may write an order for a respiratory care practitioner to follow up on the patient at home.

SUMMARY OF SCENARIO

Michael has become very adept at performing respiratory diagnostic procedures and treatments for ambulatory patients. He enjoys interacting with this special group of patients and works at maintaining an up-to-date file on educational and resource assistance in the community. Michael especially enjoys the patient education aspect of caring for people with respiratory diseases. Many of these patients have chronic diseases that require long-term care by a physician, and Michael attempts to use available "teaching moments" to reinforce healthy lifestyle habits and confirm patients' understanding of the treatments.

He also continues to take advantage of local meetings of the American Association of Medical Assistants (AAMA) to keep up with recent practice trends, and he took a medical terminology refresher course at the local community college to improve his patient interviewing and charting skills. He is investigating starting a Smoke Stoppers group out of Dr. Samuelson's office to encourage patients to develop a healthier lifestyle, and he emphasizes to his patients who work in the area's coal mines and construction businesses the importance of consistently wearing respirators.

SUMMARY OF LEARNING OBJECTIVES

1. **Define, spell, and pronounce the terms listed in the vocabulary.**
Spelling and pronouncing medical terms correctly bolster the medical assistant's credibility. Knowing the definitions of these terms promotes confidence in communication with patients and co-workers.

2. **Apply critical thinking skills in performing the patient assessment and patient care.**
Completing the Critical Thinking Application exercises throughout the chapter can help the student medical assistant become more adept at critical analysis of real-life situations.

3. **Describe the organs of the respiratory system and their functions.**
The respiratory system exchanges oxygen for carbon dioxide waste through external and internal respiration and helps maintain acid-base balance in the body. It works with the circulatory system to supply body cells with oxygen and remove metabolic wastes. The upper respiratory tract transports air through the nose, pharynx, and larynx. The lower respiratory tract consists of the trachea, bronchial tubes, and lungs.

4. **Explain the process of ventilation.**
Ventilation is the process by which the bronchioles deposit oxygenated air into the alveoli. A network of pulmonary capillaries surround the alveoli, and oxygenated air moves out of the single-celled walls of the alveoli and into the capillaries. Carbon dioxide is forced out of the capillaries, into the alveoli, and then out through the bronchioles. Inspiration is the movement of oxygen from the atmosphere into the alveoli; expiration is the movement of carbon dioxide from the alveoli into the atmosphere.

5. **Implement correct respiratory system terminology when documenting in the medical record.**
Table 46-1 defines common terms related to the respiratory system that should be used when charting a patient's signs and symptoms.

6. **Describe the major diseases of the respiratory system.**
URIs include the common cold, which is caused by a virus; sinusitis, which may be a result of an infection or allergic reaction; allergic rhinitis, which is triggered by multiple factors and causes nasal symptoms; and pneumonia, an infection of the lungs that can be caused by multiple pathogens and that may range from a minor infection to a life-threatening disease.

7. **Explain the diagnosis and treatment of tuberculosis.**
TB, caused by *M. tuberculosis,* can be either active or latent. Individuals with active TB are infectious and show the symptoms of the disease; those with latent TB have activated tubercles because of a weakened immune system. TB is diagnosed by a combination of PPD testing, chest x-ray studies, blood tests, and sputum cultures. It is treated with multiple medications, depending on the type and stage of the disease.

8. **Summarize the disorders associated with chronic obstructive pulmonary disease and their treatments.**
COPD is a group of diseases with the common characteristic of chronic airway obstruction. They include chronic bronchitis, bronchiectasis, asthma, pneumoconiosis, emphysema, and sleep apnea. The mechanism of obstruction may vary, but all these patients are unable to ventilate the lungs freely, which results in ineffective exchange of respiratory gases. Treatments include bronchodilator and corticosteroid inhalers,

evaluation of peak flow values, nebulizer treatments, oxygen, chest therapy, and CPAP machines.

9. **Teach a patient how to use a peak flow meter.**
Procedure 46-1 outlines the procedure for teaching a patient how to obtain an accurate peak flow reading.

10. **Administer a nebulizer treatment.**
Procedure 46-2 outlines the procedure for administering a nebulizer treatment.

11. **Detail patient teaching for the use of a metered-dose inhaler.**
The patient first shakes the container and then places it in the dispenser. The person opens the mouth, and holding the dispenser about 1 inch away, pushes the container down while inhaling deeply. The breath is held for a count of 10, and then the person slowly exhales. If a second dose is required, the patient should wait at least 1 minute before administering it. The patient can use a spacer, if needed, to administer the dose.

12. **Describe the cancers associated with the pulmonary system.**
Lung cancer is the leading cause of cancer-related deaths for both men and women; the lung also is a common site of metastatic tumors. The prognosis is very poor for lung cancer, because early symptoms mimic chronic conditions present in long-term smokers. Carcinoma of the larynx is linked to smoking and chronic alcohol consumption. Most laryngeal tumors are discovered in the early stages and are associated with a good prognosis.

13. **Summarize the medical assistant's role in assisting with pulmonary procedures.**
Preparing a patient for a respiratory examination includes having the patient disrobe to the waist and put on a gown with the opening in the front or back, depending on the physician's preference. The medical assistant is responsible for assisting the physician throughout the examination, providing the privacy and support for the patient, and performing diagnostic tests as ordered.

14. **Distinguish among common diagnostic procedures for the respiratory system.**
Respiratory diagnostic procedures include the Mantoux intradermal test for TB; PFTs, in which a spirometer is used to diagnose pulmonary abnormalities; pulse oximetry, a noninvasive method of evaluating both the pulse rate and the oxygen saturation of hemoglobin in the arterial blood; culturing of expectorated sputum; and bronchoscopy, in which a flexible fiberoptic instrument is used to view the larynx, trachea, and bronchi endoscopically.

15. **Perform a volume capacity spirometry test.**
Procedure 46-3 summarizes the steps in spirometry testing.

16. **Correctly use a pulse oximeter.**
The oximeter probe is placed on the patient's earlobe or finger. An infrared light passes through the tissue, and the machine measures the amount of light absorbed by oxygenated hemoglobin, which is displayed on the digital screen as a percentage. The patient's pulse rate also is displayed.

17. **Collect a sputum sample for culture.**
Procedure 46-4 explains how to collect a sputum sample for culture.

18. **Discuss legal and ethical issues associated with pulmonary medicine.**

    If the pulmonary test ordered is an invasive test, written informed consent must be obtained from the patient and filed in the patient's medical record. If the patient is to see another specialist, a consent form must be signed giving permission to copy and forward patient information to the consultant. If oxygen therapy is ordered, the physician must write a prescription that specifies the amount of oxygen to be given and the type of device to be used for delivery. The physician also may write an order for a respiratory care practitioner to follow up on the patient at home.

CONNECTIONS

Study Guide Connection: Go to the Chapter 46 Study Guide. Read and complete the activities.

Evolve Connection: Go to the Chapter 46 link at *evolve.elsevier.com/kinn* to complete the Chapter Review and Chapter Quiz. Check out the other resources listed for this chapter to make the most of what you have learned from Assisting in Pulmonary Medicine.

47

ASSISTING IN CARDIOLOGY

SCENARIO

Adam Stern, CMA (AAMA), has been working for more than 3 years as a medical assistant in a variety of physicians' offices. Adam recently was hired to work at City Hospital in the cardiology department. His job description includes working in the clinical area of the practice and assisting the attending physicians with patient education and follow-up. Because Adam has never worked for a cardiologist, he is concerned about his knowledge base and competency in cardiac patient care. Part of Adam's responsibilities will be to help evaluate patient education materials about the warning signs of a heart attack, especially the differences between the symptoms seen in men and those seen in women. The practice also is in the process of updating its policy and procedures manual, and Adam has been asked to create scenarios for telephone screening of patients who call in with symptoms of chest pain.

While studying this chapter, think about the following questions:

- Why is it important that Adam understand the normal anatomy and physiology of the cardiovascular system if he is going to work in a cardiologist's practice?
- What are some of the common diseases and disorders of the cardiovascular system with which Adam should be familiar?
- What are the common cardiovascular diagnostic procedures that Adam should be prepared to discuss and explain to patients?
- How should he go about developing scenarios for the management of telephone inquiries based on the physicians' preferences?

LEARNING OBJECTIVES

1. Define, spell, and pronounce the terms listed in the vocabulary.
2. Apply critical thinking skills in performing the patient assessment and patient care.
3. Illustrate the anatomy and physiology of the heart and its significant structures.
4. Summarize risk factors for the development of heart disease.
5. Describe the signs, symptoms, and medical procedures used in the diagnosis and treatment of coronary artery disease and myocardial infarction.
6. Explain the signs and symptoms of myocardial infarction in women.
7. Compare and contrast the treatment protocols for hypertension.
8. Outline the causes and results of congestive heart failure.
9. Summarize the effects of inflammation and valvular disorders on cardiac function.
10. Describe the anatomy and physiology of the vascular system.
11. Differentiate among the various types of shock.
12. Summarize the characteristics of common vascular disorders.
13. Outline typical cardiovascular diagnostic procedures.
14. Describe patient education topics for cardiovascular patients.

VOCABULARY

chordae tendineae (kor'-duh/ten'y-din-uh) The tendons that anchor the cusps of the heart valves to the papillary muscles of the myocardium, preventing valvular prolapse.

intermittent claudication Recurring cramping in the calves caused by poor circulation of blood to the muscles of the lower leg.

ischemia (is-ke'-mia) A decreased supply of oxygenated blood to an area or body part.

Marfan syndrome An inherited condition characterized by elongation of the bones, joint hypermobility, abnormalities of the eyes, and the development of an aortic aneurysm.

scleroderma (skluh-rah-der'-muh) An autoimmune disorder that affects the blood vessels and connective tissue, causing fibrous degeneration of the major organs.

vegetations Abnormal growth of tissue surrounding a valve consisting of fibrin, platelets, and bacteria.

Cardiac disease, in the past, was frequently seen in men but seldom in women. That has changed, and today the most common cause of illness and death, regardless of gender, is cardiovascular disease. Medical assistants in all specialties often care for patients with heart disorders. Seldom does the cardiologist discover the heart problem. Most patients who see this specialist already have been diagnosed with a suspected heart disorder and were referred to the cardiologist for verification of the initial diagnosis and specialized treatment.

Because of the overwhelming number of people with cardiovascular problems, all medical assistants must understand the cardiovascular system, be able to recognize early symptoms of potential disorders, perform basic screening tests when ordered by the physician, and assist the physician in the examination of the heart and blood vessels.

ANATOMY AND PHYSIOLOGY OF THE HEART

The heart is a hollow, muscular organ situated in the thoracic cavity in the mediastinal region, between the right and left pleural spaces. It weighs about 9 ounces and is about the size of a fist; approximately two thirds of it is located to the left of the sternum (Figure 47-1). The heart is a pump that provides the force needed to push blood through all the arteries of the body; the blood circulates a continuous supply of oxygen and nutrients to the cells and picks up the metabolic waste products from them. If deprived of these vital functions, the cells die. At the same time, the heart pushes deoxygenated blood through the pulmonary artery to the lungs for oxygen saturation and receives oxygenated blood back through the pulmonary veins into the left side of the heart. The average adult heart pumps about 5 L of blood every minute. If the heart loses its pumping action for even a few brief minutes, death or permanent damage can result.

Layers of the Heart

The heart is enclosed in a double-membrane sac called the *pericardium*. The outer layer of the pericardial sac, the parietal pericardium, is a tough membrane that connects the heart to the diaphragm and serves as a physical barrier to protect the heart against infection or inflammation from the lungs or pleural space. The inner layer, the visceral pericardium or epicardium, forms the first layer of the heart. Between the two membranes is a small space, the pericardial cavity, which contains about 30 mL of pericardial fluid; this fluid lubricates the internal surfaces of the pericardial membranes, enabling them to slide across each other during heart contractions. The middle layer of the heart, the myocardium, is the muscle layer that constitutes the largest percentage of the heart wall. Contractions of this muscle layer force the blood from the heart into the vessels. The inner layer

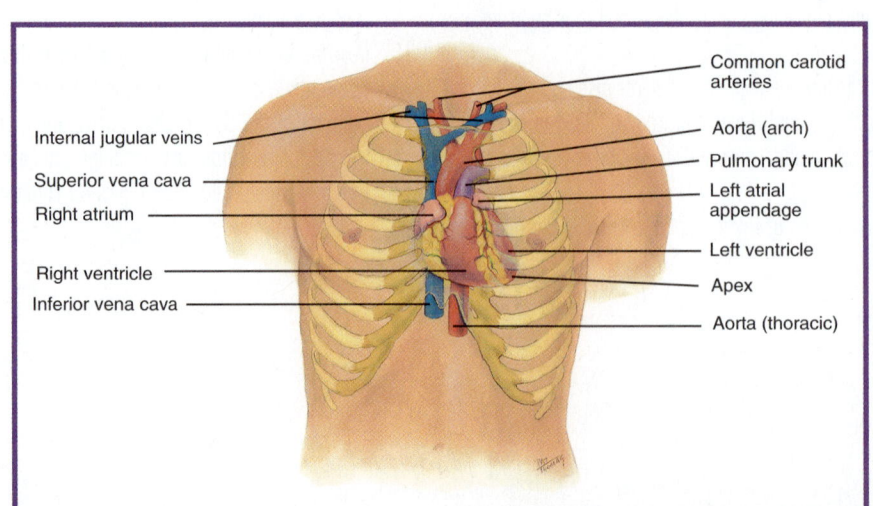

FIGURE 47-1 Location of the heart in the thoracic cavity. (From Applegate EJ: *The anatomy and physiology learning system,* ed 4, St Louis, 2010, Saunders.)

of the heart, the endocardium, includes the heart valves that separate the chambers of the heart and provide a means of blocking the flow of blood from major blood vessels entering and exiting the heart (Figure 47-2).

Heart Chambers and Arteries

The heart is divided into four chambers (Figure 47-3). The atria, the top chambers, receive blood, and the ventricles, the bottom chambers, pump the blood out. The blood flow through the heart begins in the right atrium, which receives deoxygenated blood from the inferior and superior venae cavae. The atria contract, and blood passes through the tricuspid valve into the right ventricle; the

ventricles contract, and blood passes from the right ventricle to the lungs via the pulmonary artery (the only artery in the body that contains deoxygenated blood). Oxygenation occurs in the alveoli of the lungs, and the now oxygenated blood returns to the left atria through the pulmonary veins (the only veins in the body that carry oxygen-rich blood). The atria contract, and blood passes through the mitral (bicuspid) valve into the left ventricle; the ventricles contract, and oxygen-rich blood is sent out to the body through the aorta (the largest artery in the body).

The myocardium requires a continuous supply of oxygen and nutrients, which are delivered through two coronary arteries that branch off the aorta above the aortic valve (Figure 47-4). The right coronary artery nourishes the anterior and posterior myocardium on the right side of the heart, and the left coronary artery does the same on the left side. The left coronary artery quickly divides and forms the left anterior descending artery and the left circumflex artery. Smaller branches of the coronary arteries feed the myocardium and the endocardium. Any interference in blood flow in any of the coronary vessels alters the action of the heart.

Heart Conduction

A sophisticated electrical conduction system operated by specialized cells located at various sites in the myocardium stimulates contractions. These muscle contractions move blood through the chambers of the heart and out through the aorta to the rest of the body. Each electrical impulse passes through the heart muscle in a twisting, spiral motion. These rhythmic waves stimulate the cardiac cells to beat, which causes the heart to contract.

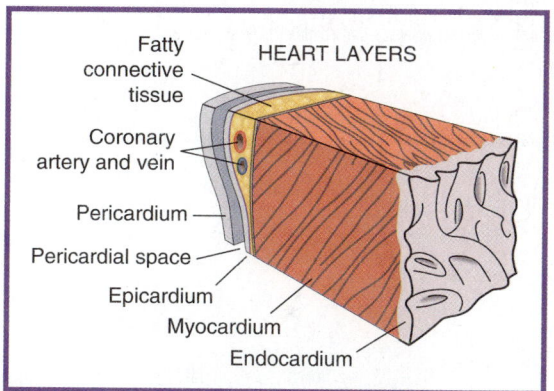

FIGURE 47-2 Layers of the heart. (From Damjanov I: *Pathology for the health-related professions,* ed 4, St Louis, 2012, Saunders.)

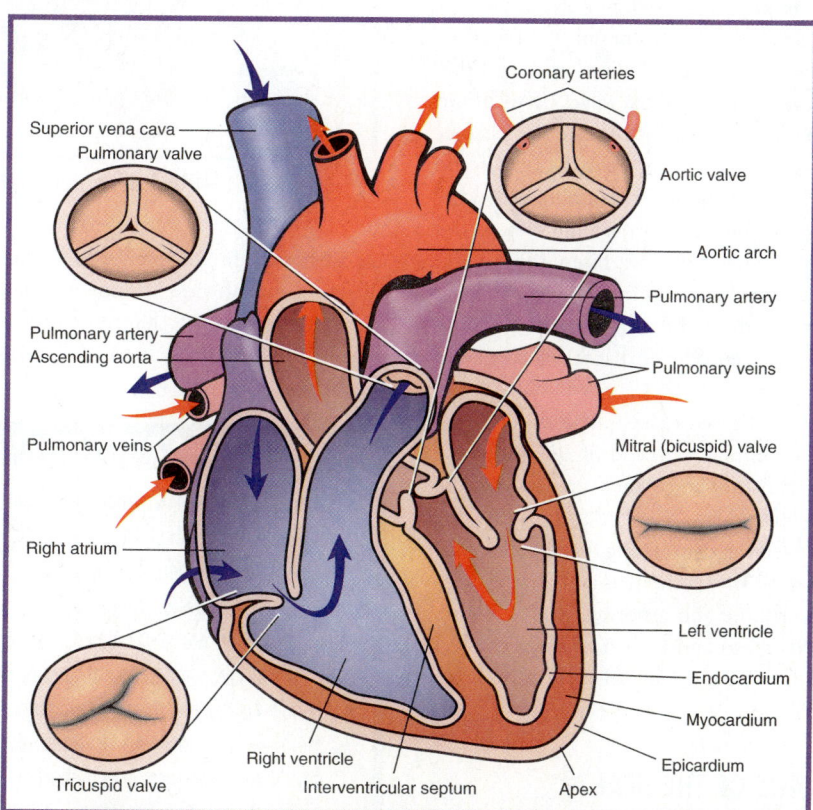

FIGURE 47-3 Chambers of the heart. (From Damjanov I: *Pathology for the health-related professions,* ed 4, St Louis, 2012, Saunders.)

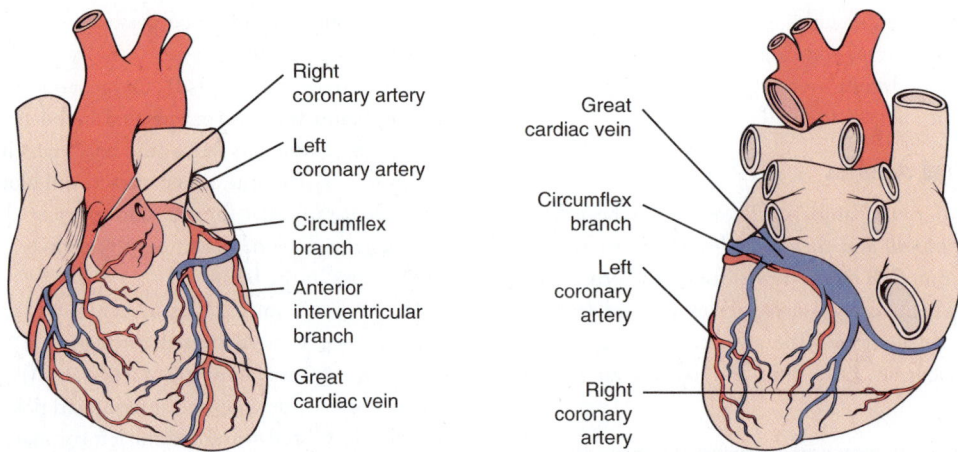

FIGURE 47-4 Coronary arteries. (From Frazier MS, Drzymkowski JW: *Essentials of human diseases and conditions,* ed 5, St Louis, 2013, Saunders.)

The cardiac impulse originates in specialized muscle tissue called the *sinoatrial (SA) node.* The SA node rhythmically initiates impulses 70 to 80 times a minute; because it creates the basic rhythm, it is the pacemaker of the heart. It is located in the posterior, superior wall of the right atrium, at the junction of the superior vena cava and the atrium and just above the tricuspid valve. When the SA node discharges its rhythm pattern into the myocardium, it passes across both atria, resulting in atrial contraction and forcing blood through the valves and into the ventricles. The wave then passes through a second area of specialized muscle tissue on the septal wall between the right atrium and right ventricle, called the *atrioventricular (AV) node.* The AV node holds the impulse for a fraction of a second to prevent inappropriately high atrial rates and to permit the blood to empty from the atria through the tricuspid and mitral valves. At this moment the **chordae tendineae** tightly close the valves between the atria and the ventricles. The AV node then releases the charge, sending it down through the bundle of His, which is located in the septum between the right and left ventricles. This bundle is divided into two main branches: the right bundle, on the right side of the septum, and the left bundle, on the left side. From the bundle branches, transmission of the cardiac wave continues through a mass of cardiac muscle fibers known as the *Purkinje fibers.* The Purkinje fibers totally encase both ventricles, and the cardiac wave causes the ventricles to contract (Figure 47-5).

Contraction of the atria and the ventricles is also called *depolarization.* After the chambers contract, a period of electric recovery occurs *(repolarization),* and the heart then returns to the resting phase *(polarization),* which starts the entire cycle again. The normal cardiac cycle consists of atrial contraction, ventricular contraction, recovery, and heart rest. This cycle maintains the average range of 60 to 100 beats per minute and a normal heart rhythm. It is this electrical force that is traced and evaluated when an electrocardiogram (ECG) is done. (Chapter 49 discusses ECGs in more detail.)

DISEASES AND DISORDERS OF THE HEART

Many diseases and disorders affect the heart and its blood vessels. Disorders that occur when the rhythm of the heart becomes irregular

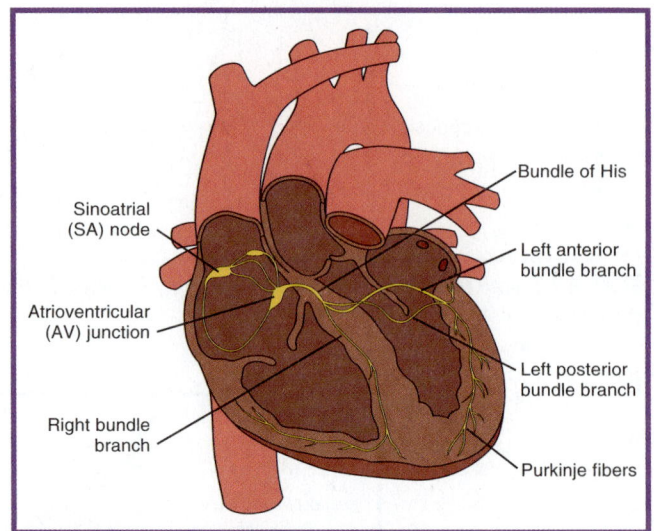

FIGURE 47-5 Cardiac conduction system.

are addressed in Chapter 49. Cardiac disease has multiple risk factors; some of these cannot be changed, and others people can change or seek to have treated. The more risk factors a person has, the greater his or her risk of developing cardiovascular disease.

RISK FACTORS FOR HEART DISEASE

Risk Factors That Cannot Be Changed

- *Advancing age:* Most people who die of heart disease are age 65 or older; older women are more likely to die of myocardial infarctions (MIs) than are older men.
- *Gender:* Men are at greater risk of MIs and experience heart attacks earlier in life; women are at greater risk after menopause.
- *Family history and race:* The children of parents with heart disease are more likely to develop it; African-Americans are at greater risk of developing hypertension and heart disease associated with it; Mexican-Americans, Native Americans, native Hawaiians, and some Asian-Americans also are at greater risk.

Lifestyle Risk Factors That Can Be Modified or Treated

- *Smoking:* Male smokers develop heart disease three times more often than women; female smokers develop heart disease six times more often than those who have never smoked. Smoking is associated with sudden cardiac death. Exposure to secondhand smoke also increases the risk.
- *High blood cholesterol:* The risk of heart disease rises with rising blood cholesterol levels.
- *Hypertension:* Hypertension increases the amount of work the heart must do to circulate blood throughout the body.
- *Sedentary lifestyle:* Regular exercise helps prevent cardiovascular disease.
- *Obesity and overweight:* Excess weight, especially increased body fat at the waist, is associated with an increased risk of heart disease and stroke; losing as little as 10 pounds can lower the risk.
- *Diabetes mellitus:* The risk of heart disease is even greater if blood glucose levels are not controlled; almost 75% of people with diabetes die of some form of heart or blood vessel disease.

From the American Heart Association. Accessed 7/10/2012. Available at www.heart.org/HEARTORG/Conditions/HeartAttack/UnderstandYourRiskofHeartAttack/Understand-Your-Risk-of-Heart-Attack_UCM_002040_Article.jsp.

Coronary Artery Disease and Myocardial Infarction

Coronary artery disease (CAD) causes more than 1 million deaths in the United States every year. In CAD, the formation of atherosclerotic plaques narrows the arteries supplying the myocardium. Atherosclerotic plaque buildup is primarily related to cholesterol blood levels (see Chapter 30, Table 30-2). Cholesterol blood testing is explained in Chapter 54. Medications that may be prescribed to treat hypercholesterolemia are described in Table 47-1. An atherosclerotic plaque originates at the site of a chronic injury to the endothelial lining of the artery caused by risk factors associated with heart disease (e.g., smoking or hypertension). Platelets attach to the site of the endothelial injury, and lipids continue to accumulate. Eventually an atheroma forms, which is made up of a tough collagen shell covering a fatty center that extends out into the lumen of the vessel, restricting blood flow past the plaque. Inflammation at the site attracts platelets to the surface of the atheroma, resulting in the formation of a clot (thrombus) that can completely occlude the lumen of the vessel, depriving the myocardium of an adequate nutritious blood supply (Figure 47-6). The cardinal symptom of myocardial **ischemia** is angina pectoris. Anginal chest pain is pain behind the sternum that is precipitated by exertion but that can be relieved either by rest or by sublingual nitroglycerin.

Patients may be asymptomatic until the disease becomes fully developed. The first symptom may be angina, followed by pressure or fullness in the chest, syncope, shortness of breath, edema, unexplained coughing spells, and fatigue. A patient reporting any of these symptoms should be seen by the physician immediately.

In recent years the rate of heart disease has declined in men but not in women. Traditional risk factors negatively affect both genders; however, women are at greater risk if they have metabolic syndrome (a combination of hypertension, elevated insulin levels, excess body fat around the waist, and high blood cholesterol levels); if they have

TABLE 47-1 Prescription Medications to Lower Blood Cholesterol Levels

CLASSIFICATION	ACTION	SIDE EFFECTS AND CAUTIONS
Statins Altoprev (lovastatin) Crestor (rosuvastatin) Lescol (fluvastatin) Lipitor (atorvastatin) Mevacor (lovastatin) Pravachol (pravastatin) Zocor (simvastatin)	Lower LDL and triglycerides; slightly increase HDL	Constipation, nausea, diarrhea, stomach pain, cramps, muscle soreness, pain and weakness; possible interaction with grapefruit juice
Bile acid–binding resins Colestid (colestipol) Questran (cholestyramine sucrose) Welchol (colesevelam)	Lower LDL	Constipation, bloating, nausea, gas; may increase triglycerides
Cholesterol absorption inhibitors Zetia (ezetimibe)	Lower LDL; slightly decrease triglycerides; slightly increase HDL	Fatigue, gas, constipation, abdominal pain, cramps, muscle soreness; possible interaction with grapefruit juice
Fibrates Lofibra (fenofibrate) Lopid (gemfibrozil) TriCor (fenofibrate)	Decrease triglycerides; increase HDL	Nausea, stomach pain, gallstones
Combination statin and niacin Advicor (niacin-lovastatin)	Decrease LDL and triglycerides; increase HDL	Facial and neck flushing, dizziness, heart palpitations, shortness of breath, sweating, chills; possible interaction with grapefruit juice

HDL, High-density lipoprotein; *LDL,* low-density lipoprotein.

increased levels of stress and/or depression; if they smoke (female smokers are at much greater risk than male smokers); and if they have reduced estrogen production before menopause. The difference in female risks and symptoms is associated with the method of plaque buildup in women; the plaque tends to develop as an evenly spread layer along the entire lumen of the blood vessels rather than as a localized plaque buildup, as is seen in men. Women with heart disease typically experience this diffuse atheroma buildup in smaller vessels, which causes more subtle symptoms than the crushing chest pain associated with classic myocardial infarctions (MIs).

The major concern in heart disease is the lack of blood to the myocardium, which occurs when a vessel becomes totally blocked. Ischemia over a prolonged period leads to necrosis (death) of a

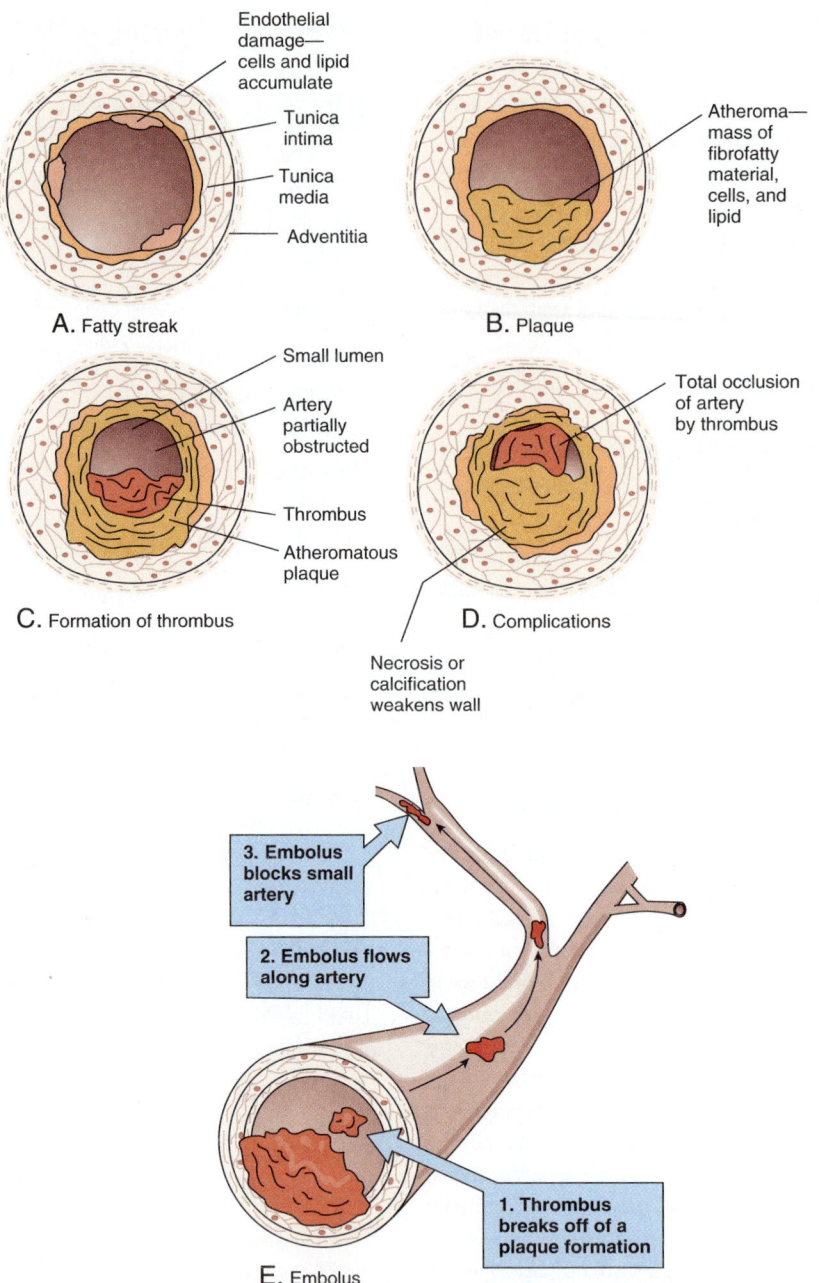

FIGURE 47-6 Development of an atheroma, leading to arterial occlusion. (From Gould BA: *Pathophysiology for the health professions,* ed 3, Philadelphia, 2002, WB Saunders.)

portion of the myocardium, resulting in an MI, or heart attack. Symptoms of an MI are similar to those of angina; however, an MI is identified by pain that lasts longer than 30 minutes and is not relieved by rest or nitroglycerin tablets. An MI is a life-threatening event; intervention must begin within the first hour, or death may occur.

CRITICAL THINKING APPLICATION   47-1

A patient who is scheduled for an appointment in 2 days calls the office and reports that she is not feeling well. She complains that she has a feeling of fullness in the chest, her arms ache, and she is very tired. Although this patient does not have a history of myocardial infarction, what should Adam do?

Diagnostic and Therapeutic Procedures

An MI is diagnosed by ECG changes and elevated cardiac enzymes. The blood test most often ordered to confirm myocardial damage is the creatine kinase (CK) level. CK levels begin to increase approximately 6 hours after the start of a heart attack and reach their peak in about 18 hours; they return to normal in 24 to 36 hours. The more severe the cardiac damage, the longer it takes for CK levels to peak and then return to normal. Determination of the troponin levels is a more sensitive blood test that can detect minor myocardial damage not evident with CK levels. Troponins increase in the bloodstream within 4 to 6 hours after the initial myocardial damage and peak in 10 to 24 hours. In the case of minor myocardial damage, troponin levels remain elevated up to 10 to 14 days, allowing for later diagnosis of the event. Patients diagnosed with an MI typically are hospitalized immediately, started on oxygen, and continuously monitored by ECG. Additional diagnostic procedures, such as an echocardiogram and heart catheterization, are discussed later in this chapter.

Medical treatment includes the use of thrombolytic medications, such as alteplase (Activase) and reteplase (Retavase), to dissolve coronary artery blockage and prevent permanent myocardial damage. To be most effective, this treatment must be started within 3 hours of the episode; however, it is still helpful if administered within 12 hours of initial symptoms. This timetable makes it extremely important that patients be diagnosed and treated as soon as possible. Thrombolytic medications are administered intravenously (IV) along with heparin to prevent clots that are being dissolved from reforming. Aspirin also is used to prevent the formation of blood clots in affected blood vessels. Additional pharmaceutical treatment includes the use of nitroglycerin to dilate the coronary arteries so that more blood can be delivered to the myocardium; beta blockers (atenolol [Tenormin], metoprolol [Lopressor], or propranolol [Inderal]) to slow the heart rate and lower blood pressure; anticoagulants (warfarin [Coumadin]) for 3 to 6 months to prevent thrombus formation; and anticholesterol agents to lower blood cholesterol levels and prevent subsequent formation of atherosclerotic plaques.

When the coronary arteries that supply blood to the myocardium are blocked, or occluded, either percutaneous transluminal coronary angioplasty (PTCA) or coronary artery bypass grafting (CABG) may be indicated. (These surgical procedures are discussed later in this chapter.)

After discharge from the hospital, patients with CAD that has resulted in an MI face multiple lifestyle changes to prevent another episode. Recommendations include no smoking; regular light exercise, such as walking 30 minutes a day, 5 days a week; a diet low in salt, fat, and cholesterol; maintaining a healthy weight; controlling hypertension; reducing stress; and limiting alcohol intake to one or two drinks a day. The medical assistant should be prepared to provide encouragement and to reinforce the importance of lifestyle changes to prevent future heart problems. If ordered by the physician, professional referrals to a cardiac rehabilitation program and dietitian can also be helpful.

SIGNS AND SYMPTOMS OF MYOCARDIAL INFARCTION IN WOMEN

In addition to angina, the signs and symptoms of a heart attack in women may start weeks before the actual cardiac injury and could include the following:

- Abdominal, neck, shoulder, or upper back pain
- Jaw pain
- Shortness of breath
- Vertigo (dizziness)
- Sweating
- Indigestion or nausea and vomiting
- Extreme fatigue
- Aching in both arms

CRITICAL THINKING APPLICATION   47-2

Adam receives a telephone call from a patient who complains of nausea and difficulty taking a deep breath and who says that he feels as if he is going to faint. What questions should Adam ask to determine the seriousness of the problem?

Hypertensive Heart Disease

Chronic elevated blood pressure can result in left ventricular hypertrophy (enlargement), angina, MI, or heart failure. Hypertension also is a major cause of stroke and nephropathy (kidney disease). Some of the risk factors for hypertension include a family history of hypertension or stroke, hypercholesterolemia (high blood cholesterol), smoking, high sodium intake, diabetes, excessive alcohol intake, sedentary lifestyle, obesity, aging, prolonged stress, and race (African-Americans have a higher incidence than Caucasians). Hypertension has an insidious onset, and the patient shows few, if any, signs and symptoms until permanent damage has occurred. Initial symptoms may include general malaise and headache; epistaxis (nosebleed), vertigo, nausea, or syncope can occur with prolonged hypertension.

The two types of hypertension are primary hypertension and secondary hypertension. Secondary hypertension occurs because of a disease process in another body system, such as renal disease or an endocrine disorder. Before secondary hypertension can be properly treated, the underlying disease process must be resolved.

Primary, or essential, hypertension is idiopathic (of unknown cause) and is diagnosed if the patient's blood pressure is persistently higher than 119 mm Hg systolic and/or 79 mm Hg diastolic at two or more office visits over several weeks or months. If the medical assistant first notes that a patient's blood pressure is elevated, the pressure should be checked in both arms with the patient seated and after the patient has been standing for at least 2 minutes with a cuff that is the proper size for the patient's arm. If the pressure readings are different, the physician uses the higher value for diagnostic purposes. The patient's blood pressures should be checked again after at least 2 minutes. All of these readings must be documented in the patient's record. Some patients have "white coat hypertension," which appears only when they visit the physician. If the patient has a history of this problem, have him or her lie down on the examination table and rest for a few minutes before the blood pressure is taken; this may help in obtaining a more accurate reading (Table 47-2).

The medical assistant can play an important role in antihypertensive therapy by teaching the patient how to take his or her own blood pressure at home, providing literature that reinforces the necessity of monitoring the blood pressure, and helping the patient understand that this condition cannot be cured but can be controlled for the rest of his or her life. Continued encouragement and support are needed, because compliance with the treatment regimen is difficult for a patient who is not showing any symptoms of disease. Table 47-3 summarizes some of the medications that may be prescribed to manage hypertension. The goal of treatment is to maintain blood pressure below 140/90 mm Hg or below 130/80 mm Hg in adults with diabetes or chronic kidney disease.

TABLE 47-2 Stages and Treatment of Hypertension

BLOOD PRESSURE	TREATMENT
Prehypertension 120 to 139/80 to 89 mm Hg	Lifestyle modification (reduced sodium, low-fat diet; regular aerobic activity; moderate alcohol intake; smoking cessation; weight loss; stress reduction) Drug therapy for patients with diabetes mellitus or chronic kidney disease
Stage 1 hypertension 140 to 159/90 to 99 mm Hg	Consider coexisting conditions Thiazide-type diuretics (e.g., furosemide [Lasix] or hydrochlorothiazide plus triamterene [Dyazide]) for most patients
Stage 2 hypertension 160/100 mm Hg	Consider coexisting conditions Two-drug combination for most patients

Recommendations from the Joint National Committee on Prevention, Detection, Evaluation, and Treatment of High Blood Pressure. Accessed February 14, 2012. Available at www.nhlbi.nih.gov/health/health-topics/topics/hbp/.

TELEPHONE SCREENING FOR CHEST PAIN

The medical assistant should activate emergency medical services if the patient reports any of the following:

- Current chest pain that is crushing, pressing, or radiating to the arms, upper back, or jaw
- Sweating, difficulty breathing, nausea, indigestion, or dizziness
- Any of these symptoms along with a history of coronary artery disease, myocardial infarction, or angina
- A change in the pattern of the angina
- Chest pain that occurs when resting or with minimum exertion

CRITICAL THINKING APPLICATION   47-3

Essential hypertension is a common problem for patients seen in the cardiology department where Adam works. What could Adam do to help patients with primary hypertension? What informational materials or community resources would be helpful in gaining patient compliance with treatment?

Congestive Heart Failure

Congestive heart failure (CHF) occurs when the myocardium is unable to pump an adequate amount of blood to meet the body's needs. Although the onset can be acute, the condition typically develops over time because of weakness in the left ventricle as a result of chronic hypertension, MI of the ventricular wall, valvular heart disease, or pulmonary complications. Typically, heart failure initially occurs on one side of the heart and then on the other side. Left-sided heart failure usually results from essential hypertension or left ventricular disease, whereas right-sided heart failure can develop as a result of lung disease. Right-sided heart failure that occurs because of pulmonary hypertension associated with chronic obstructive pulmonary disease (COPD) is called *cor pulmonale*.

TABLE 47-3 Medications Used to Treat Hypertension

CLASSIFICATION	ACTION	TREATMENT PROTOCOL
Thiazide diuretics (Hydrodiuril, Lasix, Lozol, Aldactone)	Act on kidneys to increase elimination of sodium and water to reduce blood volume	First drug of choice in hypertensive treatment; enhance the action of other blood pressure (BP) medications; used in patients with diabetes and those with chronic kidney disease with prehypertension
Beta blockers (Tenormin, Sectral, Lopressor, Ziac, Inderal)	Reduce the heart rate and cardiac output; reduce the workload of the heart and open blood vessels	May be used with a diuretic for stage 1 and stage 2 hypertension
Angiotensin-converting enzyme (ACE) inhibitors (Lotensin, Capoten, Vasotec, Monopril, Prinivil, Zestril)	Cause vasodilation and reduced vascular resistance; reduce the workload of the heart	May be used with a diuretic for stage 1 and stage 2 hypertension; also may be used for hypertension in patients with coronary artery disease, heart failure, or kidney failure
Angiotensin II receptor blockers (Cozaar, Atacand, Avapro, Diovan)	Block the action of chemicals that cause vasoconstriction	May be used with a diuretic for stage 1 and stage 2 hypertension; also may be used for hypertension in patients with coronary artery disease, heart failure, or kidney failure
Calcium channel blockers (Norvasc, Lotrel, Cardizem, Plendil, Procardia, Vascor)	Interrupt the movement of calcium into the heart and vessel cells, causing vasodilation	May be used with a diuretic for stage 1 and stage 2 hypertension; also used to treat angina and/or some arrhythmias

In left-sided heart failure, the left ventricle cannot empty completely, and blood backs up in the left atria and ultimately the lungs, resulting in pulmonary edema, or the collection of fluid in the lungs. Signs and symptoms include dyspnea, orthopnea, nonproductive cough, rales, and tachycardia. In right-sided heart failure, the right ventricle cannot maintain complete output, and blood backs up in the right atrium; this prevents complete emptying of the vena cava, resulting in systemic edema, especially in the legs and feet. Both types of heart failure cause fatigue, weakness, exercise intolerance, dyspnea, and sensitivity to cold temperatures.

Nonpharmaceutical treatment for CHF includes limiting physical activity so that the heart does not have to work so hard, restricting salt, not smoking, reducing stress, and controlling weight. Patient education for an individual with CHF must stress the importance of monitoring weight gain, because a sudden increase in weight may indicate fluid retention. Patients should weigh themselves once or twice a week and report any gain of more than 3 pounds to the physician.

Drug therapy for CHF begins with diuretics to treat dyspnea and orthopnea and control edema. Other medications may include an angiotensin-converting enzyme (ACE) inhibitor, a type of vasodilator that widens blood vessels to lower blood pressure and reduce the workload of the heart. Examples of ACE inhibitors include enalapril (Vasotec), lisinopril (Prinivil, Zestril) and captopril (Capoten). Digoxin often is prescribed to increase the strength of myocardial contractions, and beta blockers (carvedilol [Coreg] and metoprolol [Lopressor]) are used to slow the heart rate and improve heart function. Because potassium loss is a common side effect of diuretics and digitalis, patients may also be prescribed a potassium (KCl) supplement. Routine monitoring of serum electrolytes is ordered to determine the need for a potassium supplement so that potential complications can be prevented.

CRITICAL THINKING APPLICATION 47-4

Kate Glasgow, a 76-year-old patient with a history of CHF, is in the office today for a checkup. She does not understand why she must stop using salt and start weighing herself regularly at home. What can Adam do to help this patient understand the importance of her treatment regimen?

Orthostatic Hypotension

Orthostatic, or postural, hypotension is diagnosed if the patient experiences a drop in blood pressure when standing, especially when quickly changing from a prone or seated position to an upright one. When we stand, our blood pressure quickly adapts to the pull of gravity by reflexively increasing the heart rate and constricting systemic arterioles. In a patient with orthostatic hypotension, the blood pressure adjusts sluggishly or not at all to rapid changes in position. An acute episode of orthostatic hypotension may be caused by blood pooling in the lower extremities, a reaction to antihypertensive or antidepressant medication, or prolonged immobility. This is a common problem in elderly people and may contribute significantly to falls and related injuries. Patients need to be evaluated for secondary causes and encouraged to adjust from a prone position by sitting on the side of the bed for a bit before standing.

To evaluate orthostatic hypotension, the physician may ask the medical assistant to check the patient's blood pressure while the person is seated, leave the cuff in place, then have the patient stand and immediately check the blood pressure again. Both blood pressure readings should be recorded in the patient's chart for the physician to evaluate. Include in your note any patient complaints after standing, including dizziness or a feeling of lightheadedness.

Inflammations and Valvular Disorders

Rheumatic Heart Disease

Rheumatic heart disease develops because of an unusual immune reaction that occurs within 5 weeks after an untreated beta-hemolytic streptococcal infection. The infection typically starts as "strep" throat or an upper respiratory infection but progresses to the creation of antibodies that react with collagen to cause inflammation in the joints, skin, brain, and heart. During a first rheumatic fever attack, about half of those affected develop heart inflammation, but most have a complete recovery. However, in some people the heart valves are damaged and scars form. The disease process in the heart can involve all layers of heart tissue.

Pericarditis, or inflammation of the outer layer of the heart, causes reduced cardiac activity and pericardial effusion (the collection of blood or fluid in the pericardium). Myocarditis, or inflammation of the muscular lining of the heart, usually is self-limiting but may lead to acute heart failure because of weakening of the myocardial wall. Endocarditis, or inflammation of the inner lining of the heart and the heart valves, is the most common heart complication. **Vegetations** form along the outer edges of the valve cusps, causing scarring and stenosis and preventing the damaged heart valve from closing or opening completely. The valvular damage may be asymptomatic at first but eventually can cause serious problems. The mitral valve is affected most frequently, which impairs the ability of the left ventricle to function normally.

Treatment includes the use of antibiotics (penicillin) to eliminate the streptococcal infection completely and antiinflammatory agents for the inflammatory reaction. In 2007 the American Heart Association changed its guidelines regarding the prophylactic use of antibiotics before a dental or some other invasive procedure. No research links dental, gastrointestinal, or genitourinary tract procedures with the development of endocarditis. Therefore, prophylactic use of antibiotics now is recommended only for patients with the highest risk of complications from endocarditis, such as those with artificial heart valves, or certain types of congenital heart disease.

Valvular Disorders

Disorders of the valves of the heart may be caused by a congenital defect or an infection such as endocarditis. Two specific problems can occur with valve disease. The valve can be stenosed, or hardened, which restricts the forward flow of blood, or it can be incompetent, which means that it does not close completely, so blood can leak backward, or regurgitate. The most common valve defect is mitral valve prolapse (MVP), an incompetence in the mitral valve caused by a congenital defect or vegetation and scarring from endocarditis.

Valve disorders ultimately can lead to ventricular hypertrophy and cardiomegaly (enlargement of the heart). Severely damaged valves or serious congenital defects may necessitate surgical replacement of the affected valve.

BLOOD VESSELS

Blood vessels are divided into two systems that begin and end with the heart (Figure 47-7). The pulmonary system carries deoxygenated blood from the right ventricle to the lungs and oxygenated blood back to the left atrium. The systemic system carries blood from the left ventricle throughout the entire body and back to the right atrium. The vessels are classified according to their structure and function: *arteries* carry oxygenated blood away from the heart; *capillaries* are the microscopic vessels responsible for the exchange of oxygen and carbon dioxide in the tissue; and *veins* are the vessels that carry deoxygenated blood back to the heart.

Arteries

All arteries except the pulmonary artery carry oxygenated blood away from the heart to all the cells of the body. The largest of these vessels is the aorta, which starts at the left ventricle and travels through the center of the body into the lower abdomen, where it bifurcates into the right and left femoral arteries with arteries branching off this system down to the feet. As the aorta passes through the body, arteries branch off from it into smaller and smaller vessels, which ultimately become microscopic. These vessels are called *arterioles,* which terminate into tissue capillaries, the smallest and most plentiful of the blood vessels. Capillaries are a single epithelial cell thick so that nutrients and gases can pass through the vessel wall for exchange at the cellular level. Arterioles deliver erythrocytes (red blood cells [RBCs]), which carry oxygen attached to hemoglobin molecules to surrounding tissues. When the blood leaves the capillary bed, the oxygen supply has been depleted, and the return portion of the blood cycle now begins.

Veins

As the blood leaves the capillary beds, it enters the smallest veins, called *venules.* From this point on, the blood flows into larger and larger veins until it reaches the largest veins in the body, the inferior and superior venae cavae. The venae cavae deposit deoxygenated blood into the right atrium, where the blood again begins its trip through the heart through the tricuspid valve, into the right ventricle then through the pulmonary arteries to the lungs, where gas exchange occurs at the alveoli level. Oxygen-rich blood is returned to the left atrium via the pulmonary veins. The walls of veins are thinner than those of arteries because they do not have a muscular lining. Instead, veins have valves that open and close to prevent the backflow of blood. The valves operate by the contraction of muscles around the veins; these contractions massage the blood in the direction of venous flow back to the heart. Venous valves are especially important in the arms and legs, because they prevent pooling of blood in the extremities.

VASCULAR DISORDERS

The vascular system constantly supplies blood containing oxygen and nutrients to all the body's tissues and picks up waste from tissue metabolism. For tissues to receive an adequate amount of oxygen and nutrients, the arterial vessels must maintain elasticity, and their linings must remain smooth to prevent occlusion and reduced blood flow.

Shock

Shock can occur in many different situations (Table 47-4), but they all result in the same signs and symptoms and possible complications. Shock is the general collapse of the circulatory system, including reduced cardiac output, hypotension, and hypoxemia (decreased oxygen in the blood). The initial signs of shock are extreme thirstiness, restlessness, and irritability. The body attempts to compensate for circulatory collapse with constriction of peripheral blood vessels, allowing blood to pool in the vital organs. This vasoconstriction causes a generalized feeling of cool, clammy skin; pallor; tachycardia; and reduced urinary output. Symptoms progress to a rapid, weak, thready pulse; tachypnea; and altered levels of consciousness. If the process is not reversed, the central nervous system becomes depressed, and acute renal failure may occur.

The cause of the shock must be treated for the patient to survive. If the medical assistant identifies a patient in shock, emergency treatment should be started at once. Do not wait for the first indicators of shock to worsen before calling for help. If the physician is not available, call 911 for emergency medical care. Place the patient in a supine position, assess the vital signs frequently, keep the patient warm, administer oxygen, and elevate the legs (if there is no indication of head or neck trauma) to encourage the flow of blood back to the heart.

Vein Disorders

Varicose Veins

Varicose veins are dilated, tortuous, superficial veins in the legs (Figure 47-8). Varicosities can be caused by congenitally defective valves in the saphenous veins and the veins branching off them. Other contributing factors are pregnancy, obesity, prolonged standing or sitting, and heavy lifting. Whatever the cause, the vein valves do not close completely; this allows blood to flow backward, causing the vein to distend from the increased pressure.

Treatment includes consistent aerobic exercise and limiting heavy lifting. The legs should be elevated when possible, and compression stockings should be worn by those who must stand for long periods. Varicose veins may need surgical intervention, which consists of laser treatments, saline injections, or surgical ligation and stripping. Although treatment may be successful, varicosities can recur over time. Patients should be warned to investigate insurance coverage of treatment costs, because many insurance companies consider treatment of varicose veins cosmetic surgery. However, if the patient has documented proof of a health risk associated with the varicosities, insurance companies are more likely to pay for treatment.

Deep Vein Thrombosis

Phlebitis is an inflammation of a vein, most commonly seen in the lower legs. When a vein becomes inflamed, a blood clot, or thrombus, may develop at the site. A thrombus is a clot formed by the collection of platelets that attaches to the interior wall of a vessel. Deep vein thrombosis (DVT) is a thrombus with inflammatory changes that has attached to the deep venous system of the lower legs, causing partial or complete obstruction of the vessel. The calf veins are the most common sites of DVT, but it also can develop in the iliac and femoral veins. Risk factors for the formation of a DVT are recent surgery, immobilization, older age (an increased risk is

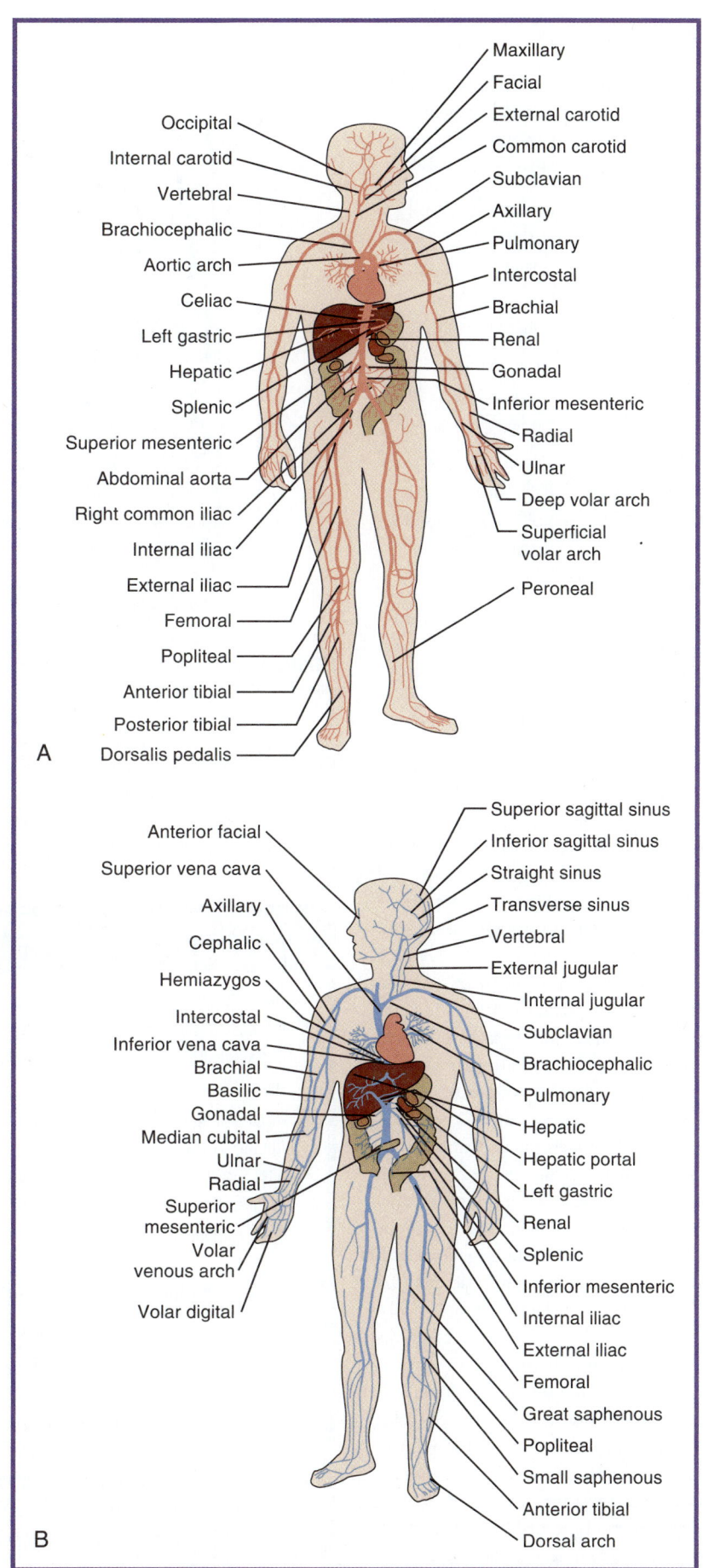

FIGURE 47-7 A, Systemic arteries. **B,** Systemic veins.

TABLE 47-4 Types and Causes of Shock

TYPE	DEFINITION	CAUSE
Cardiogenic	Low cardiac output caused by inability of the heart to pump	Acute MI, arrhythmias, pulmonary embolism, CHF
Hypovolemic	Excessive loss of blood or body fluids	GI bleeding, internal or external hemorrhage, excessive loss of plasma or body fluids, burns
Neurogenic	Peripheral vascular dilation resulting from neurologic injury or disorder	Spinal cord injury, emotional stress, drug reaction
Anaphylactic	Systemic hypersensitivity to an allergen, causing respiratory distress and vascular collapse	Drug, vaccine, shellfish, nuts, insect venom, or chemical allergies
Septic (septicemia)	Systemic vasodilation caused by the release of bacterial endotoxins	Systemic infection or bacteremia

CHF, Congestive heart failure; *GI*, gastrointestinal; *MI*, myocardial infarction.

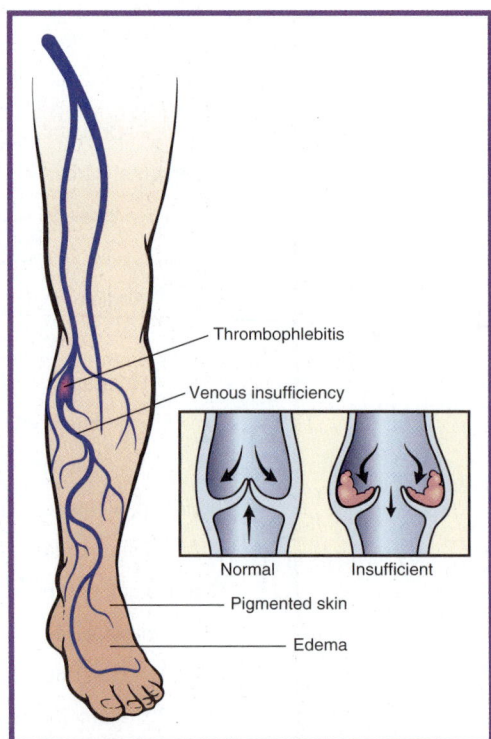

FIGURE 47-8 Varicose veins of the calf. (From Damjanov I: *Pathology for the health-related professions*, ed 4, St Louis, 2012, Saunders.)

seen after age 50), trauma, obesity, use of oral contraceptives, varicose veins, pancreatic cancer, and pregnancy.

In the early stages, approximately 50% of patients with DVT are asymptomatic. Some patients complain of calf pain or cramping and edema of the affected leg, with warmth and erythema at the site. A thrombus that dislodges and begins to move through the general circulation is called an *embolus*. A pulmonary embolism (PE), which is a thrombus that breaks loose and is carried to the lungs, causing blockage of a pulmonary artery, is the most serious complication and may be the first indication that the thrombus was present. Signs and symptoms of PE include an acute onset of chest pain that worsens with a deep breath or cough; unexplained shortness of breath; vertigo or syncope; hemoptysis; and a feeling of anxiety. Patients with any of these indicators should seek immediate medical attention.

DVT typically is diagnosed with venous Doppler studies, which use ultrasound to measure the rate of blood flow through the vessel and can accurately detect venous obstruction. Ultrasound can be used to create an image of the blood flow through the targeted vessel, allowing visualization of the thrombus. Venography also may be ordered; in venography a dye is injected into a large vein of the foot or ankle and x-ray films of the veins are taken. Once the diagnosis has been confirmed, patients usually are hospitalized for IV anticoagulant therapy (heparin) or enoxaparin sodium (Lovenox) subcutaneous (SQ) injections. Anticoagulant therapy does not dissolve existing clots but prevents clots from increasing in size and reduces the potential for additional clots. Oral anticoagulant treatment (warfarin [Coumadin]) is continued for several months. Patients require regular follow-up, including prothrombin time analysis. The medical assistant may perform venipuncture on these patients, and if so,

should follow the office policy for blood draws on patients taking anticoagulants. The medical assistant also should reinforce the physician's recommendations regarding the prevention of further thrombi and precautions about anticoagulant use.

PATIENT EDUCATION FOR PREVENTION OF DEEP VEIN THROMBOSIS

- Take your prescribed medications as directed.
- If you have been prescribed anticoagulants, eat foods high in vitamin K in small amounts (e.g., dark green, leafy vegetables and canola and soy oils).
- Avoid sitting still for long periods; walk around several times during the day or move your legs frequently.
- Alter lifestyle factors such as obesity, smoking, and hypertension, because they increase the risk of DVT.
- Wear compression stockings as ordered by the physician.

CRITICAL THINKING APPLICATION   47-5

Alitza Lincoln, a 43-year-old patient, has large varicose veins in both legs and a history of phlebitis. She is a checkout clerk at the local Wal-Mart, so she stands for extended periods. The physician is concerned about the development of a DVT, and she instructs Ms. Lincoln in the prevention, signs, and symptoms of a thrombus. Ms. Lincoln asks Adam what she can do to prevent further problems with the veins in her legs. Adam uses a picture to illustrate the valves in the leg veins and explains preventive measures. What measures should Adam include?

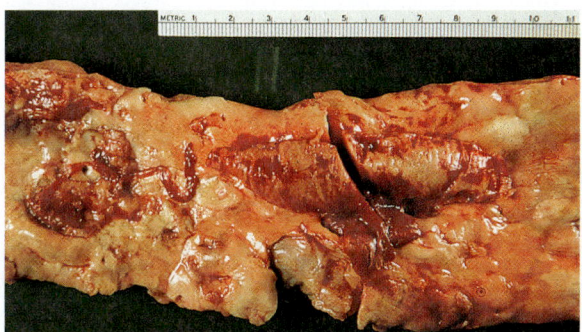

FIGURE 47-9 Atherosclerotic vessel. (From Damjanov I: *Pathology for the health-related professions,* ed 4, St Louis, 2012, Saunders.)

Arterial Disorders

Arteriosclerosis and Atherosclerosis

Arteriosclerosis is a general term for the thickening and loss of elasticity of the arterial walls that is associated with aging. Other conditions that can lead to hardening of the arterial wall are hypertension, **scleroderma**, and diabetes mellitus. Arteriosclerosis can occur in arteries throughout the body and causes systemic ischemia and necrosis over time.

Atherosclerosis is a form of arteriosclerosis marked by the formation of an atheroma, a buildup of cholesterol, cellular debris, and platelets along the inside vessel wall (Figure 47-9). (Cholesterol was discussed in Chapter 30, with recommendations for high-density lipoprotein [HDL] and low-density lipoprotein [LDL] levels.) Cholesterol is a nonessential nutrient that can be produced in the liver and that forms the base for many of the hormones created in the body. Problems arise from dietary and lifestyle factors that elevate blood cholesterol levels to a dangerous point, causing the formation of atheromas, which ultimately block arteries and cause such disorders as heart attacks and strokes.

Treatment of elevated blood cholesterol levels consists of dietary reductions in saturated fats and foods high in cholesterol, in addition to aerobic exercise to elevate HDL levels. Patients are encouraged to stop smoking. (See Table 47-1 for prescription medications for hypercholesterolemia.) The medical assistant can help by educating the patient about risk factors and promoting changes in lifestyle. Referrals to a dietitian may be helpful for patients having a difficult time controlling their fat intake.

Aneurysm

An aneurysm is a ballooning or dilation of a blood vessel wall (Figure 47-10). The patient may have an inherited factor for the development of aneurysms, such as in **Marfan syndrome**, but a common cause is the buildup of atherosclerotic plaques, which weaken the vessel wall. Aneurysms can occur in any artery but usually develop in either the abdominal aorta or the cerebral arteries. In either case, the patient seldom has any signs or symptoms. Occasionally the patient describes a pounding or pulsating pain in the area of the aneurysm.

An aneurysm can be diagnosed when auscultation of the affected vessel over the area of the aneurysm reveals turbulent blood flow sounds, or a bruit. Radiologic studies, sonography, and computed tomography (CT) all help confirm the diagnosis. Patients are

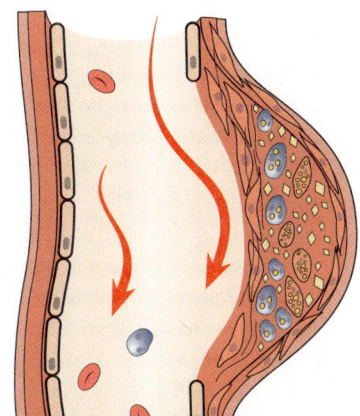

FIGURE 47-10 Aneurysm caused by weakening of the vessel wall. (From Damjanov I: *Pathology for the health-related professions,* ed 4, St Louis, 2012, Saunders.)

monitored on a routine basis for changes in the size of the aneurysm. Surgical repair is recommended for all aneurysms 6 cm or larger, but smaller ones also can rupture. If an aneurysm is tender and known to be enlarging rapidly, surgery is essential, no matter the size. If a rupture occurs, immediate lifesaving intervention is required.

The medical assistant may aid the physician by observing the patient for signs of pain, mental changes, and changes in pulse and respirations. If any of these signs is observed, the physician must be notified immediately. As with any serious condition, the patient may have a high level of anxiety, and the medical assistant's role is to support the patient and family while encouraging consistent follow-up.

Peripheral Arterial Disease

Peripheral arterial disease develops because of widespread atherosclerotic plaque buildup in the arteries outside the heart, especially in the legs. Plaque deposits reduce the size of the lumen of the blood vessel, thereby reducing the amount of oxygenated blood delivered to the tissues. This lack of oxygen causes symptoms, most notably leg pain when walking, a condition called **intermittent claudication**. Other signs and symptoms of peripheral arterial disease are leg numbness or weakness; persistently cold extremities; sores on the feet or legs that do not heal; and hair loss on the extremities. The most effective treatments for intermittent claudications are regular exercise and smoking cessation. Bypass surgery or angioplasty may be necessary if exercise does not improve blood flow to tissues.

DIAGNOSTIC PROCEDURES AND TREATMENTS

The cardiovascular examination begins with the medical assistant obtaining the patient's height and weight, temperature, radial and apical pulses, respirations, and blood pressure in both arms. Most cardiologists also want a complete list of the prescription and over-the-counter medications the patient is taking, including the strength and frequency of use for each. A large part of the physician's examination focuses on subjective symptoms. The physical examination covers the chest, heart, and vascular systems. General appearance, color of the skin, symmetry, clubbing of the fingers, jugular vein distention, temperature of the extremities, and breathing patterns are a few of the notations made by the cardiologist.

A very common diagnostic test for the cardiovascular system performed in the ambulatory care setting is the electrocardiogram, which records the electrical activity of the heart. An ECG is a routine part of many physical examinations, and it also may be ordered if the physician is trying to rule out an MI or to diagnose a cardiac arrhythmia. (ECG techniques and interpretations are covered in detail in Chapter 49.) If the physician wants to evaluate potential cardiac problems in patients over a specific period, a Holter monitor may be ordered. The Holter monitor is worn for a specified time (usually 24 hours), and the patient is instructed to record any symptoms that occur during this period. (Holter monitoring also is discussed in Chapter 49.)

Patient support and education are two very important areas in which medical assistants are deeply involved. When patients understand their condition and are encouraged to take an active role in their treatments, they are inclined to comply with the physician's orders in a more precise and orderly way. Although cardiovascular diagnostic procedures are not typically done in the ambulatory care setting, medical assistants should be familiar with the purpose of the tests so that they can answer patients' questions knowledgeably.

Doppler Studies

Doppler studies can identify occlusions of both veins and arteries from thrombi, emboli, or atherosclerotic plaques. The physician may order arterial Doppler studies for patients with intermittent claudication, lack of a pedal pulse, or leg ulcers that refuse to heal. Venous sonography is ordered to assess patients with pronounced varicosities or those with a swollen, painful leg to rule out the possibility of DVT. For a continuous wave Doppler study, a conductive gel is applied to the skin over the test site. The Doppler transducer is moved over the site, directing an ultrasound beam at the vessel being checked (Figure 47-11). The sonographic beam picks up the speed

of the RBCs as they travel through the vessel as a "swishing" sound. The physician listens to the change in the pitch of the sound produced by the transducer to evaluate the blood flow through an area that may be blocked or narrowed. Variations in RBC velocity indicate either partial or complete occlusion of the blood vessel. A two-dimensional image of an artery can be produced with a duplex Doppler scan that directly shows stenosis or occlusion of the artery. These studies usually are conducted in a vascular laboratory but may be done in a vascular surgeon's office as an initial assessment of the patient or follow-up after bypass grafting. The medical assistant working in this type of practice requires additional training to perform this procedure.

Angiography

Angiography (arteriography) can be used to evaluate any of the arterial pathways in the body (Figure 47-12). A catheter is inserted into a major artery (usually the femoral artery) and advanced to the artery under study. A radiopaque contrast medium is rapidly injected while x-ray films are taken. The study is used to identify abnormal blood vessels, determine blood flow through the vessel, and diagnose arterial anomalies. Angiography also can be used to identify and locate occlusions of the aorta and arteries of the lower extremities. If the radiopaque substance does not pass through or only partially passes through the vessel, the distal end of the artery will not be visualized or will be only partly visible on the x-ray films. Arteriosclerotic disease can create a total or partial occlusion; emboli typically cause total occlusion of the artery. The study also can diagnose dilation of a vessel caused by an aneurysm.

Echocardiography

Echocardiography is a noninvasive, sonographic procedure that assesses the structure and movement of the various parts of the heart. High-frequency sound waves from a transducer held against the chest wall penetrate the heart. The sound waves bounce off the heart and echo back through the transducer into the machine, where they are converted into a picture that shows the exact size and movement of the parts of the heart being measured. Two-dimensional echocardiography also can be done to provide a spatial picture of the

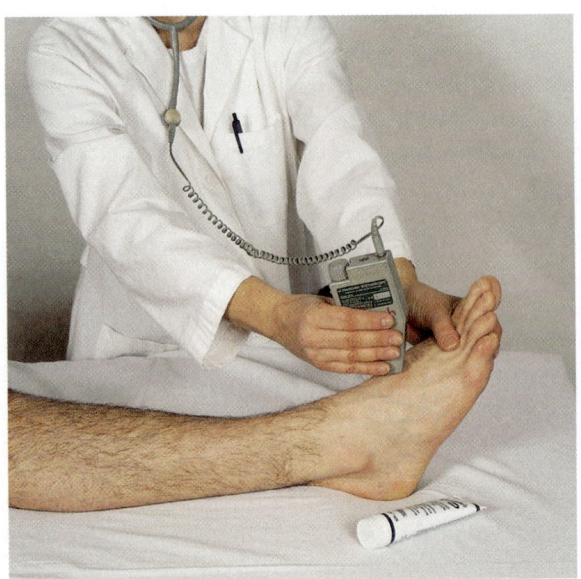

FIGURE 47-11 Doppler study. (From deWit S: *Fundamental concepts and skills for nursing,* ed 3, St Louis, 2009, Saunders.)

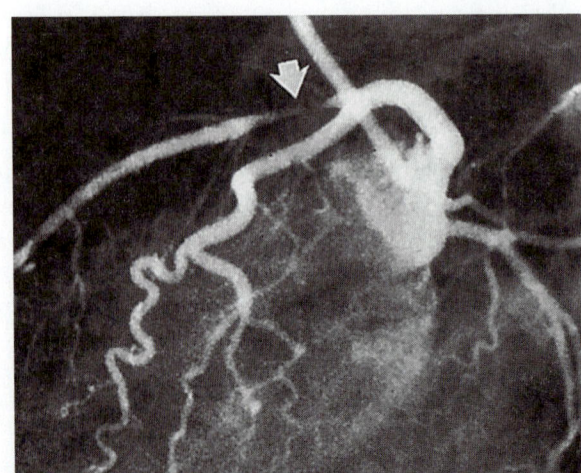

FIGURE 47-12 Coronary angiography showing stenosis *(arrow)* of the left anterior descending coronary artery. (From Braunwald E: *Heart disease: a textbook of cardiovascular medicine,* ed 4, Philadelphia, 1992, Saunders.)

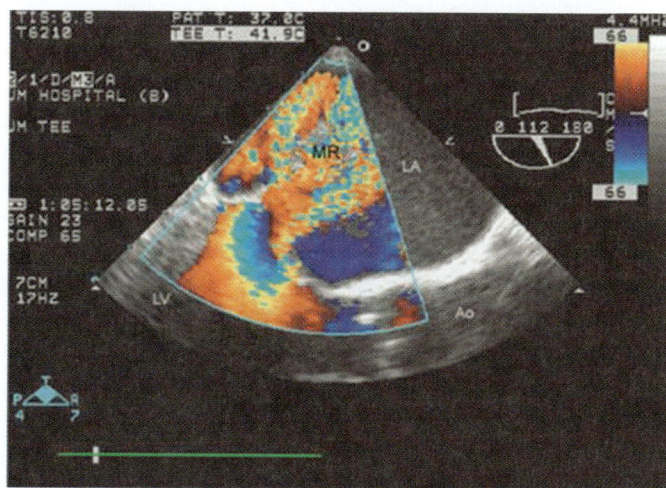

FIGURE 47-13 Transesophageal echocardiogram recorded in a patient with an acute myocardial infarction. Color flow imaging demonstrates the presence of severe mitral regurgitation. *Ao,* Aorta; *LA,* left atrium; *LV,* left ventricle. (From Mann D, Zipes D, Libby P et al: *Braunwald's heart disease,* ed 7, Philadelphia, 2005, Saunders.)

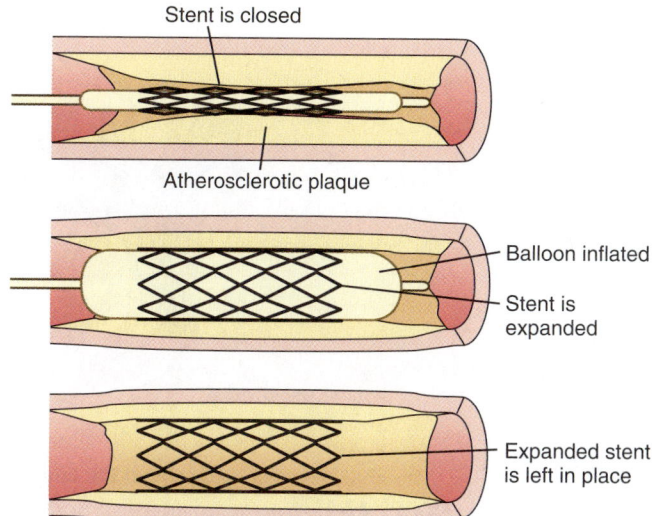

FIGURE 47-14 Angioplasty with stent placement. (From LaFleur Brooks M: *Exploring medical language,* ed 7, St Louis, 2008, Mosby.)

anatomic structures of the heart. Echocardiography usually includes color Doppler studies to show the pattern and velocity of blood flow within the heart and in the great vessels. Backflow of blood, as with a valve that is incompetent, can be identified by changes in color (Figure 47-13).

A transesophageal echocardiogram (TEE) uses a long tube with a microphone-like device mounted on one end that the patient swallows into the esophagus. Once in place, the device is very close to the heart, and sound waves emitted by the microphone create high-quality views of the heart and heart valves. Before the patient swallows the device, the mouth and throat are sprayed with medication that numbs the area. The patient may be given a sedative to help him or her relax and remain still during the procedure. Echocardiography is used to diagnose pericardial effusion, valvular heart disease, aneurysms, and myocardial wall abnormalities seen in CHF or MI.

Cardiac Catheterization and Angioplasty

Cardiac catheterization is used to diagnose or evaluate a variety of heart disorders. Patients who have chronic shortness of breath, vertigo or syncope, chest pain, heart palpitations, arrhythmias, or abnormal stress test or echocardiography results or who have recently had an MI all are considered likely candidates for a heart catheterization procedure.

In this procedure, a catheter is passed into the heart through a peripheral vein or artery. If the right side of the heart is to be evaluated, the catheter usually is passed through the subclavian, brachial, or femoral vein; for left-sided views, the right femoral artery usually is used. As the catheter is passed through the vessels into the heart and coronary arteries, pressures are monitored, oxygen levels are measured, and cardiac output is determined. Once the catheter has reached the desired position, a contrast medium is injected and fluoroscopy is used to visualize the heart chambers, valves, and coronary arteries. The cardiologist evaluates the condition of these structures, and any deviation from normal is noted. Cardiac catheterization is performed in a hospital and usually takes 2 to 3 hours. Patients are required to remain immobile and under observation for 4 to 6 hours after the procedure.

During a heart catheterization procedure, if atherosclerotic plaques are discovered to be occluding the coronary arteries, PTCA may be performed. The goals of angioplasty are to restore blood flow to ischemic myocardial tissue, reduce the need for cardiac medication, and eliminate or reduce the number of episodes of angina. When the area of plaque is found, a balloon that surrounds the upper portion of the catheter is inflated and the atherosclerotic material is pressed against the vessel walls, relieving the obstruction. More than one blockage can be treated during a single session, depending on the location of the blockages and the patient's condition. The procedure can take 30 minutes to several hours, depending on the number of blockages treated.

Lasers also may be used to dissolve the obstruction, or a coronary arterial stent, which is a mesh wire that stretches and molds to the arterial wall, may be inserted and left in place in the vessel to keep it open (Figure 47-14). If multiple coronary artery occlusions are present, the patient may need a CABG procedure. In this surgery, either part of the saphenous vein or an artificial Dacron graft is used to bypass the occluded, diseased section of the coronary artery. The blood flows through the graft to bring nourishment to the ischemic myocardium.

Cardiac Pacemakers

A cardiac pacemaker is a small, battery-powered device that is implanted in the chest wall to generate an electrical impulse, which is sent to the heart along flexible lead wires (Figure 47-15). Current pacemakers are designed to monitor several different types of data, including blood pressure, temperature, and breathing rate, to determine whether the heart needs to be stimulated to contract more frequently. Patients who require the external electrical stimulation of a pacemaker have an arrhythmia (most often bradycardia) either because of injury to the myocardium or as a consequence of the aging process. Biventricular pacemakers, which deliver electrical impulses to both of the ventricles so that they contract and empty at the same time, are the most recent types.

Pacemakers continually get smaller, from the size of a pack of cigarettes in previous years to models that now are as small as a

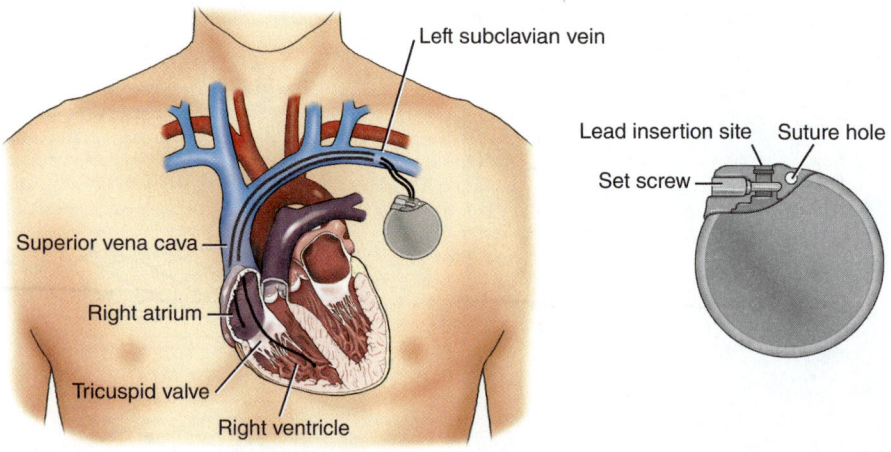

Dual Chamber Pacemaker

FIGURE 47-15 Pacemaker and placement in the chest. (From Aehlert B: *Paramedic practice today: above and beyond,* St Louis, 2009, Mosby/JEMS.)

quarter. The pacemaker must be replaced when the battery pack wears out, and the typical battery life ranges from 5 to 10 years.

Implantable Cardioverter-Defibrillator

An implantable cardioverter-defibrillator (ICD) is a cell phone–sized device implanted in the chest under the skin and attached to the heart with small wires. It continuously monitors the heart rhythm and is designed to deliver a measured electric shock to the myocardium to correct life-threatening arrhythmias, such as ventricular tachycardia or ventricular fibrillation. ICDs have become the standard treatment for any patient with a serious arrhythmia who is at risk of sudden death from cardiac arrest.

CLOSING COMMENTS

Patient Education

Heart disease and stroke account for more than one third of all deaths in the United States. Genetics, predisposition, and lifestyle factors, such as smoking, lack of exercise, and poor diet, play significant roles in the development of heart disease. Successful

management of cardiovascular disease requires major lifestyle changes for most patients. The medical assistant can help by providing encouragement and support and by using community resources to help the patient find assistance with these changes.

Sources for information include the American Heart Association (*www.heart.org/*); workshops and conferences; professional organizations, such as the American Association of Medical Assistants (AAMA); and reputable Internet sites.

Because many patients learn best through visual aids, providing them with pictures, brochures, and pamphlets is an effective means of helping them in this learning process. Always document education interventions so that the physician and/or medical assistant can clarify or expand upon the information on a return visit.

Legal and Ethical Issues

Diagnostic procedures can have a marked effect on the patient's treatment. When entrusted with performing testing procedures, the medical assistant assumes responsibility for the test's accuracy and for performing the test precisely. This is an important role, because the results submitted could strongly influence the plan of treatment.

SUMMARY OF SCENARIO

Adam enjoys his new position but recognizes the challenges of interacting with patients who have cardiovascular problems. Most individuals seen at the clinic must make significant changes in their lifestyle to improve their health or prevent further complications. Adam has found it difficult at times to try to help patients who refuse to quit smoking, who do not exercise regularly, and who continue to eat a diet high in fat. He relies on the hospital dietitian for educational support, and he encourages patients who have had an MI to follow the cardiologist's advice and participate actively in the cardiac rehabilitation program offered by the department. He also works hard to stay up to date on

cardiovascular medications and treatments, because so many of the department's patients have complicated therapeutic plans.

Adam has attended several workshops recently to help him choose patient education materials that meet the needs of the patients in his practice. With the approval of the practice's physicians, he has developed a basic policy and procedures manual for managing common telephone scenarios. He recognizes the need to continue his education in the area of cardiology to stay current with the rapid developments in medication and treatments.

SUMMARY OF LEARNING OBJECTIVES

1. **Define, spell, and pronounce the terms listed in the vocabulary.**
Spelling and pronouncing medical terms correctly bolster the medical assistant's credibility. Knowing the definitions of these terms promotes confidence in communication with patients and co-workers.

2. **Apply critical thinking skills in performing the patient assessment and patient care.**
Completing the Critical Thinking Application exercises throughout the chapter can help the student medical assistant become more adept at critical analysis of real-life situations.

3. **Illustrate the anatomy and physiology of the heart and its significant structures.**
The heart is a muscular organ that pumps blood through all the arteries of the body. It has three layers of tissue surrounded by a double-membrane sac (the pericardium): the epicardium, or first, layer; the myocardium, the middle, muscular layer; and the endocardium, the inner layer, which forms the heart valves. Blood flow through the heart begins in the right atrium, which receives deoxygenated blood from the inferior and superior venae cavae. The atria contract, and blood passes through the tricuspid valve into the right ventricle; the ventricles contract, and the blood passes from the right ventricle to the lungs via the pulmonary artery. Oxygenation occurs in the lungs, and the blood returns to the left atria through the pulmonary veins; the atria contract, and blood passes through the mitral (bicuspid) valve into the left ventricle; the ventricles contract, and oxygen-rich blood is sent out to the body through the aorta.

4. **Summarize risk factors for the development of heart disease.**
Risk factors for the development of cardiovascular disease that cannot be changed are familial history, aging, and race; factors that can be altered are hypertension, diabetes, elevated blood cholesterol levels, smoking, obesity, lack of exercise, and stress.

5. **Describe the signs, symptoms, and medical procedures used in the diagnosis and treatment of coronary artery disease and myocardial infarction.**
In CAD, the arteries supplying the myocardium become narrowed by atherosclerotic plaque, resulting in ischemia of the myocardium. The cardinal symptom is angina pectoris, followed by pressure or fullness in the chest, syncope, unexplained coughing spells, and fatigue; however, women may have a different clinical picture. Ischemia leads to necrosis of a portion of the myocardium, resulting in an MI. An MI is characterized by pain that lasts longer than 30 minutes and is unrelieved by rest or nitroglycerin tablets. It is diagnosed by ECG changes and elevated cardiac enzymes. Medical treatment includes thrombolytic medications, aspirin, beta blockers, ACE inhibitors, anticoagulants, and anticholesterol agents. With occlusion, either PTCA or CABG surgery may be indicated. (Table 47-1 reviews medications prescribed to treat hypercholesterolemia.)

6. **Explain the signs and symptoms of myocardial infarction in women.**
The signs and symptoms of a heart attack in women may start weeks before the actual cardiac injury and could include abdominal, neck, shoulder, or upper back pain; jaw pain; shortness of breath; vertigo; sweating; indigestion or nausea and vomiting; extreme fatigue; and/or aching in both arms.

7. **Compare and contrast the treatment protocols for hypertension.**
The two types of hypertension are primary and secondary hypertension. Secondary hypertension occurs because of a disease process in another body system. Primary hypertension is idiopathic and is diagnosed when the patient's blood pressure is consistently above 119 mm Hg systolic and/or 79 mm Hg diastolic. Table 47-2 summarizes how the varying stages of hypertension are identified and treated, and Table 47-3 lists antihypertensive medications. Chronic elevated blood pressure can result in left ventricular hypertrophy, angina, MI, heart failure, cerebrovascular accident, and nephropathy. Risk factors for hypertension include a family history of hypertension or stroke, hypercholesterolemia, smoking, high sodium intake, diabetes, excessive alcohol intake, aging, prolonged stress, and race.

8. **Outline the causes and results of congestive heart failure.**
CHF occurs when the myocardium is unable to pump an adequate amount of blood to meet the body's needs. It typically develops over time and initially involves one side of the heart and then the other side. Left-sided heart failure causes a backup of blood in the left atria and lungs, resulting in pulmonary edema with dyspnea, orthopnea, nonproductive cough, rales, and tachycardia. Right-sided heart failure causes a backup of blood in the right atrium, preventing emptying of the vena cava, resulting in systemic edema, especially in the legs and feet. Both types of heart failure cause fatigue, weakness, exercise intolerance, dyspnea, and sensitivity to cold temperatures.

9. **Summarize the effects of inflammation and valvular disorders on cardiac function.**
Rheumatic heart disease develops because of an unusual immune reaction that occurs approximately 2 weeks after an untreated beta-hemolytic streptococcal infection; endocarditis is the most common heart complication, with valvular damage. Disorders of the heart valves may be caused by a congenital defect or an infection. Two specific problems can occur with valve disease. The valve can be stenosed, which restricts the forward flow of blood, or it can be incompetent, which allows blood to leak backward. The most common valvular defect is MVP, which results from a congenital defect or vegetation and scarring caused by endocarditis.

10. **Describe the anatomy and physiology of the vascular system.**
Blood vessels are divided into two systems that begin and end with the heart. Vessels are classified according to their structure and function as arteries, which carry oxygenated blood away from the heart; capillaries, the microscopic vessels responsible for the exchange of oxygen and carbon dioxide in the tissue; and veins, the vessels that carry deoxygenated blood back to the heart.

11. **Differentiate among the various types of shock.**
Table 47-4 outlines the various types of shock. All result in the same signs and symptoms and possible complications. Shock is the general collapse of the circulatory system, marked by reduced cardiac output, hypotension, and hypoxemia. Symptoms progress to a rapid, weak, thready pulse; tachypnea; and altered levels of consciousness. If the process is not reversed, the central nervous system becomes depressed and acute renal failure may occur.

12. **Summarize the characteristics of common vascular disorders.**

   Varicose veins are dilated, tortuous, superficial veins in the legs that develop because the valves do not completely close, allowing blood to flow backward, thus causing the vein to distend from the increased pressure. *Phlebitis* is an inflammation of the veins most commonly seen in the lower legs. *DVT is* a thrombus with inflammatory changes that has attached to the deep venous system of the lower legs and has caused a partial or complete obstruction of the vessel. A thrombus that dislodges and begins to circulate through the general circulation is an *embolus*. *Arteriosclerosis* is a general term for the thickening and loss of elasticity of arterial walls; it can occur in arteries throughout the body and cause systemic ischemia and necrosis over time. *Atherosclerosis* is a form of arteriosclerosis in which an atheroma develops. An *aneurysm* is a ballooning or dilation of the wall of a vessel caused by weakening of the vessel wall. *Peripheral arterial disease* affects the vessels outside of the heart, especially the legs and feet, in which circulation is reduced and ischemia can occur.

13. **Outline typical cardiovascular diagnostic procedures.**

   Cardiovascular diagnostic procedures include Doppler studies of the patency of blood vessels; angiography to visualize arterial pathways; echocardiography to assess the structure and movement of the parts of the heart, especially the valves; and cardiac catheterization to show the heart chambers, valves, and coronary arteries.

14. **Describe patient education topics for cardiovascular patients.**

   Successful management of cardiovascular disease requires major lifestyle changes for most patients. The medical assistant can help by providing encouragement and support and by using community resources to help the patient find assistance with these changes. Sources for information include the American Heart Association, workshops and conferences, professional organizations, and reputable Internet sites.

CONNECTIONS

📖 **Study Guide Connection:** Go to the Chapter 47 Study Guide. Read and complete the activities.

🄴 **Evolve Connection:** Go to the Chapter 47 link at *evolve.elsevier.com/kinn* to complete the Chapter Review and Chapter Quiz. Check out the other resources listed for this chapter to make the most of what you have learned from Assisting in Cardiology.

ASSISTING IN GERIATRICS

48

SCENARIO

Bill Novelli, CMA (AAMA), works for Dr. Sara Kennedy, a primary care physician in a small town close to where he grew up. Although patients of all ages are seen in the practice, most patients are age 65 or older. Bill has learned to recognize the unique communication needs of aging individuals and the importance of using family and community resources to maintain optimum health in this special population.

While studying this chapter, think about the following questions:

- Do myths about aging and stereotypes about aging people negatively affect older individuals?
- What are the most common changes that occur in the aging body and what recommendations can be made for health promotion in this age group?
- What suggestions can be made to aging patients and their families to optimize the older adults' health and protect them from injury and disease?
- How is Alzheimer's disease diagnosed and what are the stages of its development?
- Why is depression so common in aging individuals and how is it diagnosed and treated?
- How can the medical assistant most effectively communicate with an older person?
- Why is the use of community resources such an important factor in the care of aging people?

LEARNING OBJECTIVES

1. Define, spell, and pronounce the terms listed in the vocabulary.
2. Apply critical thinking skills in performing the patient assessment and patient care.
3. Discuss the impact of a growing aging population on society.
4. Identify the stereotypes and myths associated with aging.
5. Role-play the effect of the sensorimotor changes of aging.
6. Explain the changes in the anatomy and physiology of the body systems caused by aging.
7. Summarize the major diseases and disorders faced by older patients.
8. Describe various screening tools for dementia, depression, and malnutrition.
9. Explain the effect of aging on sleep.
10. Differentiate among independent, assisted, and skilled nursing facilities.
11. Summarize the role of the medical assistant in caring for aging patients.
12. Determine the principles of effective communication with older adults.
13. Identify legal and ethical issues associated with aging patients.

VOCABULARY

collagen (kah'-luh-jen) The protein that forms the inelastic fibers of tendons, ligaments, and fascia.

costal Pertaining to the ribs.

decubitus ulcers Sores or ulcers that develop over a bony prominence as the result of ischemia from prolonged pressure; also called *bed sores*.

elastin An essential part of elastic connective tissue; when moist, it is flexible and elastic.

lacrimation (la-krihm-a'-shun) The secretion or discharge of tears.

According to the Administration on Aging, an agency of the U.S. Department of Health and Humans Services, the aging population—those age 65 or older—numbered more than 40 million in 2011. By 2030 almost 1 of every 5 Americans (about 72 million people) will be 65 years or older. The fastest growing segment of the U.S. population are those age 85 or older.

The average life expectancy of an individual who reaches age 65 is an additional 18.7 years (20 years for women, 17.1 years for men). A child born in 2010 has a projected life expectancy of 80.8 years, more than 30 years longer than a child born in 1900. Older women outnumber older men; 22.9 million women are older than age 65, as are 17.4 million men. About 30% of older people who live outside of institutions live alone; half of women over age 75 live alone. More than half a million grandparents over the age of 65 are the primary caregivers for their grandchildren who live with them. Most older people have at least one chronic medical condition, and many have multiple conditions. Hypertension, arthritis, heart disease, cancer, and diabetes are the health problems most commonly seen in the elderly, and a significant number also suffer from strokes, asthma, emphysema and chronic bronchitis.

What does all this mean to those who have chosen careers in healthcare? As the aging population expands, it will affect all aspects of society. One area in particular will be these individuals' increased use of health services. To provide better services to the aging patient, the medical assistant must understand the aging process, which includes the physical and sensory changes with which older people must cope (Procedure 48-1). This knowledge enables medical assistants to recognize the special needs of the aged and to develop therapeutic management and communication skills that can help them effectively care for the older patient. Ongoing research and education about the aging process have dispelled many of the old stereotypes.

Aging is a complex physiologic, psychological, and social process. Old age is not an illness but a normal life process that people experience in different ways. Lack of exercise, poor nutrition, substance abuse, continual stress, and air pollutants all are factors that cause a person to show the effects of aging decades earlier than someone who has practiced healthy living habits.

As people age, changes occur in their physical appearance and abilities, along with sensory changes in vision, hearing, taste, and smell. These changes do not occur at the same time in everyone; however, sensorimotor changes can have a profound effect on the individual's ability to interact with his or her environment.

STEREOTYPES AND MYTHS ABOUT AGING

- *Most aging people will develop dementia.* Dementia is not part of the normal aging process. However, the older the person, the greater the risk of dementia. About 6% of those over age 65 and 40% of those over age 85 are diagnosed with significant memory and disorientation issues.
- *Disease is a normal and an unavoidable part of the aging process.* Recent research verifies that individuals who have established healthy lifestyles as they age remain healthy well into their older years. Aging people are more likely to have health issues, but these are not inevitable for all persons over age 65.
- *Older workers are less productive than younger ones.* Individuals with a strong work ethic will continue to perform in this way. It may take aging people longer to learn new material, but they continue to be capable of learning and applying new knowledge.
- *Most older people end up in long-term care facilities.* At any given time, approximately 5% of the aging population lives in long-term care facilities; 80% of aging individuals live alone with or without a partner.
- *Most aging people have no interest in or capacity for sexual relations.* Sexual interest does not change significantly with age; a decrease in sexual activity is usually related to the loss of a partner.
- *Damage to health because of lifestyle factors is irreversible.* It is never too late to benefit from healthy lifestyle choices.

CRITICAL THINKING APPLICATION   48-1

When Bill first started working with aging patients, he believed many of the stereotypes about people over age 65. Through his work with Dr. Kennedy, he has come to realize that many of these myths have no foundation in actual practice. Based on the myths mentioned in the text, what do you think about these beliefs on aging?

CHANGES IN ANATOMY AND PHYSIOLOGY

The aging process brings about changes in all of the body's systems. Table 48-1 summarizes these changes and what can be done to promote healthy aging.

PROCEDURE 48-1

Instruct Individuals According to Their Needs: Understand the Sensorimotor Changes of Aging

GOAL: *To role-play an older adult so as to better understand the needs of aging people.*

EQUIPMENT and SUPPLIES

- Yellow-tinted glasses, ski goggles, or laboratory goggles
- Pink, white, yellow "pills" (e.g., various colors of Tic Tacs)
- Vaseline
- Cotton balls
- Eye patches
- Tape
- Thick gloves
- Utility glove
- Tongue depressors
- Elastic bandages
- Medical forms in small print
- Pennies
- Button shirts
- Walker

PROCEDURAL STEPS

1. Role-play vision and hearing loss:
   - Put two cotton balls in each ear and an eye patch over one eye. Follow your partner's instructions.
   - *Partner:* Stand out of the line of vision (to prevent lip-reading). Without using gestures or changing your voice volume, tell your partner to cross the room and pick up a book.
2. Role-play yellowing of lens:
   - Line up "pills" of different pastel colors.
   - *Partner:* Pick out the different colors while wearing the yellow-tinted glasses.

3. Role-play difficulty with focusing:
   - Put on goggles smeared with Vaseline and follow your partner's directions.
   - *Partner:* Stand at least 3 feet in front of your partner and motion for him or her to come to you (your partner is deaf, so talking will not help).
4. Role-play loss of peripheral vision:
   - Put on goggles with black paper taped to the sides.
   - *Partner:* Stand to the side, out of the field of vision, and motion for your patient to follow you.
5. Role-play aphasia and partial paralysis:
   - You are unable to use your right arm or leg. Place tape over your mouth. Let your partner know you need to go to the bathroom.
   - *Partner:* Stand at least 3 feet away with your back to your partner and wait for instructions.
6. Role-play problems with dexterity:
   - Put thick gloves on your hands and try to sign your name, button a shirt, tie your shoes, and pick up pennies.
7. Role-play problems with mobility:
   - Use the walker to cross the room.
   - *Partner:* After your partner starts to use the walker, hand him or her a book to carry.
8. Role-play changes in sensation:
   - Put a rubber utility glove on; turn on hot water; test the difference in temperature between the gloved hand and ungloved hand.
9. Summarize and share with the group your impressions of the effect of age-related sensorimotor changes.

TABLE 48-1 System Changes with Aging and Measures to Promote Health

BODY SYSTEM	AGE-RELATED CHANGES	HEALTH PROMOTION
Cardiovascular system	Arteriosclerosis and atherosclerotic plaque buildup reduces blood flow to major organs; 50% of the aging population have hypertension; CVD is the number one killer of women and men in their 60s.	Regular exercise; weight control; diet rich in fruits, vegetables, and whole grains; cholesterol, blood glucose monitoring
Central nervous system	Brain shrinks by 10% between ages 30 and 90; takes longer to learn new material; attention span and language remain the same; signs and symptoms may be caused by depression, vascular disease, and drug reactions.	Aerobic exercise to increase blood flow to CNS; maintaining mental activities (e.g., reading, interacting with others)
Endocrine system	After age 50, women have a sharp decline in estrogen; men have a more gradual decline in testosterone.	Possible hormone replacement therapy or natural soy supplements
Gastrointestinal system	Decline in gastric juices and enzymes by age 60; decreased peristalsis with increased constipation; some nutrients are not absorbed as well.	High-fiber diet and adequate fluid intake; regular exercise to prevent constipation

Continued

TABLE 48-1 System Changes with Aging and Measures to Promote Health—Cont'd

BODY SYSTEM	AGE-RELATED CHANGES	HEALTH PROMOTION
Musculoskeletal system	Muscle mass decreases; tendency to gain weight; gradual loss of bone density; deterioration of joint cartilage.	Strength training to increase muscle mass; stretching to remain limber; exercise; vitamin D and calcium supplements
Pulmonary system	At age 55 the lungs become less elastic and the chest wall gradually stiffens, making oxygenation more difficult.	Quit smoking; regular aerobic exercise
Sensory organs	Hearing is intact through the mid-50s but declines by 25% by age 80; oral problems are common; skin thins and loses elasticity; presbyopia after age 40; cataracts common after age 60.	Avoid exposure to loud noise, use of hearing aids; good dental hygiene; prevention of sun damage to the skin; annual eye examinations; diet rich in dark green, leafy vegetables to prevent cataracts and macular degeneration
Urinary system	Kidneys become less efficient; bladder muscles weaken; one third of seniors experience incontinence; prostate enlargement is common.	Pelvic exercises, drugs, or surgery for incontinence; annual PSA with digital rectal exam monitoring for men
Sexuality	Men: Impotence is not a symptom of normal aging; men over age 50 may have some altered function. Women: Menopause causes vaginal narrowing and dryness, resulting in painful intercourse.	Men: Maintenance of cardiovascular health with exercise, weight control, no smoking, diabetes management Women: Use of vaginal lubricants or estrogen cream

CNS, Central nervous system; *CVD,* cardiovascular disease; *PSA,* prostate-specific antigen.

Cardiovascular System

Cardiovascular disease is the most frequent cause of illness and disability in the aging population, and congestive heart failure (CHF) is the most common reason for hospitalization. Age-related changes occur in the cardiovascular system, but disease and lifestyle habits such as lack of exercise, poor diet, and stress contribute to these changes. Heart disease is ranked as the leading cause of death among men and women; therefore, proper management of cardiovascular disease can help maintain the health of an aging population and reduce mortality rates.

The aging process causes structural changes in the heart. Myocardial cells enlarge, and deposits of fat and connective tissue increase; these combine to make the myocardial wall stiffer and to lengthen the amount of time needed for the relaxation phase of the cardiac cycle. As a result, cardiac output declines, making aging people more susceptible to CHF. The reduction in cardiac output leads to pooling of blood in the legs, cold extremities, and edema (Table 48-2). In addition, the heart cannot respond as quickly or as forcefully to an increased workload, so exercise, sudden movements, and changes in position can result in dizziness and loss of balance. Aging also brings with it an increase in blood pressure, requiring the heart to work harder to pump blood into the systemic circulation. Hypertension increases the workload of the left ventricle, and this may result in hypertrophy of the chamber and weakening of the myocardial wall. The valves of the heart tend to thicken and become more rigid, making it more difficult for blood to circulate through the cardiopulmonary vessels. With these cardiovascular problems, arrhythmias become more common.

Aging causes the walls of the veins to weaken and stretch. This damages the valves, especially in the veins of the legs, where the walls are subject to greater pressure as blood struggles to return to the heart against the force of gravity. As a result, edema and varicose

TABLE 48-2 Normal Changes in Cardiac Output with Age

AGE	BLOOD PUMPED BY RESTING HEART (quarts/min)	MAXIMUM HEARTBEAT DURING EXERCISE (beats/min)
30	3.6	200
40	3.4	182
50	3.2	171
60	2.9	159
70	2.6	150

From the American Heart Association. Accessed 7/20/2012. Available at www.americanheart.org.

veins of the lower extremities are common in the elderly, increasing the risk of phlebitis and the formation of thrombi in the deep veins, or deep vein thrombosis (DVT).

Arteriosclerosis is considered part of the aging process. The vessel walls thicken and become less elastic as a result of the calcification and buildup of connective tissue. In addition, the artery's ability to dilate and contract diminishes. To maintain an adequate blood supply throughout the body, the heart must work harder to overcome the resistance caused by stiffened vessels. Older adults have a higher incidence of orthostatic hypotension. The clinical criterion for alterations in blood pressure from sitting to standing is a drop of more than 20 mm Hg in the systolic pressure or more than 10 mm Hg in the diastolic pressure when the position is changed. Such a decrease typically is caused by a drop in the volume of circulating blood, and it can be an important diagnostic sign in aging patients. The physician may have the medical assistant take orthostatic blood pressures as part of the routine intake protocol for aging patients.

Endocrine System

Hormonal changes that occur with aging are related to a general decrease in hormone production combined with changes in tissue receptor binding. The most common endocrine system disorder seen in aging patients is diabetes mellitus (DM) type 2. As a person ages, insulin production by the beta cells in the pancreas decreases and insulin resistance at the tissue level increases. According to the National Institutes of Health, more than half of the 16 million Americans diagnosed with diabetes type 2 are over age 65. Elderly patients with diabetes are at increased risk of developing vascular disease, including renal disorders, retinopathy, neuropathy, myocardial ischemia, angina, myocardial infarction, cerebrovascular accidents, and peripheral vascular disease, such as lower extremity ulcers.

Older patients do not always experience the classic symptoms of diabetes, which are polyuria, polydipsia, and polyphagia. They may show a variety of problems, including unexplained weight loss, slow wound healing, recurrent bacterial or fungal infections, changes in mental state, cataracts, macular disease, muscle weakness and pain, angina, foot ulcers, and uremia. The range of symptoms is due to the insidious onset of diabetes in older people, who may have gradually developing hyperglycemia for years before diagnosis.

The treatment protocol for aging patients with diabetes is the same as for other age groups; however, special consideration must be given to the patient's ability to understand and comply with the therapeutic plan. In addition, because the person may have other health problems that are being treated with medications, an aging patient newly diagnosed with diabetes may face a complicated treatment regimen that requires explicit instruction and continual follow-up in the ambulatory care setting.

The medical assistant must be aware of any sensory abnormalities, such as diminished vision or problems with fine motor skills, which may interfere with the patient's ability to follow treatment guidelines. Teaching and treatment plans must be adapted to meet the individual needs of each patient.

FACTORS THAT CAN AFFECT DIABETES MANAGEMENT IN OLDER PEOPLE

- Modifying lifestyle risk factors may be more difficult because of poor nutrition, inability to exercise, and long-standing habits such as smoking and a diet high in fat and calories.
- Previously diagnosed health conditions, such as hypertension and heart disease, in addition to an age-related decline in kidney and liver function, increase the challenge of treating diabetes.
- Older people are more likely to be prescribed multiple medications (polypharmacy), which increases the risk of adverse drug interactions.
- Elderly patients with diabetes are more prone to hypoglycemia and may not recognize and respond quickly to the signs of low blood glucose levels.
- Diabetic complications can develop quickly because of a long history of prediabetes before diagnosis.

- Older people may have decreased physical and/or mental abilities that make it difficult for them to understand and adhere to a complicated treatment regimen.
- Older patients may not be able to afford the medications and supplies needed to maintain health.

Gastrointestinal System

Age-related changes in the gastrointestinal system begin in the mouth with dental problems, a decrease in the number of taste buds and the production of saliva, and a diminishing sense of smell. Older people generally find eating less pleasurable, have a reduced appetite, and are unable to chew and lubricate their food as well as younger people; this makes dysphagia (difficulty swallowing) a common age-related problem. Aging also brings a decrease in the production of hydrochloric acid, which affects the digestion of calcium and iron. Secretion of intrinsic factor, a protein that is needed for the absorption of vitamin B_{12}, also declines, which affects the function of the nervous system and the formation of red blood cells, resulting in excessive fatigue. It is not unusual for aging patients to be seen in the physician's office regularly for vitamin B_{12} injections.

Food passes more quickly through the small intestine, resulting in poorer absorption of vitamins and minerals. Peristalsis in the colon decreases, making aging patients more susceptible to constipation and diverticular disease. Poor eating habits, a reduced fluid intake, and some medications (e.g., antidepressants, diuretics, antacids containing aluminum or calcium, and medications for Parkinson's disease) also contribute to constipation. The liver decreases in size and weight after age 70. It is still able to perform vital functions, but more time is required to metabolize drugs and alcohol. All of these factors combine to increase the potential for adverse drug reactions in older adults.

Aging individuals have a higher incidence of several gastrointestinal system diseases, such as gastroesophageal reflux disease (GERD), peptic ulcers, diverticulosis (related to lack of dietary fiber and constipation), cholelithiasis, and colorectal cancer. Dietary counseling and annual screenings should be part of the routine care of aging patients.

Integumentary System

The skin is the body's first line of protection against infection, and it also is responsible for preventing the loss of body fluid and regulating body temperature. Changes in the appearance and function of the integumentary system usually are caused by a combination of ordinary age-related changes and environmental factors, especially the amount of sun exposure over time. Exposure to ultraviolet light from the sun frequently is the cause of wrinkles, age spots, blotches, and leathery, dry, loose skin, all of which are associated with aging. Changes caused by the ultraviolet light from the sun or by the normal aging process can affect all three layers of the skin: the epidermis, dermis, and subcutaneous tissue.

The cells in the epidermis reproduce more slowly as people age, and this slower regeneration causes the skin to appear thinner. The skin becomes more prone to tearing and blistering. The risk of infections increases, the healing process takes longer, and older people are more susceptible to bruising. Because the skin can be easily torn, it is important to be very careful when performing phlebotomy or covering a wound on an older patient. Vitamin D synthesis, a major function of the epidermis, significantly declines in aged skin, and a decrease in the number of melanocytes increases photosensitivity.

The dermis loses 20% of its mass during the aging process, resulting in the paper-thin or transparent skin seen in older adults. The number of **collagen** cells in the dermis also declines with age, causing the skin to sag and wrinkle. Because both sweat and sebaceous glands decrease in number, aging people have difficulty tolerating higher temperatures because they perspire less. At the same time, the blood supply to the dermis decreases; this makes it difficult to regulate the body temperature and leads to an increased susceptibility to both hypothermia and heat stroke in aging individuals. Any situation in which an older adult would be exposed to extremes of cold or heat should be avoided. Make sure a blanket is available in the examining room if the air conditioning is on. Ask the person if he or she is too cold or too hot and take the necessary steps to make the patient feel more comfortable.

Atrophy of the subcutaneous layer increases the skin's susceptibility to trauma, so patients bruise much more easily. The skin is denied natural lubrication, and dry skin is one of the most common complaints among older people. In addition, fat deposits increase in the abdomen in men and in the abdomen and thighs in women as they age.

Suggestions that might help older people prevent and treat dry skin include:

- Using a room humidifier to moisten the air
- Bathing less frequently and using warm rather than hot water
- Using a mild soap or cleansing cream (e.g., Aveeno, Basis, or Dove)
- Wearing protective clothing in cold weather
- Moisturizing dry skin
- Applying creams and moisturizers after getting out of the bathtub or shower to reduce the chance of falls

Pain receptors are distributed throughout the skin. Because of age-related changes in the receptors, older people have a higher pain threshold. They may not notice a cut or burn as quickly as a younger person would, so a more serious burn may occur before it is noticed. In addition, wound healing becomes a problem because of decreased blood flow to dermal tissues.

Other changes occur in the skin's appendages. Hair changes in color, growth, and distribution. Hair grays because of the decreased rate of melanin production and the replacement of pigmented hair with nonpigmented hair. Women lose hair on the trunk and have increased facial hair. Although alopecia (male balding) is caused by an inherited trait, aging also causes hair loss. Hair on the eyebrows, nose, and ears becomes coarser and longer in men. The nails of older people take longer to grow and are more brittle. Nails, particularly toenails, thicken as a result of trauma or nutritional deficiencies. It is not unusual for nails to split, making them more susceptible to fungal infections.

Seborrheic keratoses, usually referred to as "age spots," are one of the most common benign skin disorders found in the aging population. They appear as waxy, greasy papules that vary from tan to dark brown (Figure 48-1) and typically are found in areas of sun exposure, such as the trunk, back, face, neck, extremities, and scalp. They are not dangerous but may be removed for cosmetic purposes.

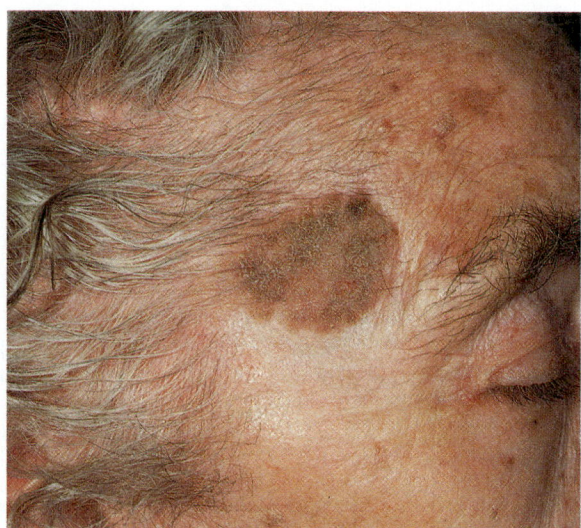

FIGURE 48-1 Seborrheic keratosis. (From Habif TP: *Clinical dermatology: a color guide to diagnosis and therapy*, ed 4, St Louis, 2004, Mosby.)

SHINGLES RISK REDUCTION

The U.S. Food and Drug Administration (FDA) has approved a vaccine, Zostavax, to reduce the risk of shingles in people age 50 or older. The varicella-zoster virus causes both shingles and chickenpox. After an active chickenpox infection, the virus lies dormant in a nerve dermatome. As people age, their risk increases that the virus will reactivate, causing the formation of blisters and varying degrees of pain along the affected nerve pathway. It is estimated that 2 in 10 people will develop shingles in their lifetime. Zostavax, a live virus vaccine, boosts immunity against the varicella-zoster virus. The vaccine is administered as a single subcutaneous injection. Studies have shown that the vaccine reduces the number of shingles cases by 50% in all individuals over age 50, but it is most effective in those age 50 to 69. For individuals who develop shingles even though they were immunized, the duration of symptoms is shorter. It is recommended that all individuals over age 50 receive the Zostavax vaccine.

CRITICAL THINKING APPLICATION   48-2

Rose Deluca, a 71-year-old patient of Dr. Kennedy's, is unhappy about the changes in her skin that have occurred in the past several years. Based on what Bill knows about the normal changes that occur in the skin as people age, how can he explain these changes to Mrs. Deluca, and what can he suggest to help with dryness and other typical aging changes?

Musculoskeletal System

As the body ages, changes occur in the muscles, bones, and joints that affect the individual's appearance, strength, and mobility. The amount of change depends on diet, exercise, and heredity. Cartilage loss and degeneration, producing osteoarthritis, commonly occur in the weight-bearing joints of older people. Joint range of motion is affected, and the intervertebral disc spaces are decreased, causing loss of height as a person ages. A breakdown in joint structures may lead to inflammation, pain, stiffness, and deformity.

Aging brings a decrease in the strength and speed of muscle contractions in the extremities but only a slight decline in overall muscle endurance. Muscular changes in the aging patient are directly related to the individual's activity level. Research shows that musculoskeletal disease is not an inevitable result of the aging process; however, 40% to 50% of women over age 50 have a serious problem with bone demineralization. Men also experience bone loss but at a later age and a much slower rate than women.

SUGGESTIONS FOR HELPING THE OLDER ADULT WITH MOBILITY, DEXTERITY, AND BALANCE

- Use assistive devices, such as adaptive silverware, tub seat or shower chair, electric razor, and reaching devices.
- Assist with gripping devices as needed (wait for the patient to place his or her hand around a cup or help him or her with it before letting go).
- Older adults may need more time to complete tasks but prefer to do so independently, so slow down.
- Stroke victims should be supported on the weak side when walking or transferring from a chair to the examination table.
- The physician may recommend physical therapy for range-of-motion exercises.
- Encourage activity; lack of activity causes a decline in the ability to function.

Osteoporosis

Osteoporosis (see Chapter 43) is the primary cause of hip fractures, which can lead to a loss of independence and complications that ultimately can end in death. The spinal vertebrae also can collapse, producing the stooped posture associated with "dowager's hump." Sometimes bones break because of the sheer weight of the body on them. Often people say they fell and broke a bone, when in reality the bone fractured, causing them to fall. Multiple factors contribute to the development of osteoporosis, but it is most common in postmenopausal women. Risk factors for osteoporosis include:

- Female gender (women have a five times greater risk than men)
- Small-boned frame, thin
- Family history of osteoporosis
- Estrogen deficiency before age 45 either from early menopause or oophorectomy
- Estrogen deficiency resulting from an abnormal absence of menses (eating disorders, excessive aerobic exercise, fibrocystic ovaries)
- Racial background (Caucasian and Asian women have the highest risk)
- Aging
- Extended use of anticonvulsant drugs, prednisone, and excessive thyroid hormone medications
- Sedentary lifestyle, smoking, excessive alcohol intake, lack of calcium and vitamin D when growing up

Weight-bearing exercises and calcium and vitamin D supplements are recommended to prevent demineralization of the bones.

Medications used to prevent and/or treat osteoporosis include alendronate (Fosamax) and risedronate (Actonel), which reduce the rate of demineralization; raloxifene (Evista), which slows bone thinning and causes some increase in bone thickness; and calcitonin (Calcimar, Miacalcin), which is either injected or inhaled as a nasal spray and results in a decrease in the rate of bone thinning and relieves the pain associated with spinal compression. The U.S. Food and Drug Administration (FDA) recently approved an intravenous (IV) medication, zoledronic acid (Reclast), for the once-yearly treatment of postmenopausal women with osteoporosis. Reclast helps increase bone density in the spine and hip, thus reducing the risk of fractures.

Falls

The risk of injuries from falls increases with age; falls cause the greatest number of injuries in people over age 70. Aging individuals are at greater risk of falling because of sensorimotor changes in vision and mobility, osteoporosis, and cerebrovascular accidents. Falls in older patients usually result in fractures, because a large percentage of them have osteoporosis. Serious fractures, such as those of the hip, require the patient to be immobile for extended periods, and this opens the door to a wide range of debilitating complications, such as **decubitus ulcers**, pneumonia, placement in long-term care facilities, and even death. Falls are largely preventable. The medical assistant can play an active role in helping family members and patients become aware of risk factors and safety measures. Suggestions that can help patients prevent falls are:

- Have regular hearing and vision tests.
- Understand the side effects of medications, especially those that cause vertigo.
- If you experience orthostatic hypotension, rise slowly and stand still for a moment with support before moving.
- Limit the use of alcohol.
- If needed, consistently use assistive devices, such as a cane or walker, for support.
- Wear low-heeled, rubber-soled shoes with good support.
- Avoid going outside in icy weather.
- Engage in regular weight-bearing exercise for muscle and bone strength.
- Keep hallways, stairs, and bathrooms well lit.
- Assess the home for possible danger areas; remove throw rugs; use handrails on steps and grab bars in bathrooms; keep emergency numbers handy.

CRITICAL THINKING APPLICATION   48-3

The family of Rita Schaeffer, a 73-year-old patient, is concerned about the risk of falls. Mrs. Schaeffer recently was diagnosed with osteoporosis, and she lives alone. What information should Bill give the family to help them prevent accidents in their mother's home? Also, Mrs. Schaeffer's 43-year-old daughter is concerned about developing osteoporosis. What steps should the daughter take to prevent the disease?

Nervous System

Cognitive ability, the ability of a person to think, is influenced by many factors, including a person's general state of health, educational background, and genetic code. The normal process of aging may contribute to a change in the thinking process. The brain begins to get smaller at approximately age 50 and continues to do so as we age because of a loss of fluid within the neurons and the shrinkage of dendrites. Thinning of the dendrites makes transmitting messages from one neuron to the next more difficult. As a result of all of these factors, the aging brain weighs less, is smaller, and has started to pull away from the sheath or cortical mantle. Older neurons process information more slowly, so retrieving old information and learning new information takes longer. Reaction time also slows, and aging individuals are distracted more easily; however, recent research shows that the loss of brain cells is minimal and that the older brain is still capable of generating new neurons. Researchers believe that continued, moderate physical and mental activity can maintain the cognitive abilities of aging individuals.

Dementia, the severe loss of intellectual ability, is not an inevitable part of aging but rather the result of an organic disorder. Most men and women remain mentally competent until the end of their lives. Sudden loss of memory, disorientation, and trouble performing the daily tasks of life indicate a problem that should be investigated. Many conditions can cause signs and symptoms of dementia, including depression; reactions to prescription and over-the-counter drugs; alcoholism; malnutrition; thyroid, liver, heart, and vascular disorders; and Parkinson's disease. Multiple factors can interfere with mental judgment and motor skills, giving the impression of decreased mental status.

The best way to ensure mental functioning in later life is to remain mentally and physically stimulated. Exercise improves memory and thinking because of its positive effect on vascular health, increasing the amount of oxygen delivered to the aging brain. Other ways to maintain mental function are to keep socially active; practice stress-reduction activities; quit smoking; drink alcohol in moderation; use hearing aids and glasses if needed to stay in touch with the world; and receive treatment for depression, diabetes, hypertension, and high cholesterol levels. Risk factors for cognitive decline include:

- Hypertension, diabetes, and heart disease (these reduce blood flow to the brain)
- Environmental exposure to lead
- High stress levels
- Sedentary lifestyle and lack of social interaction
- Low education level
- Smoking and substance abuse

One of the most frequently used screening tools for dementia is the Mini-Mental State Examination, a 5-minute test designed to evaluate basic mental function in a number of different areas. The test assesses the patient's ability to recall facts, write, and calculate numbers. It gives the physician a quick way to determine whether more in-depth testing is needed. Each area of the examination is given a score, and these scores show whether the person is functioning within the expected range for his or her age (Figure 48-2). The medical assistant may be expected to administer this examination.

Alzheimer's Disease

Alzheimer's disease (AD) is a progressive deterioration of the brain caused by the destruction of central nervous system (CNS) neurons, leading to problems with memory, language, thinking, and behavior. Cellular destruction is related to the buildup of amyloid plaques and neurofibrillary tangles in the brain. Patients who show signs and symptoms of dementia are first evaluated for organic causes, such as systemic disease or depression. AD has no definitive diagnostic test because it can be confirmed only through examination of the brain at autopsy. If the patient shows a gradual onset of progressive difficulty with memory, functional abilities, and behavior and has no evidence of other causes of these disturbances, the physician makes the diagnosis of AD. Imaging studies, including computed tomography (CT), magnetic resonance imaging (MRI), and positron emission tomography (PET), may help show the structural and functional changes in the brain that are associated with Alzheimer's disease.

Researchers believe that as many as 5.4 million Americans suffer from AD. The disease typically begins after age 60, and the risk of developing the disorder increases with age, although younger people can be diagnosed with AD. An estimated 5% of people age 65 to 74 have AD, and almost half of people age 85 or older are diagnosed with the disease. Despite these statistics, AD is not considered a normal part of the aging process. Alzheimer's disease is the seventh leading cause of death (across all ages) in the United States and the fifth leading cause of death for those age 65 or older.

SIGNS AND SYMPTOMS OF ALZHEIMER'S DISEASE

- Repeatedly asking the same questions
- Inability to remember common words or mixing up words when describing something
- Inability to complete simple tasks and misplacing items
- Becoming lost when driving familiar routes
- Sudden mood swings for no apparent reason
- Difficulty following simple directions

AD is a slowly progressive disease that begins with mild memory problems and ends with severe brain damage. The course the disease takes and how fast changes occur varies among individuals, but on average, patients live for 8 to 10 years after they are diagnosed. Currently, no treatment can stop the progression of the disease. However, a great deal of research on the diagnosis and treatment of AD is underway.

STAGES OF ALZHEIMER'S DISEASE

- *First stage—Mild AD:* Occurs during the 2 to 4 years leading up to diagnosis; memory loss affects job performance; confusion and disorientation are common. Patient experiences mood or personality changes, difficulty making decisions, and paying bills; gets lost easily; withdraws from others; loses things.
- *Second stage—Moderate AD:* Lasts 2 to 10 years after diagnosis; increased memory loss and confusion, shorter attention span, restlessness. Patient makes constant repetitive statements; has problems with reading, writing, and numbers; may be irritable or suspicious; experiences motor problems; has difficulty recognizing close friends and family members.
- *Terminal stage—Severe AD:* Lasts 1 to 3 years. Patient does not recognize family; experiences weight loss; is unable to care for self; is incontinent of bladder and bowel; requires complete care.

Patient _____   Examiner _____   Date _____

Maximum Score	Score	
		Orientation
5	( )	What is the (year) (season) (date) (day) (month)?
5	( )	Where are we: (state) (county) (town) (hospital) (floor)
		Registration
3	( )	Name three objects: (Apple, Penny, Table) 1 second to say each. Then ask the patient all three after you have said them. Give 1 point for each correct answer. Then repeat them until he or she learns all three. Count trials and record.

Trials _____

		Attention and Calculation
5	( )	Serial 7's. 1 point for each correct. Stop after five answers. Alternatively spell "world" backwards.
		Recall
3	( )	Ask for the three objects repeated above. Give 1 point for each correct.
		Language
9	( )	Name a pencil, and watch (2 points)

Overlapping pentagons

Repeat the following "No ifs, ands, or buts." (1 point)
Follow a three-stage command:
"Take a paper in your right hand, fold it in half, and put it on the floor." (3 points)
Read and obey the following:
CLOSE YOUR EYES (1 point)
Write a sentence (1 point)
Copy design (overlapping pentagons) (1 point)
Total Score
ASSESS level of consciousness along a continuum _____

Alert   Drowsy   Stupor   Coma

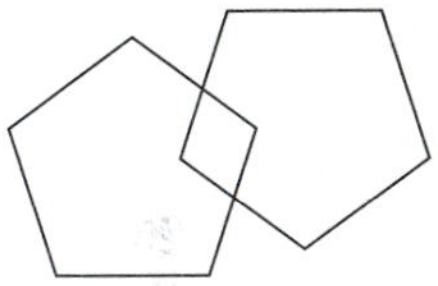

Instructions for Administration of Mini-Mental State Examination

Orientation

(1) Ask for the date. Then ask specifically for parts omitted, e.g., "Can you also tell me what season it is?" One point for each correct.
(2) Ask in turn "Can you tell me the name of this hospital?" (town, country, etc.). One point for each correct.

Registration

Ask the patient if you may test his or her memory. Then say the names of three unrelated objects, clearly and slowly, about 1 second for each. After you have said all three, ask him or her to repeat them. This first repetition determines his or her score (0–3), but keep saying them until he or she can repeat all three, up to six trials. If he or she does not eventually learn all three, recall cannot be meaningfully tested.

Attention and Calculation

Ask the patient to begin with 100 and count backwards by 7. Stop after five subtractions (93, 86, 79, 72, 65). Score the total number of correct answers.
If the patient cannot or will not perform this task, ask him or her to spell the word "world" backwards. The score is the number of letters in correct order, e.g., dlrow = 5, dlorw = 3.

Recall

Ask the patient if he or she can recall the three words you previously asked him or her to remember. Score 0–3.

Language

Naming: Show the patient a wrist watch and ask him or her what it is. Repeat for pencil. Score 0–2.
Repetition: Ask the patient to repeat the sentence after you. Allow only one trial. Score 0 or 1.
Three-stage command: Give the patient a piece of plain blank paper and repeat the command. Score 1 point for each part correctly executed.
Reading: On a blank piece of paper print the sentence "Close your eyes," in letters large enough for the patient to see clearly. Ask him or her to read it and do what it says. Score 1 point only if he or she actually closes his or her eyes.
Writing: Give the patient a blank piece of paper and ask him or her to write a sentence for you. Do not dictate a sentence, it is to be written spontaneously. It must contain a subject and verb and be sensible. Correct grammar and punctuation are not necessary.
Copying: On a clean piece of paper, draw intersecting pentagons, each side about 1 inch, and ask him or her to copy it exactly as it is. All 10 angles must be present, and 2 must intersect to score 1 point. Tremor and rotation are ignored.
Estimate the patient's level of sensorium along a continuum, from alert on the left to coma on the right.

FIGURE 48-2 Mini-Mental State Examination. (Redrawn from Folstein M et al: Mini mental state, *J Psychiatry Res* 12:196, 1975.)

The goal of treatment is to maintain normal activities as long as possible. Cholinesterase inhibitors may be prescribed to improve the production of neurotransmitters in the brain. These drugs include donepezil (Aricept), rivastigmine (Exelon), galantamine (Reminyl), and tacrine (Cognex) to help prevent memory loss from becoming worse for a limited time. However, these drugs do not help everyone; as many as 50% of patients show no improvement in mental function. Memantine (Namenda) is the first drug to be approved for the treatment of moderate to severe AD, although it, also, has limited effects. Individuals with AD frequently experience changes in behavior, so medications may be prescribed to help control sleeplessness, agitation, wandering, anxiety, and depression. Treating these problems helps make the patient more comfortable while easing the burden on caregivers.

Supportive care for family members is absolutely essential, because they are faced with caring for a loved one who is suffering progressive memory loss. The medical assistant can be especially helpful in recommending educational workshops, support groups, and stress management skills for caregivers. Multiple resources are available, including online information and support groups, which family members may find helpful.

CRITICAL THINKING APPLICATION   48-4

Maria Angelone, an 86-year-old patient of Dr. Kennedy's, is in the second stage of AD. Her husband and children are showing signs of stress from the continuous care Mrs. Angelone requires. Her family still does not understand what is happening to her and what to expect in the future. What information can Bill share with them about the disease, and what resources could be helpful to the family in dealing with the stress of caring for a loved one with dementia?

Pulmonary System

Maximum lung function decreases with age. The rate of airflow through the bronchi slowly declines after age 30, and the maximum force one is able to achieve on inspiration and expiration declines. The lungs lose their elasticity because of changes in **elastin** and collagen. They become smaller and flabbier. The alveoli enlarge, their walls become thinner, and the number of capillaries is reduced. As a result, the effective area for gas exchange in the lungs is reduced. The chest wall may stiffen from osteoporosis of the ribs and vertebrae and calcification of the **costal** cartilage. The respiratory muscles become weaker, making it harder to move air into and out of the lungs. To compensate, older adults rely more on accessory muscles, such as the diaphragm. Weakening of the respiratory muscles and stiffening of the chest wall make it harder to cough deeply enough to clear mucus from the lungs. Pulmonary function tests reveal a decrease in vital capacity and an increase in residual volume. The incidence of sleep apnea and sleep disorders increases, causing a potential problem with nocturnal hypoxemia. All these factors combine to put the older adult at greater risk for pneumonia and aspiration and for reactivation of tuberculosis.

The larynx also changes with aging, causing a change in the pitch and quality of the voice. The voice sounds quieter and slightly hoarse. The individual's voice may sound weaker, but it should not interfere with the ability to communicate effectively.

Sensory Organs

Vision

By the time a person reaches age 50, structural and functional changes in the eye become noticeable (Table 48-3). The eyebrows and eyelashes start to gray. The skin around the eyelids wrinkles, and the loss of orbital fat allows the eye to sink deeper into the orbit. The cornea increases in thickness and has reduced refractive power. A yellow-gray ring (arcus senilis) may develop on the periphery of the cornea. The iris loses pigmentation, and as a result most older people appear to have gray eyes.

The lens of the eye continues to grow. As new lens fibers grow, old lens fibers are compressed and pushed to the center, causing the lens to become denser. The lens becomes flatter, thicker, less elastic, and more opaque, progressively yellowing with age. By age 70, the lens has tripled in mass. Clouding of the lens causes light rays to scatter, creating glare.

The pupil is designed to adjust to control the amount of light entering the eye. The ciliary muscle that causes the pupil to dilate weakens during the aging process. As a result, a reduction in the size of the pupil occurs, limiting the amount of light available to reach the retina. Tear production normally decreases. Tear glands do not make enough tears, or the tears are of poor quality and do not keep the eyes wet enough. Eye irritation and excessive tearing are a result of decreased **lacrimation**.

During the fourth decade of life, presbyopia develops, which makes it difficult to focus on detailed objects close at hand. This requires the use of corrective lenses to accommodate age-related farsightedness. The ability to refocus quickly from far to near or

---

TABLE 48-3   Age-Related Changes in the Anatomic Structures of the Eye

STRUCTURE	AGE-RELATED CHANGE	EFFECTS
Lens	Thickens, becomes more opaque	Decreased refraction, causing blurred vision; decreased color acuity; cataracts
Anterior chamber	Decrease in size and volume	May develop increased intraocular pressure and glaucoma
Ciliary muscles	Affects pupil constriction and dilation	Limits light accommodation; night blindness
Cornea	Thickens, curve decreases	Problems with refraction
Retina	Decrease in number of rods and nerves	Decreased clarity; requires increase in minimum amount of light needed to see clearly

near to far decreases. Also, the ability to follow a moving object is decreased. The yellowing of the lens causes it to act like a filter, making it difficult to distinguish certain color intensities. Blues, greens, and violets are hard to differentiate, whereas yellows, reds, and oranges are easier to identify. The loss in the ability to discriminate closely related colors can affect the older person's ability to judge distances or his or her depth perception. This increases an aging person's susceptibility to falls and accidents. Stairs become a potential hazard because the edges of the steps cannot be seen clearly.

Older people need as much as six times more light to read; however, increasing the level of light does not completely compensate for visual decline, because the elderly also experience an increased sensitivity to glare. Glare is probably one of the most painful experiences for the aging eye. Exposed light bulbs, such as those used in chandeliers, and light from highly reflective surfaces, such as glass tables and floors, can produce excessive glare. The eye has a decreased ability to respond to abrupt changes from light to dark or dark to light. Going from a well-lit waiting room into a dim hallway or negotiating the way down dimly lit aisles in a movie theater could be treacherous for an older person.

Cataracts, Glaucoma, and Macular Degeneration. Eye diseases and disorders that occur frequently in older individuals are cataracts, glaucoma, and macular degeneration. Cataracts are cloudy or opaque areas in the lens that cause blurring of vision; rings or halos around lights and objects; and a blue or yellow tint to the visual field. Surgical lens extraction and implantation with an artificial lens improves vision in 95% of the cases. The procedure is performed in an outpatient facility using a small incision to remove the lens, laser therapy, or phacoemulsification (ultrasonic vibrations), which breaks up the lens and removes it without the need for an incision. Postoperatively patients must avoid bending or lifting heavy objects for 3 to 4 weeks; wearing an eye shield at night and glasses during the day helps protect the eye until it heals.

Glaucoma is a result of blockage of the outflow of aqueous humor, which causes an increase in intraocular pressure and damage to the optic nerve. If not treated, glaucoma can cause progressive loss of peripheral vision and ultimately lead to blindness; however, it can be treated with medication.

The macula is the part of the eye responsible for sharp vision and color. Damage to or breakdown of the macula is called *macular degeneration,* which causes progressive loss of the central field of vision. Macular degeneration is the leading cause of blindness in aging people, and at this time there is no effective treatment or cure. (All three of these eye disorders are discussed in more detail in Chapter 37.)

SUGGESTIONS FOR HELPING THE VISUALLY IMPAIRED OLDER ADULT

- When escorting an older person, regardless of whether he or she is visually impaired, allow the patient to place his or her hand above your elbow. It is easier for the person to follow your movements. This method also provides a source of support and security.
- Use high levels of evenly distributed, glare-free light.

- Ask the pharmacist to use large lettering when labeling medicine bottles.
- Use paper that has a nonglare finish and large print for forms and educational materials.
- Make distinct differences (e.g., size of containers or color coding with bright primary colors) for pills that are similar in size and color.
- Place all objects within the visual field and prevent clutter.

Hearing

Hearing loss can have a profound psychological effect on aging people, causing depression, social withdrawal, and feelings of isolation. Hearing loss occurs gradually over a long period and may go undetected by the older person and healthcare providers. Lack of attention when addressed, inappropriate responses, asking to have statements repeated, and speaking too loudly or too softly often are signs of hearing loss. Changes in auditory ability begin around age 30; by age 65, 25% have a hearing impairment, and the number increases to 65% of those over age 80. Age-related hearing loss usually is caused by a dysfunction or loss of cochlear cilia, resulting in an inability to hear high-frequency sounds and difficulty understanding speech. Hearing impairment is compounded by impacted cerumen, otitis media, otosclerosis, Ménière's disease, long-term exposure to intense noise, and certain ototoxic drugs, such as aspirin.

Presbycusis (see Chapter 37) is associated with normal aging and causes a decreased ability to hear high frequencies and to discriminate sounds. Parts of a conversation may be missed because the sound of the word goes above the 2000-cycle frequency. Often words that sound similar are difficult to differentiate. Consonants such as *g, f, s, sh, t,* and *z* produce high-pitched sounds that are more difficult to hear and differentiate. Low-frequency pitched sounds, such as the vowels *a, e, i, o,* and *u,* may be more easily heard by people with presbycusis. Inability to hear different frequencies combined with low background noise from groups of people talking, noise from appliances, or busy public places compromises an older person's ability to hear clearly. Hearing aids, which can be used to amplify speech, may increase background noises, resulting in sensory overload.

Another hearing disorder common among older people is tinnitus, a ringing or buzzing in the ear. It can be caused by impacted cerumen, an ear infection, use of antibiotics, a reaction to a medication, or a nerve disorder. Tinnitus can cause difficulty understanding conversational speech and can make sleeping difficult because of the continuous sensation of ringing in the ears.

Hearing loss, with its resultant isolation, is directly related to the development of depression in older adults. Treatable depression often is overlooked in elderly people because of coexisting physical illnesses that mask the symptoms of depression. The medical assistant may be able to contribute to information about depression in elderly patients through conversations with the individual and family members. The physician may use or may train the medical assistant to use the Geriatric Depression Scale short form, which includes questions for the patient about daily activities, interests, and feelings to help diagnose depression in the ambulatory setting (Figure 48-3).

GERIATRIC DEPRESSION SCALE (SHORT FORM)

Choose the best answer for how you have felt over the past week:

1. Are you basically satisfied with your life? YES / **NO**
2. Have you dropped many of your activities and interests? **YES** / NO
3. Do you feel that your life is empty? **YES** / NO
4. Do you often get bored? **YES** / NO
5. Are you in good spirits most of the time? YES / **NO**
6. Are you afraid that something bad is going to happen to you? **YES** / NO
7. Do you feel happy most of the time? YES / **NO**
8. Do you often feel helpless? **YES** / NO
9. Do you prefer to stay at home, rather than going out and doing new things? **YES** / NO
10. Do you feel you have more problems with memory than most? **YES** / NO
11. Do you think it is wonderful to be alive now? YES / **NO**
12. Do you feel pretty worthless the way you are now? **YES** / NO
13. Do you feel full of energy? YES / **NO**
14. Do you feel that your situation is hopeless? **YES** / NO
15. Do you think that most people are better off than you are? **YES** / NO

Answers in **bold** indicate depression. Although differing sensitivities and specificities have been obtained across studies, for clinical purposes a score >5 points is suggestive of depression and should warrant a follow-up interview. Scores >10 are almost always depression.

FIGURE 48-3 Geriatric Depression Scale.

SUGGESTIONS FOR HELPING THE HEARING-IMPAIRED OLDER ADULT

- Stand in the patient's direct line of vision and gently touch the person to get his or her attention.
- Use gestures, pictures, and large, bold print to communicate.
- Talk in short sentences into the ear with better hearing.
- Do not increase the volume of your speech; this also raises the frequency of the voice, which is the hearing most impaired in aging people. Use expanded speech; lower the tone of your voice and talk in distinct syllables.
- Avoid background noise. Give instructions in a quiet room with the door closed. If the patient has a hearing aid, make sure it is on.

Taste and Smell

During the aging process the abilities to taste and smell decline subtly. Deterioration and atrophy of the taste buds are part of the aging process. The ability to taste salt and sweet flavors is reduced, whereas the ability to detect bitter and sour flavors remains relatively the same. As a result, food frequently tastes bland and unappetizing. Patients on salt-restricted diets and patients with diabetes must be cautioned about the use of excessive amounts of salt and sugar. A decrease in the sense of smell accompanies the decrease in taste. Not only does this affect the individual's enjoyment of food; it also exposes the person to environmental dangers, such as gas leaks, smoke, and other dangerous odors that may go undetected. Checking for gas leaks around stoves and heaters and using smoke alarms reduce some of the danger. Also, dating food when it is put in the refrigerator is a good idea.

Nutritional Status. Because of the many environmental, social, economic, and physical changes of aging, older people are at greater risk for poor nutrition, which can adversely affect their health and energy level. It is estimated that 25% of the aging population suffers from malnutrition. Nutrition screening should be part of routine primary care to identify nutritional deficiencies and correct them before a disease process develops or to assist in the treatment of chronic disease. Patients with chronic conditions, such as cardiovascular disease, hypertension, and diabetes, can benefit from nutrition assessments and interventions. Malnourished older patients get more infections; their injuries take longer to heal; surgery is riskier for them; and their hospital stays are longer and more expensive.

The most effective method of assessing a patient's nutritional status is through a comprehensive patient interview that considers all potential stumbling blocks to adequate nutrition. The medical assistant can help determine the nutritional status of older patients by considering the following factors when conducting patient interviews.

- *Oral health:* Does the patient wear dentures and if so, do they fit properly? Does the patient have mouth pain? Can he or she swallow without difficulty?
- *Gastrointestinal complaints:* Does the patient have anorexia, nausea, vomiting, diarrhea, or constipation? Is the patient lactose intolerant (the incidence increases with age)?
- *Sensorimotor changes:* Does the patient have loss of vision or hearing or changes in taste and smell? Can the patient feed herself or himself? Does the patient need adaptive utensils?
- *Diet influences:* Can the patient afford, shop for, and prepare food? Are ethnic or religious influences a factor? Does the patient have any disease-related diet restrictions? What is the patient's alcohol consumption?
- *Social and mental influences:* Is the patient depressed, lonely, or isolated? Are support systems available?

CRITICAL THINKING APPLICATION   48-5

Multiple sensory changes occur as people age. Dr. Kennedy asks Bill to develop a handout for patients and family members to help them understand these normal, age-related sensorimotor changes and also adaptations that can improve communication. What information should Bill include?

Urinary System

As the body ages, structural changes in the kidneys cause the urinary system to become less efficient. Between the ages of 40 and 80, the kidney loses about 20% of its mass. The number of functional nephron units decreases. Blood flow to the kidneys is reduced because of a decrease in cardiovascular efficiency. Because of the reduction of blood flow to the kidneys and the decreased number of nephrons, the kidneys become less efficient at filtering waste from the blood. This results in a more diluted, less concentrated urine.

The kidneys require more water to excrete the same amount of waste. Medication takes longer to be removed from the body. Older adults are at increased risk for toxic levels of medication in the bloodstream because of this reduced filtration rate.

Fibrous connective tissue replaces the smooth muscle and elastic tissue in the bladder. This thickening of the bladder wall reduces the bladder's ability to expand. The bladder's capacity to store fluid comfortably is reduced from 400 to 250 mL. These structural changes lead to increased frequency of urination and urinary retention. Older adults are at increased risk of urinary tract infections because of residual urine. Sleep is interrupted by the need to void during the night. The sensation of bladder fullness is not recognized as quickly by the older brain. Reduced time between awareness of the need to void and involuntary urination can cause anxiety. Often older adults reduce their fluid intake to prevent possible embarrassment. Unfortunately, this causes dehydration and an increased risk of urinary tract infections. Another change is loss of muscle tone in the urethra. In addition, the pelvic floor muscles in an aging woman relax as a result of decreased estrogen levels or previous pregnancy and childbirth.

Despite these changes, the kidneys have great reserve capacity and are able to continue functioning normally. Urinary incontinence, the involuntary loss of urine, is a significant problem for aging patients but is not a normal part of the aging process. Changes in the urinary system make older people more vulnerable to incontinence, but factors such as infection, confusion, difficulty with mobility, and side effects of medications contribute to the development of the problem. Incontinence is both an emotional and a physical problem. To avoid the risk of an embarrassing accident, people with this problem may avoid social occasions or activities they enjoy. Often people are too embarrassed to admit they have this condition, or they believe it is just part of aging. Once the condition has been diagnosed by a urologist, pelvic floor muscle exercises, medication, or surgery may be recommended.

Reproductive System

Menopause is discussed in Chapter 41. Aging brings a decrease in circulating levels of the female hormones estrogen and progesterone, whereas androgen levels increase. The results of this decrease are changes in the genital tract. The vagina diminishes in width and length and becomes less elastic. The cervix, uterus, and ovaries decrease in size. Vaginal secretions decline; therefore, lubrication diminishes, resulting in vaginal dryness. Bacterial or yeast infections may occur because vaginal secretions are less acidic. Estrogen cream applied to vaginal tissue may be prescribed by the physician for help with dryness and thinning of the vaginal tissue. The patient should discuss the benefits and risks of estrogen replacement therapy with the physician to determine whether it should be used.

Even though sperm production may decline in men over age 50, men remain virile well into old age. However, they experience a change in hormonal levels of testosterone, and these changes can affect the prostate gland (see Chapter 40). The prostate enlarges over time and presses down on the urethra, causing difficulty with urination. Surgery may be required to remove excess portions of the gland. Unfortunately, the operation may cause impotence, which can be treated medically with erectile dysfunction medications.

Men experience some changes in sexual functioning as they age. It takes longer for the penis to become erect, longer for an orgasm to occur, and longer to recover. Direct stimulation may be required before an erection occurs, and when it does, it may be less firm than in younger years.

Some drugs and illnesses can interfere with sexual function. Drugs used to control high blood pressure, antihistamines, antidepressants, and some stomach acid blockers, in addition to the diseases diabetes, arthritis, and arteriosclerosis, can have an adverse effect on sexual function. Often people who have had heart surgery or a heart attack are concerned about sexual activity. Patients need to feel comfortable and should not be embarrassed to discuss their concerns openly with their physician. It is important for healthcare providers to dismiss the myth that older patients have lost the desire for and interest in sexual intercourse.

Sleep Disorders

Complaints of sleeping difficulties increase with age. The amount of time spent sleeping may be slightly longer than in a younger person, but the quality of sleep declines. Older people often are light sleepers and have periods of wakefulness in bed. Rapid eye movement (REM) sleep is the stage of sleep when people experience dreaming. Non-REM sleep is the period of deepest sleep. The amount of time spent in the deepest stages of sleep decreases with age. Sleep that is disturbed or that leaves the person feeling tired is not part of the aging process and may indicate some underlying emotional or physical problem. Lack of sleep can result in restlessness, disorientation, "thick" speech, and mispronounced words. Often these symptoms are mistaken as signs of dementia. Other factors that might influence sleep patterns are medications, caffeine, alcohol, depression, and environmental or physical changes.

Common sleep problems in older adults include dyssomnias, such as periodic limb movement disorder (PLMD), in which periodic jerking of the legs occurs during sleep, and sleep apnea, which is common among overweight individuals and can occur frequently during the night, interrupting sleep. Numerous medical conditions can interfere with sleep, including joint and bone pain; Parkinson's disease (because of difficulty changing positions); CHF; chronic obstructive pulmonary disease; diabetes mellitus, which increases nocturia; depression; and certain medications (e.g., beta blockers can cause nightmares, antidepressants increase PLMD, and barbiturates may result in nightmares or hallucinations).

It is important to be aware of the effect of sleep problems because often these can be confused with dementia. Patients who are experiencing difficulty with sleeping should be encouraged to document their sleeping patterns, napping patterns, medications, diet, exercise routines, and any events that have resulted in a change of lifestyle. They should discuss this problem with their physician. Simple modification of behavioral patterns may resolve the problem. Taking fewer naps, completing exercise several hours before bedtime, changing eating times, reducing the amount of alcohol and caffeine ingested, drinking a glass of milk before bedtime, or changing medications or the time they are taken all are suggestions that might alter the factors responsible for sleep disturbances.

If behavioral approaches are not effective, medications may be considered for short-term use only, because they have a high incidence of physical and psychological dependence. Elderly people are especially susceptible to side effects from these drugs, such as next-day drowsiness and temporary memory loss. Sedatives or hypnotics that may be prescribed include zolpidem (Ambien), eszopiclone (Lunesta), zaleplon (Sonata), and temazepam (Restoril).

Living Arrangements

At any given time, only 5% of the elderly population lives in long-term care facilities. According to information published by the National Institute on Aging, most older people live close to their children and are in frequent contact with them. People prefer to age in place; that is, they want to live in their own home environment as long as possible. Individuals are admitted to nursing homes because they are no longer able to perform activities of daily living, such as bathing, dressing, eating, walking, and maintaining bladder and bowel continence. They also have difficulty with grocery shopping, housekeeping, and money management. Chronic health conditions and accidents interfere with the older person's ability to perform these tasks.

Many resources are available to help seniors to maintain their independence. Outreach programs, such as Meals on Wheels, deliver nutritious meals to the homes of older adults. Senior centers serve as a focal point for many activities and as a source of information. Transportation services provide rides to doctors' appointments, day care centers, shopping centers, and community events. Home health agencies provide several types of services, including personal care, shopping, transportation, and meal preparation. Some home health agencies provide a range of activities, from patient education to IV therapy; medical-social services; physical, speech, and occupational therapies; and nutrition and dietary counseling. Advanced technology allows people to receive services at home that formerly were provided only at a hospital or a physician's office.

Adult day care centers provide socialization, recreation, meals and, in some centers, physical therapy, occupational therapy, and transportation. These centers offer supervision for older adults who may be taken care of by family members in the evening but need care during the day. They also serve as respite for a caregiver.

Assisted-living facilities can be retirement homes or board and care homes. These facilities are appropriate for older adults who need assistance with some activities of daily living, such as bathing, dressing, and walking. Skilled nursing facilities provide 24-hour medical care and supervision. In addition to medical care, residents receive care that may include physical, occupational, and speech therapies. The objective of treatment is to improve or maintain the person's abilities.

THE MEDICAL ASSISTANT'S ROLE IN CARING FOR THE OLDER PATIENT

Elderly patients in the ambulatory care setting present a specific set of needs that require a certain amount of accommodation by the staff. For example, aging patients typically require more time to perform tasks and have questions answered. The office staff may want to hurry them so that the day's schedule can be maintained. In the best interests of the patient, however, he or she should be treated with respect and given whatever time is needed to prepare for examinations, ask questions and receive answers, and have procedures explained. A system that is sensitive to the needs of older patients schedules longer periods for appointments; has adequate lighting in the waiting room; provides forms in large print; has an examination room equipped with furniture, magazines, and treatment folders especially designed for older adults; and invites a professional in the management of older patients for in-service training.

The primary issue in elder care is effective communication. How you communicate with people is often influenced by what you know or do not know about them. Older people are subject to many changes that affect how they are able to interact with their environment. It is important to recognize these changes and to investigate one's personal perception of older people to break down the barriers that prohibit effective communication.

As people age, they frequently experience a loss of control over their lives because of physical disabilities, economic constraints, and institutional living. Part of our job is to help aging people maintain their dignity and independence while in the ambulatory care setting. Remember, each patient, regardless of his or her education, socioeconomic status, or age, deserves to be treated with compassion and respect. Ask the patient directly what is wrong rather than discussing the patient with family members. It also is important to listen carefully and to be specific and sincere when responding. When a patient is talking, take time to allow him or her to complete the sentence; do not finish it for the person. Give the patient your full attention rather than continuing with other tasks while he or she is speaking. Older people may take a little longer to process information, but they are capable of understanding. Do not hurry through explanations or questions; rather, take time to review a form or give instructions as needed.

SUGGESTIONS FOR EFFECTIVE COMMUNICATION WITH AGING PATIENTS

- Address the patient by Mr., Mrs., or Miss unless the patient has given you permission to use his or her first name.
- Introduce yourself and explain the purpose of a procedure before performing the procedure.
- Face the aging person and softly touch the individual to get his or her attention before beginning to speak.
- Use expanded speech, gestures, demonstrations, or written instructions in block print.
- If the message must be repeated, paraphrase or find other words to say the same thing.
- Observe the patient's nonverbal behavior for cues indicating whether he or she understands.
- Provide adequate lighting without glare.
- Allow patients time to process information and take care of themselves unless they ask for assistance.
- Conduct communication in a quiet room without distractions.
- Involve family members as needed for continuity of care.
- When leaving a telephone message, remember to speak slowly and clearly and repeat the message in the same manner. It is difficult to interpret a message, and even more difficult to write it down, if the message was delivered in a hurried manner.
- Use referrals and community resources for support, such as the following:
  - Alzheimer's Association (1-800-272-3900)
  - American Council of the Blind (1-800-424-8666) — provides referrals to state and other organizations that provide services and equipment for the blind

- American Speech-Language-Hearing Association (1-800-638-8255)—offers information on hearing aids, hearing loss, and communication problems in older people and provides a list of certified audiologist and speech pathologists.
- Arthritis Foundation Information Line (1-800-283-7800)—makes referrals to local chapters and provides information
- Eldercare Locator (1-800-677-1116)—run by the National Association of Area Agencies on Aging; help line provides information on contacting local chapters that oversee services to older adults
- National Institute on Aging Information Center (1-800-222-2225)—provides information on geriatric health issues
- National Meals-on-Wheels Foundation (1-800-999-6262)
- Hospice Helpline (1-800-658-8898)—provides information about hospice care and makes referrals to local hospices

---

CRITICAL THINKING APPLICATION 48-6

New staff members in the practice are complaining of having to repeat information to older patients, who they say do not pay attention when procedures are explained. Dr. Kennedy has decided to invite a gerontologist from the local university to present an in-service workshop on healthy aging. She asks Bill to coordinate the in-service workshop and prepare materials requested by the guest speaker. What information about caring for the ambulatory aging patient should be included in the workshop?

CLOSING COMMENTS

Patient Education

The medical assistant must keep the sensorimotor changes that accompany aging and respectful patient communication in mind when conducting patient education with older patients. Remember, the aging process does not affect a person's ability to learn; it just may take longer to process the information, and the material may need to be repeated for understanding. Showing sensitivity to the needs of aging learners ensures successful patient education and improves compliance with prescribed treatment plans. The current aging population generally is respectful toward authority; therefore, if the medical assistant cannot gain the patient's cooperation, the physician may be able to provide authoritative reinforcement of material. General guidelines for effective patient education with older adults include the following:

- The patient may have short-term memory loss, so you may need to repeat the information using different words.
- The patient may be distracted more easily, so learning in a group may be difficult.
- The patient may take longer to process information, so teach at a pace that matches the patient's needs.
- Provide the patient with handouts that have large print and block letters for reviewing information at home.
- Involve family members as needed for continuity of care.

Legal and Ethical Issues

All patients have the right to know about the medications, treatments, and alternatives available to them. The Patients' Bill of Rights (see Chapter 7) informs the patient of those rights in a healthcare setting. They include the right to privacy about personal and medical information and the right to informed consent, which holds the physician accountable for explaining clearly the advantages and risks of any procedures, tests, or treatments. The patient must give permission for medical care and has the right to refuse treatment. The patient has the right to be informed about his or her condition and treatment and the chances of recovery. The patient also has the right to have advance directives explained to him or her.

Consent must be given by the individual undergoing the procedure as long as he or she is judged to be competent; that is, as long as the patient is able to understand the consequences of the procedure. In an emergency situation or if a court has ruled that the patient is incompetent, someone else must give consent. This may be a person who already was designated to hold the durable power of attorney, a close family member (spouse, adult child, parent, sibling), or a court-appointed guardian.

Most states have legal documents available that provide written instructions specifying the type of medical care a person wants in the event she or he becomes incapacitated; these are called *advance directives.* The document designates a person who has a durable power of attorney; this is an authorization for making medical decisions on an individual's behalf if he or she is unable to make treatment decisions. The document provides a list of specific instructions for the proxy to follow.

Various issues may be covered in these documents. A "do not resuscitate" (DNR) order allows a patient to refuse attempts to restore a heartbeat. The patient also may decide to withdraw life-sustaining treatment, such as respirators or feeding tubes. A copy of the directive should be kept on file as part of the patient's medical record. It is important to check the laws of the state in which you practice with regard to advance directives, because they vary from state to state (Figure 48-4).

Another legal issue in the care of aging patients is the possibility of elder abuse. Mistreatment of aging people occurs at all social, racial, and economic levels. The abuse may be physical, mental, sexual, material, or financial; it may involve neglect or failure to provide adequate care, or it may involve self-neglect when aging people are unable or refuse to care for themselves. Abuse of elders by their caregivers may be difficult to identify. The aging victim could feel embarrassed, guilty, or afraid to report the abuse. Indications that a patient may be a victim of elder abuse are:

- Poor general appearance and poor hygiene
- Pattern of changing doctors and frequent emergency department visits
- Skin lesions, signs of dehydration, bruises (signs of new and old bruising together), abrasions, welts, burns, or pressure sores
- Recurrent injuries caused by accidents
- Signs of malnutrition and weight loss without related illness
- Any injury that does not fit the given history

If abuse is suspected, interviewing the caregiver and questioning the demands of care and self-reported perceptions of stress levels may help the physician detect the problem. Many states now have laws that require reporting of suspected elder abuse. Check your state laws to determine the requirements for healthcare workers.

Directive made this _____ th day of _____ in the year _____ .
                          (day)   (month)   (year)

I, _____ , being of sound mind, willfully and voluntarily make known my desire that my life shall not be artificially prolonged under the circumstances set forth in this directive.

If at any time I should have

— an incurable or irreversible condition caused by injury,
— disease,
— or illness certified to be a terminal condition by two physicians

and if the application of life-sustaining procedures would serve only to artificially postpone the moment of my death, and if my attending physician determines that my death is imminent or will result within a relatively short time without the application of life-sustaining procedures. I direct that those procedures be withheld or withdrawn, and that I be permitted to die naturally.

In the absence of my ability to give directions regarding the use of those life-sustaining procedures, it is my intention that this directive be honored by my family and physicians as the final expression of my legal right to refuse medical or surgical treatment and accept the consequences from that refusal.

If I have been diagnosed as pregnant and that diagnosis is known to my physician, this directive has no effect during my pregnancy. This directive is in effect until it is revoked.

I understand the full import of this directive and I am emotionally and mentally competent to make this directive. I understand that I may revoke this directive at any time.

I request that only comfort care be provided to me, no antibiotics, no artificial nutrition, no mechanical ventilation, and no hydration. It is my strong preference to be allowed to die outside of a care facility if possible, even if that preference is determined by my physician to shorten my period of dying. The only condition under which I desire these preferences for end of life care to be altered is in the case of possible organ and tissue donation. I request that any and all organs and tissue that may be salvaged be provided for transplant. My remains may then be cremated.

Signed _____ in the City of _____ etc.

I am not a person designated by the declarant to make a treatment decision. I am not related to the declarant by blood or marriage. I would not be entitled to any portion of the declarant's estate on the declarant's death. I am not the attending physician of the declarant or an employee of the attending physician.

I have no claim in against any portion of the declarant's estate on the declarant's death. Furthermore, if I am an employee of the health care facility in which the declarant is a patient, I am not involved in providing direct patient care to the declarant and am not an officer, director, partner, or business office employee of the heath care facility or of any parent organization of the health care facility.

Witness _____

Witness _____

FIGURE 48-4 Sample advance directive.

SUMMARY OF SCENARIO

Through his work with Dr. Kennedy, Bill has learned to understand the special needs of aging patients. He used to think that most older people were chronically sick and would ultimately end up in long-term care facilities. Now he understands that most aging people lead healthy, active lives and that the disorders that occur in later life usually are the result of lifestyle factors, such as diet and lack of exercise. Bill also has learned how to communicate effectively with older patients and to conduct patient interviews so as to evaluate the patient's physical, mental, emotional, and nutritional health.

SUMMARY OF LEARNING OBJECTIVES

1. **Define, spell, and pronounce the terms listed in the vocabulary.**
   Spelling and pronouncing medical terms correctly bolster the medical assistant's credibility. Knowing the definitions of these terms promotes confidence in communication with patients and co-workers.

2. **Apply critical thinking skills in performing the patient assessment and patient care.**
   Completing the Critical Thinking Application exercises throughout the chapter can help the student medical assistant become more adept at critical analysis of real-life situations.

3. **Discuss the impact of a growing aging population on society.**
   More than 40 million Americans are 65 years of age or older. The most rapidly growing age group is the "oldest old," those older than 85. By the middle of the twenty-first century, more than 72 million people will be older than 65. Most older people have at least one chronic medical condition, and many have multiple conditions. The aging population will affect all aspects of society.

4. **The stereotypes and myths associated with aging are false assumptions that frequently result in age discrimination.**
   They include the likelihood of developing dementia, aging and disease development, productivity of older workers, long-term care, sexual activity, and significance of lifestyle factors.

5. **Role-play the effect of the sensorimotor changes of aging.**
   Procedure 48-1 outlines the steps in role-playing the sensorimotor changes that accompany aging.

6. **Explain the changes in the anatomy and physiology of the body systems caused by aging.**
   Table 48-1 summarizes changes associated with aging that occur across all body systems. Normal age-related changes are expected, and the individual can compensate for them. However, these changes intensify with poor health habits and chronic disease. Age-related changes can be managed through regular exercise, a healthy diet, prevention of sun damage, and annual physical examinations with health screening.

7. **Summarize the major diseases and disorders faced by older patients.**
   Major health issues of older people are related to an increase in atherosclerosis and potential cardiovascular disease; hypertension; diabetes mellitus type 2; integumentary system changes; arthritis; osteoporosis; an increased risk of injury from falls; dementia attributable to metabolic or cardiovascular disease or AD; pneumonia, aspiration, and reactivation of tuberculosis; cataracts, glaucoma, and macular degeneration; depression; malnutrition; urinary tract abnormalities; menopausal changes; and sleep disorders.

8. **Describe various screening tools for dementia, depression, and malnutrition.**
   A commonly used screening tool for dementia is the Folstein Mini-Mental State Examination, a 5-minute screening test that is designed to evaluate basic mental function. The physician may use the Geriatric Depression Scale short form, which questions the patient about daily activities, interests, and feelings. Nutritional status can be assessed through a comprehensive patient interview that considers all potential problems preventing adequate nutrition.

9. **Explain the effect of aging on sleep.**
   Complaints of sleeping difficulties increase with age. The amount of time spent in the deepest stages of sleep declines with age. Factors that might influence sleep patterns are medications, caffeine, alcohol, depression, and environmental or physical changes. Common sleep problems in older adults include PLMD and sleep apnea.

10. **Differentiate among independent, assisted, and skilled nursing facilities.**
    Aging people prefer to remain in their home environment for as long as possible. Adult day care centers can provide supervision for older adults who may be taken care of by family members in the evening but need care during the day. Assisted-living facilities are appropriate for older adults who need assistance with some activities of daily living. Skilled nursing facilities provide 24-hour medical care and supervision.

11. **Summarize the role of the medical assistant in caring for aging patients.**
    The medical assistant's role in caring for the older patient is to develop effective communication skills that accommodate age-related sensorimotor changes; to allow time for longer appointments; to provide adequate lighting and forms in large print; and to develop appropriate in-service training as requested by the physician. Examination rooms should have furniture and treatment folders especially designed for the elderly patient. Referrals and community resources should be used for patient and family support.

12. **Determine the principles of effective communication with older adults.**
    Effective communication with aging patients includes addressing the patient with an appropriate title; introducing yourself and explaining the purpose of a procedure before touching the patient; establishing eye contact and getting the patient's attention before beginning to speak; using expanded speech, gestures, demonstrations, or written instructions in block print; repeating the message as needed for understanding; observing the patient's nonverbal behaviors for cues that indicate whether he or she understands; allowing time to process information; preventing distractions; and involving family members as needed.

13. **Identify legal and ethical issues associated with aging patients.**
    Legal and ethical issues associated with aging patients include adequate informed consent, the use of advance directives, and staying alert for signs of possible elder abuse.

CONNECTIONS

📖 **Study Guide Connection:** Go to the Chapter 48 Study Guide. Read and complete the activities.

ⓔ **Evolve Connection:** Go to the Chapter 48 link at *evolve.elsevier.com/kinn* to complete the Chapter Review and Chapter Quiz. Check out the other resources listed for this chapter to make the most of what you have learned from Assisting in Geriatrics.

49

PRINCIPLES OF ELECTROCARDIOGRAPHY

Martha Reyes has worked for almost 4 years at a local family practice office, but she has decided to take a new position in the cardiology practice next door, where she will be working for Dr. Julie Lee. Martha is very enthusiastic about the new position, but she realizes that she has a great deal to learn to provide the best patient service possible in Dr. Lee's practice. Although Martha is familiar with general cardiology practices from her previous employment, she must understand and be able to perform procedures performed for cardiac patients, especially electrocardiography.

While studying this chapter, think about the following questions:

- To fulfill her job description with Dr. Lee, what does Martha need to know about the electrical conduction system of the heart?
- How does an electrocardiography (ECG) machine work?
- How should a patient be prepared for an electrocardiogram?
- How will Martha perform an ECG diagnostic procedure?
- What is the normal appearance of ECG complexes?
- What are the characteristics of common ECG arrhythmias that Martha must be able to recognize?
- What additional cardiac tests should Martha be prepared to assist with and explain to patients?

LEARNING OBJECTIVES

1. Define, spell, and pronounce the terms listed in the vocabulary.
2. Apply critical thinking skills in performing the patient assessment and patient care.
3. Illustrate the electrical conduction system through the heart.
4. Explain the concepts of cardiac polarization, depolarization, and repolarization.
5. Identify the PQRST complex on an electrocardiographic tracing.
6. Summarize the properties of the electrocardiograph.
7. Describe the electrical views of the heart recorded by the 12-lead electrocardiograph.
8. Discuss the process of recording an electrocardiogram.
9. Perform an accurate recording of the electrical activity of the heart.
10. Compare and contrast electrocardiographic artifacts and the probable cause of each.
11. Identify a typical electrocardiograph tracing.
12. Describe common electrocardiographic arrhythmias.
13. Summarize cardiac diagnostic tests.
14. Fit a patient with a Holter monitor.
15. Discuss the legal and ethical issues involved when performing ECGs.

VOCABULARY

atria The two upper chambers of the heart.

atrioventricular (AV) node The part of the cardiac conduction system between the atria and the ventricles.

bundle of His Specialized muscle fibers that conduct electrical impulses from the AV node to the ventricular myocardium.

cardiac arrest A condition in which cardiac contractions stop completely.

cardioversion The use of electroshock to convert an abnormal cardiac rhythm to a normal one.

defibrillator A machine that delivers an electroshock to the heart through electrodes placed on the chest wall.

diastole The relaxation of the chambers of the heart during which blood enters the heart from the vascular system and the lungs.

ectopic (ek-tohp'-ik) Originating outside the normal tissue.

infarction An area of tissue that has died from lack of blood supply.

ischemia (is-ke'-mia) Decreased blood flow to a body part or organ, caused by constriction or blockage of the supplying artery.

myocardial (my-oh-kar'-de-uhl) Pertaining to the heart muscle.

palpitations A pounding or racing of the heart; may or may not indicate a serious heart disorder.

sinoatrial (SA) node The pacemaker of the heart; it is located in the right atrium.

systole The contraction of the heart.

ventricles The two lower chambers of the heart.

Electrocardiography is a painless, safe procedure and is the test most frequently used for the diagnosis of heart disease in the ambulatory care setting. In electrocardiography, electrodes are attached to the patient's skin and connected to wires that go to the electrocardiograph. Electrocardiography amplifies the electrical impulses from the beating heart, and a pattern of these impulses is recorded on electrocardiographic paper. This record is called the *electrocardiogram* (ECG). The ECG is read and evaluated by the physician and becomes a part of the patient's medical record (Figure 49-1). Medical practices using electronic medical records can record an ECG tracing directly into the patient's electronic record.

To accurately represent the true cardiac activity, the ECG must be performed with a high degree of accuracy and skill. A medical assistant must have an understanding of both the normal cardiac function and the relationship of the ECG recordings to cardiac function. The medical assistant is responsible for ensuring that the patient is prepared mentally and physically for the test and that the equipment is set up properly. When performing electrocardiography, the medical assistant must be able to recognize problems with the recording and make appropriate corrections so that the physician has a clear record of the patient's cardiac activity. The goal is to obtain the most accurate ECG possible.

HISTORY OF ELECTROCARDIOGRAPHY

Dutch physiologist Willem Einthoven developed techniques to record the electrical activity of the heart in the late 1800s. He called this recording an Electro Kardio Gramm; hence the acronym EKG. Many physicians and other health care providers still call the recording an EKG, although the newer, preferred term for an electrocardiogram is ECG.

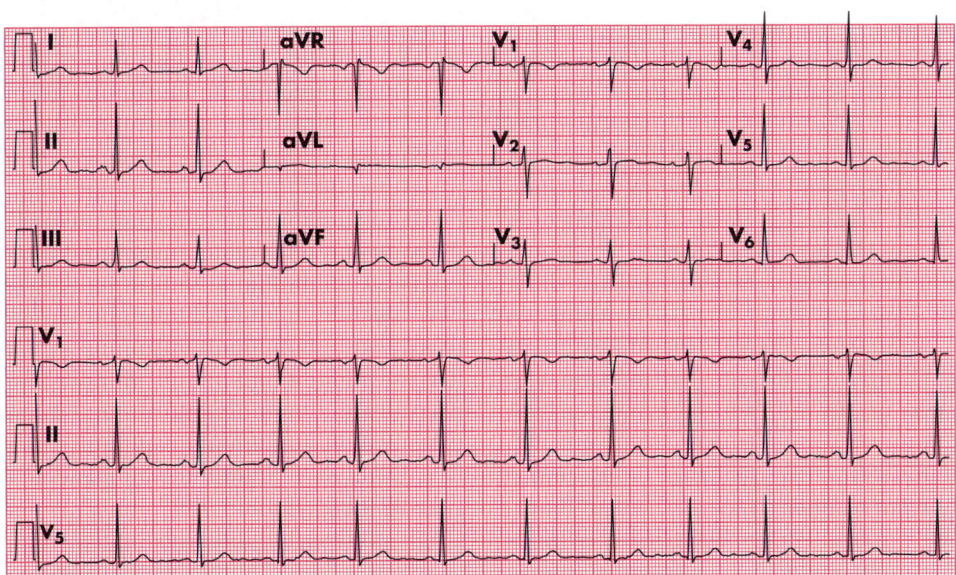

FIGURE 49-1 Example of a 12-lead ECG. (From Aehlert B: *ECGs made easy*, ed 3, St Louis, 2006, Mosby.)

THE ELECTRICAL CONDUCTION SYSTEM OF THE HEART

The Cardiac Cycle

The cardiac cycle includes all the events that occur in the heart during one single heartbeat. Each chamber of the heart goes through two phases during the cardiac cycle: **systole** and **diastole**. During systole, both the **atria** and the **ventricles** contract and empty of blood. During diastole, the relaxation phase of the heart, the chambers refill with blood. Venous blood from the inferior and superior venae cavae empties into the right atrium during atrial diastole. As the right atrium fills, increased pressure in the chamber causes the tricuspid valve to open, and the right ventricle begins to fill. At the same time, blood returning from the lungs via the pulmonary veins fills the left atrium, causing the mitral valve to open, emptying blood into the left ventricle. Before systole occurs, the ventricles are already 70% filled. The cardiac cycle for a healthy adult lasts approximately 0.8 second. However, the amount of time it takes for the heart to empty and refill depends on many factors, including the condition of the myocardium and the heart's electrical system.

The electrocardiograph records both the intensity of the electrical impulses and the actual time it takes for each part of the cardiac cycle to occur. It measures the electrical conductive impulses of the heart muscle, allowing the physician to see any disturbances or disruptions in normal heart activity. In addition to being recorded as an ECG, the cardiac cycle can appear as a continuously moving pattern on a monitor screen, accompanied by a sound for each beat.

The specialized electrical conduction system of the heart (Figure 49-2) initiates each heartbeat. The main part of this system is the **sinoatrial (SA) node**, which is located in the upper back wall of the right atrium at the junction of the superior vena cava and the right atrium. The SA node controls the rate of heart contractions by initiating electrical impulses 60 to 100 times per minute. Each cardiac cycle, or heartbeat, starts with the SA node generating an electrical impulse that travels in a wavelike pattern across the cardiac muscle of the atria, causing them to contract almost simultaneously. This electrical impulse then stimulates the **atrioventricular (AV) node**, which is located in the posterior, superior portion of the right atrial septal wall, directly behind the tricuspid valve. A slight delay in conduction at this point allows the atria to empty completely. The electrical impulse then is transmitted to a special group of conduction fibers, the **bundle of His**, in the upper part of the interventricular septal wall. The bundle of His divides into two branches; the right bundle branch carries electrical impulses to the right ventricle, and the left bundle branch carries impulses to the left ventricle. The right and left bundle branches divide into smaller and smaller branches, ending in the Purkinje fibers, which spread across the apex of the heart and through the myocardium, stimulating ventricular contraction. The ventricles contract in a twisting sort of action, forcing the blood out of the chambers and into the pulmonary artery on the right side of the heart and the aorta on the left side.

Normal sinus rhythm (NSR) refers to a regular heart rate that falls within the average range of 60 to 80 beats per minute (beats/min). Sinus bradycardia is a heart rate below 60 beats/min; sinus tachycardia is a rate above 100 beats/min. In both of these conditions, the rhythm remains even, but the rate is pathologic. An irregular cardiac rhythm is called an *arrhythmia*. Conditions that interrupt the conduction pathway, SA node to AV node to bundle of His to right and left bundle branches, can cause arrhythmias.

Polarization, Depolarization, and Repolarization

Polarization is the resting state of the **myocardial** wall; no electrical activity occurs in the heart during this phase, which is recorded on the ECG strip as a flatline. In this state the myocardial cells are ready for stimulation. When the electrical system of the heart stimulates a myocardial cell, depolarization occurs, resulting in the contraction of the stimulated heart muscle. After depolarization the heart muscle cells must return to a resting state before they can be electrically stimulated again. The process of reaching this resting state is called *repolarization.*

The electrocardiograph records a series of waves, or deflections, above or below a baseline on the ECG paper. Each deflection corresponds to a particular part of the cardiac cycle (Table 49-1). The normal ECG cycle consists of waveforms that are labeled the P wave, the Q wave, the R wave, the S wave, and the T wave. The Q, R, and S waves usually are grouped together; this is called the *QRS complex.* One entire cardiac cycle can be called the *PQRST complex.* In the next section, each part of the ECG is discussed in more detail.

PQRST Complex

The *P wave* occurs during the contraction of the atria and shows the beginning of cardiac depolarization. The P wave is the first deflection from the baseline; it typically is smooth and rounded and should occur before each QRS complex. Atrial repolarization is not recorded on the ECG strip, because its electrical impulse is small and is hidden in the QRS complex. The *PR segment* is the return to baseline after atrial contraction. The *PR interval* is the time from the beginning of atrial contraction to the beginning of ventricular contraction. It contains the P wave (depolarization of the atria) and the spread of the electrical impulse through the AV node, bundle of His, right and left bundle branches, and Purkinje fibers. As the heart rate increases, the PR interval typically shortens. The *QRS complex* shows the contraction of both ventricles and also reflects the completion of cardiac depolarization. Repolarization of the atria also occurs during this time, but it cannot be seen on the ECG because the recording of the much stronger QRS activity overshadows it. Depolarization of the ventricles results in the contraction of a much larger muscle mass than does depolarization of the atria. Therefore, the QRS complex is recorded as a much more significant electrical activity than the P wave.

The *ST segment* reflects the time between the end of ventricular contraction and the beginning of ventricular recovery. The *T wave* represents ventricular recovery or repolarization of the ventricles. After the T wave comes a period of complete heart rest, also called *polarization,* which is indicated on the ECG as a straight line. The *QT interval* is the time between the beginning of the QRS complex through the T wave. During this time the ventricles contract and relax. A *U wave* occasionally can be seen as a small waveform just after the T wave in patients with a low serum potassium level or other metabolic disorders.

By measuring the actual configuration and location of each wave in relation to the other waves and to the baseline, in addition to the intervals between waves and segments, the physician is able to detect

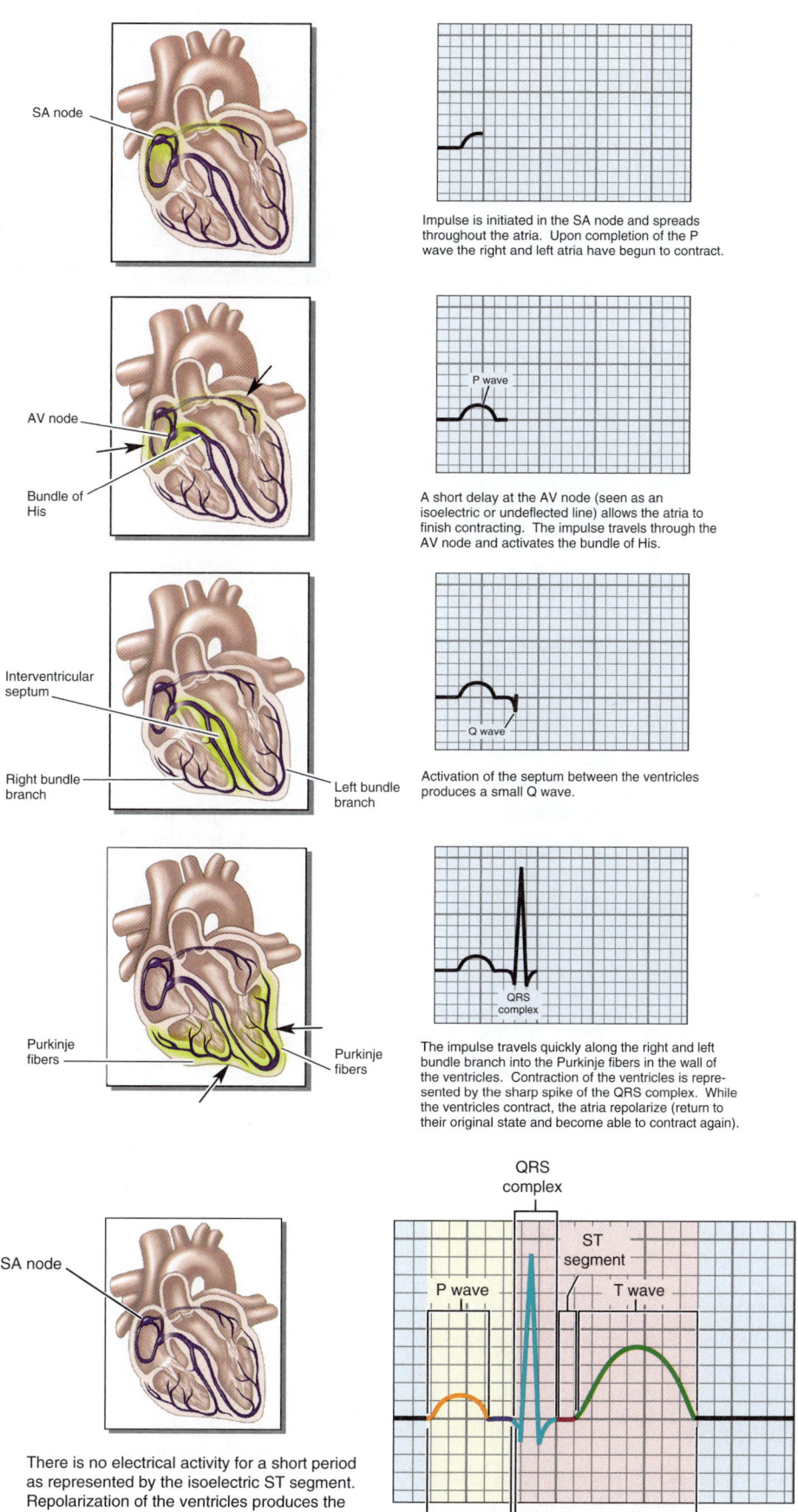

FIGURE 49-2 Electrical conduction system of the heart. (From Hunt SA: *Saunders fundamentals of medical assisting*, Philadelphia, 2002, WB Saunders.)

TABLE 49-1 The Cardiac Cycle

STAGE	HEART ACTIVITY	ELECTRICAL CURRENT
P wave*	Atrial contraction	Atrial depolarization
PR interval†	Contraction traversing the atrioventricular (AV) node	Depolarization traversing the AV node
QRS complex‡	Ventricular contraction	Ventricular depolarization
ST segment	Time interval between ventricular contraction and the beginning of ventricular recovery	Time interval between ventricular depolarization and ventricular repolarization
T wave	Ventricular contraction subsides	Ventricular repolarization (electric recovery)
U wave (not always present)	Associated with further ventricular relaxation	Associated with further ventricular repolarization
Baseline§	The heart at rest	Polarization
PR interval	Time interval between atrial contraction and ventricular contraction	Time interval between atrial depolarization and ventricular depolarization
QT interval	Time interval between the beginning of ventricular contraction and the subsiding of ventricular contraction	Time interval between the beginning of ventricular depolarization and ventricular repolarization (electric recovery)

*Wave: A uniformly advancing deflection (upward or downward) from a baseline on a recording.

†Interval: The lapse of time between two different electrocardiographic events; represents the time needed for an electrical current to move on.

‡Complex: The portion of the ECG tracing that represents the sum of three waves (contraction of the ventricles).

§Baseline: A neutral line against which waves are valued as they deflect upward (positive) or downward (negative) from the line.

rhythmic disturbances of the heart and identify different types of cardiac disorders.

THE ELECTROCARDIOGRAPH

Electrocardiograph machines (Figure 49-3) record 12 leads simultaneously and are also referred to as six-channel ECG machines. Limb and chest electrodes must be placed on the patient at specific anatomic locations before the recording starts. When the ECG is started, the machine records all 12 leads automatically and marks each lead

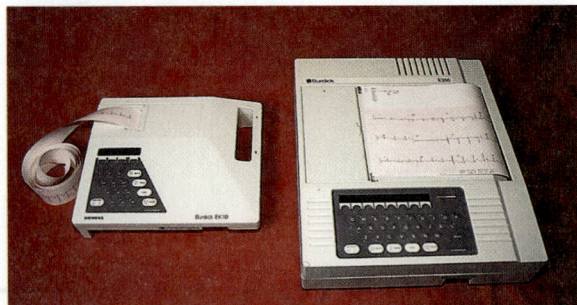

FIGURE 49-3 Many types of ECG machines are available, including single channel and multichannel models. (From Chester GA: *Modern medical assisting,* Philadelphia, 1999, WB Saunders.)

with identifying letters. These multichannel ECG tracings take seconds to perform and can be placed in the patient's medical record without mounting or can be recorded directly into the patient's electronic medical record.

CRITICAL THINKING APPLICATION   49-1

Martha has not yet been taught how to use the ECG machine in Dr. Lee's office. What steps should she take to learn how to use this machine and to feel comfortable and confident using it to obtain ECGs?

Electrocardiograph Paper

Electrocardiograph paper is heat and pressure sensitive, which means that either heat or pressure can cause a mark to appear. The stylus on an ECG machine makes the image on the ECG paper. When the machine is on, the stylus becomes hot and burns a marking on the paper as it moves horizontally past the stylus. Because the paper is pressure sensitive, it must be handled carefully to prevent any additional markings that would blemish the tracing.

ECG paper is graph paper that has horizontal and vertical lines at 1-mm intervals. This is an agreed-on international standard that allows physicians anywhere in the world to interpret a patient's ECG in the same manner. A medical assistant needs to know both the size and the meaning of each square on the ECG paper to understand its significance.

The horizontal axis represents time, and the vertical axis represents amplitude. Each small square measures 1 mm on each side. Every fifth line, both vertically and horizontally, is darker than the other lines and creates a larger square measuring 5 mm on each side. When the electrocardiograph runs at normal speed, one small 1-mm square passes the stylus every 0.04 second, which means that one large 5-mm square passes the stylus every 0.2 second. Continuing this logic, in 1 second, five large squares pass the stylus. Therefore, five sequential large squares show the record of what occurred in the heart during a time span of 1 second (5 large squares · 0.2 seconds = 1 second). Another way to say this is that at normal speed, the ECG paper travels past the stylus at a rate of 25 mm per second (Figure 49-4).

The voltage, or strength, of the heartbeat also is recorded on the paper. Voltage can be displayed as either a positive or a negative deflection. One millivolt (mV) of electrical activity moves the stylus upward over 10 mm (two large squares). This is the standard

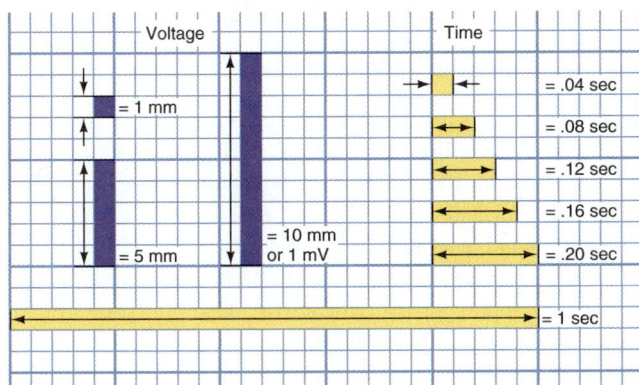

FIGURE 49-4 ECG paper. (From Chester GA: *Modern medical assisting*, Philadelphia, 1999, WB Saunders.)

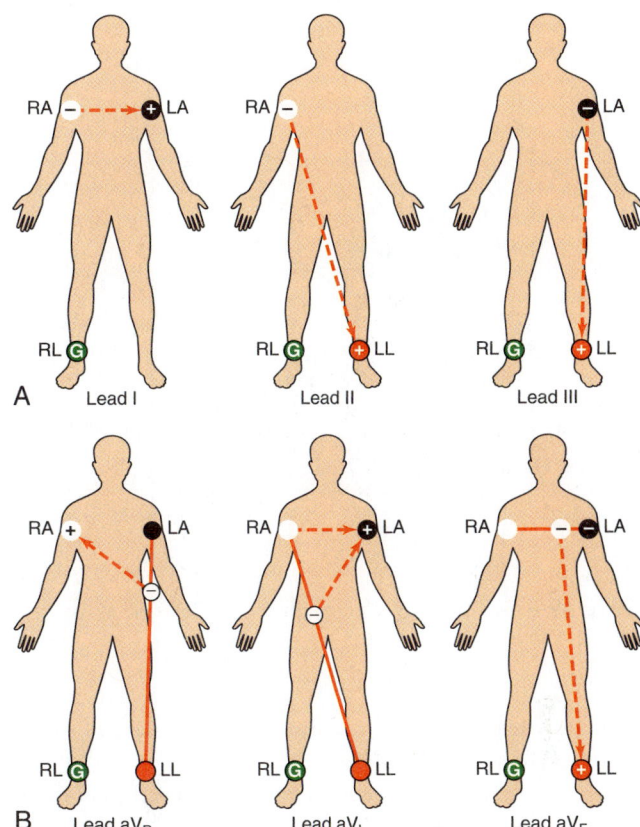

FIGURE 49-5 Standard **(A)** and augmented **(B)** limb leads. (From Chester GA: *Modern medical assisting*, Philadelphia, 1999, WB Saunders.)

normally used for obtaining an ECG, and it can be adjusted to match the strength of the electrical activity of the heart. The machine must be calibrated so that 1 mV of electrical activity produces a deflection that is 10 mm either above or below the baseline. When properly calibrated, the ECG records both the strength of the electrical activity of the heartbeat in millivolts and the speed of the heartbeat over time.

Electrodes and Leads

Ten sensors, called *electrodes,* are placed on the patient's arms (two), legs (two), and chest (six) to pick up the electrical activity of the heart. Electrodes must be applied to specific locations to record the heart's electrical activity from different angles and planes. Ten color-coded and labeled lead wires that end in a small metal clip are attached to the electrodes. The lead wires carry the signal of the heart's electrical activity to the ECG machine. Most machines require single-use, self-stick, disposable electrodes that are packaged with conductive jelly in the center.

The *leads* to the electrocardiograph carry the cardiac electrical impulses into the machine, where they are magnified by an amplifier. These amplified impulses are converted into mechanical action, which is recorded on the ECG paper by the stylus and/or shown on a monitor. A single lead records the electrical activity of the heart between two different electrodes, one positive and one negative. The placement of the positive electrode determines the particular view of the heart recorded. If depolarization occurs toward the positive electrode, the deflection is upright; if it moves toward the negative electrode, the waveform is deflected downward. Each lead records the average electrical flow at a specific time in a specific location of the heart. The ECG records views of the heart on both a frontal and a transverse plane. The frontal leads include leads I, II, III, aV_R, aV_L, and aV_F. Horizontal plane leads include the six precordial, or chest, leads (V_1 to V_6).

Lead Recordings

The standard ECG consists of 12 separate leads, or recordings of the electrical activity of the heart, from different angles.

Standard Leads

The first three leads recorded are called the *standard* or *bipolar leads,* because they each use two limb electrodes to record the heart's

electrical activity (Figure 49-5, *A*). The right arm electrode is the negative pole, and the left leg or left arm electrodes are the positive poles. Roman numerals I, II, and III are used to designate these leads.

- Lead I records tracings between the right arm and left arm, recording the electrical activity of the lateral part of the left ventricle.
- Lead II records tracings between the right arm and left leg, recording the electrical activity of the inferior surface of the left ventricle; this is the lead recorded on a cardiac monitor or on the rhythm strip at the bottom of the 12-lead ECG.
- Lead III records tracings between the left arm and left leg which reflects the electrical activity of the inferior surface of the left ventricle.

Augmented Leads

The next three leads are the augmented, or combined, leads (Figure 49-5, *B*). These are designated augmented voltage right arm (aV_R), augmented voltage left arm (aV_L), and augmented voltage left leg (aV_F). Because the electrical activity recorded by these leads is relatively small, the ECG machine amplifies (or augments) the electrical potential when recorded. These are all unipolar leads with a single positive electrode that uses the right leg for grounding.

- aV_R records the electrical activity of the atria from the right shoulder; P waves and QRS complexes are deflected below the baseline.

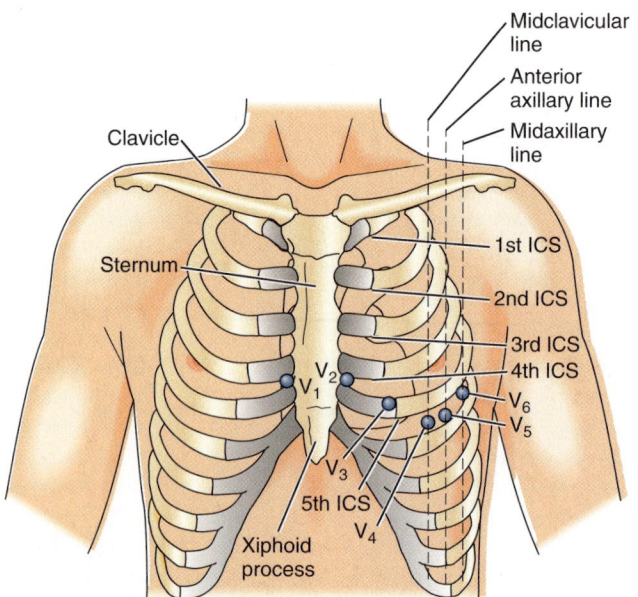

FIGURE 49-6 Chest leads. *ICS,* Intercostal space. (From Chester GA: *Modern medical assisting,* Philadelphia, 1999, WB Saunders.)

- aV_L records the electrical activity of the lateral wall of the left ventricle from the left shoulder.
- aV_F records the electrical activity of the inferior surface of the left ventricle from the left leg.

Precordial Leads

The precordial, or chest, leads are unipolar and provide a transverse plane view of the heart. They are designated V_1, V_2, V_3, V_4, V_5, and V_6. The V means chest, and each of the numbers represents a specific location on the chest. The QRS complex shows as a negative deflection in V_1 and V_2, and views with each subsequent lead become more positive. Precordial leads measure the electrical activity among six specific points on the chest wall and a point within the heart (Figure 49-6). It is important to avoid placing electrodes directly over a bony prominence.

- V_1—The electrode is placed in the fourth intercostal space, just to the right of the sternum.
- V_2—The electrode is placed in the fourth intercostal space, just to the left of the sternum.
- V_3—The electrode is placed midway between V_2 and V_4.
- V_4—The electrode is placed in the fifth intercostal space, at the left midclavicular line.
- V_5—The electrode is placed horizontal to V_4 in the left anterior axillary line.
- V_6—The electrode is placed horizontal to V_4 in the left midaxillary line.

CRITICAL THINKING APPLICATION   49-2

Dr. Lee has asked Martha to perform her first ECG on a patient who just came into the office. Martha is not confident that she knows how to place the chest leads properly in the correct locations. How should she handle this situation? Should she perform the ECG procedure as best she can? Why or why not?

PERFORMING ELECTROCARDIOGRAPHY

Preparation of the Room and Patient

The room should be in the quietest location in the office and should be as far as possible from all other electrical equipment, including x-ray machines, diathermy devices, laboratory equipment, centrifuges, fans, refrigerators, and air conditioners. The room should be warm and should have adjustable lighting.

The treatment table should be comfortable and wide enough to provide full support for the patient. The table should be wood or should have an electrically insulated surface. Position the table so that you can work from the side of the patient that is most comfortable for you. Electrocardiographers most often work on the patient's left side, but as long as the electrodes are placed in the proper position, it really makes no difference which side you use.

Small pillows are helpful for helping the patient relax and providing maximum comfort during the procedure. Offer a pillow for the head and one for under the knees. If a head pillow is used, it should not elevate the patient's shoulders.

The patient should disrobe to the waist and put on the patient gown with the opening in the front; easy access to the patient's extremities must be available. Pantyhose must be removed.

Place the patient in a supine position with the arms comfortably at the sides and the legs not touching one another. If the patient has dyspnea or orthopnea, a semi-Fowler's position should be used, or alternatively the patient can be seated on a wooden chair. However, make sure you check with the physician before obtaining an ECG in an alternative position. If a seated position is used, the patient's feet must rest comfortably on the floor or on a footstool. Note any alternative position on the ECG recording.

The patient should empty the bladder and then rest for at least 10 minutes before the ECG recording is made. Check to see whether the patient followed all the instructions provided in Figure 49-7. Record the patient's vital signs and current medications on the patient's chart. This information can be programmed into some ECG machines and automatically printed on the ECG recording.

Explain to the patient the nature and purpose of the ECG. Attempt to answer all questions and make the patient as comfortable as possible during the procedure. Stress the importance of not moving during the entire procedure, and assure the patient that there is no danger of shock. Soften the lighting in the room to obtain maximum patient comfort. When you tell the patient to lie still, observe that he or she is breathing normally. Patients often hold their breath when asked to lie still.

Attaching Leads to the Patient

Disposable, single-use electrodes are placed on the patient's limbs and chest in very specific locations (Figure 49-8). The lead wires from the machine then are connected to the electrodes. Making the proper connections is facilitated by specific lead markings or color coding on the end of each lead wire (Figure 49-9).

- RA lead is attached to the electrode on the patient's right arm.
- LA lead is attached to the electrode on the patient's left arm.
- RL lead is attached to the electrode on the patient's right leg.
- LL lead is attached to the electrode on the patient's left leg.
- The labeled lead wires then are placed on each precordial electrode.

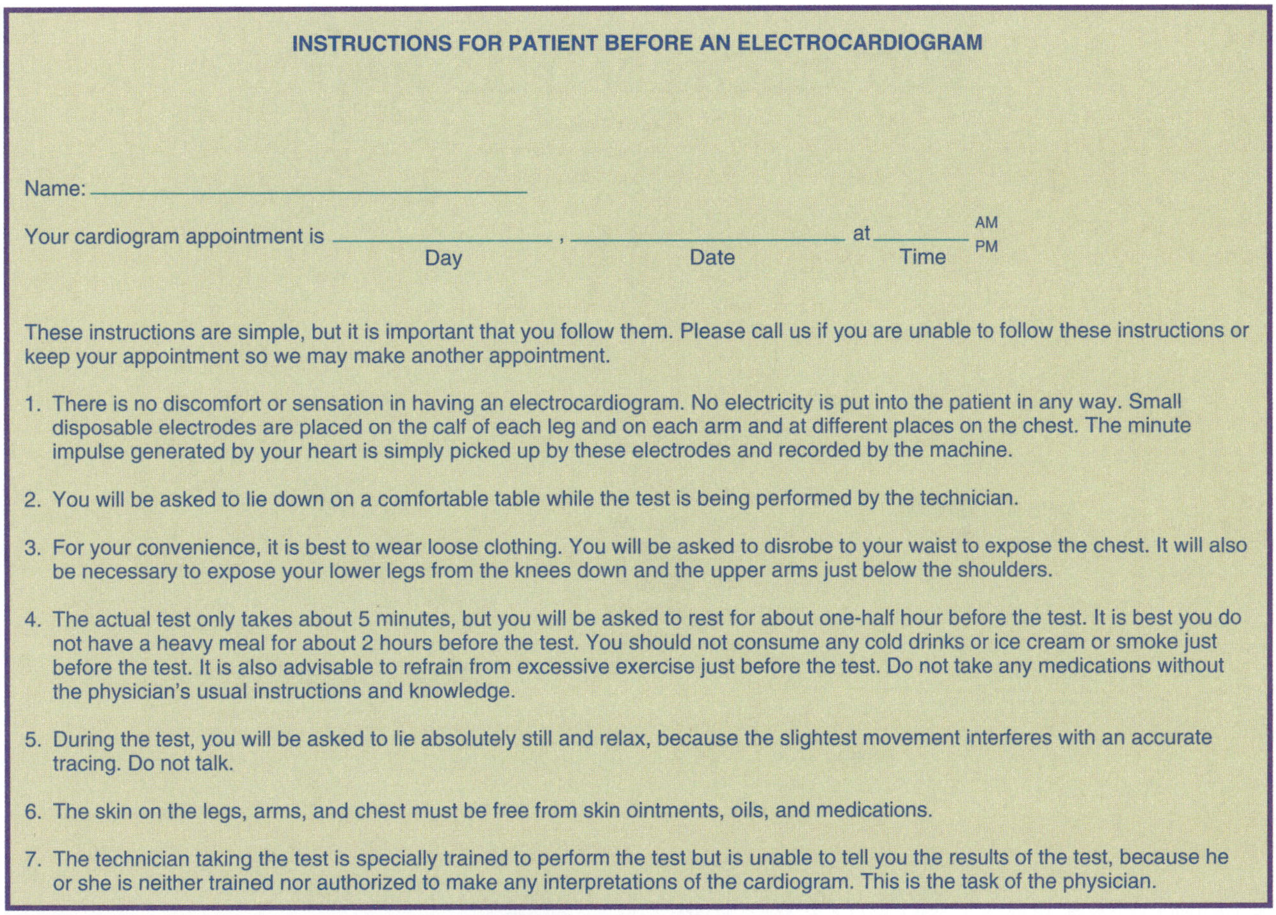

INSTRUCTIONS FOR PATIENT BEFORE AN ELECTROCARDIOGRAM

Name: _____

Your cardiogram appointment is _____ , _____ at _____ AM / PM
　　　　　　　　　　　　　　　　　Day　　　　　　　　　　　Date　　　　　　Time

These instructions are simple, but it is important that you follow them. Please call us if you are unable to follow these instructions or keep your appointment so we may make another appointment.

1. There is no discomfort or sensation in having an electrocardiogram. No electricity is put into the patient in any way. Small disposable electrodes are placed on the calf of each leg and on each arm and at different places on the chest. The minute impulse generated by your heart is simply picked up by these electrodes and recorded by the machine.

2. You will be asked to lie down on a comfortable table while the test is being performed by the technician.

3. For your convenience, it is best to wear loose clothing. You will be asked to disrobe to your waist to expose the chest. It will also be necessary to expose your lower legs from the knees down and the upper arms just below the shoulders.

4. The actual test only takes about 5 minutes, but you will be asked to rest for about one-half hour before the test. It is best you do not have a heavy meal for about 2 hours before the test. You should not consume any cold drinks or ice cream or smoke just before the test. It is also advisable to refrain from excessive exercise just before the test. Do not take any medications without the physician's usual instructions and knowledge.

5. During the test, you will be asked to lie absolutely still and relax, because the slightest movement interferes with an accurate tracing. Do not talk.

6. The skin on the legs, arms, and chest must be free from skin ointments, oils, and medications.

7. The technician taking the test is specially trained to perform the test but is unable to tell you the results of the test, because he or she is neither trained nor authorized to make any interpretations of the cardiogram. This is the task of the physician.

FIGURE 49-7 ECG patient instructions.

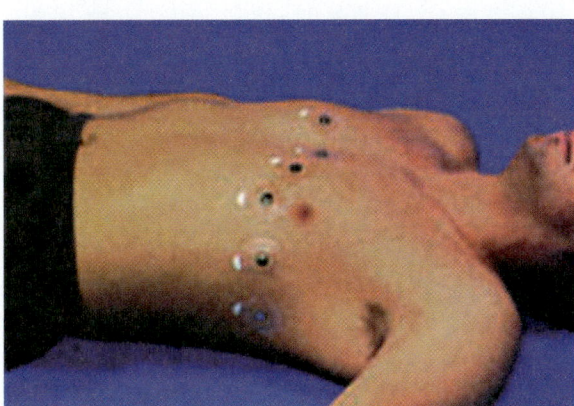

FIGURE 49-8 Chest lead locations. (From Aehlert B: *ECGs made easy,* ed 3, St Louis, 2006, Mosby.)

CRITICAL THINKING APPLICATION　　**49-3**

Two weeks later, after Martha feels much more confident in her skills at electrode placement and in recording an ECG, a new patient, Mr. Sonderford, comes to the office complaining of mild chest pain that he noted when he got out of bed this morning. What concerns might Martha have about Mr. Sonderford? His vital signs are: P 104 beats/min, weak and irregular; R 24 breaths/min and quite shallow. Mr. Sonderford is sweating profusely. What should Martha do? Why?

Recording the Electrocardiogram

Procedure 49-1 explains how to record an ECG. It is important that you become familiar with the type of machine used in your practice. Machines vary according to the age and make of the model, but most electrocardiographs currently in use perform standardization functions and labeling automatically. You may have the option of entering specific information about the patient, such as age, gender, prescriptions, and so on. Follow office protocol when performing the procedure. After the machine has been programmed, remind the patient to lie still and press the appropriate key to run the ECG strip. Six-channel machines print and label all 12 leads, with a rhythm strip across the bottom of the paper in lead II, in a matter of seconds. Review the printout for clarity, and if it is acceptable, give the recording to the physician for review. Once approved, remove the leads and electrodes from the patient, assist him or her into a sitting position, and provide assistance in getting off the table and dressing if necessary.

Standardization, Sensitivity, and Speed

Standardization has been determined by international agreement so that an ECG can be interpreted in the same way anywhere in the world. This requires the electrocardiograph to be calibrated according to universal measurements. Each time you record an ECG, you must make sure the machine is correctly standardized.

When a machine is in standard mode or set at 1 STD, 1 mV of electricity causes the stylus to move vertically 10 mm, or two large

ECG ELECTRODE PLACEMENT

Midclavicular line
Anterior axillary line
Midaxillary line

Note leads V5 and V6 remain on this dashed line level with V4.

RL ○   ● LL

RA   LA

V1 V2 V3 V4 V5 V6

Right leg: **GREEN**
Left leg: **RED**

V1: **RED**
V2: **YELLOW**
V3: **GREEN**
V4: **BLUE**
V5: **ORANGE**
V6: **PURPLE**

Right arm: WHITE
Left arm: **BLACK**

IMPORTANT
See section on AC Interference
in CompuMed Instruction Guide
● Clean and abrade skin at electrode contact site
● Clean electrodes after each use.

COMPUMED
Supporting medical excellence through technology

FIGURE 49-9 Color codes. (Courtesy CompuMed, San Diego, Calif.)

PROCEDURE 49-1

Perform Electrocardiography: Obtain a 12-Lead ECG

GOAL: *To obtain an accurate, artifact-free recording of the electrical activity of the heart.*

EQUIPMENT and SUPPLIES

- ECG machine with patient lead cable and labeled lead wires
- 10 disposable, self-adhesive electrodes
- Patient gown and drape
- Patient's medical record

PROCEDURAL STEPS

1. Sanitize your hands.
   PURPOSE: To ensure infection control.
2. Explain the procedure to the patient.
   PURPOSE: To alleviate apprehension and gain the patient's cooperation.
3. Ask the patient to disrobe to the waist (including the bra for women) and remove belts, jewelry, socks, stockings, or pantyhose as necessary.
   PURPOSE: Electrodes must be applied to bare skin without interference from clothing.
4. Position the patient supine on the examination table and drape appropriately.
   PURPOSE: To ensure the patient's modesty and comfort.
5. Turn on the machine to allow the stylus to warm up (may not be necessary with newer machines).
   PURPOSE: To ensure proper performance of the machine.

6. Label the beginning of the tracing paper with the patient's name, the date, the time, and the patient's current cardiovascular medications or input this information into the machine.
   PURPOSE: To identify the ECG recording properly.
7. At each location where an electrode will be placed, clean the skin with an alcohol wipe (Figure 1).

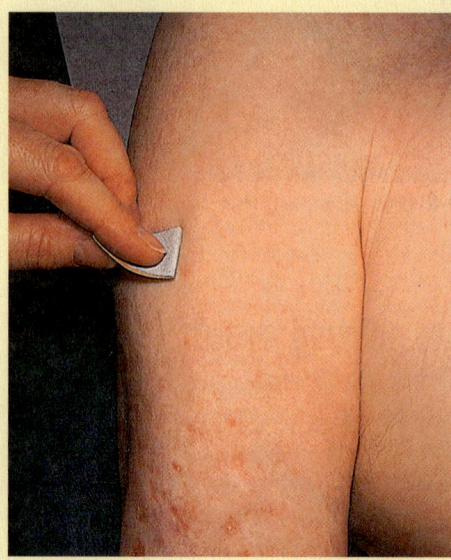

PURPOSE: To obtain good electrode adhesion to the skin.

PROCEDURE 49-1—cont'd

8. Apply the self-adhesive electrodes to clean, dry, fleshy areas of the extremities (Figure 2). Extremely hairy areas may need to be shaved to achieve adequate electrode attachment, or place a piece of tape over the electrode to make sure it is secure.

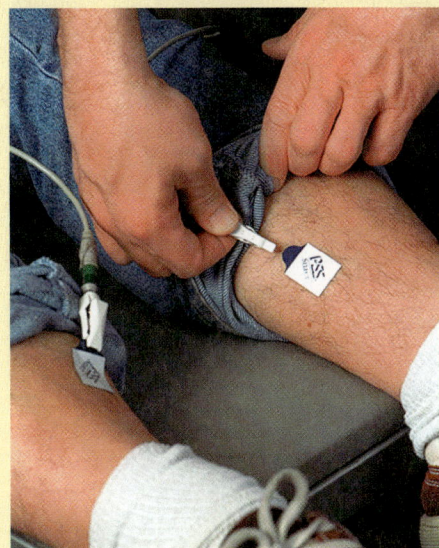

9. Apply the self-adhesive electrodes to the clean areas on the chest (Figure 3).

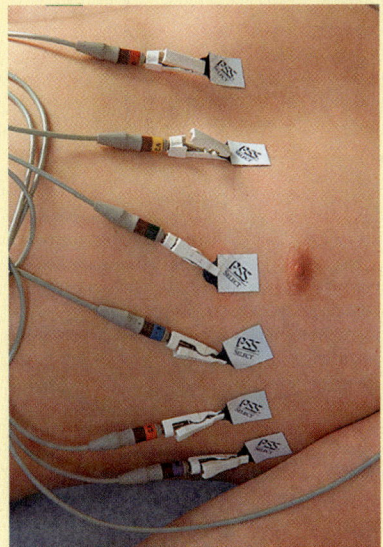

10. Carefully connect the lead wires to the correct electrode with the alligator clips on the end of each lead. Make sure the lead wires are not crossed.
    PURPOSE: To prevent artifacts.
11. Press the AUTO button on the machine and run the ECG tracing. The machine automatically places the standardization at the beginning, and the 12 leads then follow in the three-channel matrix with a lead II rhythm strip across the bottom of the page.
12. Watch for artifacts during the recording. If artifacts are present, make appropriate corrections and repeat the recording to get a clean reading.
13. Remove the lead wires from the electrodes and then remove the electrodes from the patient.
14. Assist the patient with getting dressed as needed. Clean and return the ECG machine to its storage area.
15. Place the ECG recording in the patient's medical record for physician review.
16. Sanitize your hands.
17. Document the procedure in the patient's medical record.
    PURPOSE: Procedures are not considered done until they are documented in the patient's medical record.

9/22/XX 3:10 PM 12-lead ECG recorded without incident. Martha Reyes, CMA (AAMA)

---

squares. When the machine has been properly set in this way, electrical voltages can be calculated by measuring the vertical movement of the stylus on the paper. The stylus should deflect exactly 10 mm when the standardization button is depressed with a quick pecking motion. The recording of the standardization would be 2 mm wide and rectangular. Each manufacturer's manual explains the exact method of adjustment to obtain a perfect standardization.

At minimum, standardization must be performed before the first lead is recorded. Some physicians require a separate standardization in each of the individual 12 leads.

Most machines have three sensitivity standards that can be selected: ½ STD, which deflects the stylus 5 mm, or one large square; 1 STD, which deflects the stylus 10 mm, or two large squares; and 2 STD, which deflects the stylus 20 mm or four large squares. The appropriate standard is selected as follows: if the QRS complex is too tall and is causing the stylus to move off the paper, the STD should be set to ½ STD. If the QRS complex is too short, the STD should be set to 2 STD. Figure 49-10 shows the three sensitivity standards as they appear when recorded on the ECG paper.

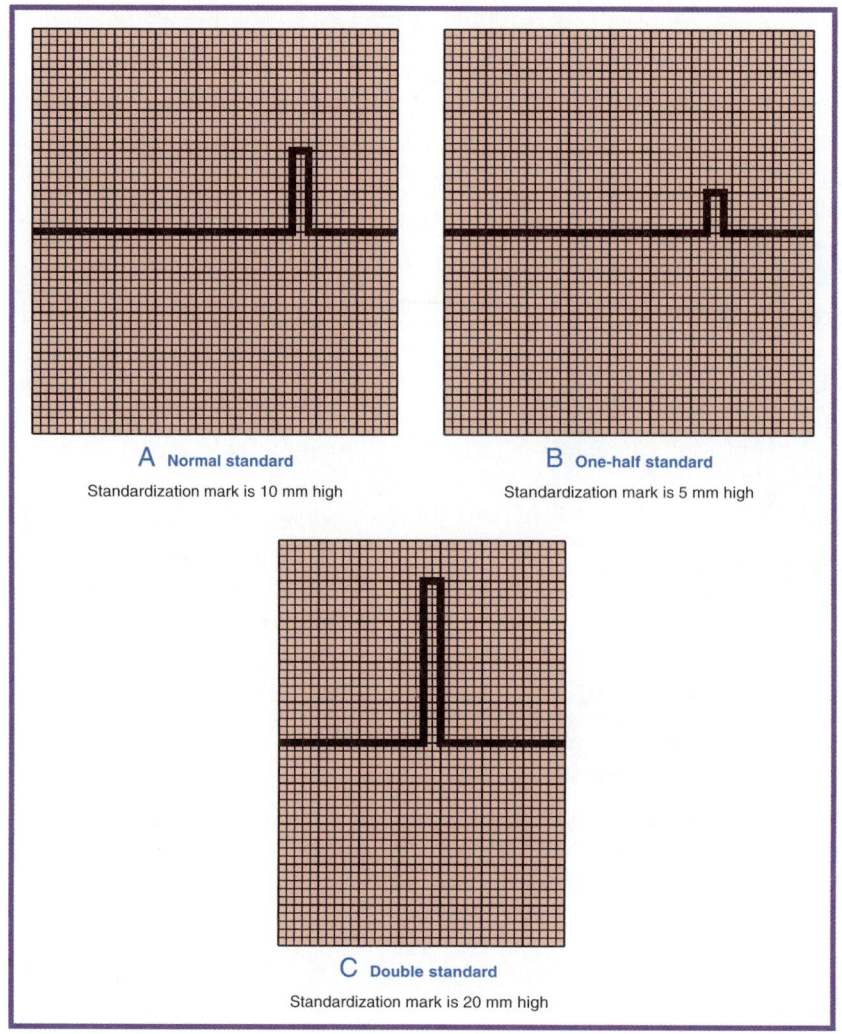

A **Normal standard**
Standardization mark is 10 mm high

B **One-half standard**
Standardization mark is 5 mm high

C **Double standard**
Standardization mark is 20 mm high

FIGURE 49-10 Sensitivity standards.

The usual speed for an ECG recording is 25 mm/sec. If the patient's heart rate is very rapid or if certain parts of the complex are too close together, the paper may need to be adjusted to run at double speed, or 50 mm/sec. This extends the recording to twice the normal length. Any change in the speed must be noted on the ECG.

The ECG Tracing and the Medical Record

ECG tracings usually are retained in medical records for many years to provide a history of patient cardiac activity. Paper clips and staples are never used, because they scratch and mark a tracing. Clear tape should not be used, because it can become sticky or yellow with age. A single photocopy of the ECG can be made without damaging the original. Many offices routinely put a photocopy in the patient's medical record because it is less likely to be damaged by handling. If the practice has electronic medical records, the tracing is scanned into the patient's electronic chart or recorded directly into the patient's medical record.

Regardless of the particular method used, each ECG should be labeled with the following information:

- Patient's full name
- Gender
- Age
- Date and time of ECG

- List of all medications and/or supplements the patient takes
- Variations from normal sensitivity and normal speed

Additional notations should be recorded for any variation from the routine, such as the following:

- Very nervous or anxious patient
- Lack of rest before the test
- Smoking immediately before the test
- Failure to follow any pretest instructions

Telephone Transmission

An electrocardiograph with phone transmission capabilities can transmit a recording over a telephone to an ECG data interpretation center. The machine is equipped with a direct ECG fax transmitter. The recording is interpreted by a computer at the data center and verified by a cardiologist. Patient information that may be important to the interpretation, such as medications and vital signs, is sent with the ECG data. A printout with the computer-assisted interpretations is returned to the sender by fax or e-mail.

Interpretive Electrocardiographs

Interpretive electrocardiographs are equipped with a computer that analyzes the recording as it is being run. With this capability, immediate information on the heart's activity is available, which can be

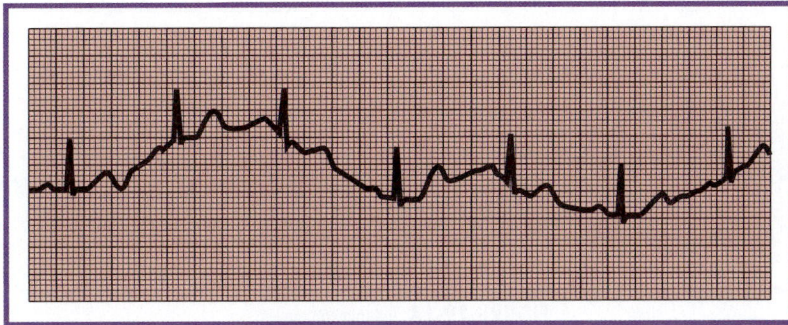

FIGURE 49-11 Wandering baseline.

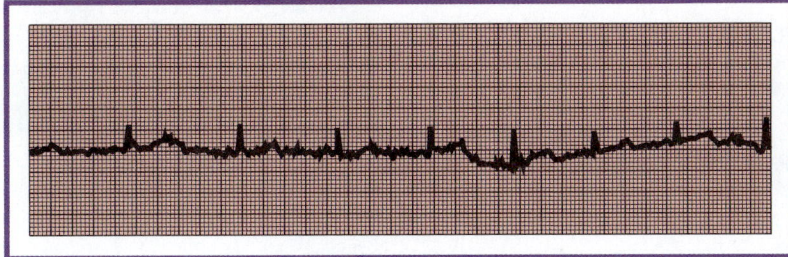

FIGURE 49-12 Somatic tremor.

valuable for reaching an early diagnosis and initiating immediate treatment. Patient baseline data must be entered into the computer before the ECG is recorded. The computer analysis of the ECG and the reason for each interpretation are then printed on the top of the recording.

Artifacts

An artifact is an unwanted, erratic movement of the stylus on the paper caused by outside interference. The electrocardiograph is extremely sensitive to any kind of nearby electrical activity. Electrical artifacts on the tracing make accurate interpretation of the ECG difficult. The medical assistant should have a thorough understanding of the causes of and remedies for these artifacts. The main types of artifacts are wandering baseline, somatic tremor, alternating current (AC) interference, and interrupted baseline.

Wandering Baseline

With a wandering baseline, the stylus gradually shifts away from the center of the paper. This usually happens because of slight movement of the patient during the tracing or poor electrode attachment (Figure 49-11). A wandering baseline is resolved by reminding the patient to remain as still as possible; this can be facilitated by keeping the patient comfortable. Make sure electrodes are completely attached to each specific site to eliminate this artifact.

Somatic Tremor

The term *somatic tremor* means muscle movement. Any muscle movement, including movement of skeletal muscle, produces a measurable electrical impulse. This additional input causes unwanted stylus movement during the tracing; this shows up on the recording as jagged peaks of irregular height and spacing with a shifting baseline (Figure 49-12). The most common causes include patient discomfort, apprehension, movement, or talking or a condition that causes uncontrollable body tremors. A patient with uncontrolled

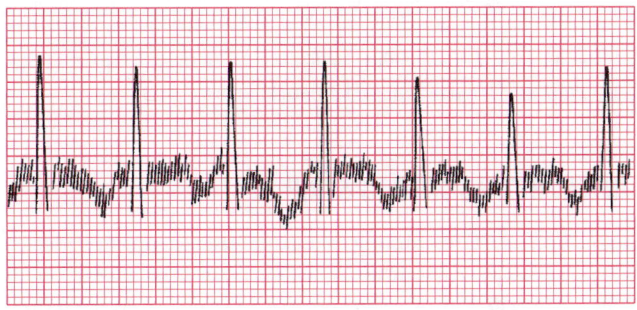

FIGURE 49-13 Sixty-cycle interference. (From Aehlert B: *ECGs made easy,* ed 3, St Louis, 2006, Mosby.)

tremors must be as calm and comfortable as possible to minimize the somatic tremor artifact. The other causes all can be resolved after they have been identified correctly.

Alternating Current (AC) Interference

AC interference appears as a series of uniform small spikes on the paper (Figure 49-13). Electrical currents in nearby equipment or wiring can leak small amounts of electrical energy into the area where the ECG machine is located. The very sensitive electrocardiograph can easily pick up this additional electrical energy signal. This can be minimized by making sure the machine is plugged into a three-pronged, grounded outlet; keeping lead wires uncrossed; unplugging other electrical appliances in the room; moving the table away from the wall; and perhaps even turning off overhead fluorescent lights. If all these measures fail, you may need to move to another examination room for the procedure. The last step is to call the manufacturer or your local service representative.

Interrupted Baseline

Baseline interruption occurs when the electrical connection has been interrupted. The stylus moves onto the margin of the paper

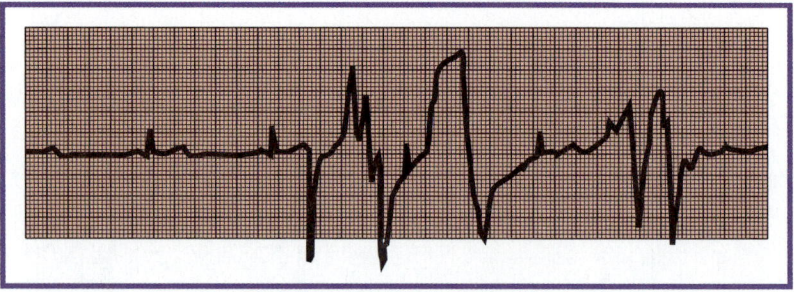

FIGURE 49-14 Interrupted baseline.

erratically (Figure 49-14). It moves violently up and down across the paper, or it may record a straight line across the top or bottom of the paper. Noticeable patient movement that dislodges the electrodes causes most baseline interruptions. This cause is virtually eliminated by using disposable, stick-on electrodes. Other causes include a broken cable wire and cable tips that are attached too loosely to the electrodes.

CRITICAL THINKING APPLICATION   49-4

Dr. Lee asks Martha to explain the causes of artifacts and the methods for correcting ECG recordings that show outside interference. Based on what you have learned about ECG artifacts, what are the typical causes and how would you recommend correcting each?

INTERPRETING AN ECG STRIP

The medical assistant working in a cardiovascular practice must be able to recognize rhythm abnormalities that may appear on the tracing. Alerting the physician to the presence of an arrhythmia while the patient is still connected to the machine may give the physician the opportunity to observe the patient while the machine is running or immediately institute some type of therapeutic or prophylactic intervention. The physician can determine two important heart functions when interpreting the ECG: heart rate and heart rhythm.

Normal Appearance of ECG Complexes

When you examine the ECG recording, first look at the characteristics of each of the waves in the recording (Table 49-2). Are the P waves, QRS complexes, and T waves clearly present? Do they have a consistent appearance and do they occur at regular intervals? Are any odd beats present that do not fit in with the others? Is the rate normal, fast, or slow? Is the rhythm regular or irregular?

In NSR (see Figure 49-1), each beat of the heart is initiated by an impulse from the SA node that travels without interruption along the normal conduction pathway of the heart. In NSR each beat on the ECG shows a P wave followed by a QRS complex.

Rate

To calculate the heart rate from the ECG recording, count the number of P waves in a 6-second strip (30 large squares) and multiply by 10. In the same manner, you can count the number of P waves in a 3-second strip (15 large squares) and multiply by 20. To get the ventricular contraction rate, you can count the number of

---

TABLE 49-2 Normal Appearance of ECG Waveforms and Complexes

WAVE OR COMPLEX	DURATION (SEC OR AMPLITUDE)	CHARACTERISTICS TO EXAMINE
P wave	0.06-0.11	Are P waves present? Are they normal shape (not notched or peaked) and normal size (<3 mm)? Do all deflect upward (positive)? Is there one for each QRS? Are they evenly spaced from the QRS?
PR interval	0.12-0.20	Is it constant?
QRS complex	0.08-0.12	Are they evenly spaced from T waves? Do all point in the same direction? Do all QRS complexes appear the same? Is each preceded by a P wave? Does the Q wave have a pronounced negative deflection?
ST segment	On baseline (isoelectric line)	Is it on baseline? Is it constant? Is it elevated above the baseline?
T wave	≤5 mm in leads I, II, III ≤10 mm in V₁-V₆	Is T wave present? Are all the same? Do all show upward deflection (positive)?
QT interval	Should not be more than half the RR interval* if patient has a regular rhythm	Is it constant?
U wave	Rounded, upright deflection	Is it present?

*RR interval: from onset of one QRS complex to onset of next QRS complex.

complete QRS complexes that occur within 6 seconds and multiply that number by 10 to get the number of ventricular contractions in 1 minute.

The heart rate also can be calculated by counting the number of small squares between two R waves and then dividing that number into 1,500 (1 minute on an ECG strip passes 1,500 small boxes). When the number of boxes from one cardiac event to the next same event is divided into 1,500, the result is the patient's heart rate. You can use the ECG strips in Figures 49-1 and 49-11 to practice these techniques.

Rhythm

The rhythm of a patient's heartbeat is either regular or irregular. You may pick up an irregular heartbeat when taking the patient's pulse. This same patient will show an irregularity (i.e., a difference in the length of time between cardiac cycles) when an ECG is recorded. If the patient's heart is beating in a regular rhythm, each cardiac cycle occurs within the same time frame, and individual cardiac cycles occur exactly the same length of time apart. To check for ventricular rhythm, you can measure the distance between two consecutive RR intervals. Atrial rhythm is determined by measuring the distance between two consecutive PP intervals. If the heart rhythm is regular, each of these interval measurements is the same.

CALCULATING A PATIENT'S HEART RATE

To calculate the patient's heart rate from an ECG strip, remember the following:
- 5 large boxes on the graph paper = 1 second
- 15 large boxes = 3 seconds
- 30 large boxes = 6 seconds

ANALYZING AN ECG STRIP

The ECG rhythm strip (lead II view) is evaluated from left to right. Each strip should be assessed for the following:
- Rate
- Rhythm
- P waves: There should be one P wave before each QRS complex; each is a positive deflection and similar in size and shape.
- Intervals: Assess for duration and distance.
- Appearance of the segments and waveforms: Are rhythmic PQRST cycles present? Are there any abnormalities, such as more than one P wave, QRS segments without a previous P wave, or an elevated ST segment? All of these abnormalities should be brought to the physician's attention immediately.

TYPICAL ECG RHYTHM ABNORMALITIES

Abnormalities in cardiac rhythm are called *arrhythmias*. These can result from disturbances anywhere along the electrical conduction pathway in the heart from the SA node through the right and left bundle branches. The best way to determine whether an arrhythmia is present is to know what the NSR looks like on an ECG. Study the NSR in the ECG in Figure 49-1. NSR is a heart rate between 60 and 100 beats/min. Any deviations from this should be recognized during the ECG recording, and the medical assistant should notify the physician immediately.

Cardiac arrhythmias commonly fall into one of four broad categories: sinus arrhythmias, atrial arrhythmias, ventricular arrhythmias, and biochemical arrhythmias. The characteristics of several arrhythmias in each of these categories are compared in Table 49-3.

Sinus Arrhythmias

Sinus rhythm is considered normal; the heart's electrical activity begins in the SA node and follows through the electrical system, ending in atrial and ventricular depolarization. In sinus arrhythmias, the pathway of the electrical charge is normal but the rate or rhythm of the heartbeat is altered. Sinus arrhythmias may be caused by the SA node firing too slowly or too quickly. In sinus bradycardia, the heart rate is below 60 beats/min. This can be a normal heart rate in well-conditioned athletes, but it is abnormal in other individuals. In sinus tachycardia, the heart rate is above 100 beats/min. This can be a normal heart rate in a person doing aerobic exercise, but it can be abnormal in a resting individual (Figure 49-15).

Atrial Arrhythmias

Problems with electrical discharge of the atria are caused by faulty electrical impulse formation or conduction defects within the atria. Premature atrial contraction (PAC) occurs when the atria contract before they should for the next cardiac cycle. This can appear on the ECG as an abnormally shaped P wave or an extra P wave. PACs can be seen in smokers and people who consume large amounts of caffeine. Occasional PACs are not abnormal, but they become a medical concern if they regularly occur more than six times a minute. In this situation, the PACs can indicate developing cardiac abnormalities.

Atrial flutter occurs when the atria beat at an extremely rapid rate, up to 300 beats/min. In atrial flutter the impulses come from many **ectopic** atrial locations but are blocked at the AV node, which prevents ventricular fibrillation. Atrial flutter is reversed with medication to slow the heart or with **cardioversion** (electrical shock).

Ventricular Arrhythmias

Premature ventricular contractions (PVCs; Figure 49-16, *A* and *B*) occur when the ventricles contract before they should for the next cardiac cycle; that is, a QRS complex appears before a P wave. PVCs occur when an electrical charge originates in either ventricle. This can appear on the ECG as an absent P wave, an abnormally shaped T wave, and a widened QRS complex. This is followed by a pause before the initiation of the next cardiac cycle (see Figure 49-15). PVCs can result from the use of tobacco, alcohol, medications containing epinephrine, and occasionally from anxiety. Infrequent PVCs are not abnormal, but they become a medical concern if they regularly occur more than six times a minute. Pathologic PVCs occur in patients with hypertension, coronary artery disease, and lung disease.

Ventricular tachycardia (commonly referred to as *V-tach*; Figure 49-16, *C*) is diagnosed when the ventricles beat at extremely rapid rates. It may be seen when multiple PVCs occur in a row or as a short run of fast beats, or it may persist longer than 30 seconds. The patient's heart rate may range from 101 to 250 beats/min. V-tach can precede ventricular fibrillation if not reversed with drugs, cardioversion, or both. V-tach always reflects a pathologic state.

TABLE 49-3 Characteristics of Arrhythmias

TYPE	SIGNS AND SYMPTOMS	CAUSE	ECG CHANGES
Sinus Arrhythmias			
Bradycardia	<60 beats/min	Vagal nerve stimulation; sleep; SA node ischemia; digitalis toxicity; drugs Can be normal in athletes	Essentially "normal" appearing, but slow
Tachycardia	Nonpathologic; heart rate >100 beats/min is pathologic	Increased demand for cardiac output; ectopic pacemaker	P wave can be obscured by ST segment (increasing the ECG speed can reduce this problem)
Atrial Arrhythmias			
PAC	Not pathologic if only several per minute	Increased SA node excitability, causing premature beats of atria Can be caused by nicotine or caffeine	"Extra" P waves
Flutter	200-350 beats/min	Many ectopic atrial pacemakers; normally unstable and progresses to atrial fibrillation if not corrected	Multiple, sawtoothed P waves before essentially normal-appearing QRS complexes
Ventricular Arrhythmias (see Figure 49-16)			
PVC	Generally none	Ectopic pacemakers originating in ventricles from electrolyte imbalance, hypoxia, acute MI	Widened QRS complex
V-tach	Heart rate >100 beats/min, always pathologic	Damaged tissue around one of the "bundles," causing a difference in conduction speed between the two branches or ectopic pacemaker cells	Rapid rate, irregular pattern that includes "extra" or erratic, irregular, or wide QRS complexes
V-fib*	Shock, loss of consciousness, no pulse	Complete loss of synchronization of conduction system	Erratic deflections on the ECG (can be either coarse or fine) No identifiable ECG waves
Asystole	<5 beats/min	Death imminent	Flatline
Biochemical Arrhythmias			
Digitalis toxicity	Abnormal bradycardia, abnormal tachycardia	Digitalis dose that is too high	"Swooping" ST segment depression and/or extended PR intervals
Hypokalemia	Malaise, fatigue, weakness, muscle cramps	Potassium too low, usually from unsupplemented diuresis, from IV fluid administration, or from excessive vomiting	Prominent U waves, T wave and U wave together look like a two-hump camel
Hyperkalemia†	May have none	Potassium too high, usually from IV supplementation	Peaked T wave (can be as tall as R wave) with widening of all waveforms

IV, Intravenous; *MI*, myocardial infarction; *PAC*, premature atrial contraction; *PVC*, premature ventricular contraction; *SA*, sinoatrial.
*Most life-threatening arrhythmia; frequently precedes asystole if not reversed.
†Life-threatening situation that must be corrected immediately.

Ventricular fibrillation (commonly referred to as *V-fib*; Figure 49-16, *D*) is the most critical, life-threatening arrhythmia; it quickly results in death if not treated. V-fib is estimated to precede 85% of cases of **cardiac arrest** in adults. In V-fib, the electrical conduction system of the heart is in total dysfunction. The heart muscle quivers uncontrollably and is essentially ineffective at pumping any blood; therefore, there is no pulse, and the patient is unresponsive and not breathing. Cardioversion with a **defibrilla-tor** is necessary to restore normal function of the electrical conduction system.

Asystole is the result of absence of a heartbeat, or cardiac cessation, which shows as a flatline on the ECG (Figure 49-16, *E*).

Biochemical Arrhythmias

Digitalis, frequently called *dig* (pronounced *dij*), is a common cardiac drug used to slow and strengthen the heartbeat. The heart is

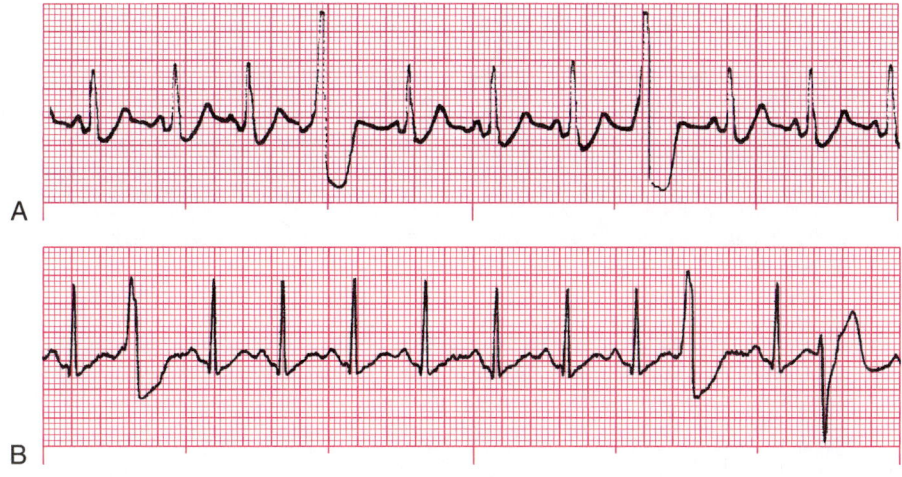

FIGURE 49-15 Sinus tachycardia with frequent, uniform PVCs **(A)** and with multiform PVCs **(B)**. (From Aehlert B: *ECGs made easy,* ed 3, St Louis, 2006, Mosby.)

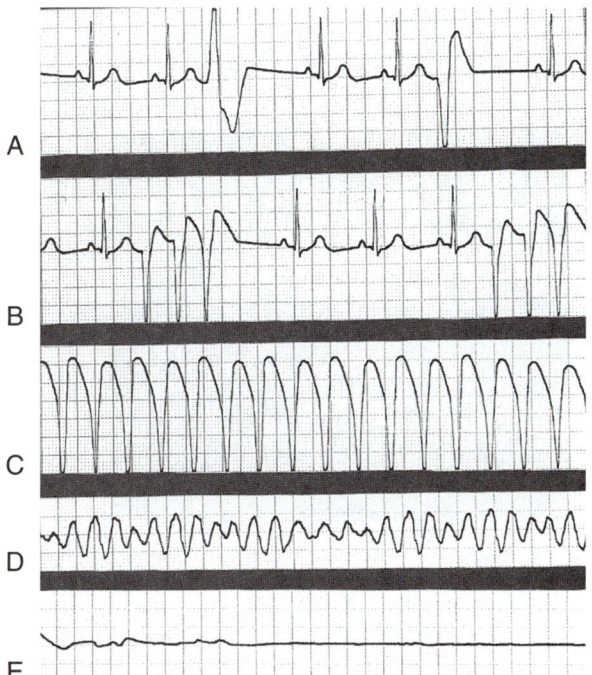

FIGURE 49-16 Ventricular arrhythmias. **A,** PVC. **B,** Three PVCs in a row. **C,** V-tach. **D,** V-fib. **E,** Asystole. (From Chester GA: *Modern medical assisting,* Philadelphia, 1999, WB Saunders.)

quite sensitive to digitalis, and too much can prove toxic and cause changes in the ECG (Figure 49-17). This condition can be reversed by reducing the dosage of digoxin or digitoxin (both are forms of digitalis).

Potassium is a critical mineral for normal cardiac function. Too much potassium in the blood (hyperkalemia) or too little (hypokalemia) can both cause life-threatening arrhythmias that must be corrected quickly. Intravenous administration of potassium can reverse hypokalemia. Administration of a diuretic that does not effectively spare potassium can reverse hyperkalemia.

Pacemaker Rhythms

A pacemaker is a device implanted under the skin that stimulates the electrical activity of the heart. It consists of a small metal pulse generator with a battery and electronic leads that extend from the generator to the myocardium. The entire pulse generator is replaced when the battery wears out, usually every 5 to 10 years. Current pacemakers are rate responsive, which means that they speed up or slow the heart rate based on such factors as the breathing rate and body temperature. Biventricular pacemakers, which stimulate both the right and left ventricles to enable more efficient cardiac contractions, may be implanted in patients with congestive heart failure.

Pacemakers are implanted in a hospital setting, and local anesthesia is used. Before the patient is discharged, the device is programmed to fire according to the needs of the individual patient. The patient is instructed to telephone the physician's office periodically to transmit pacemaker readings across the phone lines. The patient may use a transmission device attached to a wristband or a wand that is placed over the pacer. Pacemakers cause wide variations in the appearance of an ECG (Figure 49-18).

Implanted Cardioverter-Defibrillator

An implanted cardioverter-defibrillator, or ICD, monitors the heart rhythm and delivers a shock to the heart if it detects a dangerous tachycardia or fibrillation (Figure 49-19). It is a small, battery-operated device that is implanted under the skin in the chest or abdomen. An ICD can be used to reverse V-tach and V-fib, especially after the patient has previously had a myocardial **infarction** (MI), or heart attack. The generator is programmed specifically to treat the patient's particular or potential cardiac arrhythmia. Just as with pacemakers, the device is programmed to meet the needs of each individual patient, the patient can telephone in periodic readings, and the device must be replaced every 4 to 7 years.

Myocardial Infarction

Sudden heart attack, or MI, occurs in more than 1.2 million Americans each year, according to the American Heart Association. Approximately 20% of these patients die before reaching the hospital, and approximately 30% die within 30 days of the heart attack. An MI occurs when a portion of the heart muscle becomes ischemic because the blood supply to that area has been interrupted. **Ischemia** eventually leads to tissue necrosis, or infarction.

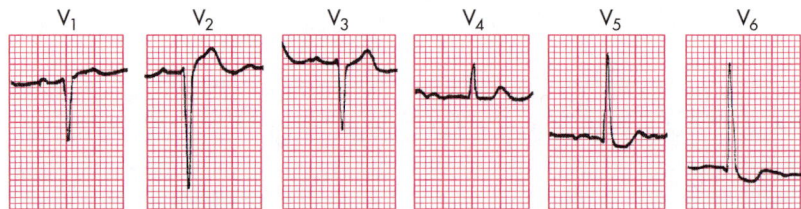

FIGURE 49-17 ECG showing the effects of digitalis. Note the "scooping" of the ST segment, as seen in leads V_5 and V_6. (From Aehlert B: *ECGs made easy*, ed 3, St Louis, 2006, Mosby.)

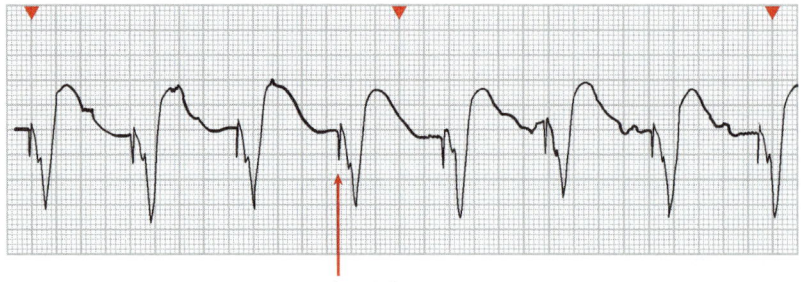

Pacemaker spike

FIGURE 49-18 Pacemaker rhythm strip. (From Lewis S et al: *Medical-surgical nursing*, ed 7, St Louis, 2007, Mosby.)

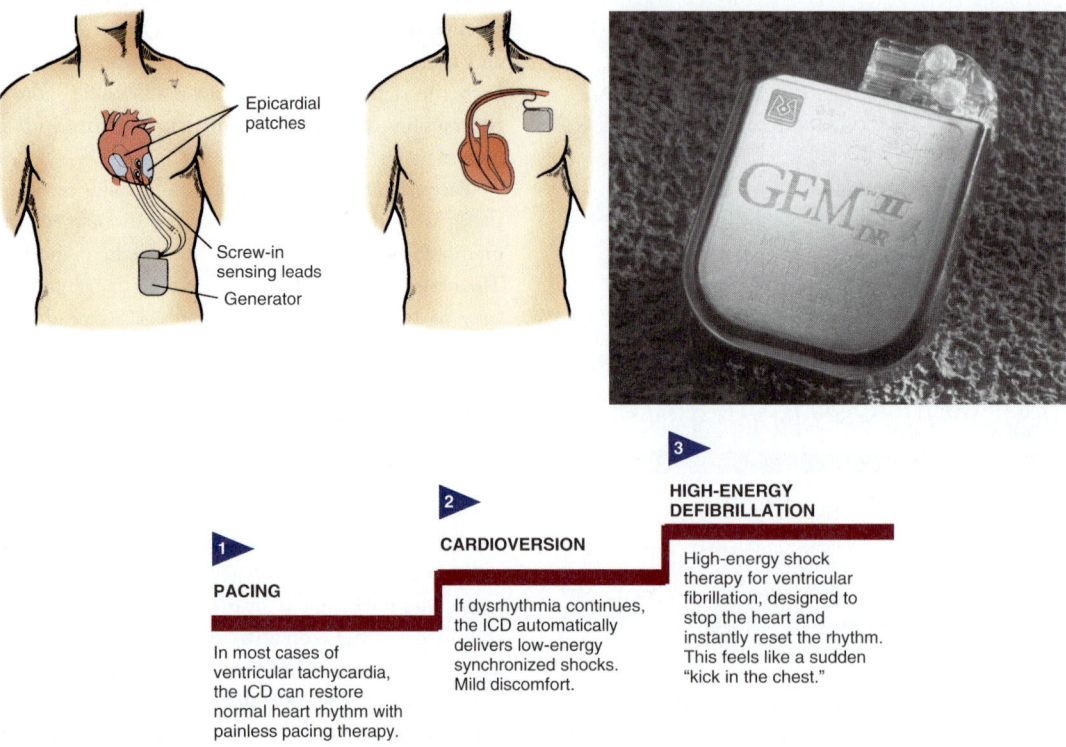

Epicardial patches

Screw-in sensing leads

Generator

1
PACING

In most cases of ventricular tachycardia, the ICD can restore normal heart rhythm with painless pacing therapy.

2
CARDIOVERSION

If dysrhythmia continues, the ICD automatically delivers low-energy synchronized shocks. Mild discomfort.

3
HIGH-ENERGY DEFIBRILLATION

High-energy shock therapy for ventricular fibrillation, designed to stop the heart and instantly reset the rhythm. This feels like a sudden "kick in the chest."

FIGURE 49-19 Implanted cardioverter-defibrillator. (From Urden L, Stacy K, Lough M: *Thelan's critical care nursing: diagnosis and management*, ed 5, St Louis, Mosby.)

The heart muscle, the myocardium, receives its oxygen supply from a network of coronary arteries (Figure 49-20) on the surface of the heart. The right coronary artery supplies much of the right side of the heart. The left coronary artery bifurcates into two main branches: the left circumflex artery, which supplies blood principally to the left lateral and posterior walls of the left ventricle, and the left anterior descending coronary artery, which supplies principally the anterior wall of the left ventricle and the interventricular septum. The left anterior descending coronary artery is sometimes called the "sudden death artery," because it feeds such a large portion of the left ventricle.

MI causes specific, recognizable changes on the ECG recording, based on the phase the patient is in when the ECG is recorded (Table 49-4). The three most common changes are elevated ST segments, inverted (upside-down) T waves, and abnormal (pathologic) Q waves (Figure 49-21).

The sooner treatment is initiated after the patient's first awareness of a heart attack, the more effective treatment is and the better the

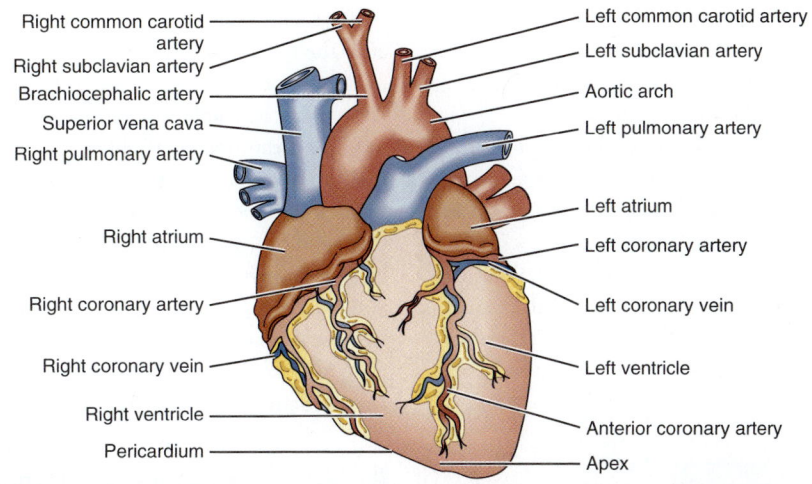

FIGURE 49-20 Coronary vessels. (From Chester GA: *Modern medical assisting,* Philadelphia, 1999, WB Saunders.)

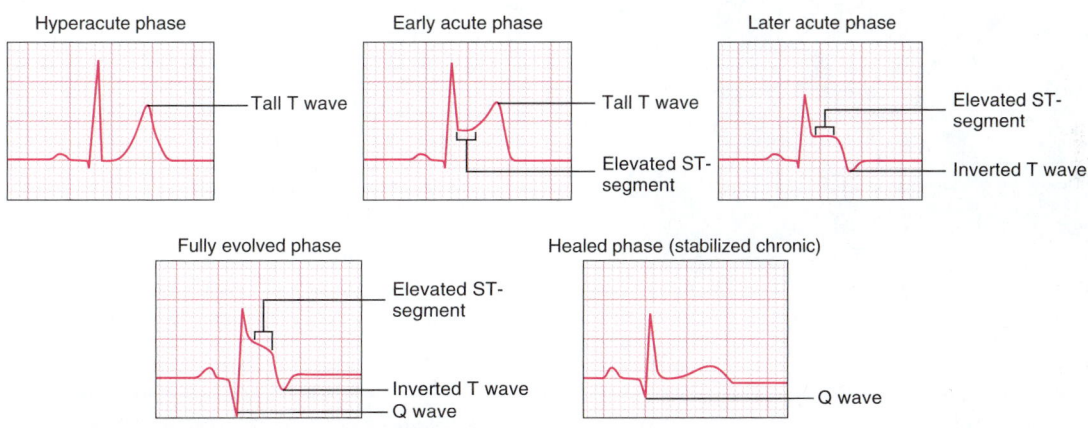

FIGURE 49-21 Changes in the PQRST segment associated with a myocardial infarction. (From Aehlert B: *ACLS study guide,* ed 3, St Louis, Mosby, 2006.)

TABLE 49-4	Phases of Myocardial Infarction with Electrocardiographic Changes	
PHASE	**APPEARANCE OF ECG CHANGES**	**SPECIFIC CHANGES SEEN ON ECG**
I (hyperacute)	Occurs in first few hours	ST segment elevated from baseline (earliest indication on ECG); peaked "hyperacute" T waves
II (fully evolved)	After hours or days	Deep T waves; pathologic Q waves appear (negative deflection)
III (resolution)	Days to weeks	ST segment returns to normal position; T waves return to normal
IV (stabilized chronic)	Permanent	Negative Q wave deflection remains

chances for the patient's survival. Immediate treatment for a heart attack includes administration of nasal oxygen, sublingual nitroglycerin (to dilate the coronary arteries), a narcotic analgesic (to eliminate pain), aspirin (to reduce inflammation and decrease clotting time), and possibly a thrombolytic agent to dissolve the clot causing the coronary artery obstruction. Early administration of thrombolytic agents enhances the likelihood of restoring circulation to the myocardium distal to the occluding thrombus (blood clot). After discharge from the hospital, the patient should quit smoking, modify the diet as instructed by a nutritionist, and enter a cardiac rehabilitation program to improve cardiac strength and recovery through exercise.

Complications of acute MI include a sudden episode of atrial fibrillation, V-fib, or bradycardia that may necessitate implantation of a pacemaker.

RELATED CARDIAC DIAGNOSTIC TESTS

Stress Test

Cardiac stress testing is performed to observe and record the patient's cardiovascular response to measured exercise challenges (Figure 49-22). Stress testing is done to accomplish the following:

- Diagnose cardiac disease that cannot be detected by a standard resting ECG
- Determine an individual's energy performance capacity
- Prescribe a specially designed exercise plan

A stress test is performed while the patient is exercising on either a bicycle or a treadmill, under careful supervision. The patient must be given the appropriate information explaining the purpose, preparation, and procedure for the test (Figure 49-23).

Cardiac arrest is a serious risk with a cardiac stress test. The medical assistant must be able to recognize symptoms of dyspnea, vertigo, extreme fatigue, severe arrhythmia, and other abnormal ECG readings that may develop during the stress test or immediately after the test during the rest period. All members of a cardiac stress testing team must be prepared to terminate testing immediately if the patient is unable to continue or if abnormalities appear on the monitor. Team members also must be certified in cardiopulmonary resuscitation (CPR) and emergency intervention. The physician must always be present during this procedure. In addition to the routine monitoring equipment, the team must have oxygen, a defibrillator, an endotracheal intubation tray, an artificial breathing bag, and emergency cardiac medications available in case of cardiac crisis. Because of the potential for life-threatening incidents, most physicians have stress tests performed in a hospital setting, where personnel are trained and ready to assist if a cardiac emergency occurs.

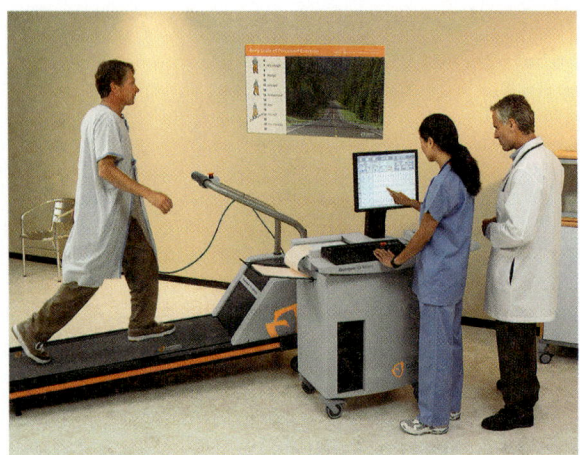

FIGURE 49-22 Cardiac stress test. (Courtesy Cardiac Science, Bothell, Wash.)

CRITICAL THINKING APPLICATION   49-5

Mr. Sonderford actually had an MI when he was previously at Dr. Lee's office. He now has completed cardiac rehabilitation and is at the office for a checkup. Dr. Lee wants him to be scheduled for a stress test. Mr. Sonderford has never had one before. He confides to Martha that he is afraid if he takes the test, he will die from another heart attack. How should Martha handle this situation?

Holter Monitor

A Holter monitor is a portable system for recording a patient's cardiac activity over a 24-hour period or longer (Procedure 49-2). The monitor is a small, lightweight device that the patient wears

---

Cardiac Stress Test

Cardiac stress testing (also known as an exercise tolerance test or treadmill test) is a means of observing, evaluating, and recording your heart's response during a measured exercise test. This test determines your capacity to adapt to physical stress.

There are various reasons that your physician may suggest this test for you:

1. To aid in determining the presence of suspected coronary heart disease.
2. To aid in the selection of therapy.
   a. For angina pectoris (tightness or pain in the chest).
   b. Following a myocardial infarction (heart attack).
   c. Following coronary bypass surgery (open heart surgery).
3. To determine your physical work capacity.
4. To authorize participation in a physical exercise program.

Preparation for the Test

1. Avoid eating a heavy meal within 2 hours of your appointment.
2. Take your medications as you usually do, unless your doctor advises you not to take them.
3. Wear a shirt or blouse that buttons down the front with slacks, a skirt, jogging pants, or shorts.
4. Do not wear one-piece undergarments, jumpsuits, or dresses.
5. Tennis shoes are ideal if you have them. Otherwise, wear comfortable flat or low-heeled shoes. Do not wear clogs, sling-backs, crepe soles, boots, or high heels, as they make walking on the treadmill more difficult.

The Procedure

When you arrive in the Cardiology Department, areas of your chest may be shaved (men only) to allow the electrodes to adhere tightly to your chest. A blood pressure cuff will be wrapped around your arm, and an electrocardiogram (ECG) is taken while you are at rest. The technician will then demonstrate how to walk on the treadmill and will answer any questions you may have.

You will then perform a graded exercise test on a motor-driven treadmill. You will begin walking very gradually at a rate you can easily accomplish.

Progressively throughout the test, the speed and grade of the treadmill will be increased, and you will be walking at a faster pace up a slight incline. At no time will you be asked to jog or run, nor will you be asked to exercise beyond your capabilities.

At all times during the test, trained personnel are in the room with you, monitoring your heart rate and blood pressure and observing you for signs of fatigue or discomfort. We do not wish to exercise you to a level that is medically unsafe or physically distressing.

An ECG is taken again when you finish walking. Your cardiologist will immediately interpret the results of the test and explain his or her findings to you. If necessary, medications or treatment will be discussed. A letter with the results of the stress test will be sent to your referring physician.

The entire procedure will take 1 to 1 1/2 hours. If you have any questions regarding the cardiac stress test or any problems with your appointment, please contact us.

FIGURE 49-23 Patient information for a cardiac stress test.

PROCEDURE 49-2

Assist the Physician with Patient Care: Fit a Patient with a Holter Monitor

GOAL: *To establish a possible correlation between coronary disorders and the patient's 24-hour daily activities.*

EQUIPMENT and SUPPLIES

- Holter monitor with new batteries
- Disposable electrodes
- Razor
- Gauze pads or abrasive tool as needed
- Activity diary
- Carrying case with belt or shoulder strap
- Alcohol swabs
- Cloth tape (nonallergenic)
- Patient's medical record

PROCEDURAL STEPS

1. Sanitize your hands.
   <u>PURPOSE:</u> To ensure infection control.
2. Assemble the needed equipment.
3. Install batteries in the monitor (Figure 1).

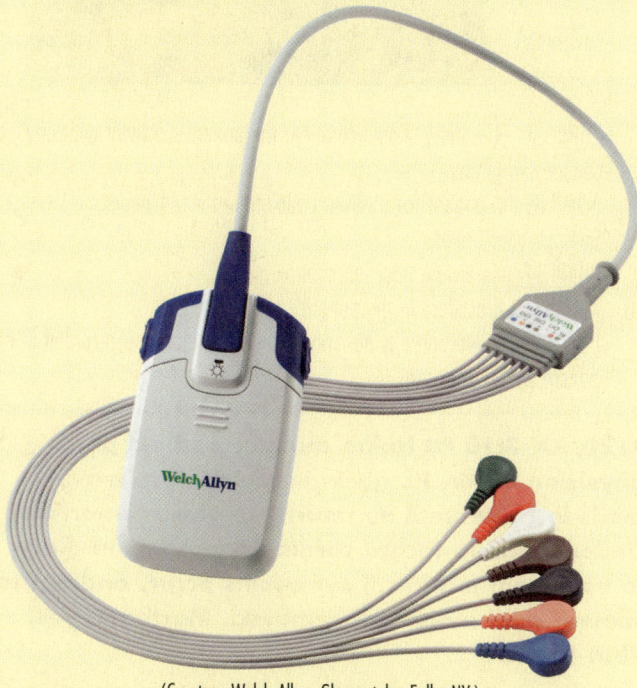

(Courtesy Welch Allyn, Skaneateles Falls, NY.)

<u>PURPOSE:</u> New or fully charged batteries ensure accurate monitor function for a 24-hour period.

4. Greet the patient and explain the procedure.
   <u>PURPOSE:</u> An informed patient helps ensure testing accuracy.
5. Ask the patient to disrobe to the waist and to sit at the end of the examination table or to lie down.
   <u>PURPOSE:</u> This places the patient at the best working level for the medical assistant.
6. Clean each electrode application site with the alcohol swab and allow the sites to air dry.

<u>PURPOSE:</u> To remove all surface skin oil to ensure maximum electrode adherence. Clean before shaving to prevent irritation and patient discomfort.

7. If the patient has a hairy chest, dry shave the area at each of the electrode sites.
   <u>PURPOSE:</u> The skin must be hairless to provide maximum electrode adherence.
8. Fold a gauze pad over your index finger and briskly rub the sites or use an abrasive tool as indicated (Figure 2).

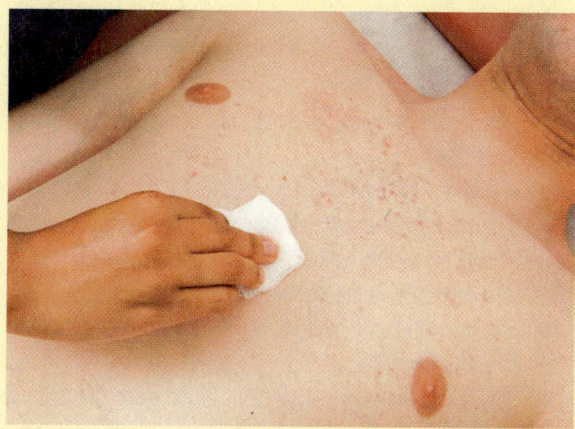

<u>PURPOSE:</u> To help electrodes stick more tightly to the skin.

9. Apply the electrodes to the sites recommended by the manufacturer; use enough pressure to make sure they adhere completely to the skin. Rub the edges of each electrode a second time to make sure the electrode will stay in place (Figures 3 and 4).

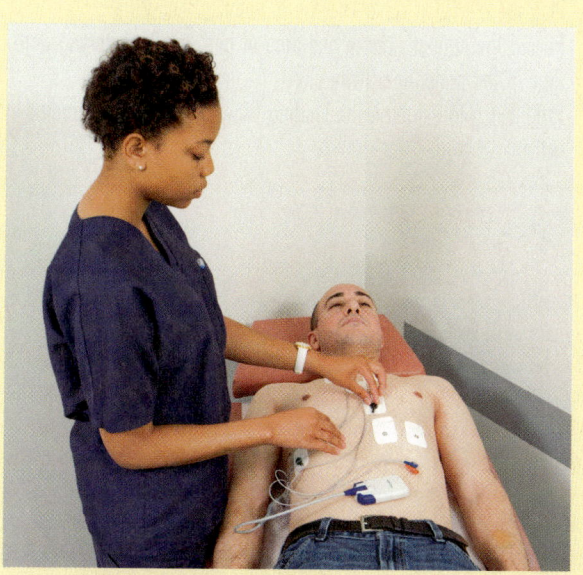

PROCEDURE 49-2—cont'd

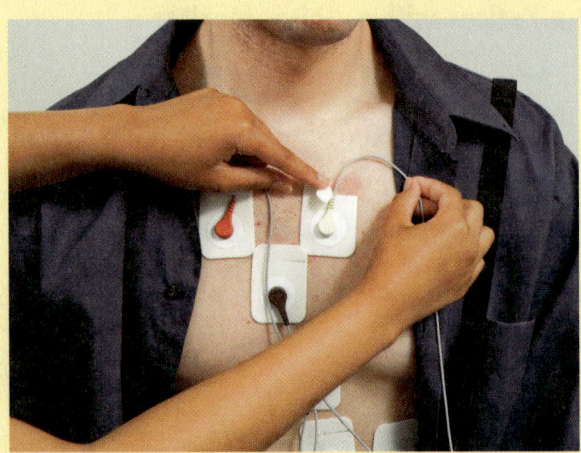

PURPOSE: Secure attachment of the electrodes is absolutely necessary to produce an accurate tracing.

10. Attach the lead wires to the electrodes and connect the end terminal to the patient cable.

11. Place a strip of cloth tape over each electrode.
    PURPOSE: To help secure the electrodes in place in case the wires are pulled during the testing period.

12. Attach the test cable to the monitor and plug it into the electrocardiograph. Run a baseline test tracing as directed by the manufacturer's guidelines.
    PURPOSE: To ensure proper connections of the electrodes and running of the monitor.

13. Help the patient get dressed without disturbing the connected electrodes. Make sure the cable extends through the buttoned front or out the bottom of the shirt or blouse.

14. Place the monitor in the carrying case and attach it to the patient's belt or pocket or place it over the shoulder. Be sure the wires are not being pulled or bent.
    PURPOSE: Taut or badly bent wires may loosen or malfunction.

15. Plug the electrode cable into the monitor.

16. Record the patient's name and date of birth and the starting date and time in the patient's activity diary.
    PURPOSE: To establish the starting time of the test and cardiac activity.

17. Give the patient the activity diary and advise him or her to begin by writing in his or her present activity (Figure 5). Include patient education information on the importance of continually recording activities in the diary; using the event marker on the monitor if he or she experiences any symptoms; and correlating the event with a recording in the diary, including the time and details of the related activity before or during the event.

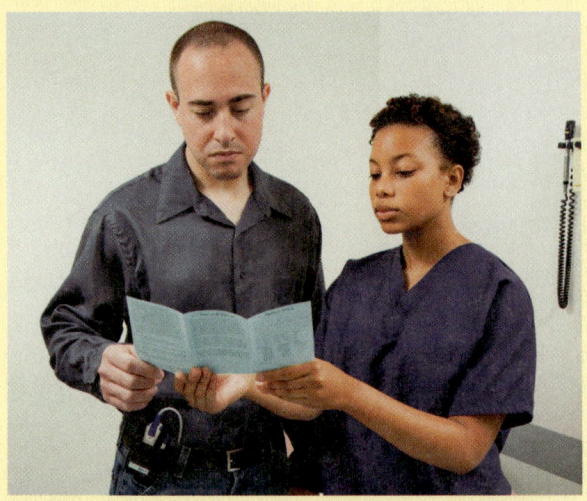

PURPOSE: The diary should correlate the patient's activity with any cardiac symptoms.

18. Schedule the patient for a return appointment in 24 hours.

19. Sanitize your hands.
    PURPOSE: To ensure infection control.

20. Record the procedure in the patient's medical record.
    PURPOSE: A procedure is not considered done until it is recorded in the patient's medical record.

9/29/XX 3:10 PM Holter monitor applied per physician order. Pt. given instructions to leave leads in place until he returns to office tomorrow. Understands to record cardiac symptoms in diary, to use event marker if symptoms occur, and not to shower until monitor is removed. Martha Reyes, CMA (AAMA)

---

while going about usual daily activities. The Holter monitor can be programmed to record cardiac information continuously or periodically, when activated by the patient if symptoms occur, or during periods of stress.

The entire time the monitor is worn, the patient must keep a journal of all stressful events and activities (and also specific details about activities when any cardiac symptoms occur). Journal entries include the time, duration, and specific activity during the cardiac event, such as rush hour traffic, bowel movements, intercourse, climbing stairs, and periods of anger or emotional distress. Some monitors can even record the patient's voice describing a symptom or event so that it can later be correlated with the ECG recording in the same time frame.

Many cardiologists routinely use Holter monitors in their practices. A medical assistant often is responsible for fitting the monitor on the patient and for removing it after the test period. The patient must have a full understanding of what is required during monitoring, particularly how to use the event marker in case a significant symptom is experienced. The patient also must know how to record the event in a written diary when the event marker is used. The patient may take only sponge baths during the 24 hours of the test. The number of electrodes and leads varies with the number of channels on the particular monitor. Electrode placement is determined by the physician or by the manufacturer's guidelines and should be followed precisely. The skin of male patients may need to be shaved so that the electrodes can be firmly attached. The lead wires are attached to the electrodes and to the Holter monitor, which is worn around the waist or on a belt or in a pouch slung over the shoulder.

At the end of the monitoring period, the patient returns to the office, the monitor is disconnected, and electrodes are removed. The recording is placed in a Holter scanner or computer, and the results are analyzed. Any part of the recording can be printed for further study.

CRITICAL THINKING APPLICATION   **49-6**

Mrs. Jamison was fitted with a Holter monitor at the office yesterday at 4 PM. When Martha arrived at the office at 8 o'clock this morning, she found that Mrs. Jamison had left a message with the answering service to call her as soon as possible. When Martha returns the call, Mrs. Jamison tells her that she had taken a shower last night, and she noticed that when she got up to go to the bathroom, "the light was not on" on the monitor. How should Martha handle this situation?

Cardiac Event Monitor

The cardiac event monitor is a small recording device that can be worn up to 30 days to catch events that are difficult to record in a 24-hour period on a Holter monitor, such as vertigo, weakness, and **palpitations**. Patients are instructed to trigger the recording when they feel any indication of a cardiac event. Using the information gathered during the recording period, the physician can diagnose heart abnormalities and design the most effective treatment. The monitor must be removed during bathing, so the patient must be taught how to remove and reapply the electrodes throughout the test period. Patient education for using an event monitor includes the following instructions:

- Protect the monitor from damage and wear it at all times except when bathing.
- Do not alter your lifestyle; regular activities need to be maintained to reflect the cause of cardiac symptoms.
- Trigger the recording by pushing the event monitor when symptoms occur.
- Use the diary to record activities when events occur.
- Change the electrodes daily and the batteries at the same time each day.
- To prevent skin irritation, do not put replacement electrodes in the same spot.
- Put the electrodes on the rib cage under the left breast and in the midaxillary region under the right shoulder.
- Most event monitor recordings can be transmitted by telephone; you will be given instructions for transmitting recordings.

- If you have any questions, use the contact information provided.

Heart Scan

A noninvasive method of assessing possible cardiac risk is a specialized type of computed tomography (CT) called an *electron beam tomography (EBT) heart scan* (also called an *ultrafast CT*). The heart scan takes less than 5 minutes and does not require any needles or injections. It is a screening tool that allows physicians to see the amount of plaque in the coronary arteries by showing the presence of calcium deposits. Calcium makes up approximately 20% of arterial plaque deposits. The EBT heart scan is read, and the physician assigns the patient a calcium score that can be a predictor of future cardiac problems.

CLOSING COMMENTS

Patient Education

Heart disease and stroke account for more than one third of all deaths. Genetic predisposition and detrimental lifestyle habits, such as smoking, lack of exercise, high-fat diets, and obesity, play significant roles in the development of heart disease. The medical assistant should talk to the patient about factors that can be changed or modified and should encourage any attempt by the patient to make these changes.

Before you can successfully counsel a patient to change a habit, you need to familiarize yourself with possible techniques and approaches to use. Such information can be obtained from the American Heart Association and reputable Internet sites.

Many patients like visual aids when they are learning new information, and brochures with pictures or posters in the office are effective means of promoting learning and eliciting questions from patients. Make a note in the medical record of the educational items you give the patient on each visit. On a subsequent visit, ask about the helpfulness of the information, whether the patient tried any modifications, and what the results were. Ask for any suggestions that might help another patient in a similar situation.

Legal and Ethical Issues

An ECG is a valuable diagnostic tool, and it continues to be one of the most common procedures used in the diagnosis of cardiac diseases and conditions. The cardiologist measures the heart's activity and compares the results with known values by analyzing the ECG tracing. Comparing an ECG tracing with previous tracings can identify changes in the condition of the patient's heart.

The physician must be able to interpret the ECG tracing accurately and to establish its value in correctly diagnosing the patient's condition; the medical assistant, therefore, has the ethical obligation to complete the task as accurately and carefully as possible. Diagnostic procedures have a profound effect on a patient's subsequent treatment. When you are entrusted with performing testing procedures, you assume full responsibility for the accuracy and precision of each test you perform. This is a critical role in the medical assisting profession. The results you submit strongly influence each patient's therapeutic treatment plan. No test is ever just routine.

SUMMARY OF SCENARIO

Martha has worked in Dr. Lee's office for almost 8 months. She has become quite confident in her ability to perform electrocardiography quickly and accurately. She also has learned to communicate effectively with patients about their fears and concerns about various cardiac diagnostic tests. She never forgets to emphasize to a patient the importance of not taking a shower during the 24-hour Holter monitoring period. In 2 months she and Dr. Lee will attend a national meeting of cardiologists in Chicago. Two days of continuing education classes will be offered for medical assistants who work in cardiology. Martha is very excited to be able to continue learning and to sharpen her skills as a medical assistant in cardiology.

SUMMARY OF LEARNING OBJECTIVES

1. **Define, spell, and pronounce the terms listed in the vocabulary.**
   Spelling and pronouncing medical terms correctly bolster the medical assistant's credibility. Knowing the definitions of these terms promotes confidence in communication with patients and co-workers.

2. **Apply critical thinking skills in performing the patient assessment and patient care.**
   Completing the Critical Thinking Application exercises throughout the chapter can help the student medical assistant become more adept at critical analysis of real-life situations.

3. **Illustrate the electrical conduction system through the heart.**
   The heart beats in response to an electrical signal that originates in the SA node in the right atrium, spreads over the atria, and causes atrial contraction. This impulse continues to the AV node, through the bundle of His, through the right and left bundle branches, and into the Purkinje fibers, eventually causing ventricular contraction.

4. **Explain the concepts of cardiac polarization, depolarization, and repolarization.**
   Polarization is the resting state of the myocardial wall, when there is no electrical activity in the heart. When the electrical system of the heart stimulates a myocardial cell, *depolarization* occurs, resulting in contraction of the stimulated heart muscle. The heart muscle cells must then return to a resting state; the process of reaching this resting state is *repolarization*.

5. **Identify the PQRST complex on an electrocardiograph tracing.**
   The *P wave* shows atrial contraction, the beginning of cardiac depolarization; the *PR segment* is the return to baseline after atrial contraction; the *PR interval* is the time from the beginning of atrial contraction to the beginning of ventricular contraction; the *QRS complex* shows the contraction of both ventricles and the completion of cardiac depolarization; the *ST segment* is the time between the end of ventricular contraction and the beginning of ventricular recovery; the *T wave* is repolarization of the ventricles; the *QT interval* is the time between the beginning of the QRS complex through the T wave; a *U wave* occasionally can be seen as a small waveform just after the T wave in certain patients.

6. **Summarize the properties of the electrocardiograph.**
   A six-channel ECG machine records all 12 leads simultaneously within seconds. Limb and chest electrodes with leads must be placed on the patient at specific anatomic locations before the recording starts. ECG paper is standardized to represent amplitude and time. The horizontal lines allow determination of the intensity of the electrical activity, and the vertical lines represent time; each of the large squares represents 0.2 second; five of them equals 1 second.

7. **Describe the electrical views of the heart recorded by the 12-lead electrocardiograph.**
   Lead I records the electrical activity of the lateral part of the left ventricle; leads II and III record the electrical activity of the inferior surface of the left ventricle. The augmented lead aV_R records the electrical activity of the atria with negative deflection of the P waves and QRS complexes; aV_L records the electrical activity of the lateral wall of the left ventricle; and aV_F records the electrical activity of the inferior surface of the left ventricle. The precordial leads provide a transverse plane view of the heart. They include V_1, V_2, V_3, V_4, V_5, and V_6, with each number representing a specific location on the chest. The QRS complex is a negative deflection in V_1 and V_2 views, and each subsequent lead becomes more positive.

8. **Discuss the process of recording an electrocardiogram.**
   Recording an ECG requires a knowledge of where to place the electrodes and connect the leads to obtain the most accurate recording possible; the ability to recognize and correct the most common types of artifacts on the ECG recording; and proper use of the machine available.

9. **Perform an accurate recording of the electrical activity of the heart.**
   Procedure 49-1 outlines the steps for performing a 12-lead ECG recording.

10. **Compare and contrast electrocardiographic artifacts and the probable cause of each.**
    An artifact is an unwanted, erratic movement of the stylus on the paper caused by outside interference. The main types include wandering baseline artifacts, in which the stylus gradually shifts away from the center of the paper because of slight movement or poor electrode attachment. Somatic tremor artifacts are a result of muscle movements in the patient that cause jagged peaks of irregular height and spacing and a shifting baseline. AC interference causes a series of uniform, small spikes on the paper because of electrical energy in the area. Interrupted baseline artifacts occur when the electric connection between the electrode and the lead is interrupted.

11. **Identify a typical electrocardiograph tracing.**
    Table 49-2 summarizes the normal appearance of ECG waveforms and complexes. The ECG tracing is made up of repeated cardiac cycle (PQRST) recordings. The heart rate is calculated from the ECG recording by counting the number of P waves in a 6-second strip (30 large

squares) and multiplying by 10. For the ventricular contraction rate, the number of complete QRS complexes within 6 seconds is counted and multiplied by 10 to get the number of ventricular contractions in 1 minute. The rhythm of the patient's heartbeat indicates whether it is regular. If the patient's heart is beating at a regular rhythm, each cardiac cycle occurs within the same time frame and individual cardiac cycles occur exactly the same length of time apart.

12. **Describe common electrocardiographic arrhythmias.**
In sinus rhythm, the heart's electrical activity begins in the SA node and follows through the electrical system, ending in atrial and ventricular depolarization. In sinus bradycardia, the heart rate is less than 60 beats/min; in sinus tachycardia, the rate is more than 100 beats/min. A PAC occurs when the atria contract before they should for the next cardiac cycle. Atrial flutter occurs when the atria beat at an extremely rapid rate, up to 300 beats/min. PVCs occur when the ventricles contract before they should for the next cardiac cycle. V-tach causes the ventricles to beat at an extremely rapid rate, from 101 to 250 beats/min. V-fib is the most critical, life-threatening arrhythmia and results in death if not effectively treated. Asystole is the result of no heartbeat. Biochemical systemic problems also can cause arrhythmias.

13. **Summarize cardiac diagnostic tests.**
Cardiac diagnostic tests include an ECG; a stress test to determine the patient's cardiac response to exercise; a 24-hour Holter monitor to pick up abnormalities during the patient's routine day; a 30-day event monitor to record infrequent cardiac symptoms; and a heart scan to provide noninvasive diagnostic information.

14. **Fit a patient with a Holter monitor.**
Procedure 49-2 explains how to fit a patient with a Holter monitor.

15. **Discuss the legal and ethical issues involved when performing ECGs.**
Diagnostic procedures have a profound effect on a patient's subsequent treatment. When the medical assistant is entrusted with performing testing procedures, he or she assumes full responsibility for the accuracy and precision of tests performed. This is a critical role in the medical assisting profession. The results you submit strongly influence each patient's therapeutic treatment plan. No test is ever just routine.

CONNECTIONS

Study Guide Connection: Go to the Chapter 49 Study Guide. Read and complete the activities.

Evolve Connection: Go to the Chapter 49 link at *evolve.elsevier.com/ kinn* to complete the Chapter Review and Chapter Quiz. Check out the other resources listed for this chapter to make the most of what you have learned from Principles of Electrocardiography.

50

ASSISTING WITH DIAGNOSTIC IMAGING

SCENARIO

Sara Elwood, CMA (AAMA), is employed by Metro Urgicenter, an urgent care clinic in an urban setting. Metro is staffed around the clock and sees patients with urgent problems that are not immediately life-threatening. Facilities at the center include an x-ray department where films of the spine and the extremities are taken to evaluate injuries for possible fractures. Chest films also are taken to aid the diagnosis of patients with respiratory complaints. The center's staff physicians read the x-ray films as they are taken. Afterward, the films are sent to a local hospital for formal interpretation by a radiologist.

Sara often assists David Swain, the radiographer, by preparing patients for x-ray examinations and processing the films. Sometimes she is responsible for sending the films to the hospital for interpretation and then filing them when they are returned. Sara is in the process of helping the clinic switch to electronic medical records, which will make the transmission of radiology results much more efficient. When a patient is sent to some other facility for special imaging studies, Sara makes the arrangements and provides the patient with a preliminary explanation of the procedure.

While studying this chapter, think about the following questions:

- To fulfill her job description at Metro Urgicenter, what does Sara need to know about preparing patients for routine x-ray examinations?
- How should a film be processed so that it has no handling artifacts?
- What should Sara know about various diagnostic procedures so that she can effectively provide patient education and answer patient's scheduling questions?

LEARNING OBJECTIVES

1. Define, spell, and pronounce the terms listed in the vocabulary.
2. Apply critical thinking skills in performing the patient assessment and patient care.
3. Identify the principal components of radiographic equipment.
4. Describe the cassette and film image receptor system and explain its function in radiography.
5. Recognize the precautions to be taken when unloading, loading, and processing radiographic film and cassettes.
6. Distinguish among the three body planes and use these terms correctly when discussing radiographic positions.
7. Identify anteroposterior (AP), posteroanterior (PA), lateral, oblique, and axial radiographic projections.
8. Compare and contrast radiography and fluoroscopy and give examples of appropriate applications of each.
9. List and describe imaging modalities that do not involve x-rays.
10. Explain the patient preparation guidelines for typical diagnostic imaging examinations.
11. Outline the general procedure for assisting with an x-ray examination.
12. Summarize guidelines for scheduling multiple diagnostic procedures.
13. Apply patient education principles when providing instructions for preparing for diagnostic procedures.
14. Describe the health risks associated with low doses of x-ray exposure, such as those used in radiography.
15. Describe precautions for ensuring the safety of equipment operators and staff members during x-ray procedures.
16. Summarize the steps for ensuring that patients receive the least possible exposure during x-ray procedures.
17. Explain the legal responsibilities associated with x-ray procedures and the administrative management of diagnostic images.

VOCABULARY

angiocardiography (an-je-o-kahr-de-og'-ruh-fe) Radiography of the heart and great vessels using an iodine contrast medium.

angiography (an-je-og'-ruh-fe) Radiography of blood vessels using an iodine contrast medium.

angioplasty (an'-je-o-plas-te) An interventional technique in which a catheter is used to open or widen a blood vessel to improve circulation.

anteroposterior (AP) (an-tuhr-o-pos-ter'-e-ohr) A frontal projection in which the patient is supine or facing the x-ray tube.

aortogram (a-or'-ti-gram) Radiography of the aorta using an iodine contrast medium.

arteriography (ahr-ter-e-og'-ruh-fe) Radiography of arteries using an iodine contrast medium.

arthrogram (ahr'-thro-gram) Fluoroscopic examination of the soft tissue components of joints with direct injection of a contrast medium into the joint capsule.

axial projections Radiographs taken with a longitudinal angulation of the x-ray beam; sometimes referred to as *semiaxial projections.*

bucky A moving grid device that prevents scatter radiation from fogging the film.

cathartics Laxative preparations.

computed tomography (CT) A computerized x-ray imaging modality that provides axial and three-dimensional scans.

contrast media Radiopaque substances used to enhance the visibility of soft tissues in imaging studies.

coronal plane The plane that divides the body into anterior and posterior parts.

coulombs per kilogram (C/kg) The international unit of radiation exposure.

dosimeter A badge for monitoring radiation exposure of personnel.

embolization An interventional technique in which a catheter is used to block off a blood vessel to prevent hemorrhage.

fluoroscopy (floo-ros'-kuh-pe) Direct observation of an x-ray image in motion.

frontal projection A radiographic view in which the coronal plane of the body or body part is parallel to the film plane; AP or PA.

gantry A doughnut-shaped portion of a scanner that surrounds the patient and functions, at least partly, to gather imaging data.

Gray (Gy) The international unit of radiation dose.

intravenous urogram (IVU) Radiographic examination of the urinary tract using intravenous injection of an iodine contrast medium.

latent image Invisible changes in exposed film that become an image when the film is processed.

lateral projections Radiographic views in which the sagittal plane of the body or body part is parallel to the film.

limited radiography Limited-scope radiography practice, usually in an outpatient setting, that does not require the same

credentials as for professional radiologic technology; also called *practical radiography.*

lower gastrointestinal series Fluoroscopic examination of the colon, usually using rectal administration of barium sulfate as a contrast medium; also called a *barium enema.*

magnetic resonance imaging (MRI) An imaging modality that uses a magnetic field and radiofrequency pulses to create computer images of both bones and soft tissues in multiple planes.

myelography (mi-uh-log'-ruh-fe) Fluoroscopic examination of the spinal canal with spinal injection of an iodine contrast medium.

NPO Nothing by mouth, from the Latin *nil per os.*

nuclear medicine An imaging modality that uses radioactive materials injected or ingested into the body to provide information about the function of organs and tissues.

oblique projections Radiographic views in which the body or part is rotated so that the projection is neither frontal nor lateral.

phosphors (fos'-fors) Fluorescent crystals that give off light when exposed to x-rays.

posteroanterior (PA) A frontal projection in which the patient is prone or facing the x-ray film or image receptor.

rad The conventional unit of radiation dose.

radiograph An x-ray image.

radiographer A person qualified to perform radiographic examinations.

radiography The process of taking diagnostic images using x-rays.

radiologist A physician who specializes in medical imaging or therapeutic applications of radiation.

radiolucent (ra-de-o-loo'-suhnt) Pertaining to a substance that is easily penetrated by x-rays; these substances appear dark on radiographs.

rem The conventional unit of radiation dose equivalent.

roentgen (R) (rent'-gen) The conventional unit of radiation exposure.

sagittal plane The plane that divides the body into right and left parts.

Sievert (Sv) (se'-vuhrt) The international unit of radiation dose equivalent.

sonography (suh-nog'-ruh-fe) An imaging modality that uses sound waves to produce images of soft tissues; also called *diagnostic ultrasound.*

tracers Radioactive substances administered to patients for nuclear medicine imaging procedures.

transducer The part of the sonography machine that is in contact with the patient; the transducer sends high-frequency sound waves and receives the sound echoes from the patient's body.

transverse plane The plane that divides the body into superior and inferior parts.

upper gastrointestinal (UGI) series Fluoroscopic examination of the esophagus, stomach, and duodenum using oral administration of barium sulfate as a contrast medium.

Physicians have been using x-ray images for more than 100 years to examine the internal structures of the body. The fascinating field of medical imaging now includes a wide variety of diagnostic imaging methods. This chapter provides an overview of imaging modalities and introduces you to **radiography**. Emphasis is placed on x-ray examinations, because these are the procedures most commonly performed in the medical assistant's practice setting.

BASIC PRINCIPLES OF RADIOGRAPHY

Radiography

Radiography is the process of making an x-ray image called a **radiograph**. X-rays are produced in a vacuum tube when electrons traveling at high speed strike certain materials, such as tungsten. When the x-rays are emitted from the tube, they diverge into space, forming the cone-shaped x-ray beam. The cross section of the x-ray beam at the point of use is called the *radiation field* (Figure 50-1). The patient or part to be x-rayed is placed in the radiation field, between the x-ray tube and the image receptor or film.

X-rays can penetrate most substances to some degree, but some substances, such as metals and bones, are more difficult to penetrate and are said to be *radiopaque*. Air, gases, and soft tissues such as fat, skin, and lungs are much easier to penetrate than bone and are said to be **radiolucent**. During the exposure, x-rays from the tube pass through the patient. Some of the x-rays are absorbed by the patient and others are not, resulting in a pattern of varying intensity in the x-ray beam that exits on the opposite side of the patient and exposes the film. The film then has a pattern of exposure, a **latent image**, and must be processed to develop the latent image into one that is visible. On the finished radiograph, radiopaque objects appear light and radiolucent objects appear dark or black (Figure 50-2).

Routine plain films are simple radiographs taken of specific body structures, such as the chest or the bones of the extremities or spine. These are the examinations most often performed in ambulatory care centers and most likely to be performed by medical assistants qualified to practice radiography.

X-Ray Exposure

Prime Factors

The **radiographer** must take a number of factors into consideration in determining the proper technique and exposure factors for an x-ray examination. The four principal exposure factors are called the *prime factors of exposure*. The interaction of these factors determines the level of x-ray production and ultimately the amount of the patient's x-ray exposure. Prime factors include the following:

- *Milliamperage* (mA)—the electrical control setting that determines how rapidly the radiation is produced; the higher the mA setting, the more x-rays produced per second.
- *Exposure time* (seconds)—the duration of the patient's x-ray exposure; most exposures are less than 1 second, so the total time a patient is exposed to the x-ray is measured in milliseconds. The amount of x-rays produced depends on the length of exposure.
- *Kilovoltage* (kVp)—the electrical control setting that determines the penetrating power of the x-ray beam; voltage controls the speed and power of x-ray beams; the higher the voltage, the shorter the x-ray wavelengths and the greater the energy of the x-ray beam.
- *Source-to-image distance* (SID)—the distance between the x-ray tube and the film or other image receptor; the greater the distance, the more widely the x-ray beam will spread and the lower the intensity of the beam.

The total amount of radiation in an exposure is indicated by the milliampere-seconds (mAs), which is determined by multiplying the rate of x-ray current flow (milliamperage) by the exposure time.

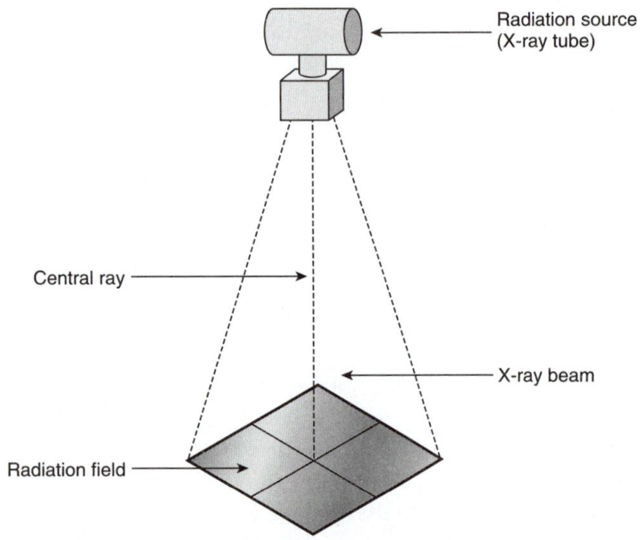

FIGURE 50-1 The primary x-ray beam leaves the x-ray tube and diverges into space. The center of the beam is called the *central ray*, and the cross section of the beam at the point of use is called the *radiation field*. (From Long BW, Frank ED, Ehrlich RA: *Radiography essentials for limited practice*, ed 3, Philadelphia, 2010, Saunders.)

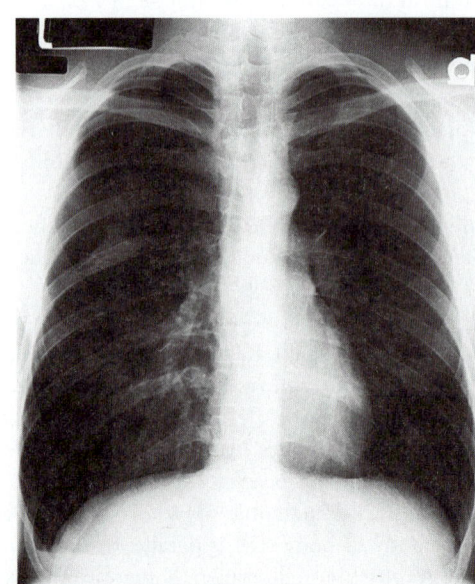

FIGURE 50-2 Chest radiograph demonstrating dark, radiolucent lungs with a light, radiopaque shadow of the spine and heart in the center. (From Long BW, Frank ED, Ehrlich RA: *Radiography essentials for limited practice*, ed 3, Philadelphia, 2010, Saunders.)

The total amount of x-ray exposure used to perform a particular diagnostic study is a combination of kilovoltage, milliamperage, exposure time, and source-to-image distance.

Technique Charts

A technique chart located near the control console provides the radiographer with a listing of recommended milliampere-seconds, kilovoltage, and source-to-image distance settings for x-ray studies of various body parts in patients of different sizes. The radiographer must refer to technique charts before performing the ordered radiographic procedure. Some control consoles have computerized units that are preprogrammed with the required exposure settings for the selected body part and size.

Radiographic Equipment

X-Ray Tube and Housing

The x-ray tube, where the x-rays form, is surrounded by a lead-lined, protective housing (Figure 50-3). The housing absorbs any radiation that is not part of the x-ray beam. The housing protects and insulates the x-ray tube itself while providing a base for attachments that allow the radiographer to manipulate the x-ray tube and to control the size and shape of the x-ray beam.

The principal attachment to the tube housing is the collimator, a boxlike device mounted beneath the opening of the housing. Collimators allow the radiographer to vary the size of the radiation field and to indicate with a light beam the size, location, and center of the field. Usually a centering light also helps align the cassette tray (Figure 50-4).

X-Ray Tube Support

The tube housing may be attached to a ceiling mount or a tube stand. Both types of mountings provide support and mobility for the heavy tube. The ceiling mount moves on a system of tracks to allow positioning of the tube at locations throughout the room. A tube stand (Figure 50-5) is a vertical support with a horizontal arm that suspends the tube over the radiographic table. The tube stand rolls along a track that is secured to the floor (and sometimes also the ceiling), allowing horizontal motion. Outpatient x-ray departments are more likely to have a tube stand.

Radiographic Table

The radiographic table is a specialized unit that is more than just a support for the patient. Some tables are adjustable in height for easy patient access, and some are designed to tilt into upright and Trendelenburg positions. A floating tabletop is a feature that assists in aligning the patient to the tube and film. Using the table to move the patient allows for x-ray imaging in a variety of angles and positions.

Grids and Bucky Devices

Beneath the table surface is a moving grid device called a **bucky** (Figure 50-6). X-ray film is placed in a cassette tray, which is then put in the bucky device under the radiographic table. This allows the cassette inside the bucky to be moved up and down the table to a point directly under the area to be x-rayed. The grid is situated between the tabletop and the film inside the cassette. It is a plate made of tissue-thin lead strips that are mounted on edge to protect the film from being fogged by scatter radiation that is displaced when the x-ray study is performed. Because the strips must be carefully

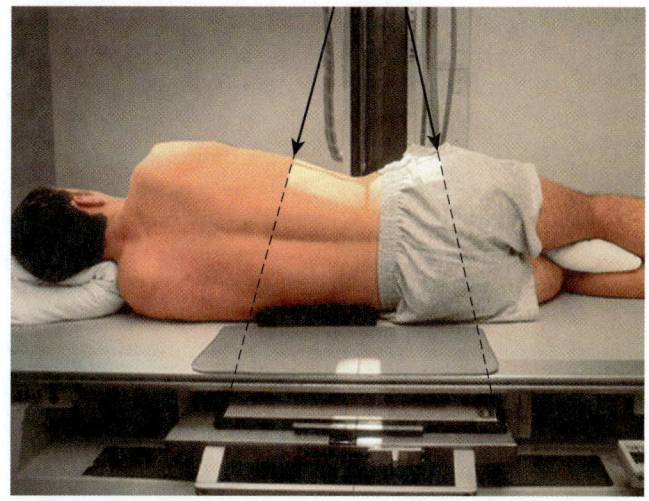

FIGURE 50-4 The collimator's light beam demonstrates the radiation field and aids alignment of the cassette tray. (From Bontrager KL, Lampignano J: *Textbook of radiographic positioning and related anatomy,* ed 7, St Louis, 2009, Mosby.)

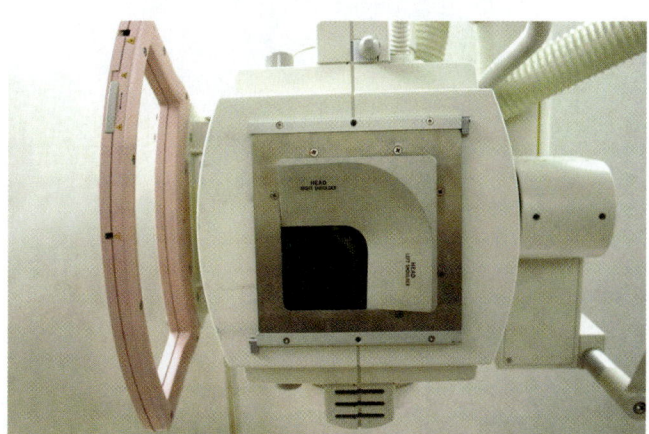

FIGURE 50-3 X-ray tube housing and collimator. (From Frank ED, Long BW, Smith BJ: *Merrill's atlas of radiographic positioning and procedures,* ed 11, St Louis, 2007, Mosby.)

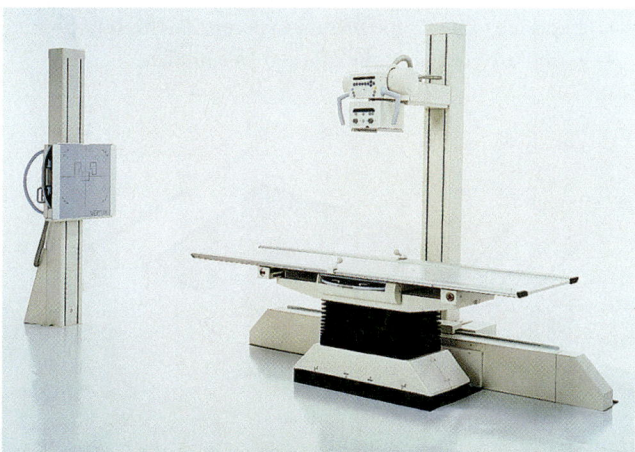

FIGURE 50-5 Tube stand. (From Long BW, Frank ED, Ehrlich RA: *Radiography essentials for limited practice,* ed 3, Philadelphia, 2010, Saunders.)

aligned with the path of the x-ray beam, precise alignment of the x-ray tube in relation to the bucky is essential. When the x-ray image is actually taken, the bucky automatically moves the grid so that it is not visible on the radiograph. Bucky grids generally are used only for body parts that are more than 10 to 12 cm thick (about the size of an adult's neck or knee). When a grid is not needed, the cassette is placed on the tabletop.

Upright Cassette Holder

The upright cassette holder, as its name implies, is a device that holds the film in an upright position for radiography. It usually is placed against a wall, and its height is adjustable. It may incorporate a bucky or stationary grid. When a grid is included, the unit may be referred to as a *grid cabinet* or *upright bucky*. When the patient is sitting or standing at the upright cassette holder for radiography, such as for a chest x-ray, the tube is angled to face the wall and cassette holder. The distance from the tube to the film may be adjusted to 40 or 72 inches, depending on the requirements of the procedure.

Control Console

The control console, located in the control booth, is the access point for the radiographer to determine exposure factors and to take the x-ray image (Figure 50-7). Radiographic control consoles have buttons, switches, dials, or digital readouts for some or all of the following functions:

- Off/On—controls the power to the control panel
- mA—allows the operator to set the milliamperage, the rate at which the x-rays are produced
- kVp—controls the kilovoltage, determining the penetrating power of the x-ray beam
- Timer—controls the duration of the exposure
- mAs—some units have an mAs control instead of mA and time settings
- Bucky—activates the motor control of the bucky device so that the grid moves during the exposure
- Automatic exposure controls—special settings available on certain units that allow termination of exposure when a certain amount of radiation has reached the film
- Meters or digital readouts—indicate the status of the settings
- Prep (ready or rotor) switch—prepares the tube for exposure
- Exposure switch—initiates the exposure and must be continuously activated until the exposure is complete

Image Receptor Systems

Cassettes and Intensifying Screens

The cassette (Figure 50-8) serves as the film holder during the x-ray procedure. It provides a light-tight, rigid structure to protect the film and also houses intensifying screens. Most cassettes have two intensifying screens, one front and one back, with the film sandwiched between them. Intensifying screens are plates coated with **phosphors** (fluorescent crystals) that give off light when exposed to x-rays. Their purpose is to reduce the amount of exposure required. Without intensifying screens, as much as 50 to 100 times more exposure would be needed. Intensifying screens greatly reduce the exposure of a patient to radiation during an x-ray procedure.

Each cassette has a small area where there is no intensifying screen and where exposure is blocked from the film by lead foil. This area is reserved for the photographic imprint of the patient identification. Its location is indicated on the front of the cassette by the position of the identifying label.

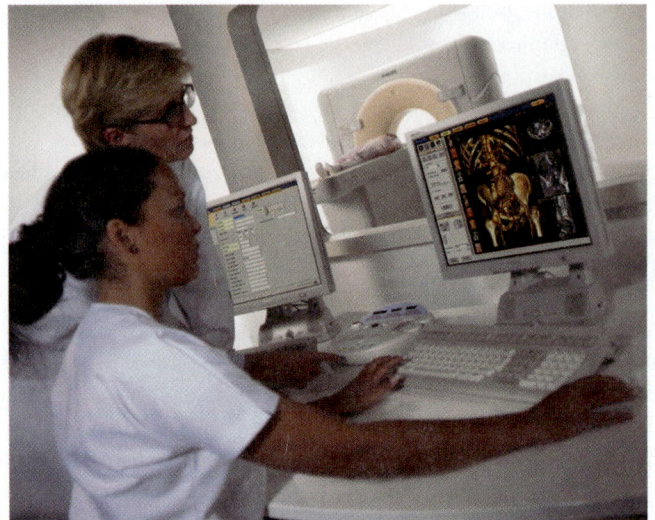

FIGURE 50-7 X-ray control console. (Courtesy Philips Electronics Corp.)

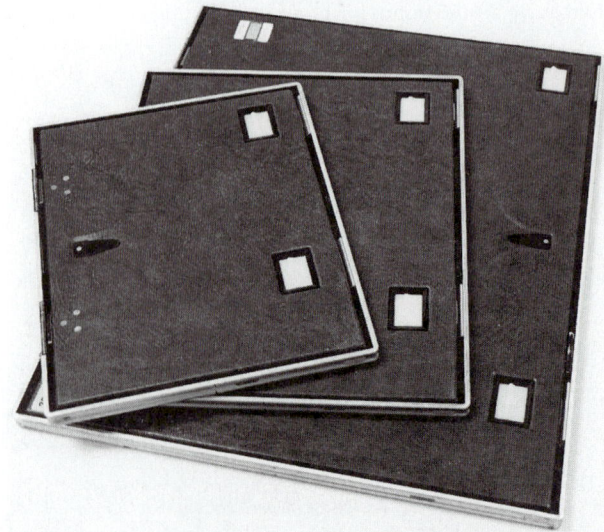

FIGURE 50-8 X-ray cassettes. (From Long BW, Frank ED, Ehrlich RA: *Radiography essentials for limited practice*, ed 3, Philadelphia, 2010, Saunders.)

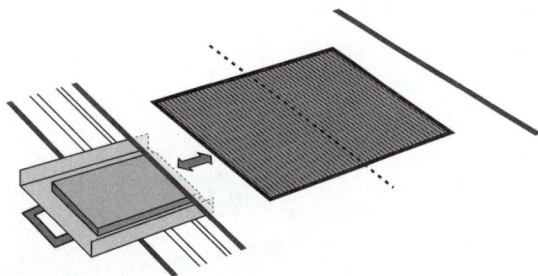

FIGURE 50-6 Bucky grid in place under the surface of the x-ray table. (From Long BW, Frank ED, Ehrlich RA: *Radiography essentials for limited practice*, ed 3, Philadelphia, 2010, Saunders.)

Intensifying screens are expensive and easily damaged. Damaged areas, dirt, or stains on the screens prevent light from exposing the film and result in artifacts on the image. For these reasons, it is important to avoid touching the screens and to keep the film processing area free of dust and dirt.

Film

Radiographic film is manufactured with a particular sensitivity to the light emitted by intensifying screens. Green-sensitive film is used with screens that emit green light, and blue-sensitive film is matched with blue-emitting screens. Film for routine radiography is coated on both sides so that the film responds to light from both intensifying screens. This double-emulsion system reduces the exposure required by half. Because both sides of the film are identical, a sheet of double-emulsion film does not have a "right" or "wrong" side. Film and cassettes come in standard sizes.

Film Care and Handling. Film must be stored correctly to prevent fog, a generalized exposure that reduces image quality. A good storage area is clean, cool, and dry and is protected from radiation and processing chemical fumes. Film boxes should stand on edge with the expiration date visible. This date is checked to ensure that older film is used before its expiration date.

To prevent artifacts from improper film handling, be sure your hands are clean and dry and touch only the corner of the film when removing it from the cassette. Prevent bending, crimping, and scraping of the film by allowing it to hang vertically when holding it with only one hand (Figure 50-9). To place it horizontally, use both hands and hold by opposite corners.

Film Processing. Comprehensive darkroom orientation is needed before you try to develop patients' films. It is especially important to know how to turn on the processor properly and to recognize when it has warmed up sufficiently for correct processing.

The exposed cassette is taken to the darkroom for processing under safelight conditions. Safelights provide a red or orange light that is quite dim but provides just enough illumination for you to see where things are located. Make sure the darkroom door is locked so that no one will open it while you are processing the film.

Film identification is essential for knowing the identity of the patient represented in the image and the date and location of the examination. Serious errors in diagnosis and treatment might occur if films are not correctly identified. The identification information is typed on a card that is inserted into the photographic printer in the darkroom. The printer is used to stamp the information on the film after it has been removed from the cassette and before it is processed (Figure 50-10).

The film then is fed into the automatic processor. The cassette is reloaded with a single sheet of fresh film (Figure 50-11) from the film bin, a storage unit located under the counter. A tone or a red light on the processor indicates when it is safe to feed another film or to turn on the lights.

The reloaded cassette should be returned immediately to the proper place so that it is ready for use. Correct locations for cassettes are essential, because you cannot determine by looking at the cassette

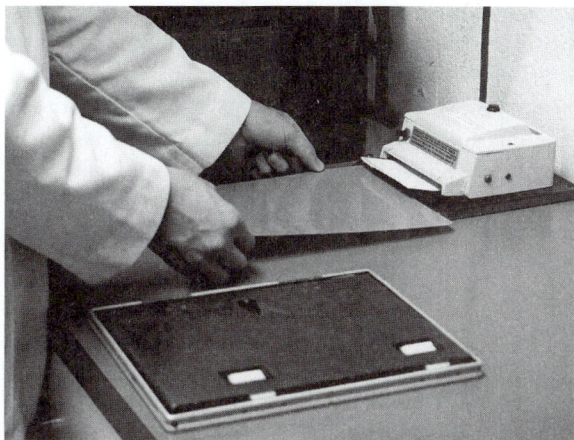

FIGURE 50-10 Film is inserted into the printer to stamp it with identification from the printer card. (From Long BW, Frank ED, Ehrlich RA: *Radiography essentials for limited practice,* ed 3, Philadelphia, 2010, Saunders.)

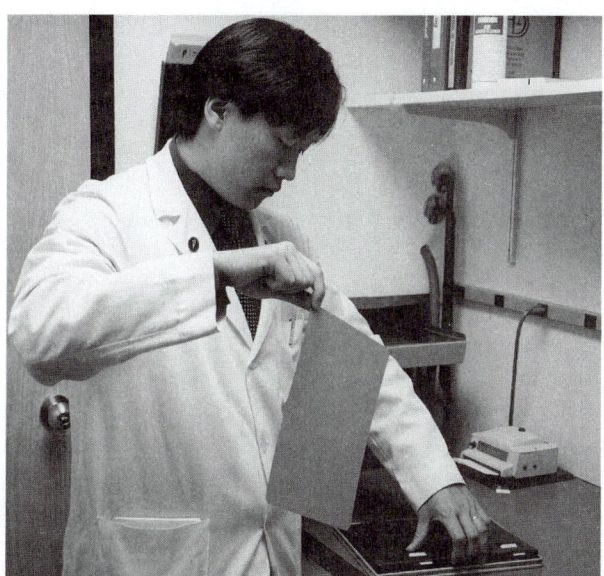

FIGURE 50-9 When holding the film with one hand, let it hang vertically. (From Long BW, Frank ED, Ehrlich RA: *Radiography essentials for limited practice,* ed 3, Philadelphia, 2010, Saunders.)

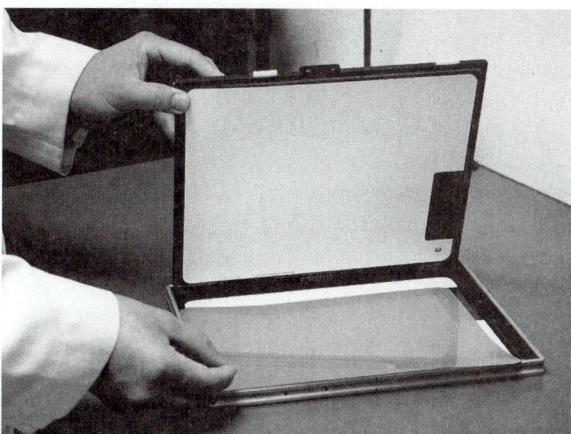

FIGURE 50-11 Reload the cassette promptly with fresh film. Make sure the film is properly situated and secure both latches. (From Long BW, Frank ED, Ehrlich RA: *Radiography essentials for limited practice,* ed 3, Philadelphia, 2010, Saunders.)

whether the film has been exposed. Only by following established routines and facility policies can you be confident that a cassette is unexposed and ready for use.

Daylight Processing. Some departments have a "daylight" system for processing film without a darkroom. These systems include a special film processor and a daylight film identification camera that uses special cassettes. Films can be identified while still in the cassette, and the entire cassette then is fed into the processor. The processor automatically removes and processes the film and then reloads the cassette with fresh film.

Computed and Digital Radiography

Computed radiography (CR) is a radiographic imaging system that does not use film. An image receptor, similar to an intensifying screen, is exposed in a special cassette using conventional x-ray equipment. The radiographer inserts the exposed cassette into a special processor and selects the type of examination from a menu so that the image is processed correctly. A small beam from a high-intensity laser in the processor converts the latent image to a visible image that is converted into an electronic signal and stored in a computer. The image then can be displayed on a high-resolution monitor. Hard copies can be produced with a laser film printer.

Digital radiography is another type of filmless imaging system. Special radiographic tables and upright cabinets contain digital receptors that react to the pattern of the radiation from the patient and transmit a digital signal directly to the computer system. No cassettes and no processing are involved. Although digital radiography has been used for some time for special applications, such as **fluoroscopy** and **angiography**, technical limitations and cost factors have prevented widespread adoption of digital systems for general radiography.

Once stored in the computer system, digital images from either computed or digital radiography are organized and cataloged and can be accessed on screen from multiple locations connected to the system network. These digital images can be manipulated electronically to enhance visibility. Conventional radiographs can be added to the system by scanning them with a laser device called a *film digitizer.*

The computer hardware and software technology used to manage digital images in hospitals and large health care systems is called a *picture archiving and communication system* (PACS). These systems provide image storage, connect images with patient database information, facilitate laser printing of images, and display both images and information at workstations throughout the network as needed. PACS may include transmission equipment for teleradiology, allowing images to be viewed in remote locations, such as a physician's home, and receiving images from remote locations, such as outlying clinics. PACS technology can transmit images directly over telephone lines and via the Internet. These advanced technologies will become more commonplace as computerized medical record systems become more widespread.

▌RADIOGRAPHIC POSITIONING

The medical assistant may be involved in explaining x-ray positions to a patient or in actually helping the patient into various positions, so it is important that you become familiar with commonly used

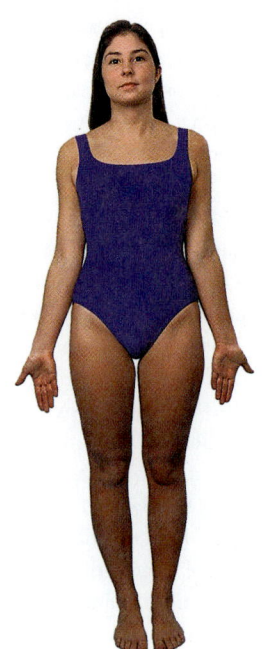

FIGURE 50-12 Anatomic position. (From Frank ED, Long BW, Smith BJ: *Merrill's atlas of radiographic positioning and procedures,* ed 11, St Louis, 2007, Mosby.)

terms. Terms that indicate the surfaces, directions, and planes of various body locations are based on the anatomic position.

Anatomic position (Figure 50-12) is a view of the body in which the individual is standing, facing the observer, with the palms of the hands forward. Terms that describe locations on and within the body include the following:

- *Anterior:* Forward or front portion of the body or body part.
- *Cephalic:* Pertaining to the head; toward the head.
- *Caudal:* Toward the tail or end of the body; away from the head; the opposite of cephalic.
- *Distal:* Away from the source or point of origin. For example, the wrist is distal to the elbow, the elbow distal to the shoulder.
- *External:* To the outside, at or near the surface of the body or a body part.
- *Inferior:* Below, farther from the head. For example, the diaphragm is inferior to the lungs.
- *Internal:* Deep, near the center of the body or a part; the opposite of external.
- *Lateral:* Referring to the side, away from the center to the left or right.
- *Medial:* Toward the center of the body or body part; the opposite of lateral.
- *Palmar:* Referring to the palm (anterior surface) of the hand.
- *Plantar:* Referring to the sole of the foot.
- *Posterior:* Backward or back portion of the body or body part; the opposite of anterior.
- *Proximal:* Toward the source or point of origin; the opposite of distal. For example, the part of the femur that is attached at the hip is the proximal end of the femur, and the part of the bone that is located at the knee is the distal end of the femur.

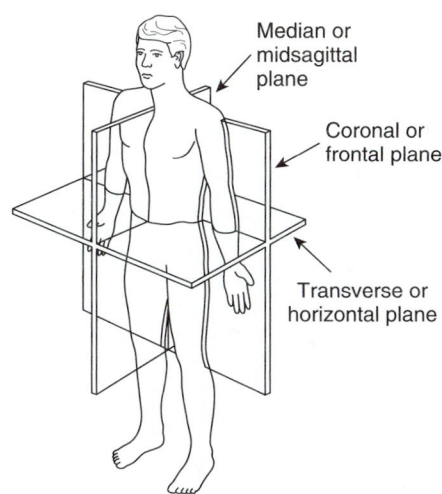

FIGURE 50-13 Body planes. (From Long BW, Frank ED, Ehrlich RA: *Radiography essentials for limited practice,* ed 3, Philadelphia, 2010, Saunders.)

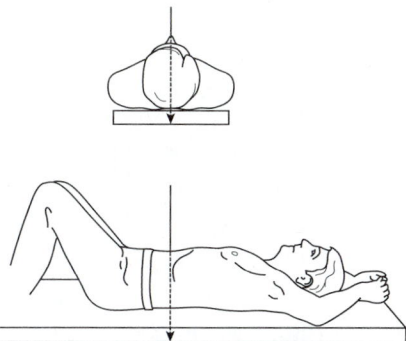

FIGURE 50-14 Anteroposterior (AP) projection. (From Long BW, Frank ED, Ehrlich RA: *Radiography essentials for limited practice,* ed 3, Philadelphia, 2010, Saunders.)

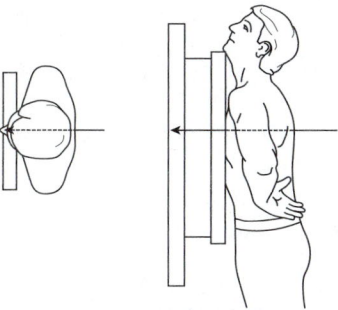

FIGURE 50-15 Posteroanterior (PA) projection. (From Long BW, Frank ED, Ehrlich RA: *Radiography essentials for limited practice,* ed 3, Philadelphia, 2010, Saunders.)

- *Superior:* Above, toward the head; the opposite of inferior. For example, the esophagus is superior to the stomach.

Besides anatomic positional terms, procedures for radiographic positioning also are described using the planes of the body (Figure 50-13). The **sagittal plane** divides the body into right and left parts, and the midsagittal plane divides the body into equal right and left parts. The **coronal plane** (sometimes called the *frontal plane*) divides the body into anterior and posterior parts. The midcoronal or midfrontal plane divides the body into relatively equal parts; it passes through the external auditory meatus (the opening of the ear), the center of the shoulder, the greater trochanter (the bony prominence in the lateral hip area), and the lateral malleolus (the bony prominence on the lateral surface of the ankle). The **transverse plane** divides the body into superior and inferior portions. It may be drawn at any level.

The medical assistant may assist with radiographic procedures by helping position the patient for a particular x-ray view. These positions can be used as follows in x-ray positioning:

- *Prone:* Lying face down
- *Recumbent:* Lying down; the position may be further described by adding the name of the body surface on which the patient is lying:
- *Dorsal recumbent:* Lying on the back (supine) with the knees bent and the feet flat on the table
- *Lateral recumbent:* Lying on the side
- *Ventral recumbent:* Lying face down, prone
- *Supine:* Lying on the back face up
- *Upright:* Standing or seated

Projections

A radiographic projection indicates the relative positions of the body part to be x-rayed, the film, and the placement of the x-ray tube.

For a **frontal projection**, the coronal plane of the body or body part is parallel to the film plane and the central ray is perpendicular to both. If the patient is supine, or facing the x-ray tube, the projection is said to be **anteroposterior (AP)** (Figure 50-14). If the patient is prone, or facing the film, the projection is said to be **posteroanterior (PA)** (Figure 50-15). Note that these terms indicate the direction of the x-ray beam, from front to back or back to front.

Lateral projections are those in which the sagittal plane of the body or body part is parallel to the film. Lateral projections are always named for the side of the patient that is nearest the film; that is, either left or right lateral (Figure 50-16).

Oblique projections are those in which the body or part is rotated so that the projection is neither frontal nor lateral. Oblique projections also are named for the part of the body nearest the film. For example, in a right anterior oblique (RAO) projection, the patient's right, anterior aspect is closest to the film. Figure 50-17 illustrates all four oblique projections: RAO, right posterior oblique (RPO), left anterior oblique (LAO), and left posterior oblique (LPO).

Axial projections, sometimes referred to as *semiaxial projections,* are radiographs taken with a longitudinal angulation of the x-ray beam. The x-ray beam is projected at an angle, either cephalad (toward the head) or caudad (away from the head) (Figure 50-18).

DIAGNOSTIC IMAGING MODALITIES

Fluoroscopy and Contrast Media

Fluoroscopy

Fluoroscopy is a technique in which special equipment is used to allow the **radiologist** to view x-ray images in motion. Fluoroscopy also allows the physician to survey an area quickly, without the delay involved in taking and processing films. Most fluoroscopic units are

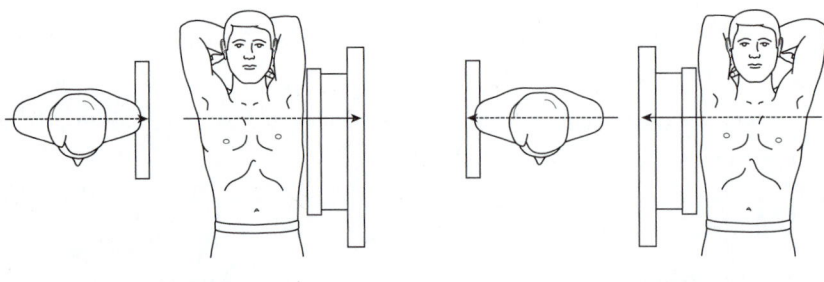

Left lateral   Right lateral

FIGURE 50-16 Lateral projections are named for the side of the body nearer the film. (From Long BW, Frank ED, Ehrlich RA: *Radiography essentials for limited practice*, ed 3, Philadelphia, 2010, Saunders.)

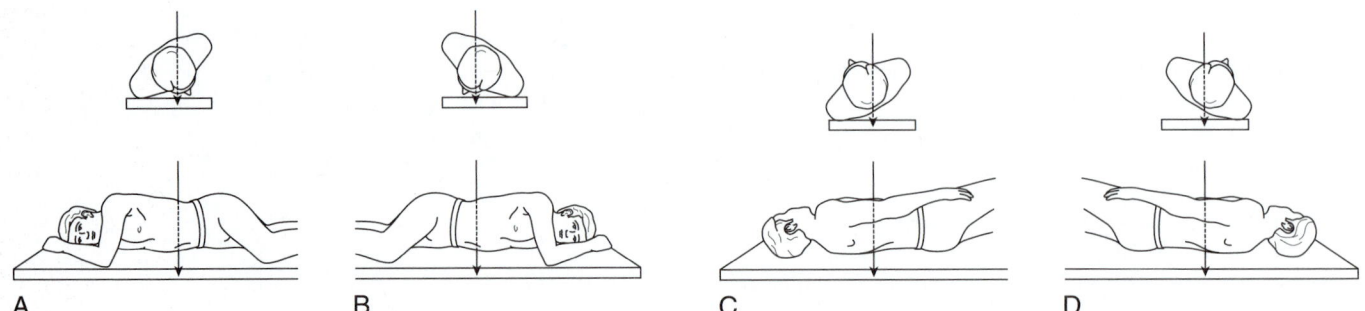

FIGURE 50-17 Oblique projections. **A,** Right anterior oblique (RAO). **B,** Left anterior oblique (LAO). **C,** Left posterior oblique (LPO). **D,** Right posterior oblique (RPO). (From Long BW, Frank ED, Ehrlich RA: *Radiography essentials for limited practice*, ed 3, Philadelphia, 2010, Saunders.)

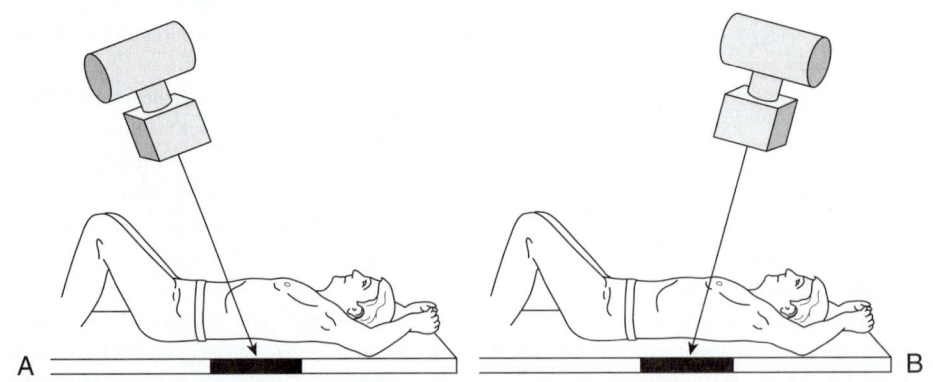

FIGURE 50-18 In axial projections, the x-ray tube is angled to direct the central ray along the long axis of the body or part. **A,** Cephalad angulation. **B,** Caudad angulation. (From Long BW, Frank ED, Ehrlich RA: *Radiography essentials for limited practice*, ed 3, Philadelphia, 2010, Saunders.)

properly called *radiographic/fluoroscopic* (R/F) units, because they are designed to take both x-ray images and fluoroscopic views. The x-ray films taken during a fluoroscopic procedure, which are called *spot films*, record the image as seen on the fluoroscope; sometimes the entire fluoroscopic examination is recorded digitally. After the fluoroscopic portion of the study is complete, larger radiographs usually are taken for comprehensive visualization of the entire anatomic region.

An example of a fluoroscopic diagnostic procedure is a barium swallow. If the physician suspects that the patient has difficulty swallowing, a fluoroscope is used to visualize the actual movement of the substance down the esophagus and into the stomach while the patient is in the act of swallowing. Fluoroscopic procedures typically require the use of a contrast medium, such as barium.

X-Ray Studies Using Contrast Media

Although the lungs and bony structures of the body produce clear x-ray images on plain film radiographs, internal organs, such as the stomach and the kidneys, are difficult to see because they absorb radiation to the same degree as the tissues that surround them. To enhance visibility of these structures, special agents, called **contrast media**, can be used to fill hollow organs and demonstrate their inner contours. Although gases such as air and carbon dioxide sometimes are used as contrast media, the use of radiopaque substances, such as

TABLE 50-1 Radiographic Procedures Using Contrast Media

EXAMINATION	CONTRAST MEDIUM	ROUTE OF ADMINISTRATION	STRUCTURES SHOWN
Angiocardiography	Iodine compounds	Intra-arterial injection via femoral or brachial catheter	Heart and large vessels
Angiography	Iodine compounds	Intra-arterial or intravenous injection	Blood vessels
Arteriography	Iodine compounds	Intra-arterial injection via catheter	Arteries
Arthrography	Iodine compounds	Direct injection into joint capsule	Joints, especially knee, shoulder, and ankle
Barium swallow	Barium sulfate suspension	Oral	Esophagus
Hysterosalpingography	Iodine compounds	Direct injection via cannula	Uterus and fallopian tubes
Intravenous urography	Iodine compounds	Intravenous injection	Kidneys, ureters, and urinary bladder
Lower gastrointestinal (GI) series (barium enema)	Barium sulfate suspension, sometimes also with air	Rectal catheter	Colon
Lymphangiography	Iodine compounds	Direct injection into lymphatic vessels in the feet	Lymphatic vessels and lymph nodes
Myelography	Iodine compounds	Intrathecal injection (spinal tap)	Spinal canal
Upper GI series	Barium sulfate suspension	Oral	Esophagus, stomach, and duodenum

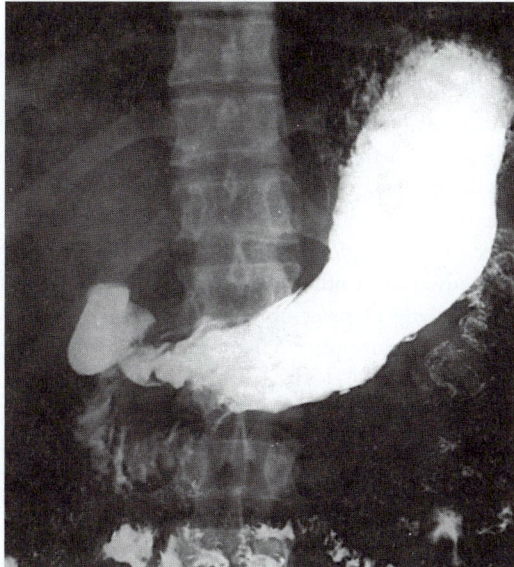

FIGURE 50-19 Radiographic image of the stomach, part of an upper gastrointestinal (UGI) series using oral administration of barium sulfate to provide contrast. (From Ballinger PW, Frank ED: *Merrill's atlas of radiographic positions and radiologic procedures,* ed 10, vol 2, St Louis, 2003, Mosby.)

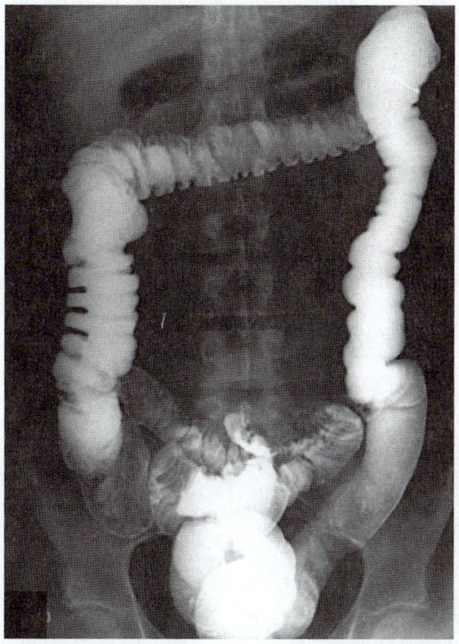

FIGURE 50-20 Lower gastrointestinal (GI) series. Radiograph of the colon filled with barium sulfate administered by barium enema. (From Ballinger PW, Frank ED: *Merrill's atlas of radiographic positions and radiologic procedures,* ed 10, vol 2, St Louis, 2003, Mosby.)

barium sulfate or iodine compounds, is far more common. The agent and the technique vary with the structures to be viewed (Table 50-1).

Among the most common fluoroscopic examinations are studies of the upper and lower gastrointestinal (GI) tract using barium sulfate as a contrast medium. Both require careful patient instruction and advance preparation for a successful study. For an **upper gastrointestinal (UGI)** series (Figure 50-19), the patient swallows a barium sulfate suspension; this study is performed to aid the diagnosis of ulcers, tumors, and other abnormalities of the esophagus, stomach, and duodenum.

A **lower gastrointestinal series** (Figure 50-20) involves a barium enema that fills the colon and aids visualization of its inner surfaces. This procedure is especially useful in the diagnosis of polyps, tumors, and diverticulosis. For this examination the inner lining of the large intestine must be clean and free of all fecal matter. The physician prescribes commercial bowel preparation kits to ensure complete emptying of the large intestine. If the preparation is not adequate, the examination must be rescheduled.

Water-soluble iodine compounds are used as contrast media for a wide variety of applications. When injected intravenously (IV), the contrast agent circulates in the blood and is excreted by the kidneys, causing the urine to become radiopaque. Radiography of the kidneys, ureters, and bladder after IV injection of a contrast medium is called an **intravenous urogram (IVU)** (it previously was called an *intravenous pyelogram,* or *IVP*); this study is useful for identifying kidney stones, tumors, and other abnormalities of the urinary tract. Preparation for an IVU involves fasting and bowel cleansing, because material in the colon can obstruct a clear picture of the urinary system.

Iodine contrast agents also can be injected into joint capsules to produce an **arthrogram**, an image of the soft tissue components of joints, especially the knee and the shoulder. **Myelography** involves injection of iodine compounds into the spinal canal to demonstrate pathologic spinal conditions, such as tumors and herniated intervertebral disks. This diagnostic technique is being replaced by MRI and CT studies that are less invasive and do not carry the potential complications of a myelogram.

Part of the screening process for diagnostic procedures that use iodine contrast injections is careful questioning of the patient regarding a history of iodine allergy. All patients who are allergic to shellfish also will be allergic to iodine dye and are at risk for a serious anaphylactic reaction if the contrast agent is injected. The medical assistant is responsible for clarifying allergies with the patient and/or family members and alerting the diagnostic facility if the patient has an iodine allergy. In addition, patients need to understand that it is normal to feel flushed or a heat rush when the dye is injected and that some patients initially experience waves of nausea. However, both of these sensations pass quickly.

Cardiovascular and Interventional Radiography

The highly specialized radiographic procedures that display blood vessels are collectively known as *angiography*. A cerebral angiogram, for example, demonstrates the vessels of the brain (Figure 50-21), and renal angiograms show the arteries and veins of the kidneys. An

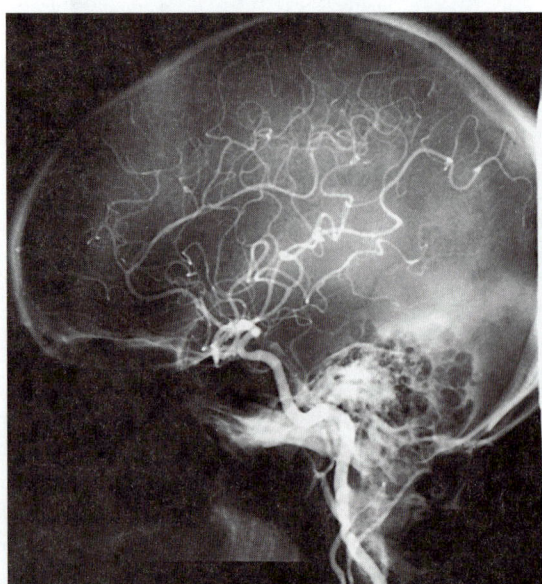

FIGURE 50-21 Cerebral angiogram showing the circulation of the brain enhanced by iodine contrast medium. (From Ballinger PW, Frank ED: *Merrill's atlas of radiographic positions and radiologic procedures,* ed 10, vol 2, St Louis, 2003, Mosby.)

angiocardiogram is a contrast study that shows the interior of the heart chambers and the great vessels that enter and exit the heart, and an **aortogram** demonstrates the aorta. Selective **angiocardiography**, or cardiac catheterization, is used to display the coronary arteries. Arteriograms are pictures of specific arteries, and venograms are studies of veins.

For all these examinations, iodine compounds are injected for radiographic contrast and a rapid series of films is taken or fluoroscopy is used to show the area of concern. Direct injection may be used for some angiographic studies, such as those of the extremities, but the preferred injection method for angiocardiography, aortography, and most **arteriography** procedures is to use a special catheter. A large artery (usually the femoral or brachial artery) is entered with a large-bore needle, and a guidewire is threaded through the needle and into the artery under fluoroscopic control. The needle is removed, the guidewire is left in the vessel, and the catheter is threaded over the wire. The wire is then removed, and the catheter remains in the artery for the duration of the examination. Further manipulation of the catheter may be needed to ensure correct placement in the vessel before injection of the iodine compound. For selective catheterization of smaller vessels, the catheter tip is maneuvered into the root of the vessel of interest, such as the coronary, celiac, renal, or carotid artery.

A timed sequence of images is taken during and after injection of the contrast medium, usually with the aid of an automatic power injector that is electronically coordinated with a programmable film changer and automated exposure control. Digital receptors are replacing film and film changers, and for some studies, such as angiocardiograms, digital fluoroscopy equipment may be used to record the images.

Because these procedures are expensive and involve a relatively high degree of risk, angiography has been replaced somewhat by technologic advances in other imaging modalities discussed in this chapter, particularly Doppler ultrasound, **nuclear medicine**, magnetic resonance angiography (MRA), and computed tomography angiography (CTA).

Despite these advances, angiography continues to be used extensively because it provides the best anatomic view of structures within the circulatory system and also offers the opportunity for immediate therapeutic interventions to treat vascular problems as they are identified. Specialized catheter techniques are used for vessel repair, called **angioplasty**, to widen or open arteries that are narrowed or occluded. **Embolization** is a therapeutic intervention technique that reduces or stops blood flow to control hemorrhage, cut off the blood supply to a tumor, or reduce blood loss during surgery.

Computed Tomography

Computed tomography (CT), formerly called *computerized axial tomography (CAT)* scanning, uses a special x-ray scanner to produce detailed pictures of a cross section of tissue. The x-ray studies are taken in the transverse plane and also can be "reconstructed" by the computer to display anatomic structures in other planes. The images are viewed in a variety of formats, called *windows*, which are designed to enhance the views of specific tissues (Figure 50-22). Multiple levels of pictures can be taken in a very short period, with up to 25 continuous images recorded in the time it takes the patient to hold a single breath. Most CT examinations are noninvasive, painless, and

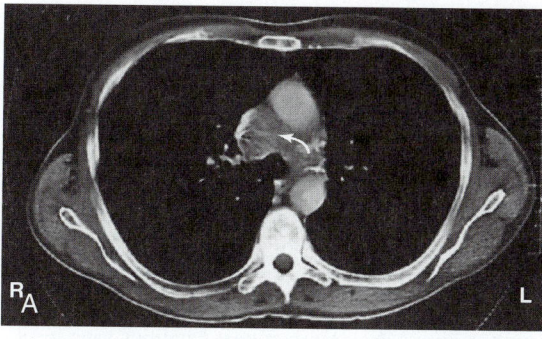
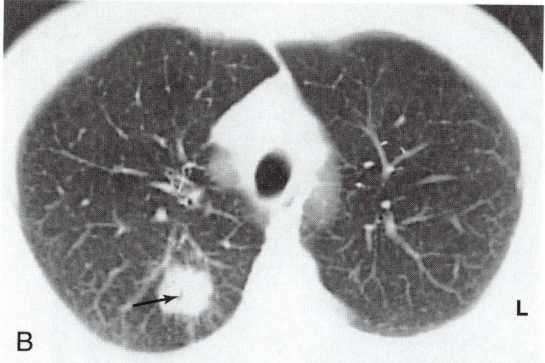

FIGURE 50-22 Two computed tomography windows demonstrating structures of the chest from the same image. **A,** Mediastinal structures are demonstrated in the center of the field, but the lungs are not well seen. **B,** "Lung window" demonstrates the blood vessels of the lungs and a lung tumor *(arrow)*. (From Seeram E: *Computed tomography: physical principles, clinical applications, and quality control,* ed 2, Philadelphia, 2001, WB Saunders.)

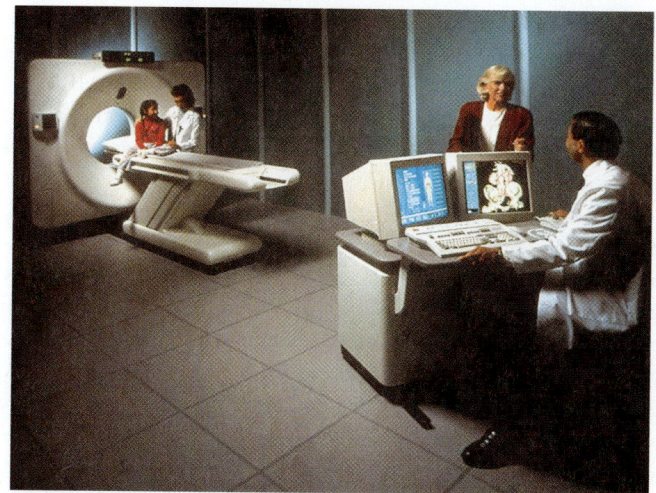

FIGURE 50-23 A computed tomography (CT) technologist monitors the patient while performing a CT scan of the brain. (Courtesy GE Healthcare, a division of General Electric Co.)

do not require any special patient preparation. However, patients may feel apprehensive about the equipment, because standard machines require the patient enter a tube for the procedure. Careful explanations are necessary to achieve the patient's cooperation and a satisfactory outcome of the study.

The CT scanner (Figure 50-23) consists of a movable table with remote control, a circular **gantry** structure that supports the x-ray tube and detectors, an operator console with a monitor, and a supporting computer system. The CT unit also includes both hardware and software to archive and manage data and to produce hard copies of images. During a scan the x-ray tube rotates around the patient to collect data. In conventional CT units, the tube makes a complete rotation to gather data for each slice. The table then moves, and the tube rotates again to obtain the next slice. A newer generation of equipment, designated as *spiral* or *helical scanners,* scans a spiral path around the patient and can collect data on a larger volume of tissue. These scanners can reconstruct views to create three-dimensional images.

The versatility of CT is illustrated by its wide range of applications, including studies of the brain, spine, abdomen, pelvis, chest, neck, and paranasal sinuses. CT is a valuable tool for emergency use,

especially in the detection of intracerebral or intraabdominal hemorrhage. It also is used for orthopedic examinations of the extremities and for contrast-enhanced vascular studies. CT is useful for localizing both lesions and needle position during needle aspiration biopsy, a nonsurgical method of obtaining cells for laboratory examination, and it often is used with myelography to expand the range of information available.

Although many CT examinations do not require contrast media, the use of contrast agents vastly increases the scope of CT imaging. Studies of the abdomen usually use oral contrast media to help differentiate the GI tract from the surrounding tissues. The patient ingests a special barium compound or an oral iodine preparation over a specified period before the study. The amount of contrast medium and the time period vary, depending on whether the examination includes only the upper abdomen or the entire abdomen and pelvis. For these studies, the patient is instructed not to eat for 12 hours and to report to the facility early to drink the contrast preparation before the procedure is scheduled. Some departments have the patient take the contrast medium home with instructions to drink it before reporting for the appointment.

IV injection of an iodine contrast medium also may be used to increase the contrast level of the patient's tissues. This is advantageous for studies of the chest, abdomen, and soft tissues of the neck, because it highlights blood vessels and enhances the visibility of vascular organs such as the liver and spleen. The contrast defines the internal structures of the kidneys, ureters, and bladder as the agent is excreted in the urine. In selected cases, IV contrast agents are used in CT scans of the head to demonstrate brain lesions.

Magnetic Resonance Imaging

Magnetic resonance imaging (MRI) is a noninvasive diagnostic modality that allows visualization of anatomic structures without the use of radioactive x-rays. A powerful magnetic field and radiofrequency pulses are combined to produce a radio signal in the body that can be detected and processed electronically to provide images on a computer monitor. The images can be managed in a computer database and can also be stored on magnetic tape and photographed with a special camera to produce film copies that appear similar to x-ray images.

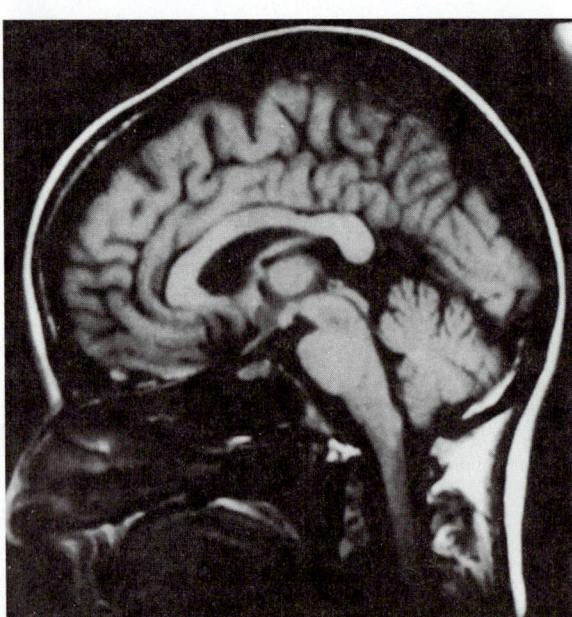

FIGURE 50-24 Midsagittal magnetic resonance image (MRI) of the brain. (From Ehrlich RA, McCloskey ED, Daly JA: *Patient care in radiography,* ed 6, St Louis, 2004, Mosby.)

The MRI gantry houses the magnet and the main radiofrequency coil. Conventional gantries are tubular, 5 to 8 feet long, and typically require the body part being studied to be placed in the tube during the scanning process. An open gantry design, the open MRI, provides better accommodation for large or claustrophobic patients, but it does not always provide image quality equal to that produced by conventional units.

MRI provides excellent imaging of the soft tissues of the nervous system (Figure 50-24). It is useful in the diagnosis of many types of pathology, including brain and spinal cord tumors and diseases such as multiple sclerosis. MRI also is used for the diagnosis of herniated intervertebral disks and to obtain images of the soft tissue components of joints, particularly the knee, shoulder, and temporomandibular joint. A more recent advance in MRI is MRA, which uses magnetic resonance technology to study the cardiovascular system. MRA aids in the diagnosis and treatment of heart disorders, stroke, and blood vessel diseases.

The typical scan time for a series of slicelike images ranges from 1 to 10 minutes, and several series demonstrating different body planes and using a variety of radiofrequency pulse sequences may be included in an examination. The average time for an MRI study is 30 to 45 minutes. It is critical that the patient remain still, maintaining the desired position, throughout the procedure.

Although contrast media are not required for most MRI studies, special paramagnetic agents sometimes are injected intravenously. These agents provide contrast enhancement of certain lesions, particularly brain and spinal cord tumors, and help differentiate disk material from scar tissue in postoperative spinal examinations. Contrast injections also are used in MRA studies. Typically, a series of images is recorded, the contrast agent is injected intravenously, and a second series of images is taken.

The unique MRI environment requires special safety precautions. Conditions that affect patient safety involve both the powerful magnetic field in the gantry and the thermal effects of radiofrequency pulses on certain materials that could overheat and possibly burn the patient. The principal means of ensuring patient safety during an MRI is careful patient screening before the procedure. Although extensive patient interviews are conducted in the magnetic resonance department, preliminary screening of patients should be conducted by the medical assistant before the appointment is made. The magnetic field or the rapid radiofrequency pulses may be hazardous for patients with artificial heart valves, aneurysm clips, neurostimulators, middle ear prostheses, or intrauterine devices. Cardiac pacemakers are a particular hazard, and patients with pacemakers cannot have MRI examinations. Fatalities have resulted from overheating of these implanted devices when patients with pacemakers were scanned.

Other factors that would prohibit the use of MRI technology include patients with orthopedic pins and screws and metal fragments or shrapnel in the soft tissues. Metalworkers who might have steel slivers in their tissues must have a screening x-ray or CT head examination to detect fragments that could damage the eyes or brain, because the pull of the magnetic field is so strong that it could cause the fragments to move. Although the energies involved in MRI have not been demonstrated to cause complications with pregnancy, the current philosophy is to avoid examination of pregnant patients except in urgent cases, especially during the first trimester.

Patients should be assured that everything possible will be done to provide assistance in dealing with both physical and emotional discomfort. Few people are completely comfortable for any length of time in a tightly enclosed space. Even patients with no history of claustrophobia may feel anxious when entering a conventional tubular MRI gantry. Occasionally, this anxiety is so severe that it creates panic, preventing the patient from continuing the examination.

Patients may be reassured if they know what to expect in advance. The procedure requires that the patient lie down on the MRI table, which then automatically moves into the gantry. Plenty of air is available, and there is no physical discomfort except for the need to lie still. The machine makes a very loud "knocking" noise during the scanning process (similar to a jack hammer or heavy machinery). Earplugs or earphones with recorded music may be offered. Patients can communicate with the technologist through an intercom, and the technologist is watching and listening from an adjacent area throughout the procedure. The patient is given a "panic button" to push in case the procedure needs to be stopped because of patient discomfort or anxiety. Because no radiation danger exists, a friend or family member can sit in the room if the patient feels more comfortable with company. Severely claustrophobic patients may be scheduled at a facility with an open gantry MRI or may be given an antianxiety medication before the procedure. Analgesic medications may be administered to patients whose pain makes it impossible to lie still for the duration of the study.

Sonography

Diagnostic medical **sonography** is a noninvasive procedure that is considered very safe for the patient. Sonography was introduced in Chapter 41, because it is used extensively for fetal imaging. This imaging modality, often referred to as *diagnostic ultrasound,* uses high-frequency sound waves to produce echoes in the body. As the echoes return to the sending point, or **transducer,** their strength and

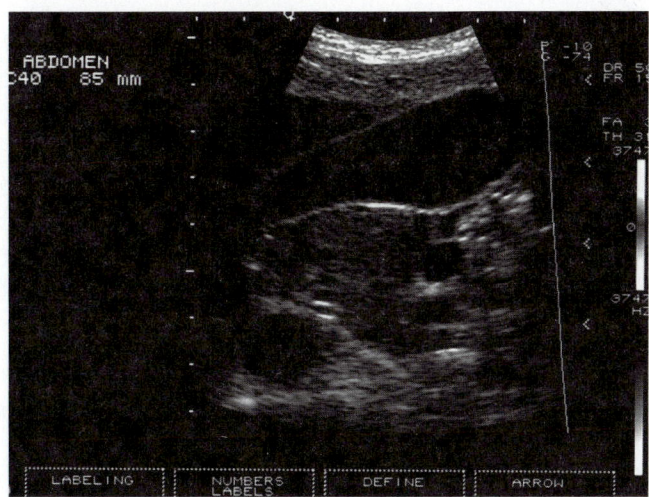

FIGURE 50-25 Abdominal sonogram. (From Ballinger PW, Frank ED: *Merrill's atlas of radiographic positions and radiologic procedures*, ed 10, vol 2, St Louis, 2003, Mosby.)

TABLE 50-2 Common Nuclear Medicine Procedures

PROCEDURE	PURPOSE
Bone scan	Helps detect fractures, tumors, and inflammation; used to determine bone growth
Brain scan	Often used with other imaging methods to detect tumors and vascular problems
Liver scan	Useful for diagnosing cirrhosis and hepatitis and for detecting tumors and liver abscesses
Lung scan	Often done to detect emboli, blood clots that have traveled through the bloodstream to the lungs
Positron emission tomography (PET) scan	Done for cancer investigation, evaluation of myocardial blood supply, investigation of central nervous system disorders
Thallium stress test	Used to evaluate cardiac condition and response to stress
Thyroid scan	Rate of contrast uptake is an indicator of thyroid function and also is useful for detecting tumors

timing are interpreted by a computer to produce a map or graphic image of the echo distribution.

The transducer is covered with a lubricant and moved over the surface of the body so that the image can be viewed in real time on a computer monitor. Special transducer probes can be inserted into body cavities such as the rectum and the vagina to obtain more detailed examinations of the prostate gland and the uterus. Any interface between substances or tissues of varying density produces an ultrasound echo, which makes sonography an effective technique for showing the shape, size, and condition of organs such as the heart, spleen, gallbladder, breast, and pancreas (Figure 50-25). Sonography, therefore, can be used to diagnose or investigate gallstones or suspicious masses in the breast. For example, if a woman has a suspicious breast mass, the mass can be visualized with a sonogram, and while the radiologist has a clear view of the location of the mass, a needle biopsy sample of the suspicious tissue is collected and sent to the pathologist for examination. This procedure limits the need for invasive surgical biopsies.

Sonography can also be used to detect an abscess, a cyst, or a tumor in adipose tissue. Recent advances in ultrasound technology include computer integration of data to produce three-dimensional images. In addition, Doppler ultrasound is used to detect vascular disease, such as atherosclerosis in the carotid arteries and venous thrombosis of the lower extremities.

Nuclear Medicine

Nuclear medicine images are created by scanning the patient after special radioactive materials, called **tracers**, have been swallowed or injected intravenously (Table 50-2). Tracers are similar to substances that are commonly used by the body, so they enter into the same chemical reactions and are metabolized in a similar way. They are taken up in the target organ or tissue over a period that may vary from half an hour to several days. The tracer then can be detected and its location recorded by a special nuclear medicine scanner called a *gamma camera*. Two types of tracers used in diagnostic studies are radioactive iodine and radioactive carbon.

Nuclear medicine scans do not provide clear images of anatomic structures. They are used to obtain information about the function of organs and tissues. Abnormal tissues are demonstrated on the image because the tracer is metabolized at a different rate, at a different location, or to a greater or lesser extent than in normal tissue.

Figure 50-26 is an example of a nuclear medicine bone scan. The tracer is absorbed by the bones and appears in greater or lesser amounts, depending on the level of metabolic activity within the bone. In this scan, the region of the right shoulder shows a high level of radioactivity, which indicates an inflammatory process. Tumors of the bone can be diagnosed by "hot spots" in the x-ray image; these show up much more brightly because of rapid cellular division, which results in a higher level of metabolic activity.

Structures visualized with nuclear medicine techniques include the thyroid gland, liver, lungs, brain, skeletal system, kidneys, heart, and blood vessels. Thallium stress studies of the heart are nuclear medicine examinations that permit the physician to view the coronary arteries to diagnose or rule out blockage. Incomplete visualization of the myocardium after administration of a nuclear tracer indicates lack of blood supply to the area and damage to the muscle of the heart.

The radioisotopes used in nuclear medicine decay within a short time, from a few hours to a few days, and are eliminated in the urine or feces. They have a very low level of radioactivity and involve less patient exposure than most x-ray examinations. Positron emission tomography (PET) and single photon emission computed tomography (SPECT) are highly specialized nuclear medicine techniques that use different types of tracers and scanners than conventional nuclear medicine, but the basic principle is the same. Radioactive substances from within the body are detected and mapped by specialized equipment to obtain information about the function of organs, tissues, or systems. Most PET scans today are combined with

CT to merge the technology of nuclear medicine procedures with the multiplane view of CT scanners. PET/CT scans are ordered for the following purposes:

- To diagnose a cancerous tumor, evaluate its spread, or determine whether cancer has returned after treatment
- To evaluate the blood flow to the heart
- To determine the extent of damage to the myocardial wall after a heart attack

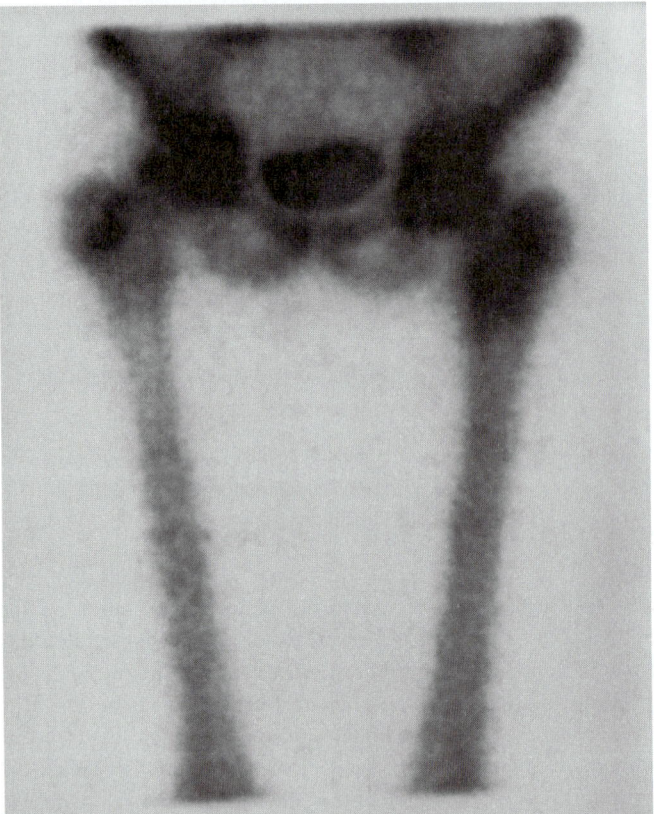

FIGURE 50-26 Bone scan showing increased tracer uptake in the proximal femur. (From Boker A, MacNicol M: Haematogenous osteomyelitis in children; epidemiology, classification, aetiology, and treatment, *Paediatr Child Health* 18:2, 2008.)

- To investigate lung lesions visualized with traditional x-rays
- To diagnose central nervous system disorders, including epilepsy, Alzheimer's disease, Parkinson's disease, and strokes, and to locate brain tumors

DEXA Scan

Dual energy x-ray absorptiometry (DEXA) scans use x-ray technology to evaluate a patient's bone density level. A decrease in bone density is diagnostic proof of osteoporosis; evidence of bone density loss (osteopenia) may indicate the individual's risk of developing osteoporosis over time. The test typically evaluates the bone density of the hip. For the examination, the patient lies prone on an x-ray table with the knees flexed and the lower legs elevated (Figure 50-27). The DEXA scanner directs an x-ray from two different sources toward the hip. The greater the mineral density of the bone, the longer the x-ray image is transmitted, the higher the test number that is recorded. The scan is completed within a few minutes and can be used to evaluate the density of the spine and legs as well. The patient's density results are compared with standard bone density tables to determine the presence and/or level of demineralization. These numbers are used to predict the patient's risk of an osteoporosis-related fracture. DEXA scans are recommended for the following individuals:

- Women with multiple risk factors for osteoporosis
- Women with long-term estrogen deficiencies
- Individuals taking steroids for an extended period
- Individuals taking osteoporosis medications (to evaluate the effectiveness of treatment)
- Patients with unexplained fractures and/or deformities of the vertebra

■ BASIC RADIOGRAPHIC PROCEDURE

▮ Patient Preparation and Explanation

Before a patient undergoes x-ray studies, a physician examines the individual and orders one or more specific x-ray procedures to help

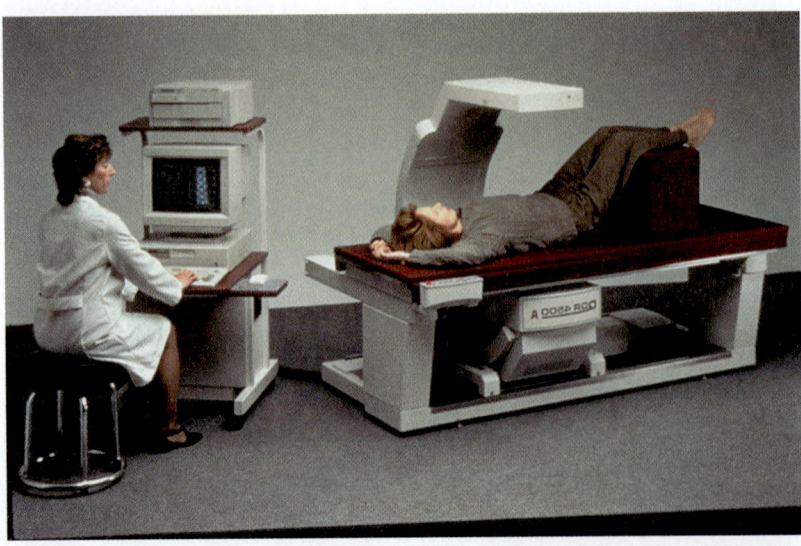

FIGURE 50-27 Patient undergoing a bone density test, or dual energy x-ray absorptiometry (DEXA or DXA).

diagnose the patient's problem or to follow up on a previously diagnosed condition. The physician is responsible for getting the patient's informed consent for any procedure, but he or she may ask the medical assistant to make sure the consent form is signed. The patient may not have to sign a consent form for noninvasive diagnostic studies, because acceptance of the procedure is adequate evidence of consent. In some facilities, however, patients may be asked to sign a consent form regardless of the type of radiographic procedure. If it is your duty to answer patients' questions about the procedure or to assist with obtaining consent, make sure you are prepared to do so.

Patients often express concern about radiation exposure. You can assure them with confidence that the risks are extremely small and outweigh the health risks of treatment without the information the examination will provide. It may help to point out that the radiographer is well trained in radiation safety and that the equipment is designed to provide good images with the least possible exposure. You can explain that the amount of radiation involved in the procedure is less than the exposure to natural background radiation that people in general receive every year.

Patient preparation for routine radiography involves having the patient remove the outer clothing from the area to be radiographed and instructing the person to wear a gown if appropriate. Underwear usually is not a problem. No metal objects should be included in the radiation field, because these items appear as artifacts on the images. This includes jewelry; zippers, snaps, and other clothing fasteners; underwire bras; and the contents of pockets. Nonmetal objects that are thick or heavy should also be removed. Buttons and the heavy seams in jeans are examples of other clothing items that can cause artifacts on radiographs if they are in the imaging field. Metal items that are not in the radiation field are not a problem, so patients need not remove jewelry or clothing from areas that will not be included in the radiograph.

When the patient is ready, the next step is to assist the patient into the general position required for the x-ray examination (Figure 50-28). For example, if a hand is to be imaged, the patient can be seated at the end of the x-ray examination table (Figure 50-28, *A*). For a spinal examination, the patient may need to lie on the table (Figure 50-28, *B*). If a chest examination has been ordered, the patient stands at an upright film holder (Figure 50-28, *C*).

The radiographer then selects the correct cassette, places a lead marker on it to identify the patient's right or left side, and places the cassette in position for the exposure (Figure 50-29). Next, the patient is positioned precisely and the x-ray tube is aligned with the body

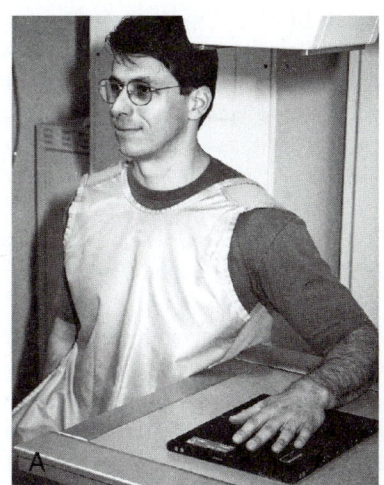
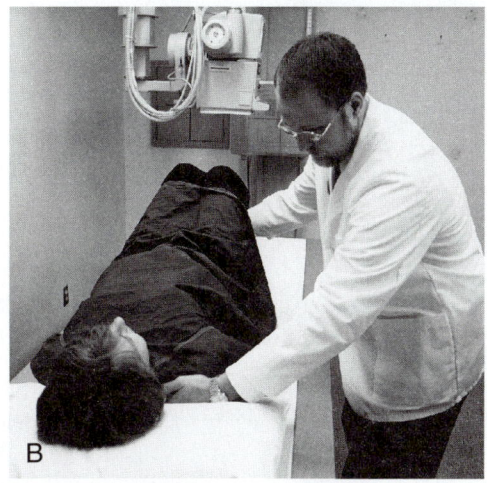
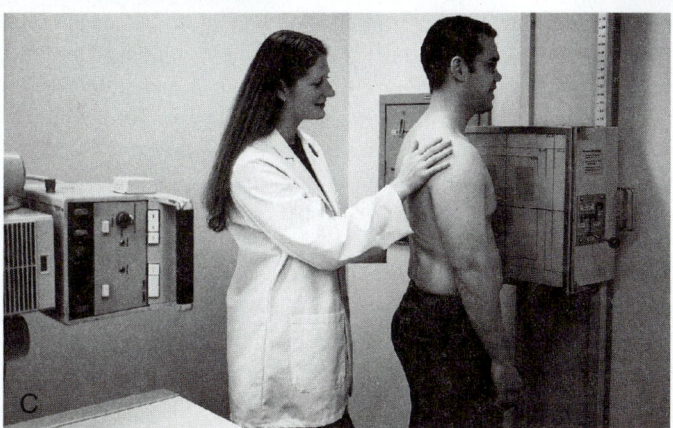

FIGURE 50-28 General positions for radiography. **A,** The patient may be seated at the x-ray table for some upper extremity examinations. **B,** The radiographer helps the patient lie down for spine radiography. **C,** The radiographer assists the patient into position at an upright bucky for chest radiographs. (From Long BW, Frank ED, Ehrlich RA: *Radiography essentials for limited practice,* ed 3, Philadelphia, 2010, WB Saunders.)

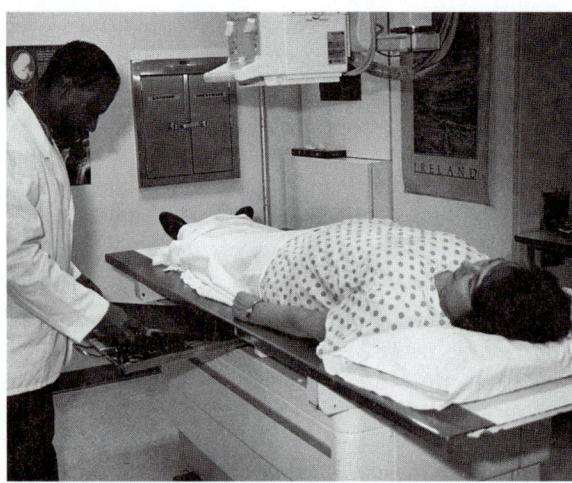

FIGURE 50-29 The cassette must be latched securely in the bucky tray, and the tray must be aligned to the anatomy of interest. (From Ehrlich RA, McCloskey ED, Daly JA: *Patient care in radiography*, ed 6, St Louis, 2004, Mosby.)

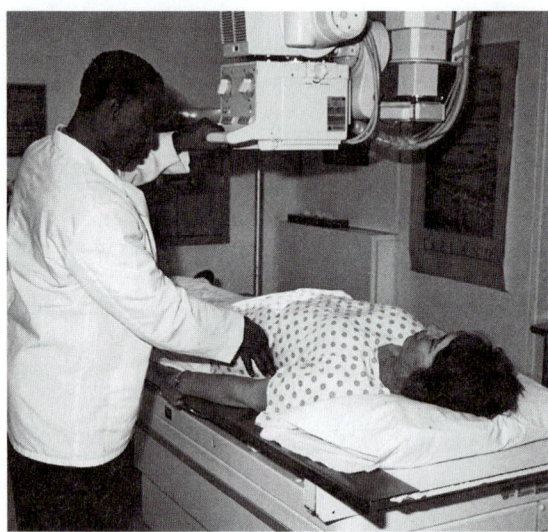

FIGURE 50-30 The x-ray tube must be aligned with the patient and cassette at the proper distance. (From Ehrlich RA, McCloskey ED, Daly JA: *Patient care in radiography*, ed 6, St Louis, 2004, Mosby.)

part and the film at a specific distance (Figure 50-30). The body part must be measured to determine the proper exposure factors according to a technique chart. At this point, lead shields are positioned for radiation protection. The radiographer then goes to the control booth, consults the technique chart, and sets the x-ray control panel to the desired exposure. Final instructions are given to the patient (typically that the patient must remain still during the x-ray procedure), and the exposure is made. If more than one exposure is needed, the film is changed, the patient is repositioned, and the steps are repeated until the examination is complete.

After the patient's safety and comfort have been ensured, the film is taken to the darkroom for processing. Film processing usually requires less than 10 minutes before the film can be evaluated. If the film is satisfactory and no further exposures are needed, the patient is returned to an examination room or dressing room. The radiographer or the medical assistant then readies the x-ray room for the next examination and prepares the films for interpretation.

The films are kept together and given to the physician with the appropriate paperwork. Films are kept in large file envelopes that may contain more than one set of films for the same patient. These envelopes must be accurately identified for proper filing. When images are added to the file, notations often are added to the envelope. After the films have been read, they are promptly filed so that they can be retrieved quickly when needed for future reference. Radiology reports also must be filed. Usually the original is filed in the patient's chart; copies may be filed separately or with the films.

SCHEDULING AND SEQUENCING DIAGNOSTIC IMAGING PROCEDURES

One of the most important communications between medical assistants and imaging departments involves the scheduling of multiple diagnostic procedures that may all be ordered at one time by the physician. Consultation often is needed to decide how many procedures can be done in one day and to sequence them in such a way that they will not interfere with one another. For example, a UGI series usually results in barium sulfate scattered throughout the intestinal tract for several days. Even tiny amounts of residual barium cause complications in radiographic examinations of the urinary tract and biliary system, where tiny opacifications are diagnostically significant. Residual barium in the digestive tract also causes unacceptable artifacts on abdominal CT scans. For this reason, barium studies are scheduled last in any series of procedures.

Some imaging departments schedule a series of several examinations in one day for patients who are able to tolerate this approach. Radiologists prefer various scheduling practices. For example, some departments schedule gallbladder and upper and lower GI studies on the same day. Others may insist on 2 or 3 days to complete the same examinations. You should become familiar with the practice in the institution where you usually schedule patients.

Scheduling several examinations on the same day may be less stressful for the patient, resulting in a single bowel preparation, a single period of fasting, and a single trip to the imaging center. However, the number of examinations an individual patient can tolerate varies, especially if the patient is elderly or ill. Make sure you discuss scheduling options with the patient and/or family before planning more than one examination per day.

When fiberoptic studies, such as gastroscopy or colonoscopy, are ordered in conjunction with radiographic examinations requiring barium as a contrast medium, the fiberoptic studies are done first. This avoids the possibility that the barium will interfere with visual assessment during the fiberoptic examination. Patients undergoing gastroscopy usually receive sedation and a muscle relaxant before the physician inserts the gastroscope. When a UGI series is to follow, it should be delayed to allow sufficient time for the patient to become responsive and alert before the UGI series, because oral administration of barium to a sedated patient increases the risk that the patient may choke on the barium.

Another study to be considered when sequencing diagnostic procedures is any thyroid assessment test that involves iodine uptake. Because the administration of a contrast medium containing iodine causes inaccurate results in such tests for at least 3 weeks, thyroid assessment tests (T_3 or T_4) or nuclear medicine thyroid scans must be performed before any contrast medium with iodine is administered.

An additional consideration in patient scheduling involves deciding which patients need early morning appointments and which can be scheduled later in the day. Imaging departments always begin the daily routine with patients who must fast in preparation for examination so that they do not have to go too long without food. When scheduling, request early priority for pediatric and geriatric patients, because they have the most difficulty maintaining nothing by mouth (**NPO**) status for long periods, and extended fasting may actually interfere with their recovery. Patients with diabetes who must postpone their insulin until their morning meal also need priority in scheduling. Outpatients who are diabetic should be reminded to postpone their morning insulin until the examination is complete, even if they have been scheduled for an early appointment. If an emergency should cause a delay, the patient who has had insulin may suffer a reaction. Paperwork done in the office for diagnostic studies needs to include information about patients with diabetes so that the radiology staff is aware of their status.

When instructing the patient about preparing for an examination, it is important to have printed instructions prepared in advance. If more than one alternative is printed on any given paper, be sure to indicate, both orally and in writing, which instructions are to be followed. Review the sheet with the patient slowly, explaining any words or procedures that may not be familiar. Have the patient explain back to you what is to be done (remember the importance of feedback in establishing whether the patient understands). If the patient is too young, too ill, confused, or incapable of understanding

and following the instructions, give the instructions (oral and written) to the person who will be responsible for assisting the patient. Be sure to include the telephone numbers of your clinical facility and of the imaging department so that the patient or the patient's family may call if any questions arise after the patient leaves the office.

In preparation for a UGI series, the patient must fast, avoiding water, smoking, and chewing gum. The NPO order is instituted for a limited period, usually 8 to 12 hours, before the procedure. This ensures that the stomach is empty at the time of examination so that an accurate radiographic image of its inner surfaces can be produced. Chewing gum and smoking are avoided because they tend to increase gastric secretions.

The preparation for a barium enema involves the use of a bowel cleansing kit. These kits usually contain one or more types of **cathartics**, a suppository, a low-volume enema, and illustrated instructions in several languages. Research has demonstrated that increased fluid intake enhances the effectiveness of cathartics and helps minimize the patient's discomfort. For this reason, instructions for cathartics are accompanied by a fluid intake schedule that suggests at least 8 ounces of water or clear liquid every 2 hours between noon and midnight on the day preceding the examination. The medical assistant should emphasize the importance of fluid intake. The required doses of cathartics have a strong, thorough action that occasionally cause patients to experience painful spasms of the bowel and irritation of the intestinal lining. Persistent diarrhea may last through the night, preventing sleep. Although patients may find this preparation uncomfortable and inconvenient, its effectiveness in cleansing the bowel usually outweighs these considerations. Caution must be exercised in implementing an aggressive preparation for elderly or frail patients who are likely to be adversely affected. A gentler alternative should be available for these debilitated patients. Those with chronic or acute diarrhea may require a lower dose or less active preparation than is usually given. When the routine strength or amount of cathartics is reduced, several days of a low-residue diet and an increased fluid intake become critical to the success of preparation. Patients should always be advised of the nature of the action expected from the cathartic when it is given. Table 50-3 summarizes common diagnostic procedures and the patient preparation required for each.

RADIATION SAFETY

Radiation Units

Two systems are used to measure radiation and radiation dose: the conventional (British) system and the international system (Système

TABLE 50-3 Diagnostic Procedures and Patient Preparation

STUDY	PURPOSE	PROCEDURE	PATIENT PREPARATION
Arteriogram	To aid diagnosis of arterial occlusion, aneurysm, hemorrhage, abnormal vessels, and transient ischemic attacks	Catheter is inserted into femoral or brachial artery and advanced under fluoroscopy to site; dye is injected, and x-ray images are taken.	Clear liquids 24 hr before test; nothing by mouth (NPO) 8 hr before test; if abdominal vasculature is to be imaged, patient may need laxative and enemas
Arthrogram	To detect damage to joint connective tissue and structures	Fluoroscopic and radiographic examination of a joint after injection of air or contrast dye.	NPO 8 hr
Barium enema	To detect bowel obstruction, celiac sprue, colon cancer, polyps, diverticulitis, irritable bowel syndrome	Fluoroscopic and radiographic examination of the colon after barium enema to find internal structural abnormalities; takes approximately 1 hr.	Bowel must be emptied before procedure; clear liquid diet 24 hr before test; laxatives day before test; enemas morning of test
Barium swallow	To detect dysphagia, esophageal varices, hiatal hernia, pyloric stenosis, stomach cancer, ulcers	Fluoroscopic and radiographic examination as barium is swallowed to detect abnormalities of the pharynx, esophagus, and stomach; takes about 15 min.	NPO 8 hr
Bone scan	To detect bone cancer, bone infection, osteoarthritis, osteomyelitis	Nuclear medicine: Radioactive isotope is injected intravenously (IV), body is scanned, and levels of isotope are recorded on film. Areas of high metabolism show as "hot spots"; scan is done 1-3 hr after isotope injection.	NPO 4 hr; must void before scan; radioactive material is excreted in urine within 48 hr and is not harmful to others
Computed tomography (CT)	Provides detailed, cross-sectional views of all types of tissue; one of the best tools for studying the chest and abdomen	Special x-ray equipment and computers are used to obtain image data from different angles around the body, and multiple cross-sectional views (tomographs) are produced.	NPO after midnight if IV contrast medium used; no metal objects; must lie very still; advise of confined space and possible claustrophobia
Intravenous urogram (IVU) or intravenous pyelogram (IVP)	To evaluate structure and function of kidneys, ureters, and bladder	IV contrast medium is injected, and x-ray films are taken of renal structures.	Bowel cleansing 24 hr before with laxatives and enema is important to prevent obstruction of views; NPO 8 hr
Magnetic resonance imaging (MRI)	To aid diagnosis of intracranial and spinal lesions, aneurysms, heart defects, multiple sclerosis, and soft tissue abnormalities throughout the body	Magnetic field and radiofrequency energy are transmitted to a computer, which produces cross-sectional images of soft tissue; it may eliminate the need for arthrography and myelography. No radiation exposure is involved. Patient lies on a flat table that moves into a tunnel-shaped scanner; takes 45-90 min.	May have fluid restriction; radioactive contrast dye may be used; must remove all metal; contraindications include any metallic implants with iron (e.g., pacemakers, artificial heart valves, aneurysm clips, material associated with metal-related occupation); patient hears loud tapping noise during test and must remain still
Myelogram	To aid diagnosis of spinal lesions, ruptured disk, spinal stenosis	Fluoroscopic and radiographic examination of the spinal column after injection of contrast medium into the subarachnoid space; takes about 1 hr.	NPO 8 hr

International [SI]) established in 1981. The conventional system is still the most commonly used in the United States. The reason for the measurement determines which unit is most appropriate.

The **roentgen (R)** is the conventional unit of radiation exposure. It represents a measurement of radiation intensity and is determined by the interaction of the x-ray beam with air. For example, an x-ray machine might produce 0.01 R during the exposure for a chest radiograph. The corresponding SI unit is **coulombs per kilogram (C/kg)**, which specifies the electrical charge in coulombs produced by the exposure of 1 kg of dry air.

The roentgen is not a useful dose unit because dose varies with the depth of measurement and the amount of radiation energy absorbed in the exposed tissue. The conventional unit used to measure both therapeutic radiation doses and specific tissue doses received in diagnostic applications is the **rad**, which stands for *radiation absorbed dose*. It usually is qualified by the specific body part to which it applies. For example, a radiation oncologist may prescribe a treatment involving 150 rad to the pelvis. The SI unit for dose measurement is the **Gray (Gy)**.

The biologic effect of radiation exposure varies according to the type of radiation involved and its energy; equal doses of various types of radiation do not necessarily result in equal biologic effects. To measure occupational dose or other exposure that may involve more than one type of radiation, the dose equivalent unit used is the **rem**, which stands for *roentgen equivalent in man*. Dose equivalents usually are assumed to represent whole body dose or the dose to unspecified tissues. The SI unit for dose equivalent is the **Sievert (Sv)**.

Because the radiation quantities involved in diagnostic radiology are so small, units may be used that represent $\frac{1}{1,000}$ of the common units: milliroentgen (mR), millirad (mrad), and millirem (mrem). It may be confusing to determine which units should be used in a given situation. This is made more difficult by the tendency of many radiographers to use the traditional roentgen, rad, and rem units interchangeably. This practice does not cause serious inaccuracy when speaking only of diagnostic x-ray studies, because exposure to 1 roentgen of x-ray energy results in approximately 1 rad of absorbed dose, which is equal to a dose equivalent of 1 rem.

Effects of Low-Dose Radiation Exposure

Cellular Response to Exposure

Most cellular effects of radiation exposure are extremely short lived, because chemical alterations within the cells are quickly repaired. Even if a cell dies, cell death is an insignificant injury unless the number of cells involved is massive. Some cells may sustain damage that requires several days for the body to repair. The body produces special enzymes that function to repair DNA protein molecules. Sometimes a cell may be damaged in such a way that its DNA "programming" is changed and the cell no longer behaves normally. This type of injury eventually may result in the runaway production of new, abnormal cells, causing a tumor or malignant blood disease.

The relative sensitivity of different types of cells is summarized in the laws of Bergonié and Tribondeau, which state that cell sensitivity to radiation exposure depends on four characteristics of the cell:

- *Age:* Younger cells are more sensitive than older ones.
- *Differentiation:* Simple cells are more sensitive than highly complex ones.

- *Metabolic rate:* Cells that use energy rapidly are more sensitive than those that have a slower metabolism.
- *Mitotic rate:* Cells that divide and multiply rapidly are more sensitive than those that replicate slowly.

According to these laws, blood cells and blood-producing cells are very sensitive. Cells that are in contact with the environment are quite simple, have relatively short lives, and are quite sensitive. These include the cells of the skin and the mucosal lining of the mouth, nose, and GI tract. Some glandular tissue also is particularly sensitive, especially that of the thyroid gland and the female breast. The tissues of embryos, fetuses, infants, children, and adolescents tend to be more sensitive than those of adults because of their young age and higher metabolic and mitotic rates. Nerve cells, which have a long life and are quite complex, are much less vulnerable to radiation injury.

Somatic Effects

Radiation effects can be classified as somatic or genetic. Somatic effects are those that occur to the body of the person who is irradiated. Whereas the effects of relatively high doses of radiation are immediate and predictable, the effects of the very low doses associated with radiography produce long-term effects. They are not easily identified as a result of radiation exposure, because they occur 3 to 30 years after treatment and because the same problems can occur in the absence of radiation exposure. Only extensive research with large populations can demonstrate the role of radiation in causing these effects. In other words, radiation causes increased risk for health problems, but the complications cannot be predicted with respect to any one individual. Although the individual risk is extremely small, increasing exposure to the entire population poses public health risks that require the attention and concern of everyone involved in applying ionizing radiation to human beings.

The documented latent effects of low doses of ionizing radiation include the following:

- *Cataract formation:* This is a risk for radiologists and radiographers who work extensively in fluoroscopy and those who perform other work that involves repeated exposure to the eyes.
- *Carcinogenesis:* Increased risk of malignant disease, particularly cancer of the skin, thyroid, breast, and leukemia.
- *Shortened life span:* A study of the life span of radiologists who died before 1945 showed that they had shorter life spans than physicians who did not use radiation in their practices. This group included radiologists who had used radiation since the early days of x-ray science. More recent studies show that occupational exposure no longer has a measurable effect on the life span of radiologists. Nevertheless, because radiation exposure has been linked to shortening of the life span, it is a public health concern and another reason to practice a high level of radiation safety.

Radiation and Pregnancy

Radiation exposure poses risks to the developing embryo or fetus. Research has demonstrated that excessive radiation during pregnancy may result in spontaneous abortion, congenital defects in the child, growth retardation, increased risk of cancer and leukemia in childhood, and an increase in significant genetic abnormalities in the children of parents who were exposed in utero. Studies of women exposed to radiation as a result of diagnostic and therapeutic procedures confirm that radiation to the uterus in excess of 5 rad is cause for concern. This is more exposure than is received with most x-ray examinations, but these levels may be encountered with direct exposure to the pelvis, especially with CT examinations or fluoroscopic studies.

Genetic Effects

Genetic effects in the form of changes or mutations in the hereditary material of reproductive cells may occur if the ovaries or testes are exposed to radiation. In the female, all the ova cells the individual will ever produce are present at birth. Because no new egg cells are created as the individual ages, the effect of radiation exposure to the ovaries accumulates over time. In addition, the genetic effects of radiation to the testes may include damage to stem cells that produce sperm, resulting in the production of sperm with a genetic mutation. Most genetic mutations threaten the survival of an individual. Even when these changes are recessive (not apparent in the offspring), they may be passed on to future generations.

GUIDELINES FOR PEDIATRIC X-RAY EXAMINATIONS

- Provide age-appropriate explanations about the procedure and instructions for patient compliance.
- Inform the parents about the procedure and answer questions.
- Give the patient or parents written information when needed about preparation for the examination.
- Explain that allowing parents in the x-ray room will be up to the facility.
- When possible, use commercial immobilization devices to position the child (e.g., restraint board with Velcro closures, papoose board, positioning chair [Figure 50-31]).
- Have a parent help the child maintain a particular position when immobilization devices are not available or are ineffective. The parent must wear the appropriate lead shielding equipment.

Radiation Protection

Clearly, exposure to x-rays creates some risk for both patients and radiographers; therefore, it is essential that those performing radiographic studies are knowledgeable about and diligently practice radiation safety. All unnecessary radiation exposure to patients, co-workers, and oneself must be prevented.

PERSONNEL SAFETY

In diagnostic x-ray departments, radiation hazards exist from exposure to the primary x-ray beam and to scatter radiation caused by an interaction between the primary beam and the patient or other material in its path. Scatter radiation is present throughout the x-ray room during an exposure. X-rays travel at the speed of light. They do not linger in the room after the exposure, and they are not capable of making the objects in the room radioactive. Therefore, the only time a radiation hazard exists is during the x-ray exposure itself.

Because radiographers are considered occupationally exposed individuals, they are prohibited from activities that would result in direct exposure to the primary x-ray beam. This means that they are not allowed to hold patients or cassettes during x-ray exposures and must stand clear of the path of the primary x-ray beam during fluoroscopic and mobile radiographic examinations. Whenever possible, patients should be immobilized without someone holding them. When infants or children must be held, a parent (as long as the parent is not pregnant) usually is the appropriate person to perform this duty, with the required lead covering.

Medical assistants may or may not be considered occupationally exposed persons, depending on their work assignments and the frequency with which they are involved with radiation use. Medical assistants who are not routinely exposed occasionally may assist with procedures by holding patients or cassettes. When this is the case, the medical assistant should wear a lead apron and should avoid direct exposure to the primary x-ray beam if possible (Figure 50-32). If the hands will be in the primary beam, lead gloves should also be worn.

Personnel are not exposed to any significant amount of radiation when standing well behind the protective lead barrier of the control booth. X-rays travel in straight lines and do not turn corners. Scatter

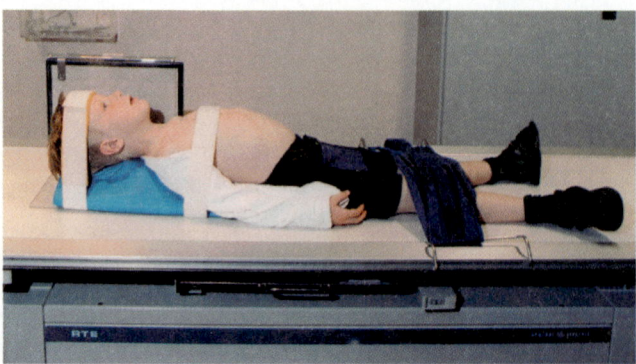

FIGURE 50-31 Immobilization device for a pediatric patient. (From Frank ED, Long BW, Smith BJ: *Merrill's atlas of radiographic positioning and procedures*, ed 11, St Louis, 2007, Mosby.)

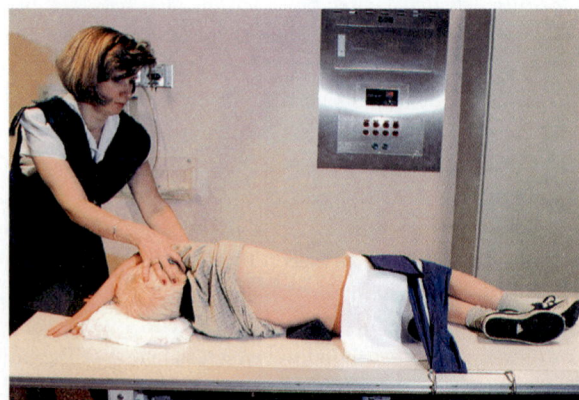

FIGURE 50-32 When holding a child for a radiographic procedure, wear a lead apron and stay as far from the primary x-ray beam as possible. (From Ballinger PW, Frank ED: *Merrill's atlas of radiographic positions and radiologic procedures*, ed 10, vol 2, St Louis, 2003, Mosby.)

radiation is not powerful enough to generate additional radiation of concern when it interacts with matter, so the control booth need not be sealed.

Occupational exposure increases when assisting with fluoroscopic procedures or using mobile x-ray equipment. The three principal methods used to protect personnel from unnecessary radiation exposure are time, distance, and shielding.

Because the amount of exposure received is directly proportional to the time spent in a radiation area, dose is decreased when this time is minimized. For example, you might shorten the time of exposure by stepping into the control booth during fluoroscopic procedures when not required to be near the patient.

The second method involves using distance. Increasing the distance between yourself and a radiation source reduces your exposure in proportion to the square of the distance; therefore, small increases in distance have a relatively large effect. Mobile x-ray units have long cords on the exposure switches, which allows the radiographer to get as far from the radiation source as possible while making an exposure.

The third method, shielding, is the most common type of personnel protection used in outpatient radiography settings. The lead wall of the control booth provides a radiation safety barrier and is the principal defense for personnel. Other types of shielding include lead aprons, gloves, goggles, and thyroid shields. These types of shielding are worn during fluoroscopic procedures and mobile radiographic examinations.

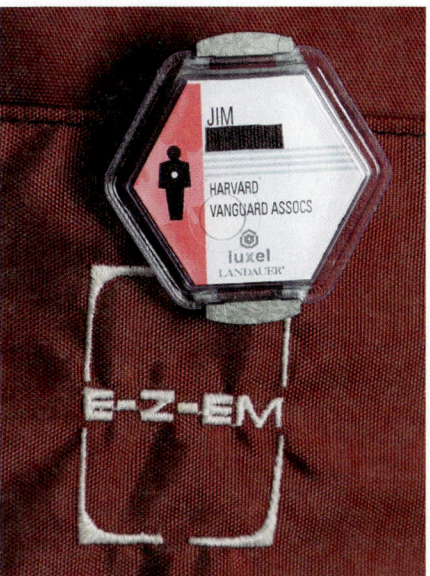

FIGURE 50-33 Optically stimulated luminescence (OSL) dosimeter.

PRE-EXPOSURE SAFETY CHECK

Before taking an x-ray, make sure of the following:
- The x-ray room door is closed; a closed door indicates that an exposure is in progress and no one may enter the room.
- No nonessential persons are in the x-ray room; all essential individuals outside the lead barrier are appropriately shielded.
- All those in the control booth are completely behind the lead barrier.
- The only cassette in the room is the one in use.

Personnel Monitoring

A device for monitoring radiation exposure to personnel is called a **dosimeter**. Dosimeters should be worn in the region of the collar and should be outside a lead apron if it is used. The three basic types of dosimeters are film badges, thermoluminescent dosimeters (TLDs), and optically stimulated luminescence dosimeters (OSLs). A film badge consists of one or two pieces of dental film that is paper wrapped and enclosed in a badgelike holder that incorporates several filters. The disadvantage of this type of dosimeter is that the dental film is subject to fog when exposed to heat or fumes, and this exposure could result in a false reading. TLD badges have one or more lithium fluoride crystals that absorb radiation energy and then emit the energy in the form of light when heated. They are more durable than film badges and respond only to ionizing radiation exposure. OSLs, the most recently developed monitoring dosimeter (Figure 50-33), use aluminum oxide as the radiation detector. OSLs provide greater stability and precision plus the ability to reanalyze and confirm results.

Your facility will contract with a radiation monitor badge service laboratory to provide badges, processing services, and reports. The laboratory also is responsible for maintaining permanent records of the radiation exposure of each person monitored. Depending on facility policy, badges are sent for evaluation of radiation exposure on a weekly, monthly, or quarterly basis. Personnel who receive relatively high doses of occupational exposure change their badges most frequently. Occupationally exposed personnel who are always or nearly always in a control booth during exposures usually are monitored with quarterly service. Monthly service is a better choice for those who work in fluoroscopy or use mobile x-ray equipment.

Service companies provide an extra badge in every batch that is marked CONTROL. This badge's purpose is to measure any radiation exposure to the entire batch while in transit. Any amount of exposure measured from the control badge is subtracted from the amounts measured from the other badges in the batch. The control badge should be kept in a safe place, away from anywhere x-ray exposure could occur. *It should never be used to measure occupational dose or for any other purpose.*

Exposure reports are sent to the facility for each batch with an annual summary of personnel exposure. The report sent by the laboratory that processes the personnel dosimeters reports occupational dose in rem. Personnel should be advised of the radiation exposure reported from their badges and should be provided with copies of the annual reports for their own records. Employers are required to provide a complete record of an employee's radiation exposure history to all employees who have radiation exposure records before the individual leaves the employment of that facility.

Effective Dose Equivalent Limits

The ALARA principle is the guiding philosophy associated with all radiation use that involves exposure to humans, both patients and workers. It states that all radiation exposure to humans should be limited to levels that are *as low as reasonably achievable.*

The effective dose equivalent (EDE) limiting system is used to calculate the upper limit of permitted occupational exposure. For occupationally exposed personnel, the EDE limit is 5 rem (50 mSv) per year. This applies to workers over age 18 who are not pregnant and is assumed to be a whole body dose. These limits apply to occupational exposure only and do not include diagnostic imaging exposure that the worker may receive as a result of tests related to their own healthcare.

The established EDE limits ensure that the safety of radiation workers is comparable to that of workers in other, safe occupations. The allowable exposure is considered to be so low as to pose an insignificant risk. The occupational exposure received by radiographers usually is well below the established limit.

Occupational Precautions During Pregnancy

Radiation exposure during pregnancy must be closely monitored because of possible complications for the developing fetus. The EDE limit of whole body radiation for the pregnant worker is 0.5 rem over the 9-month course of the pregnancy. The worker first must submit a written document to her employer declaring the pregnancy. The employer then is responsible for providing fetal radiation monitoring and for ensuring that the occupational dose does not exceed the EDE limit for pregnant workers. Here again, the ALARA principle is important. Every effort should be made to minimize exposure, keeping the dose as far below the limit as possible.

For a pregnant radiographer, the safest work assignment would be one in which a permanent lead barrier (control booth) always shields the worker during exposures. Pregnant radiographers, or those of childbearing age who may be pregnant, should pay particular attention to personal safety measures when assisting with fluoroscopy or using mobile x-ray equipment.

Patient Protection

Patients must be consistently protected from unnecessary radiation exposure. The following methods are used to minimize the radiation dose to patients:

- Avoid errors. Double-check requisitions and patient identification so that the right patient gets the right examination.
- Establish good routine procedures and follow them strictly so that careless errors do not necessitate repeat exposures.

- Collimate. Use the smallest radiation field needed to fulfill the physician's order. The size of the radiation field should always be less than the size of the film.
- Use the highest kVp consistent with acceptable film quality. This permits use of the least possible mAs to obtain an acceptable exposure.
- Use an SID of at least 40 inches. This limits patient exposure from tube housing leakage and collimator scatter.
- Use the fastest films and screens consistent with the necessary film quality.
- Provide shielding for gonads, eyes, breasts, and thyroid as appropriate.

Gonad Shielding

Lead shields that prevent unnecessary radiation exposure to the reproductive organs are required when the patient is of reproductive age or younger, whenever the gonads are within the primary radiation field, and when the shield will not interfere with the examination. This applies to most patients under age 55. A shield device consisting of at least 0.5 mm of lead or equivalent is placed between the x-ray tube and the patient. Shields attached to the collimator (shadow shields) may be positioned by viewing their shadows within the collimator light field. Shields placed on or near the patient's body are referred to as *contact shields* and are more effective than shadow shields. Both types meet the legal requirements for gonad shielding. The female shield is placed with its lower margin at the level of the pubic symphysis (Figure 50-34). The male shield is positioned with its upper margin about 1 inch below the pubic symphysis (Figure 50-35). It is helpful to note that the pubic symphysis is at about the same level as the greater trochanter of the femur, which prevents the need to palpate the pubic symphysis for proper shield placement.

Pregnant or Possibly Pregnant Patients

The greatest risks for spontaneous abortion, fetal death, and significant birth defects exist when significant levels of exposure occur during the first trimester of pregnancy. The embryo is most vulnerable to radiation insult while tissues are in the process of differentiation. Unfortunately, this creates the greatest hazard at a time when a woman may not yet be aware she is pregnant.

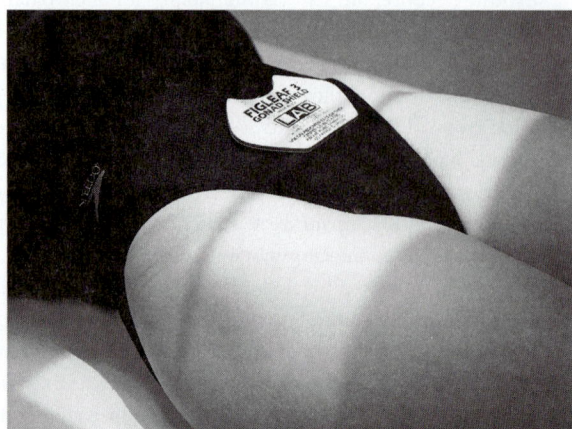
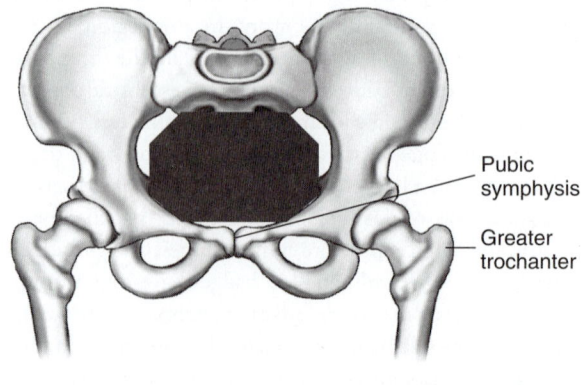

Pubic symphysis

Greater trochanter

FIGURE 50-34 When precise gonad shielding is required for female patients, place the lower margin of the shield on the upper margin of the pubic symphysis. (From Long BW, Frank ED, Ehrlich RA: *Radiography essentials for limited practice,* ed 3, Philadelphia, 2010, Saunders.)

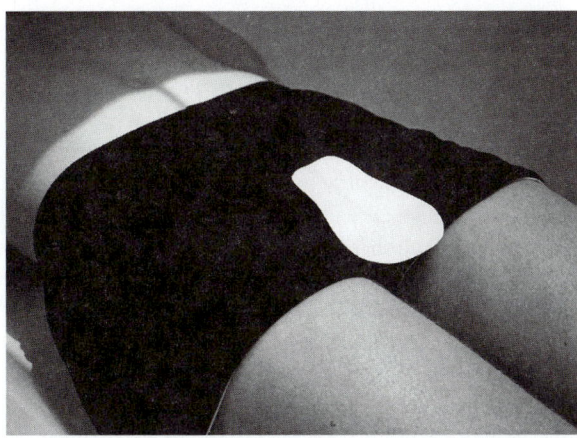
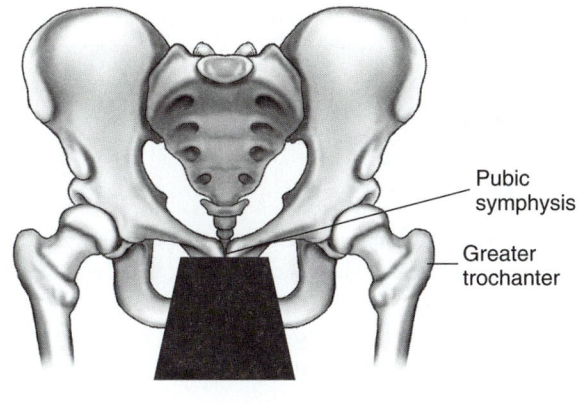

Pubic symphysis

Greater trochanter

FIGURE 50-35 When precise gonad shielding is required for male patients, place the upper margin of the shield 1 inch below the pubic symphysis. (From Long BW, Frank ED, Ehrlich RA: *Radiography essentials for limited practice*, ed 3, Philadelphia, 2010, WB Saunders.)

The public is generally aware that x-rays should be avoided during pregnancy, and this may lead to irrational fears on the part of pregnant women or their families. The chance is extremely remote that a routine x-ray examination of the chest or an extremity would harm the developing child. On the other hand, examinations requiring direct radiation to the pelvis, especially relatively high-dose fluoroscopy studies or CT scans of the abdomen or lumbar spine, may be cause for concern.

Radiation control regulations require that female patients of childbearing age be advised of potential radiation hazards before an x-ray examination. This requirement usually is met by posting signs in the radiology department advising women to tell the radiographer before the examination if they may be pregnant. These signs should be written in all languages commonly used in the community.

The medical assistant should ask specific questions to rule out pregnancy when taking a medical history. If pregnancy is a possibility, an early pregnancy test should be done to rule out the possibility. If the patient is pregnant and the proposed x-ray examination involves direct pelvic radiation, the physician must weigh the potential risks and benefits of the examination and discuss them with the patient before proceeding with the study. In the case of minor or chronic complaints, the examination typically is delayed until after the child is born. In practice, however, the possibility of pregnancy may not even be considered. This is especially true with accident or injury, when the patient is being cared for by unfamiliar physicians in an emergency situation. For this reason, it is essential to consider the possibility of pregnancy in any female of childbearing age and to ask specific questions to determine whether the physician has addressed the issue of pregnancy before proceeding with scheduling or assisting with an x-ray examination.

If an x-ray examination of a pregnant patient must be done, modifications in procedure can help minimize the dose to the embryo or fetus. If the part to be examined is not the abdomen or pelvis, this area can be shielded with a lead apron. If the abdomen or pelvis is to be evaluated, the number of views or the size of the radiation field may be minimized, resulting in less radiation exposure than that required for a routine procedure.

CRITICAL THINKING APPLICATION   **50-3**

Ingrid White is gowned and ready for a lumbar spine x-ray examination when Sara asks her whether there is any possibility she might be pregnant. Mrs. White confides that she and her husband have been trying to conceive for several months, and she is not sure whether she currently is pregnant. What should Sara do?

THE ROLE OF THE MEDICAL ASSISTANT

Depending on your location, you may or may not be legally permitted to take x-ray films. Most states require some sort of license or permit to practice radiography. Some, such as New York and New Jersey, grant licenses only to professional radiologic technologists who have completed at least a 2-year education program and obtained certification in radiography from the American Registry of Radiologic Technologists (ARRT).

Limited radiography, sometimes called *practical radiography,* is practiced primarily in clinics and physicians' offices. This field developed as nurses, medical assistants, chiropractic assistants, and other healthcare office personnel were trained to perform basic x-ray procedures in addition to their primary duties. It is called *limited* because the scope of practice is restricted compared with that of registered radiologic technologists. Limited practice does not usually involve the use of contrast media, and additional restrictions may be applied, depending on the scope of practice permitted in the states where limited radiography can be legally practiced.

However, even if you are not qualified as a radiographer, it may be helpful to understand the general procedures involved in an x-ray examination and to identify areas where the medical assistant might be of help to the patient or radiographer, or both. The exact nature of your duties will vary with your qualifications, your place of employment, the size of the staff, and the equipment available.

The process of radiography involves validation of orders, patient preparation, proper selection of cassettes and film, correct positioning of patient and equipment, measurement of the part to be examined, protective shielding, correct setting of the exposure controls, and identification and processing of the film. These basic procedures vary considerably, depending on the body part to be examined.

CLOSING COMMENTS

Legal and Ethical Issues

Only licensed health practitioners are permitted to order x-ray examinations. Interpretation of diagnostic images is part of the professional practice of making a diagnosis and is solely the privilege of physicians. Although you may learn to recognize certain conditions represented in diagnostic images, you must never discuss your observations with the patient.

In most states, x-ray machines must be licensed, and personnel operating this equipment must have a current license or permit. In all states that regulate radiography, the practice is defined as more than simply pushing the exposure button. If you position the x-ray equipment, position the patient, or set the exposure controls, even though you do not make the exposure, you are probably practicing radiography as defined by law. Practicing without a valid license or permit or practicing outside the scope of one's credentials may result in fines, imprisonment, or both. Employers may also be penalized if their employees practice radiography in violation of regulations. Everyone who practices radiography must be aware of the legal standards that apply to them and take care that their practice conforms to these standards. Even if you work in a state that currently has no requirements for practicing radiography, you should be aware that the safe practice of radiography requires additional education and experience beyond that provided in this chapter.

X-ray films and other diagnostic images are the property of the institution or facility where they are taken. Even though the patient may pay for the procedure, this does not mean the patient owns the films. They are considered part of the medical record and are subject to the same kinds of requirements with respect to confidentiality, retention, and availability to the patient. The retention period varies from state to state; usually it is 5 to 7 years. Images may be loaned or transferred to other healthcare providers to assist in the patient's care. The patient should sign a release when images or copies of images are to be sent to another healthcare provider, and a record of the date and the name and address of the borrower must be kept when original images are loaned to another facility. The patient may deliver the films when referred to another physician, but the preferable course is to send the films directly to the provider. This process is much less complicated in practices with electronic medical records. When the patient must carry the films, it is best that the physician review the films with the patient in advance so that the patient does not misinterpret the images and reach an incorrect conclusion.

> **CRITICAL THINKING APPLICATION   50-4**
>
> One of the new medical assistants at Metro Urgicenter, Carla O'Neal, tells Sara she is not qualified to practice radiography in the office's jurisdiction. David has instructed her to position a patient and set up the equipment for an x-ray examination. When Carla stated that she was not yet qualified to practice radiography, David replied, "Don't worry. I'll come by in a few minutes and make the exposure." What should Sara and Carla do about this?

SUMMARY OF SCENARIO

David Swain and the physicians at Metro Urgicenter depend on Sara's assistance to keep the x-ray department running smoothly. Today, for example, she instructed four patients to gown and prepare for routine x-ray examinations. Greg Nolan had PA and lateral views of the chest because of a persistent cough and fever. Margaret and Jeff Barge both needed spine x-ray studies to rule out possible fractures from a car accident. Dr. Farnsworth ordered AP and lateral views of Ella Jackson's left hip. Sara processed the films and was proud to see that they had no handling artifacts. This afternoon, Sara made an appointment for Cecile Marsden to have a bone scan at University Imaging Center. She was able to describe the procedure for Ms. Marsden so that she would know exactly what to expect. Sara recognizes that she must remain up to date on the current radiologic diagnostic procedures to provide assistance when needed and to answer patients' questions. Sara enjoys her work in the x-ray department and is attending evening classes to become certified as a limited radiographer.

SUMMARY OF LEARNING OBJECTIVES

1. **Define, spell, and pronounce the terms listed in the vocabulary.**
   Spelling and pronouncing medical terms correctly bolster the medical assistant's credibility. Knowing the definitions of these terms promotes confidence in communication with patients and co-workers.
2. **Apply critical thinking skills in performing the patient assessment and patient care.**
   Completing the Critical Thinking Application exercises throughout the chapter can help the student medical assistant become more adept at critical analysis of real-life situations.

3. **Identify the principal components of radiographic equipment**
   The main component of the x-ray machine is the tube in its barrel-shaped tube housing. The collimator is mounted on the tube housing. The tube housing, with its attachments, is mounted on the tube support. The radiographic table and an upright cassette holder provide support for the patient and the film and incorporate a grid device. At the control console the operator selects the exposure settings and makes the exposure.
4. **Describe the cassette and film image receptor system and explain its function in radiography.**

The image receptor system usually consists of a cassette with two intensifying screens that give off light when stimulated by x-ray energy and double-emulsion film that lies between the intensifying screens. The film is exposed on both sides, principally by the light emitted from the screens. This system greatly reduces the amount of radiation and the exposure time compared with direct exposure of film by x-rays.

5. **Recognize the precautions to be taken when unloading, loading, and processing radiographic film and cassettes.**

Cassettes are unloaded and reloaded in the darkroom under safelight illumination only. Precautions include ensuring that the door is locked; that the hands are clean and dry; and that the film is not creased, bent, or scraped in the process of loading and unloading. Care must be taken to reload the cassette with fresh film and to latch the cassette securely. The loading bench must be kept clean to prevent dirt from getting into the cassette.

6. **Distinguish among the three body planes and use these terms correctly when discussing radiographic positions.**

The three body planes are the sagittal plane, which divides the body into right and left parts, the coronal plane, which divides the body into anterior and posterior parts, and the transverse plane, which divides the body into superior and inferior parts. For a frontal projection (AP or PA), the coronal plane is parallel to the film and the sagittal plane is perpendicular to it. For a lateral projection, the sagittal plane is parallel to the film and the coronal plane is perpendicular to it. Neither the sagittal plane nor the coronal plane is parallel to the film on an oblique projection.

7. **Identify anteroposterior (AP), posteroanterior (PA), lateral, oblique, and axial radiographic projections.**

In an AP projection, the patient is supine and facing the x-ray tube. In a PA projection, the patient is facing the film, and the coronal plane is parallel to the film. In a lateral projection, the coronal plane is perpendicular to the film. In an oblique projection, neither the coronal nor the sagittal plane is parallel to the film. In an axial or semiaxial projection, the x-ray beam is angled toward the patient's head or feet along the long axis of the body.

8. **Compare and contrast radiography and fluoroscopy and give examples of appropriate applications of each.**

Radiography and fluoroscopy are both x-ray imaging procedures with a wide variety of applications. Radiography produces still images, usually on photographic film; fluoroscopy enables the radiologist to view the x-ray image directly and to observe motion.

9. **List and describe imaging modalities that do not involve x-rays.**

MRI uses a strong magnetic field and radiofrequency pulses to produce images of all parts of the body, including bone, soft tissue, and blood vessels. Nuclear medicine studies demonstrate the function of organs and tissues by mapping the radiation given off within the body when radioactive tracers have been ingested or injected into the patient. Sonography is a very safe imaging method that demonstrates soft tissues using high-frequency sound waves.

10. **Explain the patient preparation guidelines for typical diagnostic imaging examinations.**

Table 50-3 summarizes patient preparation.

11. **Outline the general procedure for assisting with an x-ray examination.**

The patient is prepared with education and appropriate gowning and positioning. Lead shields are used as needed. The medical assistant assists with film processing if trained to do so. The procedure is documented in the medical record, and radiology reports are filed.

12. **Summarize the guidelines for scheduling multiple diagnostic procedures.**

When possible, several examinations should be scheduled on the same day if the patient is strong enough. Diagnostic imaging that does not require contrast media or nuclear medicine should be scheduled first. Next are examinations of the urinary tract and biliary system. Fiberoptic studies (e.g., colonoscopy) and CT studies of the abdomen and pelvis should be scheduled before any GI studies that require barium. CT and MRI can be scheduled anytime unless they require IV contrast; if iodine dye is needed, the procedure is scheduled after examinations that do not require visualization. Barium studies are always scheduled last, and a UGI series (barium swallow) is the final procedure.

13. **Apply patient education principles when providing instructions for preparation for diagnostic procedures.**

Table 50-3 summarizes patient preparation guidelines for diagnostic imaging procedures. The patient must be informed of the purpose of the study, how the procedure will be performed, and any important patient preparation steps needed to make sure the examination can be completed successfully. The healthcare facility should have instruction sheets ready to distribute to patients scheduled for diagnostic studies. The medical assistant must understand diagnostic procedures so that the patient's questions can be answered and informed consent can be obtained. The medical assistant should review instruction sheets with the patient to make sure the preparation is done as recommended.

14. **Describe the health risks associated with low doses of x-ray exposure, such as those used in radiography.**

The health risks associated with radiography are extremely small and consist of a slightly increased likelihood of developing cataracts, cancer, or leukemia. The potential also exists for a minimal decrease in life span and for a negative outcome if the abdominal area is exposed to radiation during pregnancy. Exposure to the reproductive organs may cause genetic changes that can be passed on to future generations.

15. **Describe precautions for ensuring the safety of equipment operators and staff members during x-ray procedures.**

The principal safety precaution for x-ray equipment operators and staff is to stay completely behind the lead barrier of the control booth during exposures. Occupationally exposed individuals must not hold patients or cassettes during exposures. Any staff member required to be in the x-ray room during an exposure should be shielded by a lead apron, should stay as far from radiation sources as possible, and should minimize the time spent in the room during exposures.

16. **Summarize the steps for ensuring that patients receive the least possible exposure during x-ray procedures.**

To ensure that patients receive the least possible exposure during x-ray procedures, radiology personnel should avoid errors that could require repeat exposures; establish good routine procedures and follow them strictly; collimate to the smallest radiation field; use the highest kVp possible; use an SID of at least 40 inches; use the fastest films and screens consistent with the necessary film quality; and shield the reproductive organs and other sensitive organs (e.g., eyes, thyroid, and breasts).

17. **Explain the legal responsibilities associated with x-ray procedures and the administrative management of diagnostic images.**

Diagnostic images are the property of the facility in which they are made. Images may be loaned or transferred to other healthcare providers to assist in the patient's care, in which case the patient should sign a release, the images should be sent directly to the borrowing provider if possible, and a record must be kept of the loan. Only licensed healthcare practitioners are permitted to order x-ray examinations and/or to interpret x-ray images.

CONNECTIONS

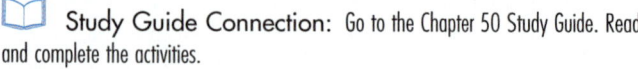

Study Guide Connection: Go to the Chapter 50 Study Guide. Read and complete the activities.

Evolve Connection: Go to the Chapter 50 link at *evolve.elsevier.com/kinn* to complete the Chapter Review and Chapter Quiz. Check out the other resources listed for this chapter to make the most of what you have learned from Assisting and Diagnostic Imaging.

ASSISTING IN THE CLINICAL LABORATORY

51

SCENARIO

Marsha Rollins has been employed for 3 years as a certified medical assistant in a medical practice. The physicians have a medical laboratory on site, and Marsha has become experienced in collecting specimens, performing laboratory tests, and reporting results. Recently she was offered a position in a smaller practice closer to home; she has accepted the position, knowing that her experience will benefit the practice because the physicians would like to expand their on-site medical laboratory testing, and Marsha will be required to equip the laboratory.

While studying this chapter, think about the following questions:

- What agencies can assist Marsha as she researches the feasibility of setting up a laboratory in the physicians' office?
- What regulations will guide the testing that will be performed in the lab?
- What equipment will she need and how will she ensure that it remains in good working order?

LEARNING OBJECTIVES

1. Define, spell, and pronounce the terms listed in the vocabulary.
2. Apply critical thinking skills in performing the patient assessment and patient care.
3. Discuss the role of the clinical laboratory in patient care and the medical assistant's role in coordinating laboratory tests and results.
4. Describe the Clinical Laboratory Improvement Amendments (CLIA) and how they influence laboratory testing.
5. Explain the three CLIA regulatory categories.
6. Describe the divisions of the clinical laboratory and give an example of a test performed in each division.
7. Compare and contrast the agencies that govern or influence practice in the clinical laboratory.
8. Summarize techniques to minimize physical, chemical, and biologic hazards in the clinical laboratory.
9. Describe the essential elements of a laboratory requisition.
10. Display sensitivity to patients' rights and feelings in collecting specimens.
11. Explain chain of custody and illustrate why it is important.
12. Compare and contrast quality assurance and quality control.
13. Describe the differences between Greenwich time and military time.
14. Identify the Fahrenheit temperature and the Celsius temperature of common laboratory equipment.
15. Name the metric units used for measuring liquid volume, distance, and mass.
16. Describe the proper use of pipets.
17. Explain how dilutions are prepared.
18. Name the parts of a microscope, and describe their functions.
19. Summarize selected microscopy tests that can be performed in the ambulatory care setting.
20. Demonstrate proper use of the microscope.
21. Describe the safe use of a centrifuge.
22. Identify legal and ethical issues in the clinical laboratory setting.

VOCABULARY

aliquot (a'-luh-kwaht) A portion of a well-mixed sample removed for testing.

analyte The substance or chemical being analyzed or detected in a specimen.

anticoagulants Chemicals added to a blood sample after collection to prevent clotting.

caustic (kos'-tik) Capable of burning, corroding, or damaging tissue by chemical action.

cytology (si-tah'-luh-je) The study of cells using microscopic methods.

diluent (dil-yuh'-wunt) A liquid used to dilute a specimen or reagent.

exudates (ek'-syu-dats) Fluids with high concentrations of protein and cellular debris that have escaped from the blood

vessels and have been deposited in tissues or on tissue surfaces.

hemolyzed Term used to describe a blood sample in which the red blood cells have ruptured.

preservatives Substances added to a specimen to prevent deterioration of cells or chemicals.

referral laboratory A private or hospital-based laboratory that performs a wide variety of tests, many of them specialized; physicians often send specimens collected in the office to referral laboratories for testing.

specimen A sample of body fluid, waste product, or tissue that is collected for analysis.

Laboratory medicine, or clinical pathology, is the medical discipline that applies clinical laboratory science and technology to the care of patients. The laboratory is the place in which a collected **specimen** is analyzed and evaluated. Tests are performed manually (by hand) or through automation (with the use of specialized instruments).

ROLE OF THE CLINICAL LABORATORY IN PATIENT CARE

Personnel in the Clinical Laboratory

Medical laboratories are located in hospitals or in facilities such as physicians' offices, clinics, public health departments, health maintenance organizations, and private referral laboratories. The director of a laboratory may be a pathologist, a physician specially trained in the nature and cause of disease, or a clinical laboratory scientist with a doctorate. The laboratory is staffed by various professionally trained individuals, including certified medical technologists (MTs), who have earned a baccalaureate degree, have had additional formal training, and have passed a national certification examination. Other personnel include certified medical laboratory technicians (MLTs) or medical laboratory assistants (MLAs) and certified medical assistants (CMAs). These employees have completed a 1- to 2-year specialized training program and have passed a registry examination. Laboratory assistants and phlebotomists, who have received specialized training in the collection and preparation of laboratory specimens, also work in laboratories. The agencies granting certifications and titles are described in Table 51-1.

The medical assistant is trained to perform certain testing procedures, as well as in methods of collecting specimens that are sent to outside reference laboratories for testing. Laboratory tests are an essential part of a medical diagnosis, and they help the physician determine the most appropriate treatment. In addition, they may be performed to help the physician decide which medication to prescribe and to monitor the effects of medications. Only healthcare practitioners may request laboratory testing for a patient. The

medical assistant may be responsible for a number of these testing procedures. To assume this responsibility, the medical assistant must know proper patient preparation, the procedures for each test, and the normal range of results for the test. The medical assistant must carefully follow all laboratory instructions in obtaining and labeling specimens and sending them to the laboratory. Good communication among the patient, the office staff, and laboratory personnel is important. The medical assistant should make the patient feel at ease with these procedures and thus gain the patient's cooperation.

Clinical Laboratory Testing

Clinical laboratory testing is used in conjunction with a thorough health history and physical examination to obtain essential data for the diagnosis and management of a patient's condition. The body is considered to be healthy when a state of equilibrium exists in the internal environment. In this state, called *homeostasis,* the physical and chemical characteristics of body substances (e.g., fluids, secretions, excretions) are within a certain acceptable range, known as the *normal* or *reference range.* A change in homeostasis results in abnormal test values (i.e., outside the reference range). Abnormal values for a particular test may be seen with more than one pathologic condition. For example, a decrease in hemoglobin levels in red blood cells (RBCs) is seen in iron-deficiency anemia, but also in hyperthyroidism and cirrhosis of the liver. Therefore, physicians cannot rely solely on laboratory tests to make a diagnosis; they must use a combination of data obtained from the health history and physical examination, and a number of diagnostic and laboratory results.

Tests performed in a clinical laboratory range from simple screening tests to complex profile testing. A screening test examines a particular specimen for the presence of a substance that may indicate a disease state. These types of tests are not diagnostic for any particular disease, but rather indicate that the disease state may exist. Screening tests are done routinely on patients on the basis of their age, history, or gender. They often are qualitative in that a numeric value is not attached to the result; results may simply be

TABLE 51-1 Certifying Agencies for Laboratory Personnel

CERTIFYING AGENCY	TITLE	POSITION
American Society for Clinical Pathologists	MT (ASCP)	Medical technologist
	MLT (ASCP)	Medical laboratory technician — certificate
	MLT-AD (ASCP)	Medical laboratory technician — associate's degree
American Medical Technologists	MT (AMT)	Medical technologist
	MLT (AMT)	Medical laboratory technician
	MLA	Medical laboratory assistant
	RMA	Registered medical assistant
Department of Health and Human Services	CLT (HHS)	Clinical laboratory technologist
National Certification Agency for Medical Laboratory Personnel	CLS (NCA)	Certified laboratory scientist
	CLT (NCA)	Certified laboratory technician
International Society for Clinical Laboratory Technology	RMT (ISCLT)	Registered medical technologist
	RLT (ISCLT)	Registered laboratory technician
American Association of Medical Assistants (AAMA)	CMA (AAMA)	Certified medical assistant
California Certifying Board for Medical Assistants	CCMA-C (CCBMA)	California certified medical assistant–clinical
National Healthcareer Association (NHA)	CCMA	Certified clinical medical assistant
	CPT	Certified phlebotomy technician
	CML	Certified medical laboratory assistant

per given volume of specimen, and it is essential that the results be reported with the units of measure. For example, in a complete blood cell count for a healthy adult, the RBCs number 5 million per cubic millimeter ($5 \times 10^{6}/mm^{3}$), the hemoglobin value is 15 grams per deciliter (15 g/dL), and the hematocrit is 45%. Generally the units are printed on the laboratory report, but the medical assistant must always make sure that the values are consistent with the test performed.

CRITICAL THINKING APPLICATION 51-1

The referral laboratory telephones to report the values on several tests performed on the urine of a patient, Cecelia Roberts. Marsha jots down the following: Total protein, 0.12; Occult blood, positive; Albumin, 50; Glucose, 120. What is wrong with the notations she has just made? Are these tests qualitative or quantitative?

Clinical Laboratory Improvement Amendments

In 1988 Congress passed the Clinical Laboratory Improvement Amendments (CLIA), establishing quality standards for all laboratory testing to ensure the accuracy, reliability, and timeliness of patient test results regardless of where the test is performed. A laboratory is defined as any facility that performs laboratory testing on specimens derived from humans for the purpose of providing information about the diagnosis, prevention, and treatment of disease or impairment in or assessment of health. The CLIA program is user-fee funded; therefore, all costs of administering the program must be covered by the regulated facilities. CLIA requires that all entities that perform even one test, including waived tests, must meet certain federal requirements and must register as a laboratory. An application must be submitted that reports information about a laboratory's operation. The type of certificate to be issued and the fees to be assessed are determined from this information.

The CLIA categorization of commercially marketed in vitro diagnostic tests is now the responsibility of the U.S. Food and Drug Administration (FDA). The FDA has assumed primary responsibility for performing the CLIA complexity categorization functions, which include the process of assigning commercially marketed in vitro diagnostic test systems to one of three CLIA regulatory categories on the basis of their potential risk to public health: waived tests, moderate-complexity tests, and high-complexity tests.

Waived Tests

Waived tests (Table 51-2) include the following:

Laboratory examinations and procedures that have been approved by the Food and Drug Administration for home use or that, as determined by the Secretary, are simple laboratory examinations and procedures that have an insignificant risk of an erroneous result, including those that (A) employ methodologies that are so simple and accurate to render the likelihood of erroneous results by the user negligible, or (B) the Secretary has determined pose no unreasonable risk of harm to the patient if performed incorrectly.

A CLIA database is available to the public on the Internet. This database contains the commercially marketed in vitro test systems categorized by the FDA since January 31, 2000, and tests categorized

reported as positive or negative. The fecal occult blood test for hidden or microscopic blood in the stool is an example of a screening test. Blood is not normally found in the stool, and its presence may indicate a cancerous lesion in the colon. A positive test result indicates that blood is present, but additional testing is required to determine the source of the blood. For example, further testing or examination may reveal that the patient had her menstrual period at the time of collection of the specimen, or that she had bleeding hemorrhoids.

In a quantitative test, units of measure are attached to numeric values. These values often are represented as the amount of **analyte**

TABLE 51-2 CLIA-Waived Tests and Their Purposes

CPT CODE(S)	TEST	PURPOSE
81002, 81003QW	Dipstick or tablet reagent urinalysis (nonautomated) for bilirubin, glucose, hemoglobin, ketone, leukocytes, nitrite, pH, protein, specific gravity, urobilinogen	Urine screening to assess or diagnose diseases such as diabetes mellitus, kidney disease, and urinary tract infection
81025	Urine pregnancy tests: visual color comparison tests	Diagnosis of pregnancy
81002	Urine chemistry analyzer: automated urine dipstick analysis	Urine screening to assess or diagnose diseases such as diabetes mellitus, kidney disease, and urinary tract infection
81002	Urine chemistry analyzer for microalbumin and creatinine	Detection of kidney disease
84830	Ovulation tests: visual color comparison tests for luteinizing hormone	Detection of ovulation
82270 82272	Fecal occult blood	Colorectal screening to detect hidden blood in the stool
85651	Erythrocyte sedimentation rate, nonautomated	Diagnosis of inflammatory process; increases in presence of arthritis, infection, leukemia, and most cancers
83026	Hemoglobin-copper sulfate, nonautomated	Measurement of blood hemoglobin levels
82947QW, 82950QW	HemoCue Hemoglobin System	Measurement of hemoglobin level in whole blood
82962	Blood glucose by glucose-monitoring devices cleared by the FDA specifically for home use	Monitoring of blood glucose levels
85018QW	HemoCue B	Measurement of glucose levels in whole blood
85013	Spun microhematocrit	Measurement of blood count; screening for certain types of anemia
82947QW, 82950QW, 82951QW	STAT-CRIT hematocrit	Screening for certain types of anemia
83036QW	Hemoglobin and hemoglobin A_{1c} by single analyte instruments with self-contained or component features to perform specimen-reagent interaction	Measurement of A_{1c} levels to assess and manage long-term care of patients with diabetes
82465QW	Cholestech LDX	Measurement of total blood cholesterol, triglycerides, HDL, and glucose levels
86308QW	Blood mononucleosis antibodies	Rapid, qualitative test to detect antibodies to help diagnose infectious mononucleosis
86318QW	*Helicobacter pylori* antibodies	Rapid whole-blood test to detect *H. pylori* antibodies to determine the cause of peptic ulcer
86618QW	*Borrelia burgdorferi* antibodies	Rapid whole-blood test to detect *B. burgdorferi* antibodies to diagnose Lyme disease
86701QW	Whole-blood OraSure HIV-1 test	Detection of HIV-1 in blood specimen
87804QW	Nasal influenza A and B	Quick qualitative diagnosis of influenza antigens in nasal secretions or swab
87449QW; 87880QW	Streptococcus A throat swab	Rapid strep test
80047QW 82330QW 82374QW	Whole-Blood i-STAT Chem8+ Cartridge	Measures ionized calcium, carbon dioxide, chloride, creatinine, glucose, potassium, sodium, urea nitrogen, and hematocrit in whole blood
G0434QW	Urine and/or blood	Multiple tests for the presence of a variety of substance abuse agents
83001QW	Urine fertility and menopause	Detects follicle-stimulating hormone in urine
84443QW	Whole-blood thyroid-stimulating hormone (TSH) assay	Qualitative determination of TSH in whole blood

From Centers for Medicare and Medicaid Services. http://www.cms.gov/CLIA/downloads/waivetbl.pdf.
FDA, U.S. Food and Drug Administration; *HDL,* high-density lipoprotein; *HIV-1,* human immunodeficiency virus type 1.

by the Centers for Disease Control and Prevention (CDC) before that date. The records can be searched by test system name, specialty or subspecialty, analyte, document number, qualifier, effective date, and complexity.

Moderate- and High-Complexity Tests

The CLIA program oversees the quality of nearly 200,000 different laboratory procedures. An estimated 10,000 different laboratory tests are performed in the United States every day; 75% of them are categorized by the FDA as moderate-complexity tests. Some of these tests are performed in physician's office laboratories (POLs), including hematology and chemistry testing done on an automated analyzer, Gram staining, and microscopic analysis of urine sediment. High-complexity tests usually are not performed in a POL; these include Papanicolaou (Pap) smear analysis, blood typing and cross-matching, and cytologic testing.

Laboratories that perform moderate- to high-complexity testing must meet CLIA regulations and are subject to unannounced inspections every 2 years. Each laboratory that performs these tests must establish a system to maintain the integrity and identification of patients' specimens throughout the testing process and to ensure accurate reporting of results. The laboratory also must have established and must follow written quality control (QC) and quality assurance (QA) procedures and must participate in proficiency testing, a form of external quality control. Three times a year, the laboratory must test samples provided by an approved proficiency testing agency using the same tests the laboratory would use to test a patient's sample. Finally, CLIA regulations specify qualifications and responsibilities for personnel in the laboratory, from directors to testing personnel. Personnel requirements are most stringent for high-complexity testing.

Medical assistants may perform all CLIA-waived tests and some moderately complex tests, depending on the certification of the laboratory or POL in which they are employed. Although medical assistants may not perform high-complexity tests, they often are involved in collecting the specimens required, preparing the patient for the test, and recording the results in the medical record.

DIVISIONS OF THE CLINICAL LABORATORY

The laboratory is divided into various departments, which may include hematology, chemistry, microbiology, specimen collection and processing, blood bank, coagulation, serology, histology, **cytology**, toxicology, urinalysis, and special chemistry. The laboratory in the physician's office usually performs procedures in urinalysis, hematology, chemistry, and microbiology.

Urinalysis

Urinalysis includes the physical, chemical, and microscopic examination of urine. In the physical examination, the color, clarity, and specific gravity are noted. Chemical analysis is performed to measure levels of such analytes as glucose, protein, ketones, blood, bilirubin, urobilinogen, nitrites, and pH. Microscopically the urine is examined for the presence of red, white, and epithelial cells, mucus, casts, crystals, yeasts, parasites, and bacteria. Additional quantitative tests may be performed in the urinalysis department to confirm routine screening tests.

Hematology

Tests performed in the hematology division may be qualitative or quantitative. Blood cell counts determine the exact number of RBCs or erythrocytes, white blood cells (WBCs, or leukocytes), or platelets (thrombocytes) either by manual or automated counting. Qualitative tests determine the characteristics of cells, such as size, shape, and maturity. In addition, the hematology department performs tests to determine the coagulating ability of blood components.

Chemistry

The clinical chemistry department analyzes blood, cerebrospinal fluid (CSF), urine, and joint fluid (synovial fluid). Procedures may include single tests or profiles, which include tests for a number of related analytes. Lipid profiles, for example, include assessments of total cholesterol, triglycerides, and low-density lipoprotein (LDL) and high-density lipoprotein (HDL) cholesterol.

Microbiology

Microbiology involves the study of bacteria, fungi, yeasts, parasites, and viruses. In the microbiology laboratory, microorganisms are grown (cultured) from blood, urine, sputum, CSF, and wound specimens and are identified. Sensitivity testing then is performed on these organisms to determine the proper antibiotic therapy. Specimens for microbiology must be collected aseptically in sterile containers.

CRITICAL THINKING APPLICATION   51-2

Dr. Watkins has ordered a routine urinalysis (UA), a urine culture and sensitivity (C&S) test, a blood glucose test, and a complete blood count (CBC) for his patient. Which division of the laboratory is responsible for analyzing the specimens for each test?

LABORATORY SAFETY

The importance of safety in the laboratory cannot be overemphasized. Most laboratory accidents can be prevented through the use of proper techniques and common sense. Following safe practices in the laboratory requires a personal commitment and concern for others; an unsafe act may harm an innocent bystander without harming the person who performs the act.

Safety Standards and Governing Agencies

Safety standards for laboratories are initiated, regulated, and reviewed by several agencies or committees. These include the U.S. Department of Labor's Occupational Safety and Health Administration (OSHA); the Clinical and Laboratory Standards Institute (CLSI, formerly the National Committee for Clinical Laboratory Standards), a nonprofit educational organization that provides a forum for the development, promotion, and use of national and international standards; the CDC, an agency of the U.S. Department of Health and Human Services; the College of American Pathologists (CAP), a leader in providing laboratory quality improvement programs; and the Environmental Protection Agency (EPA), a government agency charged with protecting human health and safeguarding the natural environment.

Through OSHA the government created a system of safeguards and regulations under the Occupational Safety and Health Act of 1970. This system affects nearly every worker in the United States, because the regulations apply to all businesses with one or more employees. (The regulations are discussed in detail in Chapter 27.) Two programs have been mandated by OSHA to ensure the safety of personnel working in clinical laboratories. One covers occupational exposure to chemical hazards; the other covers exposure to blood-borne pathogens. Both of these programs, as they relate to safety in the medical laboratory setting, are discussed later in this chapter.

LABORATORY HAZARDS

Physical Hazards

Physical hazards in the laboratory can be classified as electrical, fire, and mechanical hazards. Electric shock is a threat when any electrical equipment is in use. It is imperative to keep all electrical equipment in proper repair and always to follow manufacturers' instructions.

Use surge protectors, inspect all cords and plugs frequently, never use extension cords, and avoid overloading circuits. Unplug the electrical device before servicing, and never operate electrical instruments with wet hands. If a sink is nearby, make sure electrical cords do not come in contact with the water supply. Signs and labels should be placed on specific electrical hazards (Figure 51-1).

Open flames are rarely used in a laboratory, but the potential for fire still exists. Fires may be ignited by smoking, heating elements, and sparks. Flammable materials should not be stored near any source of ignition. All laboratory personnel should be familiar with the locations of fire extinguishers and fire safety blankets. Fire extinguishers should be the carbon dioxide (CO_2), dry chemical, or halon type, known as the ABC type of extinguisher. ABC extinguishers can be used on all types of fires. These extinguishers should be inspected regularly by a licensed inspector and replaced or recharged if used. The medical assistant may be responsible for maintaining records on the care and maintenance of fire extinguishers.

Fire safety blankets should be used to smother flames on burning clothing. However, a victim should not be wrapped in a fire blanket, because this may intensify burns. Instead, the flames should be patted out or the victim directed to roll on the blanket.

Emergency phone numbers should be posted on the wall near the telephone, and all personnel should know the locations of fire alarms, the fire escape routes, and procedures to follow if exits are blocked. Periodic fire drills should be conducted, and hallways and exits should be kept free of clutter.

Mechanical hazards arise from the use of laboratory equipment. Special care should be exercised when using equipment with moving parts, such as centrifuges, and those that rely on pressure, including autoclaves. Centrifuges, devices that separate liquids from solids, present a hazard not only from moving parts but also from glassware that might break during centrifugation and from aerosols that might be created if tubes are not capped tightly. Pressurized types of equipment, such as autoclaves used in sterilization, present a danger if opened prematurely. Although centrifuges and autoclaves often have built-in safeguards, such as locks that prevent entry until the environment is safe, improper care of the equipment can result in failure of the safety measures.

Chemical Hazards

The clinical laboratory is home to chemicals that are flammable, **caustic**, poisonous, carcinogenic, and/or teratogenic. Exposure to these dangerous chemicals can occur through inhalation, direct absorption through the skin, ingestion, entry through a mucous membrane, or entry through a break in the skin. OSHA is involved in regulating the standards directed at minimizing occupational exposure to hazardous chemicals in laboratories. The OSHA hazard communication standard (known as the employee "right to know" rule) became law in 1991 and ensures that laboratory workers are fully aware of the hazards associated with their workplace. The law requires the development of a comprehensive plan to implement safe practice throughout the laboratory with regard to chemicals. This chemical hygiene plan must outline the specific work practices and procedures needed to protect workers from any health hazards that may arise from working with in-stock chemicals. All workers must be provided with information and training, and a material safety data sheet (MSDS) must be on file for all chemicals used in the laboratory. OSHA requires the manufacturer of the chemical to make these sheets available, usually as a package insert.

OSHA recommends that each MSDS sheet follow the 16-section format developed by the American National Standards Institute (ANSI). When this format is used, information about the hazardous material that affects the worker the most is identified at the beginning of the form and the more technical information about the product is given later. The 16-section MSDS template includes the following (Figure 51-2):

- Identification of the product
- Hazard(s) identification
- Composition/information on ingredients
- First-aid measures
- Fire-fighting measures
- Accidental release measures
- Handling and storage
- Exposure controls/personal protection
- Physical and chemical properties
- Stability and reactivity
- Toxicologic information
- Ecologic information
- Disposal considerations

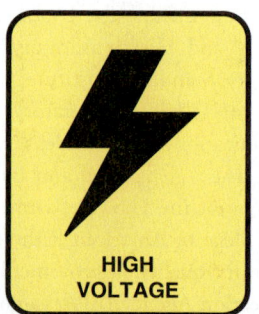
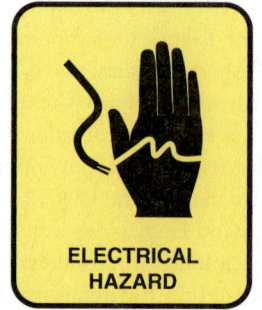

FIGURE 51-1 High-voltage and electrical hazard labels. (From Stepp CA, Woods MA: *Laboratory procedures for medical office personnel*, Philadelphia, 1998, Saunders.)

Text continued on p. 1092

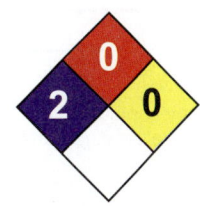
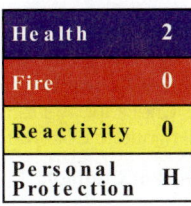

Health	2
Fire	0
Reactivity	0
Personal Protection	H

Material Safety Data Sheet
Glutaraldehyde Solution, 50% MSDS

Section 1: Chemical Product and Company Identification

Product Name: Glutaraldehyde Solution, 50%

Catalog Codes: SLG2182

CAS#: Mixture.

RTECS: MA2450000

TSCA: TSCA 8(b) inventory: Glutaraldehyde; Water

CI#: Not available.

Synonym: Glutaraldehyde Solution, 50%; Petanedial; Glutaric Dialdehyde, 50% in water

Chemical Name: Not applicable.

Chemical Formula: C5-H8-O2

Contact Information:

Sciencelab.com, Inc.
14025 Smith Rd.
Houston, Texas 77396

US Sales: **1-800-901-7247**
International Sales: **1-281-441-4400**

Order Online: ScienceLab.com

CHEMTREC (24HR Emergency Telephone), call:
1-800-424-9300

International CHEMTREC, call: 1-703-527-3887

For non-emergency assistance, call: 1-281-441-4400

Section 2: Composition and Information on Ingredients

Composition:

Name	CAS #	% by Weight
Glutaraldehyde	111-30-8	50
Water	7732-18-5	50

Toxicological Data on Ingredients: Glutaraldehyde: ORAL (LD50): Acute: 134 mg/kg [Rat]. 100 mg/kg [Mouse]. DERMAL (LD50): Acute: >2500 mg/kg [Rat]. >5840 mg/kg [Mouse]. VAPOR (LC50): Acute: 480 mg/m 4 hours [Rat].

Section 3: Hazards Identification

Potential Acute Health Effects:
Hazardous in case of skin contact (irritant), of eye contact (irritant), of ingestion, of inhalation (lung irritant, lung sensitizer). Slightly hazardous in case of skin contact (sensitizer, permeator). Liquid or spray mist may produce tissue damage particularly on mucous membranes of eyes, mouth and respiratory tract. Skin contact may produce burns. Inhalation of the spray mist may produce severe irritation of respiratory tract, characterized by coughing, choking, or shortness of breath. Severe over-exposure can result in death.

Potential Chronic Health Effects:
CARCINOGENIC EFFECTS: Classified A4 (Not classifiable for human or animal.) by ACGIH [Glutaraldehyde]. MUTAGENIC EFFECTS: Mutagenic for mammalian somatic cells. [Glutaraldehyde]. Mutagenic for bacteria and/or yeast. [Glutaraldehyde]. TERATOGENIC EFFECTS: Not available. DEVELOPMENTAL TOXICITY: Classified Reproductive system/toxin/female, Reproductive system/toxin/male [SUSPECTED] [Glutaraldehyde]. The substance may be toxic to blood, the reproductive system, liver, mucous membranes, spleen, central nervous system (CNS), Urinary System. Repeated or prolonged exposure to the substance can produce target organs damage. Repeated or prolonged contact with spray mist may produce chronic eye irritation and severe skin irritation. Repeated or prolonged exposure to spray mist may produce respiratory tract irritation leading to frequent attacks of bronchial infection. Repeated exposure to a highly toxic material may produce general deterioration of health by an accumulation in one or many human organs.

FIGURE 51-2 Sixteen-section medical safety data sheet (MSDS). (From http://www.sciencelab.com/msds.php?msdsId=9924161. Accessed August 2012.)

Continued

Section 4: First Aid Measures

Eye Contact:
Check for and remove any contact lenses. In case of contact, immediately flush eyes with plenty of water for at least 15 minutes. Cold water may be used. Get medical attention immediately.

Skin Contact:
In case of contact, immediately flush skin with plenty of water. Cover the irritated skin with an emollient. Remove contaminated clothing and shoes. Cold water may be used.Wash clothing before reuse. Thoroughly clean shoes before reuse. Get medical attention.

Serious Skin Contact:
Wash with a disinfectant soap and cover the contaminated skin with an anti-bacterial cream. Seek immediate medical attention.

Inhalation:
If inhaled, remove to fresh air. If not breathing, give artificial respiration. If breathing is difficult, give oxygen. Get medical attention immediately.

Serious Inhalation:
Evacuate the victim to a safe area as soon as possible. Loosen tight clothing such as a collar, tie, belt or waistband. If breathing is difficult, administer oxygen. If the victim is not breathing, perform mouth-to-mouth resuscitation. WARNING: It may be hazardous to the person providing aid to give mouth-to-mouth resuscitation when the inhaled material is toxic, infectious or corrosive. Seek immediate medical attention.

Ingestion:
If swallowed, do not induce vomiting unless directed to do so by medical personnel. Never give anything by mouth to an unconscious person. Loosen tight clothing such as a collar, tie, belt or waistband. Get medical attention immediately.

Serious Ingestion: Not available.

Section 5: Fire and Explosion Data

Flammability of the Product: Non-flammable.

Auto-Ignition Temperature: Not applicable.

Flash Points: Not applicable.

Flammable Limits: Not applicable.

Products of Combustion: When heated to decomposition, it emits acrid smoke and fumes.

Fire Hazards in Presence of Various Substances: Not applicable.

Explosion Hazards in Presence of Various Substances:
Risks of explosion of the product in presence of mechanical impact: Not available. Risks of explosion of the product in presence of static discharge: Not available.

Fire Fighting Media and Instructions: Not applicable.

Special Remarks on Fire Hazards: Not available.

Special Remarks on Explosion Hazards: Not available.

Section 6: Accidental Release Measures

Small Spill:
Dilute with water and mop up, or absorb with an inert dry material and place in an appropriate waste disposal container.

Large Spill:
Poisonous liquid. Stop leak if without risk. Do not get water inside container. Do not touch spilled material. Use water spray to reduce vapors. Prevent entry into sewers, basements or confined areas; dike if needed. Call for assistance on disposal. Be careful that the product is not present at a concentration level above TLV. Check TLV on the MSDS and with local authorities.

FIGURE 51-2, cont'd

Section 7: Handling and Storage

Precautions:
Keep locked up.. Do not ingest. Do not breathe gas/fumes/ vapor/spray. Wear suitable protective clothing. In case of insufficient ventilation, wear suitable respiratory equipment. If ingested, seek medical advice immediately and show the container or the label. Avoid contact with skin and eyes. Keep away from incompatibles such as oxidizing agents, alkalis.

Storage:
Light Sensitive. Refrigerate. Store in light-resistant containers. Keep containers tightly closed. Keep containers in a cool, well-ventilated area.

Section 8: Exposure Controls/Personal Protection

Engineering Controls:
Provide exhaust ventilation or other engineering controls to keep the airborne concentrations of vapors below their respective threshold limit value. Ensure that eyewash stations and safety showers are proximal to the work-station location.

Personal Protection:
Splash goggles. Lab coat. Vapor respirator. Be sure to use an approved/certified respirator or equivalent. Gloves.

Personal Protection in Case of a Large Spill:
Splash goggles. Full suit. Vapor respirator. Boots. Gloves. A self contained breathing apparatus should be used to avoid inhalation of the product. Suggested protective clothing might not be sufficient; consult a specialist BEFORE handling this product.

Exposure Limits:
Glutaraldehyde TWA: 0.2 (ppm) [Australia] TWA: 0.82 (mg/m3) [Australia] TWA: 0.25 CEIL: 0.2 (ppm) from NIOSH CEIL: 0.2 (ppm) from OSHA (PEL) [United States] TWA: 0.05 STEL: 0.05 (ppm) [United Kingdom (UK)] Consult local authorities for acceptable exposure limits.

Section 9: Physical and Chemical Properties

Physical state and appearance: Liquid.

Odor: Pungent. Like rotten apples

Taste: Not available.

Molecular Weight: Not applicable.

Color: Colorless to light yellow.

pH (1% soln/water): Not available

Boiling Point: 101°C (213.8°F)

Melting Point: -6°C (21.2°F) - -7

Critical Temperature: Not available.

Specific Gravity: 1.062 - 1.124 (Water = 1)

Vapor Pressure: 0 kPa (@ 20°C)

Vapor Density: 1.05 (Air = 1)

Volatility: Not available.

Odor Threshold: 0.04 ppm

Water/Oil Dist. Coeff.: Not available.

Ionicity (in Water): Not available.

Dispersion Properties: See solubility in water, diethyl ether.

Solubility:
Easily soluble in cold water. Soluble in diethyl ether. Soluble in benzene, ethanol and other organic solvents.

FIGURE 51-2, cont'd

Continued

Section 10: Stability and Reactivity Data

Stability: The product is stable.

Instability Temperature: Not available.

Conditions of Instability: Conditions to avoid: exposure to air, and excess heat. (Glutaraldehyde)

Incompatibility with various substances: Reactive with oxidizing agents, alkalis.

Corrosivity: Non-corrosive in presence of glass.

Special Remarks on Reactivity:
Also incompatible with amines, ammonia and other caustics (e.g. ammonium hydroxide, calcium hydroxide, potassium hydroxide, and sodium hydroxide). Alkaline solutions react with alcohol, ketones, amines, hydrazines and proteins. (Glutaraldehyde)

Special Remarks on Corrosivity: Not available.

Polymerization: Will not occur.

Section 11: Toxicological Information

Routes of Entry: Absorbed through skin. Eye contact. Inhalation. Ingestion.

Toxicity to Animals:
WARNING: THE LC50 VALUES HEREUNDER ARE ESTIMATED ON THE BASIS OF A 4-HOUR EXPOSURE. Acute oral toxicity (LD50): 100 mg/kg [Mouse]. Acute dermal toxicity (LD50): >2500 mg/kg [Rat]. Acute toxicity of the vapor (LC50): 480 mg/m 4 hours [Rat]. 3

Chronic Effects on Humans:
CARCINOGENIC EFFECTS: Classified A4 (Not classifiable for human or animal.) by ACGIH [Glutaraldehyde]. MUTAGENIC EFFECTS: Mutagenic for mammalian somatic cells. [Glutaraldehyde]. Mutagenic for bacteria and/or yeast. [Glutaraldehyde]. DEVELOPMENTAL TOXICITY: Classified Reproductive system/toxin/female, Reproductive system/toxin/male [SUSPECTED] [Glutaraldehyde]. Contains material which may cause damage to the following organs: blood, the reproductive system, liver, mucous membranes, spleen, central nervous system (CNS), Urinary system.

Other Toxic Effects on Humans:
Hazardous in case of skin contact (irritant), of ingestion, of inhalation (lung irritant, lung sensitizer). Slightly hazardous in case of skin contact (sensitizer, permeator).

Special Remarks on Toxicity to Animals:
Acute Toxicity: LD50 [Rabbit] dermal: Dose: 560 ul/kg. Reproductive Effects: TDL [male Rat] oral: Dose: 875 mg/kg given 35 days prior to mating TDL [female rat] oral: Dose 4370 mg/kg given 35 days prior to mating. (Glutaraldehyde)

Special Remarks on Chronic Effects on Humans:
May affect genetic material. Reproductive Effects in animals (rat): Paternal effects: testes, epididymis, sperm duct, prostate, seminal vesicle, Cowper's gland, accessory. Maternal effects: uterus, cervix, vagina (Glutaraldehyde)

Special Remarks on other Toxic Effects on Humans:
Potential Health Effects: Eye: Causes severe eye irritation. May cause eye injury or chemical conjunctivitis. Skin: Causes moderate to severe skin irritation. It may be absorbed through the skin, although poorly. May cause allergic contact dermatitis with itching and skin rash. May cause staining of the skin and nails to a brown or golden brown color. Ingestion: Harmful if swallowed. May cause severe irritation of the digestive tract with burning sensation in the chest, abdominal pain, cramping, vomiting, diarrhea (perhaps bloody diarrhea), vascular collapse, and coma. May also affect liver (increased liver enzymes, liver damage), spleen, blood (normocytic anemia), metabolism (weight loss), behavior (somnolence, excitement, dizziness, lethargy, ataxia, seizures), metabolism (weight loss), urinary system (abnormal reneal function, anuria) Inhalation: Harmful if inhaled. Can cause respiratory tract irritation and sudden headaches, nausea, and

Section 12: Ecological Information

Ecotoxicity: Not available.

BOD5 and COD: Not available.

Products of Biodegradation:
Possibly hazardous short term degradation products are not likely. However, long term degradation products may arise.

Toxicity of the Products of Biodegradation: The products of degradation are less toxic than the product itself.

Special Remarks on the Products of Biodegradation: Not available.

FIGURE 51-2, cont'd

Section 13: Disposal Considerations

Waste Disposal:
Waste must be disposed of in accordance with federal, state and local environmental control regulations.

Section 14: Transport Information

DOT Classification: CLASS 6.1: Poisonous material.

Identification: : Toxic Liquid, Organic, n.o.s (Glutaraldehyde solution) UNNA: 2810 PG: III

Special Provisions for Transport: Not available.

Section 15: Other Regulatory Information

Federal and State Regulations:
Pennsylvania RTK: Glutaraldehyde Florida: Glutaraldehyde Massachusetts RTK: Glutaraldehyde New Jersey: Glutaraldehyde California Director's list of Hazardous Substances: Glutaraldehyde TSCA 8(b) inventory: Glutaraldehyde; Water TSCA 8(a) PAIR: Glutaraldehyde TSCA 8(d) H and S data reporting: Glutaraldehyde: 9/30/91 to 9/30/01

Other Regulations:
OSHA: Hazardous by definition of Hazard Communication Standard (29 CFR 1910.1200). EINECS: This product is on the European Inventory of Existing Commercial Chemical Substances.

Other Classifications:

WHMIS (Canada):
CLASS D-1A: Material causing immediate and serious toxic effects (VERY TOXIC). CLASS D-2B: Material causing other toxic effects (TOXIC). CLASS E: Corrosive liquid.

DSCL (EEC):

HMIS (U.S.A.):

   Health Hazard: 2

   Fire Hazard: 0

   Reactivity: 0

   Personal Protection: h

National Fire Protection Association (U.S.A.):

   Health: 2

   Flammability: 0

   Reactivity: 0

   Specific hazard:

Protective Equipment:
Gloves. Lab coat. Vapor respirator. Be sure to use an approved/certified respirator or equivalent. Wear appropriate respirator when ventilation is inadequate. Splash goggles.

Section 16: Other Information

References: Not available.

Other Special Considerations: Not available.

Created: 10/09/2005 05:38 PM

Last Updated: 06/09/2012 12:00 PM

The information above is believed to be accurate and represents the best information currently available to us. However, we make no warranty of merchantability or any other warranty, express or implied, with respect to such information, and we assume no liability resulting from its use. Users should make their own investigations to determine the suitability of the information for their particular purposes. In no event shall ScienceLab.com be liable for any claims, losses, or damages of any third party or for lost profits or any special, indirect, incidental, consequential or exemplary damages, howsoever arising, even if ScienceLab.com has been advised of the possibility of such damages.

FIGURE 51-2, cont'd

- Transport information
- Regulatory information
- Other information

Following principles of proper handling reduces the risk of harmful effects. Harmful exposure can be reduced by using proper devices for pipetting; never pipet by mouth. If a chemical produces toxic or flammable vapors, work under a fume hood that exhausts air to the outside. In case of accidental exposure of the skin, rinse the affected area under running water for at least 5 minutes. Remove any contaminated clothing. If chemicals are splashed in the eyes, flush the eyes with water from an eyewash station for a minimum of 15 minutes. Prompt medical attention must be given to victims of chemical exposure.

Chemicals should be tightly sealed and properly labeled. A hazard identification system has been developed by the National Fire Protection Association that provides information at a glance on the potential health, flammability, and chemical reactivity hazards of materials. This identification system consists of four small, colored, diamond-shaped symbols grouped into a larger diamond shape. The top diamond is red and indicates a flammability hazard. The diamond on the left is blue and indicates hazards to health. The bottom diamond is white and provides special hazard information, including radioactivity, special biohazards, and other dangerous situations. The diamond on the right is yellow and indicates a reactivity or stability hazard. The system indicates the severity of the hazard by using numbers imprinted in the diamonds from 0 to 4, with 0 representing no hazard and 4 representing an extremely hazardous substance (Figure 51-3).

Biologic Hazards and Infection Control

Biologic hazards, or biohazards, are materials or situations that present risk or potential risk of infection. Infection with biohazardous material can occur during specimen collection, handling, transportation, or testing. Potentially infective specimens include blood, body tissue biopsy specimens, urine, **exudates**, and bacterial cultures and smears. Infection can occur through aspiration of a pathogen, accidental inoculation by a needlestick, aerosols created by uncapping specimen tubes, centrifuge accidents, and entry of pathogens through cuts and scratches.

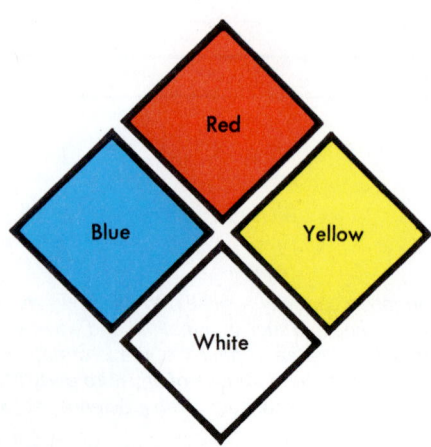

FIGURE 51-3 Identification system of the National Fire Protection Association.

One of the most important OSHA regulations covers exposure to biologic hazards. The OSHA-mandated program, Occupational Exposure to Bloodborne Pathogens, must be in place and has been law since 1992 as part of a general infection control policy. In addition, the CDC recommends safety precautions regarding handling of all patient specimens. Previously known as *Universal Precautions,* they are now referred to as *Standard Precautions* and are published on the organization's Web page and in the publication *Morbidity and Mortality Weekly Report.* Chapter 27 covers the specifics of the OSHA-mandated programs.

Recommendations from the CDC include an infection control plan, engineering and work practice controls, personal protective clothing and equipment, sufficient training and education, provision of vaccination against hepatitis B, and medical intervention after exposure incidents. The CLSI also has guidelines for the laboratory worker with regard to protection from blood-borne illness caused by contact with patients' specimens. The CAP offers a voluntary accreditation program for clinical laboratories that includes biosafety measures. One important precaution that can be taken is labeling of potentially biohazardous material, as described in Chapter 27.

Standard Precautions

Hepatitis B virus (HBV), hepatitis C virus (HCV), and human immunodeficiency virus (HIV) are a constant threat to the health and safety of clinical laboratory personnel. HBV, HCV, and HIV are transmitted through exposure to blood and body fluids. Blood and body fluids are the primary substances handled in the laboratory. OSHA mandated the Bloodborne Pathogens (BBP) Standard, which covers all employees who could be "reasonably anticipated as the result of performing their job duties to face contact with blood and other potentially infectious materials." The BBP standard requires that the laboratory employer have a written exposure control plan.

In addition to blood and blood products, the BBP standard includes "other potentially infectious materials" (OPIM). Urine is the only fluid not specifically included in the BBP standard. However, because blood and blood elements frequently are associated with urine, it must be included and considered as a possible source of exposure.

Washing or sanitizing the hands is the most effective means of preventing infection. It is the single most effective way of preventing the spread of all infections. Proper hand sanitation protects you, your patient, and your co-workers, because it removes organisms. In the laboratory area, it is absolutely essential to cleanse your hands in the following situations:

- When entering and before leaving the area
- Before and after every patient procedure
- After contact with body fluid, even if gloves were worn
- Before and after eating
- Before and after using the restroom

Every laboratory should have a safety manual that covers all safety practices and precautions. The manual should clearly explain procedures to be followed in the event of an accident. A section of the manual should prominently list emergency numbers for ambulance, fire, police, and other security services, as well as evacuation plans. Emergency numbers also should be posted near the telephone, and plans for evacuation must be posted. Second, the manual should give instructions for reporting and documenting accidents and should have an accident log for recording the names and persons involved, the type of accident, and the date it occurred. Copies of this incident report form should be included in the manual, along with an example of a properly completed form. It is important to note that such a form documents not only the accident, but also the steps taken to prevent the recurrence of such an accident.

SAFETY GUIDELINES FOR OTHER POTENTIALLY INFECTIOUS MATERIALS

- Handle and process all specimens as if they contain infectious material.
- Wipe the outside of specimen containers with a germicide.
- Dispose of all infectious materials according to state and federal guidelines.
- Clean up spills using a disinfectant (see Chapter 27).
- Immediately dispose of any chipped or broken glassware in a sharps disposable container.

SPECIMEN COLLECTION, PROCESSING, AND STORAGE

Laboratory Requisitions and Reports

A patient's medical record should be maintained in an organized manner to promote easy access to the desired information. Various methods are used to file laboratory reports in a patient's medical record. Many offices compile records in a set order so that the laboratory report sheets follow entry A and precede entry B. Another method is to use standard-sized sheets of a specific color and stagger the reports from the bottom of the sheet upward.

As discussed in Chapter 28, in the source-oriented medical record, all like reports are filed in one section. For example, all laboratory reports are together, all surgical reports are together, and all electrocardiograph reports are together. The latest test is placed on top, because it is the most important for the patient's current care and treatment. In the problem-oriented medical record, all test results are entered and recorded in the objective part of the progress notes, preceded by the number and title of the particular problem. With electronic medical records, laboratory reports are typically sent directly from the referral laboratory to the patient's medical record, or they are received electronically in a general electronic record source and then are transferred to the correct patient record by practice staff.

The medical assistant's responsibility is to make sure that all reports are received for diagnostic tests performed on the patient outside the physician's office. Only after the physician reviews the test results should they be filed in the patient's record.

When the physician requests laboratory testing that must be done outside the office, a written requisition for the work must be sent to the laboratory with the patient or with the specimen (Figure 51-4). These forms are preprinted, and the most commonly requested tests are indicated in logical sequence. Patient information must be complete, accurate, and legible.

Specimen Collection

The medical assistant is responsible for the collection of many different types of specimens. It is important to recognize that all clinical laboratory results are only as good as the specimen received. The importance of specimen collection cannot be overemphasized. If test results are to be accurate indicators of the patient's state of health, it is imperative that the concepts of specimen collection be understood and followed exactly. The most common specimens are blood, urine, and swab samples collected from wounds or mucous membranes. Less often, feces, gastric contents, CSF, tissue samples, semen, and aspirates, such as synovial fluid, are submitted for testing. These specimens are analyzed for levels of many chemicals and drugs, types and numbers of cells present, and the presence of microorganisms.

Initial identification of the patient is essential, as is collection of the specimen in an appropriate collection container. For example, blood may be collected using a vacuum tube system. These tubes are available in a variety of sizes, with and without **preservatives** and **anticoagulants**. The tubes are color-coded so that the color of the stopper denotes which, if any, additive is present (Figure 51-5). Collection in an incorrect tube results in an unacceptable specimen, and re-collection is necessary. If the specimen is to be tested for the presence of microorganisms, a sterile container must be used. If the patient is to collect the specimen at home, he or she should be provided with the appropriate container and complete instructions for collection. Bear in mind the principles of patient education, as discussed in Chapter 29, and be sensitive to individual patient factors, which sometimes can affect the patient's understanding of the instructions, as well as the person's ability to follow through on those instructions.

The medical assistant should always check the laboratory's specimen requirements manual for any unfamiliar tests. The manual lists all information on specimen collection. Any unanswered questions should be resolved by calling the laboratory before collecting the specimen. The container must be labeled properly at the time of collection; unlabeled containers will not be accepted for laboratory testing. Labels should include the patient's full name, the date and time of collection, and the type of specimen. Label information typically required when specimens are sent to a reference laboratory includes the following:

- Physician's name, account number, address, and phone number
- Patient's full name, surname first; age, date of birth, and gender; address and insurance information
- Source of specimen
- Date and time of collection
- Specific test (or tests) requested
- Medications the patient is taking
- Whether the patient fasted or followed dietary restrictions if required; time of last intake
- Possible diagnosis
- Indication of whether the test is to be performed stat

If the specimen is to be mailed, it must be carefully packaged to prevent breakage, damage, or contamination by all persons handling it. Place specimens in unbreakable tubes with safe-top lids and wrap the containers in absorbent material. Tape lids shut so that no leakage occurs if the specimen container breaks. Place all specimens

Lab Services

IMPORTANT
Patient instructions
and map on back

PHYSICIAN ORDERS

M ☐ Patient
F ☐ SS# _____ - _____ - _____

Patient _____ D.O.B. _____
        Last Name   First   M.I.

Address _____ City _____ Zip _____ Phone # _____

Physician _____
          ATTACH COPY OF INSURANCE CARD

Date & Time of Collection:
_____
Drawing
Facility:

Diagnosis/ICD-9 Code _____
                        (Additional codes on reverse)

☐ ROUTINE   ☐ PHONE RESULTS TO: #
☐ ASAP   ☐ FAX RESULTS TO: #
☐ STAT   ☐ COPY TO: _____

☐ 789.00 Abdominal Pain   ☐ 414.9 Coronary Artery Disease (CAD)   ☐ 244.9 Hypothyroidism
☐ 285.9 Anemia (NOS)   ☐ 250.0 DM (diabetes mellitus)   ☐ 272.4 Hyperlipidemia
                           ☐ 780.7 Fatigue/Malaise   ☐ 401.9 Hypertension
                           ☐ 272.0 Hypercholesterolemia   ☐ 485.9 URI (upper respiratory infection)

HEMATOLOGY	CHEMISTRY	CHEMISTRY	MICROBIOLOGY
☐ 1021 CBC, Automated Diff (incl. Platelet Ct.)	☐ 5550 Alpha Fetoprotein, Prenatal	☐ 5232 HBaAg	
☐ 1023 Hemoglobin/Hematocrit	☐ 3000 Amylase	☐ 3175 HIV (Consent required)	Source _____
☐ 1020 Hemogram	☐ 3153 B12/Folate	☐ 3581 Iron & Iron Binding Capacity	☐ 7240 Culture, AFB
☐ 1025 Platelet Count	☐ 3156 Beta HCG, Quantitative	☐ 3195 LH	☐ 7200 Culture, Blood x _____
☐ 1150 Pro Time Diagnostic	☐ 3321 Bilirubin, Total	☐ 3590 Magnesium	☐ Draw Interval _____
☐ 1151 Pro Time, Therapeutic	☐ 3324 Bilirubin, Total/Direct	☐ 3527 Phenobarbital	☐ 7280 Culture, Fungus
☐ 1155 PTT	☐ 3009 BUN	☐ 3095 Potassium	☐ Culture, Routine
☐ 1315 Reticulocyte Count	☐ 3159 CEA	☐ 3689 Pregnancy Test, Serum (HCG, qual)	☐ 7005 Culture, Stool
☐ 1310 Sed Rate/Westergren	☐ 3348 Cholesterol	☐ 3653 Pregnancy Test, Urine	☐ 7010 Culture, Throat
	☐ 3030 Creatinine, Serum	☐ 3197 Prolactin	☐ 7000 Culture, Urine
URINE	☐ 3509 Digoxin (recommend 12 hrs., after dose)	☐ 3199 PSA	☐ 7300 Gram Stain
☐ 1059 Urinalysis	☐ 3515 Dilantin	☐ 3339 SGOT/AST	☐ 7355 Occult Blood x _____
☐ 1082 Urinalysis w/Culture if indicated	☐ 3168 Ferritin	☐ 3342 SGPT/ALT	☐ 7365 Ova & Parasites x _____
Urine-24 Hr _____ Spot _____	☐ 3193 FSH	☐ 3093 Sodium/Potassium, Serum	☐ 7400 Smear & Suspension
Ht. _____ Wt. _____	☐ 3066 ▼ Glucose, Fasting	☐ 3510 Tegretol	(includes Gram Stain/Wet Mount)
☐ 3033 Creatinine	☐ 3061 Glucose, 1ª Post 50 g Glucola	☐ 3551 Theophylline	☐ 7060 Rapid Strep A Screen (Negs confir by cult)
☐ 3036 Creatinine Clearance (also requires blood)	☐ 3075 ▼ Glucose, 2ª Post Glucola	☐ 3333 Uric Acid	☐ 7065 Rapid Strep A Screen only
☐ 3398 Protein	☐ 3060 Glucose, 2ª Post Prandial (meal)		☐ 7030 Beta Strep Culture
☐ 3096 Sodium/Potassium	☐ 3049 ▼ Glucose Tolerance Oral GTT		☐ 5207 GC by DNA Probe
☐ Microalbumin 24 Hr ____ Spot ____	☐ 3047 ▼Glucose Tolerance Gestational GTT		☐ 5130 Chlamydia by DNA Probe
	☐ 3650 Hemoglobin, A1C		☐ 5555 Chlamydia/GC by DNA Probe
SEROLOGY			☐ 7375 Wright Stain, Stool
☐ 8020 ANA (Antinuclear Antibody)			
☐ 8040 Mono Spot			
☐ 3494 Rheumatoid Factor			
☐ 8010 RPR			
☐ 5365 Rubella	Additional Tests _____		

PANELS & PROFILES

☐ ✗ 3309 CHEM 12
Albumin, Alkaline Phosphatase,
BUN, Calcium, Cholesterol, Glucose,
LDH, Phosphorus, AST, Total
Bilirubin, Total Protein, Uric Acid

☐ ▼ 3315 CHEM 20
Chem 12, Electrolyte Panel,
Creatinine, Iron, Gamma GT, ALT,
Triglycerides

☐ ▼ 3357 CARDIAC RISK PANEL
Cholesterol, HDL, LDL, Risk Factors,
VLDL Triglycerides

☐ ✗ 3042 CRITICAL CARE PANEL
BUN, Chloride, CO2, Glucose,
Potassium, Sodium

☐ 3046 ELECTROLYTE PANEL
Chloride, CO2, Potassium, Sodium

☐ ▼ 3399 EXECUTIVE PANEL
Chem 20, Iron, Cardiac Risk Panel,
CBC, RPR, Thyroid Cascade

☐ 5242 HEPATITIS PANEL, ACUTE
HAVgMAb, HBsAg, HBeAb, HBcAb, HCVAb

☐ ▼ 3355 LIPID MONITORING PANEL
Cholesterol, Triglycerides, HDL, LDL, VLDL,
ALT, AST

☐ 3312 LIVER PANEL
Alkaline Phosphatase, AST, Total Bilirubin,
Gamma GT, Total Protein, Albumin, ALT

☐ ✗ 3083 METABOLIC STATUS PANEL
BUN, Osmolality (calculated), Chloride, CO2
Creatinine, Glucose, Potassium, Sodium,
BUN/Creatinine, Ratio, Anion Gap

☐ ✗ 3376 PANEL B
Chem 12, CBC, Electrolyte Panel

☐ ▼ 3382 PANEL D
Chem 20, CBC, Thyroid Cascade

☐ ✗ 3388 PANEL F
Chem 12, CBC, Electrolyte Panel,
Thyroid Cascade

☐ ▼ 3391 PANEL G
Chem 20, Cardiac Risk Panel, CBC,
Thyroid Cascade

☐ ▼ 3389 PANEL H
Chem 20, CBC, Cardiac Risk Panel
Rheumatoid Factor, Thyroid Cascade

☐ ▼ 3397 PANEL J
Chem 20, Cardiac Risk Panel

☐ 5351 PRENATAL PANEL
Antibody Screen ABO/Rh, CBC
Rubella, HBsAg, RPR
☐ 1059 with Urinalysis, Routine
☐ 1082 with Urinalysis w/Culture
if indicated

☐ ✗ 3102 RENAL PANEL
Metabolic Status Panel, Calcium,
Phosphorus

☐ 3168 THYROID CASCADE
TSH, Reflex Testing

▼ - patient **required** to fast
for 12-14 hours

✗ - patient **recommended** to
fast 12-14 hours

LAB USE ONLY		INIT	
☐ SST		☐ PLASMA	
☐ PURPLE		☐ SERUM	
☐ YELLOW		☐ SWAB	
☐ BLUE		☐ SLIDES	
☐ GREEN		☐ DNA PROBE	
☐ GREY		☐ B. CULT BTLS	
☐ URINE			
☐ BLACK			
☐ OTHER:			
RECV. SPECIMEN:	☐ FROZEN		
☐ AMBIENT	☐ ON ICE		

Special Instructions/Pertinent Clinical Information _____

Physician's Signature _____ Date _____
These orders may be FAXed to: 449-5288   7060-500 (7/96)

LAB

FIGURE 51-4 Laboratory requisition form.

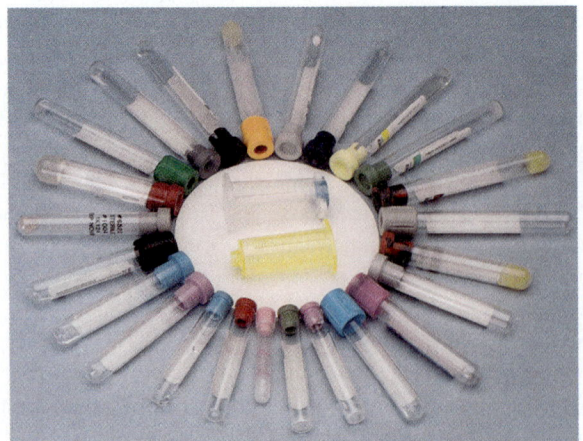

FIGURE 51-5 Vacutainer tubes; note the color-coded tops.

in a second container, such as an impervious biohazard bag, for transport. The completed requisition goes inside the outermost wrap. Usually Styrofoam mailers (Figure 51-6) are used, because they cushion the sample and provide insulation. Styrofoam inserts can be shaped to fit around the specimen container. A warning label specifying the etiologic agent or biologic specimen is placed on the outside of the container. Most offices have a laboratory courier service that picks up specimens periodically throughout the day. Specimens should be properly stored (some require refrigeration) until the courier arrives. Instructions for properly obtaining, processing, and preparing a specimen for transport usually are supplied by the testing laboratory. If the instructions are not clear, or if you have a question about a particular collection, the laboratory can answer your question over the phone. Criteria for safe shipping of specimens include length of time that is acceptable for transit, recommended temperature ranges to maintain the integrity of the specimen, and whether light can affect the specimen.

Preventing Contamination

Medical assistants must take care to prevent contamination of the specimen and of themselves. Expiration dates on swabs, tubes, transport media, and other collection containers should be checked before these items are used. An improperly handled specimen may become contaminated or may contaminate the surrounding environment. Standard Precautions should be followed. All blood and other body fluids from all patients should be considered infectious.

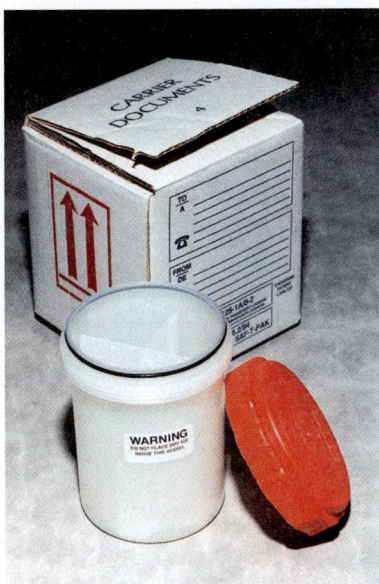

FIGURE 51-6 Specimen mailers.

Sufficient samples should be collected for the tests requested by the physician. Amounts may vary on the basis of methods used. A report returned from the laboratory marked "QNS" (quantity not sufficient) indicates a request for an additional specimen. Make sure to clarify any questions about the previous specimen by calling the laboratory before collecting a new one.

The specimen collected must be a true representative sample. A swab for a wound culture collected from the surface of the wound generally does not yield the same results as one taken from the depths of the wound. A **hemolyzed** blood specimen or one taken from an atypical area, such as a hematoma or the area above or below an intravenous drip, shows marked differences in many tests. If a large volume of specimen is collected, such as a 24-hour urine specimen, the total volume or weight must be carefully measured and recorded. The specimen must be well mixed before an **aliquot** is removed and submitted for testing.

PROPER HANDLING, PROCESSING, AND STORAGE

The specimen must be handled, processed, and stored according to individual guidelines to avoid causing any alterations that would affect test results. The medical assistant should determine whether the specimen needs to be kept warm or cool. Specimens such as urine require chilling if testing will not be performed immediately. Some cultures or specimens need to be kept at body temperature after collection. Samples for gonorrhea cultures and semen analysis are two such examples, because cooling kills micro-organisms and sperm. When required, serum must be separated from the cells as soon as possible after the specimen has clotted to prevent changes caused by the metabolism of the cells. Specimens for bilirubin testing must be protected from light. Some specimens need to be frozen to prevent chemical constituents from changing. Laboratory specimen requirements should be consulted to ensure that each specimen is handled and processed properly.

Chain of Custody

When a specimen may be needed as evidence in a court case, certain procedures must be followed in collecting and handling the specimen. Forensic or medicolegal implications require that any results gathered on testing of a specimen should be obtained in such a fashion that they are recognized by a court of law. Specimen processing must be documented meticulously, ensuring that no tampering with evidence has occurred. *Chain of custody* refers to the stepwise method used to collect, process, and test a specimen. The documentation must be signed by every person who has contact with the specimen, from collection to final reporting of results. Blood alcohol level testing and drug screening often require chain of custody handling. Everything needed for collection of the specimen is provided in a kit—even the gloves, the vacuum tube, and the needle used to collect the blood specimen. Documentation is included and must be signed by all personnel. Medical assistants and phlebotomists have been subpoenaed to testify in court about specimens they have collected; therefore, it is in your best interest to follow chain of custody procedures rigorously.

COLLECTING SPECIMENS FOR LABORATORY TESTS AND INFORMING THE PATIENT OF THE RESULTS

1. The healthcare practitioner orders laboratory tests on the basis of physical examination findings and/or to diagnose a disorder.
2. Complete a lab requisition.
3. Collect the specimen after receiving the physician's order or instruct the patient on how to collect the ordered specimen at home.
4. Label the appropriate container.
5. Process the specimen as trained or prepare the specimen for transport to a reference laboratory.
6. Properly dispose of specimens collected and tested in the office in biohazard waste containers after tests are completed.
7. The laboratory report shows the results of the test. Reference laboratory results are filed in the patient's medical record after the physician has reviewed and signed them. The results of tests performed in the office are recorded in the patient's record.
8. Confidentially notify the patient of test results according to office policy, and document in the patient's record that test results were received.

QUALITY ASSURANCE AND QUALITY CONTROL

Quality Assurance Guidelines

Quality assurance (QA) is the pledge of healthcare professionals to work to achieve the highest degree of excellence in the healthcare given every patient. QA encompasses a comprehensive set of policies and procedures developed to ensure the reliability of laboratory testing. It includes quality control (QC), personnel orientation, laboratory documentation, knowledge of laboratory instrumentation, and enrollment in a proficiency testing program. QA focuses on establishing a series of operating procedures to produce reliable laboratory results for the benefit of the patient, the physician, and the medical assistant who does the laboratory testing.

These policies benefit the physician by reducing the liability for inaccurate reporting of test results. When a physician uses a laboratory test in diagnosing, the results must be compared with reference values. Reference values also are useful for assessing the efficacy of a patient's course of treatment. The QA system enables the laboratory to assess, verify, and document the quality of the test results. This documentation is a way of comparing "what is" with "what should be." QC is covered in *Subpart K* of the February 28, 1992, CLIA regulations, published in the *Federal Register*. POLs are required to have a procedure manual that describes the processes for testing and reporting patients' results. Personnel are required to calibrate laboratory instruments and to verify the calibrations at least every 6 months. In addition, they must run two levels of control material each day of testing and document the results, and they must perform and document remedial action when errors or problems are identified. Finally, preventive maintenance schedules must be followed and documented.

CRITICAL THINKING APPLICATION   51-3

As part of her daily routine, Marsha performs quality control on the lab's glucometer before patient testing. According to the package insert, the value of the control sample should be 160 mg/dL ± 3 mg/dL. Marsha performs the test, and the glucometer reads 140 mg/dL. She repeats the test three times, obtaining values of 141, 140, and 139 mg/dL. Is the instrument accurate? Is the instrument reliable? Can she proceed with the day's testing? If not, what should she do?

GUIDELINES FOR A PREVENTIVE MAINTENANCE PROGRAM

- Follow the manufacturer's instructions for calibrating instruments.
- Read and understand the instructions for routine instrument care.
- Perform all preventive maintenance specified by the manufacturer's instructions.
- Keep spare parts available for immediate use.
- Record the name, address, and phone number of a contact person for maintenance or repair.
- Create a maintenance form or use the one provided.

Quality Control Guidelines

The objective of QC in the laboratory is to ensure the accuracy and reliability of test results while detecting and eliminating error. *Accuracy* refers to how close the obtained value is to the real, true value, and *reliability* refers to the reproducibility of the test procedure. POLs play a vital part in QC, because patient treatment often is based on or is reinforced by the results of laboratory tests. As mandated by law, QC programs monitor all aspects of laboratory activity, from specimen collection through processing, testing, and reporting steps. Programs check supplies, reagents, machinery, personnel, and actual test performance. Without a QC program, laboratory error is difficult to detect unless the physician notices test results inconsistent with a patient's history. Undetected laboratory errors may result in harm to the patient.

Specially prepared QC samples are tested daily, along with patient samples. The results of testing performed on QC samples must be within a pre-established range before patient results can be reported. QC samples, called *controls,* usually are supplied with prepackaged kits intended for use in the small laboratory. These controls should be analyzed at specified intervals. For example, positive and negative controls supplied with pregnancy test kits should be performed with each patient specimen. Urinalysis dipsticks (used for chemical examination of urine) should be checked daily and each time a new container is opened. Controls for automated chemistry analyses should be performed at specified intervals during the day. Consistent results of controls ensure constant conditions throughout the testing sequence.

Standardization of laboratory instruments is important to ensure proper operation and accurate test results. Standardization involves testing samples with specific, known values and adjusting the instrumentation until it displays those values. These samples are known as *standards*. Preventive maintenance prolongs the life of equipment and reduces breakdown; it includes daily cleaning and adjustment and replacement of parts when necessary. Each instrument should have a log or worksheet for recording all changes, including daily maintenance details.

Accurate record keeping is one of the key responsibilities of a medical assistant. Various forms are available to assist in the recording of laboratory information, although much of this information now can be found online and recorded in an electronic format. If your office uses hard copies, the primary record is the laboratory master logbook, in which each procedure performed in the POL is entered with the dates clearly shown. On every day that patient tests are performed, QC tests must also be performed. The results of standardization tests and the dates when new control vials are begun must be entered, along with the expiration dates of the controls. These records must be retained for several years; the exact number of years is determined by state law and CLIA mandates.

CRITICAL THINKING APPLICATION   51-4

Marsha is performing a blood urea nitrogen (BUN) test on a sample using an automated BUN analyzer. First she performed QC by using a test sample and made adjustments to the equipment as needed. Then she tested the patient's sample and recorded the value. Explain why she ran the control sample and why the patient sample was the last to be tested.

LABORATORY MATHEMATICS AND MEASUREMENT

All laboratory testing, from specimen collection through reporting of results, relies on accurate use of values and measurements. For example, values are used for reporting the time the sample was collected, the amount of analyte found in a specimen, the volume of the specimen, and dilutions used in sample preparation and for recording QC results.

Measuring Time

Time of day often is a critical factor in patient care. Medications must be administered, diets must be followed, and specimens must be collected on a particular schedule. Many clinical laboratories use the 24-hour clock when recording time; this method avoids the confusion that comes with the Greenwich clock, which uses AM (morning) and PM (afternoon) designations.

The 24-hour clock system, also known as *military time,* is expressed with four digits in terms of "hundred hours." Noon is referred to as 1200 ("twelve hundred") hours; midnight is 0000 ("zero hundred") or 2400 hours. The military clock is based on a 60-minute hour, as is the Greenwich clock; therefore, 5:35 PM is expressed as 1735 ("seventeen thirty-five") hours (Table 51-3).

Measuring Temperature

Two scales currently are used for measuring temperature (Table 51-4); each is divided into units called *degrees.* The Fahrenheit scale is considered part of the English system of measurement and is the scale most commonly used in the United States. The Celsius scale, formerly called the *centigrade scale,* is used in countries that apply the metric system. On the Celsius (C) scale, water freezes at 0°C and boils at 100°C. On the Fahrenheit (F) scale, water freezes at 32°F and boils at 212°F. The method for converting temperatures from one scale to the other is found in Chapter 31.

TABLE 51-3 Greenwich and Military Times

GREENWICH TIME	MILITARY TIME
1:00 AM	0100 hours
3:00 AM	0300 hours
5:00 AM	0500 hours
7:00 AM	0700 hours
9:00 AM	0900 hours
11:00 AM	1100 hours
1:00 PM	1300 hours
3:00 PM	1500 hours
5:00 PM	1700 hours
7:00 PM	1900 hours
9:00 PM	2100 hours
11:00 PM	2300 hours
12:00 AM (midnight)	2400 hours

TABLE 51-4 Common Laboratory Temperatures

	FAHRENHEIT	CELSIUS
Refrigerator temperature	35°-46°	2°-8°
Freezer temperature	32°	0°
Room temperature	59°-86°	15°-30°
Incubator temperature	98.6°	37°
Body temperature	98.6°	37°
Autoclave temperature	254°	121°

Units of Measurement

The units of measurement that we commonly use in the United States differ from those used in the clinical laboratory. In everyday life we use the English system of measurement, in which weight is measured in ounces and pounds, length is measured in inches and feet, and volume is measured in cups and quarts. In the laboratory, the metric system and the Système International (SI) are used. It is important that the medical assistant memorize and practice these systems so that he or she can communicate professionally.

The metric system is based on a decimal system, which consists of basic units and prefixes that indicate a system of division in multiples of ten. The basic units of the metric system are the gram (g) for weight, the meter (m) for length, and the liter (L) for volume. Prefixes are added to each symbol to reduce or enlarge them by units of ten. This information was already discussed in Chapter 34. The most common metric units used in the laboratory are millimeters (mm), centimeters (cm), micrograms (mcg), milligrams (mg), grams (g), microliters (mcL), milliliters (mL), liters (L), and cubic centimeters (cc). The cubic centimeter and the milliliter are used interchangeably in the clinical laboratory.

Quantitative test results are reported using the appropriate units of measurement. Some commonly used designations for reporting analytes are mg, μ, g, dL, and L. Blood glucose, for example, is reported in milligrams per deciliter (mg/dL); hemoglobin levels are reported as grams per deciliter (g/dL).

The Système Internationale, or SI units, is a system of reporting numbers that has been recognized by international organizations such as the World Health Organization (WHO). Many countries have adopted its use; the United States has not completely converted to the SI system.

The SI is an adaptation of the metric system that uses several of the basic units, although many are different for reporting results. For example, blood glucose is reported in millimoles per liter (mmol/L), and hemoglobin is reported in grams per liter (g/L). Therefore, it is very important that the medical assistant double-check the laboratory's standard and include the appropriate units of measurement when reporting test values.

Measuring Liquid Volume

Most vessels used to measure volume in the laboratory are plastic and disposable for infection control purposes. Beakers are wide, straight-sided cylindric vessels that are used for mixing or reagent preparation. They are not calibrated to hold an exact volume but can be used for estimating volume. Erlenmeyer flasks are used for reagent preparation and have a narrower mouth than a beaker. Like beakers, they are not calibrated.

Test tubes come in many sizes and are typically disposable. Test tubes may be sterile, and some may be calibrated. Graduated cylinders are used for measuring exact amounts of a liquid. The size of the cylinder should be matched as closely as possible to the volume of liquid being measured to obtain the most accurate reading. In other words, a 50-mL graduated cylinder should not be used to measure 10 mL—a 10-mL cylinder should be used. For the most accurate measurement, a volumetric flask is used. Volumetric glassware, including flasks and pipets, must go through rigorous calibration to ensure the accuracy of the measurement. They are calibrated to single, specific amounts, such as 100 mL or 500 mL, and cannot be used to measure volumes other than those indicated. Figure 51-7 shows the glassware used in a laboratory.

Pipets (Figure 51-8) also are used extensively in the laboratory. These cylindric, calibrated tubes are used to deliver or transfer specified volumes of liquid. Drawing liquid into the pipet requires a bulb or a vacuum pump–type device; pipetting by mouth is forbidden. For most general laboratory procedures, two main types of manual pipets are used: the volumetric pipet, which is used for transferring, and the graduated pipet, which is used for measuring. The graduated pipet is classified according to whether it contains or delivers the amount specified. A "to deliver" (TD) pipet delivers the specified volume by drawing the liquid up to the calibration mark and then allowing it to drain out vertically, unassisted. A small amount of liquid always remains in the tip of the pipet. A "to contain" (TC) pipet must be emptied completely to deliver the specified amount. When mouth pipetting was routinely practiced, these pipets were said to be "blown out," meaning that all the liquid was to be forcibly expelled from the pipet. This is now an unacceptable practice.

A serologic pipet is much like the graduated pipet in appearance. However, the tip opening is large, which permits fast flow of liquid but less accuracy. This pipet is calibrated into the tip. Serologic pipets are used to prepare dilutions of serum but should not be used in the preparation of reagents.

When measuring liquid in a narrow vessel, such as a pipet or a graduated cylinder, you will notice that the liquid has a curvature at the surface. This is called the *meniscus*, and it should be adjusted so that at eye level the bottom of the curve is at the calibration line (Figure 51-9).

Micropipettors (Figure 51-10) are used to deliver very small amounts of liquid, from 1 to 1,000 microliters (mcL). It is important

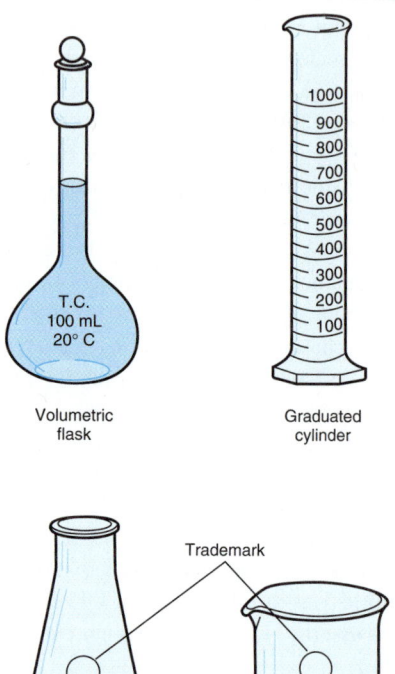

FIGURE 51-7 Laboratory glassware. *T.C.,* To contain. (Redrawn from Linne JJ, Ringsrud KM: *Clinical laboratory science: the basics and routine techniques,* ed 5, St Louis, 2007, Mosby.)

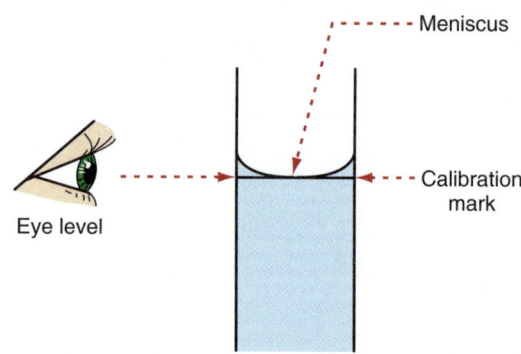

FIGURE 51-9 Reading the meniscus. (From Linne JJ, Ringsrud KM: *Clinical laboratory science: the basics and routine techniques,* ed 5, St Louis, 2007, Mosby.)

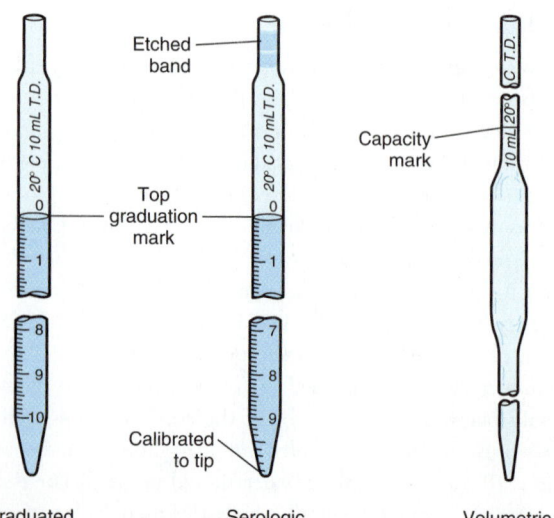

FIGURE 51-8 Types of manual pipets. (Redrawn from Linne JJ, Ringsrud KM: *Clinical laboratory science: the basics and routine techniques,* ed 5, St Louis, 2007, Mosby.)

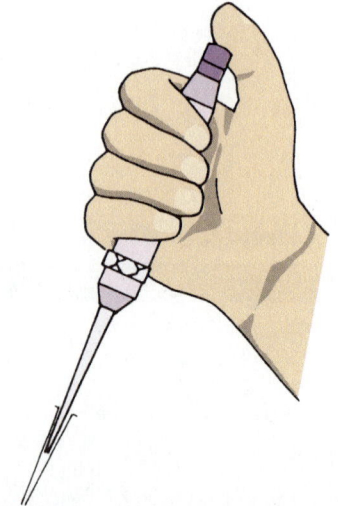

FIGURE 51-10 Piston-type automatic micropipettor. (Modified from Linne JJ, Ringsrud KM: *Clinical laboratory science: the basics and routine techniques,* ed 5, St Louis, 2007, Mosby.)

to follow the manufacturer's instructions for the device, because each may be slightly different. These pipetting devices must be fitted with an appropriate disposable tip. The tips may be sterile, depending on their use. The device is fitted with a piston at the top, which must be depressed before the pipet is filled and when the pipet is drained.

Preparing Dilutions

When the medical assistant performs laboratory tests, he or she may find it necessary to dilute a body fluid sample with a **diluent**, such as water, saline solution, or a buffer. For example, dilutions must be made when testing for the presence and strength of antibodies in serum, or when a patient's analyte level is grossly elevated and cannot be read by the instrument.

The term *dilution* refers to parts in total volume; it is a statement of relative concentration and represents expressions of concentration, not expressions of volume. For example, a 1:10 dilution can be prepared by measuring 1 mL of sample and diluting it with diluent to 10 mL. This means that 9 mL of diluent is added. The same 1:10 dilution can be prepared by mixing 2 mL of sample and 18 mL of diluent or 0.5 mL of sample and 4.5 mL of diluent. Note that the final volume is not the same in each of the above examples, yet each is a 1:10 dilution. Any volume of a dilution can be made as long as the relative amounts of the components remain the same.

CLINICAL LABORATORY EQUIPMENT

Microscope

Nearly every medical laboratory is equipped with a microscope. This indispensable instrument is used to view objects too small to be seen with the naked eye (Figure 51-11). The microscope is used to evaluate stained blood smears, urine sediment, vaginal secretions, and smears made from body fluids or microbiologic cultures. Typically, no QC procedures are used for these tests (Table 51-5). Provider-performed microscopy procedures (PPMP) laboratories must meet the same quality standards as laboratories that perform moderate-complexity tests; laboratories that perform only CLIA-waived tests may perform certain microscopic tests through a certificate of waiver (COW). In a physician's office laboratory with a COW, only a physician, a physician's assistant, a dentist, or other highly trained personnel can perform microscopic analysis. If the laboratory is CLIA certified to perform moderate-complexity testing, personnel other than physicians can perform microscopic analysis, provided that they are trained and supervised by a qualified individual and the laboratory maintains its CLIA certification.

Microscopes have three components: the magnification system, the illumination system, and the framework, which includes all components responsible for positioning the slide and focusing. The magnification system includes the ocular and the objective lenses.

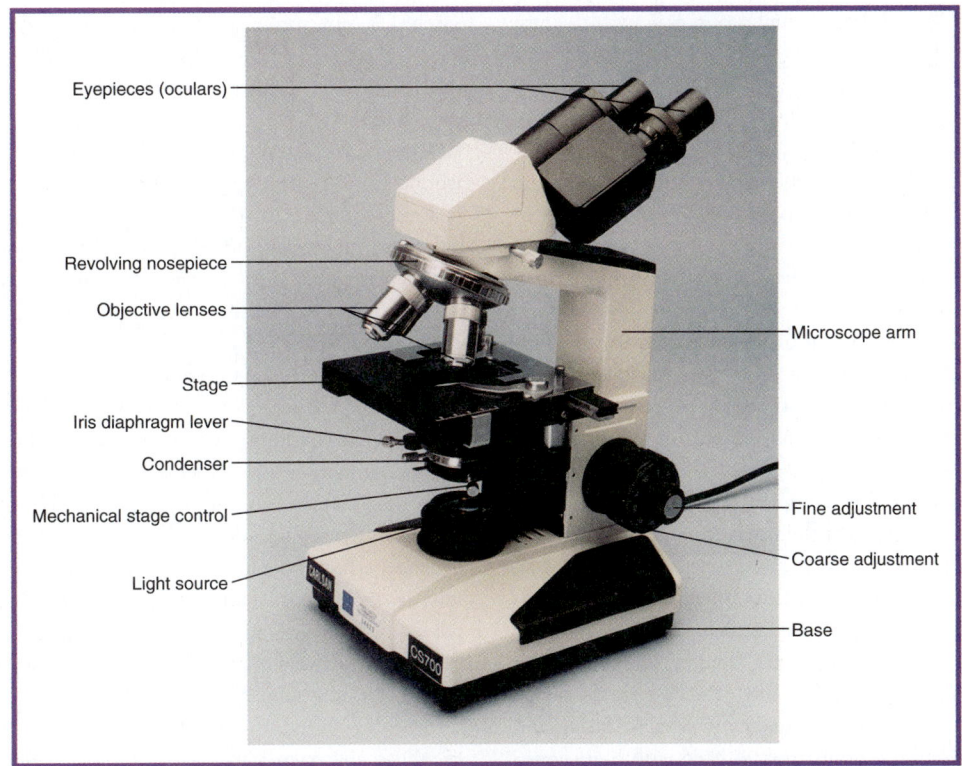

FIGURE 51-11 The parts of a microscope. (Courtesy Cynmar, Carlinville, Illinois.)

TABLE 51-5 Selected Microscopy Tests Performed by Providers

TEST NAME	DESCRIPTION	EXAMPLE
Direct wet mount	Examination of specimens for presence or absence of bacteria, fungi, parasites, and human cellular elements	Observing vaginal secretions for presence of yeast to assist with diagnosis of vulvovaginal candidiasis
KOH preparation	Any preparation using potassium hydroxide	Observing skin scrapings for the presence of fungi
Fecal leukocyte examination	Simple stain of fecal specimen; assists in diagnosis of diarrheal disease	Leukocytes are found in stool in antibiotic-associated colitis, ulcerative colitis, shigellosis, and salmonellosis
Pinworm examination	Preparations are observed for the presence or absence of *Enterobius vermicularis* eggs	See **Procedure 55-7**, Performing a Cellulose Tape Collection for Pinworms
Postcoital direct, qualitative examinations	Vaginal or cervical mucus is examined 4-10 hours after intercourse for presence of live, motile sperm	Assists in the diagnosis of infertility
Qualitative semen analysis	Semen is examined for presence or absence of spermatozoa; motility of the sperm is noted	Assists in postvasectomy semen analysis and in the diagnosis of infertility
Urine sediment examination	Urine sediment is examined for presence or absence of formed elements	Part of a routine urinalysis; see **Procedure 52-6**, Preparing a Urine Specimen for Microscopic Examination

Microscopes may be monocular or binocular. A monocular microscope has one eyepiece for viewing, and a binocular has two. The eyepiece, or ocular, is located at the top of the microscope and contains a lens to magnify what is being viewed. The usual magnification is 10 times (10×). In addition to the ocular, compound microscopes have objective lenses that increase the magnification of the specimen. The objectives are attached to the revolving nosepiece. Most microscopes have four objectives, each with a different magnifying power. The shortest objective has the lowest power (4×) and is called the *scanning lens.* This lens is used to scan the field of interest and then focus on a particular object. Greater detail is observed with the next longest objective, which is low power (10×). The high or high dry objective usually has a magnification of 40× or 45×, and the longest objective, oil immersion (100×), allows the finest focusing of the object and requires the use of a special oil that is placed directly on the slide. This special oil, called *immersion oil,* prevents refraction of the light and improves the resolution (clarity) of the magnified image. Oil immersion is used to view cells and extremely small materials, such as bacteria and platelets, and to examine stained specimens.

To determine the total magnification of the specimen, multiply the magnification of the objective lens by 10 (the magnification of the ocular). Therefore, if you have the 10× objective in place when you are observing blood cells, you are magnifying the image 100 times.

The arm of the microscope connects the objectives and the oculars to the base, which supports the microscope and contains its light source. The stage of the microscope holds the slide to be viewed. Together, the light source, the condenser, and the iris diaphragm compose the illumination system. The condenser directs light up through the stage, and the iris diaphragm regulates the amount of light passing through the specimen. Just above the base are the focusing knobs. The coarse adjustment is used only with scanning and low-power lenses, and the fine adjustment is used with high-power and oil immersion lenses.

Microscopes are very precise and expensive instruments that require careful handling. The amount of routine maintenance required depends on the amount of daily use. Dirt is the enemy of the microscope, which must be kept scrupulously clean at all times. Oil, makeup, dust, and eye secretions all can obstruct vision through the lens and may transmit infective organisms. The microscope should always be stored in a plastic dust cover when not in use. Lenses should be cleaned before and after each use with lens paper and lens cleaner. Any other type of tissue scratches the lenses or leaves lint residue behind. Routine use of solvent cleaners, such as xylene, is not recommended, because these cleaners may loosen lenses. However, xylene can be used to remove oil that has dried on the lenses. The body of the microscope should be dusted with a soft cloth.

The microscope should be placed in a permanent location in the laboratory on a sturdy table in an area where it cannot be bumped. If a microscope must be moved, it should be carried securely, with one hand supporting the base and the other holding the arm. When the microscope is stored, it should be left covered and with the low-power objective in the lowest position. The stage should be centered.

Using a microscope involves focusing and illumination (Procedure 51-1). The image is focused by moving the objective closer to the specimen, and illumination is accomplished by raising or lowering the condenser and by moving the specimen closer to or farther from the objective.

The microscope is focused through movement of the objective or stage, which is controlled by round knobs on both sides of the microscope. Proper focusing begins with the objective at lowest power. The coarse adjustment moves the objective very quickly. This knob is used first to bring the specimen into approximate focus. The fine adjustment focus knob then brings the specimen into precise focus. The fine focus moves the objective more slowly to allow the viewer to zero in on the specimen with greater accuracy.

PROCEDURE 51-1

Use the Microscope

GOAL: *To focus the microscope properly using a prepared slide under low power, high power, and oil immersion.*

EQUIPMENT and SUPPLIES

- Microscope
- Lens cleaner
- Lens tissue
- Slide containing specimen
- Immersion oil

PROCEDURAL STEPS

1. Sanitize your hands.
2. Gather the needed materials.
3. Clean the lenses with lens tissue and lens cleaner.
   PURPOSE: Dust on lenses can obscure elements in the microscopic field.
4. Adjust the seating to a comfortable height.
5. Plug the microscope into an electrical outlet and turn on the light switch.
6. Place the slide specimen on the stage and secure it.
7. Turn the revolving nosepiece to engage the 4× or 10× lens.
   PURPOSE: Always begin microscopic observations at low power.
8. Carefully raise the stage while observing with the naked eye from the side.
   PURPOSE: Observing the side of the slide will prevent the possibility of breaking the slide because the adjustment knob is advanced too far.
9. Focus the specimen using the coarse adjustment knob.
   PURPOSE: The coarse adjustment knob quickly brings the specimen into focus.
10. Adjust the amount of light by closing the iris diaphragm or by adjusting the light from the source.
    PURPOSE: Too much light when the low-power objective is used can be irritating to the microscopist's eyes.
11. Switch to the 40× lens. Use the fine adjustment knob to focus the specimen in detail.
12. Turn the revolving nosepiece to the area between the high-power objective and oil immersion.
13. Place a small drop of oil on the slide.
    PURPOSE: Immersion oil has nearly the same refractive index as glass and prevents refraction of the light, thus improving resolution.
14. Carefully rotate the oil immersion objective into place. The objective will be immersed in the oil.
15. Adjust the focus with the fine adjustment knob.
    PURPOSE: The fine adjustment knob moves the objective slowly, preventing damage to the microscope and the slide.
16. Increase the light by opening the iris diaphragm and raising the condenser.
    PURPOSE: Lighting is crucial to microscopy; the higher the magnification, the more light that is needed.
17. Identify the specimen.
18. Return to low power but do not drag the 40× lens through the oil.
19. Remove the slide and dispose of it in a biohazard container.
20. Lower the stage.
21. Center the stage.
    PURPOSE: Returning the microscope to this position protects it during storage.
22. Switch off the light and unplug the microscope.
23. Clean the lenses with lens tissue and remove oil with lens cleaner.
    PURPOSE: Dust and oil must be removed from the lenses after a procedure.
24. Wipe the microscope with a cloth.
25. Cover the microscope.
26. Sanitize the work area.
27. Sanitize your hands.

If the microscope is a binocular model, the eyepieces may need to be adjusted to accommodate the distance between the pupils and the individual's point of greatest visual acuity. A gentle push inward or pull outward adjusts the distance between the eyepieces.

Centrifuge

Centrifugation, which is used when solids must be separated from liquids, involves the application of increased gravitational force achieved by rapid spinning. Centrifugation is used to separate blood cells from serum and also solid materials, such as cells and crystals, from urine; it is used in many areas of the clinical laboratory.

Centrifuges (Figure 51-12) are designed for specific uses. They may be bench-top or floor models; some may be refrigerated. Some may have rotors or heads that are interchangeable. A typical clinical centrifuge may have a rotor that is set at a fixed angle, in which the specimen cups are held in a rigid position at a fixed angle; one that has a horizontal head with swinging buckets that swing out horizontally during centrifugation; and a third that is used for centrifuging capillary tubes for microhematocrit determination (see Chapter 53). Centrifuges also may be equipped with timers to automatically stop centrifugation at a set time.

Directions for using a centrifuge usually are given in terms of revolutions per minute (rpm). Spinning generates centrifugal force. General laboratory centrifuges operate at up to 6,000 rpm, generating a relative centrifugal force of up to 7,300 times the force of gravity (G). Conventional horizontal centrifuges attain speeds of up to 3,000 rpm; angle-head centrifuges can attain higher speeds (up to 7,000 rpm).

Centrifuges can be dangerous if not used correctly. The most important rule is to ensure that the centrifuge is balanced so that

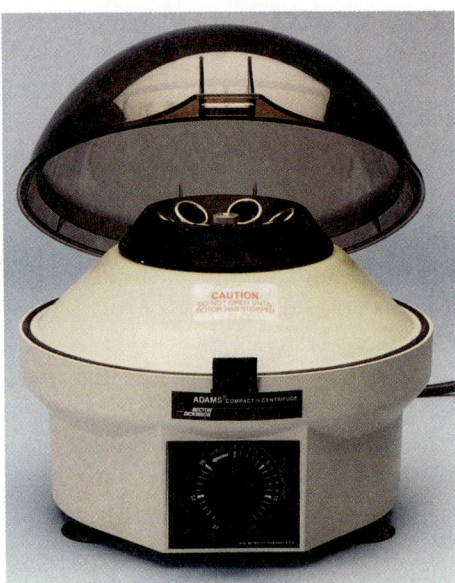

FIGURE 51-12 A centrifuge.

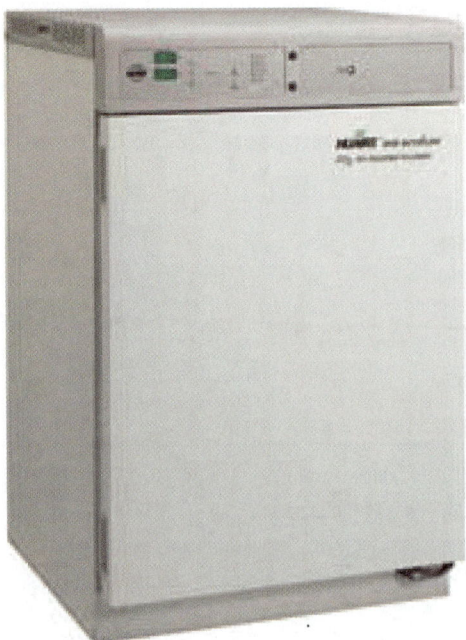

FIGURE 51-13 An incubator. (Courtesy NuAire, Inc., Plymouth, Minnesota.)

tubes of equal size and containing equal volume are directly across from one another in the rotor holders. Therefore, there will always be an even number of tubes in the centrifuge. If a second specimen of the same volume in the same-sized tube is not available for balance, a tube of water may be used to balance the load. Tubes being centrifuged should be capped to prevent emission of aerosols. Rubber cups should be placed in the bottom of the carrier cups to prevent breakage of glass tubes.

Centrifuges should never be opened while they are in operation, nor should you attempt to slow a centrifuge with your hands. Most models are equipped with a brake, which should be used only in an emergency, the most common of which is a broken glass tube. In this case, wait until the centrifuge comes to a complete stop and follow the manufacturer's instructions for disinfecting the unit; also follow Standard Precautions to prevent injury and disease transmission.

Centrifuges should be checked, cleaned, and lubricated regularly to ensure proper operation. A certified technician must use a photoelectric device or a strobe tachometer to ensure the centrifuge's speed to comply with quality assurance guidelines set forth by CAP.

Incubator

Incubators are cabinets that maintain constant temperatures (Figure 51-13). Generally used in the microbiology laboratory, they maintain a constant temperature of 95°F to 98.6°F (35°C to 37°C), although other temperatures may also be appropriate. Some incubator interiors may be enriched with carbon dioxide (CO_2) gas to enhance the growth of pathogenic bacteria; a pressurized tank of CO_2 gas is attached to the cabinet, and the concentration is maintained at 10%. Incubators may have warning alarms that sound if the temperature exceeds or falls below a specified range. The temperature should be checked daily, and the cabinets should be cleaned regularly with a disinfectant approved by the manufacturer.

Autoclave

The autoclave is an instrument that uses steam under pressure to sterilize materials that can withstand high temperatures. The principles of operation are explained in Chapter 57.

It is essential that strict QA methods be followed when an autoclave is used. A certified technician should regularly examine the autoclave, and biologic and chemical indicators should be checked daily. Biologic indicators include spore preparations that are wrapped in the autoclave load. At the end of the sterilization period, they are incubated and checked for germination. If spores fail to germinate, the autoclave reached the appropriate temperature.

CLOSING COMMENTS

Patient Education

For many testing procedures, patients must be given a specific set of instructions to follow. For example, patients may be required to fast 8 to 12 hours before blood and urine samples are collected. They may need to follow a high-carbohydrate diet for several days before they are given a glucose tolerance test. The consumption of some foods and medication must be discontinued. The physician discusses medication alternatives with the patient. In some cases discontinuing the medication may not be medically advisable, and this must be noted on the laboratory requisition. The laboratory then is alerted to the possibility of drug interference, and an alternative test method may be used.

Often the medical assistant is responsible for explaining to the patient the measures to be taken before laboratory testing. Make sure you have interpreted the physician's orders correctly before explaining the procedure to the patient. The patient should be given written instructions, with a phone number included on the instruction sheet so the patient can call if he or she has questions.

Legal and Ethical Issues

If disease did not exist, there would be little need for clinical laboratories. The fact that the human body is susceptible to disease necessitates the existence of laboratory testing. All health and safety risks cannot be anticipated or eliminated, but the risks are greatly reduced when everyone who works in the laboratory is conscious of safety guidelines.

Use common sense and document everything. If you are in doubt about the safety of a procedure, ask your supervisor. If you are aware of a potential safety problem, report it to the person in charge. Your welfare, the welfare of the patient, and the welfare of your co-workers may depend on your commitment to safety.

Before the patient receives test results, the medical assistant must make sure the physician has reviewed and signed the results and has given permission for the patient to be told the results of testing. Most physicians personally inform patients of laboratory results, but some physicians may delegate this duty to office staff. Regardless of who informs the patient of test results, the individual must make sure the specific guidelines for communication are followed as stipulated in the patient's Health Insurance Portability and Accountability Act (HIPAA) release form. Maintaining a patient's privacy and confidentiality are crucial factors that must be considered when communicating with the patient about test results.

SUMMARY OF SCENARIO

Marsha's experience in clinical laboratory testing has made her a valuable asset to her new employer. A thorough understanding of government rules and regulations, including specifics about CLIA, and of the guidelines published by CDC, EPA, and OSHA helped Marsha implement laboratory testing in the clinic. Marsha helped the physicians design a safe, efficient laboratory space with a refrigerator, a centrifuge, and a biohazard waste station. She developed a rigorous QA program and is now training other medical assistants to perform CLIA-waived testing.

Marsha found it most challenging to determine how to comply with proper medical waste disposal regulations. She had to make several phone calls to state environmental protection agencies, but her diligence was rewarded when the laboratory received certification. Marsha pays close attention to CLIA regulations and receives regular updates on the tests that can be performed in a POL. She currently is determining the feasibility of performing drug screenings for local businesses. Her employers are pleased with her efforts, and the patients appreciate the convenience of on-site testing.

SUMMARY OF LEARNING OBJECTIVES

1. **Define, spell, and pronounce the terms listed in the vocabulary.**
   Spelling and pronouncing medical terms correctly bolsters the medical assistant's credibility. Knowing the definitions of these terms promotes confidence in communication with patients and co-workers.

2. **Apply critical thinking skills in performing patient assessment and patient care.**
   Completing the Critical Thinking Application exercises throughout the chapter can help the student medical assistant become more adept at critical analysis of real-life situations.

3. **Discuss the role of the clinical laboratory in patient care and the medical assistant's role in coordinating laboratory tests and results.**
   The clinical laboratory is responsible for analyzing blood and body fluids and for providing the physician with test results that become part of the essential data needed to diagnose and manage a patient's condition. Medical assistants are responsible for collecting specimens, instructing patients, and performing CLIA-waived and some moderately complex testing.

4. **Describe the Clinical Laboratory Improvement Amendments (CLIA) and how they influence laboratory testing.**
   CLIA established the standards of quality for laboratory testing. Medical assistants can perform all CLIA-waived and some CLIA moderate-complexity laboratory procedures. Table 51-2 summarizes CLIA-waived tests.

5. **Explain the three CLIA regulatory categories.**
   A CLIA-waived test is one that is approved by the FDA for over-the-counter sales, or one that has been determined to pose no unreasonable risk or harm if performed incorrectly. Other levels of tests require more training or education to perform and can be performed only in CLIA-certified laboratories.

6. **Describe the divisions of the clinical laboratory and give an example of a test performed in each division.**
   Most physicians' offices that perform laboratory testing do so in the areas of urinalysis, hematology, chemistry, and microbiology. Routine urinalysis, complete blood counts, and throat cultures are some of the tests that might be performed in a POL.

7. **Compare and contrast the agencies that govern or influence practice in the clinical laboratory.**
   Federal agencies that regulate the laboratory include the U.S. Department of Labor, the U.S. Department of Health and Human Services, and the EPA. Professional agencies that provide guidelines include CLSI and CAP. Although all these agencies provide recommendations for operational procedures in the clinical laboratory, not all have the power to enforce them. The Department of Labor and the EPA can impose significant fines for failing to follow regulations, but the Standard Precautions set forth by the CDC are recommended but not enforceable.

8. **Summarize techniques to minimize physical, chemical, and biologic hazards in the clinical laboratory.**

   Risks can be minimized in all areas of the laboratory by using common sense and by having a formal safety training program and an up-to-date safety manual. Safety equipment such as fire blankets, fire extinguishers, and eyewash stations should be accessible to employees. Chemicals should be clearly marked with the National Fire Protection Association diamond, and MSDSs should be bound in an accessible manual. Standard Precautions should be observed when any biologic material is handled.

9. **Describe the essential elements of a laboratory requisition.**

   The laboratory requisition must include all information needed to identify the patient, the ordering physician, the test ordered, and the specific details of collection of the specimen (e.g., time and source).

10. **Display sensitivity to patients' rights and feelings in collecting specimens.**

    Initial identification of the patient is essential. If the patient is to collect the specimen at home, he or she should be provided with the appropriate container and complete instructions for collection. Bear in mind the principles of patient education, and be sensitive to individual patient factors that can affect the individual's understanding of the instructions for specimen collection and the person's ability to follow through on those instructions.

11. **Explain chain of custody and illustrate why it is important.**

    Chain of custody is a method used to ensure that a specimen provided by a patient who may be involved in a legal matter is handled in a fashion that does not compromise the test results. All individuals who handle or test the specimen must be identified in writing and must provide a signature.

12. **Compare and contrast quality assurance and quality control.**

    QA involves procedures undertaken to ensure that each patient is provided excellent care. QC, which ensures that laboratory testing is accurate and reliable, is part of a QA program.

13. **Describe the differences between Greenwich time and military time.**

    Greenwich time uses the designations AM and PM, whereas military time uses the 24-hour clock: 3:15 PM is equivalent to 1515 hours. Table 51-3 compares Greenwich and military time.

14. **Identify the Fahrenheit temperature and the Celsius temperature of common pieces of laboratory equipment.**

    Although the Celsius (Centigrade) thermometer is used in the clinical laboratory, in everyday life we commonly use the Fahrenheit system. The incubator is usually set at 37°C (98°F), the autoclave sterilizes at 121°C (254°F), and the refrigerator temperature is 2°C to 8°C (35°F to 46°F) (see Table 51-4).

15. **Name the metric units used for measuring liquid volume, distance, and mass.**

    Liquid volume is measured in liters, distance is measured in meters, and mass is measured in grams. Prefixes commonly used in the clinical laboratory include *milli-* (0.001), *centi-* (0.01), *micro-* (0.000001), *deci-* (0.1), and *kilo-* (1,000).

16. **Describe the proper use of pipets.**

    Pipets must be chosen according to the job they are to perform. A pipetting device, such as a bulb or a pump, should be attached, and particular attention must be given to emptying the pipet. The mouth should never be used in pipetting.

17. **Explain how dilutions are prepared.**

    Dilutions are prepared by mixing volumes of sample, such as blood, body fluids, or reagents, and volumes of diluent, such as water, saline solution, or buffer. The term *dilution* refers to parts in total volume and is an expression of concentration.

18. **Name the parts of a microscope, and describe their functions.**

    The parts of the microscope can be divided into the illumination system (light source, condenser, and iris diaphragm lever), the frame (base, adjustment knobs, arm, stage, and stage control), and the magnification system (objective lenses on the revolving nosepiece and oculars). The illumination system controls the light that passes through the specimen to the eye, the frame provides the structure for the instrument and the components that allow for adjustment of the sample, and the magnification system provides the ground-glass lenses that magnify the specimen.

19. **Summarize selected microscopy tests that can be performed in the ambulatory care setting.**

    Refer to Table 51-5.

20. **Demonstrate the proper use of the microscope.**

    Procedure 51-1 outlines the steps for using a microscope.

21. **Describe the safe use of a centrifuge.**

    For safe use of a centrifuge, the proper tube must be used and it must be protected from breakage. Centrifuge loads must be carefully balanced. Specimens must be capped to prevent aerosols. Under no circumstances should centrifuges be opened while they are in operation.

22. **Identify legal and ethical issues in the clinical laboratory setting.**

    If you are aware of a potential safety problem, report it to the person in charge. Make sure the physician has reviewed and signed test results and has given permission for the patient to be told the results of testing. Follow specific guidelines for communication as stipulated in the patient's Health Insurance Portability and Accountability Act (HIPAA) release form. Maintaining a patient's privacy and confidentiality is a crucial factor that must be considered when one is communicating with the patient about test results.

CONNECTIONS

📖 **Study Guide Connection:** Go to the Chapter 51 Study Guide. Read and complete the activities.

🅮 **Evolve Connection:** Go to the Chapter 51 link at *evolve.elsevier.com/kinn* to complete the Chapter Review and Chapter Quiz. Peruse other resources listed for this chapter to increase your knowledge of Assisting in the Clinical Laboratory.

ASSISTING IN THE ANALYSIS OF URINE

52

SCENARIO

As part of her duties as a CMA (AAMA), Rosa Gonzales performs tests on patients' urine ordered by her employer, Dr. Ronald Hill. Rosa knows that urinalysis is a very important part of patient care, and a number of urinary tests are performed in the laboratory in Dr. Hill's busy practice. Dr. Hill most commonly orders routine urinalysis testing, but Rosa also performs some specialized tests. Today, Dr. Hill has ordered a urinalysis (UA) on a specimen from Mr. Parks, a UA and pregnancy test on a specimen from Mrs. Carpenter, and a UA and culture and sensitivity (C&S) on a specimen from Ms. Hillman.

While studying this chapter, think about the following questions:

- What is involved in a routine urinalysis?
- What quality assurance measures will Rosa take when performing laboratory tests on urine?
- How are pregnancy and drug tests performed on urine?
- How will Rosa instruct patients in the collection of urine for a routine urinalysis, a urine culture, and other specialized tests such as pregnancy tests and drug tests?

LEARNING OBJECTIVES

1. Define, spell, and pronounce the terms listed in the vocabulary.
2. Apply critical thinking skills in performing the patient assessment and patient care.
3. Understand the purpose of routine urinalysis.
4. Describe the physiology of urine formation.
5. Display sensitivity to patient rights and feelings when collecting specimens.
6. Explain the various means and methods used to collect urine specimens.
7. Instruct a patient in the collection of a 24-hour urine specimen.
8. Instruct a patient in the collection of a clean-catch midstream urine specimen.
9. Describe the components of the physical and chemical examination of urine.
10. Measure the urine specific gravity.
11. Perform a complete urinalysis using a chemical reagent strip.
12. Recognize and correctly identify the formed elements found in a microscopic examination of urine sediment.
13. Prepare a urine specimen for microscopic examination.
14. Perform quality control measures to determine the reliability of chemical reagent strips.
15. Conduct glucose testing using the Clinitest method.
16. Explain the principle of lateral flow technology in pregnancy testing.
17. Perform a pregnancy test.
18. Describe methods for determining fertility and menopause using Clinical Laboratory Improvement Amendments (CLIA)-waived urine tests.
19. Explain the principle of lateral flow technology in drug testing on urine.
20. Demonstrate a method of drug testing on a urine specimen.
21. List the means by which urine could be adulterated before drug testing.
22. Demonstrate a method of detecting adulterating substances in a urine sample for drug testing.
23. Describe patient education factors that are pertinent to urine sample collection.
24. Discuss the legal and ethical responsibilities of the medical assistant who is assisting with urinalysis.

VOCABULARY

amorphous (a-mohr´-fuhs) Lacking a defined shape.

bilirubinuria (bi-li-roo´-bin-yuhr-e-uh) The presence of bilirubin in the urine.

colony-forming units (CFUs) A term used when reporting bacteriuria; one CFU represents one bacterium present in the urine sample.

crenate Forming notches or leaflike, scalloped edges on an object.

culture and sensitivity (C&S) A procedure performed in the microbiology laboratory in which a specimen is cultured on artificial media to detect bacterial or fungal growth, followed by appropriate screening for antibiotic sensitivity.

cystoscopy Visual examination of the urinary bladder using a fiberoptic instrument.

enzymatic reaction A chemical reaction controlled by an enzyme.

filtrate The fluid that remains after a liquid is passed through a membranous filter.

gold standard The paragon of excellence; the diagnostic test against which all others are compared.

metabolite The product of the metabolism of a substance, such as a drug.

mononuclear white blood cells Leukocytes with an unsegmented nucleus; monocytes and lymphocytes in particular.

myoglobinuria The abnormal presence of a hemoglobinlike chemical of muscle tissue in the urine; it is the result of muscle deterioration.

phenylalanine (fe-nehl-ah´-luh-nen) An essential amino acid found in milk, eggs, and other foods.

polymorphonuclear white blood cells Leukocytes with a segmented nucleus; also known as *polymorphonuclear neutrophils* (PMNs) or *segmented neutrophils.*

refractile (re-frak´-tuhl) Causing light to refract or bend, thus creating a sharp boundary or image.

renal thresholds Levels above which substances cannot be reabsorbed by the renal tubules and therefore are excreted in the urine.

sediment Insoluble material that settles to the bottom of a urine specimen.

supravital Of, related to, or capable of staining living cells after their removal from a living or recently dead organism.

A routine urinalysis (UA) is one of the more common laboratory examinations used in the diagnosis and treatment of disease. It is easily and quickly performed, and invasive techniques generally are not needed to collect the specimen. The results of a routine UA can reveal diseases of the bladder or kidneys; systemic metabolic or endocrine disorders, such as diabetes; and diseases of the liver, such as hepatitis or cirrhosis, or obstruction of the bile ducts. UA is routinely performed on all patients undergoing physical examination and on those entering the hospital for treatment.

PHYSIOLOGY OF URINE FORMATION

For centuries abnormalities in the urine have been recognized as possible indicators of a disruption of homeostasis. One of the earliest known tests of urine involved pouring it on the ground to see whether it attracted insects. Such attraction indicated "honey urine," which was known to be excreted by people with skin eruptions. Today, urine is still checked for glucose as a means of detecting diabetes.

Historically, examination of the urine became a game for quacks and charlatans. Paintings from the Middle Ages show physicians peering into round-bottomed flasks of urine, claiming not only to be able to diagnose disease, but also to see into the future by simply looking at the fluid. These charlatans became known as "pisse prophets." During the twentieth century, UA became a practical laboratory procedure, and today urine is the most commonly analyzed body fluid in the clinical laboratory.

Urine is analyzed for several reasons—first to detect extrinsic conditions, in which the kidneys are functioning normally but abnormal end products of metabolism are excreted as a result of an imbalance in homeostasis. For example, individuals with diabetes mellitus may excrete glucose in the urine when they are experiencing hyperglycemia. The second reason is to detect intrinsic pathologic conditions that involve the kidneys or the urinary tract, such as the presence of kidney stones or of a urinary tract infection. In addition, because chemicals are excreted through the kidneys, urinalysis can be used to determine the effectiveness of medications and/or the possibility of urinary system side effects from prescribed drugs.

Anatomy of the Urinary Tract

Medical assistants must have a basic knowledge of kidney structure and urine formation to understand the results of a UA. The urinary tract consists of two kidneys, two ureters, one bladder, and one urethra. The functional unit of the kidney is the nephron. Each kidney has more than 1 million nephrons, and each nephron is composed of five distinct areas, each playing a role in urine formation (Figure 52-1). Each nephron consists of a glomerulus, which acts in filtering, and a tubule, through which the **filtrate** passes. As the filtrate passes through, various changes occur. Certain solutes are reabsorbed, and others are secreted into the kidney for eventual excretion. Nearly all of the water that passes through the glomeruli is reabsorbed.

The glomerulus is composed of a network of capillaries surrounded by a membrane called *Bowman's capsule.* The afferent arteriole carries blood from the renal artery into the glomerulus, where it then divides to form a capillary network. Where they reunite, the capillaries form the efferent arteriole, through which blood exits the glomerulus.

The tubular portion of the nephron is composed of the proximal convoluted tubule, the thin-walled segment, and the distal convoluted tubule. The thin-walled descending portion forms a loop known as the *loop of Henle.* Filtrate from several nephrons drains into a collecting tubule, several of which join to form a collecting duct. The collecting ducts join to form the papillary ducts, which empty at the tips of the papillae into the calyces. The filtrate then

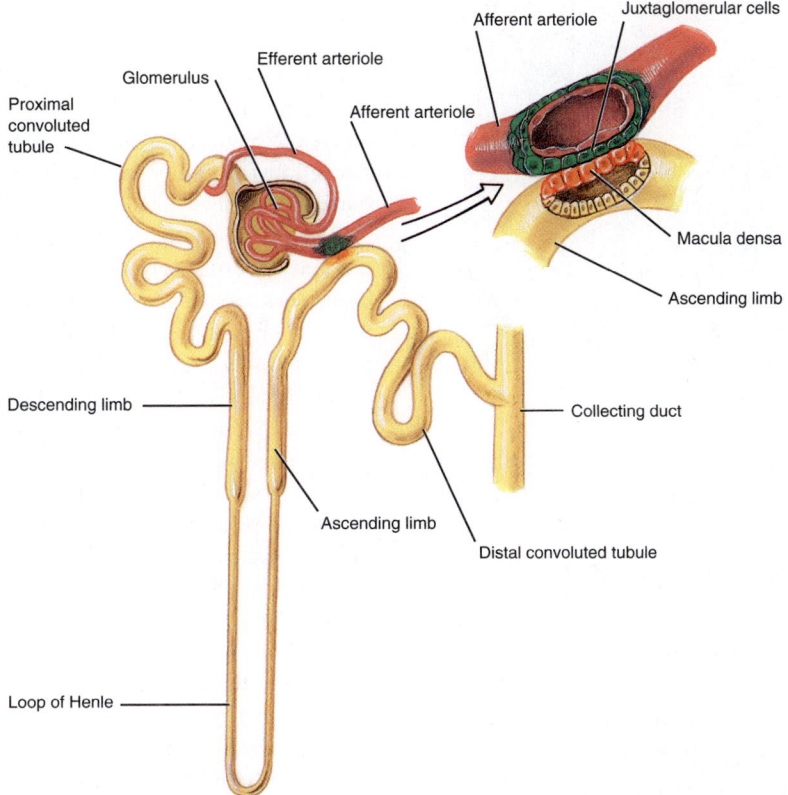

FIGURE 52-1 A nephron. (From Applegate EJ: *The anatomy and physiology learning system,* ed 3, Philadelphia, 2006, Saunders.)

drains into the renal pelvis and is now called *urine.* Urine passes from the pelvis of the kidney down the ureter and into the bladder, where it remains until it is voided through the urethra.

Formation of Urine

The kidney selectively excretes or retains substances according to the body's needs and **renal thresholds**. Approximately 1,200 mL of blood flows through the kidneys each minute. The blood enters the glomerulus through the afferent arteriole. The capillary walls of the glomerulus are highly permeable to water and to the low-molecular-weight solutes of the plasma, and they filter through into Bowman's space and then into the tubules. Many components of the filtrate, including glucose, water, and amino acids, are partially or completely reabsorbed by the capillaries surrounding the proximal tubules. More water is absorbed, and hydrogen and potassium ions are secreted in the distal tubules. Urine is concentrated in the system of collecting tubules and the loop of Henle. The kidneys convert nearly 180,000 mL of filtered plasma per day into a final urine volume of 750 to 2000 mL—approximately 1% of the filtered plasma volume. The largest component of urine is water; the solutes consist mostly of urea, chloride, sodium, potassium, phosphate, sulfate, creatinine, and uric acid.

COLLECTING A URINE SPECIMEN

Patient Sensitivity

The request for a urine specimen may create an embarrassing moment for the patient. The request should be made in private, such

as after the patient is seated in the examination room, and the individual should be given explicit instructions so that he or she understands what is expected. The medical assistant should use therapeutic communication to explain the details of the procedure to the patient and should be observant for indications of confusion. If a language barrier exists, be creative but respectful of the patient's need to follow through correctly on the instructions for collection of the specimen.

Containers

The most important requirement for a collection container is scrupulous cleanliness. The physician's office laboratory should provide a container; patients should not use jars from home. Disposable, nonsterile, plastic, or coated paper containers are the most common and are available in many sizes with tight-fitting lids. If the sample is being sent to the laboratory for a culture, the specimen must be collected in a sterile container, and the patient must understand how to collect the specimen and how to handle the sterile specimen cup. Special pliable polyethylene bags with adhesive (see Chapter 42) are used to collect urine from infants and children who are not toilet trained. For specimens that must be collected over a specified period, large, wide-mouth plastic containers with screw-cap tops are used. Most routine UA testing, pregnancy testing, and tests for abnormal analytes are performed on urine collected in nonsterile containers.

As mentioned, when a urine culture is ordered, the specimen must be collected in a sterile container. Such containers are packaged with an intact paper seal over the cap and/or in sterile envelopes (Figure 52-2). The label on all specimens must include the patient's

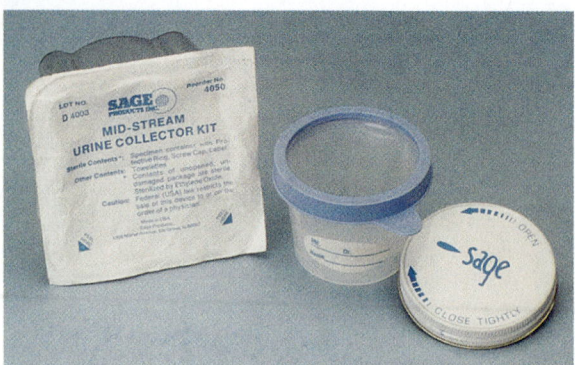

FIGURE 52-2 A sterile container for a midstream specimen.

name, the date and time of collection, and the type of specimen. Always put on gloves before handling filled specimen containers.

CRITICAL THINKING APPLICATION   52-1

It is 9 AM, and Rosa has received three urine specimens in the laboratory. One of the specimens is in a cup with a paper tab, indicating that the container was sterile, and the other two are in nonsterile containers. What procedures do you think might be performed on the urine collected in the sterile container? What might Rosa do with the other urine specimens? What information should she look for on the label of each specimen?

Methods of Specimen Collection

Most analyses are performed on freshly voided urine collected in clean containers; this is called a *random specimen.* If the specimen is ordered to be collected when the patient arises in the morning, it is called a *first morning specimen.* These specimens are most concentrated and are best for nitrite and protein determination, bacterial culture, pregnancy testing, and microscopic examination. Two-hour postprandial urine specimens, collected 2 hours after a meal, are used in diabetes screening and for home diabetes testing programs. The 24-hour urine specimen is collected over 24 hours to provide a quantitative chemical analysis, such as hormone levels and creatinine clearance rates (a procedure for evaluating the glomerular filtration rate of the kidneys) (Procedure 52-1).

A second-voided specimen usually is collected to determine glucose levels; the first void of the morning is discarded, and the second void of the day is collected. For a catheterized specimen, the physician, the physician's assistant, or the nurse must insert a sterile catheter into the bladder to collect the specimen. A suprapubic specimen is collected with a needle inserted directly into the bladder.

The minimum volume for a routine UA usually is 12 mL, but 50 mL is preferred. For any type of collection, it is imperative that the patient receive adequate verbal and/or written instructions. The easiest directions for the patient are to ask the person to fill the container halfway.

PROCEDURE 52-1

Explain the Rationale for Performing a Procedure: Instruct a Patient in the Collection of a 24-Hour Urine Specimen

GOAL: *To collect a 24-hour urine sample for creatinine clearance.*

EQUIPMENT and SUPPLIES

- 3-L urine collection container
- Printed patient instructions
- Laboratory requisition
- Patient's medical record

PROCEDURAL STEPS

1. Greet the patient by name.
   <u>PURPOSE:</u> To make sure you have the right patient.
2. Label the container with the patient's name and the current date, identify the specimen as a 24-hour urine specimen, and include your initials.
   <u>PURPOSE:</u> Labeling the container prevents a possible mix-up of specimens.
3. Explain the following instructions to adult patients or to the guardians of pediatric patients.
4. After explaining the following instructions, give the patient the specimen container with written instructions to confirm understanding.

Patient Instructions for Obtaining a 24-Hour Urine Specimen

1. Empty your bladder into the toilet in the morning without saving any of the specimen. Record the time you first emptied your bladder.

2. For the next 24 hours, each time you empty your bladder, the urine should be voided directly into the large specimen container (Figure 1).

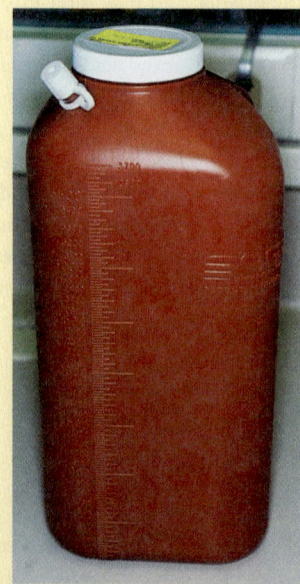

3. Put the lid back on the container after each urination and store the container in the refrigerator or in an ice chest throughout the 24 hours of the study.
   PURPOSE: To inhibit microbial growth in the specimen.
4. If at any time you forget to empty your bladder into the specimen container, or if some urine is accidentally spilled, the test must be started all over again with an empty container and a newly recorded start time.
   PURPOSE: The test will be inaccurate if the patient fails to collect all urine produced during the designated 24-hour period.
5. The last collection of urine should be done at the same time as the first specimen on the previous day so that exactly 24 hours of urine collection is completed. The collection ends with the first voided morning specimen that completes the 24-hour collection period.
6. As soon as possible after collection is completed, return the specimen container to the physician's office.

7. Give the patient the specimen container with written instructions to confirm understanding.
8. Document the details of the patient education intervention in the patient's record.

Processing a 24-Hour Urine Specimen

1. Ask the patient whether he or she collected all voided urine throughout the 24-hour period or whether any problems occurred during the collection process.
   PURPOSE: To confirm the accuracy of the specimen.
2. Complete the laboratory request form and prepare the specimen for transport.
3. Store the specimen in the refrigerator until it is picked up by the laboratory.
4. Document that the specimen was sent to the laboratory, including the type of test ordered, the date and time, and the type of specimen.

A clean-catch midstream specimen (CCMS) is ordered when the physician suspects a urinary tract infection and therefore orders a urine culture for examination of microorganisms. The clean-catch technique is used to remove microorganisms from the urinary meatus by thoroughly cleansing the area around the meatus and to flush out the distal portion of the urethra. Because the specimen is collected in the medical office by the patient, the medical assistant needs to give complete, understandable instructions to the patient on the method of collection (Procedure 52-2). Failure to do so may mean that the patient will have to return to the office to provide another specimen. For a urine culture, the urine is collected either by catheterization or by the clean-catch method in a sterile container.

Handling and Transportation of a Specimen

Proper handling of specimens is essential. The chemical and cellular components of urine change if the urine is allowed to stand at room temperature (Table 52-1). Urine specimens should be kept refrigerated and should be processed within 1 hour of collection. If the specimen must be transported to a referral laboratory, evacuated transport tubes are available; these contain preservatives and look much like blood collection tubes (Figure 52-3). The vacuum in the tube allows for the delivery of 7 to 8 mL of urine, using a transfer straw or a urine collection cup with an integrated sampling device. Alternatively, the urine can be poured into the tube after the stopper

---

PROCEDURE 52-2

Instruct Patients According to Their Needs: Instruct a Patient in the Collection of a Clean-Catch Midstream Urine Specimen

GOAL: *To collect a contaminant-free urine sample for culture or analysis using the clean-catch midstream specimen (CCMS) technique.*

EQUIPMENT and SUPPLIES

- Sterile container with lid and label
- Antiseptic towelettes
- Patient record

PROCEDURAL STEPS

1. Label the container and give the patient the supplies (Figure 1).
   PURPOSE: Labeling the container prevents a possible mix-up of specimens.

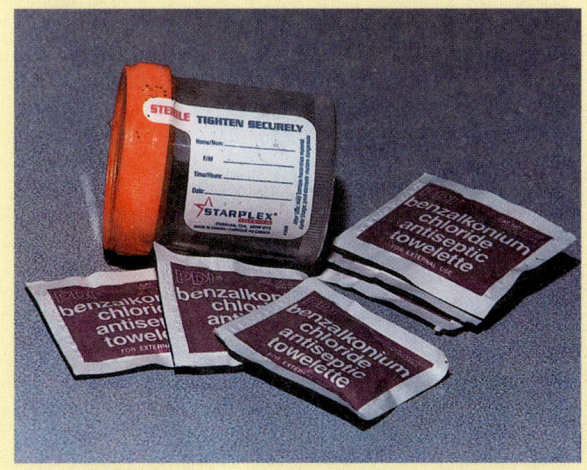

2. Explain the following instructions to adult patients or to the guardians of pediatric patients, being sensitive to privacy issues.

Obtaining a Clean-Catch Midstream Specimen (Female Patient)

1. Wash your hands and open the towelette packages for easy access.
2. Remove the lid from the specimen container, being careful not to touch the inside of the lid or the inside of the container. Place the lid, facing up, on a paper towel.
   PURPOSE: The lid and the container must be handled carefully to maintain the sterility of the container and prevent contamination of the urine sample.
3. Remove your underclothing and sit on the toilet.
4. Expose the urinary meatus by spreading apart the labia with one hand (Figure 2, *A*).

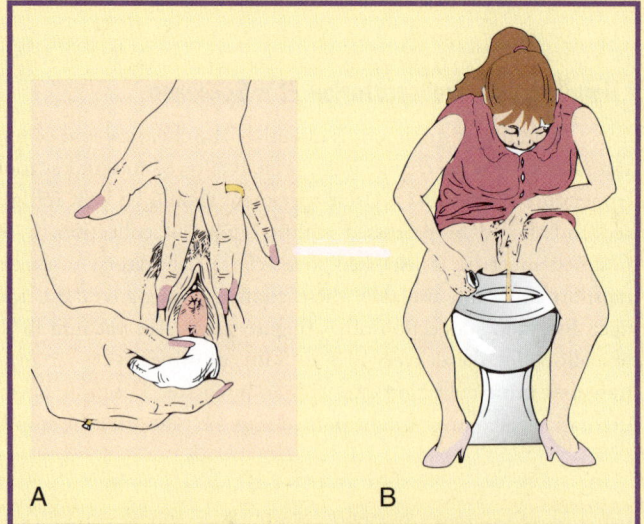

A   B

5. Cleanse each side of the urinary meatus with a front-to-back motion, from the pubis to the anus. Use a separate antiseptic wipe to cleanse each side of the meatus.
   PURPOSE: Cleansing the area around the urinary meatus prevents contamination of the urine sample. Wiping in one stroke from front to back prevents the passage of microorganisms from the anal region to the area around the urinary meatus.
6. Cleanse directly across the meatus, front-to-back, using a third antiseptic wipe (see Figure 2, *A*).
7. Hold the labia apart throughout this procedure.
8. Void a small amount of urine into the toilet (Figure 2, *B*).
   PURPOSE: Allowing the initial flow of urine to pass into the toilet flushes the opening of the urethra.
9. Move the specimen container into position and void the next portion of urine into it. Fill the container halfway. Remember, this is a sterile container. Do not put your fingers on the inside of the container.
10. Remove the cup and void the last amount of urine into the toilet. (This means that the first part and the last part of the urinary flow have been excluded from the specimen. Only the middle portion of the flow is included.)
11. Place the lid on the container, taking care not to touch the interior surface of the lid. Wipe in your usual manner, redress, and return the sterile specimen to the place designated by the medical facility.

Obtaining a Clean-Catch Midstream Specimen (Male Patients)

1. Wash your hands and expose the penis.
2. Retract the foreskin of the penis (if not circumcised).
3. Cleanse the area around the glans penis (meatus) and the urethral opening by washing each side of the glans with a separate antiseptic wipe (Figure 3, *A*).

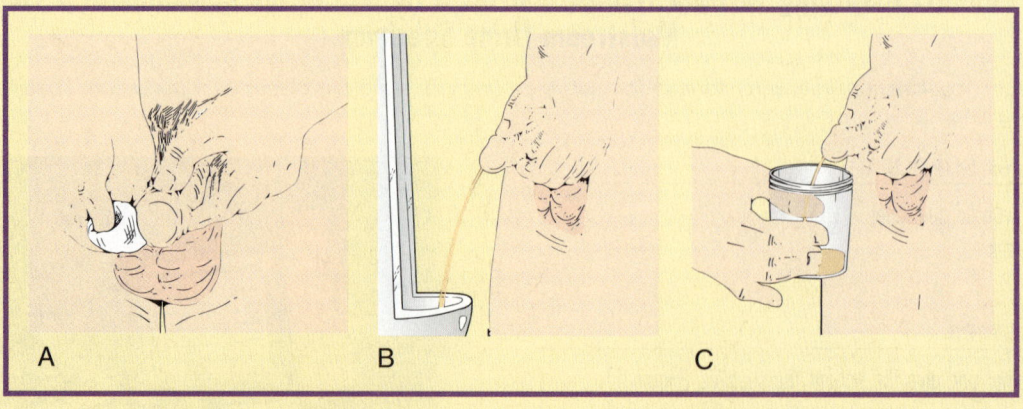

A   B   C

PROCEDURE 52-2—cont'd

4. Cleanse directly across the urethral opening using a third antiseptic wipe.
5. Void a small amount of urine into the toilet or urinal (Figure 3, *B*).
6. Collect the next portion of the urine in the sterile container, filling the container halfway without touching the inside of the container with the hands or the penis (Figure 3, *C*).
7. Void the last amount of urine into the toilet or urinal.
8. Place the lid on the container, taking care not to touch the interior surface of the lid. Wipe and redress.
9. Return the specimen to the designated area.
   <u>PURPOSE:</u> Instructions must be understood if they are to be followed correctly. By talking to the patient, you can determine whether the patient understands or has any questions.

Processing a Clean-Catch Urine Specimen
1. Document the date, time, and collection type.
2. Process the specimen according to the physician's orders. Perform urinalysis in the office or prepare the specimen for transport to the laboratory. If it is to be sent to an outside laboratory, complete the following steps:
   - Make sure the label is properly completed with patient information, date, time, and test ordered.
   - Place the specimen in a biohazard specimen bag.
   - Complete a laboratory requisition and place it in the outside pocket of the specimen bag.
   - Keep the specimen refrigerated until pickup.
   - Document that the specimen was sent.

TABLE 52-1   Changes in Urine at Room Temperature

CONSTITUENT	CHANGE
Clarity	Becomes cloudy as crystals precipitate and bacteria multiply
Color	May change if pH becomes alkaline
pH	Becomes alkaline as bacteria form ammonia from urea
Glucose	Decreases as it is metabolized by bacteria
Ketones	Decrease because of evaporation
Bilirubin and urobilinogen	Undergo degradation in light
Blood	May hemolyze; false-positive results are possible because of bacterial peroxidase
Nitrite	May become positive as bacteria multiply and reduce nitrate
Casts	Lyse or dissolve in alkaline urine
Cells	Lyse or dissolve in alkaline urine
Bacteria	Multiply twofold approximately every 20 minutes
Yeasts	Multiply
Crystals	Precipitate as urine cools; may dissolve if pH changes

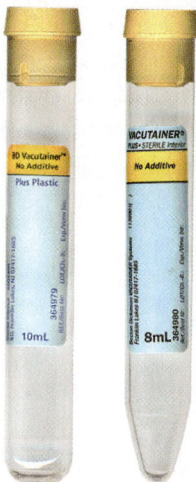

FIGURE 52-3 BD Vacutainer urine preservation tubes. (Courtesy Becton, Dickinson & Company, Franklin Lakes, New Jersey.)

is removed. The preservatives in the BD Vacutainer cherry red/yellow-stoppered tube—chlorhexidine, ethylparaben, and sodium propionate—prevent the overgrowth of bacteria and inhibit changes in the urine that can affect test results. Chemical reagent strip testing can be performed on preserved specimens; however, it should be performed within 72 hours. Tubes may be held at room temperature during this time.

A different preservative must be used for urine specimens slated for culture. The BD Vacutainer urine collection kit contains the preservatives sodium formate and boric acid to help preserve the level of bacteria present at the time of collection. This transport system should be used only for urine specimens that will be cultured. Results on the chemical reagent strip may be altered by these preservatives. **Culture and sensitivity (C&S)** testing should be performed within 72 hours. Tubes may be held at room temperature.

A laboratory request form must be completed for all specimens that will be transported to another site for analysis. Typical forms include the patient's name and the date, the type of urinalysis ordered, the name of the physician requesting the examination, the appropriate *International Classification of Diseases, Ninth Revision,*

Clinical Modification (ICD-9-CM) code for the diagnosis that warranted the test, and a line for the physician to sign after he or she has reviewed the results. Specimens are sent to the laboratory in a plastic biohazard bag that zips closed and has an outside pocket, where the laboratory request is placed.

GUIDELINES FOR CARING FOR A URINE SPECIMEN OBTAINED AT HOME

- Do not put anything but your urine into the bottle.
- Do not pour out any liquid or powdered preservative from the container.
- If you accidentally spill some of the preservative on yourself, immediately wash with water and call the testing center or designated laboratory.
- Always keep the collection bottle cool. Refrigerate or keep the bottle in an ice-filled cooler or pail.
- Keep the cap on the container.

CRITICAL THINKING APPLICATION 52-2

Dr. Hill has ordered a UA on the specimen from Mr. Parks, a UA and pregnancy test on the specimen from Mrs. Carpenter, and a UA and C&S on the specimen from Ms. Hillman. After reviewing the requisitions and entering the patient information into the daily logbook, Rosa notes that Mrs. Carpenter's specimen was collected at 6 AM—3 hours ago. Is this acceptable? Explain your answer. Rosa also notes that the specimen collected in the sterile container from Ms. Hillman is marked "CCMS." Why is this important?

ROUTINE URINALYSIS

Physical Examination of the Urine

The first part of a complete UA is assessment of the physical properties of the urine and measurement of selected chemical constituents that are diagnostically important (Table 52-2 and Procedure 52-3).

Appearance

Color. Normal urine is a shade of yellow, ranging from pale straw to yellow to amber. The color depends on the concentration of the pigment urochrome and the amount of water in the specimen. A dilute specimen should be pale, and a more concentrated specimen should be a darker yellow. Variations in color may be caused by diet, medication, and disease. Abnormal colors may be related to pathologic or nonpathologic factors (Table 52-3).

Turbidity. Both normal and abnormal urine specimens may range in appearance from clear to very cloudy. Cloudiness may be caused by cells, bacteria, yeast, vaginal contaminants, or crystals. Often a urine specimen that was clear when voided becomes cloudy as it cools, as crystals form and precipitate.

Volume

The amount of urine is rarely measured in a random specimen. With a timed specimen, volume is measured by pouring the entire

TABLE 52-2 Components of Macroscopic Urinalysis

PHYSICAL PROPERTIES	CHEMICAL PROPERTIES
Color	Protein
Clarity	Glucose
Specific gravity	Ketones
Volume*	Bilirubin
Odor*	Blood
Foam*	Nitrite
	pH
	Urobilinogen
	Leukocyte esterase

*Not always assessed.

TABLE 52-3 Causes of Urine Colors

COLOR	PATHOLOGIC CAUSE	NONPATHOLOGIC CAUSE
Straw	Diabetes	Diuretics; high fluid intake (coffee, beer)
Amber	Dehydration	Excessive sweating; low fluid intake
Bright yellow		Carotene, vitamins
Red	Blood, porphyrins	Menstruation, beets, drugs, dyes
Orange-yellow	Bile, hepatitis	Pyridium (phenazopyridine hydrochloride), dyes, drugs
Greenish yellow	Bile, hepatitis	Senna, cascara, rhubarb
Reddish brown	Old blood, methemoglobin	
Brownish black	Methemoglobin, melanin	Levodopa
Salmon pink		Amorphous urates
White (milky)	Fats, pus	Amorphous phosphates
Blue-green	Biliverdin, infection with *Pseudomonas* organisms	Vitamin B, drugs, dyes

collection into a large, graduated cylinder. Generally, it is not accurate enough to use the markings on the side of the collection container. Once the volume has been measured and recorded, a portion of well-mixed specimen, called an *aliquot,* is removed for testing. The remainder is discarded or stored, depending on the preference of the laboratory.

The normal volume of urine produced every 24 hours varies according to the age of the individual. Infants and children produce smaller volumes than adults. The normal adult volume is 750 to 2,000 mL in 24 hours; the average amount is about 1,500 mL.

PROCEDURE 52-3

Perform a Urinalysis and Patient Screening Using Established Protocols: Assess the Urine for Color and Turbidity—the Physical Test

GOAL: *To assess and record the color and clarity of a urine specimen.*

EQUIPMENT and SUPPLIES

- Urine specimen
- Centrifuge tube
- Disposable gloves
- Biohazard container
- Patient's record

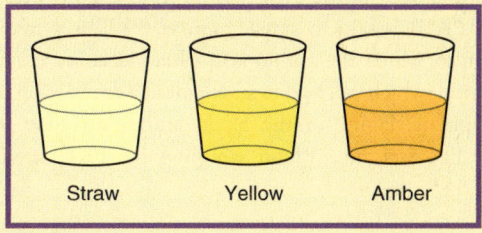

Straw   Yellow   Amber

PROCEDURAL STEPS

1. Sanitize your hands and put on gloves.
2. Mix the urine by swirling.
   PURPOSE: Suspended substances settle when urine stands. If urine is not mixed before assessment of appearance, the finding will be incorrect.
3. Label a centrifuge tube if a complete urinalysis is being done.
   PURPOSE: If a complete urinalysis is to be done, a portion of the specimen will be centrifuged for microscopic examination. The centrifuged specimen must be labeled to prevent specimen confusion.
4. Pour the specimen into a standard-sized centrifuge tube.
   PURPOSE: Standard-sized containers are better for assessing color and clarity results.
5. Assess and record the color (Figure 1):
   - Pale straw
   - Yellow
   - Amber

6. Assess the clarity:
   - Clear—no cloudiness
   - Slightly turbid—can see light print through tube
   - Moderately turbid—can see only dark print through tube
   - Very turbid—cannot see through tube
7. Clean the work area, remove your gloves, dispose of the gloves and procedure supplies in a biohazard waste container, and sanitize your hands.
   PURPOSE: To ensure infection control.
8. Record the results in the patient's record.
   PURPOSE: A procedure is considered not done until it is recorded.

Excessive production of urine is called *polyuria*. This is common in diabetes and in certain kidney disorders. Oliguria is insufficient production of urine, which can be caused by dehydration, decreased fluid intake, shock, or renal disease. The absence of urine production, anuria, occurs in renal obstruction and renal failure.

Foam

Normally the presence of foam is not recorded, but careful observation of this property can be a significant clue to an abnormality. Foam is seen as small bubbles that persist for a long time after the specimen has been shaken; they must not be confused with any bubbles that rapidly disperse. White foam can indicate the presence of increased protein (Figure 52-4). Greenish yellow foam can mean **bilirubinuria**. Care should be taken in handling such urines, because the color of the foam may indicate that the patient has viral hepatitis.

Odor

As with foam, odor is not normally recorded but can be an important clue to metabolic disorders. Normal urine is said to be aromatic. Changes in the odor of urine may be caused by disease, the presence of bacteria, or diet. The odor of the urine of a patient

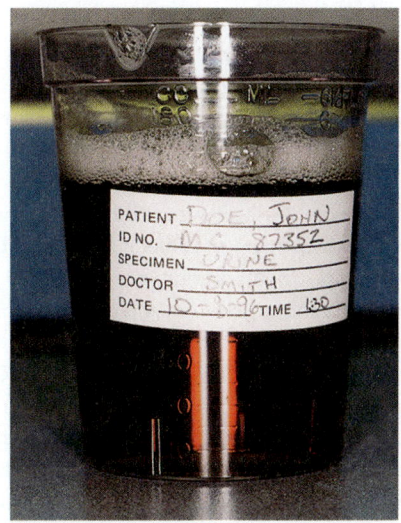

FIGURE 52-4 Dark amber urine with foam indicates possible increased protein and possible hematuria.

with uncontrolled diabetes is described as fruity because of the presence of ketones, which are the products of fat metabolism. An ammonia or putrid smell in the urine can be caused by an infection or may be noted in urine that has been allowed to stand before it is tested. The bacteria break down the urea in the urine to form ammonia. Foods such as asparagus and garlic also can produce an abnormal odor in the urine. Urine from a child with phenylketonuria (PKU) is said to smell "mousy." PKU is a rare hereditary condition in which the amino acid **phenylalanine** is not properly metabolized, which can lead to severe mental retardation. Accumulation of phenylalanine in the blood and urine gives body fluids an odor like wet fur. (Blood sampling for PKU is discussed in Chapter 54.)

Specific Gravity

Specific gravity is the weight of a substance compared with the weight of an equal volume of distilled water. In UA, it is the rough measurement of the concentration, or amount, of substances dissolved in urine. The specific gravity of distilled water is 1.000. The normal specific gravity of urine ranges from 1.005 to 1.030, depending on the patient's fluid intake. Most samples fall between 1.010 and 1.025. The urine specific gravity indicates whether the kidneys are able to concentrate the urine and is one of the first indications of kidney disease. The presence of glucose, protein, or an x-ray contrast medium used in diagnostic studies also may increase the specific gravity of urine. To measure the specific gravity of urine, laboratories may use a urinometer, a refractometer, or a chemical reagent strip.

A urinometer is a sealed glass float with a calibrated paper scale in its stem (Figure 52-5). According to guidelines established by the Occupational Safety and Health Administration (OSHA), urinometers containing mercury must be replaced, because mercury is a hazardous waste. With a slight spinning motion, the urinometer is placed in a cylinder containing a urine sample, and the value is read at the meniscus of the urine. Enough urine must be used to suspend the float freely—usually about 20 to 25 mL. If the sample is insufficient to float the urinometer, a refractometer can be used, or "QNS" (quantity not sufficient) can be recorded.

A urinometer is fragile, and jarring can cause the paper scale in the stem to shift, resulting in erroneous readings. Because a damaged urinometer occasionally loses its calibration, the calibration should be checked daily with distilled water. The specific gravity of the distilled water should calibrate at 1.000 at 20°C (68°F; room temperature). For example, if the urinometer reads 1.002 in distilled water, 0.002 must be subtracted from the urine readings. However, it is better to replace the instrument. For each 3°C (37.4°F) the water temperature measures above 20°C (68°F), 0.001 must be added to the reading. For each 3°C (37.4°F) the water temperature measures below 20°C (68°F), 0.001 must be subtracted from the reading. Use a laboratory thermometer to determine the water temperature. The urinometer method, although considered the **gold standard** of specific gravity testing, uses a large volume of urine and results in contamination of several pieces of glassware. For these reasons, it is rarely used in modern laboratories.

A refractometer measures the refraction of light through solids in a liquid. The result is called the *refractive index,* which for our purposes is the same as specific gravity (Figure 52-6). The refractometer

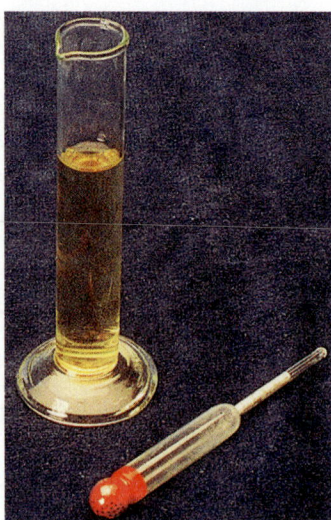

FIGURE 52-5 A urine-filled cylinder and urinometer.

is both faster and easier to use than the urinometer and requires only a drop of urine. One drop of well-mixed urine is placed under the hinged cover of the instrument, and the value is read directly from a scale viewed through an ocular. The refractometer must be calibrated daily with distilled water, which should read 1.000 (Procedure 52-4). Note that the measurement of specific gravity carries no unit of measure after the number.

The reagent strip (dipstick) test is the method most commonly used in the physician's office laboratory (POL), and it is considered a Clinical Laboratory Improvement Amendments (CLIA)-waived test. The pad on the strip contains a chemical that is sensitive to positively charged ions, such as sodium (Na^+) and potassium (K^+). The strip detects specific gravity in the range of 1.005 to 1.030.

> ## CRITICAL THINKING APPLICATION 52-3
>
> - The requisitions accompanying the urine specimens indicate that all three require a UA. Rosa performs the physical analysis and notes that Mrs. Carpenter's urine, which requires the pregnancy test, is amber, whereas the other two specimens are pale yellow. What are possible explanations for Rosa's observations? Should Rosa be concerned about the darker color of Mrs. Carpenter's urine?
> - Ms. Hillman's urine is turbid, whereas Mr. Parks's urine is clear. What might be causing the cloudiness in Ms. Hillman's urine? Is a cloudy urine cause for concern?

Chemical Examination of Urine

Tests can be performed on urine to detect the presence of certain chemicals, which can provide valuable information to the physician. In certain situations, these chemical test results can be critical to the diagnosis.

Reagent strip testing is the most widely used technique for detecting chemicals in the urine (Procedure 52-5); these strips are available in a variety of types (Figure 52-7). Generally, they are plastic strips to which one or more pads containing chemicals are attached. Tests are available for pH, specific gravity, vitamin C, leukocyte esterase,

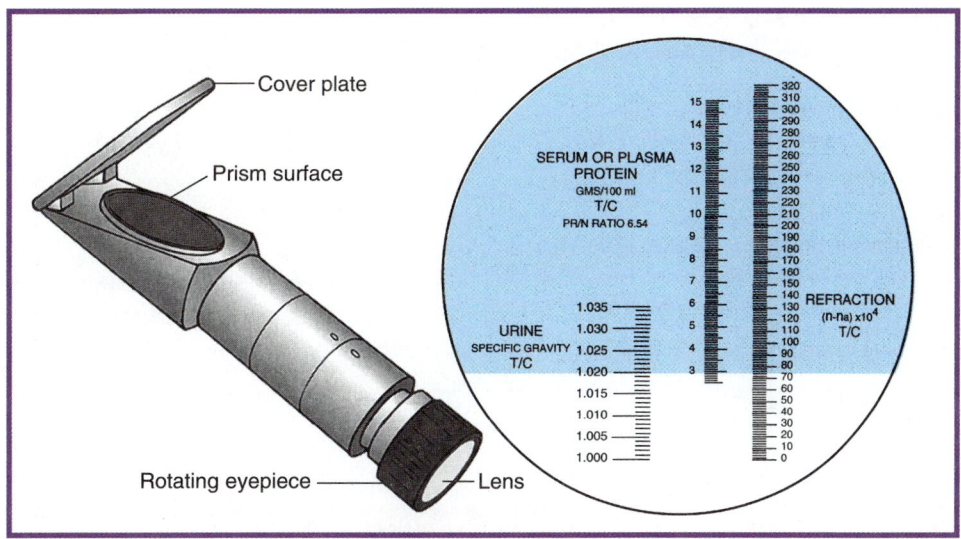

FIGURE 52-6 A refractometer.

PROCEDURE 52-4

Perform Quality Control Measures: Measure the Urine Specific Gravity with a Refractometer

GOAL: *To calibrate a refractometer and measure the refractive index of urine. A refractometer is also known as a total solids (TS) meter.*

EQUIPMENT and SUPPLIES

- Urinary refractometer
- Distilled water
- Disposable pipet
- Biohazard waste container
- Disposable gloves
- Patient's record

PROCEDURAL STEPS

1. Sanitize your hands and assemble the equipment while the urine specimen reaches room temperature.
   PURPOSE: Measuring the specific gravity of cold or warm urine may alter the results.
2. Put on gloves and mix the urine specimen in the collection container.
   PURPOSE: Mixing the urine resuspends solids that have settled during storage.
3. Using a disposable pipet, apply a drop of water to the prism of the refractometer (see Figure 52-6) by lifting the plastic cover. Close the cover and point the device toward a light source, such as a window or a lamp. Look into the refractometer and rotate the eyepiece so that the scale can be clearly read. The scale reads from 1.000 to 1.035 in increments of 0.001.
4. Calibrate the refractometer by inserting the small screwdriver provided by the manufacturer into the screw on the underside of the instrument. Turn the screw so that the line is positioned over 1.000 (Figure 1).
   PURPOSE: This step ensures that the refractometer has been calibrated properly and must be performed daily.

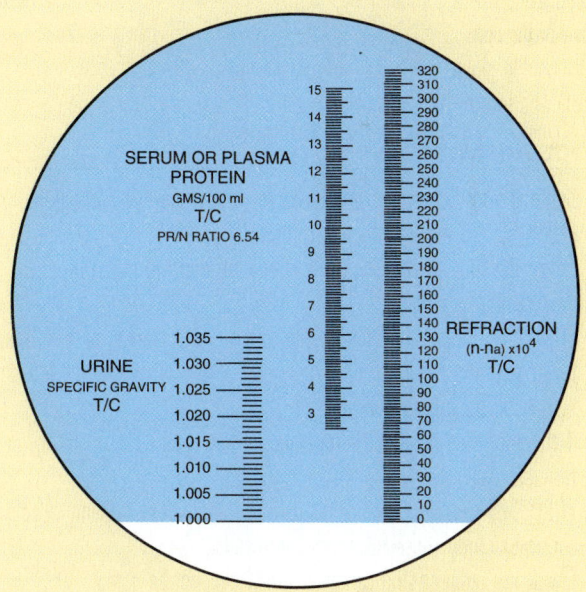

(From Stepp CA, Woods MA: *Laboratory procedures for medical office personnel*, Philadelphia, 1998, Saunders.)

5. Wipe the prism with a soft, lint-free tissue and apply a drop of mixed urine. Close the cover, point the device at a light source, and read the specific gravity on the scale. Discard the pipet in a biohazard waste container. The value for the specific gravity shown in Figure 52-7 is 1.020. Note that specific gravity has no units after the value.
   PURPOSE: A soft cloth should be used to prevent scratching of the glass prism.

PROCEDURE 52-4—cont'd

6. Wipe the urine from the prism with a disposable, soft, lint-free tissue between samples. When finished, clean with tissue moistened with alcohol or with a disposable alcohol wipe. Discard these tissues in a biohazard waste container.
   PURPOSE: Urine, a biohazardous material, must be removed from the prism. The prism must be decontaminated after use.
7. Discard the urine sample. Remove and discard your gloves in the biohazard container and sanitize your hands.

8. Document the results in the patient's record.
   PURPOSE: A procedure is not considered finished until it is recorded.

10/1/XX 9:28 AM SG: 1.010 Rosa Gonzales, CMA (AAMA) _____

PROCEDURE 52-5

Perform a Urinalysis and Patient Screening Using Established Protocols: Test Urine with Chemical Reagent Strips—the Chemical Urinalysis

GOAL: *To perform chemical testing on a urine sample.*

EQUIPMENT and SUPPLIES

- Urine specimen
- Reagent strips
- Timer
- Biohazard waste container
- Eye protection
- Disposable gloves
- Patient's record

PROCEDURAL STEPS

1. Sanitize your hands. Put on nonsterile gloves and eye protection.
   PURPOSE: To ensure infection control.
2. Check the time of collection, the container, and the mode of preservation.
   PURPOSE: Proper specimen identification and screening of specimens for appropriate collection containers and collection procedures prevent testing of inappropriate specimens.
3. If the specimen has been refrigerated, allow it to warm to room temperature.
   PURPOSE: Certain tests are temperature dependent. Testing of cold specimens may cause false-negative results.
4. Check the reagent strip container for the expiration date.
   PURPOSE: Do not use expired reagents.
5. Remove the reagent strip from the container. Hold it in your hand or place it on a clean paper towel. Recap the container tightly.
   PURPOSE: Test strips are sensitive to moisture and light and must be stored in tightly sealed containers. Contamination from chemical residues on countertops can affect results.
6. Compare nonreactive test pads with the negative color blocks on the color chart on the container.
   PURPOSE: Discolored pads indicate that the product has not been properly stored and must not be used for testing.

7. Thoroughly mix the specimen by swirling.
   PURPOSE: If settling occurs, certain elements may not be detected.
8. Following the manufacturer's directions, note the time, dip the strip into the urine, and then remove it.
   PURPOSE: Tests are time dependent. Some pads darken over time.
9. Quickly remove the excess urine from the strip by touching the side of the strip to a paper towel or to the side of the urine container.
   PURPOSE: Excess urine on the strip or prolonged dipping time affects test results.
10. Hold the strip horizontally. At the required time, compare the strip with the appropriate color chart on the reagent container (Figure 1). Document on the reagent strip flow sheet each result as it is read. Alternately, the strip can be placed on a paper towel.
    PURPOSE: Holding the strip horizontally prevents runover from one test pad to another and prevents interference from mixing of chemicals in the test pads.

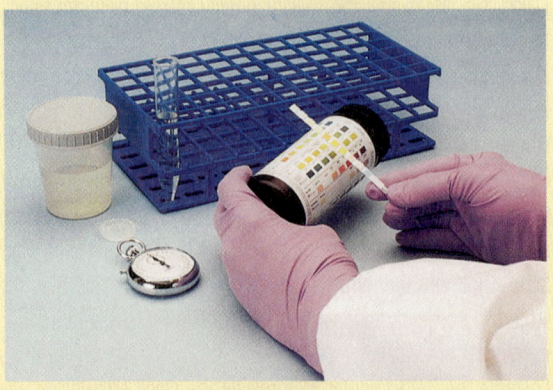

11. Read the concentration by comparing the strip with the color chart on the side of the bottle (Figure 2). *Do not touch the strip to the bottle.*
    PURPOSE: Timing is critical. Allowing the strip to come in contact with the bottle contaminates the bottle.

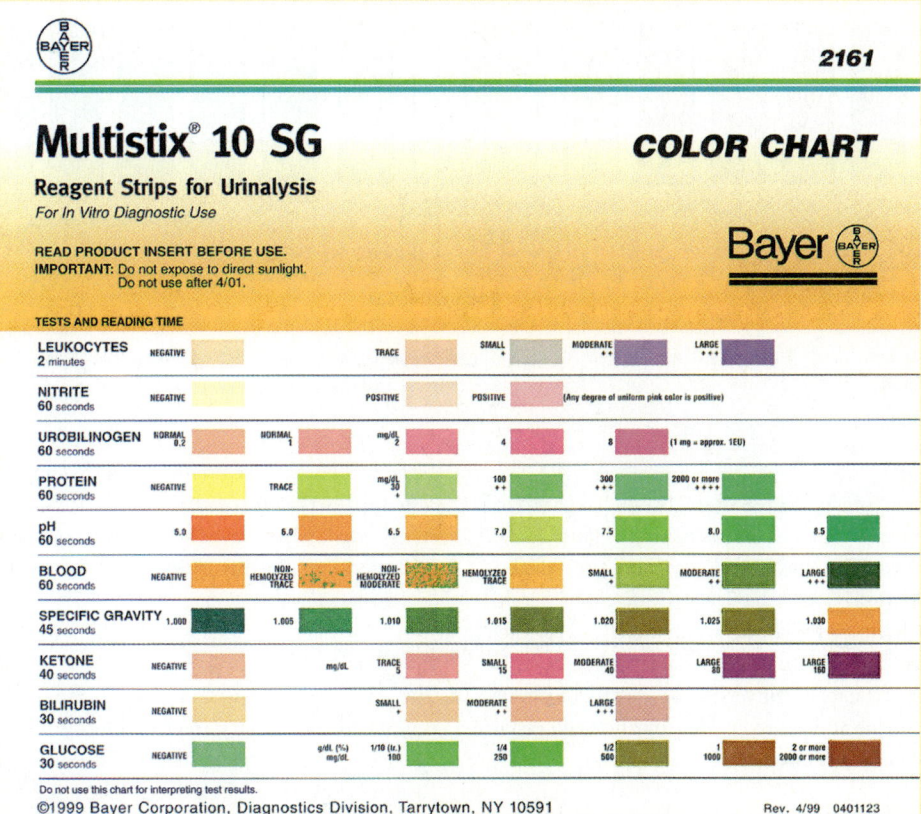

(From Bonewit-West K: *Clinical procedures for medical assistants*, ed 8, St. Louis, 2012, Saunders.)

12. Clean the work area, remove your gloves, and sanitize your hands. If a paper towel was used, dispose of it, the reagent strip, and your gloves in the biohazard container.
    <u>PURPOSE:</u> To ensure infection control.

13. Document the results in the patient's record.
    <u>PURPOSE:</u> A procedure is considered not done until it is recorded.

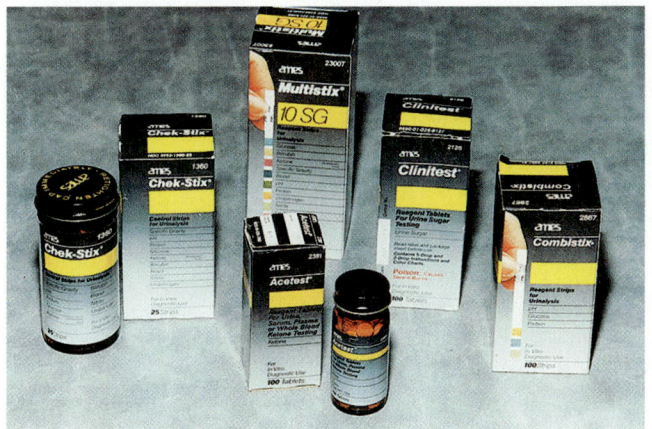

FIGURE 52-7 Examples of reagent strips.

protein, ketones, glucose, blood, bilirubin, nitrite, urobilinogen, phenylketones, and other chemicals. The presence or absence of these chemicals in the urine provides information on the status of carbohydrate metabolism, liver and kidney function, and the patient's acid-base balance.

Reagent strips are designed to be used once and then discarded. The directions for each strip are included inside the package, and these instructions must be followed exactly if accurate results are to be obtained. A color comparison chart is provided on the label of the container. In addition to reagent strips, various tablet tests are available.

All strips and tablets must be kept in tightly closed containers in a cool, dry area and should be removed immediately before testing. To prevent contamination of the bottle, never touch a strip that has been exposed to urine against the color comparison chart. If both a UA and a C&S have been ordered for a specimen, the urine must be cultured before the UA is started, because introducing a reagent strip into the urine contaminates it.

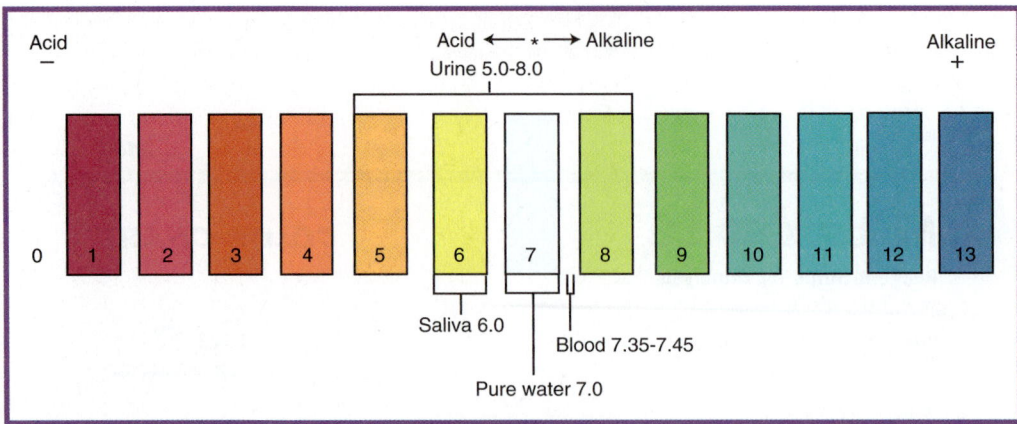

FIGURE 52-8 The pH scale. (From Stepp CA, Woods MA: *Laboratory procedures for medical office personnel*, Philadelphia, 1998, Saunders.)

pH

The pH is a measurement of the degree of acidity or alkalinity of the urine. A urine specimen with a pH of 7 is neutral (Figure 52-8). A value below 7 indicates acidity, and one above 7 indicates alkalinity. Normal, freshly voided urine may have a pH range of 5.5 to 8. The urinary pH varies with an individual's metabolic status, diet, drug therapy, and disease. In the case of gross bacteriuria, the urine pH is alkaline as a result of bacterial conversion of urea to ammonia. Knowing the pH of the urine also assists in identification of crystals if they are found in the urine **sediment.**

Glucose

Glucose is filtered at the glomerulus, but under normal conditions most of it is reabsorbed in the tubules. The minute quantities normally present in the urine are not detected by reagent strips and tablets. Detectable glycosuria occurs whenever the renal tubules cannot reabsorb the filtered glucose load. A positive glucose finding is common in urine from patients with diabetes and may be the first indication of the disease. The reagent strip glucose testing method is based on an **enzymatic reaction.** It detects only glucose; in other words, it is specific for glucose.

Protein

Protein in the urine in detectable amounts is called *proteinuria* and is one of the first signs of renal disease. We normally excrete a small amount of protein every day; proteinuria may be light to heavy, constant or sporadic. It may be affected by posture; in orthostatic proteinuria, protein is excreted only when the patient is in an upright position. Generally, first morning specimens from these patients are negative, but protein is found in urine passed throughout the day. Proteinuria is a common finding in pregnancy. It also is almost always present after heavy exercise. The reagent strip is highly sensitive to urinary albumin and is less sensitive to hemoglobin, immunoglobulin, and mucoproteins.

Ketones

Ketones are the end product of fat metabolism in the body. Acetoacetate, acetone, and beta-hydroxybutyric acid are collectively called *ketone bodies,* or *ketones.* Ketonuria is common with starvation, low-carbohydrate diets, excessive vomiting, and diabetes mellitus. Because ketones evaporate at room temperature, urine should be tested immediately, or the specimen should be tightly covered and refrigerated. The reagent strip detects only acetoacetate. The Acetest, discussed later in this chapter, can be used to detect both acetone and acetoacetate.

Blood

The presence of blood in the urine may indicate infection or trauma to the urinary tract or bleeding in the kidneys. The blood test pad on the reagent strip reacts with three different blood constituents: intact red blood cells, hemoglobin from red blood cells, and myoglobin, a hemoglobinlike molecule that transports oxygen in muscle tissue.

Hematuria is the presence of intact red blood cells in urine. The color reaction on the reagent strip ranges from yellow through green to dark green when hematuria is present, revealing a speckled appearance. Hematuria can be caused by irritation of the ureters, bladder, or urethra. It also is a common finding in cystitis and in individuals passing kidney stones. A random specimen may contain blood from vaginal contamination if the woman is menstruating.

Hemoglobinuria is the presence of hemolyzed red blood cells. True hemoglobinuria is rare. It occurs as a result of intravascular red blood cell destruction and can be caused by transfusion reactions, malaria, drug reactions, snake bites, and severe burns. **Myoglobinuria** occurs when muscle tissue is damaged or injured, as in crushing injuries, myocardial infarctions, and contact sports. Patients with muscular dystrophy often have myoglobinuria. Hemoglobinuria cannot be distinguished from myoglobinuria by reagent strip testing; both cause a uniform change in color from light green to dark green on the strip.

Bilirubin and Urobilinogen

Bilirubin is a product of the breakdown of hemoglobin. Hemoglobin is released from old red blood cells and is gradually converted to bilirubin in the liver, then further to urobilinogen in the intestines. Bilirubin is a bile pigment not normally found in urine. Its presence in urine is one of the first signs of liver disease or other disease in which the liver may be involved, such as infectious mononucleosis.

Bilirubinuria can occur even before jaundice or other symptoms of liver disease are evident. It is the result of liver cell damage or obstruction of the common bile duct by stones or neoplasms (tumors). Excessive bilirubin colors the urine yellow-brown to greenish orange. Because direct light causes decomposition of bilirubin, urine samples must be protected from light until testing is complete.

Urobilinogen normally is present in urine in small amounts. Increases are seen with increased red blood cell destruction and in liver disease. With total obstruction of the bile duct, no urobilinogen is formed in the intestines, none is reabsorbed into the circulation, and therefore none is present in the urine. Reagent strip methods cannot detect a decrease in urobilinogen.

Nitrite

Nitrite occurs in urine when bacteria break down nitrate, a common component of urine. A positive nitrite test result may indicate the presence of a urinary tract infection (UTI). However, not all bacteria are able to reduce nitrate to nitrite. Negative nitrite test results also can occur when bacteria are insufficient, or when the urine has not incubated in the bladder long enough for the reaction to occur. *Escherichia coli,* the organism that causes most UTIs, reduces nitrate to nitrite. False-positive results can occur if a specimen is allowed to sit at room temperature and contaminating bacteria multiply. False-negative results may occur if the bacteria further metabolize the nitrite they have produced to ammonia.

Leukocyte Esterase

Leukocytes (white blood cells) occur in urine with infections of the urinary tract. They also can be contaminants from the vagina. The leukocyte esterase test on reagent strips detects intact and lysed **polymorphonuclear white blood cells.** However, it does not detect **mononuclear white blood cells,** which occasionally are present during infection. The test does not react with the small numbers of white blood cells found in normal urine.

Limitations of Reagent Strip Testing

The reagent strip is a reliable method of chemical analysis of urine if used properly. The normal urine reference ranges for a reagent strip can be found in Table 52-4. Error can arise from a number of sources, for example, if the strip is soaked excessively in the specimen, chemicals in the pads may be diluted. If the strip is not held horizontally while read, colors from one pad may bleed onto another. Finally, certain chemicals, such as ascorbic acid, may affect the results of nitrite, glucose, bilirubin, and occult blood tests. Normal levels of vitamin C do not interfere, but if a person consumes large amounts of the vitamin, a special strip can be used to detect interfering levels of vitamin C. If an elevated level is found, the patient should be instructed to discontinue vitamin C intake for 24 hours and then another urine specimen should be collected for testing.

Visual interpretation of color on the reagent strip pads is likely to vary among individuals, and some laboratories use automated instruments to read the strips. Several companies manufacture instruments that use the principle of reflectance photometry in the analysis of reagent strip color. Once the strip has been placed in the instrument, a microprocessor controls the movement of the strip into the reflectometer. There, light of specific wavelengths is beamed onto the strip. Some light is absorbed, and some scatters or is reflected. The amount of reflected light is analyzed by the

microprocessor and is converted into a digital reading, and the result is printed out (Figure 52-9). The advantage of this method is that timing and color interpretation are consistent. The disadvantage is that the instrument is not able to identify and compensate for highly pigmented urine, leading to false-positive results. The medical assistant should be aware of this and should manually test urine specimens that are darkly pigmented.

TABLE 52-4	Normal Urine Reference Ranges for Reagent Strips
REFERENCE	**RANGE**
Color	Pale yellow to straw
Clarity	Clear to slightly turbid
Specific gravity	1.001-1.035
pH	4.6-8
Protein (mg/dL)	NEG
Glucose (mg/dL)	NEG
Ketone (mg/dL)	NEG
Bilirubin (mg/dL)	NEG
Blood (mg/dL)	NEG
Nitrite (mg/dL)	NEG
Urobilinogen (Ehrlich units)	0.1-1
White blood cells	NEG

CRITICAL THINKING APPLICATION 52-4

- Rosa prepares to do the chemical examination of the three urine specimens. Remember, Dr. Hill has ordered a UA on the specimen from Mr. Parks, a UA and pregnancy test on the specimen from Mrs. Carpenter, and a UA and C&S on the specimen from Ms. Hillman. Should Rosa proceed with the chemical analysis of each specimen in exactly the same manner? Explain your answer.
- On completing the chemical analysis of the three specimens, Rosa notes several differences among the samples. Mrs. Carpenter's sample has a high specific gravity. Ms. Hillman's sample reveals an elevated nitrite level, a pH of 8, and an elevated leukocyte esterase reading. Mr. Parks's test results reveal elevated glucose and ketone levels and a specific gravity of 1.035. Based on this information, what are the probable reasons each of these patients visited Dr. Hill today?

Microscopic Examination of Urine Sediment

Microscopic examination of urine (Procedure 52-6) consists of categorizing and counting cells, casts, crystals, and miscellaneous constituents of the sediment obtained when a measured portion of urine is centrifuged. The test is not categorized as CLIA waived; therefore, it would not be performed by a medical assistant without additional training and rigid compliance with CLIA quality assurance protocols for the laboratory, including periodic proficiency testing. However,

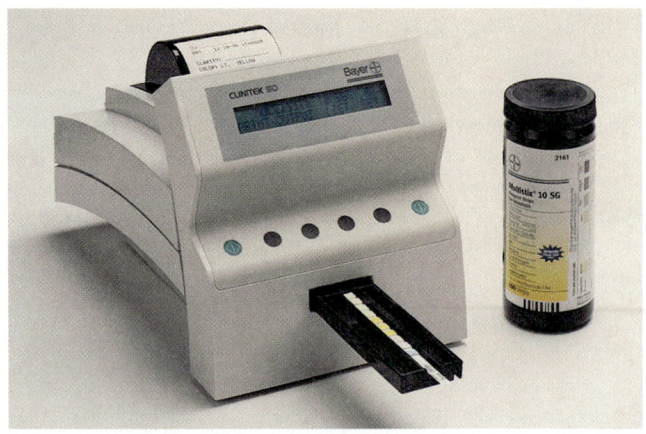

ID: _____*Erika Seager*_____
       11-16-XX   5:37 PM
CLARITY: _____*Clear*_____
COLOR: YELLOW

MULTISTIX 10 SG

GLU	NEGATIVE
BIL	NEGATIVE
KET	NEGATIVE
SG	1.025
BLO	TRACE-LYSED
pH	5.5
PRO	NEGATIVE
URO	0.2 E.U./dl
NIT	NEGATIVE
LEU	NEGATIVE

FIGURE 52-9 Sample printout from a Clinitek 50 Urine Chemistry Analyzer.

PROCEDURE 52-6

Perform a Urinalysis: Prepare a Urine Specimen for Microscopic Examination

GOAL: *To perform a microscopic examination of urine to determine the presence of normal and abnormal elements.*

EQUIPMENT and SUPPLIES

- Urine specimen
- Centrifuge tube
- Centrifuge
- Disposable pipet
- Microscope slide and coverslip
- Microscope
- Permanent marker
- Disposable gloves
- Face protection
- Biohazard waste container
- Patient's record

PROCEDURAL STEPS

1. Sanitize your hands. Put on nonsterile gloves and face protection.
   PURPOSE: To ensure infection control.
2. Gently mix the urine specimen.
   PURPOSE: If the urine is not well mixed, elements that have settled to the bottom of the specimen container will be missed.
3. Pour 10 mL of urine into a labeled centrifuge tube and cap the tube.
4. Place the tube in the centrifuge (Figure 1).

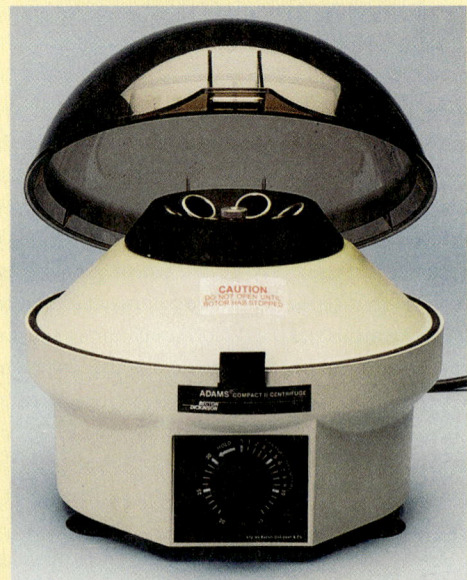

(From Stepp CA, Woods MA: *Laboratory procedures for medical office personnel*, Philadelphia, 1998, Saunders.)

PROCEDURE 52-6—cont'd

5. Place another tube containing 10 mL of water in the opposite cup.
   PURPOSE: For proper operation, centrifuges must be carefully balanced. If not properly balanced, damage to the instrument can occur.
6. Secure the lid and centrifuge for 5 minutes or for the time specified for your instrument.
   PURPOSE: Timing varies according to the speed and the size of the centrifuge head.
7. Remove the tube from the centrifuge after the instrument has come to a full stop.
8. Pour off the clear supernatant from the top of the specimen by inverting the centrifuge tube over the sink drain. Do not turn the tube upright until the supernatant has been fully decanted (Figure 2).

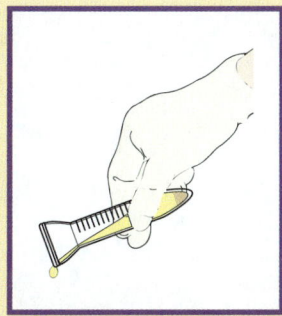

(From Stepp CA, Woods MA: *Laboratory procedures for medical office personnel*, Philadelphia, 1998, Saunders.)

9. Prevent the loss of sediment down the drain.
   PURPOSE: The sediment is what will be examined under the microscope.
10. Thoroughly mix the sediment by grasping the tube near the top and rapidly flicking it with the fingers of the other hand until all sediment is thoroughly resuspended (Figure 3).
    PURPOSE: Elements centrifuge at different rates. Failure to mix the entire sediment completely will cause errors in quantification.

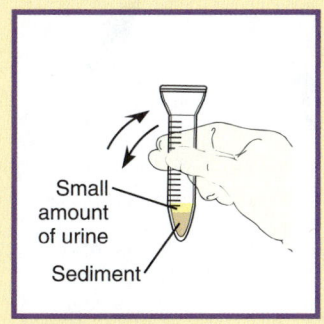

Small amount of urine

Sediment

(From Stepp CA, Woods MA: *Laboratory procedures for medical office personnel*, Philadelphia, 1998, Saunders.)

11. Transfer one drop of sediment to a clean, labeled slide using a clean, disposable transfer pipet.
12. Place a clean coverslip over the drop and place the slide on the microscope stage. Remove face protection.
    The remaining steps typically are performed by the healthcare practitioner. Medical assistants should not perform the microscopic examination unless they are specially trained to do so.
13. Focus under low power and reduce the light.
    PURPOSE: Mucus and casts are easily missed if reduced light is not used. Constant focusing helps locate them.
14. First, scan the entire coverslip for abnormal findings.
    PURPOSE: Casts tend to migrate to the edges of the coverslips.
15. Examine five low-power fields. Count and classify each type of cast seen, if any, and note mucus if present.
    PURPOSE: Choose five fields so that one is selected from each corner of the coverslip and the last one is chosen from the middle of the coverslip. If you move to an area and nothing is there, record a zero.
16. Switch to high-power magnification and adjust the light.
    PURPOSE: As magnification increases, more light is needed.
17. In five high-power fields, count the following elements: red blood cells, white blood cells, and round, transitional, and squamous epithelial cells.
18. In the same five fields, report the following as few, moderate, or many: crystals (identify and report each type seen separately), bacteria (identify as rods or cocci), sperm, yeast, and parasites.
    PURPOSE: *Few, moderate,* and *many* are more easily and universally understood than are exact numbers.
19. Average the five fields and report the results.
    NOTE: Steps 13 to 19 are performed only by qualified personnel.
20. Disinfect the work area, dispose of contaminated materials in a biohazard container, remove and dispose of gloves, and sanitize your hands.
21. Document the results in the patient's record.
    PURPOSE: A procedure is not considered finished until it is recorded.

medical assistants should be familiar with preparing the urine for this test and with the possible results. The clear upper portion of the specimen is called the *supernatant*. It is poured off, and a drop of the well-mixed sediment is examined under a microscope. The sediment may be stained with a **supravital** sediment stain to give greater contrast to the formed elements. The most commonly used stain is the Sternheimer-Malbin stain, which consists of crystal violet and safranin. This stain assists in the identification of formed elements by enhancing the detail of internal cellular structure.

Microscopic observation is performed with a bright field, phase contrast, or polarizing microscope. With a traditional bright field microscope, correct light adjustment is essential. The light must be reduced by closing the condenser iris diaphragm to increase the contrast. The condenser should be lowered slightly. Bright field microscopy is enhanced by the use of stains. Phase contrast microscopy converts variations in the refractive index into variations in contrast by fitting a bright field microscope with a special device known as an *annular ring*, which enhances contrast in living cells and low refractive index components. The polarizing microscope is used most often in the UA laboratory to confirm the presence of fat, specifically cholesterol, and to identify crystals.

Many formed elements are found in the urine. Some are significant; others are not. Most important, the microscopic examination should correlate with the physical and chemical analyses. For example, if the presence of red blood cells is confirmed on the reagent strip, red blood cells should be visible on the microscopic examination, and the urine may appear pink or red tinged.

Casts

Casts are formed when protein accumulates and precipitates in the kidney tubules and is washed into the urine. The protein takes on the size and shape of the tubules, hence the term *casts*. Casts are cylindric, with flat or rounded ends, and are classified according to the substances observed in them. Certain types of casts are associated with renal pathologic conditions; others are physiologic and are generally caused by strenuous exercise.

Casts are counted and reported under low-power magnification, but occasionally high-power magnification is needed to identify the type. Because casts tend to migrate to the edges of the coverslip, this area should be examined closely. Because casts dissolve in alkaline urine on standing, examination of a fresh urine specimen is very important.

Hyaline casts are pale, transparent, cylindric structures that have rounded ends and parallel sides (Figure 52-10). Hyaline casts will be missed entirely if the light is not reduced at the condenser. They are formed when urine flow through individual nephrons is diminished. They can be found in the urine of individuals with kidney disease but also in the urine of people without such disease who have exercised heavily. Occasionally, hyaline casts have granular or cellular inclusions.

White blood cell casts are hyaline casts that contain leukocytes. White blood cells usually have a multilobed nucleus, which differentiates them from renal tubular epithelial cells, which have single, round nuclei. White blood cell casts are seen in pyelonephritis (Figure 52-11).

Finely and coarsely granular casts may be caused by exercise, but the presence of increased numbers may indicate renal disease.

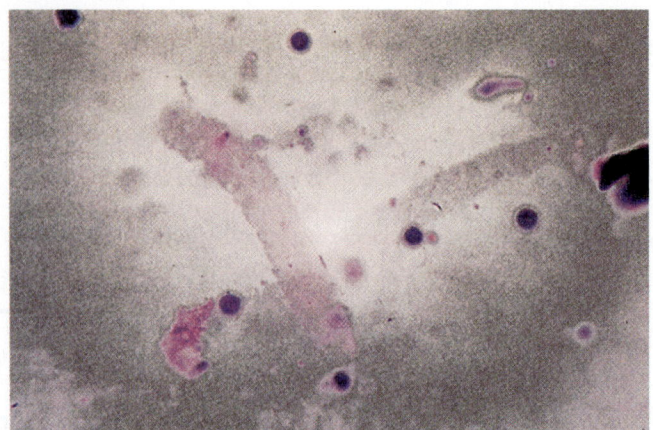

FIGURE 52-10 Hyaline casts (Sedi-Stain, 400×). (Modified from Bonewit-West K: *Clinical procedures for medical assistants*, ed 7, St Louis, 2008, Saunders.)

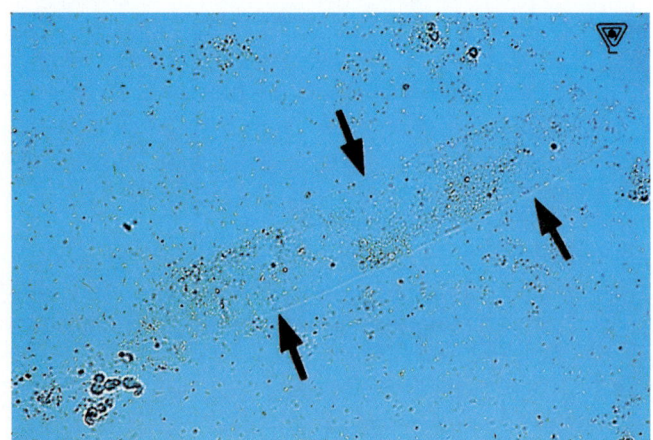

FIGURE 52-11 White blood cell casts. (From Stepp CA, Woods MA: *Laboratory procedures for medical office personnel*, Philadelphia, 1998, Saunders.)

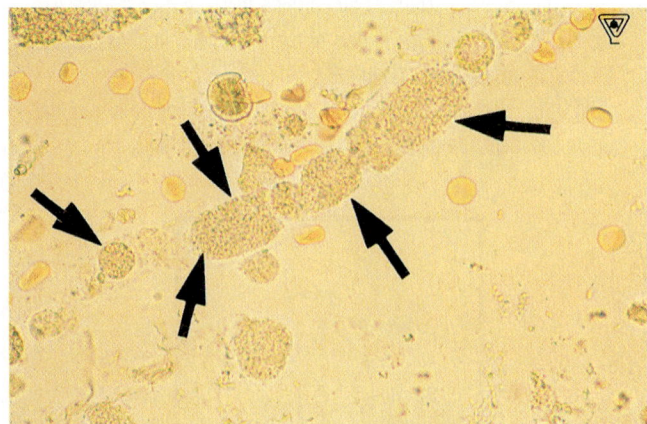

FIGURE 52-12 Granular casts. (From Stepp CA, Woods MA: *Laboratory procedures for medical office personnel*, Philadelphia, 1998, Saunders.)

On close examination, granular casts show a hyaline matrix with coarse or fine granular inclusions. The granules are thought to be caused by protein aggregation or degeneration of cellular inclusions (Figure 52-12).

Red blood cell casts always indicate a pathologic condition and are highly diagnostic. These casts occur in glomerulonephritis. They

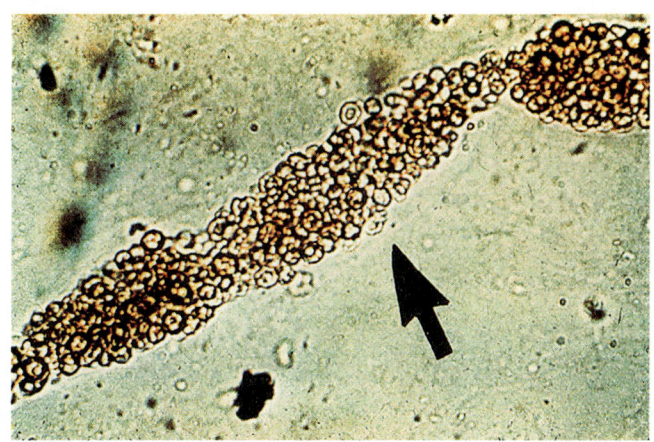

FIGURE 52-13 Red blood cell casts. (From Stepp CA, Woods MA: *Laboratory procedures for medical office personnel*, Philadelphia, 1998, Saunders.)

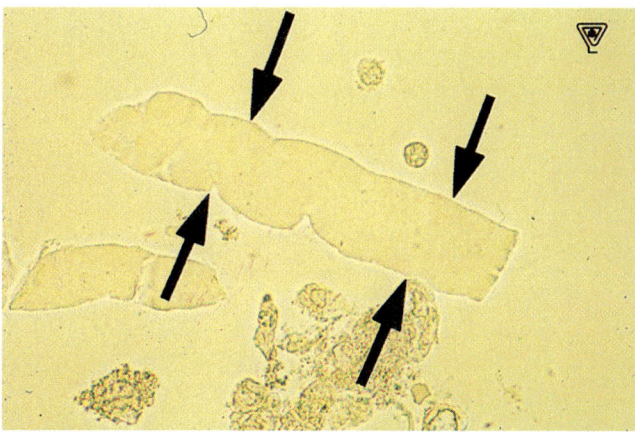

FIGURE 52-15 Waxy casts. (From Stepp CA, Woods MA: *Laboratory procedures for medical office personnel*, Philadelphia, 1998, Saunders.)

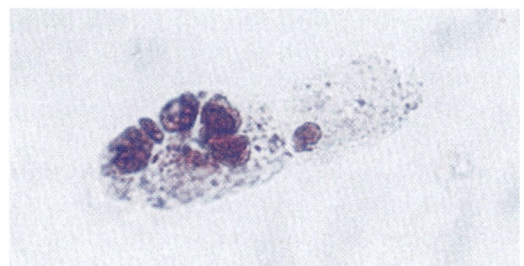

FIGURE 52-14 A renal tubular cell cast, seen with bright field microscopy (Sedi-Stain, 400×). (From Brunzel NA: *Fundamentals of urine and body fluid analysis*, ed 2, St Louis, 2004, Saunders.)

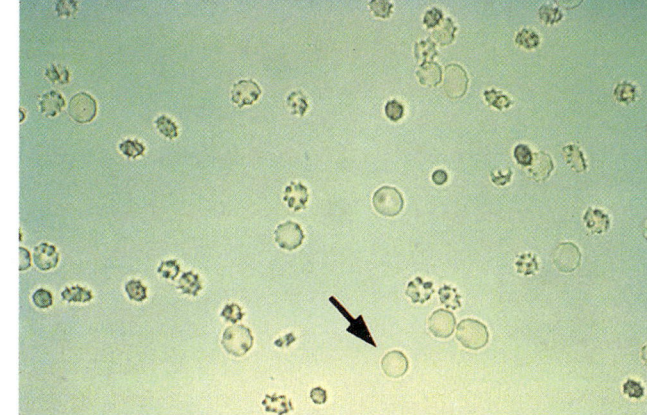

FIGURE 52-16 Red blood cells in the urine. (From Stepp CA, Woods MA: *Laboratory procedures for medical office personnel*, Philadelphia, 1998, Saunders.)

are hyaline casts with embedded red cells, and their presence indicates damage to the glomerular membrane. They may appear brown as a result of the color of the red blood cells present (Figure 52-13).

Renal tubular epithelial cell casts contain embedded renal tubular epithelial cells. These casts are easily confused with white blood cell casts, particularly if the cells have started to degenerate. Renal tubular epithelial cell casts are found when excessive damage has occurred. Causes are shock, renal ischemia, heavy-metal poisoning, certain allergic reactions, and nephrotoxic drugs (Figure 52-14).

Waxy casts are rarely seen. They appear as glassy, brittle, smooth, homogeneous structures. They usually are yellowish, have cracks or fissures, and have squared or broken ends. They are considered to be degenerated cellular casts and are found in individuals with severe renal disease (Figure 52-15).

Occasionally more than one type of cell is found in a single cast. Mixed cellular casts have been reported, and absolute identification of the cell types present may be difficult.

Cells

Cells found in the urine include epithelial cells, which are derived from the lining of the genitourinary tract, and red blood cells and white blood cells from the bloodstream. Cells are classified and counted under high-power magnification.

Red blood cells may enter the urinary tract at any point of inflammation or injury. They may be found in normal urine in small numbers—usually fewer than one or two per high-power field. Persistent hematuria should be investigated. Red blood cells are pale,

round, nongranular, and flat or biconcave (Figure 52-16). They are smaller than white blood cells and have no nucleus. In hypotonic (dilute) urine, they swell and burst. In hypertonic (concentrated) urine, they may **crenate** and wrinkle. When they crenate, they can be mistaken for white blood cells, because the wrinkled surface makes them appear granular. They often are confused with yeast (see Figure 52-23), oil droplets, and droplets of lens cleaner.

White blood cells, also called *leukocytes,* occasionally may be found in normal urine, but increased numbers (usually more than five cells per high-power field) are associated with inflammation or contamination of the specimen during collection. White blood cells are larger than red blood cells, have a granular appearance, and usually have a multilobed nucleus, although nuclear detail may not be evident. Most white blood cells in the urine are neutrophils (Figure 52-17).

Renal tubular or round epithelial cells are somewhat larger than white blood cells, are round or oval, and have a nucleus that is single, large, oval, and sometimes eccentric. A few may be found in normal urine specimens, but their presence in increased numbers indicates tubular damage (Figure 52-18).

Transitional epithelial cells line the urinary tract from the renal pelvis to the upper portion of the urethra. They vary from slightly

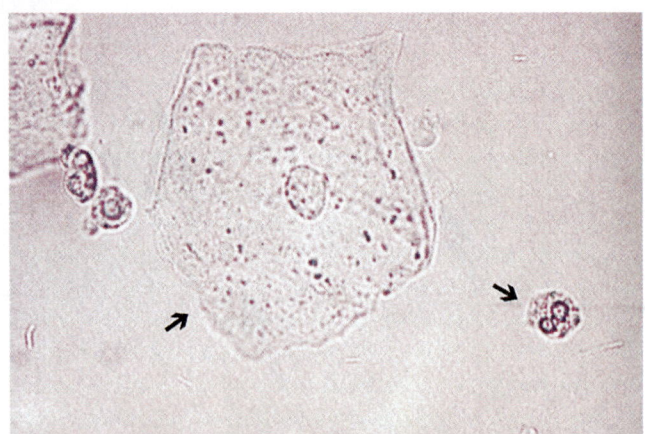

FIGURE 52-17 A white blood cell and a squamous epithelial cell (Unstained, 640×). (From Ringsrud KM, Linne JJ: *Urinalysis and body fluids: a color text and atlas,* St Louis, 1995, Mosby.)

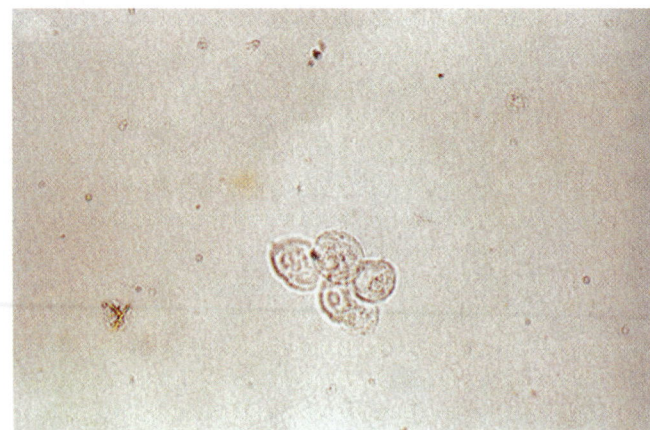

FIGURE 52-19 A cluster of small, unstained transitional epithelial cells (400×). (From Ringsrud KM, Linne JJ: *Urinalysis and body fluids: a color text and atlas,* St Louis, 1995, Mosby.)

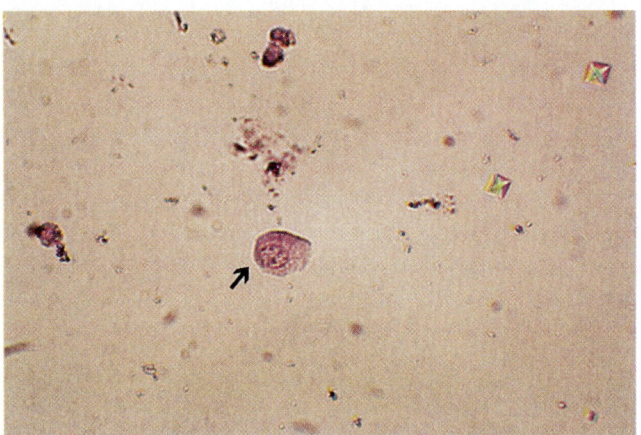

FIGURE 52-18 A renal epithelial cell *(arrow)* (Sedi-Stain, 400×). (From Ringsrud KM, Linne JJ: *Urinalysis and body fluids: a color text and atlas,* St Louis, 1995, Mosby.)

larger than a round epithelial cell to smaller than a squamous epithelial cell. They are round or oval and may have a tail. Occasionally, two nuclei are seen. When transitional cells are present in large numbers, a pathologic condition may exist (Figure 52-19).

Squamous epithelial cells line the lower portion of the genitourinary tract. When present in large numbers in female patients, they usually indicate vaginal contamination. Squamous epithelial cells are large, flat, irregular cells and are easily recognized under low-power magnification. They have a single, small, round, centrally located nucleus and often occur in sheets or clumps. Because of their flat nature, the edges of the cells often are rolled or folded (see Figure 52-19).

When identifying epithelial cells, it is helpful to remember the appearance of eggs; round epithelial cells resemble hard-boiled eggs that have been cut in half. Transitional forms resemble poached eggs, and squamous cells resemble fried eggs with large, runny whites.

Crystals

Crystals are common in urine specimens, particularly if the specimen has been allowed to cool. Cooling causes the solid crystals to precipitate out of the urine. The presence of most crystals is not clinically significant unless they are found in large numbers. With only very rare exceptions, abnormal crystals are seen in acidic urine. Abnormal crystals may be of metabolic origin and are present because of certain disease states or an inherited metabolic condition, or they may be of iatrogenic origin and are present as a result of medication or treatment. Identification of crystals begins with determination of the pH of the urine to ascertain whether the sample is acidic or alkaline. Next, the color, shape, and refractivity are observed. Viewing with a polarized or phase microscope or using a supravital stain can assist in identification. Often a history of medication intake and recent diagnostic testing is helpful.

Crystals are identified with low-power and high-power lenses, and their presence is reported as *occasional, few, moderate,* or *many* per high-power field (Table 52-5). At times crystals can be amorphous. Amorphous urates (Figure 52-20) are salts of uric acid and are seen as shapeless granulation in acidic urine. Amorphous phosphates (Figure 52-21) are found in alkaline urine and are seen as fluffy white precipitate. Amorphous crystals often are so profuse that they obscure other formed elements in the sediment. Frequently crystals are difficult to identify without additional chemical testing, such as solubility testing in acid and base.

Miscellaneous Findings

Oval fat bodies are formed when renal tubular epithelial cells or macrophages absorb fats. The fat droplets in the cells vary in size and are quite **refractile.** Oval fat bodies are characteristic of nephrotic syndrome and are best distinguished by using Sudan III stain, because they are easily confused with other elements (Figure 52-22).

Yeast in the urine may indicate vaginal contamination or infection of the urine with yeast (Figure 52-23). Yeast is common in the urine of patients with diabetes. Yeasts are easily confused with red blood cells; they usually are oval, may show budding, and are more refractile. To differentiate yeast from red blood cells, a drop of sediment is placed on the blood test pad of a reagent strip. Yeast does not react, but red blood cells do. Red blood cells dissolve when a drop of dilute acetic acid (regular white vinegar) is added to the sediment, but the yeast remains intact.

A few bacteria may be found in normal urine specimens. Heavy bacterial concentrations in the absence of white blood cells may

TABLE 52-5 Normal and Abnormal Crystals Found in the Urine

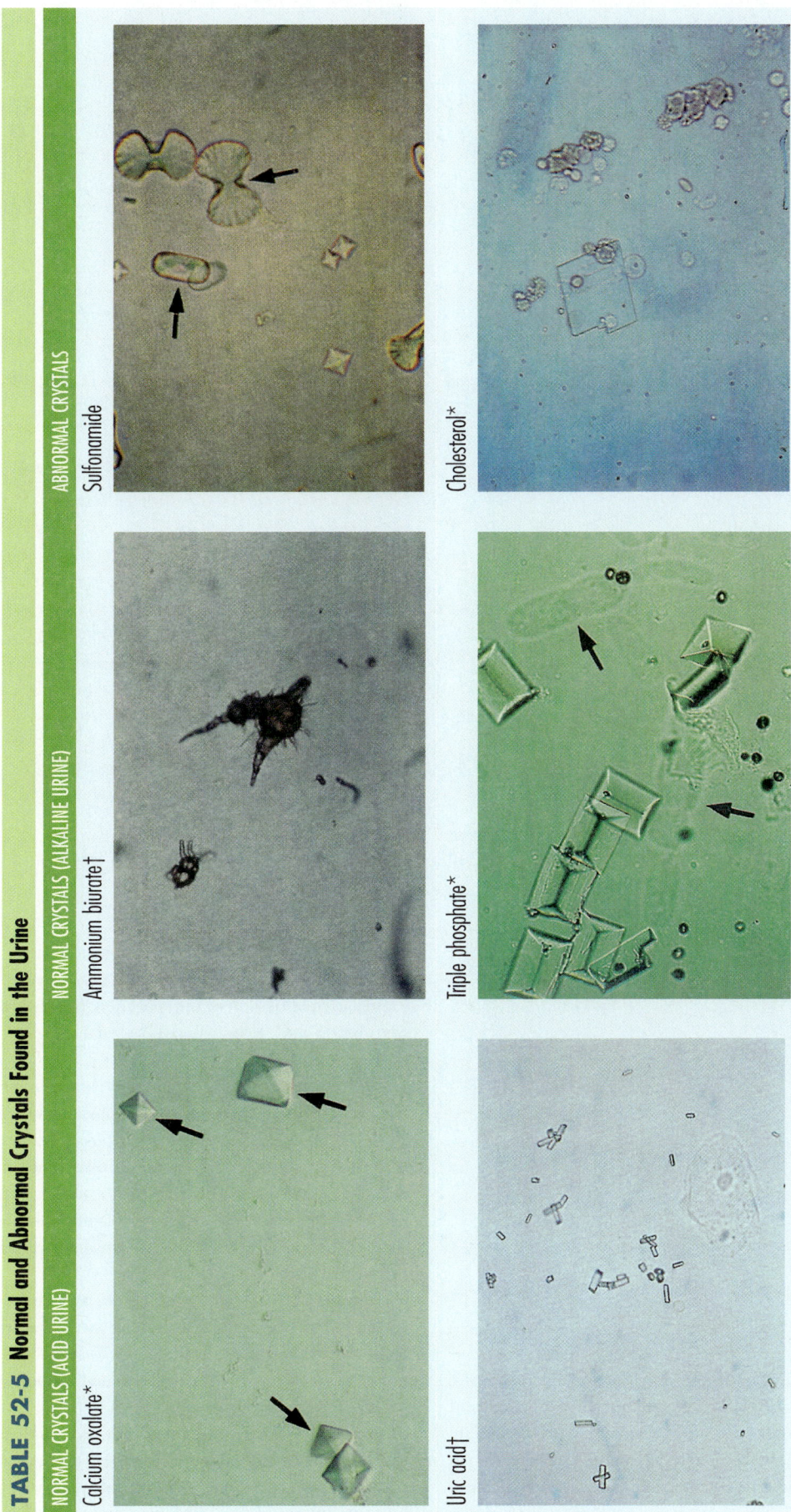

NORMAL CRYSTALS (ACID URINE)

Calcium oxalate*

Uric acid†

NORMAL CRYSTALS (ALKALINE URINE)

Ammonium biurate†

Triple phosphate*

ABNORMAL CRYSTALS

Sulfonamide

Cholesterol*

*From Stepp CA, Woods MA: *Laboratory procedures for medical office personnel,* Philadelphia, 1998, Saunders.
†From Ringsrud KM, Linne JJ: *Urinalysis and body fluids: a color text and atlas,* St Louis, 1995, Mosby.

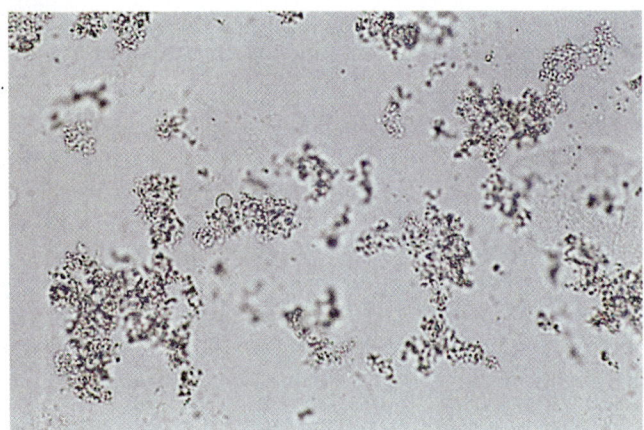

FIGURE 52-20 Amorphous urates (400×). (From Ringsrud KM, Linne JJ: *Urinalysis and body fluids: a color text and atlas*, St Louis, 1995, Mosby.)

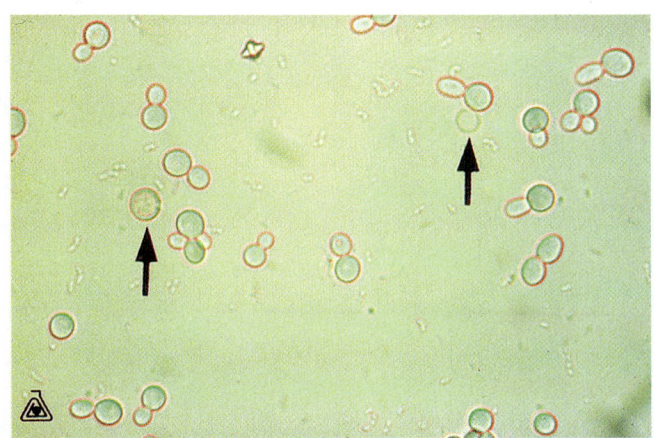

FIGURE 52-23 Yeast in the urine. (From Stepp CA, Woods MA: *Laboratory procedures for medical office personnel*, Philadelphia, 1998, Saunders.)

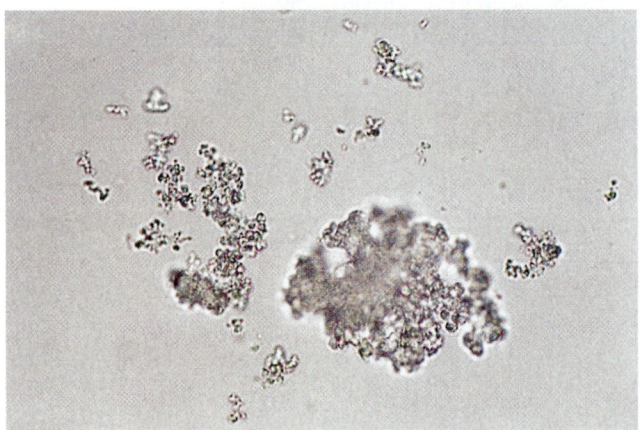

FIGURE 52-21 Amorphous phosphates (400×). (From Ringsrud KM, Linne JJ: *Urinalysis and body fluids: a color text and atlas*, St Louis, 1995, Mosby.)

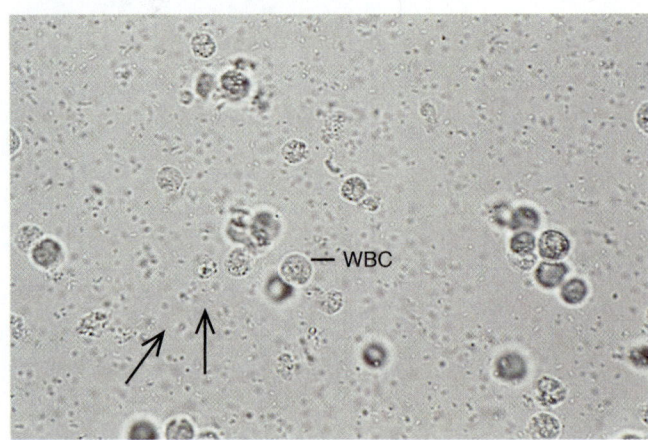

FIGURE 52-24 These small, rod-shaped bacteria *(arrows)* appear like possible cocci and white cells (Unstained, 400×). (From Ringsrud KM, Linne JJ: *Urinalysis and body fluids: a color text and atlas*, St Louis, 1995, Mosby.)

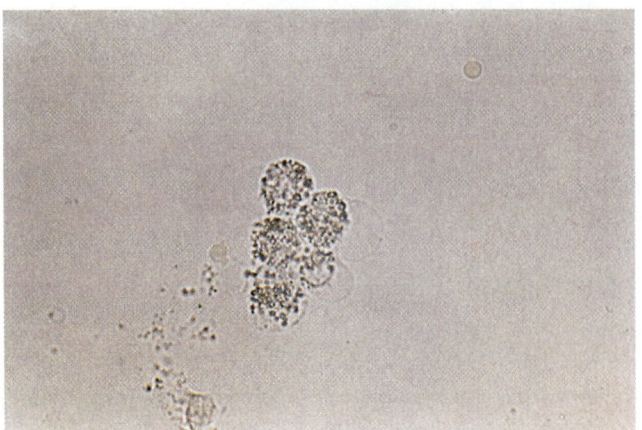

FIGURE 52-22 A small cluster of oval fat bodies (Unstained, 400×). (From Ringsrud KM, Linne JJ: *Urinalysis and body fluids: a color text and atlas*, St Louis, 1995, Mosby.)

indicate that the specimen was allowed to sit at room temperature and the bacteria multiplied. Urine specimens with a putrid odor, numerous white blood cells, and bacteria (Figure 52-24) are common with UTIs. The bacteria may be bacilli (rod shaped) or cocci (spheric) and are identified under high-power magnification. They are often motile.

Spermatozoa can be found in the urine specimens of both male and female patients. In the latter case, their presence represents vaginal contamination of the specimen. Sperm usually have pointed, oval heads and long, threadlike tails. They may be motile in fresh urine.

The most commonly encountered parasite in urine is *Trichomonas vaginalis* (Figure 52-25). It is usually a vaginal contaminant but may also be found in urine specimens from male patients. When urine is fresh and warm, *Trichomonas* organisms may be motile and may dart about rapidly. *Trichomonas* organisms are pear-shaped protozoa with four flagella. They are larger than round epithelial cells but smaller than squamous cells. *Trichomonas* organisms die when the specimen is cooled.

Mucous threads can be found in most urine specimens. They appear as pale, irregular, threadlike structures with tapered ends. Beginners often confuse hyaline casts with mucous threads. Increased numbers are seen with inflammation and in specimens contaminated with vaginal secretions (Figure 52-26).

Artifacts and contaminants often are found in urine sediment; training is required to differentiate them and to learn to ignore them. As a rule, structures that are apparent when you first view the sediment are unimportant. Starch granules are common artifacts simply

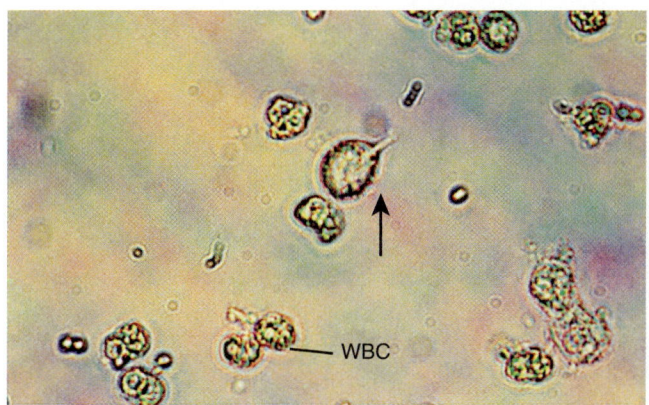

FIGURE 52-25 *Trichomonas organisms (arrow)* in the urine. (From Stepp CA, Woods MA: *Laboratory procedures for medical office personnel,* Philadelphia, 1998, Saunders.)

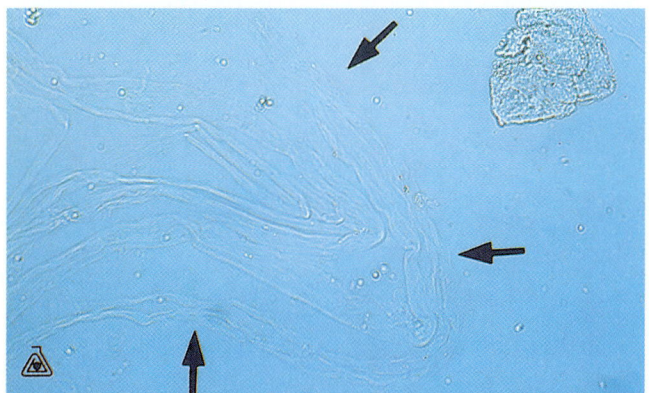

FIGURE 52-26 Mucous threads in the urine. (From Stepp CA, Woods MA: *Laboratory procedures for medical office personnel,* Philadelphia, 1998, Saunders.)

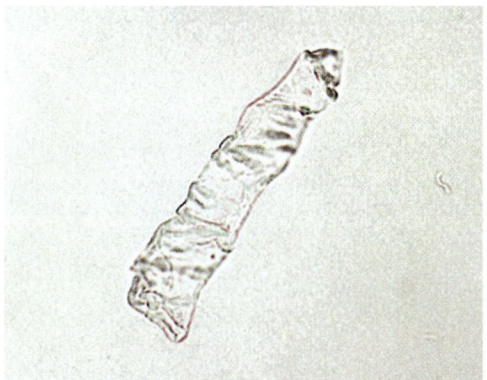

FIGURE 52-27 Diaper fibers. (From Ringsrud KM, Linne JJ: *Urinalysis and body fluids: a color text and atlas,* St Louis, 1995, Mosby.)

because of the extensive use of powdered gloves in the laboratory. The granules are highly refractile and dimpled, resembling a pillow with a center button. Fibers also are common in the sediment and come from clothing, diapers, or digested plant material. Clothing fibers often are long and twisted and sometimes are colored. Diaper fibers can be confused with casts (Figure 52-27). Plant fibers appear in the urine as a result of fecal contamination (Figure 52-28). Hair is distinguishable not only because of the visible rough and

fragmented cuticle, but also because of the size (Figure 52-29). Air bubbles are common if the coverslip was improperly placed over the sediment. Air bubbles are structureless and refractile and have a dark outline (Figure 52-30).

Interpretation of the Microscopic Examination

The medical assistant should understand how the findings of a microscopic examination of the sediment are reported. First, the sediment is examined under the low-power objective and low light to locate casts, which generally are found around the edges of the coverslip. Ten to 15 low-power fields are scanned, and the number of casts is counted and reported. The high-power objective and increased light then are used to identify red and white blood cells, epithelial cells, yeasts, bacteria, and crystals. Ten to 15 high-powered fields should be scanned and the number counted, averaged, and reported. The method of counting varies considerably among laboratories. It is important that all workers in the same laboratory use the same counting and reporting systems. Report the results of the microscopic examination as follows:

1. Separately total the number for each element counted, then average. (Casts, white blood cells, red blood cells, and the three categories of epithelial cells are counted, totaled, and averaged.) Casts, white blood cells, and red blood cells are reported using numeric ranges based on the average:

   0
   0-1
   1-2
   2-5
   5-10
   10-20 and so forth
   TNTC: too numerous to count

   Epithelial cells are reported as *occasional, few, moderate,* or *many,* as follows:

0	
0-3	Occasional
3-6	Few
6-12	Moderate
≥12	Many

2. Estimate the remaining elements as occasional, few, moderate, or many, as follows:

Occasional	Not seen in every field
Few	Covers less than a quarter of the field
Moderate	Covers approximately half of the field
Many	Covers the entire field

Do not report fibers, hair, talc granules, oil droplets, or other artifacts. These may be identified as amorphous debris on the laboratory report form.

Table 52-6 presents an example of the calculating and reporting of a microscopic UA examination.

Quality Assurance and Quality Control in Urinalysis

The U.S. Food and Drug Administration (FDA) categorizes the chemical analysis of urine performed by an instrument or a reagent strip as a CLIA-waived test. The chemical analysis includes the reagent strip (dipstick) tests for bilirubin, glucose, hemoglobin or

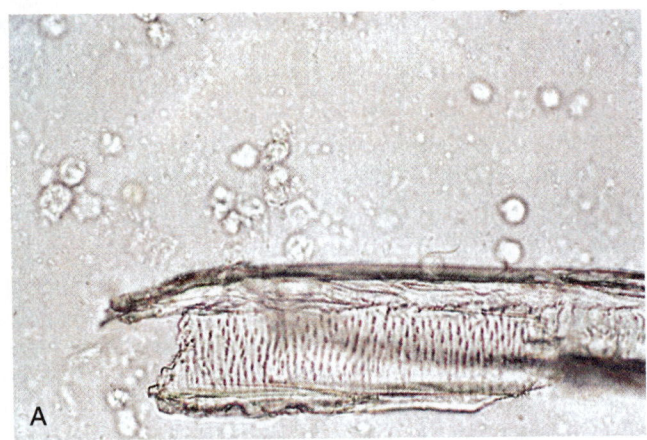
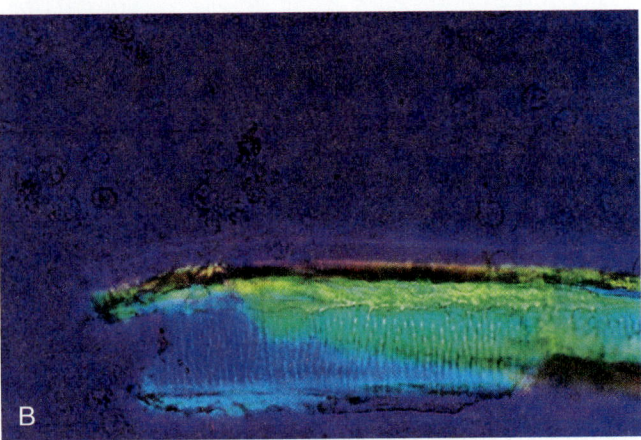

FIGURE 52-28 Plant fiber from fecal contamination; cells and bacteria also are present (400×). **A,** Bright field. **B,** Compensated polarized light showing birefringence. (From Ringsrud KM, Linne JJ: *Urinalysis and body fluids: a color text and atlas,* St Louis, 1995, Mosby.)

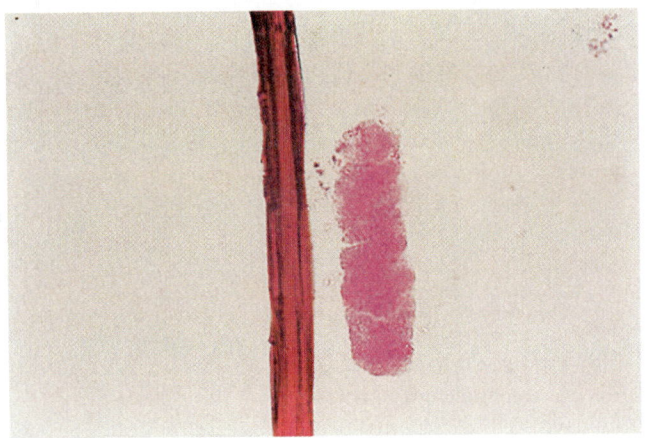

FIGURE 52-29 Fiber, probably hair *(left);* a waxy cast *(right)* (Sedi-Stain, 400×). (From Ringsrud KM, Linne JJ: *Urinalysis and body fluids: a color text and atlas,* St Louis, 1995, Mosby.)

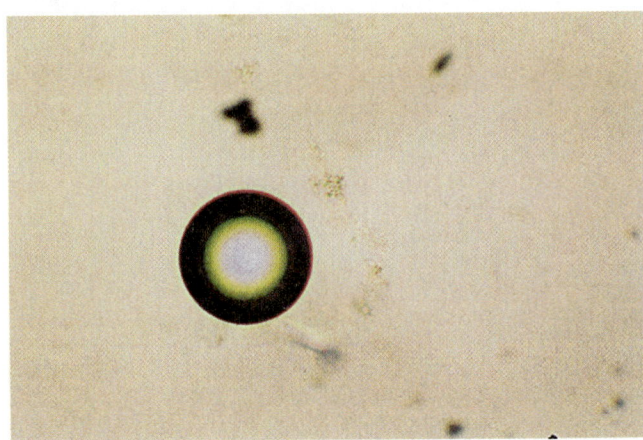

FIGURE 52-30 A large air bubble (400×). (From Ringsrud KM, Linne JJ: *Urinalysis and body fluids: a color text and atlas,* St Louis, 1995, Mosby.)

TABLE 52-6 Calculating a Microscopic Urinalysis

	PER LOW-POWER FIELD					PER HIGH-POWER FIELD					
FIELD	CASTS	MUCUS	SQUAMOUS EPITHELIAL CELLS	WBC	RBC	TRANSITIONAL EPITHELIAL CELLS	ROUND EPITHELIAL CELLS	BACTERIA	CRYSTALS	OTHER
1	0	Few	1	16	1	0	0	Moderate (rods)	Calcium oxalate—few Uric acid—few	—
2	1 hyaline	Few	3	32	0	0	0	Many	Calcium oxalate—few	Yeast
3	1 coarse granular	Moderate	3	21	2	0	0	Many	Calcium oxalate—few	Yeast
4	1 coarse granular	Few	5	12	1	0	1	Moderate	Uric acid—few	—
5	0	Few	4	25	0	0	0	Many	—	—
Total	1 hyaline 2 coarse granular	Few	16	106	4	0	1	Many	Calcium oxalate—few Uric acid—few	Yeast

TABLE 52-6 Calculating a Microscopic Urinalysis—Cont'd

		PER LOW-POWER FIELD				PER HIGH-POWER FIELD				
FIELD	CASTS	MUCUS	SQUAMOUS EPITHELIAL CELLS	WBC	RBC	TRANSITIONAL EPITHELIAL CELLS	ROUND EPITHELIAL CELLS	BACTERIA	CRYSTALS	OTHER
Average	0.2 hyaline 0.4 coarse granular	Few	3.2	21.2	0.8	0	0.2	Many	Calcium oxalate—few Uric acid—few	Yeast
Report	0-1 hyaline 0-1 coarse granular	Few	Few	20-30	0-1	0	Occasionally	Many (rods)	Calcium oxalate—few Uric acid—few	Yeast

RBC, Red blood cells; *WBC,* white blood cells.

PROCEDURE 52-7

Perform Quality Control Measures: Determine the Reliability of Chemical Reagent Strips

GOAL: *To reconstitute a control sample and test the reliability of the urinalysis chemical testing strip.*

EQUIPMENT and SUPPLIES

- Chek-Stix Control Strips for Urinalysis (Bayer)
- Distilled water
- Capped tube with milliliter markings
- Test tube rack
- Forceps
- Timer
- Chemical strips for urine testing
- Color chart for chemical strips
- Disposable gloves
- Biohazard waste container

PROCEDURAL STEPS

1. Assemble the equipment and supplies. Record the lot number and the expiration date of the Chek-Stix.
   PURPOSE: Chek-Stix cannot be used if they are past the expiration date. Recording the lot number and expiration date is an important part of quality assurance.
2. Sanitize your hands and put on nonsterile gloves.
   PURPOSE: To ensure infection control.
3. Place a conical tube in the rack and remove the cap.
4. Pour 15 mL of distilled water into the tube.
5. Using forceps, remove one strip from the bottle. Inspect the strips for mottling or discoloration.

PURPOSE: Mottling or discoloration may mean that the strips have been exposed to moisture, light, or solvents. Improperly stored control strips should not be used.
6. Place the strip into the water and tightly cap the tube.
7. Invert the tube for 2 minutes.
   PURPOSE: Chemicals embedded in the pads must be thoroughly dissolved in the water.
8. Allow the tube to sit in the rack for 30 minutes.
9. Invert the tube one time and remove the strip with forceps.
10. Discard the strip in a biohazard waste container. Once reconstituted, the control solution is stable for 8 hours at room temperature.
    PURPOSE: To ensure infection control.
11. Perform quality control of the chemical reagent strip by dipping it into the control solution according to Procedure 52-5.
12. Read and record the results.
13. Compare the results with the Chek-Stix package insert or chart on the bottle provided by the manufacturer.
    PURPOSE: Results should fall within a given range provided by the manufacturer. If they do not, the chemical reagent strips cannot be used to test patients' urine.
14. Discard the chemical reagent strip and the control solution into the biohazard container.
15. Clean up the work area, remove your gloves, and sanitize your hands.
    PURPOSE: To ensure infection control.

---

blood, ketones, leukocyte esterase, nitrite, pH, protein, specific gravity, and urobilinogen. To perform a microscopic UA procedure, a laboratory must be certified to perform moderate-complexity tests. Such a laboratory can also perform waived tests if it meets those qualifications (Procedure 52-7).

A commercially available control strip should be used to determine the reliability of the reagent strip used in chemical analysis. One such control strip is the Chek-Stix (Bayer, Tarrytown, New York). The plastic control strip has seven pads (Figure 52-31), each of which contains synthetic ingredients that mimic human urine

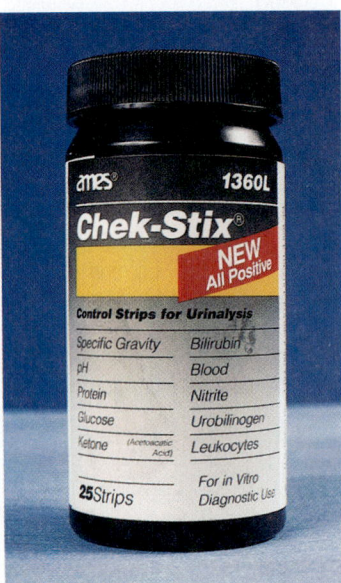

FIGURE 52-31 Chek-Stix control strips. (From Bonewit-West K: *Clinical procedures for medical assistants,* ed 7, St Louis, 2008, Saunders.)

when reconstituted in water. After reconstitution, a reagent strip is immersed in the solution and the results are compared with a chart that accompanies the Chek-Stix. Both positive and negative Chek-Stix strips are available (see Procedure 52-7).

Quality control is as important in the microscopic examination as in the chemical analysis of urine. To ensure consistency, standardized, commercially available systems can be used, such as the KOVA System (Hycor Biomedical, Garden Grove, California) or the UriSystem (Fisher Scientific, Hampton, New Hampshire). These systems may include specially designed, graduated centrifuge tubes with devices or pipets that allow easy decanting of supernatant and retention of an exact amount of sediment. They also use specially designed plastic slides with wells or coverslips that accept only a given amount of sediment. Whatever system is used, the Clinical and Laboratory Standards Institute (CLSI) recommends the following:

- The urine volume should be 12 mL.
- The specimen should be centrifuged for 5 minutes at a relative centrifugal force of 400 g (i.e., 400 times normal gravity).
- A standardized slide should be used to view the sediment.
- A consistent reporting format should be used.

Additional Tests Performed on Urine

Clinitest

The glucose test on the reagent strip detects only glucose, the most common sugar found in the urine. However, sugars other than glucose also can appear in the urine. Certain metabolic disorders can result in the excretion of sugars such as galactose, fructose, lactose, maltose, or pentoses. Galactosemia, a rare pathologic condition, is a congenital deficiency in the body's ability to metabolize galactose to glucose; galactosemia results in excretion of galactose in the urine. Seen in infants, it results in failure to thrive, vomiting, and diarrhea. If detected early, galactose can be eliminated from the diet, and the child develops normally. Lactose may be found in the urine of pregnant women or premature infants. In rare cases, urine may contain fructose or pentoses (e.g., xylose, arabinose) as a result of excessive consumption of honey or fruit. Maltose may be excreted in patients with diabetes. Of the many sugars, only the presence of glucose or galactose signifies a pathologic condition.

The Clinitest (Bayer), which is based on the chemical reduction of copper, is commonly used to screen and confirm glycosuria and to detect other sugars in urine (Procedure 52-8). Copper reduction tests are based on the principle that reducing substances can chemically convert cupric sulfate to cuprous oxide, resulting in a color change. A sugar's reducing ability is determined by the presence of a "chemical reducing group" present in all monosaccharides. The Clinitest tablet is dropped directly into a test tube containing diluted urine. A heat-releasing reaction occurs, and after the boiling stops, the color of the tube's contents is compared with a chart provided by the manufacturer.

Acetest

Acetest reagent tablets provide an alternative to strip testing when urine must be tested for the presence of ketones. Ketonuria results when the body metabolizes stored fat because of inadequate cellular uptake of carbohydrates. This is common with diabetes, starvation, and excessive vomiting. The Acetest tablet test (Bayer) is based on the same chemical reaction as the reagent strip test, but its advantage lies in the fact that the tablet can be used with specimens other than urine, and it detects both acetone and acetoacetate.

Urine Pregnancy Testing

The phrase "the rabbit died" came to be a euphemism for a positive pregnancy test in the late 1920s and early 1930s. About 1927, it was discovered that if the urine of a pregnant woman was injected into a rabbit, hemorrhaging occurred in the rabbit's ovaries. These bulging masses could not be seen without killing the rabbit to inspect the ovaries, so invariably, every rabbit died, even if the woman was not pregnant. All pregnancy tests detect the presence of human chorionic gonadotropin (hCG), a hormone produced by the placenta and present in urine during pregnancy. After implantation of the fertilized egg in the uterus, the hCG levels in serum double every few days. This rapid rise occurs for approximately 7 weeks, and then the level begins to decline. Within 72 hours of delivery, the hormone disappears.

Nowadays no rabbits are needed to confirm a pregnancy. The most common type of test for pregnancy is the lateral flow immunoassay test. Many brands are available for laboratory use and are also available over the counter. These tests can be sensitive enough to detect the presence of hCG as early as 1 week after implantation or 4 to 5 days before a missed menstrual period. The tests can be performed in as little as 5 minutes, and the results are easy to interpret—usually as easy as reading a color change. For optimum results, the test should be performed on the first morning voided specimen. The test is based on reactions that occur between antibodies and antigens. Antibodies are proteins formed in response to antigens. When they come in contact, the antibody binds to the antigen, as long as the two are present in sufficient quantity and the antibody is specific for the antigen (e.g., as with a lock and key).

The pregnancy test cartridge contains a membrane with an absorbent pad overlapping a strip of fiberglass paper that is impregnated with a freeze-dried conjugate of gold particles and antibodies to hCG

PROCEDURE 52-8

Perform a Urinalysis: Test Urine for Glucose Using the Clinitest Method

GOAL: *To perform confirmatory testing for glucose in the urine using the Clinitest procedure for reducing substances.*

EQUIPMENT and SUPPLIES

- Urine specimen
- Clinitest tablet, tube, and dropper
- Distilled water
- Test tube rack
- Color chart
- Timer
- Disposable gloves
- Eye protection
- Biohazard waste container
- Patient record

PROCEDURAL STEPS

1. Sanitize your hands and put on nonsterile gloves and eye protection.
2. Holding a Clinitest dropper vertically, add 10 drops of distilled water and then 5 drops of urine to a Clinitest tube.
   PURPOSE: Holding the dropper vertically prevents alteration of the size of the drops.
3. Place the prepared tube in the rack (Figure 1).
   PURPOSE: The tube will become too hot to hold when the tablet is placed in the tube.

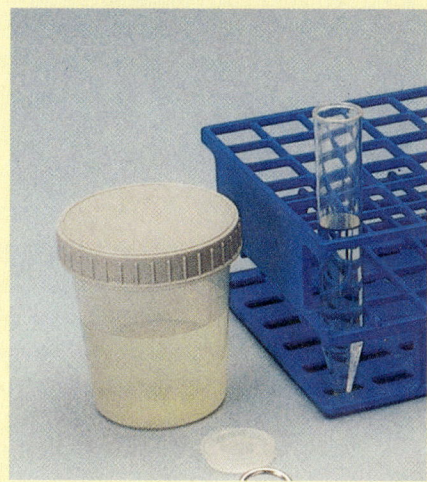

4. With dry hands, remove a Clinitest tablet from the bottle by shaking a tablet into the bottle cap.
   PURPOSE: Clinitest tablets react with moisture and became caustic. Handling tablets with moist hands could result in hydroxide burns.

5. Tap the tablet into the test tube and recap the container.
6. Observe the entire reaction to detect the rapid pass-through phenomenon, which indicates that the glucose level in the urine is very high. (See Step 9.)
   PURPOSE: If pass-through occurs but is not detected, the reading will be falsely low.
7. When boiling stops, time exactly 15 seconds and then gently shake the tube to mix the entire contents.
8. Immediately compare the color of the specimen with the five-drop color chart and record your findings (Figure 2).
   PURPOSE: Color darkens with time. For accurate results, time carefully.

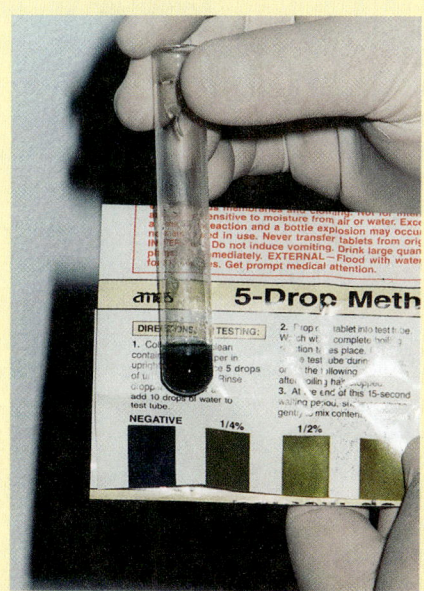

9. If an orange color briefly develops during the reaction, rapid pass-through has occurred, and the test must be repeated using the two-drop color chart.
10. Record the results.
11. Clean up the work area, remove your gloves, and sanitize your hands.
    PURPOSE: To ensure infection control.
12. Record the results in the patient's record.
    PURPOSE: A procedure is not considered finished until it is recorded.

A. Before the addition of urine

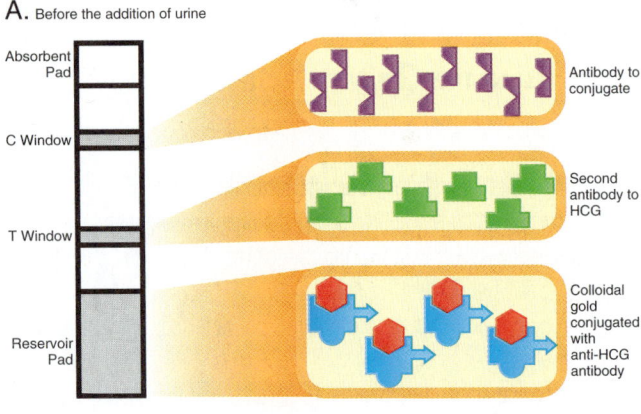

B. After the addition of urine containing HCG

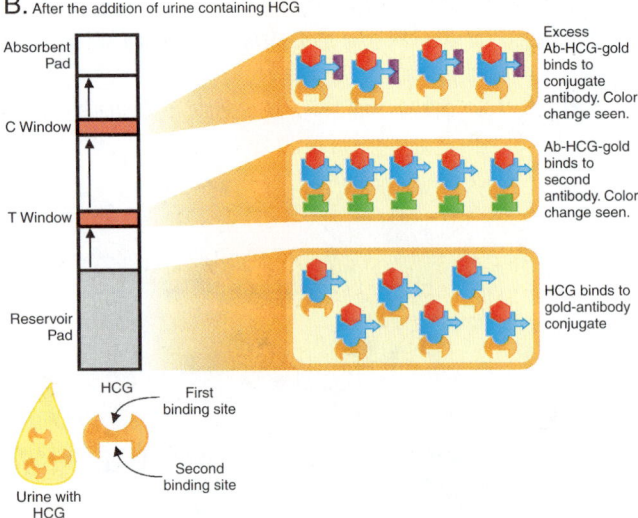

C. After the addition of urine without HCG

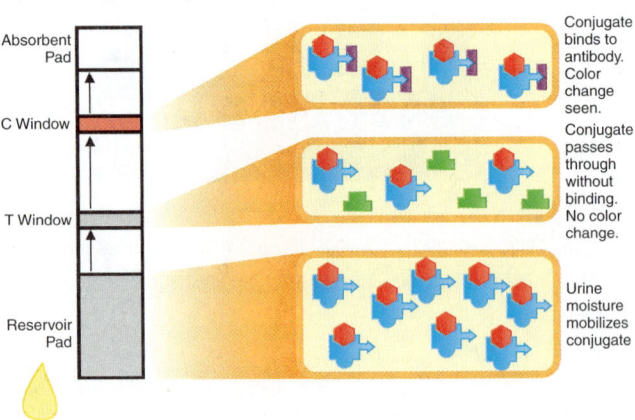

FIGURE 52-32 Lateral flow assay pregnancy test.

(Figure 52-32). The urine sample is introduced into the device, and it wicks through the absorbent pad, reaching a chromatographic membrane (color-coded reservoir pad). As it contacts the membrane, the urine dissolves the freeze-dried conjugate. In a positive sample, the hCG antigen attaches to the antibodies in the colloidal solution. As the conjugate moves forward on the membrane, anti-hCG monoclonal antibodies affixed on the test zone ("T") bind the hCG-gold conjugate complex, where the gold particles accumulate, forming a pink line. All samples cause the "C" line to turn pink. The "C" line contains antibodies that bind to the colloidal gold conjugate regardless of whether they have bound to hCG. The presence of this line indicates that the test has been carried out correctly. The QuickVue test is a lateral flow pregnancy test that can be performed on urine (Procedure 52-9). It is used routinely in many physicians' office laboratories.

Ovulation Testing

CLIA-waived lateral flow urine tests are available to assist in the prediction of ovulation for women attempting to conceive either naturally or using artificial insemination. During the menstrual cycle, human luteinizing hormone (LH) remains at a relatively stable level. Approximately 14 days before menstruation, the body experiences the "LH surge"—a brief, rapid increase in LH. This surge triggers the release of the ovum from the ovary. Two to 3 days after the surge, the LH level returns to the base level. Conception is most likely to occur within 36 hours after the LH surge. The principle of this test is similar to that of the pregnancy test: The reservoir pad contains anti-LH antibodies conjugated to colloidal gold. A positive test result indicates a urine LH level of 20 mIU/mL or higher. Testing usually is performed for 5 consecutive days in the middle of the cycle. Once the surge is detected, ovulation can be expected within 2 to 3 days.

Menopause Testing

A woman is said to have reached menopause when menstruation has not occurred for at least 12 months. The time before menopause, called *perimenopause,* can last for years, bringing with it uncomfortable symptoms such as irregular periods, hot flashes, vaginal dryness, or sleep problems. Some of this may be due to an increase in follicle-stimulating hormone (FSH). Levels of FSH, which is produced by the pituitary gland, increase temporarily each month to stimulate the ovaries. When a woman enters menopause, the ovaries stop producing eggs, and the levels of FSH rise. CLIA-waived lateral flow tests detect FSH in the urine. A positive test result indicates that a woman may be in a stage of menopause; a negative test result, along with symptoms of menopause, may indicate that a woman is in perimenopause. The qualitative lateral flow test should never be used to direct a woman to stop using birth control methods if she does not want to conceive, because pregnancy is still possible during perimenopause.

Bladder Tumor–Associated Antigen Testing

The most reliable test for identifying bladder cancer is **cystoscopy;** however, this is an invasive test. Urine cytology is noninvasive and is accurate at detecting high-grade bladder cancer and carcinoma in situ, but its ability to detect low-grade cancer is limited. Therefore, urine-based marker tests have been developed that are noninvasive

PROCEDURE 52-9

Perform a Urinalysis: Perform a Pregnancy Test

GOAL: To perform a pregnancy test on urine using the QuickVue pregnancy test method.

EQUIPMENT and SUPPLIES

- Urine specimen
- QuickVue test kit (Quidel, San Diego, California)
- Disposable gloves
- Biohazard waste container
- Patient's record

PROCEDURAL STEPS

1. Sanitize your hands. Put on nonsterile gloves.
2. Prepare the testing equipment (Figure 1).

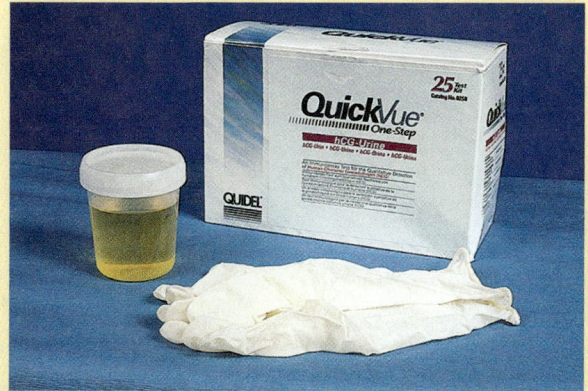

(From Bonewit-West K: *Clinical procedures for medical assistants*, ed 7, St Louis, 2008, Saunders.)

3. Collect the specimen.
4. Remove the test cassette from the foil pouch.
5. Add three drops of urine using the dropper that accompanies the kit (Figure 2). Dispose of the dropper in a biohazard bag.
   UPURPOSE: To ensure accurate test results, the specimen amount must be exact.

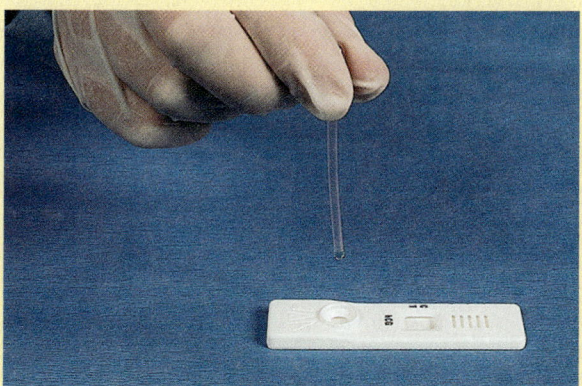

(From Bonewit-West K: *Clinical procedures for medical assistants*, ed 7, St Louis, 2008, Saunders.)

6. Wait 3 minutes and read the test results.
   UPURPOSE: To ensure accurate test results, timing must be exact.
7. Interpret the results (Figure 3).
   - Negative: A blue control line is next to the letter C; no line is seen next to the letter T.
   - Positive: A blue control line is next to the letter C, and a pink line is next to the letter T.

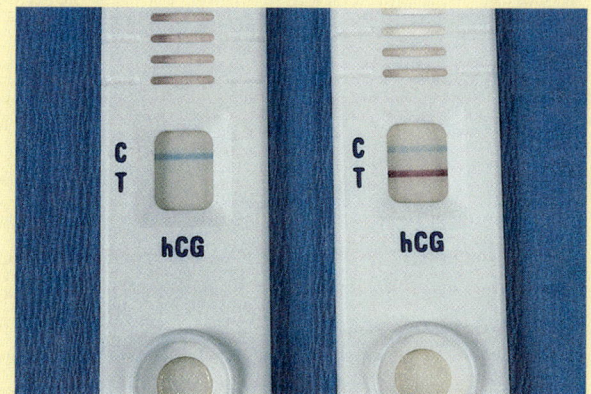

(From Bonewit-West K: *Clinical procedures for medical assistants*, ed 7, St Louis, 2008, Saunders.)

8. If a blue line does not appear in the C area, the test is invalid and the specimen must be retested using another kit. Check the expiration date of the kit before proceeding.
9. Discard the cassette into a biohazard waste container, remove your gloves, and sanitize your hands.
   UPURPOSE: To ensure infection control.
10. Record the results in the patient's record as either positive or negative.
    UPURPOSE: A procedure is not considered finished until it is recorded.

10/2/XX 3:47 PM LMP 9/16/XX. QuickVue pregnancy test: Positive. Rosa Gonzales, CMA (AAMA) _____

and accurate in detecting low-grade bladder cancer. In addition, they are useful for monitoring for recurring bladder cancer.

The BTA Stat Test (Bion Diagnostics, Woburn, Massachusetts) is a rapid, single-step immunoassay. The disposable test device, which looks much like the device used for pregnancy testing, contains two monoclonal antibodies that detect the presence of human complement factor H–related protein (hCFHrp), which is shed by cancerous bladder cells but not by normal bladder epithelial cells. When the BTA Stat Test is used, freshly voided urine is placed in the sample well of the test device, and positive or negative results are obtained in 5 minutes. Bladder cancer is one of the most common forms of cancer in the United States. About 53,000 Americans are diagnosed with the disease each year, and approximately 500,000 people are routinely monitored for it. The cancer is most common in men over age 50, in smokers, and in workers exposed to chemicals in the rubber, leather tanning, metal, and dye industries.

CRITICAL THINKING APPLICATION   52-6

After centrifugation of the three urine specimens, Rosa prepares to view the sediment. She knows that she must correlate the findings from the visual and chemical examinations she has already performed on these specimens. She reviews the results and notes that Mr. Parks's and Mrs. Carpenter's specimens were clear, but Ms. Hillman's specimen was turbid. Given the results of the chemical analysis, during which Rosa noted an alkaline pH, an elevated nitrite level, and an elevated leukocyte esterase reading, what might she find when she examines Ms. Hillman's specimen microscopically?

URINE TOXICOLOGY

Toxicology is the study of poisonous substances and their effects on the body. The clinical laboratory performs testing on body fluids and tissues to monitor the use of therapeutic drugs such as digoxin (a cardiac medication) or to detect poisoning by herbicides, metals, animal toxins, and poisonous gases (e.g., carbon monoxide).

Laboratory testing for illegal drugs or alcohol also is done, most commonly as an employment, insurance, or legal requirement (Table 52-7). Although serum (blood) tests are more accurate for determining current impairment or the time of ingestion, urine is the specimen of choice for most routine screening procedures. For routine screening, a random specimen usually is collected. Often, safeguards are used to ensure that a specimen is fresh and is truly from the patient. Water may be temporarily unavailable in the restroom, bluing agents may be added to the toilets, a container with a temperature-sensitive strip may be provided, and someone may accompany the patient into the restroom. In some cases a strict chain of custody is required. The substance for which the test is performed or its **metabolite** often remains in urine much longer than the impairment or intoxication lasts. This is one reason urine screening is favored over serum or blood screening.

As a medical assistant, you may be responsible for collecting specimens for toxicology tests and for performing certain tests. Rapid drug screening devices are about the size and shape of a credit card (Figure 52-33). The device is dipped into a urine sample, or urine is directly applied to the device. The results are read according

TABLE 52-7   Commonly Abused Drugs and Body Retention Times

DRUG	RETENTION TIME
Alcohol	2-10 hours
Amphetamine	24-48 hours
Methamphetamine	3-5+ days
Barbiturates	
Phenobarbital	2-6 days
Secobarbital	24 hours
Cocaine, cocaine metabolites	12 hours-3 days
Opiates, heroin, morphine	3-4 days
Phencyclidine (PCP)	3-7+ days
Marijuana (tetrahydrocannabinol metabolites)	2 days-11 weeks

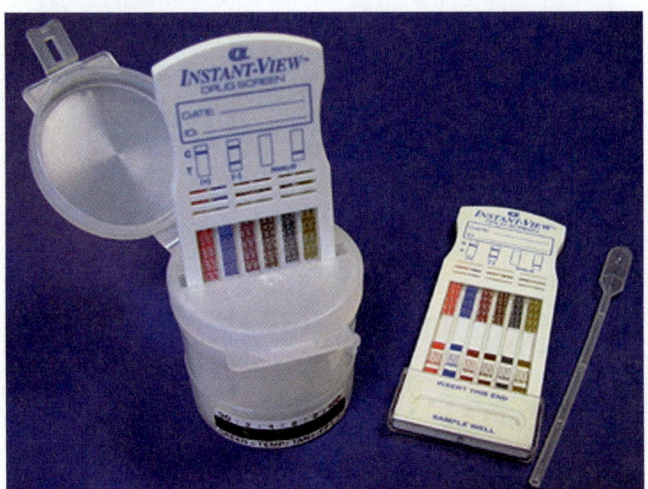

FIGURE 52-33 Instant-View Drug Test. (Courtesy Alfa Scientific, Poway, California.)

to the manufacturer's instructions in just minutes. "Negative" results indicate that none of the targeted drugs were detected in the urine sample at specified cutoff levels; "inconclusive" results indicate that the device reacted with something in the urine and confirmation testing is required.

The Instant-View Multi-Drug Screen (Alfa Scientific, Poway, California) urine test is a lateral flow chromatographic immunoassay that tests for urine metabolites of a variety of drugs, including amphetamines, barbiturates, benzodiazepines, cocaine, morphine, methadone, phencyclidine (PCP), tricyclics, marijuana, Ecstasy, and methamphetamines. Available in cartridges that test from two to six drugs, the test is a competitive binding immunoassay in which drug and drug metabolites in a urine sample compete with immobilized drug conjugate for limited labeled antibody binding sites. By using antibodies specific to different drug classes, the test permits independent, simultaneous detection of up to six drugs from a single sample in 5 minutes.

In the procedure, urine mixes with a labeled antibody-dye conjugate and migrates along a porous membrane. If the concentration of a given drug is below the detection limit of the test, the antibody-dye conjugate that did not bind to a drug metabolite binds to antigen conjugate immobilized on the membrane, producing a rose-pink–colored band in the appropriate band for that drug. If the level of the drug in the urine is at or above the detection limit, free drug competes with the immobilized antigen conjugate on the membrane by binding to the antibody-dye conjugate, forming an antigen-antibody complex and preventing the development of a rose-pink band (Procedure 52-10). Note that unlike the lateral flow test for pregnancy, ovulation, and menopause, with a drug screening test, the appearance of a line in the T band indicates a negative test result.

Drug testing has legal ramifications; therefore additional testing often is necessary to ensure that samples have not been adulterated (Procedure 52-11). Adulteration is the intentional manipulation of a urine sample to allow someone to falsely pass a drug screening test. It may involve using urine from another person or an animal, diluting the sample with water, or adding substances such as bleach, vinegar, eye drops, baking soda, drain openers, soft drinks, or hydrogen peroxide. Urine collection cups with built-in thermometer panels often are used to ensure that urine has been freshly voided from the bladder. A temperature of 32° C to 38° C (90° F to 100° F) within 4 minutes of collection is expected. Test strips that detect human immunoglobulins (antibodies) in urine can determine whether the specimen is human in origin and if it is naturally dilute or has been diluted. Human immunoglobulin G (IgG) is exclusive to humans and is always found at certain levels in urine, even if it is dilute. The addition of chemicals to the urine will prevent the reaction on the test strip.

PROCEDURE 52-10

Perform a Urinalysis and Patient Screening Using Established Protocols: Perform a Multidrug Screening Test on Urine

GOAL: *To screen a urine specimen for drugs or drug metabolites at their specified cutoff levels.*

EQUIPMENT and SUPPLIES

- Instant-View Multi-Drug Screen Urine Test in a sealed pouch
- Freshly voided urine sample
- Timer
- Biohazard container
- Disposable gloves
- Patient's record

PROCEDURAL STEPS

1. Sanitize your hands and assemble the equipment and specimen. Check the expiration date on the test kit.
   <u>PURPOSE:</u> An expired test strip may yield inaccurate results.
2. Determine the temperature of the urine (within 4 minutes of voiding). The temperature should be between 32° C and 38° C (90° F and 100° F).
   <u>PURPOSE:</u> If the urine temperature is below or above this range, the sample may have been adulterated. Once it has been determined that the sample is at the correct temperature, it may be stored at room temperature for 8 hours or in the refrigerator for up to 3 days before testing.
3. Bring the specimen and the testing device to room temperature.
   <u>PURPOSE:</u> Both the specimen and the device must be at room temperature to ensure accurate results.
4. Remove the device from the foil pouch and label it with the specimen identification.

Dip Method

5. Remove the cap of the specimen and dip the device into the specimen for 10 seconds. The surface of the urine must be above the sample well and below the arrowheads in the window (Figure 1).
   <u>PURPOSE:</u> The pads must be saturated with urine.

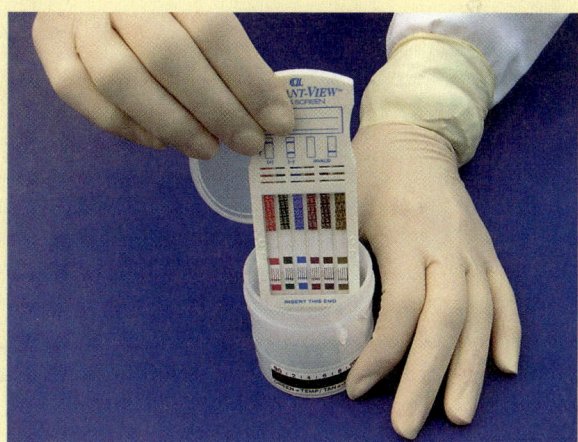

(Courtesy Alfa Scientific, Poway, California.)

Alternate Method

6. Remove the pipet from the pouch and fill the pipet to the line on the barrel with urine. Dispense the entire volume onto the sample well on the testing device (Figure 2).

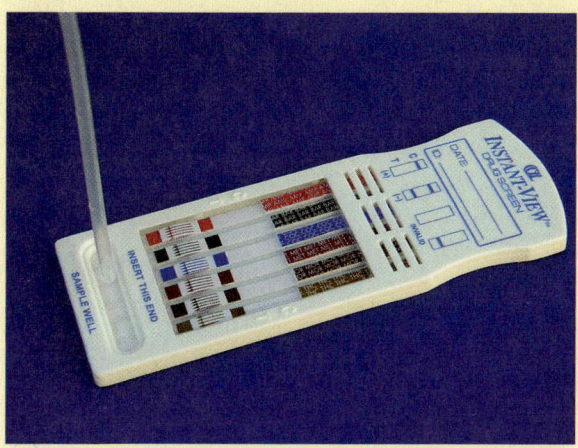

(Courtesy Alfa Scientific, Poway, California.)

PROCEDURE 52-10—cont'd

<u>PURPOSE:</u> If insufficient urine is available in the cup to use the dip method, this method applies urine to the device.

7. Recap the urine specimen.
8. Set the timer for 4 to 7 minutes. Do not read the results after 7 minutes.
   <u>PURPOSE:</u> Correct timing is essential for reliable, accurate results.
9. Interpret the results (Figure 3):

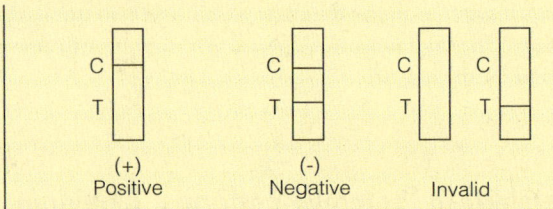

(+)
Positive   (-)
Negative   Invalid

- Positive: If the C line appears and no T line is present, the test indicates a positive result for that drug.

- Negative: If both the C line and the T line appear, the test indicates that the level for the drug or its metabolites is below the cutoff level.

- Invalid—If no C line develops within 5 minutes on any test strip, the assay is invalid. Make sure the urine has not been adulterated (see Procedure 52-11) and/or repeat the assay with a new test device.

10. Color photocopying provides a permanent record of results, but the copy must be made within 7 minutes of adding the urine. Make sure the photocopier does not become contaminated; wipe the glass with alcohol or another manufacturer-approved disinfectant after making the copy.
11. Discard the urine and the device into the biohazard container. Disinfect the area.
12. Remove your gloves and sanitize your hands.
    <u>PURPOSE:</u> To ensure infection control.
13. Record the results in the patient's record.
    <u>PURPOSE:</u> A procedure is not considered complete until it is recorded.

PROCEDURE 52-11

Perform a Urinalysis: Assess a Urine Specimen for Adulteration Before Drug Testing

GOAL: *To assess a urine specimen for additive adulteration.*

EQUIPMENT and SUPPLIES

- Quik Test Adulterant Strips (Quik Test USA, Boca Raton, Florida)
- Urine sample (freshly voided; urine should be stored at room temperature for no longer than 2 hours or at refrigerator temperature for no longer than 4 hours before testing)
- Paper towels
- Timer
- Biohazard waste container
- Disposable gloves
- Patient's record

PROCEDURAL STEPS

1. Sanitize your hands and assemble the equipment and the specimen. Check the expiration date on the test kit.
   <u>PURPOSE:</u> An expired test strip may yield inaccurate results.
2. Put on gloves. Remove one strip from the container and recap tightly.
3. Dip the test strip briefly into the urine and then remove it.
4. Blot the strip by touching the side of the strip to a paper towel.
   <u>PURPOSE:</u> Oversaturated strips may not react consistently.
5. Read the results within 1 minute by comparing each pad with the color strips on the canister (Figure 1). These results are for the Quik Test Adulterant Strips. Because the monitor color may vary from manufacturer to manufacturer, please refer to the package for the specific product for accurate color reference.
   <u>PURPOSE:</u> Exceeding the allotted time may result in error.

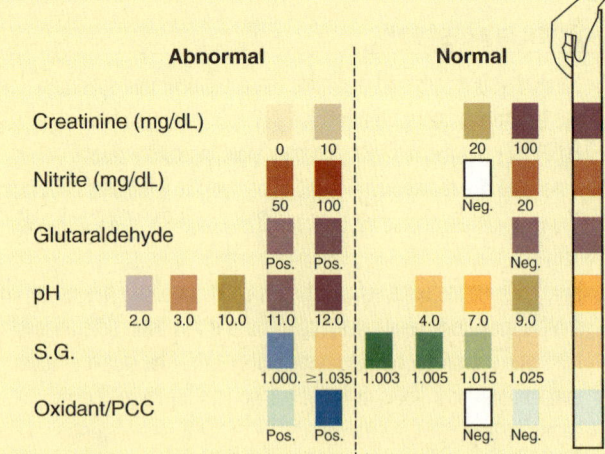

	Abnormal				Normal		
Creatinine (mg/dL)	0	10			20	100	
Nitrite (mg/dL)	50	100			Neg.	20	
Glutaraldehyde	Pos.	Pos.				Neg.	
pH	2.0	3.0	10.0	11.0	12.0	4.0	7.0	9.0
S.G.	1.000	≥1.035	1.003	1.005	1.015	1.025
Oxidant/PCC	Pos.	Pos.			Neg.	Neg.	

6. Dispose of the paper towels and the strip in the biohazard container.
7. Disinfect the area. Remove your gloves and dispose of them in the biohazard container; sanitize your hands.
   <u>PURPOSE:</u> To ensure infection control.
8. Record the results in the patient's record.
   <u>PURPOSE:</u> A procedure is not considered complete until it is recorded.

BASICS OF DRUG TESTING AND CHAIN OF CUSTODY

- The individual being tested must provide photo identification.
- Indirect observation of specimen collection is important to make sure the sample is actually provided by the patient being tested. Indirect methods of observation include measuring the specimen's temperature; securing water faucets in the restroom so that urine cannot be diluted; and having the patient remove outer clothing and leave personal belongings in the examination room.
- Water cannot be run in the restroom during the collection, and the toilet should not be flushed.
- If it is suspected that the sample has been adulterated, the patient can be asked to provide another specimen.
- Within 4 minutes of receiving the specimen, check its temperature (range is 32° C to 38° C/90° F to 100° F) and volume (30 to 45 mL is required), and inspect it for any indications of adulteration (e.g., an unusual color, the presence of foreign materials).
- Pour the specimen into a specimen bottle and seal the lid with the tamper-evident label/seal provided at the bottom of the chain of custody form with the donor present; include the date and your initials on the label (Figure 52-34).
- Ship the specimen to the testing laboratory as soon as possible; it must be sent the same day it is collected.
- Individual results may vary, making some results positive at lower substance levels; also, diet, the volume of urine flow, and the amount of substance used can alter results.
- Because of the legal implications of drug testing, chain of custody must be strictly followed. Each step from collection of the specimen to reporting of test results to the patient must be strictly monitored. Requirements include sealed specimen containers; supervised laboratory analysis throughout the process; and authorized signatures at each step.

Other test strips are available that detect creatinine, nitrite, pH, specific gravity, glutaraldehyde, and oxidants. Creatinine is always present in normal urine, because it is excreted from the body at a constant rate. Low or absent levels indicate diluted or substituted nonhuman samples. Urine can be diluted if the person being tested drinks abnormally large amounts of water before the test, or if water or another liquid is added to the sample. Creatinine levels usually are checked in conjunction with the specific gravity to screen for dilution or substitution adulteration. Specific gravity readings also determine whether substances such as table salt have been added to the urine.

Nitrites are oxidizing substances that react with the drug or drug metabolite molecules in the urine. Nitrites primarily interfere with antibody binding in lateral flow tests. Nitrates must be added to the urine after voiding. Commercial adulterants, such as Whizzies, Klear, and UrineLuck, are tablets or powders that can be added to voided urine. They do not change the color or temperature of the urine. The level of nitrites found in urine with gross bacteriuria or from therapeutic drug metabolites (e.g., nitroglycerin) is below the cutoff for adulteration screening tests.

The pH of the sample can affect enzymatic and antibody reactions in lateral flow drug tests. Levels higher than 9.5 or lower than 3.0 may hamper the enzymatic rate. Alteration of the pH may also affect the stability of the drug or its metabolite. Adulteration of a sample with bleach, drain cleaners, or baking soda changes the pH, but this type of tampering can be detected by an adulteration strip test.

Glutaraldehyde can mask the presence of illegal drugs. Commercially available products such as UrinAid and Clear Choice contain glutaraldehyde intended to adulterate urine. In addition, a 10% solution of glutaraldehyde is sold over the counter for the treatment of warts. This chemical prevents the enzymes in lateral flow tests from reacting properly.

Sensitivity limits for drug screening are set by the U.S. Substance Abuse and Mental Health Services Administration (SAMHSA), the National Institute on Drug Abuse (NIDA), and the U.S. Department of Health and Human Services. Positive results on urine samples tested for substances should be confirmed by more specific chemical methods, such as gas chromatography (GC), mass spectrometry (MS), and enzyme-multiplied immunoassay (EMIT).

Alcohol Testing

Alcohol testing is not performed on urine, but CLIA-waived tests are available to detect alcohol using saliva. Saliva-based tests have a high degree of correlation to blood alcohol analysis. The saliva alcohol test manufactured by STC Technologies (Bethlehem, Pennsylvania) uses a Dacron swab saturated with saliva to detect ethanol. The test is used primarily for workplace testing, including the federally mandated testing of transportation workers, but also in private company "drug-free workplace" programs and by emergency departments.

CULTURING THE URINE

Urine cultures are performed to assist in the diagnosis of a UTI and to assess the effectiveness of certain antibiotics in treatment of the infection. Rapid detection systems and culturing of specimens using Petri dishes are addressed in Chapter 55.

CLOSING COMMENTS

Patient Education

Frequently a medical assistant is called on to explain collection techniques to the patient. Patients want to do the procedure correctly but often lack the knowledge of urinary terminology and are embarrassed to or do not know how to ask questions regarding cleaning of the genital area. When explaining a urinary collection procedure, use pictures and words that the patient will understand. As you explain the procedure in terms that the patient knows, he or she will feel comfortable telling you or asking you pertinent details that may have a definite impact on treatment of the problem. Providing the patient with a clearly written instruction sheet is also helpful. The instruction sheet should be personalized with his or her name, the time to begin collection or testing (if applicable), what supplies should be used, and a phone number to call if questions arise.

FEDERAL DRUG TESTING CUSTODY AND CONTROL FORM

SPECIMEN ID NO.   **1234567**   LAB ACCESSION NO.

OMB No. 0930-0158

STEP 1: COMPLETED BY COLLECTOR OR EMPLOYER REPRESENTATIVE

A. Employer Name, Address, I.D. No.   B. MRO Name, Address, Phone and Fax No.

C. Donor SSN or Employee I.D. No. _____

D. Reason for Test: ☐ Pre-employment   ☐ Random   ☐ Reasonable Suspicion/Cause   ☐ Post Accident
                       ☐ Return to Duty   ☐ Follow-up   ☐ Other (specify)_____

E. Drug Tests to be Performed: ☐ THC, COC, PCP, OPI, AMP   ☐ THC & COC Only   ☐ Other (specify)_____

F. Collection Site Address:

Collector Phone No. _____

Collector Fax No. _____

STEP 2: COMPLETED BY COLLECTOR

Read specimen temperature within 4 minutes. Is temperature between 90° and 100° F?   ☐ Yes   ☐ No, Enter Remark

Specimen Collection: ☐ Split   ☐ Single   ☐ None Provided (Enter Remark)   ☐ Observed (Enter Remark)

REMARKS

STEP 3: Collector affixes bottle seal(s) to bottle(s). Collector dates seal(s). Donor initials seal(s). Donor completes STEP 5 on Copy 2 (MRO Copy)

STEP 4: CHAIN OF CUSTODY - INITIATED BY COLLECTOR AND COMPLETED BY LABORATORY

I certify that the specimen given to me by the donor identified in the certification section on Copy 2 of this form was collected, labeled, sealed and released to the Delivery Service noted in accordance with applicable Federal requirements.

X_____   Time of Collection   AM PM   ▶

SPECIMEN BOTTLE(S) RELEASED TO:

Signature of Collector

_____   Date (Mo./Day/Yr.)   ▶
(PRINT) Collector's Name (First, MI, Last)   Name of Delivery Service Transferring Specimen to Lab

RECEIVED AT LAB:

X_____   ▶
Signature of Accessioner

Primary Specimen Bottle Seal Intact   **SPECIMEN BOTTLE(S) RELEASED TO:**

☐ Yes

_____   Date (Mo./Day/Yr.)   ▶   ☐ No, Enter Remark Below
(PRINT) Accessioner's Name (First, MI, Last)

STEP 5a: PRIMARY SPECIMEN TEST RESULTS - COMPLETED BY PRIMARY LABORATORY

☐ NEGATIVE   ☐ POSITIVE for: ☐ MARIJUANA METABOLITE   ☐ CODEINE   ☐ AMPHETAMINE   ☐ ADULTERATED
☐ DILUTE   ☐ COCAINE METABOLITE   ☐ MORPHINE   ☐ METHAMPHETAMINE   ☐ SUBSTITUTED
☐ REJECTED FOR TESTING   ☐ PCP   ☐ 6-ACETYLMORPHINE   ☐ INVALID RESULT

REMARKS _____

TEST LAB (if different from above)_____

I certify that the specimen identified on this form was examined upon receipt, handled using chain of custody procedures, analyzed, and reported in accordance with applicable Federal requirements.

X_____   _____   _____
Signature of Certifying Scientist   (PRINT) Certifying Scientist's Name (First, MI, Last)   Date (Mo./Day/Yr.)

STEP 5b: SPLIT SPECIMEN TEST RESULTS - (IF TESTED) COMPLETED BY SECONDARY LABORATORY

☐ RECONFIRMED   ☐ FAILED TO RECONFIRM - REASON_____

_____   I certify that the split specimen identified on this form was examined upon receipt, handled using chain of custody procedures, analyzed,
Laboratory Name   and reported in accordance with applicable Federal requirements.

X_____

_____   _____   _____   _____
Laboratory Address   Signature of Certifying Scientist   (PRINT) Certifying Scientist's Name (First, MI, Last)   Date (Mo./Day/Yr.)

PRESS HARD - YOU ARE MAKING MULTIPLE COPIES

PEEL   **1234567**   A   SPECIMEN ID NO.

PLACE OVER CAP

1234567
SPECIMEN BOTTLE SEAL

Date (Mo. Day Yr.)
Donor's Initials

PEEL   **1234567**   B (SPLIT)   SPECIMEN ID NO.

PLACE OVER CAP

1234567
SPECIMEN BOTTLE SEAL

Date (Mo. Day Yr.)
Donor's Initials

COPY 1 - LABORATORY

0000-0000-0225

FIGURE 52-34 First page of a five-page Federal Drug Testing Custody and Control form.

LEGAL AND ETHICAL ISSUES

Similar to all other procedures, the test is only as valid as the specimen and the procedure performed on that specimen. You, as the physician's agent, are responsible for that validity when you instruct the patient and when you perform the test.

A medical assistant who is responsible for office laboratory testing must clearly understand the basic concepts of laboratory medicine. To do this, you must stay current with the rapid technologic advances in laboratory medicine and assist in establishing a protocol of the tests best suited to your physician-employer.

You have the responsibility for properly collecting specimens and accurately testing them. In addition, you are responsible for strict adherence to protocol when collecting and testing specimens when legal ramifications are associated with the test results. Patient confidentiality is paramount when drug testing is performed, as is rigid conformation to all established rules and regulations.

SUMMARY OF SCENARIO

Rosa's capabilities in the laboratory analysis of urine are highly valued by Dr. Hill. Because tests can be performed in the office laboratory, Dr. Hill has the results immediately. Dr. Hill's patients also appreciate the convenience of office laboratory testing, in which physical and chemical analysis is performed by Rosa and other medical assistants, and microscopic UA is performed by Dr. Hill. Mrs. Carpenter knows the results of her pregnancy test on her first morning urine without waiting for a call from the laboratory, and urinalysis of Ms. Hillman's CCMS urine sample will help Dr. Hill diagnose a UTI within minutes. Rosa knows that the laboratory services and the quality control measures she takes when performing the complete UA or lateral flow tests are an integral part of the excellent patient care provided by Dr. Hill.

SUMMARY OF LEARNING OBJECTIVES

1. **Define, spell, and pronounce the terms listed in the vocabulary.**
   Spelling and pronouncing medical terms correctly bolsters the medical assistant's credibility. Knowing the definitions of these terms promotes confidence in communication with patients and co-workers.

2. **Apply critical thinking skills in performing the patient assessment and patient care.**
   Completing the Critical Thinking Application exercises throughout the chapter can help the student medical assistant become more adept at critical analysis of real-life situations.

3. **Understand the purpose of routine urinalysis.**
   Routine UA is performed primarily as a screening test to detect metabolic and physiologic disorders. Urine is easily obtained, making it an ideal specimen for testing. Urine is analyzed for detection of extrinsic and intrinsic pathologic conditions.

4. **Describe the physiology of urine formation.**
   Urine is formed through a filtration mechanism in the kidney via the nephrons. As the filtrate passes through the tubules, various changes occur. Urine is stored in the bladder and is voided through the urethra.

5. **Display sensitivity to patient rights and feelings when collecting specimens.**
   Requesting a urine specimen from a patient may be an embarrassing moment for the patient. The request should be made in private, and the patient should be given explicit instructions so that he or she understands what is expected.

6. **Explain the various means and methods used to collect urine specimens.**
   Some urine collections, such as the 2-hour postprandial specimen, must be timed around meals or fasts. Routine UA requires no special preparation, whereas a CCMS requires cleansing of the external genitalia. Only urine that will be cultured must be collected in a sterile container. Urine to be sent to a referral laboratory may require the addition of preservatives.

7. **Instruct a patient in the collection of a 24-hour urine specimen.**
   Timed urine specimens are collected to determine the amount of a particular analyte in the urine during a given time frame. Proper patient instruction is necessary to obtain an acceptable specimen (see Procedure 52-1).

8. **Instruct a patient in the collection of a clean-catch midstream urine specimen.**
   Proper patient instruction is necessary for an acceptable CCMS. Both men and women are given instructions in cleaning the external genitalia to prevent contamination of the urine. Urine must be collected in a sterile container and refrigerated if it cannot be tested within 1 hour (see Procedure 52-2).

9. **Describe the components of the physical and chemical examination of urine.**
   Physical examination of the urine involves determination of the color, turbidity, and specific gravity. Odor and foam color may be noted (see Procedure 52-3). The chemical examination of urine involves determination of the pH level and the levels of glucose, protein, ketones, blood, bilirubin, urobilinogen, and nitrite, as well as specific gravity and leukocyte esterase, with the use of a reagent strip.

10. **Measure the urine specific gravity.**
    Refer to Procedure 52-4.

11. **Perform a complete urinalysis using a chemical reagent strip.**
    A complete UA involves physical, chemical, and microscopic assessment. The results of the three must correlate with one another. Most urine

testing requires reagent strips or tablets. It is essential that these supplies be stored in dark, cool, moisture-free areas (see Procedure 52-5).

12. **Recognize and correctly identify the formed elements found in a microscopic examination of urine sediment.**
Formed elements in the urine sediment include casts, cells, and crystals. Artifacts may be present but are not reported.

13. **Prepare a urine specimen for microscopic examination.**
Refer to Procedure 52-6.

14. **Perform quality control measures to determine the reliability of chemical reagent strips.**
Refer to Procedure 52-7.

15. **Conduct glucose testing using the Clinitest method.**
The Clinitest detects reducing sugars in the urine, including glucose and galactose. It is superior to the reagent strip test because it detects sugars other than glucose (see Procedure 52-8).

16. **Explain the principle of using lateral flow technology in pregnancy testing.**
Pregnancy tests detect hCG, a hormone produced by the placenta. Anti-hCG antibodies embedded in test cartridges bind to hCG and initiate color changes in test areas. Urine moves through lateral flow devices by capillary action.

17. **Perform a pregnancy test.**
Refer to Procedure 52-9.

18. **Describe methods for determining fertility and menopause using Clinical Laboratory Improvement Amendments (CLIA)-waived urine tests.**
Fertility can be assessed using lateral flow tests that detect LH, a hormone that increases in concentration in the urine shortly before ovulation. Menopause can be assessed using lateral flow tests that detect FSH, which increases as menopause approaches.

19. **Explain the principle of lateral flow technology in drug testing on urine.**
Drug testing with lateral flow technology is similar to pregnancy testing except that it uses a competitive binding principle. Unlike with the pregnancy test, a line in the T region indicates a negative test.

20. **Demonstrate a method of drug testing on a urine specimen.**
Refer to Procedure 52-10.

21. **List the means by which urine could be adulterated before drug testing.**
Consuming excessive water before urinating, adding water to a urine specimen, and adding chemicals or products sold specifically to adulterate urine all could render a drug test invalid. Adulteration test strips can detect most methods of adulteration.

22. **Demonstrate a method of detecting adulterating substances in a urine sample for drug testing.**
Refer to Procedure 52-11.

23. **Describe patient education factors that are pertinent to urine sample collection.**
Comprehensive patient education that is sensitive to the patient's learning needs will ensure the urine collection process.

24. **Discuss the legal and ethical responsibilities of the medical assistant who is assisting with urinalysis.**
Laboratory tests are only as valid as the specimen and the procedure performed on that specimen. The medical assistant is responsible for ongoing education to maintain standards and skills in the physician office laboratory. Patient confidentiality is paramount when drug testing is performed.

CONNECTIONS

📖 **Study Guide Connection:** Go to the Chapter 52 Study Guide. Read and complete the activities.

🅔 **Evolve Connection:** Go to the Chapter 52 link at *evolve.elsevier.com/kinn* to complete the Chapter Review and Chapter Quiz. Peruse other resources listed for this chapter to increase your knowledge of Assisting in the Analysis of Urine.

ASSISTING IN PHLEBOTOMY

53

SCENARIO

Leah Barney, a recent graduate of a CMA (AAMA) program, is a new employee at the Health Alliance Medical Clinic. The class on medical laboratory procedures was Leah's favorite in her medical assisting program at the community college; in that class, she learned the principles of phlebotomy and performed several phlebotomy procedures both in the school's laboratory and at her externship site. Her employer has arranged for Leah to spend time with an experienced phlebotomist at the clinic so that she is prepared to perform phlebotomy duties in her new position. Nervous but excited, she begins her training.

While studying this chapter, think about the following questions:

- How will Leah know which tubes or which needle size to use?
- How will Leah approach phlebotomy on a child or an elderly person?
- What conditions will require a capillary puncture?
- How can Leah make the clinic patients comfortable and at ease?
- How will Leah handle a difficult "stick"?

LEARNING OBJECTIVES

1. Define, spell, and pronounce the terms listed in the vocabulary.
2. Apply critical thinking skills in performing the patient assessment and patient care.
3. List the equipment needed for venipuncture.
4. Explain the purpose of a tourniquet.
5. Explain how to apply a tourniquet and the consequences of improper application.
6. Explain why the stopper colors on evacuated tubes differ.
7. State the correct order in which samples for various types of tubes should be collected.
8. Describe the types of sharps used in phlebotomy.
9. Explain why a syringe rather than an evacuated tube would be chosen for blood collection.
10. Discuss the use of sharps with engineered sharps injury protection.
11. Summarize postexposure management of needlesticks.
12. Detail patient preparation for venipuncture that shows sensitivity to the patient's rights and feelings.
13. Describe and name the veins that may be used for blood collection.
14. List in order the steps of a routine venipuncture.
15. Collect a venous blood sample using the syringe method.
16. Collect a venous blood sample using the evacuated tube method.
17. Explain why a winged infusion set (butterfly needle) would be chosen over an evacuated tube.
18. Perform a venipuncture using a winged infusion set.
19. Summarize typical problems that may be associated with venipuncture.
20. Identify the major causes of hemolysis during venous blood collection.
21. List situations in which capillary puncture would be preferred over venipuncture.
22. Discuss proper dermal puncture sites.
23. Describe containers that may be used to collect capillary blood.
24. Explain why the first drop of blood is wiped away when a capillary puncture is performed.
25. Perform a capillary puncture.
26. Differentiate whole blood, serum, and plasma and give an example of a test performed with each.
27. Describe handling and transport methods for blood after collection.
28. Explain chain of custody procedures when drawing blood samples.
29. Discuss the role of the medical assistant in patient education when performing phlebotomy.

VOCABULARY

hemoconcentration A condition in which the concentration of blood cells is increased in proportion to the plasma.

hemolysis (hi-muh′-luh-sis) The destruction or dissolution of red blood cells, with subsequent release of hemoglobin.

plasma The liquid portion of whole blood that contains active clotting agents.

serum The liquid portion of whole blood that remains after the blood has clotted.

thixotropic gel A material that appears to be a solid until subjected to a disturbance, such as centrifugation, whereupon it becomes a liquid.

Phlebotomy, the practice of drawing blood, has its roots in the ancient practice of restoring the four body humors: blood, phlegm, yellow bile, and black bile. The foundation of all medical treatment was to keep these humors in balance by purging, starving, vomiting, or bloodletting.

The art of bloodletting was flourishing by the Middle Ages, and both barbers and surgeons performed it. Barbers advertised with a red and white striped pole; red represented blood, and white represented the tourniquet. The pole itself represented the stick the patient squeezed during the procedure. Typically, 16 to 30 ounces (1 to 4 pints) of blood was drained to treat an illness. When the patient became faint, the "treatment" was stopped. Often, bleeding over large areas of the body was accomplished by multiple incisions. George Washington is reported to have died in 1799 after being drained of 9 pints of blood within 24 hours to cure a throat infection. In Washington's day, it was believed that the blood was a carrier of the impurities of disease, and with bleeding, new and healthy blood would replace what was lost. By the end of the nineteenth century, bloodletting was declared quackery.

Today phlebotomy is performed primarily to diagnose and to monitor a patient's condition. According to the American Society of Clinical Pathologists (ASCP), nearly 80% of physicians' decisions are based on laboratory tests, most of which are blood tests. Phlebotomy involves highly developed procedures and equipment to ensure the patient's comfort and safety. The high standards necessary for the proper practice of phlebotomy led to the creation of different organizations that develop standards for training. Medical assistants are trained to perform phlebotomy. To be certified as a phlebotomist, they must complete course work and training at an accredited institution and then pass a national examination. Some medical assistant programs include this specialized training in their curriculum.

Certifying agencies include ASCP, the International Academy of Phlebotomy Sciences, the National Certification Agency (NCA), and the National Phlebotomy Association (NPA). Continuing education often is required to maintain certification. California and Louisiana were the first states to create state certification requirements. It is important that medical assistants become familiar with the guidelines of their home states, because not all states require a certificate to perform phlebotomy.

The most common method of obtaining blood is venipuncture, in which the blood is taken directly from a surface vein. The vein is punctured with a needle, and the blood is collected either in a syringe or in a stoppered tube. The procedure is safe when performed by a trained professional, but it must be performed with care. Much practice is required to become skilled and confident in the technique of venipuncture.

VENIPUNCTURE EQUIPMENT

Proper collection of blood requires specialized equipment. A complete list of materials used in routine venipuncture is shown in the box. Phlebotomists generally carry the equipment in a portable tray (Figure 53-1). A physician's office laboratory often has a permanent location where venipuncture is performed. In such cases, you likely will seat the patient in a venipuncture chair, which has an adjustable locking armrest to protect the patient if he or she should faint (Figure 53-2). However, if the patient has a history of syncope, it is best to perform phlebotomy while the patient is lying on an examination table.

EQUIPMENT USED IN ROUTINE VENIPUNCTURE

- Double-pointed safety needles
- Evacuated, stoppered tubes
- Needle holder
- Sharps container
- Syringes
- Winged infusion sets (butterfly needles)
- Tourniquet
- Marking pen
- Alcohol swabs
- Gauze pads
- Bandages
- Gloves

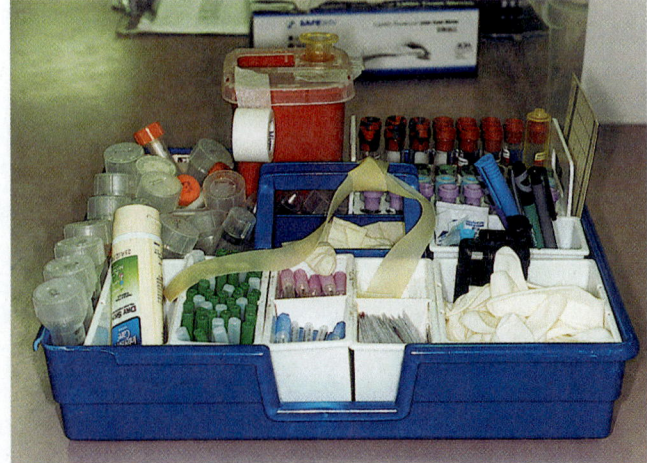

FIGURE 53-1 A fully stocked venipuncture tray. (From Stepp CA, Woods MA: *Laboratory procedures for medical office personnel,* Philadelphia, 1998, Saunders.)

Gloves

Employers must provide employees with gloves, including the hypoallergenic, powderless, and vinyl types, as needed. Remember, even though an employee may not have a latex allergy, the patient may be allergic. Therefore, it is important to ask patients about allergies each time they visit the office. If the patient is allergic to latex, alternative gloves (e.g., vinyl) must be worn; in addition, the medical assistant must consider other necessary supplies, such as tourniquets and adhesive bandages, which may have to be exchanged for versions that do not contain latex. Many facilities stock only latex-free supplies because of the potential for allergic responses in workers and patients.

The Occupational Safety and Health Administration (OSHA) requires healthcare workers to wear gloves during venipuncture; however, the agency does not specify when during the course of the procedure the gloves must be put on. Because veins can be difficult to locate with gloved fingertips, the site may be palpated before gloves are put on. The standard procedure for venipuncture established by the Clinical and Laboratory Standards Institute (CLSI) states that gloves should be put on after vein palpation but before preparation of the site. Those who need the final assurance of one last palpation before the needle is inserted must remember that touching the prepared site, even with gloves, contaminates the area. To help find the vein after cleansing the area, make note of certain skin markers, such as creases, freckles, or scars. If the area is touched, it must be cleansed again. Keep in mind that the tourniquet should be tied for no longer than 1 minute at a time.

Tourniquets

Before blood can be drawn, a vein must be located. Application of a tourniquet (Figure 53-3) is the most common way to do this; it prevents venous flow out of the site, causing the veins to bulge. The tourniquet is tied around the upper arm so that it is tight but not uncomfortable and can be released easily with one hand. Latex tourniquets are inexpensive, but they may become contaminated, and some patients are allergic to latex. Other tourniquets with Velcro closures are available and may be more comfortable for the patient, but they are difficult to release. Single-use, nonlatex tourniquets are available and currently are recommended for reducing cross-contamination between patients and healthcare workers, preventing nosocomial infection, and preventing latex exposure.

Tourniquets are tied 3 to 4 inches above the elbow immediately before the venipuncture procedure begins. Because a tourniquet impedes blood flow, leaving it on for longer than 1 minute greatly increases the possibility of **hemoconcentration** and altered test results. The tourniquet should not be tied so tightly as to impede arterial blood flow; this restricts venous blood return, resulting in poor venous distention. Checking the pulse at the wrist ensures that arterial flow is not restricted. Tourniquets also are used when blood is drawn from hand and foot veins and are tied on the wrist or ankle, respectively.

Tourniquets can be uncomfortable for patients, especially those with heavy-set or hairy upper arms, if they are not applied correctly. Make sure the tourniquet is flat against the skin, and if necessary, tie it over the clothing if it is causing the patient discomfort. This may be especially important when blood is drawn in an aging individual because of the fragility of the skin.

Antiseptics

To prevent infection, a venipuncture site must be cleansed with an antiseptic. The most commonly used is 70% isopropyl alcohol, also known as *rubbing alcohol*. Prepackaged alcohol "prep pads" are the

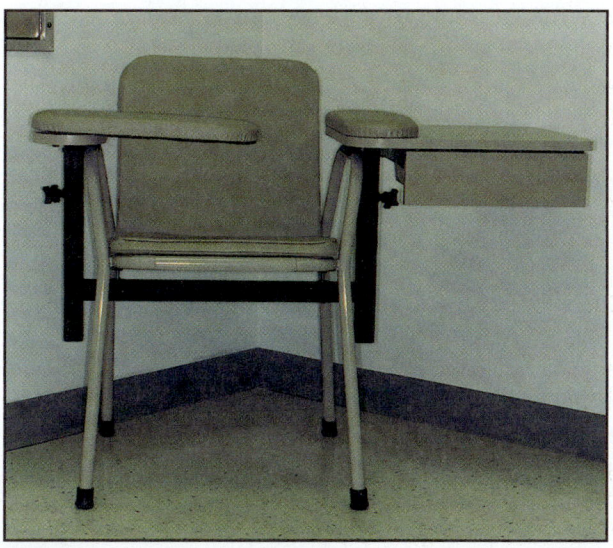

FIGURE 53-2 A phlebotomy chair. (From Stepp CA, Woods MA: *Laboratory procedures for medical office personnel*, Philadelphia, 1998, Saunders.)

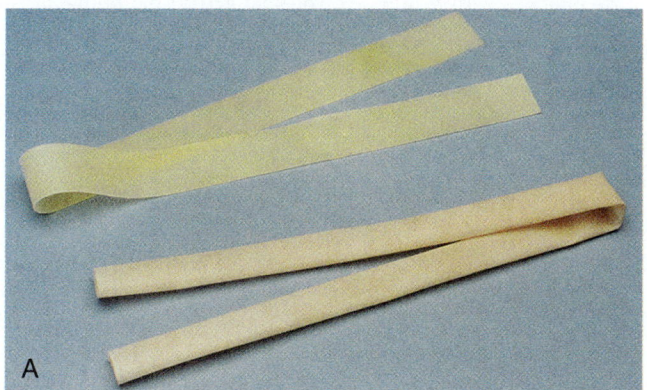
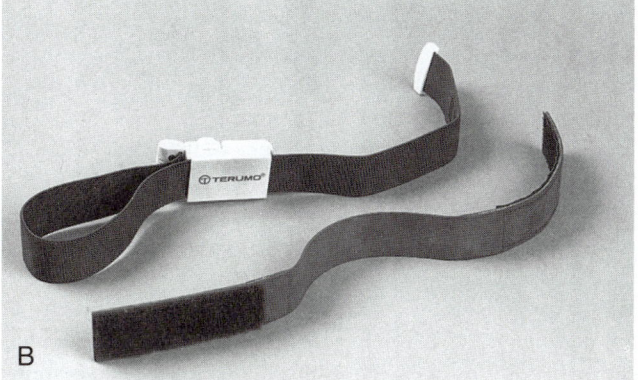

FIGURE 53-3 Examples of tourniquets. (**B,** From Flynn JC Jr: *Procedures in phlebotomy*, ed 3, Philadelphia, 2005, Saunders.)

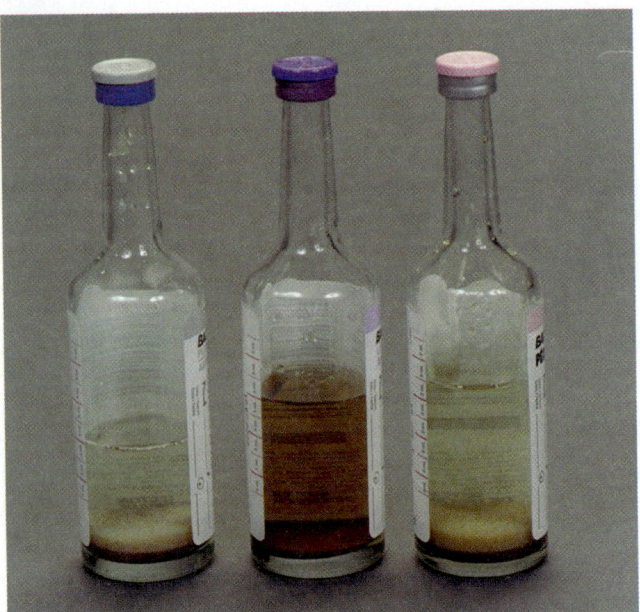

FIGURE 53-4 Bactec blood culture bottles.

most commonly used product. The square prep pad is rubbed on the skin in a circular motion, and the alcohol is allowed to dry. Alcohol does not sterilize the skin; it inhibits the reproduction of bacteria that might contaminate the sample. To be most effective, the alcohol should remain on the skin 30 to 60 seconds. However, isopropyl alcohol should not be used when a sample for a blood alcohol test is drawn. Sterile soap pads, benzalkonium chloride, or povidone-iodine (Betadine) can be used instead.

If a blood culture is ordered, additional preparation is needed at the venipuncture site to eliminate contaminating bacteria. Povidone-iodine solution commonly is used, and chlorhexidine gluconate or benzalkonium chloride can be used for patients allergic to iodine. More vigorous cleansing is required for a blood culture sample than for a routine venipuncture. Blood cultures must be drawn into a sterile tube or a bottle specifically designed for the test (Figure 53-4).

Evacuated Collection Tubes

The evacuated tube (Vacutainer) system is the most common collection system in use. It consists of evacuated tubes of various sizes that have color-coded tops, which indicate the tube's contents (Table 53-1). Tubes are available in both glass and shatter-resistant glass. The tube contents include anticoagulants, clot activators, and/or **thixotropic gel.** The vacuum in each tube draws a measured amount of blood into the tube. Tube volumes range from 2 to 15 mL. Be sure to match the needle gauge to the size of the tube; the larger the tube, the greater the vacuum and the more likely it is that the blood will hemolyze if a high-gauge needle with a small lumen is used.

The size of the tube to be used depends on several factors. Each test performed in the laboratory requires a specific amount of blood. Consult the manual provided by the laboratory to make sure you are drawing the right amount of blood for the test. Tests can often be combined, which reduces the number of tubes that must be drawn. For example, both a complete blood count and an

erythrocyte sedimentation rate test (discussed in Chapter 54) are performed on a sample from a lavender-topped tube; you need not draw two tubes, because the 7-mL volume is sufficient for both tests. When in doubt, call the laboratory. Keep in mind that blood is approximately half cells and half liquid. If a test requires 3 mL of **serum,** 6 mL of blood must be collected.

Patients often express great concern when several tubes of blood must be drawn. You can allay their fears by explaining that the average adult has a little less than 10 pints of blood (5 L). Most adults can relate to donating a unit of blood, which is around a pint (400 to 500 mL). Because the red-topped tube contains 10 mL, you would have to draw 40 to 50 tubes before you have removed a pint.

Tube Additives

All tubes except the red-topped one contain an additive. Anticoagulants are added to prevent blood from clotting. Tubes may be glass or plastic, and the additive may be a powder, a liquid visible in the tube, or a liquid sprayed inside the tube by the manufacturer and allowed to dry. The choice of anticoagulant depends on the test to be done.

Ethylenediaminetetraacetic acid (EDTA), found in the lavender-topped tube, prevents platelet clumping and preserves the appearance of blood cells for microscopic examination; however, it is incompatible with the testing reagents used in coagulation studies. Consult the manual provided by the laboratory before obtaining a specimen from the patient.

Clot activators promote blood clotting. Silica particles enhance clotting, for example, by providing a surface for platelet activation. Thrombin quickly promotes clotting and is used in tubes drawn for stat chemistry testing or in the event a sample is needed from a patient taking a prescribed anticoagulant, such as heparin.

Anticoagulants prevent blood from clotting, which allows the contents of the tube to be used in two ways. First, the sample can be used as whole blood; second, the sample can be centrifuged, and the liquid portion, called **plasma,** can be retrieved. Whole blood is used for tests such as complete blood counts and blood typing, whereas plasma is used for stat chemistry testing and coagulation studies.

If blood is allowed to clot and then is centrifuged, the liquid portion is referred to as *serum.* Without a clot activator, blood clots in 30 to 60 minutes, after which it must be centrifuged. The serum must be separated from the cells quickly, because cells may continue to metabolize substances such as glucose or may release metabolites that interfere with testing. Thixotropic gel can be found in some tubes, including the serum separation tube (SST) red-gray and the plasma separation tube (PST) green-gray (marbled) topped tubes by Becton, Dickinson (Franklin Lakes, New Jersey). This synthetic gel has a density between that of red cells and plasma or serum, and it settles between the two during centrifugation, forming a barrier that facilitates retrieval of the liquid portion without cellular contamination.

It is important to mix the contents of the tube well after collection by inverting it several times (do not shake the tube) and also to avoid a short draw (i.e., a tube that is not completely filled) (Table 53-2). Having the proper ratio of blood to additive is crucial. Always be sure to check the tube for an expiration date. Outdated tubes may have diminished vacuum, or the additive may have degraded.

TABLE 53-1 Common Stoppers and Additives and Their Laboratory Uses

VACUTAINER COLOR*	COLOR	HEMOGARD COLOR†	ADDITIVE AND ITS FUNCTION‡	LABORATORY USE	OPTIMUM VOLUME/MINIMUM VOLUME
Adult Tubes					
Yellow		Yellow	SPS prevents blood from clotting and stabilizes bacterial growth	Blood or body fluid cultures	5 mL/NA
Red		Red	None	Serum tests; chemistry studies, blood bank, serology	10 mL/NA
Red-gray (marbled)		Gold	None, but contains silica particles to enhance clot formation	Serum tests	10 mL/NA
Light blue		Light blue	Sodium citrate; removes calcium to prevent blood from clotting	Coagulation testing	4.5 mL/4.5 mL
Green		Green	Heparin (sodium/lithium/ammonium); inhibits thrombin formation to prevent clotting	Chemistry tests	10 mL/3.5 mL
Green-gray (marbled)		Light green	Lithium heparin and gel for plasma separation	Plasma determinations in chemistry studies	2 mL/2 mL
Yellow-gray (marbled)		Orange	Thrombin	Stat serum demonstrations in chemistry studies	2 mL/2 mL
Lavender		Lavender	EDTA; removes calcium to prevent blood from clotting	Hematology tests	7 mL/2 mL
Gray		Gray	Potassium oxalate and sodium fluoride; removes calcium to prevent blood from clotting; fluoride inhibits glycolysis	Chemistry testing, especially glucose and alcohol levels	10 mL/10 mL
Royal blue		Royal blue	Sodium heparin (also sodium EDTA); inhibits thrombin formation to prevent clotting	Chemistry trace elements	7 mL
Pediatric Tubes					
Red		Red			2 mL/NA 3 mL/NA 4 mL/NA
Lavender		Lavender			2 mL/0.6 mL 3 mL/0.9 mL 4 mL/1 mL
Green		Green			2 mL/2 mL
Light blue		Light blue			2.7 mL/2.7 mL

Modified from Rodak BF: *Diagnostic hematology*, Philadelphia, 1995, Saunders.

EDTA, Ethylenediamine tetraacetic acid; *SPS,* sodium polyanetholsulfonate.

*Stopper colors are based on Becton-Dickinson Vacutainer tubes.

†Hemogard closures provide a protective plastic cover over the rubber stopper as an additional safety feature.

‡Additives, additive functions, and laboratory uses are the same for both pediatric and adult tubes.

TABLE 53-2 Effects of Underfilling Collection Tubes

STOPPER COLOR	EFFECT
Yellow	Reduces possibility of bacterial recovery
Red	Insufficient sample
Red-gray	Poor barrier formation; insufficient sample
Light blue	Coagulation test results falsely prolonged
Green	False results because of excess heparin
Green-gray	False results because of excess heparin
Lavender	Falsely low blood cell counts and hematocrits; morphologic changes to red blood cells; staining alteration
Yellow-gray	False results
Gray	False results
Royal blue	False results

TABLE 53-3 Stopper Color and Inversion Mixing

STOPPER COLOR	MIX BY INVERSION
Yellow	8-10 times
Light blue	3-4 times
Red or red speckled	5 times
Green	8-10 times
Lavender	8-10 times
Gray	8-10 times

CRITICAL THINKING APPLICATION   53-1

- Melissa Machen has been assigned to orient Leah to the clinic and her duties as a certified medical assistant. Melissa takes Leah to the laboratory in the clinic, which has a small room with a blood collection chair and a table. What supplies should be on the table for performing venipuncture?
- What else might Leah find in this room?

Order of Collection

If samples for more than one tube must be drawn during a venipuncture, a specified order must be followed so that material from a previous tube is not transferred to the next tube. Carryover of additives from one tube to the next could cause sample alteration and erroneous results. The CLSI (formerly the National Committee for Clinical Laboratory Standards [NCCLS]) developed a set of standards outlining the order of draw for a multitube draw. The same order applies to the filling of tubes when blood is collected in a syringe and takes into account the use of newer plastic tubes:

1. *Yellow* blood culture tubes are filled first, because they are sterile.
2. *Light blue*–topped tubes with sodium citrate are next, because other anticoagulants might contaminate the sample collected for coagulation studies. If no blood culture has been ordered, CLSI recommends that blood for the light blue–topped tube should be drawn first if routine coagulation testing has been ordered (i.e., prothrombin time [PT] and activated partial thromboplastin time [APTT]; see Chapter 54). For testing other than routine PT and APTT, a red-topped "waste" tube may be filled. When a winged infusion set is used, CLSI currently recommends that blood be drawn into a red-topped tube even if the order does not call for it. This is done to fill the tubing's dead space with blood and to prevent any thromboplastin released during venipuncture from contaminating the light blue–topped tube and interfering with coagulation testing. It is not necessary to fill the tube to be discarded.
3. *Red* serum tubes without clot activator (red stopper) or with clot activator (*red-gold* or *speckled stopper*) are filled next. Although CLSI notes that glass, nonadditive serum tubes can be drawn before the light blue–topped tubes, the draw order has been simplified to function for all serum tubes, regardless of their composition.
4. *Green*-topped tubes are next, because heparin is less likely to interfere with EDTA than vice versa.
5. *Lavender*-topped tubes follow. Because EDTA binds with calcium, blood for this tube is drawn near the end.
6. The *gray*-topped tube is last, because the contents can elevate electrolyte levels or damage cells if passed into another tube (Table 53-3).

Types of Sharps and Supplies Used in Phlebotomy

A critical part of phlebotomy is the knowledge of which needle and which tube or syringe should be used in each situation. All needles used in phlebotomy are sterile, disposable, and used only once. Each is housed in a cover, which should be inspected before use to ensure that sterility has not been compromised (i.e., the seal should be intact), and that the needle has no manufacturing defects, such as burrs or nicks. Needles have two parts: the hub and the shaft. Shafts differ in length, ranging from ¾ to 1½ inches. The length of the shaft has no bearing on the venipuncture procedure, but some prefer a longer needle because it is less likely to slip out of the vein, whereas others prefer a shorter needle because it makes patients less uneasy. One end of the shaft is cut at an angle and forms the bevel, which creates a very sharp point. The hole in the bevel is called the *lumen*.

Lumen size is important in venipuncture and is referred to as the *gauge*. The gauge is designated by a numeric value; the higher the number, the smaller the lumen. A blood bank uses a 16-gauge needle to collect pints of blood for transfusions, because the lumen is wide, which reduces the chance of **hemolysis.** The smallest-gauge needles (23 gauge) are used to collect blood from small or fragile veins, such as those found in elderly and very young patients. Routine adult venipuncture requires a 20- to 21-gauge needle. The hub is the point where the needle attaches to the syringe or the needle holder.

Multisample Needles

Multisample needles are commonly used in routine adult venipuncture. They are so called because they are used when several tubes are to be drawn during a single venipuncture. These needles are double-pointed (Figure 53-5). One point enters the patient's vein, and the other punctures the rubber stopper of the collection tube. The point that enters the tube is sheathed with a retractable rubber sleeve that allows tubes to be changed without blood leaking into the needle holder or tube holder.

Syringes

Syringes are used when there is concern that the strong vacuum in a stoppered tube might collapse the vein. The syringe needle fits on the end of the barrel and comes in different gauges. The amount of blood drawn into the barrel depends on how much is to be transferred to stoppered tubes. When blood is drawn into a syringe, it must be transferred immediately to another tube, because the blood will clot in the syringe barrel. In these situations a syringe with an engineered sharps injury prevention feature and safe work practices should be used. The blood must be transferred from the syringe to the test tube with a needleless blood transfer device, as required by OSHA. A special transfer tube adapter is used to transfer the blood to the Vacutainer tube. The adapter connects to the top of the syringe once the needle cover is in place and the needle is removed. The adapter contains an enclosed needle that punctures and delivers the blood into the Vacutainer tube (Figure 53-6).

Winged Infusion Sets (Butterfly Needles)

Butterfly needles (Figure 53-7) are designed for use on small veins, such as those in the hand or in pediatric patients. The most common needle size is 23 gauge; the needle is ½ to ¾ inch long and has a plastic, flexible, butterfly-shaped grip attached to a short length of tubing. One end is fitted into the syringe or the vacuum tube adapter. Often a syringe is used, because the vacuum can be controlled more easily. Smaller evacuated tubes, with a less powerful vacuum, are preferable when a butterfly set is used.

Needle Holders

Double-pointed needles must be firmly placed into a needle adapter or tube holder (Figure 53-8). Usually they are translucent cylinders, and they come in different sizes to accommodate the tube used. The cylinders often have a ring that indicates how far the tube can be pushed onto the needle without losing the vacuum. OSHA requires that, to prevent accidental needle sticks, needle holders must be discarded after a single use. In most cases the entire needle and holder are disposed of simultaneously; needles are not removed from the needle holder, and the safety feature on the needle must be activated before disposal.

Needle Safety

Healthcare workers who use or may be exposed to needles are at increased risk of needlestick injury. Such injuries can lead to serious or fatal infections with blood-borne pathogens such as hepatitis B virus (HBV), hepatitis C virus (HCV), or human immunodeficiency virus (HIV). An estimated 600,000 needlestick injuries occur each year, and nursing staff members are most frequently injured. Needlestick injuries account for up to 80% of accidental exposures to blood. As discussed in Chapter 27, used needles should never be recapped.

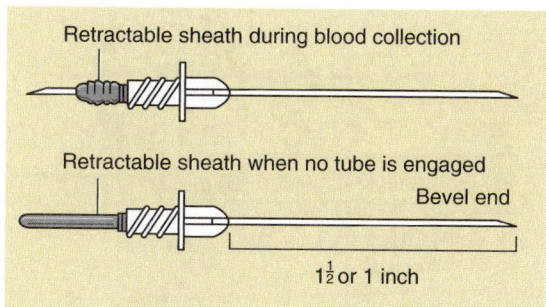

FIGURE 53-5 Multisample needles.

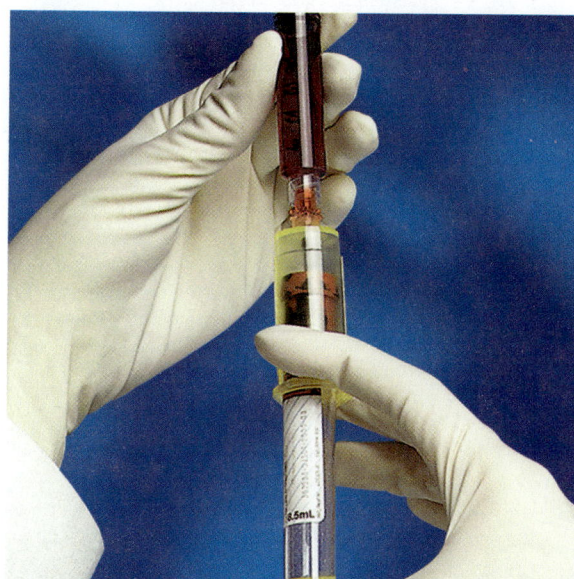

FIGURE 53-6 BD Vacutainer blood transfer device. (Courtesy Becton, Dickinson, Franklin Lakes, New Jersey.)

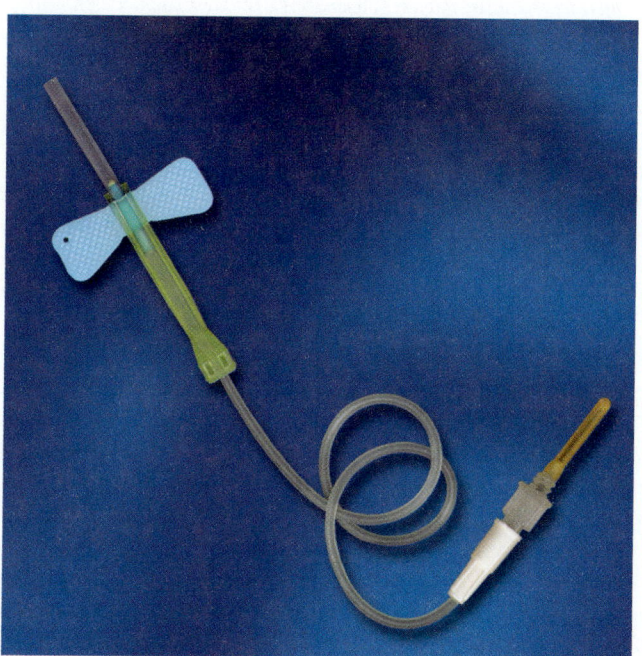

FIGURE 53-7 Winged infusion set attached to an evacuated tube holder with a Luer needle holder. (Courtesy and © Becton, Dickinson and Company, Franklin Lakes, New Jersey.)

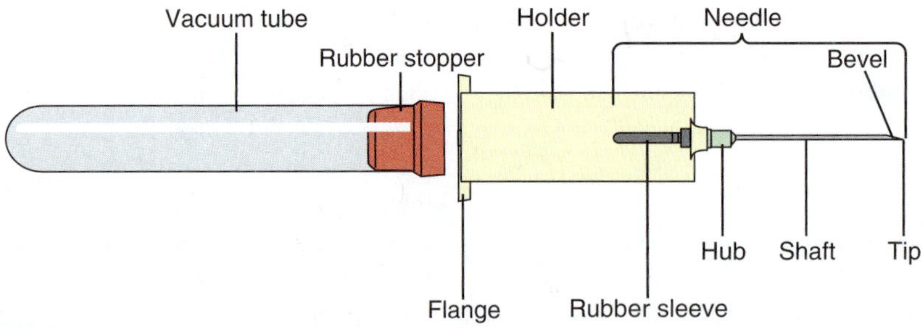

FIGURE 53-8 *Vacuum system with needle and needle holder. (From Hunt SA: Saunders fundamentals of medical assisting-revised reprint, St Louis, 2007, Saunders.)*

According to OSHA, the best practice for preventing needlestick injuries after phlebotomy is to use a sharp with engineered sharps injury protection (SESIP) attached to a needle holder. SESIPs, or safety needles, eliminate the need to remove the needle from the needle holder and in some way shield the needle immediately after use. The U.S. Food and Drug Administration (FDA), which is responsible for approving medical devices marketed and sold in the United States, recommends devices that provide a barrier between the hands and the needle after use in which the phlebotomist's hands remain behind the needle at all times. Safety shields that can be activated before or immediately after removal of the needle from the vein and that remain in effect after disposal also should be an integral part of the device. Finally, these devices should be as simple as possible, requiring little or no training to use. Some examples of SESIPs include the following:

- *Self-sheathing safety devices* (Figure 53-9): These devices have sliding needle shields attached to disposable syringes and vacuum tube holders. Before activation, the sleeve is positioned over the barrel of the syringe. After the procedure, the phlebotomist slides the sleeve forward over the needle, where it locks into place, protecting the needle.
- *Retractable safety devices* (Figure 53-10): After the needle has been used and removed from the vein, a plunger is pushed to retract the needle into the syringe or needle holder. The entire unit is disposed of in the sharps container.
- *Needle-blunting safety mechanisms* (Figures 53-11 and 53-12): After the venipuncture, a blunt tube is moved through the needle, covering the sharp point. With the needle in the needle holder, the vacuum tube is removed and then is pushed forward again while the needle is still in the vein. This moves the blunt-tipped needle forward through the needle, past the sharp needle point. The blunt point tip of the needle can be activated before it is removed from the patient.

When a butterfly set is used, a third "wing" is rotated after collection and before removal of the needle from the vein. As the third wing is rotated, it moves the blunt needle down the shaft before it is removed from the patient.

- *Hinged or sliding safety mechanisms* (Figure 53-13): These devices, which are attached to the phlebotomy needle or to a winged infusion needle, are manually engaged after the needle has been removed from the vein. The plastic sheath covers the needle, and the entire unit is disposed of in the sharps container.

The following steps should be taken to protect against needlestick injuries:

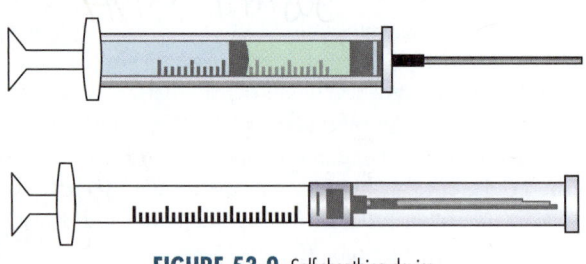

FIGURE 53-9 Self-sheathing device.

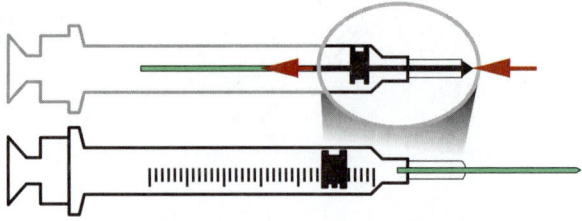

FIGURE 53-10 Retractable safety device.

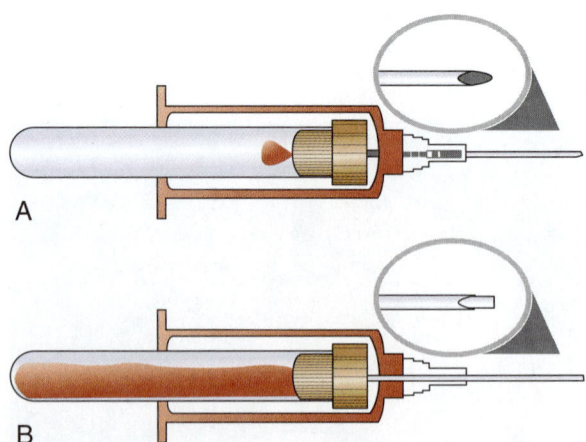

FIGURE 53-11 Needle-blunting sharp with engineered sharps injury protection (SESIP) for the needle holder. **A,** Needle while collecting specimen before activation. **B,** Needle with blunting device activated.

- Do not use needles when safe, effective alternatives are available.
- Help your employer select and evaluate devices with safety features.
- Use devices with safety features provided by your employer.

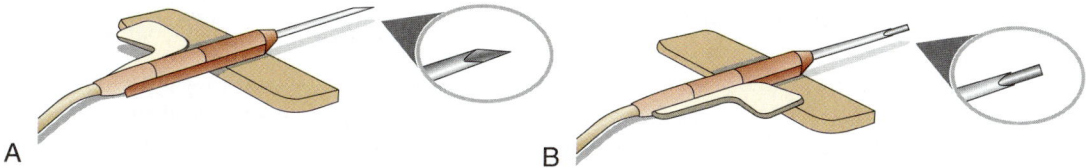

FIGURE 53-12 Needle-blunting sharp with engineered sharps injury protection (SESIP) for winged infusion sets. **A,** Before activation, with needle in vein. **B,** After activation.

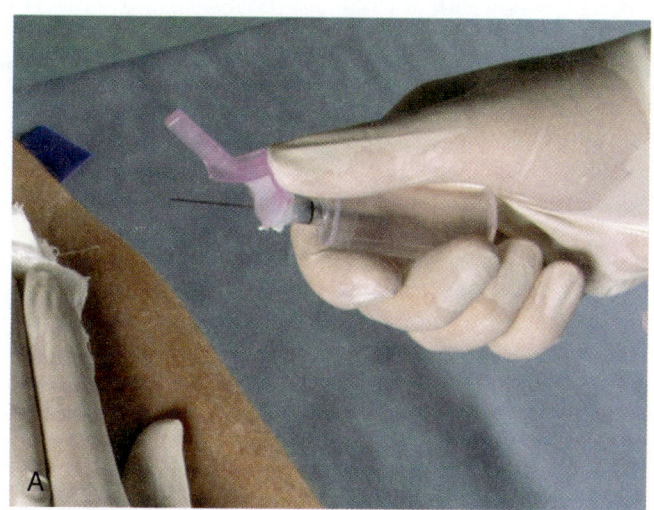
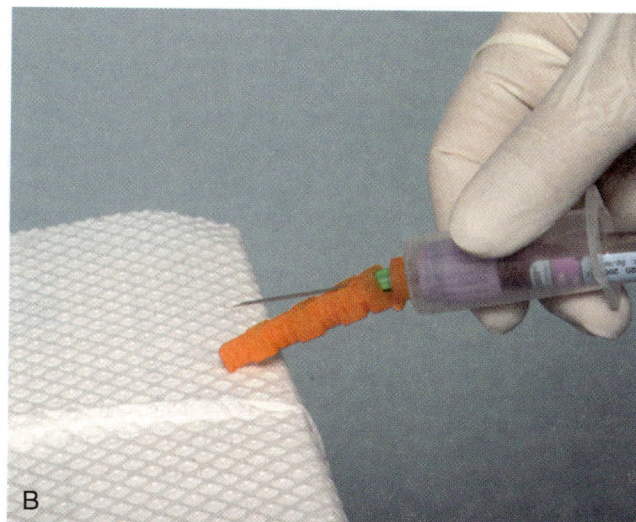

FIGURE 53-13 Hinged or sliding sharp with engineered sharps injury protection (SESIP). **A,** Before venipuncture. **B,** After activation. (Modified from Garrels M, Oatis C: *Laboratory testing for ambulatory settings,* ed 2, St Louis, 2011, Saunders.)

- Never recap a contaminated needle.
- Plan for safe handling and disposal before beginning any procedure using needles.
- Dispose of used needles and needle holders promptly in appropriate sharps disposal containers.
- Report all needlestick and other sharps-related injuries promptly to ensure that you receive appropriate follow-up care.
- Tell your employer about hazards from needles that you observe in your work environment.
- Participate in blood-borne pathogen training and follow recommended infection prevention practices, including obtaining hepatitis B vaccination.

As detailed in Chapter 27, OSHA requires employers to establish and maintain a sharps injury log for recording injuries from contaminated sharps. This log should contain information about the device involved in the incident and the department or work area where the incident occurred, as well as an explanation of the incident. Employee confidentiality must be maintained.

Postexposure Management of Needlesticks

An accidental needlestick is a medical emergency. (OSHA-recommended management procedures are discussed in detail in Chapter 27.) Effective management of an accidental sharps exposure includes the following:

- Immediately after injury, the wound is inspected for foreign material, which is removed. The site is washed for 10 minutes with an antimicrobial soap, 10% iodine solution, or chlorine-based antiseptic.
- The injury is reported to the supervisor and an incident report is completed.
- The employee is referred to a physician for confidential assessment and follow-up. Baseline testing for HBV, HCV, and HIV is recommended for both the employee and the source individual. If the employee has been immunized for HBV and has a positive postimmunization titer, there is no risk of acquiring HBV and no source testing is needed. If the worker has not been immunized, source testing for infection with HBV is recommended if the source is known and can be located. If the source patient tests positive for HBV, the employee should receive HBV immune globulin (HBIG), and the series of HBV immunizations should be initiated. If the source tests negative, no treatment is indicated. If the source patient cannot be tested, the employee should be treated as if the source patient were positive for HBV. The source should also be tested for HCV. If positive, the employee should be monitored for signs and symptoms of hepatitis for 6 months. No postexposure prophylaxis is recommended for HCV infection. For HIV exposure, most employers recommend a 4-week regimen of antiretroviral drugs. To best protect the victim, antiretroviral therapy should be administered within hours of exposure. HIV treatment involves potentially serious side effects; therefore, the employee decides whether medications are started. If the

source is found to be negative, antiretroviral therapy can be discontinued.

- Interim testing may be performed if the healthcare worker experiences symptoms of acute HIV exposure or hepatitis. For HIV, antibody testing should be repeated at 6 weeks, 12 weeks, and 6 months if either the source was HIV positive or the source's status remains unknown. Confidential follow-up care must include provisions for emotional support and counseling for the healthcare worker.

CRITICAL THINKING APPLICATION   **53-2**

- During her lunch break, Leah meets some of her co-workers. The conversation in the lunchroom involves an accident that occurred several years ago when a former employee was performing venipuncture on a recovering intravenous drug addict and was accidentally stuck with the needle. Describe the procedure for follow-up of an accidental needlestick incident.
- What measures are available to prevent accidental needlesticks?

ROUTINE VENIPUNCTURE

Your appearance and actions reflect your laboratory or facility. A patient's first impression of the facility often comes from you. Clean laboratory coats or scrubs tell the patient the facility is clean; wearing gloves tells the patient you will treat him or her with care; and speaking knowledgeably provides the impression that the facility is staffed with professionals.

Venipuncture involves several important steps with which the medical assistant must be thoroughly familiar before attempting the procedure. The first step is to select the proper method for venipuncture (syringe or evacuated tube). Next, the patient must be prepared for the procedure. Patient preparation is followed by the actual venipuncture and specimen collection. The final step is care of the puncture site before the patient is discharged.

Patient Preparation

All blood collections begin with a requisition, a form from the patient's physician requesting a test. Requisitions may be computer generated or handwritten and at minimum must include the following information:

- Patient's name
- Date of birth
- Identification number
- Name of the physician making the request
- Type of test requested
- Test status (timed, fasting, stat, and so forth)

Venipuncture begins with greeting and identifying the patient. According to CLSI, proper identification includes asking outpatients to provide their full name and address, and an identification number or birth date. This information must be compared with the written information on the requisition. With inpatients, CLSI recommends asking for the same information and comparing it with the information on the requisition and on the identification bracelet. If the patient speaks a different language, has limited language skills (such as a child), or is otherwise unable to communicate, a family member or caregiver must provide the information. The name of this person should be documented.

Introduce yourself and briefly explain the purpose and procedure of the venipuncture. If the patient has questions about the ordered tests, politely request that the patient speak to the physician, and ask whether the individual would like to do so before you collect the sample. Obtain verbal consent to perform the procedure simply by asking whether you have permission to take some blood from the patient's arm. Always ask the patient whether he or she has experienced problems during routine venipuncture in the past, and take steps to prevent such problems. Your self-confidence in the procedure will be evident to the patient and will help allay any fears. Instilling confidence in your patients means acting and speaking professionally. Refer to the patient as "sir" or "ma'am" or Mr. Jones or Ms. Smith, not "honey," "sweetie," Bill, or Margaret. Being friendly is important, but make sure your patients feel respected and understand that you take your role in their care seriously.

Preparing for the Venipuncture

Seat the patient in a chair or have the person lie down on an examination table, if the patient has a history of syncope, and ask the patient to extend the arm. Inspect both arms and ask whether the patient has a preference. Generally, veins in the forearm or the elbow (antecubital area) are used for venipuncture (Figure 53-14). The puncture site should be carefully selected after both arms have been inspected. Alternative sites may be indicated if the area is cyanotic, scarred, bruised, edematous, or burned. You may use veins on the lower forearm, the back of the hand, or the wrist. Use foot or ankle veins only if the patient has good circulation in the legs and you have received permission from your supervisor or the physician. Never draw blood from this area if the patient is diabetic.

To apply a tourniquet, place the tourniquet 3 to 4 inches above the patient's elbow, making sure it is not twisted (Figure 53-15). Grasp the tourniquet ends, one in each hand, at the part of the tourniquet that is closest to the patient's skin. Pull the ends apart to

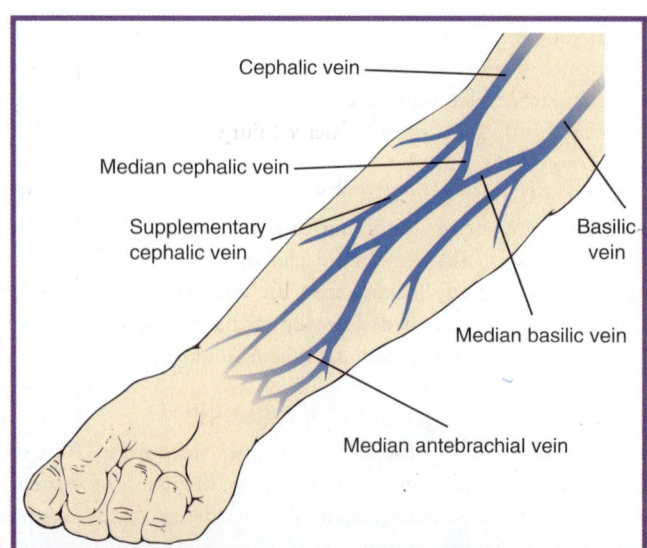

FIGURE 53-14 The veins of the forearm. (From Stepp CA, Woods MA: *Laboratory procedures for medical office personnel*, Philadelphia, 1998, Saunders.)

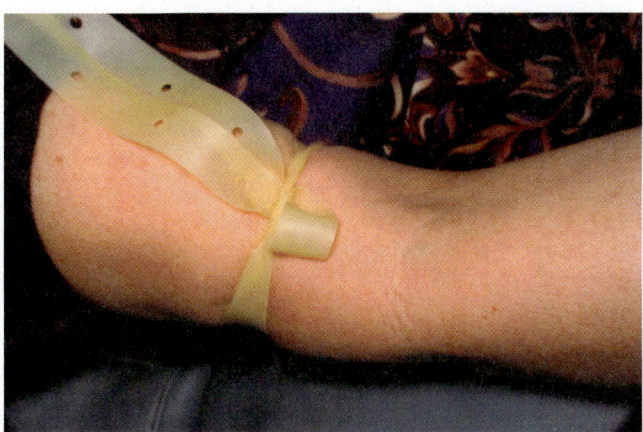

FIGURE 53-15 Placement of a tourniquet. (From Rose L et al: *Periodontics*, St Louis, 2004, Mosby.)

stretch the rubber material, then cross one end over the other while maintaining the tension. Tuck the top end of the tourniquet underneath the bottom piece, creating a loop with the upper flap free so it can be released with one hand. The tourniquet should be tight without being twisted or pinching the patient's skin. Both ends of the tourniquet should be pointing upward so that they do not contaminate the blood draw site.

When the tourniquet is in place, ask the patient to make a fist, and palpate for an acceptable vein using your ungloved index finger. If you are able to palpate the vein through gloved fingers, you can continue with the phlebotomy process. A thorough survey of both arms should be done before the venipuncture site is chosen. Veins bounce lightly when palpated. The medial veins generally run parallel or at a slight angle to the fold in the antecubital area, whereas the cephalic veins run lateral or to the outside of the antecubital area. These veins are the veins of choice. The basilic vein, which lies on the inside part of the antecubital area, is very close to the brachial artery and median nerves and should be used only if the medial or cephalic veins are inaccessible. The most common injury patients suffer from phlebotomy is nerve injury. If the patient complains of tingling, numbness, or a shooting pain, discontinue the procedure and choose another site before continuing. Do not probe with the needle under this condition; any attempt at relocating the needle puts the patient at great risk of nerve injury.

Performing the Venipuncture

When you have located a vein, remove the tourniquet. A tourniquet can remain in place for 1 minute. After its removal, you must wait 2 minutes before reapplying it. Assemble the appropriate equipment, making sure everything is within easy reach, that the sterile packets are torn open, and that the contents are easily accessible. Sanitize your hands.

Reapply the tourniquet and quickly relocate the vein. Put on your gloves and cleanse the antecubital area with the alcohol, working outward in a circular motion. Do not touch this area after cleansing. Ask the patient to clench the hand into a fist. Do not have the patient pump the fist, because this may temporarily increase the level of potassium and ionized calcium in the blood. Anchor the vein by stretching the skin downward below the collection site with the

thumb of the nondominant hand, and swiftly insert the needle into the vein at a 15-degree angle. The bevel should be facing up. If the needle is inserted at an angle greater than 15 degrees, it quickly penetrates the other side of the vein and enters other structures, such as nerves or the brachial artery, and very likely will cause a hematoma or an injury. Pull back on the syringe plunger or push the evacuated tube into the double-pointed needle. When blood enters the tube or barrel, ask the patient to unclench the fist.

Completing the Venipuncture

Continue to draw the specimen, checking periodically on the patient's condition. As you remove each tube from the needle holder, gently invert it several times before you place it in the rack. Tubes with clot activator should be inverted five times, light-blue–topped tubes for coagulation studies should be inverted three or four times, and all other anticoagulant tubes should be inverted eight to ten times. If the tubes are not inverted immediately after collection, small clots can form in the specimen. When you are nearing the end of the draw and the last tube to be collected has been filled, carefully release the tourniquet without jarring the needle, and remove the final vacuum tube. Remove the needle quickly and apply gauze with pressure to the puncture site. Ask the patient to apply direct pressure to the gauze but not to bend the arm. Immediately activate the safety device to cover the needle, and dispose of the entire needle/needle holder unit into a sharps container. Before putting on the bandage, perform a two-point check to make sure the vein is not leaking. Observe the site for 5 to 10 seconds after releasing pressure and removing the gauze. If visible bleeding occurs, or if the tissue around the puncture site rises, continue applying pressure until the bleeding has stopped. Special precautions must be taken for patients receiving anticoagulants, because the phlebotomy site will bleed longer than is the norm. Put on a bandage and dispose of the gauze in a biohazard waste container. Clean gauze, not a cotton ball, can be taped over the site in lieu of a bandage. Label all tubes by the patient's side. Never leave the room or release an outpatient until the tubes have been labeled. Assess the patient's status one last time, then dismiss the patient or leave the room.

Procedures 53-1 and 53-2 outline the proper procedures for venipuncture using a syringe and the evacuated tube method. Certain patients, such as those with narrow veins, young children, and aging adults, may require a winged infusion set (butterfly needle) rather than the previously mentioned methods. Butterfly units also can be used to draw blood from the hands of adults. As mentioned, the needle in a winged infusion unit is shorter, and the wings help you grasp and guide the needle more easily. The tubing also minimizes the strength of the vacuum, thus preventing the collapse of fragile veins, which is a common problem in phlebotomy on elderly patients (Procedure 53-3).

PROBLEMS ASSOCIATED WITH VENIPUNCTURE

Failure to obtain blood can occur because of a number of factors. Determining the cause of the problem may help you decide whether a second attempt would be successful. The first rule is to remain calm so that you can think clearly and can systematically determine the possible cause of the problem.

Text continued on p. 1159

PROCEDURE 53-1

Perform Venipuncture:

Collect a Venous Blood Sample Using the Syringe Method

GOAL: *To collect a venous blood specimen using the syringe technique.*

EQUIPMENT and SUPPLIES

- Needle, syringe with 21- or 22-gauge safety needle
- Vacutainer tubes appropriate for tests ordered
- 70% isopropyl alcohol pads
- Sterile gauze pads
- Tourniquet
- Syringe adapter for transfer to Vacutainer tubes
- Hypoallergenic tape or bandage
- Permanent marking pen or printed labels
- Biohazard bag and sharps container
- Disposable gloves
- Patient's record

PROCEDURAL STEPS

1. Check the requisition form to determine the tests ordered. Gather the appropriate tubes and supplies.
   PURPOSE: To collect the specimen properly.
2. Sanitize your hands and put on nonsterile gloves.
   PURPOSE: To ensure infection control.
3. Identify the patient, explain the procedure, and obtain permission to perform the venipuncture.
   PURPOSE: To make sure you have the right patient; explanations help to gain the patient's cooperation.
4. Assist the patient to sit with the arm well supported in a slightly downward position.
   PURPOSE: The veins of the antecubital fossa are more easily located when the elbow is straight.
5. Assemble the equipment. The choice of syringe barrel size and needle size depends on your inspection of the patient's veins and the amount of blood required for the ordered tests. Attach the needle to the syringe. Pull and depress the plunger several times to loosen it in the barrel. Keep the cover on the needle.
   PURPOSE: Using the smallest syringe possible minimizes the chance of hemolysis. Engaging the plunger ensures that you will not have to use as much force to pull the blood into the barrel, thereby minimizing the chance of hemolysis.
6. Apply the tourniquet around the patient's arm 3 to 4 inches above the elbow. The tourniquet should never be tied so tightly that it restricts blood flow in the artery (Figure 1). The tourniquet should remain in place no longer than 1 minute.
   PURPOSE: The tourniquet is used to make the veins more prominent. A quick check of the radial pulse ensures that the tourniquet has not been applied too tightly.

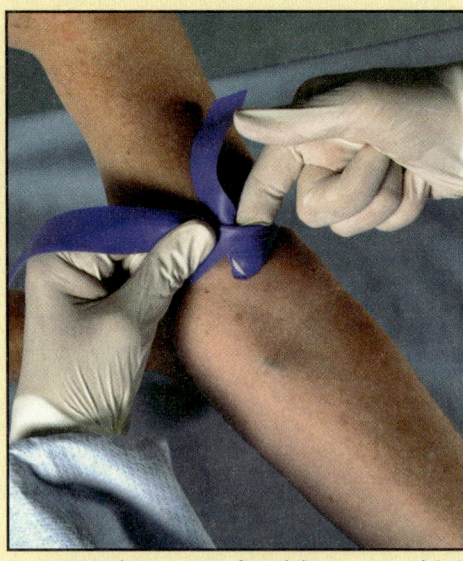

(From Garrels M, Oatis C: *Laboratory testing for ambulatory settings*, ed 2, St Louis, 2011, Saunders.)

7. Ask the patient to make a fist.
   PURPOSE: Clenching the fist produces engorgement of the vein.
8. Select the venipuncture site by palpating the antecubital space (if you have difficulty palpating the vein with gloves, you can remove the gloves, palpate the vein and visibly mark its location, then put on new gloves before continuing); use your index finger to trace the path of the vein and to judge its depth. The vein most often used is the median cephalic vein, which lies in the middle of the elbow (Figure 2).

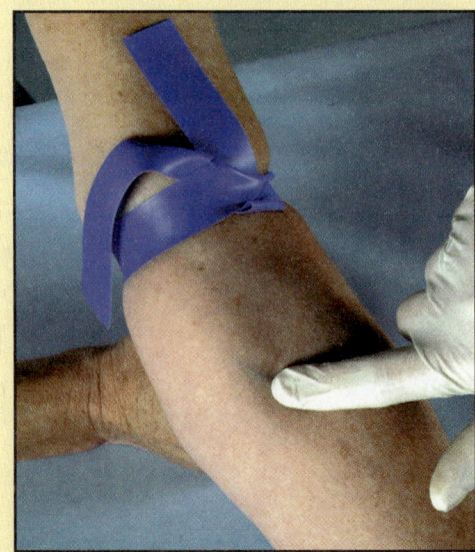

(From Garrels M, Oatis C: *Laboratory testing for ambulatory settings*, ed 2, St Louis, 2011, Saunders.)

PURPOSE: The index finger is most sensitive for palpating. Do not use the thumb, because it has a pulse of its own, which may confuse you.

PROCEDURE 53-1—cont'd

9. Cleanse the site, starting in the center of the area and working outward in a circular pattern with the alcohol pad (Figure 3). Allow the area to dry before proceeding.

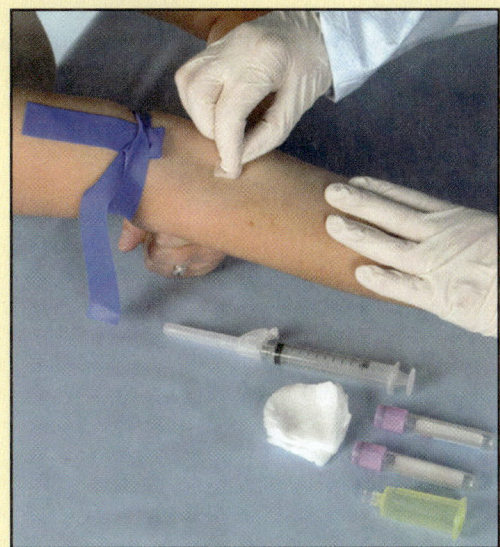

(From Garrels M, Oatis C: *Laboratory testing for ambulatory settings*, ed 2, St Louis, 2011, Saunders.)

PURPOSE: The circular pattern helps prevent recontamination of the area. Puncturing a wet area stings and can cause hemolysis of the sample.

10. Hold the syringe in your dominant hand. Your thumb should be on top and your fingers underneath. Remove the needle sheath.

11. Grasp the patient's arm with the nondominant hand and anchor the vein by stretching the skin downward below the collection site with the thumb of the nondominant hand.
    PURPOSE: Failure to anchor the vein makes puncturing more difficult and painful and may result in a missed vein.

12. With the bevel of the needle up, aligned parallel to the vein, and at a 15-degree angle, insert the needle through the skin and into the vein rapidly and smoothly (Figure 4). Observe for a "flash" of blood in the hub of the syringe. Ask the patient to release the fist.

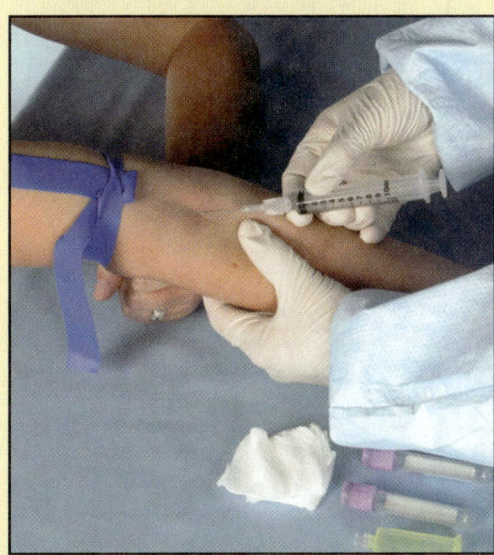

(From Garrels M, Oatis C: *Laboratory testing for ambulatory settings*, ed 2, St Louis, 2011, Saunders.)

PURPOSE: The sharpest point of the needle is inserted first. The angle ensures that the needle does not penetrate through the vein. The appearance ("flash") of blood in the hub ensures that the needle is in the vein.

13. Slowly pull back the plunger of the syringe with the nondominant hand. Do not allow more than 1 mL of head space between the blood and the top of the plunger. Make sure you do not move the needle after entering the vein. Fill the barrel to the needed volume (Figure 5).

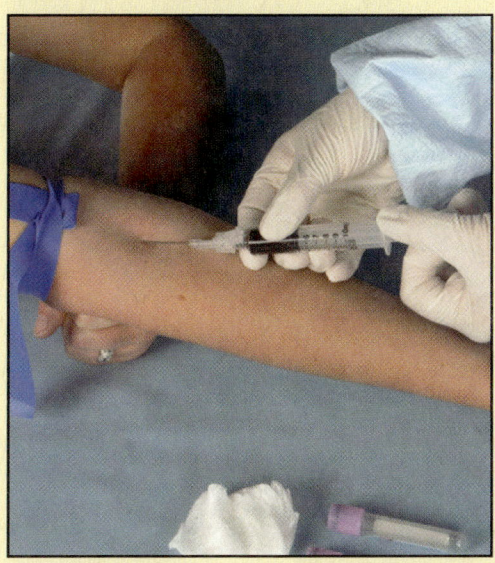

(From Garrels M, Oatis C: *Laboratory testing for ambulatory settings*, ed 2, St Louis, 2011, Saunders.)

14. Release the tourniquet when venipuncture is complete. It must be released before the needle is removed from the arm (Figure 6).

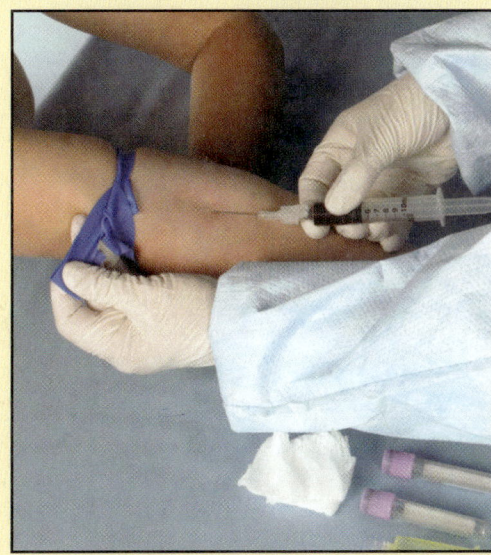

(From Garrels M, Oatis C: *Laboratory testing for ambulatory settings*, ed 2, St Louis, 2011, Saunders.)

PURPOSE: Removal of the tourniquet releases pressure on the vein and helps prevent blood from getting into adjacent tissues and causing a hematoma.

15. Place sterile gauze over the puncture site at the time of needle withdrawal (Figure 7). Immediately activate the needle safety device.

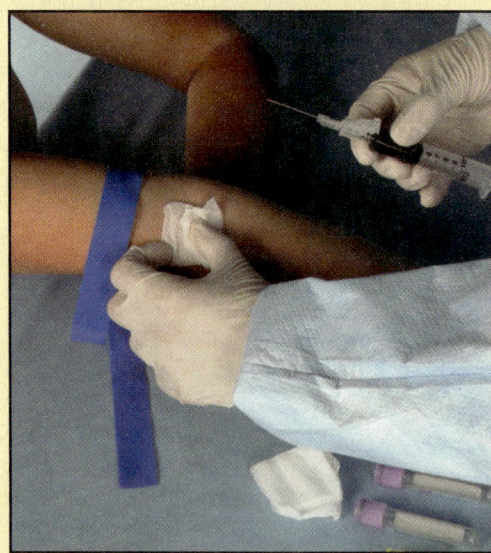

(From Garrels M, Oatis C: *Laboratory testing for ambulatory settings*, ed 2, St Louis, 2011, Saunders.)

16. Instruct the patient to apply direct pressure on the puncture site with sterile gauze. The patient may elevate the arm but should not bend it.
    <u>PURPOSE:</u> Direct pressure is the best method to stop bleeding. Elevating the arm above the heart also stops bleeding.

17. Transfer the blood immediately to the required tube or tubes using a syringe adapter. Do not push on the plunger during transfer. Discard the entire unit in the sharps container when transfer is complete. Invert the tubes after the addition of blood and label them with the necessary patient information (Figure 8).

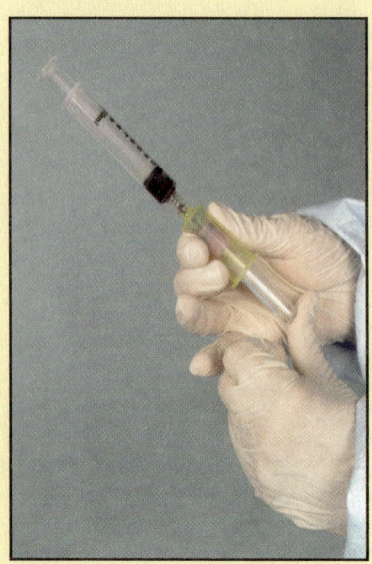

(From Garrels M, Oatis C: *Laboratory testing for ambulatory settings*, ed 2, St Louis, 2011, Saunders.)

<u>PURPOSE:</u> The syringe adapter protects against accidental needlesticks and allows the correct amount of blood to be delivered into the tube by vacuum. Pushing the plunger hemolyzes the blood. Blood begins to clot shortly after collection, so it must be transferred into the vacuum tube and mixed with anticoagulant immediately after collection. Inverting the tubes ensures anticoagulation.

18. Inspect the puncture site for bleeding or hematoma.

19. Apply a hypoallergenic bandage (Figure 9).

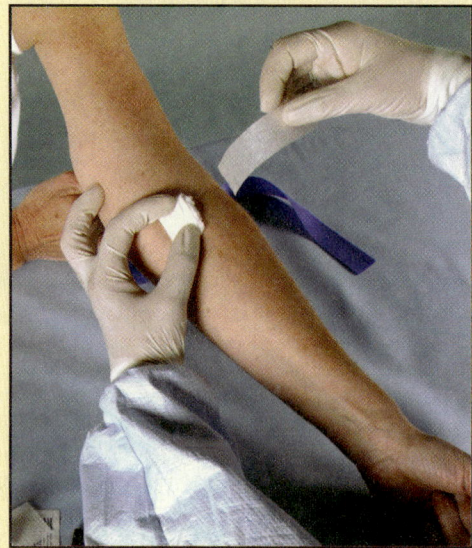

(From Garrels M, Oatis C: *Laboratory testing for ambulatory settings*, ed 2, St Louis, 2011, Saunders.)

20. Disinfect the work area, dispose of any blood-contaminated materials (e.g., gauze) in the biohazard container, remove your gloves, and sanitize your hands.
    <u>PURPOSE:</u> To ensure infection control.

21. Complete the laboratory requisition form and route the specimen to the proper place. Record the procedure in the patient's record.
    <u>PURPOSE:</u> A procedure is not considered complete until it is recorded.

PROCEDURE 53-2

Perform Venipuncture: Collect a Venous Blood Sample Using the Evacuated Tube Method

GOAL: *To collect a venous blood specimen by the evacuated tube technique.*

EQUIPMENT and SUPPLIES

- Vacutainer needle, needle holder, and proper tubes for requested tests
- 70% isopropyl alcohol pads
- Sterile gauze pads
- Tourniquet
- Hypoallergenic tape or bandage
- Permanent marking pen or printed labels
- Biohazard bag and sharps container
- Disposable gloves
- Patient's record

PROCEDURAL STEPS

1. Check the requisition form to determine the tests ordered. Gather the appropriate tubes and supplies.
   <u>PURPOSE:</u> To perform specimen collection properly.
2. Sanitize your hands and put on nonsterile gloves.
   <u>PURPOSE:</u> To ensure infection control.
3. Identify the patient, explain the procedure, and obtain permission for the venipuncture.
   <u>PURPOSE:</u> To make sure you have the right patient; explanations help gain the patient's cooperation.
4. Assist the patient to sit with the arm well supported in a slightly downward position.
   <u>PURPOSE:</u> The veins of the antecubital fossa are more easily located when the elbow is straight.
5. Assemble the equipment. The choice of needle size depends on your inspection of the patient's veins. Attach the needle firmly to the Vacutainer holder. Keep the cover on the needle.
   <u>PURPOSE:</u> If the needle is loose, air can enter the tube, causing frothing and subsequent hemolysis.
6. Apply the tourniquet around the patient's arm 3 to 4 inches above the elbow. The tourniquet should never be tied so tightly that it restricts blood flow in the artery (Figure 1). Tourniquets should remain in place no longer than 60 seconds.
   <u>PURPOSE:</u> The tourniquet is used to make the veins more prominent. A quick check of the radial pulse ensures that the tourniquet has not been applied too tightly.

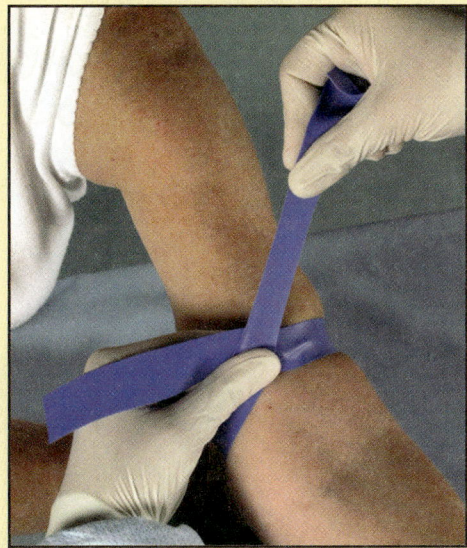

(From Garrels M, Oatis C: *Laboratory testing for ambulatory settings*, ed 2, St Louis, 2011, Saunders.)

7. Ask the patient to make a fist.
   <u>PURPOSE:</u> Clenching the fist produces engorgement of the vein. Do not ask the patient to pump the fist, because this may disrupt the blood's electrolyte balance.
8. Select the venipuncture site by palpating the antecubital space and use your index finger to trace the path of the vein and to judge its depth. The vein most often used is the median cephalic vein, which lies in the middle of the elbow (Figure 2).

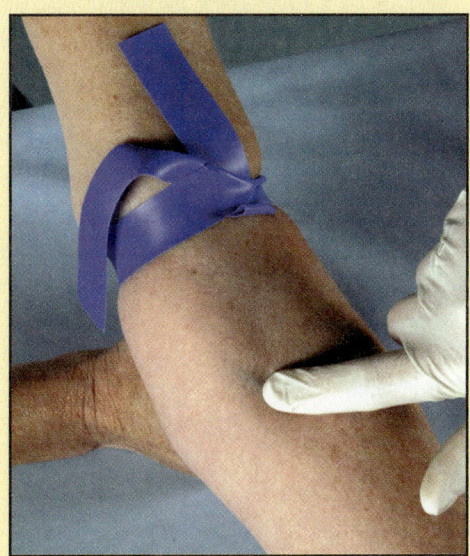

(From Garrels M, Oatis C: *Laboratory testing for ambulatory settings*, ed 2, St Louis, 2011, Saunders.)

<u>PURPOSE:</u> The index finger is most sensitive for palpating. Do not use the thumb, because it has a pulse of its own, which may confuse you.

9. Cleanse the site, starting in the center of the area and working outward in a circular pattern with the alcohol pad (Figure 3).

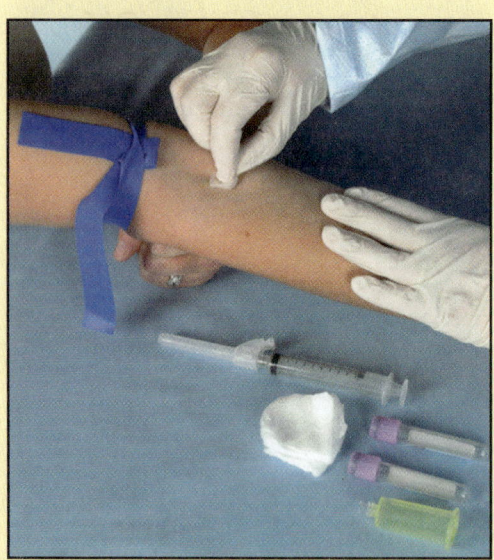

(From Garrels M, Oatis C: *Laboratory testing for ambulatory settings*, ed 2, St Louis, 2011, Saunders.)

10. Dry the site with a sterile gauze pad or allow the area to dry before proceeding.
    PURPOSE: The circular pattern helps prevent recontamination of the area. Puncturing a wet area stings and can cause hemolysis of the sample.

11. Hold the Vacutainer assembly in your dominant hand. Your thumb should be on top and your fingers underneath. You may want to position the first tube to be drawn into the needle holder, but do not push it onto the double-pointed needle past the marking on the holder. Remove the needle sheath.
    PURPOSE: Positioning the hand in this manner provides the best visibility of the needle entering the site. Pushing the tube onto the double-pointed needle causes air to rush into the tube, destroying the vacuum.

12. Grasp the patient's arm with the nondominant hand and anchor the vein by stretching the skin downward below the collection site with the thumb of the nondominant hand.
    PURPOSE: Failure to anchor the vein makes puncturing more difficult and painful and may result in a missed vein.

13. With the bevel of the needle up, aligned parallel to the vein, and at a 15-degree angle, insert the needle through the skin and into the vein rapidly and smoothly (Figure 4).
    PURPOSE: The sharpest point of the needle is inserted first. Inserting the needle quickly minimizes pain.

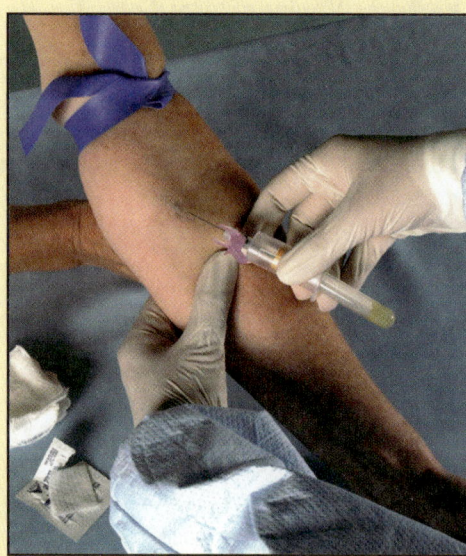

(From Garrels M, Oatis C: *Laboratory testing for ambulatory settings*, ed 2, St Louis, 2011, Saunders.)

14. Place two fingers on the flanges of the needle holder and use the thumb to push the tube onto the double-pointed needle. Make sure you do not change the needle's position in the vein. When blood begins to flow into the tube, ask the patient to release the fist.
    PURPOSE: The thumb has the strength necessary to push the needle swiftly through the stopper. However, if you are not careful, the needle can easily be pushed farther into the site when the tube is pushed.

15. Allow the tube to fill to maximum capacity. Remove the tube by curling the fingers underneath and pushing on the needle holder with the thumb. Take care not to move the needle when removing the tube.
    PURPOSE: Tubes must be full to ensure the proper anticoagulant-to-blood ratio. Moving the needle may result in inadvertent penetration of the other side of the vein or slipping of the needle out of the vein.

16. Insert the second tube into the needle holder, following the instructions in the previous steps. Continue filling tubes until the order on the requisition has been filled. Gently invert each tube immediately after removing it the needle holder to mix anticoagulants and blood. As the last tube is filling, release the tourniquet.
    PURPOSE: The tourniquet should remain in place for no longer than 1 minute to prevent hemoconcentration. Gentle inversion prevents clotting of blood, whereas vigorous mixing may cause hemolysis.

17. Remove the last tube from the holder. Place gauze over the puncture site (Figure 5) and quickly remove the needle, engaging the safety device. Dispose of the entire unit in the sharps container.
    PURPOSE: To ensure infection control.

PROCEDURE 53-2—cont'd

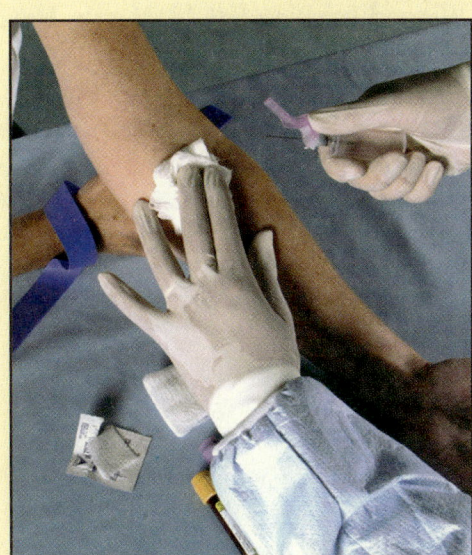

(From Garrels M, Oatis C: *Laboratory testing for ambulatory settings*, ed 2, St Louis, 2011, Saunders.)

18. Apply pressure to the gauze or instruct the patient to do so. The patient may elevate the arm but should not bend it.
    PURPOSE: Applying direct pressure is the best method to stop bleeding. Elevating the arm above the heart also stops bleeding.
19. Label the tubes with the patient's name, the date, and the time, or apply the preprinted tube labels (Figure 6).

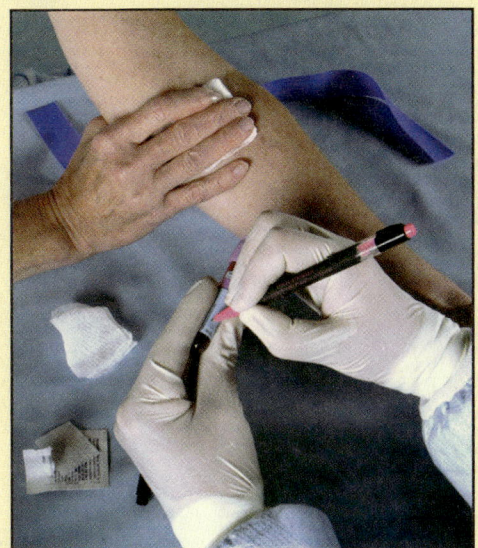

(From Garrels M, Oatis C: *Laboratory testing for ambulatory settings*, ed 2, St Louis, 2011, Saunders.)

20. Check the puncture site for bleeding and hematoma formation.
21. Apply a hypoallergenic bandage (Figure 7).

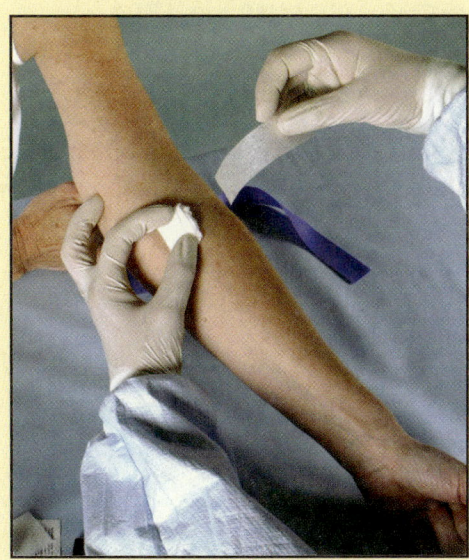

(From Garrels M, Oatis C: *Laboratory testing for ambulatory settings*, ed 2, St Louis, 2011, Saunders.)

22. Disinfect the work area, dispose of any blood-contaminated materials (e.g., gauze) in the biohazard container, remove your gloves, and sanitize your hands.
    PURPOSE: To ensure infection control.
23. Complete the laboratory requisition form and route the specimen to the proper place. Record the procedure in the patient's record.
    PURPOSE: A procedure is considered not done until it is recorded.

10/5/XX 1:45 PM Venous blood drawn from antecubital space of ® arm for CBC with differential and SMA 12. Placed for pick-up by Health Alliance Labs. Leah Barney, CMA (AAMA) _____

PROCEDURE 53-3

Performing Venipuncture: Obtain a Venous Sample with a Winged Infusion Set (Butterfly Needle)

GOAL: *To obtain a venous sample accurately from a hand vein using a winged infusion set.*

EQUIPMENT and SUPPLIES

- Tourniquet
- Alcohol pads or other antiseptic preps
- Sterile gauze pads
- Winged infusion (butterfly) needle set
- Appropriate tubes with a needle and needle adapter
- Syringe with needle
- Sharps disposal container
- Hypoallergenic bandage
- Permanent marking pen or printed labels
- Biohazard waste container
- Disposable gloves
- Patient record

PROCEDURAL STEPS

1. Check the requisition and gather the appropriate tubes for the needed tests. Assemble the balance of your supplies.
   PURPOSE: For efficiency in preparation.
2. Sanitize your hands and put on gloves.
   PURPOSE: To ensure infection control.
3. Identify the patient, and explain the procedure.
   PURPOSE: To make sure you have the right patient; explanations help to gain the patient's cooperation.
4. Remove the butterfly device from the package and stretch the tubing slightly. Take care not to activate the needle-retracting safety device accidentally.
   PURPOSE: To keep the tube from recoiling.
5. Attach the butterfly device to the syringe (Figure 1) or needle holder.

6. Seat the first tube in the evacuated tube holder and place the unit carefully where it will not roll away.
7. Apply a tourniquet to the patient's wrist just proximal to the wrist bone. Do not apply the tourniquet so tightly that blood flow in the arteries is impeded.
8. Hold the patient's hand in your nondominant hand with the fingers lower than the wrist.
   PURPOSE: This position aids identification of the veins and draw site.
9. Select a vein and cleanse the site at the bifurcation (forking) of the veins.
10. Using your thumb, pull the patient's skin taut over the knuckles.
    PURPOSE: Stretching the skin prevents the veins from rolling underneath.
11. With the needle at a 10- to 15-degree angle, bevel up, align it with the vein.
12. Insert the needle by holding the wings or the rear of the set. After insertion the wings are never touched again. Make sure the safety device is not activated.
    PURPOSE: Inserting the needle by holding the wings gives a greater sense of control. If the sides are held, the safety shield slides forward over the needle when the point of the needle makes contact with the skin.
13. Draw blood into the syringe or push the blood collecting tube onto the end of the holder (Figure 2). Note the position of the hands while drawing the blood. When drawing blood into the syringe, make sure the vacuum you create is slow and steady, and that no more than 1 mL of head space exists between the blood and the plunger.

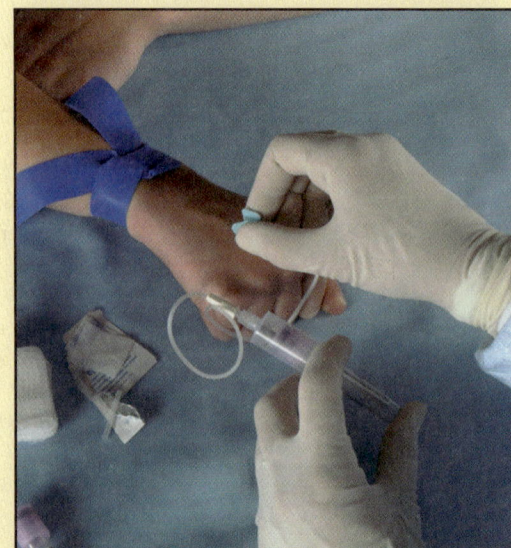

(From Garrels M, Oatis C: *Laboratory testing for ambulatory settings*, ed 2, St Louis, 2011, Saunders.)

PURPOSE: Drawing blood too forcefully into the syringe may collapse the vein or hemolyze the blood.

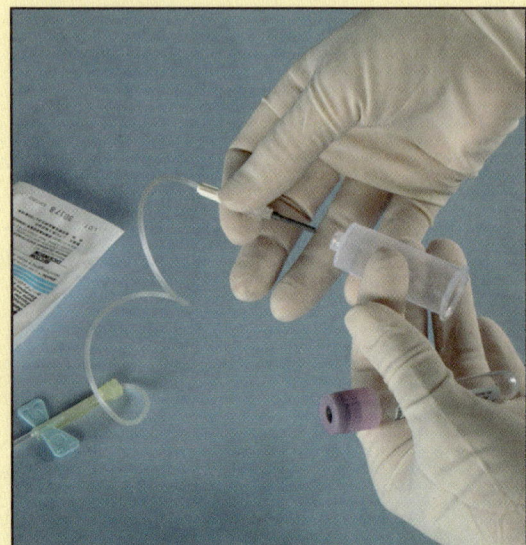

(From Garrels M, Oatis C: *Laboratory testing for ambulatory settings*, ed 2, St Louis, 2011, Saunders.)

PROCEDURE 53-3—cont'd

14. Release the tourniquet when the blood appears in the tube or a "flash" of blood is seen in the hub of the syringe.

    <u>PURPOSE:</u> To prevent hemoconcentration, the tourniquet should remain in place no longer than 1 minute.

15. Always keep the tube and the holder in a downward position so that the tube fills from the bottom up.

16. Place a gauze pad over the puncture site and gently remove the needle engaging the safety device. Dispose of the entire unit in the sharps container (Figure 3).

17. Complete the procedure as you would for an antecubital draw (see Procedure 53-2, Steps 19 through 23).

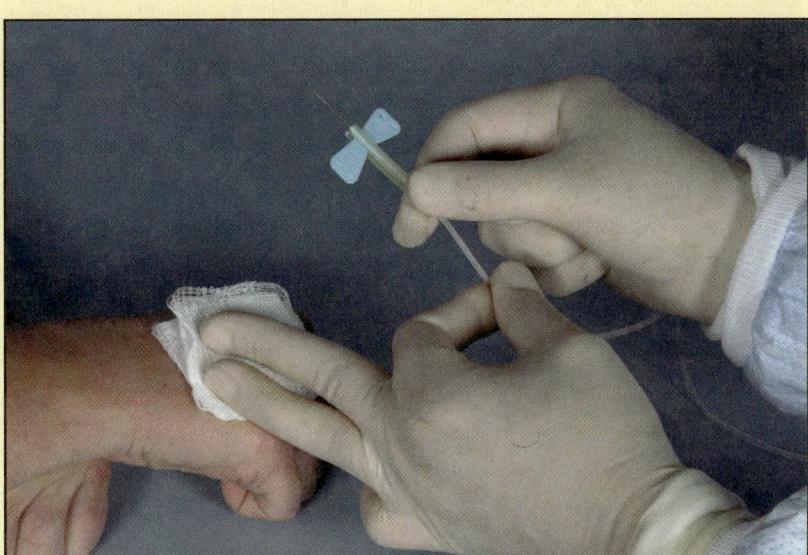

(From Garrels M, Oatis C: *Laboratory testing for ambulatory settings*, ed 2, St Louis, 2011, Saunders.)

A hematoma is a large, painful, bruised area at the puncture site caused by blood leaking into the tissue, which causes the tissue around the puncture site to swell. The most common causes of hematoma formation during the draw are excessive probing with the needle to locate a vein, failure to insert the needle far enough into the vein, and a needle that goes through the vein. A hematoma also can form after a draw if you fail to remove the tourniquet before removing the needle, fail to withdraw the vacuum tube before the needle is withdrawn, or fail to apply adequate pressure on the puncture site, or if the elbow is bent while pressure is applied. If a hematoma forms, discontinue the procedure stat, apply pressure to the area for a minimum of 3 minutes, and then apply an ice pack to the area. Notify the physician and observe the site to determine whether the bleeding has stopped. Depending on the facility's policy, an incident report may have to be completed and recorded in the patient's record.

Fainting, or syncope, can have serious consequences, and the phlebotomist must always be prepared. Securing the patient in a blood collection chair prevents bodily injury if the person faints. Constant conversation with the patient during the procedure can help identify an impending episode, as can observing the patient's face and breathing rate.

FAINTING

According to the Clinical and Laboratory Standards Institute (CLSI), the procedure for a fainting patient or one who is nonresponsive is as follows:

- If the patient begins to faint, quickly remove the tourniquet and needle from the arm and immediately dispose of the unit in a sharps container to prevent an accidental exposure.
- Notify staff members for assistance.
- Lay the patient flat or lower the head if the patient is sitting.
- Loosen tight clothing.
- Do not use ammonia inhalants/capsules because these are associated with adverse effects and are no longer recommended.
- Apply a cold compress or washcloth to the patient's forehead and back of the neck.
- Stay with the patient until recovery is complete.
- Document the incident according to facility policies.
- When the patient regains consciousness, he or she must remain in the facility for at least 15 minutes and should not operate a vehicle for at least 30 minutes.

TABLE 53-4 Managing Blood Draw Complications

POSSIBLE COMPLICATION	STRATEGIES
Burned area	Choose another site, because these areas are prone to infection.
Convulsions	Stay calm. Remove the needle and quickly dispose of it in a sharps container, then help guide the patient to the floor, protecting him or her from injury. Call for help.
Damaged or scarred veins or infected areas	Look for an alternative site; do not draw blood from scarred or infected areas.
Edema	Avoid the area; look for an alternative site.
Hematoma	Adjust the depth of the needle or remove the needle and apply pressure.
Intravenous (IV) therapy or blood transfusion sites	Blood samples should not be drawn from an arm that is also the site for IV infusion or blood transfusion because of the dilution factor.
Mastectomy	Do not draw blood from the side of the mastectomy, because mastectomy surgery causes lymphostasis, which may produce false results.
Nausea	Place a cold cloth on the patient's forehead, give the patient a basin in case of vomiting, and instruct him or her to take deep breaths. Alert the physician.
No blood	Manipulate the needle slightly or remove the Vacutainer and perform the blood draw again using a syringe or butterfly setup.
Petechiae	Loosen the tourniquet, because this complication usually results from the tourniquet being in place for longer than 2 minutes.
Syncope	Position the patient's head between the knees (if in a sitting position). Check and record the patient's pulse, blood pressure, and respiration rate, and continue to observe the patient. Never leave the patient unattended.

Nerve damage can be a consequence of venipuncture, albeit an unlikely one. Preventive measures include avoiding the basilic vein and refraining from blind probing if the vein is missed.

Table 53-4 lists some probable solutions to complications. As a general rule, it is wise to limit yourself to two attempts to obtain blood from any one patient. If you fail on the second attempt, ask the patient whether he or she would prefer having someone else try, or whether it would be better to come back at another time. This maneuver lets the patient feel that he or she is in control of the situation. At one time or another, everyone is unsuccessful in obtaining a needed blood sample, so do not feel that you are a failure.

CRITICAL THINKING APPLICATION   53-3

Leah is in her second week at the clinic, and she is confident that she can perform phlebotomy on her own. Melissa has been a good mentor, and Leah has done quite a few successful "sticks" without any problems. Today, however, she is just having a bad day. Mr. Godfrey Lawrence has come to the clinic with numerous problems, and Dr. Gupta has ordered several blood tests. Mr. Lawrence is uncooperative when he sees that Leah must draw four tubes of blood. He angrily tells her that she cannot take that much blood out of him; she is a vampire and she will drain him. How should Leah deal with this problem?

SPECIMEN RE-COLLECTION

Sometimes problems with a sample cannot be determined until the specimen is analyzed in the laboratory. Rejected specimens must be

re-collected. The laboratory may reject a specimen for reasons that include the following:

- Unlabeled or mislabeled specimen
- Insufficient quantity
- Defective tube
- Incorrect tube used for the test ordered
- Hemolysis
- Clotted blood in an anticoagulated specimen
- Improper handling

Hemolysis is the major cause of specimen rejection. Because it cannot be detected until the blood cells separate from the plasma or serum, it is crucial to take steps to prevent red blood cell damage during collection. Hemolyzed serum or plasma appears rosy to bright red in color because of the release of hemoglobin from the cells. Some of the more routine tests that are adversely affected by hemolysis are chemistry tests for electrolytes (e.g., potassium, sodium), bilirubin, total protein, and numerous liver enzymes (e.g., alkaline phosphatase, gamma glutamyl transferase). Table 53-5 reviews the major causes of hemolysis during collection.

CRITICAL THINKING APPLICATION   53-4

- Leah next must draw a sample from Ms. Danielle Rollins. Ms. Rollins indicates that she has a history of bruising after venipuncture, and sure enough, a hematoma begins to rise shortly after Leah inserts the needle. She then notices that Ms. Rollins has become pale and is perspiring. What should Leah do first?
- What other steps should Leah take? Can she still obtain the sample?

TABLE 53-5 Major Causes of Hemolysis During Collection

CAUSE OF HEMOLYSIS	EXPLANATION	PREVENTION
Alcohol preparation	Transfer of alcohol into the specimen causes hemolysis.	Allow venipuncture site to dry completely.
Incorrect needle size	A high-gauge needle causes the blood to be forced through a small lumen with great force, shearing the cell membranes; a very-low-gauge needle allows a large amount of blood to suddenly enter the tube with great force, causing frothing.	Choose the correct needle for the job, aiming for a 19- to 23-gauge needle.
Loose connections on the vacuum tube assembly	If the connection between the needle holder and the double-pointed needle or the syringe and the needle is loose, air can enter the sample and cause frothing.	Make sure all connections are tight before beginning the venipuncture.
Removing the needle from the vein with the tube intact	The remaining vacuum in the tube can cause air to be drawn forcefully into the tube, causing frothing.	Remove the final tube from the needle holder before withdrawing the needle from the patient's vein.
Underfilled tubes	Underfilling tubes leads to an improper blood/additive ratio. Certain additives in disproportionate amounts (e.g., sodium fluoride) can cause hemolysis.	Permit blood to flow into the tubes until no more movement can be seen.
Syringe collections	Pulling back forcibly on the plunger draws blood too quickly through the needle, shearing cell membranes; transferring blood into a vacuum tube further traumatizes red blood cells.	Pump the plunger several times before use to loosen it in the barrel. Use the smallest syringe possible. Pace the aspiration rate so that no more than 1 mL of air space is present at any time. Transfer blood into the vacuum tube immediately, preferably using a transfer device. *Never* push on the plunger when transferring to a vacuum tube. Angle the syringe so that the blood runs gently down the side of the tube, preventing the cells from hitting the bottom of the tube with force.
Mixing tubes too vigorously	All tubes except the red-topped tube must be mixed.	Gently invert tubes immediately after the draw. Anything other than gentle inversion (e.g., shaking) can hemolyze cells.
Temperature and transport problems	Trauma and temperature extremes can damage cells. Freezing results in ice crystals that puncture cell membranes.	Tubes should be transported in the upright position with as little trauma as possible. Temperature should be controlled—not too hot and too cold.
Separation of plasma or serum from red blood cells	Removing the serum or plasma from the cells minimizes the risk of contaminating the specimen with red blood cell contents.	Blood samples should be centrifuged, when applicable, as soon as possible and serum or plasma removed from the cells.
Prolonged tourniquet time	While the tourniquet restricts blood flow, interstitial fluid can leak into the veins and hemolyze red blood cells.	Adhere to the 1-minute rule for tourniquet application.
Poor collection; blood flowing too slowly into the tube	The needle lumen may be blocked because it is too close to the inner wall of the vein.	Withdraw the needle slightly to center it within the vein.

CAPILLARY PUNCTURE

Capillaries are small blood vessels that connect small arterioles to small venules. A capillary, or dermal, puncture is an efficient means of collecting a blood specimen when only a small amount of blood is required, or when a patient's condition makes venipuncture difficult. Because the requisition will not indicate that the collection is to be made in this manner, you must be familiar with the advantages, limitations, and appropriate uses of this technique. Capillary puncture is warranted in the following situations:

- Older patients
- Pediatric patients (especially younger than age 2)
- Patients who require frequent glucose monitoring
- Patients with burns or scars in venipuncture sites
- Obese patients
- Patients receiving intravenous therapy

- Patients who have had a mastectomy
- Patients at risk for venous thrombosis
- Patients who are severely dehydrated
- Tests that require a small volume of blood

Because capillaries are bridges between arteries and veins, capillary blood is a mixture of the two. Small amounts of tissue fluid also are present in capillary blood, especially in the first drop. Analyte levels are usually the same in capillary and venous blood, with a few exceptions. Hemoglobin and glucose values are higher in capillary blood; potassium, calcium, and total protein are higher in venous blood.

Equipment

Skin Puncture Devices

The device used to perform a dermal puncture is the lancet, which delivers a quick puncture to a predetermined depth (Figure 53-16). OSHA has directed that lancets must have retractable blades; they also must have locks that prevent accidental puncture after use and that prevent the device from being reused (Table 53-6). Skin puncture devices should always be discarded in a sharps container.

Collection Containers

Different types of collection devices and containers are available, and the ones used depend on the test to be performed (Figure 53-17). Microcollection, or Microtainer, tubes hold up to 750 L (0.75 mL) of blood and are available with a variety of anticoagulants and additives. The tops are color-coded in the same fashion as evacuated tubes. Blood is collected drop-wise into these tubes through a funnel-like device. Capillary tubes are another means of collecting blood from a dermal puncture. These are glass or plastic tubes that draw blood by capillary action, that is, the blood fills into these narrow tubes without the need for suction. If the capillary tube is coated with the anticoagulant heparin, a red band will be seen at the top. A common, heparin-coated capillary tube is the microhematocrit tube used for determining the percentage of packed red blood cells in the microhematocrit test (see Chapter 54).

Manufacturers also provide various collection devices for obtaining small amounts of blood for "point-of-care" testing, such as for glucose, hemoglobin A_{1c}, and cholesterol (see Chapter 54). The blood is pulled into the collecting device by capillary action after puncture, or it is dropped onto a reagent strip, which is inserted into the instrument to be analyzed.

Blood from a capillary puncture also can be deposited on paper cards. One such card, the Guthrie card, is used to test neonates for

TABLE 53-6   Lancet Blade Recommendations

DEVICE DEPTH AND DIMENSION	BLOOD VOLUME	APPLICATION
2.25-mm, 28-gauge needle	Single drop	Fingersticks
2.25-mm, 23-gauge needle	Single drop	Fingersticks, glucose test
1 × 1.5-mm blade	Low blood flow	Fingersticks, microhematocrit tube, or drop of blood for glucose or cholesterol test
1.5 × 1.5-mm blade	Medium blood flow	Fingersticks; to fill a single Microtainer tube
2 × 1.5-mm blade	High blood flow	Fingersticks; to fill multiple Microtainer tubes

Modified from Beckton, Dickinson, and Company, at http://www.bd.com/vacutainer/faqs/#urine_faq

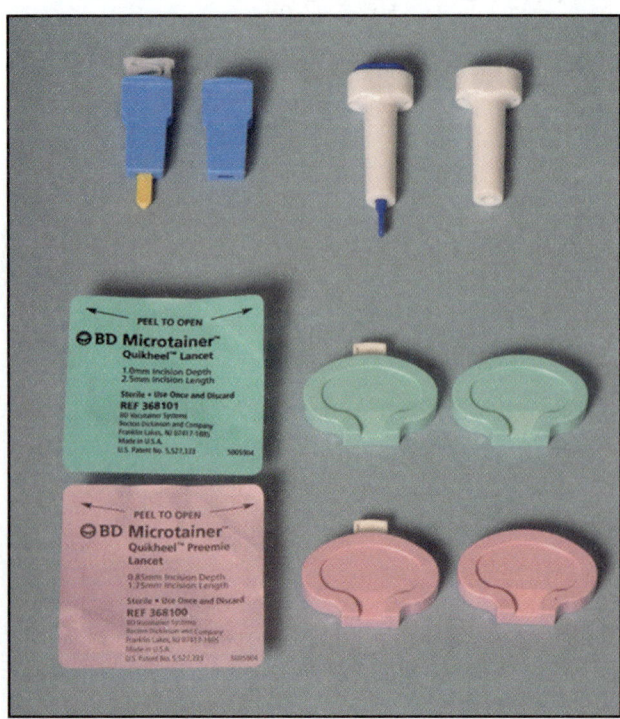

FIGURE 53-16 Skin puncture devices include simple lancets and automated devices that control the depth and width of the incision. (Courtesy Becton, Dickinson and Company, Franklin Lakes, New Jersey.)

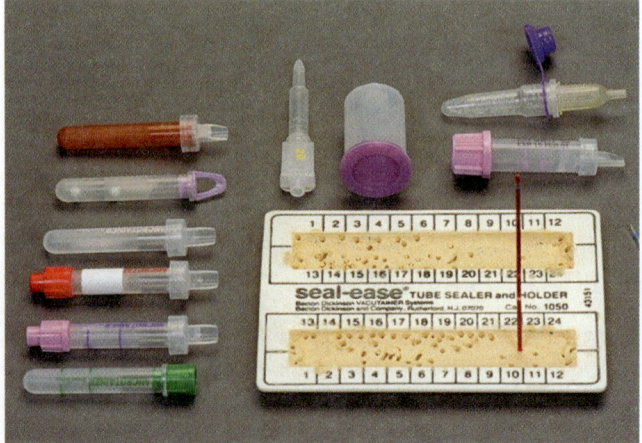

FIGURE 53-17 Microsample containers: Microtainer tubes and a capillary tube in sealing clay.

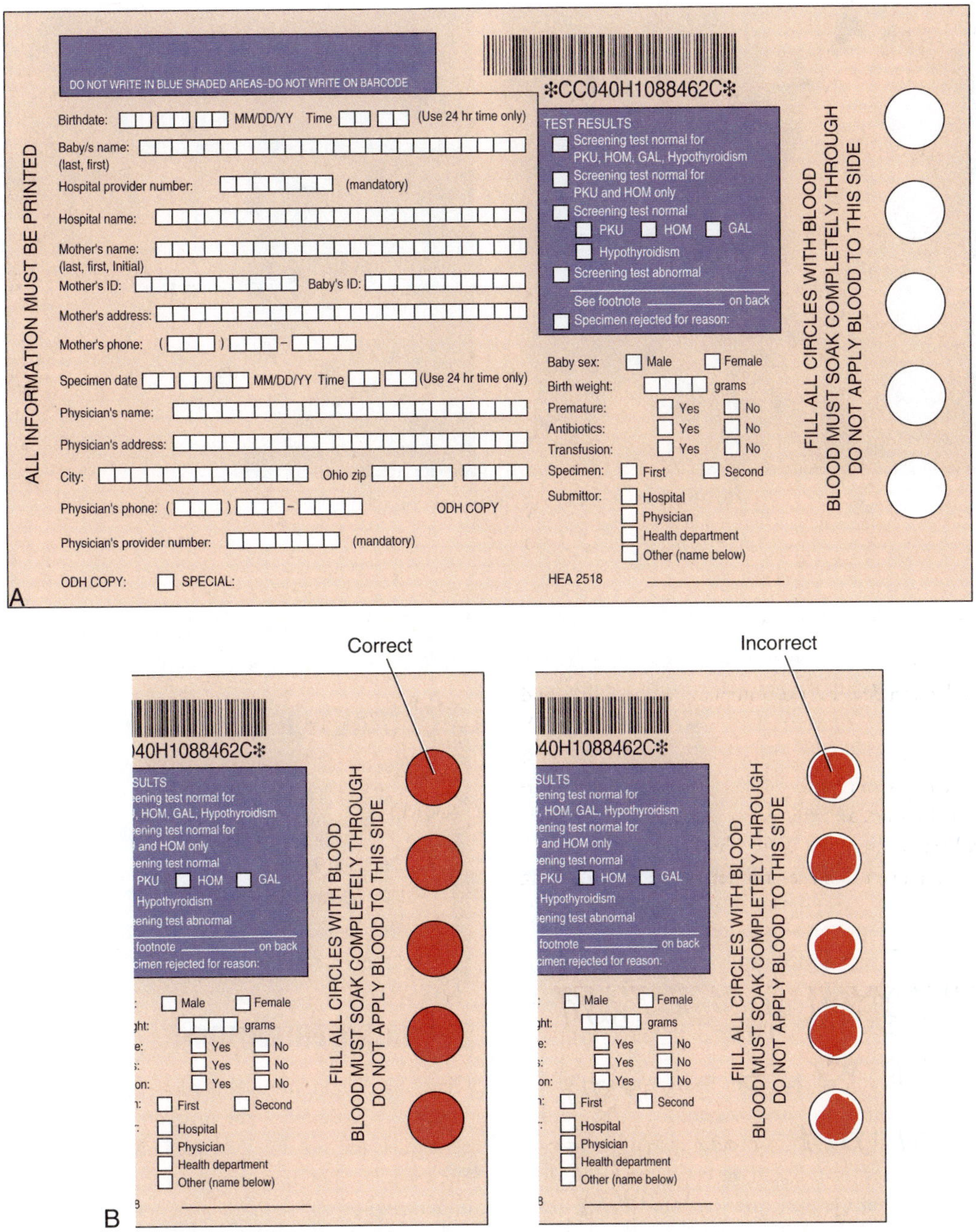

FIGURE 53-18 A, A Guthrie card used in neonatal screening. **B,** Correct and incorrect ways to fill in the circles. (From Sommer SR, Warekois RS: *Phlebotomy: worktext and procedures manual,* Philadelphia, 2002, Saunders.)

certain metabolic disorders, such as phenylketonuria (PKU). Blood is deposited into circles on biologically inactive filter paper and is sent to a referral laboratory for analysis within 24 hours of sampling. Federal postal regulations for the mailing of biohazardous material must be followed (Figure 53-18).

Routine Capillary Puncture

Site Selection

In adults and children, the usual puncture site is the ring finger, but capillary blood can be obtained from the middle finger or heel (Figure 53-19). The thumb usually is too callused, and the index finger has extra nerve endings that make the puncture more painful. The fifth finger has too little tissue for a successful puncture. The

puncture is made at the tip and slightly to the side of the finger. Be sure to puncture a fleshy area closer to the center of the finger to prevent damage to underlying bone. Avoid areas that are callused, scarred, burned, infected, cyanotic, or edematous.

For children younger than 1 year, dermal puncture is performed on the medial and lateral surfaces of the plantar surface (bottom) of the heel. Areas other than these are unsafe, and bone or nerve damage to an infant may occur. Blood flow from an infant's heel can be increased as much as sevenfold by applying a warm, moist towel (or other warming device) at a temperature no higher than 42°C (108°F) for 3 to 5 minutes. Never place bandages on the heel or anywhere on infants younger than age 2, because they may peel off and become a choking hazard.

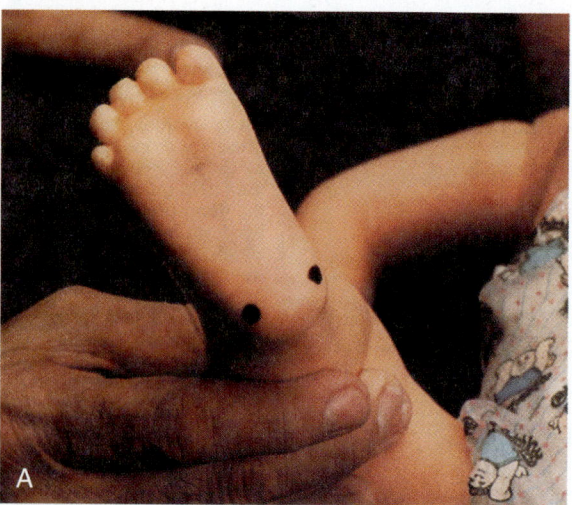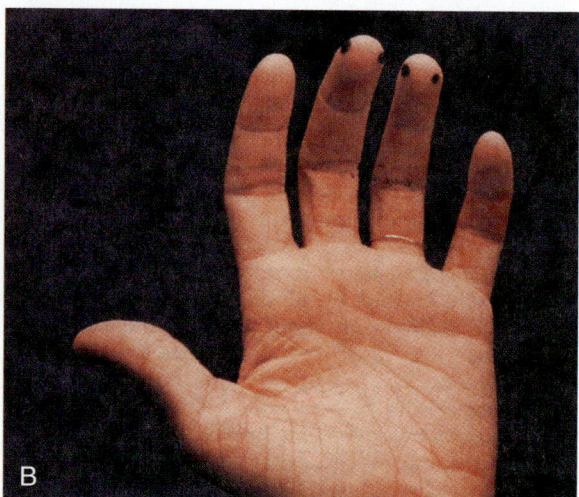

FIGURE 53-19 Capillary puncture sites on the heel and on the fingers.

Patient Preparation

Preparation for a capillary puncture is similar to that for venipuncture. Put on gloves and cleanse the finger well with an alcohol prep pad. If the patient's hands are excessively soiled, ask the person to wash them before the procedure. If the patient's hands are cold, warm them in warm water and dry them thoroughly, or ask the person to rub or shake them vigorously.

Generally, you must work very efficiently when performing a capillary puncture, because blood flow stops quickly. Be sure to have your supplies organized and within easy reach. Grasp the finger firmly and apply gentle, intermittent pressure, but do not squeeze or "milk" it. Press the puncture device firmly against the skin and quickly depress the plunger.

Collecting the Specimen

After the dermis is punctured, it is important to wipe away the first drop of blood with sterile gauze. This drop contains tissue fluid that could interfere with test results. Fill the sampling containers according to the manufacturer's directions. Touch the container to the drop of blood as it is released from the puncture site, but do not touch the skin. If blood flow stops, wiping the site with sterile gauze may restart the flow. Be prepared for blood to contaminate your gloves or surfaces by having spare gloves, extra gauze pads, and disinfectant nearby. After the containers have been filled, ask the patient to apply pressure to the gauze you have placed over the puncture site if he or she is able. Seal containers as recommended by the manufacturer if necessary.

Specimen Handling

Capillary collection containers often are too small for a label to be applied. The most efficient way to transport capillary tubes is to remove the stopper from a red-topped tube, insert the capillary tubes, sealed-end down, replace the stopper, and label the tube. Microtainer tubes have plastic plugs that fit over the top. They may be placed in a labeled tube or in a labeled zipper-lock bag for transport. Always decontaminate collection containers before delivering them to the laboratory if blood was deposited on the surface during collection. The procedure for routine capillary collection is outlined in Procedure 53-4.

PEDIATRIC PHLEBOTOMY

Obtaining blood from children and infants may be difficult and potentially hazardous. The procedure should be performed only by personnel trained in the techniques for pediatric phlebotomy. Successfully obtaining blood from children requires skill and an understanding of pediatric psychological development, as well as appropriate communication skills. The phlebotomist must gain the child's confidence and often that of the parent as well. Parents often ask the phlebotomist to explain the tests being done and why. You should be very careful when divulging information; never tell the parents what disease or condition a specific blood test detects. Refer questions to the child's physician. A parent or guardian may or may not be an asset during the procedure. Ask the parent about the child's previous phlebotomy experiences and how cooperative the child is likely to be. Tactfully determine whether the parent is comfortable with assisting in restraining an uncooperative child. Parental behavior greatly influences the child's behavior during the procedure. Children should never be restrained in a way that might cause physical injury. If the parent is unable or unwilling to assist with necessary restraint, always refer to the office or laboratory policy on restraints and procedural holds. Table 53-7 provides information on the typical fears and concerns of children during the procedure and suggested parental involvement.

PROCEDURE 53-4

Perform Capillary Puncture: Obtain a Capillary Blood Sample by Fingertip Puncture

GOAL: *To collect a capillary blood specimen suitable for testing using the fingertip puncture technique.*

EQUIPMENT and SUPPLIES

- Sterile disposable safety lancet
- 70% alcohol prep pads
- Sterile gauze pads
- Nonallergenic tape
- Appropriate collection containers (e.g., capillary tubes, Microtainer devices)
- Sealing clay or caps for capillary tubes
- Permanent marking pen or printed labels
- Biohazard waste container and sharps container
- Disposable gloves
- Patient's record

PROCEDURAL STEPS

1. Read the requisition and gather all needed supplies on the basis of the physician's requisition.
   PURPOSE: To perform the procedure efficiently. Once the skin has been punctured, the collection must proceed as rapidly as possible so that the blood does not clot before the entire specimen has been collected.
2. Sanitize your hands. Put on nonsterile gloves.
3. Identify the patient and explain the procedure.
   PURPOSE: To make sure you have the right patient; explanations help gain the patient's cooperation.
4. Select a puncture site depending on the patient's age and the sample to be obtained (side of middle or ring finger of nondominant hand, medial or lateral curved surface of the heel for an infant).
   PURPOSE: The nondominant hand may have fewer calluses. The side of the finger is less sensitive, and the skin usually is not as thick. Use great caution when performing capillary puncture on infants.
5. Gently rub the finger along the sides.
   PURPOSE: To promote circulation. If the finger is very cold, you may immerse it in warm water or moisten it with warm towels.
6. Clean the site with alcohol, allow it to air dry, or dry it with sterile gauze (Figure 1).
   PURPOSE: Puncturing skin that is wet with alcohol is painful and can hemolyze the specimen.

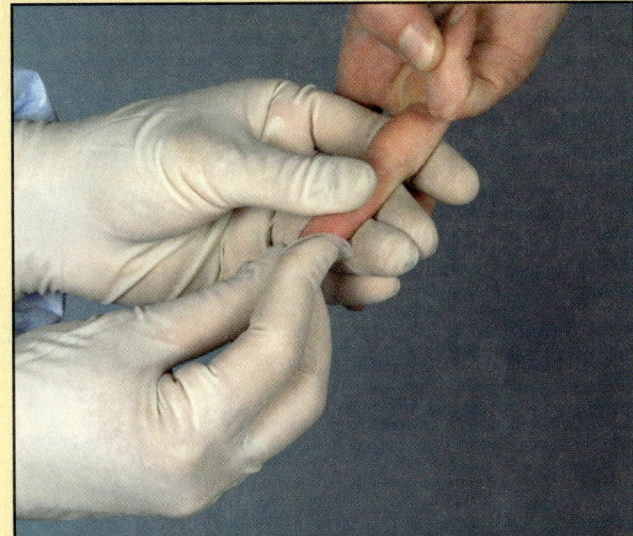

(From Garrels M, Oatis C: *Laboratory testing for ambulatory settings*, ed 2, St Louis, 2011, Saunders.)

7. Grasp the patient's finger on the sides near the puncture site with your nondominant forefinger and thumb.
   PURPOSE: Firmly holding the site allows control of the puncture.
8. Hold the lancet at a right angle to the patient's finger and make a rapid, deep puncture on the side of the patient's fingertip (Figure 2).

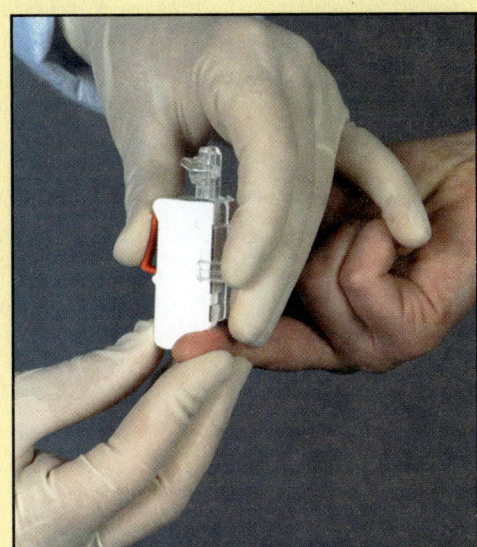

(From Garrels M, Oatis C: *Laboratory testing for ambulatory settings*, ed 2, St Louis, 2011, Saunders.)

PURPOSE: Lancets are designed to puncture at specific depths that permit the free flow of blood.

PROCEDURE 53-4—cont'd

9. Dispose of the lancet in the sharps container. Wipe away the first drop of blood with clean, sterile gauze.
   <u>PURPOSE:</u> The first drop of blood contains tissue fluid, which may alter test results.
10. Apply gentle pressure to cause the blood to flow freely (Figure 3).

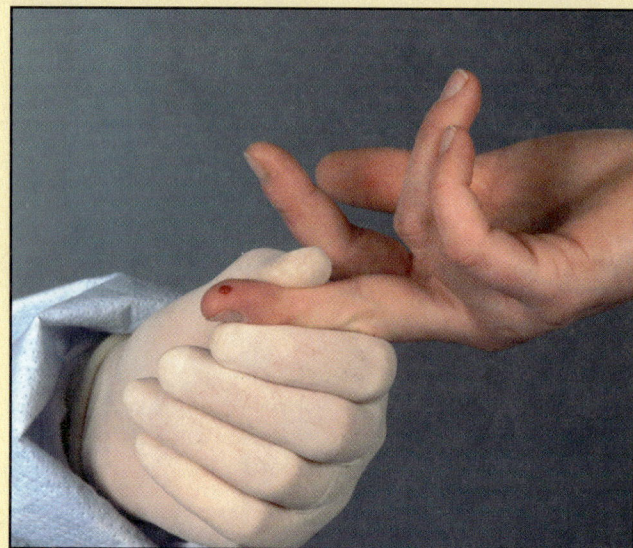

(From Garrels M, Oatis C: *Laboratory testing for ambulatory settings*, ed 2, St Louis, 2011, Saunders.)

<u>PURPOSE:</u> Forceful squeezing liberates fluid that dilutes the blood and causes inaccurate results.

11. Collect blood samples.
    a. Express a large drop of blood, touch the end of the tube to the drop of blood (not the finger), fill the capillary tubes (Figure 4), place the finger over the blood-free end of the tube, and seal the other end of the tube by inserting it into the sealing clay. The tube should be approximately three quarters full before it is sealed.

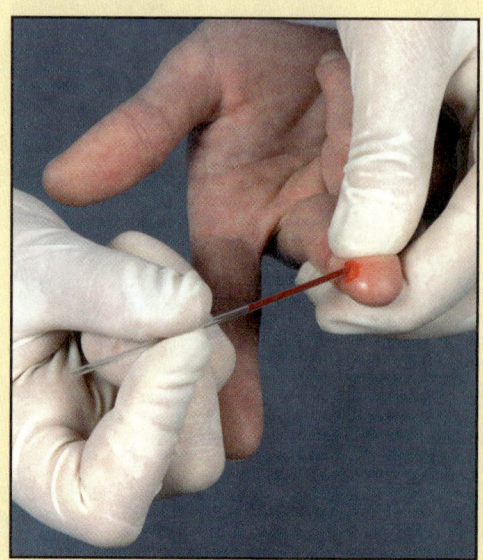

(From Garrels M, Oatis C: *Laboratory testing for ambulatory settings*, ed 2, St Louis, 2011, Saunders.)

<u>PURPOSE:</u> Placing the finger over the capillary tube prevents the blood from dripping onto the sealing clay.

b. Wipe the finger with a clean, sterile gauze pad, express another large drop of blood, and fill a Microtainer (Figure 5). Do not touch the container to the finger. If more blood is needed, wipe the puncture with clean gauze and gently squeeze another drop. Cap the tube when the collection is complete.

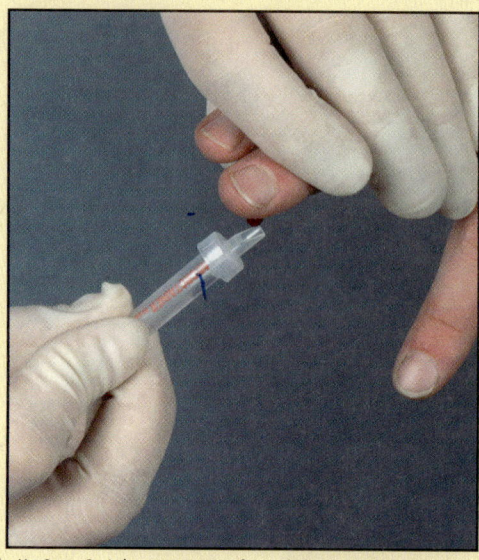

(From Garrels M, Oatis C: *Laboratory testing for ambulatory settings*, ed 2, St Louis, 2011, Saunders.)

<u>PURPOSE:</u> Touching the container to the finger irritates the puncture site and may cause infection.

12. When collection is complete, apply pressure to the site with clean sterile gauze (Figure 6). The patient may be able to assist with this step.
13. Select an appropriate means of labeling the containers. Capillary tubes can be placed in a red-topped tube, which is subsequently labeled. Microtainers can be placed in zipper-lock bags that are subsequently labeled.
14. Check the patient for bleeding, clean the site if traces of blood are visible, and apply a nonallergenic bandage if indicated.
15. Dispose of used materials in the proper containers.
16. Disinfect the work area. Dispose of any blood-contaminated materials (e.g., gauze) in the biohazard container. Remove your gloves and sanitize your hands.
    <u>PURPOSE:</u> To ensure infection control.
17. Record the procedure in the patient's record.
    <u>PURPOSE:</u> A procedure is considered not done until it is recorded.

PROCEDURE 53-4—cont'd

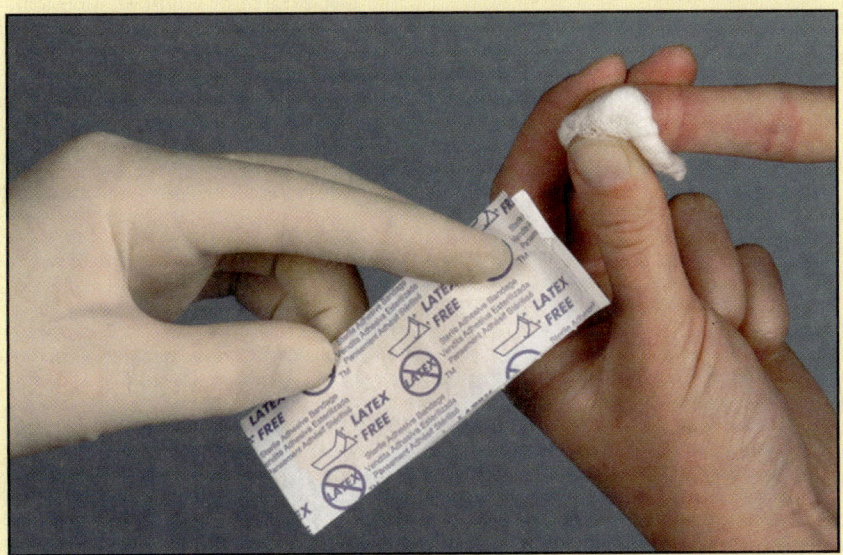

(From Garrels M, Oatis C: *Laboratory testing for ambulatory settings*, ed 2, St Louis, 2011, Saunders.)

TABLE 53-7 **Childhood Behavior and Parental Involvement During Phlebotomy**

AGE	TYPICAL MENTAL STATE	SUGGESTED PARENTAL INVOLVEMENT
Newborns (0-12 months)	Trust that adults will respond to their needs.	Parent should assist by cradling and comforting child.
Infants and toddlers (1-3 years)	Minimal fear of danger but fear of separation. Limited language and understanding of procedure.	Parent should assist by holding the child and providing emotional support.
Preschoolers (3-6 years)	Fearful of injury to body; still dependent on parent.	Parent may be present to provide emotional support and to assist in obtaining child's cooperation.
School-aged children (7-12 years)	Less dependent on parent and more willing to cooperate; fear of loss of self-control (crying).	Child may not want parent present.
Teenagers (13-18 years)	Fully engaged in the process; embarrassed to show fear and may show hostility to cover emotions.	Teen may not want parent present.

Removing large amounts of blood, especially from premature infants, may result in anemia (Table 53-8). The amount of blood withdrawn must be recorded in the child's chart. Puncturing deep veins in children may result in cardiac arrest, hemorrhage, venous thrombosis, damage to surrounding tissues, or infection. In addition, the child could be harmed during forceful restraint. To prevent these problems, blood should be collected only by dermal puncture from children younger than age 2 unless the procedure warrants venous collection (lead levels or blood culture). Venipuncture on children younger than age 2 should be performed only on surface veins, including the dorsal hand vein, using a 23-gauge winged infusion set coupled to a syringe or a pediatric vacuum tube collection set.

When the medical assistant is required to perform pediatric phlebotomy, wearing a colorful smock, being truthful about the discomfort the child will feel, and providing tokens and praise for bravery go a long way toward allaying the child's fears. Topical anesthetics, such as ethyl chloride (EC) spray or amethocaine gel (Ametop), may

TABLE 53-8 **General Guidelines for Pediatric Venipuncture**

WEIGHT (lb)	LIMIT DURING A SINGLE DRAW
8-10	3.5 mL
11-15	5 mL
16-40	10 mL
41-60	20 mL
61-65	25 mL
66-80	30 mL

be used to reduce pain at the puncture site. In most cases a calm, professional phlebotomist who understands the developmental needs of the child and relates to the child on that level can gain the acceptance necessary to perform a successful venipuncture or dermal puncture with a minimum of restraint and frustration.

Postcollection Specimen Handling

It has been said that the results of laboratory testing are only as good as the specimen sent for testing. Specimens handled improperly after collection may provide erroneous results and unnecessarily compromise the patient's health. From the moment the specimen is collected, analytes in the blood begin to decay, and it is a race against time to provide results that accurately represent a patient's condition at the time of the blood collection. After collection, blood may need to be processed before the sample is sent to its final destination. For most samples, this involves separation of the plasma or serum from the red blood cells. If the tube contains no anticoagulant, blood begins to clot when it comes in contact with the glass tube. Plastic tubes require the addition of a clot activator; the SST speckle-topped tube has silica additives to accelerate clotting. "Clot" tubes should be allowed to sit upright in a rack for 30 to 60 minutes at room temperature while a solid clot forms. Tubes with clot accelerator should form a dense clot within 30 minutes. The presence of anticoagulants in the blood, such as warfarin (Coumadin) or heparin, may delay clotting. Once the clot has formed, every effort should be made to remove the clot from the serum within 2 hours.

Removal of the clot from the serum requires centrifugation. For the thixotropic gel to form the barrier between the clot and the serum, certain g-force, time, and temperature requirements must be met. A minimum g-force of 1,000 g must be achieved by centrifugation; the gel must be at 25°C (77°F), and the tube must be centrifuged for 10 to 15 minutes. The serum does not have to be removed from the tube after centrifugation, because the gel has formed a barrier over the red blood cells. Once a tube with thixotropic gel has been centrifuged, it cannot be centrifuged again. The serum, however, can be decanted and centrifuged in another tube.

For tests that require plasma, the plasma should be removed from the cells as soon as possible. This can be accomplished with centrifugation followed by aspiration of the plasma and transfer to another tube using a disposable pipet. The green-gray marbled-topped tube, with lithium heparin anticoagulant, has a thixotropic gel, which forms the necessary barrier when centrifuged as described previously. Certain blood tests, such as the complete blood count, require whole blood. It is wise to check the requirements of the laboratory that will perform the test as to how the specimen should be transported and stored. The College of American Pathologists recommends that whole blood for automated blood counts be refrigerated and tested within 72 hours.

Often specimens must be transported by courier to other facilities. The Hazardous Materials Shipping Regulations established by the Department of Transportation apply to the packaging or shipping of hazardous materials by ground transportation. Those who ship human specimens must be trained in all aspects of handling, packing, and shipping of biohazardous materials.

CHAIN OF CUSTODY

As discussed in Chapter 52, blood samples may be collected as evidence in legal proceedings. Blood may be drawn for drug and alcohol testing, DNA analysis, or parentage testing. These samples must be handled according to special procedures to prevent tampering, misidentification, or interference with the test results.

Chain of custody is a legal term that refers to the ability to guarantee the identity and integrity of the specimen from collection to reporting of test results. It is a process used to maintain and document the chronologic history of a specimen. (Documents should include the name or initials of the individual collecting the specimen, each person or entity subsequently having custody of it, the date the specimen was collected or transferred, the employer or agency, the specimen number, the patient's or employee's name, and a brief description of the specimen.)

Collection kits are available that contain everything needed for the venipuncture, including the tube, the needle, the chain of custody forms and seals, the antiseptic, and even the tourniquet. Familiarize yourself with these kits before you are required to use them. You may be required to testify at a legal proceeding if you are involved in the collection or testing of a sample involved in a legal proceeding.

CLOSING COMMENTS

Patient Education

Medical assistants who work as phlebotomists must maintain a professional attitude, yet remain sympathetic to the patient's fears and anxiety about being "stuck with a needle." Establishing an environment that encourages the person to relax can minimize the patient's pain and discomfort during the procedure.

Always remember to identify your patient and explain what you are going to do. Answer any questions the patient may have, and perform the procedure skillfully before anxiety has time to set in.

Provide as much explanation as needed to ease the patient's anxiety. Often the patient can help by identifying the site of the last successful blood draw. Follow the patient's suggestion in choosing the site for obtaining a blood specimen. When a patient is allowed to become an active participant in the procedure, he or she remains more relaxed, talkative, and confident in your expertise as a phlebotomist.

The atmosphere can change dramatically if the patient has had an unpleasant experience and associates pain and discomfort with venipuncture. Such a patient usually is ill at ease and apprehensive. In this case, you need to make every effort to perform the procedure quickly, efficiently, and effectively. Once the blood has been drawn and the patient has relaxed, you can help the patient develop a positive attitude.

If your patient has a history of syncope when blood is drawn, or if you suspect the patient may faint during the procedure, have the person lie down. Assemble your equipment and alert the physician before beginning the procedure. This type of professional care may help the patient get through the procedure without a traumatic effect.

Legal and Ethical Issues

Venipuncture and microcapillary blood collection are invasive procedures in which a sterile needle or a lancet is inserted through the skin. Because the skin is penetrated, drawing blood becomes a surgical procedure and is subject to the laws and regulations of surgery.

When venipuncture is performed, the rules and regulations must be enforced with no deviations. Be sure to follow the procedures as written and to become familiar with the regulations and standards established by local and state agencies, as well as the CLSI and OSHA. Deviations leave the medical assistant open to accusations of malpractice. Document any situations that arise in which observation of the standard of care comes into question.

On rare occasions, patients who have scarred veins as a result of intravenous drug use may ask to draw their own blood. You should never permit this and should always take precautions that your supplies are secure.

SUMMARY OF SCENARIO

Leah has learned that phlebotomy is truly an art. Although she was nervous at first, she has become quite proficient with this new skill. She discovered that her nervousness was "contagious," and that if she remains calm and organized, her patients are more likely to feel at ease with the procedure. She has learned that it is necessary to talk with patients before drawing their blood, not only to allay their fears, but also to get clues about past problems or the best site for the draw. She has learned that she is responsible for explaining the tests ordered and how much blood she will draw, but that she is not responsible for explaining the reasons the tests are being done. Effective communication is the most important aspect of phlebotomy.

Through practice and careful attention, Leah has come to recognize the proper equipment to use in phlebotomy, and she never hesitates to call the referral laboratory used by her employer if she has a question about proper collection of a specimen. Communicating with children and adults is as different as the equipment she uses for venipuncture; the small veins of children and the elderly require special care, and she has become proficient in the use of winged infusion sets and syringes to prevent vein collapse. Leah is well aware of the dangers of phlebotomy, and through education and the use of approved safety devices, she is confident that she can provide excellent care for her patients at the Health Alliance Medical Clinic.

SUMMARY OF LEARNING OBJECTIVES

1. **Define, spell, and pronounce the terms listed in the vocabulary.**
   Spelling and pronouncing medical terms correctly bolsters the medical assistant's credibility. Knowing the definitions of these terms promotes confidence in communication with patients and co-workers.

2. **Apply critical thinking skills in performing the patient assessment and patient care.**
   Completing the Critical Thinking Application exercises throughout the chapter can help the student medical assistant become more adept at critical analysis of real-life situations.

3. **List the equipment needed for venipuncture.**
   Venipuncture requires a double-pointed safety needle, evacuated collection tubes, a needle holder or a syringe fitted with a safety needle, a tourniquet, an alcohol prep pad, gauze or cotton, a sterile bandage, latex gloves, and a biohazard disposal container.

4. **Explain the purpose of a tourniquet.**
   A tourniquet is used to prevent venous flow out of the site, which causes the veins to bulge. The tourniquet makes veins easier to locate and puncture.

5. **Explain how to apply a tourniquet and the consequences of improper application.**
   Tourniquets are applied snugly around the upper arm (or wrist for a hand draw) in a fashion that permits easy release. Leaving the tourniquet on a prolonged time results in hemoconcentration; applying the tourniquet too tightly results in unnecessary discomfort to the patient and the release of tissue fluid into the blood.

6. **Explain why the stopper colors on evacuated tubes differ.**
   The various colors of vacuum tube stoppers indicate the contents of the tube. Certain additives are compatible with certain laboratory tests. The phlebotomist must be knowledgeable about blood tests and the types of tubes needed. Consulting literature provided by the manufacturer ensures the proper choice of a collection tube.

7. **State the correct order in which samples for various types of tubes should be collected.**
   (1) Sterile or SPS, (2) light blue, (3) red or red speckled, (4) green, (5) lavender, and (6) gray. Evacuated tubes should be collected in a specific order to prevent carryover of tube additives.

8. **Describe the types of sharps used in phlebotomy.**
The venipuncture needle has a shaft with one end cut at an angle (bevel). The other end (the hub) attaches to the syringe or to a needle holder. The opening in the tip, the lumen, is measured in gauge numbers. Double-pointed needles are used for the evacuated tube method. Needles with special adapters are used with disposable syringes. Lancets are used for dermal puncture.

9. **Explain why a syringe rather than an evacuated tube would be chosen for blood collection.**
Syringes are more commonly used for blood collection from elderly patients, whose veins tend to be more fragile; from children, whose veins tend to be small; and from obese patients, whose veins tend to be deep. Using a syringe allows a more controlled draw. Syringes commonly are used with winged infusion sets.

10. **Discuss the use of sharps with engineered sharps injury protection.**
OSHA requires that all sharps used for phlebotomy should be engineered with safety devices, such as retractable needles, self-sheathing needles, and blunting devices. Needles should never be recapped, and in most cases they are not removed from the venipuncture unit. All sharps must be disposed of in an approved sharps container.

11. **Summarize postexposure management of needlesticks.**
OSHA requires employers to have a postexposure plan in place for accidental sharps exposures. These plans generally include a means to cleanse the wound with an appropriate antiseptic cleanser; evaluation of the exposure to determine whether the employee is at risk for contracting HBV, HCV, or HIV, depending on the circumstance of the injury; gathering of information about the source of the blood involved; prophylactic care if necessary; confidential counseling for the injured; and follow-up on the exposure.

12. **Detail patient preparation for venipuncture that shows sensitivity to the patient's rights and feelings.**
The medical assistant must be sensitive to the needs and concerns of patients both before and during the phlebotomy procedure. The procedure should be explained to the patient, and all questions should be answered. The patient should be observed for any problems during the procedure, and the medical assistant should use therapeutic communication techniques throughout the intervention.

13. **Describe and name the veins that may be used for blood collection.**
The median cephalic vein is the vein of choice for phlebotomy, but blood can be drawn from the cephalic vein and the median basilic vein. The basilic vein should not be used if possible. The dorsal vein on the hand may be used.

14. **List in order the steps of a routine venipuncture.**
A routine venipuncture begins with greeting and identifying the patient. The medical assistant then assembles the equipment, locates the vein, draws the blood, removes and properly disposes of the needle, tends to the puncture site, labels the tubes, and delivers them to the laboratory. Standard Precautions are followed during the procedure.

15. **Collect a venous blood sample using the syringe method.**
Refer to Procedure 53-1.

16. **Collect a venous blood sample using the evacuated tube method.**
Refer to Procedure 53-2.

17. **Explain why a winged infusion set (butterfly needle) would be chosen over an evacuated tube.**
A winged infusion set (butterfly needle) is used on blood draws from the hand and from children. The needle is shorter, and the wings assist with holding and guiding the needle. The tubing minimizes the vacuum and prevents collapse of fragile veins. Using a syringe can control the vacuum to a greater extent than using vacuum tubes.

18. **Perform a venipuncture using a winged infusion set.**
Refer to Procedure 53-3.

19. **Summarize typical problems that may be associated with venipuncture.**
Refer to Table 53-4.

20. **Identify the major causes of hemolysis during venous blood collection.**
Refer to Table 53-5.

21. **List situations in which capillary puncture would be preferred over venipuncture.**
Capillary puncture is preferred over venipuncture for certain tests, such as hematocrit or hemoglobin analysis. It is performed routinely on children younger than age 2.

22. **Discuss proper dermal puncture sites.**
The middle two fingers (the lateral sides of each) generally are used for capillary puncture. In infants, the heel is the site of choice. The center of the heel must be avoided.

23. **Describe containers that may be used to collect capillary blood.**
Capillary blood can be collected in Microtainer devices, in capillary tubes, or on paper test cards. The Microtainer devices may contain anticoagulants and have stopper colors consistent with vacuum tubes.

24. **Explain why the first drop of blood is wiped away when a capillary puncture is performed.**
The first drop of blood contains tissue fluid that could affect the test results.

25. **Perform a capillary puncture.**
Refer to Procedure 53-4.

26. **Differentiate whole blood, serum, and plasma and give an example of a test performed with each.**
Whole blood coagulates unless mixed with an anticoagulant. The anticoagulant must be matched with the test so as not to interfere with the results. Whole blood is required for the complete blood count and differential. When clotted blood is centrifuged, the cells and the liquid separate; the liquid portion is the serum. Most chemistry and serology testing is performed on serum. When anticoagulated blood is centrifuged, the liquid that remains is plasma. Plasma may be used for coagulation studies and for blood glucose testing.

27. **Describe handling and transport methods for blood after collection.**
Blood cells can easily hemolyze, which alters test results; therefore, serum or plasma should be separated from the cells as soon as possible after collection. This is done by centrifugation. Blood samples to be transported must be packaged securely and sent according to regulations set forth by governmental agencies.

28. **Explain chain of custody procedures when blood samples are drawn.**
    Chain of custody is a legal term that refers to the ability to guarantee the identity and integrity of the specimen from collection to reporting of the test results. It is a process used to maintain and document the chronologic history of a specimen. Collection kits are available that contain everything needed for the venipuncture.

29. **Discuss the role of the medical assistant in patient education when performing phlebotomy.**

Medical assistants who work as phlebotomists must maintain a professional attitude, yet remain sympathetic to the patient's fears and anxiety about being "stuck with a needle." Establishing an environment that encourages the person to relax can minimize the patient's pain and discomfort during the procedure. Answer any questions the patient may have and perform the procedure skillfully before anxiety has time to set in. Provide as much explanation as needed to ease the patient's anxiety.

CONNECTIONS

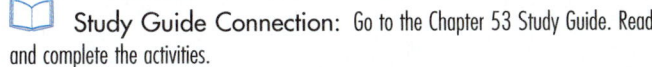

Study Guide Connection: Go to the Chapter 53 Study Guide. Read and complete the activities.

Evolve Connection: Go to the Chapter 53 link at *evolve.elsevier.com/kinn* to complete the Chapter Review and Chapter Quiz. Peruse other resources listed for this chapter to increase your knowledge of Assisting in Phlebotomy.

Dana Cummings is a certified medical assistant working in the Westhills Family Practice Center. She is preparing to collect blood from Mr. Corrigan, who recently underwent renal transplantation because of complications from diabetes type 1. He has come to the office today for a routine examination. Dr. Fischbach suspects that Mr. Corrigan is anemic and orders an anemia panel in addition to a renal panel; a hemoglobin A_{1c} level; a complete blood count, including hemoglobin, hematocrit, and differential; prothrombin time (PT); and alanine aminotransferase/aspartate aminotransferase (ALT/AST) testing.

While studying this chapter, think about the following questions:

- Why are so many tests being performed for Mr. Corrigan?

- Which of these tests probably will be completed today in the office laboratory?

LEARNING OBJECTIVES

1. Define, spell, and pronounce the terms listed in the vocabulary.
2. Apply critical thinking skills in performing the patient assessment and patient care.
3. Name the main functions of blood.
4. Identify the role of the hematology laboratory in patient care.
5. Describe the appearance and function of erythrocytes.
6. Describe the appearance and function of granular and agranular leukocytes.
7. Differentiate between T cells and B cells.
8. Describe the appearance and function of thrombocytes.
9. Explain the process of clot formation.
10. Identify the anticoagulant of choice for hematology testing.
11. Explain the purpose of the microhematocrit test.
12. Perform a microhematocrit test.
13. Explain the role of hemoglobin in the body.
14. Perform a hemoglobin test.
15. Identify the tests included in a complete blood count (CBC) and their reference ranges.
16. Explain the process of automated blood cell counting.
17. Distinguish between normal and abnormal test results.
18. Describe the red blood cell (RBC) indices and how they are calculated.
19. Explain the reasons for performing a white blood cell (WBC) differential.
20. Discuss Wright's stain sequence.
21. Describe the appearance of normal erythrocytes.

22. Describe the appearance of the five different types of leukocytes seen in a normal Wright-stained differential.
23. Cite the reasons for performing an erythrocyte sedimentation rate test.
24. Describe the sources of error for the erythrocyte sedimentation rate test.
25. Determine an erythrocyte sedimentation rate using a modified Westergren method.
26. Describe the tests performed to assess coagulation.
27. Differentiate between the ABO blood groupings and the Rh blood groupings.
28. Secure a capillary blood sample and determine the ABO and Rh groupings of the sample.
29. Discuss rare blood types and the implications of having a rare blood type when transfusion is necessary.
30. Describe the method behind the clinical chemistry testing methods used in the physician's office laboratory.
31. Explain the reasons for testing blood glucose, blood cholesterol, hemoglobin A_{1c}, thyroid hormone levels, and liver enzymes.
32. Perform a cholesterol test using a cholesterol monitor approved by the U.S. Food and Drug Administration (FDA).
33. Summarize typical chemistry panels, the reason for performing each panel, and the individual tests performed in those panels.
34. Describe the medical assistant's responsibility for legally preparing a patient for a blood transfusion.

VOCABULARY

anemia A condition marked by deficiency of red blood cells (RBCs).

artifacts Structures or features not normally present but visible as a result of an external agent or action, such as in a microscopic specimen after fixation or in a radiographic image.

centrifuge (sen′-truh-fuhj) An apparatus consisting essentially of a compartment that spins about a central axis to separate contained materials of different specific gravities or to separate colloidal particles suspended in a liquid.

enzymes Complex proteins produced by cells that act as catalysts in specific biochemical reactions.

polycythemia vera (pah-le-si-the′-me-uh/veh′-rah) A condition marked by an abnormally large number of red blood cells (RBCs) in the circulatory system.

type and cross-match Tests performed to assess the compatibility of blood to be transfused.

urea The major nitrogenous end product of protein metabolism and the chief nitrogenous component of the urine.

The average body holds 10 to 12 pints of blood. The heart circulates the blood through the circulatory system more than 1,000 times every day. More than 70,000 miles of passageways, most of which are narrower than a human hair, carry blood throughout the body. The blood is contained in a closed system of vessels; the largest is the aorta, and the smallest are the capillaries. The capillaries are only one cell layer thick, and their thin, permeable walls allow certain substances to move back and forth between blood vessels and surrounding tissue. The circulating blood contains more than 25 trillion cells, and every second the body replaces 8 million old red blood cells (RBCs) with 8 million new RBCs.

Besides supplying body cells with nutrients and oxygen, the blood carries away carbon dioxide and **urea,** the waste products of normal cell activity. If the blood did not carry away these waste products, they would accumulate and damage the cell. Carbon dioxide is carried in the blood to the lungs, where it is exhaled as part of normal breathing. The blood carries urea to the kidneys, where it is excreted in the urine along with other body wastes. The blood also distributes **enzymes,** hormones, and other chemicals needed for control and regulation of body activities. In addition, the blood functions to maintain the body at a uniform temperature, to keep other body fluids in a state of pH balance, and to carry hormones from the secreting gland to the tissues where they are needed.

Blood testing is done routinely in the hematology, immunology (serology), immunohematology (blood banking), and chemistry sections of the laboratory. The degree of blood testing performed by medical assistants depends on the level of service offered by the physician's office and the regulations established by the Clinical Laboratory Improvement Amendments (CLIA). As a medical assistant, you will not perform all the procedures described here. Some have been replaced by automated procedures, and others are considered highly complex by CLIA standards and therefore are not performed by medical assistants. Nevertheless, this chapter explains these procedures to provide background information critical to an understanding of the analysis of blood, from collection of the specimen, through testing, to recording of the results.

HEMATOLOGY

The hematology section of a laboratory deals with counting RBCs, white blood cells (WBCs), and platelets; differentiating WBCs on stained blood smears; measuring the percentage of RBCs in the blood (hematocrit); and determining the oxygen-carrying capacity of the blood (hemoglobin).

The complete blood cell count (CBC) is the laboratory procedure most frequently ordered for blood specimens. It gives a fairly complete look at the components of blood and can provide a wealth of information about a patient's condition. It routinely includes the following:

- RBC count
- WBC count
- Hemoglobin determination
- Hematocrit determination
- Differential WBC count
- Estimation of platelet numbers
- Red cell indices

> **CRITICAL THINKING APPLICATION   54-1**
> - Dana will collect the specimen for Mr. Corrigan's CBC. What tests are included in the CBC? Can any of these tests be performed by capillary puncture? Explain.
> - Which vacuum tube will Dana use to collect the CBC sample?

Whole blood is composed of formed elements suspended in a clear, yellow, liquid portion called *plasma*. Plasma makes up approximately 55% of blood by volume. The remaining 45% consists of formed cellular elements: erythrocytes (RBCs), leukocytes (WBCs), and thrombocytes (platelets). All of these cellular elements have special functions.

Erythrocytes

RBCs, or erythrocytes, are formed in the red bone marrow of the ribs, sternum, pelvis, and skull and in the ends of long bones in adults. The nucleus of the immature form of the RBC disintegrates as the cell matures. Loss of the nucleus results in the familiar shape of the RBC: a biconcave disk that is thicker at the rim than in the middle. Erythrocytes transport oxygen from the lungs to the body cells and carry carbon dioxide away from cells, back to the lungs to be exhaled. The main constituent is the red pigment hemoglobin, which is composed of iron and protein. Hemoglobin actually carries oxygen and some carbon dioxide throughout the body.

The life span of an erythrocyte is approximately 120 days. As the cell nears the end of its life, it becomes more fragile and eventually ruptures and breaks. The iron is reused for the formation of new RBCs, and the protein is converted into a bile pigment.

Leukocytes

WBCs, or leukocytes, have a nucleus and are larger than erythrocytes. The prime function of the leukocyte is to protect the body against infection and disease. The five types of leukocytes are classified as granular or agranular. Granular leukocytes, or polymorphonuclear leukocytes, include neutrophils, eosinophils, and basophils. They are characterized by their heavily granulated cytoplasm and segmented nuclei. Agranular leukocytes are the lymphocytes and monocytes, both of which have clear cytoplasm and a solid nucleus.

Granular leukocytes are phagocytic, that is, they engulf invading bacteria and viruses. Unlike erythrocytes, leukocytes function in the tissues. During inflammation, the blood carries the WBCs through dilated vessels to the site of injury. Capillary walls become more permeable, and granular cells squeeze through by ameboid motion. Once at the site of infection or injury, the cells engulf the invading microorganism, creating pus, which contains dead leukocytes, bacteria, and tissue cells.

Agranular leukocytes produce antibodies. The lymphocytes are classified as T cells or B cells, on the basis of their functional characteristics.

T Cells

T cells make up about 65% to 80% of circulating lymphocytes and have a life span of months to years. This is important for conferring long-lasting immunity to microbial infections. T cells mount the immune response to intracellular parasites, viruses, fungi, and bacteria. Delayed hypersensitivity reactions, such as the response to poison ivy, are controlled by T-cell defenses, as is organ transplant rejection. T cells are subdivided into several types, according to their function:

- *Cytotoxic (killer) T cells:* These cells kill foreign, virus-infected, and tumor cells. They produce proteins called *perforans* that induce cell death by punching holes in the cell membrane.
- *Helper T cells:* These are the most numerous type of T cell. They stimulate the activity of other T cells.
- *Suppressor T cells:* These cells inhibit the activity of other T cells.
- *Memory T cells:* These cells, which have a long life span, respond quickly to presentation of the same antigen at a later date.
- *Natural killer cells:* These cells kill virus-infected cells and tumor cells without previous sensitization.

B Cells

B cells are formed in bone marrow and then migrate to other lymph organs, where they multiply and reside. When stimulated, B cells differentiate into plasma cells that produce specific antibodies to an antigen. Antibodies circulate in the plasma or are present in secretions. Some antibodies cause cells to clump and precipitate, whereas others activate the complement system. The complement system is a series of reactions between plasma proteins that amplifies the immunologic response to foreign molecules. Activation of the complement system leads to lysis of microorganisms or their phagocytosis by neutrophils.

Antibodies are protein molecules that attach to antigens. Very small antigens, such as toxins and viruses, can be directly neutralized by antibodies; larger antigens, such as bacteria, require the help of agranular leukocytes. Three steps are required to destroy these pathogens:

1. *Antigen processing:* When a macrophage phagocytizes bacteria, proteins (antigens) from the bacteria are broken down into smaller molecules, which are then "displayed" on the surface of the macrophage, attached to special molecules called *major histocompatibility complex class II* (MHC II) molecules. Bacterial proteins are similarly processed and displayed on MHC II molecules on the surface of B lymphocytes.

2. *Lymphocyte stimulation:* When a T lymphocyte "sees" the same peptide on the macrophage and on the B cell, the T cell stimulates the B cell to turn on antibody production.

3. *Antibody production:* The stimulated B cell undergoes repeated cell divisions, enlargement, and differentiation to form a clone of antibody-secreting plasma cells. Hence, through specific antigen recognition of the invader, clonal expansion, and B-cell differentiation, an effective number of plasma cells are acquired, all secreting the same needed antibody. That antibody then binds to the bacteria, making them easier for the white cells to ingest. Antibody combined with a plasma component called *complement* may also kill the bacteria directly.

Thrombocytes

Thrombocytes are not true cells, but rather cytoplasmic fragments of a megakaryocyte, a large cell in the bone marrow. They are the smallest formed elements of the blood. They typically have a discoid shape; however, when activated, they become globular and form fingerlike cytoplasmic extensions called *pseudopodia.*

Clot Formation

In minor injuries, thrombocytes tend to collect and form plugs in blood vessel openings. To control bleeding from vessels larger than capillaries, a clot must form at the point of injury. Coagulation of the blood also is initiated by blood platelets. The platelets produce a substance that combines with calcium ions in the blood to form thromboplastin, which in turn converts the protein prothrombin into thrombin through a complex series of reactions. Thrombin, an enzyme, converts fibrinogen, a protein substance, into fibrin, an insoluble protein that forms an intricate network of minute, threadlike structures called *fibrils,* and causes the blood plasma to gel. The blood cells and plasma become enmeshed in the network of fibrils, forming a clot.

Blood clotting can be initiated by the extrinsic mechanism, in which substances from damaged tissues are mixed with the blood, or by the intrinsic mechanism, in which the blood itself is traumatized. More than 30 substances in blood have been found to affect clotting; whether blood will coagulate depends on a balance between the substances that promote coagulation (procoagulants) and those that inhibit it (anticoagulants). Coagulation of blood within blood vessels in the absence of injury can cause serious illness or death, especially when a clot forms in the coronary arteries (thrombosis) or in the cerebral arteries (stroke).

Hemophilia, a bleeding disorder, occurs when a person has a mutation in one of the clotting factor genes. It is a hereditary, gender-linked disorder that affects males of all races and ethnic groups. The mutated gene is on the X chromosome inherited from the mother. Approximately one in 4,000 males is born with the disorder; it is rare, but possible, for a female to have hemophilia. People with hemophilia are treated with intravenous (IV) purified clotting factor to prevent bleeding episodes. Internal bleeding, particularly in the joints, is a problem despite treatment and leads to painful arthritis.

Plasma

Plasma is a highly complex liquid that is the carrier for formed elements and other substances, such as proteins, carbohydrates, fats, hormones, enzymes, mineral salts, gases, and waste products. Plasma is composed of approximately 90% water, 9% protein, and 1% various other chemical substances. When plasma proteins and other components are used up during the clotting process, the remaining liquid is called *serum*.

COLLECTION OF BLOOD SPECIMENS

For most hematology tests, an adequate blood sample can be obtained from capillaries by finger puncture. If a larger sample is required, blood can be obtained from a vein by venipuncture. For a CBC, venous blood is collected in a tube containing an anticoagulant that prevents clotting. Ethylenediaminetetraacetic acid (EDTA) is the anticoagulant of choice for hematology testing. It is important to prevent blood from being hemolyzed during collection for hematology testing.

Hematocrit

The hematocrit (Hct) is a measurement of the percentage of packed RBCs in a volume of blood. The spun microhematocrit test is based on the principle of separating the cellular elements from plasma by centrifugation (Procedures 54-1 and 54-2). Two or three drops of blood are collected from a capillary puncture in two capillary tubes and are placed in a specially designed microhematocrit **centrifuge** (Figure 54-1). Alternatively, the capillary tubes can be filled with EDTA-anticoagulated blood from a lavender-topped vacuum tube. Capillary tubes can either be preplugged or open and may be made of glass or plastic. If the tube is not plugged, it must be sealed with special clay before centrifugation.

After centrifugation, packed RBCs are at the bottom of the tube, WBCs and platelets are in the center buffy coat, and plasma is on top (Figure 54-2). From this separation the microhematocrit is

---

PROCEDURE 54-1

Perform Hematology Testing: Perform a Microhematocrit Test

GOAL: *To perform a microhematocrit test accurately.*

EQUIPMENT and SUPPLIES

- Fresh sample of blood collected in a tube containing ethylenediaminetetraacetic acid (EDTA) anticoagulant
- Capillary tubes
- Sealing clay
- Centrifuge
- Disposable gloves
- Protective eyewear
- Biohazardous waste and sharps containers
- Patient's record

PROCEDURAL STEPS

1. Sanitize your hands. Put on nonsterile gloves and protective eyewear.
   <u>PURPOSE:</u> To ensure infection control.
2. Assemble the materials needed.
3. Fill two plain (blue-tipped) capillary tubes two thirds to three fourths full with well-mixed blood by tipping the blood tube slightly and touching the capillary tube end opposite the blue band to the blood. If the capillary tube and the blood tube are held almost parallel to the table, the capillary tube fills easily by capillary action.
   <u>PURPOSE:</u> Duplicates should always be done as a means of quality control. Tubes are not filled completely to provide space for the sealing clay.
4. Wipe the outside of the tube with clean gauze without touching the wet open end of the tube.

<u>PURPOSE:</u> Wiping the capillary tube removes any blood. Touching the blood with absorbent material removes more plasma than blood cells and can alter the hematocrit.

5. Tip the tube until the blood runs toward the end with the colored band.
   <u>PURPOSE:</u> This prevents blood from accidentally being removed from the tube.
6. Seal the end with the blue band with sealing clay by holding the tube horizontally and inserting the tube. Insert the tube as many times as needed to achieve a plug up to the blue band (Figure 1).

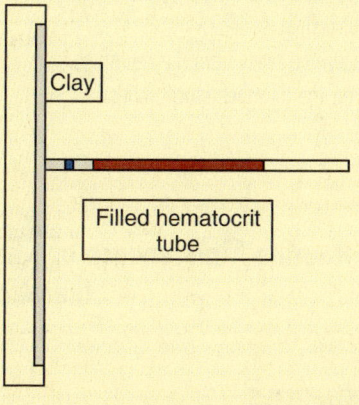

(From Rodak B: *Hematology: clinical principles and applications,* ed 3, St Louis, 2007, Saunders.)

PROCEDURE 54-1—cont'd

PURPOSE: This prevents the clay from becoming contaminated with blood, helps prevent leakage of blood, and keeps the gasket in the centrifuge from being cut by the capillary tubes.

7. Place the tubes opposite each other in the centrifuge with the sealed ends securely against the gasket (see Figure 54-1).
   PURPOSE: The centrifuge must always be balanced to prevent damage. If the clay ends of the capillary tubes are not outermost against the gasket, the sample will spin out of the tubes, contaminating the centrifuge.

8. Note the numbers on the centrifuge slots and record them.
   PURPOSE: The sample must be identified throughout the entire procedure.

9. Secure the locking top, fasten the lid down, and lock.
   PURPOSE: If the locking top is not firmly in place during the spinning cycle, the tubes will come out of their slots and break. The lid is always locked during centrifugation for safety purposes, that is, to prevent aerosols or broken glass from being ejected.

10. Set the timer and adjust the speed as needed.
    PURPOSE: The prescribed time is 3 to 5 minutes at 11,000 to 12,000 rpm. Check the manufacturer's instructions for time and speed.

11. Allow the centrifuge to come to a complete stop. Unlock the lids.
    PURPOSE: Opening the centrifuge before it has stopped could result in harm to the user.

12. Remove the tubes immediately and read the results. If this is not possible, store the tubes in an upright position.
    PURPOSE: Tubes left in the centrifuge will show altered results, because the red blood cell (RBC) layer spreads horizontally.

13. Determine the microhematocrit values using one of the following methods:
    a. Centrifuge with built-in reader using calibrated capillary tubes.
       • Position the tubes as directed by the manufacturer's instructions.
       • Read both tubes.
       • The average of the two results is reported.
       • The two values should not vary by more than 2%.
    b. Centrifuge without built-in reader.
       • Carefully remove the tubes from the centrifuge.
       • Place a tube on the microhematocrit reader.

• Align the clay-RBC junction with the zero line on the reader. Align the plasma meniscus with the 100% line. The value is read at the junction of the red cell layer and the buffy coat. The buffy coat is not included in the reading (Figure 2).

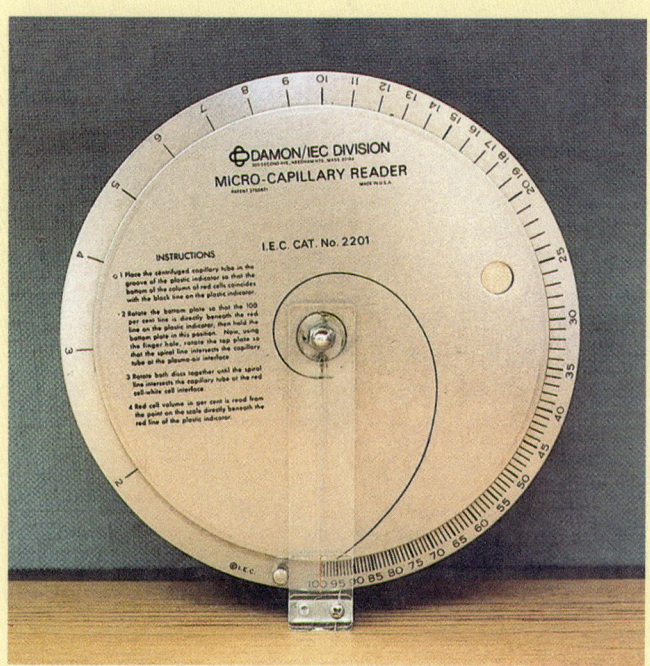

(From Rodak B: *Hematology: clinical principles and applications*, ed 3, St Louis, 2007, Saunders.)

• Read both tubes.
• The average of the two results is reported.
• The two values should not vary by more than 2%.

14. Dispose of the capillary tubes in a sharps container.

15. Disinfect the work area and properly dispose of all biohazard materials. Remove your gloves and eyewear and sanitize your hands.
    PURPOSE: To ensure infection control.

16. Record the results in the patient's medical record.
    PURPOSE: A procedure is not considered done until it is charted.

10/7/XX 11:25 AM Hct: 44 Dana Cummings, CMA (AAMA)

PROCEDURE 54-2

Perform Routine Maintenance of Clinical Equipment: Perform Preventive Maintenance for the Microhematocrit Centrifuge

GOAL: *To perform daily, monthly, and quarterly quality control on a microhematocrit centrifuge.*

EQUIPMENT and SUPPLIES

- Microhematocrit centrifuge
- Quality control logbook
- High-, normal-, and low-quality control samples
- Utility gloves

- Disposable gloves
- Face shield, moisture-proof gown as needed
- Disinfectant
- Biohazardous waste container
- Maintenance logbook

PROCEDURE 54-2—cont'd

PROCEDURAL STEPS

<u>NOTE:</u> These are generic recommendations. Always check the manufacturer's guidelines for specific instructions. Always unplug the power cord before cleaning or servicing the centrifuge. Wear protective clothing and gloves, as well as a face shield.

Daily Maintenance

1. Clean the inside of the centrifuge and the gasket with a disinfectant recommended by the manufacturer. Plastic and nonmetal parts may be cleaned with a fresh solution of 5% sodium hypochlorite (bleach) mixed 1:10 with water (one part bleach plus nine parts water).
<u>PURPOSE:</u> To remove any dried blood or shattered glass. Do not use bleach on the gasket, because it may harden the rubber.

Monthly Maintenance

1. Check the reading device. Misuse and zeroing of the reading devices can promote considerable error. Always use a second, simple reading device as a cross-check. Use a ruler or a flat plastic card specially made for this purpose. To use these cards, lay the spun hematocrit tube on the card and align the red cells with a line on the card to obtain the reading.
2. Check the rotor for cracks or corrosion and check the interior for signs of white powder.
<u>PURPOSE:</u> Cracks, corrosion, or powder may indicate impending rotor failure; they require the immediate attention of a service technician.
3. Record all preventive maintenance in the laboratory logbook.
<u>PURPOSE:</u> Recording maintenance is necessary to maintain warranties and to comply with regulations established by the Clinical Laboratory Improvement Amendments (CLIA) and other regulatory agencies.

Semiannual Maintenance

1. Check the gasket for cuts and breaks.
<u>PURPOSE:</u> Cut gaskets allow tubes to leak and must be replaced.
2. Check the timer with a stopwatch.
3. Perform a maximum cell pack to verify the time required for complete packing by reading a sample after centrifugation and then recentrifuging for 1 minute. The results should be the same. If they are not, perform preventive maintenance and/or call the service technician.
<u>PURPOSE:</u> If the cells compact further during recentrifugation, the centrifuge is not rotating at the proper speed, and hematocrit results will be falsely elevated.
4. Record all preventive measures in the laboratory logbook.
<u>PURPOSE:</u> Recording maintenance is necessary to maintain warranties and to comply with regulations established by CLIA and other regulatory agencies.

Annual Maintenance (or maintenance performed as needed)

1. The centrifuge functions and maintenance verification should be performed by qualified personnel. This includes checking the centrifuge mechanism, rotors, timer, speed, and electrical leads.
2. Record all professional service calls in the laboratory logbook.

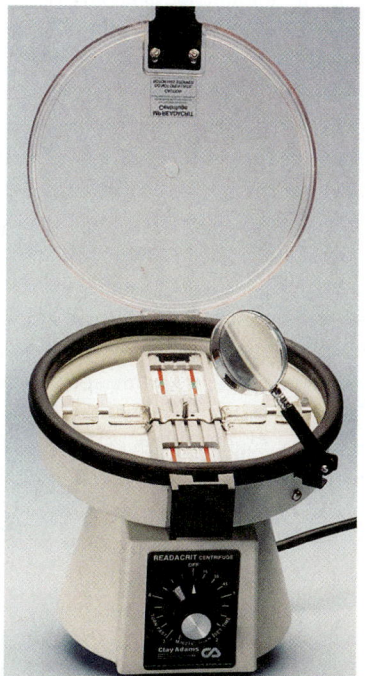

FIGURE 54-1 Centrifuge with capillary tube placement indications.

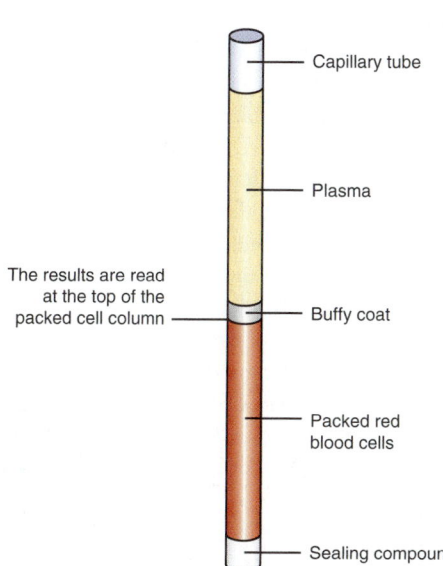

FIGURE 54-2 Hematocrit test results. Cellular elements are separated from plasma by centrifuging an anticoagulated blood specimen, and the results are read at the top of the packed cell column. (From Bonewit-West K: *Clinical procedures for medical assistants*, ed 7, St Louis, 2008, Saunders.)

TABLE 54-1   Hematocrit (Hct) Reference Values

AGE AND/OR GENDER	Hct VALUE (%)
Neonate	44-64
Infant	
1 mo	35-49
6 mo	30-40
Child, 1-10 yr	35-41
Adult	
Men	42-52
Women	36-45

From Stepp CA, Woods MA: *Laboratory procedures for medical office personnel,* Philadelphia, 1998, Saunders.

determined by comparing the concentration of RBCs with the total volume of the whole blood sample. The percentage is read by placing the tubes on a special microhematocrit reader. Some microhematocrit centrifuges have a built-in reading scale that reads calibrated capillary tubes. Microhematocrits should be performed in duplicate and the average of the two results reported.

Inverness Medical Professional Diagnostics (formerly Wampole, Princeton, New Jersey) manufactures a CLIA-waived instrument that uses electrical conductivity to determine the hematocrit. The STAT-CRIT Hct is a self-contained, portable unit that determines the hematocrit in 30 seconds. The testing method is based on the principle that blood is a conducting medium in which RBCs act as resistors. The plasma conducts electricity based on temperature. The greater the number of erythrocytes in a sample, the greater is the resistance recorded. A blood sample is introduced into the sample carrier, which has a thin, plastic membrane that permits rapid equilibration of the temperature of the blood and the measuring port. This instrument is best used with fresh blood obtained from a fingerstick; anticoagulants can interfere with conductivity, and heparin, not EDTA, is the anticoagulant of choice.

The hematocrit also can be calculated using RBC count and RBC size values from an automated cell counter.

Normal Hct values vary with gender and age (Table 54-1). They range from a low of 36% in women to a high of 52% in men. Low microhematocrit values can indicate **anemia** or the presence of bleeding; high values may be caused by dehydration or by a condition such as **polycythemia vera**. Values can be influenced by physiologic or pathologic factors and by collection techniques.

The microhematocrit is a commonly performed test requested by physicians separately or as part of the CBC. Because it is a simple procedure that requires only a small amount of blood, it is an ideal screening test and often is part of a routine physical examination.

◼ HEMOGLOBIN

The hemoglobin (Hgb) determination is a rough measure of the oxygen-carrying capacity of blood. The hemoglobin concentration can be determined as part of the CBC or as an individual test. Many methods of determining the hemoglobin concentration have been used over the years. The earliest measures simply involved comparing

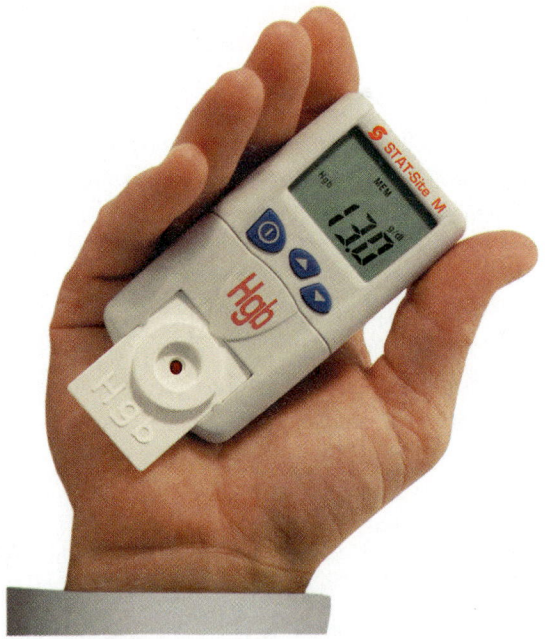

FIGURE 54-3 Handheld instruments, such as the Stat-Site System, can analyze hemoglobin quickly and accurately. (Courtesy Stanbio Laboratory, Boerne, Texas.)

the color of a drop of blood against a chart. Dark red blood has more hemoglobin than pale red blood. The international reference, or "gold standard," method for hemoglobin determination is the hemiglobincyanide or cyanmethemoglobin (HiCN) method. A sample of whole blood is diluted in Drabkin's reagent, which contains cyanide. The RBCs lyse, releasing hemoglobin, which reacts with cyanide to form hemiglobincyanide. Then the sample is placed in a colorimeter, and the amount of light absorbed by the sample at a 540-nm wavelength is determined.

A hemoglobinometer is a colorimeter that determines hemoglobin by measuring the amount of light absorbed by a sample of blood in which the hemoglobin has been released and chemically modified.

CLIA-waived methods include the STAT-Site M Hgb (Stanbio Laboratories, Boerne, Texas), a completely portable, battery-operated hemoglobin analyzer that fits in the palm of the hand (Figure 54-3), and the HemoCue (HemoCue AB, Angelgolm, Sweden) (Procedure 54-3). The HemoCue uses plastic cuvettes that contain sodium deoxycholate, sodium nitrite, and sodium azide. The sodium deoxycholate lyses the erythrocytes in the sample, releasing hemoglobin, which reacts with sodium nitrite to form methemoglobin. The methemoglobin reacts with the sodium azide to form azidemethemoglobin, which can be detected at two different wavelengths: 570 nm and 880 nm. Two wavelengths are used to compensate for possible turbidity in the sample. Capillary, venous, or arterial blood can be used in the cuvette, and cuvettes have a long shelf life.

The copper sulfate method is a CLIA-waived manual method of hemoglobin determination that is often used to screen blood donors. It is based on the principle of specific gravity; when a drop of blood from a patient with normal hemoglobin values is dropped into a copper sulfate solution, it falls rapidly to the bottom (Figure 54-4). If the drop falls slowly or not at all, hemoglobin levels are below reference range.

PROCEDURE 54-3

Perform Hematology Testing: Perform a Hemoglobin Test

GOAL: *To determine accurately the level of hemoglobin present in a blood sample using the HemoCue B-Hemoglobin System.*

EQUIPMENT and SUPPLIES

- HemoCue (HemoCue, Lake Forest, California)
- HemoCue cuvette
- Autolet or blood lancet
- Alcohol prep pads
- Gauze squares
- Disposable gloves
- Biohazardous waste container and sharps container
- Patient's record

PROCEDURAL STEPS

1. Perform instrument quality control by inserting the control cuvette into the instrument. Make sure the reading is within acceptable limits before proceeding.
   PURPOSE: Only instruments that record values within acceptable control limits can be used for patient testing. If the value is outside the control limits, refer to the troubleshooting guide for the instrument or contact the manufacturer.
2. Sanitize your hands.
   PURPOSE: To ensure infection control.
3. Collect and assemble all equipment and supplies needed.
4. Explain the procedure to the patient.
   PURPOSE: Explaining the reason for a diagnostic procedure helps gain the patient's compliance and addresses the person's questions and concerns.
5. Put on gloves.
6. Examine the fingers and choose the site to be used to obtain the blood sample.
   PURPOSE: The site must be free of trauma, calluses, and scarring.
7. Clean the site with alcohol or another recommended antiseptic preparation.
8. Perform a capillary puncture and obtain the blood sample.
9. Wipe away the first drop of blood.
   PURPOSE: This drop may contain tissue fluid.
10. Touch the microcuvette to the drop of blood. Do not touch the finger. The correct volume is drawn into the cuvette by capillary action. Wipe off any excess blood from the sides of the cuvette (Figures 1 and 2).

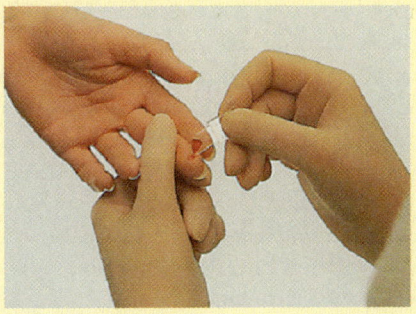

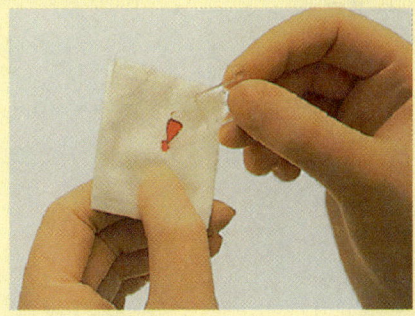

PURPOSE: Blood on the cuvette may alter the readings or contaminate the instrument.

11. Place the cuvette in the cuvette holder and insert it into the instrument (Figure 3).

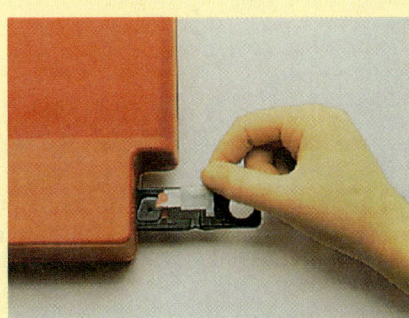

12. Read the result and record it on the patient's medical record.
    PURPOSE: A procedure is not completed until the results are recorded.
13. Dispose of biohazardous waste in the correct containers and properly disinfect the work area. Turn the instrument off and return it to the proper storage location.
14. Remove gloves and sanitize your hands.
    PURPOSE: To ensure infection control.

10/9/XX 9:30 AM Hgb 15.5 g/dL Dana Cummings, CMA (AAMA) _____

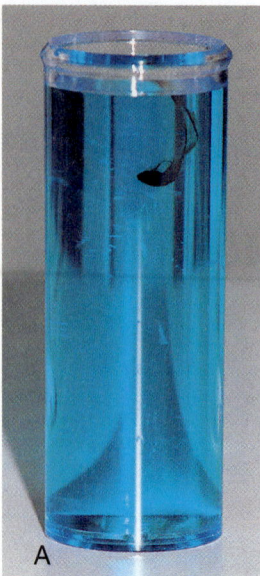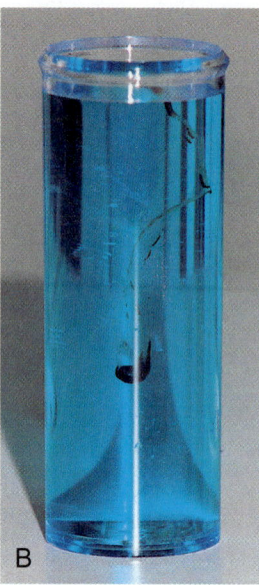

FIGURE 54-4 Copper sulfate specific gravity method for determining hemoglobin values. **A,** A drop of the patient's blood is placed in copper sulfate. The rate and distance it drops determine the level of hemoglobin present. **B,** The level indicates that this patient's hemoglobin is within reference range. (From Stepp CA, Woods MA: *Laboratory procedures for medical office personnel,* Philadelphia, 1998, Saunders.)

TABLE 54-2 Hemoglobin (Hgb) Reference Values

AGE AND/OR GENDER	Hgb LEVEL (g/dL)
Neonate	17-23
Infant (2 mo)	9-14
Child	11-16
Female	12-16
Male	15-17

From Stepp CA, Woods MA: *Laboratory procedures for medical office personnel,* Philadelphia, 1998, Saunders.

Normal hemoglobin values vary throughout life. They normally are quite high at birth, decline during childhood, and then increase through the teens until adult levels are reached (Table 54-2). Values range from a low of 12 g/dL in women to a high of 17.5 g/dL in men. The various factors that affect the hemoglobin level include age, gender, diet, altitude, and disease.

Hemoglobin and hematocrit tests often are performed together and are referred to as an "H&H." A quick mental calculation should always be done before H&H results are reported: Hemoglobin value × 3 ± 3 should equal the hematocrit value. For example, if the hemoglobin is 15 g/dL, the hematocrit should be 42% to 48%.

CRITICAL THINKING APPLICATION   54-2

Mr. Corrigan's hematocrit value is 37%. What does Dana calculate as the expected hemoglobin value? Does this test confirm the doctor's suspicions of anemia?

RED BLOOD CELL COUNT

The RBC count is a commonly performed procedure and is part of the CBC (Table 54-3). It approximates the number of circulating RBCs. The function of RBCs is to transport oxygen to tissues. The condition in which the oxygen-carrying capacity of blood is below normal is called *anemia.* The RBC count often is decreased in anemia. Increases are found in people with dehydration, polycythemia vera, or severe burns, and in those who live at high altitudes, in whom it reflects an adaptation to the lower oxygen content of the air.

Normal RBC values range from 4 million to 6 million cells/mm^3. RBC counts usually are higher in males than in females.

WHITE BLOOD CELL COUNT

The WBC count gives an approximation of the total number of leukocytes in circulating blood. The count is performed to help the physician determine whether an infection is present or to aid in the diagnosis of leukemia. It also may be used to follow the course of a disease and as an indication of whether the patient is responding to treatment.

The normal WBC count varies with age. It is higher in newborns and decreases throughout life. The average adult range is 4,000 to 11,000 cells/mm^3. Many factors can affect the WBC count. An increase in the number of normal WBCs is a condition called *leukocytosis.*

Physiologic increases in the WBC count are seen with pregnancy, stress, anesthesia, exercise, and exposure to temperature extremes, and after treatment with corticosteroids. Pathologic causes of leukocytosis include many bacterial infections, leukemia, appendicitis, and pneumonia. A decrease in the WBC count is called *leukopenia.* This condition may be caused by viral infection or by exposure to radiation and certain chemicals and drugs.

Determining the Red Blood Cell and White Blood Cell Counts

In the past, blood counts were performed by diluting the blood with special pipets and diluting fluid, placing the sample on a counting slide called a *hemacytometer,* and manually counting the cells using a microscope. This method was time-consuming and often inconsistent and therefore has largely been replaced by automated cell counting.

The current availability of many different types of cell counters has made it possible for the physician's office to become fully automated. Modern instruments range from relatively simple, inexpensive counters to very complex, expensive instruments. Automation improves the accuracy of cell counting and results in greater efficiency. In addition, it reduces the frequency of handling of individual blood specimens and the risk of exposure to blood-borne pathogens. The operation of the typical counters used in a physician's office laboratory is considered moderately complex by CLIA standards. It is essential that strict standardization procedures and quality control methods be followed when automated instruments are used to perform blood cell counts.

Most automated cell counters operate first by diluting the cells in a fluid that conducts an electrical current. These diluted cells then

TABLE 54-3   Reference Ranges for Complete Blood Count Values

TEST	NEONATES	INFANTS (6 mo)	CHILDREN	MEN	WOMEN
RBCs	4.8-7.1 million/mm³	3.8-5.5 million/mm³	4.5-4.8 million/mm³	4.5-6 million/mm³	4-5.5 million/mm³
Hematocrit (Hct)	44%-64%	30%-40%	35%-41%	42%-52%	36%-45%
Hemoglobin (Hgb)	17-23 g/dL	9-14 g/dL	11-16 g/dL	15-17 g/dL	12-16 g/dL
WBCs	9,000-30,000/mm³	6,000-16,000/mm³	5,000-13,000/mm³	4,000-11,000/mm³	
RBC Indices					
MCV	96-108 fL			82-99 fL	
MCH	32-34 pg			26-34 pg	
MCHC	31-33 g/dL			31-37 g/dL	
WBC Differential					
Neutrophils	≥45% by age 1 wk	32%	60% for children 2 yr or older	50%-65%	
Bands	—	—	—	0%-7%	
Eosinophils	—	—	0%-3%	1%-3%	
Basophils	—	—	1%-3%	0%-1%	
Monocytes	—	—	4%-9%	3%-9%	
Lymphocytes	≥41% by age 1 wk	61%	59% for children 2 yr or older	25%-40%	
Platelets	140,000-300,000/mm³	200,000-473,000/mm³	150,000-450,000/mm³	150,000-400,000/mm³	

From Stepp CA, Woods MA: *Laboratory procedures for medical office personnel,* Philadelphia, 1998, Saunders.
MCH, Mean corpuscular hemoglobin; *MCHC,* mean corpuscular hemoglobin concentration; *MCV,* mean corpuscular volume; *RBC,* red blood cell; *WBC,* white blood cell.

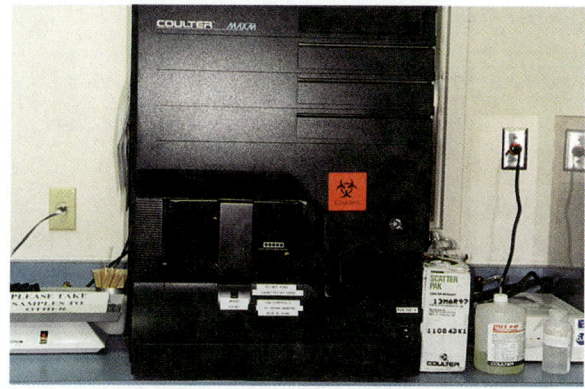

FIGURE 54-5 Automated cell counter. (Courtesy Coulter, Los Angeles, California.)

the RBCs. Hemoglobin usually is determined using the cyanmethemoglobin method, and hematocrit is determined mathematically using red cell counts and red cell volumes. With this information, an on-board computer determines certain parameters, known as *red cell indices,* which are included on the printout of the patient's results. When taken together, these results make up the CBC.

It is important that medical assistants understand hematology laboratory results and that they are able to distinguish between normal and abnormal levels. After combining what you have learned from hematology diagnostic reference ranges in Table 54-3 and from Figure 54-6, which is a sample lab report that identifies this particular lab's reference ranges, complete the following critical thinking exercise.

pass through a special narrow opening in the instrument. The passing cells interrupt the flow of current, and each interruption is counted. Some instruments use a laser beam instead of an electrical current (Figure 54-5). Red cells and white cells are counted in separate diluting chambers or channels. In the white cell counting area, the red cells are first lysed, usually with acetic acid, to make the white cells easier to count. Platelets usually are counted in the same channel as red cells, and the cells are differentiated by size. All cells are reported in units per volume of whole blood.

In addition to counting RBCs, WBCs, and platelets, the instruments analyze hemoglobin, hematocrit, and the size and shape of

CRITICAL THINKING APPLICATION   54-3

Distinguish between normal and abnormal test results in the following patients:

- Maggie McGuire, age 6, has a hematocrit of 38%. Is that normal?
- Carlos Santiago, age 54, has a WBC count of 13,000/mm³, and Dr. Fischbach asks to see his previous blood work. Why?
- Angelina Washington, age 23, has an Hct of 32% and an Hgb of 10 g/dL. Why would she be diagnosed with anemia?
- Rose Conrad has a platelet count of 142,000/mm³. Why is Dr. Fischbach concerned about a bleeding disorder?

DATE & TIME RECEIVED		ACCESSION NUMBER	
10/ 20/ 2013 20: 45			
LOCATION		DATE REPORTED	
		10/ 21/ 2000	

PHYSICIAN		PATIENT INFORMATION	

TEST		RESULTS	REFERENCE RANGE	UNITS
HEMOGRAM	LO	2. 9	4. 5-10. 5	CU. MM.
WHITE BLOOD COUNT	LO	2. 39	4. 40-5. 90	CU. MM.
RED BLOOD COUNT	LO	7. 4	14. 0-18. 0	GM/ 100 ML
HEMOGLOBIN	LO	22. 3	40. 0-52. 0	%
MEAN CORPUSCULAR VOLUME		93	80-100	fL
MEAN CORPUSCULAR HGB		31. 0	27. 0-32. 0	PG
MEAN CORPUSCULAR HGB CONC		33. 2	31. 0-36. 0	%
DIFFERENTIAL, WBC				
SEGMENTED NEUTROPHILS		57	38-80	%
LYMPHOCYTE		29	15-45	%
MONOCYTES		7	1-10	%
EOSINOPHILS		1	0-4	%
BAND NEUTROPHILS	HI	6	0-5	%
ANISOCYTOSIS	ABN	SLIGHT		
HYPOCHROMIA	ABN	SLIGHT		
PLATELET ESTIMATE	ABN	DECREASED		
PARTIAL THROMBOPLASTIN TIME				
PARTIAL THROMBOPLASTIN TIME		31.7	20. 0-40. 0	SECONDS
CONTROL PTT		30. 4	20. 0-40. 0	SECONDS
PROTHROMBIN TIME				
PROTHROMBIN TIME		12. 2	10. 0-13. 5	SECONDS
CONTROL PT		12. 0	11. 0-13. 0	SECONDS
FINAL Report		(Summary)		

FIGURE 54-6 A sample laboratory report. (From Zakus S: *Mosby's clinical skills for medical assistants*, ed 4, St Louis, 2001, Mosby.)

RED CELL INDICES

A variety of calculations can be performed using the information obtained from the CBC to produce indices that provide information about RBC disorders. Opinions vary about the clinical value of red cell indices. They are used to classify anemias and to select additional tests to determine the cause of anemia. They also may be used to monitor the treatment of anemia, because they may change in response to treatment. The standard indices are as follows:

- *Mean corpuscular volume (MCV):* On automated cell counters, the MCV is computed using the measurements of each red cell. With manual methods, it is calculated by dividing the hematocrit by the red cell count and multiplying by 10; the unit of measurement is the femtoliter (fL). The MCV measures the size of RBCs and is the most important index for classifying anemias as macrocytic (higher than normal MCV) or microcytic (low MCV). The normal reference range is 82 to 108 fL.

- *Mean corpuscular hemoglobin (MCH):* MCH = Hemoglobin ÷ RBC count. The MCH is calculated to give the average weight of hemoglobin in an individual RBC; the unit of measurement is the *picogram (pg)*. The reference range is 26 to 34 pg.

- *MCH concentration or content (MCHC):* MCHC = Hemoglobin ÷ Hematocrit. The MCHC indicates the average weight of hemoglobin compared with the cell size. It traditionally is a calculated value, but some instruments may measure the density of the cells as they are counted and compare this value with the calculated value. The reference range is 32 to 37 g/dL. With a decreased MCHC, the RBCs appear pale, or hypochromic, in a stained blood smear. An increased MCHC is rarely a true value and probably represents an error in measurement of the hemoglobin or hematocrit.

- *Red cell distribution width (RDW):* The RDW is the degree of red cell size variation, or how much difference exists between the largest and smallest red cells. The RDW is calculated to provide

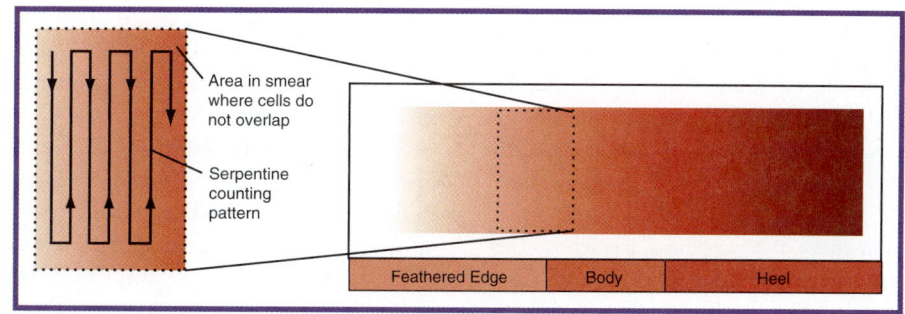

FIGURE 54-7 Appearance of a properly prepared wedge smear and serpentine (winding) pattern used to count cells. (From Stepp CA, Woods MA: *Laboratory procedures for medical office personnel*, Philadelphia, 1998, Saunders.)

a measure of the anisocytosis, or variation in size, of the RBCs. The reference range is 9 to 14.5.

DIFFERENTIAL CELL COUNT

The purpose of the differential, or "diff," is to analyze and quantitate the types of WBCs found in a sample of blood. The differential can be performed manually using a stained blood smear and a microscope or with an automated instrument. A number of automated cell counters have integrated differential analyzers that use high-frequency conductivity to gather information about cell size, internal structure, and density; they also have helium-neon lasers coupled with multiple-angle light scatter that provide information about a cell's internal structure, granulation, and surface characteristics.

Preparation of Blood Smears for the Differential

A blood smear enables the examiner to view the cellular components of blood in as natural a state as possible. The morphology of leukocytes, erythrocytes, and platelets can be studied, and their size, shape, and maturity can be evaluated.

A blood smear is prepared by spreading a drop of blood on a clean glass slide. The slide must be free of dust and grease. The best specimen for a blood smear is capillary blood that has no anticoagulant added. EDTA-anticoagulated blood can be used, provided the smear is made within 2 hours of collection.

The three kinds of blood smears are the coverglass smear, the spun smear, and the wedge smear. The coverglass smear is often used for bone marrow aspirations and involves placing a drop of blood between two coverslips and quickly pulling them apart. The spun smear uses a centrifuge to distribute the blood on a slide and often has the advantage of being a closed system, in that the blood tube is punctured by the instrument and does not have to be handled by the technician. The wedge smear is used most frequently and involves placing a small drop of blood ½ inch from the right end of a glass slide. The end of a second glass spreader slide is placed in front of the drop of blood at an angle of 30 to 35 degrees. The spreader slide is brought back into the drop until the blood spreads along the edge of the spreader slide. This is done with a quick but smooth gliding motion. The spreader slide then is pushed to the left with a quick, steady motion, spreading the blood across the slide.

A good wedge smear should cover half to three fourths of the slide. It should show a gradual transition from a thick to a thin end with a feathered edge. It should have a smooth appearance with no

ridges, holes, lines, streaks, or clumps (Figure 54-7). On microscopic examination, the cells should be distributed evenly.

After the smear has been made, it should be allowed to dry. The slide should be propped up to dry with the thick end (heel) down. Do not blow on the slide to dry it. This can cause **artifacts** in the RBCs from the moisture in your breath. Once dry, the patient's name is written on the frosted end of the slide with a pencil or marker.

After labeling, the slide is fixed in methanol, a fixative that preserves and prevents changes or deterioration of the cellular components. Many of the quick stains available on the market contain the fixative in the stain.

Staining of Blood Smears

Stains commonly used in the examination of blood cells are described as *polychromatic,* because they contain dyes that stain various cell components different colors. The stains usually contain methylene blue, a blue stain, and eosin, a red-orange stain. These stains are attracted to different parts of the cell, which makes the cells and their structures easier to see and differentiate. The most commonly used differential blood stain is Wright's stain. The traditional Wright's stain dates from the early 1890s and was an alcoholic solution of methylene blue and eosin Y. The traditional stain must be diluted 1:2 with buffer before use; this dilution generally was achieved by flooding the slide with Wright's stain, applying the buffer with a dropper, and blowing on the slide to mix. Many modifications of the original Wright's stain have been produced, most involving a chemical alteration in the methylene blue to improve polychroming. Most Wright's stains today contain mixtures of methylene blue, azure A, thionin, and eosin Y. In the quick stain, the buffer already is dissolved in the stain.

Identification of Normal Blood Cells

Much useful information can be gathered from microscopic identification and evaluation of blood cells in a stained smear. A great deal more information can be acquired from observation of these blood cells than from actual cell counts.

The features of blood cells that the medical assistant may observe and evaluate are cell size, nuclear appearance, and cytoplasmic characteristics. These three features allow cells to be identified, although much practice is required for recognition and classification of all the blood cells that may be seen in various disease states. A medical assistant might perform the differential analysis if employed in a laboratory that complies with certain CLIA regulations and if he or she is specifically trained to perform the analysis.

Cells are examined with the oil immersion objective of the microscope. The light should be bright to facilitate the visualization of colors and small structures. The slide is examined near the feathered end of the smear, where cells are barely touching one another and are easiest to identify.

RBCs are the most numerous of the cellular elements. They are biconcave disks with no nuclei. The red cells should appear pinkish tan as a result of staining of the hemoglobin in the cells (Figure 54-8).

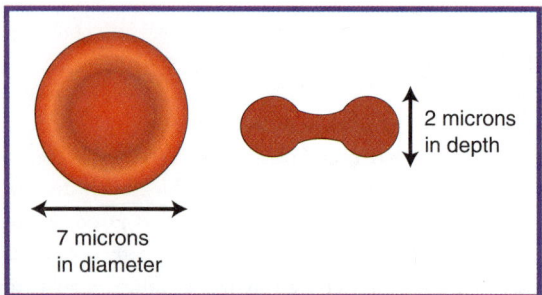

FIGURE 54-8 Red blood cell morphology. (From Stepp CA, Woods MA: *Laboratory procedures for medical office personnel,* Philadelphia, 1998, Saunders.)

Thrombocytes, or platelets, the smallest of the cellular elements, may be round or oval. They have no nucleus, because a platelet is just a fragment of cytoplasm from a large bone marrow cell. Platelets stain blue.

Leukocytes are the largest of the normal circulating blood cells (Table 54-4). Each of the five types has a characteristic appearance. As has been mentioned, the granulocytes include neutrophils, eosinophils, and basophils. Granulocytes have distinctive granules in the cytoplasm and may have segmented nuclei. The agranulocytes include lymphocytes and monocytes. They have few, if any, granules and nonsegmented nuclei. The nuclei of the leukocytes should appear purple, and their cytoplasm may vary from pink to blue or blue-gray. Neutrophils are known by a variety of names, including polymorphonuclear neutrophils (PMNs), segmented neutrophils, "polys," and "segs" (Figure 54-9). They are the most numerous WBCs in circulation in adults. They are produced in bone marrow, are released into the circulation, and eventually enter tissue to fight off invading microorganisms by engulfing them (phagocytosis). Many types of bacterial infection stimulate increased production of neutrophils.

The segmented neutrophil nucleus is segmented into two to five lobes connected by a strand. The nucleus stains a dark purple. The cytoplasm is pale pink and contains fine pink or lilac granules.

TABLE 54-4 Characteristics of Leukocytes

	GRANULOCYTES				AGRANULOCYTES	
	Neutrophil segmented (mature)	**Neutrophil band (immature)**	**Eosinophil**	**Basophil**	**Lymphocyte**	**Monocyte**
Cell size	10-15 mcL	10-15 mcL	10-15 mcL	10-15 mcL	6-15 mcL	12-20 mcL
Nucleus shape	Two to five lobes connected by threadlike filaments	Band or U-shaped	Bilobed or band	Slightly segmented, granular, or band	Round or oval	Round, indented, or superimposed lobes
Nucleus structure	Coarse	Coarse	Coarse	Obscured by granules	Smudged, lumpy, or clumped	Brainlike convolutions or folded
Cytoplasm amount	Abundant	Abundant	Abundant	Abundant	Scant	Abundant
Cytoplasm color	Colorless to light pink	Colorless to light pink	Colorless to light pink	Colorless to light pink	Sky blue to dark blue	Dull gray to blue-gray
Cytoplasm inclusions	Many tiny tan, pink, or red-purple granules	Many tiny tan, pink with increased red-purple granules	Large, rounder oval red to red-orange granule	Large, coarse blue-black granules	None to few round red-purple granules	Ground-glass appearance, fine red-purple granules, rare blue granules

From Stepp CA, Woods MA: *Laboratory procedures for medical office personnel,* Philadelphia, 1998, Saunders.

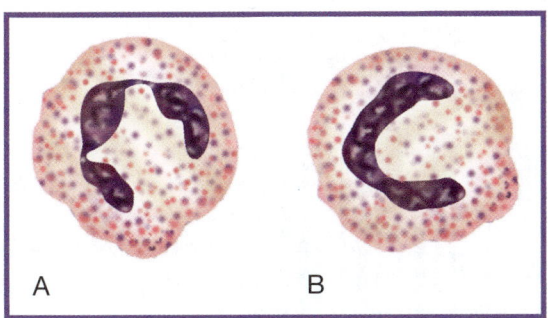

FIGURE 54-9 Neutrophilic cells. **A,** Segmented. **B,** Band. (From Stepp CA, Woods MA: *Laboratory procedures for medical office personnel*, Philadelphia, 1998, Saunders.)

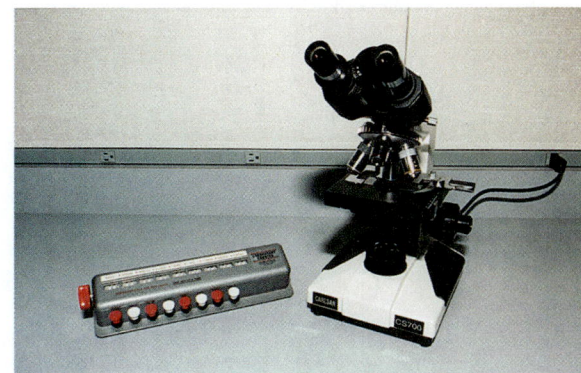

FIGURE 54-10 Microscope with differential cell counter. (Courtesy Cynmar, Carlinville, Illinois.)

An immature form of a neutrophil is called a *band* or *stab*. Instead of having a segmented nucleus in which the lobes are separated by a thin filament, the band has an unsegmented nucleus shaped like a horseshoe or a banana. The staining is the same as in the segmented neutrophil. An increase in bands is called a *shift to the left* and is seen in infections such as bacterial meningitis, pneumonia, appendicitis, strep throat, and abscesses and in chronic granulocytic leukemia.

The nucleus of an eosinophil is divided into two or three lobes that stain purple. The cytoplasm stains pink and has large round or oval, red-orange granules. Eosinophils are phagocytic and are closely associated with allergies such as hay fever and with asthma, as well as with certain parasitic infestations such as tapeworm and amebic dysentery.

The nucleus of a basophil is segmented and stains light purple. The large, dark, blue-black granules contain histamine, heparin, and other compounds that are part of the allergic response. Basophils are associated with the immediate immune response to external antigens, such as occurs with asthma, hay fever, and anaphylaxis.

Lymphocytes are the second most numerous type of WBC in adults. In children they usually are the most numerous. Their purple-staining nucleus usually is large, oval or round, and smooth. The cytoplasm stains blue. "Lymphs," as they are commonly called, are responsible for recognizing foreign antigens and producing circulating antibodies for immunity to disease. Increased numbers of lymphocytes are found with most viral diseases; with some bacterial infections, such as syphilis and tuberculosis; with leukemias; and in young children who are actively making antibodies. In many viral infections, stimulated or reactive lymphocytes, called *atypical lymphocytes,* are found. These are common in infectious mononucleosis.

Monocytes are the largest type of WBC in circulation. The nucleus may be oval, indented, or horseshoe shaped. The cytoplasm stains a dull gray-blue and may contain vacuoles, which appear as clear spaces in the cytoplasm filled with fluid or air. Monocytes are called *macrophages* when they enter tissues and ingest bacteria and debris of cellular breakdown. They are increased in patients with certain viral infections, such as hepatitis and mumps; rickettsial infections, such as Rocky Mountain spotted fever; and bacterial infections, such as tuberculosis and typhoid fever.

Differential Examination

A specific area of a stained smear must be examined microscopically when the differential count is done. This area must be where RBCs are touching but are not clumped when viewed microscopically. For manually prepared smears, this area would be the feathered edge. The entire slide is acceptable for viewing when the smear is prepared by automation. After you have located an appropriate area under low power of the microscope, focus using the oil immersion lens. The differential examination consists of counting and classifying 100 consecutive WBCs while moving in a specific winding pattern through the smear (see Figure 54-7). This pattern must be followed to avoid counting the same cells twice. A tally of the cells observed is kept on a differential cell counter or a computer (Figure 54-10).

Normal values for a differential vary with age. The reference ranges for adults are as follows:
- Neutrophils: 40% to 60%
- Lymphocytes: 20% to 40%
- Monocytes: 2% to 8%
- Eosinophils: 1% to 4%
- Basophils: 0.5% to 1%
- Band: 0% to 3%

Many disease states alter the ratios of the different types of leukocytes, and the differential can be very useful in assisting with the physician's diagnosis. A differential examination typically is performed in a reference laboratory.

Red Blood Cell Morphology

After the differential cell count has been determined, the RBCs are observed and evaluated. Normally, stained RBCs are the same size and shape and are well filled with hemoglobin. Any variations from the normal state are reported (Figure 54-11). The appearance of the RBCs should correlate with the RBC indices.

Size

Normal-sized RBCs are said to be *normocytic*. If the cells are larger than normal, they are *macrocytic;* if smaller, they are *microcytic*. The condition in which different sizes of RBCs are present is called *anisocytosis*.

Shape

Normal RBCs are round or slightly oval. Cells may be shaped like sickles, targets, crescents, or burrs. Poikilocytosis is a significant variation in the shape of RBCs.

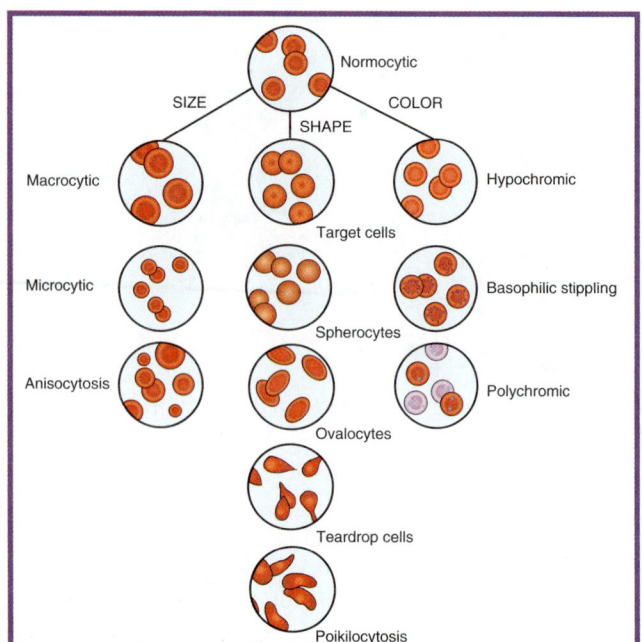

FIGURE 54-11 Abnormal erythrocytes. (Modified from Stepp CA, Woods MA: *Laboratory procedures for medical office personnel,* Philadelphia, 1998, Saunders.)

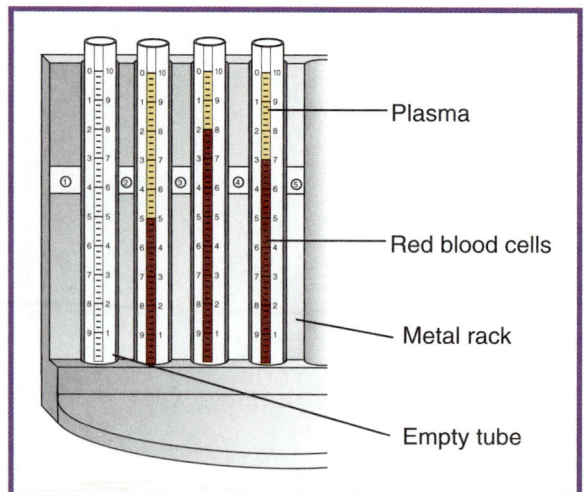

FIGURE 54-12 Wintrobe sedimentation rate system. (From Stepp CA, Woods MA: *Laboratory procedures for medical office personnel,* Philadelphia, 1998, Saunders.)

TABLE 54-5	Erythrocyte Sedimentation Rate Reference Values	
	WINTROBE METHOD (mm/hr)	**WESTERGREN METHOD (mm/hr)**
Men	0-10	≤50 yr: 0-15
		>50 yr: 0-20
Women	1-20	≤50 yr: 0-20
		>50 yr: 0-30

From Stepp CA, Woods MA: *Laboratory procedures for medical office personnel,* Philadelphia, 1998, Saunders.

Content

An RBC with a normal amount of hemoglobin is said to be *normochromic.* Pale-staining cells are *hypochromic* and have less hemoglobin than normal. Any inclusions in red cells should be reported.

Platelet Analysis

On a stained smear, the morphology of platelets is observed for any abnormalities. Platelets are small and irregularly shaped, and may vary considerably in size. The average number of platelets seen in 10 to 15 fields is reported. The normal platelet count is 150,000 to 400,000/mm³. An increase in platelets is called *thrombocytosis,* and a decrease is called *thrombocytopenia.* Excessive clumping of platelets is reported.

In the past 10 years, the hematology laboratory has seen great advancements in the use of automation, and many procedures have become "closed tube" operations. Not only are cell counts performed by instruments that sample the tube without opening it, but slide preparation and staining can be performed by instruments that sample the specimen and make thin, consistent films or smears without ever opening the tube. These instruments are so sensitive that they can adjust the film preparation on the basis of the calculated hematocrit of the CBC. The advantages are many; closed-tube systems are safer for personnel, and results are more consistent. Still, laboratory personnel must watch closely for "flagged" or inconsistent values, and they must be prepared to perform backup tests to verify the results of the automated tests.

ERYTHROCYTE SEDIMENTATION RATE

The erythrocyte sedimentation rate (ESR) is a laboratory test that measures the rate at which erythrocytes gradually separate from plasma and settle to the bottom of a specially calibrated tube in an hour. The test is not specific for a particular disease but is used as a general indication of inflammation. Increases are found in such conditions as acute and chronic infections, rheumatoid arthritis, tuberculosis, hepatitis, cancer, multiple myeloma, rheumatic fever, and lupus erythematosus.

Normal values vary slightly with age and gender (Table 54-5). Only increased ESR rates are significant. Several methods of measuring the ESR are used, including the Wintrobe (Figure 54-12), Westergren (Procedure 54-4), and Landau-Adams methods. These methods are based on the same principle and differ only in the amount of blood needed and the tube size and calibration used.

The International Committee for Standardization in Hematology has selected Westergren's method as the recommended method. A straight glass tube 30 cm long and 2.55 mm (±0.15 mm) in diameter with a bore uniform to 0.05 mm throughout is used. Blood is obtained by clean venipuncture in an EDTA tube and is diluted accurately with one volume of 109 mmol/L trisodium citrate to four volumes of blood. The test should be performed within 2 hours of collection, or within 6 hours if the blood is stored at 4°C (39.2°F). The diluted blood sample is drawn to the 200-mm mark in the tube by means of a mechanical device or an aspiration bulb. The tube is placed vertically in a vibration- and draft-free environment, away from direct sunlight. After 1 hour the ESR is measured in millimeters as the height of clear plasma above the column of sedimented cells.

PROCEDURE 54-4

Perform Hematology Testing: Determine the Erythrocyte Sedimentation Rate Using a Modified Westergren Method

GOAL: *To fill a Westergren tube properly and to observe and record an erythrocyte sedimentation rate (ESR) obtained by using the Westergren method.*

EQUIPMENT and SUPPLIES

- Ethylenediaminetetraacetic acid (EDTA)-anticoagulated blood specimen
- Safety tube decapper
- Sediplast erythrocyte sedimentation rate (ESR) system
- Sediplast rack
- Timer
- Disposable gloves
- Face protector/shield
- Biohazardous waste container
- Patient's record

PROCEDURAL STEPS

1. Sanitize your hands. Put on face protection and nonsterile gloves.
   PURPOSE: To ensure infection control.
2. Assemble the materials needed.
3. Check the leveling bubble of the Sediplast rack.
   PURPOSE: The rack must be horizontal on the table or bench to ensure that the tube is vertical.
4. Bring the blood sample to room temperature if it has been refrigerated and mix the sample well by inverting the tube gently several times, making sure the tube has no bubbles.
   PURPOSE: Cells settle when a specimen stands, and blood must always be well mixed before sampling. Test results will be altered if refrigerated blood is used.
5. Remove the stopper on the blood sample using a tube decapper and on the prefilled Sediplast vial.
   PURPOSE: Removing the cap with a protective device blocks blood splashes and helps prevent aerosolization of the specimen.
6. Fill the vial to the indicated line, replace the stopper on the prefilled vial, and invert several times to mix. Recap the blood collection tube (Figure 1).

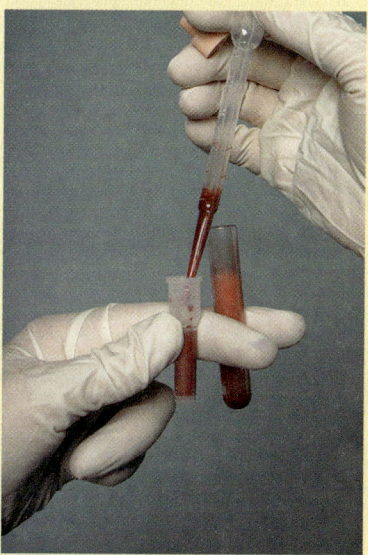

PURPOSE: This dilutes the blood in accordance with the Westergren procedure.
7. Insert the Sediplast pipet through the pierceable stopper on the vial and push down until the pipet touches the bottom of the vial. The pipet automatically draws the blood up to the zero mark.
8. Insert the pipet and the vial into the rack, making sure the pipet is vertical (Figure 2).

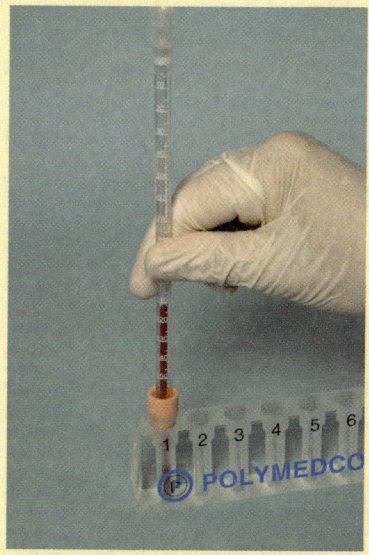

(Courtesy Polymedco, Cortland Manor, New York.)

PURPOSE: A pipet that is not vertical produces erroneous results.
9. Allow the tube to stand undisturbed for 60 minutes.
   PURPOSE: Jarring increases the sedimentation rate.
10. Measure the distance the erythrocytes have fallen. The scale reads in millimeters; each line is 1 mm.
11. Disinfect the work area and properly dispose of all biohazard materials. Dispose of the pipet in a biohazard container. Remove your face protection and gloves and sanitize your hands.
12. Record the findings in the patient's medical record.
    REMEMBER: The Westergren ESR is reported in millimeters per hour.
    PURPOSE: A procedure is considered not done until it is recorded.

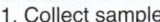
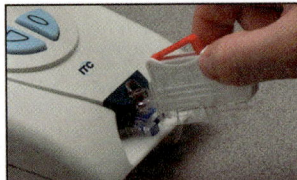
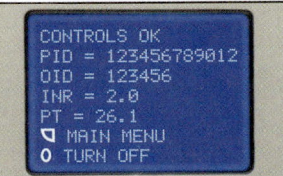

1. Collect sample   2. Attach Tenderlett Plus   3. Read results

FIGURE 54-13 ProTime microcoagulation system.

Variations on the standard method have been developed using plastic and disposable glass tubes and capillary tubes for infants. One such method is the Sediplast (Polymedco, Redmond, Washington). This closed system incorporates a pierceable stopper that ensures a leakproof seal when pierced by a pipet. An automatic self-zeroing cap and reservoir accurately bring the blood level to the zero mark and prevent overfilling. A prefilled vial of sodium citrate diluent is provided for dilution of blood before testing (see Procedure 54-4).

Rapid automated systems also have been developed. Strek Laboratories (LaVista, Nebraska) manufactures the ESR-10, a nonautomated, CLIA-waived test that uses ESR vacuum tubes. The tubes automatically draw the correct amount of sample and then are placed in the rack for 30 minutes. Although not CLIA-waived, analyzers that force readings are also manufactured by Strek Laboratories and allow results as quickly as 10 minutes.

Becton, Dickinson & Company (Franklin Lakes, New Jersey) has introduced the Seditainer, an ESR tube that fits the Vacutainer system. This self-contained tube contains a buffered sodium citrate solution, which provides a proper dilution of buffer to blood when the tube is filled from the venipuncture. The specimen need not be transferred to another tube for analysis. The Seditainer is placed in a calibrated stand from which the ESR is read after 60 minutes. The Seditainer tube has a black stopper, and it should be filled after the light blue–topped and red-topped tubes, along with any other additive tubes, are filled. It should be inverted eight times after filling.

Many factors can affect the ESR. The tube must be completely filled with blood and must not have air bubbles. The tube must be allowed to sit in a vertical position, undisturbed, for a full hour. Minor degrees of tilting may increase the sedimentation rate; careful timing is important. Jarring or vibrations from nearby machinery will falsely increase the ESR. If testing cannot be performed immediately, the blood should be stored at room temperature, and testing must be performed within 62 hours.

COAGULATION TESTING

Coagulation testing usually is performed in the hematology laboratory. The medical assistant may be asked to perform a test to determine prothrombin time (PT) using a handheld, CLIA-waived instrument that uses whole blood or citrated plasma. The PT is a method of measuring how well the blood clots. Generally, the PT is considered prolonged if it is more than 1.2 times the control time. Patients who have problems with delayed blood clotting are given a number of tests to determine the cause of the problem. The prothrombin test specifically evaluates the presence of factors VIIa, V, and X, prothrombin, and fibrinogen. Prothrombin is a protein in the liquid part of blood (plasma) that is converted to thrombin as

part of the clotting process. Fibrinogen is a type of blood protein called a *globulin;* it is converted to fibrin during the clotting process. With a drop in concentration of any of these factors, the blood takes longer to clot.

The PT is used in combination with the partial thromboplastin time (PTT) to screen for hemophilia and other hereditary clotting disorders. The PT also is used to monitor the condition of patients taking the drug warfarin (Coumadin). Warfarin is given to prevent clots in the deep veins of the legs and to treat pulmonary embolism. It interferes with blood clotting by lowering the liver's production of certain clotting factors.

The ProTime Microcoagulation System (ITC, Edison, New Jersey) measures PT according to the time it takes the blood to form a fibrin clot. A precise amount of blood is drawn from the fingerstick into channels in the testing strip, where it is mixed with a thromboplastin reagent (Figure 54-13). The blood is pumped back and forth in the channel, and a series of light-emitting diodes (LEDs) detect formation of the clot when movement of the blood stops.

PT test results are reported as the number of seconds the blood takes to clot when mixed with a thromboplastin reagent. The international normalized ratio (INR) was created by the World Health Organization (WHO) because PT test results can vary, depending on the thromboplastin reagent used. The INR is a conversion unit that takes into account the different sensitivities of available reagents. It is widely accepted as the standard unit for reporting PT results rather than the time in seconds. Normal PT values are 10 to 13 seconds, or an INR of 1 to 1.4. The warfarin (Coumadin) dosage in people treated to prevent the formation of blood clots and in those with artificial heart valves usually is adjusted so that the PT is about 1.5 to 2.5 times the normal value (or INR values 2 to 3).

It is important that the medical assistant know how to accurately document INR follow-up and related Coumadin dosages on a laboratory flow sheet. The physician will balance repeated INR levels with Coumadin doses so the INR is maintained at 2 throughout the anticoagulant treatment period (Figure 54-14).

IMMUNOHEMATOLOGY

Formerly called the *blood bank,* the immunohematology division of the laboratory is responsible for blood typing. The major reason for performing immunohematologic tests is to prevent problems caused by incompatibility of blood types. Compatibility testing (cross-matching) is performed to prevent transfusion reactions in patients receiving blood transfusions and to identify potential Rh-incompatibility problems in expectant mothers. Rh incompatibility between an expectant mother and the unborn child may result in hemolytic disease of the newborn.

Westhills Family Practice Center
Coumadin Anticoagulant Record

Patient's Name: _____   DOB: _____
Address: _____   SSN: _____
_____
Patient's Phone: _____
Dx for Anticoagulation: _____   ICDM Code: _____
Date Coumadin Started : _____   INR Goal: _____
Phone for Outside Lab: _____

Date	Warfarin Dose Pre-Test	PT	INR	Warfarin Dose Order	Next INR/PT	Signature

FIGURE 54-14 Coumadin flow sheet.

TABLE 54-6 Blood Type Distribution in the United States

TYPE	CAUCASIAN	AFRICAN-AMERICAN	HISPANIC	ASIAN
O+	37%	47%	53%	39%
O−	8%	4%	4%	1%
A+	33%	24%	29%	27%
A−	7%	2%	2%	0.5%
B+	9%	18%	9%	25%
B−	2%	1%	1%	0.4%
AB+	3%	4%	2%	7%
AB−	1%	0.3%	0.2%	0.1%

Data from the American Red Cross at http://www.redcrossblood.org/learn-about-blood/blood-types

Blood Grouping

The two major blood antigen systems are the ABO (or Landsteiner) system and the Rh system. The ABO system has four major blood groups: A, B, O, and AB. A person is either Rh positive or Rh negative. Certain blood types are more common in certain countries. In China more than 99% of the population has Rh-positive blood. In the United States, about 85% of the population is Rh positive. Blood type, like eye color, is inherited. Racial and ethnic differences in blood type and composition exist as a result of inheritance and populations that have migrated and mixed over time. Different kinds of animals also have different kinds of blood. Dogs have four blood types; cats have 11; cows have about 800. Table 54-6 shows the

distribution of blood types of the peoples of the United States for which data are available.

Determination of ABO Blood Group

Determination of ABO blood groups is a simple test that can easily be performed (Procedure 54-5), but because of the implications of performing the test incorrectly, blood typing is not CLIA waived. The test detects the presence of A or B antigens on RBCs on the basis of the presence or absence of agglutination with a known antiserum. When the antigen on a patient's RBCs corresponds to the test antibody, agglutination occurs. If the corresponding antigen is not present on the cells, agglutination does not occur.

In addition to the blood antigens found on RBCs, naturally occurring antibodies are found in plasma. These antibodies appear shortly after birth, and the body never produces an antibody that can combine with its own blood antigen. Because of the blood group antibodies, blood transfusions ideally should be specific: Type A blood should receive type A blood in a transfusion. In emergencies, if there is no time for the laboratory to perform a **type and cross-match**, type O negative (O−) blood is administered. Type O negative is referred to as the "universal donor," because there are no circulating antibodies to the ABO antigen, nor are there Rh antigens that might sensitize an Rh-negative recipient. Table 54-7 shows the compatibility among blood types for transfusion.

Determination of Rh Factor

Determination of the Rh type is another simple test (although it is not CLIA waived) that can be performed with a minimum amount of equipment (Procedure 54-6). The Rh factor is so called because it was first discovered in rhesus monkeys. Later this same protein

PROCEDURE 54-5

Perform Hematology Testing: Determine the ABO Group Using a Slide Test

GOAL: *To determine a patient's ABO group accurately using the slide test technique.*

EQUIPMENT and SUPPLIES

- Glass slides with frosted ends
- Anti-A and anti-B serum (Figure 1)

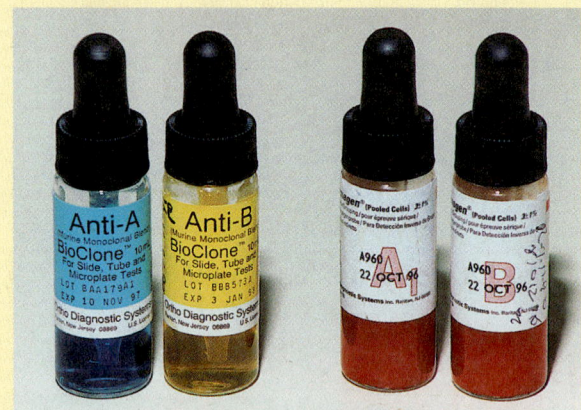

(From Stepp CA, Woods MA: *Laboratory procedures for medical office personnel,* Philadelphia, 1998, Saunders.)

- Applicator sticks
- Lancet and automatic finger puncture device
- Alcohol preps
- Sterile gauze squares
- Adhesive bandage strip
- Laboratory marking pen or pencil
- Disposable gloves
- Face protector/shield
- Biohazardous waste container and sharps container
- Patient's record

PROCEDURAL STEPS

1. Assemble all of the supplies and equipment needed to complete the testing procedure.
2. Sanitize your hands and put on face protection and gloves.
   PURPOSE: To ensure infection control.
3. Explain the procedure to the patient.
   PURPOSE: Explaining the reason for a diagnostic procedure helps gain the patient's compliance and addresses the person's questions and concerns.

4. Label the slides in the frosted area with the patient's name.
   PURPOSE: To ensure proper identification of test results.
5. Place one drop of anti-A serum on slide 1, one drop of anti-B serum on slide 2, and one drop of anti-A and anti-B serum on slide 3.
6. Select the puncture site, cleanse the site with an alcohol pad, and perform a finger puncture.
7. Wipe away the first drop of blood.
   PURPOSE: The first drop of blood may contain tissue fluid.
8. Place one large drop of blood on each of the three prepared slides, close to but not touching the drop of antiserum.
9. Cover the puncture site with a sterile gauze square, and instruct the patient to apply gentle pressure to the site.
10. Mix the antiserum and blood thoroughly, using a clean applicator stick for each slide. Rock the slide after mixing to check for agglutination. The mixture should be spread over an area measuring approximately 20 × 40 mm.
11. Read and interpret the results of the reaction for all slides (Figure 2).

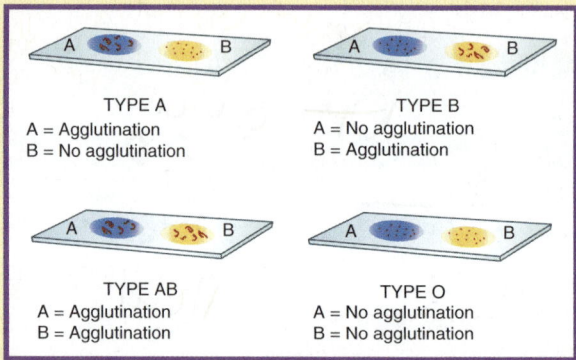

12. Make sure the patient has stopped bleeding and apply a bandage strip to the puncture site if necessary.
13. Discard all biohazard testing waste in the appropriate container.
   PURPOSE: To ensure infection control.
14. Disinfect the testing area and sanitize your hands.
15. Record the testing results in the patient's record.
   PURPOSE: A procedure is not considered done until it is recorded.
   NOTE: Because of the serious implications of incorrect blood typing, ABO and Rh typing is not routinely performed in a physician's office laboratory. Instead, these tests are performed in a hospital or blood bank.

was found on the RBCs of some humans. This test detects the presence of proteins (D antigens) on the surface of RBCs on the basis of the presence or absence of agglutination with anti-D antiserum. When the D antigen is present, agglutination occurs when the anti-D antiserum is mixed with RBCs. If the D antigen is not present, agglutination does not occur. Rh-positive blood agglutinates in the presence of anti-D antiserum but not in the presence of the Rh control. Rh-negative blood does not agglutinate in the presence of anti-D antiserum, nor does it agglutinate in the presence of the Rh control.

TABLE 54-7 Blood Compatibility

	RECIPIENT BLOOD*	
RBC ANTIGEN	PLASMA ANTIBODIES	COMPATIBLE WITH DONOR TYPES†
Type O (no antigens)	Anti-A and anti-B	O
Type A (type A antigen)	Anti-B	O and A
Type B (type B antigen)	Anti-A	O and B
Type AB (type AB antigen)	None	O, A, B, and AB

From Stepp CA, Woods MA: *Laboratory procedures for medical office personnel*, Philadelphia, 1998, Saunders.
RBC, Red blood cell.
*Patients with type AB blood are considered universal recipients.
†Patients with type O blood are considered universal donors.

BLOOD AGGLUTINATION PRINCIPLES

- Type A blood agglutinates in the presence of anti-A antiserum but does not agglutinate in the presence of anti-B antiserum.
- Type B blood agglutinates in the presence of anti-B antiserum but not in the presence of anti-A antiserum.
- Type O blood does not agglutinate in the presence of either anti-A antiserum or anti-B antiserum.
- Type AB blood agglutinates in the presence of both anti-A antiserum and anti-B antiserum.

PROCEDURE 54-6

Perform Hematology Testing: Determine the Rh Factor Using the Slide Method

GOAL: *To determine accurately the presence or absence of anti-D agglutinations.*

EQUIPMENT and SUPPLIES

- Two glass slides with frosted ends
- Anti-D serum (Figure 1)

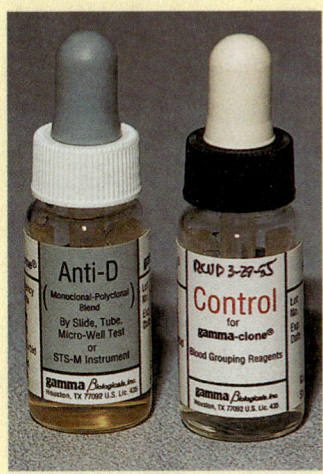

(From Stepp CA, Woods MA: *Laboratory procedures for medical office personnel*, Philadelphia, 1998, Saunders.)

- Applicator sticks
- Lancet and automatic finger puncture device
- Alcohol preps
- Sterile gauze squares
- Laboratory marker or pencil
- Disposable gloves
- Face protector/shield
- Biohazardous waste and sharps containers
- Patient's record

PROCEDURAL STEPS

1. Assemble all the equipment and supplies needed to perform the test.
2. Sanitize your hands and put on face protection and gloves.
   PURPOSE: To ensure infection control.
3. Label one slide "D" and one slide "C."
   PURPOSE: To differentiate between the anti-D slide and the control slide.
4. Place one drop of anti-D serum on the D slide.
5. Place one drop of the appropriate control reagent on the C slide.
6. Perform a capillary puncture to secure a blood specimen.
7. To each slide, add one large drop of the patient's blood, close to but not touching the antiserum.
8. Thoroughly mix the blood with the anti-D serum and the control, using a clean applicator stick for each slide, and spread the reaction mixture over an area measuring approximately 20 × 40 mm on each slide.
9. Place the slide on an Rh view box.
   PURPOSE: The view box provides warmth, which promotes agglutination, and also provides extra illumination for viewing.
10. Read the results immediately.
    PURPOSE: Drying of the reaction mixture must not be confused with agglutination.
11. Discard all disposable equipment in the proper biohazardous waste containers.
12. Disinfect the area. Remove your gloves and face protection and sanitize your hands.
    PURPOSE: To ensure infection control.
13. Record the test results.
    PURPOSE: A procedure is not considered done until it is recorded.
    NOTE: Because of the serious implications of incorrect blood typing, ABO and Rh typing is not routinely performed in a physician's office laboratory. Instead, these tests are performed in a hospital or blood banking facility.

There are no naturally occurring antibodies to the Rh factor as there are to the A and B antigens. A person develops antibodies to the D antigen only in the event of exposure to the antigen. This is possible if an incompatible transfusion is administered, or if an Rh-negative mother is exposed to the Rh-positive blood of her infant during pregnancy, a miscarriage, abortion, or delivery. If this occurs, the mother may develop antibodies to the D antigen. This usually does not cause a problem during the first pregnancy. However, in a subsequent pregnancy with an Rh-positive fetus, the woman's immune system begins to produce more antibodies, because she was sensitized during the first pregnancy. These antibodies cross the placenta and destroy the RBCs of the fetus, which can lead to anemia, heart failure, or brain damage in the infant and may even cause death. These events are collectively called *hemolytic disease of the newborn* (HDN). The disease sometimes is also called *hydrops* or *blue baby syndrome.* Until 1968, no preventive measure could be taken for this problem. Exchange transfusion, in which all of the infant's blood is replaced, was the only option. Today, however, HDN can be prevented by the administration of Rh immune globulin products. Rho(D) immune globulin is a protein solution containing large numbers of Rh(D) antibodies. It is given to the Rh-negative mother by injection after a miscarriage or abortion, or after the delivery of an Rh-positive baby. In most cases it now is also given during pregnancy. The immune globulin prevents the infant's Rh-positive cells from stimulating the mother's immune system, thus preventing HDN.

The source of Rho(D) immune globulin is plasma from women who have had children affected by HDN or from Rh-negative men who are voluntarily injected with Rh-positive RBCs.

Other Blood Types

In addition to the A and B antigens that characterize the ABO blood grouping, more than 600 antigens and more than 20 other blood type systems are known. Many are named after the person or family in which the blood type system was discovered. Table 54-8 describes other blood systems. The letters and symbols used to describe a blood type can be confusing. Generally, an abbreviation is followed by a

TABLE 54-8 Other Blood Typing Systems

SYSTEM	REMARKS
Diego	Found only among East Asians and Native Americans.
MNS	Useful in maternity and paternity testing.
Duffy	The malarial parasite requires the Duffy antigen to enter the red blood cells. Lack of the antigen confers resistance to malaria. Duffy-negative blood is found only in descendants of African populations.
Lewis	Antigens are soluble in blood rather than attached to the red blood cells. These are the only blood group antibodies that have never been implicated in hemolytic disease of the newborn.

Other blood group systems include Colton, M, Kell, Kidd, Lewis, Landsteiner-Wiener, P, Yt or Cartwright, XG, Scianna, Dombrock, Chido/Rodgers, Kx, Gerbich, Cromer, Knops, Indian, Ok, Raph, and JMH.

negative (−) or a positive (+) symbol; the negative symbol indicates that the antigen represented by the letters is lacking; a plus sign indicates that the antigen is present on the RBCs. For example, AB+ indicates that the red cells have the A and B antigens and the Rh(D) antigen, whereas the blood type O−K−Fy+ lacks the A, B, Rh, and K (Kell) antigens and has the Fy (Duffy) antigen.

Rare Blood Types

Approximately 1 person in 1,000 has a rare blood type. Because blood types are inherited, certain rare blood types are more common among certain ethnic groups. Finding compatible blood for lifesaving transfusions can become more difficult for those with a rare blood type. The Duffy system is particularly important. The Duffy antigens are represented as Fy(a) and Fy(b). The blood types Fy(a−b+), and Fy(a+b+), are very common among the U.S. Caucasian population; Fy(a−β−) is very rare in the Caucasian population but is present in 68% of the African-American population in the United States.

These blood type systems generally are not significant for blood donations but can be troublesome for individuals who have had numerous transfusions and may have developed atypical antibodies, making future cross-matching more of a challenge. The American Red Cross, in collaboration with the American Association of Blood Banks (AABB), maintains a rare donor database as part of the American Rare Donor Program. When a rare blood type is needed, those in the registry can be contacted to make a donation. In addition, blood of a rare type can be frozen to ensure availability when needed.

CRITICAL THINKING APPLICATION   54-4
Before Mr. Corrigan's kidney transplant, he had a type and cross-match and was determined to be type O+. Explain how the test was performed and what the technician observed with the anti-A, anti-B, and anti-D antisera.

CLINICAL CHEMISTRY

Most clinical chemistry methods are classified as moderately complex according to CLIA guidelines, and only people with documented training in the method are permitted to perform testing, which must be done under the supervision of the director of the physician's office laboratory. Increasingly, however, clinical chemistry tests are being granted CLIA-waived status.

BLOOD GLUCOSE TESTING

Glucose is used as a fuel by many body cells; under normal circumstances, it is the only substance used to nourish brain cells. Maintenance of blood glucose levels within a normal range is vital to homeostasis of the human body. Understanding the importance of glucose can help the medical assistant understand why glucose is the most frequently tested analyte.

Elevated blood glucose levels most often are associated with diabetes mellitus, but they also may indicate pancreatitis, endocrine disorders, or chronic renal failure. Diabetes mellitus is a disorder of carbohydrate metabolism that results in elevated blood and urine glucose levels secondary to the inability of the pancreas to produce sufficient insulin. (Diabetes is discussed in Chapter 45.)

To check a patient for diabetes mellitus, the physician may request a blood glucose tolerance test (GTT). For this test the fasting patient receives an adequate carbohydrate meal of 100 g of glucose by mouth. This usually is given to the patient as a drink that is similar to a sweet fruit punch. The amount may be adjusted according to the patient's weight. If the glucose level does not exceed 100 g/dL at the onset of the testing period, or 180 g/dL 1 hour after ingestion of the glucose drink, the patient is believed to have a normal glucose level. If the blood glucose level exceeds 200 g/dL, glucose escapes into the urine, because the renal tubules no longer are able to absorb the excessive amount present in the glomerulus.

Self-monitoring of blood glucose levels has become an important part of the treatment of diabetes. Testing methods have evolved over the past 20 years. The earliest test methods available were urine reagent strips (see Chapter 52) that detected glucose and ketones. Although simple to use, they lacked the precision to be useful for adjusting insulin dosage. In the 1970s similar strips for testing glucose levels in the blood were introduced. A drop of blood from a capillary puncture was applied to the strip, and the excess was wiped away. After careful timing, the color of the pad on the reagent strip was compared with a chart. The results were highly dependent on the user.

The first handheld devices were marketed shortly after this and were designed to read the test strips electronically rather than visually using reflectance photometry. Although this technology still required wiping and timing, the devices were precise enough to monitor blood glucose and assist with insulin adjustment.

In the 1980s, blood glucose monitors using electrochemistry and devices that used reflectance photometry joined the market. The need for wiping and timing was eliminated. These technologies use an enzyme to convert glucose to measurable products. Enzymes commonly used are glucose oxidase, glucose dehydrogenase, and hexokinase.

The medical assistant can screen a patient's blood glucose levels by using a glucometer cleared for home use by the U.S. Food and Drug Administration (FDA). This procedure was described in Chapter 45 (see Procedure 45-1). The blood glucose level is routinely monitored by patients with diabetes mellitus type 1 or type 2. Glucose levels also may be monitored by women with gestational diabetes, a condition seen during pregnancy in which the effect of insulin is partially blocked by a variety of other hormones made in the placenta.

Hemoglobin A$_{1c}$ Testing

During the past two decades, diabetes researchers have developed several new laboratory tests that aid in the evaluation of blood glucose levels. These tests measure glycohemoglobin, fructosamine, and glycosylated protein. The tests are not substitutes for monitoring of blood glucose levels; rather, they give different information about the health of the patient with diabetes and add a new dimension to the evaluation of the disease.

The glycohemoglobin test was developed in the late 1970s. Other names that have been used to describe the same test are *glycosylated hemoglobin* and *hemoglobin A$_{1c}$*. This test gives information about the average blood glucose level during the past 2 or 3 months. In the

TABLE 54-9	Relationship Between Glycosylated Hemoglobin Levels and Blood Glucose Levels
GLYCOSYLATED HEMOGLOBIN (%)	**BLOOD GLUCOSE (mg/dL)**
14.0	380
13.0	350
12.0	315
11.0	280
10.0	250
9.0	215
8.0	180
7.0	150
6.0	115
5.0	80
4.0	50

blood, glucose binds irreversibly to hemoglobin molecules in RBCs. The amount of glucose that is bound to hemoglobin is directly tied to the concentration of glucose in the blood.

Because RBCs have a life span of approximately 120 days, measuring the amount of glucose bound to hemoglobin can provide an assessment of average blood sugar control during the 60 to 90 days preceding the test. This is the purpose of the glycohemoglobin tests, most commonly the hemoglobin A$_{1c}$ (HbA$_{1c}$) measurement. Because the test results give feedback on the previous 2 to 3 months, an HbA$_{1c}$ test every 3 months provides data on the patient's average blood glucose level. If the glycohemoglobin value is higher than the normal range, the average blood sugar has been elevated during the past 2 months. The normal HbA$_{1c}$ level for a person without diabetes ranges from 4% to 6%. For patients with diabetes, the goal is to maintain the glycosylated hemoglobin level below 7%. Table 54-9 associates glycosylated hemoglobin levels with blood glucose levels. If the HbA$_{1c}$ levels are 9% or higher, the patient's treatment should be reassessed, or the physician may question the patient's compliance with treatment. HbA$_{1c}$ levels of 7% to 8% are considered good, and those below 7% demonstrate excellent blood glucose control.

Several methods can be used to measure the HbA$_{1c}$, and the medical assistant can perform HbA$_{1c}$ testing using several CLIA-waived devices. The DCA 2000, made by Bayer Diagnostics (Tarrytown, New York), provides HbA$_{1c}$ values in 6 minutes from one drop of capillary blood obtained from a fingerstick. Patients also can perform HbA$_{1c}$ testing at home using FDA-approved instrumentation, including the A1CNow by Metrika (Sunnyvale, California) and the Micromat II from Bio-Rad (Hercules, California).

The fructosamine test was developed more recently. *Fructosamine* is a term that refers to the linking of blood sugar onto protein molecules in the bloodstream. Fructosamine levels change more rapidly than glycohemoglobin levels. The fructosamine value depends on the average blood sugar level during the past 3 weeks; therefore, this test might be able to detect changes in diabetic control earlier than the glycohemoglobin test. The fructosamine test could be viewed as complementary to the glycohemoglobin test, because the two tests are different reflections of diabetes control: The glycohemoglobin test looks back approximately 8 weeks, and the fructosamine test looks back approximately 3 weeks.

Other tests similar to the fructosamine test have been proposed, such as the glycosylated protein test. Unfortunately, these newer tests are less reliable than was originally hoped, and it seems unlikely that either the fructosamine test or the glycosylated protein test will ever become as widely used for monitoring diabetes as the glycohemoglobin level test.

> ### CRITICAL THINKING APPLICATION   54-5
> Mr. Corrigan routinely monitors his blood sugar. Why is Dr. Fischbach also interested in his hemoglobin A_{1c} levels? What complications of diabetes led to Mr. Corrigan's need for a transplant?

CHOLESTEROL TESTING

Cholesterol is a fatlike substance (lipid) present in cell membranes. It is needed to form bile acids and steroid hormones. Cholesterol travels in the blood in distinct particles containing both lipid and proteins. These particles are called *lipoproteins*. The cholesterol level in the blood is determined partly by inheritance and partly by acquired factors, such as diet, calorie balance, and level of physical activity.

Patients often are confused by cholesterol testing. The confusion is caused partly by the way some people use the term *cholesterol*, which often is a catchall term for both the cholesterol a person eats and the cholesterol that is maintained in the body. A high level of low-density lipoprotein, or LDL, cholesterol reflects an increased risk of heart disease, which is why LDL cholesterol is often called "bad" cholesterol. Lower levels of LDL cholesterol reflect a lower risk of heart disease. When too much LDL cholesterol circulates in the blood, it can slowly build up in the walls of arteries that feed the heart and brain. Together with other substances, it can form plaque, a thick, hard deposit that can clog those arteries. This condition is known as *atherosclerosis*. If a clot (thrombus) forms at the site of plaque, blood flow can be blocked to part of the heart muscle, causing a heart attack. If a clot blocks blood flow to part of the brain, a stroke results.

About one third to one fourth of blood cholesterol is carried by high-density lipoprotein (HDL). HDL cholesterol is known as the "good" cholesterol, because a high level of HDL cholesterol seems to protect against heart attack. Medical experts think that HDL tends to carry cholesterol away from the arteries and back to the liver, where it is passed from the body. Some experts believe that excess cholesterol is removed from atherosclerotic plaque by HDL, which slows the buildup; however, low HDL cholesterol levels (i.e., lower than 35 mg/dL) may result in a greater risk of heart disease.

Adults older than 20 years of age should have a cholesterol test at least once every 5 years. Total cholesterol, the combination of HDL and LDL, typically is measured (Procedure 54-7); however, the physician may order an HDL determination separately. Both tests are considered screening tests, and elevated results always require additional testing before a diagnosis can be made. In general, total cholesterol levels under 200 mg/dL are considered normal.

Results over 240 mg/dL are considered elevated and, on the basis of confirmed testing, place a person in the high-risk category for coronary heart disease. An HDL cholesterol level of 35 mg/dL is considered acceptable. Values below 35 mg/dL place a person in the high-risk category.

Although total cholesterol and HDL cholesterol levels are not significantly affected by food consumption, you should follow office policy for patient education in preparation for the test. Most physicians prefer that patients fast for 12 hours before cholesterol levels are checked. If the total cholesterol is elevated, the physician is likely to order a lipid profile, which is a series of tests that measures the total cholesterol, triglyceride, and HDL and LDL cholesterol levels. Triglyceride levels are affected by food consumption, and the patient must be instructed to fast before the test.

CLIA-waived cholesterol monitors can measure HDL cholesterol, total cholesterol, and triglycerides. The Cholestech LDX analyzer (Cholestech, Hayward, California), uses enzymatic reactions to produce products that are quantified by reflectance photometry using blood from a fingerstick.

THYROID HORMONE TESTING

The thyroid gland is located anterior to the trachea in the throat. It produces the hormones triiodothyronine (T_3) and thyroxine (T_4). These hormones are essential for life and have many effects on body metabolism, growth, and development. The thyroid gland is influenced by hormones produced by two other organs found in the brain: the pituitary gland and the hypothalamus. The pituitary gland produces thyroid-stimulating hormone (TSH), and the hypothalamus produces thyrotropin-releasing hormone (TRH). (Regulation of thyroid hormone production and thyroid disorders are discussed in Chapter 45.)

CLIA-waived rapid diagnostic tests to qualitatively measure TSH are available for point-of-care testing. Using whole blood from a fingerstick, these tests screen patients for hypothyroidism by detecting elevated levels of TSH, which constitutes a sign of hypothyroidism. The tests use lateral flow chromatographic immunoassay technology housed in a plastic cassette similar to the pregnancy test discussed in Chapter 52. One such commercially available test is the ThyroTest (ThyroTek, Honeybrook, Pennsylvania).

ALANINE AMINOTRANSFERASE AND ASPARTATE AMINOTRANSFERASE TESTING

Certain drugs can impair liver function and require monitoring of liver enzymes. These drugs include statins and fibrates, pharmaceutical agents used to lower blood cholesterol, and certain antidiabetic and antihypertensive drugs. Liver function also must be monitored during therapy with drugs that have the potential to cause liver malfunction. Two liver enzymes, aspartate aminotransferase (AST) and alanine aminotransferase (ALT), can be useful for monitoring homeostasis during drug therapy. The first liver enzyme testing to be CLIA waived was the Cholestech ALT/AST test, which is performed on the Cholestech LDX System (Cholestech). This system also analyzes glucose, total cholesterol, HDL, and triglycerides using a combination of enzymatic reactions and reflectance photometry to detect the resulting color changes.

PROCEDURE 54-7

Perform Chemistry Testing: Determine Cholesterol Level Using a ProAct Testing Device

GOAL: *To perform a ProAct test for total cholesterol level and accurately report the results.*
ORDER: *Perform a total blood cholesterol level on Connie Lange stat.*

EQUIPMENT and SUPPLIES

- ProAct testing device
- Sterile gauze
- Lithium heparin
- Alcohol preps
- Capillary tube and capillary pipet
- Lancets and lancet device
- Disposable gloves
- Biohazardous waste container and sharps container
- Patient's record

PROCEDURAL STEPS

1. Reread the physician's order and assemble all the supplies and equipment needed to complete the test.
2. Sanitize your hands and put on gloves.
   PURPOSE: To ensure infection control.
3. Explain the procedure to the patient.
4. Load the lancet device with a sterile lancet.
5. Examine the patient's index and ring fingers and pick a puncture site.
   PURPOSE: The puncture site must be free of trauma.
6. Cleanse the chosen puncture site with alcohol and allow the site to air dry.
7. Puncture the site and wipe away the first drop of blood with a sterile gauze square.
   PURPOSE: The first drop of blood may contain tissue fluid.
8. Hold the capillary tube horizontally by the colored end of the tube and allow the tube to fill. Do not allow air bubbles to enter the tube; if this occurs, discard the capillary tube and continue drawing the sample with a new tube.
   PURPOSE: Air bubbles may cause erroneous test results.
9. Give the patient a sterile gauze square and ask the person to apply pressure to the puncture site.
10. Remove a cholesterol testing strip from the container and close the container immediately (Figure 1).
    PURPOSE: Closing the container prevents possible exposure of the unused strips.

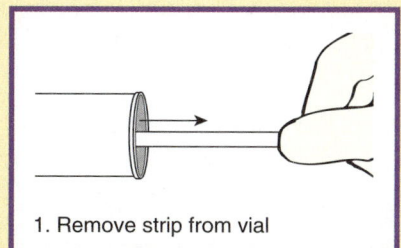

1. Remove strip from vial

(From Stepp CA, Woods MA: *Laboratory procedures for medical office personnel*, Philadelphia, 1998, Saunders.)

11. Remove the foil protecting the test area of the strip and place the strip on a dry, hard, flat surface (Figure 2).

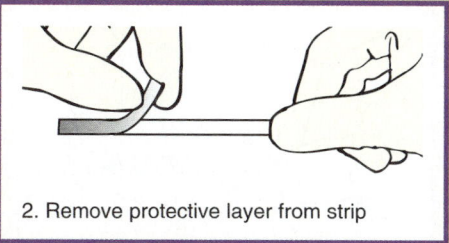

2. Remove protective layer from strip

12. Attach the capillary tube filled with blood to the pipet.
13. Squeeze the plunger of the pipet completely to allow a drop of blood to form at the end of the capillary tube.
14. Allow the drop of blood to fall onto the center of the red mesh application zone. Make sure the tip of the capillary tube does not touch the test strip and that all blood is dispensed (Figure 3).
    PURPOSE: To obtain the best test results, the strip must be saturated with blood.

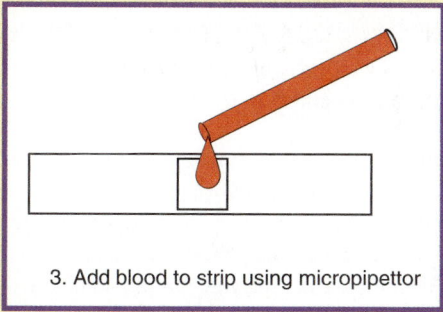

3. Add blood to strip using micropipettor

15. Allow the sample to soak into the red mesh for 3 to 15 seconds.
16. Insert the cholesterol strip into the test port. The ProAct device counts down approximately 160 seconds (Figure 4).

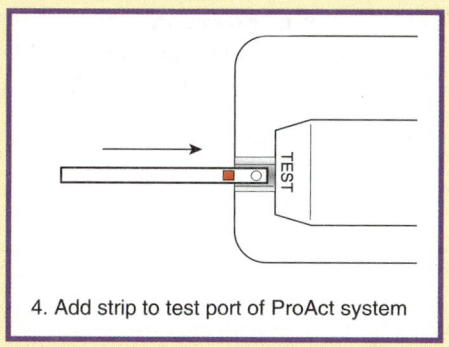

4. Add strip to test port of ProAct system

PROCEDURE 54-7—cont'd

17. Remove the capillary tube from the pipet and discard it in a biohazardous waste container.
    <u>PURPOSE:</u> To ensure infection control.
18. When the measurement time is complete, REMOVE STRIP appears in the LED display window. Remove the used test strip; the test result will appear on the display (Figure 5).

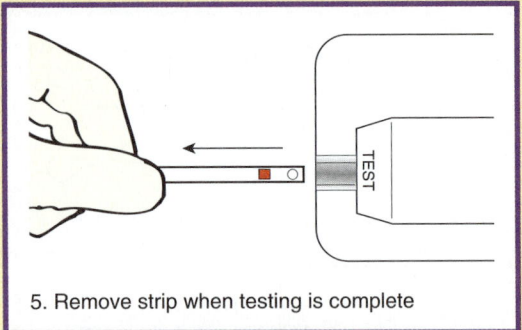

5. Remove strip when testing is complete

19. Examine the test area of the used testing strip for uneven color development before discarding it in the biohazardous waste container.
    <u>PURPOSE:</u> If the color appears mottled, the test may not be valid, and it is advisable to repeat the entire test process.
20. Discard all biohazardous waste in the appropriate containers, disinfect the test area, remove your gloves, and sanitize your hands.
    <u>PURPOSE:</u> To ensure infection control.
21. Record the test results in the patient's medical record.
    <u>PURPOSE:</u> A procedure is not considered done until it is recorded.

5/25/XX 9:30 AM Total cholesterol test performed as ordered. ProAct test results 247. D. Cummings, CMA (AAMA)

CRITICAL THINKING APPLICATION   54-6

For what reason might Dr. Fischbach want to evaluate Mr. Corrigan's liver enzymes? What clinical chemistry tests might he order from the referral laboratory? What Vacutainer tube would be needed for these tests? What tests for liver enzymes might Dana be able to perform in the physician's office laboratory? What sample will she need for those tests?

CHEMISTRY PANELS

Automated blood chemistry analyzers often are used to perform blood chemistry testing. It is not uncommon for several analytes to be detected at once. A physician may order a chemistry panel, such as a renal or liver panel, that determines the levels of several related analytes (Figure 54-15). Analytes commonly detected in the chemistry laboratory are listed in Table 54-10. In general, serum is needed for these tests. Typical panels are shown in Table 54-11.

CRITICAL THINKING APPLICATION   54-7

What tests are routinely done as part of the renal panel? What information will these tests give Dr. Fischbach about the status of Mr. Corrigan's kidney?

CLOSING COMMENTS

Legal and Ethical Issues

The Blood Safety Act was passed in 1991 to ensure that all donor blood is tested for HIV and other viral diseases. The Act also requires physicians to provide patients with information about blood transfusion options such as the exclusive use of the donor's own blood (autologous transfusion) or possible donations made by family or friends This information must be provided before surgery and before any medical procedure in which the possibility exists that blood transfusion may be necessary. Physicians also are required to note on each patient's medical record that a written summary was given to the patient. As the physician's agent, you share this responsibility. If a blood transfusion may be required for a particular patient, every member of the healthcare team is responsible for ensuring that (1) the patient is provided with the information; (2) this is noted on the patient's chart and initialed; and (3) the written summary is formally prepared (copies of the official form can be requested from the state department of health services).

PHYSICIAN'S MEDICAL CENTER
77332 E. CAPITAL DRIVE
ANYTOWN, USA 11123

PMC

Ronald J. Haldor M.D.
Kaye M. Jones M.D.
Nicholas C. Stepp M.D.

PATIENT – PLEASE NOTE

If this box is checked, don't eat or drink anything, except water, for 14 hours before going to the lab.

PATIENT NAME _____
LAST   FIRST   M.I.
ADDRESS _____ DOB _____
CITY _____ STATE _____ ZIP _____ SEX: M F
TELEPHONE # _____ SOCIAL SECURITY # _____ – _____ – _____
ORDERING PHYSICIAN _____ DATE _____
BILLING: ☐ HMO ☐ MEDICARE ☐ MEDI-CAL ☐ OTHER # _____
(Please attach copy of eligibilty card.)
GUARANTOR (If other than patient) _____
☐ PHONE RESULTS TO _____
☐ SEND ADDITIONAL COPIES OF REPORT TO _____

Patient Diagnosis _____

☐ 906 ARTERIAL BLOOD GASES
  ROOM AIR _____
  RESP. ASSIST _____
☐ 105 BLOOD CELL PROFILE (Hgb + Hct)
☐ 862 BILIRUBIN (NEONATAL)
☐ 868 BILIRUBIN (TOTAL & DIRECT)
☐ 100 CBC (Complete Blood Count & Diff)
☐ 3000 ELECTROLYTES
☐   (NA, K, CO2, Cl)
☐   FANA
☐   GLUCOSE
☐ 915 GLUCOSE, PRE-NATAL DIABETIC SCR.
  (1 Hour Post-Glucola)
☐   GLUCOSE TOLERANCE TEST
  # OF HOURS _____ DOSE _____
☐ 3398 HEPATITIS PANEL
  (B-Surf Ag/Ab, B-Core Ab, A-Ab)
☐ 988 LIPID PROFILE
  (Chol, Trig, HDL, LDL, Cardiac Risk)
☐ 3380 LIVER PANEL
  (Alk Phos, Bili, TP, Alb, GGT, SGOT (AST)
  SGPT (ALT), & Consult)
☐ 3006 METABOLIC 7
  (Na, K, CO2, Cl, Glu, Mg)

☐ 3035 PANEL 17
  (Panel 13 + Na + K + Cl + CO2)
☐ 3020 METABOLIC 10
  (Na, K, CO2, Cl, Glu, BUN, Creat)
☐ 3015 METABOLIC 11
  (Met 10 & Phos)
☐ 3160 OBSTETRICAL PANEL 1
  (CBC, UA, ABO/Rh, Antibody Screen,
  Rubella, RPR)
☐ 3172 OBSTETRICAL PANEL 3
  (CBC, ABO/Rh, Antibody Screen,
  Rubella, RPR)
☐ 3445 OBSTETRICAL PANEL 7
  (ABO/Rh, Antibody Screen, Rubella,
  RPR)
☐ 3447 OBSTETRICAL PANEL 7A
  (ABO/Rh, Antibody Screen, Rubella,
  RPR, Hepatitis B Surt Ag)
☐ 3025 PANEL 13
  (Glu, BUN, Creat, Uric Acid, Ca, Tp,
  Alb, Bili, Chol, Alk, Phos, SGOT (AST),
  LDH, Phos)
☐ 3030 PANEL 15
  (Panel 13 + Na + K)

☐ 3010 METABOLIC 8
  (Na, K, CO2, Cl, Glu, BUN)
☐ 3040 PANEL 20 - SMAC
  (Panel 17 + SGPT (ALT) + GGT +
  Osmolality)
☐ 3043 S-1 Panel (Panel 20 + Triglyceride)
☐ 500 PROTHROMBIN TIME (PT)
☐ 505 Partial Thromboplastin Time (PPT)
☐ 7500 RPR
☐ 7515 RUBELLA
☐ 2030 THYROID SCREEN
  (T4, T3, Uptake, Adj T4)
☐ 704 URINALYSIS

BACTERIOLOGY

SPECIMEN SOURCE (REQUIRED) _____
COLLECTION DATE _____
☐ _____ ROUTINE CULTURE
☐ 8919 AFB CULTURE
☐ 8921 FUNGAL CULTURE

ADDITIONAL LABORATORY TESTS:

LABORATORY OUTPATIENT REQUEST

2804 (4/93)

OFFICE USE ONLY
Telephone Order per _____
Order Received by _____

FIGURE 54-15 Panel request form. (From Stepp CA, Woods MA: *Laboratory procedures for medical office personnel*, Philadelphia, 1998, Saunders.)

TABLE 54-10 Blood Chemistry Tests

TEST	ABBREVIATION	NORMAL VALUES	DESCRIPTION	PURPOSE
Alanine aminotransferase	ALT (SGPT)	<45 U/L	Enzyme found predominantly in the liver but also in the kidney	To detect liver disease
Albumin		3.5-5 g/dL	Protein	To assess kidney function
Alkaline phosphatase	ALP	20-70 U/L	Enzyme found in several tissues	To detect liver and bone disease
Aspartate aminotransferase	AST (SGOT)	<40 U/L	Enzyme found in several tissues	To detect tissue damage
Blood urea nitrogen	BUN	7-18 mg/dL; 2.5-6.4 mmol/L	Metabolic products of protein catabolism	To detect renal disease
Calcium	CA	8.4-10.2 mg/dL; 2.1-2.6 mmol/L	Mineral	To assess parathyroid function and calcium metabolism
Chloride	Cl	98-106 mmol/L	Electrolyte	To determine acid-base and water balance
Cholesterol	CH, Chol	*Total:* <200 mg/dL; <5.18 mmol/L *LDL:* <130 mg/dL; <3.37 mmol/L *HDL:* >35 mg/dL; >0.91 mmol/L	Lipid	Screening for atherosclerosis related to heart disease
Creatine phosphokinase	CPK	Specific to testing method used	Enzyme found in several tissues	To assess source of muscle damage (myocardial infarct)
Creatinine	creat	0.2-0.8 mg/dL	Metabolic product of protein catabolism	To screen for renal function
Ferritin		20-50 ng/mL	Iron-carrying protein	To detect amount of iron stored in the body
Gamma glutamyl transferase	GGT	0-45 U/L	Enzyme found mainly in liver cells	To detect liver disease
Globulin	glob, Ig	Varies according to type	Protein	To detect abnormalities in protein synthesis and removal
Glucose fasting blood sugar	FBS	70-100 mg/dL; 3.9-6.1 mmol/L	Carbohydrate	To detect disorders of glucose metabolism (diabetes)
Glucose tolerance test	GTT	Varies with time	Carbohydrate	To detect disorders of glucose metabolism (diabetes)
Iron	Fe	35-140 mcg/dL	Mineral	To assist in diagnosis of anemia
Lactate dehydrogenase	LDH	<240 U/L	Enzyme found in several tissues	To assist in confirmation of myocardial or pulmonary infarct
pH	pH	7.35-7.45		To assess acidity or alkalinity of blood
Phosphorus	P	3-4.5 mg/dL; 0.97-1.45 mmol/L	Mineral	To assist in proper evaluation of calcium levels and to detect endocrine system disorders
Potassium	K	3.5-5.1 mmol/L	Mineral	To assist in diagnosis of acid-base and water balance

TABLE 54-10 Blood Chemistry Tests—Cont'd

TEST	ABBREVIATION	NORMAL VALUES	DESCRIPTION	PURPOSE
Sodium	Na	135-146 mmol/L	Mineral	To assist in diagnosis of acid-base and water balance
Total bilirubin	TB	0.2-1 mg/dL; 3.4-17.1 mmol/L	Metabolic product of hemoglobin catabolism	To evaluate liver function and to aid in diagnosis of anemia
Total iron-binding capacity	TIBC	245-400 µg/dL		A measure of the potential to transport iron
Total protein	TP	6-8 g/dL; 60-80 g/L		To assess the state of hydration; to screen for diseases that alter protein balance
Troponin I and T		<0.4	Cardiac-specific protein found only with heart muscle damage	To aid in diagnosis of myocardial infarct
Thyroid-stimulating hormone (thyrotropin)	TSH	5-6 mU/L	Hormone produced by the pituitary	To assess thyroid and pituitary gland function
Thyroxine	T_4	5-12 mcg/dL; 64-155 mmol/L	Hormone produced by the thyroid gland	To assess thyroid function
Triglycerides	Trig	30-190 mg/dL; 0.34-2.15 mmol/L		Screening for atherosclerosis related to heart disease
Triiodothyronine	T_3	27%-47%	Hormone produced by the thyroid gland	To assess thyroid function
Uric acid	UA	*Male*: 3.4-7 mg/dL; 202-416 µmol/L *Female*: 2.4-6 mg/dL; 143-357 µmol/L	Metabolic product of protein catabolism	To evaluate renal failure, gout, and leukemia

TABLE 54-11 Typical Chemistry Panels

PANEL	COMPONENT	PANEL	COMPONENT
Liver	Alkaline phosphatase (ALP) Gamma glutamyl transferase (GGT) Aspartate aminotransferase (AST) Alanine aminotransferase (ALT) Lactate dehydrogenase (LDH)	Cardiac	Creatinine phosphokinase (CPK) Troponin I Troponin T
Anemia	Iron Total iron-binding capacity Ferritin Transferrin	Electrolyte	Sodium Potassium Chloride
Thyroid	Thyroid-stimulating hormone (TSH) Thyroxine (T_4) Triiodothyronine (T_3)	Renal	Creatinine Blood urea nitrogen Uric acid Glucose

SUMMARY OF SCENARIO

Dana knows the important role laboratory analysis of blood plays in patient care. Often many different tests are needed to assess a patient's health. Mr. Corrigan appreciates that he can have many of these tests done during his routine visits with a simple fingerstick, such as the hemoglobin A_{1c} level, hemoglobin and hematocrit, PT, and ALT/AST testing. The anemia panel, CBC and differential, and hemoglobin and hematocrit provide Dr. Fischbach with essential information for diagnosing anemia, and the hemoglobin A_{1c} level is used to monitor Mr. Corrigan's diabetes. The prothrombin time, which monitors coagulation, and the liver enzyme tests assure Dr. Fischbach that Mr. Corrigan's liver is functioning properly while he is taking medication to treat his diabetes and to manage the transplant.

SUMMARY OF LEARNING OBJECTIVES

1. **Define, spell, and pronounce the terms listed in the vocabulary.**
   Spelling and pronouncing medical terms correctly bolsters the medical assistant's credibility. Knowing the definitions of these terms promotes confidence in communication with patients and co-workers.

2. **Apply critical thinking skills in performing the patient assessment and patient care.**
   Completing the Critical Thinking Application exercises throughout the chapter can help the student medical assistant become more adept at critical analysis of real-life situations.

3. **Name the main functions of blood.**
   Blood supplies cells with needed nutrients, delivers oxygen to tissues through hemoglobin, and removes waste.

4. **Identify the role of the hematology laboratory in patient care.**
   In the hematology laboratory, blood cells are enumerated, WBCs are differentiated, and the oxygen-carrying capacity of blood is determined. Hematology testing provides an excellent overview of homeostasis.

5. **Describe the appearance and function of erythrocytes.**
   Erythrocytes are also called *red blood cells* because of their red color, which comes from hemoglobin. The biconcave disks lack a nucleus and are responsible for transporting oxygen and carbon dioxide to and from tissues.

6. **Describe the appearance and function of granular and agranular leukocytes.**
   Leukocytes are also called *white blood cells*. Agranular leukocytes lack granules in the cytoplasm, and granular leukocytes have granules. All leukocytes function in fighting infection.

7. **Differentiate between T cells and B cells.**
   T lymphocytes are important in immunity and play roles in killing foreign, virus-infected, and tumor cells; they also assist in antibody production and keep the immune system in check. B cells are responsible for antibody production.

8. **Describe the appearance and function of thrombocytes.**
   A thrombocyte (platelet) is a fragment of a larger cell (megakaryocyte) found in the bone marrow. Thrombocytes play an important role in clot formation, both physically and chemically.

9. **Explain the process of clot formation.**
   Clot formation begins with the aggregation of thrombocytes, which release a substance that initiates the clotting cascade, resulting in a network of minute threads that trap plasma and blood cells.

10. **Identify the anticoagulant of choice for hematology testing.**
    The anticoagulant required for most hematology testing is ethylenediaminetetraacetic acid (EDTA). The lavender-topped vacuum tube used in phlebotomy contains this anticoagulant.

11. **Explain the purpose of a microhematocrit test.**
    A microhematocrit (or hematocrit) test is performed to assess the volume of erythrocytes in relationship to total blood volume by centrifuging a small amount of whole blood in a capillary tube. Whole blood normally consists of slightly less than 50% RBCs. Hematocrit is reported as a percentage and is roughly three times that of hemoglobin.

12. **Perform a microhematocrit test.**
    Refer to Procedure 54-1.

13. **Explain the role of hemoglobin in the body.**
    Hemoglobin is the RBC protein responsible for oxygen transport from the lungs to the tissues. It gives the blood its red color.

14. **Perform a hemoglobin test.**
    Refer to Procedure 54-3.

15. **Identify the tests included in a complete blood count (CBC) and their reference ranges.**
    The CBC involves an erythrocyte count, leukocyte count, thrombocyte count, hemoglobin and hematocrit determination, differential examination of leukocytes, and calculation of red cell indices.

16. **Explain the process of automated blood cell counting.**
    Blood first is diluted in a fluid that conducts an electrical current. The diluted sample passes through a narrow opening in the blood counting instrument, interrupting the flow of electrical current, and each interruption is counted.

17. **Distinguish between normal and abnormal test results.**
    Refer to the hematology diagnostic reference ranges in Table 54-3 and Figure 54-6.

18. **Describe the red blood cell (RBC) indices and how they are calculated.**
    RBC indices are calculated using values obtained from the CBC, namely, RBC count, hemoglobin, and hematocrit. They assist the physician in diagnosing blood disorders such as anemia.

19. **Explain the reasons for performing a white blood cell (WBC) differential.**
    A differential WBC count is performed to assess the numbers and types of WBCs in the blood. A thin smear of whole blood is stained, typically

with Wright's stain, and is examined microscopically. In addition, the red cells and platelets are examined for distribution and abnormalities.

20. **Discuss the Wright's stain sequence.**

Stains commonly used in blood tests are attracted to different parts of the cell; thus the cells and their structures are more easily seen and differentiated. The most commonly used differential blood stain is Wright's stain. Most Wright's stains today contain mixtures of methylene blue, azure A, thionin, and eosin Y.

21. **Describe the appearance of normal erythrocytes.**

A normal erythrocyte is circular, is evenly stained red-purple, and appears to have a hole or depression in the center.

22. **Describe the appearance of the five different types of leukocytes seen in a normal Wright-stained differential.**

The typical leukocytes seen in the differential examination are (1) the segmented neutrophil, which has a segmented blue nucleus and lavender granules in the cytoplasm; (2) the eosinophil, which resembles the neutrophil but has orange granules; (3) the basophil, which resembles the neutrophil but has blue-black granules; (4) the lymphocyte, which is a smaller cell with a light-blue cytoplasm and a large dark-blue nucleus; and (5) the monocyte, the largest cell, which has a cerebriform blue nucleus and a light-blue cytoplasm that appears to have bubblelike inclusions.

23. **Cite the reasons for performing an erythrocyte sedimentation rate test.**

An ESR test is performed to assess inflammation and often is used to monitor rheumatoid arthritis. This test measures the rate at which RBCs fall in a calibrated tube in a 60-minute period.

24. **Describe the sources of error for the erythrocyte sedimentation rate test.**

An ESR test result may be erroneous if a tube is not standing vertically in the rack; bubbles are present in the Westergren or Wintrobe tube; dilutions are incorrect; vibrations or jarring occurs; the blood is at a temperature other than room temperature; and the blood has hemolyzed.

25. **Determine an erythrocyte sedimentation rate using a modified Westergren method.**

Refer to Procedure 54-4.

26. **Describe the tests performed to assess coagulation.**

PT and PTT are the tests most commonly performed to assess coagulation capacity. The PT test also is routinely performed to assess a patient's response to anticlotting drugs such as warfarin (Coumadin).

27. **Differentiate between the ABO blood groupings and the Rh blood groupings.**

Both the ABO blood type and the Rh type result from antigens on the surfaces of RBCs, and both groups are crucial when it comes to transfusion. There are four different ABO types (A, AB, B, and O), but only two Rh types (positive and negative). Corresponding antibodies are present in the blood for the ABO type (e.g., anti-A antibody is found in type B and type O blood); corresponding antibodies are not normally found in the Rh system.

28. **Secure a capillary blood sample and determine the ABO and Rh groupings of the sample.**

Refer to Procedures 54-5 and 54-6.

29. **Discuss rare blood types and the implications of having a rare blood type when transfusion is necessary.**

A rare blood type is one in which the blood group antigen (or lack thereof) is not common in a population. More than 20 blood types other than the ABO and Rh systems exist. Individuals with rare blood types are at risk of developing atypical antibodies when transfused with incompatible blood. These atypical antibodies make future cross-matching more challenging.

30. **Describe the method behind the clinical chemistry testing methods used in the physician's office laboratory.**

Four methods generally are used in the physician's office laboratory:

- *Lateral flow immunoassay:* Antigen-antibody reactions result in the deposition of a colored molecule or particle on a solid-phase membrane.
- *Reflectance photometry:* A chemical reaction produces a colored product, which has an absorbed wavelength that is detected by an instrument.
- *Amperometry (electrochemistry):* An instrument detects the number of electrons generated by a chemical reaction.
- *Chemiluminescence:* Electrons generated from a chemical reaction react with a luminescing compound on a test strip, producing a flash of light, which is detected by an instrument.

31. **Explain the reasons for testing blood glucose, blood cholesterol, hemoglobin A_{1c}, thyroid hormone levels, and liver enzymes.**

The blood glucose level is monitored routinely in patients with diabetes type 1 or type 2 and in women who have gestational diabetes during pregnancy. Cholesterol testing generally refers to assessing levels of HDL cholesterol and LDL cholesterol; it is done to help determine a patient's susceptibility to coronary artery disease. Hemoglobin A_{1c} levels are measured to determine the average blood glucose level during the 2 to 3 months before the test; this test assists in management of diabetes. Thyroid testing is performed in the physician's office laboratory to detect elevated TSH levels and to assist with the diagnosis of hypothyroidism. Liver enzyme testing (ALT and AST) is performed in the physician's office laboratory primarily to monitor the side effects of certain therapeutic drugs, such as those used to treat elevated cholesterol and diabetes. Refer to Table 54-9.

32. **Perform a cholesterol test using a cholesterol monitor approved by the U.S. Food and Drug Administration (FDA).**

Refer to Procedure 54-7.

33. **Summarize typical chemistry panels, the reason for performing each panel, and the individual tests performed in those panels.**

Certain tests that provide information about a disease or syndrome are grouped together in panels. For example, a liver panel detects abnormalities in a number of different liver enzymes (see Tables 54-10 and 54-11).

34. **Describe the medical assistant's responsibility for legally preparing a patient for a blood transfusion.**

The medical practice must comply with the stipulations of the Blood Safety Act if a patient may require a blood transfusion during a procedure.

CONNECTIONS

Study Guide Connection: Go to the Chapter 54 Study Guide. Read and complete the activities.

Evolve Connection: Go to the Chapter 54 link at *evolve.elsevier.com/kinn* to complete the Chapter Review and Chapter Quiz. Peruse other resources listed for this chapter to increase your knowledge of Assisting in the Analysis of Blood.

ASSISTING IN MICROBIOLOGY AND IMMUNOLOGY

55

SCENARIO

Infectious diseases are a continuing threat for everyone. Anna McIntyre, CMA (AAMA), knows that some diseases have been effectively controlled with the help of modern technology, but new diseases are constantly appearing, such as the avian flu and West Nile virus infection. In addition, other familiar infectious diseases, such as malaria, tuberculosis, and bacterial pneumonias, now are appearing in forms that are resistant to drug treatment. Anna knows that it is important to identify pathogens quickly so that the proper treatment can begin. The identification of pathogens, she has discovered, can involve many different types of tests, many of which can be performed in the physician office laboratory (POL) where she works.

While studying this chapter, think about the following questions:

- How can Anna protect herself and other patients in the practice from infectious microorganisms?
- How can body fluids or other samples be tested for the presence of pathogenic organisms?
- How are pathogenic organisms differentiated from normal, nonpathogenic species?
- What role do laboratory healthcare workers play in the identification and treatment of infections caused by microorganisms?

LEARNING OBJECTIVES

1. Define, spell, and pronounce the terms listed in the vocabulary.
2. Apply critical thinking skills in performing the patient assessment and patient care.
3. Cite the protocols for the collection, transport, and processing of specimens.
4. Identify the elements needed for microbial growth.
5. Compare bacteria with viruses.
6. Describe the characteristics of common viral diseases.
7. Describe the bacterial structures used in identification.
8. Describe various bacterial morphologies.
9. Explain the characteristics of common diseases caused by bacteria.
10. Compare bacteria with fungi, parasites, and protozoa.
11. Describe the unusual characteristics of *Chlamydia, Rickettsia,* and *Mycoplasma* organisms.
12. Identify the characteristics of common diseases caused by fungi, protozoa, and parasites.
13. Perform patient education on the collection of a stool specimen for ova and parasite testing.
14. Describe the equipment needed in a microbiology laboratory.
15. List the different growth media used for culturing.
16. Perform the procedure for inoculating a blood agar plate.
17. Perform a urine culture.
18. Perform a screening urine culture test.
19. Prepare a direct smear or culture smear for staining.
20. Compare and contrast the throat culture for *Streptococcus pyogenes* with the rapid strep test.
21. Perform a rapid strep test.
22. Describe three microbiologic tests that use a rapid identification technique.
23. Describe the method used for antimicrobial susceptibility testing.
24. Explain how pinworm testing is done and when it must be performed.
25. Perform a cellulose tape collection for pinworms.
26. Discuss the purpose of immunologic testing.
27. Describe three rapid immunologic tests that could be done in the physician office laboratory.
28. Perform the Mono-test for mononucleosis.
29. Discuss legal and ethical issues involved in laboratory testing.

VOCABULARY

antimicrobial agents Drugs used to treat infection.

arthropods (ahr'-throh-pods) Members of a class of invertebrate animals that includes insects, crustaceans, and arachnids.

broad-spectrum antimicrobial agents Drugs used to treat a wide range of infectious microorganisms.

cysts Small, capsulelike sacs that enclose certain organisms in their dormant or larval stage.

eukaryotes (yoo-kar'-e-ohts) Single-celled or multicellular organisms with cells that contain a distinct membrane-bound nucleus.

fastidious Requiring specialized media or growth factors to grow.

flora Microbes that live on or in the body that perform vital functions and protect the body against infection.

genus A breakdown of a family of microorganisms.

interleukin (in-tehr-loo'-kin) A protein produced by certain white blood cells that regulates immune responses by activating lymphocytes and initiating fever.

in vitro Referring to conditions outside of a living body.

macromolecules The molecules needed for metabolism: carbohydrates, lipids, proteins, and nucleic acids.

microorganisms Organisms of microscopic or submicroscopic size.

molecules Groups of like or different atoms held together by chemical forces.

nanometers Units measuring 1 billionth (10^{-9}) of a meter.

organelles (or-guh-nels') Differentiated structures within a cell (e.g., mitochondria, vacuoles, and chloroplasts) that perform a specific function.

pathogens Disease-causing microorganisms.

prokaryote (pro-kar'-e-oht) A unicellular organism with cells that lack a membrane-bound nucleus.

prostaglandins (prahs-tih-glan'-dins) Chemicals released from cells that cause smooth muscle contraction and pain.

pure culture A bacterial or fungal culture that contains a single organism.

species A category of microorganisms that is below genus in rank; a genetically distinct group.

tissue culture The technique or process of keeping tissue alive and growing in a culture medium.

transport medium A medium used to keep an organism alive during transport to the laboratory.

turbidity Cloudiness in a liquid caused by the presence of suspended particles; it increases with the concentration of particles present.

viable Capable of living, developing, or germinating under favorable conditions.

wet mount A slide preparation in which a drop of liquid specimen or the like is covered with a coverslip and observed with a microscope.

Microorganisms get a lot of publicity. Bioterrorism became a reality in the United States in the fall of 2001, when *Bacillus anthracis* spores sent through the mail caused anthrax, killing three people. Products line our grocery store shelves declaring their ability to keep us germ free. The evening news reports on the latest outbreaks of "flesh-eating bacteria," contaminated water supplies, and antibiotic-resistant microbes. No wonder most people have the impression that all microorganisms are harmful. In reality, less than 1% of known microorganisms are **pathogens**. In fact, without microorganisms, we could not survive.

Microorganisms are responsible for decomposition of waste and natural recycling. The organisms that are normally present on and in our bodies ensure that our food is digested, that our blood clots properly as a result of vitamin K production by the organisms inhabiting our intestines, and that pathogens are prohibited from invading our skin, mucous membranes, and gastrointestinal and genitourinary tracts. When the normal **flora** are disrupted, such as by antibiotic use or hormonal changes, certain organisms that are present normally in low numbers overgrow, causing a superinfection. For example, vulvovaginal candidiasis, a yeast infection of the vaginal tract, is common in women taking **broad-spectrum antimicrobial agents**.

The study of immunology, or the immune system, is closely tied to microbiology. Microorganisms induce an immune response, leading to the production of a variety of **molecules** that come to our defense. These molecules include antibodies and mediators of inflammation such as **interleukin**, **prostaglandins**, and interferon. Often a bacterial or viral infection must be diagnosed indirectly by testing for antibodies to the infectious agent rather than by isolating the pathogen itself.

As a medical assistant, you need to understand the role of microorganisms in both health and disease. The main objective of microbiology procedures is to identify the organisms responsible for illness so that the physician can properly treat the patient. In addition, your responsibilities will include preventing nosocomial infections and assisting with infection control in the physician office laboratory (POL) and in the patients the POL serves. Microbiology procedures may be performed in the POL or in the microbiology department of a medical referral laboratory.

Chapter 27 discussed the chain of infection and how it can be broken using infection control procedures such as proper hand sanitization, antiseptics and disinfectants, and sterilization methods. This chapter covers the cultivation of microorganisms; detection of infecting organisms by microscopy; detection of specific products of infecting organisms using chemical, immunologic, or molecular techniques; and detection of antibodies produced by the patient in response to an infecting organism (immunodiagnosis).

▌ SPECIMEN COLLECTION AND TRANSPORT

Specimen collection and handling are among the most critical considerations in patient care, because any results the laboratory generates are directly dependent on the quality of the specimen and its condition on arrival in the laboratory. Specimens for microbiology testing must be collected in such a way as to prevent the introduction of any contaminating microorganisms. This means not only using special sterile collection and transport devices, but also taking steps to prevent environmental and patient contamination. Such steps include using antiseptics on the skin before drawing blood, instructing a patient in the collection of a urine sample using the clean catch midstream (CCMS) technique (see Chapter 52), and avoiding the teeth and tongue when collecting a throat culture specimen on a swab.

When collecting specimens for microbiologic analysis, medical assistants should ask themselves two questions: "In what ways can I prevent contamination of this sample?" and "What can I do to protect myself from becoming infected while I collect this sample?" Answers to the first question include cleansing the area to be sampled with an antiseptic, opening sterile containers only when necessary, and never touching a sterile swab or collection device to a nonsterile surface. Answers to the second question include wearing gloves and a disposable surgical mask or face shield while collecting a throat or sputum culture and wearing gloves when receiving a urine specimen from a patient who has just voided.

Ideally, specimens should be collected during the acute phase of an illness and before antibiotics are prescribed. Many types of samples can be collected. Sterile swabs can be used to collect samples from wounds and the upper respiratory tract. Serum or whole blood can be used to test for infectious organisms. Urine and feces can be collected in containers by patients at home. If patients are expected to collect specimens, it is crucial that they receive clear instructions on how to perform the procedure without contaminating the sample. The referral laboratory is responsible for providing a manual of written instructions to the POL, and the POL is responsible for providing clear instructions (preferably written) to the patient, especially if the patient will be collecting the sample in private or at home.

The transport of specimens is also crucial. Many different types of transport devices are available, and close attention must be given to their proper use. Microorganisms are living organisms and must be provided with conditions that permit their survival but do not permit their multiplication. If microorganisms are allowed to multiply after specimen collection, the culture results will not reflect the true disease state. Specialized transport media, such as modified

Stuart's medium or Amie's medium, often are used in the swabbing devices used for specimen collection (Figure 55-1). These collection devices typically are made of a plastic tube that encases a sterile Dacron swab and a sealed vial of **transport medium**. After the specimen is obtained on the swab, it is placed in the plastic tube and the transport medium is released, usually by crushing the internal vial. It is essential to follow the manufacturer's directions to prevent drying of the swab and specimen.

Ideally a specimen should be transported to the laboratory and cultured immediately after collection. In most situations, however, this is not possible, and the transport device must be handled by a courier en route to a referral laboratory or held in the POL until it can be cultured. For specimens that will be transported by a courier, make sure the specimens are safely packaged in leakproof containers marked with warning labels (Figure 55-2). Proper temperature and time of storage are crucial. Most pathogenic organisms prefer temperatures around 37°C (98.6°F) and will remain **viable** for up to 72 hours if held at room temperature or refrigerator temperature (4°C [39.2°F]). However, some organisms die if exposed to cold temperatures. Always check the referral laboratory's procedure manual for directions on duration and temperature of storage before plating. Likewise, microorganisms have oxygen requirements; some, called *aerobes,* require oxygen to stay alive; others, called *anaerobes,* die if exposed to oxygen. Devices are available for both aerobic and anaerobic collection. Table 55-1 lists the collection, transport, and

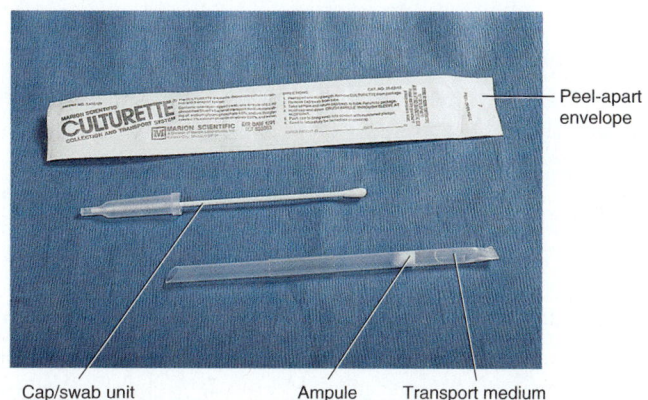

Cap/swab unit   Ampule   Transport medium

FIGURE 55-1 Culturette collection and transport system. (From Bonewit-West K: *Clinical procedures for medical assistants,* ed 7, St Louis, 2008, WB Saunders.)

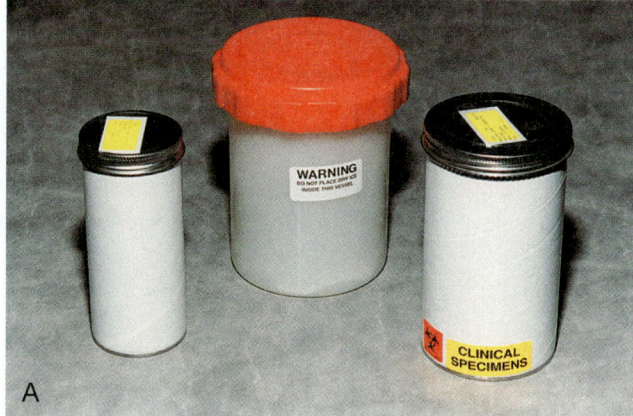
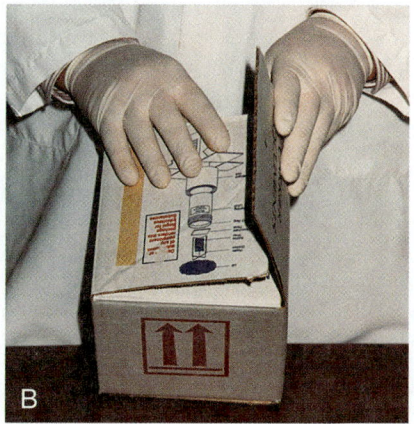

FIGURE 55-2 A, Appropriate containers for transport. **B,** Appropriate packaging for transport.

TABLE 55-1 Collection, Transport, and Processing of Specimens Commonly Submitted to the Physician Office Laboratory

SPECIMEN	CONTAINER	PATIENT PREPARATION	SPECIAL INSTRUCTIONS	STORAGE BEFORE PROCESSING
Blood	Blood culture media set or Vacutainer brand blood culture tube with SPS	Disinfect venipuncture site with alcohol swab and Betadine	Draw blood during febrile episodes; draw two sets from right and left arms	Deliver to laboratory within 2 hr; incubate at 37° C (98.6° F) on receipt in the laboratory
Body fluids (e.g., peritoneal, synovial, pleural)	Sterile, screw-cap container or anaerobic transporter	Disinfect aspiration site with alcohol swab and Betadine	Needle aspirations are preferable to swab collections	Transport immediately and plate specimen immediately on receipt in the laboratory
Eye	Aerobic transport swab		Moisten swab with Amie's or Stuart's medium before collection	May be stored up to 24 hr at room temperature
Stool	Clean, leakproof container		Transport to laboratory within 24 hr if storing at 4° C (39.2° F)	Plate within 72 hr if storing at 4° C (39.2° F)
Rectal swab	Swab placed directly in enteric transport medium		Insert swab approximately 1 inch past anal sphincter	Store at 4° C (39.2° F), transport within 24 hr to laboratory and plate within 72 hr
Gonorrhea culture	Jembec transport system or transport device with Stuart's or Amie's medium	Wipe away exudate before obtaining culture specimen, obtain culture specimen with swab	Do not refrigerate	Transport to laboratory within 2 hr
Chlamydia culture	Specialized *Chlamydia* transport medium containing antibiotics	Urogenital swabs preferred; necessary to obtain epithelial cells, not exudate	Transport immediately on ice to laboratory	Store up to 24 hr at 4° C (39.2° F); inoculate cultures within 15 min of collection if swab is not on ice
Skin scraping (fungal culture)	Clean, screw-top tube	Wipe skin with alcohol prep pad	Scrape skin at leading edge of lesion	Can be held indefinitely at room temperature but best to process within 72 hr of collection
Sputum	Sterile, screw-cap container	Patient should rinse or gargle with mouthwash before collection	Have patient collect from deep cough; do not collect saliva	Store at 4° C (39.2° F), and plate within 24 hr
Throat	Transport swab	Moisten swab with Stuart's or Amie's transport medium	Swab pharynx and tonsils, not mouth, tongue, or teeth	Transport and plate within 24 hr; room temperature storage
Ova and parasite (O&P)	O&P transport device (with formalin and PVA)	Three specimens collected every other day at a minimum for outpatients	Wait 7-10 days if patient has been taking Pepto-Bismol, Kaopectate, or Milk of Magnesia	Store at room temperature and deliver to laboratory within 24 hr
Urine	Sterile, screw-cap container	Instruct patient in clean catch midstream collection	Hold at 4° C (39.2° F) and deliver to laboratory within 24 hr	Hold at 4° C (39.2° F) and plate within 24 hr
Superficial wound	Aerobic transport swab	Wipe area with sterile saline or alcohol prep pad before collection	Moisten swab with Amie's or Stuart's medium before collection	Transport and plate within 24 hr; room temperature storage
Deep wound or abscess	Anaerobic transport device	Wipe area with sterile saline or alcohol prep pad before collection	Aspirate material, excise tissue, or insert swab deep into wound	Transport and plate within 24 hr; room temperature storage

Modified from Forbes BA, Sahm DF, Weissfeld AS: *Bailey and Scott's diagnostic microbiology,* ed 11, St Louis, 2002, Mosby.
SPS, Sodium polyanetholsulfonate; *PVA,* polyvinyl alcohol.

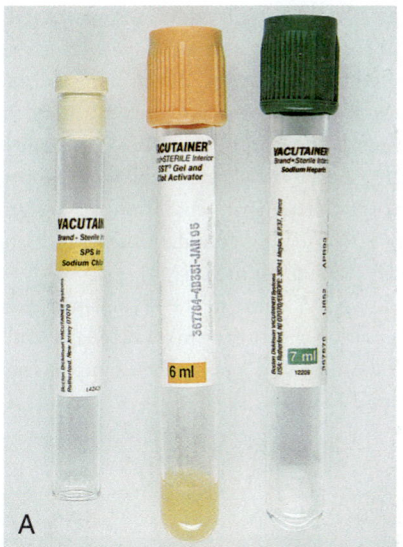
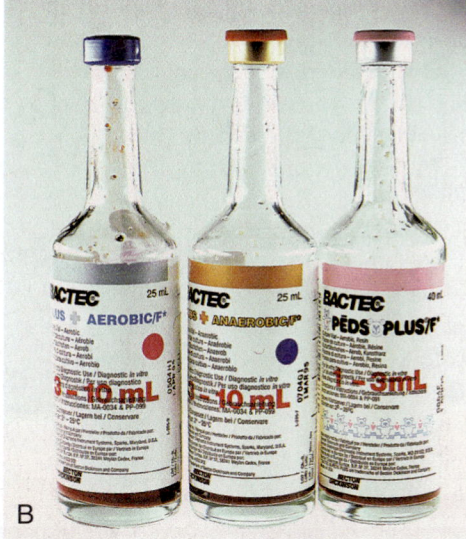
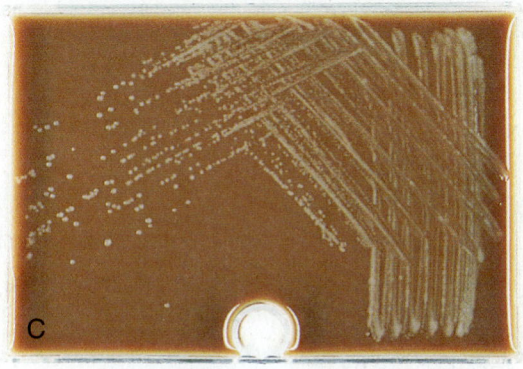
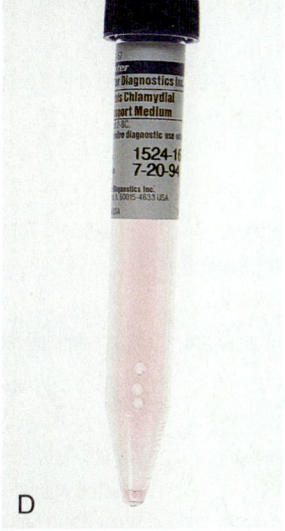

FIGURE 55-3 A, Blood collection Vacutainer tubes. **B,** Bactec blood culture bottles. **C,** Jembec plate. **D,** Viral-chlamydial transport medium. (From De la Maza LM, Pezzlo MT, Baron EJ: *Color atlas of diagnostic microbiology,* St Louis, 1997, Mosby.)

storage of specimens commonly collected or handled by medical assistants. Figure 55-3 shows some commonly used collection devices.

> **CRITICAL THINKING** APPLICATION   55-1
>
> Aaron Mitchell, age 9, was brought into the clinic this morning at 9 o'clock with scabbing sores on his upper lip. Dr. Chowdry suspects impetigo and orders a wound culture. How will Anna collect this culture? What device might she use? How should she store this specimen until the courier, who does not come until 3 PM, arrives? Anna knows that impetigo is highly contagious. How can she protect herself from becoming infected?

CLASSIFICATION OF MICROORGANISMS

Once the specimen reaches the microbiology laboratory, it is analyzed for the presence of infectious microorganisms or their components. Although the medical assistant is not responsible for

identifying microorganisms, a working knowledge of the terminology used in the classification of microorganisms is essential.

Most cultures handled by the medical assistant have been ordered to diagnose bacterial infections. Bacteria are one type of microorganism; other microorganisms include fungi and protozoa. Parasitic worms are studied in the microbiology laboratory but are not considered microorganisms.

Many microbiologists do not consider viruses to be microorganisms simply because they are not, by definition, alive. Viruses consist of a core of either ribonucleic acid (RNA) or deoxyribonucleic acid (DNA) covered by a protein shell. Alone, they neither metabolize nor reproduce; however, once inside a host cell, viruses use the host cell's **organelles** and **macromolecules** to multiply. Because of this absolute need for a host cell for replication, viruses are called *obligate intracellular parasites,* and they cannot be cultured on artificial media such as those used to culture bacteria.

Viruses must be cultured in fertilized eggs or in **tissue culture,** which is done by referral or hospital laboratories. Often, instead of culturing a specimen for a virus, antigenic products of the virus or antibodies made by a patient to a virus are detected. For example, in the diagnosis of hepatitis B virus infection, the serum is tested for hepatitis B surface antigen (HBsAg), a protein found in the shell of the virus. Table 55-2 lists common diseases caused by viruses.

Naming of Microorganisms

Scientists have used the binomial system of nomenclature developed by Swedish botanist Carl von Linné to name all living organisms: animals, plants, fungi, protozoa, and bacteria. This binomial system assigns two names; the first name is the **genus**, and the second is the **species**. Both names are either italicized or underlined when written. The genus begins with a capital letter, the species with a lowercase letter. Often the name reveals some characteristic about the organism. For example, *Neisseria gonorrhoeae* is a bacterium that was studied extensively by Albert Neisser, and it causes the sexually transmitted disease gonorrhea. When culture results are reported, it is essential that both the genus and species names be recorded. Different species may cause different symptoms or require different antibiotic treatment. For example, *N. gonorrhoeae* causes disease, whereas *N. sicca* is found in the mouth and does not cause disease under normal conditions.

The genus name of the organism may be represented by a single letter after the organism's full genus and species name has been written once in a report. For example, *Escherichia coli* is commonly referred to as *E. coli*.

TABLE 55-2 Common Diseases Caused by Viruses

DISEASE	VIRUS	TRANSMISSION	SYMPTOMS	TESTS	PREVENTION
Smallpox	Variola major	Direct contact; fomites	Vesicles on entire body, including soles and palms		Eradicated (vaccine is still available)
Infectious mononucleosis	Epstein-Barr virus	Direct and airborne	Sore throat, fever, malaise, lymph gland involvement; hepatitis, enlarged spleen	Serology testing for heterophile antibodies; CBC	Avoid direct contact with known cases
Influenza	Myxovirus—influenza A and B	Droplet and fomites	Fever, body aches, cough	Nasopharyngeal swab, nasal wash	Immunization for the old, young, and debilitated
Warts (verruca)	Human papilloma virus	Direct and indirect contact	Circumscribed outgrowths on skin; most common on hands and feet		
Rabies	Rhabdovirus	Contact with saliva of infected animal (dog, cat, skunk, fox, bat are usual)	Fever, uncontrollable excitement, spasms of the throat, profuse salivation	DFA from brain or hair follicle tissue	Vaccine available; vaccinate pets
Mumps	Paramyxovirus—mumps virus	Direct contact	Pain, swelling of salivary glands; fever	Acute and convalescent titers	MMR vaccine
Measles	Paramyxovirus—measles virus	Direct contact; droplets	Fever, nasal discharge, red eyes; Koplik's spots, rash	Serologic titer	MMR vaccine
Rubella (German measles)		Direct contact; droplets; congenital	Rash, swollen lymph glands; causes severe birth defects	Serologic titer	MMR vaccine
Common cold	Rhinovirus and many others	Direct; droplets; fomites	Headache, fever, runny nose, congestion		Good hygiene (hand washing)
Polio	Poliovirus	Direct contact; carriers enter via mouth	Fever, headache, stiff neck and back, paralysis of muscles		IPV; SC or IM; four doses
Molluscum contagiosum warts	Molluscipox virus	Direct contact with infected individual	Small pink or white domes found in clusters	Microscopic evaluation	Avoid contact with infected individual; have existing warts removed

Courtesy Kathleen Moody.
CBC, Complete blood count; *DFA,* direct fluorescent antibody; *IM,* intramuscular; *IPV,* inactivated polio vaccine; *MMR,* measles, mumps, rubella; *SC,* subcutaneous.

CRITICAL THINKING APPLICATION   **55-2**

While preparing to collect the specimen from Aaron, Anna receives a telephone call from BioStatLab, the referral laboratory the clinic uses. The results from Ms. Tina Walker's urine culture and from Mr. Robert Livore's abscess culture are complete.

- Anna listens carefully to the technician's report on Mr. Livore's abscess culture, and she jots down "*staphylococcus*" on the reporting form. She asks the technician what species of "staph." Why is this important?
- The technician also reports Ms. Walker's test results. She says that the organism causing Ms. Walker's urinary tract infection was identified as *Escherichia coli.* How could *E. coli* have infected the urinary tract?

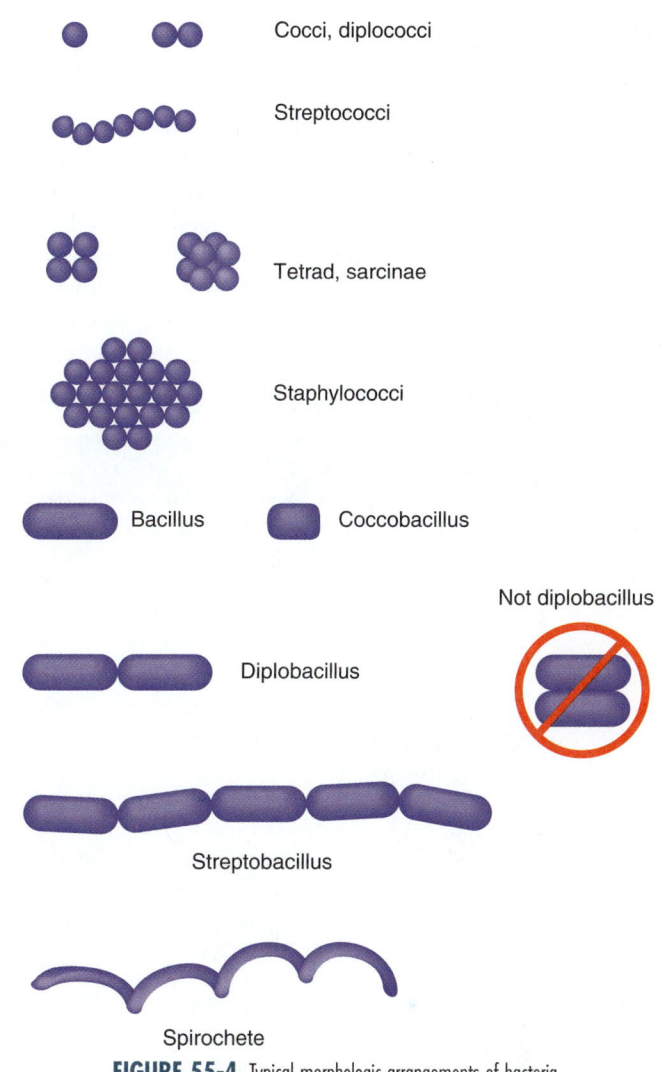

FIGURE 55-4 Typical morphologic arrangements of bacteria.

Typical Pathogenic Bacteria

Bacteria are single-celled **prokaryote** organisms that reproduce by binary fission, a process that involves duplication of the chromosome and subsequent fission (splitting in half) of the cell. This process of asexual reproduction results in tremendous numbers of bacteria from a single cell and explains why bacterial infections can quickly overwhelm a person's immune system. Some bacteria reproduce in as little as 14 minutes, whereas others take days to divide. Theoretically, a single *E. coli* cell, which has a reproduction time of about 30 minutes, produces 351,843,724,088,831 offspring in 24 hours if it is able to enter the urinary bladder.

Bacteria often are classified according to their shape, their staining characteristics, and the environmental conditions in which they thrive. Both shape and staining characteristics are direct results of the cell wall composition. Three types of cell wall structures are found among pathogenic bacteria: gram positive, gram negative, and acid fast. These designations are based on reactions in specialized stains used to see the bacteria under the microscope. The bacterial cell wall is composed of peptidoglycan (PG), a molecule composed of carbohydrate and protein. The gram-positive cell has a thick layer of PG with no lipid layer surrounding it; the gram-negative cell has a thin layer of PG with a lipid layer surrounding it; and the acid-fast cell has a thin layer of PG surrounded by a thick layer of waxlike lipids. Acid-fast bacteria do not stain well with Gram stain, and gram-positive and gram-negative bacteria both stain negative with the acid-fast stain. With Gram stain, gram-positive bacteria stain purple, and gram-negative bacteria stain pink. With the acid-fast stain, acid-fast–positive bacteria (AFB) stain pink and acid-fast–negative bacteria stain blue.

Bacterial Shapes

Pathogenic bacteria assume three different morphologic shapes. Spheric bacteria are called *cocci* (singular, *coccus*), rod-shaped bacteria are *bacilli* (singular, *bacillus*), and spiral bacteria are *spirilla* (singular, *spirillum*). Tightly coiled spirilla are called *spirochetes.* Certain arrangements are also seen in different genera and species. When bacteria are in a chain formation, the prefix *strepto-* is used. When bacteria are found in pairs, the prefix *diplo-* is used, and when they are found in grapelike clusters, the prefix *staphylo-* is used. Cocci in

packets of four are called *tetrads* and in packets of eight or 16 are called *sarcinae* (Figure 55-4).

CRITICAL THINKING APPLICATION   **55-3**

Anna knows that impetigo is caused by *Staphylococcus aureus.* Without using a microscope, she knows what the organism looks like. How does she know?

Bacterial Oxygen Requirements

Bacteria are also classified according to oxygen requirements. As mentioned, those that require oxygen to live are called *aerobes;* those that die in the presence of oxygen are *anaerobes.* Some bacteria are flexible concerning oxygen requirements and, although they are anaerobes, can survive in the presence of oxygen. These organisms are called *facultative anaerobes. Mycobacterium tuberculosis* thrives in white blood cells in the lungs, causing tuberculosis; it is an aerobe. *Bacteroides fragilis* is the predominant bacterium found in the intestines. This gram-negative bacillus is an anaerobe. *E. coli,* also an inhabitant of the intestines and the most common cause of urinary tract infections, is a facultative anaerobe.

Bacterial Physical Structures

Bacteria can be classified and identified according to physical structures. Some bacteria have thin, long structures called *flagella* that aid in propulsion. *Proteus vulgaris* is a gram-negative bacillus with many flagella surrounding the cell. It can propel itself into the bladder and is the primary cause of nosocomial urinary tract infections. Some bacteria may have thick, gelatinous coats surrounding the cell wall; these are called *capsules*. *Streptococcus pneumoniae* is nonpathogenic if it is not producing a capsule; however, it is the most common cause of pneumonia in older adults when it is encapsulated. The Pneumovax vaccine, which is given to older patients and those at high risk for respiratory complications (e.g., patients with asthma), is composed of highly purified capsular polysaccharides from 23 strains of *S. pneumoniae*. Certain bacteria are able to form intracellular structures called *endospores* that allow the cell to remain viable when environmental conditions are not favorable. *Bacillus anthracis* produces such spores, as does *Clostridium tetani*. If spores of *C. tetani* enter a wound and germinate, they cause the disease known as *tetanus*. Tables 55-3 to 55-5 list some important infectious diseases caused by typical pathogenic bacteria.

TABLE 55-3 Common Diseases Caused by Bacilli

DISEASE	ORGANISM	DESCRIPTION	TRANSMISSION	SYMPTOMS	TESTS AND SPECIMENS	PREVENTION AND IMMUNIZATION
Tuberculosis	*Mycobacterium tuberculosis*	Acid-fast branching bacilli	Inhalation	Pulmonary—cough, hemoptysis, sweats, weight loss; may affect other systems	Sputum for culture; x-ray; skin tests	BCG vaccine (not routinely given in the United States)
Urinary tract infections	*Escherichia coli, Proteus* spp., *Klebsiella* spp., *Pseudomonas aeruginosa*	Gram-negative bacilli, many flagellated	Ascends urethra; catheterization	Cystitis—frequency, burning bloody urine Pyelonephritis—flank pain, fever	Clean catch urine for culture and analysis	Good personal hygiene; always wipe from front to back
Legionnaires disease	*Legionella pneumophila*	Gram-negative bacillus (stains poorly with usual methods)	Grows freely in water (air conditioning systems)	Pneumonia-like symptoms	Sputum; blood	Avoid smoking
Tetanus (lockjaw)	*Clostridium tetani*	Gram-positive spore-forming bacilli, anaerobic	Open wounds, fractures, punctures	Toxin affects motor nerves; muscle spasms, convulsions, rigidity	Blood	DTaP in childhood; T or Td every 10 yr
Gas gangrene	*Clostridium perfringens*	Gram-positive spore-forming bacilli, anaerobic	Wounds	Gas and watery exudate in infected wound	Swab, aspirate of wound for culture	Proper wound care
Botulism	*Clostridium botulinum*	Gram-positive spore-forming bacilli, anaerobic	Improperly cooked canned foods	Neurotoxin affects speech, swallowing, vision; paralysis of respiratory muscles, death	Contaminated food; blood	Botulinus antitoxin; boil canned goods 20 min before tasting or eating
Diphtheria respiratory secretions	*Corynebacterium diphtheriae*	Gram-positive bacilli, club shaped		Sore throat, fever, headache, gray membrane in throat	Swabs; Gram stain, culture; Schick test for immunity	DTaP in childhood
Whooping cough	*Bordetella pertussis*	Gram-negative bacilli	Respiratory secretions	Upper respiratory tract symptoms; high-pitched, crowing whoop	Swabs for culture	DTaP in childhood
Plague	*Yersinia pestis*	Gram-negative bacilli	Flea bite from infected rodents	Fever and chills, delirium, enlarged, painful lymph nodes	Sputum for culture; blood	Vaccine available; rodent control

Courtesy Kathleen Moody.

BCG, Bacille Calmette-Guérin vaccine; *DTaP*, diphtheria-tetanus-acellular pertussis vaccine; *T*, tetanus (toxoid); *Td*, tetanus and diphtheria (toxoids).

TABLE 55-4 Common Diseases Caused by Cocci

DISEASE	ORGANISM	DESCRIPTION	TRANSMISSION	SYMPTOMS	SPECIMENS	TESTS	PREVENTION
Pneumonia	*Streptococcus pneumoniae*	Gram-positive encapsulated cocci in pairs	Direct contact, droplets	Productive cough, fever, chest pain	Sputum; bronchoscopy secretions	Culture, Gram stain	Vaccine
Strep throat	*Streptococcus pyogenes* (group A streptococcus)	Gram-positive cocci in chains	Direct contact, droplets, fomites	Severe sore throat, fever, malaise	Direct swab	Rapid strep test, throat culture	Good personal hygiene
Wound infection, abscesses, boils	*Staphylococcus aureus*	Gram-positive cocci in clusters	Direct contact, fomites, carriers; poor hand washing	Area red, warm, swollen; pus; pain; ulceration or sinus formation	Deep swab; aspirate of drainage	Culture and sensitivity (aerobic and anaerobic)	Good personal hygiene
Staphylococcal food poisoning	*Staphylococcus aureus*	Gram-positive cocci in clusters	Poor hygiene and improper refrigeration of foods	Vomiting, abdominal cramps, diarrhea	Suspected food, stool	Culture of food (organism is not found in stool)	Refrigerate food to prevent toxin production
Toxic shock	*Staphylococcus aureus*	Gram-positive cocci in clusters	Use of absorbent packing materials (e.g., tampons, nasal packs)	Fever, headache, nausea, vomiting, delirium, low blood pressure	Swab, blood	Culture and serology	Change tampon, packing material often
Gonorrhea	*Neisseria gonorrhoeae*	Gram-negative cocci in pairs; intracellular in white blood cells	Sexually transmitted	*Females:* Pelvic pain, discharge; may be asymptomatic *Males:* Urethral drip, pain on urination	Swab of cervix, urethra; rectal and pharyngeal swabs in homosexual men	Gram stain; culture	Avoid unprotected sex
Meningococcal meningitis	*Neisseria meningitidis*	Gram-negative diplococci	Respiratory tract secretions	High fever, headache, projectile vomiting, delirium, neck and back rigidity, convulsions, petechial rash	Nasopharyngeal swabs, cerebrospinal fluid, blood	Gram stain; culture; cell counts and chemistries	Vaccine; prophylactic antibiotics

Unusual Pathogenic Bacteria: Chlamydiae, Mycoplasmas, and Rickettsiae

In the small scale used to measure microorganisms, viruses range from 10 to 100 **nanometers** (nm). Typical pathogenic bacteria measure 1,000 to 5,000 nm. Chlamydiae, mycoplasmas, and rickettsiae are tiny, unusual bacteria that fall between the size ranges of viruses and typical pathogenic bacteria.

The rickettsiae are tiny gram-negative bacteria that are transmitted by blood-sucking **arthropods**. They cannot multiply outside a host cell, and once inside the host cell, they are able to perform only some of the life-sustaining metabolic reactions on their own. Chlamydiae also are tiny bacteria that require host cells for growth and once were considered viruses. Unlike rickettsiae, chlamydiae are not transmitted by arthropod vectors.

TABLE 55-5 Common Diseases Caused by Spirilla

DISEASE	ORGANISM	DESCRIPTION	TRANSMISSION	SYMPTOMS	TESTS AND SPECIMENS	PREVENTION AND IMMUNIZATION
Syphilis	*Treponema pallidum*	Spirochete	Sexually; congenitally	*Primary:* Painless sore (chancre) *Secondary:* Generalized rash involving palms and soles of feet *Congenital:* birth defects	Blood for serologic tests: VDRL, RPR, FTA-ABS	Avoid unprotected sex
Lyme disease	*Borrelia burgdorferi*	Spirochete	Tick bite	Fever, joint pain, red bull's-eye rash	Blood	Avoiding tick-infested areas
Pyloric ulcers	*Helicobacter pylori*	Gram-negative, spiral shaped	Unknown; possibly food and water	Burning pain in stomach, especially between meals	Stomach biopsy for staining and culture; stool for EIA testing	None known
Food poisoning (most common cause in United States)	*Campylobacter jejuni*	Paired, gram-negative, curved rods forming a seagull shape	Contaminated food, water, and milk	Bloody or watery diarrhea	Stool for dark field microscopy and culture	Sanitary food preparation and control of water and milk supplies

Courtesy Kathleen Moody.
EIA, Enzyme immunoassays; *FTA-ABS,* fluorescent treponemal antibody absorption (test); *RPR,* rapid plasma reagin (test); *VDRL,* Venereal Disease Research Laboratory.

TABLE 55-6 Diseases Caused by Rickettsiae, Mycoplasmas, and Chlamydiae

DISEASE	ORGANISM	TRANSMISSION	SYMPTOMS	TESTS AND SPECIMENS
Rocky Mountain spotted fever	*Rickettsia rickettsii*	Tick bite	Headache, chills, fever, characteristic rash on extremities and trunk	Blood for serologic tests; skin biopsy for direct fluorescent microscopy
Typhus	*Rickettsia prowazekii*	Tick bite	Fever, rash, confusion	Blood for serology
Atypical (walking) pneumonia	*Mycoplasma pneumoniae*	Respiratory secretions	Fever, cough, chest pain	Blood, sputum for culture
Nongonococcal urethritis and vaginitis	*Chlamydia trachomatis*	Sexual	May be asymptomatic	Swabs for DNA probe and serologic testing
Inclusion conjunctivitis, pneumonia	*Chlamydia trachomatis*	During birth	Severe conjunctivitis or afebrile pneumonia in newborns	Swabs for DNA probe and serologic testing

Courtesy Kathleen Moody.

Mycoplasmas are unusual in that they have no PG in the cell wall, but they are not obligate parasites as are rickettsiae and chlamydiae. Rickettsiae and chlamydiae do not grow on artificial media in the laboratory; tissue culture or serologic testing is required to identify them. Mycoplasmas can be cultivated from a patient specimen in the laboratory (Table 55-6).

Fungi

Mycology is the study of fungi and the diseases they cause. Fungi (singular, *fungus*) are **eukaryotes** that are larger than bacteria; they include unicellular yeasts and multicellular molds. Fungi are present in the soil, air, and water, but only a few species cause disease. They are transmitted by direct contact with infected persons, by prolonged exposure to a moist environment, and by inhalation of contaminated dust or soil. Fungal infections may be superficial, affecting only the skin, hair, or nails. However, some fungi can penetrate the tissues of the internal body structures and produce serious diseases of the mucous membranes, heart, lungs, and other organs. Fungal infections are resistant to the antibiotics used in the treatment of bacterial infections, and fungi must be treated with drugs active against their unusual cell walls.

A superficial fungal infection often is referred to as a *tinea* (Latin for "ringworm"). Tinea pedis, for example, is athlete's foot; tinea barbae is a fungal infection of the facial hair follicles. The term *ringworm* arose because the infected area is often circular and appears wrinkled in the center as a result of the healing process. Diagnosis of fungal infections usually is based on culturing or microscopic observation of skin scrapings, hair samples, or samples of sputum or mucous membranes. Usually the samples are treated with potassium hydroxide before microscopic observation to dissolve away nonfungal material, making the fungal elements easier to observe (Table 55-7).

Parasites

Parasitology includes the study of all parasitic organisms that live on or in the human body. In parasitic relationships the host is harmed as the parasite thrives. Parasites are transmitted by ingestion during the infective stage, direct penetration of the skin by infective larvae, and inoculation by an arthropod vector. A parasite cannot be identified accurately on the basis of a single test or specimen. Most parasites are identified in urine, sputum, tissue fluids, or tissue biopsy samples (Table 55-8).

Helminths

Helminths are eukaryote parasites called *worms*. Helminths live on or within another living organism and nourish themselves at the expense of the host organism. They can live in animals or humans and usually are transmitted through the soil, by infected clothing or fingernails, or through contact with infected persons or contaminated food or water. Helminths go through the same life cycle as other worms. The adult worm lays eggs (ova). The ova develop into larvae. Larvae grow into adult worms, which lay eggs, and the cycle begins again. Diagnosis usually is based on microscopic examination of feces for ova and parasites and on the patient's signs and symptoms (Figure 55-5).

Protozoa

Protozoa (singular, *protozoon*) are single-celled parasitic eukaryotes that range in size from microscopic to macroscopic (visible to the naked eye). They are present in moist environments and in bodies of water such as lakes and ponds. Protozoa are transmitted through

TABLE 55-7 Common Diseases Caused by Fungi

DISEASE	ORGANISM	PREDISPOSING CONDITIONS AND TRANSMISSION	SYMPTOMS	TESTS AND SPECIMENS
Thrush (oral yeast), vulvovaginal candidiasis, or monilia (vaginal yeast)	*Candida* spp. (yeast)	*Oral:* During birth *Other:* After antibiotic therapy, oral birth control, severe diabetes	White, cheesy growth	Swab for KOH prep, culture
Athlete's foot, jock itch, ringworm (tinea)	*Trichophyton* spp., *Microsporum* spp., and others (skin fungi)	Opportunist; direct contact; clothing; prolonged exposure to moist environment	Hair loss, thickening of skin, nails; itching; red, scaly patches	Skin scraping for KOH prep; skin, hair for culture
Histoplasmosis	*Histoplasma capsulatum*	Inhalation of dust contaminated with bird or bat droppings	Mild, flulike to systemic	Serologic; culture of biopsy material
Cryptococcosis	*Cryptococcus neoformans*	Contact with poultry droppings	Cough, fever, malaise; can become systemic	Sputum culture; cerebrospinal fluid culture, India ink direct examination
Sporotrichosis	*Sporothrix schenckii*	Farmers, florists, people exposed to soil	Skin lesions that spread along lymphatics; can become systemic	Skin scraping for KOH prep; serologic
Pneumocystis pneumonia	*Pneumocystis carinii*	Widely prevalent in animals; occurs in debilitated or immunosuppressed individuals; common in patients with AIDS	Pneumonia-like	Biopsy of lung tissue with microscopic examination

Courtesy Kathleen Moody.
AIDS, Acquired immunodeficiency syndrome; *KOH,* potassium hydroxide.

TABLE 55-8 Common Diseases Caused by Protozoa and Parasites

DISEASE	ORGANISM	TRANSMISSION	SYMPTOMS	TESTS AND SPECIMENS
Malaria	*Plasmodium* spp. (protozoa)	Bite of the *Anopheles* mosquito	Chills, fever (cyclic)	Blood: examination of stained blood for parasites
Toxoplasmosis	*Toxoplasma gondii* (protozoon)	Fecal contamination (cat litter); congenital	Febrile illness, rash; congenital: jaundice, enlarged liver and spleen, brain abnormalities	Skin test for screening blood, fluid, or tissue for confirmation
Amebic dysentery	*Entamoeba histolytica* (protozoon)	Fecal contamination of food and water	Bloody diarrhea, cramping, fever	Stool for O&P
Giardiasis	*Giardia lamblia* (protozoon)	Common in intestinal tract, opportunist; contaminated surface water	Asymptomatic to severe diarrhea and abdominal discomfort	Stool for O&P; intestinal biopsy
Trichinosis	*Trichinella spiralis* (roundworm)	Ingestion of undercooked pork, bear meat	Nausea, fever, diarrhea, muscle pain and swelling, edema of face	Biopsy; blood tests
Tapeworm	*Taenia* spp.	Undercooked meat (beef and pork)	Abdominal discomfort, diarrhea, weight loss	Stool for O&P
	Diphyllobothrium latum	Undercooked fish; common among Norwegians, Japanese	As above; may become anemic	Stool for O&P
Pinworm	*Enterobius vermicularis* (roundworm)	Fecal-oral	Severe rectal itching, restlessness, insomnia	Scotch tape applied to perianal region for ova
Scabies	*Sarcoptes scabiei*—itch mite	Direct contact; clothing, bedding	Nocturnal itching; skin burrows	Skin scrapings for parasites
Lice	*Pediculus humanus; Pthirus pubis* (crabs)	Direct contact; clothing, bedding, furniture (can transmit other diseases via bite)	Intense itching; skin lesions	Finding adult lice or eggs (nits) on body or hair

Courtesy Kathleen Moody.
O&P, Ova and parasites.

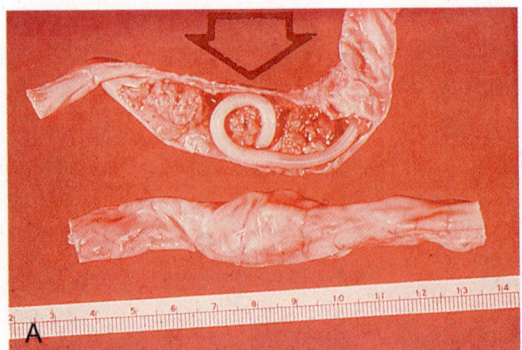
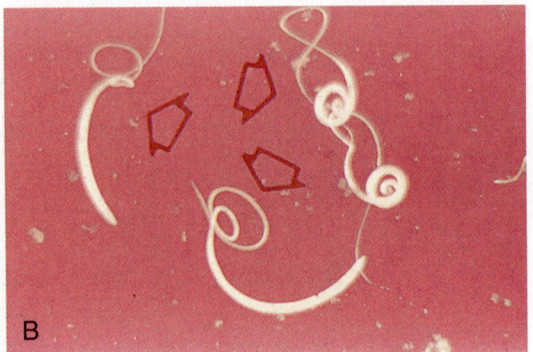

FIGURE 55-5 A, Roundworms. **B,** Whipworms. (From Stepp CA, Woods MA: *Laboratory procedures for medical office personnel,* Philadelphia, 1998, WB Saunders.)

contaminated feces, food, and drink. Some pathogenic protozoa inhabit the bloodstream, whereas others inhabit the intestines and genital tract. Diagnosis usually is based on the patient's signs and symptoms and on the microscopic examination of stool and blood (see Table 55-8).

Stool specimens commonly are examined for parasitic protozoa and helminths. The stool specimen is collected and placed into two vials, each with a preservative. Most commonly, sodium acetate acetic acid formalin (SAF) and polyvinyl alcohol (PVA) are used. From these preparations, a **wet mount** is made to observe motile organisms, a stained smear is made to provide contrast to the existing debris in the stool, and the specimen is concentrated either by sedimentation or flotation to allow recovery of protozoan **cysts** and helminth eggs. The medical assistant should always consult the procedure manual provided by the referral laboratory when an ova and parasites stool examination (O&P) is ordered to ensure proper collection and transport of the specimen (Procedure 55-1).

MICROBIOLOGY LABORATORY

The equipment and supplies in a microbiology laboratory vary with the size of the facility. Most laboratories have a refrigerator, an autoclave, a safety cabinet, a microscope, and an incubator (discussed in Chapter 51). In addition, you are likely to find the following equipment and supplies.

Inoculating Equipment

Cultivation and identification of microbes require the use of certain tools. Inoculating loops and needles (Figure 55-6) are needed to transfer samples or microbes to growth media or to slides for staining. Loops and needles may be disposable and presterilized, or they may be made of wire and can be heat sterilized before and after use. An inoculating loop is shaped like a bubble wand, and a thin film of liquid adheres to the loop. The amount of fluid held by the loop can be calibrated; for a urine culture, a 1-mcL sample must be applied to the culture medium, and special loops are available that

---

PROCEDURE 55-1

Instruct Patients According to Their Needs: Instruct Patients in the Collection of Fecal Specimens to Be Tested for Ova and Parasites

GOAL: *To instruct a patient in the proper collection of stool for an ova and parasite microscopic examination.*

EQUIPMENT and SUPPLIES

- Clean, dry container for stool collection
- Parasitology collection vials*
- Plastic biohazard zipper-lock bag

PROCEDURAL STEPS

1. Instruct the patient not to take any antacids, laxatives, or stool softeners before collecting the specimen.
   <u>PURPOSE:</u> Laxatives increase fecal transit time and may result in a false-negative test result.
2. Instruct the patient to urinate before collecting the specimen.
   <u>PURPOSE:</u> This eliminates the possibility of contaminating the stool with urine.
3. The patient then collects the specimen.
   a. From adults: Instruct the patient to defecate into the container. Stool cannot be retrieved from the toilet bowl.
   b. From children: Loosely drape the toilet rim with plastic wrap and lower the seat. The child should have a bowel movement into the toilet, onto the wrap. Remove the stool using a disposable plastic spoon.
      <u>PURPOSE:</u> The stool cannot be contaminated by or diluted with water.
   c. From infants: Fasten a "diaper" made of plastic wrap over the child using tape. Remove the plastic wrap immediately after a bowel movement and remove the stool using a plastic spoon. *Never leave the child unattended with the plastic wrap in place, as it could cause suffocation should it be removed.*
      <u>PURPOSE:</u> Stool cannot be collected in a diaper.
4. Instruct the patient to add stool to the collection container.
   a. If the stool is formed, use the scoop on the lid of the container to add a large, jelly bean–sized piece of stool to the liquid in the containers (Figure 1).

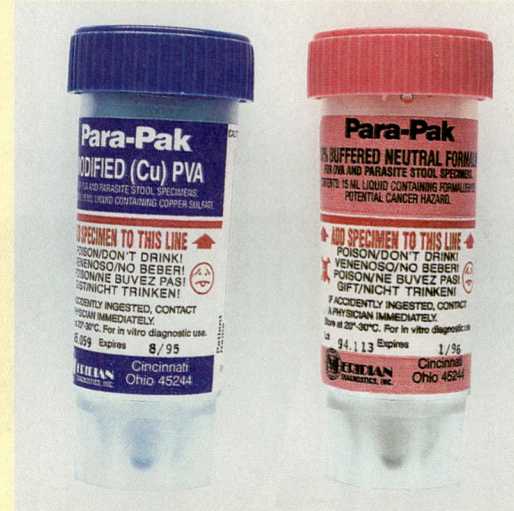

(From Meridian Bioscience, Cincinnati, Ohio.)

   b. If the stool is liquid, pour it into the container until the preservative in the vial reaches the indicated level on the containers.
5. Instruct the patient to tighten the caps completely and wipe the outside of the vials with rubbing alcohol or to wash carefully with soap and water.
   <u>PURPOSE:</u> To ensure infection control.
6. The vials should be labeled, placed in a biohazard bag with a zipper closure, and transported to the laboratory immediately if possible. Do not refrigerate the vials.
7. Instruct the patient to wash his or her hands after the procedure.
   <u>PURPOSE:</u> To ensure infection control.

---

*Several types of preservatives are available. Check with the referral laboratory to make sure the patient is given the proper vials for collection. Preservatives include low-viscosity polyvinyl alcohol (LV-PVA), zinc sulfite polyvinyl alcohol (ZN-PVA), sodium acetate acetic acid formalin (SAF), and 10% neutral buffered formalin.

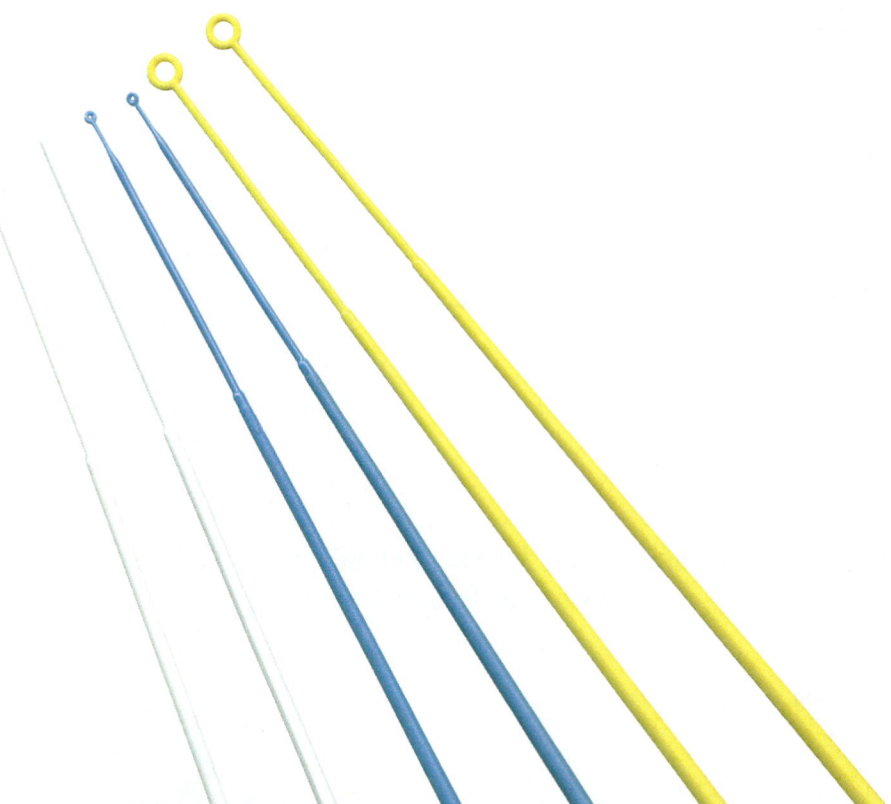

FIGURE 55-6 Inoculating loop and needle. (Courtesy Simport Plastics, Beloeil, Quebec, Canada.)

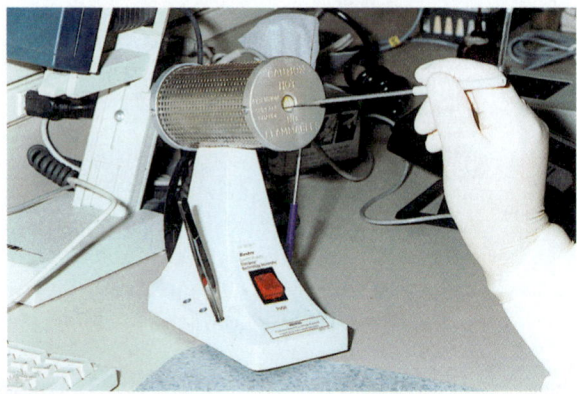

FIGURE 55-7 Loop incinerator. (From Stepp CA, Woods MA: *Laboratory procedures for medical office personnel*, Philadelphia, 1998, WB Saunders.)

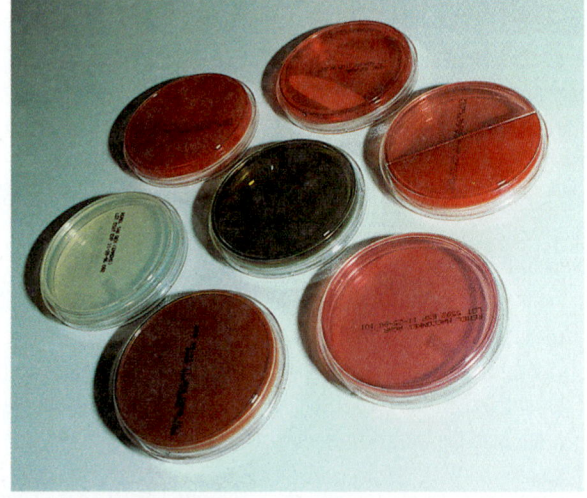

FIGURE 55-8 Media used in cultures. (From Stepp CA, Woods MA: *Laboratory procedures for medical office personnel*, Philadelphia, 1998, WB Saunders.)

deliver this amount. An inoculating needle is thin and pointed and is ideal for sampling single colonies.

Incineration Equipment

Incineration is the fastest way to sterilize reusable equipment (e.g., wire loops, needles, and metal forceps) that must be sterilized before and after use. Some laboratories use a Bunsen burner connected to a natural gas supply, but most use an electric incinerator because of the reduced fire hazard (Figure 55-7). An incinerator can also be used to heat-fix smears for a bacterial stain.

Culture Media

Once a specimen has been properly collected, it must be inoculated onto an appropriate medium (Figure 55-8). Under the proper incubation conditions, the bacteria or fungi in the sample metabolize and reproduce using the nutrients in the medium and become visible as colonies. Media can be solid, liquid, or semisolid. A liquid medium is called a *broth*. The addition of a powdered extract of seaweed called *agar* to a boiling liquid medium allows it to solidify and remain solid at 37° C (98.6° F). The molten medium can be poured into Petri dishes (a plastic dish with a lid) or into tubes. Four types of media typically are used in a microbiology laboratory:

- *All-purpose* or *nutritive media*. All-purpose media are used to support the growth of a wide variety of bacteria; however, they do not support the growth of **fastidious** bacteria.

- *Selective media.* Selective media support the growth of one type of organism while inhibiting the growth of others through the addition of a salt, dye, antibiotic, or chemical. For example, phenyl ethanol agar contains alcohol, which inhibits the growth of gram-negative bacteria and permits gram-positive bacteria to flourish.
- *Differential media.* Differential media contain chemicals or dyes that alter the appearance of certain types of bacteria. Many differential media are also selective. For example, mannitol salt agar contains a higher level (7.5%) of sodium chloride (salt), which selects for staphylococci. It also contains mannitol, a carbohydrate that can be fermented to an acid end-product by *Staphylococcus aureus* but not by *Staphylococcus epidermidis.* The medium contains a pH indicator that turns yellow in the presence of acid. Therefore, if the colony is yellow on the agar medium, it is presumptively *S. aureus.* Differential media are used in biochemical testing.
- *Enriched media.* An enriched medium contains complex organic materials that certain fastidious species must have to multiply. Blood agar, which is needed for the growth of *Streptococcus pyogenes,* is made by adding sterile sheep's blood to an all-purpose medium. It is widely used in clinical microbiology to cultivate pathogens.

All media should be inspected for contamination before use. New batches of media should be inoculated with control microorganisms to ensure quality. The manufacturer provides a list of organisms that can be used for this purpose.

Inoculation of Media

Once the specimen has been collected, it must be "plated," or inoculated onto the appropriate medium. If the specimen was collected with a swab, the swab is rolled onto a portion of the agar medium in a Petri dish, and a sterile inoculating loop is used to spread the sample. If the sample is liquid, such as sputum or urine, a sterile inoculating loop is used to spread it.

Several techniques can be used to spread the sample. For the quadrant streak, a loop is used to spread the sample thinly over the agar medium in several directions. This effectively separates the bacteria so that they can grow in individual colonies. The lawn, or spread, streak is used when an antibiotic's effectiveness must be assessed or colonies counted. This involves using a swab or loop to spread the sample continuously over the entire plate.

Once the sample has been inoculated onto the plates, the plates are incubated in an inverted position so that any condensation that accumulates on the underside of the lid does not fall down onto the growth. The temperature and conditions of incubation depend on the source of the specimen and the suspected pathogens. Most cultures are incubated in an aerobic atmosphere enriched with 5% carbon dioxide at 37°C (98.6°F). Cultures for fungi are incubated both at room temperature and at 37°C (98.6°F) to promote dimorphism, a characteristic of some fungi in which they appear as a budding yeast at 37°C (98.6°F) and as a filamentous mold at room temperature.

Cultures for anaerobes must be incubated in an atmosphere devoid of oxygen. Special jars called *anaerobe jars* chemically remove oxygen from the environment and are small enough to place in an incubator (Figure 55-9).

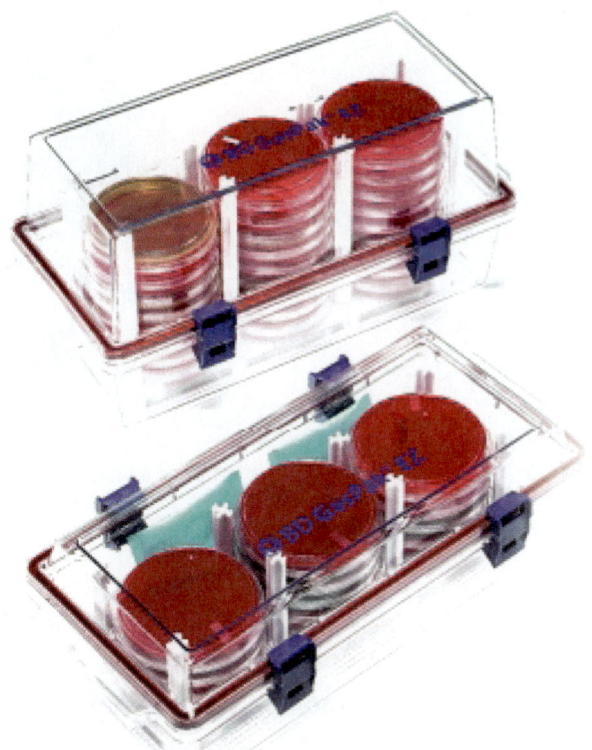

FIGURE 55-9 GasPak anaerobe jar. (Courtesy Becton, Dickinson, & Co.)

IDENTIFICATION OF PATHOGENS IN THE MICROBIOLOGY LABORATORY

Assessing a Culture

When the original (primary) culture has incubated at the appropriate temperature for 18 to 24 hours, it is examined for evidence of pathogens. Because normal floras often are present in samples in addition to pathogens, a trained eye is required to spot the organisms that might be causing an infection. Suspicious colonies are subcultured onto the appropriate medium to isolate them in **pure culture**. When the organism is in pure culture, staining and additional biochemical testing can be done to identify it at the genus and species level. Throat and urine cultures may be performed in POLs that have been certified to perform moderately complex testing.

Throat Culture

Streptococcus pyogenes, also known as *group A beta-hemolytic streptococcus,* causes septic sore throat ("strep throat"). If not diagnosed and treated promptly, this organism can caused severe complications, including scarlet fever, rheumatic fever, and glomerulonephritis. A swab of the throat is streaked on a sheep's blood agar plate, and then a differentiation disk is placed on the most heavily streaked first quadrant. This disk contains an antibiotic (bacitracin), which inhibits the growth of *S. pyogenes* and is used for differential diagnosis. Complete clearing of the agar around the colonies indicates beta hemolysis as a result of a toxin produced by the organism; the toxin lyses the sheep red blood cells in the agar, hence the name *beta-hemolytic "strep"* (Figure 55-10 and Procedure 55-2). The presence of beta-hemolytic colonies and a zone of no growth around the disk

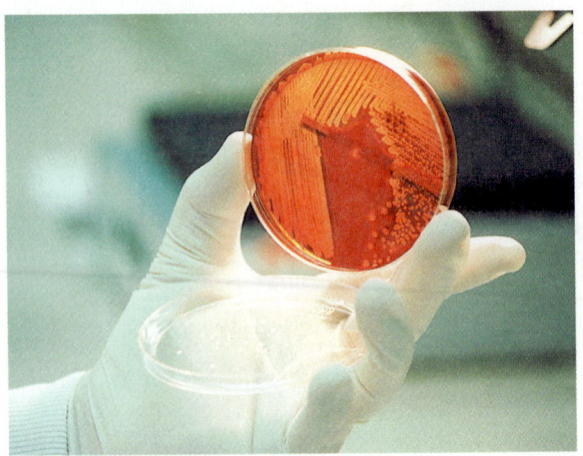

FIGURE 55-10 Beta hemolysis, seen as a clear area around the streptococci colonies. (From Stepp CA, Woods MA: *Laboratory procedures for medical office personnel*, Philadelphia, 1998, WB Saunders.)

indicates that the patient has strep throat. Additional testing may be needed to confirm the identity of the organism.

Urine Cultures

With urine cultures, the number of bacterial colonies present in a sample are counted. Most laboratories use a variety of differential and selective media, along with an all-purpose medium to which 1 mcL ($\frac{1}{1,000}$ mL) of urine is applied. By the standards established by the Clinical Laboratory Improvement Amendments (CLIA), this is a moderately complex test. A calibrated inoculating loop is dipped into a well-mixed urine sample that has been collected by the CCMS method (described in Chapter 52) or by catheterization. The urine from the loop is spread on the medium and incubated for 18 to 24 hours at 37°C (98.6°F). Each colony that grows on the plate represents 1,000 colony-forming units (cfu) per milliliter. A system of numeric values has been devised to assess the possibility of a urinary tract infection (Procedure 55-3).

PROCEDURE 55-2

Inoculate a Blood Agar Plate to Culture *Streptococcus pyogenes*

GOAL: *To inoculate a blood agar plate to detect the etiologic agent for strep throat.*

EQUIPMENT and SUPPLIES

- Blood agar plate
- Bacitracin disk or strep A disk
- Incinerator
- Inoculating loop
- Permanent marker or printed label
- Swab from patient's throat (see Procedure 37-8)
- Forceps
- Bacti-Cinerator
- Disposable gloves
- Face protection
- Biohazardous waste container

PROCEDURAL STEPS

1. Sanitize your hands. Put on face protection and gloves.
   PURPOSE: To ensure infection control.
2. Remove the swab from the transport device. Grasp the plate by the bottom (media side) and lift the base from the cover, or lift the cover while the plate is on the table.
   PURPOSE: To make handling the plate easier and to prevent contamination of the plate.
3. Roll the swab down the middle of the top half of the plate, then use the swab to streak back and forth on the same half of the plate. Dispose of the swab properly (Figure 1).
   PURPOSE: Rolling the swab ensures contact with the surface of the agar.

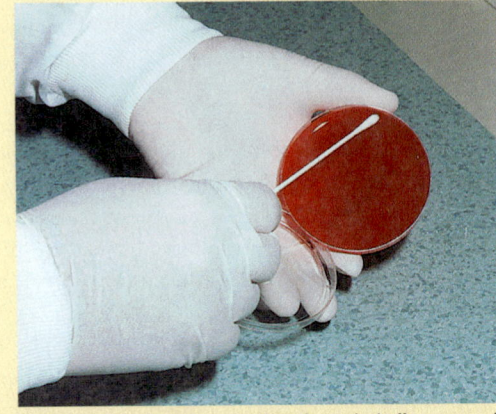

(From Stepp CA, Woods MA: *Laboratory procedures for medical office personnel*, Philadelphia, 1998, WB Saunders.)

4. Sterilize the loop in the Bacti-Cinerator and allow it to cool (Figure 2).
   PURPOSE: Loops must be sterilized before and after use to prevent cross-contamination of specimens.

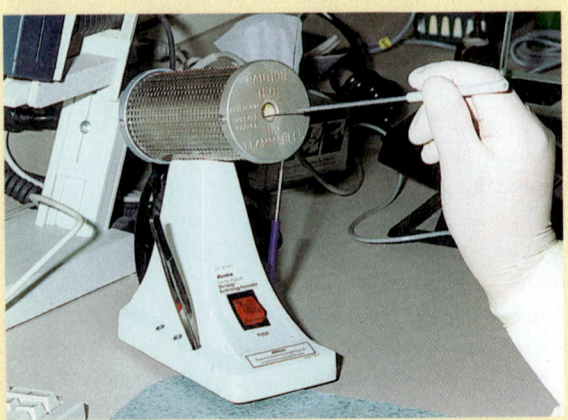

PROCEDURE 55-2—cont'd

5. Use the loop to streak for isolation of colonies in the second, third, and fourth quadrants. Pull the loop over the surface of the agar, pulling some of the inoculum into the uninoculated portion of the plate, and spread it around. Flame the loop again and pull some of the inoculum from the second area into the third area, and so on (Figure 3).

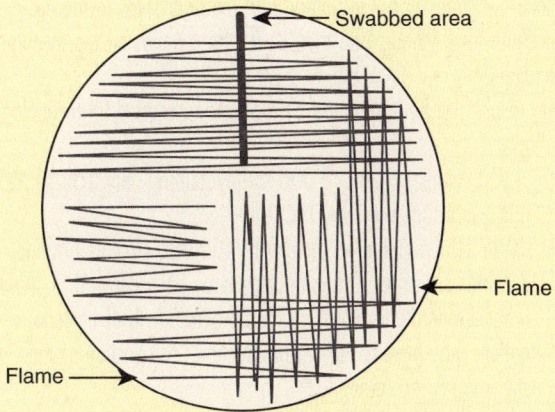

6. Use the loop to make three slices approximately 1 cm long in the agar in the heavy inoculum—swabbed area. Sterilize the loop (see Figure 2).
PURPOSE: Isolated colonies are needed for observation of colony morphology. The agar is sliced to allow for detection of subsurface hemolysis.

7. Sterilize the forceps and remove one disk from the bacitracin vial. Place the disk on the agar in the first quadrant. Sterilize the forceps.
PURPOSE: Group A beta-hemolytic streptococci are presumptively identified by their sensitivity to the bacitracin.

8. With permanent marker, label the agar side of the plate with the patient's name and identification number and the date or apply a printed label.
PURPOSE: Labeling the agar side of dish rather than the lid prevents mixing up of specimens.

9. Place the plate in the incubator in an inverted position.
PURPOSE: Placing the plate with the agar side up prevents the accumulation of moisture on the surface of the agar.

10. Incubate for 24 hours. Beta-hemolytic colonies are shown in Figure 4.

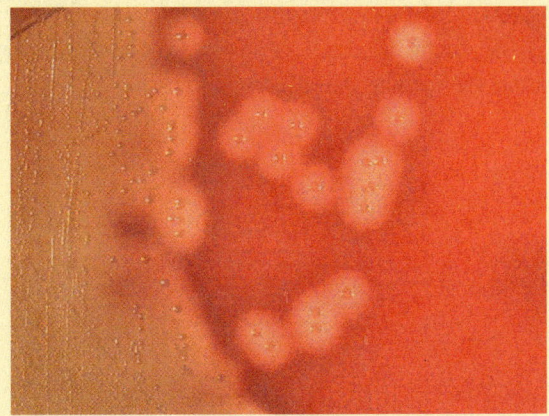

11. Incubate negative cultures for an additional 24 hours.
PURPOSE: Some hemolysis patterns are not well defined after 24 hours of growth.

12. Disinfect the work area and properly dispose of all biohazardous waste.

13. Remove your gloves and sanitize your hands.

PROCEDURE 55-3

Perform a Urine Culture

GOAL: *To inoculate three plates with 1 mcL of urine to quantitate the number of bacteria and aid in the diagnosis of a urinary tract infection.*

EQUIPMENT and SUPPLIES

- Urine specimen, collected clean catch midstream (CCMS) in a sterile container
- Bacti-Cinerator
- 1-mcL calibrated inoculating loop
- Blood agar plate, MacConkey agar plate, and Columbia nutrient agar plate (or an appropriate selection of all-purpose, differential, and selective media)
- Permanent marker or printed label
- Disposable gloves
- Face protection
- Biohazardous waste container

PROCEDURAL STEPS

1. Sanitize your hands. Put on face protection and gloves.
PURPOSE: To ensure infection control.

2. With the screw-cap lid in place, mix the urine specimen thoroughly by swirling.
PURPOSE: When a specimen is allowed to stand, microorganisms settle to the bottom.

PROCEDURE 55-3—cont'd

3. Sterilize the calibrated loop, cool it, and dip the tip into the specimen.
   PURPOSE: The loop must be allowed to cool, or the heat will destroy the microorganisms as the loop comes in contact with the urine specimen, resulting in falsely low colony counts on the culture. Urine on the shaft of the loop will run down the shaft and increase the size of the specimen deposited on the plate, resulting in a falsely elevated colony count on the culture.

4. Spread the urine on the plate by "painting" the specimen down the center of the plate and then streaking thoroughly at right angles (Figure 1).
   PURPOSE: Careful streaking of the plates is necessary for an accurate count of the organisms present.

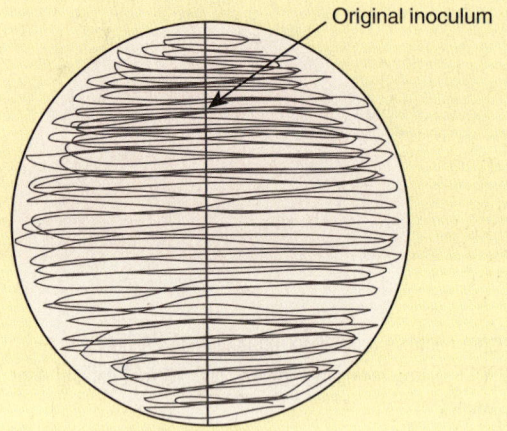

Original inoculum

5. Inoculate the second and third plates in the same manner.

6. With permanent marker, label the bottom of the plates with the patient's name and identification number and the date or apply the printed label.
   PURPOSE: Labeling the bottom of the plates prevents mixing up of the specimens.

7. Place the plates in the incubator with the agar sides facing up.

8. Incubate for 24 hours and then count the colonies on the all-purpose medium.

9. The results will be interpreted by a physician or medical technologist as follows:
   - >100 colonies = >100,000 colony-forming units (cfu)/mL of urine; indicates a urinary tract infection.
   - 10 to 100 colonies = 10,000 to 100,000 cfu/mL of urine; indicates suspicion. The urine may have been allowed to stand at room temperature, which facilitated overgrowth of bacteria, or the patient may have a subclinical infection. Recollection of the specimen is recommended.
   - <10 colonies = 10,000 cfu/mL of urine; indicates normal urethral microbiota.
   PURPOSE: Because the urine was collected by passing through the urethra, some normal bacteria should be present. This system of quantitation accounts for the presence of normal flora.

10. Disinfect the work area, dispose of all biohazardous waste, remove your gloves, and sanitize your hands.

Several self-contained, convenient culture systems for urine are available. These systems are ideal for the smaller laboratory that does not want to buy plate media and that has been certified to perform moderately complex tests. Examples of these systems include the Diaslide (Diatech Diagnostics, Boston, Massachusetts), Bacturcult (Carter-Wallace, Wampole Division, Cranbury, New Jersey), and Uri-Kit (Culture Kits, Norwich, New York). These devices contain culture media either on a paddle or on the walls of a container. The paddle is dipped into the urine, or the urine is poured into the container, swirled, and discarded. The device then is incubated (often at room temperature), and the number of colonies that form on the media is compared with a colony density chart to determine the level of bacteria (Procedure 55-4).

CRITICAL THINKING APPLICATION   55-4
The technician from the referral laboratory indicated that Ms. Walker had a urinary tract infection. Anna recorded the test results as ">100,000 cfu/mL" in the patient's record. What does this number mean?

CHOOSING AN APPROPRIATE ANTIMICROBIAL AGENT

The appropriate antimicrobial agent meets the following criteria:
- Demonstrates the most activity against the infectious agent
- Has the least toxicity to the patient
- Has the least impact on the normal microbiota of the body
- Has the desired pharmacologic characteristics
- Is the most economic

Staining

Pathogenic microorganisms generally are colorless, and a microscope is needed to see them. Special differential stains, such as the Gram stain and the acid-fast stain, often are used to differentiate bacteria based on biochemical differences. As discussed previously, the Gram stain differentiates bacteria into two categories according to cell wall thickness, and the acid-fast stain differentiates bacteria into two categories based on the presence or absence of a waxy lipid in the cell wall.

Before staining can be done, the bacteria must be applied to a labeled slide. A direct smear from a swab can be made, or a culture can be stained. Individual colonies growing on the culture medium can be spread into a drop of sterile saline on a glass slide, or material directly from the site of infection can be spread on the slide from the swab used to collect it. The slide then is air dried and fixed. Either heat or methanol can be used to fix the slide, which results in the material adhering to the slide. Both heat (e.g., from a Bunsen burner or an incinerator) and methanol cause protein in the sample to denature and stick to the slide, much as egg white sticks to a hot frying pan (Procedure 55-5).

Gram Stain

The Gram stain, developed by Dr. Hans Christian Gram more than 100 years ago, is still the most commonly used stain in the microbiology laboratory. It involves applying a sequence of primary dye, mordant, decolorizer, and counterstain to the slide. The dyes are taken up differently according to the chemical composition of the cell walls. Bacteria react best in the Gram stain when they are 24 hours old or less. Gram-positive bacteria stain purple, and gram-negative bacteria stain pink or red (Figure 55-11). Although Gram staining is considered a CLIA moderately complex test, it is useful for the medical assistant to understand the procedures and the microscopic results obtained.

PROCEDURE 55-4

Perform Microbiologic Testing: Perform a Screening Urine Culture Test

GOAL: *To assess the level of bacteriuria using a dip and count method so as to aid in the diagnosis of urinary tract infections.*

EQUIPMENT and SUPPLIES

- Clean catch midstream (CCMS) urine specimen
- Uricult test kit
- Incubator
- Biohazardous waste container
- Disposable gloves
- Patient's record

PROCEDURAL STEPS

1. Sanitize your hands, assemble the equipment and the specimen, and put on gloves. Check the expiration date on the test kit. Label the vial with the patient information (Figure 1).

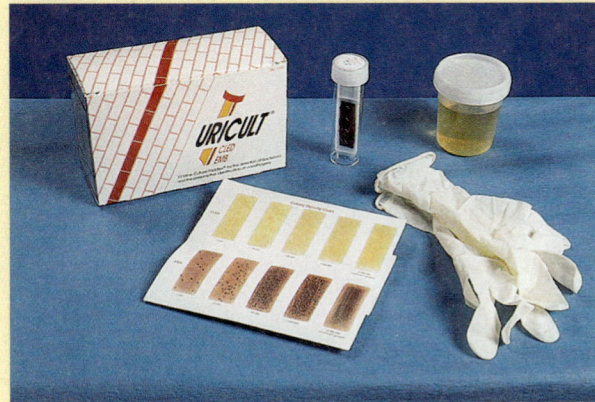

(From Bonewit-West K: *Clinical procedures for medical assistants,* ed 5, Philadelphia, 2000, WB Saunders.)

PURPOSE: An expired test kit may yield inaccurate test results.
2. Remove the slide from the test kit. Do not touch the slide or lay it down.
PURPOSE: Touching the slide or laying it down contaminates the slide.
3. Dip the slide into the urine specimen, tipping the cup carefully if necessary. Alternatively, the urine may be poured over the slide and caught in another container (Figure 2).

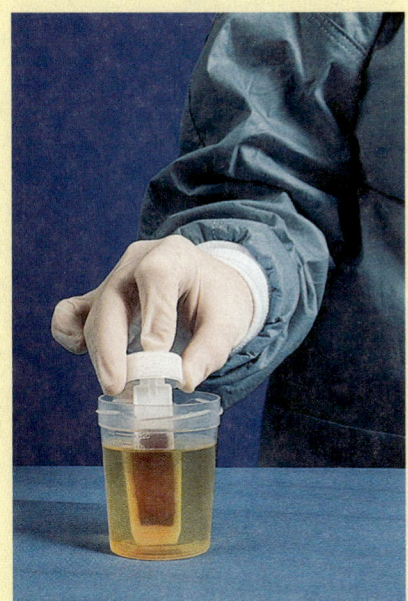

(From Bonewit-West K: *Clinical procedures for medical assistants,* ed 5, Philadelphia, 2000, WB Saunders.)

PURPOSE: The entire slide must be covered with urine for accurate results.
4. Allow excess urine to drain and then replace the slide in the protective vial. Screw the cap on loosely.
PURPOSE: The cap must be loose to allow gas exchange in the tube.
5. Incubate the vial upright in an incubator at 35° to 37° C (90° to 98.6° F) for 18 to 24 hours.
PURPOSE: Incubation for less or more time may produce erroneous results. Disease-causing bacteria grow best at body temperature, which is 35° to 37° C (90° to 98.6° F).
6. After incubation, the test results are interpreted by removing the slide from its protective vial, assessing the bacterial colony density, and comparing the density on the slide with the density chart provided. No actual colony counting is necessary (Figure 3).

PROCEDURE 55-4—cont'd

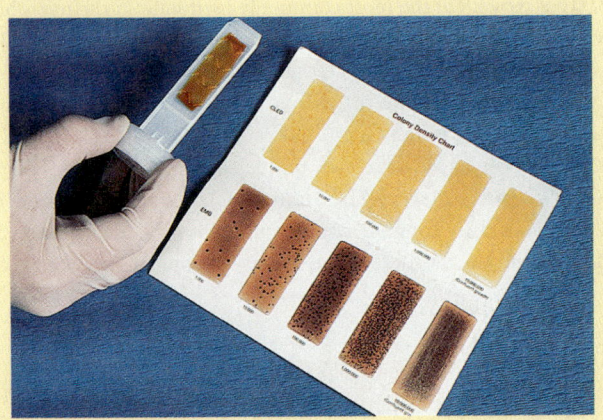

(From Bonewit-West K: *Clinical procedures for medical assistants,* ed 5, Philadelphia, 2000, WB Saunders.

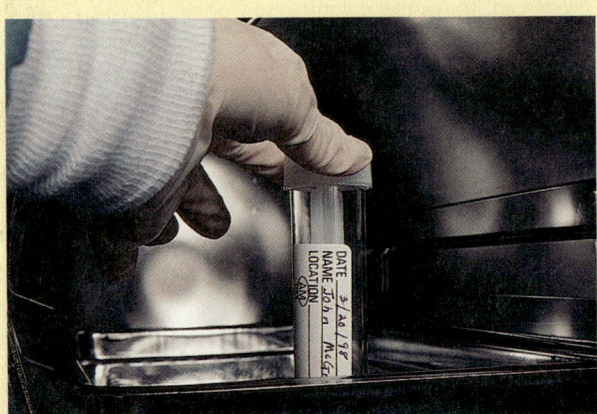

(From Bonewit-West K: *Clinical procedures for medical assistants,* ed 5, Philadelphia, 2000, WB Saunders.)

7. The results are interpreted as follows:
   - Normal: <10,000 colony-forming units (cfu)/mL of urine; no urinary tract infection (UTI) is present.
   - Borderline: 10,000 to 100,000 cfu/mL of urine; a chronic or relapsing infection may be present, and the test should be repeated.
   - Positive: >100,000 cfu/mL of urine; a UTI is likely.
8. Return the vial to the protective case and replace the cap.
9. Dispose of the test in a biohazardous waste container (Figure 4).

PURPOSE: The slide is contaminated. Alternatively, the protective case may be filled with a disinfectant, such as 1:10 chlorine bleach, before the slide is reinserted.

10. Remove your gloves and sanitize your hands.
    PURPOSE: To ensure infection control.
11. Record the results in the patient's medical record.
    PURPOSE: A procedure is not considered done until it is recorded.

PROCEDURE 55-5

Prepare a Direct Smear or Culture Smear for Staining

GOAL: *To prepare a smear for staining from a clinical specimen or from a culture medium.*

EQUIPMENT and SUPPLIES

- Clean glass slides
- Permanent marker
- Incinerator
- Normal saline solution
- Specimen collected on a smear
- 24-hour culture on agar
- Biohazardous waste container
- Disposable gloves
- Face protection

PROCEDURAL STEPS

Direct Smear
1. Sanitize your hands. Put on face protection and gloves.
2. Label the slide with a permanent marking pen.
   PURPOSE: Other labels are destroyed in the staining process.
3. Prepare a thin smear by rolling the swab on the slide. Make sure all areas of the swab touch the slide (Figure 1).

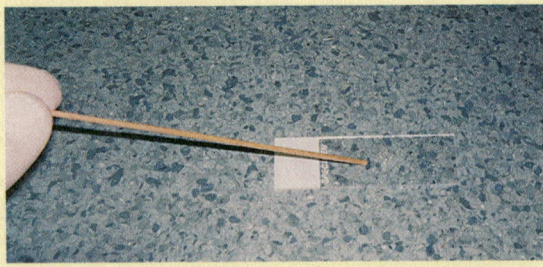

PURPOSE: Rolling the swab ensures that all parts of the swab come in contact with the slide so that the organisms collected are deposited on the slide. Thin smears are needed for evaluation.

4. Allow the smear to air dry. Do not wave it or heat dry it.
   PURPOSE: Waving the slide spreads pathogens. Overheating organisms distorts them.
5. Hold the slide with the smear up. Heat-fix the slide using an incinerator. Check the heating process by touching the slide to the back of the gloved hand (Figure 2). The slide should feel warm, not hot. Check it often by

touching the back of the slide to the back of the gloved hand. Cool the slide.
PURPOSE: Heat-fixing causes materials to adhere to the slide.

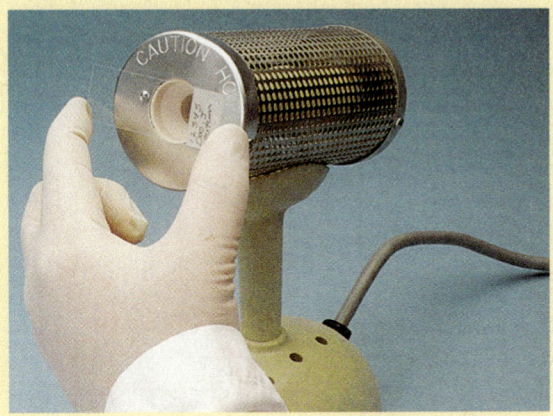

Culture Smear

1. Sanitize your hands. Put on face protection and gloves.
2. Identify the colonies to be stained by circling them on the back of the plate and numbering them with a permanent marker. Label the slide accordingly.
   PURPOSE: This allows accurate identification of colonies.
3. Using a loop, apply a small drop of saline solution to the slide.
   PURPOSE: Liquid is needed to emulsify the colony. Large drops require a longer drying time.
4. Using a sterile loop, touch only the top of the colony chosen. Transfer the material picked up to the appropriate area of the slide and spread it in a circular motion to the size of a dime. Repeat for each colony chosen using a separate slide.
   PURPOSE: Only a small amount of colony is needed for staining.
5. Allow the smear to air dry.
6. Heat-fix the smear as described for a direct smear.
7. Properly dispose of all biohazardous materials and clean the work area.
8. Remove your gloves and sanitize your hands.

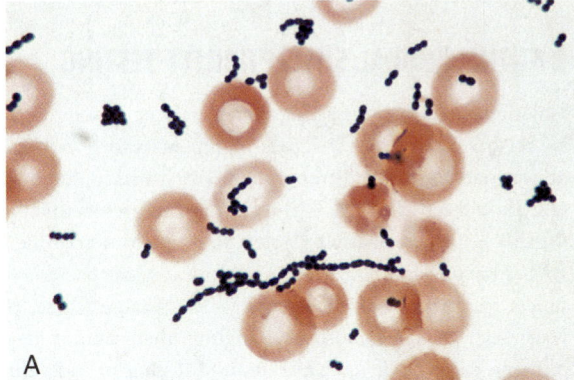
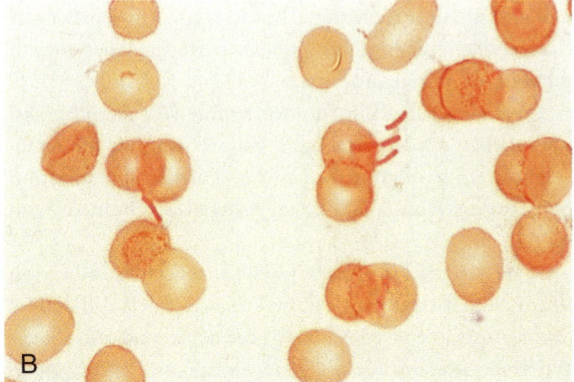

FIGURE 55-11 Gram stain. **A,** Red blood cells (RBCs) and gram-positive cocci. **B,** RBCs with gram-negative bacilli. (From De la Maza LM, Pezzlo MT, Baron EJ: *Color atlas of diagnostic microbiology,* St Louis, 1997, Mosby.)

Acid-Fast Stain

The acid-fast stain is used in the identification protocol for *Mycobacterium* species. *M. tuberculosis* and *M. avium* complex (MAC) are two important species of mycobacteria. The former causes tuberculosis and can be isolated from sputum or tissue samples from infected patients; the latter is a common soil organism that enters through the respiratory tract and disseminates throughout the body. MAC is the third most common cause of death among patients with acquired immunodeficiency syndrome (AIDS). For the acid-fast stain, a sequence of primary dye (carbolfuchsin), decolorizer (acid-alcohol), and counterstain (methylene blue) is applied. Two procedures can be used, both of which help disrupt the waxy cell wall to facilitate staining. In the Ziehl-Neelsen protocol, the primary dye is applied in the presence of heat; in the Kinyoun protocol, the primary dye is mixed with a detergent. Acid-fast–positive bacilli often are referred to as *AFB* (Figure 55-12).

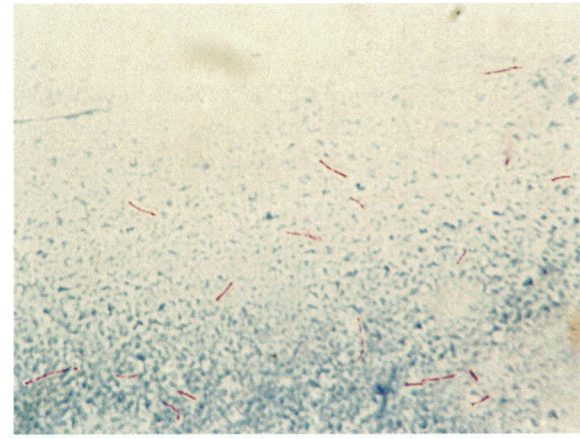

FIGURE 55-12 The acid-fast stain. Pink acid-fast bacilli (AFB) are seen in this smear. (From De la Maza LM, Pezzlo MT, Baron EJ: *Color atlas of diagnostic microbiology,* St Louis, 1997, Mosby.)

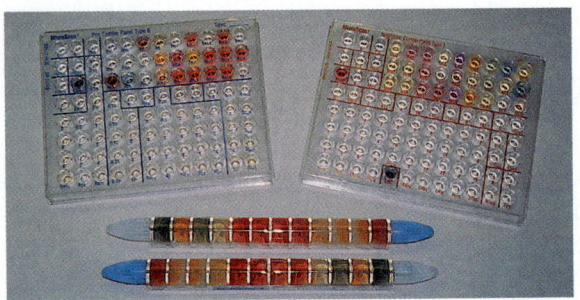

FIGURE 55-13 Enterotube II and Microscan identification tests. (From Stepp CA, Woods MA: *Laboratory procedures for medical office personnel*, Philadelphia, 1998, WB Saunders.)

Biochemical Testing

Once a suspected pathogen has been isolated and is in pure culture, biochemical testing must be performed to identify the genus and species. Some of these tests, such as a catalase rapid enzyme test or an oxidase test, take only a few minutes. Others, such as fermentation testing using various carbohydrates, take up to 24 hours. Hundreds of tests are available to identify an organism biochemically, and manufacturers have developed miniaturized multitest systems that speed inoculation and identification (Figure 55-13).

Rapid Identification Methods

POLs with appropriate CLIA certification can perform many rapid culture and identification tests. The tests used in a particular laboratory depend on the number of tests performed per month and the amount of refrigerator space available for storage. Dry media tests have a long shelf life, do not require refrigeration, and occupy little incubator space. The rapid culture methods offer presumptive identification of most organisms. Further specialization and sensitivity testing require additional materials, equipment, and procedures.

Rapid tests are designed to give the physician a positive indication of the problem so that treatment can be initiated. For a differential or a specific diagnosis, the physician may need additional tests. Some of the rapid tests available detect *Neisseria* species, *Haemophilus* species, and anaerobes. CLIA-waived tests include rapid detection tests for *S. pyogenes*, influenza A and B, and respiratory syncytial virus (RSV) in clinical samples.

Rapid Strep Testing

Rapid strep testing is commonly performed in the POL and can be completed while the patient waits. The patient's throat is swabbed (see Procedure 37-8), the swab is placed in an extraction tube, and the extract is tested for proteins found on the surface of *S. pyogenes* (Procedure 55-6) using an immunochromatographic assay. Negative test results should be confirmed with a throat culture; the rapid strep tests are highly specific but not as highly sensitive. This means that if the test results are positive, there is a high degree of confidence that *S. pyogenes* is in the sample; if the test results are negative, the organism may not have been present in sufficient numbers to be detected.

Influenza a and B Testing

Influenza virus causes influenza, or "the flu," a highly contagious, acute viral infection of the respiratory tract. The infection is highly communicable through the respiratory route, and outbreaks typically are seen in the fall and winter. Type A viruses usually are more prevalent than type B viruses; type A viruses typically are associated with epidemics, and type B viruses cause a milder infection. Rapid diagnosis of influenza can assist with decisions to administer antiviral medications, which must be given early in the course of the infection if they are to be effective. CLIA-waived rapid immunochromatographic assays detect both influenza A and influenza B antigens from nasopharyngeal swabs or nasal washes. If a swab is used, the sample is removed from the swab using saline, a transport medium, or a solution provided by the manufacturer. Nasal washings can be used directly in the test kit.

Respiratory Syncytial Virus Testing

RSV is a major cause of upper and lower respiratory tract infections and the major cause of bronchiolitis and pneumonia in children and infants. Outbreaks typically occur yearly in the fall, winter, and spring and can be severe for very young children. The CLIA-waived rapid immunochromatographic assay for RSV uses a nasopharyngeal swab specimen or nasal washings to detect a protein the virus uses to fuse to human cells. Because antiviral agents are available to treat RSV infection, rapid diagnosis can lead to shorter hospital stays, a reduced need for antibiotic therapy to treat secondary bacterial infection, and a lower cost for hospital care. The tests are intended for children under age 5.

ANTIMICROBIAL SUSCEPTIBILITY TESTING

Isolating the infectious agent from a patient is only the first step in successful treatment. When a physician wants to determine the appropriate antibiotic through laboratory testing, he or she orders a culture and sensitivity (C&S) test. "Culture" refers to cultivating the organisms, and "sensitivity" refers to a test to determine the organism's susceptibility to certain antibiotics. Most bacteria show resistance to **antimicrobial agents**, and because these patterns of resistance are continuously changing, they cannot be predicted. Shifting patterns of resistance require testing of individual bacteria against the appropriate antimicrobial agent.

The clinical microbiology laboratory can recommend antimicrobial agents based only on their **in vitro** activity. The healthcare practitioner must decide which medication to order based on test results and a physical examination.

Whenever specimens are inoculated, asepsis must be strictly observed to ensure safety and good results. The organism being tested must also be isolated in pure culture before the test. The test, often referred to as the *Kirby-Bauer Antimicrobial Susceptibility Test*, is performed by inoculating sterile water with the pure culture of bacteria to a specified degree of **turbidity**. This suspension is spread with a swab in a lawn pattern on the surface of the appropriate agar medium. Disks that each contain an antimicrobial agent, such as penicillin or tetracycline, are placed on the agar with forceps or an automatic dispenser. After incubation, the zone of inhibition (area of no growth) around each disk is measured in millimeters and compared with values provided by the manufacturer of the disks (Figure 55-14). Three determinations are possible: S, R, or I. S means that the pathogen is "susceptible," or that the antibiotic is effective against the organism in that particular concentration in

PROCEDURE 55-6

Screen Test Results: Perform a Rapid Strep Test

GOAL: *To perform a rapid strep screening test to assist in the diagnosis of strep throat and to follow up negative results by performing a throat culture collection.*

EQUIPMENT and SUPPLIES

- Directigen Strep A test kit
- Timer or wristwatch with sweep second hand
- Throat swab specimen (see Procedure 37-8)
- Biohazardous waste container
- Disposable gloves
- Face protection
- Patient's record

PROCEDURAL STEPS

1. Collect all necessary supplies and equipment. Bring all reagents and reaction disks to room temperature (minimum of 30 minutes).
2. Sanitize your hands. Put on gloves and face protection.
   PURPOSE: To ensure infection control.
3. Position all bottles vertically and dispense reagents slowly as free-falling drops. Avoid reagent contact with your eyes, because the reagent is an irritant (Figure 1).

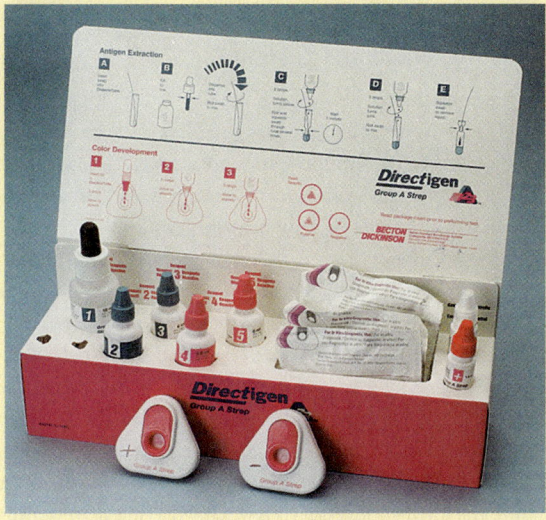

4. Add three drops of reagent 1 to an extraction tube. This solution is pink.
5. Add three drops of reagent 2 to the same tube. The solution should turn yellow.
6. Place the specimen swab in the tube, twirling the swab in the mix.
7. Let stand for exactly 1 minute.
8. Add three drops of reagent 3 to the same tube, again twirling the swab in the tube to mix. This solution should be pink.
9. Express the liquid from the swab by squeezing the tube with the thumb and forefinger and rotating the swab as it is withdrawn. The liquid must be thoroughly removed from the swab. Best results are achieved when the liquid reaches or exceeds the line on the tube.
10. Discard the swab in a biohazardous waste container.
11. Remove the reaction disk from the pouch and place it on a dry, flat surface.
12. Pour the entire contents of the tube into the reaction disk.
13. Read the test results when the entire end of the assay window turns red (5 to 10 minutes).
14. Properly dispose of all contaminated waste.
    PURPOSE: Items that come in contact with samples are considered potentially infectious.
15. Disinfect the work area, remove your gloves, and sanitize your hands.
    PURPOSE: To ensure infection control.
16. Record the test results in the patient's medical record.
    PURPOSE: A procedure is considered not done until it is properly recorded.
17. If the test results are negative, a second throat swab should be obtained and a throat culture should be performed. Often two swabs are used simultaneously when the sample is collected from the throat to prevent the need to recollect a specimen.
    PURPOSE: Negative rapid strep test results should be confirmed with a throat culture.

---

vitro; R means that the organism is "resistant" to the antibiotic; I means "intermediate"; that is, additional testing must be performed to determine the dosage of antimicrobial necessary for therapeutic treatment.

CRITICAL THINKING APPLICATION   55-5

Anna has recorded the results of Ms. Walker's urine culture. She notes that 10 antimicrobial agents had been tested, but the *Escherichia coli* was susceptible to only five of them. How will Dr. Ling determine which of these five antibiotics would be best for Ms. Walker?

MISCELLANEOUS MICROBIOLOGIC TESTING

Testing for Pinworms

Enterobius vermicularis, commonly called the pinworm, is a species of parasite that infests primarily young children. Humans are infected by ingesting mature eggs through hand-to-mouth transfers, feces-contaminated fingers, or feces-contaminated foods or liquids or by inhaling eggs in air currents from infected areas. The eggs hatch in the small intestine, and the females migrate out of the anus, usually at night, to deposit the eggs. The eggs adhere to the skin, perianal hairs, sleeping garments, and other clothing. This results in itching

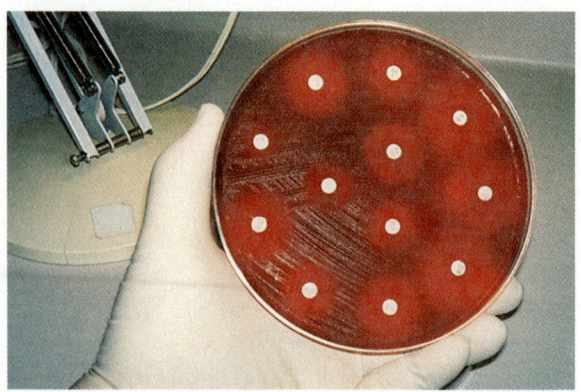

FIGURE 55-14 Antimicrobial susceptibility test. Note the zones of inhibition around 11 of the 12 disks.

of the anal area, which causes the eggs to come in contact with the hands and fingernails of the host.

In children, specimens are best collected late at night or early in the morning before a bowel movement, urination, or bathing. Paraffin swabs impregnated with petroleum jelly or cellulose tape may be used to collect the eggs deposited by the adult worm during the night. The diagnosis is based on laboratory detection of the eggs in fecal smears. If the parent does not feel comfortable about obtaining the needed specimen, instruct the parent to bring the child to the office as soon as he or she awakens in the morning. Instruct the parent not to change the child's clothing or the child's diaper before coming to the office, but to bring the child immediately on waking. When the child arrives, have all the needed supplies ready to use and perform the procedure immediately (Procedure 55-7).

Immunologic Testing

Immunologic testing provides information about past or present infections with bacteria or viruses and also is done to detect certain types of cancers. Testing done in the immunology laboratory is designed to demonstrate the reaction between antigen and antibody. Antibodies are formed when the body encounters a foreign agent. In the acute phase of a disease, the antibody level is high; during the convalescent stage, the antibody level declines. Once an antigen has been recognized by the immune system and antibodies have been made, the level of antibody to that particular antigen remains at a low but detectable level indefinitely. The amount of antibody at any given time can be measured with serologic testing and is referred to as the *titer*.

The reaction between antigen and antibody is demonstrated in vitro through several means, most commonly agglutination, precipitation, and immunochromatographic assay. In agglutination and precipitation reactions, latex beads or red blood cells (RBCs) from an animal such as a rabbit are needed. The antigen or antibody is chemically bound to the bead or cell by the manufacturer. When the corresponding antibody or antigen molecule comes into contact with the bead or cell, they link and clump (agglutinate). If this reaction occurs in a test tube, the clumps precipitate to the bottom of the tube. If the reaction occurs on a glass or paper surface, such as a slide, the clumps are visible to the naked eye. Antigen and antibody must be present in roughly equal proportions for clumping to occur, because the linking is much like latticework. If markedly more

antigen than antibody is present, or vice versa, the lattice cannot form properly; this is a false-negative reaction and is called the *prozone reaction.*

Immunochromatographic assays are replacing many of the precipitation and agglutination tests in the serology laboratory because of their enhanced specificity and sensitivity. Solid-phase immunoassay, described in Chapter 52, involves the immobilization (attachment) of antigens or antibodies on solid surfaces such as beads, wells in plastic dishes, or plastic cartridges. Generally, when an antigen-antibody reaction occurs, a color change is visible. With some tests, the more intense the color, the higher the concentration of the antibody being measured.

Most serologic testing performed in the physician's office is done with individual testing kits. When a serologic test is performed, the first step is to review the package insert provided by the manufacturer. This review provides valuable information about the test, the principle on which the test is based, the reagents and equipment required, proper specimen collection techniques, preparation requirements, test procedures, and any precautions or warnings that pertain to the procedure. In addition, the inserts provide information about quality control, interpretation of results, limitations of the procedure performance characteristics, and references.

CLIA-waived tests that can be performed by a medical assistant to detect antibody to a pathogen include those for infectious mononucleosis, *Helicobacter pylori*, human immunodeficiency virus (HIV), and Lyme disease.

Infectious Mononucleosis Testing

Infectious mononucleosis, also called "mono" or the "kissing disease," is an acute infectious disease caused by the Epstein-Barr virus (EBV). EBV is one of the most common human viruses. The virus occurs worldwide; it is especially common in teenagers and occasionally in adults, but it is found most frequently in people between the ages of 10 and 25. Most people are infected with EBV at some time during their lives. In the United States, as many as 95% of adults between 35 and 40 years of age have already been infected.

In children the infection may pass unrecognized or result in a mild illness lasting only a few days, with sore throat, fever, swollen tonsils, and enlarged lymph nodes in the neck. These signs and symptoms can be indistinguishable from those of other mild illnesses of childhood. In young people, some of the most common complications include the abrupt onset of fatigue, headaches, aching muscles, faint rash, fever, very swollen tonsils, enlarged lymph glands, and loss of appetite often associated with nausea. There may be a short or prolonged period (days or weeks) after the initial illness when the fatigue continues. Occasionally, complications occur, including the development of a swollen spleen or liver. Heart problems or any involvement of the central nervous system (CNS) is rare, and infectious mononucleosis is almost never fatal.

Testing for mononucleosis involves a complete blood count (CBC) and serologic tests. The CBC reveals an increased number of lymphocytes that appear atypical on the differential examination. The infected lymphocytes undergo a cellular transformation, causing them to take on an appearance similar to a monocyte (hence the name *mononucleosis*). Most patients exposed to EBV develop a nonspecific antibody response to the virus. The antibodies react with surface antigens of horse erythrocytes, causing agglutination

Obtain a Specimen for Microbiologic Testing: Perform a Cellulose Tape Collection for Pinworms

GOAL: *To obtain a rectal sample with cellulose tape for testing for pinworm eggs.*

EQUIPMENT and SUPPLIES

- Glass slide
- Clear cellulose tape
- Wooden tongue depressor
- Toluene
- Microscope
- Gauze or cotton balls
- Biohazardous waste container
- Disposable gloves
- Face protection
- Patient's record

PROCEDURAL STEPS

1. Ask the patient to assist you with this procedure.
2. Gather and prepare the necessary supplies and equipment.
3. Place a strip of cellulose tape on a glass slide, starting ½ inch from one end and running toward the same end. Continue around this end lengthwise. Tear off the strip so that it is even with the other end (Figure 1).
   NOTE: Do not use Magic transparent tape; use regular clear cellulose tape.

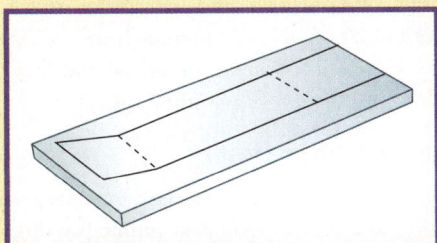

(From Stepp CA, Woods MA: *Laboratory procedures for medical office personnel*, Philadelphia, 1998, WB Saunders.)

4. Place a strip of paper measuring ½ × 1 inch between the slide and the tape at the end where the tape is torn flush; this is the specimen-labeling area. As soon as the child arrives, place the child with the attending parent in the prepared examination room.
5. Sanitize your hands and put on gloves and face protection.
   PURPOSE: To ensure infection control.
6. Remove the child's clothing and diaper and lay the child in a prone position, over the parent's lap, with the buttocks in a superior plane.
7. To obtain the perianal sample, first peel back the tape on the slide by gripping the label (Figure 2). With the tape looped (adhesive side outward) over a wooden tongue depressor that is held against the slide and extended about 1 inch beyond it, press the tape firmly against the right and left anal folds (Figure 3).

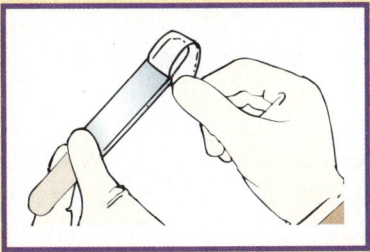

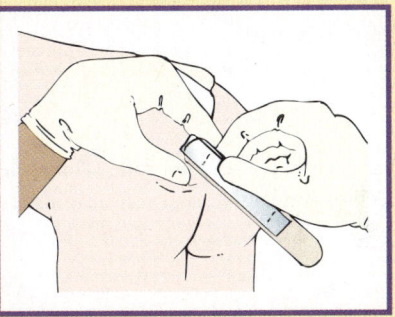

8. Spread the tape back on the slide, adhesive side down (Figure 4).

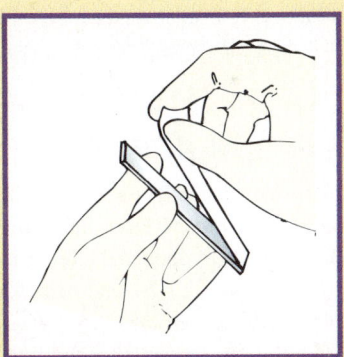

9. Smooth the tape using a cotton ball or gauze square (Figure 5).

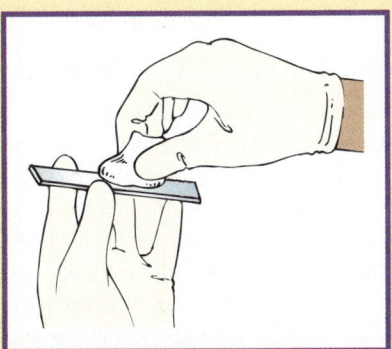

PROCEDURE 55-7—cont'd

10. Write the patient's name and date on the slide label.
11. Advise the parent that the child can be dressed or assist with dressing the child if needed.

Testing the Sample

1. Lift one side of the tape and apply one drop of toluene before pressing the tape back down on the glass slide.
   PURPOSE: This clears the specimen so that any eggs are visible.
2. Place the prepared slide under the microscope's low-power objective for examination by a physician or medical technologist under low illumination (Figure 6).
3. Record the results in the patient's record.
4. Dispose of all biohazardous waste, clean the work area, remove your gloves, and sanitize your hands.

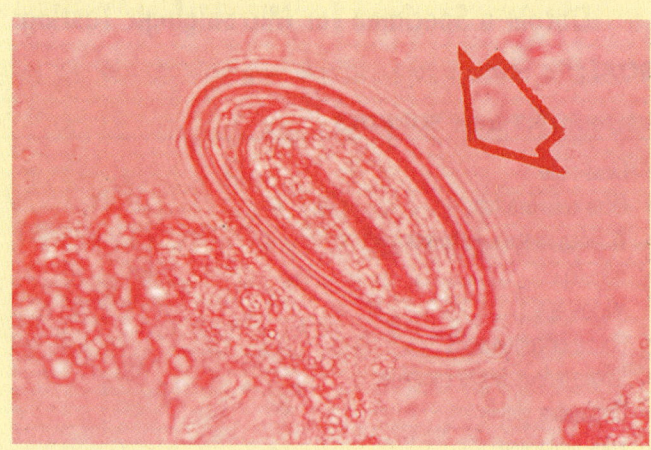

(clumping) that is visible on the test slide (Procedure 55-8). Solid-phase immunochromatographic assay tests may also be used to diagnose EBV.

CRITICAL THINKING APPLICATION   55-6

Tiffany Warhola, a seventh grade student, visits Dr. Chowdry complaining of extreme fatigue and a sore throat. Dr. Chowdry orders a rapid strep test and a mononucleosis test. What sample will Anna need for the rapid strep test? What sample will she need for the mononucleosis test?

Helicobacter Pylori Antibody Testing

H. pylori is a spiral-shaped bacterium that can infect the gastric mucous layer or adhere to the epithelial lining of the stomach. *H. pylori* causes more than 90% of duodenal ulcers and more than 80% of gastric ulcers (see Chapter 39). Several methods can be used to diagnose *H. pylori* infection. Serologic tests that measure specific *H. pylori* IgG antibodies can determine whether a person has been infected. CLIA-waived rapid qualitative immunochromatographic assay tests use whole blood applied to a well in a test cartridge. After the blood migrates through the cartridge, lines appear in the window, indicating the presence of antibodies to the pathogen.

Human Immunodeficiency Virus Antibody Testing

The OraQuick Advance Rapid HIV-1/2 Antibody Test (Ora-Sure Laboratories, Bethlehem, Pennsylvania) is a single-use, qualitative, two-step immunochromatographic assay to detect antibodies to HIV type 1 (HIV-1) and type 2 (HIV-2) in oral fluid and whole blood. It is a CLIA-waived screening test for HIV-1, the virus that causes AIDS (see Chapter 40). However, the test does not detect HIV-1 infection in people who contracted the virus within 3 months (approximately) before taking the test, because it can take that long for detectable antibodies to HIV-1 to appear in the blood. Because this is a screening test, the results must be confirmed by additional, more specific tests. All individuals taking this test must receive the "Subject Information" pamphlet before specimen collection and counseling after receiving their test results.

The test kit (Figure 55-15) includes a testing device with a flat pad that is rubbed once over the upper and lower gums. It then is inserted into the test vial, which is placed in a plastic stand that holds the device at the proper angle. The test results are read in 20 minutes. If whole blood is used, it can be obtained from a finger stick or venipuncture. A specimen loop is dipped into the drop of blood obtained by finger stick or into the venipuncture tube. The blood is mixed into the collection vial, and the testing device is inserted. Results are read in 20 minutes. The test includes an internal control band that verifies that a specimen was added and that the test was run correctly.

Lyme Disease Antibody Testing

Lyme disease is the most common insect-borne infectious disease in North America, and it is a significant public health concern. The spirochete bacterium, *Borrelia burgdorferi*, is the causative agent in Lyme disease.

The disease is contracted from the bite of a tick with saliva that contains the bacteria. These ticks typically are found on deer, mice, dogs, horses, and birds. Infection occurs after the bacteria enter the wound, and a characteristic bull's-eye rash, known as *erythema migrans* (EM), may develop at the bite site in 60% to 80% of patients. Lyme disease progresses in three stages, which have unclear transition and overlapping symptoms. As the disease progresses, the spirochete bacterium invades the skin, joints, CNS, heart, eyes, bones, spleen, and kidneys. Arthritic or CNS syndromes often accompany late-stage disease and may be the only clinical, symptomatic indications of infection.

Early detection of Lyme disease can be accomplished using a CLIA-waived test such as the Wampole PreVue *B. burgdorferi* test (MedPointe Co., Princeton, New Jersey). This immunochromatographic assay tests for IgG and IgM antibodies in whole blood. A sample of blood is applied to a test cartridge, a diluent is added, and the results are read in 20 minutes. Positive results should be verified by confirmatory testing.

PROCEDURE 55-8

Perform Immunologic Testing: Perform the Mono-Test for Infectious Mononucleosis

GOAL: *To perform and interpret a slide test for infectious mononucleosis.*

EQUIPMENT and SUPPLIES

- Mono-Test kit
- Blood specimen (serum or plasma)
- Timer or wristwatch with sweep second hand
- Biohazardous waste container
- Disposable gloves
- Face protection
- Patient's record

PROCEDURAL STEPS

1. Remove the test kit from the refrigerator and allow the reagents to warm to room temperature. Check the expiration date of the kit.
   <u>PURPOSE:</u> Outdated or cold reagents do not react as expected.
2. Sanitize your hands. Put on face protection and gloves.
   <u>PURPOSE:</u> To ensure infection control
3. Fill a disposable capillary tube to the calibration mark with serum or plasma (see Chapter 53 for collection of blood). Using the rubber bulb included in the kit, deposit the specimen in the first circle of the clean glass or paper slide also provided in the kit (Figure 1).
   <u>PURPOSE:</u> The capillary tube measures the exact amount of sample for accurate testing.

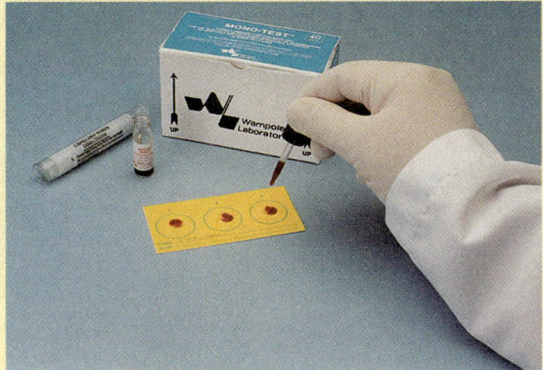

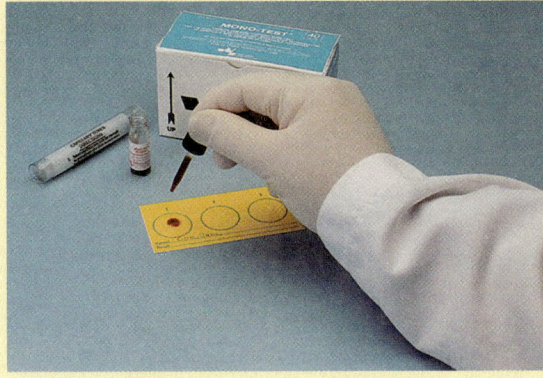

4. Place one drop of negative control in the second circle and one drop of positive control in the third circle (Figure 2).
   <u>PURPOSE:</u> Known controls ensure that reagents are functioning properly.

5. Thoroughly mix the Mono-Test reagent by rolling the bottle gently between the palms of the hands. Squeeze the enclosed dropper to mix all the contents of the bottle.
   <u>PURPOSE:</u> Reagent RBCs settle on standing and must be mixed before use.
6. Hold the dropper in a vertical position and add one drop of Mono-Test reagent to each area of the slide. Do not touch the dropper to the slide.
   <u>PURPOSE:</u> Holding a dropper vertically ensures delivery of the same size drop. If the dropper touches other materials, it becomes contaminated, and the results will be inaccurate.
7. Using separate stirrers, quickly and thoroughly mix each area, spreading each area out to 1 inch in diameter.
   <u>PURPOSE:</u> Failure to use a clean stirrer for each area would invalidate the test because of cross-contamination.
8. Rock the slide gently for exactly 2 minutes; observe immediately for agglutination. A dark background is best for viewing.
   <u>PURPOSE:</u> Timing is always important.
9. Interpret the test results and record them. Agglutination is positive, and no agglutination is negative.
10. Disinfect the work area, remove your gloves, and sanitize your hands.
11. Record the test results in the patient's medical record.
    <u>PURPOSE:</u> A procedure is not considered done until it is properly recorded.

▌CLOSING COMMENTS

▌Patient Education

Microorganisms such as bacteria, viruses, fungi, and parasites are responsible for most human diseases. Patient education plays an important role in helping the patient and family control the spread of infection. The following list of teaching topics can help you educate a patient in infection control:

- An explanation of the patient's type of infection—bacterial, viral, fungal, or parasitic
- How infection spreads
- Normal barriers to infection
- Risk factors for infection
- Patient preparation for cultures and serologic, hematologic, and imaging tests, as necessary
- The patient's role in specimen collection

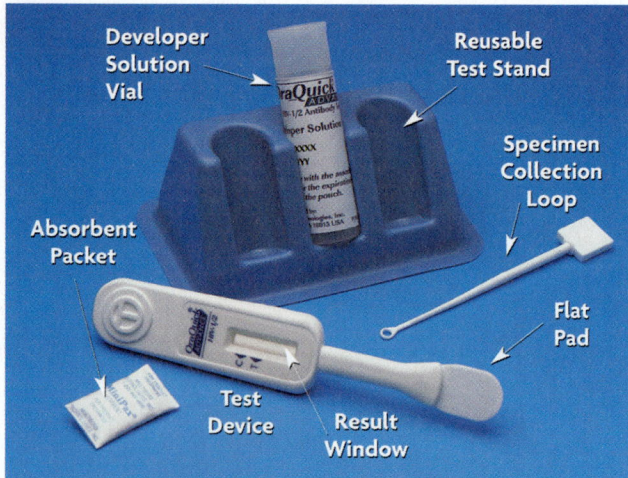

FIGURE 55-15 HIV test kit. (Courtesy OraSure Technologies, Bethlehem, Pa.)

- Hand sanitization, proper storage and cleaning of personal items, and disposal of contaminated supplies

Explain to the patient that infection does not always occur at the entry site; for example, measles can be transmitted through the respiratory tract. Reinforce the need for strict adherence to the prescribed antimicrobial therapy by pointing out the possible complications of noncompliance, such as relapse or systemic involvement. Explain to the patient that inadequate drug therapy (not taking the medication as prescribed) may cause the infection to worsen and spread.

Above all, always listen to the patient; be sure to answer all questions. However, do not try to answer a question if you are unsure of the answer. Notify the physician of the patient's concerns so that he or she can provide further detail before the patient leaves the facility.

CRITICAL THINKING APPLICATION   55-7

Aaron's culture was confirmed as *Staphylococcus aureus*. What information can Anna give Aaron and his mother about the contagiousness of this infection?

Legal and Ethical Issues

Maintaining a laboratory in the office increases the physician's liability. By testing patients' specimens in the office, the physician assumes responsibility for the interpretation and accuracy of the results. As the person in the office who runs the tests and notes the results in the patient's record, you are responsible for maintaining optimum accuracy in testing results. A quality assurance (QA) program for POLs may reduce the risks involved and still allow the patient to benefit from the convenience of office testing. Strict confidentiality is essential. Never release information to anyone other than the patient or legal guardian; however, certain infectious diseases must be reported to the Centers for Disease Control and Prevention (CDC) or local board of health. Each state legislature determines how the data is to be reported and what diseases must be reported. The data for nationally notifiable diseases is published weekly by the CDC in the *Morbidity and Mortality Weekly Report* (MMR). An annual report is available on the Internet at *www.cdc.gov*. The 2012 summary lists the following conditions as notifiable.

Nationally Notifiable Infectious Conditions

- Anthrax
- Arboviral neuroinvasive and non-neuroinvasive diseases
- Babesiosis
- Botulism
- Chancroid
- *Chlamydia trachomatis,* genital infections
- Cholera
- Coccidioidomycosis
- Cryptosporidiosis
- Cyclosporiasis
- Dengue
- Diphtheria
- Ehrlichiosis/anaplasmosis
- Giardiasis
- Gonorrhea
- *Haemophilus influenzae,* invasive disease
- Hansen's disease (leprosy)
- Hantavirus pulmonary syndrome
- Hemolytic uremic syndrome, postdiarrheal
- Hepatitis, viral, acute (A, B, C)
- Hepatitis, viral, chronic
- HIV infection (acquired immunodeficiency syndrome [AIDS] is now classified as HIV stage III)
- Influenza-associated pediatric mortality
- Legionellosis
- Listeriosis
- Lyme disease
- Malaria
- Measles
- Meningococcal disease
- Mumps
- Novel influenza A virus infections
- Pertussis
- Plague
- Poliomyelitis, paralytic
- Poliovirus infection, nonparalytic
- Psittacosis
- Q fever (acute and chronic)
- Rabies
- Rocky Mountain spotted fever and spotted fever rickettsioses
- Rubella (German measles)
- Rubella, congenital syndrome
- Salmonellosis
- Severe acute respiratory syndrome–associated *Coronavirus* (SARS)
- Shiga toxin–producing *Escherichia coli* (STEC)
- Shigellosis
- Smallpox
- Streptococcal toxic shock syndrome
- *Streptococcus pneumoniae* invasive disease
- Syphilis (all stages and congenital)
- Tetanus
- Toxic shock syndrome (other than streptococcal)
- Trichinellosis (Trichinosis)
- Tuberculosis
- Tularemia
- Typhoid fever

- Vancomycin-intermediate *Staphylococcus aureus* (VISA)
- Vancomycin-resistant *Staphylococcus aureus* (VRSA)
- Varicella (morbidity)
- Varicella (deaths only)
- Vibriosis
- Viral hemorrhagic fever (VHF)
- Yellow fever

Nationally Notifiable Noninfectious Conditions

- Cancer
- Elevated blood lead levels (child: <16 years; adult: ≥16 years)
- Foodborne disease outbreak
- Pesticide-related illness, acute
- Silicosis
- Waterborne disease outbreak

SUMMARY OF SCENARIO

It seems to Anna that she sees something new about harmful bacteria on the television or in the newspaper every day. Outbreaks on cruise ships and bio-warfare have become common topics, yet Anna knows that most bacteria are harmless. People can protect themselves from infection by using a few simple techniques, such as frequently sanitizing the hands and keeping the hands away from the face. Anna makes a point of explaining this to the patients she sees at the family clinic. Prevention, she knows, is the key to controlling infection.

Anna realizes that the POL can play a vital role in the diagnosis and treatment of infectious disease. She knows that proper specimen collection is of the utmost importance in microbiology testing and that contamination could mean vital time lost in identifying pathogens. Rapid testing allows for quick diagnosis, which is important when dealing with infectious organisms that reproduce quickly. Anna has learned that certain microbiology tests are CLIA waived,

whereas others can be performed in a POL that has obtained a certificate for CLIA moderate-complexity testing. As a CMA (AAMA) she is qualified to perform waived tests, and with the appropriate documented training, she may perform moderately complex tests. Testing, she has discovered, may not always involve detection of the pathogen itself. Culturing on artificial media may be performed on urine, wound, or throat specimens, and sometimes the pathogen is detected by demonstrating its presence using a rapid identification test, such as the rapid strep test. At other times, however, antibodies made in response to the pathogen must be detected to diagnose the disease, such as with the mononucleosis test.

Anna knows that the technology for rapid testing is evolving quickly, and she is aware that she can easily check the FDA's Web site for new tests that could be performed in the POL.

SUMMARY OF LEARNING OBJECTIVES

1. **Define, spell, and pronounce the terms listed in the vocabulary.**
   Spelling and pronouncing medical terms correctly bolster the medical assistant's credibility. Knowing the definitions of these terms promotes confidence in communication with patients and co-workers.

2. **Apply critical thinking skills in performing the patient assessment and patient care.**
   Completing the Critical Thinking Application exercises throughout the chapter can help the student medical assistant become more adept at critical analysis of real-life situations.

3. **Cite the protocols for the collection, transport, and processing of specimens.**
   Specimens for the microbiology laboratory must be collected in sterile containers. Transport systems are available if the specimen cannot be plated immediately. These systems often contain a transport medium that keeps the organisms alive but does not let them multiply (see Table 55-1).

4. **Identify the elements needed for microbial growth.**
   All microbes require nutrients and water to stay alive. Aerobes require oxygen; anaerobes die in the presence of oxygen. Most pathogens prefer an incubation temperature of 37° C (98.6° F) and a pH of 7.

5. **Compare bacteria with viruses.**
   Viruses differ from bacteria in that they are not cells. Viruses have a core of nucleic acid surrounded by a protein coat. Unlike bacteria, they do not metabolize, and they cannot replicate on their own.

6. **Describe the characteristics of common viral diseases.**
   Refer to Table 55-2.

7. **Describe the bacterial structures used in identification.**
   Some bacteria have flagella protruding from the cell wall. These structures aid in propulsion. Some bacteria produce gelatinous capsules that enhance their virulence. Bacteria in the genera *Bacillus* and *Clostridium* produce endospores that allow them to survive harsh conditions.

8. **Describe various bacterial morphologies.**
   Identification of bacteria begins with the observation of their morphology. Cocci are spheric organisms, bacilli are rod-shaped organisms, and spirilla are spiral-shaped organisms. Staphylococci are cocci in clusters; streptococci and streptobacilli are organisms arranged in chains, and diplococci and diplobacilli are organisms arranged in pairs.

9. **Explain the characteristics of common diseases caused by bacteria.**
   Refer to Tables 55-3 to 55-5.

10. **Compare bacteria with fungi, parasites, and protozoa.**
    Bacteria are prokaryotic; fungi, protozoa, and parasites are eukaryotic. Bacteria, fungi, and protozoa must be observed microscopically; helminths, or worms, can be seen with the naked eye (see Tables 55-3 to 55-8).

11. **Describe the unusual characteristics of *Chlamydia*, *Rickettsia*, and *Mycoplasma* organisms.**
    Chlamydia and *Rickettsia* organisms are tiny bacteria, but unlike most bacteria, they require a host cell for replication. *Rickettsia* organisms are transmitted by arthropods. *Mycoplasma* organisms are bacteria without cell walls (see Table 55-6).

12. **Identify the characteristics of common diseases caused by fungi, protozoa, and parasites.**
Refer to Tables 55-7 and 55-8.

13. **Perform patient education on the collection of a stool specimen for ova and parasite testing.**
Stool is collected in special transport devices that contain preservatives and fixatives that will assist the microscopic examination of the specimen. Explicit instructions must be given to the patient to ensure proper collection (see Procedure 55-1).

14. **Describe the equipment needed in a microbiology laboratory.**
Cultivation equipment includes inoculating loops and needles, Petri dishes with agar media, and incubators. Viewing equipment includes slides, stains, and microscopes. Sterilizing equipment includes incinerators and autoclaves.

15. **List the different growth media used for culturing.**
Growth media consists of nutrients selected for certain species. Media can be liquid or can be made solid by the addition of agar. Solid media can be prepared as Petri plates or as tube media. Media can be all purpose and support the growth of many species. It also can be selective, permitting only a certain type of microbe to grow. Media can be differential, allowing differentiation of species based on color changes caused by different biochemical reactions. Enriched media support the growth of fastidious bacteria.

16. **Perform the procedure for inoculating a blood agar plate.**
Refer to Procedure 55-2.

17. **Perform a urine culture.**
Refer to Procedure 55-3.

18. **Perform a screening urine culture test.**
Refer to Procedure 55-4.

19. **Prepare a direct smear or culture smear for staining.**
Refer to Procedure 55-5.

20. **Compare and contrast the throat culture for *Streptococcus pyogenes* with the rapid strep test.**
The throat culture involves obtaining a swabbing of the throat and culturing it on a sheep's blood agar plate. The throat culture is observed for beta hemolysis and susceptibility to bacitracin, both of which indicate the presence of group A beta-hemolytic streptococci. The rapid strep test does not involve culturing but is an immunochromatographic assay that assesses the presence of *Streptococcus* antigen in the sample. A negative rapid strep test should be confirmed with a throat culture.

21. **Perform a rapid strep test.**
Refer to Procedure 55-6.

22. **Describe three microbiologic tests that use a rapid identification technique.**
The rapid strep test detects *S. pyogenes* and is used in the diagnosis of streptococcal pharyngitis. The influenza A and B rapid tests detect surface antigens of the virus that causes influenza. The RSV rapid test detects antigens from RSV, which causes pneumonia and bronchiolitis in young children.

23. **Describe the method used for antimicrobial susceptibility testing.**
Antimicrobial susceptibility testing uses disks impregnated with antimicrobial agents dropped onto the surface of an agar plate inoculated with a pathogen. The pathogen displays susceptibility, resistance, or an intermediate reaction to the antimicrobial agent. These determinations are made by measuring the zone of inhibition around each disk and comparing them with a chart provided by the manufacturer.

24. **Explain how pinworm testing is done and when it must be performed.**
Pinworm testing detects the eggs of the pinworm, *E. vermicularis*. The worm deposits eggs in the anal folds at night. The eggs can be retrieved by using a sticky collection device either late in the evening or in the morning before a bowel movement. The diagnosis is made if the eggs are found microscopically.

25. **Perform a cellulose tape collection for pinworms.**
Refer to Procedure 55-7.

26. **Discuss the purpose of immunologic testing.**
Often cultivation of a pathogen is difficult, or demonstrating the presence of the pathogen with antigen testing is difficult. Immunologic testing detects antibodies to a pathogen.

27. **Describe three rapid immunologic tests that could be done in the physician office laboratory.**
Mononucleosis testing detects the heterophile antibodies made in reaction to infection with the Epstein-Barr virus. Serum, plasma, or whole blood can be used, depending on the test. *H. pylori* testing detects antibodies to the bacterium, which is a common cause of stomach ulcers. Whole blood is used for the test. Rapid HIV testing detects the two viruses, HIV-1 and HIV-2, that cause AIDS. Either oral swabbings or whole blood can be used.

28. **Perform the Mono-test for mononucleosis.**
Refer to Procedure 55-8.

29. **Discuss legal and ethical issues involved in laboratory testing.**
The medical assistant must be aware that patient confidentiality is of utmost importance; however, certain infections must be reported to the CDC and to the local board of health.

CONNECTIONS

📖 **Study Guide Connection:** Go to the Chapter 55 Study Guide. Read and complete the activities.

ⓔ **Evolve Connection:** Go to the Chapter 55 link at *evolve.elsevier.com/kinn* to complete the Chapter Review and Chapter Quiz. Check out the other resources listed for this chapter to make the most of what you have learned from Assisting in Microbiology and Immunology.

SURGICAL SUPPLIES AND INSTRUMENTS

56

SCENARIO

Tom Anderson, CMA (AAMA), works for Dr. Sheila Samanski, a dermatologist who frequently performs minor surgical procedures in the office. Tom assists Dr. Samanski with procedures and is also responsible for maintaining stock supplies in the minor surgery room, including solutions and medications, and for cleaning, maintaining, and inspecting the surgical instruments. Because there are no procedures scheduled for today, Tom is planning to compile an inventory of supplies and equipment and perform routine maintenance activities.

While studying this chapter, think about the following questions:

- What solutions and medications should be available in the surgical area of a medical office?
- What are the typical instruments used in minor surgical procedures?
- How are surgical instruments identified and classified?
- How should surgical instruments be cared for and handled before, during, and after a surgical procedure?
- What types of sutures and needles are used in minor surgical procedures?

LEARNING OBJECTIVES

1. Define, spell, and pronounce the terms listed in the vocabulary.
2. Apply critical thinking skills in performing the patient assessment and patient care.
3. Describe typical solutions and medications used in minor surgical procedures.
4. Summarize methods for identifying surgical instruments used in minor office surgery.
5. Outline the general classifications of surgical instruments.
6. Identify surgical instruments.
7. Describe the care of surgical instruments.
8. Identify types of sutures and surgical needles.
9. Explain the medical assistant's responsibility to help ease patients' concerns about procedures.

VOCABULARY

abscesses Localized collections of pus that may be under the skin or deep within the body and that cause tissue destruction.

cannula (kan'-yoo-lah) A rigid tube that surrounds a blunt trocar or a sharp, pointed trocar inserted into the body; when withdrawn, fluid may escape from the body through the cannula, depending on where it was inserted.

curettage (kyur'-eh-tahjz) The act of scraping a body cavity with a surgical instrument, such as a curette.

dilation The opening or widening of the circumference of a body orifice with a dilating instrument.

dissect To cut or separate tissue with a cutting instrument or scissors.

fascia A sheet or band of fibrous tissue deep in the skin that covers muscles and body organs.

fornix A recess in the upper part of the vagina caused by the protrusion of the cervix into the vaginal wall.

obturator A metal rod with a smooth, rounded tip that is placed in hollow instruments to reduce injury to body tissues during insertion.

patency Open condition of a body cavity or canal.

stylus A metal probe that is inserted into or passed through a catheter, needle, or tube used for clearing purposes or to facilitate passage into a body orifice.

Office surgery is restricted to the management of minor problems and injuries. The medical assistant is expected to prepare the patient and the sterile field, assist the physician as needed, take care of the patient after the procedure, properly disinfect the area, and document appropriately. Some medical assistants are employed in outpatient surgical facilities and are expected to assist with procedures that once were performed in the hospital. Although these more difficult operations may involve complete gowning and gloving with surgical masks and caps, the two surgical chapters in this text limit discussion and descriptions to the routines necessary to prepare for and assist in minor surgery only. This chapter includes a discussion of surgical supplies and instruments, the care and handling of instruments, and the different types of surgical sutures and needles. It prepares you for Chapter 57, which presents sterilization, preparation of the sterile field, specific minor surgical procedures, and care of the patient.

MINOR SURGERY ROOM

When minor surgery is routinely performed, the medical office is designed to include a changing room and a minor surgery room that are separate from the other examining rooms. Larger surgery centers have recovery rooms and family waiting areas. The minor surgery room in the physician's office setting should be near a workroom with a sink and an autoclave if the room does not have its own. It should be easy to disinfect and uncluttered to allow easy movement and minimal dust collection. In addition to the operating table, equipment should include a clock with a second hand, an operating light, sitting stools, and Mayo stands (Figure 56-1). Cabinets with countertops are necessary to serve as a side or back table during the surgery. All surgical supplies are stored in these cabinets. Supplies used in this room should not be used elsewhere, and supplies used elsewhere should not be brought into this room.

SURGICAL SOLUTIONS AND MEDICATIONS

Treatment room supplies include standard solutions and medications that are used in minor surgery and dressing changes. Although the solutions and medications listed here are basic, every physician's office practice has preferred items and methods of applying them. The medical assistant is responsible for their care and for maintaining up-to-date supplies.

Sterile water is kept in two forms. Multiple-dose vials are used as a diluent for medications; larger containers of sterile water are for rinsing instruments that have been in a chemical disinfectant solution.

Sterile physiologic saline solution (0.9%) is also stocked in two sizes. The small multiple-dose vial is used for injection. A larger container of sterile saline is used for rinsing and irrigating wounds. These commercially prepared products are ordered from a medical supply company.

The surgical site on the patient must be prepared preoperatively with an antiseptic skin cleansing preparation to reduce the number of pathogens. Although it is not possible to remove all microorganisms from the skin, it is important to prepare the surgical site to remove transient and pathogenic microorganisms on the skin's surface and to reduce resident flora. In addition, the surgeon's hands and those of the medical assistant require disinfection to reduce the chances of wound contamination even though hands will be covered with sterile gloves. Surgical scrub preparations should have a broad antimicrobial action effective against bacterial spores; they also should work rapidly to reduce transient bacteria, show evidence of persistent activity on the skin, and work despite the presence of organic matter such as blood or wound drainage. Research indicates that chlorhexidine (Hibiscrub or Hibiclens) and povidone-iodine (Betadine) are safe and effective antiseptics.

Even minor surgical procedures require the use of anesthetics, which either are injected locally at the site of the procedure or may be sprayed on the skin as a preinjection anesthetic. For patients who find injections of local anesthesia painful or traumatic, the physician may first spray the injection area with a topical anesthetic, such as Fluori-Methane 15%, which is supplied in 3.5-ounce amber glass bottles for either fine or medium spray. Immediately after spraying the site, the physician makes a series of injections around the area with a local anesthetic.

Another topical anesthetic spray is ethyl chloride, a vapocoolant that controls pain associated with minor surgical procedures, such as lancing boils or incision and drainage of small **abscesses**, by

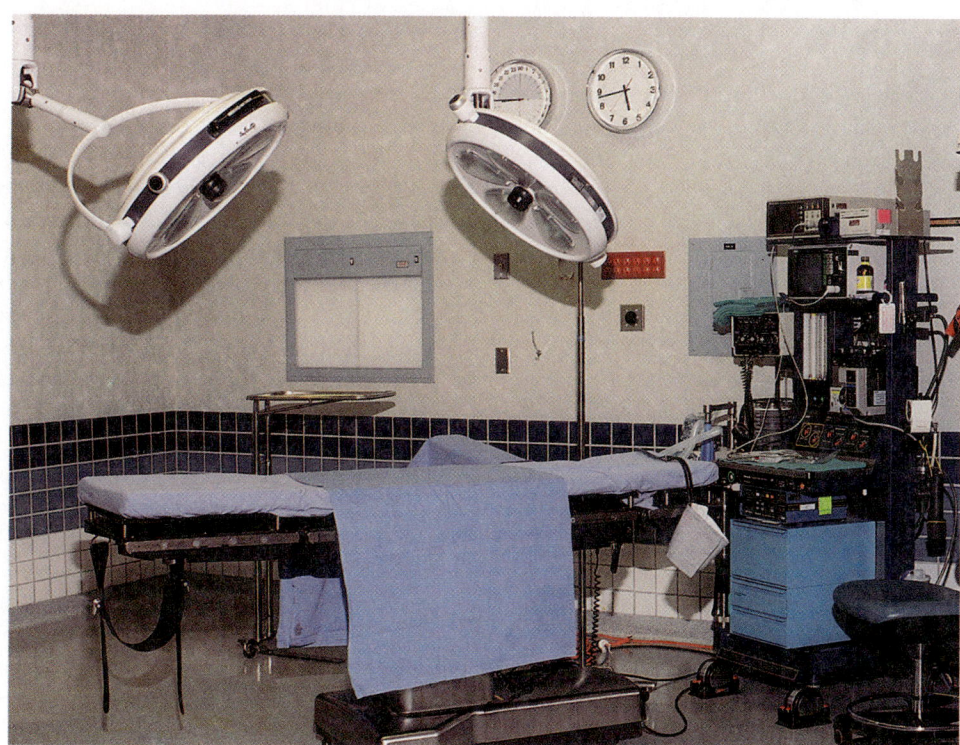

FIGURE 56-1 Operating room and equipment. (Courtesy Fresno Surgery Center, Fresno, Calif.)

causing localized freezing of the affected area. Because ethyl chloride is highly flammable, it should never be used in the presence of electrical cauterizing equipment, and it requires the application of petroleum jelly to surrounding areas to protect them from the cooling action of the spray. It has a short duration, so all equipment must be prepared and the physician must be ready to perform the procedure before it is applied.

Local anesthetics are injected into the subcutaneous tissue. These produce a temporary cessation of feeling at the site of injection by blocking the generation and conduction of nerve impulses. Many different types of local anesthetics are available, but all share the same suffix, *-caine.* Those used most frequently include lidocaine (Xylocaine), chloroprocaine (Nesacaine), and bupivacaine (Sensorcaine). Local anesthetics are purchased in multiple-dose vials of 30 to 50 mL and in varying strengths, such as 0.5%, 1%, and 2%. They begin acting relatively quickly, within 5 to 15 minutes; the duration of action depends on the type of anesthetic, but they usually last 1 to 3 hours. When highly vascular areas are involved, local anesthetics containing epinephrine may be used. Epinephrine causes vasoconstriction at the site, which keeps the anesthetic in the tissues longer, prolonging its effect. It also minimizes local bleeding. However, epinephrine is not used in areas where decreased circulation may cause problems with healing, such as fingertips or toes.

All tissues removed, or biopsied, from the patient are sent to the pathology laboratory for analysis. A 10% formalin solution typically is used to preserve excised tissue for specimens. Specimen bottles are purchased with preservatives included and should be part of the supplies prepared for a surgical procedure if a biopsy is to be done. The physician places the specimen in the container, and the medical assistant is responsible for accurately labeling the container with the patient's name, the date of collection, and the type of specimen.

Sometimes the physician may want to use topical silver nitrate ($AgNO_3$) solution or coated applicator sticks to stop localized bleeding, such as with epistaxis (nosebleed) or capillary bleeding at the site of a wound. The applicators must be kept in lightproof brown containers, and the most commonly used strength is 20%. The applicator sticks are convenient for use in the mouth or nose.

CRITICAL THINKING APPLICATION   56-1

Tom is ready to do an inventory of supplies in the minor surgery room. What solutions, medications, and miscellaneous supplies should he make sure are on hand for the busy surgical schedule planned for next week?

ADDITIONAL SURGICAL SUPPLIES

- Wound drains (Penrose drains)—rubber drains placed in a wound at the end of a surgical procedure to drain excess fluid
- Sterilized gauze squares or strips saturated with petroleum jelly or petrolatum—used to pack wounds
- Sterilized iodoform gauze strips, ¼ inch to 2 inches wide and impregnated with iodoform iodine—used to pack abscesses to act as a wick to draw out the infection; also used as a local antibacterial agent (Figure 56-2)
- Surgical sponges—used to absorb blood and protect tissues during surgery
- Syringes and needles—used to inject local anesthetics and irrigate wounds

SURGICAL INSTRUMENTS

The medical assistant must know which instruments are used for each procedure and should be able to identify and understand the function of the surgical instruments preferred by the physician. Instruments have clearly identifiable parts and can be visually differentiated from one another (Procedure 56-1). The basic components are the handle, the closing mechanism, and the part that comes in contact with the patient, commonly called the *jaws*.

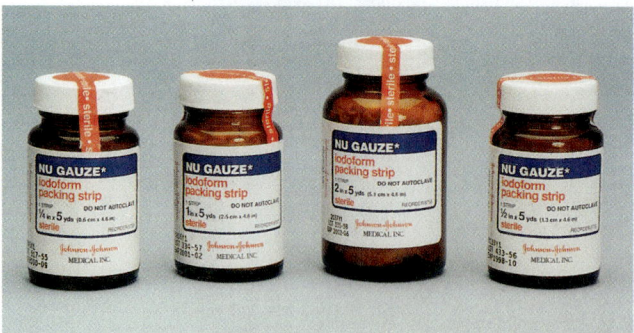

FIGURE 56-2 Iodoform gauze. (Courtesy Johnson & Johnson Medical, Arlington, Texas.)

Many instruments can be ordered with either straight or curved tips, depending on the operator's preference and the task to be performed.

Instruments have either ring handles (finger rings; Figure 56-3, *A* and *B*) or spring handles (Figure 56-3, *C*; these sometimes are called *thumb-handled* or *thumb grasp* instruments). Scissors are an example of a ring-handled instrument; tweezers have spring handles. Some instruments have a hinge type of mechanism called a *box lock*.

Ratchets resemble gears and are located just below the ring handle (see Figure 56-3, *A* and *B*). They are used to lock an instrument into position. Most ratchets can be closed at three or more positions, depending on the thickness of the tissue or materials being grasped.

The inner surfaces of the jaws on some instruments have ridged teeth called *serrations*, and both ring-handled and thumb-type instruments may have them. These serrations may be crisscross, horizontal, or lengthwise (Figure 56-4). Serrations prevent small blood vessels and tissue from slipping out of the jaws of the instrument.

Instrument tips or jaws may be plain tipped or mouse toothed (Figure 56-5, *A*). If the tooth is large, the tip is called *rat toothed* (Figure 56-5, *B*). Tissue forceps usually are toothed instruments and are identified by the number of intermeshing teeth (e.g., 12, 23, 34). Allis forceps (Figure 56-5, *C*) are used to grasp delicate, soft tissues,

---

PROCEDURE 56-1

Identify Surgical Instruments

GOAL: *To identify, correctly spell the names of, and determine the use or uses of standard office surgical instruments or those selected by your instructor.*

EQUIPMENT and SUPPLIES

- Curved hemostat
- Straight hemostat
- Dressing (thumb) forceps
- Paper and pen
- Disposable scalpel and blade
- Dissecting scissors
- Towel clamp
- Vaginal speculum
- Bandage scissors
- Allis tissue forceps

PROCEDURAL STEPS

1. Look for the following parts that determine use: box lock, serrations, finger rings, cutting edge, noncutting edge, thumb type, teeth ratchets, and electric attachments.
   <u>PURPOSE:</u> To determine the combination of features and parts for each instrument.
2. Consider the general classification of the instrument: cutting and dissection, grasping and clamping, retracting, or probing and dilating.
   <u>PURPOSE:</u> The clue to the name of the instrument may be found by determining the classification.

3. Carefully examine the teeth and serrations.
   <u>PURPOSE:</u> The clue to the name of the instrument may be found by determining its distinctive parts.
4. Consider the length of the instrument to determine the area of the body for which it is used.
   <u>PURPOSE:</u> The clue to the name of the instrument may be found by determining where it can reach.
5. Try to remember whether the instrument was named for a famous physician, university, or clinic.
   <u>PURPOSE:</u> Many instruments are named for the inventor.
6. If the instrument is a pair of scissors, look at the points and determine whether the tips are sharp-sharp, sharp-blunt, or blunt-blunt.
7. Carefully compare the instrument with similar instruments with which you are familiar to determine whether it is in the same category or has the same name.
   <u>PURPOSE:</u> A clue to the name of an instrument may be found in the knowledge you already have.
8. Write, with correct spelling, the complete name of each instrument, including its category and use.

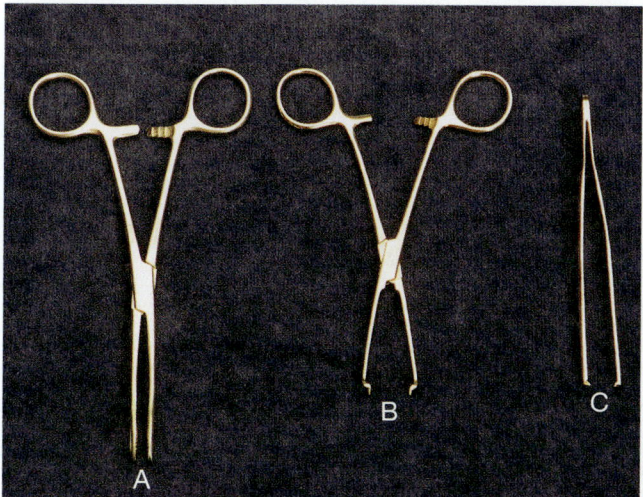

FIGURE 56-3 A and **B,** Ring-handle forceps. **C,** Spring-handle thumb forceps.

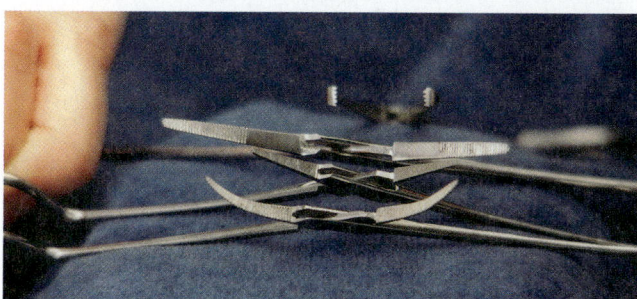

FIGURE 56-4 Instruments with serrations.

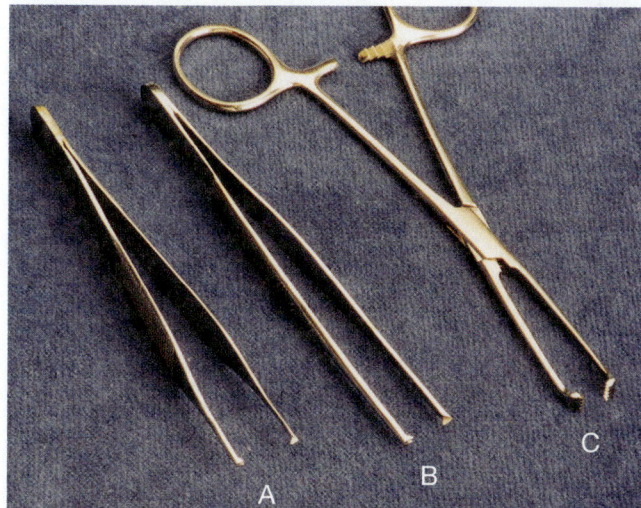

FIGURE 56-5 A, Mouse-toothed jaws. **B,** Rat-toothed jaws. **C,** Teeth of Allis tissue forceps.

An instrument is usually named for its use (e.g., splinter forceps, for removing splinters) or after the person or people who developed it (e.g., Mayo-Hegar needle holder). Many general instruments are identified by the part of the body on which they are used (e.g., rectal speculum and nasal speculum).

There are thousands of surgical instruments with multiple name variations. The same instrument may have two or three different names, depending on the physician identifying it or the part of the country in which the practice is located. A physician may ask for a clamp or forceps when a Kelly hemostat is wanted. It is important to learn the physician's preference in terminology. Learn to recognize the distinctive parts of instruments and the reasons for each part, and you will quickly build a working knowledge of hundreds of instruments.

CLASSIFICATIONS OF SURGICAL INSTRUMENTS

Surgical instruments generally are classified according to their use, and most belong to one of four groups:
- Cutting
- Grasping
- Retracting
- Probing and dilating

Cutting and Dissecting Instruments

Cutting and dissecting instruments, which are used for cutting, incising, scraping, punching, and puncturing, include scissors, scalpels, chisels, elevators, curettes, punches, drills, and needles. Instruments with a sharp blade or surface can cut, scrape, or **dissect**.

Bandage Scissors (Figure 56-6, A)
- Blunt probe tip
- Easily inserted under bandages with relative safety
- Used to remove bandages and dressings

Operating (Surgical) Scissors
Metzenbaum (Metz) Scissors (Figure 56-6, B)
- Most frequently used length is 5¼ inches
- Used to cut and dissect tissue
Mayo Scissors (Figure 56-6, C and D)
- 5 to 6 inches long
- Curved or straight blade tips
- Used to cut and dissect fascia and muscle
- Straight Mayo scissors can be used as suture scissors
Iris Scissors (Figure 56-6, E and F)
- Usual length is 4 inches
- Curved or straight blade tips
- Straight tips usually are used for suture removal

Littauer Stitch or Suture Scissors (Figure 56-7)
- Blade has beak or hook to slide under sutures
- 4 to 5 inches long
- Used to remove sutures

Disposable Scalpels (Figure 56-8)
- *Handles:* No. 3 is the standard handle; No. 3L and No. 7 are used in deeper cavities

so the teeth are finer, shallower, and more rounded. Other forceps have teeth that are sharper and deeper. Still others have sharp, hook-like, single or double teeth, such as a tenaculum or vulsellum. Usually, the tenaculum has a single, sharp hook on each jaw. The vulsellum has a double hook that resembles the fangs of a snake (see Figure 56-18, *F*). Toothed instruments commonly have ratchets for locking into towels or human tissues. Instrument tips may also be either straight or curved, depending on their use.

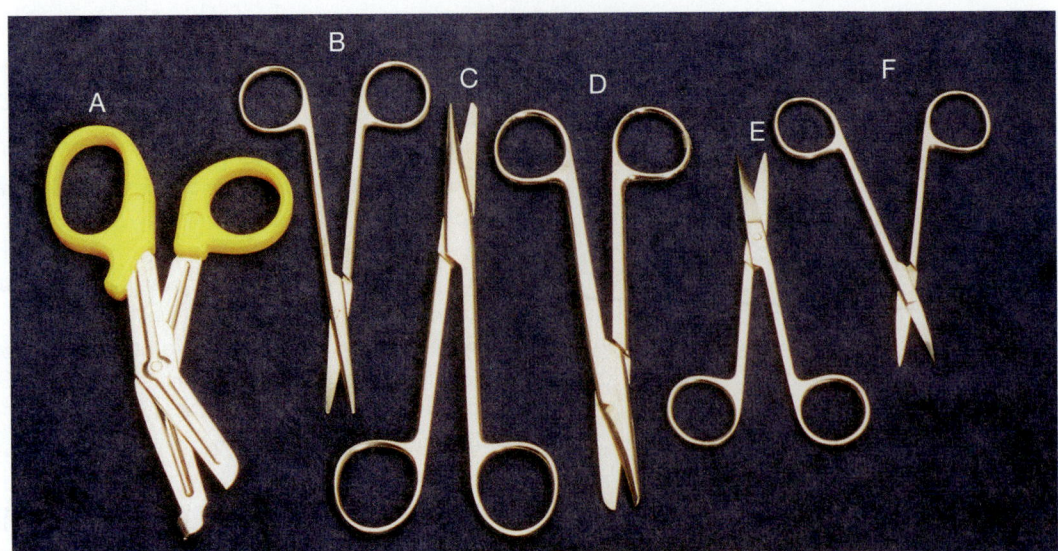

FIGURE 56-6 Operating scissors. **A,** Bandage scissors. **B,** Metzenbaum ("Metz") scissors. **C,** Curved Mayo scissors. **D,** Straight Mayo scissors. **E,** Straight iris scissors. **F,** Curved iris scissors.

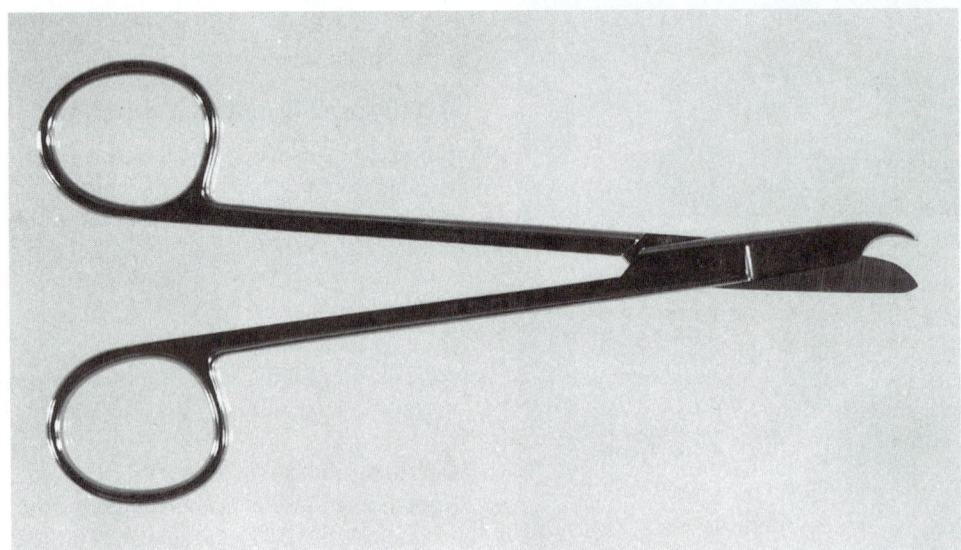

FIGURE 56-7 Suture scissors. (From Wells, MP: *Surgical instruments: a pocket guide,* ed 4, St Louis, 2011, Saunders.)

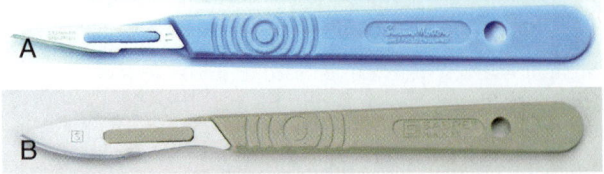

FIGURE 56-8 Disposable scalpels.

- *Blades:* No. 15 is commonly used; No. 10, 11, and 12 are used for specialty incisions

Grasping and Clamping Instruments

Clamping instruments are used for many different tasks. Many have a sharp tooth or teeth and are used to retract, hold, and manipulate fascia. The most common clamping instruments are hemostats, which originally were designed to stop bleeding or to clamp severed blood vessels. Some clamping instruments are used to grasp other instruments or sterilized materials. Sometimes hemostats and other clamping instruments are used interchangeably.

Hemostat Forceps (Figure 56-9, A and B)

- Jaws may be fully or partly serrated, without teeth
- May be curved or straight
- Used to clamp small vessels or hold tissue
- Mosquito forceps (4 inches) are smaller and used for very small vessels
- Crile forceps (5 inches) are medium sized
- Kelly forceps (6 to 7 inches) are larger

Needle Holders (Figure 56-9, C and D)

- Jaws are shorter and stronger than hemostat jaws
- Jaws may be serrated or may have a groove in the center

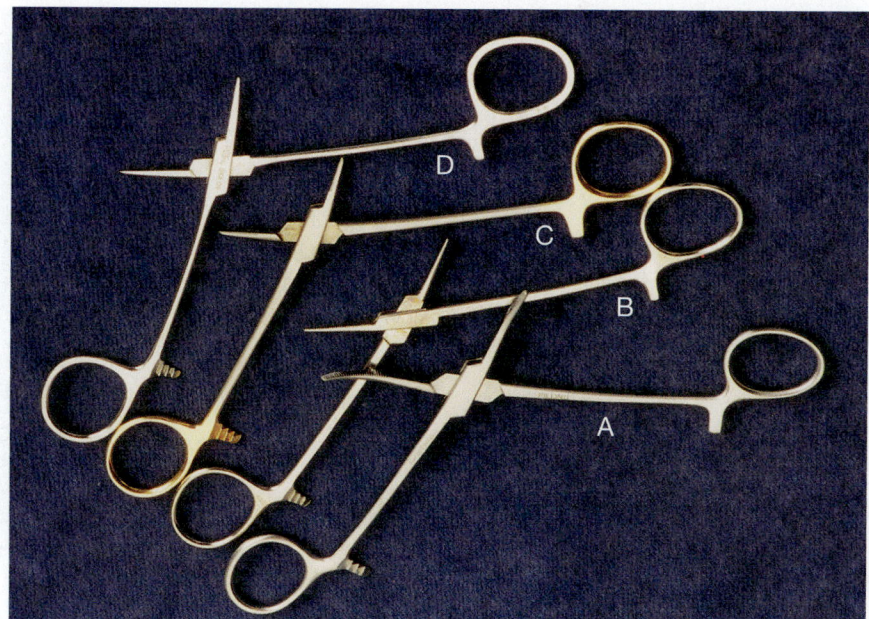

FIGURE 56-9 **A,** Kelly hemostat forceps. **B,** Mosquito hemostat forceps. **C,** Needle holder. **D,** Smooth-tip needle holder.

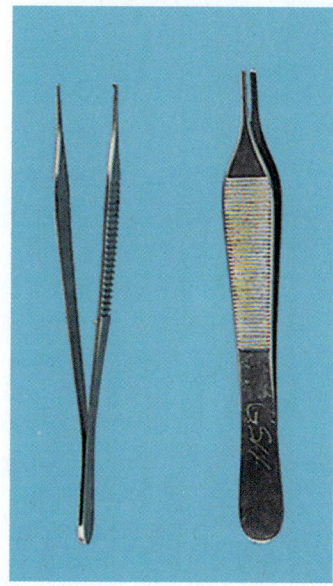

FIGURE 56-10 Adson forceps. (From Tighe SM: *Instrumentation for the operating room: a photographic manual,* ed 7, St Louis, 2007, Mosby.)

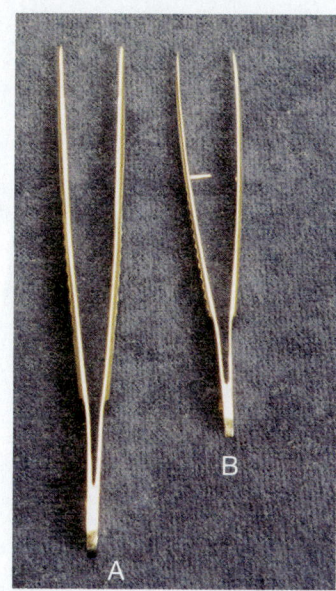

FIGURE 56-11 **A,** Long plain-tip forceps. **B,** Short plain-tip forceps.

- Are 4 to 7 inches in length
- Used to grasp a suture needle firmly

Splinter Forceps
- Design and construction vary
- Fine tip for foreign object retrieval

Adson Forceps (Figure 56-10)
- Used to grasp tissue and in suturing

Plain Thumb (Dressing) Forceps (Figure 56-11)
- Manufactured in lengths from 4 to 12 inches
- Varying types of serrated jaws but no teeth

- Used to insert packing into or remove objects from deep cavities

Towel Forceps (Towel Clamp) (Figure 56-12)
- May have sharp or atraumatic tips
- Various lengths from 3 to 6½ inches
- Used to hold drapes in place during surgery

Allis Tissue Forceps (Figure 56-13, *A*)
- Available in different lengths and jaw widths
- Used to grasp tissue, muscle, or skin surrounding a wound

Foerster Sponge Forceps (Figure 56-13, *B*)
- Used to hold gauze squares to sponge the surgical site

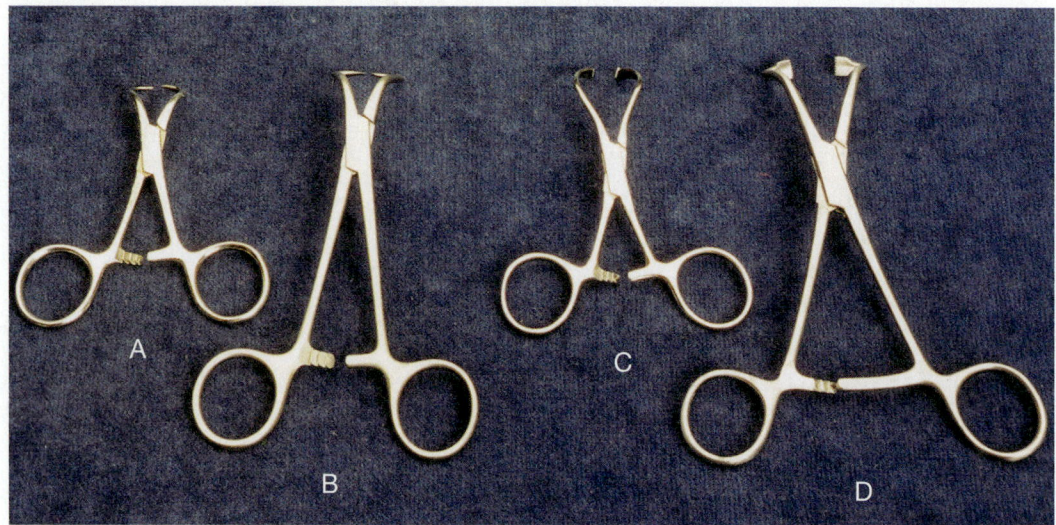

FIGURE 56-12 **A,** Small sharp towel forceps. **B,** Large sharp towel forceps. **C,** Small atraumatic towel forceps. **D,** Large atraumatic towel forceps.

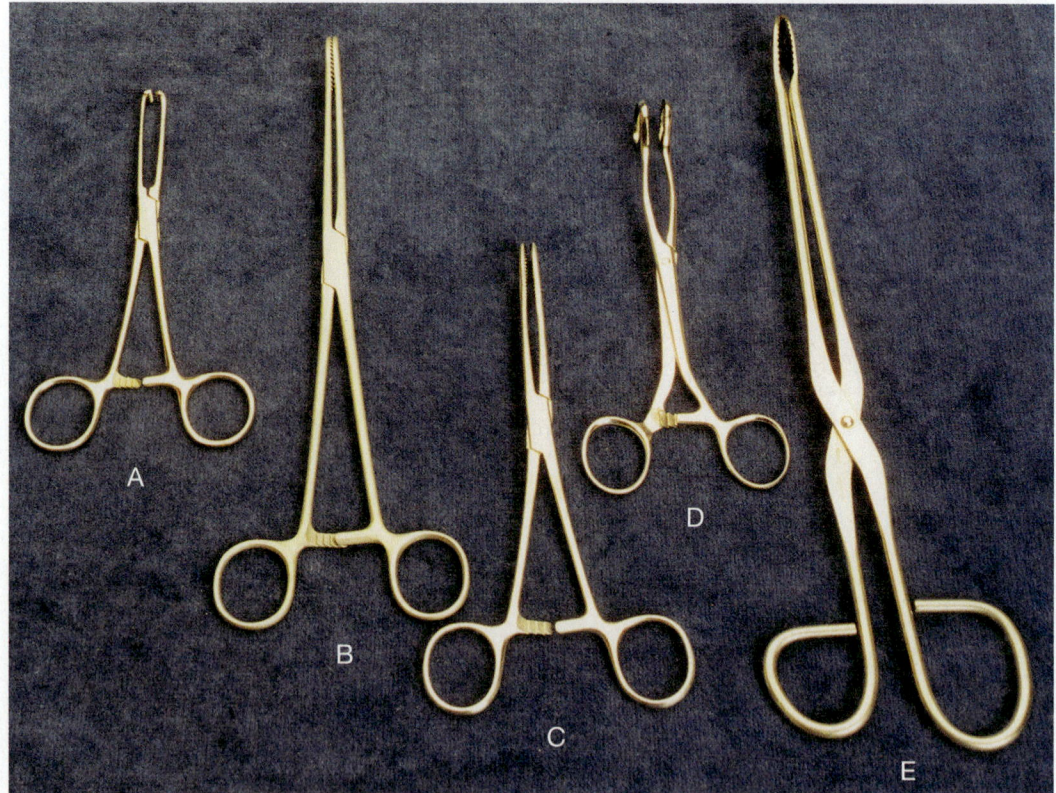

FIGURE 56-13 **A,** Allis forceps. **B,** Foerster sponge forceps. **C,** Straight transfer forceps. **D,** Short transfer forceps. **E,** Long transfer forceps.

Transfer Forceps (Figure 56-13, *C* to *E*)
- Many sizes and lengths available
- Sterile transfer forceps may be used to arrange items on a sterile tray

Adson Thumb Forceps (Figure 56-14, *A* and *B*)
- Usual length is 4 inches
- Manufactured with or without teeth
- Used to grasp tissue and in suturing

Bayonet Forceps (Figure 56-14, *C* to *E*)
- Manufactured in different lengths
- Smooth tipped
- Used to insert packing into or remove objects from the nose and ear

Plain-Tip Tissue Forceps (Figure 56-14, *F*)
- Manufactured in different lengths
- Atraumatic for tissue
- Used to grasp tissue, muscle, or skin surrounding a wound

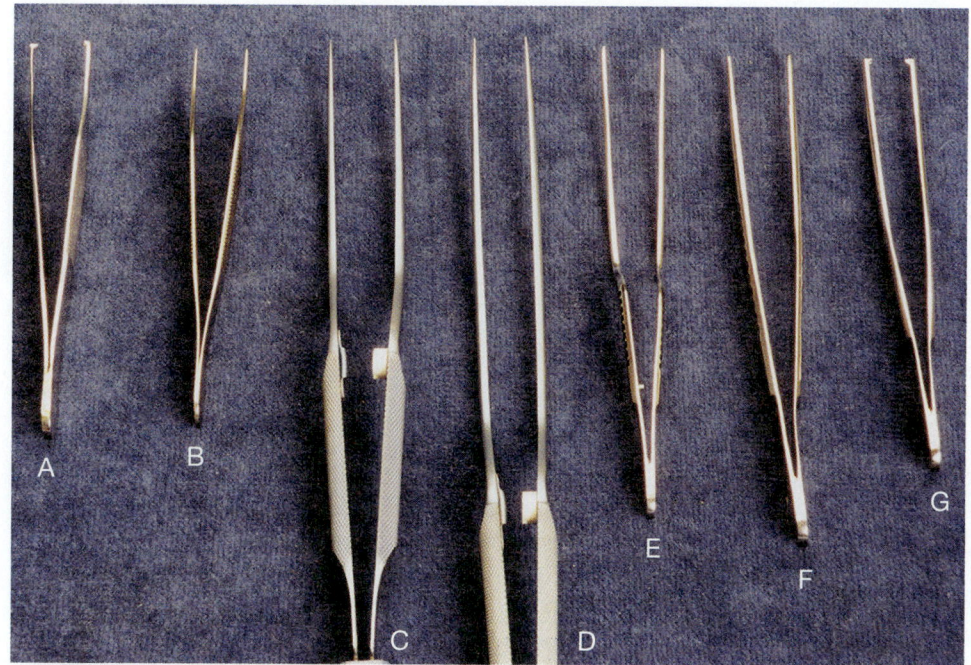

FIGURE 56-14 A, Toothed Adson forceps. **B,** Smooth Adson forceps. **C,** Medium long bayonet forceps. **D,** Long bayonet forceps. **E,** Short bayonet forceps. **F,** Plain-tip tissue forceps. **G,** Toothed tissue forceps.

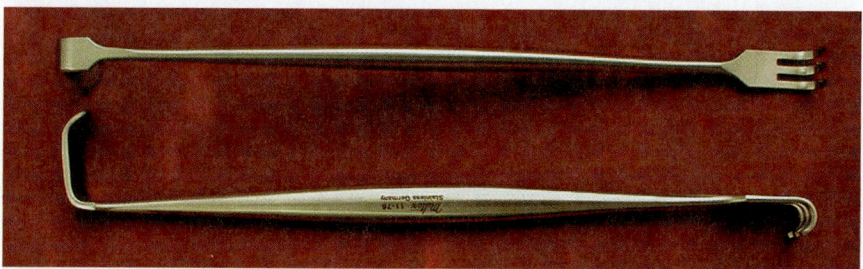

FIGURE 56-15 Senn retractor.

Toothed Tissue Forceps (Figure 56-14, G)
- Manufactured in 4- to 18-inch lengths
- Pincher grip
- Used to grasp tissue, muscle, or skin surrounding a wound

Retractors

Retracting instruments hold tissue away from the surgical wound (incision). Depending on the physician's preference, skin hooks and Senn retractors are used to retract during most minor surgical procedures. These instruments are handheld and are used for skin retraction.

Senn Retractor (Figure 56-15)
- Used to retract small incisions or to secure a skin edge for suturing
- Flat end is a blunt retractor
- Three-prong end may be sharp or dull

Probes and Dilators

Probes and dilators are used for both surgery and examinations. Probes can be used to search for a foreign body in a wound or to enter a fistula. Dilators are used to stretch a cavity or opening for examination or before inserting another instrument to obtain a tissue specimen.

Probes (Figure 56-16, A to C)
- Length ranges from 4 to 12 inches; available with or without bulbous tip
- May be smooth or may have a grooved director
- Used to find foreign bodies embedded in dermal tissue or muscle or to trace a wound tract

Trocars and Obturators (Figure 56-16, D to G)
- Consist of a sharply pointed **stylus** (**obturator**) contained in a **cannula** (outer tube)
- Available in various sizes
- Used to withdraw fluids from cavities or for draining and irrigating with a catheter

Specula (Figure 56-17)
- Most common dilator used
- Valves are spread apart, dilating the opening
- Used to open or distend a body orifice or cavity

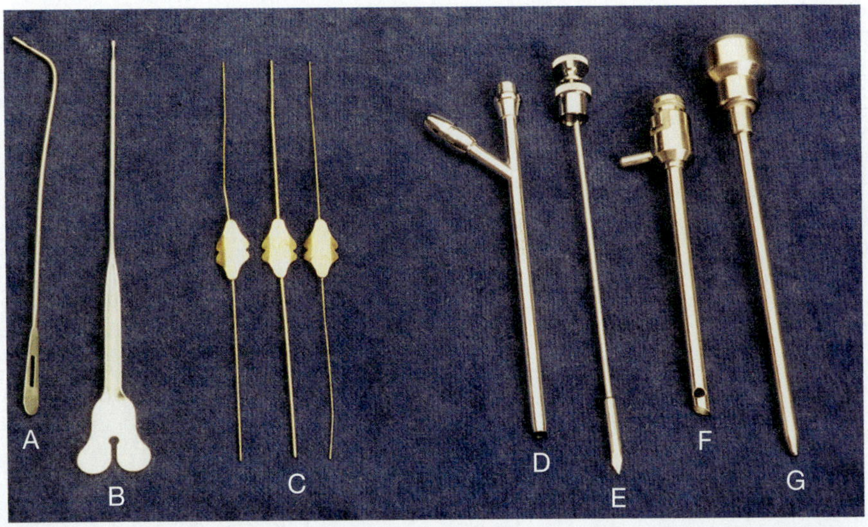

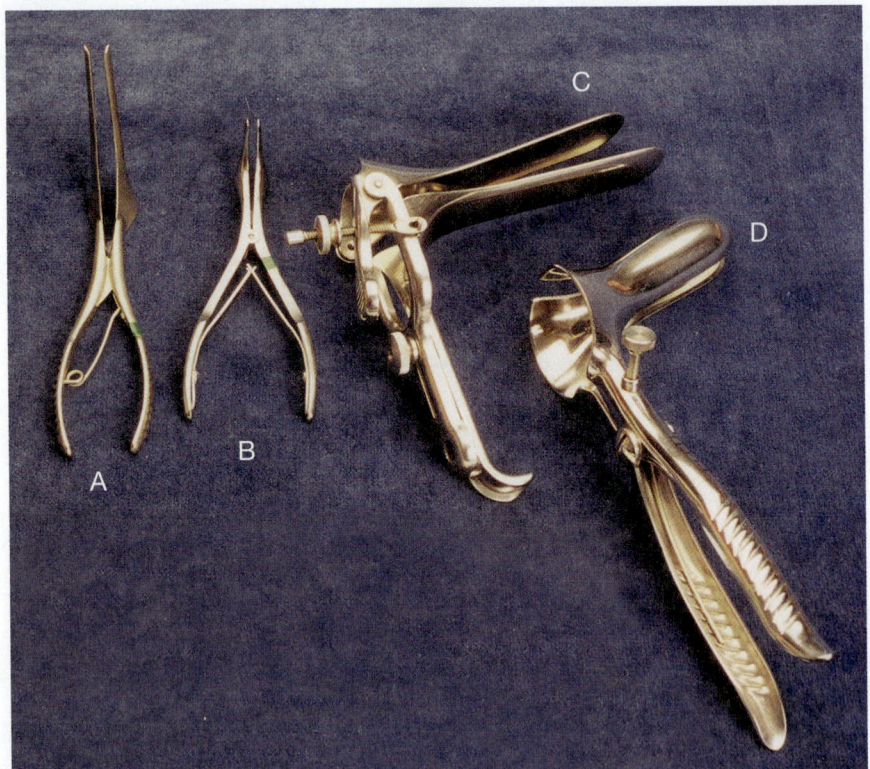

FIGURE 56-16 **A,** Probe. **B,** Grooved director. **C,** Lacrimal duct probes. **D,** Double-ended cannula: **E,** Sharp trocar. **F,** Cannula. **G,** Blunt-tip obturator.

FIGURE 56-17 **A,** Long nasal speculum. **B,** Short nasal speculum. **C,** Graves vaginal speculum. **D,** Anal speculum, self-retaining.

Nasal Specula (see Figure 56-17, A and B)
- Valves can be spread to facilitate viewing
- Applicator or snare can be introduced through the valves
- Used to spread the nostrils for examination

SPECIALTY INSTRUMENTS

Although all instruments fall under the same four categories as the surgical instruments just discussed, the remaining instruments are organized into specialty groupings. Presenting the instruments in this manner makes it easy to see how the instruments relate to particular examinations. In addition to recognizing the name and use of each instrument, the medical assistant must organize and set out the instruments needed for each particular examination in what is called a *tray setup*.

Gynecologic Instruments

Foerster Sponge Forceps (Figure 56-18, A)
- Round and serrated tips
- Used in the same way as the dressing forceps

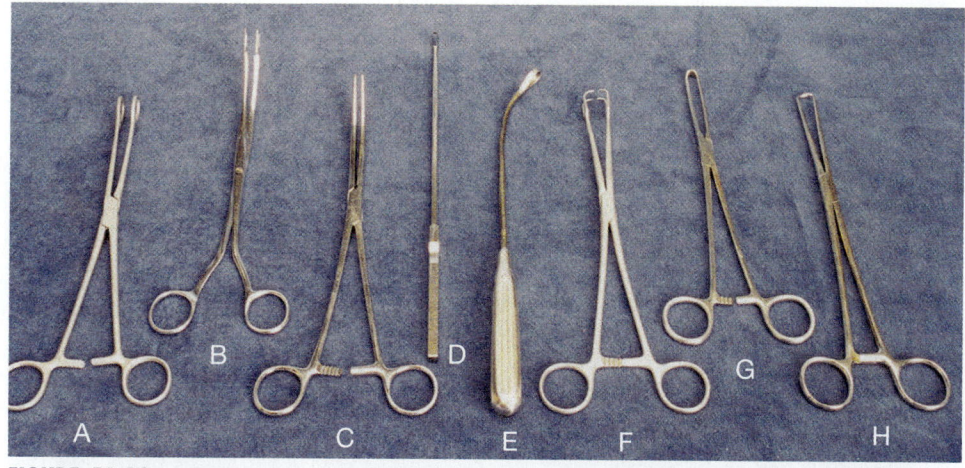

FIGURE 56-18 A, Foerster sponge forceps. **B,** Placenta forceps. **C,** Bozeman uterine dressing forceps. **D,** Endocervical curette. **E,** Sims uterine curette. **F,** Schroeder uterine vulsellum forceps. **G,** Long Allis forceps. **H,** Schroeder uterine tenaculum forceps.

Placenta Forceps (Figure 56-18, *B*)

- Used to remove tissue from the uterus

Bozeman Uterine Dressing Forceps (Figure 56-18, *C*)

- Designed to hold sponges or dressings
- Capable of reaching the cervix through the vagina
- Used to swab the area or apply medication

Endocervical Curette (Figure 56-18, *D*)

- Smaller than the uterine curette
- Used in the same way as the uterine curette

Sims Uterine Curette (Figure 56-18, *E*)

- Available in several sizes
- Hollow and spoon shaped; used for scraping
- Used to remove polyps, secretions, and bits of placental tissue

Schroeder Uterine Vulsellum Forceps (Figure 56-18, *F*)

- Used to hold tissue (e.g., the cervix) while a tissue specimen is obtained or to lift the cervix to view the **fornix**

Long Allis Forceps (Figure 56-18, *G*)

- Same as Allis forceps
- Used in deeper body cavities

Schroeder Uterine Tenaculum Forceps (Figure 56-18, *H*)

- Very sharp, pointed tips
- Used to hold tissue (e.g., the cervix) while a tissue specimen is obtained or to lift the cervix to view the fornix

Hegar Uterine Dilators (Figure 56-19, *A*)

- Available in sets
- Double or single ended
- Used to dilate the cervix for **dilation** and **curettage**

Sims Uterine Sounds (Figure 56-19, *B*)

- Used to check the patency of the cervical os or the urethral meatus

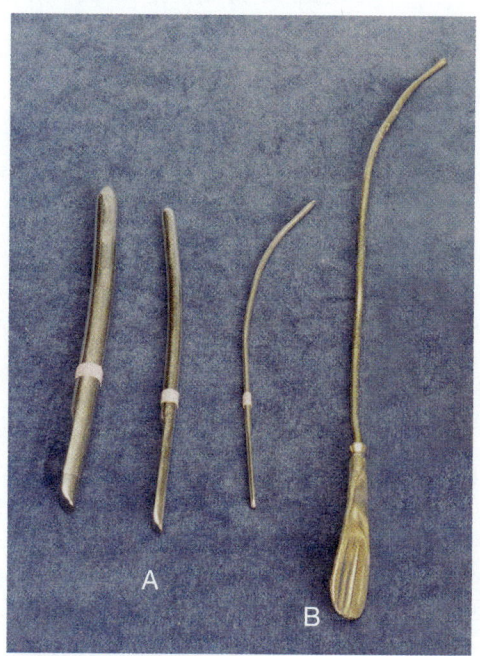

FIGURE 56-19 A, Uterine dilators. **B,** Sims uterine sounds.

Ophthalmologic and Otolaryngologic Instruments

Krause Nasal Snare (Figure 56-20, *A*)

- Wire loop at the tip that can be tightened
- Used to remove polyps from the nares

Metal Tongue Depressor (Figure 56-20, *B*)

- Used to depress the tongue for oral examinations

Hartmann "Alligator" Ear Forceps (Figure 56-20, *C*)

- Has a 3½-inch shaft and is made in a variety of styles
- Action of the jaw similar to that of an alligator's jaws
- Used to remove foreign bodies or polyps

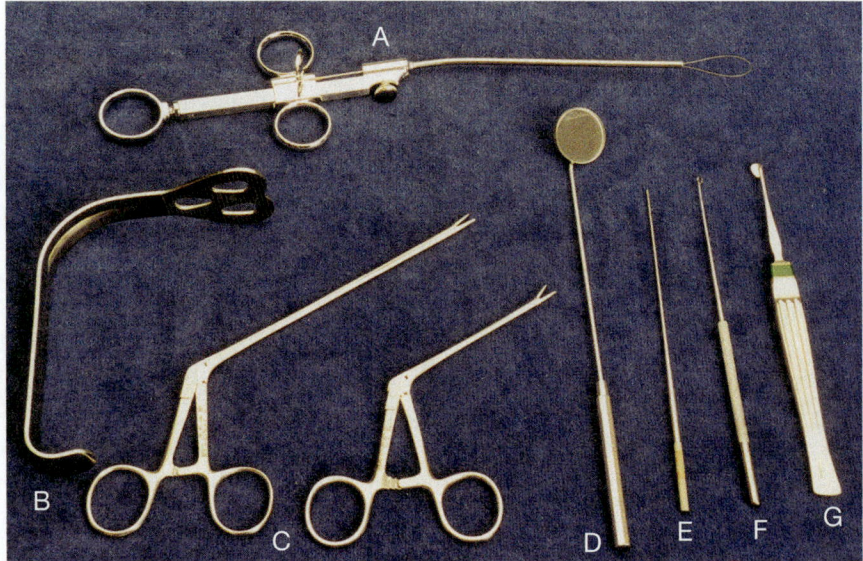

FIGURE 56-20 A, Krause nasal snare. **B,** Metal tongue depressor. **C,** Long and short alligator forceps. **D,** Laryngeal mirror. **E,** Ivan metal applicator. **F,** "Buck" ear curette. **G,** Sharp ear dissector.

Laryngeal Mirror (Figure 56-20, *D*)
- Made in various sizes
- May have a nonfogging surface
- Used for examination of the larynx and postnasal area

Ivan Laryngeal Metal Applicator (Figure 56-20, *E*)
- Holds cotton in place with its roughened end; used to swab or sponge throat or postnasal tissue
- Six to 9 inches long with curved end for use in throat or postnasal areas
- Used to remove foreign bodies imbedded in the pharynx

"Buck" Ear Curette (Figure 56-20, *F*)
- Has a stainless steel loop at the end
- Made with sharp or blunt scraper ends
- Manufactured in various sizes
- Used to remove foreign matter from the ear canals

Sharp Ear Dissector (Figure 56-20, *G*)
- Used to remove debris from the ear canal

Biopsy Instruments

Cervical Biopsy Forceps (Figure 56-21, *A*)
- Available with or without teeth
- Used to obtain cervical specimens for diagnostic examination

Rectal Biopsy Punch (Figure 56-21, *B*)
- Manufactured with interchangeable stems
- Available in different lengths and styles
- Used through a proctoscope or sigmoidoscope

Silverman Biopsy Needle
- Manufactured with a split cannula
- Stylus is removed, and cannula is inserted to retrieve the specimen
- Needle biopsy can eliminate the need for surgical incision

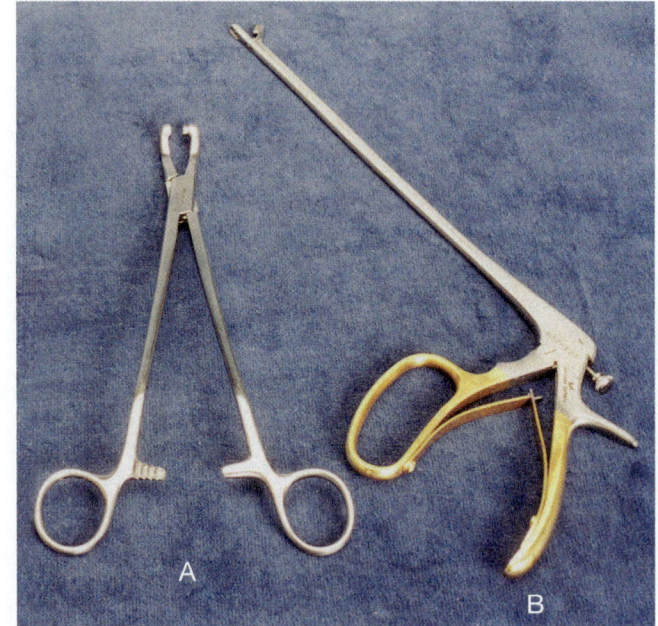

FIGURE 56-21 A, Cervical biopsy forceps. **B,** Rectal biopsy punch.

Genitourinary Instruments

Catheter Guide (Figure 56-22, *A*)
- Metal guide
- Used with extreme caution
- Used by the physician when a catheter cannot be inserted by usual means

Foley Catheter with Inflated Balloon (Figure 56-22, *B*)
- Manufactured in sizes 8 to 32 French with a double rubber lining toward the tip (each French unit is equal to 1.32 mm; the higher the number, the larger the lumen)
- After insertion, sterile solution is injected into the inner lining (inflating the balloon) to hold it in the bladder
- Used as an indwelling catheter

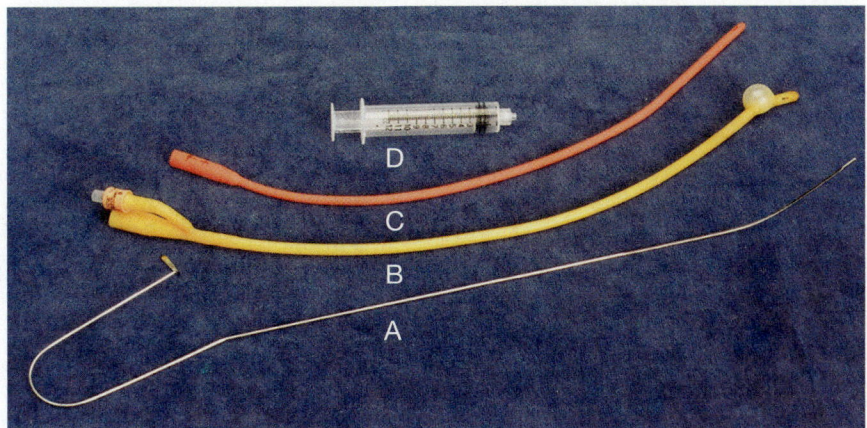

FIGURE 56-22 A, Metal catheter guide. **B,** Foley catheter with inflated balloon. **C,** Red Robinson catheter. **D,** 12-mL Luer-Lok syringe.

Red Robinson Catheter (Figure 56-22, C)

- Soft rubber urethral catheter in sizes 8 to 32 French
- Inserted temporarily into the bladder for drainage or to obtain a specimen

12-mL Luer-Lok Syringe (Figure 56-22, D)

- Used for injecting amounts greater than 5 mL
- Typically used to inject sterile saline into a catheter to inflate the balloon at the tip of an indwelling catheter

> **CRITICAL THINKING APPLICATION   56-2**
>
> Tom is preparing instrument and supply packs for specific procedures performed by Dr. Samanski. One of the packs he is preparing for the autoclave is for removal of a nasal polyp. Based on your understanding of typical and specialty instruments and supplies, what items should Tom include in the instrument pack?

CARE AND HANDLING OF INSTRUMENTS

Because instruments are expensive and the physician's skill depends on their quality, the medical assistant must properly care for each instrument to maximize its life and ensure that every part is in safe working order.

Most instruments are made of fine-grade stainless steel. The term *stainless* usually is taken too literally. Although stainless steel does resist rust and keeps a fine edge and tip longer, even the best stainless steel may develop water spots and stains, especially if water with a high mineral content is used. Proper hardness and flexibility are important. Inexpensive instruments that are chrome plated may be too brittle or too soft. In addition, mistreatment of chrome-plated instruments can cause minute breaks in the finish, which may become a source of contamination or may tear the surgeon's gloves.

All instruments should be carefully examined when they are purchased. Scissors should be tested to see whether they shear the full length of the blades completely to the tip. If the scissors cut a piece of cloth cleanly and do not chew at any point, even at the tip, they are functioning correctly. Teeth and serrations should be checked to see whether they intermesh completely and whether the jaws are even on the sides and tip. Each instrument should be felt over its entire surface for any rough areas that may tear or snag the surgeon's gloves or act as a future source of contamination. Box locks and hinges must work freely but should not be too loose. Thumb- and spring-handled instruments must have the correct tension and meet evenly at the tips. After inspection, instruments should be cleaned and checked again for possible faulty workmanship before sterilization.

Under no circumstances should instruments be bundled together or allowed to become entangled. Do not mix stainless steel instruments with others made of different metals, including chrome-plated instruments, because this may cause electrolysis and result in etching. If an instrument is accidentally dropped, it may be permanently damaged. If scissors are dropped with the blades partly open, there may be a nick at the point where the blades cross. Any damaged or malfunctioning instrument must be disposed of to prevent complications during a surgical procedure.

After a surgical procedure, contaminated instruments should be placed in a basin of disinfectant solution with heavier instruments on the bottom of the basin and lighter, more delicate instruments on top. Always unlock each instrument before immersion in the chemical decontaminant to permit sanitization of the entire surface area. Never allow blood or other coagulable substances to dry on an instrument, because they will be difficult to remove. If immediate sanitization and disinfection is not possible, the instruments should be rinsed well and placed in a cold water solution with a blood solvent and mild detergent. The detergent increases the wetting ability of the water, giving the instrument surfaces better exposure to the solution. It is best to use a detergent that has a neutral pH and low suds and can be rinsed off easily. The manufacturer's recommendations for the correct dilution and time of immersion of the various sanitizing agents, disinfectants and blood solvents must be strictly followed for the chemicals to be effective.

When the surgical procedure is completed, the receiving basin for instruments should be transferred from the surgical area to the disinfection and sterilization room. It is important to remove used instruments from the patient's view as soon as possible. After sanitization is complete, instruments should be rinsed thoroughly and either washed by hand or washed mechanically using an ultrasonic device.

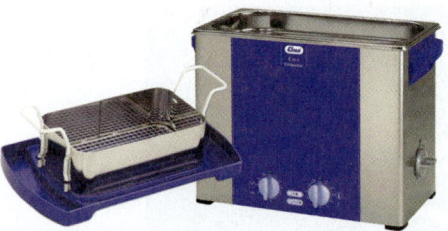

FIGURE 56-23 Elmasonic E ultrasonic cleaner unit. (Courtesy Tovatech, South Orange, NJ.)

Some delicate instruments, such as microsurgical and lensed instruments, should be washed by hand with a mild, low sudsing, neutral pH detergent solution and a soft brush. The instruments should be cleaned while submerged to prevent the airborne spread of microorganisms. Throughout the sanitization process, the medical assistant should wear heavy utility gloves to prevent possible exposure to contaminants. Instruments then should be rinsed with distilled water, dried with a lint-free cloth, and inspected for proper functioning before they are packed for sterilization.

Mechanical washing, such as with an ultrasonic device, can be used for most instruments and is an especially good method for sanitizing sharp instruments to prevent injuries (Figure 56-23). With an ultrasonic cleaning unit, the instruments are immersed in a cleaning solution and the device produces sound waves that clean contaminants from the instruments' surfaces. The unit then rinses and dries the instruments, leaving them ready for the sterilization process. However, manufacturers' guidelines should be followed for rubber and plastic materials.

After disinfection and inspection, the instruments are ready for the sterilization process. This procedure is discussed in Chapter 57.

Commercially prepared, disposable packs are available for most minor surgical procedures. They save time and eliminate the need for sanitization, disinfection, and sterilization of reusable stainless steel instruments, but they may be too costly for individual practices.

CRITICAL THINKING APPLICATION   56-3

Tom is responsible for inspecting and caring for all the surgical instruments in the minor surgery room and for sanitizing, disinfecting, and preparing contaminated instruments for autoclaving. He is in the process of writing an addition to the office policies and procedures manual on the management of surgical instruments. Based on what you know about the care and handling of surgical instruments, what should Tom include in the policy?

DRAPES, SUTURES, AND NEEDLES

Disposable surgical drapes are available in several different materials and sizes and typically have an opening (fenestration) for the operative site (Figure 56-24). The drape is placed over the operative area using sterile technique after the patient's skin preparation has been completed. This procedure is presented in Chapter 57.

Sutures

The word *suture* is used as both a noun and a verb. As a noun it refers to a surgical stitch or to the material used to close a wound.

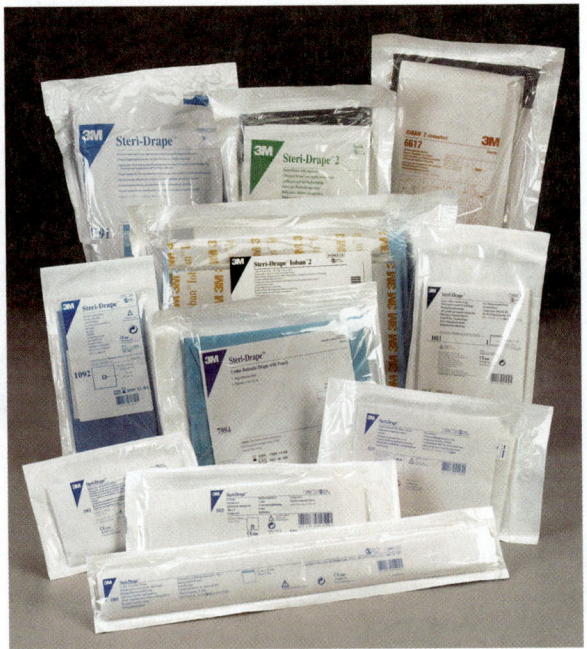

FIGURE 56-24 Sample surgical drapes. (Courtesy 3M, St. Paul, Minn.)

As a verb it refers to the act of stitching. Modern surgery and the use of sutures began in 1865, when Lister developed antisepsis and the disinfection of suture materials. Many kinds of materials have been used over the centuries, including precious metals, horse hair, animal tendons, and cotton and linen cord. Most of the improvements in suture materials and techniques have occurred in the past 50 years. The primary purpose of a suture is to hold the edges of a wound together until natural healing occurs.

A suture may also be used as a ligature. This is a strand of suture material used to tie off a blood vessel or to strangulate tissue. If a ligature is used to tie off an internal tubular structure, it must last permanently or long enough for the structure itself to disintegrate. The ideal suture material has certain characteristics:

- Easy to handle and makes a secure knot
- Does not induce a localized tissue reaction and is nonallergenic
- Has adequate strength without cutting through tissue
- Can be sterilized

The physician will request a certain type of suture based on the specific properties of the suture material, the desirable rate of absorption, the size of the suture, and the type of needle the physician prefers. Both natural and synthetic suture materials are available. Sutures may be classified as either absorbable or nonabsorbable. Many different suture materials are available, each having its advantages and disadvantages. Suture materials commonly used in minor surgical procedures are described in the following paragraphs (Figure 56-25).

Absorbable Sutures

Absorbable sutures are dissolved by the body's enzymes during the healing process. They are used when deep incisions or lacerations require inner layers of sutures to close the wound. Absorbable suture material is also used in areas where suture removal is difficult, as in oral surgery. An example of an absorbable suture material is surgical

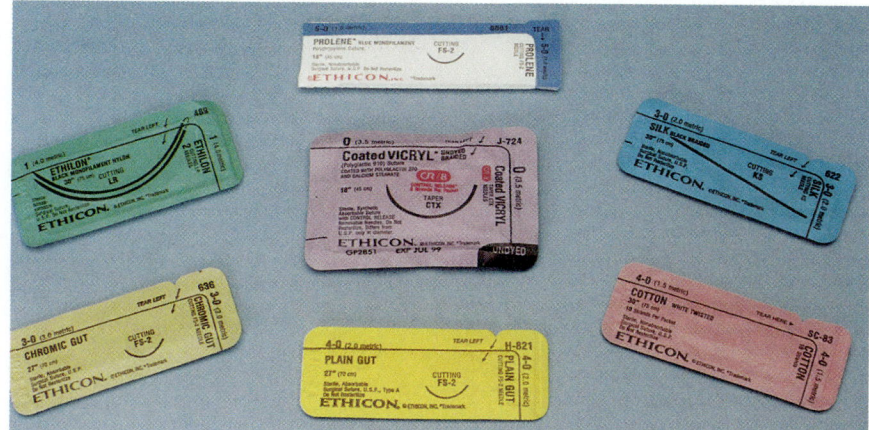

FIGURE 56-25 Suture packets labeled according to size, type, length, and type of needle point and shape.

catgut, which is obtained from sheep, cattle, or pig intestine. Plain catgut is used in tissues that heal most rapidly, such as mucous membranes and subcutaneous tissues, because it is broken down within a week. Chromic catgut is coated with chromic salts, which delays the absorption of the suture material up to 80 days.

Catgut once was the absorbable suture material of choice, but it has been replaced in recent years by Vicryl, a synthetic absorbable suture made of polyglactin. Other synthetic absorbable suture materials include Dexon, PDS, and Maxon. These materials remain stable longer than natural catgut (up to 11 weeks), allowing the wound to heal completely before absorption occurs.

Nonabsorbable Sutures

Nonabsorbable suture material is left in the wound site until healing is complete. It frequently is used in minor surgical procedures performed in the medical office, because most of the suturing required is superficial, and it can be used in areas where sutures can be removed after healing has taken place. A common, nonabsorbable suture material is silk, because it is strong and easy to tie. It is treated with a coating to prevent tissue drag and flaking. Polyester fiber sutures, such as Dacron and Prolene, are among the strongest non-absorbable sutures, along with surgical steel. These fine filaments are braided and have great tensile strength. Nylon suture is strong and has a high degree of elasticity. It is primarily used for skin closure. Owing to its elasticity and stiffness, many knots must be used, because the knots tend to untie if placed incorrectly.

Surgical staples can also be used for skin closure. They are made of stainless steel or titanium and are available in different sizes. They are applied and removed with specific staple instruments (Figure 56-26). Other techniques of wound closure include Steri-Strips, which are self-adhesive tapes that are placed over the wound, pulling the wound edges together. Steri-Strips can be used to support a wound if there is potential tension at the site or for superficial wounds such as a laceration of the forehead (Figure 56-27). Tissue adhesives, similar to glue, can also be used for superficial wounds.

Suture Sizing and Packaging

Suture material is available in a variety of diameters and lengths. The diameter of the suture strand determines its size; the smaller gauges are numbered below 0 (pronounced *aught*), and the larger gauges

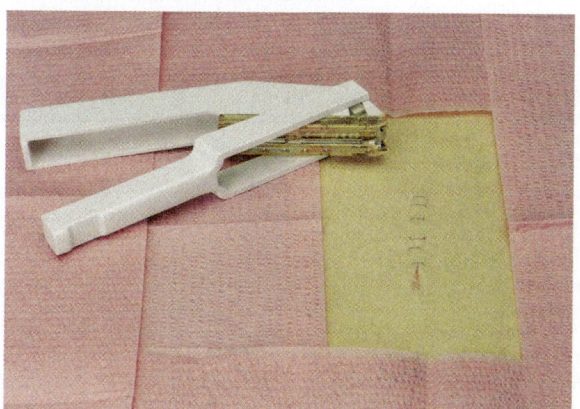

FIGURE 56-26 Disposable skin stapler.

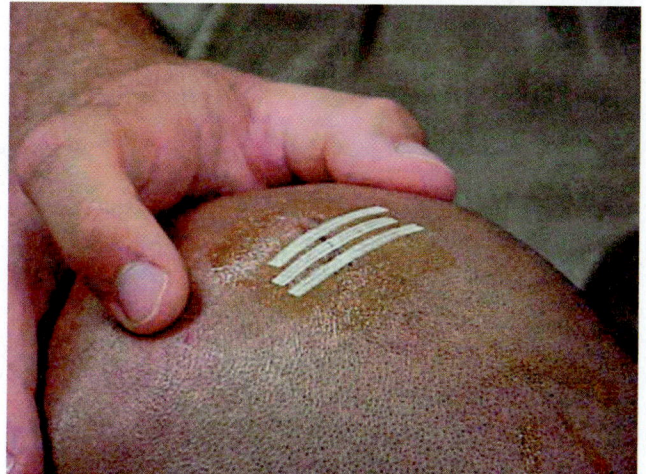

FIGURE 56-27 Wound closed with Steri-Strips. (From Cummings N: *Perspectives in athletic training*, St Louis, 2008, Mosby.)

are identified with numbers above 0. For instance, 2-0 suture is thinner than size 0, which is thinner than size 2. The sizes from 2-0 to 6-0 are used most frequently in the medical office. The length of the suture material may vary, with strands precut in 18-, 24-, 54-, and 60-inch lengths (Figure 56-28).

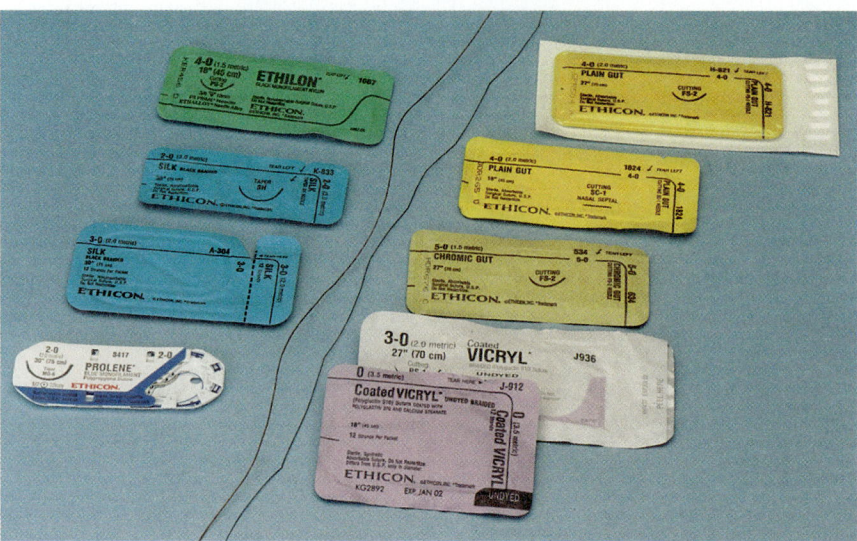

FIGURE 56-28 Suture packets (and opened suture strands) with and without needles.

SUTURE SIZES

Sutures are sized according to the U. S. Pharmacopoeia (USP) scale.

Suture Size	Diameter
6-0	0.07 mm
5-0	0.10 mm
4-0	0.15 mm
3-0	0.20 mm
2-0	0.30 mm
0	0.35 mm
1	0.40 mm
2	0.50 mm

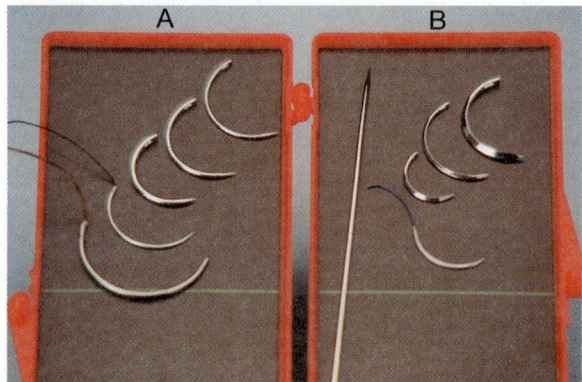

FIGURE 56-29 Surgical needle shapes. **A,** Taper point. **B,** Cutting point.

Needles

Surgical needles are chosen according to the area in which they are to be used and the depth and width of the desired suture. They are classified according to shape, which may be straight or curved (Figure 56-29). Most sutures are applied with curved needles, because they allow the physician to penetrate the surface and then come back up on the other side. The sharper the curve of the needle, the deeper the surgeon can pass it into the tissue. The point of a needle can be a taper or a cutting edge. A taper is used on delicate tissues. The cutting edge needle is used on the skin. It lacerates the skin as the needle is passed through. This is advantageous on tougher tissues, such as connective tissue.

Needles are manufactured with the suture material attached, or *swaged,* to the needle. These atraumatic needles do not have an eyelet and cause the least amount of trauma as they are passed through the tissues. Manufacturers package suture strands with the suture needle attached in peel-apart sterile, disposable packages. These may be obtained as single, individually packed or as multipack sutures in a variety of needle types and sizes with a wide range of suture materials and lengths. The most common needle type for minor skin repair is the curved, cutting edge, swaged needle.

CLOSING COMMENTS

Patient Education

Patients may have questions about the instruments the surgeon will use, and the medical assistant can help allay patients' fears by answering these questions. Explaining the patient preparation for the procedure, how the procedure will be performed, and what to expect afterward helps make the procedure go more smoothly and encourages the patient to follow the physician's advice and orders.

Legal and Ethical Issues

An awareness of legal responsibilities is imperative for surgical procedures done in the medical office. The medical assistant must know what surgery is planned and whether the patient has been informed about the procedure. In the surgical setting, the medical assistant must realize the full extent of his or her role as the patient's advocate and the physician's agent.

The medical assistant should confirm that the physician has explained the surgery to the patient and that the patient has signed informed consent. Clarify that the patient understands all aspects of the procedure. The better the patient understanding, the greater the likelihood that he or she will comply with presurgical preparations and postsurgical care.

SUMMARY OF SCENARIO

Tom has worked for Dr. Samanski for 2 years and is familiar with her preference in surgical solutions, local anesthesia, suture materials, and the typical instruments used in her practice. He also has worked hard to update the policy and procedures manual to include standards for instrument care so other medical assistants in the office will know how instruments should be sanitized, disinfected, inspected, and prepared for the autoclave. Tom realizes he needs to

continue his education in surgical procedures and takes advantage of professional workshops on the topic. He and Dr. Samanski work well together in the minor surgery area of the office, and Tom consistently attempts to stay up-to-date on the surgical advances, medications, and instruments Dr. Samanski uses in her practice.

SUMMARY OF LEARNING OBJECTIVES

1. **Define, spell, and pronounce the terms listed in the vocabulary.**

   Spelling and pronouncing medical terms correctly bolster the medical assistant's credibility. Knowing the definitions of these terms promotes confidence in communication with patients and co-workers.

2. **Apply critical thinking skills in performing the patient assessment and patient care.**

   Completing the Critical Thinking Application exercises throughout the chapter can help the student medical assistant become more adept at critical analysis of real-life situations.

3. **Describe typical solutions and medications used in minor surgical procedures.**

   Solutions used in minor surgery include sterile water for mixing with medications or rinsing instruments; sterile saline for injection or wound irrigation; antiseptic skin cleansers, such as Betadine or Hibiclens, for site preparation; and local anesthetics, including ethyl chloride or Fluori-Methane topical applications, in addition to lidocaine, Nesacaine, or Sensorcaine injectables. These local anesthetics may come packaged with or without epinephrine. The physician also may use topical silver nitrate to control local bleeding.

4. **Summarize methods for identifying surgical instruments used in minor office surgery.**

   Refer to Procedure 56-1.

5. **Outline the general classifications of surgical instruments.**

   Surgical instruments are classified according to their use as cutting, grasping, retracting, probing, or dilating tools. The components of the instrument include the type of handle, the closing mechanism, and the jaws. Instrument tips may be either straight or curved and toothed or not toothed. The instruments used in minor surgical procedures depend on the type of procedure and the physician's preference.

6. **Identify surgical instruments.**

   Refer to Procedure 56-1.

7. **Describe the care of surgical instruments.**

   Surgical instruments are expensive and must be cared for properly to maintain function and maximize life. Instruments must be examined when purchased for proper working order and possible faults with mechanisms. Stainless steel instruments should be kept separate from other metal types. Each instrument must be cleaned according to the manufacturer's guidelines, unlocked, and disinfected immediately after use. Most instruments can be cleaned with an ultrasonic washer, which helps prevent injuries.

8. **Identify types of sutures and surgical needles.**

   Suture material is available as absorbable, for internal sutures, and nonabsorbable, for skin closure. Catgut and Vicryl are the two most popular absorbable materials; nonabsorbable sutures can be made of silk or nylon, or staples can be used. Suture materials range in size from smaller gauges (i.e., below 0 [aught], used for finer tissues) to thicker gauges (above 0) and are available in various lengths. Surgical needles are either straight or curved. Most needles are manufactured with swaged suture material.

9. **Explain the medical assistant's responsibility to help ease patients' concerns about procedures.**

   The medical assistant can help ease the patient's fears by answering his or her questions. Explaining the patient preparation for a procedure, how the procedure will be performed, and what to expect afterward helps make the procedure go more smoothly and encourages the patient to follow the physician's advice and orders. In the surgical setting, the medical assistant must realize the full extent of his or her role as the patient's advocate and the physician's agent.

CONNECTIONS

 Study Guide Connection: Go to the Chapter 56 Study Guide. Read and complete the activities.

Evolve Connection: Go to the Chapter 56 link at *evolve.elsevier.com/kinn* to complete the Chapter Review and Chapter Quiz. Check out the other resources listed for this chapter to make the most of what you have learned from Surgical Supplies and Instruments.

57

SURGICAL ASEPSIS AND ASSISTING WITH SURGICAL PROCEDURES

SCENARIO

Melissa Gelbart, CMA (AAMA), works for a dermatologist, Dr. Susan Armstrong, who frequently performs minor surgical procedures in the office. Melissa was hired to work as an administrative medical assistant at the front desk, but one of the clinical medical assistants has unexpectedly quit, and the office manager has offered Melissa her position. Melissa is excited about this opportunity, but she also is concerned about her skill level in sterile procedures. At least she is familiar with a number of the patients, most of the staff, and the types of outpatient surgeries performed in the facility. Surgical asepsis and assisting with surgery were her favorite topics when she was in medical assisting school. However, before she can assist with surgeries, Melissa must demonstrate her ability to set up a sterile field without contaminating the site. She also must show that she can apply a sterile dressing properly and change sterile bandages.

While studying this chapter, think about the following questions:

- What are the crucial steps Melissa must follow to set up and maintain a sterile field?
- How does an autoclave work and what are the important rules to remember when preparing surgical trays for the autoclave and correctly operating the machine?
- How will Melissa know whether surgical trays processed in the autoclave are actually sterile?
- What techniques must Melissa follow to prepare for and assist with a surgical procedure?

- What are common surgical procedures performed in an ambulatory care facility?
- What is the medical assistant's role in preparing the patient, equipment, and room for a surgical procedure?
- Why is it important that Melissa understand and be prepared to answer patients' questions about the process of wound healing?
- What bandaging techniques should Melissa be prepared to perform?

LEARNING OBJECTIVES

1. Define, spell, and pronounce the terms listed in the vocabulary.
2. Apply critical thinking skills in performing the patient assessment and patient care.
3. Define the concepts of aseptic technique.
4. Explain the differences among sanitization, disinfection, and sterilization.
5. Summarize tips for improving autoclave techniques.
6. Demonstrate how to wrap instrument packs for autoclave sterilization.
7. Explain the types and uses of sterilization indicators.
8. Summarize the correct methods of loading, operating, and unloading an autoclave.
9. Demonstrate how to operate an autoclave.
10. Summarize common minor surgical procedures.
11. Detail the medical assistant's role in minor office surgery.
12. Perform a skin prep for surgery.
13. Perform a surgical hand scrub.
14. Outline the rules for setting up and maintaining a sterile field.
15. Open a sterile pack to create a sterile field.
16. Transfer sterile instruments and pour solutions into a sterile field.
17. Put on sterile gloves without contaminating them.
18. Demonstrate how to assist with a minor surgical procedure and suturing.
19. Summarize postoperative instructions and care of wounds.
20. Demonstrate how to remove sutures and the technique for removing surgical staples.
21. Explain the process of wound healing.
22. Properly apply dressings and bandages to surgical sites.
23. Conduct patient education in aseptic technique and surgical procedures.
24. Discuss the legal and ethical concerns regarding surgical asepsis and infection control.

VOCABULARY

cicatrix Early scar tissue that appears pale, contracted, and firm.
dehiscence The separation of wound edges or rupture of a wound closure.

infection Invasion of body tissues by microorganisms, which then proliferate and damage tissues.
sterilization Complete destruction of all forms of microbial life.

Asepsis is the condition of being free of **infection** or infectious material. *Medical asepsis* is the destruction of organisms after they leave the body. The principles of medical asepsis are implemented to prevent reinfection of a patient and cross-infection of another patient or ourselves. To prevent cross-contamination, potential microorganisms and pathogens must be isolated by following standard blood and body fluid precautions and by disinfecting or sterilizing objects as soon as possible after they become contaminated. As discussed in Chapter 27, medical asepsis is the process of either reducing the number of pathogens or destroying them; this creates an environment that is clean but not sterile (free of microorganisms).

Surgical asepsis is the complete destruction of organisms on instruments or equipment that will enter the patient's body. This technique is mandatory for any procedure that invades the body's skin or tissues, such as surgery. Everything that comes in contact with the patient must be sterile, including surgical gowns, drapes, and instruments, in addition to the gloved hands of the surgeon and surgical assistants. Anytime the skin or a mucous membrane is punctured or pierced, as in venipunctures or injections, aseptic techniques must be practiced. Urinary catheterizations, biopsies, and dressing changes on open wounds are performed using sterile technique.

A medical assistant must develop an inner sense of sterile procedures. It is important that these techniques be performed on such a routine basis that they become an unbreakable habit. Conscientious attention must be given to sterilizing all items at all times. Frequent checking and rechecking of procedures helps ensure that they are effective and are used without any "breaks" in technique. Single-use, disposable items offer the best method of infection control, and they are being used more frequently in medical offices. However, when disposable equipment is used, the assistant must know the specific disposal guidelines for contaminated instruments and supplies.

STERILIZATION

Before an instrument or piece of equipment can be used in a surgical procedure, it first must be sanitized, then disinfected, and finally sterilized to remove all forms of microorganisms. Sanitization and disinfection were described in Chapter 27. It is essential that you understand these two concepts, so review them if necessary before learning **sterilization** methods.

Instruments and other items used in office surgery, examination, or treatment must be carefully cleaned before proceeding with the steps of disinfection or sterilization. *Sanitization* is the cleansing process that reduces the number of microorganisms to a safe level as dictated by public health guidelines. This cleansing process removes debris such as blood and other body fluids from instruments or equipment. Blood and debris must be removed so that later disinfection with chemicals or sterilization with steam, heat, or gases can

penetrate to all the instrument's surfaces (see Procedure 27-5). The procedure should be completed immediately after the instruments are used. If this is not possible, rinse the used items under cold water immediately after the surgical procedure and place them in a low-sudsing, rust-inhibiting, enzyme-containing, detergent solution. Never allow blood or other substances that can coagulate to dry on an instrument.

The medical assistant should always wear gloves while performing sanitization (thick utility gloves if the instruments have sharp or pointed edges) to prevent possible personal contamination with potentially infectious body fluids that may be present on the articles being cleaned. When you are ready to sanitize instruments, drain off the soak solution and rinse each instrument in cold, running water. Separate the sharp instruments from the others, because metal instruments may damage the cutting edges, and sharp instruments may damage the other instruments or injure you. Clean all sharp instruments at one time, when you can concentrate on preventing injury to yourself. Open all hinges and scrub serrations and ratchets with a small scrub brush or toothbrush. Rinse the instruments in hot water, then check them carefully for proper working order before they are disinfected or sterilized. The items should be hand dried with a towel to prevent spotting.

Disinfection is the process of killing pathogenic organisms or of rendering them inactive. However, it is not always effective against spores, the tubercle bacilli, and certain viruses. Disinfectant chemicals may kill microbes within a short time but are usually very hard on instruments. Some chemicals, such as Cidex, are effective enough to kill all organisms, but the usual immersion time for these sterilants is 10 hours or longer. Many types of disinfecting agents are available and have varying degrees of effectiveness. It is important to follow the manufacturer's guidelines on the proper use of each product and also to understand the product's advantages and disadvantages and the possible sources of error.

To ensure proper sterilization for surgical aseptic procedures, an area (usually a utility room) should be set aside in each office for just this purpose. The area should be divided into two sections, one dirty and one clean. The dirty section is used for receiving contaminated instruments and other materials at the conclusion of surgical procedures. This area should have a sink, receiving basins, proper cleaning agents, brushes, utility gloves, autoclave wrapping paper or cloth, autoclave envelopes and tape, sterilizer indicators, and disposable gloves. Designated biohazardous waste containers are needed for gloves worn when handling contaminated items. Personal protective equipment (PPE) for autoclave procedures includes:

- Heat-resistant autoclave gloves for loading and unloading
- Fluid-resistant gloves to prevent contact with contaminants
- A laboratory coat or impervious gown, if needed, to protect against splashes
- A face shield and/or goggles if a splash hazard exists

The clean section of the utility room should be reserved for receiving the sterile items after they have been removed from the sterilizer. Clear, clean plastic bags in which to store sterile packs may be kept in the clean area. Both areas should be spotlessly clean and well organized. Sterilization can be achieved by moist heat in an autoclave, by gas, or with chemicals. Most medical offices use the autoclave method. A written sterilization procedure should be in place for each workplace.

> ### CRITICAL THINKING APPLICATION   57-1
> The office manager told Melissa she needs to review the office policy and procedures manual on surgical supplies and sterilization methods. Why is this important before Melissa starts performing sterilization procedures? What information in this manual would be most important to Melissa as she starts this new position? Why?

Autoclave

Steam under pressure in the autoclave (Figure 57-1) is the best method of sterilization, because it kills all pathogens and spores. Pressurized steam is fast, convenient, and dependable. The pressure allows for heat higher than the boiling point, and when combined with moisture, these two factors create a very effective mechanism for killing all microorganisms. When steam is admitted into the autoclave chamber, it simultaneously heats and wets the object, coagulating the proteins present in all living organisms. When the cycle is complete and the chamber has cooled, the steam condenses and explodes the cells of microorganisms, thus destroying them. To be effective, the steam moisture must come in contact with all surfaces being sterilized. Steam under pressure is capable of much faster penetration of fabrics and textiles than dry heat, but its use has definite limitations if the proper techniques are not followed.

The recommended temperature for sterilization in an autoclave is 121° to 123° C (250° to 255° F). Unwrapped items should be sterilized for 20 minutes, small wrapped items for 30 minutes (Table 57-1), and large or tightly wrapped items for 40 minutes. Processing time starts *after* the autoclave reaches normal operating conditions of 121° C (250° F) and 15 pounds per square inch (psi) pressure.

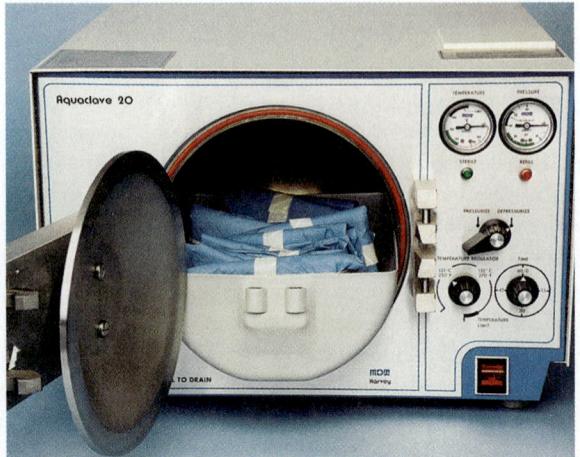

FIGURE 57-1 Steam autoclave. (Courtesy Aquaclave by Medtronic, Cincinnati, Ohio.)

The three basic autoclave cycles are as follows:

- Gravity (*"fast exhaust"*) cycle: This cycle is used to sterilize stainless steel instruments, glassware, and so on. The autoclave fills with steam and is held at a set temperature for a set period. When the cycle is complete, a valve opens and the chamber rapidly returns to atmospheric pressure. Drying time may be added to the end of the cycle. This is the cycle most often used in the physician's office setting.
- *Liquid ("slow exhaust") cycle:* This cycle is used to prevent sterilized liquids from boiling. Steam is exhausted slowly at the end of the cycle, allowing the liquids to cool.
- *Prevacuum cycle:* This cycle is used for porous materials. The chamber is partially evacuated before the introduction of steam for greater steam penetration; this is not available on all machines.

Incorrect operation of an autoclave may result in superheated steam. If steam is brought to too high a temperature, it is literally dried out, and the advantage of a higher heat is diminished. Wet steam is another cause of incomplete sterilization. Wet steam results

TABLE 57-1 Sterilization Chart*

ARTICLE	METHOD	TEMPERATURE (° F)	TIME
Gauze, small, loosely packed	Autoclave	250°	30 min
Gauze, large, loosely packed	Autoclave	270°	30 min
Gauze, small, tightly packed	Autoclave	250°	40 min
Gauze, large, tightly packed	Autoclave	270°	40 min
Gauze, tightly packed	Dry heat	320°	3 hr
Gauze, loosely packed	Dry heat	320°	2 hr
Glass syringes in tubes	Autoclave	250°	30 min
Glass syringes in muslin	Dry heat	320°	1 hr
Instruments on tray, muslin under and over	Dry heat	320°	1 hr
Instruments on tray, muslin under and over	Autoclave	250°	15 min
Solutions in flasks with gauze plug	Autoclave	250°	30 min
Glassware unwrapped	Dry heat	320°	1 hr
Glassware wrapped	Autoclave	250°	30 min
Petroleum jelly, 1-ounce jar	Dry heat	340°	1 hr
Petroleum jelly, 2-ounce jar	Dry heat	320°	2 hr
Petroleum gauze in instrument tray	Dry heat	320°	150 min
Powder, 1-ounce jar	Dry heat	320°	2 hr
Powder, small glove packs	Autoclave	250°	15 min

*Remember always to place a sterilization indicator in areas where there is doubt the steam will penetrate. Do not assess effectiveness by chamber pounds per square inch; a thermometer and sterilization indicator are the reliable methods of judging a killing temperature.

from failing to preheat the chamber, which causes excessive condensation in the interior of the chamber. Condensation is necessary, but too much prevents the sterilization process from being completed properly. It can be compared with taking a hot shower in a cold bathroom, which results in heavily steamed mirrors, walls, and towels. If packs become too saturated to dry during the drying cycle, the packs pick up and absorb bacteria from the air or any surface on which they are placed after removal from the autoclave. Placing cold instruments in a hot chamber also increases condensation. Other causes of wet steam include opening the door too wide at the end of the cycle or allowing a rush of cold air into the chamber. Overfilling the water reservoir may produce this same effect.

The main cause of incomplete sterilization in the autoclave is the presence of residual air. Without the complete elimination of air, an adequately high temperature cannot be reached. Air and steam do not mix. Because air is heavier than steam, it pools wherever possible. One tenth of 1% (0. 1%) residual air trapped around an instrument prevents complete sterilization. This is especially dangerous in older autoclaves that do not have a chamber thermometer separate from the pressure gauge. Adequate chamber pressure does not guarantee a proper chamber temperature. Table 57-2 provides tips for improving autoclave techniques.

Wrapping Materials

Maintenance of sterility depends completely on the wrapper and method of wrapping (Procedure 57-1). The wrapping material must be permeable to steam but impervious to contaminants. Acceptable wrapping materials for autoclaving should be made of a substance that allows the steam to penetrate while preventing pathogens from entering during storage and handling. A wrapper should not be used if it is torn or has a hole in it. Clean muslin, disposable autoclave paper, and polypropylene bags are examples of autoclave instrument wraps (Figure 57-2).

Wrapping Instruments

The method used to wrap instruments for autoclave sterilization must allow the pack to be opened without becoming contaminated. The rules for protecting package contents include the following:

- Inspect muslin wrappers for holes before each use and discard if any holes are found.
- Wrap all hinged instruments in the open position to allow full steam penetration of the joint.
- Place a gauze sponge around the tips of sharp instruments to prevent them from piercing the wrapping material.
- If a number of instruments are to be placed on a stainless steel tray for wrapping, first place a double-folded towel on the tray, then position the instruments. This helps to protect them.
- Polypropylene is a plastic capable of withstanding autoclaving but is resistant to heat transfer. Therefore, materials in a polypropylene pan take longer to autoclave than the same materials in a stainless steel pan.
- When using sterilizing bags, insert the jaws of the instruments first to ensure that the grasping end of the instrument can be reached easily when the bag is opened.

TABLE 57-2 Tips for Improving Autoclave Techniques

PROBLEM	CAUSES	CORRECTION
Damp linens	Clogged chamber drain; goods removed from chamber too soon after cycle; improper loading	Remove strainer; free openings of lint. Allow goods to remain in sterilizer an additional 15 min with door slightly open. Place packs on edge; arrange for least possible resistance to flow of steam and air.
Stained linens	Dirty chamber	Clean chamber with Calgonite solution; never use strong abrasives, such as steel wool; rinse thoroughly after cleaning.
Corroded instruments	Poor cleaning; residual soil; exposure to hard chemicals (e.g., iodine, salt, and acids); inferior instruments	Improve cleaning; do not allow soil to dry on instruments; sanitize first. Do not expose instruments to these chemicals; if exposure occurs, rinse immediately. Use only top-quality instruments.
Spotted or stained instruments	Mineral deposits on instruments; residual detergents from cleaning; mineral deposits from tap water	Wash with soft soap and detergent with good wetting properties. Rinse instruments thoroughly with distilled water.
Instruments with soft hinges or joints	Corrosion or soil in joint; instrument parts out of alignment	Clean with warm, weak acid solutions (10% nitric acid solution); rinse thoroughly. Have instrument realigned by qualified instrument repair professional.
Ebullition, or caps that blow off solutions	Too rapid exhausting of chamber	Use slow exhaust, cool liquids, or turn autoclave off and let cool on its own; that is, let the pressure drop at its own rate.
Steam leakage	Worn gasket; door closes improperly	Replace gasket; reopen door and shut carefully; have serviced if unable to close door properly.
Chamber door does not open	Vacuum in chamber (check chamber pressure gauge)	Turn on controls to starting steam pressure; wait until equalized, then vent and open door.

PROCEDURE 57-1

Prepare Items for Autoclaving: Wrap Instruments and Supplies for Sterilization in an Autoclave

GOAL: *To place dry, checked, sanitized, and disinfected supplies and instruments inside appropriate wrapping materials for sterilization and storage without contamination.*

EQUIPMENT and SUPPLIES

- Dry, checked, sanitized, and disinfected items
- Autoclave paper or cloth wrapping material
- Autoclave tape
- Sterilization indicator
- Waterproof, felt-tipped pen
- Disposable gloves (if part of office policy)

PROCEDURAL STEPS

1. Sanitize your hands. Collect and assemble already sanitized and disinfected items to be wrapped. Gloves may be worn.
2. Place the wrapping material on a clean, flat surface.
3. Place the item (or items) diagonally at the approximate center of the wrapping material. Make sure the size of the square is large enough for the items (Figure 1).

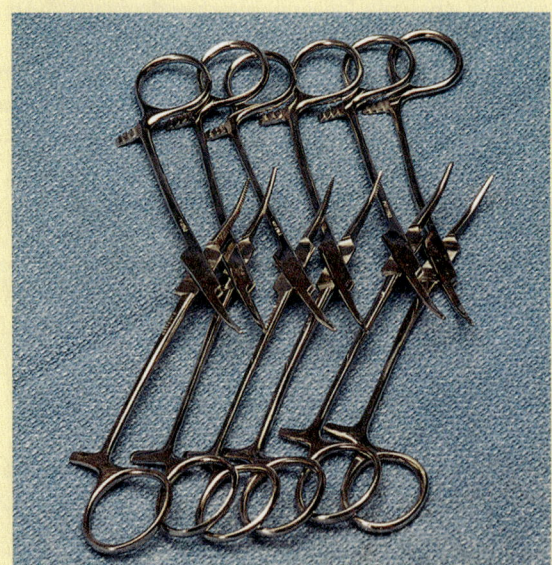

   <u>PURPOSE:</u> Each of the four corners must fold over and completely cover the items, with a few extra inches of overlap for folding.
4. With the squares that are cloth fabric, use two pieces if the cloth is single layered; follow the manufacturer's recommendation when using commercial autoclave wrapping paper.
   <u>PURPOSE:</u> To ensure sterility until the sterile item is needed for use.
5. Open any hinged instruments. If the instrument is sharp, its teeth or tip should be shielded with cotton or gauze.
   <u>PURPOSE:</u> To prevent puncture of the package or injury to the operator.
6. If the package is to contain several items, place a commercial sterilization indicator inside the package at the approximate center.
   <u>PURPOSE:</u> To ensure that the autoclave is reaching effective levels of heat and pressure.

7. Bring up the bottom corner of the wrap and fold back a portion of it.
   <u>PURPOSE:</u> This folded-back flap is the only part of each wrapper corner that can be touched when a sterile package is opened (Figure 2).

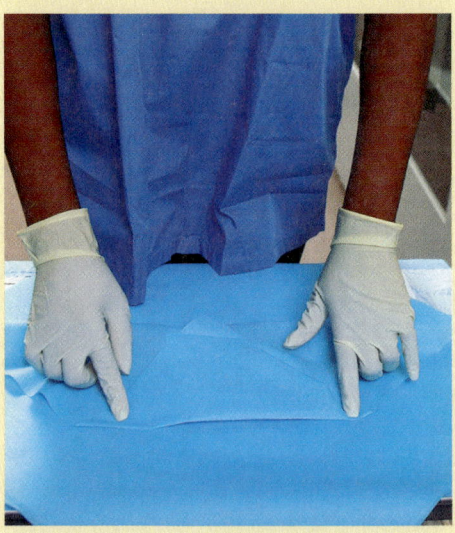

8. Repeat the above step with each corner, making sure to turn back a portion each time (Figures 3 and 4).

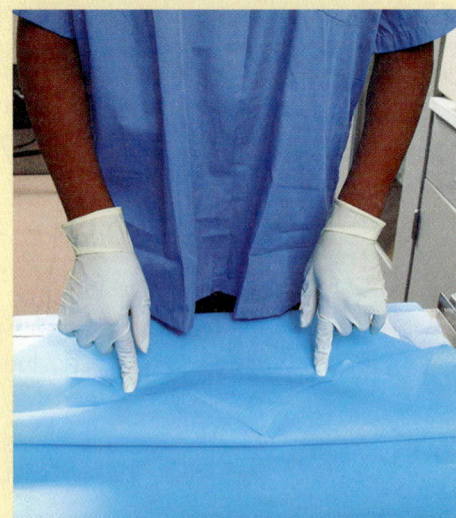

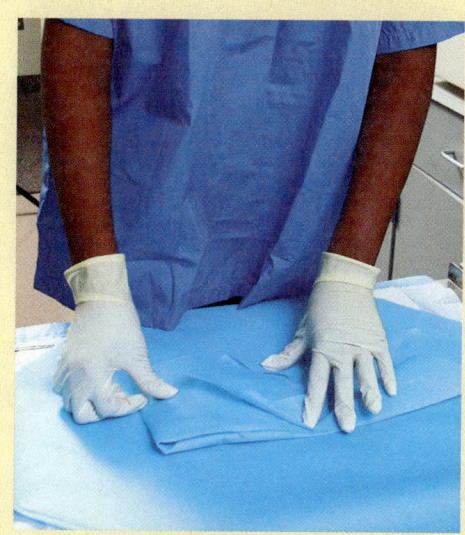

9. Fold the last flap over (Figure 5).

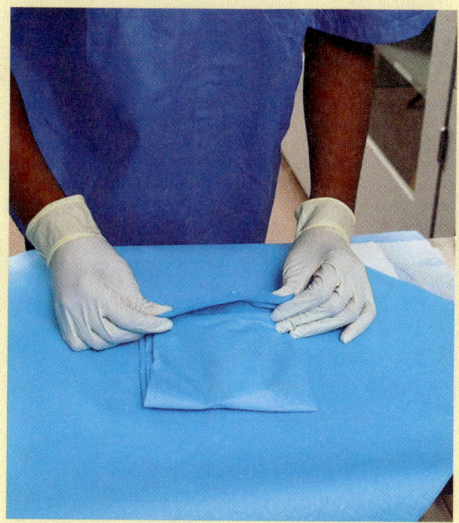

10. Secure with autoclave tape (Figure 6).

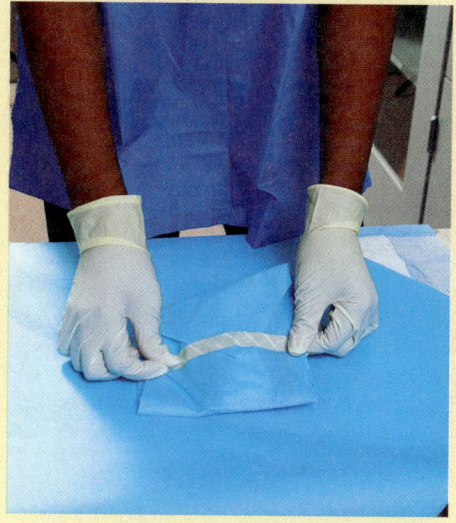

11. Secure with autoclave tape and label the package with the date, including the year, contents, and your initials (Figure 7).

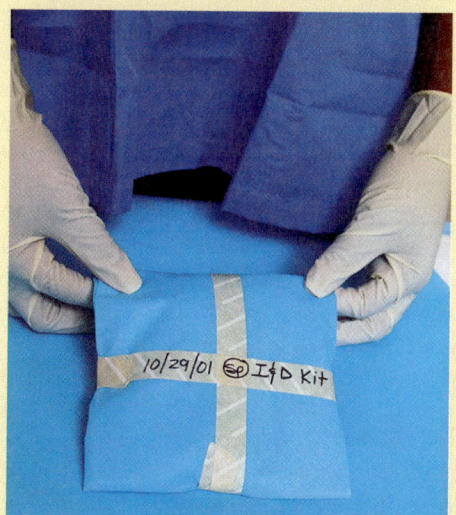

<u>PURPOSE:</u> So that staff members will know what is in the pack at a later date, whether the shelf life has expired (expiration date), and who performed the task. As a general rule, most office-autoclaved packs are considered sterile (usable) for up to 28 days.

- Indicate on the wrapper what is in the package or label it with a code. This code should correspond with a list of instruments that are stored with the pack after sterilization.
- Label each pack according to the instrument contents, sterilization date, and your initials. Use a permanent marker, never a ballpoint pen.
- Whether you are wrapping one item or many items together on a tray as a surgical pack, the procedure is the same; be sure the wrapper is large enough to cover the items to be sterilized.

CRITICAL THINKING APPLICATION **57-2**

Melissa is processing instruments and trays when she notices that one of her co-workers never inspects a muslin wrapper before wrapping a pack. What is the significance of Melissa's observation? How should she handle this situation? Why?

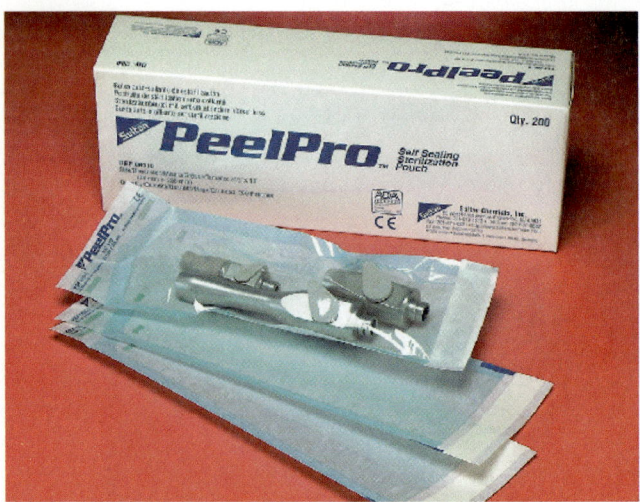

FIGURE 57-2 Sterilization pouches with sterilization indicators on the outside and inside of the envelope. The puncture-resistant, tinted plastic front is safety sealed to an autoclave paper backing. (Courtesy Practicon Dental, Greenville, NC.)

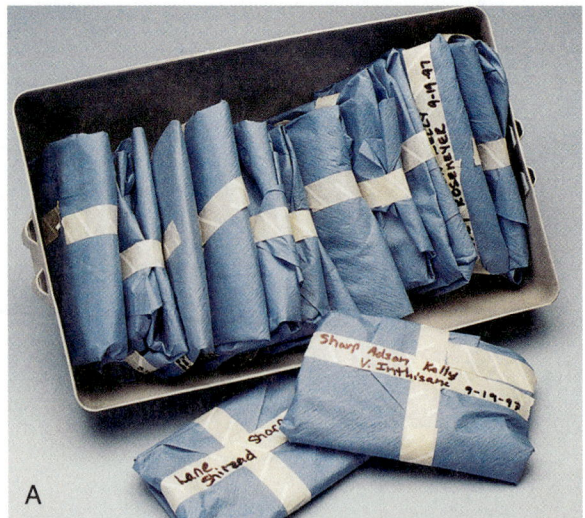

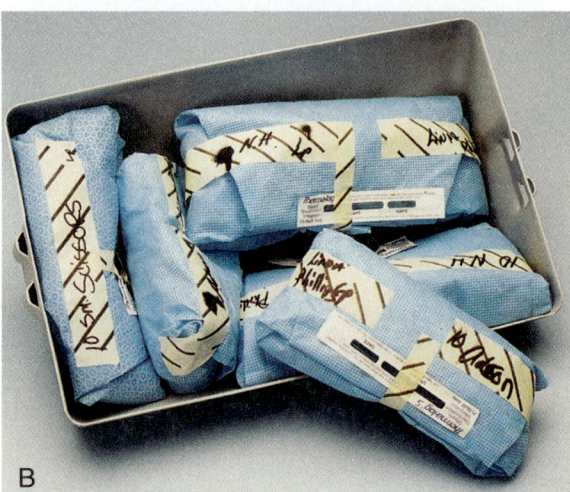

FIGURE 57-3 A, Instrument packs wrapped with autoclave paper and autoclave tape before the autoclave procedure. **B,** Instrument packs after autoclaving. Note the difference in the chemical lines on the autoclave tape.

Sterilization Indicators

Sterilization is achieved only when steam reaches the optimum temperature for a designated length of time and has penetrated to the center of the articles. Sterilization indicators must be used routinely to determine whether all microorganisms have been destroyed. The two basic types of sterilization indicators are chemical indicators (autoclave tape) and biologic indicators (bacterial spore strips).

Chemical Sterilization Indicators. Autoclave tape, a commonly used sterilization indicator, contains a chemical dye that changes color when exposed to steam (Figure 57-3). The tape is not an absolute indication that the proper sterilization time, temperature, and steam have been maintained; it merely indicates that a high temperature was reached while the article was in the autoclave. The strip must completely change color (colors vary by manufacturer) or reveal the word "autoclaved" to ensure effective operation. The main function of autoclave tape, besides holding the wrapping material together or closing a sterilization bag, is to verify that the package has been autoclaved.

Biologic Sterilization Indicators. The facility should have a policy for how frequently the autoclave is tested using biologic methods. One type, a spore strip indicator, contains a temperature-sensitive dye that changes color when the proper combination of steam, temperature, and time has been achieved. An indicator strip should be placed in the center of the largest pack that typically would be autoclaved in the facility to determine the accuracy of the autoclave and autoclave procedures. Test indicator kits are available that use ampules of *Bacillus stearothermophilus,* which is destroyed at 121° C (250° F). On completion of the cycle, the ampule is sent to the laboratory for analysis of any type of microbial growth, which would indicate that the autoclave is not sterilizing properly.

Quality Assurance Records for Office Sterilization

Every office should have specific protocols to follow for quality-assurance evaluations of the autoclave. This is done at specified intervals, depending on the volume and frequency of autoclave use. A log must be kept of the type of control test done, when it was

performed, and the testing results. If the testing results indicate that sterilization was inadequate, a report must be made and filed. The report should identify the nature of the problem and how and when it was corrected. The report also should contain proof of correction by indicating the date and time of a first, subsequent, and successful sterilization run.

Loading the Autoclave

Prepare all packs and arrange the load in a way that allows maximum circulation of steam and heat (Procedure 57-2). Articles should be resting on their edges and should not be crowded. Placing the packs in stainless steel racks prevents packing of the autoclave too tightly. Jars, bottles, and trays must be wrapped and placed on their sides if they are to be used to store sterile items. Covers on jars and containers should be put to one side or left open to allow steam to penetrate. Extreme care must be taken not to contaminate jars when replacing their lids after autoclaving.

Instruments may be autoclaved unwrapped if they do not need to be sterile when used later. For example, although vaginal speculums do not need to be sterilized for use (the vagina is a body cavity

Perform Sterilization Procedures: Operate the Autoclave

GOAL: *To sterilize properly prepared supplies and instruments using the autoclave.*

EQUIPMENT and SUPPLIES

- Autoclave
- Wrapped items ready to be sterilized
- Heat-resistant gloves

PROCEDURAL STEPS

NOTE: The specific instructions for operating an autoclave may vary based on the model number and manufacturer. Refer to the instructions that accompany the autoclave to be sure the appropriate steps are followed.

1. Check the water level in the reservoir and add distilled water as necessary.
   PURPOSE: Too much or too little water may alter the effectiveness of the equipment. Tap water leaves lime deposits in the chamber.
2. Turn the control to "Fill" to allow water to flow into the chamber. The water flows until you turn the control to its next position. Do not let the water overflow.
3. Load the chamber with wrapped items, spacing them for maximum circulation and penetration.
   PURPOSE: To ensure sterilization of all items.
4. Close and seal the door.
   PURPOSE: The door must be closed, or the heated water in the chamber evaporates.
5. Turn the control setting to "On" or "Autoclave" to start the cycle.

6. Watch the gauges until the temperature gauge reaches at least 121° C (250° F) and the pressure gauge reaches 15 pounds (lb) of pressure.
   PURPOSE: The proper temperature and pressure must be reached before sterilization can begin.
7. Set the timer for the desired time.
8. At the end of the timed cycle, turn the control setting to "Vent."
   PURPOSE: This releases the steam and pressure. The water at the bottom of the chamber drains back into the reservoir.
9. Wait for the pressure gauge to reach zero.
10. Standing behind the autoclave door, carefully open the chamber door ¼ inch.
    PURPOSE: To allow steam to escape faster. Be careful to prevent accidental burns.
11. Leave the autoclave control at "Vent" to continue releasing heat.
    PURPOSE: To dry the items faster.
12. Allow complete drying of all articles.
13. Using heat-resistant gloves, remove the items from the chamber and place the sterilized packages on dry, covered shelves or open the autoclave door and allow the items to cool completely before removal and storage.
14. Turn the control knob to "Off" and keep the door slightly ajar.
    PURPOSE: To allow the inside of the autoclave to dry completely.

---

that is naturally open to the external environment), they must be sanitized, disinfected, and sterilized to prevent cross-contamination among patients. They can be placed unwrapped on a perforated stainless steel tray in the autoclave and then stored in a clean area for future use.

Unloading Guidelines

When the autoclave's sterilization cycle is complete, release the pressure according to the manufacturer's guidelines. Once the pressure gauge reads "0," stand back from the door and, with heat-resistant gloves, open the door approximately ¼ inch. Allow the load to dry for at least 15 minutes (this time varies according to the type of autoclave and the size of the load). Capillary attraction is the action that draws moisture through the surface of materials. Packs can act like a sponge, attracting outside moisture and microorganisms. Touching a wet pack allows microorganisms on your hands to penetrate the wrappings, making the contents of the pack nonsterile. Dry, wrapped packs may be removed with clean, dry hands, but it is safer to wear heat-resistant gloves to reduce the possibility of burns from the hot instruments inside the packs. If possible, allow all packs to cool in the autoclave with the door open. Place the packs on a dry, dust-free surface inside an enclosed cupboard or drawer for storage. Do not place the packs on cold surfaces, because hot packs

may cause condensation, and moisture will contaminate the contents.

Guidelines for unloading an autoclave include the following:
- Stand behind the door when opening it to prevent accidental steam burns.
- Slowly open the door only a crack, allowing the items to cool for 15 to 20 minutes before removing them.
- If for any reason the integrity of the sterilization process is in question, the load should be considered contaminated and autoclaved again. Reasons for concern include the following:
  o Any load that fails to convert a sterilization indicator strip
  o Any loads processed after a biologic test indicates that the autoclave is not working properly

Shelf Life of Sterilized Packs. Each office has its own guidelines for the shelf life of sterile packs. Generally, muslin and autoclave paper packs are considered sterile for up to 28 days from the date of sterilization. Polypropylene autoclave bags are sterile for up to 6 months from the sterilization date. All sterile packs should be stored on dry, dust-free, covered shelves or in drawers. Fabric wrappers must be inspected for holes and laundered after each use. A damaged pack or a broken seal renders the package nonsterile; spills of any fluid onto a package also contaminate it. When a pack is no longer sterile for any reason, including the expiration date, the contents must be reprocessed as if the pack had been used for surgery. The contents must be sanitized, disinfected, wrapped, and sterilized as usual.

CRITICAL THINKING APPLICATION   57-3

Melissa discovers a number of packages of paper-wrapped sterile instruments that have no dates on them. The indicator tape shows that they have been autoclaved. What should she do with these packs? Why?

Gas Sterilization

A variety of gas sterilizers are available. Each has its own very specific operating guidelines to ensure operator safety. Because of the long processing times, the very specific requirements for gas ventilation established by the Occupational Safety and Health Administration (OSHA), and the hazards of reproductive organ damage and cancer associated with gas sterilization, it is unrealistic to use gas sterilization in the physician's office.

Chemical Sterilization

In the medical office, chemical sterilization is used for instruments that cannot be exposed to the high temperatures of steam sterilization. The sterilizing chemical solution must be mixed exactly according to the instructions on the bottle. The solution must be marked with the date of preparation and expiration. Materials to be sterilized must be submerged in this chemical bath with a closed lid for 8 hours or longer. Items are removed with sterile forceps and must be rinsed with sterile water to remove all traces of the chemical before the items are used on a patient. Removed items are then dried with a sterile towel. You must avoid skin contact with the sterilizing solution because it is very caustic.

SURGICAL PROCEDURES

Common surgical procedures that are routinely performed in the primary care office include suturing, cyst removal, incision and drainage (I&D) of abscesses, and collection of biopsy specimens. The medical assistant should be proficient in explaining each of these procedures to the patient, preparing the patient and the room, assisting the physician with the surgery, and applying a sterile dressing and bandage after the procedure is finished.

Each surgical procedure requires appropriate skin preparation and draping with a *fenestrated* drape, also called an *eye sheet*. This is a surgical drape with an opening in the center. The size of the opening depends on the size of the surgical field. The opening is placed directly over the surgical site after the site has been suitably prepared (or "prepped," as it is called in healthcare practice). A minor surgery tray is opened, and a sterile field is created on a Mayo instrument stand. Sutures, scalpel, and any other instruments needed are added to the field, according to the surgeon's preference. Have a local anesthetic ready, also according to the physician's preference.

After achieving suitable local anesthesia, the physician opens the skin with an incision. If a cyst is being removed, the physician dissects around it and usually tries to "deliver" it from the wound intact. If the procedure is an I&D, foul matter will start oozing from the wound immediately after the skin is incised. The wound is drained completely and flushed with copious amounts of sterile saline

solution. A drain may be placed in the wound and left for several days. If the procedure is a biopsy, a small amount of tissue is removed and placed in a specimen container with preservative. The specimen container must be carefully labeled with the appropriate patient information, the date, and specifics about the specimen type and location. It then is sent to the laboratory, where it is examined microscopically for changes or abnormalities.

Electrosurgery

Electrosurgery is also known as *electrocautery*. An electrosurgical unit (ESU) uses high-frequency current to cut through tissue and coagulate blood vessels. A small probe with an electric current running through it is used to *cauterize* (burn or destroy) the tissue. When the electric current comes in contact with tissue and blood cells, they are vaporized, producing carbon and steam. This process seals blood vessels, minimizing cellular oozing and bleeding. Electrosurgery may be used to destroy granulations and small polyps.

Necessary components are the ESU's power source, the grounding cable and pad, and the active electrode (a pencil-like instrument with a tip and cord). Tips are disposable and are used according to the type of procedure performed. The two most commonly used tips are the needle and flat designs.

Holding the pencil-like instrument, the surgeon touches the tissue with the tip and activates the electric current with a switch on the instrument or a foot pedal. The electric current is delivered to the tissues, and tissue is vaporized at the site of contact.

IMPORTANT TIPS ABOUT THE GROUNDING PAD

- Carefully inspect the pad, cable, and skin before the procedure.
- Place the pad close to the operative site.
- The pad must be tight against the patient's skin.
- Apply the pad to a fleshy area, such as the thigh.
- Do not place the pad over a bony area.
- Do not place the pad over body hair.
- Do not place the pad over metal implants or a pacemaker.
- Carefully inspect the pad site on the skin after the procedure.

Laser Surgery

Laser is an acronym for *l*ight *a*mplification by *s*timulated *e*mission of *r*adiation. Because a laser beam is so small and precise, it can be used to safely treat specific tissue with minimal damage to surrounding tissues and limited scar formation. Lasers were first used in medicine to treat diseases of the retina, and they now are used for many procedures, including excision of lesions, cauterization of blood vessels, removal of warts or moles, and cosmetic surgical procedures.

Several types of lasers are used, including the carbon dioxide, yttrium-aluminum-garnet (YAG), and pulsed dye lasers. Each laser has a specific use. The color of the laser light beam is directly related to the type of surgery performed.

A medical assistant must be specially trained to operate a laser before assisting with laser surgery. Laser equipment requires very careful handling, care, and maintenance. Laser light destroys tissue and can harm the patient, the physician, and you if handled improperly. The medical assistant should complete a full laser safety program before assisting in laser procedures. Once trained, the medical assistant's role during laser surgery includes:

- Observing the surgical field through safety goggles for possible contamination and protecting the patient's eyes
- Keeping wet sponges ready
- Removing any flammable item from the laser's path
- Assisting with suctioning of the plume to maintain a clear visual field
- Having a basin of sterile normal saline solution and a filled irrigating syringe ready
- Watching each application of the laser beam and anticipating the need for protective supplies, special equipment, or instruments

Microsurgery

Microsurgery involves the use of an operating microscope to perform delicate surgical procedures. One of its major uses is in ophthalmologic surgery. It also is used in otologic, rhinologic and sinus, laryngologic, neurosurgical, microvascular, gynecologic, and genitourinary procedures. A medical assistant must acquire a basic knowledge of the operation and care of a microscope before becoming qualified to assist in these types of procedures.

The basic components of an operating microscope are the light source, eyepieces (also called the *oculars*), lenses, and cord. Accessory pieces include assistant and observer lenses, cameras, video recorders, television monitors, and printers. These are all valuable for documentation and teaching purposes. Disposable sterile drapes and handle covers are used on the microscope during surgical procedures.

Surgical microscopes are expensive, delicate instruments that require extreme care in handling and cleaning. All lenses and cords should be carefully inspected before and after each use.

Endoscopic Procedures

An endoscope is a medical device consisting of a miniature camera mounted on a flexible tube with an optical system and a light source that is used to examine the area inside an organ or cavity. Many types of endoscopes are used, and they are named according to the organs or areas they are used to explore, such as the urinary bladder, bronchus, larynx, colon (Figure 57-4), stomach, uterus, abdomen, and various joints. Small instruments can be used to take samples of suspicious tissues through the endoscope.

Direct visualization with an endoscope is used for diagnostic purposes or to perform surgical procedures. Endoscopes may be rigid (e.g., laparoscope or hysteroscope), semirigid, or flexible (colonoscopes, bronchoscopes, gastroscopes). All are delicate and expensive and require extreme care in handling to protect them from damage.

Accessory equipment used with endoscopes includes fiberoptic light cables and light source; irrigators for solution instillation and suction; and a camera, monitor, printer, and video recorder. The fiberoptic light cable consists of hundreds of glass fibers. It is important to protect it from being bent, dropped, kinked, squashed, or smashed. The light source can become very hot and must be kept out of contact with the patient, the physician, the staff, and any flammable material, such as surgical draping. All equipment must

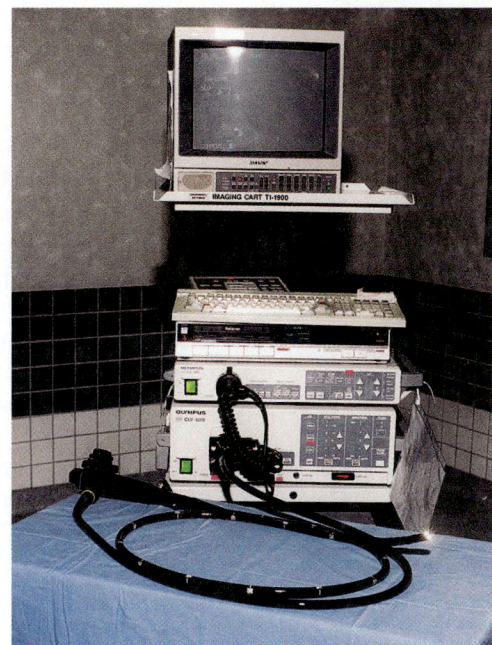

FIGURE 57-4 Flexible colonoscope with monitor and video recorder.

be checked before and after use. Always follow the manufacturer's recommendations for use, care, and maintenance of equipment.

Cryosurgery

Cryosurgery involves the use of a very-low-temperature probe to destroy tissue by freezing it on contact. The probe's temperature usually is below $-20°$ C ($4°$ F). This cold temperature is achieved by circulating liquid nitrogen through the tip of the probe. A local anesthetic usually is administered before cryosurgery. Cryosurgery is used to treat cancers of the skin, prostate, liver, pancreas, and kidney. In many situations, cryosurgery is less invasive than traditional surgery and therefore generally has fewer associated complications. Cryosurgery often is performed in an office setting or in an outpatient surgery center.

ASSISTING WITH SURGICAL PROCEDURES

Surgery performed in a medical office is restricted to the management of minor problems and injuries. The medical assistant is expected to assist with preparing the patient and setting up the sterile field. The following procedures must be used without exception when assisting with minor surgery. Individual facilities may have specific guidelines for some of these procedures; however, the theory behind sterile technique is universal, regardless of where you work.

Preparation of the Patient

Whether minor surgery is performed because of an unforeseen accident or is a planned, elective procedure, the patient needs both psychological and physical support. A patient facing a surgical procedure may be concerned about pain, disfigurement, and a possible diagnosis of cancer. An injured patient may feel anxious about medical bills or possible loss of employment. Because surgery is a frightening experience, the medical assistant must take the time, both preoperatively and at the time of surgery, to help the patient deal with fears and anxieties. The best way to help is to make sure that the patient understands the details of the procedure, that all questions are answered by the physician, and that the patient has the opportunity to talk about the procedure and voice any concerns.

Questions should be answered directly, but you should answer only the questions that are within your scope of knowledge and the policies of the office. If you cannot answer a question, assure the patient that you will relay it to the physician before the procedure and then be sure to do so. What may seem to be a minor or unimportant question to you may be a very frightening concern to the patient. The minor surgery room can be intimidating, so unless the patient is sedated, try to make conversation with him or her while you prepare for the physician's arrival.

Preoperative preparation may include blood and urine tests, completion of a consent form, and gathering of the current history concerning any recent illnesses, medications, and allergies. Patient preparations before surgery may include a shave prep, cleansing enemas, food intake restrictions, special bathing, and administration of a sedative medication. On the day of surgery, the patient is instructed to empty the bladder and undress and gown as requested. The vital signs are recorded in preparation for the procedure.

Preoperative Instructions

When office surgery is planned, certain procedures are followed before the appointment. These include the following:

- Having the necessary consent forms ready to sign
- Giving the patient the necessary preoperative instructions, such as medications to be used and special skin-cleansing instructions
- Telling the patient to bring a relative or friend to drive him or her home after the surgery
- Instructing the patient to leave jewelry and other valuables at home
- Calling the patient the day before the scheduled surgery to confirm any special instructions

Informed Consent

The physician must have the patient's written informed consent before beginning any surgical procedure. To sign an informed consent form permitting the physician to legally perform the surgery, the patient must understand what procedure will be performed, why it should be done, the potential risks and benefits of the surgery, alternative treatments (including no treatment), and the possible risks of any alternative treatment. This legal requirement is not met simply by having the patient sign an operative permit; a discussion must occur, during which the physician provides the patient or the patient's legal representative with enough information to enable the person to decide whether to proceed with the proposed surgical treatment. After this discussion, the patient either consents to or refuses the surgery. The patient then signs or refuses to sign the consent form. If the patient signs with an X, the medical assistant should write "patient's mark" beside the X and also should have a family member witness the signature. The discussion must be fully documented in the patient's medical record. A copy of the signed form must also be included in the patient's record. Treatment may not exceed the scope of the consent form.

The patient must not be under the influence of any sedative medication at the time he or she signs the consent form. This condition must *never* be violated.

Positioning

Have the patient disrobe sufficiently to expose the surgical site completely so that accidental contamination does not occur during the procedure. Clothing may also act as a tourniquet or may make applying a proper dressing or bandage difficult. In addition, the patient's clothing may be stained by the skin prep solution or may interfere with adequate site preparation.

The patient needs to be positioned as comfortably as possible for the procedure. An uncomfortable position can be held for only a limited time, and the patient may have to move, perhaps in the middle of a procedure, if you have not ensured his or her comfort from the beginning. When deciding on the correct position, consider where you and the physician will stand or sit, where the instruments will be placed, and where other needed equipment will be located. If the patient has an open wound that will need irrigation during the procedure, wear nonsterile gloves to assist the patient into position. If there is active and profuse bleeding, an impermeable gown and gloves should be worn. If there is danger of blood and body fluid contamination to your face or eyes, wear goggles, a mask, or a face shield.

Skin Preparation

The human skin is a reservoir of bacteria, but it cannot be sterilized without the risk of damaging cells and tissues. The goal of adequate skin preparation for a surgical procedure is to reduce the number of transient and resident microorganisms so that transference of harmful organisms at the incision site is limited. Cleansing the patient's skin before surgery with surgical soap and an antiseptic and shaving the area if needed is called a *skin prep* (Procedure 57-3). Sometimes the patient may be instructed to repeatedly cleanse the surgical area with bacteriostatic or antiseptic soap several days before the surgery. Disposable skin prep trays and razors are commonly used in a physician's office.

Preparation of the Room

If you are to assist in a minor surgical procedure, study the physician's care preferences, review the procedure, and note the materials needed. Next, prepare the room and gather the supplies to be used. Sterile supplies are opened just before the procedure. Opened materials that have been exposed longer than 1 hour, usually because of a delay, are considered nonsterile. Supplies should not be placed where they can be knocked over or dropped. Wrapped sterile supplies that fall to the floor must not be used. Once supplies have been opened, the sterile field should be covered with a sterile drape, and

PROCEDURE 57-3

Assist the Physician with Patient Care: Perform Skin Prep for Surgery

GOAL: *To prepare the patient's skin and remove hair from the surgical site to reduce the risk of wound contamination.*

EQUIPMENT and SUPPLIES

- A disposable skin prep kit or collect the following:
  - Gauze sponges
  - Cotton-tipped applicators
  - Antiseptic soap
  - Disposable gloves
  - Disposable razor
  - Two small bowls
  - Antiseptic or antiseptic swabs (e.g., Betadine swabs)
  - Sterile normal saline solution
  - Optional: cotton balls, nail pick, scrub brush
- Sterile drape
- Biohazardous sharps container and waste receptacle
- Patient's record

PROCEDURAL STEPS

1. Sanitize your hands.
   PURPOSE: To follow Standard Precautions.
2. Instruct the patient in the skin preparation procedure, making sure the person understands the procedure and the rationale for it.
   PURPOSE: To ensure cooperation and demonstrate awareness of possible patient concerns.
3. Ask the patient to remove any clothing that might interfere with exposure of the site and provide a gown if needed.
4. Assist the patient into the proper position for site exposure. Provide a drape if necessary to protect the patient's privacy.
5. Expose the site. Use a light if necessary.
6. Put on gloves and open the skin prep pack.
7. Add the antiseptic soap to the two bowls.
8. Start at the incision site and begin washing with the antiseptic soap on a gauze sponge in a circular motion, moving from the center to the edges of the area to be scrubbed (Figure 1).

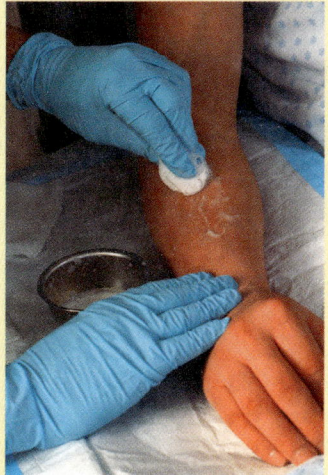

PURPOSE: A circular motion from inside to outside drags contaminants away from the incision site.

9. After one complete wipe, discard the sponge and begin again with a new sponge soaked in the antiseptic solution.
   PURPOSE: After one circular sweep, the sponge is contaminated with skin bacteria and debris.
10. When you return to the incision site for the next circular sweep, you must use clean material.
11. Repeat the process, using sufficient friction for 5 minutes (or follow office policy for the length of time required for a particular prep).
12. If hair is present, the area may need to be shaved. Hold the skin taut and shave in the direction of growth (Figure 2). Take care to prevent injury to yourself or your patient. Immediately after completion, dispose of the razor in the sharps container.

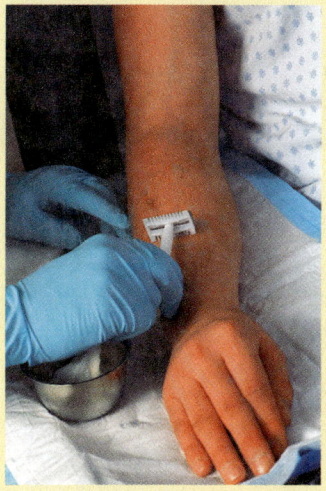

PURPOSE: Hair should be removed before any invasive procedure to limit the potential for infection; follow Standard Precautions regarding sharps.

13. After shaving, scrub the skin a second time.
14. Rinse the area with a sterile normal saline solution (Figure 3).

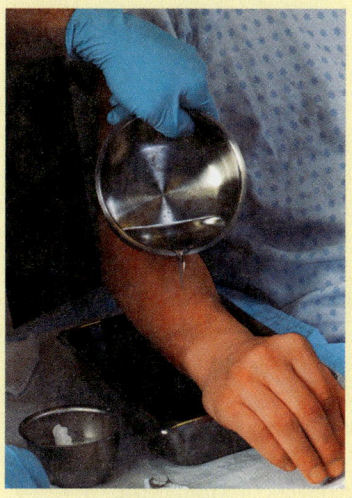

PROCEDURE 57-3—cont'd

15. Dry the area, using the same circular technique with dry sponges. The area may be dried by blotting with a sterile towel.
16. Paint on the antiseptic with the cotton-tipped applicators or gauze sponges, using the same circular technique and never returning to an area that has already been painted (Figure 4).

17. Place a sterile drape and/or towel over the area.
18. Answer all the patient's questions to relieve anxiety about the upcoming surgical procedure.
19. Document completion of the skin prep in the patient's chart.

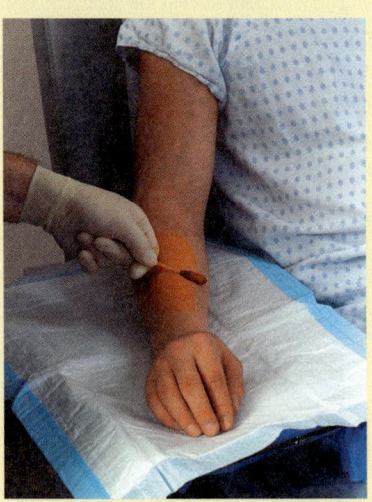

a team member should stay in the room to monitor them. Make sure the patient and family members understand that they should not approach or touch the sterile field.

Sterile Technique

Accurately performing surgical aseptic technique involves a degree of dexterity and vigilance that can come only with practice. It requires a great deal of concentration and planning of all movements and procedural steps. The procedures covered in this chapter are for minor surgery, but they are the same techniques used during major surgery. To develop a sound knowledge of sterility and sterile technique, use the following memory aid: *Everything sterile is white and everything that is not sterile is black. There is no gray!* Sterile surfaces must *never* come in contact with nonsterile surfaces. If this occurs, the sterile surface immediately is considered contaminated or nonsterile. Constant vigilance and absolute honesty are essential for maintaining sterile techniques. When a sterile surface comes in contact with a nonsterile item, this is called a "break" in sterility or a "break" in the sterile field. During any procedure, everything must stop at this point and the "break" must be corrected immediately—which usually means the assistant must start over again at the very beginning of the procedure. Any break could lead to serious wound contamination, postoperative infection, and even death.

Before assisting with minor surgery, the medical assistant must perform a series of procedures to ensure surgical asepsis (Procedures 57-4 to 57-8). These skills must be learned, practiced, and followed precisely to establish and maintain the sterile environment required during a surgical procedure. Medical asepsis directly affects the health and well-being of the patient, the physician, and the office staff and must be practiced without fail.

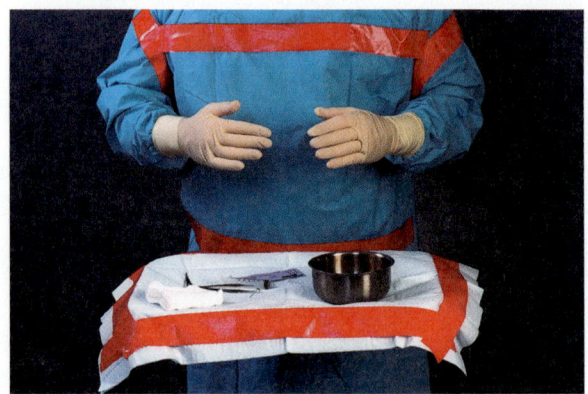

FIGURE 57-5 Sterile field (red outline).

CRITICAL THINKING APPLICATION   57-5

After completing a surgical scrub before assisting with a minor surgical procedure, Melissa sneezes. She does not touch her face, but instinctively raises her hands toward her face in the "sneeze range." Can she go ahead with putting on her sterile gloves? Why or why not?

Sterile Field

A sterile field is any sterile surface on which sterile items are placed. In the office, a sterile field most often is set up on a Mayo stand (Figure 57-5). In surgery, a sterile field is created by draping sterile towels (either disposable or from autoclaved packs) over a Mayo stand or table. The surgical site on the patient's skin is prepared and

Text continued on p. 1270

Perform Hand Washing: Perform a Surgical Hand Scrub

GOAL: *To scrub the hands with surgical soap, using friction, running water, and a sterile brush to sanitize the skin before assisting with any procedure that requires surgical asepsis.*

EQUIPMENT and SUPPLIES

- Sink with foot, knee, or arm control for running water
- Surgical soap in a dispenser
- Towels (sterile towels if indicated by office policy)
- Nail file or orange stick
- Sterile brush

Procedural Steps

1. Remove all jewelry.
   PURPOSE: Jewelry harbors bacteria and is not permitted in surgical asepsis.
2. Roll long sleeves above the elbows.
3. Inspect your fingernails for length and your hands for skin breaks.
4. Turn on the faucet and regulate the water to a comfortable temperature, being careful to stand away from the sink to prevent contamination of clothing.
5. Keep your hands upright and held at or above waist level (Figure 1).

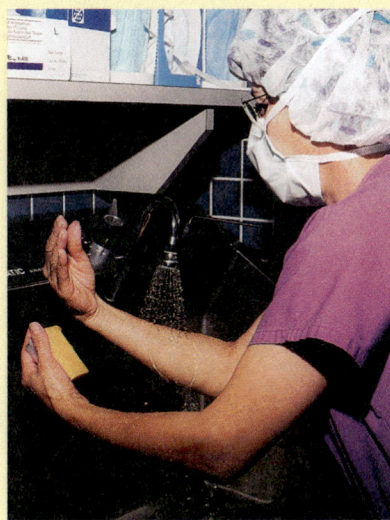

PURPOSE: Water running from the unscrubbed area above the elbow down to the hands can carry bacteria back onto the hands. All areas below the waist are considered contaminated during all surgical procedures.

6. Clean your fingernails with a file, discard it (in most situations you will drop the file into the sink and discard it later to prevent contamination by lowering your hands and/or touching a waste receptacle), and rinse your hands under the faucet without touching the faucet or the inside of the sink basin (Figure 2).

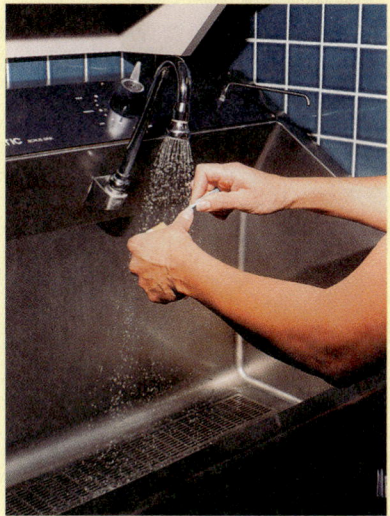

7. Allow the water to run over your hands from the fingertips to the elbows without moving the arm back and forth under the water.
   PURPOSE: Water running from the elbow down to the hands can carry bacteria back onto the hands.
8. Apply surgical soap from the dispenser to the sterile brush (or use a prepared disposable brush) and start the scrub by scrubbing the palm of the hand in a circular fashion.
9. Continue from the palm to the base of the thumb, then move on to the other fingers, scrubbing from the base, along each side, and across the nail, holding the fingertips upward and remembering to rub between the fingers (Figure 3). After the fingers have been completely scrubbed, clean the posterior surface of the hand in a circular fashion and then proceed to the wrist. The scrub process should take at least 5 minutes for each hand and arm.

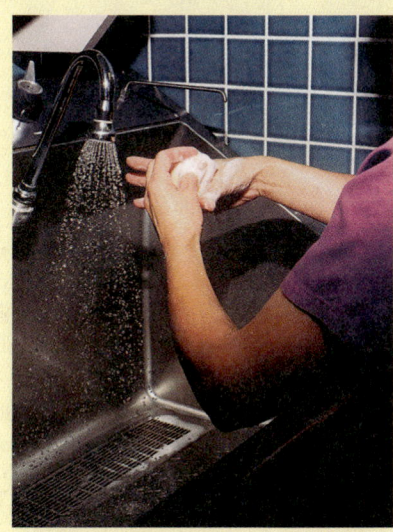

PURPOSE: The surfaces of the fingers have four sides.

10. Do not return to a clean area after you have moved to the next part of the hand.
    <u>PURPOSE:</u> Once an area has been scrubbed, it is considered surgically clean, and rubbing that area again contaminates it.

11. Wash the wrists and forearms in a circular fashion around the arm while holding your hands above waist level (Figure 4).

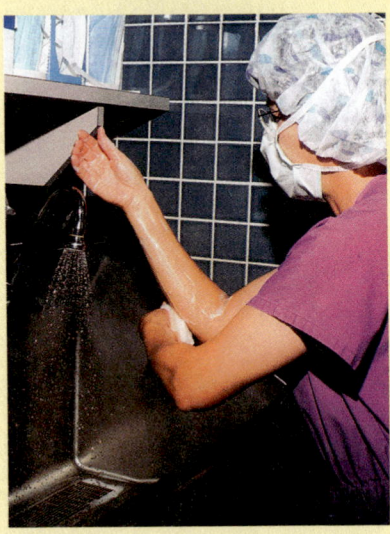

12. Rinse the arms and forearms from the fingertips upward, holding the fingers up, without touching the faucet or the inside of the sink basin (Figure 5).

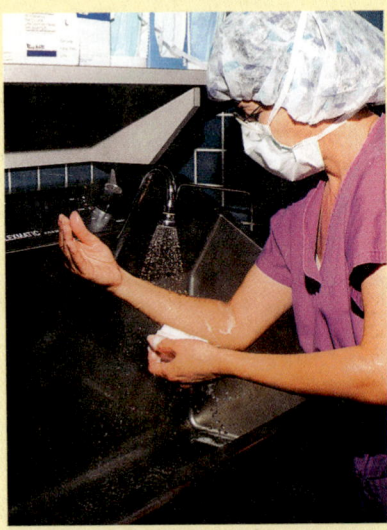

<u>PURPOSE:</u> Keep the fingers higher than the rest of the arm to prevent contamination from water running downward from the elbow. Touching the dirty faucet and/or basin causes contamination.

13. Apply more solution without touching any dirty surface and repeat the scrub on the other side, remembering to wash and use friction between each finger with a firm, circular motion.

14. Scrub all surfaces, being careful not to abrade your skin. The second hand and arm should take at least 5 minutes.

15. Rinse thoroughly, keeping your hands up and above waist level. Discard the scrub brush without lowering the arms below the waist (Figures 6 and 7).

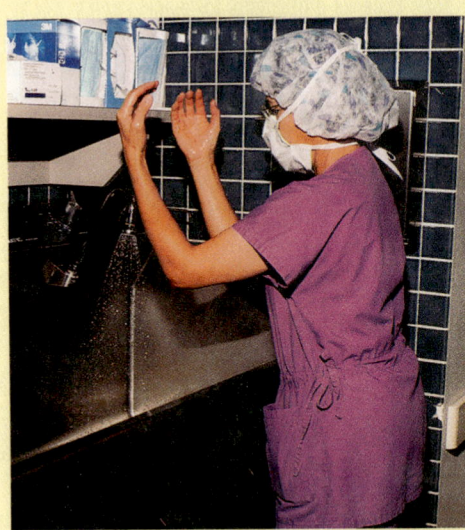

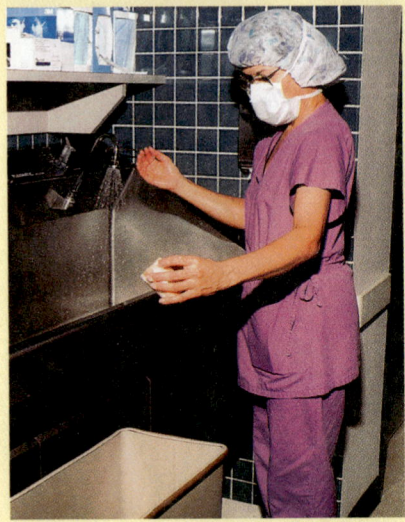

16. Turn off the faucet with the foot, knee, or forearm lever, if available.
    <u>PURPOSE:</u> To prevent clean hands from touching the contaminated faucet handles.

17. Dry your hands with a sterile towel, being careful to keep the fingers pointing upward and your hands above the waist. Do not rub back and forth, dragging contaminants from the dirtier area of the upper arm down toward the hands (Figures 8 and 9). Use the opposite end of the towel for the other hand.

PROCEDURE 57-4—cont'd

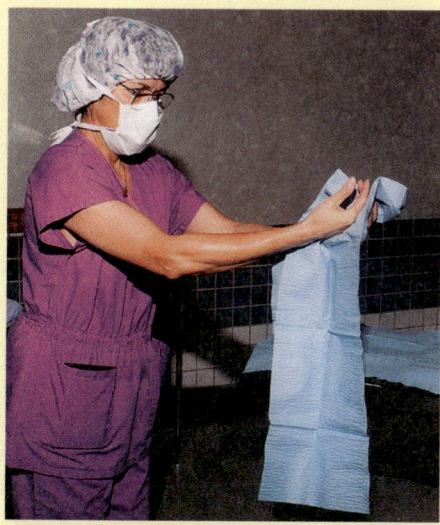

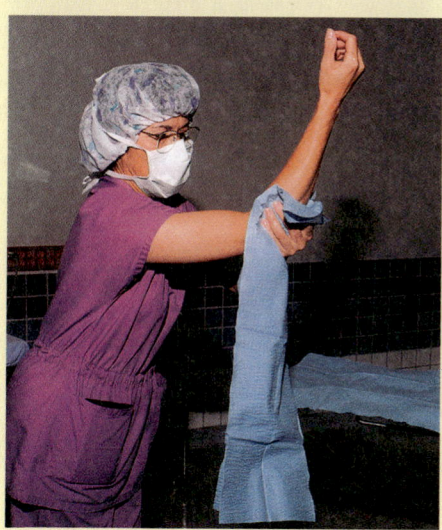

PURPOSE: To keep your clean hands from touching the part of the towel that comes in contact with your forearms, which are not as clean as your hands. If you are to gown and glove for a procedure, you must use a sterile towel.

18. Using a patting motion, continue to dry the forearms. Discard the towel and keep your hands up and above waist level (Figure 10).

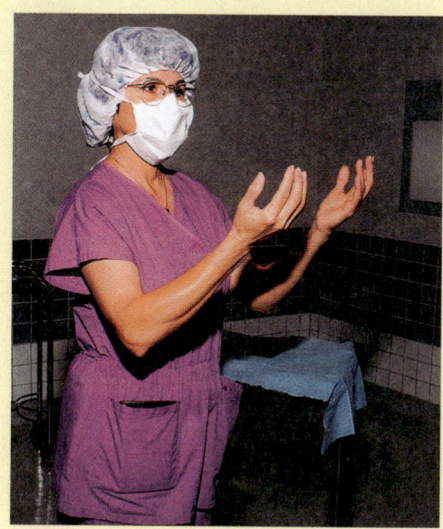

PROCEDURE 57-5

Assist the Physician with Patient Care: Open a Sterile Pack and Create a Sterile Field

GOAL: *To open a sterile instrument pack using correct aseptic technique.*

EQUIPMENT and SUPPLIES

- A sterile instrument pack wrapped with either muslin or autoclave paper that, when opened, will serve as a sterile table drape or field
- Mayo stand or countertop
- Disinfectant and gauze sponges

PROCEDURAL STEPS

1. Check that the Mayo stand or countertop is dust free and clean. If it is not, clean with 70% alcohol or another disinfectant and dry carefully.
   PURPOSE: Although some areas cannot be sterile, steps must be taken to keep contamination to a minimum; moisture on a tray contaminates the pack.

2. Sanitize your hands and make sure they are completely dry. If you will be assisting with a surgical procedure immediately after opening the sterile pack, perform the surgical hand scrub as explained in Procedure 57-4.
   PURPOSE: To reduce the number of transient and resident bacteria on your hands and forearms; moisture on your hands contaminates the pack.

3. Place the sterile pack on the Mayo stand or countertop and read the label.
   PURPOSE: Take care to open the required pack. Most medical offices have a limited supply of autoclaved packs. Opening a wrong package could mean not having enough sterile supplies for a different procedure.

4. Check the expiration date. If using an autoclaved pack, check the indicator tape for a color change.
   <u>PURPOSE:</u> An expired pack is not considered sterile. Autoclave indicator tape changes color after the sterile processing cycle.
5. Open the outside cover (Figure 1). Position the package so that the outer envelope flap is at the top and facing you.

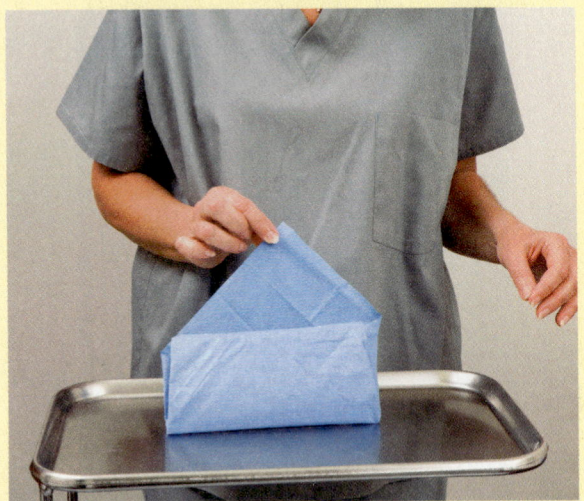

<u>PURPOSE:</u> This positions the pack for correct opening so that you do not have to cross over the sterile pack to open it.
6. Open the outermost flap (Figure 2). Next, open the first flap away from you. Do not cross over the pack.

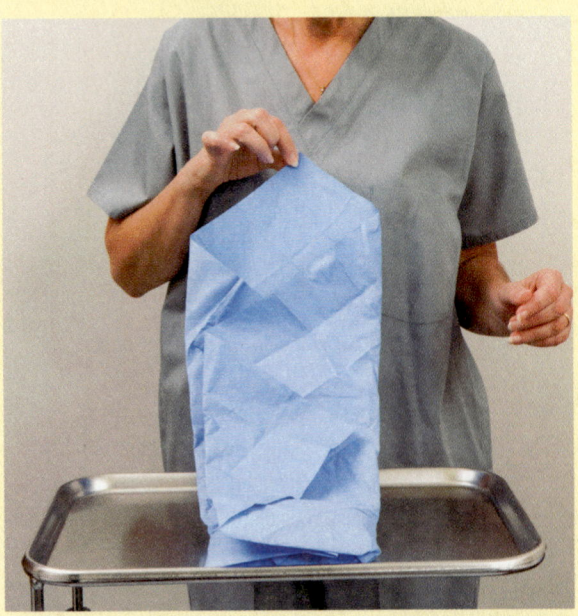

7. Open the second corner, pulling to side (Figure 3).

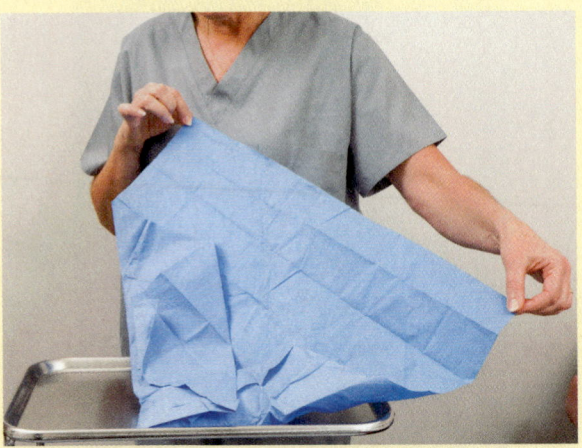

<u>PURPOSE:</u> To prevent contamination of the sterile field.
8. Be careful to lift the flaps by touching only the small, folded-back tab and without touching or crossing over the inner surface of the pack or its contents. Open the remaining two corners of the pack. (Figure 4).

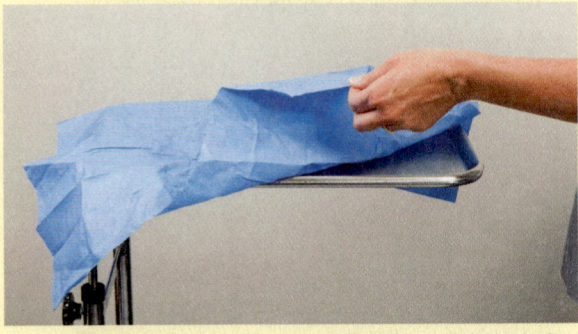

9. You now have a sterile drape as a sterile field from which to work and for the distribution of additional sterile supplies and instruments (Figure 5).

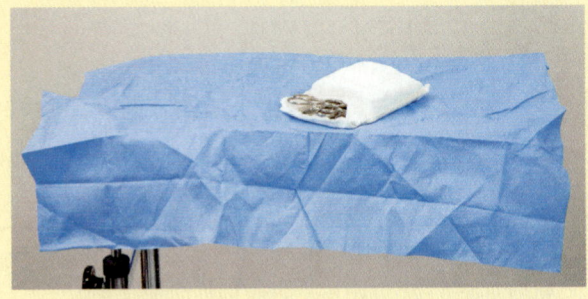

PROCEDURE 57-6

Assist the Physician with Patient Care: Use Transfer Forceps

GOAL: *To move sterile items on a sterile field or transfer sterile items to a gloved team member.*

EQUIPMENT and SUPPLIES

- Sterile item to move or transfer
- Sterile wrapped transfer forceps
- Mayo stand setup with a sterile field and sterile instruments

PROCEDURAL STEPS

1. Sanitize your hands, making sure they are completely dry. If you will be assisting with a surgical procedure immediately after this procedure, perform the surgical hand scrub as explained in Procedure 57-4.
   <u>PURPOSE:</u> To reduce the number of transient and resident bacteria on your hands and forearms; moisture on your hands contaminates the pack.

2. Open a package containing sterile transfer forceps (Figure 1).

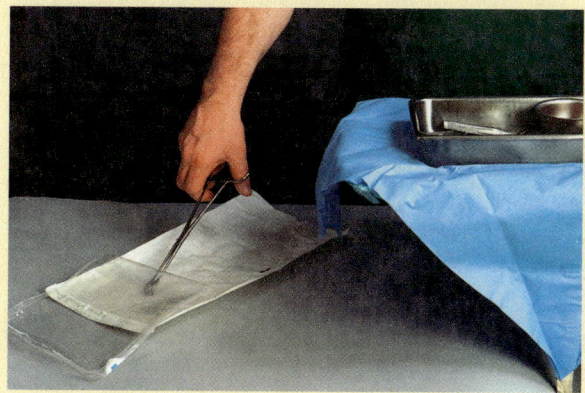

3. Using sterile technique, handle the sterile forceps by the ring handle only. Always point the forceps tips down.
   <u>PURPOSE:</u> If the tips are turned upward, any solution encountered will run onto the nonsterile area, and then back down over the sterile end when the tips are turned down again, thus contaminating the forceps.

4. Grasp an item on the sterile field with the sterile forceps, points down, and move it to its proper position for the procedure, making sure not to cross the sterile field with the hand or contaminated end of the forceps (Figure 2).

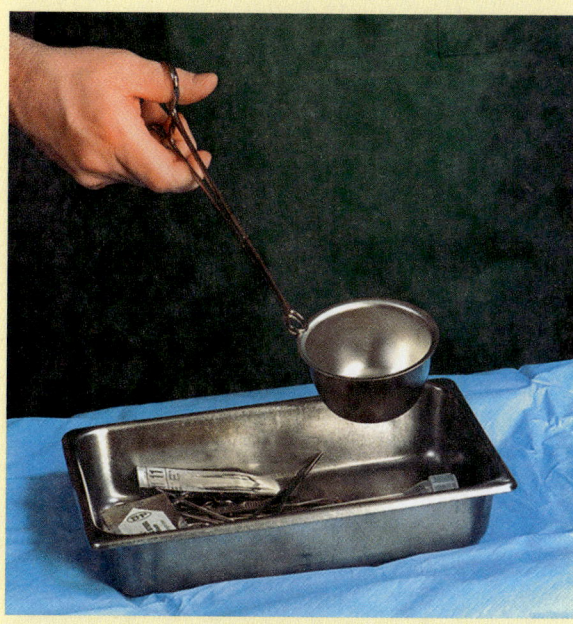

5. Alternatively, transfer an instrument from the autoclave to the sterile field.
6. Remove the transfer forceps after one-time use.

PROCEDURE 57-7

Assist the Physician with Patient Care: Pour a Sterile Solution onto a Sterile Field

GOAL: *To pour a sterile solution into a sterile stainless steel bowl or container sitting at the edge of a sterile field.*

EQUIPMENT and SUPPLIES

- Bottle of sterile solution
- Sterile bowl or container
- Sterile field
- Sink or waste receptacle
  <u>NOTE:</u> The sterile bowl should be placed, using sterile transfer forceps, near one edge of the field and the perimeter of the 1-inch barrier.

PROCEDURAL STEPS

1. Sanitize your hands, making sure they are completely dry. If you will be assisting with a surgical procedure immediately after this procedure, perform the surgical hand scrub as explained in Procedure 57-4.
   <u>PURPOSE:</u> To reduce the number of transient and resident bacteria on your hands and forearms; moisture on your hands contaminates the pack.

2. Read the label of the ordered solution.
   <u>PURPOSE:</u> Always perform the three label checks before administering any solution or medication.
3. Place your hand over the label and lift the bottle.
   <u>NOTE:</u> If the container has a double cap, set the outer cap on the counter inside up and then proceed.
4. Lift the lid of the bottle straight up and then slightly to one side; hold the lid in your nondominant hand facing downward.
   <u>PURPOSE:</u> Air currents carry contaminants that could settle on the inside of the lid.
5. Pour away from the label (Figure 1).

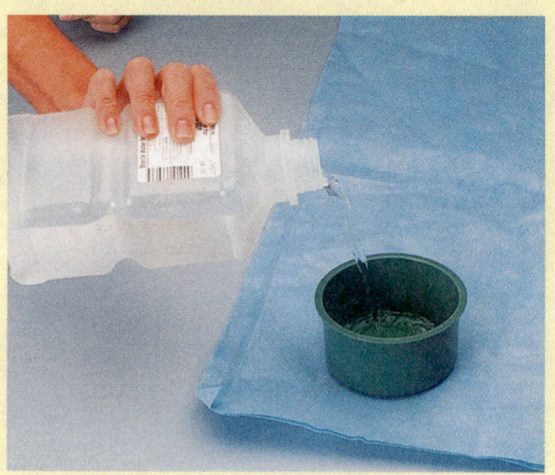

<u>PURPOSE:</u> Spills down the side of the bottle can stain the label or make it unreadable.

6. If the container does not have a double cap, before pouring the solution into the sterile container, pour off a small amount of the solution into a waste receptacle.
   <u>PURPOSE:</u> To rinse any contaminants off the bottle lip.

7. Pour away from the label, into the bowl, without allowing any part of the bottle to touch the bowl and without crossing over the sterile field (Figure 2).

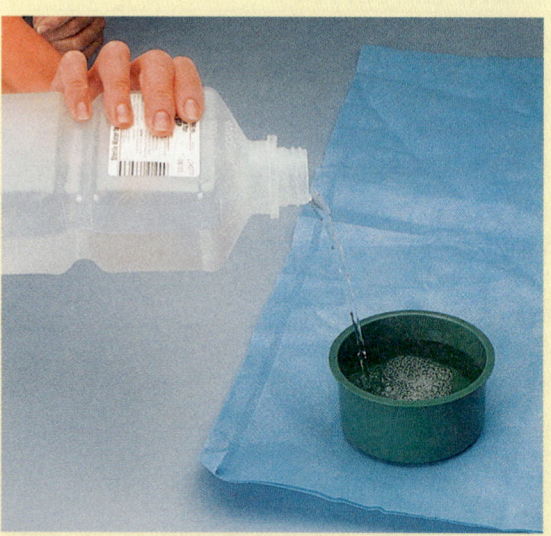

<u>PURPOSE:</u> The bottle exterior is not sterile.
8. Tilt the bottle up to stop the pouring while it is still over the bowl.
   <u>PURPOSE:</u> Solutions spilled on the sterile field may contaminate the field.
9. Replace the cap (or caps) off to the side, away from the sterile field, being careful not to touch and therefore contaminate the internal surface of the lid.

PROCEDURE 57-8

Assist the Physician with Patient Care: Put on Sterile Gloves

GOAL: *To put on sterile gloves correctly before performing sterile procedures.*

EQUIPMENT and SUPPLIES

- Pair of packaged sterile gloves in your size

PROCEDURAL STEPS

1. Perform the surgical hand scrub as explained in Procedure 57-4 before putting on sterile gloves.
2. Open the glove pack, being careful not to cross over the open area in the middle of the pack. Remember, a 1-inch area around the perimeter of the glove wrapper is considered not sterile.
   <u>PURPOSE:</u> The open glove pack is a sterile field.

3. Glove your dominant hand first.
   <u>PURPOSE:</u> This sets up your dominant hand to do the more difficult step, which is to put on the second glove.
4. With your nondominant hand, pick up the glove for your dominant hand with your thumb and forefinger, grabbing the top of the folded cuff, which is the inside of the glove, being careful not to cross over the other sterile glove (Figure 1).

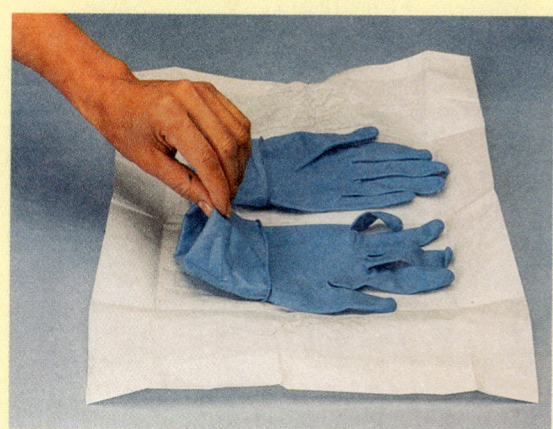

<u>PURPOSE:</u> The inside of the glove will be next to your skin and is considered not sterile.

5. Lift the glove up and away from the sterile package.
   <u>PURPOSE:</u> To prevent accidental contamination from touching the glove on the 1-inch area around the perimeter of the glove wrapper.

6. Hold your hands up and away from your body and slide the dominant hand into the glove (Figure 2).

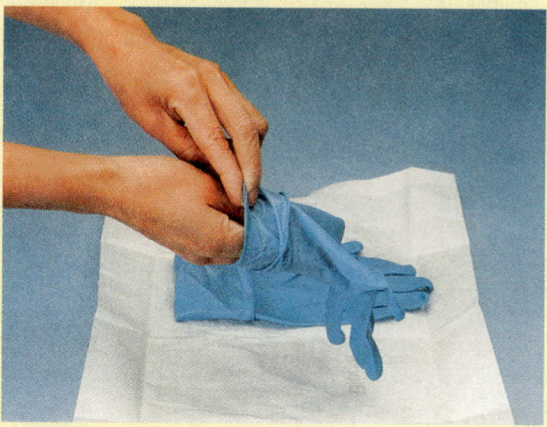

7. Leave the cuff folded (Figure 3).

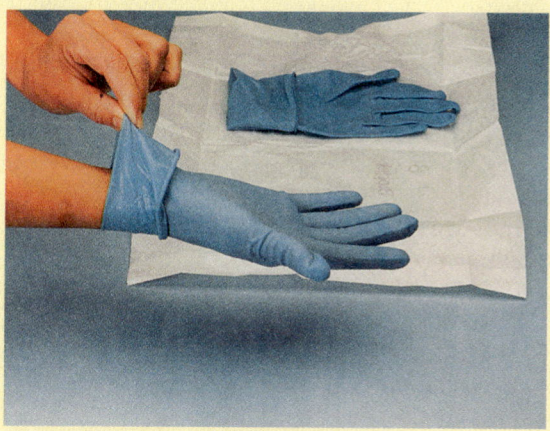

<u>PURPOSE:</u> You will unfold the cuff later.

8. With your gloved dominant hand, pick up the second glove by slipping your gloved fingers under the cuff, extending the thumb up and away from the glove, so that your gloved fingers touch only the outside of the second glove (Figure 4).

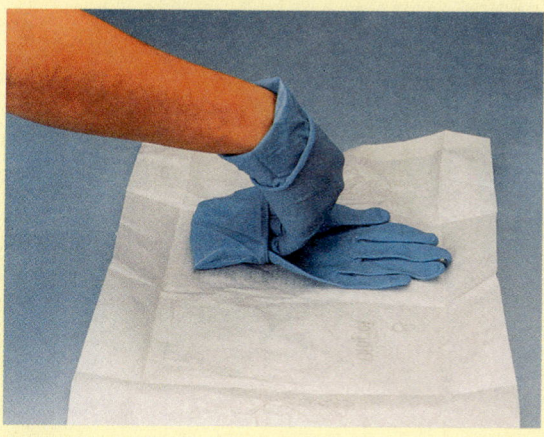

<u>PURPOSE:</u> Sterile surfaces must always touch sterile surfaces.

9. Slide your nondominant hand into the glove without touching the exterior of the glove or any part of the gloved hand (Figures 5 and 6).

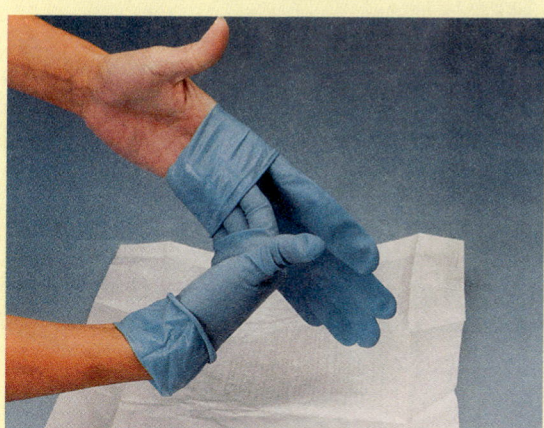

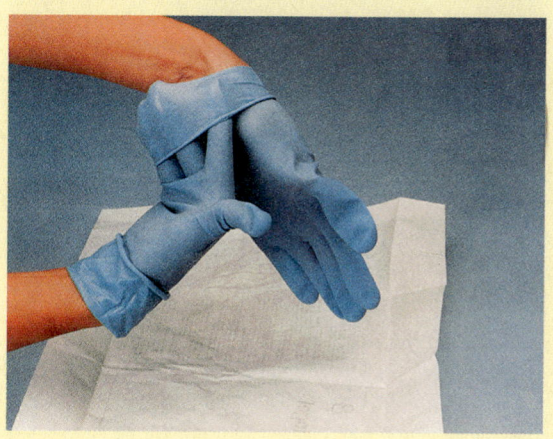

10. Still holding your hands away from you, unroll the cuff by slipping the fingers into the cuff and gently pulling up and out. Do not touch your bare arm or the internal surface of the glove with any part of the sterile glove (Figure 7).

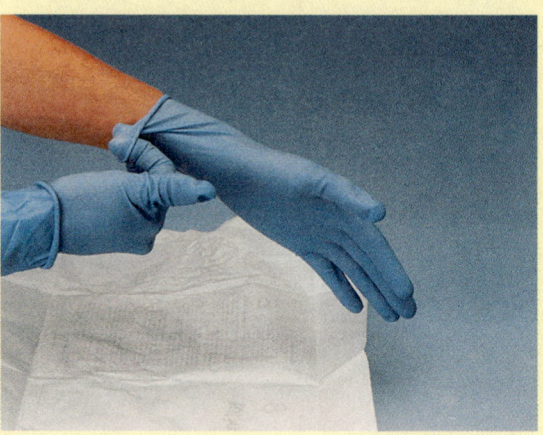

11. Now, slip your gloved fingers up under the first cuff and unroll it, using the same technique (Figure 8).

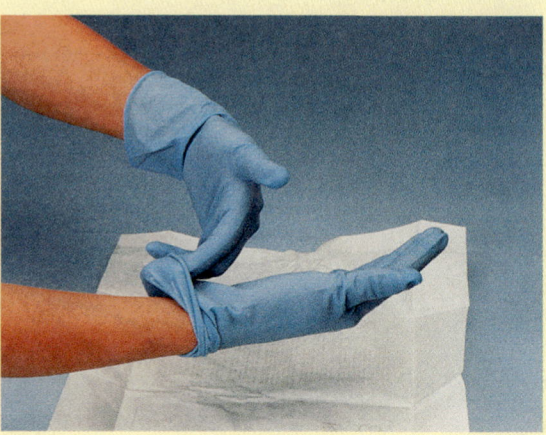

then draped with sterile towels or drapes so that it, also, becomes a sterile field.

Hands and hair are two of the greatest sources of contamination when a sterile field is set up. With practice, you will learn to know what may be touched with your hands and what must be touched only with sterile gloved hands. Hair that falls freely over the shoulders and forward gives off a cloud of bacteria with every movement. It must always be secured back and up, not touching the shoulders.

RULES FOR MAINTAINING A STERILE FIELD

- Talking should be kept to a minimum because air currents carry bacteria.
- Sterile team members should always face one another.
- Always keep the sterile field in your view. If you turn your back on a sterile field or lose sight of it, it is considered contaminated.
- Nonsterile persons or items should never cross over the sterile field.
- Tables are sterile only at table level; anything that falls below the edge of the Mayo tray is considered contaminated. A 1-inch border surrounding the tray is considered contaminated, so anything placed on the tray within that 1-inch border is contaminated.
- Consider a sterile barrier contaminated if it has been wet, cut, or torn.
- Packages placed on a clean surface are contaminated on the outside, but the inside of the sterilized package may be used as a sterile field.
- Keep sterile gloved hands above waist level at all times; do not let hands drop below the waist.
- Never remove and then replace any item in the field (e.g., using sterile forceps to cleanse a wound), or the field is contaminated.

- The inside of a sterile package remains so if the package is peeled open properly; it should be opened the entire way, and the contents then tossed onto the field without crossing over the sterile area.
- If a sterile package falls to the floor, it must be discarded.
- *If you are in doubt about the sterility of anything, consider it contaminated.*

Assisting the Physician during Surgery

The physician ultimately is responsible for the patient; however, the medical assistant is responsible for ensuring that everything the assistant and the physician will use in caring for the surgical patient is accounted for, ready for use, and prepared in a safe and sterile manner (Procedure 57-9). Every team has preferences about the sequence they follow during routine minor surgery. Once a routine has been established, it should be followed in every case. Sample setups for various types of minor surgery are provided in Table 57-3.

The medical assistant sorts and places the scalpels, hemostats, scissors, tissue forceps, and retractors on the sterile field according to their sequence and frequency of use (Figure 57-6). Scalpels and sharp instruments should be conspicuously placed so that they do not accidentally injure a team member. The physician enters the room after scrubbing and then puts on gloves. The physician drapes the patient with towels or a fenestrated drape as the medical assistant hands the drapes, one at a time. Once the site has been draped, the Mayo stand with the sterile field is positioned below the site, and the medical assistant stands opposite the physician over the patient, ready to help as needed.

Passing Instruments

During a procedure, the medical assistant must protect the sterile field from contamination. Notify the physician if a break in sterile

PROCEDURE 57-9

PROCEDURE 57-9

Assist the Physician with Patient Care: Assist with Minor Surgery

GOAL: *To maintain the sterile field and to pass instruments in a prescribed sequence during a surgical procedure that involves the making of a surgical incision and the removal of a growth.*

EQUIPMENT and SUPPLIES

- Open patient drape pack on the side counter
- Mayo stand covered with a sterile drape
- Packaged sterile gloves (two pairs)
- Needle and syringe for anesthesia medication
- Vial of local anesthetic medication
- Sterile drape
- Disposable scalpel with No. 15 blade
- Allis tissue forceps
- Skin retractor
- Three hemostats
- Supply of sterile gauze sponges
- Biohazardous waste receptacle
- Sharps container
- Needle with suture material
- Specimen cup
- Laboratory requisitions
- Patient's record

PROCEDURAL STEPS

1. Prep the patient's skin with surgical soap and antiseptic solution as explained in Procedure 57-3. Explain the prep procedure to the patient.
   PURPOSE: To ensure infection control and to demonstrate awareness of possible patient concerns.
2. Perform the surgical hand scrub as explained in Procedure 57-4.
3. Set up the sterile field with instruments and supplies, in the sequence to be used (Figure 1). If it is necessary to touch sterile supplies, put on sterile gloves (see Procedure 57-8) or use sterile transfer forceps (see Procedure 57-6). After the sterile field has been set up, cover it with a sterile drape.

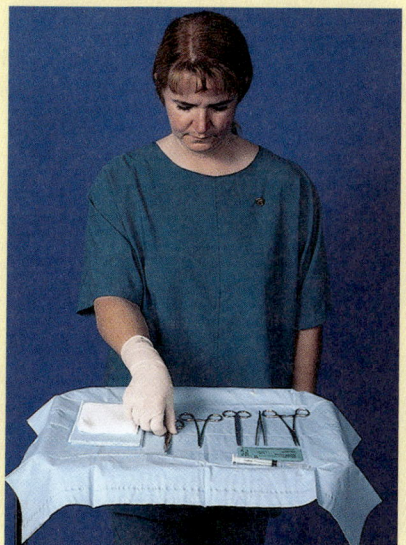

(From Bonewit-West K: *Clinical procedures for medical assistants*, ed 7, St Louis, 2008, WB Saunders.)

4. Position the Mayo stand near the patient and the operative site, making sure the patient understands not to touch the sterile field (Figure 2).

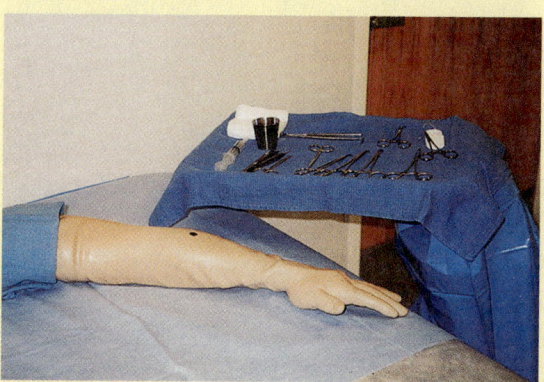

(From Bonewit-West K: *Clinical procedures for medical assistants*, ed 7, St Louis, 2008, WB Saunders.)

PURPOSE: To prevent contamination of supplies and provide easy access for the physician.
5. Put on sterile gloves using aseptic technique.
6. Grasp the patient drape by holding one edge or corner in each hand (Figure 3).

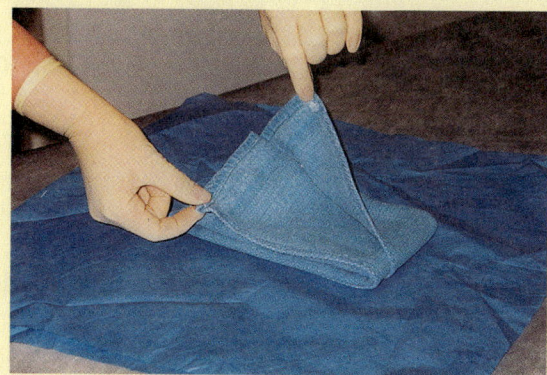

(From Bonewit-West K: *Clinical procedures for medical assistants*, ed 7, St Louis, 2008, WB Saunders.)

7. Drape the surgical site without touching any part of the patient or the operating area with your gloved hands (Figure 4).

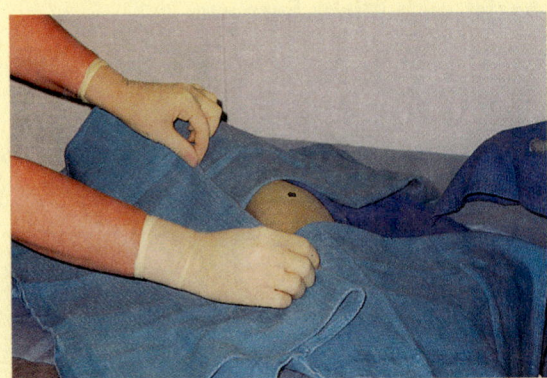

8. If the physician requests medication, such as a local anesthetic, a second circulating assistant holds the vial of local anesthetic so that the physician can read the label. The physician withdraws the desired amount using sterile technique (Figure 5).

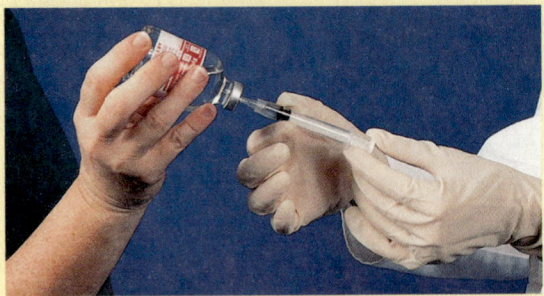

PURPOSE: The vial of local anesthetic medication must be held by the second assistant away from the sterile field to prevent crossing over the field with a nonsterile item. The medication label must be checked before a medication is dispensed or administered.

9. The surgeon injects the local anesthetic and waits a few minutes for it to take effect.
10. Position yourself across from the surgeon. Arrange the sterile field. Check the placement location on the Mayo stand (Figure 6).

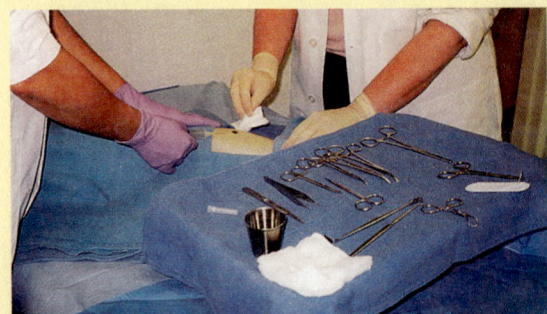

11. Place two sponges on the patient next to the wound site (Figure 7).

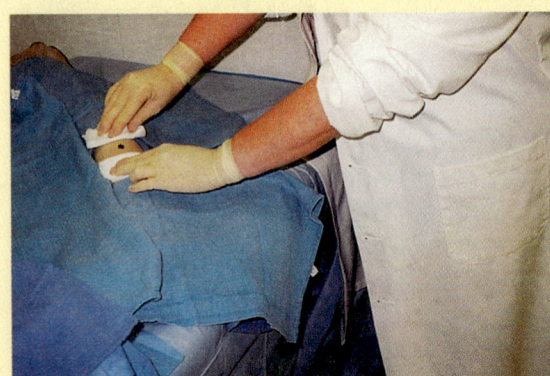

12. Keep all sharp equipment conspicuously placed on the sterile field. PURPOSE: Sharp instruments that are not clearly visible may injure a team member.
13. Pass the scalpel, blade down and handle first, to the surgeon, or the surgeon will reach for it himself or herself. The surgeon will take the scalpel with the thumb and forefinger in the position ready for use (Figure 8).

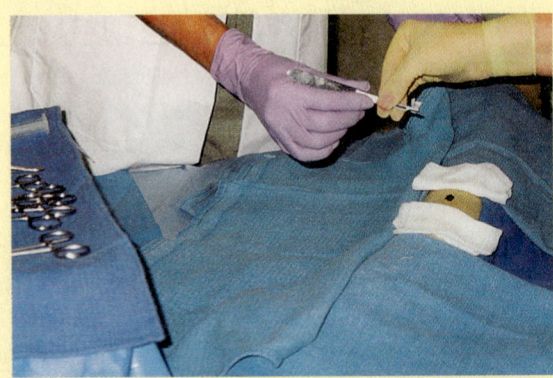

PURPOSE: To protect the surgeon and yourself from injury.
14. Grasp an Allis tissue forceps by the tips and pass it to the surgeon to grasp a piece of the tissue to be excised (Figure 9).

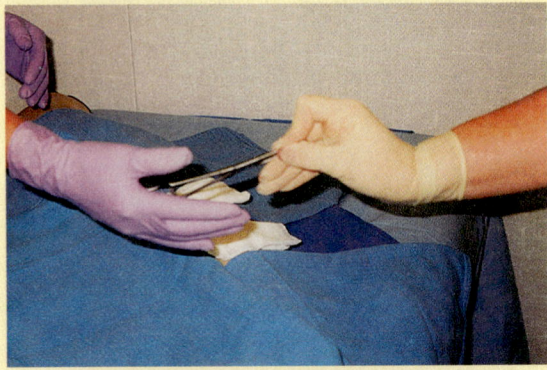

15. Pass the handles into the surgeon's open palm with a firm, purposeful motion. A gentle "snap" is heard as it comes in contact with the surgeon's gloved hand.
    <u>PURPOSE:</u> The surgeon will not have to look up to receive the instrument.

16. Dispose of soiled sponges in the biohazardous waste receptacle, being careful to keep your hands above your waist and to avoid touching any nonsterile items.

17. Hold clean sponges in your hand to pat or sponge the wound as needed (Figure 10).

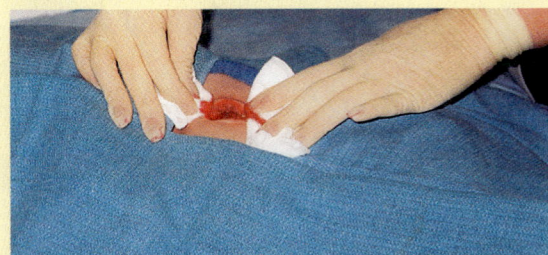

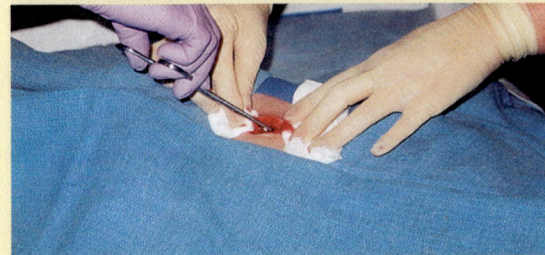

(From Bonewit-West K: *Clinical procedures for medical assistants,* ed 7, St Louis, 2008, WB Saunders.)

18. Safely position the specimen (if any) where it will not be disturbed on the sterile field (Figure 11).

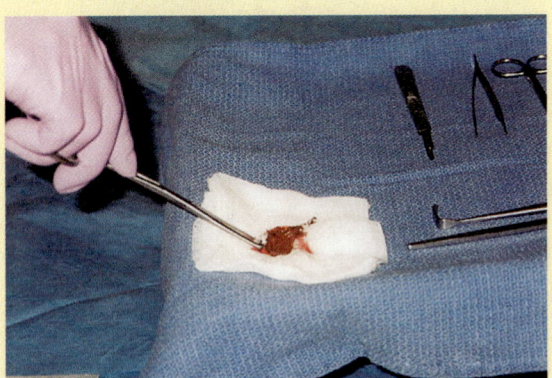

(From Bonewit-West K: *Clinical procedures for medical assistants,* ed 7, St Louis, 2008, WB Saunders.)

19. If there is a bleeding vessel or if a hemostat is requested, pass the hemostat in the manner described in steps 14 and 15.

20. Continue to sponge blood from the wound site.

21. Retract the wound edge, as needed, with a skin retractor.

22. Continue to monitor the sterile field and assist the surgeon as needed.

23. Pass the needle and suture material to close the wound and apply a sterile dressing as requested (Figure 12).

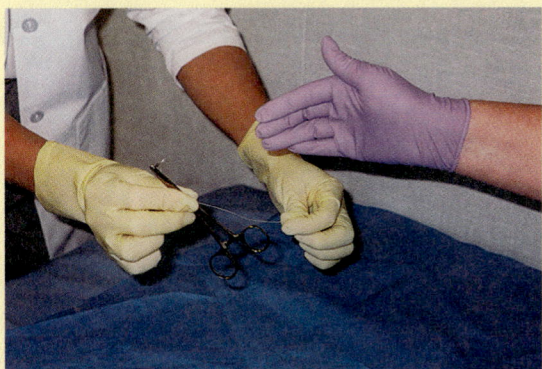

(From Bonewit-West K: *Clinical procedures for medical assistants,* ed 7, St Louis, 2008, WB Saunders.)

24. Monitor the patient and provide assistance as needed.

25. When the physician is finished, clean the area using aseptic technique.

26. Collect the specimen, place it in a labeled specimen cup, and send it to the laboratory with the proper requisitions.

27. Document the procedure, wound condition, and patient education on wound care.

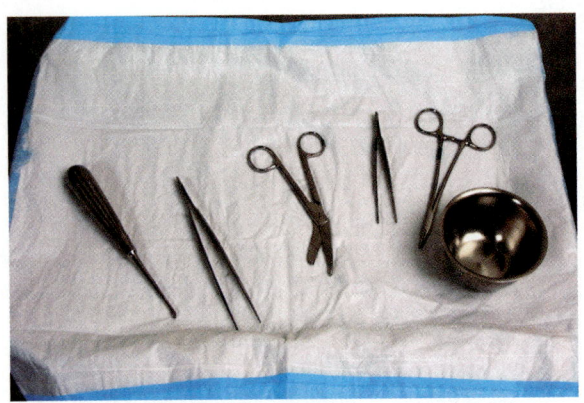

FIGURE 57-6 Mayo stand with surgical setup on sterile field.

technique occurs, dispose of soiled sponges into the biohazardous waste container, and anticipate the surgeon's need for instruments. The physician may request instruments or may use hand signals (Figure 57-7). As the team works together over time, the physician may not need to give any signals, because the assistant will be able to anticipate the instrument needed next during the procedure.

Instrumentation is logical; if the physician requests a suture, scissors will be needed next to cut the suture strand. In the case of sudden hemorrhage from a bleeding vessel, the physician will need an appropriately sized hemostat. While gaining experience, the assistant watches, listens, and learns to judge what will be needed or performed next. Pass instruments with a firm, purposeful motion so that the physician does not have to look up. Wait until you feel the

TABLE 57-3 Setups for Minor Surgeries

PROCEDURE	SIDE COUNTER	STERILE FIELD	COMMENTS	POSTOPERATIVE CARE
Suture repair	Local anesthetic, dressings and bandages, splints or guards, tape, drape, gloves, sterile normal saline solution	Syringe and needle, hemostats (three), scissors, sponges, suture material and needle, tissue forceps or skin hook, needle holder	If a patient arrives with a pressure dressing over a laceration, follow Standard Precautions. Do not remove the pressure dressing until the physician is ready to suture. If the patient's pressure cloth must be removed, have ample sterile dressings ready to apply immediately. Ask the patient the approximate length, depth, and exact location of the laceration. Follow the physician's directions regarding cleansing of the wound.	Clean lacerations in a moderately protected area; may not require a dressing. The patient is instructed to keep the area clean and dry. Some lacerations may be closed with Steri-Strips or an adhesive bond.
Needle biopsy	Specimen container with prepackaged fixative or preserving solution, laboratory form and label, local anesthetic, gloves	Biopsy needle, syringe and needle, sponges	A biopsy is the examination of tissue removed from the living body. Biopsies usually are done to determine whether a growth is malignant or benign; however, a biopsy may be done as a diagnostic aid in other diseases or infections. A needle biopsy may be done by aspiration with a needle and syringe or with a special biopsy needle. The specimen then is sent to a pathologist for either a cytologic or histologic examination.	Usually no special dressing is required after a needle biopsy. An adhesive bandage strip (e.g., Band-Aid) often is sufficient.
Cyst removal	Local anesthetic, disinfectant (skin prep), laboratory form, dressing (size depends on site), gloves, drape, specimen container with prepackaged fixative or preserving solution	Kelly hemostats (two straight and two curved), dressing forceps (two), suture and needle, scissors, dissector (physician's choice), skin hook, syringe and needle, disposable scalpel No. 11 or No. 15 blade, tissue forceps (two), Allis forceps, needle holder, sponges	A sebaceous cyst is a benign retention cyst of a sebaceous gland containing fatty substance from the gland. The cyst is attached to the skin and moves freely over the underlying tissue. For cosmetic reasons the physician makes the incision on the natural skin crease lines if possible.	See suture repair, above, or apply a small sterile dressing, depending on the size of the incision.

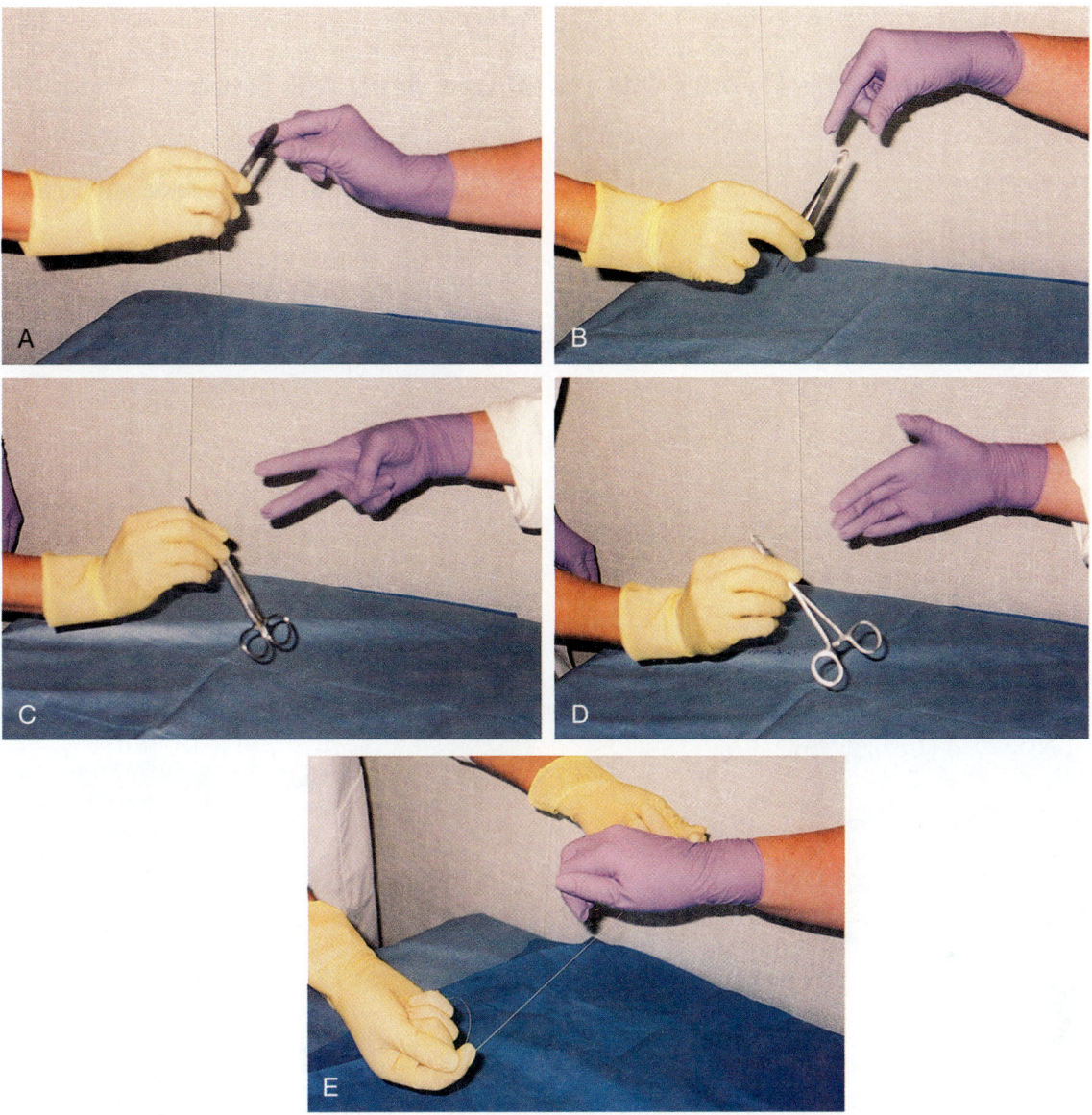

FIGURE 57-7 Passing sterile surgical instruments. **A,** Scalpel. **B,** Forceps. **C,** Scissors. **D,** Clamp. **E,** Free suture pass (free tie).

physician grasp the instrument so that it does not drop onto the patient or the floor and be careful that you and the physician are protected from injury. Pass the scalpel with the blade down and present the handle to the surgeon. Hold all instruments by their tips and pass the handle ends into the physician's palm or fingers.

CRITICAL THINKING APPLICATION 57-6

In passing the scalpel to the surgeon while assisting with an I&D, Melissa feels the blade "slice" through her glove. She quickly and secretly looks at it and notices a "very tiny" nick in her glove. Because this is a "dirty" procedure, she decides to say nothing and continues assisting with the procedure. Is her reasoning sound here? What is the best approach to handling this situation? Why?

Specimen Collection

If a specimen is collected during a procedure, it is placed in a sterile glass or basin. Do not remove the specimen from the sterile field until the physician gives the order. The surgeon may want to examine the specimen again during the surgery. After the procedure is complete, place the specimen in an appropriate container, label it, and send it to the laboratory for analysis.

Completing the Surgical Procedure

At the conclusion of the procedure, the physician begins wound closure (Procedure 57-10). The techniques and methods of tissue closure vary greatly; all of them cannot be described or illustrated here. The two basic methods of suturing are the continuous running suture and the interrupted suture, in which each knot is placed and tied one at a time, so that if one breaks, the others keep the wound closure intact (Figure 57-8). The interrupted technique is used for most skin closures in a medical office.

The physician may prefer that the medical assistant place the needle in a needle holder and pass it, handle first. As the physician closes the wound, you may assist by cutting the suture and sponging the site. The physician places the first interrupted suture at the

PROCEDURE 57-10

Assist the Physician with Patient Care: Assist with Suturing

GOAL: *To assist the surgeon in wound closure, using sterile technique.*

EQUIPMENT and SUPPLIES

- Sterile field on Mayo stand
- Surgical scissors
- Suture material
- Sterile gloves
- Needle holder
- Sterile gauze sponges
- Biohazardous sharps container and waste receptacle
- Patient's record

NOTE: This procedure may be a continuation of Procedure 57-9. If done independently, you must perform the surgical scrub and glove before beginning step 1.

PROCEDURAL STEPS

1. Hold the curved needle point in your minor hand, 4 to 5 inches over the sterile field (Figure 1).

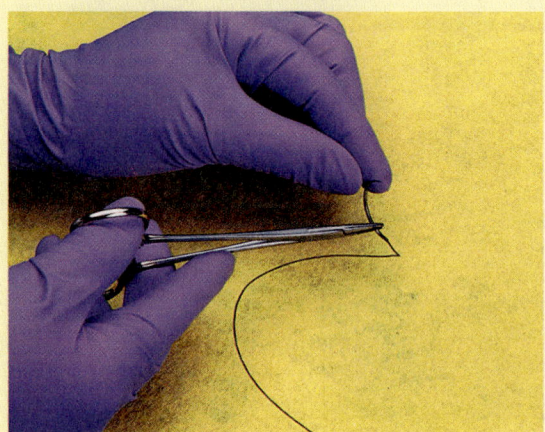

PURPOSE: Always work over a sterile field and take care not to puncture gloves with the sharp needle.

2. With the needle holder, clamp the suture needle at the upper third of its total length (Figure 2).

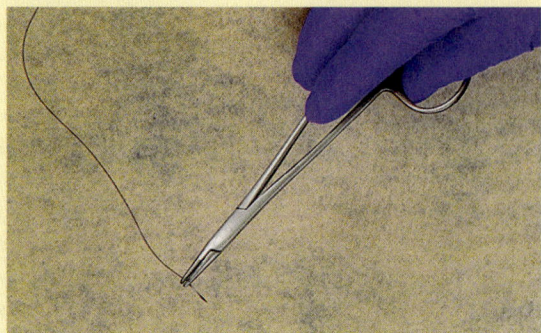

PURPOSE: Clamping in the middle weakens and may distort the shape of the needle. Clamping too near the thread may cause the suture to detach from the needle. Clamping at the tip of the needle damages the needle point.

3. With your dominant hand, hold the needle holder halfway down its shaft with the suture needle point up.

4. With your nondominant hand, hold the suture strand and pass the needle holder into the surgeon's hand (Figures 3 and 4).

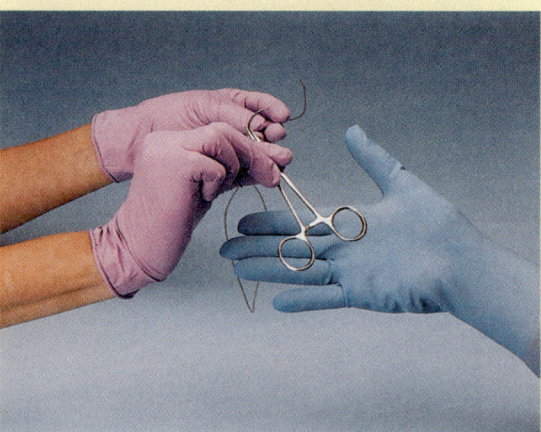

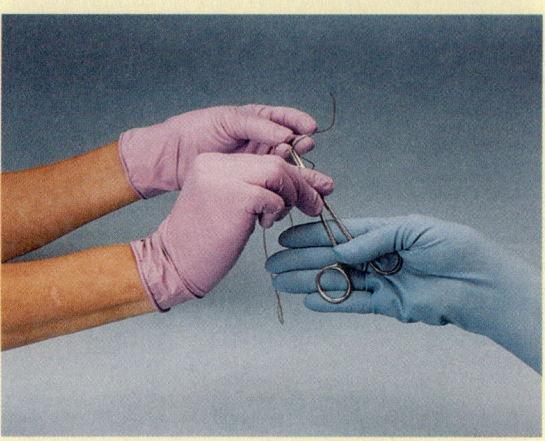

5. Pick up the surgical scissors with your dominant hand and a gauze sponge with your nondominant hand.

6. After the surgeon places a closure suture, knots it, and holds the two strands taut, cut both suture strands in one motion. Cut between the knot and the surgeon, at the length requested, approximately 1/8 inch.
   PURPOSE: Too long a suture may irritate the patient during recovery, and too short a suture may untie during recovery.

7. Gently blot the closure once with the gauze sponge in your nondominant hand.
   PURPOSE: Rubbing or friction may damage the wound edges.

8. If additional strands of suture are needed, repeat the process.

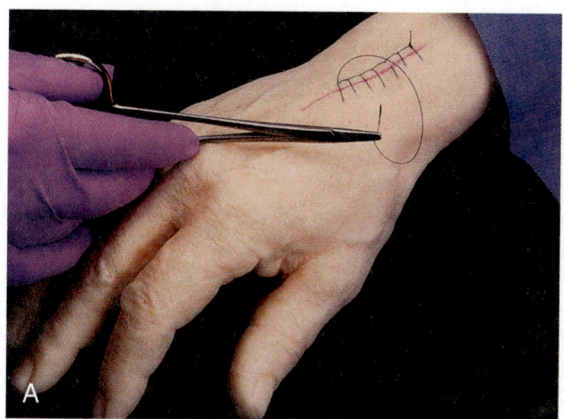 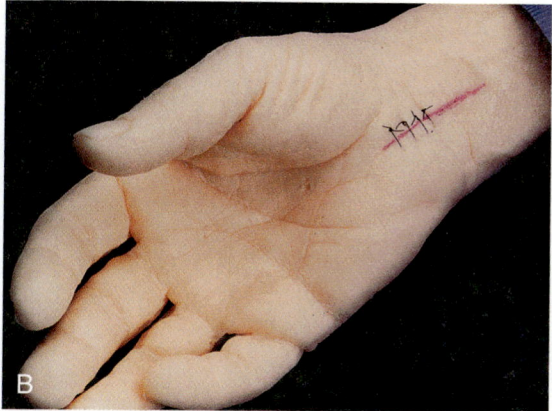

FIGURE 57-8 A, Continuous (running) suture placement. **B,** Interrupted suture placement.

PROCEDURE 57-11

Assist the Physician with Patient Care: Apply or Change a Sterile Dressing

GOAL: *To apply a sterile dressing properly at the completion of a surgical procedure.*

EQUIPMENT and SUPPLIES

- Sterile dressing material or Telfa
- Sterile gloves
- Patient's record

PROCEDURAL STEPS

1. After surgery is complete, before the sterile drape is removed and while you are still wearing sterile gloves, pick up the dressing from the sterile field, place it on the wound, and hold it there.
   PURPOSE: To prevent the introduction of microorganisms into the wound area.

2. Then remove the drape, switching hands to hold the dressing in place.
   PURPOSE: To keep the wound as clean as possible.

3. Secure the dressing with paper tape and/or an appropriate bandage.
   PURPOSE: To keep the wound covered and protected.

4. Document the procedure in the patient's medical record.
   PURPOSE: A procedure is not completed until it is recorded.

10/12/XX 2:15 PM Dressing change completed to wound on ① mid-forearm. Area slightly inflamed, mod amt serosanguineous drainage noted. Site cleansed and sterile dressing applied. Pt instructed on home wound care and to notify physician if drainage changes, inflammation increases, or fever occurs. Melissa Gelbert, CMA (AAMA)

---

midpoint of the incision. Then each side of the first suture is mentally divided in half again, and the next two sutures are placed at each of these midpoints. The rest of the sutures are placed using the same technique until the wound edges have been completely approximated. The physician may also opt to close a wound with surgical staples.

After the skin closure, the wound site is cleansed with wet (using sterile, normal saline solution) and sterile dry sponges by the surgeon or the assistant. Care must be taken not to disturb the wound edges or sutures. Next, a sterile dressing is placed over the incision (Procedure 57-11), and a bandage is applied to support the dressing.

Postoperative Responsibilities

After caring for the patient, the medical assistant clears the sterile field, following Standard Precautions. Wear disposable gloves until all contaminated materials have been properly removed and handled. Place disposable equipment and supplies in biohazardous waste containers and/or sharps containers. The room should be checked for any blood spills or other contamination and disinfected

appropriately. After completing this process, remove the contaminated gloves and sanitize your hands.

Use clean gloves to disinfect the room, including the table, Mayo stand, side and back tables, any other equipment in the room, and the floor. Used instruments must be sanitized, disinfected, and resterilized for future use. The surgeon and medical assistant both document the procedure in the patient's medical record.

SINGLE-ASSISTANT PREPARATION FOR MINOR SURGERY

1. Sanitize your hands and gather all supplies.
   - *Sterile side (Mayo tray):* Two towel packs, skin prep pack, patient drape pack, instrument pack, miscellaneous pack or packs, three glove packs, masks, goggles, aprons or gowns
   - *Nonsterile side (side counter):* Syringes, suture material, anesthesia solutions, additional sponges, dressings, bandages, transfer

forceps, waste basin, waste receptacle, nonsterile gloves, masks, goggles, aprons or gowns

2. Escort the patient into the room.
3. Greet and converse with the patient.
4. Position the patient on the table.
5. Sanitize your hands.
6. Open the first towel pack.
7. Open the skin prep pack.
8. Pour soap and antiseptic solutions.
9. Expose the site to be prepped.
10. Glove and arrange prep items within the sterile field.
11. Place sterile towels at skin scrub boundaries using sterile technique.
12. Prep the patient's skin.
13. Discard skin prep materials in appropriate sharps/biohazard containers.
14. Discard gloves; wash your hands, following the guidelines for a surgical hand scrub (Procedure 57-4) if this procedure is part of the policy of the attending physician or the facility.
15. Open the table drape pack on the Mayo stand to create the sterile field.
16. Open the instrument pack or packs and transfer the instruments to the sterile field. Add the sterile syringe unit.
17. Add sterile items as requested.
18. The physician joins you and converses with the patient.
19. Open the physician's glove pack (the physician now puts on gloves).
20. Open the patient drape pack (the physician now drapes the surgical site).
21. Cleanse and hold up the anesthesia vial for the physician to withdraw anesthesia with the sterile syringe (the physician now administers the anesthesia).
22. Repeat the surgical hand wash; reglove with a new glove pack.
23. Arrange the sterile field instruments and other materials for safety and in sequence; check the condition of each instrument.
24. Open the suture/needle pack per the physician's choice; load the first suture into the needle holder.
25. Place two gauze sponges at the site.
26. Assist with the procedure.*
   - *For the physician:* Pass the instruments; maintain the field; anticipate his or her needs; and cut sutures.
   - *For the patient:* Retract tissue; sponge blood from the wound; apply the bandage; and care for the specimen.
27. Escort the patient to the recovery area and check vital signs as instructed.
28. Record and prepare specimens.
29. Clean the room; clear materials and discard in biohazardous waste containers.
30. Chart the procedure in the patient's medical record.
31. Help the patient prepare to leave the office.
32. Sanitize, disinfect, and sterilize the equipment at the first available time.

*By law, the assistant may not clamp tissues, place sutures, or alter body tissues in any way.

Postoperative Instructions and Care

The patient should be given time to rest after the surgery. If a sedative was administered, make sure the patient has recovered sufficiently to avoid injury after the surgery or during the journey home. If the patient has been given a topical or local anesthetic, explain to the patient that the anesthesia effect will wear off and that some discomfort may be felt at the operative site. Check with the physician whether pain medication needs to be prescribed. If medication has been prescribed, review the purpose of the medication and the directions for its use with the patient and his or her companion. Make a follow-up appointment before the patient leaves the office.

Postoperative care extends for the total recovery period, not just for the time of immediate care before the patient leaves the office. Most medical assistants are responsible for teaching patients to care for themselves at home after surgery. The concentration of a postoperative patient is diminished after the stress of surgery, so all instructions should be given to the patient in writing. They should be simple in style and easily understood by both the patient and caregivers. These instructions can be preprinted forms for each type of surgery, or a general form with checked boxes for particular postoperative instructions that apply specifically to the individual patient (Figure 57-9).

Warning Signs

Explain to the patient the importance of calling the office if any questions arise or changes occur that cause the person concern. If the patient does not call within the next 24 hours, you should call the patient. Many patients tend to "ride it out" or say they did not want to disturb you. Never allow the postoperative patient to leave the office without the physician's knowledge and approval. Tell the patient to call the office immediately if he or she notes redness around the operative site, bleeding from the wound, fever, swelling, or increasing or severe pain. The wound should be kept clean and dry, and the patient should be taught how to change the dressing if needed.

Follow-Up

If the healing process is a long one or if the wound becomes infected, the patient may return for follow-up care. If the wound requires a new dressing, follow Standard Precautions; wear gloves and other protective barriers as appropriate. If at any time you determine that the wound may be infected, stop and have the physician examine it. Generally, no bandaging material should be reused, including Ace wraps. Tape applied directly to a patient's skin is not a good dressing immobilizer. If tape is used, always keep it to a minimum. If tape is holding a dressing in place, always remove it by pulling toward the wound. If it is adhering to a hairy area of the body, lift the outer tape edge with one hand and slowly and gently separate the underlying hair and skin from the tape with the thumb of your other hand. Peel the skin from the bandage, not the bandage from the skin. Never rapidly "rip" tape from the body, because this may injure the skin. If the tape is not irritating to the patient, it may be advisable to leave the tape in place until total healing has taken place. If the wound has healed, the physician may ask the medical assistant to remove the patient's sutures. If the physician closed the wound with surgical staples, the patient must return to the facility to have the staples removed (Procedure 57-12).

POSTOP INSTRUCTIONS FOR _____

☐ Elevate your arm.
☐ Elevate your leg.
☐ Limit food intake to _____.
☐ Limit activity to _____.
☐ Do not bathe or shower.
☐ Sponge bath only.
☐ Change dressing as instructed.
☐ Call the office for fever, redness, pain, swelling, or bleeding.
☐ Take_____ every 4 hours as needed for pain.
☐ Return to school/work in _____ days.
☐ Call the office tomorrow before _____ p.m.
☐ Your next appointment is on M T W Th F S_____ at _____.

FIGURE 57-9 Example of preprinted postoperative patient instructions.

PROCEDURE 57-12

Assist the Physician with Patient Care: Remove Sutures and Surgical Staples

GOAL: To remove sutures and/or surgical staples from a healed incision using sterile technique and without injuring the closed wound.

EQUIPMENT and SUPPLIES

- Sterile suture removal kit containing the following:
- Suture removal scissors
- Gauze sponges
- Thumb dressing forceps
- Steri-Strips or adhesive bandage strips (e.g., Band-Aids)
- Skin antiseptic swabs (e.g., Betadine swabs)
- Surgical staple remover with 4 × 4-inch gauze sponges
- Biohazardous waste container
- Sterile gloves
- Patient's record

PROCEDURAL STEPS

1. Assemble the necessary supplies.
2. Sanitize your hands, following Standard Precautions.
3. Explain the procedure to the patient and instruct the person to lie or sit still during the procedure.
   PURPOSE: To ensure cooperation during the procedure.
4. Position the patient comfortably and support the sutured area.
5. Place dry towels under the site.
6. Check the incision line to make sure the wound edges are approximated and there are no signs of infection, such as inflammation, edema, or drainage.
   PURPOSE: Sutures or staples should not be removed unless the site is completely healed with the wound edges together; infection at the site will interfere with the healing process; removing sutures or staples before the site is completely healed may result in wound **dehiscence**.
7. Put on disposable gloves. Using antiseptic swabs, cleanse the wound to remove exudate and destroy microorganisms around the sutures or staples. Clean the site from the inside out, starting at the top of the wound and working your way down. Use a new swab if the step must be repeated.

PURPOSE: Dried exudate on sutures or staples may make removing them without traumatizing the wound more difficult. Cleansing the wound reduces the possibility of wound infection.

8. Open the suture or staple removal pack while maintaining the sterility of the contents.
9. Place a sterile gauze sponge next to the wound site.
   PURPOSE: To receive the removed sutures or staples.
10. Put on sterile gloves.
11. Remove the sutures or staples.
    To Remove Sutures
    a. Grasp the knot of the suture with the dressing forceps without pulling.
    b. Cut the suture at skin level (Figure 1).

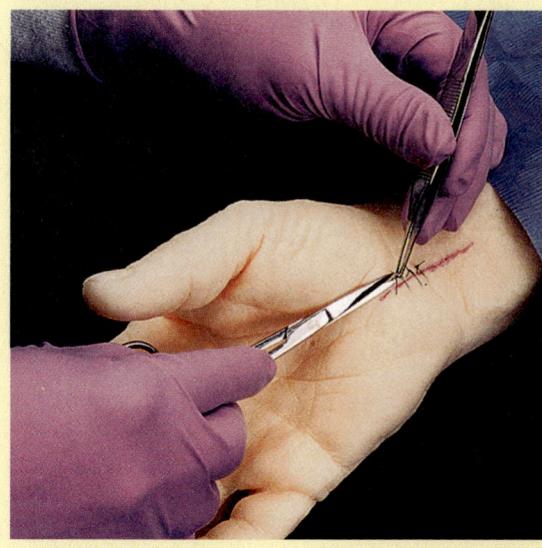

c. Lift, do not pull, the suture toward the incision and out with the dressing forceps (Figure 2).

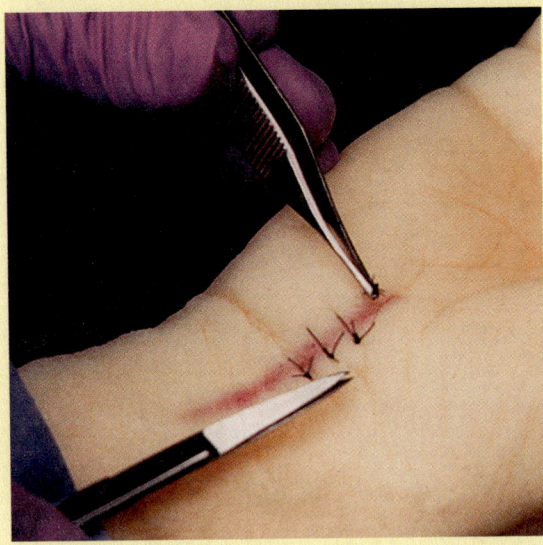

d. Place the suture on the sterile gauze sponge and check that the entire suture strand has been removed.
   <u>PURPOSE:</u> Suture fragments left in a wound may cause irritation and/or infection and may prolong the healing process.

e. If any bleeding occurs, blot the area with a sterile gauze sponge before continuing.

f. Continue in the same manner until all sutures have been removed.

To Remove Staples

a. Gently place the bottom jaw of the staple remover (Figure 3) under the first staple.

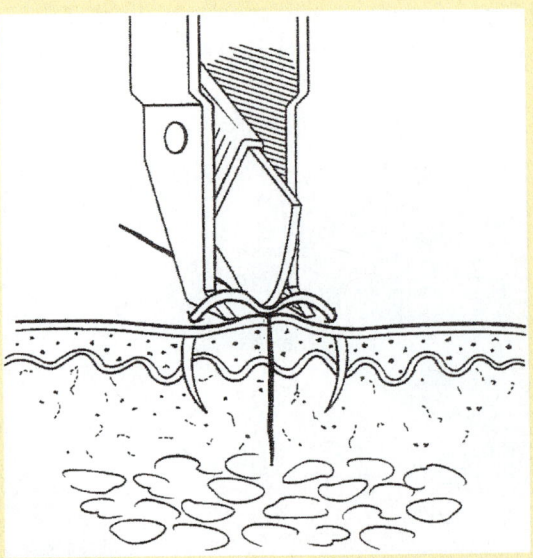

b. Tightly squeeze the staple handles together.

c. Carefully tilt the staple remover upward until the staple lifts out of the wound (Figure 4).

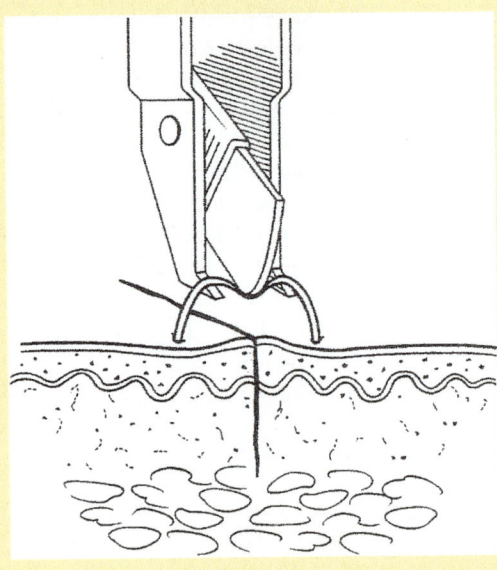

d. Place the removed staple on a 4 × 4-inch gauze square.

e. Continue the process until all staples have been removed.

12. Remove the gauze sponge holding the sutures or staples and dispose of contaminated materials in the biohazardous waste container.

13. The surgeon may apply or may have you apply Steri-Strips or an adhesive bandage strip for added support, strength, and protection.

14. Instruct the patient to keep the wound edges clean and dry and not to place excessive strain on the area.

15. Document the procedure, wound condition, number of sutures or staples removed, whether a dressing or bandage was applied, and the instructions on wound care given to the patient.
    <u>PURPOSE:</u> A procedure that is not documented was not done.

WOUND CARE

A wound can be intentional (i.e., from a surgical incision) or accidental, and it may be open or closed (Figure 57-10). An open wound has an outward opening where the skin is broken, exposing the underlying tissues. A closed or nonpenetrating wound does not have an outward opening, but the underlying tissues are damaged, as in a hematoma, contusion, or bruise. Closed wounds usually are the result of some type of blunt trauma to the body. An aseptic (clean) wound is not infected with pathogens. Septic wounds are infected with pathogens.

Open wounds may be classified according to the appearance of their openings. An incised wound has a clean edge and is made with a cutting instrument. An incised wound may be the result of surgery, an accident, or a knife wound. A lacerated wound has torn or mangled tissues and is made by a dull or blunt instrument. A penetrating or puncture wound is caused by a sharp, slender object, such as a needle or ice pick, and passes through the skin into the underlying tissues. A perforated wound is a penetrating wound that passes through to a body organ or cavity, such as a gunshot wound.

Wound Healing

All wounds go through a healing or repair process that has three phases. The *lag phase* occurs first, when the blood vessels contract to control hemorrhage, and blood platelets form a network in the wound that acts as a glue to plug the wound. After a cascade of chemical reactions, fibrin is released into the wound and clotting begins. Fibrin continues to collect red blood cells (RBCs), and the clot dries into a scab. About 12 hours later, special white blood cells (WBCs), macrophages, arrive to clear away bacteria and dead tissue. Within 1 to 4 days the fibrin threads contract and pull the edges of the wound together under the scab.

The second phase, *proliferation,* is the wound healing and new growth period, which lasts 5 to 20 days. During this phase, the tissues repair themselves. New cells form, and the wound continues to contract and seal. If the wound is a clean surgical incision, complete contraction usually takes place and a **cicatrix** forms.

The final phase, the *remodeling phase,* extends from day 21 onward. Clean, shallow wounds may contract in the first two stages; large or mangled wounds require the time and cellular activity of

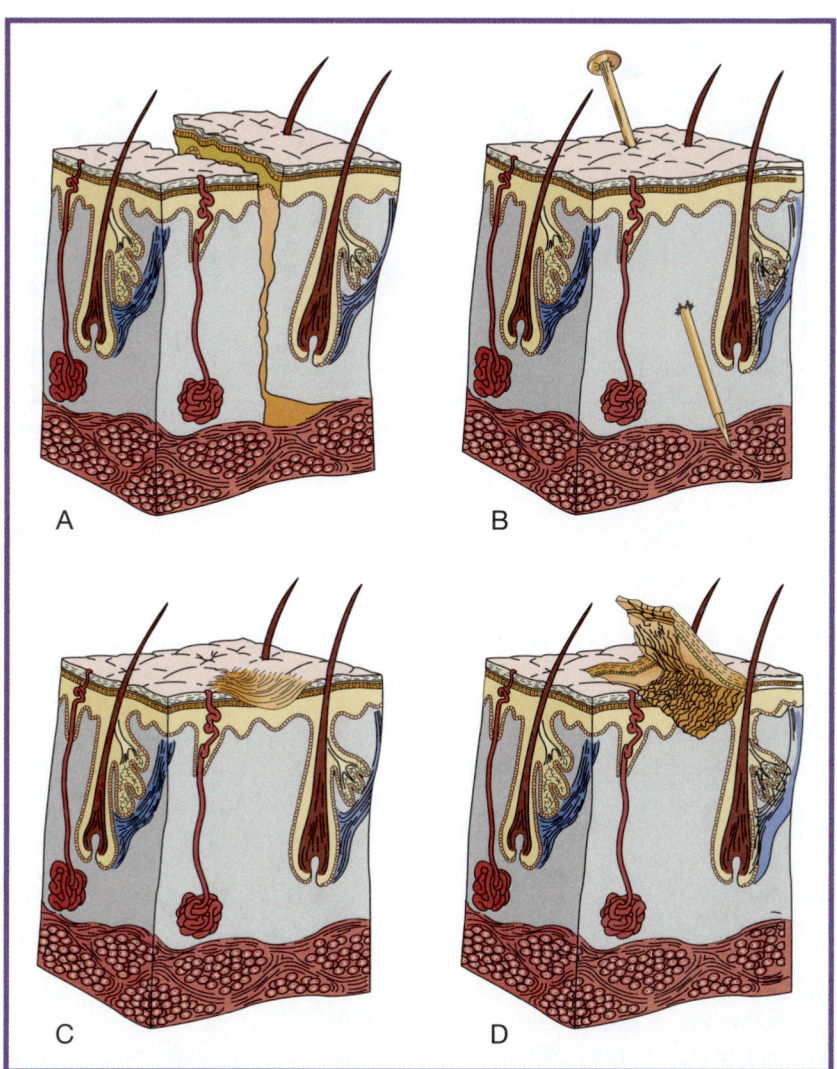

FIGURE 57-10 Types of wounds. **A,** Laceration—a jagged, irregular breaking or tearing of tissues, usually caused by blunt trauma. **B,** Puncture—piercing of the skin by a pointed object, such as a pin, nail, splinter, or bullet. **C,** Abrasion—a superficial wound made by scraping of the skin. **D,** Avulsion—tissue forcibly torn or separated, caused by accidents.

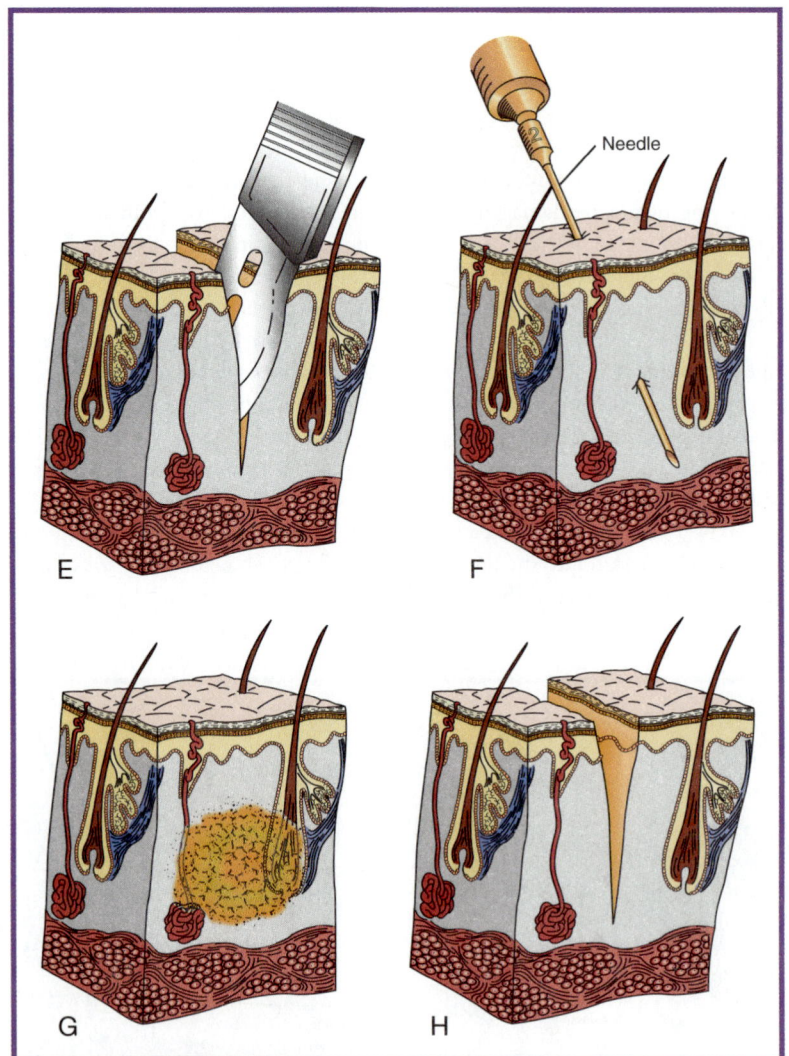

FIGURE 57-10, cont'd E, Surgical incision—a neat, clean cut. **F,** Hypodermic puncture—an injection under the skin. **G,** Contusion—a closed, nonpenetrating wound in which blood from broken vessels accumulates in tissues. **H,** Incision—a neat, clean cut from sharp objects, such as glass, knives, or metal.

this third phase to build a bridge of new tissue to close the gap of the wound. The cells produce a fibrous protein substance called *collagen* (connective tissue) that gives the wounded tissues strength and forms scar tissue. Scar tissue is not true skin; it usually is very strong, but it lacks the elasticity of normal skin tissue. Scar tissue also is devoid of a normal blood supply and nerves.

Wounds are classified by the way they repair themselves. A clean, surgical wound that has been sutured closed and heals quickly without much scarring does so by *first intention*. Tissues that are severely damaged or purposely kept open or that fail to close are said to heal by *granulation* (healing from the bottom of the wound outward), which is called *second intention.*

Several factors influence the healing process. People who are young, in good general health, and have adequate nutrition heal more rapidly. Adequate protection and rest of the injured area also enhance the healing process. Destruction or reinjury during the second phase can delay healing and increase scarring. Wounds are susceptible to infection, because the normal skin barrier is broken. If debris is present in a wound as the result of the breakdown of various cellular components, this dead (necrotic) tissue acts as a culture medium for bacterial growth. Suppuration (pus) contains

necrotic tissue, bacteria, dead WBCs, and other products of tissue breakdown. Necrotic tissue must be removed; the removal of debris is called *debridement,* which may occur naturally or may be performed surgically.

Sometimes the physician may prefer no dressing or bandage on small wounds. This is called *open wound healing.* Some advantages to open wound healing are:

- Air can circulate freely around the wound.
- The wound is not irritated or rubbed by a dressing.
- The wound stays dry, which inhibits bacterial growth, reducing the chance of infection.
- Sutures stay dry and hold together better.
- Any pre-existing infection remains localized and is not spread by the dressing or bandage.

Dressings

A dressing is a sterile covering placed over a wound for the purposes of:

- Protecting the wound from injury and contamination
- Maintaining constant pressure to minimize bleeding and swelling

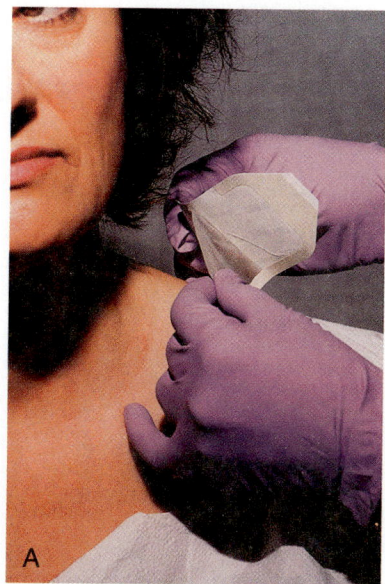
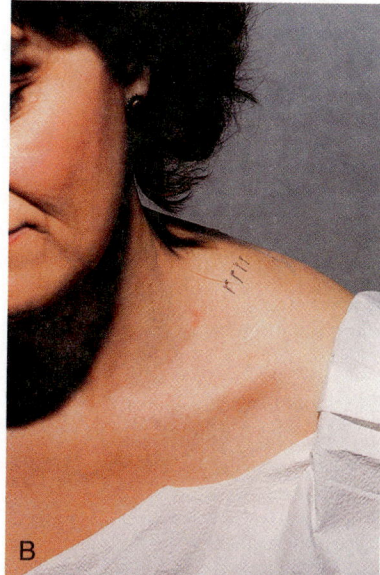

FIGURE 57-11 **A,** Placing a clear dressing on a sutured wound. **B,** Clear dressing in place over a sutured wound.

- Holding the wound edges together
- Absorbing drainage and secretions

A dressing usually consists of a strip of lubricated mesh gauze, a nonstick Telfa pad, or a clear dressing placed over a sutured wound (Figure 57-11). Gauze sponges may be placed over nonadhering material, depending on the physician's preference. Body cavities or wounds that need to remain open for a time are dressed with long, thin packing material that often is impregnated with an antiseptic or a lubricant; this sometimes is called *packing*. A good dressing must be effective and comfortable and must remain in place. If the dressing covers a hairless area, it may be anchored with tape, but no tape should touch the wound.

Frequently, small, clean lacerations may be closed with Steri-Strips (Figure 57-12). These strips reduce the chance of infection and do not leave suture scars. Steri-Strips are used on areas of the body that are protected from movement and stress. They often are used on the face. Because they are a suture replacement, only the physician should place them on a fresh wound. However, if they are applied after suture removal to provide further support for healing tissues, the medical assistant may apply them. They are placed on the wound in the same sequence and at the same intervals as interrupted sutures and are left in place until they fall off or the wound heals.

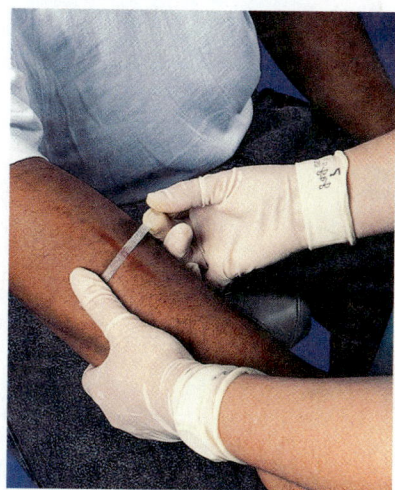

FIGURE 57-12 Steri-Strips on a wound. (From Bonewit-West K: *Clinical procedures for medical assistants,* ed 7, St Louis, 2008, WB Saunders.)

Bandages

Bandages hold dressings in place and also help maintain even pressure, support the affected part, and help protect the wound from injury and contamination. Bandages can be gauze, cloth, or elastic cloth rolls and are bound by clips, tape, or ties. Dressings and bandages frequently appear easy and simple to apply; however, special skill is required to use different types of bandaging techniques (Procedure 57-13). Bandages that are too loose fall off; those that are too tight may compromise circulation and further harm the patient.

Plain roller gauze is seldom used. It is difficult to handle, has no elasticity, and tends to bind. It also tends to slip, because it does not adhere to itself. Wrinkled crepe-type roller bandages (e.g., Kling) are preferred, because they easily conform to various shapes of the body and adhere to themselves (Figure 57-13, *A*). If the

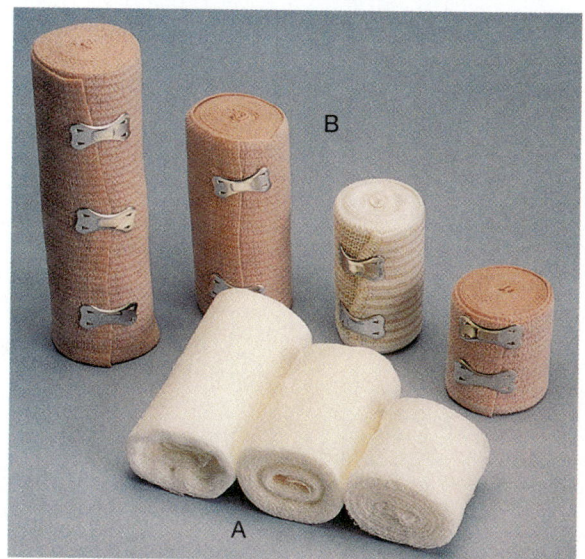

FIGURE 57-13 **A,** Kling bandages. **B,** Roller bandages.

PROCEDURE 57-13

Assist the Physician with Patient Care: Apply an Elastic Support Bandage Using a Spiral Turn

GOAL: *To apply an elastic bandage to the forearm.*

EQUIPMENT and SUPPLIES

- One 3- or 4-inch elastic bandage with clip closures

PROCEDURAL STEPS

1. Choose the proper size bandage for the size of the arm you are bandaging.
   PURPOSE: To provide proper support for the area.
2. Sanitize your hands. Perform a circular turn at the starting point, securing a turned down corner of the bandage in the first circle around the site.
   PURPOSE: To anchor the bandage at the starting point.
3. Hold the roll so that the bandage can be rolled away from you (Figure 1).

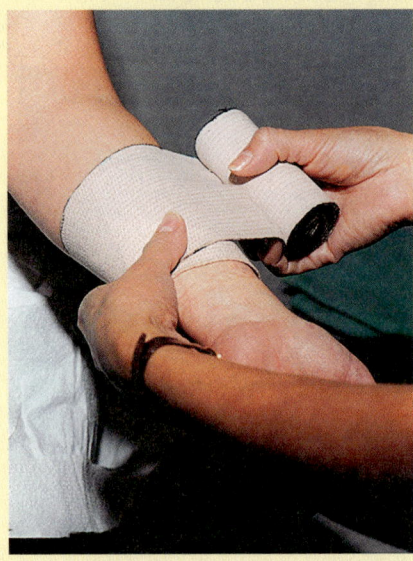

PURPOSE: To easily and securely apply the bandage.

4. Keep the roll close to the patient and keep it facing upward (Figure 2). With each successive turn, overlap the previous bandage turn by half.

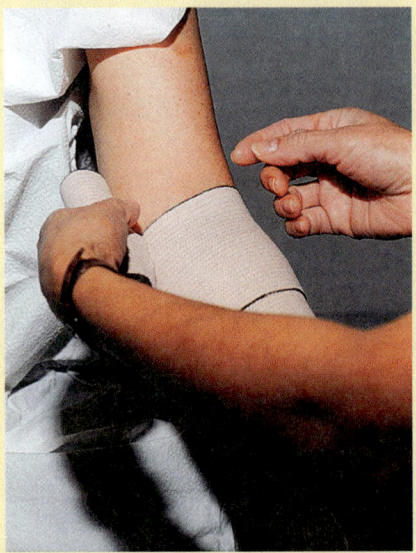

5. Maintain even tension and spacing as you continue to apply the bandage up the forearm.
   PURPOSE: To maintain even, light pressure over the entire area.
6. When crossing a joint, slightly flex the joint (Figure 3).

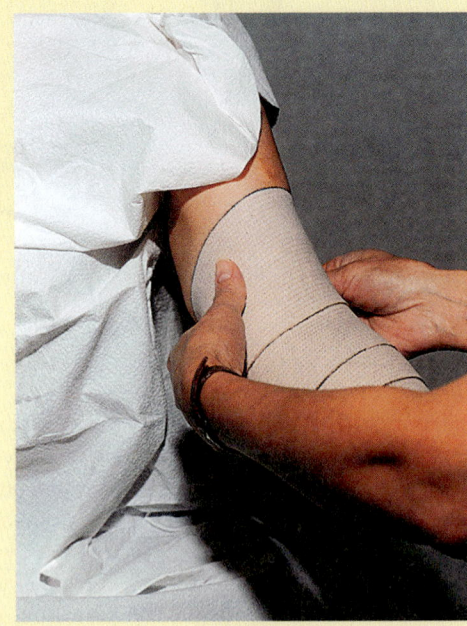

PURPOSE: To facilitate patient comfort and maintain normal circulation.

7. Fasten the end of the bandage with clips or tape (Figure 4).

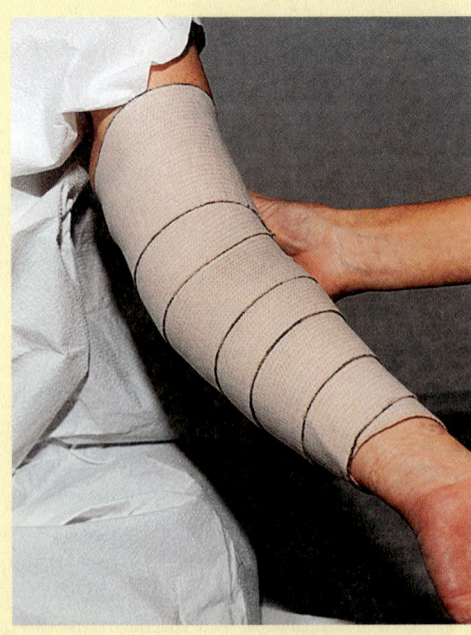

8. Check the nail beds for cyanosis; ask the patient whether the bandage is comfortable or feels too tight.
   PURPOSE: To ensure that the bandage is not acting as a tourniquet if applied too tightly.
9. Check the radial pulse.
   PURPOSE: To ensure that the bandage is not acting as a tourniquet if applied too tightly.
10. Have the patient move the fingers.
    PURPOSE: To check that nerve function is normal.

11. Document the procedure in the patient's medical record; also document instructions given to the patient about bandage care and replacement.
    PURPOSE: The procedure is not completed until it is recorded, dated, and signed.

10/22/XX 9:40 AM Spiral elastic bandage applied to ℗ forearm. Pt denies bandage too tight. Fingers warm to touch. Melissa Gelbart, CMA (AAMA)

---

bandage is to cover a wound, it should always be applied over a sterile dressing.

Plain elastic cloth (e.g., Ace) bandages or elastic roller cloth with adhesive backing make flexible, secure covers (Figure 57-13, *B*). When an Ace elastic roller bandage is applied as a pressure bandage, especially to the lower limbs, it is essential to keep the bandage consistent in spacing and tension to ensure even pressure. Even, gentle pressure stimulates circulation and healing. Uneven pressure causes constriction points that can create pressure sores, ulcers, or edema. Roller bandages usually are applied from the distal to the proximal part of the area, because it is more even and snug if it is wrapped from a smaller to a larger circumference. Elevate the limb while you are bandaging and work with the roller facing upward, close to the patient's skin. Elastic bandages are excellent for bandaging the hand and wrist (Figure 57-14) and the foot and ankle (Figure 57-15).

> ### CRITICAL THINKING APPLICATION 57-7
> Melissa applied a figure-eight elastic bandage to the hand and wrist of a patient who came into the office for suturing. She immediately sent the patient home after applying the bandage. She did not document the procedure in the patient's medical record at that time because the office was quite busy. Discuss all of your concerns regarding this situation. In what ways were safe patient practices ignored? What would be the worst-case scenario for the outcome of this situation? How can this potentially serious situation be corrected after the fact?

Seamless tubular gauze bandage, with or without elastic, is a superior material for covering round narrow surfaces such as fingers or toes. It can be used as a dressing if the gauze material is sterile or as a bandage. A tubular gauze bandage is applied with a cagelike applicator (Figure 57-16). Work with the open circle of the applicator toward the patient. Hold the applicator in the dominant hand and control the tension flow with your fingers as the applicator is gradually rotated and the material slides off. Tubular dressing may be applied with or without slight pressure. Beyond the tip of the bandaged part, give the applicator a full half-turn, place the applicator again over the part, and repeat the process, being careful not to create a tourniquet effect when you reverse the applicator. When the desired thickness of the bandage is reached, cut the gauze and anchor the final gauze application with tape or by tying at the wrist.

CLOSING COMMENTS

Patient Education

A medical assistant can help the patient in many ways. The best time to instruct your patient in aseptic techniques to be used at home is while you are performing an aseptic procedure. For example:

- While sanitizing your hands before a procedure or examination, explain to the patient that hands should be washed before meals; after sneezing, coughing, or nose blowing; after using the bathroom; before and after changing a dressing or bandage; and after changing an infant's diaper.
- Instruct the patient about the differences between sterile and clean dressings and bandages. Show the person step by step how to change a dressing properly and then how to dispose of the contaminated items.

A medical assistant's duty may include calling the patient the day before surgery to confirm the scheduled surgical procedure and appointment time. Explaining the procedure and what to expect during and after surgery prepares the patient and helps calm the person's fears or concerns. Lying still during surgery is important, and eating a light meal the night before should be encouraged. Bathing before coming to the office helps reduce the number of bacteria on the skin, and comfortable, loose clothing should be worn. Sometimes in the course of general conversation the medical assistant can pick up hints of concerns the patient may have and can direct the conversation into a discussion of these concerns.

Patients should be informed that they may need someone to accompany them home. A bandage is applied after surgery, and it must be kept clean and dry. The patient may have some pain, and the physician probably will prescribe some type of analgesic. After the procedure is complete, make sure the patient makes an appointment for a return visit and examination. Patients should also be encouraged to call the office immediately if they suspect an infection or have a sudden increase in pain at the surgical site.

Legal and Ethical Issues

Many minor surgical procedures previously performed in the hospital are now being done in a medical office, surgery center, or clinic. As insurance companies continue to recognize the cost-effectiveness

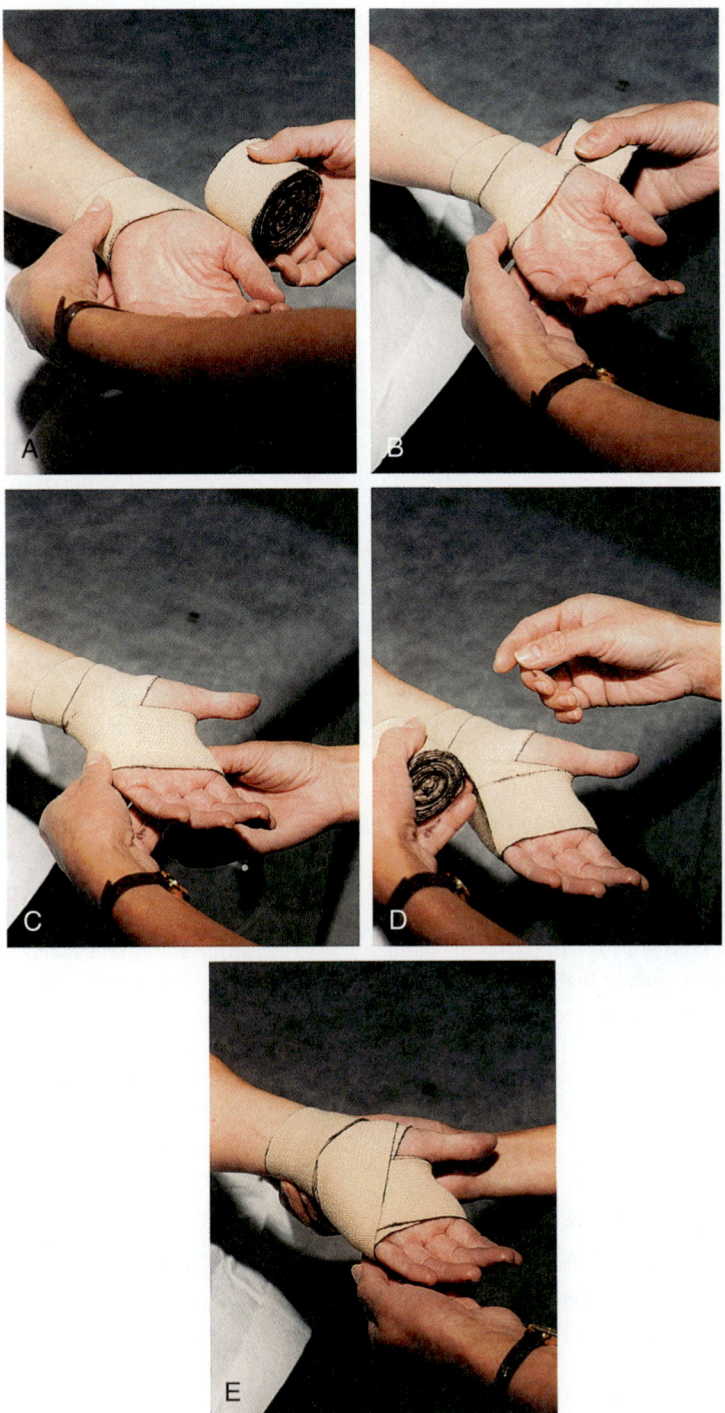

FIGURE 57-14 A, A combination of recurrent and figure-eight turns are used for the hand. **B,** Bandaging starts at the wrist. **C,** Applying a roller bandage to the hand. **D,** Roller bandage in place on the hand. **E,** Consistent tension is maintained while the bandage is applied.

of performing minor surgical procedures in these settings, the role of the medical assistant continues to expand.

Personal discipline is the primary concern in surgical asepsis. Often the assistant is alone when performing a surgical aseptic procedure; if contamination occurs, no one may know except the medical assistant. It is the surgical assistant's responsibility to begin the procedure again with clean or sterile supplies if it is possible that contamination occurred. The medical assistant's main responsibilities include carrying out sanitization, disinfection, and sterilization procedures with precision and with total effectiveness. There is no room for compromise.

Patients should have absolute assurance that they are being taken care of in an aseptic atmosphere and under the most stringent aseptic conditions. This assurance is just as important for the protection of

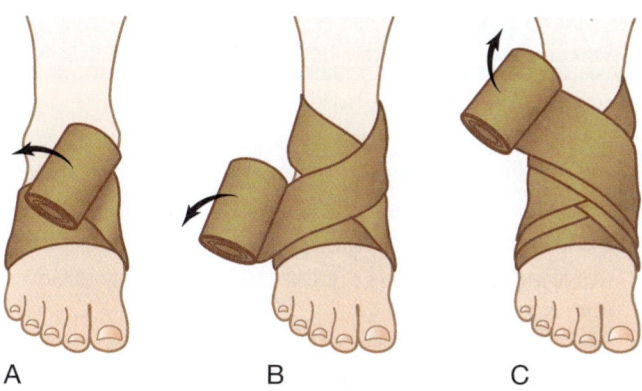

FIGURE 57-15 Using the figure-eight turn for the ankle.

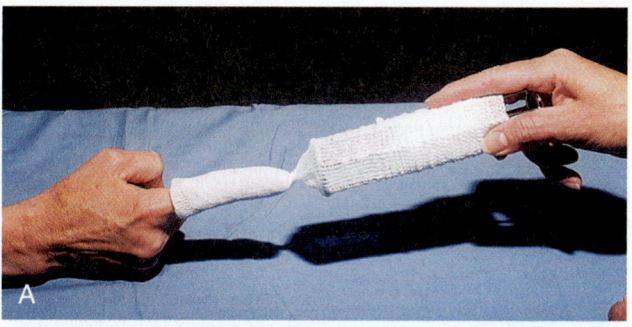

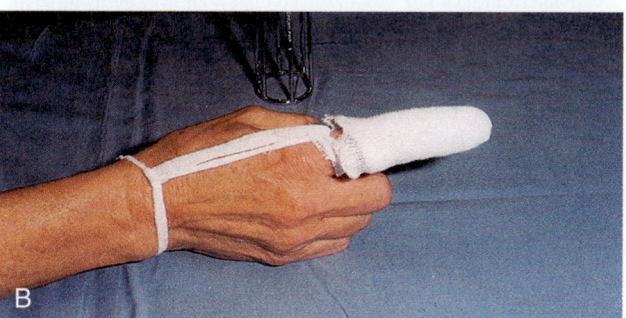

FIGURE 57-16 A, Tube gauze is applied with even tension and is twisted at the fingertip before the next layer is applied. **B,** Tube gauze bandage has been applied and secured by tying at the wrist.

the office staff as it is for the patient. Allowing the physician to assume that the correct aseptic techniques have been used in the preparation of equipment and allowing him or her to use contaminated equipment on a patient can result in claims of malpractice and charges of battery. Absolute, uncompromising honesty on the part of the assistant builds self-respect and contributes to professional achievement and satisfaction.

To have a good understanding of the subject, you must become familiar with the various techniques of sanitization, disinfection, and sterilization. Ignorance or carelessness can be dangerous and is inexcusable before the law.

The medical assistant must know what procedure is scheduled and whether the patient has been informed about the procedure. In the surgical setting, the medical assistant must realize the full extent of his or her role as the patient's advocate and the physician's agent.

Confirm that the physician has explained the procedure to the patient and that the patient fully understands all aspects of the procedure to be performed. This means that when the patient signs the consent for surgery, he or she is fully informed. Legal action can result if complications arise because of failure to complete consent

forms. The surgical procedure is expedited when the patient is given instructions and knows what to expect. Increasing the patient's understanding ensures greater compliance with presurgical preparations, and the patient is more likely to follow instructions and advice after surgery.

The medical assistant must practice perfect aseptic technique. A break in technique may invite infection and possible legal action. It is the medical assistant's duty to protect the patient. A major responsibility of the medical assistant is to adhere strictly to aseptic technique and to correct immediately any break in technique.

SUMMARY OF SCENARIO

Melissa is finding her clinical medical assisting position in Dr. Armstrong's practice rewarding, exciting, and challenging. She enjoys coming to work every day and has learned all aspects of her position much more quickly than most of her peers. Melissa frequently reads the latest information on new developments in minor surgery practice. Her concern for her patient's well-being makes her stand out, and the physician constantly gets positive comments on her level of professionalism.

Melissa has made a few errors in sterile technique since starting the clinical assistant position, but she has learned from each situation and has never

covered up a mistake. Whenever she realized that she did not follow procedure, she has discussed the issue with her supervisor and with Dr. Armstrong. In this way, errors can be corrected, if possible, and she most likely will not make the same or similar mistakes again.

Melissa is a team player who consistently tries to anticipate the needs of the physician and patient both before and during surgery. Her cooperative, supportive manner is appreciated by everyone on the clinical staff.

SUMMARY OF LEARNING OBJECTIVES

1. **Define, spell, and pronounce the terms listed in the vocabulary.**
   Spelling and pronouncing medical terms correctly bolster the medical assistant's credibility. Knowing the definitions of these terms promotes confidence in communication with patients and co-workers.

2. **Apply critical thinking skills in performing the patient assessment and patient care.**
   Completing the Critical Thinking Application exercises throughout the chapter can help the student medical assistant become more adept at critical analysis of real-life situations.

3. **Define the concepts of aseptic technique.**
   Medical asepsis is the process of reducing the number of pathogens or destroying all pathogens; surgical asepsis is the complete destruction of all organisms on instruments or equipment that will enter the patient's body. Using proper surgical aseptic technique is the primary means of preventing postoperative infections in surgical patients. Everyone on the surgical team is responsible for preventing and correcting breaks in technique.

4. **Explain the differences among sanitization, disinfection, and sterilization.**
   Sanitization is the cleaning of instruments and the environment to reduce the number of pathogens. *Disinfection* is the destruction of pathogens by physical or chemical means. *Sterilization* is the destruction of all microorganisms.

5. **Summarize tips for improving autoclave techniques.**
   Refer to Table 57-2.

6. **Demonstrate how to wrap instrument packs for autoclave sterilization.**
   Refer to Procedure 57-1.

7. **Explain the types and uses of sterilization indicators.**
   Autoclave tape contains a chemical dye that changes color when exposed to steam. Biologic sterilization indicators include a spore strip indicator, which contains a temperature-sensitive dye that changes color when the proper combination of steam, temperature, and time has been achieved. An indicator strip should be placed in the center of the largest pack.

8. **Summarize the correct methods of loading, operating, and unloading an autoclave.**
   The load is arranged for maximum circulation of steam and heat. Articles should be resting on edges; jars and bottles should be placed on their sides. When the cycle is complete, the pressure is released according to the manufacturer's guidelines. The medical assistant stands back from the door and, with heat-resistant gloves, opens the door approximately ¼ inch. The load is allowed to dry for at least 15 minutes before removal.

9. **Demonstrate how to operate an autoclave.**
   Refer to Procedure 57-2.

10. **Summarize common minor surgical procedures.**
    Typical minor surgical procedures include I&D of a cyst; electrosurgery, which uses high-frequency current to cut through tissue and coagulate blood vessels; laser surgery, which uses tiny light beams to safely treat specific tissues with minimal damage to surrounding tissues and to limit scar formation; microsurgery, which involves the use of an operating microscope to perform delicate surgical procedures; endoscopic procedures, which use a fiberoptic instrument with a miniature camera mounted on a flexible tube to examine the area within an organ or cavity and which are named according to the organs or areas they explore; and cryosurgery, which is the use of extreme cold to destroy tissues such as warts and skin lesions.

11. **Detail the medical assistant's role in minor office surgery.**
    The medical assistant is responsible for preparing the patient for surgery; performing the physician's preoperative orders; confirming that the patient has signed an informed consent form; making sure all the patient's questions and concerns have been addressed; assisting with positioning of the patient; performing skin preparation if ordered; and preparing the room for the procedure.

12. **Perform a skin prep for surgery.**
    Refer to Procedure 57-3.

13. **Perform a surgical hand scrub.**
    A surgical hand scrub is done to lower the number of transient and resident bacteria on the practitioner's hands so that the risk of wound contamination is reduced (see Procedure 57-4).

14. **Outline the rules for setting up and maintaining a sterile field.**
    Sterile surfaces must never come in contact with nonsterile surfaces. If this occurs, the sterile surface immediately is considered contaminated. The rules for maintaining a sterile field include keeping talking to a minimum; maintaining sight of the sterile field; and never crossing over the sterile field. Anything that falls below the edge of the Mayo tray and within a 1-inch border surrounding the tray is considered contaminated. A sterile barrier that is wet, cut, or torn is contaminated. Sterile gloved hands must be kept above waist level at all times. An item is never removed from and then again put into the field. A sterile package should be opened the entire way and the contents tossed onto the field without crossing over the sterile area. If a sterile package falls to the floor, it must be discarded. If any doubt exists about sterility, the field must be considered contaminated and the process must start all over again.

15. **Open a sterile pack to create a sterile field.**
    Refer to Procedure 57-5.

16. **Transfer sterile instruments and pour solutions into a sterile field.**
    Refer to Procedures 57-6 and 57-7.

17. **Put on sterile gloves without contaminating them.**
    Refer to Procedure 57-8.

18. **Demonstrate how to assist with a minor surgical procedure and suturing.**
    Refer to Procedures 57-9 and 57-10.

19. **Summarize postoperative instructions and wound care.**
    If medication is prescribed, review the purpose of the medication and directions for its use with the patient and his or her companion and make a follow-up appointment. The patient should be taught to care for himself or herself at home after surgery and should receive both verbal and written instructions. Explain to the patient the importance of calling the office if any questions arise or if he or she notes redness around the

operative site, bleeding from the wound, fever, swelling, or increasing or severe pain. If the patient does not call within the next 24 hours, the medical assistant should call the patient.

20. **Demonstrate how to remove sutures and the technique for removing surgical staples.**

Refer to Procedures 57-12.

21. **Explain the process of wound healing.**

All wounds go through a healing or repair process that has three phases. The lag phase occurs first when the blood vessels contract to control hemorrhage, platelets form a fibrin network, and a clot dries into a scab. Proliferation is a new growth period during which tissues repair themselves. During the final, or remodeling, phase, a bridge of new tissue is built to close the gap of the wound. Collagen gives the wounded tissues strength and forms scar tissue. Wounds are classified by the way they repair themselves: either by first intention, with clean, straight edges that heal quickly, or by granulation (or second intention), as in tissues that are severely damaged and are left open or fail to close.

22. **Properly apply dressings and bandages to surgical sites.**

Refer to Procedures 57-11 and 57-13.

23. **Conduct patient education in aseptic technique and surgical procedures.**

The best time for a medical assistant to instruct the patient in aseptic techniques to be used at home is during an aseptic procedure. Patient education includes the purpose and importance of hand washing; using disposable tissues to cover the nose and mouth when coughing or sneezing and properly disposing of used tissues; the differences between sterile and clean dressings and bandages; and step-by-step instructions on how to change a dressing properly and dispose of contaminated items.

24. **Discuss the legal and ethical concerns regarding surgical asepsis and infection control.**

The medical assistant must know what procedure is to be performed and whether the patient has received and provided informed consent. The medical assistant must realize the full extent of his or her role as the patient's advocate and the physician's agent. The more patients understand about their procedures, the more they comply with presurgical preparations and the more likely they are to follow instructions and advice after surgery. A major responsibility of the medical assistant is to adhere strictly to aseptic technique and to correct immediately any break in technique.

CONNECTIONS

📖 **Study Guide Connection:** Go to the Chapter 57 Study Guide. Read and complete the activities.

℮ **Evolve Connection:** Go to the Chapter 57 link at *evolve.elsevier.com/ kinn* to complete the Chapter Review and Chapter Quiz. Check out the other resources listed for this chapter to make the most of what you have learned from Surgical Asepsis and Assisting with Surgical Procedures.

58

CAREER DEVELOPMENT AND LIFE SKILLS

Lisa Walker is 1 month away from graduating from her medical assisting program. She has been an excellent student and is looking forward to beginning her career in the medical field. Lisa wants to begin her job search now so that she will be employed soon after her externship ends.

Lisa participated in several volunteer activities while she attended school. She plans to list these experiences on her resumé. She met many office managers and physicians while doing volunteer work, and she will be contacting those people in hopes of obtaining more job leads.

Lisa began saving for interview clothing when she first began school. She is on a strict budget, but she found several outfits appropriate for interviews at secondhand clothing shops and discount stores. Her best-looking suit cost only $25!

Not a person afraid to interview, Lisa looks forward to sharing her skills and experience with potential employers. She looks on each interview as a practice session for the next one, and this helps her relax more and present a true picture of herself to the office manager. She has a great smile and projects a natural friendliness and positive attitude.

Lisa has given much thought to what she wants from her first job as a medical assistant. She knows that she may not start at a high salary, but she also realizes that there are benefits and perquisites ("perks") to working in a physician's office. She plans to commit to working for 2 years on her first job, gaining experience before looking for her next job at a higher salary and with additional benefits.

Lisa is excited about her future as a medical assistant. She is ready to put the training she received to work with patients. She is determined to perform exceptionally well at her externship site and to go above and beyond her assigned duties to impress the staff in that facility, who will become references for her first paid position. Lisa is dedicated to being the best medical assistant possible and to becoming indispensable to her employer.

While studying this chapter, think about the following questions:

- How can the medical assistant prepare for his or her first job throughout the duration of training?
- What is meant by "writing your resumé every day"?
- How can the medical assistant organize the job search?
- How can the new medical assistant employee make a positive, lasting impression on co-workers and supervisors?

LEARNING OBJECTIVES

1. Define, spell, and pronounce the terms listed in the vocabulary.
2. Discuss the reasons job search training is important to a medical assistant.
3. List three expectations employers have of employees.
4. Understand the three types of employee skill strengths.
5. Explain the two best job search methods.
6. Describe some of the errors that should be avoided on a resumé.
7. List the four phases of the interview process.
8. Explain the importance of having demographic information about former jobs before appearing for an interview.
9. List and discuss legal and illegal interview questions.
10. Discuss the importance of the probationary period for a new employee.
11. List some common early mistakes of which a new employee should be aware.
12. Understand the importance of maintaining liability coverage once employed in the industry.
13. Explain why a performance appraisal rating is usually not perfect.
14. Organize a job search.
15. Prepare a resumé.
16. Complete a job application.
17. Interview for a job.
18. Negotiate a salary.

VOCABULARY

counteroffer Return offer made by one who has rejected an offer or a job.
default To fail to pay a financial debt, such as a student loan.
deferment Postponement, especially of a student loan.
genuineness Expressing sincerity and honest feeling.
intolerable Not tolerable or bearable.
mock Simulated; intended for imitation or practice.
networking Exchange of information or services among individuals, groups, or institutions; also, meeting and getting to know individuals in the same or similar career fields and sharing information about available opportunities.

pertinent (pur'-tuh-nent) Having a clear, decisive relevance to the matter at hand.
proofread To read and mark corrections.
rectify (rek'-tuh-fy) To correct by removing errors.
subtle Ingenious; artful; delicate.
succinct (suhk-sinkt') Marked by compact, precise expression without wasted words.
synopsis Condensed statement or outline.
vocation The work in which a person is regularly employed.

Each day a person exists is a small portion of a whole—a part of a person's entire lifetime. The events that happen during a day, no matter how small, shape the future. In the same way, the events that happen in the life of a medical assistant play a role in shaping his or her career. Every day, the medical assistant "writes a resumé"—through actions that reveal strengths, highlight skills, and summarize accomplishments—that builds on his or her **vocation**. Each duty performed becomes a part of the medical assistant's sum of experience and is important in the overall growth of the individual. Each action taken can have an impact on the future for the medical assistant. If the actions are professional, accurate, and performed to the individual's utmost ability, the resumé the medical assistant is writing will be one that leads to greater opportunities. If the medical assistant performs poorly, the resumé will be one that does not reflect trustworthiness and dependability. The small decisions made each day greatly affect the overall impression the medical assistant makes in the workplace.

Most people seeking employment have never had any type of formal training in the job search process. A newly graduated medical assistant should take advantage of job search training for three reasons:

- It will reduce the amount of time spent searching for a job.
- It will increase the chances of receiving better wages through negotiation.
- It will help eliminate the fears of looking for work and interviewing.

WHAT DOES THE EMPLOYER WANT?

Employers have three basic desires when they interview individuals for a job:

- They want a person who has a neat appearance and looks as if he or she fits the job (Figure 58-1).
- They want an individual who is dependable and can prove that he or she has been a reliable team member in other job positions.
- They want a person with the skills to do the job.

From the beginning of the job search process, a medical assistant's attitude is the most critical part of his or her potential success in getting a job (Figure 58-2). A good attitude is not a trait that can

be developed overnight. For this reason, a medical assistant must have a positive outlook in all situations so that the **genuineness** of his or her demeanor is clear during job interviews. The attitude displayed during training and externships is likely to be the same attitude that will be evident on the job. Make it a positive, enthusiastic one.

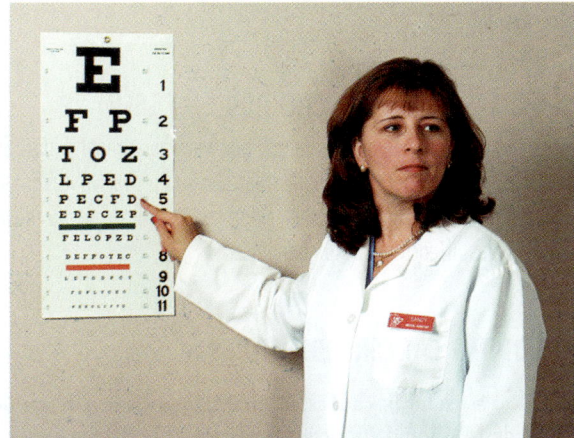

FIGURE 58-1 A professional appearance is mandatory in the medical office.

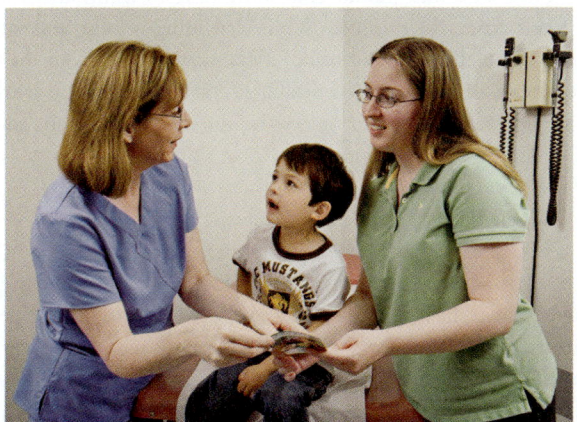

FIGURE 58-2 A great attitude is the best personal asset. Employers in the medical profession want medical assistants who have a positive attitude with patients.

CRITICAL THINKING APPLICATION   **58-1**

Lisa knows that attitude is of primary importance on a job. How can she prove to a potential employer in an interview that she has a good attitude? What exactly constitutes a good attitude? A bad attitude? What does it take to change an attitude from bad to good?

ASSESSING STRENGTHS

Before promoting himself or herself as a potential employee, a medical assistant must first determine the strengths that make him or her a valuable team member. The three types of skill strengths are job skills, self-management skills, and transferable skills.

Job skills are the abilities the medical assistant needs to perform the job. These include such skills as performing venipuncture, billing insurance, answering the telephone, scheduling appointments, giving injections, and handling other tasks.

Self-management skills relate to the medical assistant's personality and character traits. They include such attributes as honesty, integrity, and enthusiasm.

Transferable skills can be taken from one job to another. For instance, if the medical assistant has the ability to communicate effectively, this skill can be used on every job. Leadership is a transferable skill, as are the ability to follow directions and the ability to manage people.

CRITICAL THINKING APPLICATION   **58-2**

Lisa expects potential employers to ask her what her strengths are. She has determined six specific strengths that she can prove with examples from past positions or her externship. What six strengths can you prove? Give examples of each of these strengths.

DEVELOPING CAREER OBJECTIVES

Each medical assistant has a reason for entering the healthcare field. This basic desire should influence decisions concerning his or her career choices. Because medical assisting is such a versatile profession, a medical assistant has numerous options after graduation.

Medical assistants should take some time to think about what they want from their career. While attending school and subsequently completing an externship, ideas may surface about the area of healthcare in which the medical assistant most wants to work.

When developing career objectives, the medical assistant should start by asking several questions:

- Where am I today?
- Where do I want to be in 5 years?
- Where do I want to be in 10 years?
- What additional skills do I need to get where I want to go?

Write down the questions and answers and go into specific detail. Set realistic goals and develop a plan as to how and when they will be reached. It is helpful to put a list of goals in a prominent place at home, where you can see them each day. Some people use a spiral notebook, the front of the refrigerator, or Post-it notes attached to a mirror in the area where they get dressed. Keep goals in a visible place to keep them in mind even on the more difficult days, when they seem far from sight.

CRITICAL THINKING APPLICATION   **58-3**

Lisa knows that goals are important when a person is attempting to achieve in life. She has written down five goals for her job search and her first position as a medical assistant. What are some realistic goals for the job search? What realistic goals could be developed for the first position as a medical assistant?

KNOWING PERSONAL NEEDS

When searching for a job, the medical assistant must evaluate all of his or her needs. Most people have a minimum salary they require, in addition to certain benefits. For example, if the medical assistant is a single mother, she may require a moderate salary and insist on health insurance benefits. We also have intrinsic needs, which are internal desires important to us personally.

A helpful activity is to write a **synopsis** of a typical day on an ideal medical assisting job. Imagine the type of office, the job title, the daily duties, and the salary and benefits that would be a part of the ideal job (Figure 58-3). This can help you develop a focus and a goal to work toward as your career develops.

FINDING A JOB

Many people have misconceptions about the job market that exists today. Fortunately, the medical field is not an industry that sees high levels of unemployment. Usually, healthcare percentages remain high even in a poor economy. Graduation from a medical assisting program does not guarantee that the student will obtain employment. Completion of the program gives the medical assistant the job skills needed to work, but a good attitude and positive outlook are essential for success in the job search. In addition, the medical assistant should always be open to new and better opportunities.

Some job seekers assume that potential employers will not interact with students until they graduate. However, prospecting before graduation is a smart idea, and there are **subtle** ways of introducing

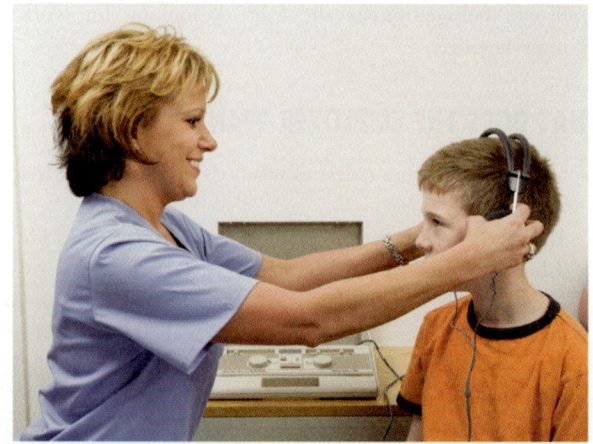

FIGURE 58-3 Enjoyment of the job is paramount. Medical assistants should enjoy their work and give compassionate, friendly care to all patients.

oneself to a facility without bluntly asking for employment. Many also think they must have work experience to be hired, but employers are more interested in attitude and "teachability" than a long resumé full of experience. In fact, many physicians like hiring students fresh from school so that they can teach them specifically how they want procedures done before the new graduate gets used to doing them another way.

Two Best Job Search Methods

Although there are many ways to find employment, two methods have proved to be the best and most effective: networking and direct contact with employers.

Networking is the exchange of information or services among individuals, groups, or institutions. When related to a job search, networking involves meeting and getting to know individuals in the same or similar career fields and sharing information about available opportunities. A medical assistant should begin to form a network of friends, business associates, co-workers, and acquaintances early in training, and he or she should stay in contact with these people throughout the job search effort and beyond (Figure 58-4). E-mail, Facebook, MySpace, and other electronic advances make staying in touch with former classmates and instructors very easy.

How does one network? One way is by joining professional medical assisting organizations. The members who attend regular meetings often know about job leads in the area. The medical assistant should also tell his or her personal physician or physicians about being in school and the approximate time of graduation. Friends and family members can be on the lookout for potential opportunities and may help by asking their personal physicians if they are aware of positions that will open for applications soon. Always keep a few resumés on hand; the opportunity to network could come at any time.

Networking is not limited to job searching, and many organizations are formed to develop networks of individuals or groups that assist one another and refer clients to one another. However, these groups are useful to the person who is looking for employment, and by attending meetings and get-togethers held for networking purposes, medical assistants may happen onto the ideal job for which they have been looking.

CRITICAL THINKING APPLICATION   58-4

Lisa knows that networking is a great way to find employment. She is making a list of people with whom she can share her resumé or inform that she is now ready to seek employment as a medical assistant.
- How many relatives can you think of who are good prospects for networking?
- How many professional people can you think of who are good prospects for networking?

Direct contact with employers is also an effective method of job searching. Medical assistants often know of specific clinics or facilities they would like to investigate as job possibilities. Compile a list of these places and learn as much about them as possible. If the facility has a Web site, read it thoroughly. Ask for brochures or patient information packets offered by the employer. Some have an annual report that lists details about the organization. All this information helps the medical assistant get a good basic idea of why the facility exists and what it does for the community.

Contact with employers does not necessarily begin only after the student has graduated. Students can begin networking and contacting employers from the very start of their enrollment at school. The student can keep a file of potential employers. Take a drive around the area where your home is located and make note of the medical facilities close by. Then, determine the facilities that are good prospects for employment and begin researching them. Call to find out who supervises medical assistants in the facility. In a physician's office, this usually is the office manager. Then call the office manager and ask to make an appointment to learn about the facility. Even the busiest people usually are willing to help a student investigate healthcare facilities in the area.

Do not tell the office manager that the objective of the appointment is a job offer. The goal at this point is to learn about the facility, what it offers the community, and what roles the medical assistants in the facility perform. Suggest that the appointment be set at the office manager's convenience. Then treat the appointment like an actual job interview, dressing appropriately and arriving on time. Do not be late or cancel without calling first. Have a list of questions about the facility prepared in advance and do not take too much of the office manager's time. Take notes about what the office manager says about the facility so that you can refer to them after graduation, during the actual job search.

After the appointment with the office manager, ask for a business card and always send a thank you note or letter. Remember this critical point! This helps the office manager remember the name of the medical assistant, and it is a pleasant addition to the daily mail. Everyone enjoys being recognized for his or her efforts, and the office manager will appreciate the thank you note.

Toward time for graduation, determine the possibility of performing an externship at one of the facilities you visited early in training. Check with school regulations to determine whether this

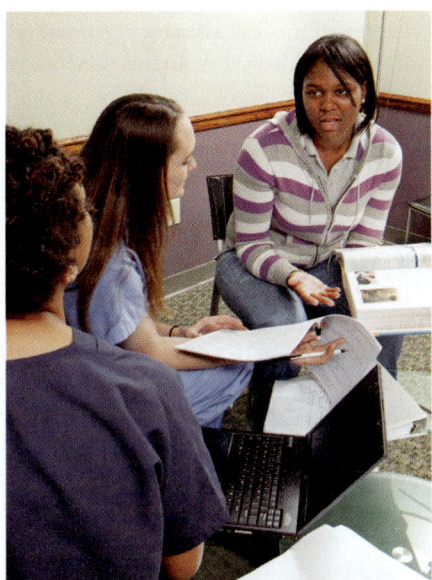

FIGURE 58-4 Stay in touch with classmates. They are excellent networking contacts and may be able to provide job leads.

is possible. Then the office manager can be approached about allowing the student to extern in the office. Be sure to follow school guidelines when investigating these possibilities. Some schools allow students to secure their own externship sites, but this must be discussed with the externship supervisor at school. Performing an externship at a medical facility usually is the first practical experience the student has in the medical field and can be used as a reference in building a resumé.

After the externship is complete, the medical assistant may want to send a resumé to all the office managers he or she met through the direct contact efforts made earlier in training. A professional resumé with a cover letter that refers to the earlier meeting will prompt the office manager to remember the student. Ask in the cover letter whether any opportunities are available in the facility. Mention that the facility and staff were impressive on the first meeting and that the facility would be an exciting place to begin a career. In the letter request that, if the office manager does not have any positions available at that time, he or she keep the resumé on file or pass it along to an acquaintance who is looking for an additional staff member.

Internet and the Job Search

The Internet opens a whole new world of opportunity when it comes to job searches. The medical assistant can find a gargantuan amount of information about writing resumés, interviewing, and follow-up methods, but perhaps most important, the Internet can provide information about who is hiring right now.

Many databases provide information about job openings. Monster, Yahoo! Jobs, and the Online Career Center are a few examples. The search can be targeted to specific geographic areas, certain career fields, or even specific job titles. Conduct a search in a selected state (or metropolitan area), then look for jobs in the medical profession, then narrow the field even more by asking for information on jobs specifically for medical assistants.

The medical assistant also can express interest in a job by perusing the company Web site and then contacting the employer directly on the "contact us" page. Anyone looking at the Web site should be able to find an e-mail address to use for gathering additional information. Mention that the school encourages quality businesses as potential employers and ask for information that could be presented to a class. Most employers are happy to get the word out about their company and may give all kinds of pamphlets and "freebies" to share with a class. By sending a thank you note and staying in touch with the company, the medical assistant creates a new lead for the job search.

Just remember, the information available to one medical assistant on the Internet is also available to every other medical assistant. The Internet is great for researching positions and companies, but networking and direct contact are still the most successful ways to obtain a job. All the elements of the medical assistant's "whole package"—the resumé, application, interview, follow-up, attitude, appearance, and job skills—combine to make an impression on the employer. Will that impression be favorable enough to result in a job offer?

Traditional Job Search Methods

The more traditional job search methods may be effective but usually are not as successful as networking and contacting employers directly.

School Career Placement Offices

Students usually have lifetime access to their school placement offices. Take advantage of the job search classes held at the school and seek advice regularly from the placement officers. They can suggest facilities that have job openings and will often make appointments for interviews. The placement office should be the first resource for the student's job search.

Newspaper Ads

Newspaper ads normally produce a huge number of applicants and resumés for the employer. A resumé or application must stand out in the crowd to be noticed when it arrives at the facility. Some applicants use clear envelopes, which draw attention to the resumé quickly in a stack of mail.

Employment Agencies

Employment agencies usually charge a fee for their services. Even when the employer pays the fee, the medical assistant may be offered a lower wage to compensate for the fee. These agencies can be useful, however, especially in salary negotiations. The agency knows the salary range the employer is willing to pay. This means that medical assistants can command a salary within that range and are not short-changed by asking for a salary that is much lower than the employer is willing to pay.

> ### CRITICAL THINKING APPLICATION   58-5
> Lisa keeps an eye on the local newspapers for ads that mention a need for medical assistants.
> - What current ads in local papers are interesting and would prompt sending a resumé?
> - What factors might the medical assistant consider in choosing ads to which he or she will respond?
> - How can the medical assistant determine which are good potential employers?

Professional Organizations

Joining local chapters of medical assistant organizations, such as the American Association of Medical Assistants (AAMA) or the American Medical Technologists (AMT), can help the student in many ways. Not only is valuable information exchanged at the meetings, but the medical assistant also may hear of positions becoming available in various medical facilities. Participating in professional organizations is a form of networking with the added benefit of continuing educational opportunities.

Volunteering

By volunteering in medical offices or facilities, the medical assistant meets other professionals who may be able to provide job leads. Volunteer activities should be added to the resumé, because these valuable experiences often can be used in the physician's office as well. It does not matter that the position was not a paid job; experience counts, whether paid or not.

Mailing Resumés

Mailing a large number of resumés is not a very effective method of searching for a job. Out of 100 resumés sent, one or two potential employers may respond with a request for an interview. It is much more effective to network first, then follow up with a good cover letter and resumé. Resumés can be used when contacting employers directly, and this approach allows the medical assistant to meet at least one employee of the facility when the document is delivered. Be sure to ask for a business card and write down the name of the person to whom the resumé was delivered. For impressive facilities, send a note of thanks to the person who accepted the resumé, asking to be considered for future positions.

Cold Calling

Cold calling is contacting employers by phone and prospecting for available positions. If the medical assistant asks, "Are you hiring?" at the beginning of the conversation, he or she should expect a negative answer and has just wasted the call. This is all but useless in the job search effort. However, an assistant who calls for information about the clinic and schedules an appointment with the office manager may have more success. Most office managers are open to talking with a medical assistant about the profession and will gladly make an appointment if it can be at their convenience. Some would not even consider interrupting their day just to talk with a student medical assistant, but most are happy to help new graduates obtain answers to questions and get started in their medical career. However, do not waste the time the person has offered. Prepare a list of questions in advance and be sure to ask about the interviewer's career in the healthcare industry. People enjoy talking about themselves and their accomplishments, and valuable information may be gleaned from hearing how the office manager started in healthcare. Never attempt to get a job over the phone. Even when interested employers call and ask questions, attempt to set up an interview to discuss your qualifications in person.

Performing Well on Externships

Performing well on externships may be one of the best ways to secure a job. If an opening exists, the medical assistant extern is already oriented to the practice and may be the perfect fit for the job. Perform duties assigned on the externship as if they were final examinations at school. Even if the office does not have a position available at that time, there may be one soon, or the office manager or physician may know of an office that has an opening. Do the best job possible, and an employment offer may be waiting at the conclusion of the externship. Be ready to learn from the moment the externship begins until the moment it ends.

Organizing the Job Search

Seeking a job is a full-time job. The new medical assistant must put forth effort, have stamina, and be persistent. Do not expect to get a job with the first practice that offers an interview. By keeping track of opportunities found, the medical assistant is more likely to obtain employment soon after graduation (Procedure 58-1).

A job lead is any information that could lead to a position, either now or in the future. Some of the most promising job leads for the newly graduated medical assistant come from the externship experience. Be friendly and meet as many people as possible while completing this part of training. Ask for business cards and stay in contact with the medical professionals you meet at the externship site and nearby hospitals. Be willing to shake hands and make introductions

at all times so that the circle of promising contacts for job leads continues to expand.

The medical assistant would be wise to keep a record of all job leads (Figure 58-5). The name and address of the facility, a contact name, and phone numbers all are important pieces of information. Keep track of where the lead was obtained; if it was provided by an individual, thank that person properly, especially if the lead results in a job offer. These records are an excellent starting place when making calls to set up job interviews. Remember, the placement office at school is a resource for job leads but should not be the only source used for obtaining leads. Each medical assistant graduate must take personal responsibility for finding and following up on job opportunities.

The job lead is not the only information that should be recorded during job search efforts. Keep a record of arrangements when an interview is secured, including information such as the following:

- Day, date, and time of the interview
- Directions to the interview site
- Name of the interviewer
- Items to bring to the interview
- Information about the company or facility

As soon as the interview is over, make a few notes about what happened during the interview. After several interviews, remembering which facility offered what salary, which had medical benefits, and which was closest to home may be difficult. By keeping accurate records, the medical assistant can follow up in the appropriate manner and send a note or letter of appreciation to the person who conducted the interview (Figure 58-6).

DEVELOPING A RESUMÉ

A resumé is a fact sheet that summarizes an applicant's qualifications, education, and experience. Medical assistants must determine what to include in the resumé, remembering that they are "selling" themselves to an employer (Procedure 58-2). The resumé should be developed before cover letters are written or job applications are completed so that strengths can be identified and highlighted on all job search documents.

Many types of resumés can be used. Three of the most common are the chronologic resumé, the functional resumé, and the targeted resumé. A chronologic resumé highlights the medical assistant's abilities in a logical order, such as most recent jobs back to the beginning of the individual's career (Figure 58-7). A functional resumé highlights specific skill sets, emphasizing the most important abilities or the most valuable experiences the medical assistant has had (Figure 58-8). A targeted resumé is perhaps the most effective; it emphasizes the skills that relate specifically to the job for which the medical assistant is applying (Figure 58-9).

The medical assistant should target the resumé to the specific job for which he or she is applying. This means that the job requirements should be compared with the skills on the resumé, and those skills should be highlighted in the document using action words (Figure 58-10). Of course, to do this effectively, the medical assistant must actually know the job requirements. Clinical and administrative duties are likely to be similar from place to place, but the ad for the position may provide further information about the scope of duties. The medical assistant should read this information carefully and

PROCEDURE 58-1

Organize a Job Search

GOAL: *To devote adequate time to and organize the job search in an efficient way so that proper follow up can be conducted.*

EQUIPMENT and SUPPLIES

- Record of a job lead form
- Record of an interview form
- Copies of your resumé
- List of interview questions
- Contact information for former employers and references
- Map of geographic area or printout from Internet mapping program
- Internet access
- Computer
- Job search Web links
- Local newspapers
- Contact information for friends and family

PROCEDURAL STEPS

1. Format the resumé as an accurate, up-to-date document.
   PURPOSE: If the resumé is kept on a computer, it can be easily updated and targeted for various job opportunities.
2. Make copies of the record of job lead and record of interview forms.
3. Research job search Web sites and newspapers for job leads.
4. Network and contact employers directly to obtain job leads.
   PURPOSE: Networking and direct employer contact are the best two methods of searching for a job.
5. Gather information on job leads and complete a record of job lead form for each one.

PURPOSE: Employers are impressed when the person being interviewed is familiar with the company; much information can be found on the company's Web site.

6. Prepare a targeted copy of the resumé for each job lead.
   PURPOSE: Targeted resumés are designed to highlight the candidate's skills for a particular job, and the resumé can easily be tailored for each specific company on a computer.
7. Take the resumé to the facility and ask to complete an application or (see step 8).
8. E-mail the resumé to the facility according to directions listed in the job advertisement.
9. Document all activity on each job lead.
   PURPOSE: The job search should be an organized process.
10. Schedule interviews for as many facilities as possible.
    PURPOSE: The more interviews, the better prepared the candidate will be.
11. Keep a record of job details on the record of the interview form for later reference.
    PURPOSE: Keeping a record of the details about each job possibility helps keep them organized and is useful for comparing job offers.
12. After an interview, send a thank you note to the interviewer.
    PURPOSE: Never fail to send a thank you note, because this gesture may be the deciding factor in securing the job.
13. Compare opportunities when making a choice between offered positions.

---

should emphasize on the resumé that those responsibilities are part of his or her skill set.

Compose the resumé and save it on the computer, a CD, or other storage device. Keep a copy on a flash drive so that the information is readily available if needed when away from the primary computer. Remember to keep the flash drive in the car or in a purse or backpack. Then, as each job opportunity presents itself, the resumé can be modified to fit the job. For instance, if the resumé lists back-office skills first and the job is for an administrative position, the administrative skills should be moved to the top to draw more attention to them. This is easy to accomplish when the resumé is on a computer, because the medical assistant can cut and paste where necessary to make changes and save several versions of the resumé. Then an original can be printed on high-quality paper for every job for which he or she applies.

A resumé is an important job search tool, but it should never be expected to get the medical assistant a job on its own merit. Resumés are one of many tools that should be used when looking for employment. Developing a professional resumé takes some effort but proves to be a good time investment. Give the document some thought and follow generally accepted guidelines for constructing it.

> ### CRITICAL THINKING APPLICATION   58-6
> Lisa has drafted her resumé and given a copy to three of her instructors. One recommended that Lisa remove the mention of her volunteer experience, because it was not in the medical field.
> - Should Lisa do this? Why or why not?
> - How can experience outside the medical field be beneficial to a new graduate?

Critical Resumé Errors

The first error that should be prevented on a resumé is just that—any error. The resumé should have no errors at all; many employers automatically disqualify a job candidate if one is found.

One medical assistant who was having trouble finding a job consulted her placement director at school. The director suggested

Record of a Job Lead

Job Title _____ Medical Office/Facility Name _____

Phone Number_____Fax Number _____

Contact Name _____ Contact Title _____

Contact Phone Number/Extension _____

Physician(s) _____Office Manager _____

Office/Facility Address _____

City _____ State _____ Zip _____

Referred By _____ Phone Number _____

Date First Contacted _____ Person Spoken To _____

Information Submitted:

☐ Cover Letter   ☐ Résumé   ☐ References

Date Sent _____   Date Sent _____   Date Sent _____

First Interview Scheduled: Day/Date _____   Time _____

Interviewer Name _____   Phone _____

Second Interview Scheduled: Day/Date _____   Time _____

Interviewer Name _____   Phone _____

Travel Directions _____

_____

_____

Office/Facility Information _____

_____

Basic Job Duties _____

_____

Miscellaneous Information _____

_____

_____

_____

(staple a business card to this form from the office/facility – use back for additional information)

FIGURE 58-5 Record of a job lead.

Record of an Interview

Job Title _____ Medical Office/Facility Name _____

Phone Number_____Fax Number _____

Contact Name _____ Contact Title _____

Contact Phone Number/Extension _____

Physician(s) _____Office Manager _____

Office/Facility Address _____

City _____ State _____ Zip _____

Interviewer Name _____ Phone _____

Travel Directions _____

_____

_____

Office/Facility Information _____

_____

Basic Job Duties _____

_____

Benefits/Salary Discussed _____

_____

Hours/Days to Work _____

General Impression of Office and Personnel _____

Questions as a result of interview _____

_____

Self-Evaluation of Interview Performance _____

_____

Thank-you sent ☐ yes ☐ no Date _____ Job Offer ☐ yes ☐ no (use back for notes)

Other Follow-up _____

_____

(staple a business card to this form from the office/facility – use back for additional information)

FIGURE 58-6 Record of an interview.

PROCEDURE 58-2

Prepare a Resumé

GOAL: *To write an effective resumé for use as a tool in obtaining employment.*

EQUIPMENT and SUPPLIES

- Scratch paper
- Pen or pencil
- Former job descriptions, if available
- List of addresses of former employers and schools and names of supervisors
- Computer or word processor
- Quality stationery and envelopes

PROCEDURAL STEPS

1. Perform a self-evaluation by making notes about your strengths as a medical assistant. Consider job skills, self-management skills, and transferable skills.
   PURPOSE: To determine the strongest aspects of your abilities so that they can be highlighted on the resumé.
2. Explore formatting and decide on a professional resumé appearance that best highlights your skills and experience. Use the templates available in word processing software or design your own.
   PURPOSE: To construct an attractive document.
3. Place your name, address, and two telephone numbers where you can be contacted at the top of the resumé.
   PURPOSE: To make sure potential employers have a means of contacting you.
4. Write a job objective that specifies your employment goals.
   PURPOSE: To give the prospective employer an idea of what you are looking for in a medical assisting position.
5. Provide details about your educational experience. List degrees and/or certifications you have obtained.

6. Provide details about your work experience. Include all contact information and names of supervisors. Do not include salary expectations or reasons for leaving former jobs. Use former job descriptions to detail work experience from previous employment.
   PURPOSE: No negative information should be put on the resumé. Salaries should not be discussed; if a certain salary is listed on the resumé, it may limit the amount the facility offers the medical assistant.
7. Include information on the resumé that exhibits dependability, punctuality, positive work ethics, initiative, the ability to adapt to change, and a responsible attitude.
8. Prepare a cover letter and a list of references. Send the references with the resumé only when requested.
9. Type the resumé carefully and make sure the document has no errors.
   PURPOSE: Resumés submitted with errors often are discarded without consideration.
10. Proofread the resumé. Allow another person to read it as well and look for missed errors.
    PURPOSE: To make sure the resumé is error free.
11. Print the resumé on high-quality paper. Review the resumé again for errors and to make sure it looks attractive on the printed page.
12. Target each resumé to a specific person or position. Do not send generic resumés to each prospective employer.
    PURPOSE: Targeted resumés get better results during the job search.
13. For all resumés that are distributed, follow up with a phone call to arrange an interview.
    PURPOSE: A resumé sent without follow-up usually is ineffective.

---

that she come in for a **mock** interview. About halfway through the interview, the placement director realized the problem. The medical assistant had worked for 2 years at a local grocery store and had misspelled the name of the store on the resumé. From an employer's point of view, a person who cannot spell the name of a facility where she worked for a length of time, even though she cashed a paycheck with the company name on it, might well make critical errors in charting or in other aspects of her duties. Within a week after this error was corrected, the medical assistant found a job.

Never list salary expectations on the resumé. If the medical assistant lists a salary of $26,620 for the last job held, the future employer might not offer more than $27,000 to $28,000, realizing that this is a step up from the last salary. If the employer had been willing to pay $32,000, the medical assistant lost an opportunity for much higher wages.

Avoid using "I" or other personal pronouns on the resumé. If abbreviations are used on the resumé, be sure to spell them out for clarity the first time they are used if they are not well-known

abbreviations. Never include personal information, such as height, weight, age, marital status, number of children, or any other information that is not **pertinent** to the job requirements.

Do not list dates along the left-hand side of the paper. This is distracting and draws attention away from the points that should be emphasized. A resumé must be visually appealing and easy to read. The medical assistant should make good use of spacing, margins, indention, capitalization, and underlining to ensure an attractive document. Proofread the document several times to be sure it has no errors. Having someone else **proofread** it can be helpful, because often the writer of a document misses errors when proofreading.

Never include a photograph with the resumé. Photographs can be a discriminatory factor in the hiring process, and the medical assistant should be wary of any employer who requests a photograph with the resumé.

One of the most senseless errors common to resumés is not including the appropriate contact information, such as an address, telephone number, and e-mail address. Two phone numbers are

Ruby Dunham
9362 Caesar Creek Road
Mytown, OH 45458
(937) 555-1899
rdunham@comcast.net

Education

• 1998: A.S. in Medical Assisting, Community College, Mytown, OH

Experience:

1995–present: Medical Transcriptionist, Community Hospital, Mytown, OH

• Transcribe 55 wpm
• Specialist in medical terminology
• Excellent attendance record
• Detail oriented
• Increased personal productivity each quarter

1990–1995: Secretary, State University School of Medicine, Mytown, OH

• Coordinated schedules of four full-time professors
• Maintained office supply and assistant budget
• Created final examination scheduling guidelines for department
• Developed excellent written communication skills
• Familiar with a variety of office machines

1986–1990: Shift Manager, Burger World, Mytown, OH

• Managed 10 employees, including hiring, training, evaluating, and firing
• Developed excellent oral communication skills and team player concept
• Improved inventory supply techniques, reducing losses by 10%
• Maintained cleanliness standards highest in chain
• Developed customer-focused service goals for store

FIGURE 58-7 Chronologic resumé.

Max Bryan
1234 Rolling View Court
Mytown, OH 45431
(937) 555-3137
maxbryan@yahoo.com

OBJECTIVE

• An entry level position in medical assisting, with the opportunity to utilize and refine skills and training

EDUCATION

• 1998: A.S. in Medical Assisting, Community College, Mytown, OH Dean's list senior year, cumulative GPA 3.5

STRENGTHS

• Possess excellent interpersonal and communication skills
• Demonstrate consistent positive attitude and high energy
• Caring and compassionate
• Responsible, self-motivated, precise in work
• Experienced in customer-focused service

ACCOMPLISHMENTS

• Tutored students in medical assisting and 12-lead EKG courses Received excellent evaluations and positive results
• Certified Medical Assistant, active member of local AAMA
• Experienced in MS Office programs
• Consistent "excellent" ratings in clinical externships

COMMUNITY ACTIVITIES

• 1995–present: Organized, recruited, and trained 20 others for church hand bell choir, direct weekly practices and monthly performances
• 1996–present: Teach community CPR twice yearly to high school students
• Vice-President Student Government, Community College, Mytown, OH. Recruited members, organized fund-raisers, campaigned successfully for policy changes

EMPLOYMENT

• 1996–present: Tutor, Community College, Mytown, OH
• Waiter, Scott's Place, Mytown, OH

FIGURE 58-8 Functional resumé.

suggested, such as a cell phone number and a home phone number, so that an office manager has a better chance of reaching the candidate to schedule an interview. Place an e-mail address on the front page so that potential employers can make contact quickly. Make sure the e-mail address is professional; do not use something like "babydoll@yahoo.com." If an interview time becomes available late in the day, having access to job candidates by e-mail may make a difference in who is scheduled and who ultimately gets the job.

Argument about Length

Professionals disagree about the acceptable length of a resumé. One page may be considered the ideal length, but a person who has worked for 10 years will never get all his or her skills and experience on a single page. A medical assistant without previous work experience may easily fit the resumé on one page.

Recent trends indicate that a good rule of thumb is to allow one page for every 6 years of experience. If a person has a 20-year career, the resumé would be approximately three pages long. This is a general guideline; the document should be as **succinct** as possible while clearly communicating the applicant's strengths and background. Make sure your contact information, such as name, phone number, and an e-mail address, are also provided on each subsequent page of the resumé. If the front page or cover letter is somehow

misplaced, the employer will be able to use the information at the top of the page to contact the applicant. Number the pages if the resumé is longer than one page.

Purpose of a Resumé

The purpose of a resumé is not to get the medical assistant a job, although this is a commonly held belief. The purpose of the cover letter is to get the employer to look at the resumé. The purpose of the resumé is to get the applicant an interview. The purpose of the interview, of course, is to get the job. Remember this and use the resumé as a tool, along with other strategies for job searching.

The medical assistant should be the one who writes the resumé, or at the very least should have a hand in its composition. Professional resumé services may be helpful, but the person who knows the most about the experience and education gained is the medical assistant.

Roscoe Patterson
3472 Vienna Woods Lane
Mytown, OH 45449
(937) 555-8874
rpatt@aol.com

Job Target:

• A long-term medical assistant position in a busy and varied medical office

Education:

• 1992: BA in Art History, State University, Mytown, OH
• 1998: AS in Medical Assisting, Community College, Mytown, OH

Capabilities:

• Excellent interpersonal skills and caring attitude
• Detail oriented, with strong analytical and problem-solving abilities
• Utilize solid organizational and time-management abilities in coordinating multiple projects
• Self-starter, take initiative to ensure jobs get done properly and efficiently
• Upbeat, personable, and highly energetic
• Ability to communicate in Spanish and American Sign Language

Accomplishments/Achievements:

• Campaigned for and raised consistent 15% annual increase in contributions and grants, allowing expansion of exhibits and needed renovations to art museum
• Maintained museum budget with 100% accountability
• Organized annual "Art Ball" for 100 contributors under budget
• Museum employee of the year 1995
• Certificates in CPR and EKG; Certified Nursing Assistant; will sit for CMA exam this November

Work History:

• 1998–present: Certified Nursing Assistant, Friendly Nursing Home, Mytown, OH
• 1992–1998: Assistant to the Curator, Mytown Museum of Art, Mytown, OH

FIGURE 58-9 Targeted resumé.

USEFUL ACTION WORDS

Accelerated	Manage
Actively	Motivated
Adapted	Organized
Administered	Originate
Analyze	Participated
Approve	Perform
Completed	Pinpointed
Conceived conduct	Plan
Control	Proficient
Coordinate	Program
Created	Proposed
Delegate	Proved
Demonstrate	Provide
Develop	Recommended
Direct	Reduced
Effect	Reinforced
Eliminated	Reorganized
Established	Responsibilities
Evaluate	Revamped
Expanded	Review
Expedite	Revise
Founded	Schedule
Generated	Significantly
Implemented	Simplify
Improved	Solve
Increased	Strategy
Influence	Streamline
Interpret	Structure
Launched	Successfully
Lead	Supervise
Lecture	Support
Maintain	Teach

FIGURE 58-10 Use action words when describing your skills on the resumé.

CRITICAL THINKING APPLICATION 58-7

Lisa has been asked by a potential employer to e-mail her resumé. She has used an unusual font on her cover letter and on the top of the resumé.

■ What concerns should Lisa have about e-mailing the document?

■ How can Lisa make sure her document arrives in a readable format?

■ How can she ensure that it will look exactly as she designed it when it is opened?

COVER LETTER

When sending a resumé, always include a cover letter (Figure 58-11). This is the introduction to the resumé and the person sending the document. A cover letter should always be sent to an individual, not to the facility or "to whom it may concern." The name of the person to whom the resumé should be sent usually can be obtained with a simple phone call. Ask for the name of the office manager, or, if this information is not obtained, address the cover letter specifically to the physician.

The purpose of the cover letter is to gain attention. Many potential employers schedule an interview with an individual based strictly on the content of the cover letter. Some are general letters that provide basic information without targeting the requirements of a specific job. An executive briefing, as described by Martin Yate in his book *Cover Letters That Knock 'Em Dead*, is a variation on the traditional cover letter. It provides a comprehensive picture of a thorough professional, plus a personalized, fast, and easy to read synopsis that details exactly how the applicant meets the major job requirements. This type of cover letter is extremely effective, but the applicant must have some idea of the job requirements in advance. To produce a dynamic executive briefing, the medical assistant should choose the most important qualifications listed in the ad for the job and then explain how he or she fits those qualifications (Figure 58-12).

Remember, direct supervisors are not always the first recipient of the resumé, so the impression made by the cover letter may make the difference in getting to the next step in the hiring process. Make it easy for screeners to find the strengths that match the job description. The cover letter should be brief but interesting. Use the same paper stock weight and color as the resumé. Be sure to include

Brutis Walter
2345 Morrow Court
Mytown, OH 45310
(937) 555-7426

May 23, 1998

Andrea Foreman, CMA
Office Manager
Family Health, Inc.
123 Timberleaf Drive
Mytown, OH 45432

Ms. Foreman:

I will be graduating from Community College with an A.S. in Medical Assisting on June 9 and am interested in an entry-level medical assistant position in your office. I will consider part-time or temporary work to gain experience in a diverse office such as yours.

My training includes hands-on experience in pediatrics, cardiology, internal medicine, obstetrics, and geriatrics. My administrative training would allow me to fill in wherever needed in the office. I am highly motivated and have supported myself and paid my own way through college. I understand responsibility and am a true team player. Belinda Mallet, RN, a fellow church member, told me the office will be short-staffed this summer owing to vacations and a maternity leave. I believe I could help your office run smoothly this summer, and beyond.

I look forward to hearing from you. I am available Tuesday and Thursday afternoons and Friday mornings until graduation. I will call you next Tuesday to set up an appointment for an interview.
Thank you for your consideration.

Very truly yours,

Brutis Walter

FIGURE 58-11 Basic cover letter.

contact information, such as an address and at least two phone numbers, even if these are on the attached resume. The supervisor may separate the two documents, so each one must include a method of contact. Never start a cover letter with the sentence, "I saw your ad in the newspaper" or a similar phrase. Be creative with the opening line and try to capture the reader's attention.

A cover letter should be one to three paragraphs long. The final section should include a call to action that prompts an interview. If the document concludes with a request for a meeting, the medical assistant should state when he or she will call for a time and date.

▍JOB APPLICATIONS

Many facilities require a job application along with a resumé (Figure 58-13). Arrive 15 minutes before the scheduled interview to allow time to fill out an application.

A job application can be considered a legal document if the person is hired; therefore, it should be filled out neatly, correctly, and completely (Procedure 58-3). Always read the application before filling it out, so that directions make sense and information is not placed in the wrong area of the form. Carry a planner or address book to the interview so that former employers' and supervisors' names, addresses, and phone numbers are handy. The medical

EXECUTIVE BRIEFING

Allison Aubrey, R.M.A.
3040 Wood Branch Drive
Austin, Texas 78716
512-434-9902

James Richardson, M.D.
Family Practice Clinic
5508 Lamar Blvd.
Austin, Texas 78752

Dear Dr. Richardson:

Although my attached resume will provide you with a general outline of my work history, my problem-solving abilities, and some of my achievements, it may take longer than a few moments to peruse. For your convenience, I have listed your specified requirements for the medical assistant position at the Lakewood office below, and the skills I have developed that match those specifications. I hope this briefing will allow you to quickly determine my eligibility for the position and will prompt you to contact me for an interview.

Your Requirements:	My Skills:
1. Two years' experience as a medical assistant.	1. Three years' experience as a registered medical assistant.
2. Ability to work with a larger supervisory team in planning, budgeting, and policy formulating.	2. Experience as employee council president, intricately involved in planning and budgeting.
3. Familiarity with HIPAA regulations.	3. Trained in HIPAA compliance and received three certificates for continuing education related to HIPAA compliance.
4. Ability to work with others as a team.	4. Awarded "Employee of the Quarter" honors twice during past year, and nominated for "Employee of the Year" by my coworkers.

I know that my experience and abilities will be of benefit to your organization. I look forward to discussing my qualifications and your requirements in person. I am confident that we can develop an exceptional working relationship and that I am the right individual for your organization. I will telephone you on Monday to arrange an interview to take place at your convenience.

Sincerely yours,

Allison Aubrey, R.M.A.

FIGURE 58-12 Executive briefing.

assistant should not have to ask for a phone book to get an address. Have all of this information ready when it is needed.

Applications often ask for a date when the medical assistant would be available for work. Be careful with this question. If the applicant currently has a job, yet writes that he or she is "immediately available," it may indicate that the applicant intends to quit without notice. On the other hand, the current employer may be aware that the person is seeking other employment and may have granted him or her permission to quit immediately once a new job is found.

Be careful on the sections that ask the reason for leaving former positions. Think about the answers to be listed in those spaces and try to put the information in as positive a light as possible. Ask the

APPLICATION FOR POSITION / Medical or Dental Office
AN EQUAL OPPORTUNITY EMPLOYER

No employee, applicant, or candidate for promotion, training or other advantage shall be discriminated against (or given preference) because of race, color, religion, sex, age, physical handicap, veteran status, or national origin.

(In answering questions, use extra blank sheet if necessary)

Date of Application

PLEASE READ CAREFULLY AND WRITE OR PRINT ANSWERS TO ALL QUESTIONS. DO NOT TYPE.

A. PERSONAL INFORMATION

Name - Last First Middle	Social Security No.	Area Code/Phone No. ( )
Present Address: - Street (Apt #) City State Zip		How Long At This Address?:
Previous Address: - Street City State Zip From: To:	Person to notify in case of Emergency or Accident - Name: Address: Telephone:	

B. EMPLOYMENT INFORMATION

For What Position Are You Applying?:	☐ Full-Time ☐ Part-Time ☐ Either	Date Available For Employment?:	Wage/Salary Expectations:
List Hrs./Days You Prefer To Work	List Any Hrs./Days You Are Not Available: (Except for times required for religious practices or observances)		Can You Work Overtime, If Necessary? ☐ Yes ☐ No
Are You Employed Now?: ☐ Yes ☐ No	If So, May We Inquire Of Your Present Employer?: ☐ No ☐ Yes, If Yes: Name Of Employer: Phone Number: ( )		
Have You Ever Been Bonded? ☐ Yes ☐ No	If Required For Position, Are You Bondable? ☐ Yes ☐ No ☐ Uncertain	Have You Applied For A Position With This Office Before? ☐ No ☐ Yes If Yes, When?:	
Referred By / Or Where Did You Learn Of This Job?:			
Can You, Upon Employment, Submit Verification Of Your Legal Right To Work In The United States?: ☐ Yes ☐ No Submit Proof That You Meet Legal Age Requirement For Employment? ☐ Yes ☐ No		Language(s) Applicant Speaks or Writes (If Use Of A Language Other Than English Is Relevant To The Job For Which The Applicant Is Applying:	

C. EDUCATIONAL HISTORY

Name & Address Of Schools Attended (Include Current)	Dates From	Dates Thru	Highest Grade/Level Completed	Diploma/Degree(s) Obtained/Areas of Study
High School				
College				Degree/Major
Post Graduate				Degree/Major
Other				Course/Diploma/License/ Certificate
Specific Training, Education, Or Experiences Which Will Assist You In The Job For Which You Have Applied.				
Future Educational Plans				

D. SPECIAL SKILLS

CHECK BELOW THE KINDS OF WORK YOU HAVE DONE:		☐ MEDICAL INSURANCE FORMS	☐ RECEPTIONIST
☐ BLOOD COUNTS	☐ DENTAL ASSISTANT	☐ MEDICAL TERMINOLOGY	☐ TELEPHONES
☐ BOOKKEEPING	☐ DENTAL HYGIENIST	☐ MEDICAL TRANSCRIPTION	☐ TYPING
☐ COLLECTIONS	☐ FILING	☐ NURSING	☐ STENOGRAPHY
☐ COMPOSING LETTERS	☐ INJECTIONS	☐ PHLEBOTOMY (Draw Blood)	☐ URINALYSIS
☐ COMPUTER INPUT	☐ INSTRUMENT STERILIZATION	☐ POSTING	☐ X-RAY
OFFICE EQUIPMENT USED: ☐ COMPUTER	☐ DICTATING EQUIPMENT	☐ WORD PROCESSOR	☐ OTHER:
Other Kinds Of Tasks Performed Or Skills That May Be Applicable To Position:		Typing Speed	Shorthand Speed

ORDER # 72-110 • © 1976 BIBBERO SYSTEMS, INC. • PETALUMA, CA. • (REV. 1/95)
TO REORDER CALL TOLL FREE: (800) BIBBERO (800-242-2376) OR FAX (800) 242-9330 MFG IN U.S.A.

(PLEASE COMPLETE OTHER SIDE)

FIGURE 58-13 Application for employment. (Courtesy Bibbero Systems, Petaluma, Calif.)

Continued

E. EMPLOYMENT RECORD

LIST MOST RECENT EMPLOYMENT FIRST   May We Contact Your Previous Employer(s) For A Reference? ☐ Yes ☐ No

1) Employer   Work Performed. Be Specific:

Address   Street   City   State   Zip Code

Phone Number
(   )

Type of Business   Dates   Mo. | Yr.   Mo. | Yr.
                          From   To

Your Position   Hourly Rate/Salary
                          Starting   Final

Supervisor's Name

Reason For Leaving

2) Employer   Worked Performed. Be Specific:

Address   Street   City   State   Zip Code

Phone Number
(   )

Type of Business   Dates   Mo. | Yr.   Mo. | Yr.
                          From   To

Your Position   Hourly Rate/Salary
                          Starting   Final

Supervisor's Name

Reason For Leaving

3) Employer   Worked Performed. Be Specific:

Address   Street   City   State   Zip Code

Phone Number
(   )

Type of Business   Dates   Mo. | Yr.   Mo. | Yr.
                          From   To

Your Position   Hourly Rate/Salary
                          Starting   Final

Supervisor's Name

Reason For Leaving

F. REFERENCES — FRIENDS / ACQUAINTANCES NON-RELATED

(1) _____
    Name   Address   Telephone Number   (☐ Work ☐ Home)   Occupation   Years Acquainted

(1) _____
    Name   Address   Telephone Number   (☐ Work ☐ Home)   Occupation   Years Acquainted

Please Feel Free To Add Any Information Which You Feel Will Help Us Consider You For Employment

READ THE FOLLOWING CAREFULLY, THEN SIGN AND DATE THE APPLICATION

"I certify that all answers given by me on this application are true, correct and complete to the best of my knowledge. I acknowledge notice that the information contained in this application is subject to check. I agree that, if hired, my continued employment may be contingent upon the accuracy of that information. If employed, I further agree to comply with Company/Office rules and regulations."

Signature: _____   Date: _____

FIGURE 58-13, cont'd

PROCEDURE 58-3

Complete a Job Application

GOAL: *To complete an accurate, detailed job application legibly so as to secure a job offer.*

EQUIPMENT and SUPPLIES

- Record of a job lead form
- Record of an interview form
- Copies of your resumé
- Contact information for former employers and references
- Contact information for friends and family

PROCEDURAL STEPS

1. Read the entire job application before completing any part of the document.
   <u>PURPOSE:</u> Reading through the entire application helps prevent errors while filling out the document.

2. Gather any information that may be necessary to answer all questions on the application.
   <u>PURPOSE:</u> The candidate should have all information available for completing a job application.

3. Begin to complete the application legibly.
   <u>PURPOSE:</u> The interviewer evaluates the candidate's handwriting to make sure it would be legible on medical records.

4. Answer each question on the document or write "not applicable."

5. Do not leave any space blank.
   <u>PURPOSE:</u> Leaving a space blank on the application may suggest that the candidate did not want to answer a certain question or accidentally overlooked it. By writing "not applicable" on such questions, the candidate demonstrates competence and attention to detail.

6. Do not write "see resumé" anywhere on the document.
   <u>PURPOSE:</u> Many supervisors view this practice as laziness. Always fill out the job application completely and do not leave blank spaces.

7. Be completely honest about every fact written on the document.

8. Include information on the resumé that exhibits dependability, punctuality, positive work ethics, initiative, the ability to adapt to change, and a responsible attitude.

9. Sign the document and date it.

10. Proofread the document and make sure none of the information conflicts with the resumé.
    <u>PURPOSE:</u> Proofreading helps the candidate to catch any errors before submitting the application.

11. Submit the application.

---

advice of your placement counselor if you are unsure what to say in these sections.

If there are sections available for listing special skills and qualifications, fill them out fully. Describe cardiopulmonary resuscitation (CPR) and first aid certifications and any professional organizations of which you are a member. If references are requested, list the name, title, employer, and a means of contact. Be sure to get permission before using someone as a reference.

One of the most common mistakes on job applications is writing "see resumé." This is an indication of laziness and must be avoided. Even if the same information is found on the resumé, the application must be completed in its entirety. If the exact information is not included on the job application, that legal document is incomplete. In addition, most job applications include a disclaimer that if a false or incomplete statement is made on the application, the individual can be dismissed from any position for which he or she was hired. So make sure all the information given is accurate.

JOB INTERVIEW

A medical assistant may interview with the office manager, the physician, or both, and other staff members may be brought in for part of the interview. This is especially true in offices with a cohesive team of employees.

The interview usually is the most stressful of the job search steps. Some individuals dread job interviews and become extremely nervous at the prospect of interviewing. Others are very comfortable and consider the interview as much for their own purposes as for the employer's. Either way, the more interviews the medical assistant has, the more comfortable he or she will be with each subsequent interview.

An interview has four phases: preparation for the interview, the interview itself, the follow-up, and the negotiation.

Preparation for the Interview

When preparing for an interview, the medical assistant should learn everything possible about the employer. Look on the Internet for information about the facility. Practice answering possible interview questions. Prepare an outfit to wear to interviews. It is wise to drive to the interview site on a day preceding the interview date if the location is unfamiliar to avoid getting lost on the day of the important event. The better prepared the medical assistant is, the more comfortable he or she will be while interviewing.

The critical part of the interview is the medical assistant's ability to present himself or herself as the best candidate for the job. By preparing to answer interview questions before the interview, the medical assistant will be much more prepared. Although no one can guess exactly what questions will be asked, some standard interview questions are very common (Figure 58-14). Review these questions thoroughly, answer them in writing, then study them before the interview. Then when the medical assistant is asked, "What are your three greatest strengths?" he or she can confidently answer, "I am professional, reliable, and honest."

When preparing on the day of the interview, be conservative with wardrobe choices. For women a skirt and blouse or business suit is appropriate. For men a business suit is the best choice. Depending

TOP 100 INTERVIEW QUESTIONS

1. Tell me about yourself.
2. Why do you want to work for this company?
3. Why should I hire you?
4. How do you work under pressure?
5. What type of job or salary do you expect to make in 5 years?
6. How do you handle criticism?
7. What do you think your co-workers think about you?
8. What is your opinion of the company you last worked for?
9. Describe your last supervisor.
10. What is your view of management?
11. What would you like to change about yourself and how would you do it?
12. What is your best asset?
13. What adjectives would you use to describe yourself?
14. What aspects of your life are you most happy with?
15. How would you describe the perfect job?
16. Why did you leave your last job?
17. Why did you choose this type of profession?
18. What salary do you expect?
19. What are your strongest and weakest personal qualities?
20. What motivates you?
21. What have you learned from some of your previous jobs?
22. What personal characteristics are necessary for success in your chosen field?
23. What do you know about this facility and our competitors?
24. What were your major courses of study in school?
25. Do you plan to continue your education?
26. Did school meet your expectations or were you disappointed?
27. How did you pay for your education?
28. Sell this pen to me.
29. To what extent do your grades reflect how much you have learned?
30. Do you feel your education was worthwhile?
31. What were the major responsibilities of your last job?
32. What has been your most rewarding experience at work?
33. What was your single most important accomplishment for the company on your last job?
34. What was the toughest problem you have ever solved and how did you do it?
35. How do you see yourself fitting in with our company?
36. What skills did you learn on your last job that can be used here?
37. What would you do if you were fired in two years?
38. What kinds of additional education do you think you need to meet your career goals?
39. How long do you plan to stay with our company?
40. What immediate contribution could you make if you came to work for us today?
41. Do you feel that you have received good general training?
42. If you were starting school all over again, what courses would you take?
43. How much money do you hope to earn in 5 years? 10 years?
44. Do you think that your extracurricular activities were worth the time spent?
45. Are you interested in making money or do you have other reasons for entering this career field?
46. Do you prefer working with others or by yourself?
47. Can you take instructions or criticism without being upset?
48. Tell me a story.
49. What do you know about the opportunities in the field in which you are trained?
50. How long do you expect to work?
51. Have you ever had any difficulty in getting along with a co-worker, classmate, or instructor?
52. Which of your school years was most difficult?
53. Do you like routine work?
54. Define cooperation.
55. Will you fight to get ahead?
56. Do you have an analytical mind?
57. Are you willing to go where the company sends you?
58. What job in this company would you choose if you could?
59. Do you think that employers should consider grades?
60. What have you done that shows initiative and willingness to work?
61. What benefits did you receive from your last employer?
62. What has been your most important accomplishment during your school years?
63. Have you ever helped to reduce operating costs, and how?
64. Have you ever developed or helped develop any programs, and how did you do this?
65. What do you think determines a person's progress in a company?
66. What would you do if a personal problem interfered with your work?
67. What would you do if you became bored with your job?
68. What would you do if you had a personality clash with a supervisor?
69. How will you be getting to work each day?
70. Do you have reliable transportation?
71. How do you feel about working with someone who is HIV positive?
72. What person has most influenced your life?
73. What is the last book you read?
74. Who do you most admire?
75. Who is your favorite relative?
76. What will previous supervisors say about you?
77. What makes a good supervisor?
78. Why would you be successful in this job?
79. Why have you held so many jobs?
80. Can you explain this gap in your employment history?
81. Have you ever been fired from a position?
82. Do you have adequate child care arrangements that will allow you to be at work when scheduled?
83. What is your philosophy of life?
84. How many other positions are you considering?
85. Why were your grades in school so low?
86. Are you a member of any professional organizations?
87. How old were you when you began to support yourself?
88. Do you participate in continuing education activities or seminars?
89. Have you had the hepatitis B injection series?
90. Where did you perform your externship?
91. How many days of school did you miss?
92. Why did you decide to attend the college/school you attended?
93. What kind of boss do you prefer?
94. How do you usually spend your weekends?
95. Why types of people seem to rub you the wrong way?
96. What planning procedures do you use?
97. What frustrates you about your current job?
98. What is unique about you?
99. What have you done that indicates you are qualified for this job?
100. Do you have any questions?

FIGURE 58-14 Top 100 interview questions.

on the office situation, one may be given very specific instructions on wardrobe. Some office managers or physicians even tell the potential employee to arrive in jeans. Is this a test? The physician may be curious as to whether the medical assistant can follow directions and actually wear jeans. Obtain a hint about clothing by visiting the office before the interview, even if it is just to ask for directions. That way, the potential employee can see what the office staff members are wearing. A similar wardrobe should be sufficient for an interview. If the staff wears scrubs, then wear neatly pressed scrubs with clean shoes; do not wear the slouchy scrubs one might find in a hospital surgical suite. Conservative business suits should always be acceptable in an interview.

Be sure clothing is fresh, wrinkle free, and well fitting and that shoes are clean and shined. It is a good idea to carry a planner or other method of taking notes during the interview; this makes a good impression and indicates interest in the job. Always arrive 15 minutes early for the interview. Do not wear heavy perfumes or colognes, do not chew gum, and do not wear excessive jewelry. Never take anyone along on a job interview, especially children, even if they are older.

Pay particular attention to other aspects of appearance (Figure 58-15). Make sure your hair is clean and styled attractively, your teeth are clean, and your breath is fresh. Nails are also important and should be clean and well groomed, because the medical assistant should give the interviewer a firm handshake. However, nails should not be excessively long or painted in highly visible colors. Remember the appearance guidelines that applied to the externship; some employers will react negatively to tattoos, extravagant hairstyles, or other excessive wardrobe choices. Always dress appropriately and conservatively for an interview. Once hired, the new employee may be allowed to wear more diverse styles but must comply with the employee handbook or procedure manual. Expect to be a little nervous. Any interview can be a stressful situation. The better prepared the medical assistant is, the more of a success the interview will be.

Take a professional binder to the interview with extra copies of your resume and reference list. Include a list of both former employees and references, as well as the dates of employment, supervisors'

names and their spelling, and any other demographic information that might be needed to accurately complete paperwork (this could also be saved into documents or applications in a smart phone). This will help to avoid the embarrassment of asking to look up an address in a phone book or calling to obtain the information.

Interview

The interviewer should not ask any illegal questions, including those that are related to age, sex, nationality, religion, marital/family status, affiliations/organizations, and disabilities. For instance, the interviewer may ask "Are you legally eligible to work in this country?" However, the interview cannot legally ask "What nationality are you?" If the job involves some travel, the interviewer cannot legally ask "What are your child care arrangements?" However, the interviewer can ask "Can you travel and work overtime if necessary?"

Employers may ask illegal questions, whether intentionally or accidentally, and the way that the medical assistant answers the questions can influence the employer's hiring decision. If the medical assistant is openly offended, then the sometimes abrasive comments that patients make may be offensive as well. If the illegal question is answered, the interviewer may use the information in the answer to weed out the medical assistant as a candidate. The best approach is to politely address the question, either by answering it directly or by redirecting the interviewer back to the job requirements. For example, if the interviewer asks if the candidate plans to put children in day care (which might be a way of determining the age of the dependent children and thus the likelihood of absenteeism due to the children's illnesses), the medical assistant could answer, "I will be able to meet the work schedule and the responsibilities that this job requires." Some questions that might normally be considered illegal, such as "What organizations are you a member of?" might be job related. The employer may be interested in knowing that the medical assistant is a member of various professional organizations, such as the American Association of Medical Assistants or the American Medical Technologists.

During the actual interview, maintain good eye contact. Many supervisors refuse to hire people who seem uncomfortable looking them directly in the eyes. Never take control of the interview. Allow the supervisor to ask questions at his or her own pace. Do not fidget in the chair and observe the interviewer's body language for clues as to how interested he or she might be. Do not volunteer any negative information; be honest and do not exaggerate experience or lengths of employment. Never speak negatively about former employers.

Be careful when answering questions such as, "Tell me about yourself." Most female medical assistants might begin to answer this question with a phrase like, "I'm a recent graduate, and I am married and have two children." The answer to this question should not reflect information about personal issues. Focus all answers on professionalism and the strengths that will be an asset to the medical office.

Remember that the interview is centered on the medical assistant, so freely discuss the skills and attributes that you would bring to the job. The better prepared the medical assistant is, the smoother the interview will go. Be able to prove the skills you claim and explain how they meet the needs of the company or facility. Avoid a "know it all" attitude, which indicates overconfidence and reluctance to take direction. Always express an interest in the employer and his or her

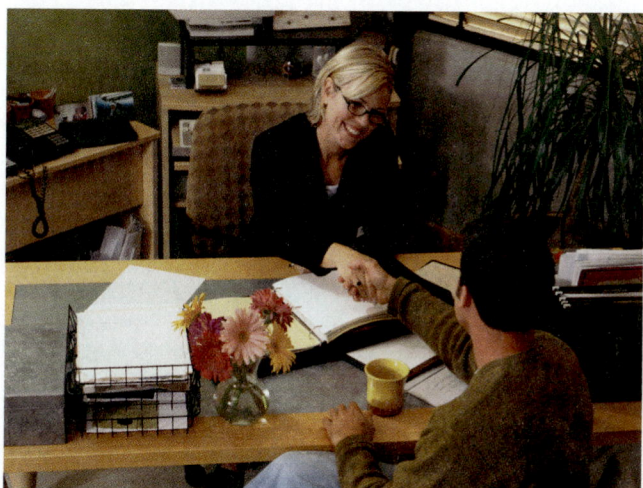

FIGURE 58-15 Present a professional appearance during the job interview and be sure to smile often. (From Yoder-Wise P: *Leading and managing in nursing,* ed 4, 2006, St Louis, Mosby.)

PROCEDURE 58-4

Interview for a Job

GOAL: *To project a professional appearance during a job interview and to be able to express the reasons the medical assistant is the best candidate for the position.*

EQUIPMENT and SUPPLIES

- Record of a job lead form
- Record of an interview form
- Job application
- Copies of your resumé
- Contact information for former employers and references
- Contact information for friends and family
- Sample interview questions

PROCEDURAL STEPS

1. Prepare for the interview by studying sample interview questions and researching basic information about the facility.
   PURPOSE: Employers are impressed by candidates who have researched the company and know some details about its operation.

2. Know all the information on the resumé so that it can be discussed confidently during the interview.

3. Prepare clothing that reflects a professional image for the facility in which the medical assistant is hoping to gain employment.
   PURPOSE: Most medical facilities prefer conservative dress.

4. Gather all materials that might be needed during the interview, such as copies of your resumé, contact information, and copies of earned certificates.
   PURPOSE: All information must be handy and prepared before the interview.

5. Arrive for the interview at least 15 minutes early.
   PURPOSE: Arrive early in case forms must be completed before the interview.

6. Stand and shake hands with the interviewer when he or she appears.
   PURPOSE: A confident, firm handshake is a positive gesture.

7. Listen intently to the interviewer as the position is described and be ready to explain how you fit the requirements for the position.
   PURPOSE: The interviewer evaluates how well the candidate listens and answers questions.

8. Answer all interview questions confidently, smiling when appropriate and displaying a positive, responsible attitude.

9. While answering interview questions, stress dependability, punctuality, positive work ethics, initiative, and the ability to adapt to change.

10. Ask intelligent questions after the interviewer finishes.
    PURPOSE: The questions asked at the end of an interview should indicate an interest in the position and should not focus on how the candidate would benefit from the job, but rather on what the candidate can do for the company.

11. Determine a day and time when the next contact will be made.

12. Express interest in the position.
    PURPOSE: Employers expect some type of confirmation that the candidate is interested in the job.

13. Send a thank you note or letter to the interviewer within 24 hours of the interview.
    PURPOSE: A thank you note is impressive and reinforces the candidate's interest in the position.

14. Follow up as appropriate on the interview.

projects, rather than in what the employer can do for the employee. Ask intelligent questions at the end of the interview if given the opportunity. Never let your first question be, "How much will I be paid?" Money, although important, cannot appear to be your primary concern.

Before the interview ends, the medical assistant should ask when a decision will be made and if it would be acceptable to call to follow up (Procedure 58-4).

CRITICAL THINKING APPLICATION   58-8

Lisa is enjoying a good interview when the interviewer, a male supervisor, asks her if she is married. When Lisa replies that she is not, he asks if she has a steady boyfriend.

- What might the supervisor's motive be with this line of questioning?
- How should Lisa respond?
- Are these questions inappropriate or do they serve a purpose?

▌Follow-Up after the Interview

Follow-up is critical after an interview. Always send a written thank you note or letter to the person who conducted the interview. Many employers wait to see who sends a thank you letter before making the final hiring decision. Limit follow-up calls to one or two a week. Most employers give an indication of when the hiring decision will be made. The company should notify all those who interviewed once a decision has been made, unless specific protocols were set during the interview about follow-up. For instance, if the office manager says a decision will be made on Friday and the final three candidates will be called for a second interview, the medical assistant knows if a call is not received to continue the job search. Although not all companies provide this type of notification, it is considered professional etiquette to tell the candidates who interviewed for the job if they are no longer under consideration. Never place all your hope in one job; continue to prospect and interview until an offer is made and accepted. In addition, always be on the watch for the next job opportunity.

REASONS PEOPLE DO NOT GET HIRED

The following is a ranked list of reasons interviewers do not hire job candidates. The list was compiled from the results of a nationwide survey of 153 companies performed by Northcentral Technical College, Wausau, Wisconsin.

1. Poor personal appearance
2. Lack of interest or enthusiasm
3. Overemphasis on money
4. Poor voice, diction, grammar
5. Lack of planning
6. No purpose or goals
7. Condemnation of past employers
8. Poor eye contact
9. "Limp fish" handshake
10. Late to interview
11. Lack of tact
12. Lack of maturity
13. Lack of courtesy
14. Asking no questions
15. Overbearing, "know-it-all" attitude
16. Lack of confidence and poise
17. Failure to participate in activities
18. Making excuses, evading unfavorable factors on record
19. Indecisiveness
20. Just shopping around
21. No interest in company
22. Sloppy application form
23. Wanting a job for a short time
24. Unwillingness to relocate
25. Cynical attitude
26. Low moral standards
27. Laziness
28. Intolerance or strong prejudices
29. No sense of humor
30. Narrow interests
31. Inability to take criticism
32. No appreciation of the value of experience
33. Radical ideas
34. Too aggressive during interview

Negotiation

The negotiation stage of job acceptance can be as stressful as the actual interviews. A medical assistant should know the lowest salary he or she can afford and should ask for a little more than that figure. Bracket salary requests: instead of asking for $13 per hour, ask for a salary in the "mid to high twenties." Let the employer mention a figure first or a range of salary. Usually the person who mentions a salary range first has the disadvantage. If the medical assistant requests $13 per hour and the facility was willing to pay $16 per hour, the medical assistant probably will get $13.

Never say "no" to a job offer on the spot. Request at least 24 hours to consider the offer (Procedure 58-5). A medical assistant should not let the salary amount be the main factor in the decision whether to accept a position. Before accepting or rejecting a job offer, consider whether the position carries any authority, the benefits, the hours, the distance from home, and the potential for advancement. People accept jobs for reasons other than the salary; remember the value of experience.

YOU GOT THE JOB!

Once the job offer has been made and accepted, a start date will be determined. Before the first day, use the computer to map several ways to get to work. If you are unsure of the traffic flow, leave home extra early the first day so that you are guaranteed to arrive on time.

Most employees are placed on a 30- to 90-day probationary period, during which employment may be terminated for unsatisfactory performance. The probationary period also provides the employer and employee an opportunity to learn about each other. The medical assistant will interact with other co-workers, patients, and providers. A new medical assistant should volunteer to help others and efficiently complete the duties assigned. Use the probationary period as a testing ground, carefully observing ways in which the office might run in a smoother manner. However, do not make numerous suggestions for change during this period. Discover why certain methods are used and make an effort to fit in with the rest of the team before suggesting that the office routine be changed. Remember, the people at the office may have been employed for a substantially longer time and may resent suggestions from a new staff member. Learn the office rhythms, procedures, and culture first and demonstrate a team-oriented attitude. After new employees prove their responsibility and good attitude, other staff members will be open to suggestions about improvements for the office.

Common Early Mistakes

Some medical assistants make mistakes early on a new job. Never be disruptive to the office by gossiping or complaining. A medical assistant must realize that procedures may be performed in many different ways and that the way he or she was taught in school probably is not the only correct way. Be open to learning new ideas, concepts, and procedures. Although some mistakes are to be expected, make sure that once a mistake has been pointed out, it is corrected. Do not make the same mistakes over and over.

Supervisors may work closely with the medical assistants. Some expect medical assistants to carry out orders on their own. Do not make too much supervision necessary or force the office manager to constantly check the work you have done. Finish all assigned duties in a timely manner and avoid procrastination. When significant problems arise, discuss them openly with the supervisor and attempt to find a quick resolution. Limit absences and tardy days to a minimum and miss work only when absolutely necessary, especially during the probationary period.

Being a Good Employee

A medical assistant can be a better employee in several ways. First and foremost, arrive 15 minutes before the scheduled shift and do not leave early. Even the best medical assistant cannot benefit an

PROCEDURE 58-5

Negotiate a Salary

GOAL: *To develop negotiation skills that will help the medical assistant obtain the salary and benefits he or she requires.*

EQUIPMENT and SUPPLIES

- Record of a job lead form
- Record of an interview form
- Information about job offers received
- Contact name at medical facility

PROCEDURAL STEPS

1. Study the job offer at hand.
2. Determine whether the offer is sufficient as it stands.
3. Make a list of what additional salary requirements and/or benefits are needed at a minimum.
   PURPOSE: Know the minimum salary and benefits you can accept when evaluating a job offer.
4. Arrive at the second or subsequent interview appointment to discuss the job with the hiring supervisor.
5. Thank the supervisor for the offer that has been presented and express interest in the position.
6. Express the additional salary and/or benefits desired.
   PURPOSE: The candidate should be able to express what he or she needs with regard to salary and benefits.
7. Discuss whether the facility would be willing to increase the offer to match your desires.
8. Express valid reasons that explain why the additional benefits should be offered, based on past performance, experience, or other valid factors.
9. Discuss reasonable compromises regarding the additional salary and/or benefits.
   PURPOSE: The ability to compromise is a valuable employee trait.
10. Ask what level of performance is expected for salary and/or benefits to be increased.
11. Be courteous and diplomatic during all negotiations.
12. Express interest in and promise serious consideration of the position.
13. Determine the next contact time with the supervisor.
14. Weigh the offer and compromises to make a good decision about the job offer.

---

office if he or she does not come to work. Be honest and demonstrate trustworthiness and professionalism. Get along with co-workers in the facility. A medical assistant should be able to resolve simple problems with others easily without involving the supervisor. Reflect a friendly attitude toward others, even if they are difficult to get along with. Arrive every single day ready to learn. The medical assistant's education does not end on graduation from school. The medical field is one of constant change, and those who work in it must learn and change along with it.

A medical assistant should constantly be performing assigned duties and should not expect frequent breaks in the medical office. Most offices are fast paced, and the supervisor expects the medical assistant to keep up with the activity. Even during slow periods, there is always a counter to clean or filing to do. Be supportive of the leadership in the facility and ask for more responsibility if necessary. Take the initiative to perform duties that are cumbersome or repetitive and get them done quickly.

Always treat patients with compassion. Remember that they are not always at their best when ill, so be kind and courteous to them and their families. The patients are the reason the facility exists. Treat them with great respect and care.

Remember that medical assistants can be held individually responsible for their actions even though they work as an agent of the physician-employer. Although the physician is usually the person against whom professional liability lawsuits are brought, the medical assistant can still be named in a lawsuit. For this reason, it is wise to carry individual professional liability coverage once employed in the medical industry. The coverage should be maintained throughout the medical assistant's career.

CRITICAL THINKING APPLICATION   58-9

On Lisa's second day at the externship site, she clearly sees a co-worker taking and using a controlled drug from the storage area.

- What should Lisa do?
- What potential problems arise with this situation?
- To whom should Lisa report this incident, if anyone?

Dealing with Supervisors

Supervisors appreciate employees who come to them when they have questions, but who are able to handle minor decisions on their own. Never hesitate to approach supervisors when an issue at hand needs their attention. Do not allow a situation to go unaddressed and then say, "I didn't want to bother you with that." The office manager is responsible for dealing with difficult issues, and these should be handled immediately when they arise.

A medical assistant should never attempt to cover up a mistake; admitting the error is a much better approach to solving the problem. When talking with the supervisor, do not hesitate to speak and do not avoid the subject. State the problem clearly and explain what routes are available to **rectify** the situation. Work with the supervisor to resolve issues and accept the advice given with a positive attitude.

Performance Appraisals

Performance appraisals usually are done after the initial probationary period and annually thereafter. The performance appraisal is designed to inform the employee of his or her strengths and weaknesses on the job, according to the supervisor's point of view. Most of these appraisals offer a scale to rate the employee's performance, such as 1 to 5. Do not expect to receive a perfect appraisal, because employees are seldom perfect in all aspects of their jobs. If the supervisor gives perfect scores to an employee, there is no room for growth or improvement. It is the rare employee who completes all duties and meets every expectation without any errors.

When asked to sit down with your supervisor for a performance appraisal, expect to address areas that need improvement. Ask questions and work with the supervisor to improve in the areas that may need more effort or a different approach.

If the employee strongly disagrees with any area of the performance appraisal, he or she should discuss this with the supervisor. There may have been a misunderstanding as to the duties involved. Clarify this calmly and patiently and strive to do better next time.

Asking for a Raise

Most facilities have some type of schedule for pay increases. Some offer a cost of living increase on an annual basis; others use a merit system, offering raises only when earned and deserved based on performance.

There may come a time when the medical assistant feels the need to ask for a raise. Before doing so, a little self-reflection is important to determine whether a raise is in order. Has attendance been exemplary? How many times was the medical assistant tardy? Does he or she work well with little supervision? Has he or she performed all the expected duties well and in a timely manner?

Approach the supervisor at a relatively calm part of the day and ask how a salary raise might be earned in the near future. Do not expect a raise of more than 3% to 5% at any given time, unless the employee is promoted to another position or given additional duties. If the supervisor is unable to grant a raise, determine whether the reasons are valid. If they are not, the medical assistant may want to pursue other employment options. The medical assistant will find that finding a job is always easier if one already has a job, so do not quit outright unless the work environment is **intolerable**. Begin networking again and discover the options available.

Leaving a Job

Always offer at least 2 weeks' notice when resigning from a job. Prepare a written notice of resignation and take it to the supervisor in person. Do not just leave it on a desk or place it in the interoffice mail.

Resigning from a job just as an attempt to get a salary increase is a dangerous practice. Once the employer doubts the employee's loyalty, the future usually is not bright for the employee at that facility. Resign only after a final decision has been made. If the medical assistant is resigning to take another position, the current employer may be expected to make a **counteroffer**. However, be wary about accepting counteroffers. What led you to look for a new job in the first place? Has the situation been resolved? Ask yourself these questions before agreeing to stay with the current employer. Often employees who accept a counteroffer and stay at their original job find that few changes are made, and the employee ends up leaving the position in the long run.

LIFE SKILLS

To be successful in the job search, the medical assistant must have the basic entry-level skills needed to perform in the workplace. Even more important, he or she must develop certain life skills that are essential to excel in any profession. If these skills are not developed and refined, the medical assistant may find fewer opportunities and advancements available, as well as less impressive salaries and benefits. Perhaps even more important, the medical assistant who does not have his or her personal life in order will not be able to offer their employer their best performance every day. He or she will be expected to give a full day's work for a full day's pay on every single shift. Although personal issues do affect work performance, the medical assistant must make a good effort to put personal problems aside when working.

The most important life skill one can have is the willingness to change. Many employees insist on doing things the same way they have always been done, and they resist any changes in policy or procedure. However, a medical assistant who does not welcome and work hard to adjust to change is a failure waiting to happen.

Personal Growth

Personal growth is a comprehensive term that applies to many aspects of a person's mental, physical, and spiritual health. This growth is a result of goals that are set for self-improvement. Without clear goals, people rarely experience personal growth that is initiated from within. Growth may happen as a result of some outside influence, but a conscious effort toward personal growth is an innate decision.

No matter how great the training or how many opportunities are placed in front of a person, fear and doubt can sabotage efforts to improve the self-image, confidence, and future potential of an individual. Personal growth involves such traits as self-control, self-esteem, problem-solving skills, decision-making skills, and stress management.

Self-Control

Self-control is a vital trait in the medical office. Some patients are not at their best because of their illness, and this may make them less than cordial toward the staff. Remember that this is usually a temporary situation. A medical assistant must exercise self-control and must not respond in kind to patients who are disagreeable.

Self-control is important in other areas of the medical office. Never remove drugs from the storage areas without permission and be careful when dealing with petty cash. A medical assistant must get enough rest during the work week that he or she can care for the patients in an enthusiastic manner.

Self-Esteem

Everyone has certain strengths and weaknesses. Good self-esteem is the result of knowing what those strengths are and overcoming the weaknesses. It is having a positive outlook about oneself and others. A person with good self-esteem is motivated, able to express love, and capable of handling criticism. A person's self-esteem improves if he or she has developed adaptive skills. Especially in the medical profession, one thing that is guaranteed in the workplace is change.

Change can be positive or negative; this depends mostly on the way it is viewed by the individual.

A person is not doomed to live with poor self-esteem forever. With a degree of effort and open mindedness, an individual can work toward better self-esteem, which can make a tremendous difference in the individual's future potential.

Problem-Solving Skills

For individuals to work together, they must have a degree of trust and be willing to make suggestions for the good of the group. The phrase "two heads are better than one" is still true when it comes to problem solving. Employees usually want to play a part in solving the problems in the workplace, and they appreciate knowing that their opinions make a difference. A medical assistant who can listen to the concerns of others and is willing to give and take will be an excellent problem solver.

Decision-Making Skills

People who know how to make good decisions usually are successful. Thinking through a decision requires logic, and it is best to take some time to think carefully of all the pros and cons. Unfortunately, a medical assistant may not always have time to consider decisions in a leisurely fashion, especially when dealing with emergencies. A good decision maker is honest in identifying the real problems and attempts to keep personal feelings isolated from the process.

There are several steps in making a sound decision. The problem must be specifically defined and evaluated so that the individual understands clearly what needs to happen to resolve the situation. Gather as much information as possible and consider all alternatives. It sometimes is helpful to choose an alternative and consider all the ramifications of making a decision using that alternative. Then, when the best alternative has been determined, the decision should be made and put into action. Care should be taken to avoid making a decision simply because it is easy and comfortable, because more problems could arise later as a result of not addressing the true problem in the beginning.

CRITICAL THINKING APPLICATION   58-10

Lisa has been on several interviews and likes the prospect of working for three different physicians. If an offer is made at each office, how can Lisa decide which to accept? What will help Lisa make this decision?

Stress Management

The demands of the medical profession make it a stressful environment at times. Stress is not always bad. In fact, some stress is a positive motivator toward a goal. A *stressor* is a stimulus that prompts a reaction from the body. Positive stress, or *eustress,* includes exhilarating activities or success, which often leads to higher expectations from the person experiencing the eustress. The opposite is distress, which includes disappointment, failure, or embarrassment. Stress management is a conscious effort to control the stressors and resulting reactions so that the body and mind operate evenly, even when stress is present in an individual's life.

By learning to recognize the signs of stressful overload, a medical assistant can possibly ward off the negative reactions that are so physically and mentally draining to the body. Many people notice a headache or fatigue when overly stressed. Breathing correctly is one way to reduce stress. Often an accelerated breathing pattern that is quick and shallow is a stress indicator. Breathing from the abdomen at a slower pace, inhaling through the nose, and exhaling through the mouth, may help reduce tension. Taking time for relaxing activities and getting plenty of exercise are other methods of stress reduction.

Planning a Budget

A newly graduated medical assistant should formulate a simple budget and live within that budget. Track spending with checkbook ledgers, bill stubs, receipts, and daily records for 3 months before developing a firm budget, so that you have a realistic accounting of where money goes when it leaves the checkbook. Use that information to design a reasonable spending plan for monthly income that accounts for monthly, quarterly, and annual expenses, as well as special expenses.

Even if you make only a small salary, building savings is important. A medical assistant should set aside 5% to 10% of the net income in a savings account. The money in savings should not be touched except in emergencies. Establish a separate emergency fund, which ideally should hold 3 to 6 months' salary. This way, enough cash is available to pay bills for 3 months in case of a sudden job loss or emergency. No one can do this immediately when beginning a new job, but it can be done over a period of time if one is committed to the effort.

Avoid going into debt whenever possible. If credit cards are used at all, they should be used conservatively and not for impulse purchases. Instead of using credit, set spending goals and save for a purchase or use layaway programs. Always make more than the minimum payment on credit cards to prevent excessive interest from accruing on the account. Even better, pay off the entire balance when the statement is received each month, avoiding charges higher than what can be paid with the monthly salary in addition to other bills. Everyone should work toward being debt free as soon as possible.

In his book *The Total Money Makeover,* author Dave Ramsey recommends avoiding credit card use altogether and paying off all debts in order from smallest to largest to become debt free. Avoiding debt helps keep finances manageable whether the economy is up or down.

Student Loans

Student loans are designed to provide the opportunity to obtain an education. They must be paid back. If an individual **defaults** on a student loan, he or she becomes ineligible for future student loans until the original loan is paid back, and amounts owed may be deducted from tax refunds involuntarily. Remember that interest is accrued on loans, so the student will owe more than was actually borrowed. Although small loans may run around $50 per month once they are due, larger loans can result in payments in excess of $1,000 per month. Never incur more student loan debt than absolutely necessary and make every effort to pay off the loan as early as possible, even if that means making extra payments or a larger lump-sum payment in addition to the required monthly amounts. If the student can avoid loans by saving for school expenses and paying for each semester in cash, the education will cost less, because no interest charges will be added to the tuition costs.

There is never a reason to default on a student loan. The medical assistant should contact the company that services the student loan and explain any problems that are preventing repayment of the debt. These companies want to work with students to clear their accounts. Often a **deferment** is available, which allows the student to postpone the payments for a period of time. Deferments may be available if the student is unemployed, attending school to continue his or her education, suffering economic hardship, completing a graduate fellowship, completing rehabilitation training, or in other situations. The medical assistant should contact the lender to find out whether he or she is eligible for a deferment. (For tips on how to avoid defaulting on a loan, along with an in-school deferment form, visit the Evolve site at *evolve.elsevier.com/kinn*.)

Guideline Budget

Dealing with personal finances can be a stressor. Developing a realistic budget helps a medical assistant plan his or her spending. When careful planning is implemented, more can be accomplished with less money if a commitment has been made to staying on budget and resisting the temptation to spend.

Start by evaluating your monthly expenses. The easiest way to do this is to save every single receipt and a copy of each bank transaction for 3 months. Then, divide the receipts into the appropriate month and determine where your money is going. Put the receipt amounts in specific categories, such as:

- Rent/mortgage
- Child care
- Utilities
- Food
- Car payments
- Car expenses
- Credit/debts
- Professional dues
- Household expenses
- Medical/dental care
- Child support
- School expenses
- Student loans

Budgets should be designed and planned to be as personal as possible. Using the information from the receipts, you can easily determine which categories fit your individual budget. Budget forms are readily accessible on the Internet or can be designed using computer programs, such as Microsoft Word or Excel. A sample budget outline is shown in Figure 58-16. Take an honest look at each item listed and determine the amount you spend monthly in each category. Compare these amounts with your monthly income and see whether your current budget is positive or negative. Remember that the gross salary is the amount earned before taxes and other deductions. The net salary is the take-home pay. Adjustments may be needed to bring the budget into balance.

Getting a Paycheck

Nothing is more exciting than receiving the first paycheck from a new job. Still, the recipient must handle finances responsibly so that financial obligations can be met. Employees who handle their personal finances well can better focus on work responsibilities and those in their personal life.

MONTHLY INCOME	AMOUNT
Net Income	
Spouse Net Income	
Child Support	
Other Income	

MONTHLY EXPENSES	AMOUNT
Rent	
Gas	
Electric	
Home/Renters Insurance	
Water/Sewage	
Trash	
Home Telephone	
Cell Telephone	
Pager	
Cable TV/Satellite	
Internet/DSL	
Child Care	
Lawn Care	
Clothing	
Food - Home	
Food - Work or School	
Food - Eating Out	
Laundry/Dry Cleaning	
Medical Expenses	
Dental Expenses	
Life Insurance	
Medical Insurance	
Dental Insurance	
Eyeglasses	
Prescriptions	
Automobile Payment	
Automobile Insurance	
Repairs	
Gas/Oil	
Furniture	
Beauty/Barber Shop	
Pet Expenses	
Student Loan	
Other Loans	
Credit Cards	
Church/Charities	
Birthdays	
Anniversaries	
Christmas	
Vacation Planning	
Entertainment	

FIGURE 58-16 The guideline budget.

Several deductions will be taken from the employee's paycheck, such as Federal Insurance Contributions Act (FICA) and Medicare contributions, in addition to optional deductions, such as those for medical and dental insurance, disability insurance, vision care, retirement funds, and others, depending upon what is offered by the employer. If the employee knows the amount of all the deductions on the paycheck, he or she can figure the FICA and Medicare contributions to estimate the net amount of the check each pay period and know the amount of money that will be available toward the budget. The current FICA deduction is 12.4% of the income earned for the period, and the Medicare deduction is 3.8%. By calculating these deductions from the gross salary for the period minus optional deductions, the net salary can be determined. Always bring questions to the attention of the payroll manager immediately so that payroll issues can be rectified quickly.

Dangerous Habits

Some individuals practice dangerous habits with regard to finances. For instance, if this month's bills are arriving and last month's have not been paid, frustration and depression may result. Some people may even avoid opening letters or bills just so they do not have to deal with seeing the balance due. Writing checks on funds that are not in the checking account is not only unwise, it is also illegal. All states have laws against writing insufficient funds checks, and most legislation considers this a form of theft. A person can be arrested for writing "hot" checks. People headed for financial disaster also purchase daily items, such as bread and milk, with a credit card. All these behaviors are signs of financial trouble.

CLOSING COMMENTS

The period surrounding graduation is a celebration, but also a busy time that requires much planning. Cooperate with the school in securing externship sites and make an effort to obtain a site that will be the most beneficial to the career you want. Do not take an externship just because it is close to home. Think about the skills that will be offered and learn as much as possible. Then perform well, so that the staff and physicians are happy to offer a good reference to potential employers. Strive to attain goals, and once they are reached, set additional goals to continue moving forward in life.

Even though the medical assistant educational experience ends, remember that there is constantly something new to learn in the medical profession. Join professional societies and participate in as many educational seminars and continuing education classes as possible. Remain in a continual state of learning and be determined to be the best medical assistant you can be.

Patient Education

Some patients assume that the people who assist the physician in the office are all nurses. The medical assistant should always specify that he or she is a medical assistant, especially when making initial introductions. There should never be any representation that the medical assistant is the "office nurse." If a patient uses that term, correct him or her in a friendly manner.

A medical assistant may find it necessary to educate the patient about the definition of a medical assistant. An occasional rare patient

may not have heard of the profession. Explain the type of training that was completed, emphasizing that medical assistants are trained specifically for work in a physician's office. If patients have any questions about the medical assistant's qualifications, refer them to the office manager or physician.

STEPS FOR ACHIEVING GOALS

- Decide what you want.
- Write down the goal.
- Set the date for accomplishment.
- Read the goal three times a day.
- Think of the goal often.
- See yourself accomplishing the goal.
- Develop a plan of action for reaching the goal.
- Do not discuss the plan with others who might be discouraging.
- Be confident.
- Act successful, and you will be!

Legal and Ethical Issues

Always be completely honest when completing a job application and offering information on a resumé. Most facilities stipulate that if an individual is not truthful on these documents, his or her employment can be terminated when the deception is discovered. Employers are more interested in honesty and a forthright explanation than in minor problems that affect the job performance.

If a medical assistant has had some brush with the law that requires disclosure on the job application, the best policy is to be honest and to deal with the ramifications of telling the truth. Most businesses can verify whether a potential employee has any type of criminal record. A solid explanation of the facts, admission of a past mistake, and excellent, current references often prompt an employer to have faith and make a positive decision about offering employment.

SUMMARY OF SCENARIO

The end of medical assistant training is a time of great excitement and perhaps a small bit of apprehension. Lisa is prepared to accept the challenges ahead as she readies herself for her future in her new career. She has begun her externship and has been expanding her network of acquaintances in the medical profession for several months. Lisa has met many office managers and a few physicians and has learned a great deal about several area medical facilities. Through her research, she has decided that she would like to work with one of three local physicians who need a medical assistant. One is a pediatrician, another is a well-known neurologist, and the third is a family practitioner just out of medical school. Lisa has gathered information about all of these professionals, and each has invited her for a job interview.

Lisa knows that she will need to be at her best, so she takes care of herself and gets plenty of rest. She has a long list of interview questions and has taken the time to write out answers to the questions in preparation for her interviews. She is careful about her grooming every day that she reports to the externship, because she knows that the physician at her site is her first reference in the medical field. In addition, she knows that she may be called for an interview any day that might be scheduled just after her workday ends. Looking professional prepares her for this each day.

Lisa is comfortable during her interviews because she is well prepared. She has identified her strengths and can share them with a potential employer. She is focused on her objectives and knows her minimum requirements to accept a position. She has a healthy self-esteem, and her good decision-making skills will help her to determine which position is right for her. Her enthusiasm and excitement show in her eyes, and she is dedicated to making a difference in the lives of her patients and co-workers.

SUMMARY OF LEARNING OBJECTIVES

1. **Define, spell, and pronounce the terms listed in the vocabulary.**

   Spelling and pronouncing medical terms correctly bolster the medical assistant's credibility. Knowing the definitions of these terms promotes confidence in communication with patients and co-workers.

2. **Discuss the reasons job search training is important to a medical assistant.**

   Because approximately 85% of individuals do not have any formal training in job search skills, taking the time to learn the best methods puts the medical assistant at an advantage. Training reduces the time spent looking for work and increases the benefits and salary offered when good negotiating skills are used. The medical assistant also is more comfortable during interviews and throughout the job search process.

3. **List three expectations employers have of employees.**

   Employers have three basic expectations of their medical assistant employees. They want an employee with a good appearance, who looks as if he or she fits in the medical profession. A medical assistant should also be dependable and have the skills to do the job for which he or she was hired.

4. **Understand the three types of employee skill strengths.**

   Three types of skill strengths may be used by employees. Job skills are those used to actually perform a job, such as venipunctures or scheduling appointments. Self-management skills usually are part of the medical assistant's personality; these include honesty and dependability. Transferable skills are those that can be taken from one job to another or used on any job. Examples include the ability to communicate effectively and to lead and manage individuals.

5. **Explain the two best job search methods.**

   Networking and contacting employers directly are the two best methods of searching for a job. Networking involves developing a network of individuals who can assist the medical assistant in finding employment. This group may include co-workers, other students, relatives, or friends who provide leads to potential employers. Contacting employers directly includes taking resumés to specific offices or making appointments to gain knowledge about the facility and then later using that knowledge during the job search. These two methods are more effective than most traditional means of finding a job.

6. **Describe some of the errors that should be avoided on a resumé.**

   Any error should be avoided on a resumé. Medical assistants must make sure everything is spelled correctly, but they cannot rely on the computer's spell-check feature alone. They must proofread the document and have someone else proofread it to catch errors that may have been overlooked. Salary expectations should never be stated on the resumé, and a photograph should not be included. Personal information, such as height and weight, also are not included.

7. **List the four phases of the interview process.**

   The four phases of the interview process include the preparation, the actual interview, the follow-up, and the negotiation. The preparation includes all efforts made before the actual interview in obtaining information about the company, deciding on the wardrobe, and making sure nails are groomed and shoes are shined. The interview itself is designed to help the employer and potential employee get to know each other and discover whether they are compatible. The follow-up is perhaps the most critical stage, wherein the medical assistant should send a thank you letter and continue to stay in touch with the facility until the job is filled. The negotiation includes discussion of the salary and benefits that will be offered to the new employee.

8. **Explain the importance of having demographic information about former jobs before appearing for an interview.**

   Demographic information on other employers should be taken to interviews and kept handy when filling out job applications. A medical assistant should never have to ask for a phone book to look up the address of a former employer. This demonstrates a lack of preparation and planning on the part of the potential employee.

9. **List and discuss legal and illegal interview questions.**

   Employers may intentionally or accidentally ask illegal interview questions, and the medical assistant has three choices in this situation: (1) refusing to answer the question, which may indicate that he or she will not tolerate difficult patients; (2) answering the question directly, which may cost the medical assistant the position; or (3) relating the question back to the position, which indicates maturity and the ability to be tactful and polite.

10. **Discuss the importance of the probationary period for a new employee.**

    The probationary period is a time for the new medical assistant to become oriented to the facility. It also allows the employer to assess whether the medical assistant fits with the team and performs the duties of the job in a satisfactory way. During this time, the medical assistant should demonstrate that he or she is a productive team member with an excellent attitude. There should never be idle time; rather, when all duties are completed, the medical assistant should look for ways to assist others.

11. **List some common early mistakes of which a new employee should be aware.**

    A new employee in the medical office should avoid arriving late or being absent, especially during the probationary period. He or she should never participate in office gossip and should make a good attempt to get along with every employee. A medical assistant should not make excessive supervision necessary and should be open to learning new ways of performing procedures. A new employee who fits in with the team finds the job more rewarding.

12. **Understand the importance of maintaining liability coverage once employed in the industry.**

    Because patients can bring professional liability suits against any personnel involved in their care, the medical assistant should maintain professional liability coverage throughout their career in the healthcare industry.

13. **Explain why a performance appraisal rating is usually not perfect.**

    No employee is perfect, so performance appraisals rarely have perfect ratings. Even an employee who is doing an excellent job has room for improvement in some area. Without comments that suggest improvement, the employee may not feel that the position offers growth potential. Constructive comments help a medical assistant perform better and take on more responsibility.

14. **Organize a job search.**
Time management and organizational skills help the medical assistant launch an effective job search (see Procedure 58-2).

15. **Prepare a resumé.**
The resumé must be accurate and error free (see Procedure 58-1).

16. **Complete a job application.**
Job applications must be filled out accurately and completely (see Procedure 58-3).

17. **Interview for a job.**
The interview is the job search step that most influences hiring decisions (see Procedure 58-4).

18. **Negotiate a salary.**
The medical assistant should develop skills in negotiating salary after he or she has determined the minimum amount in both benefits and pay that can be accepted (see Procedure 58-5).

CONNECTIONS

Study Guide Connection: Go to the Chapter 58 Study Guide. Read and complete the activities.

Evolve Connection: Go to the Chapter 58 link at *evolve.elsevier.com/kinn* to complete the Chapter Review and Chapter Quiz. Check out the other resources listed for this chapter to make the most of what you have learned from Career Development and Life Skills.

GLOSSARY

abandonment To withdraw protection or support; in medicine, to discontinue medical care without proper notice after accepting a patient.

abscesses Localized collections of pus that may be under the skin or deep in the body and that cause tissue destruction.

abstract An outline or summary of the diagnostic statement and/or procedures and services performed. In procedural coding, the outline or summary assists in ensuring that all procedures and services are included in an insurance claim submission and that nothing is omitted or added to the encounter form or charge ticket; as a verb form, *abstract* also means to compile this outline or summary for use in procedural coding.

academic degree A title conferred by a college, university, or professional school upon completion of a program of study.

accommodation Adjustment of the eye that allows a person to see various sizes of objects at different distances.

account A statement of transactions during a fiscal period and the resulting balance.

account balance The amount owed on an account.

accounts payable Debts incurred and not yet paid.

accounts receivable Amounts owed to the physician.

accounts receivable ledger A record of the charges and payments posted on an account.

accounts receivable trial balance A method of determining that the journal and the ledger are in balance.

accreditation (u-kre-duh-ta'-shun) The process through which an organization is recognized for adherence to a group of standards that meet or exceed the expectations of the accrediting agency.

accrual basis of accounting A method of accounting in which income is recorded when earned and expenses are recorded when incurred.

acronyms Abbreviations, such as ECG for electrocardiography.

act The formal action of a legislative body; a decision or determination of a sovereign state, a legislative council, or a court of justice.

adage (a'-dij) A saying, often in metaphoric form, that embodies a common observation.

add-on codes Codes that indicate additional or supplemental procedures carried out along with the primary procedure.

adhesions (ad-he'-zhuns) Bands of scar tissue that bind together two anatomic surfaces that normally are separate.

admonition Counsel or warning against fault or oversight.

adnexal (add'-neks-uhl) Pertaining to adjacent or accessory parts.

adrenocorticotropic hormone (ACTH) (uh-dren-o-cor-ti-ko-tro'-pik) A hormone that stimulates the production and secretion of glucocorticoids; it is released by the anterior pituitary gland.

advance An amount of money or credit furnished in anticipation of repayment.

advent Coming into being or use.

adverse event An injury caused by medical management rather than the underlying condition of the patient.

advocate (ad'-vuh-kat) One who pleads the cause of another; one who defends or maintains a cause or proposal.

affable Pleasant and at ease in talking to others; characterized by ease and friendliness.

agenda (ah-jen'-duh) A list or outline of things to be considered or done.

aggressive Forceful or intended to dominate; hostile, injurious, or destructive, especially when referring to a behavior caused by frustration.

albuminuria (al-byu-muh-nur-e'-uh) The abnormal presence of albumin protein in the urine.

aliquot (a'-luh-kwaht) A portion of a well-mixed sample removed for testing.

allegation (a-li-ga'-shun) A statement by a party to a legal action of what the party undertakes to prove; an assertion made without proof.

alleviate To partly remove or correct; to relieve or lessen.

allied health fields Occupational disciplines in which professionals involved with the delivery of healthcare or related services assist physicians with the diagnosis, treatment, and care of patients in many different specialty areas.

allocating (a'-luh-ka-ting) Apportioning for a specific purpose or to particular persons or things.

allopathic (al-o-path'-ik) A term used to contrast homeopathic medicine with mainstream medicine; allopathic medicine is characterized by an effort to counteract the symptoms of a disease by administration of treatments that produce effects opposite to the symptoms.

allowed charge (allowable amount) The maximum amount of money that many third-party payers allow for a specific procedure or service.

alopecia (al-o-pe'-se-uh) Partial or complete lack of hair.

alphabetic filing Any system that arranges names or topics according to the sequence of the letters in the alphabet.

Alphabetic Index Volume 2 of the ICD-9-CM coding manual; it lists conditions, injuries, illnesses, and diseases in alphabetical order by main terms, modifying terms, and subterms. It also contains the Classification of Factors Influencing Health Status and Contact with Health Service (V Codes) and the index for Supplemental Classification of External Causes of Injury and Poisoning (E Codes).

alphanumeric Of or relating to systems made up of combinations of letters and numbers.

ambiguous (am-bi'-gu-wus) Capable of being understood in two or more possible senses or ways; unclear.

amblyopia (am-ble-o′-pe-uh)   Reduction or dimness of vision with no apparent organic cause; often referred to as *lazy eye syndrome*.

ambulatory (am′-bu-la-to-re)   Able to walk about and not be bedridden.

amenities   Things that contribute to comfort, enjoyment, or convenience.

amenity (uh-me′-nuh-te)   Something conducive to comfort, convenience, or enjoyment.

amiable (a′-me-uh-buhl)   Having qualities that make one liked and easy to deal with.

amino acids   Organic compounds that form the chief constituents of protein and are used by the body to build and repair tissues.

amorphous (a-mohr′-fuhs)   Lacking a defined shape.

analyte   The substance or chemical being analyzed or detected in a specimen.

anaphylaxis (an-uh-fuh-lak′-sis)   An exaggerated hypersensitivity reaction that in severe cases leads to vascular collapse, bronchospasm, and shock.

anaplastic   Relating to an alteration in cells to a more primitive form; a term that describes cancer-producing cells.

anastomosis (uh-nas-tuh-mo′-suhs)   The surgical joining of two normally distinct organs.

ancillary (an′-suh-ler-e)   Subordinate; auxiliary.

ancillary diagnostic services   Services that support patient diagnoses (e.g., laboratory or radiologic services).

and   In the context of the ICD-9-CM, *and* should be interpreted as *and/or*.

anemia   A condition marked by deficiency of red blood cells (RBCs).

angina pectoris (an-ji′-nuh/pek′-tuh-ruhs)   Spasmlike pain in the chest caused by myocardial anoxia.

angiocardiography (an-je-o-kahr-de-og′-ruh-fe)   Radiography of the heart and great vessels using an iodine contrast medium.

angiography (an-je-og′-ruh-fe)   Radiography of blood vessels using an iodine contrast medium.

angioplasty (an′-je-o-plas-te)   An interventional technique in which a catheter is used to open or widen a blood vessel to improve circulation.

animate   To fill with life; to give spirit and support to expressions.

annotating   Furnishing with notes that are usually critical or explanatory.

annotations (a-nuh-ta′-shun)   Notes added by way of comment or explanation.

anomalies (uh-noh′-muh-lez)   Deformities or deviations from a normal condition, resulting from faulty development of a fetus.

anomaly   A congenital malformation that occurs during fetal development.

anorexia (a-nuh-rek′-se-uh)   A lack or loss of appetite for food.

anteroposterior (AP) (an-tuhr-o-pos-ter′-e-ohr)   A frontal projection in which the patient is supine or facing the x-ray tube.

antibodies (an′-ti-bah-dees)   Immunoglobulins produced by the immune system in response to bacteria, viruses, or other antigenic substances.

anticoagulants   Chemicals added to a blood sample after collection to prevent clotting.

antigen (an′-ti-juhn)   A foreign substance that causes the production of a specific antibody.

antimicrobial agents   Drugs used to treat infection.

antiseptics (an-ti-sep-tik)   Substances that inhibit the growth of microorganisms on living tissue (e.g., alcohol and povidone-iodine solution [Betadine]).

aortogram (a-or′-ti-gram)   Radiography of the aorta using an iodine contrast medium.

apnea (ap′-nee-uh)   Absence or cessation of breathing.

appeal   A legal proceeding by which a case is brought before a higher court for review of the decision of a lower court.

appellate (uh-pe′-lut)   Having the power to review the judgment of another tribunal or body of jurisdiction, such as an appellate court.

application software   Computer programs designed to perform specific tasks.

appraisal   An expert judgment of the value or merit of something; judgment as to quality.

aqueous (ak′-wee-uhs)   A term describing a waterlike substance; a medication prepared with water.

arbitration (ar-buh-tra′-shun)   The hearing and determination of a cause in controversy by a person or persons either chosen by the parties involved or appointed under statutory authority.

arbitrator (ar-buh-tra′-ter)   A neutral person chosen to settle differences between two parties in a controversy.

archived   To have filed or collected records or documents.

arrhythmia (uh-rith′-mee-uh)   An abnormality or irregularity in the heart rhythm.

arteriography (ahr-ter-e-og′-ruh-fe)   Radiography of arteries using an iodine contrast medium.

arteriosclerosis (ar-ter′-ee-o-scler-o-sis)   Thickening, decreased elasticity, and calcification of arterial walls.

arthritis   Inflammation of a joint.

arthrogram (ahr′-thro-gram)   Fluoroscopic examination of the soft tissue components of joints, for which a contrast medium is injected directly into the joint capsule.

arthropods (ahr′-throh-pods)   Members of a class of invertebrate animals that includes insects, crustaceans, and arachnids.

articular (ar-ti′-kyuh-luhr)   Pertaining to a joint.

artifacts   Structures or features not normally present but visible as a result of an external agent or action, such as in a microscopic specimen after fixation or in a radiographic image.

artificial intelligence   The aspect of computer science that deals with computers taking on the attributes of humans, such as mimicking human thought. For example, expert systems can make decisions, such as software designed to help a physician diagnose a patient, given a set of symptoms.

ascites (uh-si′-tez)   An abnormal collection of fluid containing high levels of protein and electrolytes in the peritoneal cavity.

assault   An intentional, unlawful attempt of bodily injury to another by force.

assent   To agree to something, especially after thoughtful consideration.

assessment   The physician's determination of what is or may be wrong with the patient based on the findings from the history and physical examination (H&P). The assessment includes a preliminary, interim, or final diagnosis.

assets   The entire property of a person, association, corporation, or estate applicable or subject to the payment of debts.

assignment of benefits   The transfer of the patient's legal right to collect benefits for medical expenses to the provider of those services, authorizing the payment to be sent directly to the provider.

asymptomatic   Without symptoms of a disease process.

asystole (ay-sis'-toh-le)   The absence of a heartbeat.

ataxia (uh-taks'-e-uh)   Failure or irregularity of muscle actions and coordination.

atria   The two upper chambers of the heart.

atrioventricular (AV) node   The part of the cardiac conduction system between the atria and the ventricles.

attenuated (uh-ten-yuh-wat'-ed)   Weakened or changed; refers to the virulence of a pathogenic microorganism.

audiologist (au-de-ah'-lah-jist)   Allied healthcare professional who specializes in evaluation of hearing function, detection of hearing impairment, and determination of the anatomic site of impairment.

audit   A formal examination of an organization's or individual's accounts or financial situation; a methodic examination and review. *Also,* a process performed prior to insurance claims submission to examine claims for accuracy and completeness. An audit can be performed manually or, if computer billing software is used, electronically.

audit trail   The path left by a transaction when it has been completed; often referred to when tracking medical services used by patients or researching claims.

augment   To make greater, more numerous, larger, or more intense.

aura   A peculiar sensation that precedes the appearance of a more definite disturbance.

auscultation   The act of listening to body sounds, typically with a stethoscope, to assess various organs throughout the body.

authenticated   Proved; with regard to medical records, it applies to a signature, initials, or computer keystroke by the maker of the record to verify that the record is correct.

authorization   An alphanumeric designation or a number given by the insurance company authorizing approval of a procedure or service. This does not guarantee payment.

autoimmune (o-to-im'-yuhn)   Pertaining to a disturbance in the immune system in which the body reacts against its own tissue. Examples of autoimmune disorders include multiple sclerosis, rheumatoid arthritis, and systemic lupus erythematosus.

automatic call routing   A software system that answers phones automatically and routes calls to staff after the caller responds to prompts; also used to call a large number of patients to remind them of appointments or make announcements.

avert   To see coming and ward off or avoid.

axial projections   Radiographs taken with a longitudinal angulation of the x-ray beam; sometimes referred to as *semiaxial projections.*

azotemia (a-zo-te'-me-uh)   The retention of excessive quantities of nitrogenous wastes in the blood.

backorder   An ordered item that is not delivered when promised or demanded but will be filled at a later date.

backup   Any type of storage that prevents the loss of files with hard disk failure.

bailiff   An officer of some U.S. courts who usually serves as a messenger or usher and who keeps order at the request of the judge.

balance sheet   A financial statement for a specific date that shows the total assets, liabilities, and capital of the business.

Bartholin's cyst   A fluid-filled cyst in one of the vestibular glands located on either side of the vaginal orifice.

battery   A willful and unlawful use of force or violence on the person of another. *Also,* offensive touching or the use of force on a person without his or her consent.

benchmarks   Items or factors that serve as standards against which other items or factors can be measured or judged.

beneficence (buh-ne'-fuh-sens)   The act of doing or producing good, especially performing acts of charity or kindness.

beneficiary   The individual entitled to receive benefits from an insurance policy or program or a governmental entitlement program offering healthcare benefits. Also called a *participant, subscriber, dependent, enrollee,* or *member.*

benefits   Services or payments provided under a health plan, employee plan, or some other agreement, including programs such as health insurance, pensions, retirement planning, and many other options that may be offered to employees of a company or an organization.

benign   Not cancerous and not recurring.

bevel (bev'-uhl)   The angled tip of a needle.

bifurcates   Divides from one into two branches.

bilirubin (bih-luh-roo'-bin)   An orange pigment in bile; its accumulation leads to jaundice.

bilirubinuria (bi-li-roo'-bin-yuhr-e-uh)   The presence of bilirubin in the urine.

biophysical (bi-o-fi'-zi-kuhl)   The science of applying physical laws and theories to biologic problems.

birthday rule   An insurance rule that applies as follows: when an individual is covered under two insurance policies, the insurance plan of the policyholder whose birthday comes first in the calendar year (month and day, not year) becomes the primary insurance.

bits   The smallest units of information inside the computer, each represented either by the digit "0" or "1"; 8 bits equal 1 byte.

blatant   Completely obvious, conspicuous, or obtrusive, especially in a crass or offensive manner; brazen.

bleak   Not hopeful or encouraging.

blood-brain barrier   An anatomic-physiologic structure made up of astrocyte glial cells that prevents or slows the transfer of chemicals into the neurons of the central nervous system (CNS).

bond   A durable, formal paper used for documents.

bookkeeping   The recording of business and accounting transactions.

bookmark   A command in a browser that marks the Internet protocol (IP) address of a Web site so that it can be saved and recalled quickly without typing the entire Web address.

bounding   A term used to describe a pulse that feels full because of increased power of cardiac contraction or as a result of increased blood volume.

bradycardia (brad-i-kahr'-dee-uh)   A slow heartbeat; a pulse below 60 beats per minute.

bradypnea (brad-ip-nee'-uh)   Respirations that are regular in rhythm but slower than normal in rate.

branding   The process involved in creating a unique name and image in the customer's mind, mainly through advertising campaigns with a consistent theme.

broad-spectrum antimicrobial agents   Drugs used to treat a wide range of infectious microorganisms.

bronchiectasis (brong´-ke-ek-tuh-sis) Dilation of the bronchi and bronchioles associated with secondary infection or ciliary dysfunction.

bronchoconstriction Narrowing of the bronchiole tubes.

bronchodilator (brahn-ko-di´-la-tuhr) A drug that relaxes contractions of the smooth muscle of the bronchioles to improve lung ventilation.

browsers Software programs that allow users to view Web pages on the Internet (e.g., Internet Explorer, Firefox).

bruit (broo´-it) An abnormal sound or murmur heard on auscultation of an organ, a vessel (e.g., carotid artery), or gland.

bucky A moving grid device that prevents scatter radiation from fogging the film.

budget A plan for the coordination of resources and expenditures; the amount of money available or required for a particular purpose.

bundle of His Specialized muscle fibers that conduct electrical impulses from the AV node to the ventricular myocardium.

bundled codes CPT codes designating procedures or services that are grouped together and paid for as one procedure or service, according to the National Correct Coding Initiative (NCCI) edits, established by the Centers for Medicare and Medicaid Services (CMS).

burnout Exhaustion of physical or emotional strength or motivation, usually as a result of prolonged stress or frustration.

bursae (bur´-suh) Fluid-filled, saclike membranes that provide cushioning and allow frictionless motion between two tissues.

business associates Individuals or organizations that perform or assist a covered entity in the performance of a function or activity involving the use or disclosure of individually identifiable health information.

byte A unit of data that contains 8 binary digits, or bits.

cache (kash) Special, high-speed storage that either can be part of the computer's main memory or a separate storage device. One function of a cache is to store Web sites visited in the computer memory for faster recall the next time the Web site is requested.

candidiasis (kan-duh-de-uh´-sis) An infection caused by a yeast that typically affects the vaginal mucosa and skin.

cannula (kan´-yoo-lah) A rigid tube that surrounds a blunt trocar or a sharp, pointed trocar inserted into the body; when the trocar is withdrawn, fluid may escape from the body through the cannula, depending on where it was inserted.

capitation A payment method used by many managed care organizations in which a fixed amount of money is reimbursed to the provider for patients enrolled during a specific period of time, no matter what services were received or how many visits were made.

caption A heading, title, or subtitle under which records are filed.

carcinogens (kar-si´-nuh-juhns) Substances or agents that cause the development or increase the incidence of cancer.

cardiac arrest A condition in which cardiac contractions stop completely.

cardioversion The use of electroshock to convert an abnormal cardiac rhythm to a normal one.

carriers In insurance terms, companies that assume the risk of an insurance policy.

cartilage A rubbery, smooth, somewhat elastic connective tissue that covers the ends of bones.

case management The process of assessing and planning patient care, including referral and follow-up, to ensure continuity of care and quality management.

cash basis of accounting A method of accounting in which income is recorded when received and expenses are recorded when paid.

cash flow statement A financial summary for a specific period that shows the beginning balance on hand, the receipts and disbursements during the period, and the balance on hand at the end of the period.

casts Fibrous or protein material molded to the shape of the part in which it has accumulated and thrown off into the urine in kidney disease.

categorically Placed in a specific division of a system of classification.

category In the CPT manual, the element indented one level below a subsection; it usually refers to a specific anatomic site or to procedures and/or services.

Category I codes Five-digit primary procedure or service codes, found in the Tabular Index, that are selected when performing insurance billing or statistical research.

Category II codes Special codes that can help providers track revenue and reimbursement; these codes are alphanumeric and end in the letter F.

Category III codes Codes for a new or experimental procedure or service, otherwise referred to as "Emerging Technology"; these codes are alphanumeric and end in the letter T.

cathartics Laxative preparations.

caustic (kos´-tik) Capable of burning, corroding, or damaging tissue by chemical action. *Also,* marked by sarcasm.

CD burner A device that can "write" data on a blank compact disk (CD) or copy data from one CD to a blank CD.

centrifuge (sen´-truh-fuhj) An apparatus consisting essentially of a compartment that spins about a central axis to separate contained materials of different specific gravities or to separate colloidal particles suspended in a liquid.

certification (ser-tuh-fuh-ka´-shun) The attesting of something as being true as represented or as meeting a standard; the result of having been tested, usually by a third party, and awarded a certificate based on proven knowledge.

cerumen (see-room´-men) A waxy secretion in the ear canal; commonly called *ear wax.*

cervical (ser´-vi-kuhl) Pertaining to the neck region, which has seven cervical vertebrae.

chain of command A series of executive positions in order of authority.

channels Means of communication or expression; courses or directions of thought.

characteristics Distinguishing traits, qualities, or properties.

chief complaint (CC) The reason the patient has sought medical care, usually taken down in the patient's own words. It is recorded in the history documentation in the medical record, preceded by the abbreviation CC.

chiropractic (ki´-ruh-prak-tik) A medical discipline that focuses on the nervous system and involves manual adjustment of the vertebral column to affect the nervous system, thereby treating various disorders, and also to promote patient wellness.

cholesterol (kuh-les´-tuh-rol) A substance produced by the liver and found in animal fats that can produce fatty deposits or atherosclerotic plaques in blood vessels.

chordae tendineae (kor´-duh/ten´y-din-uh) The tendons that anchor the cusps of the heart valves to the papillary muscles of the myocardium, preventing valvular prolapse.

chronic bronchitis   Recurrent inflammation of the membranes lining the bronchial tubes.

chronic obstructive pulmonary disease (COPD)   A progressive, irreversible lung condition that results in diminished lung capacity.

chronologic order   Of, relating to, or arranged in or according to the order of time.

cicatrix   Early scar tissue that appears pale, contracted, and firm.

cilia (sil'-e-uh)   Hairlike projections capable of movement; in the lungs, cilia waves move unwanted substances (e.g., mucus, dust, and pus) upward; cilia are destroyed by smoking.

circumvent (suhr-kuhm-vent')   To manage to get around, especially by ingenuity or strategy.

cirrhosis (suh-ro'-suhs)   A chronic, degenerative disease of the liver that interferes with normal liver function.

cited   Quoted by way of example, authority, or proof or mentioned formally in commendation or praise.

Civilian Health and Medical Program of the Department of Veterans Affairs (CHAMPVA)   A health benefits program run by the Department of Veterans Affairs (VA) that helps eligible beneficiaries pay the cost of specific healthcare services and supplies.

Civilian Health and Medical Program of the Uniformed Services (CHAMPUS)   See TRICARE.

clarity   The quality or state of being clear.

clauses   Groups of words containing a subject and predicate and functioning as a member of a complex or compound sentence.

clean claims   Insurance claim forms that have been completed correctly (no errors or omissions) and can be processed and paid promptly if they meet the restrictions on covered services and blocks.

clearinghouse   A centralized facility to which insurance claims are transmitted. Clearinghouses separate, check, and redistribute claims electronically to various insurance carriers and may offer additional services to the physician.

clinical trials   Research studies that test how well new medical treatments or other interventions work in the subjects, usually human beings.

clitoris (kli'-tuh-ris)   A small, elongated, erectile body above the urinary meatus at the superior point of the labia minora.

clubbing   Abnormal enlargement of the distal phalanges (fingers and toes) associated with cyanotic heart disease or advanced chronic pulmonary disease.

coagulate (ko-ag'-yuh-lat)   To form into clots.

code first   When more than one code is necessary to identify a given condition, *code first* or *use additional code* is used. A *code first* note is found at a manifestation code. A *use additional code* note is found at the etiology code when the underlying condition is sequenced first followed by the manifestation.

Code of Federal Regulations (CFR)   A coded delineation of the rules and regulations published in the *Federal Register* by the various departments and agencies of the federal government. The CFR is divided into 50 titles that represent broad subject areas and chapters that provide specific detail.

coding   Converting verbal or written descriptions into numeric and alphanumeric designations.

cognitive (kog'-nuh-tiv)   Pertaining to the operation of the mind; referring to the process by which we become aware of perceiving, thinking, and remembering.

cohesive   Sticking together tightly; exhibiting or producing cohesion.

co-insurance   A policy provision frequently found in medical insurance whereby the policyholder and the insurance company share the cost of covered losses in a specified ratio (e.g., 80/20 means that 80% is covered by the insurer and 20% by the insured).

coitus   Sexual union between male and female; also called *intercourse*.

collagen (kah'-luh-jen)   The protein that forms the inelastic fibers of tendons, ligaments, and fascia.

collect on delivery (COD)   A method of payment used when an article or item is delivered, and payment is expected before the item is released.

colloidal (kah-loid'-uhl)   Pertaining to a gluelike substance.

colonoscopy   A procedure in which a fiberoptic scope is used to examine the large intestine.

colony-forming units (CFUs)   A term used in reporting bacteriuria; one CFU represents one bacterium present in the urine sample.

colostrum (koh-lahs'-trum)   A thin, yellow, milky fluid secreted by the mammary glands a few days before and after delivery.

coma   An unconscious state from which the patient cannot be aroused.

comfort zone   A place in the mind where an individual feels safe and confident.

commensurate (ku-men'-su-rut)   Corresponding in size, amount, extent, or degree; equal in measure, proportionate.

commercial insurance plans   Plans that reimburse the insured for expenses resulting from illness or injury according to a specific fee schedule as outlined in the insurance policy and on a fee-for-service basis. Sometimes called *private insurance*.

competent   Having adequate abilities or qualities; having the capacity to function or perform in a certain way.

complainant (kuhm-pla'-nuhnt)   The person making a complaint against another person and/or organization.

complementary and alternative medicine (CAM)   A group of diverse medical and healthcare systems, practices, and products that are not generally considered part of conventional medicine. Complementary medicine is used in combination with conventional medicine (allopathic or osteopathic); alternative medicine is used instead of conventional medicine.

compression   The state of being pressed together.

computed tomography (CT)   A computerized x-ray imaging modality that provides axial and three-dimensional scans.

computerized physician/provider order entry (CPOE)   A process of electronic data entry of medical practitioner or provider instructions for the treatment of patients.

concise (kun-sice')   Expressing much in brief form.

concurrently   Occurring at the same time.

condescending   Assuming an air of superiority.

cones   Structures in the retina that make the perception of color possible.

congruence (kon-groo'-ents)   Agreement; the state that occurs when the verbal expression of the message matches the sender's nonverbal body language.

congruent (kun-gru'-unt)   Being in agreement, harmony, or correspondence; conforming to the circumstances or requirements of a situation.

connotation (kah-nuh-ta'-shun)   An implication; something suggested by a word or thing.

contaminated   Soiled with pathogens or infectious material; nonsterile.

contamination (kun-ta-mu-na´-shun) The process by which something is made impure, unclean, or unfit for use by the introduction of unwholesome or undesirable elements.

continuation pages The second and following pages of a letter.

continuing education units (CEUs) Credits for courses, classes, or seminars related to an individual's profession that are designed to promote education and to keep the professional up-to-date on current procedures and trends in the field; CEUs often are required for licensing.

continuity of care Continuation of care smoothly from one provider to another, so that the patient receives the most benefit and no interruption in care.

contraindications (kahn-truh-in-duh-ka´-shuns) Factors, such as symptoms or conditions, that make a particular treatment or procedure inadvisable.

contralateral (kon-trah-la´-tehr-uhl) Pertaining to the opposite side of the body.

contrast media Radiopaque substances used to enhance the visibility of soft tissues in imaging studies.

contributory negligence Statutes in some states that may prevent a party from recovering some damages if he or she contributed in any way to the injury or condition.

controls A standard of comparison to make sure answers obtained are accurate.

conventional medicine Medicine as practiced by holders of the Doctor of Medicine (MD) and Doctor of Osteopathy (OD) degrees and by their allied health professionals, such as physical therapists, psychologists, and registered nurses.

conventions Abbreviations, punctuation, symbols, instructional notations, and related entities that help guide the medical assistant or coder in the selection of an accurate, specific code.

cookies Messages sent to a Web browser from a Web server that identify users and can prepare custom Web pages for them, possibly displaying their name on return to the site.

co-payment A sum of money that is paid at the time of medical service; a form of co-insurance.

copulation Sexual intercourse.

coronal plane The plane that divides the body into anterior and posterior parts.

corticosteroids Antiinflammatory hormones, natural or synthetic.

costal Pertaining to the ribs.

coulombs per kilogram (C/kg) The international unit of radiation exposure.

counteroffer Return offer made by one who has rejected an offer or a job.

courier A messenger, especially one on official or diplomatic business; a service that provides delivery and transportation services for documents and/or packages.

covered entities As defined by HIPAA, organizations that transmit information in an electronic form during a transaction.

creatinine (kre´-a-tuhn-en) Nitrogenous waste from muscle metabolism that is excreted in the urine.

credentialing (kri-den´-shuh-ling) The process of extending professional or medical privileges to an individual; the process of verifying and evaluating that person's credentials.

credibility The quality or power of inspiring belief.

credit An entry on an account constituting an addition to a revenue, net worth, or liability account; the balance in a person's favor.

credit cards Devices issued by a bank or other financial institution, retail stores, and other businesses that allow the card holder to make purchases prior to paying for them; the card holder is then billed, usually after interest has been added.

crenate Forming notches or leaflike, scalloped edges on an object.

crepitation (kre-puh-ta´-shun) A dry, crackling sound or sensation.

critical thinking The constant practice of considering all aspects of a situation when deciding what to believe or what to do.

cross-training Training in more than one area so that a multitude of duties may be performed by one person or so that substitutions of personnel may be made in an emergency or at other necessary times.

cryosurgery The technique of exposing tissue to extreme cold to produce a well-defined area of cell destruction.

cryptogenic (krip-tuh-je´-nik) Pertaining to a disease with an unknown cause.

culpability Meriting condemnation, responsibility, or blame, especially as wrong or harmful.

cultivate To foster the growth of something; to improve by labor, care, or study.

culture and sensitivity (C&S) A procedure performed in the microbiology laboratory in which a specimen is cultured on artificial media to detect bacterial or fungal growth, followed by appropriate screening for antibiotic sensitivity.

curettage (kyur´-eh-tahjz) The act of scraping a body cavity with a surgical instrument, such as a curette.

cursor A symbol on the monitor screen that shows the location of the next character to be typed.

curt Marked by rude or peremptory shortness.

cyanosis (si-an-oh´-sis) A blue coloration of the mucous membranes and body extremities caused by lack of oxygen.

cyberspace The nonphysical space of the online world of computer networks in which communication takes place.

cystoscopy Visual examination of the urinary bladder using a fiber-optic instrument.

cysts Small, capsulelike sacs that enclose certain organisms in their dormant or larval stage.

cytology (si-tah´-luh-je) The study of cells using microscopic methods.

damages Loss or harm resulting from injury to person, property, or reputation; compensation in money imposed by law for losses or injuries.

database A collection of related files that serves as a foundation for retrieving information.

debit An entry on an account representing an addition to an expense or asset account or a deduction from a revenue, a net worth, or a liability account.

debit cards Cards that look like credit cards and with which money can be withdrawn, bills paid, or purchases made directly from the holder's bank account without the payment of interest.

debridement The removal of foreign material and dead, damaged tissue from a wound.

decedent (di-se´-dent) A legal term for a deceased person.

decodes Converts, as in a message, into intelligible form; recognizes and interprets.

decubitus ulcers   Sores or ulcers that develop over a bony prominence as the result of ischemia from prolonged pressure; also called *bed sores*.

deductibles   Specific amounts of money a patient must pay out of pocket before the insurance carrier begins paying. Usually this amount ranges from $100 to $500. This deductible amount is met on a yearly or per-incident basis.

default   To fail to pay a financial debt, such as a student loan.

defendant   A person required to answer in a legal action or suit; in criminal cases, the person accused of a crime.

defense mechanisms   Psychological methods of dealing with stressful situations that are encountered in day-to-day living.

deferment   Postponement, especially of a student loan.

defibrillator   A machine that delivers an electroshock to the heart through electrodes placed on the chest wall.

deficiencies (di-fi´-shun-ses)   Conditions that result with a below normal intake of particular substances.

dehiscence   The separation of wound edges or rupture of a wound closure.

demeanor (di-me´-nur)   Behavior toward others; outward manner.

demographic (de-muh-gra´-fik)   The statistical characteristics of human populations (as in age or income) used especially to identify markets.

dependents   The spouse, children, and sometimes domestic partner or other individuals designated by the insured who are covered under a healthcare plan.

depleted   Lessened markedly in quantity, content, power, or value.

detrimental (de-truh-men´-til)   Obviously harmful or damaging.

device driver   The program or commands given to a device connected to a computer that enable the device to function. For instance, a printer may come equipped with software that must be loaded onto the computer first so that the printer will work.

diabetes mellitus type 1   A disease in which the beta cells in the pancreas no longer produce insulin. The individual must rely on daily insulin administration to use glucose for energy and prevent complications.

diabetes mellitus type 2   A disease in which the body is unable to use glucose for energy as a result either of inadequate insulin production in the pancreas or resistance to insulin on the cellular level.

diagnosis   The concise, technical description of the cause, nature, or manifestations of a condition or problem. *Initial diagnosis:* The physician's temporary impression, sometimes called a *working diagnosis. Differentiated diagnosis:* A comparison of two or more diseases with similar signs and symptoms. *Clinical diagnosis:* The conclusion the physician reaches after evaluating all findings, including laboratory and other test results.

diagnostic statement   Information about a patient's diagnosis or diagnoses that has been extracted from the medical documentation.

diaphoresis (di-uh-fuh-re´-sis)   The profuse excretion of sweat.

diaphysis (di-a´-fuh-suhs)   The midportion of a long bone; it contains the medullary cavity.

diastole   The relaxation of the chambers of the heart, during which blood enters the heart from the vascular system and the lungs.

dictation (dik-tay´-shun)   The act or manner of uttering words to be transcribed.

diction   The choice of words, especially with regard to clearness, correctness, or effectiveness.

digestion   The process of converting food into chemical substances that can be used by the body.

digital subscriber line (DSL)   A high-speed, sophisticated modulation scheme that operates over existing copper telephone wiring systems; often referred to as "last-mile technologies," because DSL is used for connections from a telephone switching station to a home or office and not between switching stations.

digital video disk (DVD)   An optical disk that holds approximately 28 times more information than a CD; a DVD is most commonly used to hold full-length movies. Compared with a CD, which holds approximately 600 megabytes, a DVD can hold approximately 4.7 gigabytes. Also called a *digital versatile disk.*

dilation and curettage (D&C)   The widening of the cervix and scraping of the endometrial wall of the uterus.

dilation   The opening of the cervix through the process of labor, measured as 0 to 10 cm dilated. *Also,* the opening or widening of the circumference of a body orifice with a dilating instrument.

diluent (dil-yuh´-wunt)   A liquid used to dilute a specimen or reagent.

direct billing   A method of electronic claims submission that uses computer software to allow a provider to submit an insurance claim directly to an insurance carrier for payment.

direct filing system   A filing system in which materials can be located without consulting an intermediary source of reference.

dirty claims   Claims that contain errors or omissions; such claims must be corrected and resubmitted to an insurance carrier to obtain reimbursement.

disability income insurance   Insurance that provides periodic payments to replace income when an insured person is unable to work as a result of illness, injury, or disease.

disbursements   Funds paid out.

disbursements journal   A summary of accounts paid out.

disclaimer   A denial of responsibility; a denial of a legal claim.

discrepancies   Differences between conflicting facts, claims, or opinions.

discretion (dis-kre´-shun)   The quality of being discreet; having or showing good judgment or conduct, especially in speech.

disinfectant   A liquid chemical that is capable of eliminating many or all pathogens but is not effective against bacterial spores.

disk drives   Devices that load a program or data stored on a disk into the computer.

disparaging (dis-pahr´-uh-jing)   Slighting; having a negative or degrading tone.

disparities (di-spar´-uh-tes)   Fundamentally different and often incongruous elements; elements that are markedly distinct in quality or character.

dispense   To prepare a drug for administration.

disposition (dis-puh-zi´-shun)   The tendency of something or someone to act in a certain manner under given circumstances.

disruption   An unexpected event that throws a plan into disorder; an interruption that prevents a system or process from continuing as usual or as expected.

dissection (di-sek´-shun)   The separation into pieces and exposure of parts for scientific examination.

disseminate (di-se´-muh-nat)   To disperse throughout.

diurnal (die-ur´-nl) rhythm   A pattern of activity or behavior that follows a day-night cycle.

diverticulosis (di-vuhr-ti-kyuh-lo´-suhs) The presence of pouchlike herniations through the muscular layer of the colon.

divulge (duh-vuhlj´) To make known, as a confidence or secret.

docket A formal record of judicial proceedings; a list of legal cases to be tried.

domain name The initial part of a URL listing; the domain and name of the host or server, indicating the publisher of a Web page or site.

domestic mail Mail sent within the boundaries of the United States and its territories.

downcoding A change in a code or codes for entries submitted for reimbursement. This change usually is made by the insurance company, generally because the code submitted in some way does not match the company's specifications.

drawee A bank or facility on which a check is drawn or written.

drawer The person who writes a check.

drug of choice The drug an abuser uses most frequently to satisfy the craving for a certain feeling; the user's preferred drug.

due diligence The effort made by an ordinarily prudent or reasonable party to prevent harm to another party or oneself; doing everything possible to prevent something negative from happening; also called *due care*.

due process A fundamental constitutional guarantee that all legal proceedings will be fair; that one will be given notice of the proceedings and an opportunity to be heard before the government acts to take away life, liberty, or property; a constitutional guarantee that a law will not be unreasonable or arbitrary.

duty Obligatory tasks, conduct, service, or functions that arise from one's position, as in life or in a group.

dysplasia An alteration in cell growth, causing differences in size, shape, and appearance.

dyspnea (disp-nee´-uh) Difficult or painful breathing.

dysuria Pain or difficulty with urination.

e-banking Electronic banking via computer modem or over the Internet.

ecchymosis (e-ki-moh´-sis) A hemorrhagic skin discoloration commonly called *bruising*.

e-commerce Short for *electronic commerce;* used to describe the sale and purchase of goods and services over the Internet; doing business over the Internet.

ectopic (ek-tohp´-ik) Originating outside of the normal tissue.

edema (i-dee´-muh) An abnormal accumulation of fluid in the interstitial spaces of tissues.

editing To prepare for publication or public presentation; to alter, adapt, or refine, especially to bring about conformity to a standard or to suit a particular purpose.

effacement The thinning of the cervix during labor, measured in percentages from 0% to 100% effaced.

effective date The date on which an insurance policy or plan takes effect so that benefits are payable.

elastin An essential part of elastic connective tissue; when moist, it is flexible and elastic.

electrocardiogram (i-lek-tro-kar´-de-uh-gram) A graphic record of electrical conduction through the heart.

electrodesiccation The destruction of cells and tissue by means of short, high-frequency electrical sparks.

electronic (or digital) signature A scanned signature or other such mark that is accepted as proof of approval of and/or responsibility for the content of an electronic document.

electronic claims Claims that are submitted to insurance processing facilities using a computerized medium, such as direct data entry, direct wire, dial-in telephone digital fax, or personal computer download or upload.

electronic data interchange (EDI) The transfer of data back and forth between two or more entities using an electronic medium.

electronic fund transfer (EFT) The movement of funds between different accounts in the same or different banks using wire transfer, automated teller machines (ATMs), or computers, without the use of paper documents.

electronic health record (EHR) An electronic record of health-related information about a patient that conforms to nationally recognized interoperability standards and that can be created, managed, and consulted by authorized clinicians and staff from *more than one healthcare organization.*

electronic media The means of electronic transmission, including the Internet, private networks, dial-up phone lines, and fax modems; includes information moved from one place to another while stored on an electronic device.

electronic medical record (EMR) An electronic record of health-related information about an individual that can be created, gathered, managed, and consulted by authorized clinicians and staff *within a single healthcare organization.*

electronic remittance advice (ERA) An explanation that accompanies checks and relays details of the payment sent to the provider from the insurance company or other third-party provider.

eligibility A term that describes whether a patient's insurance coverage is in effect and eligible for payment of insurance benefits.

e-mail Short for *electronic mail;* communications transmitted via computer or computer network.

emancipated minor A person under legal age who is self-supporting and living apart from parents or a guardian; a mature minor considered by the courts to possess a sufficient understanding of self-care and responsibility.

embezzlement Stealing from an employer; to appropriate goods, services, or funds for personal use without permission.

embolus A foreign material that blocks a blood vessel; frequently a blood clot that has traveled from some other part of the body.

emetic (eh-met´-ik) A substance that causes vomiting.

empathy (em´-puh-the) Sensitivity to the individual needs and reactions of patients.

emphysema (em-fuh-ze´-muh) The pathologic accumulation of air in the alveoli, which results in alveolar destruction and overall oxygen deprivation; in the lungs, the bronchioles become plugged with mucus and lose elasticity.

Employer Identification Number (EIN) The number used by the Internal Revenue Service that identifies a business or individual functioning as a business entity for income tax reporting.

encodes Converts from one system of communication to another; converts a message into code.

encounter Any contact between a healthcare provider and a patient that results in treatment or evaluation of the patient's condition; it is not limited to in-person contact.

encroachments Actions that advance beyond the usual or proper limits.

encrypted (in-kript'-ed) Encoded; converted from one system of communication to another.

endocervical curettage The scraping of cells from the wall of the uterus.

endorser The person who signs his or her name on the back of a check for the purpose of transferring title to another person.

enteric-coated A term that refers to an oral medication that is coated to protect the drug against the stomach juices; this design is used to ensure that the medicine is absorbed in the small intestine.

entry A record or notation of an occurrence, transaction, or proceeding.

enunciate (e-nun'-se-at) To utter articulate sounds; the act of being very distinct in speech.

enunciation (e-nun-se-a'-shun) The utterance of articulate, clear sounds.

environment The state of a computer, usually determined by the programs running and hardware and software characteristics.

enzymatic reaction A chemical reaction controlled by an enzyme.

enzymes Complex proteins produced by cells that act as catalysts in specific biochemical reactions.

epiphysis (i-pi'-fuh-suhs) The end of a long bone; it contains the growth (epiphyseal) plates.

eponym A name or term for something that is based on the name of a person (or occasionally a place or thing). Traditionally in medicine, discoveries often are named after the person or people who made the discovery.

e-prescribing The use of electronic devices to communicate with pharmacies and send prescribing information, taking the place of writing a prescription by hand and physically giving it to a patient; new or refill prescriptions can be submitted electronically, cutting down on fraud and errors.

equities The monetary value of a property or of an interest in a property in excess of claims or liens against it.

erroneous (eh-ro'-ne-uhs) Containing or characterized by error or assumption.

erythropoietin (i-rith-ruh-poi-e'-tuhn) A substance released by the kidneys and liver that promotes red blood cell formation.

eschar Devitalized skin that forms a scab or a dry crust over a burn area.

esophageal varices (i-sah-fuh-je'-uhl var'-uh-sez) Varicose veins of the esophagus that occur as a result of portal hypertension; these vessels can easily hemorrhage.

essential hypertension Elevated blood pressure of unknown cause that develops for no apparent reason; sometimes called *primary hypertension.*

established patient (EP) A patient who has received professional services (face to face) from the physician, or from another physician of the *exact* same specialty *and subspecialty* who belongs to the same group practice, within the past 3 years.

etiology The science and study of the causes of disease. The cause of a disorder; a claim may be classified according to the etiology.

eukaryotes (yoo-kar'-e-ohts) Single-celled or multicellular organisms with cells that contain a distinct, membrane-bound nucleus.

euthanasia (yu-thuh-na'-zhe-uh) The act or practice of killing or permitting the death of hopelessly sick or injured individuals in a relatively painless way for reasons of mercy.

exacerbation An increase in the seriousness of a disease, marked by greater intensity of the signs and symptoms.

excludes Exclusion terms are always written in italics, and the word *excludes* often is enclosed in a box to draw particular attention to these instructions. Exclusion terms may apply to a chapter, a section, a category, or a subcategory. The applicable code number usually follows the exclusion term. An *excludes* note under a code indicates that the terms excluded from the code are to be coded elsewhere. The term *Excludes* means "DO NOT CODE HERE."

exclusions Limitations on an insurance contract for which benefits are not payable.

excoriated Skin that has been injured by scratching; abraded.

expediency (ik-spe'-de-un-se) A means of achieving a particular end, as in a situation requiring haste or caution.

expert witnesses People who provide testimony to a court as experts in certain fields or subjects to verify facts presented by one or both sides in a lawsuit, often compensated and used to refute or disprove the claims of one party.

explanation of benefits (EOB) A letter or statement from the insurance carrier describing what was paid, denied, or reduced in payment. It also contains information about amounts applied to the deductible, the patient's co-insurance, and the allowed amounts.

explanation of Medicare Benefits (EOMB) An explanation of benefits from Medicare (see *explanation of benefits [EOB]*).

external noise Sounds or factors outside the brain that interfere with the communication process.

externalization The attribution of an event or occurrence to causes outside the self.

externship (or internship) A training program that is part of the medical assisting course of study in an educational institution. This part of training is taken in the actual business setting of that field of study; the terms are interchanged in some areas of the country.

extrinsic (eks-trin'-zik) External to a thing, its essential nature, or its original character.

exudates (ek'-syu-dats) Fluids with high concentrations of protein and cellular debris that have escaped from the blood vessels and have been deposited in tissues or on tissue surfaces.

familial Occurring in or affecting members of a family more than would be expected by chance.

fascia A sheet or band of fibrous tissue deep in the skin that covers muscles and body organs.

fastidious Requiring specialized media or growth factors to grow.

febrile (feb'-ril) Pertaining to an elevated body temperature.

fecalith (fe'-kuh-lith) A hard, impacted mass of feces in the colon.

fee for service An established schedule of fees set for services performed by providers and paid by the patient.

fee profile A compilation or average of physicians' fees over a given period.

fee schedule A compilation of pre-established fee allowances for given services or procedures.

feedback The transmission of evaluative or corrective information to the original or controlling source about an action, event, or process.

felony A major crime, such as murder, rape, or burglary; punishable by a more stringent sentence than that given for a misdemeanor.

fermentation (fur-men-ta'-shun)   An enzymatically controlled transformation of an organic compound.

fervent   Exhibiting or marked by great intensity of feeling.

fibrillation   Rapid, random, ineffective contractions of the heart.

fidelity (fuh-de'-luh-te)   Faithfulness to something to which one is bound by pledge or duty.

filtrate   The fluid that remains after a liquid is passed through a membranous filter.

fine   A sum imposed as punishment for an offense; a forfeiture or penalty paid to an injured party or the government in a civil or criminal action.

fiscal agent   An organization under contract to the government (and some private plans) to act as financial representatives in handling insurance claims from providers of healthcare; also referred to as a *fiscal intermediary*.

fiscal intermediary   An organization that contracts with the government to handle and mediate insurance claims from medical facilities, home health agencies, or providers of medical services or supplies.

fiscal year   An accounting period of 12 months during which a company determines earnings and profit; the fiscal year does not necessarily begin in January; the business determines the beginning of its fiscal year.

fissures   Narrow slits or clefts in the abdominal wall.

fistula (fis'-chuh-luh)   An abnormal, tubelike passage between internal organs or from an internal organ to the body's surface.

flash drive   A small, portable device that can carry 2 to 8 gigabytes or more of information and that plugs into a USB port; also called a *thumb drive, jump drive,* or *portable drive.*

flatus   Gas expelled through the anus.

flora   Microbes that live on or in the body that perform vital functions and protect the body against infection.

fluoroscopy (floo-ros'-kuh-pe)   Direct observation of an x-ray image in motion.

flush   Directly abutting or immediately adjacent, as set even with an edge of a type page or column; having no indention.

follicle-stimulating hormone (FSH)   A hormone secreted by the anterior pituitary; it stimulates oogenesis and spermatogenesis.

fomites   Contaminated, nonliving objects (e.g., examination room equipment) that can transmit infectious organisms.

fontanelles   A space covered by thick membranes between the sutures of an infant's skull; called the baby's "soft spots"; there are both anterior and posterior fontanelles.

formulary   A list of drugs compiled by a health insurance company that identifies the drugs the insurance company will cover under benefits.

fornix   A recess in the upper part of the vagina caused by the protrusion of the cervix into the vaginal wall.

fovea centralis (fo'-ve-uhl/sen-trah'-luhs)   A small pit in the center of the retina that is considered the center of clearest vision.

free radicals   Compounds with at least one unpaired electron, which makes the compound unstable and highly reactive. Free radicals are believed to damage cell components, ultimately leading to cancer, heart disease, and other diseases.

frontal projection   A radiographic view in which the coronal plane of the body or body part is parallel to the film plane; AP or PA.

fundus   The curved, top portion of the uterus; the fundal height can be used as a measurement of fetal growth and to estimate gestation.

gait   Manner or style of walking.

gametes (ga'-meets)   Mature male or female germ cells, usually possessing a haploid chromosome set and capable of initiating formation of a new diploid individual; a sex cell, whether sperm or ovum.

gangrene   The death of body tissue as a result of loss of nutritive supply, followed by bacterial invasion and putrefaction.

gantry   A doughnut-shaped portion of a scanner that surrounds the patient and functions, at least partly, to gather imaging data.

generic   A term for a medication that is not protected by trademark.

genome (jeh'-nom)   The genetic material of an organism.

genuineness   Expressing sincerity and honest feeling.

genus   A breakdown of a family of microorganisms.

germicides (jur'-muh-sids)   Agents that destroy pathogenic organisms.

gigabyte (GB)   Approximately 1 billion bytes.

girth   A measure around a body or an item.

gleaned   Gathered bit by bit (e.g., information or material); picked over in search of relevant material.

glomerulonephritis (glo-mer'-yoo-loh-nih-fri'-tuhs)   Inflammation of the glomerulus of the kidney.

gluconeogenesis (glu-kuh-ne-uh-je'-nuh-suhs)   The formation of glucose in the liver from proteins and fats.

glycogen   The sugar (starch) formed from glucose; it is stored mainly in the liver.

glycosuria   The abnormal presence of glucose in the urine.

gold standard   The paragon of excellence; the diagnostic test to which all others are compared.

goniometer   An instrument for measuring the degrees of motion in a joint.

gonioscopy (goh-nee-os'-kuh-pee)   A procedure in which a mirrored optical instrument is used to visualize the filtration angle of the anterior chamber of the eye; the procedure is used to diagnose glaucoma.

government plans   Entitlement programs or healthcare plans that are sponsored and/or subsidized by the state or federal government, such as Medicaid and Medicare.

gradients   A change in parameters or the value of a quantity, such as temperature or pressure; a change in response with distance from the stimulus; a graded difference in physiological activity along an axis, as of the body or embryonic fluid.

grammar   The study of the classes of words, their inflections, and their functions and relations in the sentence; a study of what is preferred and what should be avoided in inflection and syntax.

Gray (Gy)   The international unit of radiation dose.

grief   Reaction to an unfortunate outcome; a deep distress caused by bereavement, a loss, or a perceived loss.

group policy   Insurance written under a policy that covers a number of people under a single master contract issued to their employer or to an association with which they are affiliated.

growth hormone (GH)   A hormone that stimulates tissue growth and restricts tissue glucose dependence when nutrients are not available. Also called *somatotropic hormone.*

guarantor   The person responsible for paying a medical bill.

guardian ad litem   Legal representative for a minor.

guidelines   Found at the beginning of each section of the coding manual, guidelines are the specific definitions of items that must be read to appropriately interpret and report the procedures and services contained in that section.

hard copy The readable paper copy or printout of information.

hardware The physical components of the computer system, such as the central processing unit (CPU), monitor, and printer.

harmonious Marked by accord in sentiment or action; having the parts agreeably related.

HCPCS *Health Care Common Procedural Coding System;* also called *Level II codes.* HCPCS codes were created by the CMS to report supplies, materials, injections, and certain procedures and services not defined in the CPT manual.

health insurance Insurance protection, provided in return for periodic premium payments, that provides reimbursement of expenses resulting from illness or injury. It includes accident, disability income, medical expense, and accidental death and dismemberment insurance. Also known as *accident and health insurance* or *disability income insurance.*

Health Insurance Portability and Accountability Act (HIPAA) A law enacted in 1996 to improve the portability and continuity of health insurance coverage; to combat waste, fraud, and abuse in health insurance and healthcare delivery; to promote the use of medical savings accounts; to improve access to long-term care services and coverage; to simplify the administration of health insurance; and to serve other purposes. As a result, standards have been created for electronic health information transactions and for the privacy of health information. Also known as the Kassebaum-Kennedy Act.

health maintenance organization (HMO) An organization that provides a wide range of comprehensive healthcare services for a specified group at a fixed periodic payment. HMOs can be sponsored by the government, medical schools, hospitals, employers, labor unions, consumer groups, insurance companies, and hospital-medical plans.

healthcare providers Providers of medical or health services, individually or as organizations, that furnish, bill for, or are paid for services or products.

hematemesis (hi-mat-uh-me´-sis) Vomiting of bright red blood, indicating rapid upper gastrointestinal (GI) bleeding; associated with esophageal varices or peptic ulcer.

hematocrit The percentage by volume of packed red blood cells in a given sample of blood after centrifugation.

hematopoiesis (hi-ma-tuh-poi-e´-suhs) The formation and development of blood cells in the red bone marrow.

hematuria (hi-ma-tuhr´-e-uh) Blood in the urine.

hemoconcentration A condition in which the concentration of blood cells is increased in proportion to the plasma.

hemoglobin (he´-muh-glo-buhn) A protein found in erythrocytes that transports molecular oxygen in the blood.

hemolysis (hi-muh´-luh-sis) The destruction or dissolution of red blood cells, with subsequent release of hemoglobin.

hemolyzed A term used to describe a blood sample in which the red blood cells have ruptured.

hepatomegaly (he-puh-to-me´-guh-le) Abnormal enlargement of the liver.

hereditary (huh-re´-duh-ter-e) Pertaining to a characteristic, condition, or disease transmitted from parent to offspring on the DNA chain.

hermetically (hur-met´-ik-lee) sealed Sealed so that no air can enter.

hertz A unit of measurement used in hearing examinations; a wave frequency equal to 1 cycle per second.

history and physical examination (H&P, HPE) At the patient's first visit with a new physician or an established provider or upon admission to a hospital, the history and physical examination (H&P) are documented. The H&P normally includes the chief complaint, a review of systems (ROS), the patient's personal and family medical history, a physical examination, an assessment of the findings from the history and physical exam, and a treatment plan for the patient, also referred to as Medical Decision Making (MDM).

holder The person who presents a check for payment.

holistic (ho-lis´-tik) A health viewpoint that considers all the systems of the body and their interdependence, rather than breaking down the body into discrete parts.

homeopathy (ho-me-uh´-puh-the) A type of alternative medicine that attempts to stimulate the body to recover by itself; a system of therapy based on the concept that disease can be treated with minute doses of drugs thought capable of producing the same symptoms in healthy people as the disease itself.

homeostasis Internal adaptation and change in response to environmental factors; multiple functions that attempt to keep the body's functions in balance.

honorarium A payment in recognition of acts or professional services, usually on a special occasion.

hospice (hos´-pus) A concept of care that involves health professionals and volunteers who provide medical, psychological, and spiritual support to terminally ill patients and their loved ones.

HTML The acronym for *hypertext markup language,* the language used to create documents for the Internet.

HTTP The acronym for *hypertext transfer protocol,* which defines how messages are formatted and transmitted over the Internet. When a URL is entered into the computer, an HTTP command tells the Web server to retrieve the requested Web page.

hub A common connection point for devices in a network with multiple ports, often used to connect segments of a local area network (LAN).

human chorionic gonadotropin (HCG) A hormone secreted by the placenta that is found in the urine of pregnant females.

hydrocephaly (hi-dro-suh´-fuh-le) Enlargement of the cranium caused by abnormal accumulation of cerebrospinal fluid within the cerebral system.

hydrogenated (hi-drah´-juh-na-ted) Combined with, treated with, or exposed to hydrogen.

hypercapnia (hi-per-kap´-ne-uh) Excess levels of carbon dioxide in the blood.

hypercholesterolemia (hi-per-kuh-les-tuh-ruh-le´-me-uh) Elevated blood levels of cholesterol.

hyperplasia An increase in the number of normal cells.

hyperpnea (hahy-perp-nee´-uh) An increase in the depth of breathing.

hypertension High blood pressure.

hyperventilation Abnormally prolonged and deep breathing, usually associated with acute anxiety or emotional tension.

hypotension Blood pressure that is below normal (systolic pressure below 90 mm Hg and diastolic pressure below 50 mm Hg).

icons Pictures, often on the monitor screen "desktop," that represent programs or objects. Clicking on an icon directs the user to the program.

idealism The practice of forming ideas or living under the influence of ideas.

idiopathic Pertaining to a condition or a disease that has no known cause.

ileostomy The surgical formation of an opening of the ileum onto the surface of the abdomen, through which fecal material is emptied.

immunosuppressant A substance that suppresses or prevents an immune system response.

immunotherapy Administration of repeated injections of diluted extracts of a substance that causes an allergy; also called *desensitization.*

impaired Being in a less than perfect or less than whole condition; it includes having handicaps or functional defects and being under the influence of drugs, alcohol, and/or controlled substances.

impenetrable Incapable of being penetrated or pierced; not capable of being damaged or harmed.

implied consent Presumed consent, such as when a patient offers an arm for a phlebotomy procedure.

implied contract A legally enforceable agreement that arises from conduct, from assumed intentions, from some relationship among the immediate parties, or from the application of the legal principle of equity.

in balance The state in which the total ending balances of patient ledgers equals the total of accounts receivable.

in vitro Referring to conditions outside of a living body.

incentives Things that incite or spur to action; rewards or reasons for performing a task.

incidental disclosure A secondary use of health information that cannot reasonably be prevented, is limited in nature, and occurs as a result of another use or disclosure that is permitted.

includes When this term appears under a subdivision, such as a category (three-digit code) or two-digit procedure code title, it indicates that the code and title include these terms. Other terms also classified to that particular code and title are listed in the Alphabetic Index.

incomplete claim A claim that is missing information and is returned to the provider for correction and resubmission. Also called an *invalid claim.*

incurred To become liable or subject to; to bring down upon oneself.

indemnity plans Traditional health insurance plans that pay for all or a share of the cost of covered services, regardless of which physician, hospital, or other licensed healthcare provider is used. Policyholders of indemnity plans and their dependents choose when and where to get healthcare services.

indicators An important point or group of statistical values that, when evaluated, indicates the quality of care provided in a healthcare facility.

indicted (in-di´-ted) Charged with a crime by the finding of a jury according to due process of law.

indigent (in´-di-junt) A needy or poor person who is unable to provide the basic necessities of life; totally lacking in something of need.

indirect filing system A filing system in which an intermediary source of reference (e.g., a card file) must be consulted to locate specific files.

individual policy An insurance policy designed specifically for the use of one person and his or her dependents. An individual policy generally does not offer some of the amenities of a group policy (e.g., lower premiums). Often called *personal insurance.*

individually identifiable health information Any part of a patient's health record that is created or received by a covered entity.

induration (in-doo-rey´-shuhn) An abnormally hard, inflamed area.

infarction An area of tissue that has died from lack of blood supply.

infection Invasion of body tissues by microorganisms, which then proliferate and damage tissues.

inferred Derived as a conclusion from facts and premises.

infertile Not fertile or productive; not capable of reproducing.

inflammation A tissue reaction to trauma or disease that includes redness, heat, swelling, and pain.

inflection (in-flek´-shun) A change in the pitch or loudness of the voice.

informed consent A consent, usually written, that states understanding of what treatment is to be undertaken and of the risks involved, why it should be done, and alternative methods of treatment available (including no treatment) and their attendant risks.

infractions (in-frak´-shuns) Breaking the law; minor offenses against the rules, usually punishable by fines.

initiative Energy or aptitude to cause or facilitate the start of something or to cause something to happen.

innate Existing in, belonging to, or determined by factors present in an individual since birth.

innocuous (i´-nuh-kyu-wus) Having no effect, adverse or otherwise; harmless.

input Information entered into and used by the computer.

instigate To goad or urge forward; to provoke.

insubordination (in-suh´-bor-din-a-shun) Disobedience to authority.

insured An individual or organization covered by an insurance policy according to the policy terms; usually, the individual or group that pays the premiums. Blue Cross/Blue Shield refers to this person or group as the *subscriber.*

intangibles (in-tan´-juh-buls) Qualities that cannot be perceived, especially by touch, or cannot be precisely identified or realized by the mind.

integral (in´-ti-grul) Essential; being an indispensable part of a whole.

integrated delivery system (IDS) A network of healthcare providers and organizations that provides or arranges to provide a coordinated continuum of services to a defined population and is willing to be held clinically and fiscally accountable for the clinical outcomes and health status of the population served.

integrated Formed, coordinated, or blended into a functioning or unified whole; to incorporate into a larger unit.

intelligent character recognition (ICR) The electronic scanning of printed blocks as images and the use of special software to recognize these images (or characters) as ASCII text for uploading into a computer database.

interaction A two-way communication; mutual or reciprocal action or influence.

intercellular A term referring to the area between cells.

intercom A two-way communication system with a microphone and loudspeaker at each station for localized use.

interferon (in´-tuhr-fir-on) A protein formed when a cell is exposed to a virus; the protein blocks viral action on the cell and protects against viral invasion.

interleukin (in-tehr-loo´-kin) A protein produced by certain white blood cells that regulates immune responses by activating lymphocytes and initiating fever.

intermittent Coming and going at intervals; not continuous.

intermittent claudication Recurring cramping in the calves caused by poor circulation of blood to the muscles of the lower leg.

intermittent pulse A pulse in which beats occasionally are skipped.

internal noise Factors inside the brain that interfere with the communication process.

***International Classification of Diseases, Ninth Revision, Clinical Modification* (ICD-9-CM)** The manual that establishes the system for classifying disease to facilitate collection of uniform and comparable health information for statistical purposes, for indexing medical records for data storage and retrieval, and to facilitate payment.

international mail Mail that is sent outside the boundaries of the United States and its territories.

***International Statistical Classifications of Diseases and Related Health Problems, Tenth Revision, Clinical Modification* (ICD-10-CM)** The current ICM rules manual, which contains the greatest number of changes in the ICD-CM system in ICD history. To allow more specific reporting of diseases and newly recognized conditions, the ICD-10-CM contains approximately 55,000 more codes than the ICD-9-CM.

interoperable The capability of a system to work with or use the parts or equipment of another system.

interval Space of time between events.

intolerable Not tolerable or bearable.

intracellular A term referring to the area within the cell membrane.

intravenous urogram (IVU) Radiographic examination of the urinary tract using intravenous injection of an iodine contrast medium.

intrinsic (in-trin´-zik) Belonging to the essential nature or constitution of a thing; indwelling, inward.

introspection (in-truh-spek´-shun) An inward, reflective examination of one's own thoughts and feelings.

invariably (in-var´-e-uh-buh-le) Consistently; not changing or capable of change.

invasive Involving entry into the living body, as by incision or insertion of an instrument.

invoice A paper describing a purchase and the amount due.

ipsilateral (ips-uh-la´-tehr-uhl) Pertaining to the same side of the body.

ischemia (is-ke´-mia) A decreased supply of oxygenated blood to an area or a body part.

jargon The technical terminology or characteristic idiom of a particular group or special activity, as opposed to lay terms.

jaundice A yellow discoloration of the skin and mucous membranes caused by deposits of bile pigments; these deposits occur because of excess bilirubin in the blood.

judicial (ju-di´-shuhl) Of or relating to a judgment, the function of judging, the administration of justice, or the judiciary.

jurisdiction (jur-uhs-dik´-shun) A power constitutionally conferred on a judge or magistrate to decide cases according to law and to carry sentence into execution; jurisdiction is original when it is conferred on the court in the first instance, called original jurisdiction; or

it is appellate when an appeal is given from the judgment of another court.

jurisprudence (jur-uhs-proo´-dens) The science or philosophy of law; a system or body of law or the course of court decisions.

justice With regard to medical ethics, the fair distribution of benefits and burdens among individuals or groups in society with legitimate claims on those benefits.

Kaposi's sarcoma A malignant tumor of endothelial cells that begins as brown or purple papules on the feet and slowly spreads in the skin.

keloid A raised, firm scar formation caused by overgrowth of collagen at the site of a skin injury.

keratin A very hard, tough protein found in the hair, nails, and epidermal tissue.

keratinocytes The skin cells that synthesize keratin.

kilobyte (KB) Approximately 1,024 bytes.

kyphotic (kahy-fot´-ik) A term referring to the normal convex curvature of the thoracic spine.

lacrimation (la-krihm-a´-shun) The secretion or discharge of tears.

language barrier Any type of interference that inhibits the communication process and is related to languages spoken by the people attempting to communicate.

laryngoscopy (lar-uhn-gahs´-kuh-pe) Visual examination of the voice box area through an endoscope equipped with a light and mirrors for illumination.

latent image Invisible changes in exposed film that become an image when the film is processed.

lateral projections Radiographic views in which the sagittal plane of the body or body part is parallel to the film.

law A binding custom or practice of a community; a rule of conduct or action prescribed or formally recognized as binding or enforceable by a controlling authority.

learning style The way an individual perceives and processes information to learn new material.

leukoderma Lack of skin pigmentation, especially in patches.

liabilities Things that are owed; debts.

liable (li´-uh-buhl) Obligated according to law or equity; responsible for an act or circumstance.

liaison A close bond or connection; a person with a connection, contract, link, or conspiracy with another person or group.

libel A written defamatory statement or representation that conveys an unjustly unfavorable impression.

ligaments Tough connective tissue bands that hold joints together by attaching to the bones on either side of the joint.

limited radiography A limited-scope radiography practice, usually in an outpatient setting, that does not require the same credentials as for professional radiologic technology; also called *practical radiography*.

lithotripsy (li´-thuh-trip-se) A procedure for eliminating a kidney stone or gallstone by crushing or dissolving it in situ through the use of high-intensity sound waves.

litigious (luh-ti´-juhs) Prone to engage in lawsuits.

loading dose A large dose administered as the first dose of a medication; it usually is used in antibiotic therapy to quickly achieve therapeutic blood levels of the drug.

lordotic (lor-do´-tik) A term referring to the normal concave curvature of the cervical and lumbar spines.

lower gastrointestinal series   Fluoroscopic examination of the colon, usually using rectal administration of barium sulfate as a contrast medium; also called a *barium enema.*

lumbar   A term referring to the lower back region, which contains the five lumbar vertebrae.

lumen   An open space, such as within a blood vessel or the intestine, or the inside of a needle or an examining instrument.

luteinizing hormone (LH) (lu-te-uh-niz'-ing)   A hormone produced by the anterior pituitary gland that promotes ovulation.

luxation   Dislocation of a bone from its normal anatomic location.

lymphadenopathy (lim-fa-duh-nah'-puh-the)   Any disorder of the lymph nodes or lymph vessels.

lymphedema (limf-uh-de'-muh)   Swelling caused by the accumulation of lymph fluid in soft tissues.

macromolecules   The molecules needed for metabolism: carbohydrates, lipids, proteins, and nucleic acids.

macular degeneration   Progressive deterioration of the macula of the eye, causing loss of central vision.

magnetic resonance imaging (MRI)   An imaging modality that uses a magnetic field and radiofrequency pulses to create computer images of both bones and soft tissues in multiple planes.

main term   The primary or key word or words abstracted from a medical record that are used to begin the code search in the Alphabetic Index. A main term can identify a procedure or service performed; an organ or anatomic site; a condition, illness, or injury; or an eponym, abbreviation, or acronym.

Main Text   See Tabular Index.

maker   Any individual, corporation, or legal party who signs a check or any type of negotiable instrument.

malaise (muh-laz')   An indefinite feeling of debility or lack of health, often indicative of or accompanying the onset of an illness.

malediction (ma-luh-dik'-shun)   Speaking evil or the calling of a curse.

malignant   Cancerous.

managed care plans   An umbrella term for all healthcare plans that provide healthcare in return for preset monthly payments and coordinated care through a defined network of primary care physicians and hospitals.

manifestation (ma-nuh-fuh-sta'-shun)   Something that is easily understood or recognized by the mind. *Also,* an indication of the existence, reality, or presence of something, especially an illness.

Marfan syndrome   An inherited condition characterized by elongation of the bones, joint hypermobility, abnormalities of the eyes, and the development of an aortic aneurysm.

marketing   The process or technique of promoting, selling, and distributing a product or service.

matrix   Something in which a thing originates, develops, takes shape, or is contained; a base on which to build.

m-banking   Banking through the use of mobile devices, such as cell phones and wireless Internet services.

media   A term applied to agencies of mass communication, such as newspapers, magazines, and telecommunications.

mediastinum (meh-de-ast'-uhn-um)   The space in the center of the chest under the sternum.

Medicaid   A federal- and state-sponsored health insurance program for the medically indigent.

medical savings accounts (MSAs)   Tax-deferred bank or savings accounts that are combined with a low-premium, high-deductible insurance policy; they are designed for individuals or families who choose to fund their own healthcare expenses and medical insurance.

medically indigent   Able to take care of ordinary living expenses but unable to afford medical care.

Medicare   A federally sponsored health insurance program for those over age 65 and for individuals under age 65 who are disabled.

Medigap   A term sometimes applied to private insurance products that supplement Medicare insurance benefits.

medullary cavity   The inner portion of the diaphysis; it contains the bone marrow.

megabyte (MB)   Approximately 1 million bytes.

megahertz (MHz)   The measuring device for microprocessors. A megahertz is 1 million cycles of electromagnetic currency alternation per second and is used as a unit of measure for the clock speed of computer microprocessors.

meniscus (meh-nis'-kus)   The curved surface of liquids in a container.

mentors   Trusted counselors or guides.

metabolic alkalosis   A condition characterized by significant loss of acid in the body or an increased amount of bicarbonate; severe metabolic alkalosis can lead to coma and death.

metabolite   The product of the metabolism of a substance, such as a drug.

meticulous (meh-tiku'-luhs)   Marked by extreme or excessive care in the consideration or treatment of details.

microcephaly   Small size of the head in relation to the rest of the body.

microfilm   A film with a photographic record of printed or other graphic matter on a reduced scale.

micromanage   To manage with great or excessive control or attention to details.

microorganisms   Organisms of microscopic or submicroscopic size.

miotic (mi-ah'-tik)   Any substance or medication that causes constriction of the pupil.

misdemeanor (mis-duh-me'-nuhr)   A minor crime, as opposed to a felony, punishable by fine or imprisonment in a city or county jail rather than in a penitentiary.

mitigating   To cause to become less harsh or hostile; to make less severe or painful.

mock   Simulated; intended for imitation or practice.

modem   Short for *modulator-demodulator;* a device that allows information to be transmitted over telephone lines at speeds measured in bits per second (bps). The modem speed generally is listed somewhere on the unit.

modifiers   Terms that serve as the means to report or indicate that a service or procedure performed has been altered by some specific circumstance but not changed in its definition or code.

modifying terms   Key words selected after the main term has been chosen to help further define or describe the procedure or service performed.

molecules   Groups of like or different atoms held together by chemical forces.

mononuclear white blood cells   Leukocytes with an unsegmented nucleus; monocytes and lymphocytes in particular.

monotone   A succession of syllables, words, or sentences in an unvaried key or pitch.

mons pubis   The fat pad that covers the symphysis pubis.

morale (mo-ral′)   The mental and emotional condition, enthusiasm, loyalty, or confidence of an individual or group with regard to the function or tasks at hand.

motivation   The process of inciting a person to some action or behavior.

multimedia   The presentation of graphics, animation, video, sound, and text on a computer in an integrated way or all at once. CD-ROMs are efficient multimedia devices.

multiparous   Pertaining to women who have had two or more pregnancies.

multitasking   Performing multiple tasks at the same time.

municipal (myu-ni′-suh-puhl) courts   Courts that sit in some cities and larger towns and that usually have civil and criminal jurisdiction over cases arising within the municipality.

mydriatic (mid-ree-at′-ik)   A topical ophthalmic medication that dilates the pupil; it is used in diagnostic procedures of the eye and as treatment for glaucoma.

myelin sheath   A segmented, fatty tissue that wraps around the axon of the nerve cell and acts as an electrical insulator to speed the conduction of nerve impulses.

myelography (mi-uh-log′-ruh-fe)   Fluoroscopic examination of the spinal canal, in which spinal injection of an iodine contrast medium is performed.

myelomeningocele   A herniation of a portion of the spinal cord and its meninges that protrudes through a congenital opening in the vertebral column.

myocardial (my-oh-kar′-de-uhl)   Pertaining to the heart muscle.

myocardium (my-oh-kar′-de-um)   The muscular lining of the heart.

myoglobinuria   The abnormal presence of a hemoglobinlike chemical of muscle tissue in the urine; it is the result of muscle deterioration.

mysticism   The experience of seeming to have direct communication with God or ultimate reality.

nanometer   Units that measure 1 billionth (10^{-9}) of a meter.

National Provider Identifier (NPI)   A lifetime number consisting of 10 digits that Medicare uses to replace the Provider Identification Number (PIN) and the Unique Physician Identification Number (UPIN).

naturopathy (na-chu-ra′-puh-the)   An alternative to conventional medicine in which holistic methods are used, in addition to herbs and natural supplements, with the belief that the body will heal itself. Naturopathic physicians currently can be licensed in 15 states, Puerto Rico, and the Virgin Islands.

near miss   A situation in which an error is caught or corrected before it affects the patient.

necrosis (neh-kroh′-sis)   The death of cells or tissues.

negligence (ne′-gli-jents)   Failure to exercise the care a prudent person usually exercises; implies inattention to one's duty or business; implies want of due or necessary diligence or care.

negotiable   Legally transferable to another party.

networking   Exchange of information or services among individuals, groups, or institutions. *Also,* meeting and getting to know individuals in the same or similar career fields and sharing information about available opportunities.

neural tube defects   Congenital malformations of the skull and spinal column caused by failure of the neural tube to close during embryonic development; the neural tube is the origin of the brain, spinal cord, and other central nervous system tissue.

new patient (NP)   A patient who has *not* received any professional services (face to face) from the physician or another physician of the *exact* same specialty *and subspecialty* who belongs to the same group practice, within the past 3 years.

nocturia   Excessive urination during the night.

nomogram   A graph on which variables are plotted so that a particular value can be read on the appropriate line.

nonmaleficence (non-mal-fe′-zens)   Refraining from the act of harming or committing evil.

nonstress tests (NSTs)   Fetal monitoring used in combination with maternal reports of fetal movement to evaluate the fetal heart rate response.

no-show   A person who fails to keep an appointment without giving advance notice.

nosocomial (no-suh-ko′-me-uhl)   Originating or taking place in a hospital.

notations   Found in both the Alphabetic Index and the Tabular Index, notations are instructions or guides in classification assignments, defining category content or the use of subdivision codes; also called *instructional notations.*

notebook   Although often used interchangeably with "laptop," this term was created to identify a smaller, thinner, and lighter device, partially designed to fit on tray tables on airplanes.

NPO   Nothing by mouth, from the Latin *nil per os.*

nuclear medicine   An imaging modality in which radioactive materials are injected or ingested into the body to provide information about the function of organs and tissues.

numeric filing   The filing of records, correspondence, or cards by number.

obesity   Excessive accumulation of body fat; defined as a body mass index (BMI) of 30 or higher.

objective information   Information gathered by watching or observing a patient.

objective   Something toward which effort is directed; aim, goal, or purpose of action.

oblique projections   Radiographic views in which the body or part is rotated so that the projection is neither frontal nor lateral.

obliteration (uh-bli-tuh-ra′-shun)   The act of making undecipherable or imperceptible by obscuring or wearing away.

obturator   A metal rod with a smooth, rounded tip that is placed in hollow instruments to reduce injury to body tissues during insertion.

occlusion   Complete obstruction of an opening.

Office for Civil Rights (OCR)   The division of the federal government that enforces privacy standards.

Office of the Inspector General (OIG)   An office of the U.S. Department of Health and Human Services that conducts audits, investigations, and inspections involving laws pertaining to health and human services.

opaque   Not translucent or transparent; murky.

opinions   Formal expressions of judgment or advice by an expert; formal expressions of the legal reasons and principles on which a legal decision is based.

opportunistic infections Infections caused by a normally nonpathogenic organism in a host whose resistance has been decreased.

optimistic Inclined to put the most favorable construction on actions and events or to anticipate the best possible outcome.

ordinance (or'-di-nens) Authoritative decree or direction; law set forth by a governmental authority, specifically, municipal regulation.

organelles (or-guh-nels') Differentiated structures within a cell (e.g., mitochondria, vacuoles, and chloroplasts) that perform a specific function.

orthopnea (or-thop'-nee-uh) A condition that requires an individual to sit or stand to breathe comfortably.

orthostatic (postural) hypotension A temporary fall in blood pressure when a person rapidly changes from a recumbent position to a standing position.

osteopathic (us-te-uh-path'-ik) A term describing the type of medicine that is based on the theory that disturbances in the musculoskeletal system affect other bodily parts, causing many disorders that can be corrected by various manipulative techniques in conjunction with conventional medical, surgical, pharmacologic, and other therapeutic procedures.

osteoporosis (ah-ste-o-puh-ro'-ses) Loss of bone density; lack of calcium intake is a major factor in its development.

other potentially infectious materials (OPIM) Substances or materials other than blood that have the potential to carry infectious pathogens, such as body fluid, urine, semen, and others.

otitis externa Inflammation or infection of the external auditory canal (swimmer's ear).

OUTfolder A folder used to provide space for the temporary filing of materials.

OUTguide A heavy guide used to replace a folder temporarily removed from the filing space.

output Information processed by the computer and transmitted to a monitor, printer, or other device.

outreach The process of using marketing and education strategies to reach and involve diverse audiences through the use of key messages and effective programs.

outsourcing The practice of subcontracting work to an outside company.

overhead The ongoing administrative expenses of a business that cannot be attributed to any specific business activity but are still necessary for the business to function (e.g., rent, utilities, insurance).

over-the-counter (OTC) drugs Medications sold without a prescription.

packing slip A list of items included in a shipment.

palliative A substance that relieves or alleviates the symptoms of a disease without curing the disease.

palpitations Pounding or racing of the heart, which may or may not indicate a serious heart disorder.

pandemic (pan-de'-mik) A condition in which most people in a country, a number of countries, or a geographic area are affected.

paper (hard copy) claims Insurance claims that have been completed manually, on paper, and sent by surface mail.

papilledema Swelling of the optic disc from increased intracranial pressure.

parameters Any set of physical properties, the values of which determine characteristics or behavior.

paraphrasing To express an idea in different wording in an effort to enhance communication and clarify meaning.

parenteral (puh-ren'-tuh-ruhl) The injection or introduction of substances into the body by any route other than the digestive tract (e.g., subcutaneous, intravenous, or intramuscular administration).

paresthesia (par-uhs-thee'-zee-uh) An abnormal sensation of burning, prickling, or stinging.

paroxysmal (par-ehk-siz'-muhl) Pertaining to a sudden, recurrent spasm of symptoms.

participating provider (PAR) A physician or other healthcare provider who enters into a contract with a specific insurance company or program and by doing so agrees to abide by certain rules and regulations set forth by that particular third-party payer.

parturition (par-too-rih'-shun) The act or process of giving birth to a child.

patency Open condition of a body cavity or canal.

pathogenic (path'-o-jen-ic) Pertaining to a disease-causing microorganism.

pathogens Disease-causing microorganisms.

patient status (PS) The state of a patient as either new or established; appears in the Evaluation and Management section of the CPT.

payables Balances due to a creditor on an account.

payee The person named on a draft or check as the recipient of the amount shown.

payer The person who writes a check in favor of the payee.

peer review organizations (PROs) Groups of medical reviewers contracted by the Centers for Medicare and Medicaid Services (CMS) to ensure quality control and the medical necessity of services provided by a facility.

pegboard system An older method of tracking patient accounts that allows the figures to be proved accurate through mathematic formulas. It is still used in some small to medium practices; also called the *write-it-once system.*

per diem By the day; per day. An allowance for daily expenses.

perceiving (pur-sev'-ing) How an individual looks at information and sees it as real.

perception A quick, acute, and intuitive cognition; a capacity for comprehension.

periosteum The thin, highly innervated, membranous covering of a bone.

peripheral (puh-rif'-er-uhl) A term referring to an area outside of or away from an organ or structure.

peristalsis The rhythmic, involuntary, serial contraction of the smooth muscles lining the GI tract.

perjured testimony The voluntary violation of an oath or vow either by swearing to what is untrue or by omission to do what has been promised under oath; false testimony.

perks Extra advantages or benefits of working in a specific job that may or may not be commonplace in that particular profession; a shortened form of perquisites.

permeable (pur'-me-uh-buhl) Allowing a substance to pass or soak through.

persona (pur-so'-nuh) An individual's social facade or front that reflects the role in life the individual is playing; the personality a person projects in public.

personal digital assistant (PDA) A handheld computer capable of functions such as mobile telephony, Web browsing, and media playing. PDAs typically include an appointment calendar, to-do list, address book, note programs, and e-mail and/ or Web capabilities.

personal health information (PHI) The patient's own information that pertains to his or her health.

personal health record (PHR) An electronic record of health-related information about an individual that conforms to nationally recognized interoperability standards and that *can be drawn from multiple sources but that is managed, shared, and controlled by the individual.*

pertinent (pur′-tuh-nent) Having a clear, decisive relevance to the matter at hand.

petechiae (peh-te′-ke-uh) Small, purplish hemorrhagic spots on the skin.

petty cash fund A fund maintained to pay small, unpredictable cash expenditures.

phenylalanine (fe-nehl-ah′-luh-nen) An essential amino acid found in milk, eggs, and other foods.

philanthropist (fu-lan′-thruh-pist) An individual who makes an active effort to promote human welfare.

philosopher A person who seeks wisdom or enlightenment; an expounder of a theory in a certain area of experience.

phlebitis (fluh-bi′-tis) Inflammation of a vein, with the possible complication of clot formation at the site (thrombophlebitis).

phlebotomy (fli-bah′-tuh-me) An invasive procedure used to obtain a blood specimen for testing, experimentation, or diagnosis of disease.

phonetic (fuh-ne′-tik) Constituting an alteration of ordinary spelling that better represents the spoken language, that uses only characters of the regular alphabet, and that is used in a context of conventional spelling.

phosphors (fos′-fors) Fluorescent crystals that give off light when exposed to x-rays.

photophobia An abnormal sensitivity to light.

phrases Groups of words with a specific grammatical function, such as a noun phrase or an adjective phrase.

physical status The physical condition of the patient.

physician office laboratories (POLs) Laboratories owned by a private physician or corporation, such as the laboratory inside a physician's office or a freestanding laboratory.

physiologic noise Internal interferences comprised of biologic factors within a speaker or listener that hinder effective and accurate communication.

pitch Highness or lowness of a sound; the relative level, intensity, or extent of some quality or state.

place of service (POS) codes Codes used on professional claims to specify the facility or location where the service or services were rendered.

plaintiff The person or group bringing a case or legal action to court.

plaque An abnormal accumulation of a fatty substance.

plasma The liquid portion of whole blood that contains active clotting agents.

policyholder A person who pays a premium to an insurance company and in whose name the policy is written in exchange for the insurance protection provided by a policy of insurance.

polycythemia vera (pah-le-si-the′-me-uh/veh′-rah) A condition marked by an abnormally large number of red blood cells (RBCs) in the circulatory system.

polydipsia Excessive thirst.

polymorphonuclear white blood cells Leukocytes with a segmented nucleus; also known as *polymorphonuclear neutrophils* (PMNs) or *segmented neutrophils.*

polyphagia (pah-le-faj′-e-uh) Increased appetite.

polyps (pah′-lips) Tumors or outgrowths found in the mucosal lining of the colon; they are considered precancerous.

polyuria (pah-le-yur′-e-uh) Excretion of an unusually large amount of urine.

portal circulation The pathway of blood flow through the portal vein from the GI system to the liver.

portal hypertension Increased venous pressure in the portal circulation caused by cirrhosis or compression of the hepatic vascular system.

portfolio A set of pictures, drawings, documents, or photographs either bound in book form or loose in a folder.

posteroanterior (PA) A frontal projection in which the patient is prone or facing the x-ray film or image receptor.

postherpetic neuralgia Pain that lasts longer than a month after a shingles infection and is caused by damage to the nerve; the pain may last for months or years.

posting Entering figures in an accounting system; transferring or carrying from a book of original entry to a ledger.

postmortem Done, collected, or occurring after death.

potentially compensable event (PCE) An adverse occurrence, usually involving a patient, that could result in a financial obligation for a business or organization.

power of attorney A legal instrument authorizing a person to act as the attorney or agent of the grantor.

practicum Another word for the externship; a training program that is a part of the medical assisting course of study in the actual business setting of a medical office or facility. (This term is used by the Commission on Accreditation of Allied Health Education Programs [CAAHEP] to designate the externship.)

preauthorization A process required by some insurance carriers in which the provider obtains permission to perform certain procedures or services or refers a patient to a specialist.

precedence (pre-sed′-ens) To surpass in rank, dignity, or importance; to be, go, or come ahead or in front of.

precedents (pre′-suh-dens) A person or thing that serves as a model; something done or said that may serve as an example or rule to authorize or justify a subsequent act of the same kind.

precertification A process required by some insurance carriers in which the provider must prove medical necessity before performing a procedure.

preclude To rule out in advance.

premium The periodic (monthly, quarterly, or annual) payment of a specific sum of money to an insurance company, for which the insurer in return agrees to provide certain benefits.

preponderance A superiority or excess in number or quantity; a majority.

preponderance of the evidence Evidence of greater weight or more convincing than the evidence offered in opposition to it; evidence that as a whole shows that the fact sought to be proven is more probable than not.

prerequisite (pre-re′-kwe-zut) Something that is necessary to an end or to carry out a function.

present illness The chief complaint, written in chronologic sequence, with dates of onset.

preservatives Substances added to a specimen to prevent deterioration of cells or chemicals.

posting Entering figures in an accounting system; transferring or carrying from a book of original entry to a ledger.

postmortem Done, collected, or occurring after death.

potentially compensable event (PCE) An adverse occurrence, usually involving a patient, that could result in a financial obligation for a business or organization.

power of attorney A legal instrument authorizing a person to act as the attorney or agent of the grantor.

practicum Another word for the externship; a training program that is a part of the medical assisting course of study in the actual business setting of a medical office or facility. (This term is used by the Commission on Accreditation of Allied Health Education Programs [CAAHEP] to designate the externship.)

preauthorization A process required by some insurance carriers in which the provider obtains permission to perform certain procedures or services or refers a patient to a specialist.

precedence (pre-sed'-ens) To surpass in rank, dignity, or importance; to be, go, or come ahead or in front of.

precedents (pre'-suh-dens) A person or thing that serves as a model; something done or said that may serve as an example or rule to authorize or justify a subsequent act of the same kind.

precertification A process required by some insurance carriers in which the provider must prove medical necessity before performing a procedure.

preclude To rule out in advance.

premium The periodic (monthly, quarterly, or annual) payment of a specific sum of money to an insurance company, for which the insurer in return agrees to provide certain benefits.

preponderance A superiority or excess in number or quantity; a majority.

preponderance of the evidence Evidence of greater weight or more convincing than the evidence offered in opposition to it; evidence that as a whole shows that the fact sought to be proven is more probable than not.

prerequisite (pre-re'-kwe-zut) Something that is necessary to an end or to carry out a function.

procurement (pro-kuhr'-ment) To get possession of, to obtain by particular care and effort.

professional behaviors Actions that identify the medical assistant as a member of a healthcare profession, including being dependable, providing respectful patient care, exercising initiative, demonstrating a positive attitude, and working as an effective team member.

professional courtesy Reduction or absence of fees to professional associates.

professionalism The conduct or qualities characterized by or conforming to the technical or ethical standards of a profession; exhibiting a courteous, conscientious, and generally businesslike manner in the workplace.

proficiency (pruh-fi'-shun-se) Competency as a result of training or practice.

profit sharing Offer of a part of a company's profits to employees or other designated individuals or groups.

progress notes Notes used in the medical record to track the patient's progress and condition.

prokaryote (pro-kar'-e-oht) A unicellular organism with cells that lack a membrane-bound nucleus.

prolactin (PRL) A hormone secreted by the anterior pituitary gland that stimulates the development of the mammary gland.

proofread To read and mark corrections.

proprioception The sensation of awareness of body movements and posture; nerve impulses that provide the central nervous system with information about the position of body parts.

prostaglandins (prahs-tih-glan'-dins) Chemicals released from cells that cause smooth muscle contraction and pain.

prosthesis (prahs-the'-suhs) An artificial replacement for a body part.

protected health information (PHI) Any individually identifiable health information that may be transmitted and/or maintained in electronic form.

provider An individual or individuals qualified by education, training, licensure or regulation, and facility privileging who perform a professional service within their scope of practice and independently report that professional service. *Also,* a company that provides medical care and services to a patient or the public.

provider identification number (PIN) A number assigned to providers by a carrier for use in the submission of claims.

provisional diagnosis A temporary diagnosis made before all test results have been received.

proxemics (prok-se'-miks) The study of the nature, degree, and effect of the spatial separation individuals naturally maintain.

prudent Marked by wisdom or judiciousness; shrewd in the management of practical affairs.

psychosocial Pertaining to a combination of psychological and social factors.

psyllium (si'-le-um) A grain found in some cereal products, in certain dietary supplements, and in certain bulk fiber laxatives; a water-soluble fiber.

public domain The realm embracing property rights that belong to the community at large, are unprotected by copyright or patent, and are subject to use or appropriation by anyone.

pulmonary consolidation In pneumonia, the process by which the lungs become solidified as they fill with exudates.

pulse deficit A condition in which the radial pulse is less than the apical pulse; it may indicate a peripheral vascular abnormality.

pulse pressure The difference between systolic and diastolic blood pressures (30 to 50 mm Hg is considered normal).

pure culture A bacterial or fungal culture that contains a single organism.

purging The process of moving active files to inactive status.

putrefaction (pyu-truh-fak'-shun) Decomposition of animal matter, which results in a foul smell.

pyemia (pi-em'-e-uh) The presence of pus-forming organisms in the blood.

pyloric sphincter A muscular ring at the distal end of the stomach that separates the stomach from the duodenum of the small intestine.

pyrexia (pi-rek'-see-a) A febrile condition or fever.

quackery The pretense of curing disease.

quality assurance (QA) Activities designed to increase the quality of a product or service through process or system changes that increase efficiency or effectiveness.

quality control An aggregate of activities designed to ensure adequate quality, especially in manufactured products or in the service industries.

queries Requests for information from a database.

rad The conventional unit of radiation dose.

radiograph An x-ray image.

radiographer A person qualified to perform radiographic examinations.

radiography The process of taking diagnostic images using x-rays.

radiologist A physician who specializes in medical imaging or therapeutic applications of radiation.

radiolucent (ra-de-o-loo'-suhnt) Pertaining to a substance that is easily penetrated by x-rays; these substances appear dark on radiographs.

radiopaque A substance that can easily be visualized on an x-ray film.

rales Abnormal or crackling breath sounds during inspiration.

ramifications (ra-muh-fuh-ka'-shuns) Consequences produced by a cause or following from a set of conditions.

range of motion (ROM) The extent of movement possible in a joint; the degree of motion depends on the type of joint and whether a disease process is present; ROM exercises are applied actively (independently) or passively (with assistance) to prevent or treat joint problems.

rapport (ra-por') A relationship of harmony and accord between the patient and the healthcare professional.

Raynaud's phenomenon Intermittent attacks of ischemia of the extremities, resulting in cyanosis, numbness, tingling, and pain.

ream A quantity of paper weighing 20 lb or consisting of, variously, 480, 500, or 516 sheets.

reasonable cause Circumstances that would make it unreasonable for the covered entity, despite the exercise of ordinary business care and prudence, to comply with the administrative simplification provision that was violated.

reasonable diligence The business care and prudence expected from a person seeking to satisfy a legal requirement under similar circumstances.

reasonable doubt Doubt based on reason and arising from evidence or lack of evidence; it is not doubt that is imagined or conjured up, but doubt that would cause reasonable persons to hesitate before acting.

receipts Amounts paid on patient accounts.

receivables Total payments received on accounts.

recipient The receiver of some thing or item.

reciprocity The mutual exchange of privileges; a recognition of one state or institution of the licenses or privileges granted by the other.

reconciliation The process of proving that a bank statement and checkbook balance are in agreement.

recourse A turning to something or someone for help or protection.

rectify (rek'-tuh-fy)

reduction The return to correct anatomic position, as in reduction of a fracture.

referral An insurance term used when a primary care provider wants to send a patient to a specialist. Typically, the provider must obtain authorization from the insurance carrier in advance to refer a patient.

referral laboratory A private or hospital-based laboratory that performs a wide variety of tests, many of them specialized; physicians often send specimens collected in the office to referral laboratories for testing.

reflection (re-flek'-shun) The process of considering new information and internalizing it to create new ways of examining information.

refractile (re-frak'-tuhl) Causing light to refract or bend, thus creating a sharp boundary or image.

registered dietitian (RD) An individual with a minimum of a bachelor's degree in food and nutrition who is concerned with the maintenance and promotion of health and the treatment of diseases through diet.

reimbursement Payment of benefits to the physician for services rendered according to the guidelines of the third-party payer.

rejected claims Claims returned unpaid to the provider for clarification of any question; these claims must be corrected before resubmission.

relapse Recurrence of the symptoms of a disease after apparent recovery.

relevant Having significant and demonstrable bearing on the matter at hand.

rem The conventional unit of radiation dose equivalent.

remission The partial or complete disappearance of the clinical and subjective characteristics of a chronic or malignant disease.

remittance advice (RA) An explanation of benefits from Medicaid (see *explanation of benefits [EOB]*).

renal thresholds Levels above which substances cannot be reabsorbed by the renal tubules and therefore are excreted in the urine.

renin An enzyme produced and stored in the glomerulus; it is released by a homeostatic response to raise the blood pressure when needed.

reparations (re-puh-ra'-shuns) Amends, acts of atonement, or satisfaction given as a result of a wrong or injury.

reprimands Criticisms for a fault; severe or formal reproofs.

reproach An expression of rebuke or disapproval; a cause or occasion of blame, discredit, or disgrace.

requisites (re'-kwuh-zuhts) Entities considered essential or necessary.

resident bacteria Bacteria that live in or on a certain part of the body, such as the skin or mucosa.

resource-based relative value scale (RBRVS) A fee schedule designed to provide national uniform payment of Medicare benefits after adjustment to reflect the differences in practice costs across geographic areas.

respondent (ri-spahn'-dunt) The person required to make answer in a civil legal action or suit; similar to a defendant in a criminal trial.

retention schedule A method or plan for retaining or keeping medical records and for their movement from active, to inactive, to closed filing.

retention The act of keeping in possession or use; keeping in one's pay or service.

reverse chronologic order Arranged in order so that the most recent item is on top and older items are filed further back.

rhinitis (rin-i'-tis) Inflammation of the mucous membranes of the nose.

rhinorrhea (ri-no-re'-uh) The discharge of nasal drainage.

rhonchi (ron'-ki) Abnormal rumbling sounds on expiration that indicate airway obstruction by thick secretions or spasms.

rider A special provision or group of provisions that may be added to a policy to expand or limit the benefits otherwise payable. It may increase or decrease benefits, waive a condition or coverage, or in any other way amend the original contract.

robotics   Technology dealing with the design, construction, and operation of robots in automation.

roentgen (R) (rent´-gen)   The conventional unit of radiation exposure.

router (rau´-ter)   A device used to connect any number of LANs, which communicate with other routers and determine the best route between any two hosts.

sagittal plane   The plane that divides the body into right and left parts.

salutation (sal-yu-ta´-shun)   An expression of greeting, goodwill, or courtesy by words or gestures.

sarcasm   A sharp and often satirical response or ironic utterance designed to cut or inflict pain.

satiety   The state of being satisfied or feeling full after eating.

scanner   A device that reads text or illustrations on a printed page and can translate the information on that page into a form the computer can understand.

scleroderma (skluh-rah-der´-muh)   An autoimmune disorder that affects the blood vessels and connective tissue, causing fibrous degeneration of the major organs.

sclerotherapy (skluh-rah-ther´-ah-pe)   The treatment of hemorrhoids, varicose veins, or esophageal varices by means of injection of sclerosing solutions.

scoliosis   An abnormal lateral curvature of the spine.

scored   Slashed (e.g., a tablet manufactured with an indentation for division through the center).

screen   Something that shields, protects, or hides; to select or eliminate through a screening process.

screening   A system for examining and separating into different groups; in the medical office, determining the severity of illness that patients experience and prioritizing appointments based on that severity.

search engines   Programs that search documents for keywords and return a list of documents containing those words.

secondary hypertension   Elevated blood pressure resulting from another condition, typically kidney disease.

section   One of the six primary divisions of the main body of the CPT.

secured   A loan or line of credit that is backed by a pledge of payment and usually obtained using collateral.

sediment   Insoluble material that settles to the bottom of a urine specimen.

see   A direction to the coder to look in another place; this instruction must always be followed. It is found in the Alphabetic Index, volumes 2 and 3.

see also   A direction to the coder to look elsewhere if the main term or subterm (or subterms) for that entry are not sufficient for coding the information. If a code number follows, *see also* is enclosed in parentheses. If there is no code number, *see also* is preceded by a dash.

see category   A direction to the coder to see a specific category (three-digit code); this instruction must always be followed.

self-insured (or self-funded) plan   An insurance plan funded by an organization having a large enough employee base that it can afford to fund its own insurance program.

self-referral   Occurs when a patient or an insured individual refers himself or herself to a specialist without requesting the referral from the primary provider (e.g., a woman seeking an annual gynecologic examination). Managed care guidelines may require the patient to report the self-referral.

sentinel events   Unexpected occurrences involving death or serious physical or psychological injury, or the risk thereof.

sequentially (si-kwen´-shuh-le)   Of, relating to, or arranged in a sequence.

serous   A term referring to a thin, watery, serumlike drainage.

serum   The liquid portion of whole blood that remains after the blood has clotted.

server   A computer or device on a network that manages shared network resources.

service benefit plans   Plans that provide benefits in the form of certain surgical and medical services rendered rather than cash. A service benefit plan is not restricted to a fee schedule.

shingling   A method of filing in which a report is laid on top of the older report, resembling the shingles of a roof.

Sievert (Sv) (se´-vuhrt)   The international unit of radiation dose equivalent.

signs   Objective findings determined by a clinician, such as a fever, hypertension, or rash.

sinoatrial (SA) node   The pacemaker of the heart; it is located in the right atrium.

sinus arrhythmia   An irregular heartbeat that originates in the sinoatrial node (pacemaker).

slander   Oral defamation; a harmful, false statement made about another person.

SOAP notes   A system of charting comprising the *s*ubjective findings, *o*bjective findings, *a*ssessment, and *p*lan for treatment.

socioeconomic   Relating to a combination of social and economic factors.

sociologic   Oriented or directed toward social needs and problems.

sonography (suh-nog´-ruh-fe)   An imaging modality that uses sound waves to produce images of soft tissues; also called *diagnostic ultrasound.*

species   A category of microorganisms that is below genus in rank; a genetically distinct group.

specific gravity   The density of urine compared with an equal volume of water.

specimen   A sample of body fluid, waste product, or tissue that is collected for analysis.

spermicide (spuhr´-muh-sid)   A chemical substance that kills sperms cells.

spirometer   An instrument that measures the volume of air inhaled and exhaled.

spore   A thick-walled, dormant form of bacteria that is very resistant to disinfection measures.

staff privileges   The permission granted by a facility to a healthcare professional to practice in that facility.

standards   Items or indicators used as a measure of quality or compliance with a statutory or accrediting body's policies and regulations. *Also,* models or examples established by authority, custom, or general consent; something set up and established by authority as a rule for the measure of quantity, weight, extent, value, or quality.

STAT   Medical abbreviation for immediately; at this moment.

statement   A request for payment.

statement of income and expense   A summary of all income and expenses for a given period.

stationers (sta´-shuh-nerz) Sellers of stationery.

statutes (sta-choots) Laws enacted by the legislative branch of a government.

stereotactic Pertaining to an x-ray procedure used to guide the insertion of a needle into a specific area of the breast.

stereotype Something conforming to a fixed or general pattern; a standardized mental picture that is held in common by many and represents an oversimplified opinion, prejudiced attitude, or uncritical judgment.

sterile (ster´-il) Free of all microorganisms, pathogenic and nonpathogenic.

sterilization Complete destruction of all forms of microbial life.

stertorous (stuh-tuh´-rus) A term describing a strenuous respiratory effort marked by a snoring sound.

stipulate To specify as a condition or requirement of an agreement or offer; to make an agreement or covenant to do or forbear from doing something.

stock options Offers of stocks for purchase to a certain group of individuals or certain groups, such as employees of a for-profit hospital.

stressors Stimuli that cause stress.

striated A term referring to muscle tissue that contains fibers divided by bands of cross stripes, or striations, because of overlapping myofilaments.

stridor A shrill, harsh respiratory sound heard during inhalation when a laryngeal obstruction is present.

stylus A metal probe that is inserted into or passed through a catheter, needle, or tube used for clearing purposes or to facilitate passage into a body orifice.

subcategory In the CPT manual, the element indented one level below a category, usually a procedure or service unique to a specific category.

subjective information Information gained by questioning the patient or taking it from a form.

subluxations (suh-blek-sa´-shuns) Slight misalignments of the vertebrae or a partial dislocation.

subordinate Submissive to or controlled by authority; placed in or occupying a lower class, rank, or position.

subpoena (suh-pe´-nuh) A writ or document commanding a person to appear in court under a penalty for failure to appear.

subpoena duces tecum A legally binding request to appear in court and provide records or documents that pertain to a particular case.

subsection In the CPT manual, the element indented one level below a section; it usually describes an anatomic site or organ system (e.g., Integumentary, Cardiology).

subsidiary Supporting other documents or records.

substance number A number based on the weight of a ream of paper containing 500 sheets.

subtle Difficult to understand or perceive; having or marked by keen insight and ability to penetrate deeply and thoroughly. *Also,* ingenious, artful, delicate.

succinct (suhk-sinkt´) Marked by compact, precise expression without wasted words.

superfluous (suh-puhr´-flu-uhs) Exceeding what is sufficient or necessary.

superuser A special account on a computer system that is used for system administration; also, a person in a facility who is able to make system-wide changes to a computer system.

suppurative Characterized by the formation and/or discharge of pus.

supravital Of, related to, or capable of staining living cells after their removal from a living or recently dead organism.

surface area The total area of the body exposed to the outside environment.

surrogate (suhr´-uh-gat) A substitute; to put in place of another.

switch In networks, a device that filters information between LAN segments and reduces overall network traffic and increases speed and bandwidth use efficiency.

symptoms Subjective complaints reported by the patient, such as pain or visual disturbances.

syncope (sing´-kuh-pee) Fainting; a brief lapse in consciousness.

synopsis Condensed statement or outline.

synovial fluid A clear fluid found in joint cavities that facilitates smooth movements and nourishes joint structures.

system software The operating system and all utility programs that allow the computer to function and perform operations.

systole The contraction of the heart.

tablet A wireless, portable personal computer with a touch screen interface, usually smaller than a notebook but larger than a smart phone (e.g., Apple iPad, Samsung Galaxy, Dell Streak).

Tabular Index Volume 1 (Main Text) of the ICD-9-CM coding manual. It contains all the diagnostic codes in alphanumeric order, which are grouped into 17 chapters of diseases and injuries.

tachycardia (tak-i-kahr´-dee-uh) A rapid but regular heart rate; one that exceeds 100 beats per minute.

tachypnea (tak-ip-nee´-uh) A condition marked by rapid, shallow respirations.

tactful Having a keen sense of what to do or say to maintain good relations with others or to prevent offense.

tangible (tan´-juh-buhl) Capable of being appraised at an actual or approximate value; capable of being precisely identified or realized by the mind.

target market A specific group of individuals toward whom the marketing plan is focused.

targeted Directed or used toward a target; directed toward a specific desire or position.

TCP/IP The acronym for *transmission control protocol/Internet protocol*; a suite of communications protocols used to connect users or hosts to the Internet.

tedious (te´-de-yus) Tiresome because of length or dullness.

telecommunications The science and technology of communication by transmission of information from one location to another via telephone, television, telegraph, or satellite.

telemedicine The use of telecommunications in the practice of medicine to compensate for the great distances that can separate healthcare professionals, colleagues, patients, and students.

teleradiology The use of telecommunication devices to enhance and improve the results of radiologic procedures.

template A predeveloped page layout used to make new pages with a similar design, pattern, or style; a standardized file type used in computer software as a preformatted example on which to base other files.

tendons Tough bands of connective tissue that connect muscle to bone.

terabyte (TB) Approximately 1 trillion bytes.

teratogen (te-rah´-tuh-jen) Any substance that interferes with normal prenatal development, resulting in a developmental abnormality.

testimony A solemn declaration usually made orally by a witness under oath in response to interrogation by a lawyer or authorized public official.

thanatology (tha-nuh-tah'-luh-je) The study of the phenomena of death and of psychological methods of coping with death.

therapeutic range The blood concentration of a drug that produces the desired effect without toxicity.

third-party administrator (TPA) An organization that processes claims and performs other business-related functions for a health plan.

third-party payers Entities that make payment on an obligation or debt but are not parties to the contract that created the debt.

thixotropic gel A material that appears to be a solid until subjected to a disturbance, such as centrifugation, whereupon it becomes a liquid.

thready A term describing a pulse that is scarcely perceptible.

thrombolytics Agents that dissolve blood clots.

thrombus A blood clot.

thyroid-stimulating hormone (TSH) A hormone secreted by the anterior pituitary gland that stimulates the secretion of hormones produced by the thyroid gland.

tickler file A chronologic file used as a reminder that something must be dealt with on a certain date.

tinea (tin'-e-uh) Any fungal skin disease that results in scaling, itching, and inflammation.

tinnitus A noise sensation of ringing heard in one or both ears.

tissue culture The technique or process of keeping tissue alive and growing in a culture medium.

tolerance The need to use more and more of a substance to get the same feeling as the body learns to tolerate the drug.

tracers Radioactive substances administered to patients for nuclear medicine imaging procedures.

tracheostomy (tra-ke-os'-tuh-me) A surgical opening made through the neck into the trachea to allow breathing.

transaction An exchange or transfer of goods, services, or funds.

transactions As defined by HIPAA, transmissions of information between two parties to carry out financial or administrative activities related to healthcare.

transcription A written copy of something made either in longhand or by machine.

transducer The part of the sonography machine that is in contact with the patient; the transducer sends high-frequency sound waves and receives the sound echoes from the patient's body.

transection Cross section; a division made by cutting across.

transient bacteria Bacteria temporarily living in or on a certain body part, such as the hands.

transient ischemic attack (TIA) Temporary neurologic symptoms caused by gradual or partial occlusion of a cerebral blood vessel.

transport medium A medium used to keep an organism alive during transport to the laboratory.

transposed Altered in sequence; interchanged.

transverse plane The plane that divides the body into superior and inferior parts.

treatises (tree'-te-ses) Systematic expositions or arguments in writing, including a methodic discussion of the facts and principles involved and the conclusions reached.

triage (tree'-azh) Identification of the severity of patients' conditions and the allocation of treatment according to a system of priorities, which is designed to maximize the number of survivors and provide treatment for the sickest patients first.

trial balance A method of checking the accuracy of accounts.

TRICARE A government-sponsored program under which authorized dependents of military personnel receive medical care. Originally called *CHAMPUS*.

triglyceride (tri-gli'-suh-rid) A fatty acid and glycerol compound that combines with a protein molecule to form high- or low-density lipoprotein.

trustee A person to whom property is legally committed to be administered for the benefit of a beneficiary or held by an administrator to be distributed to multiple individuals or businesses.

tubercle (too'-buhr-kuhl) A nodule produced by the tuberculosis bacillus.

turbid A term referring to a cloudy solution.

turbidity Cloudiness in a liquid caused by the presence of suspended particles; it increases with the concentration of particles present.

turgor A term referring to normal skin tension; it is the resistance of the skin to being grasped between the fingers and released. Turgor is decreased with dehydration and increased with edema.

type and cross-match Tests performed to assess the compatibility of blood to be transfused.

unbundled codes Codes in which the components of a major procedure are separated and reported separately.

Uniform Commercial Code (UCC) A unified set of rules covering many business transactions; it has been adopted in all 50 states, the District of Columbia, and most U.S. territories. It regulates the fields of sales of goods; commercial paper, such as checks; secured transactions in personal property; and particular aspects of banking, letters of credit, warehouse receipts, bills of lading, and investment securities.

unique identifiers Codes used instead of names to protect the confidentiality of the patient in a method of anonymous HIV testing.

Unique Provider Identification Number (UPIN) A number assigned by fiscal intermediaries to identify providers on claims for services.

unit dose A method used by the pharmacy to prepare individual doses of medication.

universal claim form The form developed by the Health Care Financing Administration (HCFA; now the Centers for Medicare and Medicaid Services [CMS]) and approved by the American Medical Association (AMA) for use in submitting all government-sponsored claims. Also known as the *CMS-1500 Health Insurance Claim Form.*

unsecured A debt that is not protected by collateral.

upcoding A deliberate increase in a CPT code, despite the lack of documentation, to the next highest reimbursable code so as to obtain higher reimbursements.

upper gastrointestinal (UGI) series Fluoroscopic examination of the esophagus, stomach, and duodenum in which oral barium sulfate is administered as a contrast medium.

urea The major nitrogenous end product of protein metabolism and the chief nitrogenous component of the urine.

urinary incontinence A sudden, compelling desire to urinate and the inability to control the release of urine.

URL The acronym for *uniform resource locator;* specifies the global address of documents or information on the Internet. The URL provides the IP address and the domain name for the Web page, such as microsoft.com.

urticaria (uhr-tuh-kar´-e-uh)   A skin eruption that creates inflamed wheals; hives.

use additional code   A *use additional code* note is found at the etiology code when the underlying condition is sequenced first, followed by the manifestation. A term that appears only in the Tabular Index (Volume 1) in subdivisions in which the user should add further information, by means of an additional code, to give a more complete picture of the diagnosis. In some cases, *if desired* follows the term. For the purpose of coding, the *if desired* phrase will not be used. When the term *use additional code if desired* appears, disregard "if desired" and assign the appropriate additional code.

utilization review   A review of individual cases by a committee to make sure that services are medically necessary and to study how providers use medical care resources.

Valsalva's maneuver   An effect created when a person strains to defecate or urinate, uses the arms and upper trunk muscles to move up in bed, or strains during laughing, coughing, or vomiting; it causes trapping of blood in the great veins, preventing it from entering the chest and right atrium, and may cause heart attack and death.

vasodilation   An increase in the diameter of a blood vessel.

vectors   Animals or insects (e.g., ticks) that transmit the causative organisms of disease.

vegetations   Abnormal tissue growths, consisting of fibrin, platelets, and bacteria, that surround a valve.

vehemently (ve´-uh-ment-le)   In a manner marked by forceful energy; intensely, emotionally.

ventricles   The two lower chambers of the heart.

veracity (vuh-ra´-suh-te)   A devotion to or conformity with the truth.

verbiage   A manner of expressing oneself in words.

verdict   The finding or decision of a jury on a matter submitted to it in trial.

versatile (vur´-suh-til)   Embracing a variety of subjects, fields, or skills; having a wide range of abilities.

vertigo   Dizziness; a sensation of faintness or an inability to maintain normal balance.

vested   Granted or endowed with a particular authority, right, or property; to have a special interest in.

viable   Capable of living, developing, or germinating under favorable conditions.

virtual reality   An artificial environment presented to a computer user that feels as if it were a real environment, often involving use of special gloves, earphones, and goggles to enhance the experience.

virulent (vir´-u-lent)   Exceedingly pathogenic, noxious, or deadly.

viscosity (vis-kos´-uh-te)   The quality of being thick and of lacking the capability of easy movement.

vocation   The work in which a person is regularly employed.

volatile (vah´-luh-til)   Easily aroused; tending to erupt in violence. *Also,* capable of vaporizing at a low temperature, such as an explosive substance.

vulva   The external female genitalia, which begins at the mons pubis and terminates at the anus.

wasting syndrome   Physical deterioration resulting in profound weight loss, fatigue, anorexia, and mental confusion.

watermark   A marking in paper resulting from differences in thickness usually produced by the pressure of a projecting design in the mold or on a processing roll; it is visible when the paper is held up to the light.

wet mount   A slide preparation in which a drop of liquid specimen or the like is covered with a coverslip and observed with a microscope.

wheal (weel)   A localized area of edema or a raised lesion.

wheezing   A high-pitched sound heard on expiration; indicates obstruction or narrowing of respiratory passages.

willful neglect   Conscious, intentional failure or reckless indifference to the obligation to comply with the administrative simplification provision violated.

with   In the context of the ICD-9-CM, the terms *with, with mention of,* and *associated with* in a title dictate that both parts of the title must be present in the diagnostic statement to allow assignment of the particular code.

work ethics   A set of values based on the moral virtues of hard work and diligence.

workers' compensation   Insurance against liability imposed employers cover medical expenses and lost wages to employees who are injured on the job and to pay benefits to dependents of employees killed in the course of or arising out of their employment.

INDEX

Page numbers followed by "f" indicate figures, "t" indicate tables, and "b" indicate boxes.